MW00446104

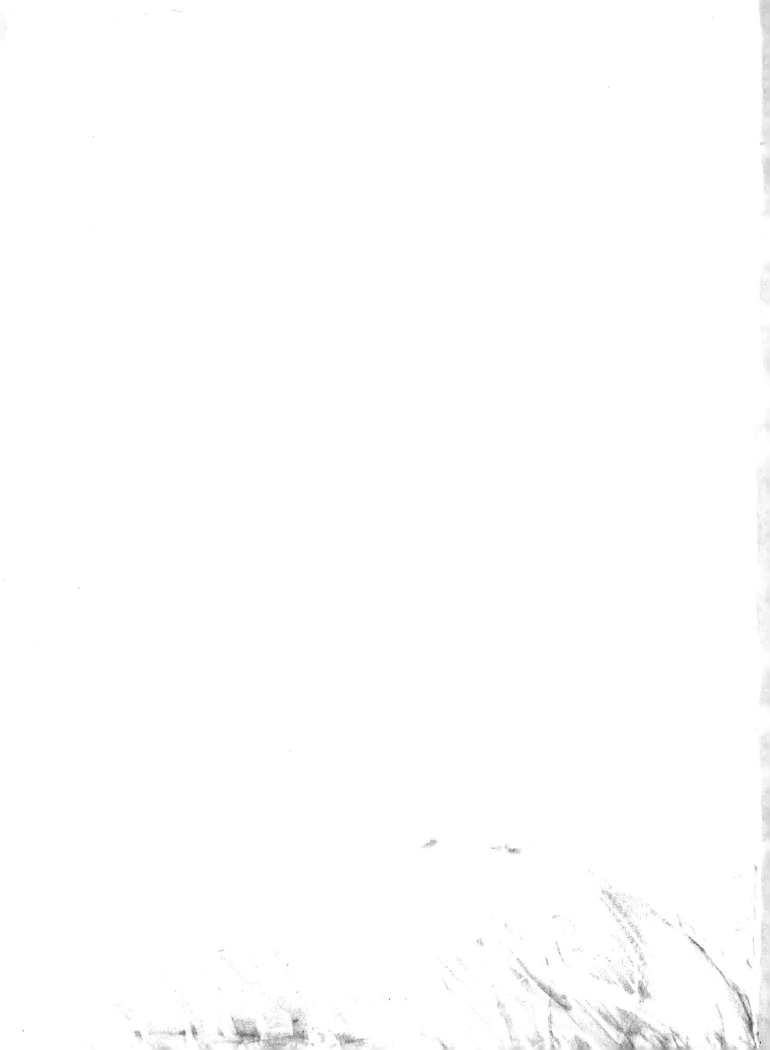

DIAGNOSTIC PATHOLOGY

HEAD AND NECK

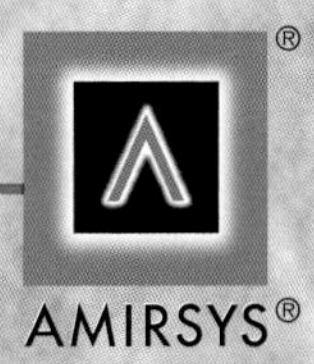

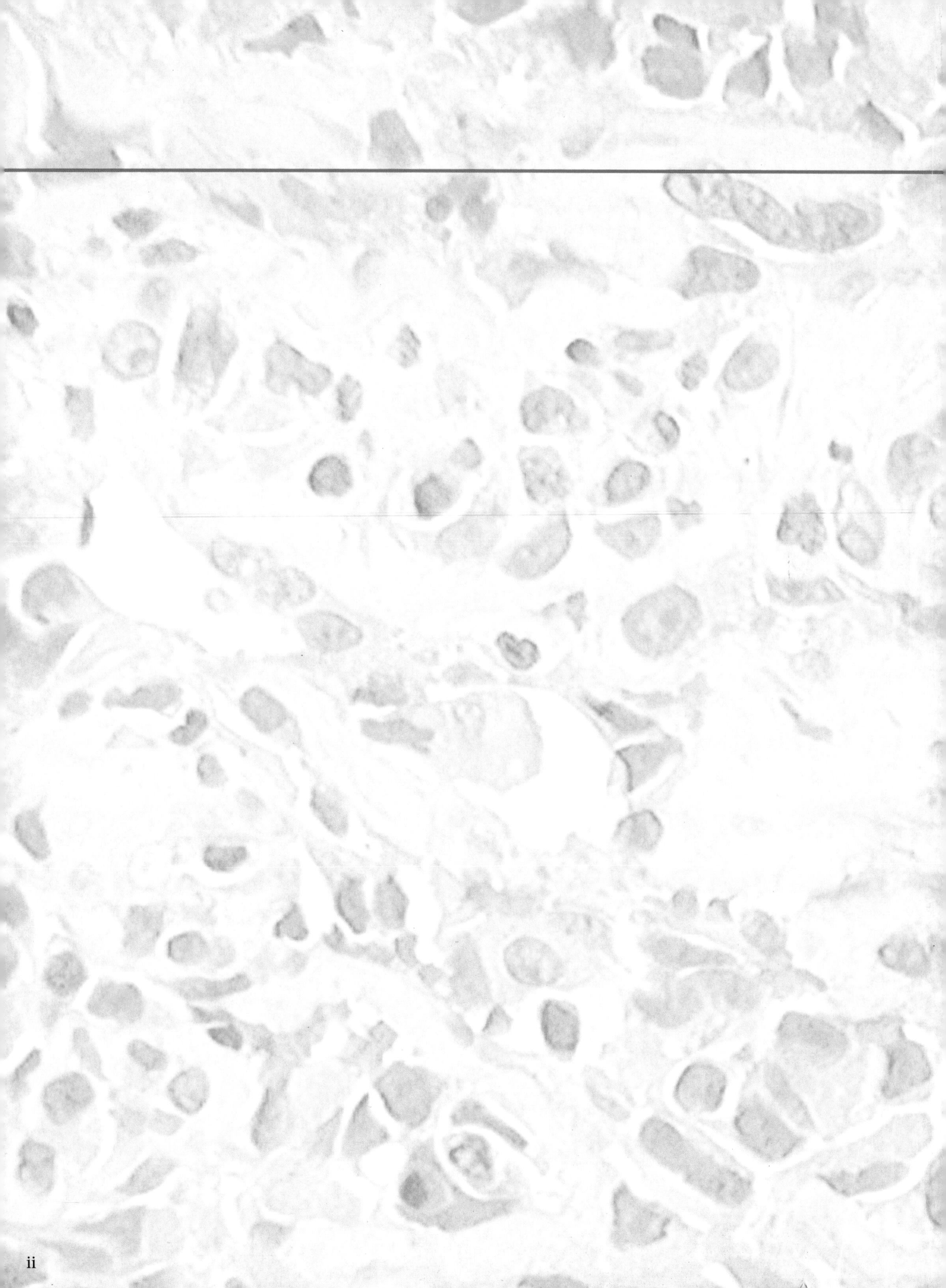

DIAGNOSTIC PATHOLOGY

HEAD AND NECK

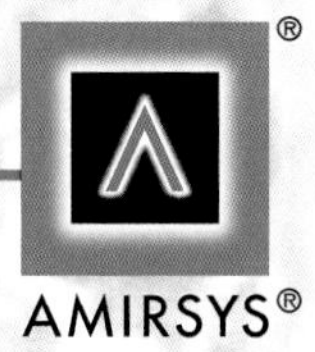

Lester D. R. Thompson, MD
Consultant Pathologist
Department of Pathology and Laboratory Medicine
Southern California Permanente Medical Group
Woodland Hills, CA

Brenda L. Nelson, DDS, MS
Head of Anatomic Pathology
Naval Medical Center San Diego
San Diego, CA

Francis H. Gannon, MD
Associate Professor of Pathology, Immunology, and Orthopedic Surgery
Director, Residency and Fellowship Programs
Deptartment of Pathology and Immunology
Baylor College of Medicine
Houston, TX

David Cassarino, MD, PhD
Consultant Dermatopathologist and Staff Pathologist
Southern California Permanente Medical Group
Los Angeles, CA
Clinical Professor
Department of Dermatology
University of California, Irvine
Irvine, CA

Bruce M. Wenig, MD
Chairman, Department of Diagnostic Pathology and Laboratory Medicine
Beth Israel Medical Center, St. Luke's-Roosevelt Hospitals
New York, NY
Professor of Pathology
Albert Einstein College of Medicine
Bronx, NY

Susan Müller, DMD, MS
Professor
Department of Pathology and Laboratory Medicine
Department of Otolaryngology, Head and Neck Surgery
Winship Cancer Institute
Emory University School of Medicine
Atlanta, GA

Kevin R. Torske, DDS, MS
Chairman and Residency Program Director
Department of Oral and Maxillofacial Pathology
Naval Postgraduate Dental School
Bethesda, MD

Nina Gale, MD, PhD
Professor of Pathology
Director of the Institute of Pathology
Faculty of Medicine
University of Ljubljana
Ljubljana, Slovenia

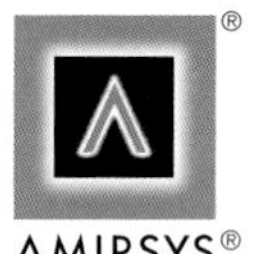

AMIRSYS®
Names you know. Content you trust.®

First Edition

Second Printing - September 2012

Printed in Canada by Friesens, Altona, Manitoba, Canada

ISBN: 978-1-931884-61-7

Notice and Disclaimer

Library of Congress Cataloging-in-Publication Data

Thompson, Lester D. R.
Diagnostic pathology. Head and neck / Lester D. R. Thompson, Bruce M. Wenig.
p. ; cm.
Head and neck
Includes bibliographical references and index.
ISBN 978-1-931884-61-7
1. Head--Cancer. 2. Neck--Cancer. 3. Head--Pathophysiology. 4. Neck--Pathophysiology. I. Wenig, Bruce M. II. Title. III. Title: Head and neck.
[DNLM: 1. Head and Neck Neoplasms. 2. Head--pathology. 3. Neck--pathology. WE 707]
RC280.H4T46 2011
616.99'491--dc22

2010050640

The course of our life's journey is determined by a myriad of seemingly small and insignificant decisions about which route to take. We do not know the itinerary, the times, places, or destinations. There is no reconnoitering. We start exploring by crawling, walking, and then running. Soon the adventure expands to biking, climbing, skating, paddling, swimming, and driving. Our wanderlust takes us on a rail ride, cruising aboard all types of water vessels, flying, trekking, bungee jumping, skydiving, ballooning, white water or black water rafting, hang gliding, parasailing, zip-lining—you name it, we try it. The odyssey includes a hop here, a jaunt there, a migration across the globe, a safari, sauntering along the beach, gallivanting to forgotten lands, an overnight outing, a weekend getaway, an extended deployment, a lazy drifting, a pilgrimage, traipsing through adversity, or even gyrating in place! Every choice—a right or left turn, a veering slightly to one direction, a flight, a spin on a roundabout, and even the occasional U-turn or stop—all determine where we are, how we got there, what we do when we are there, and where we will advance to next. No matter what is chosen, the map of life gradually fills in to reflect our expedition—and maybe even the ultimate destination. There are many people we meet along the way: trip planners, tour guides, managers, operators, agents, drivers, pilots, captains, divers, cabin attendants, crew, staff, explorers, scouts, navigators, passengers, and companions. The people in my life know which of these roles they have played or continue to play in my expedition. Early on, I learned that all travel is benefited from a map. I have studied countless maps in hundreds of cities in > 93 countries of the world. Even when written in another language, they are still invaluable in getting you where you want to be. I hope this book provides a map to head and neck pathology—but hope the journey is as much fun as the destination. As I was finishing residency, I was lucky enough to find a perfect MAP—PAM! She is all of the parts of my adventure in one—the only map I will ever need for a perfect expedition, both the journey and the destination.

I love you all the words ever written!

LDRT

To Ana, Sarah, Eli, and Jake for their love, understanding, and support, with all my love.

BMW

Thank you to my friend and mentor, Lester Thompson. To my parents, John and Carol, for their constant love and support. And to my husband, Dave, and my son, Adam, for their unconditional love and inspiration.

BLN

To my mentors, Charles Waldron, Dwight R. Weathers, and Leon Barnes, and my husband, Steven Budnick, for their guidance and support.

SM

To my family, for their love and support.

FHG

For all students of pathology.

KRT

To my wonderful wife and children for their support and inspiration.

DC

To my family.

NG

DIAGNOSTIC PATHOLOGY

HEAD AND NECK

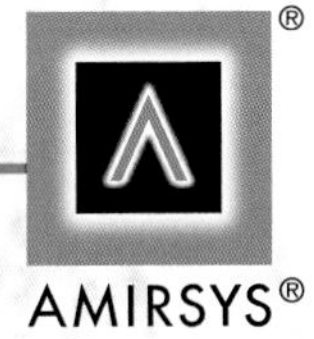

Amirsys, creators of the highly acclaimed radiology series Diagnostic Imaging, proudly introduces its new Diagnostic Pathology series, designed as easy-to-use reference texts for the busy practicing surgical pathologist. Written by world-renowned experts, the series will consist of 15 titles in all the crucial diagnostic areas of surgical pathology.

The newest book in this series, *Diagnostic Pathology: Head and Neck*, contains approximately 1,100 pages of comprehensive, yet concise, descriptions of more than 300 specific diagnoses. Amirsys's pioneering bulleted format distills pertinent information to the essentials. Each chapter has the same organization providing an easy-to-read reference for making rapid, efficient, and accurate diagnoses in a busy surgical pathology practice. A highlighted Key Facts box provides the essential features of each diagnosis. Detailed sections on Terminology, Etiology/Pathogenesis, Clinical Issues, Macroscopic and Microscopic Findings, and the all important Differential Diagnoses follow so you can find the information you need in the exact same place every time.

Most importantly, every diagnosis features numerous high-quality images, including gross pathology, H&E and immunohistochemical stains, correlative radiographic images, and richly colored graphics, all of which are fully annotated to maximize their illustrative potential.

We believe that this lavishly illustrated series, with its up-to-date information and practical focus, will become the core of your reference collection. Enjoy!

Elizabeth H. Hammond, MD
Executive Editor, Pathology
Amirsys, Inc.

Anne G. Osborn, MD
Chairman and Chief Executive Officer
Amirsys Publishing, Inc.

PREFACE

The pathology of the head and neck includes a wide array of lesions that test the acumen of even the most experienced surgical pathologist. Any textbook attempting to cover the depth and breadth of the pathologic lesions found in the head and neck is bound to fall short of accomplishing such a daunting task. It is our intent in this book to provide as comprehensive a review of head and neck pathology as possible, in a format that allows for easy access of pertinent information, richly illustrated, that allow the user to arrive at an accurate diagnosis.

Diagnostic Pathology: Head and Neck is organized into 10 sections, including Nasal Cavity and Paranasal Sinuses, Pharynx, Larynx and Trachea, Oral Cavity, Salivary Glands, Jaw, Ear and Temporal Bone, Neck, Thyroid Gland, and Parathyroid Glands. The organization within each section includes nonneoplastic lesions (e.g., congenital, infectious, inflammatory, reactive), benign neoplasms, and malignant neoplasms. Where applicable, a chapter concludes with the protocol for reporting resection specimens. Nearly all chapters follow a stylized format, written in succinct bullets and include synonym(s), definition, etiology or pathogenesis, clinical and demographic parameters, treatment, prognosis, radiographic features (if pertinent), pathologic features (macroscopic, microscopic), ancillary studies (cytology, special stains, immunohistochemistry, molecular biology, cytogenetics, and ultrastructure), and differential diagnoses. The Key Facts for each entity appear in a separate box for quick reference. Plentiful graphics and illustrations highlight the key diagnostic features of each disease. Immunohistochemical tables are included in many chapters, providing a rapid source for the key markers used in the diagnosis and differential of a given lesion.

As is true for the field of pathology in general, there is rapid expansion of our knowledge and understanding of head and neck pathology in particular as it applies to personalized medicine. We have attempted to be as current as possible relative to information contained in this book, but we are acutely aware that the rapid changes in this field will make some of this information outdated shortly following publication of the book. To this end, the Amirsys eBook Advantage™ will allow us to keep our book "fresh" and relevant with on-going timely updates.

We hope that *Diagnostic Pathology: Head and Neck* will be a useful, practical, and valuable resource for individuals with interest in diseases of the head and neck.

Bruce M. Wenig, MD
Chairman, Department of Diagnostic Pathology and Laboratory Medicine
Beth Israel Medical Center, St. Luke's-Roosevelt Hospitals
New York, NY
Professor of Pathology
Albert Einstein College of Medicine
Bronx, NY

Lester D. R. Thompson, MD
Consultant Pathologist
Department of Pathology and Laboratory Medicine
Southern California Permanente Medical Group
Woodland Hills, CA

ACKNOWLEDGMENTS

Text Editing
Ashley R. Renlund, MA
Arthur G. Gelsinger, MA
Matthew R. Connelly, MA
Lorna Morring, MS
Alicia M. Moulton

Image Editing
Jeffrey J. Marmorstone
Lisa A. Magar

Medical Text Editing
Sara Cuadra Acree, MD

Illustrations
Laura C. Sesto, MA
Richard Coombs, MS
Lane R. Bennion, MS

Art Direction and Design
Laura C. Sesto, MA

Assistant Editor
Dave L. Chance, MA

Publishing Lead
Kellie J. Heap

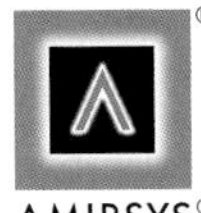

AMIRSYS®

Names you know. Content you trust.®

SECTIONS

TABLE OF CONTENTS

SECTION 1
Nasal Cavity and Paranasal Sinuses

Congenital/Genetic/Hereditary

Infectious

Inflammatory-Immune Dysfunction

Reactive

Benign Neoplasm

Borderline Neoplasm

Malignant Neoplasm

Specimen Examination, Nasal Cavity & Paranasal Sinuses

SECTION 2
Pharynx (Nasal, Oro-, Hypo-)

Congenital/Genetic/Hereditary

Infectious

Reactive

Benign Neoplasm

Malignant Neoplasm

Staging and Grading, Pharynx

SECTION 3
Larynx and Trachea

Congenital/Genetic/Hereditary

Infectious

Reactive

Benign Neoplasm

Malignant Neoplasm

SECTION 9 Thyroid Gland

Congenital/Genetic/Hereditary

Infectious

Inflammatory-Immune Dysfunction

Reactive

Benign Neoplasm

Malignant Neoplasm

Specimen Examination, Thyroid

SECTION 10
Parathyroid Glands

Nonneoplastic

Benign Neoplasm

Malignant Neoplasm

SECTION 11
Antibody Index

DIAGNOSTIC PATHOLOGY

HEAD AND NECK

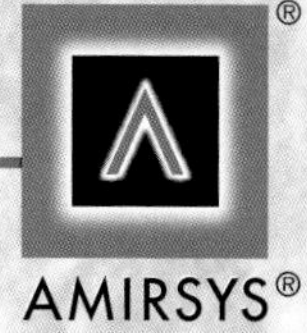

Nasal Cavity and Paranasal Sinuses

Congenital/Genetic/Hereditary

Infectious

Inflammatory-Immune Dysfunction

Reactive

Benign Neoplasm

Borderline Neoplasm

Malignant Neoplasm

Specimen Examination, Nasal Cavity & Paranasal Sinuses

NASAL GLIAL HETEROTOPIA

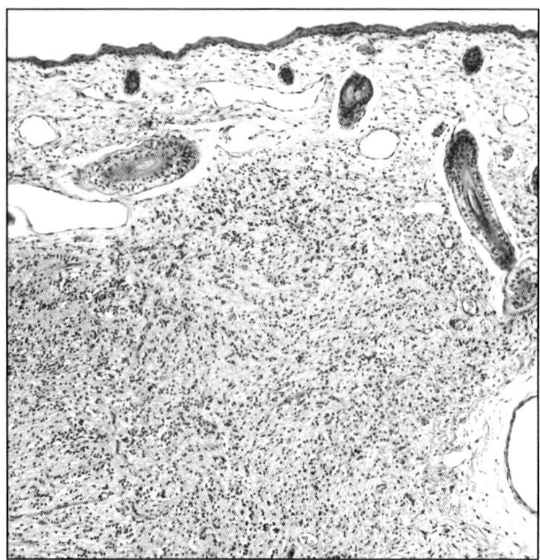

Hematoxylin & eosin shows an intact skin with adnexal structures (hair shafts) surrounding a haphazard collection of neural elements (glial tissue).

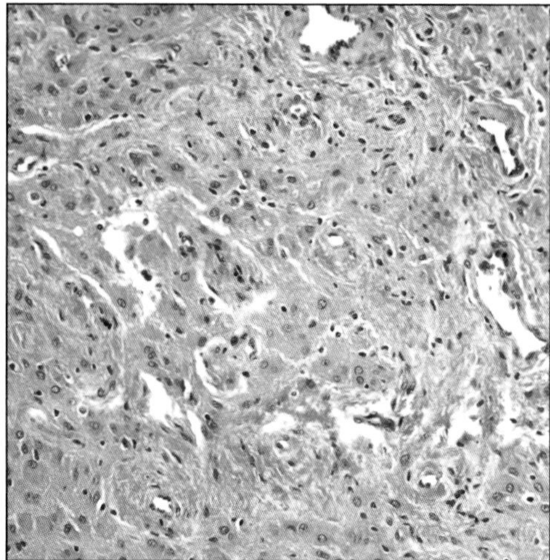

Hematoxylin & eosin shows the intermingling of glial elements with fibrosis. This is a very subtle finding, highlighting the reason for performing special studies in many cases.

TERMINOLOGY

Abbreviations

- Nasal glial heterotopia (NGH)

Synonyms

- Glioma: Implies tumor and is to be discouraged

Definitions

- Nasal glial heterotopia are congenital malformations of displaced normal, mature glial tissue (choristomas)
  - Continuity with intracranial component is usually obliterated
- Encephalocele represents herniation of brain tissue and leptomeninges through bony defect of skull
  - Continuity with cranial cavity is maintained

ETIOLOGY/PATHOGENESIS

Developmental Anomaly

- Congenital malformation of displaced normal and mature glial tissue

Iatrogenic

- Encephalocele is herniation of brain tissue through bony defect
  - Often secondary to infections, trauma, or surgery

CLINICAL ISSUES

Epidemiology

- Incidence
  - NGH is rare
  - Encephalocele is uncommon
- Age
  - NGH usually presents during infancy
  - Encephalocele may present in older children and adults
- Gender
  - Equal gender distribution

Site

- Separated into 2 types, based on location
  - Extranasal (60%): Subcutaneous bridge of nose
  - Intranasal (30%): Superior nasal cavity
  - Mixed (10%)

Presentation

- Firm, subcutaneous nodule at bridge of nose
- Polypoid mass within superior nasal cavity
- Obstruction
- Nasal polyps
- Chronic rhinosinusitis
- Nasal drainage
- Chronic otitis media
- CSF rhinorrhea represents encephalocele

Treatment

- Options, risks, complications
  - Radiographs are prerequisite to avoid post biopsy complications
    - Meningitis
    - CSF rhinorrhea
- Surgical approaches
  - Excision must be adequate

Prognosis

- Excellent
- Recurrences (up to 30%) if incompletely excised

IMAGE FINDINGS

Radiographic Findings

- Must be obtained before biopsy
- Sharply demarcated, expansile mass
- Need to document continuity with central nervous system
- Intracranial extension (tract or cribriform plate defect) must be excluded

NASAL GLIAL HETEROTOPIA

Key Facts

Etiology/Pathogenesis
- Congenital malformation of displaced normal and mature glial tissue

Clinical Issues
- Separated into extranasal and intranasal
- NGH usually presents during infancy
- Radiographs are prerequisite to avoid post biopsy complications
- Recurrences (up to 30%) if incompletely excised

Microscopic Pathology
- Gliosis pattern in glial tissue
- Fibrosis frequently obliterates or obscures glial tissue; special stains required to confirm

Ancillary Tests
- Glial tissue: S100 protein and GFAP positive

Top Differential Diagnoses
- Fibrosed nasal polyp

  - Especially difficult to document with CT or MR if defect is small

MACROSCOPIC FEATURES

General Features
- Smooth, homogeneous glistening cut surface
- Looks similar to brain tissue
- Sometimes fibrous connective tissue dominates, making it firm

Size
- Usually < 2 cm

MICROSCOPIC PATHOLOGY

Histologic Features
- Skin or surface mucosa is intact
- Glial tissue appears similar to gliosis
- Fibrous connective tissue blended with glial tissue
  - Fibrosis frequently obliterates or obscures glial tissue; special stains required to confirm
- Nests and sheets of fibrillar neuroglial tissue
- Prominent glial fibrillar network
- Gemistocytes may be noted
- Neurons are uncommon
- Choroid plexus, ependyma, and retinal pigmented cells are exceedingly rare
- Encephalocele shows glial degeneration but requires radiographic/clinical correlation

ANCILLARY TESTS

Histochemistry
- Trichrome
  - Reactivity: Positive
  - Staining pattern
    - Glial tissue: Bright red; fibrosis: Blue

Immunohistochemistry
- Glial tissue is highlighted with S100 protein and GFAP (latter more sensitive)

DIFFERENTIAL DIAGNOSIS

Fibrosed Nasal Polyp
- Lacks glial tissue
- Contains mucoserous glands
- Usually has greater amount of inflammation

SELECTED REFERENCES

1. Penner CR et al: Nasal glial heterotopia. Ear Nose Throat J. 83(2):92-3, 2004
2. Penner CR et al: Nasal glial heterotopia: a clinicopathologic and immunophenotypic analysis of 10 cases with a review of the literature. Ann Diagn Pathol. 7(6):354-9, 2003
3. Kardon DE: Nasal glial heterotopia. Arch Pathol Lab Med. 124(12):1849, 2000

IMAGE GALLERY

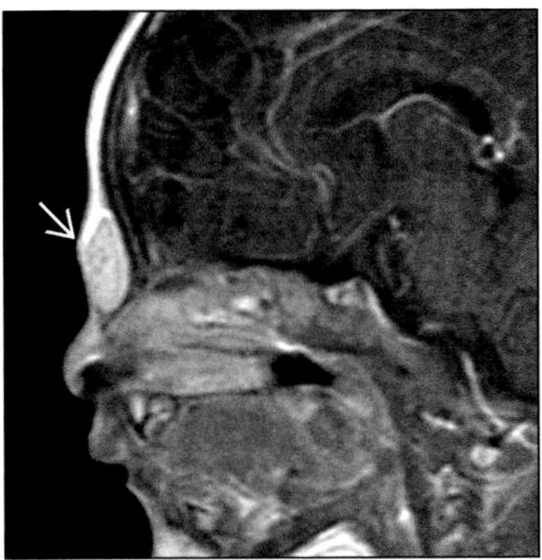

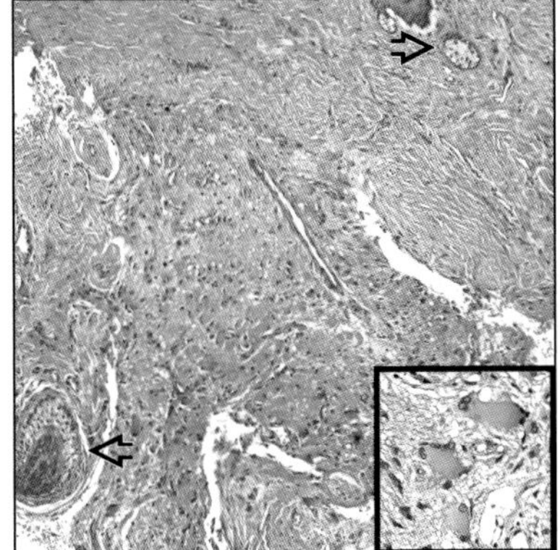

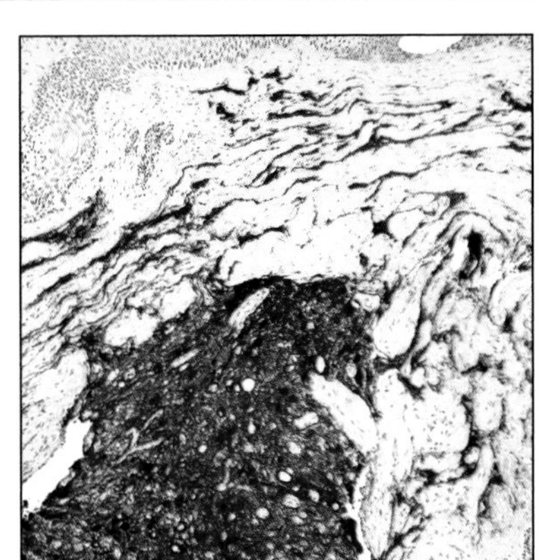

(Left) *Sagittal MR shows enhancement of the ovoid mass above the nose ➡. There is no intracranial connection.* ***(Center)*** *Hematoxylin & eosin shows pilosebaceous units ⇨, with a gemistocytic-like glial proliferation within the fibrous connective tissue. The inset shows higher power of the gemistocytes.* ***(Right)*** *GFAP highlights the glial tissue below the intact epithelium. Note the "infiltrative" appearance of the process as it is separated by reactive fibrosis.*

NASAL DERMOID CYST AND SINUS

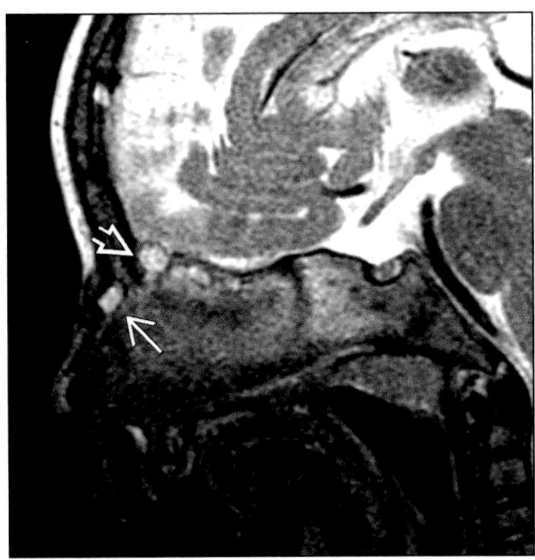

Sagittal T2WI MR shows small extracranial epidermoid ➔ under the bridge of the nose associated with 2nd intracranial epidermoid in foramen cecum area ➔.

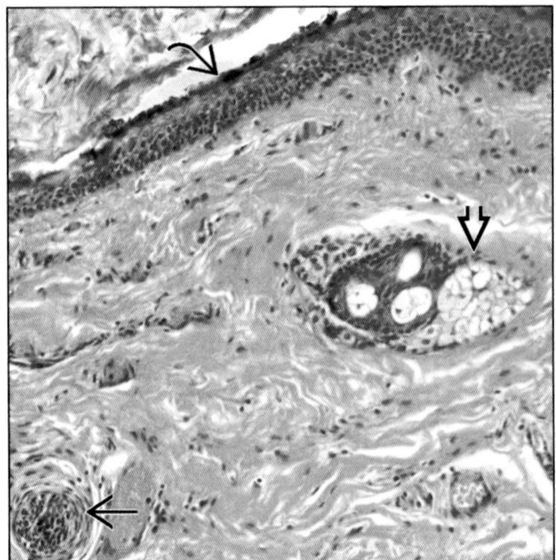

The resected cystic lesion is lined by stratified squamous epithelium ➔ with identifiable cutaneous appendages, including sebaceous glands ➔ and hair follicles ➔ in the wall of the cyst.

TERMINOLOGY

Synonyms

- Craniofacial dermoids

Definitions

- Congenital developmental lesion histologically identical to dermoid cysts found in other anatomic locations

ETIOLOGY/PATHOGENESIS

Developmental Anomaly

- May be associated with or coexist with other congenital developmental malformations
- May be familial
- Predominance as midline lesion on nasal bridge
  - Similar location as glial heterotopias suggests relationship between these lesions

CLINICAL ISSUES

Epidemiology

- Incidence
  - Represent ~ 10% of all dermoids in cervicofacial region
- Age
  - Usually infants or young children
    - May occur in adults
- Gender
  - Equal gender distribution

Site

- Majority occur at root of nose (nasal bridge)
  - May be found in lower and lateral regions of nose near nasal ala

Presentation

- Midline swelling

Treatment

- Options, risks, complications
  - Most important treatment concern is possibility of associated deeply seated cyst or related sinus tract involving anterior midline skull base
- Surgical approaches
  - Lesions with intracranial extension have traditionally been managed with
    - Lateral rhinotomy
    - Midface degloving
    - External rhinoplasty combined with frontal craniotomy
  - More recently, subcranial approach proposed
    - Offers excellent exposure
    - Minimizes frontal lobe retention
    - Reduces likelihood of cerebrospinal fluid leak
    - Provides for excellent cosmetic result
    - Shows long-term follow-up with no recurrence or negative effect on craniofacial growth

Prognosis

- Surgery is curative treatment
- Low recurrence rates

Radiographic Examination

- Preoperative evaluation essential to rule out intracranial extension
- CT &/or MR indicated in order to
  - Delineate deep tissue involvement
  - Exclude possible associated intracranial extension
- Necessary to judge deep extent of lesion

MACROSCOPIC FEATURES

General Features

- Small lesions or deeply seated cysts may not be apparent until after they become infected and inflamed
- Sinus tract with epidermal opening may be present

NASAL DERMOID CYST AND SINUS

Key Facts

Terminology
- Congenital developmental lesion virtually identical to dermoid cysts found in other anatomic locations

Clinical Issues
- Represent ~ 10% of all dermoids in cervicofacial region
- Usually infants or young children
- Majority occur at root of nose (nasal bridge)
- Surgery is curative treatment

Microscopic Pathology
- Stratified squamous epithelium lines cyst with cutaneous appendages including
  - Hair follicles, sebaceous glands, sweat glands identified in connective tissue wall

Top Differential Diagnoses
- Normal skin surface
- Nasopharyngeal dermoids
- Nasal glial heterotopia

- Intracranial extension may occur

MICROSCOPIC PATHOLOGY

Histologic Features
- Stratified squamous epithelium lines cyst with cutaneous appendages identified in connective tissue wall including
  - Hair follicles
  - Sebaceous glands
  - Sweat glands
- Lumen filled with keratin or sebaceous material
- Respiratory epithelium may be identified

DIFFERENTIAL DIAGNOSIS

Normal Skin Surface
- Clinical presentation as mass or swelling assists in differentiating dermoid cyst from normal skin

Nasopharyngeal Dermoids
- Not actually cysts but ectopic accessory auricles

Nasal Glial Heterotopia
- Glial tissue identified
  - Confirmed by immunohistochemical staining including
    - Glial fibrillary acidic protein (GFAP)
    - Neurofibrillary protein (NFP)

SELECTED REFERENCES

1. Cambiaghi S et al: Nasal dermoid sinus cyst. Pediatr Dermatol. 24(6):646-50, 2007
2. Sreetharan V et al: Atypical congenital dermoids of the face: a 25-year experience. J Plast Reconstr Aesthet Surg. 60(9):1025-9, 2007
3. Blake WE et al: Nasal dermoid sinus cysts: a retrospective review and discussion of investigation and management. Ann Plast Surg. 57(5):535-40, 2006
4. Zapata S et al: Nasal dermoids. Curr Opin Otolaryngol Head Neck Surg. 14(6):406-11, 2006
5. Charrier JB et al: Craniofacial dermoids: an embryological theory unifying nasal dermoid sinus cysts. Cleft Palate Craniofac J. 42(1):51-7, 2005
6. Meher R et al: Nasal dermoid with intracranial extension. J Postgrad Med. 51(1):39-40, 2005
7. Rahbar R et al: The presentation and management of nasal dermoid: a 30-year experience. Arch Otolaryngol Head Neck Surg. 129(4):464-71, 2003
8. Urth A et al: Nasal dermoid cyst: diagnosis and management of five cases. Acta Otorhinolaryngol Belg. 56(3):325-9, 2002
9. Pivnick EK et al: Gorlin syndrome associated with midline nasal dermoid cyst. J Med Genet. 33(8):704-6, 1996
10. Allbery SM et al: MR imaging of nasal masses. Radiographics. 15(6):1311-27, 1995
11. Posnick JC et al: Intracranial nasal dermoid sinus cysts: computed tomographic scan findings and surgical results. Plast Reconstr Surg. 93(4):745-54; discussion 755-6, 1994
12. Pensler JM et al: Craniofacial dermoids. Plast Reconstr Surg. 82(6):953-8, 1988
13. McCaffrey TV et al: Dermoid cysts of the nose: review of 21 cases. Otolaryngol Head Neck Surg. 87(1):52-9, 1979

IMAGE GALLERY

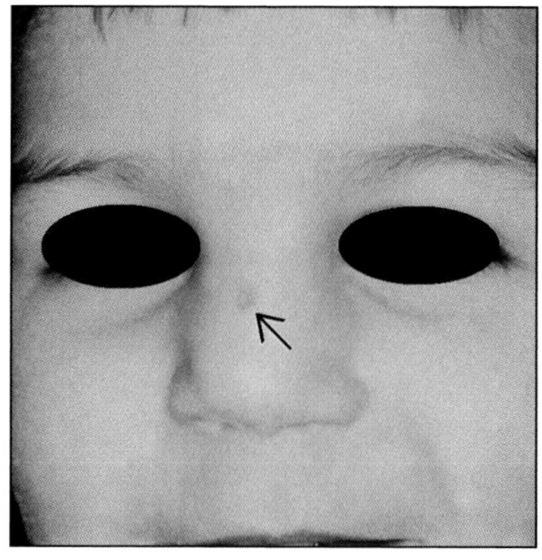

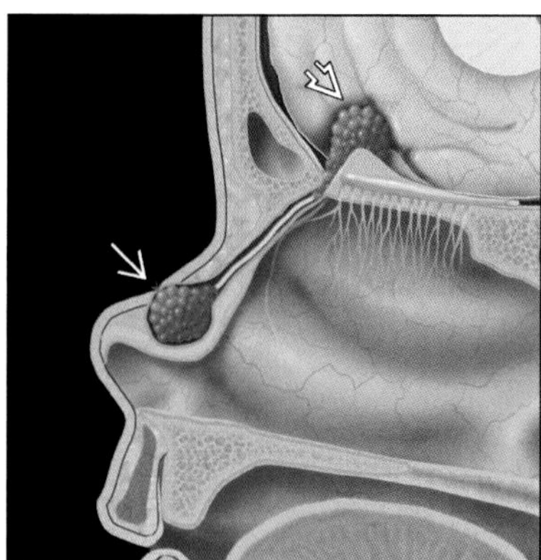

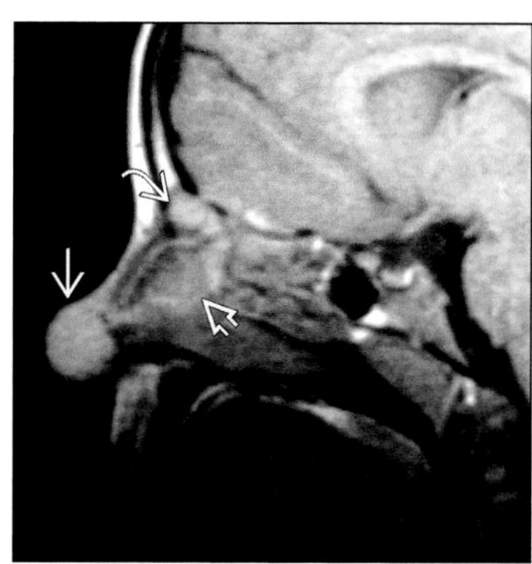

*(**Left**) Child with nasal dermal sinus shows the nasal pit ➔ on the bridge of the nose. The broad nasal bridge is secondary to growing subcutaneous dermoid. (**Center**) Lateral graphic depicts nasal dermal sinus with extracranial dermoids just below the nasal pit ➔; an intracranial dermoid ➔ splits bifid crista galli. (**Right**) Sagittal T1WI MR shows the dermoid at the nasal tip ➔. Additional dermoids are noted in the nasal septum ➔ and at the skull base ➔.*

PRIMARY CILIARY DYSKINESIA

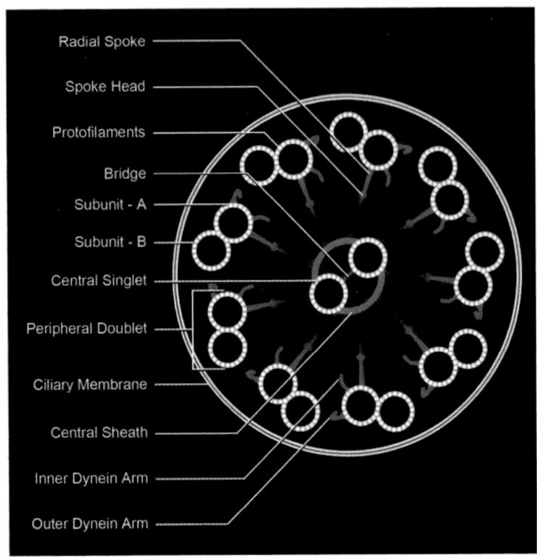

Schematic cross section shows a ciliary axoneme (main body of the organellum) detailing the normal ciliary structures, including single central couplet and 9 pairs of peripheral doublets.

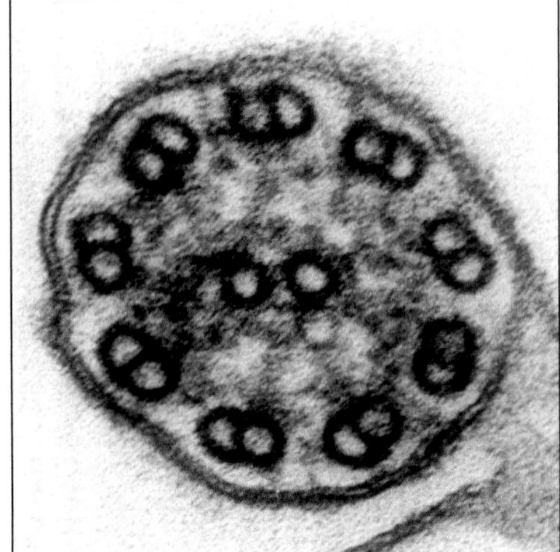

Electron microscopic evaluation of nasal biopsy in a patient suspected of having PCD shows a cilia with complete absence of dynein arms, the most confidently diagnosable ciliary structural anomaly.

TERMINOLOGY

Abbreviations

- Primary ciliary dyskinesia (PCD)

Synonyms

- Immotile cilia syndrome

Definitions

- Multisystem disease caused by ultrastructural defects of respiratory cilia and sperm tails

ETIOLOGY/PATHOGENESIS

Genetic

- Majority are inherited as autosomal recessive trait
- Different genes are involved in different patients and genetic mutations include
  - *DNAI1* (chromosome 7p21), *DNAH5* (chromosome 5p15-5p14), *DNAH11* (chromosome 7p21)

Acquired

- Referred to as secondary ciliary dyskinesia, usually result of epithelial alterations subsequent to inflammatory disease

CLINICAL ISSUES

Epidemiology

- Incidence
  - Unknown
  - Associated in approximately 50% of patients with situs inversus totalis (Kartagener syndrome)
- Age
  - Typically presents in early neonatal period

Presentation

- Characterized by recurrent respiratory tract infections, sinusitis, bronchiectasis, and male subfertility
  - Sinusitis, mucopurulent rhinorrhea, otitis media often striking, occurring in virtually all patients
- Chronic bronchitis, recurrent pneumonia, and atelectasis virtually pathognomonic for Kartagener syndrome
  - This scenario does not require cilia evaluation for diagnosis
    - Approximately 50% of patients lack situs inversus

Laboratory Tests

- Exhaled and nasal nitric oxide (NO) measurements useful to screen children and detect PCD in children
  - Nasal NO significantly lower in children with proven PCD compared to cases with negative biopsy results and healthy control subjects
  - Nasal NO below a cut-off level of < 105 ppb reported specificity of 88% for PCD and positive predictive value of 89%
  - Nasal NO above cut-off level of 105 ppb excluded PCD with 100% certainty

Treatment

- Palliative, centered on maintaining airway
- Surgery may be required for nasal polyps

Prognosis

- Not usually life-threatening
- Ciliary abnormality represents universal and permanent genetic defect

MACROSCOPIC FEATURES

Sections to Be Submitted

- Nasal cavity biopsy most easily obtained specimen
- Foci of squamous metaplasia secondary to chronic rhinitis common
  - Biopsy from this area likely contains no cilia
  - In this situation, specimen best obtained from more posterior nasal cavity

PRIMARY CILIARY DYSKINESIA

Key Facts

Terminology
- Multisystem disease caused by ultrastructural defects of respiratory cilia and sperm tails

Etiology/Pathogenesis
- Usually inherited as autosomal recessive trait

Clinical Issues
- Sinusitis, otitis media, and mucopurulent rhinorrhea often striking, occurring in virtually all patients
- Chronic bronchitis, recurrent pneumonia, and atelectasis are common

Macroscopic Features
- Nasal cavity biopsy is usually most easily obtained specimen

Ancillary Tests
- Absence of dynein arms is most confidently diagnosable structural anomaly

- Tracheal mucosal brushing or biopsy has much higher chance of producing specimen with abundant cilia

ANCILLARY TESTS

Electron Microscopy
- Ultrastructural examination of cilia required for diagnostic purposes
  - Absence of dynein arms is most confidently diagnosable structural anomaly
  - Dynein arms necessary for translational movement of ciliary peripheral doublet tubules with respect to one another
- Evaluation of dynein arm abnormality may be problematic
  - Requires sample with multiple ciliary cross sections with clear structural detail
  - Arms not seen on every tubule doublet even with the best photographic results
  - Mediocre or poor technical results make it difficult to see arms clearly
  - Diagnosis of "shortened," "defective," or "partial absent" arms extremely difficult in most instances
    - Especially true of "absent inner arms," as inner arms seen less well than outer arms

DIFFERENTIAL DIAGNOSIS

Ultrastructurally Normal Cilia
- Internal structure of axoneme of cilia has classic 9 + 2 microtubular pattern
  - Pair in center composed of single microtubules (singlets)
  - Peripheral row of 9 are double-barreled (doublets) composed of subunits A and B
  - 2 short diverging arms (dynein arms) project clockwise from subunit A of each doublet toward the next doublet
  - Radial spokes connect subunit A to central sheath surrounding central singlets

SELECTED REFERENCES

1. Baker K et al: Making sense of cilia in disease: the human ciliopathies. Am J Med Genet C Semin Med Genet. 151C(4):281-95, 2009
2. Escudier E et al: Ciliary defects and genetics of primary ciliary dyskinesia. Paediatr Respir Rev. 10(2):51-4, 2009
3. Santamaria F et al: Nasal nitric oxide assessment in primary ciliary dyskinesia using aspiration, exhalation, and humming. Med Sci Monit. 14(2):CR80-85, 2008
4. Geremek M et al: Primary ciliary dyskinesia: genes, candidate genes and chromosomal regions. J Appl Genet. 45(3):347-61, 2004
5. Mierau GW et al: The role of electron microscopy in evaluating ciliary dysfunction: report of a workshop. Ultrastruct Pathol. 16(1-2):245-54, 1992

IMAGE GALLERY

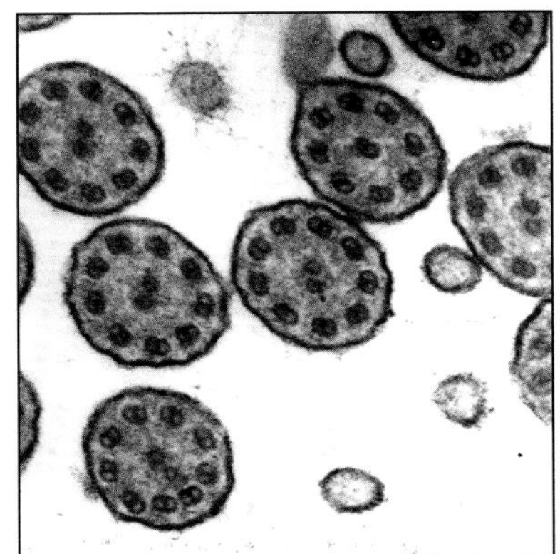

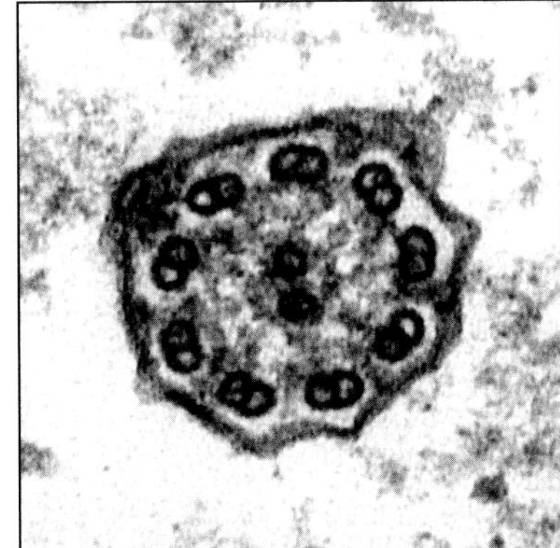

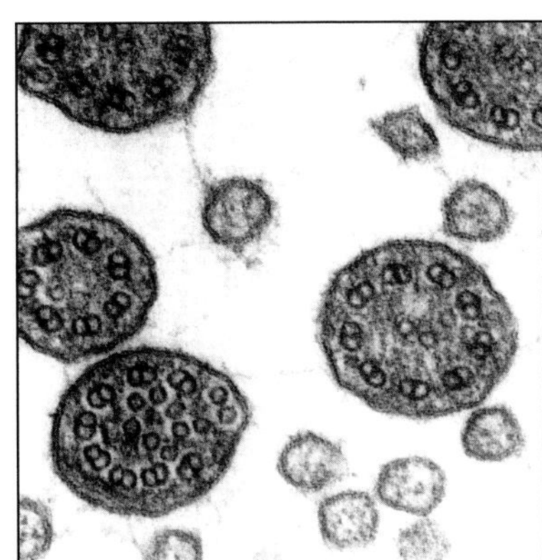

*(**Left**) Nasal cavity biopsy in a patient suspected of PCD, including well-prepared EM, shows cilia with loss of outer dynein arms. (**Center**) Patient with known Kartagener syndrome (situs inversus totalis) shows the absence of dynein arms. Evaluation of cilia is not required in a patient known to have Kartagener syndrome. (**Right**) Example of partial absence of inner and outer dynein arms is shown. Adequate preparation is critical to prevent overinterpreting structural abnormalities.*

ALLERGIC FUNGAL SINUSITIS

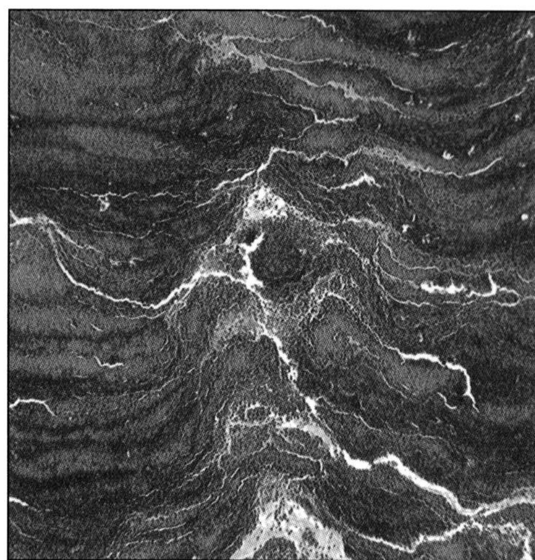

Hematoxylin & eosin shows "tide lines," "tree rings," or alternating bands of nuclear and cytoplasmic debris, findings characteristic for allergic fungal sinusitis.

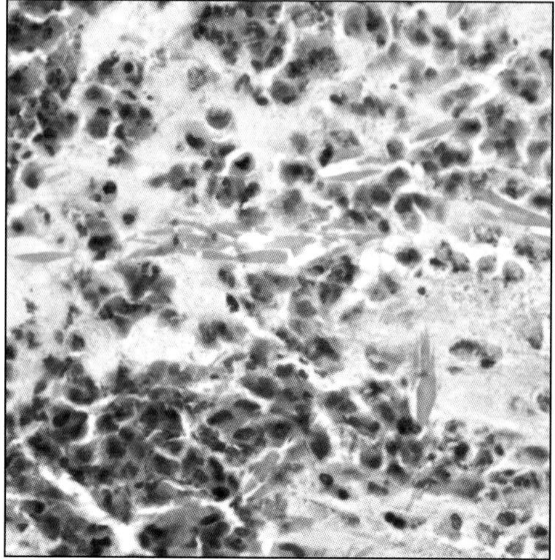

Hematoxylin & eosin shows degenerated inflammatory cells and eosinophils with Charcot-Leyden crystals (breakdown products of eosinophils).

TERMINOLOGY

Abbreviations

- Allergic fungal sinusitis (AFS)

Synonyms

- Allergic mucin
- Eosinophilic fungal rhinosinusitis (EFRS)
- Eosinophilic mucin rhinosinusitis (EMRS)
- Allergic fungal rhinosinusitis
- Hypertrophic sinus disease (HSD)
- Atopical fungal sinusitis

Definitions

- Allergic response in sinonasal tract mucosa to aerosolized fungal allergens, amplified and perpetuated by eosinophils

ETIOLOGY/PATHOGENESIS

Environmental Exposure

- Allergic reaction to inhaled fungal elements
  - Class II genes in major histocompatibility complex are involved in antigen presentation and immune response/modulation
  - Allergic reaction develops in immunocompetent people
  - *Aspergillus* species most common
  - Dematiaceous (brown-pigmented) fungi
    - Widespread in soil, wood, and decomposing plant material
    - *Alternaria*
    - *Bipolaris*
    - *Curvularia*
    - *Exserohilum*
    - *Phialophora* species
  - *Mucor* is uncommon agent

Pathogenesis

- Atopic host is exposed to finely dispersed fungi
- Inflammatory response is mediated by immunoglobulin E (IgE)
  - Type 1 hypersensitivity reaction
- Tissue edema with sinus obstruction and stasis
- Proliferation of fungus results in increased antigenic exposure
- Self-perpetuating cycle producing allergic mucin and possibly polyps

CLINICAL ISSUES

Epidemiology

- Incidence
  - Common
    - Approximately 10% of patients with chronic rhinosinusitis or nasal polyposis have AFS concurrently
    - Increased frequency in patients with asthma, allergies (atopic), and allergic bronchopulmonary aspergillosis (ABPA)
  - Increased in warmer climates
- Age
  - Usually in 3rd to 7th decades
  - Not a disease seen in children
- Gender
  - Equal gender distribution
    - Males more likely to present with bone erosion than females

Site

- Nasal cavity
- Paranasal sinuses
  - Maxillary and ethmoid sinuses most common

Presentation

- Atopy is common (allergy)
- Chronic, unrelenting rhinosinusitis
- Mass
  - May result in facial dysmorphia and proptosis

ALLERGIC FUNGAL SINUSITIS

Key Facts

Terminology
- Eosinophilic fungal rhinosinusitis (EFRS)
- Allergic response within sinonasal tract mucosa to aerosolized fungal allergens, amplified and perpetuated by eosinophils

Etiology/Pathogenesis
- Allergic reaction to inhaled fungal elements
- *Aspergillus* species most common

Clinical Issues
- Atopy is common (allergy)
- Polyps with putty-like material
- Peripheral eosinophilia
- Elevated fungal-specific IgE
- Extensive debridement and complete evacuation of impacted mucin is mainstay of therapy
- Postoperative anti-inflammatory therapy, including oral corticosteroids

Macroscopic Features
- Foul odor
- Putty or crunchy peanut butter-like consistency
- Muddy or greasy consistency

Microscopic Pathology
- "Tide lines," "tree rings," waves, or ripples of mucin material alternating with inflammatory debris

Ancillary Tests
- GMS (Gomori methenamine silver); PAS/light green

Top Differential Diagnoses
- Invasive fungal sinusitis
- Mycetoma

    - If proptosis is present, visual disturbances are reported
- Discharge
- Rhinorrhea
- Headache

Laboratory Tests
- Peripheral eosinophilia
- Elevated fungal-specific IgE
  - May also have elevated levels of fungal-specific IgG3
- Cultures performed to identify etiologic fungal agent
  - Results used to conduct desensitization treatments
  - Cultures are **not** used to provide antibiotic sensitivities since there is no invasive fungal infection

Treatment
- Options, risks, complications
  - Usually requires combination of surgery and medical therapy to yield best long-term outcome
- Surgical approaches
  - Extensive debridement and complete evacuation of impacted mucin is mainstay of therapy
  - Polypectomy and marsupialization of involved sinuses at minimum
  - Procedures may be endoscopic
    - Functional endoscopic sinus surgery (FESS)
- Drugs
  - Postoperative anti-inflammatory therapy
    - Oral corticosteroids usually yield best outcome
  - Postoperative azoles (specifically, itraconazole) may reduce recurrences
  - Medical management of allergic inflammatory disease
- Allergic desensitization (immunotherapy)

Prognosis
- Good with integrated medical and surgical approach
- Recurrences develop with fair frequency
  - Can be problematic to functional status of patient

IMAGE FINDINGS

CT Findings
- Expansile, sometimes destructive mass within nasal cavity and paranasal sinuses
- Bone remodeling or destruction
  - Orbital expansion and bony erosion are prominent features
- Bone erosion can be seen in advanced cases

MACROSCOPIC FEATURES

General Features
- Foul odor
- Polypoid fragments
- Putty or crunchy peanut butter-like consistency
- Muddy consistency
- Greasy to palpation

Size
- Range: 0.1-0.4 cm fragments of tissue
  - Mean overall aggregate: Up to 8 cm

MICROSCOPIC PATHOLOGY

Histologic Features
- Multiple polypoid fragments identified histologically
- "Mucinous" material is free floating, unattached to surrounding respiratory tissues
- "Tide lines," "tree rings," waves, or ripples
  - Appearance due to mucin material alternating with inflammatory debris
  - Yields overall "blue and pink" alternating appearance
- Degenerated material composed of neutrophils, eosinophils, and mucinous debris
  - Ghost outlines of cells common
  - Nuclear debris tends to aggregate
- Charcot-Leyden crystals (degenerated eosinophils)
  - Long, needle-shaped, or bipyramidal crystals
  - Dropped sub-stage condenser will yield refractile appearance to crystals

- Fungal elements often difficult to detect (even with special stains)
  - When fungal elements not identified, EMRS can be used instead
- Concurrent sinonasal pathology
  - Sinonasal inflammatory polyps
    - Polyps may show inflammation but not abscesses or necrotic material
  - Chronic rhinosinusitis

ANCILLARY TESTS

Histochemistry

- GMS (Gomori methenamine silver)
  - Highlights fungal hyphae (when present)
- PAS/light green
  - Highlights fungal hyphae (when present)

DIFFERENTIAL DIAGNOSIS

Invasive Fungal Sinusitis

- Fungal hyphae identified within
  - Vessel walls or vascular spaces
  - Tissue
- Significant host response within stroma
  - Inflammatory cells are identified within tissue rather than floating in lumen mucin as seen with AFS
- No alternating pattern

Sinonasal Polyps

- Polypoid structures with intact surface epithelium
- Mucinous or edema material in background mixed with inflammatory cells
  - Eosinophils may be seen but usually not degenerated or associated with Charcot Leyden crystals
- Lacks alternating pattern
- Generally contains minor mucoserous glands in stroma

Mycetoma

- Aggregation or ball of fungi (yeasts &/or hyphae)
- Fruiting heads are common in this fungal disease
- Usually no host response
  - If present, can be lymphohistiocytic or eosinophilic
- Dematiaceous fungi most common

DIAGNOSTIC CHECKLIST

Pathologic Interpretation Pearls

- Putty-like gross appearance
- Alternating "tide lines" or "tree rings"
- Eosinophils and their breakdown products
- Do not need to prove fungal elements are present

SELECTED REFERENCES

1. Wise SK et al: Antigen-specific IgE in sinus mucosa of allergic fungal rhinosinusitis patients. Am J Rhinol. 22(5):451-6, 2008
2. Aribandi M et al: Imaging features of invasive and noninvasive fungal sinusitis: a review. Radiographics. 27(5):1283-96, 2007
3. Driemel O et al: [Allergic fungal sinusitis, fungus ball and invasive sinonasal mycosis - three fungal-related diseases] Mund Kiefer Gesichtschir. 11(3):153-9, 2007
4. Ghegan MD et al: Socioeconomic factors in allergic fungal rhinosinusitis with bone erosion. Am J Rhinol. 21(5):560-3, 2007
5. Kimura M et al: Usefulness of Fungiflora Y to detect fungus in a frozen section of allergic mucin. Pathol Int. 57(9):613-7, 2007
6. Mirante JP et al: Endoscopic view of allergic fungal sinusitis. Ear Nose Throat J. 86(2):74, 2007
7. Orlandi RR et al: Microarray analysis of allergic fungal sinusitis and eosinophilic mucin rhinosinusitis. Otolaryngol Head Neck Surg. 136(5):707-13, 2007
8. Revankar SG: Dematiaceous fungi. Mycoses. 50(2):91-101, 2007
9. Ryan MW et al: Allergic fungal rhinosinusitis: diagnosis and management. Curr Opin Otolaryngol Head Neck Surg. 15(1):18-22, 2007
10. Schubert MS: Allergic fungal sinusitis. Clin Allergy Immunol. 20:263-71, 2007
11. Schubert MS: Allergic fungal sinusitis. Clin Rev Allergy Immunol. 30(3):205-16, 2006
12. Heffner DK: Allergic fungal sinusitis is a histopathologic diagnosis; paranasal mucocele is not. Ann Diagn Pathol. 8(5):316-23, 2004
13. Huchton DM: Allergic fungal sinusitis: an otorhinolaryngologic perspective. Allergy Asthma Proc. 24(5):307-11, 2003
14. Ferguson BJ: Definitions of fungal rhinosinusitis. Otolaryngol Clin North Am. 33(2):227-35, 2000
15. Kuhn FA et al: Allergic fungal rhinosinusitis: perioperative management, prevention of recurrence, and role of steroids and antifungal agents. Otolaryngol Clin North Am. 33(2):419-33, 2000
16. Mabry RL et al: Allergic fungal sinusitis: the role of immunotherapy. Otolaryngol Clin North Am. 33(2):433-40, 2000
17. Marple BF: Allergic fungal rhinosinusitis: surgical management. Otolaryngol Clin North Am. 33(2):409-19, 2000

Radiographic, Gross, and Microscopic Features

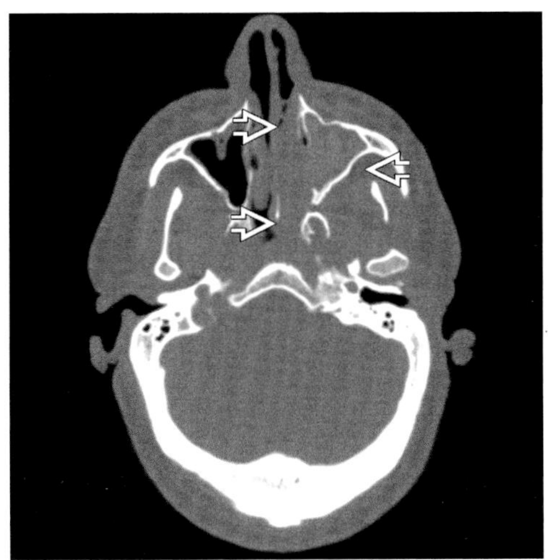

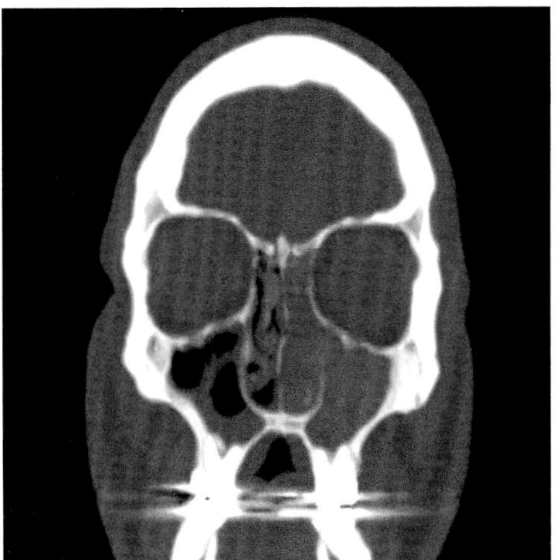

(Left) *Radiologic image shows opacification but no destruction of the nasal cavity and sinuses (left) by allergic fungal sinusitis ⮞. Polyps are noted in the contralateral maxillary sinus, a frequent concurrent finding.* **(Right)** *Radiologic image shows opacification of the sinuses and nasal cavity by a homogeneous density. Note polypoid tissue and mucosal thickening in the opposite maxillary sinus, frequently concurrently identified.*

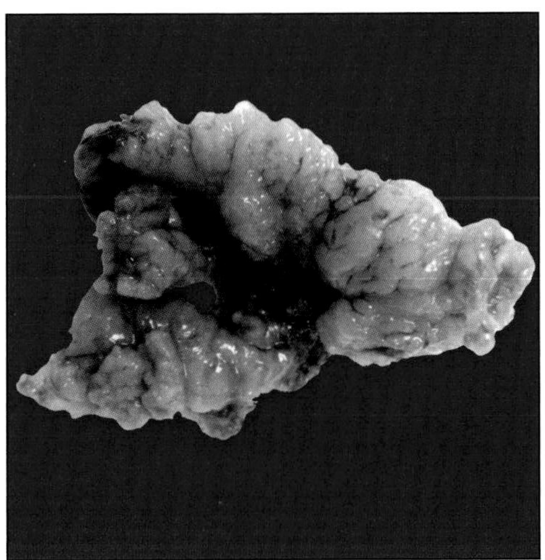

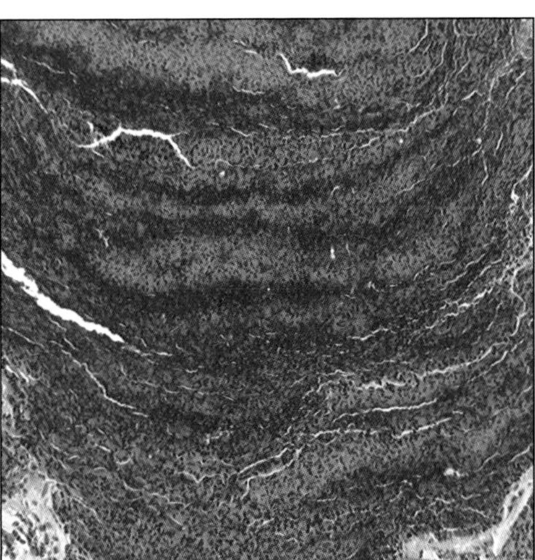

(Left) *Gross photograph shows a polypoid fragment of tissue with multiple projections. The tissue was greasy with a putty-like consistency on cut section.* **(Right)** *Hematoxylin & eosin shows alternating ripples of eosinophils and neutrophils. The mucinous to myxoid degeneration creates these "light" and "dark" rings or bands. This feature alone is quite characteristic of the disorder, seldom requiring any additional studies or evaluation.*

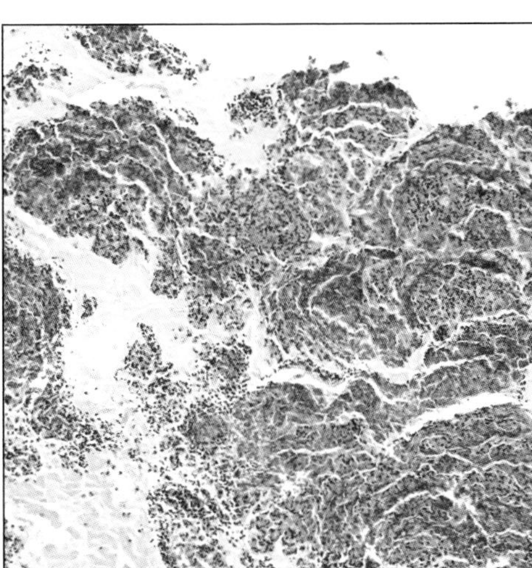

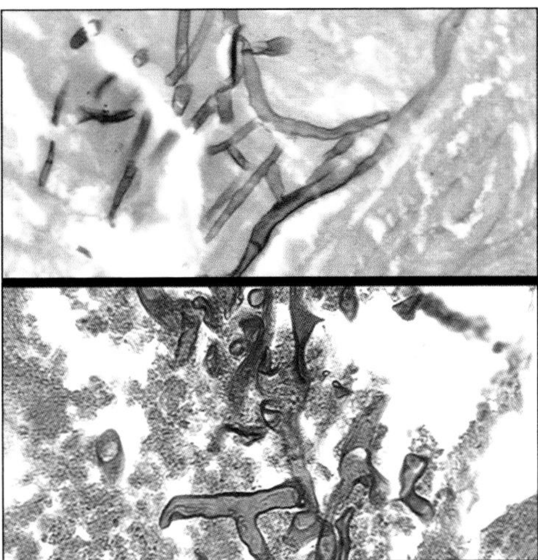

(Left) *Hematoxylin & eosin shows degenerated inflammatory cells with mucinous material and neutrophilic and eosinophilic debris. The cracking artifacts within the tissue highlight the tide-line appearance.* **(Right)** *Composite image shows fungal organisms embedded within the degenerated debris. Top: GMS highlights Aspergillus species with acute angle branching and septations. Bottom: Hematoxylin & eosin stain highlights Mucor species with wide, ribbon-like, aseptate hyphae.*

MYCETOMA

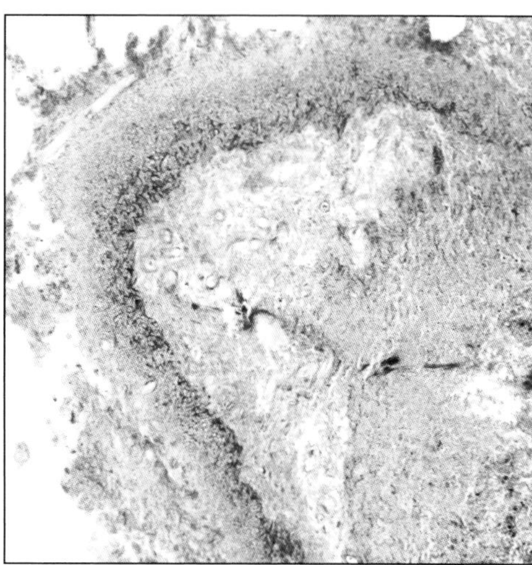

Hematoxylin & eosin shows myriad organisms aggregated to form a ball, with the yeast forming toward the periphery.

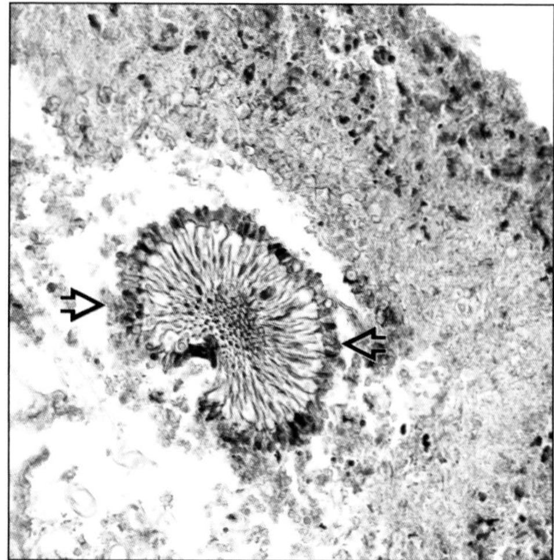

Hematoxylin & eosin shows fungal organisms surrounding a fruiting head ➢, a finding that can be seen in mycetoma.

TERMINOLOGY

Synonyms

- Sinus fungal ball, fungus ball, noninvasive fungal sinusitis, noninvasive sinus mycetoma, "snotoma"
- Extramucosal fungal sinusitis (EFS)

Definitions

- Aggregation of fungal elements in sinus lumen, eliciting limited response but not invading sinonasal tract tissues
- Noninvasive or extramucosal mycotic infection

ETIOLOGY/PATHOGENESIS

Infectious Agents

- Commensal fungi in nose may be the source
- *Aspergillus* species most common

CLINICAL ISSUES

Epidemiology

- Age
  - All ages affected
- Gender
  - Equal gender distribution

Site

- Maxillary sinus is most commonly affected (~ 85%)
- Sphenoid, ethmoid, and frontal sinuses affected less commonly

Presentation

- Unilateral nasal discharge, nasal obstruction, chronic sinusitis and stuffiness
- Rhinorrhea, often present for extended duration
- Nasal polyps and atopy may be present
- Pain is uncommon
- Patients are usually immunocompetent
- Rare: Diplopia and new onset seizures

Laboratory Tests

- Fungal cultures are usually negative
- Immunoglobulin levels normal

Treatment

- Options, risks, complications
  - Antifungal therapy is not indicated
    - Concurrent invasive fungal sinusitis: Antifungal medication required
  - Nasal lavage with topical steroids helps improve postsurgical outcome
- Surgical approaches
  - Complete surgical extraction by functional endoscopic sinus surgery (FESS) performed at sinus ostium
    - Ensures adequate access, careful removal of fungal elements, drainage and aeration
    - Gauze-assisted technique may be effective
    - Caldwell-Luc procedure can be used but alters sinus physiology adversely

Prognosis

- Excellent; rare recurrence/persistence (< 4%)

IMAGE FINDINGS

Radiographic Findings

- Heterogeneous opacification, microcalcifications, sinus expansion, and bone erosion (lysis) within sinus(es) on computed tomography
- "Foreign body" appearance may be noted

MACROSCOPIC FEATURES

General Features

- Cheesy, gray-green to yellow-white
- "Ball" may be hard or calcified

MYCETOMA

Key Facts

Terminology

- Aggregation of fungal elements in sinus lumen without invading sinonasal tract tissues

Clinical Issues

- Unilateral maxillary sinus involvement (~ 85%)

Image Findings

- Heterogeneous opacification, microcalcifications in sinuses on CT

Macroscopic Features

- Cheesy, gray-green to yellow-white material

Microscopic Pathology

- Huge aggregates of hyphae creating ball
- *Aspergillus* species most common

Top Differential Diagnoses

- Invasive fungal sinusitis
- Allergic fungal sinusitis

MICROSCOPIC PATHOLOGY

Histologic Features

- Huge aggregates of hyphae, creating "concretion" or ball
- Identified within cavity spaces and not within mucosa or soft tissue
- *Aspergillus fumigatus* is most common
- Fruiting heads identified (not in invasive sinusitis)
- Inflammatory cells usually limited

ANCILLARY TESTS

Histochemistry

- GMS (Gomori methenamine silver) positive organisms

DIFFERENTIAL DIAGNOSIS

Invasive Fungal Sinusitis

- Requires fungal hyphae within tissue, vascular spaces, or bone
- Needs to be carefully excluded

Allergic Fungal Sinusitis

- Purely luminal aggregation of alternating pattern of degenerated inflammatory cells, especially eosinophils, with mucin
- Fungal organisms hard to identify

Sinonasal Inflammatory Polyps

- Polyps may have edema and abundant inflammatory cells but not aggregates of fungal elements

SELECTED REFERENCES

1. Costa F et al: Functional endoscopic sinus surgery for the treatment of Aspergillus mycetomas of the maxillary sinus. Minerva Stomatol. 57(3):117-25, 2008
2. Costa F et al: Surgical treatment of Aspergillus mycetomas of the maxillary sinus: review of the literature. Oral Surg Oral Med Oral Pathol Oral Radiol Endod. 103(6):e23-9, 2007
3. Chao TK et al: Gauze-assisted technique in endoscopic removal of fungus balls of the maxillary sinus. Am J Rhinol. 20(4):417-20, 2006
4. Taxy JB: Paranasal fungal sinusitis: contributions of histopathology to diagnosis: a report of 60 cases and literature review. Am J Surg Pathol. 30(6):713-20, 2006
5. Dufour X et al: Paranasal sinus fungus ball and surgery: a review of 175 cases. Rhinology. 43(1):34-9, 2005
6. Schubert MS: Fungal rhinosinusitis: diagnosis and therapy. Curr Allergy Asthma Rep. 1(3):268-76, 2001
7. deShazo RD et al: A new classification and diagnostic criteria for invasive fungal sinusitis. Arch Otolaryngol Head Neck Surg. 123(11):1181-8, 1997
8. Klossek JM et al: Functional endoscopic sinus surgery and 109 mycetomas of paranasal sinuses. Laryngoscope. 107(1):112-7, 1997

IMAGE GALLERY

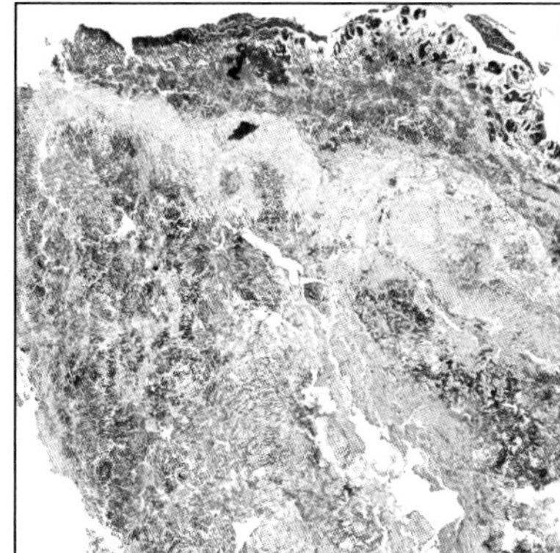

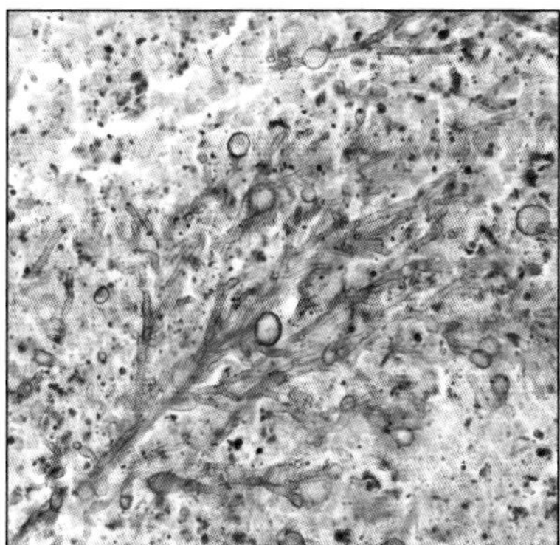

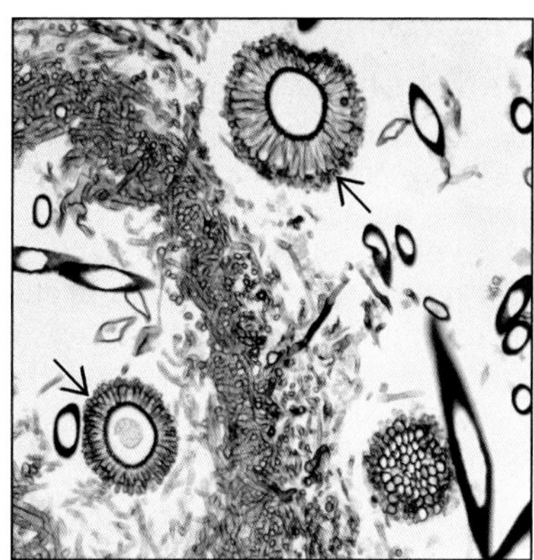

(Left) *Hematoxylin & eosin shows fungal elements (brown, rust, and purple) associated with bacterial colonies (blue material) in the upper portion of the field. Cracking artifacts are common.* ***(Center)*** *Hematoxylin & eosin shows acute angle branching of hyphae, with yeast forms attached at the end.* ***(Right)*** *GMS (Gomori methenamine silver) highlights the fungal elements and fruiting heads* ⇒ *but is usually not required for diagnosis.*

INVASIVE FUNGAL SINUSITIS

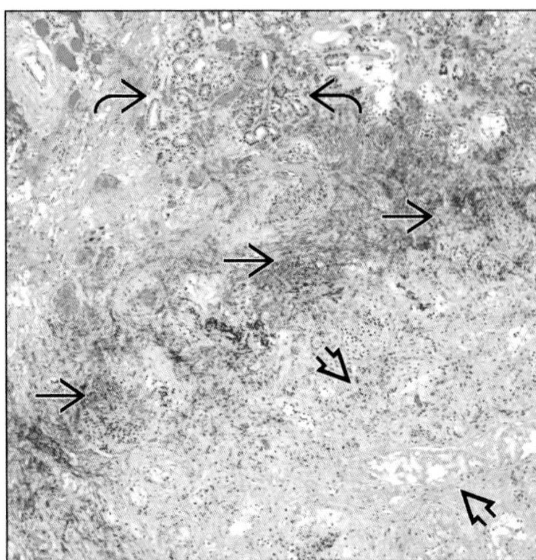

Resection material from invasive fungal sinusitis shows necrosis ⇒ and infarction ⇒ with effacement of the normal mucosal architecture, although residual mucoserous glands are present ⇒.

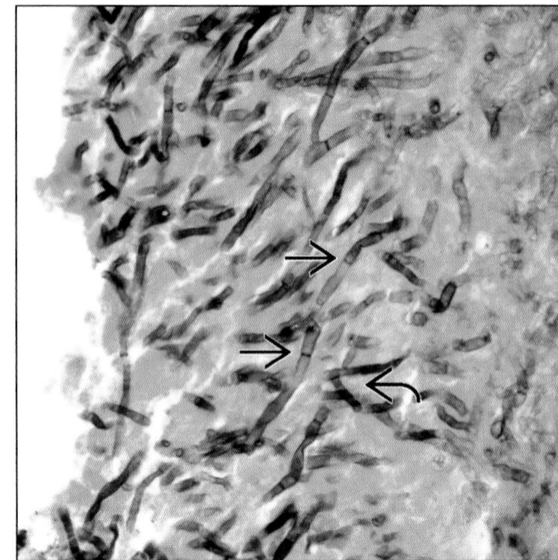

The identification of fungi is facilitated by histochemical staining. Aspergillus species are characterized by septated hyphae ⇒ and acute angle branching ⇒.

TERMINOLOGY

Synonyms

- Acute fulminant *Aspergillus* sinusitis

Definitions

- Acute, fulminant fungal infestation of sinonasal tract often resulting in destruction of involved sinus(es) within days

ETIOLOGY/PATHOGENESIS

Infectious Agents

- Most often caused by *Aspergillus* species
  - Other fungi found to be causative may include dematiaceous fungi
    - i.e., *Bipolaris, Exserohilum, Curvularia, Drechslera,* and *Alternaria*

CLINICAL ISSUES

Epidemiology

- Age
  - Most often occurs in adults but may occur in younger (immunocompromised) patients

Presentation

- Nasal discharge and sinus pain
  - Swelling of face (maxillary area and periorbital region) may be present
  - With progression of disease, blindness may occur
- Clinical picture of fulminant infection more similar to clinical picture of mucormycosis than to clinical features of other forms of sinonasal aspergillosis
- Typical clinical scenario includes occurrence in immunocompromised patients (e.g., diabetics, immunosuppression)
  - Immunosuppressed conditions may include post-transplant, malignant neoplasm
    - e.g., lymphoma
  - May occur in immunocompetent patients
- Patients may require immediate surgical debridement, often necessitating intraoperative consultation (i.e., frozen section) to determine cause of fulminant clinical picture
  - Pathologists tasked to histologically evaluate for presence of fungi
  - Intraoperative samples should be performed and sent for microbiologic cultures in order to speciate fungus

Treatment

- Options, risks, complications
  - Requires surgical debridement and antifungal chemotherapy
    - e.g., voriconazole, amphotericin B

Prognosis

- Mortality rates may be high
- Early diagnosis and treatment decreases morbidity and mortality

MICROSCOPIC PATHOLOGY

Histologic Features

- Tissue necrosis is evident, but inflammatory response often is very limited
- Fungal forms are identified throughout resected tissue
  - *Aspergillus* hyphae are thin (2-5 µm) with acute angle branching (45°) and septated
  - Fungi seen within mucosal and submucosal tissues as well as in and around vascular spaces (angioinvasion)

ANCILLARY TESTS

Histochemistry

- Gomori methenamine silver (GMS)

Key Facts

Terminology
- Acute, fulminant fungal infestation of sinonasal tract resulting in tissue destruction within days

Clinical Issues
- Typically occurs in immunocompromised patients
- Requires surgical debridement and antifungal chemotherapy (e.g., voriconazole, amphotericin B)
- Mortality rates high

Microscopic Pathology
- Tissue necrosis is evident, but inflammatory response often is very limited
- Fungal forms identified throughout resected tissue, which may include angioinvasion

Ancillary Tests
- Histochemical stains (GMS, PAS) positive

    - Positive; delineates fungal forms
- Periodic acid-Schiff (PAS)
    - Positive; delineates fungal forms

DIFFERENTIAL DIAGNOSIS

Mucormycosis
- In comparison to *Aspergillus*, *Mucor* hyphae are larger (7-20 µm), branch at haphazard angles (45-90°), and lack septations

Wegener Granulomatosis
- Absence of microorganisms and biocollagenolytic geographic-type granular necrosis
- Presence in active disease of elevated antineutrophil cytoplasmic autoantibodies &/or proteinase 3

Hematolymphoid Malignancy
- Characterized by malignant cellular infiltrate

DIAGNOSTIC CHECKLIST

Pathologic Interpretation Pearls
- Tissue necrosis with identification of fungal forms within tissue

SELECTED REFERENCES

1. Nakaya K et al: New treatment for invasive fungal sinusitis: three cases of chronic invasive fungal sinusitis treated with surgery and voriconazole. Auris Nasus Larynx. 37(2):244-9, 2010
2. Chakrabarti A et al: Fungal rhinosinusitis: a categorization and definitional schema addressing current controversies. Laryngoscope. 119(9):1809-18, 2009
3. Das A et al: Spectrum of fungal rhinosinusitis; histopathologist's perspective. Histopathology. 54(7):854-9, 2009
4. Deshazo RD: Syndromes of invasive fungal sinusitis. Med Mycol. 47 Suppl 1:S309-14, 2009
5. Anselmo-Lima WT et al: Invasive fungal rhinosinusitis in immunocompromised patients. Rhinology. 42(3):141-4, 2004
6. Granville L et al: Fungal sinusitis: histologic spectrum and correlation with culture. Hum Pathol. 35(4):474-81, 2004
7. Parikh SL et al: Invasive fungal sinusitis: a 15-year review from a single institution. Am J Rhinol. 18(2):75-81, 2004
8. Brandt ME et al: Epidemiology, clinical manifestations, and therapy of infections caused by dematiaceous fungi. J Chemother. 15 Suppl 2:36-47, 2003
9. Streppel M et al: Successful treatment of an invasive aspergillosis of the skull base and paranasal sinuses with liposomal amphotericin B and itraconazole. Ann Otol Rhinol Laryngol. 108(2):205-7, 1999
10. Gillespie MB et al: An approach to fulminant invasive fungal rhinosinusitis in the immunocompromised host. Arch Otolaryngol Head Neck Surg. 124(5):520-6, 1998
11. deShazo RD et al: A new classification and diagnostic criteria for invasive fungal sinusitis. Arch Otolaryngol Head Neck Surg. 123(11):1181-8, 1997

IMAGE GALLERY

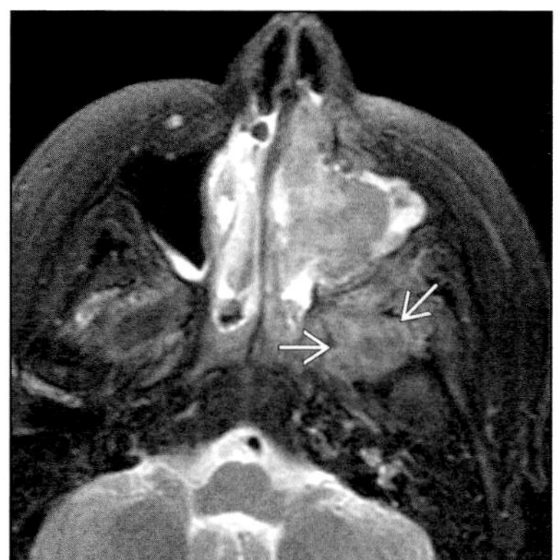

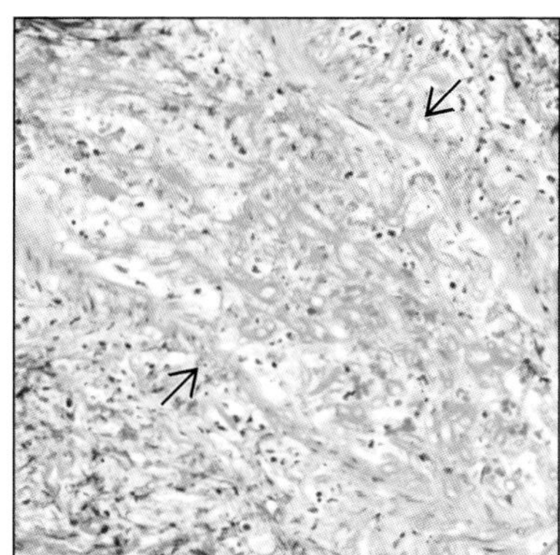

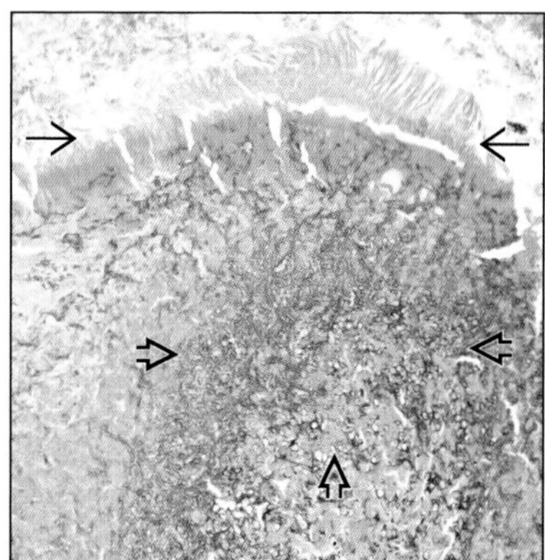

*(**Left**) The heterogeneity of the maxillary sinus contents is apparent on this T2 MR image. Abnormal signal is seen in the masticator space musculature ➡, indicative of spread beyond the sinus. (**Center**) Vascular thrombosis includes fungi, which required histochemical stains to identify (not shown); muscular wall ➡ assists in identifying the blood vessel. (**Right**) Fungal invasion and effacement of sinonasal mucosa ➡ is present. Note residual necrotic respiratory epithelium ➡.*

RHINOSCLEROMA

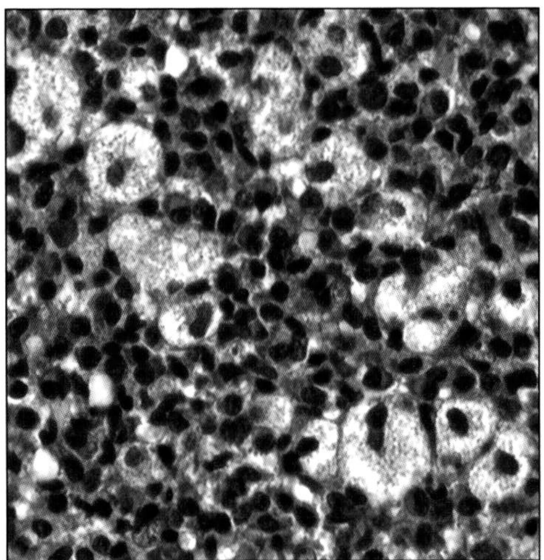

Hematoxylin & eosin shows multiple foamy macrophages (Mikulicz cells) within a background of lymphocytes.

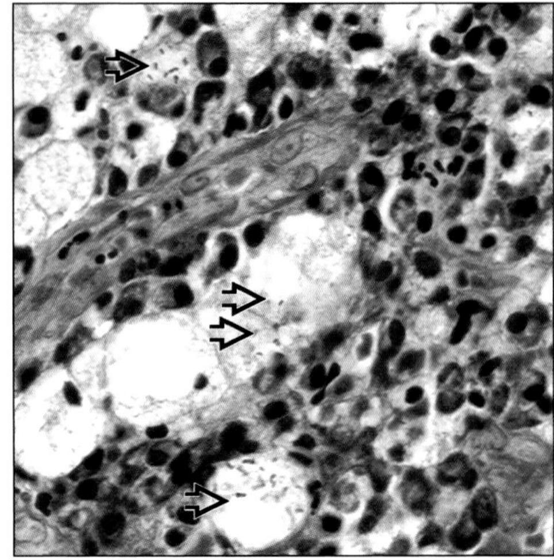

Warthin-Starry shows intracellular bacilli ➡ within the macrophages.

TERMINOLOGY

Synonyms

- Scleroma
- Hebra nose (after Hans von Hebra, who originally described the disease in 1870)
- Scrofulous lupus (no longer used)

Definitions

- Endemic, chronic, progressive, granulomatous infection of upper airways caused by bacterium *Klebsiella rhinoscleromatis*
  - Enterobacteriaceae family, also called Frisch bacillus (Anton von Frisch originally identified organisms in 1882)

ETIOLOGY/PATHOGENESIS

Infectious Agents

- *Klebsiella rhinoscleromatis*
  - Patients are immunologically competent but lack effective phagocytosis of organism by Mikulicz cells
    - Mikulicz described microscopic features in 1876

CLINICAL ISSUES

Epidemiology

- Incidence
  - Endemic within Central America, Egypt, tropical Africa, India, Indonesia, eastern Europe
    - Immigration patterns have led to increased number of patients in USA
- Age
  - Peak in 2nd and 3rd decades
- Gender
  - Female > Male
- Ethnicity
  - Central African, central American, Indian

Site

- Upper aerodigestive tract, nasal cavity specifically

Presentation

- Crowded conditions, poor hygiene & nutrition contribute to transmission
  - Tends to develop in blood-related people
  - Contracted from droplets or inhalation of contaminated material
- Any part of respiratory tract may be involved
- 3 overlapping clinical stages
  - Ozena (catarrhal phase): Includes atrophic rhinitis, with rhinorrhea
  - Granulomatous (proliferative phase): Granulomatous inflammation dominates and occludes nasal passages
  - Scleroma (cicatricial phase): Scarring and retraction of tissues

Laboratory Tests

- Relative reduction in CD4(+) cells; absolute increase in CD8(+) cells
  - Inversion of CD4(+)/CD8(+) ratio
- Culture for confirmation and antibiotic sensitivity
  - MacConkey agar, although growth seen in only ~ 50% of cases

Treatment

- Options, risks, complications
  - Long-term antibiotic therapy should be determined by age, sex, and repeat biopsies during careful monitoring for potential relapses
    - Organisms are difficult to eradicate
- Surgical approaches
  - Debridement
    - Laser (carbon-dioxide) vaporization can yield good results
    - Nasal dilation may be required to maintain physiologic nasal function
- Drugs

RHINOSCLEROMA

Key Facts

Terminology
- Chronic, progressive, granulomatous infection of upper airways caused by bacterium *Klebsiella rhinoscleromatis*

Clinical Issues
- Crowded conditions, poor hygiene, and poor nutrition contribute to transmission
- 3 overlapping clinical stages (ozena, granulomatous, scleroma)
- Treat with long-term antibiotic therapy and surgery

Microscopic Pathology
- Histiocyte and plasma cell nodules
- Vasculitis and acute inflammation
- Pseudoepitheliomatous hyperplasia, ulceration, and submucosal keratin cyst

Ancillary Tests
- Warthin-Starry stain highlights rod-shaped bacillus

- Selective prolonged antibiotic treatment
  - Tetracycline or ciprofloxacin

Prognosis
- Opportunistic infection that requires diligent follow-up due to high recurrence rate
- May cause significant disfigurement
- Antibiotic resistance needs to be evaluated
- Rarely, sepsis can be fatal

MICROSCOPIC PATHOLOGY

Histologic Features
- Sheets of inflammatory cells and histiocytes (Mikulicz cells)
  - Mikulicz cells are foamy histiocytes with organisms
  - Dominant inflammatory cells are plasma cells including Mott cells and Russell bodies
- Vasculitis, pseudoepitheliomatous hyperplasia, ulceration, and submucosal keratin cysts

ANCILLARY TESTS

Histochemistry
- Warthin-Starry stain highlights encapsulated, nonmotile, rod-shaped bacillus in Mikulicz cells
- PAS, Hotchkiss-McManis, Methenamine silver, Giemsa, Dieterle, Brown and Brenn, and Brown and Hopps do not give reliable results

Immunohistochemistry
- Highly sensitive and specific immunohistochemistry for *Klebsiella rhinoscleromatis* capsular antigen 3

DIFFERENTIAL DIAGNOSIS

Atypical Mycobacteria
- Tend to have less lymphoplasmacytic infiltrate and show granulomatous inflammation with giant cells

Lepromatous Leprosy
- Sheets of histiocytes filled with AFB organisms

Syphilis
- Plasma cells with vasculitis and spirochetes

Wegener Granulomatosis
- Biocollangenolysis with scant giant cells and vasculitis

SELECTED REFERENCES

1. Thompson LD: Rhinoscleroma. Ear Nose Throat J. 81(8):506, 2002
2. Andraca R et al: Rhinoscleroma: a growing concern in the United States? Mayo Clinic experience. Mayo Clin Proc. 68(12):1151-7, 1993
3. Meyer PR et al: Scleroma (Rhinoscleroma). A histologic immunohistochemical study with bacteriologic correlates. Arch Pathol Lab Med. 107(7):377-83, 1983
4. Shum TK et al: Clinical update on rhinoscleroma. Laryngoscope. 92(10 Pt 1):1149-53, 1982

IMAGE GALLERY

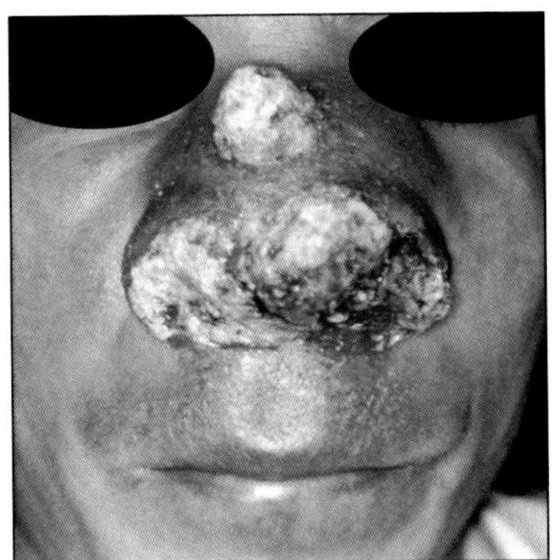

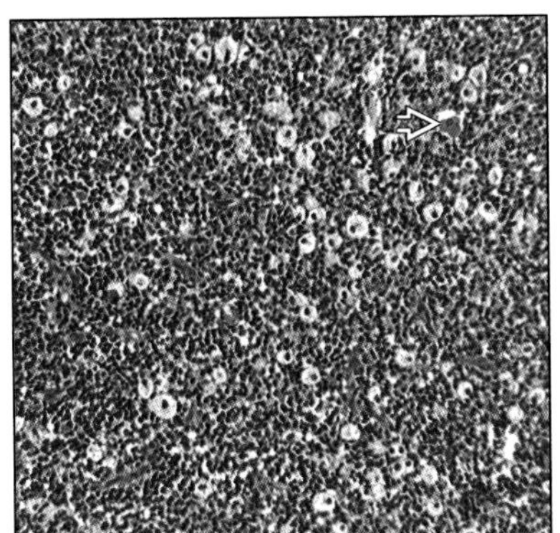

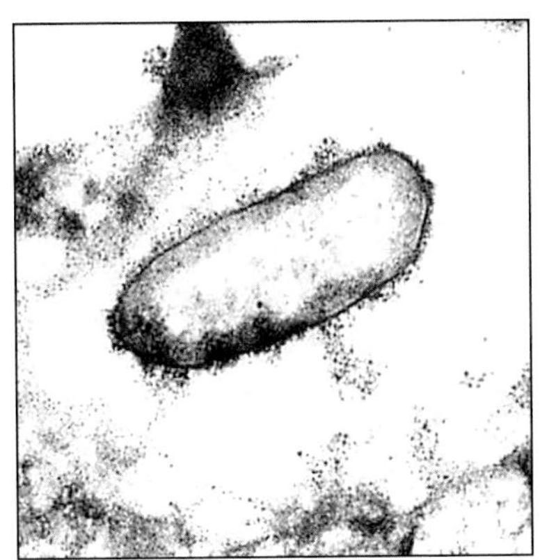

*(**Left**) Clinical photograph shows nasal destruction in a 42-year-old man with a several year history of a progressively destructive lesion. A palatal perforation was also noted. (Courtesy R. Carlos, MD.) (**Center**) Hematoxylin & eosin shows a sea of lymphoid cells with histiocytes throughout. Note the Russell body ➡. (**Right**) Ultrastructural examination shows the rod of Klebsiella rhinoscleromatis. Culture would be required to confirm the diagnosis, as the ultrastructural findings alone are insufficient.*

RHINOSPORIDIOSIS

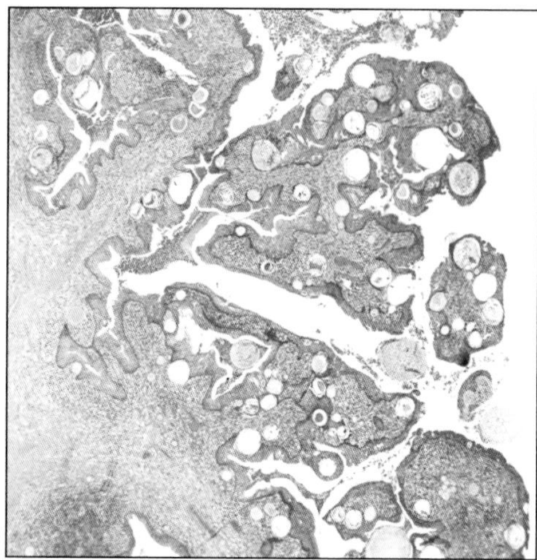

This polypoid proliferation is characterized by the presence of intraepithelial and submucosal cysts (sporangia). There is squamous metaplasia and irregular hyperplasia of the surface epithelium.

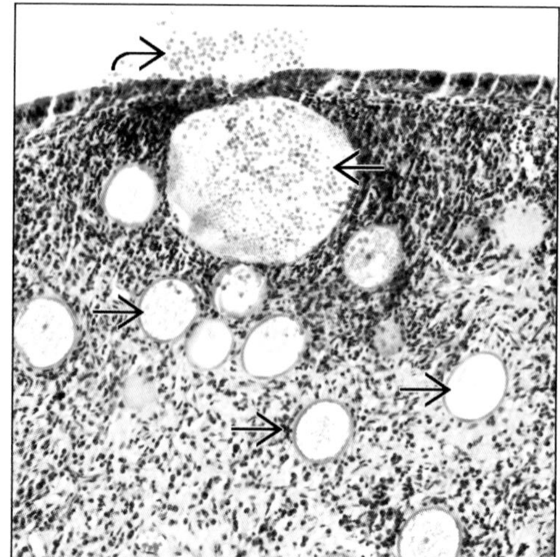

Thick-walled submucosal cysts (sporangia) ➔ of variable sizes contain endospores of varying maturation. One of the cysts ruptured with extrusion of endospores ➔ through the surface epithelium.

TERMINOLOGY

Definitions

- Chronic, indolent infection of upper respiratory tract disease caused by sporulating microorganism *Rhinosporidium seeberi*

ETIOLOGY/PATHOGENESIS

Environmental Exposure

- Thought to be zoonotic as rhinosporidiosis seen in cattle, horses, and mules
- Transmission thought to occur via water or dust
  - Endospore penetrates nasal mucosa and matures into sporangium in submucosal compartment
  - Following maturation, sporangia burst releasing endospores into surrounding tissue

Infectious Agents

- *R. seeberi*
  - Fungal organism
    - Does not grow on synthetic media
    - Has been propagated in cell culture media
    - Not considered contagious

CLINICAL ISSUES

Epidemiology

- Incidence
  - Endemic in India, Sri Lanka, and Brazil
    - Only sporadic occurrence in USA
- Age
  - All ages but common in 3rd and 4th decades
- Gender
  - Male > Female

Site

- Most commonly involves nasal cavity (inferior turbinate along lateral nasal wall) and nasopharynx
  - Infection may involve other mucosal sites
    - e.g., larynx, tracheobronchial tree, esophagus, pharynx, oral cavity, palpebral conjunctiva, ears

Presentation

- Patients are usually healthy
- Symptoms include
  - Nasal obstruction, epistaxis, rhinorrhea

Treatment

- Surgical approaches
  - Surgical excision
- Drugs
  - Antibiotic therapy not effective

Prognosis

- Recurrences necessitating additional surgical excision may occur in up to 10% of cases

MACROSCOPIC FEATURES

General Features

- Single or multiple polypoid, pedunculated, or sessile masses
  - Grossly resemble sinonasal inflammatory polyps
- Cut section shows pink- to purplish-appearing tissue with glistening mucoid surface
  - Microcysts may be seen in submucosal stroma

MICROSCOPIC PATHOLOGY

Histologic Features

- Mucosal and submucosal cysts (sporangia) ranging in size from 10-300 microns in diameter
- Sporangia contain innumerable sporangiospores (endospores) seen by hematoxylin and eosin
  - 2 sizes of sporangiospores may be seen
    - Smaller spores measuring ~ 1-2 micrometers in diameter

Key Facts

Terminology
- Chronic infectious disease caused by sporulating fungal microorganism *Rhinosporidium seeberi*

Etiology/Pathogenesis
- Transmission thought to occur via water or dust

Clinical Issues
- Most commonly involves nasal cavity and nasopharynx
- Surgical excision
- Antibiotic therapy not effective
- Recurrences in up to 10% of cases

Microscopic Pathology
- Mucosal and submucosal cysts (sporangia)
- Sporangia contain innumerable sporangiospores (endospores)
- Microorganisms stain with mucicarmine and periodic acid-Schiff

    - Larger spores measuring ~ 5-10 micrometers in diameter
  - Larger spores are the more mature forms
    - Tend to congregate toward the center with smaller being more peripheral, creating zonated appearance relative to spore size
- Smaller cystic structures (without sporangiospores) ranging from 10-100 micrometers are also seen
  - Called trophocysts
  - Considered to result from autoinfection via mature sporangiospores released from sporangia
  - Sporangia and trophocysts have eosinophilic walls measuring several micrometers in thickness
- Chronic inflammatory response consisting of lymphocytes, plasma cells, and eosinophils accompany the microorganisms
- Rupture of cysts will induce acute inflammatory response
  - Granulomatous reaction usually not seen, but cyst rupture may result in presence of multinucleated giant cells
- Overlying epithelium may be hyperplastic &/or demonstrate squamous metaplasia

ANCILLARY TESTS

Histochemistry
- Periodic acid-Schiff
  - Reactivity: Positive
- Mucicarmine
  - Reactivity: Positive

DIFFERENTIAL DIAGNOSIS

Coccidiomycosis Infection
- *R. seeberi* is usually much larger than *Coccidioides immitis*
- *C. immitis* does not stain with mucin
  - Wall of *R. seeberi* stains with mucin

Schneiderian Papilloma, Cylindrical Cell Type
- Cysts associated with schneiderian papilloma only intraepithelial
  - Cysts of rhinosporidiosis intraepithelial and submucosal

SELECTED REFERENCES

1. Makannavar JH et al: Rhinosporidiosis--a clinicopathological study of 34 cases. Indian J Pathol Microbiol. 44(1):17-21, 2001
2. Blitzer A et al: Fungal infections of the nose and paranasal sinuses. Part I. Otolaryngol Clin North Am. 26(6):1007-35, 1993
3. Batsakis JG et al: Rhinoscleroma and rhinosporidiosis. Ann Otol Rhinol Laryngol. 101(10):879-82, 1992
4. Thianprasit M et al: Rhinosporidiosis. Curr Top Med Mycol. 3:64-85, 1989
5. Satyanarayana C: Rhinosporidiosis with a record of 255 cases. Acta Otolaryngol. 51:348-66, 1960

IMAGE GALLERY

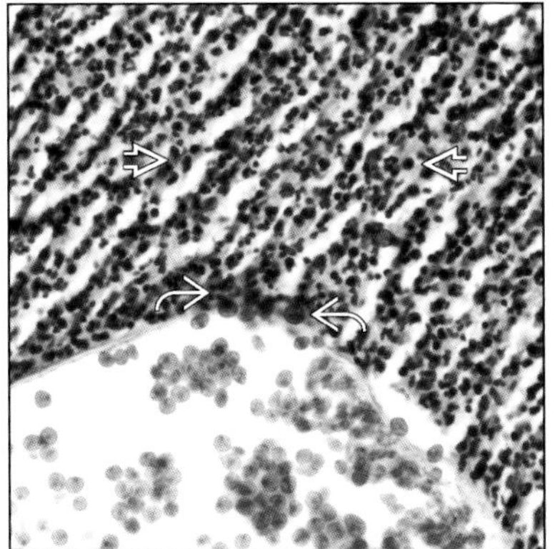

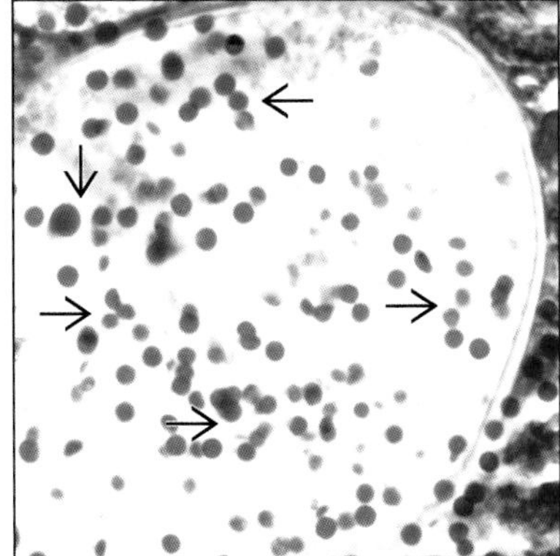

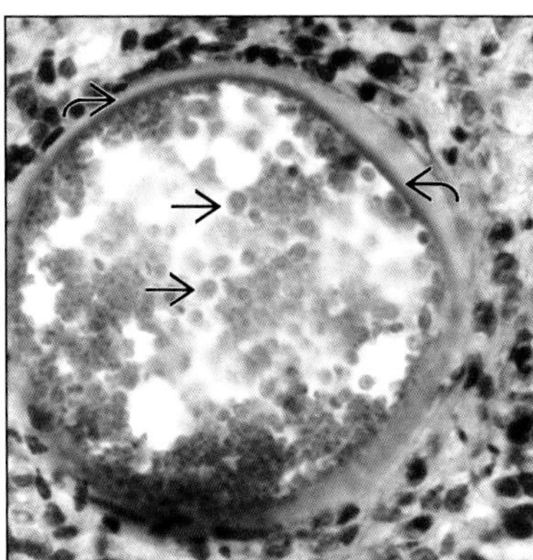

*(**Left**) Rupture of this cyst results in microabscess formation characterized by a sea of neutrophils ➡. Endospores are visible outside the cyst wall ➡. (**Center**) In addition to hematoxylin and eosin staining, the microorganisms (R. seeberi) are identifiable on histochemical staining. Periodic acid-Schiff (PAS) highlights the endospores ➡. (**Right**) The endospores ➡ are mucicarmine positive. The thick wall of the sporangium is also mucicarmine positive ➡.*

MYCOBACTERIA LEPRAE INFECTION

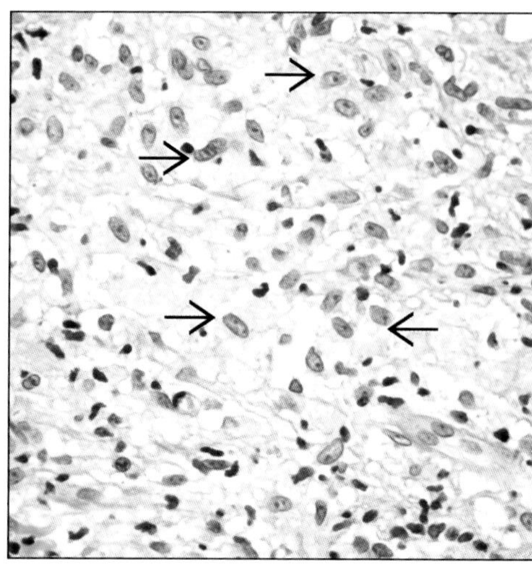

Lepromatous leprosy shows a diffuse proliferation of vacuolated histiocytes (so-called lepra cells) ⇒. In contrast to tuberculoid leprosy, well-formed granulomas are not present.

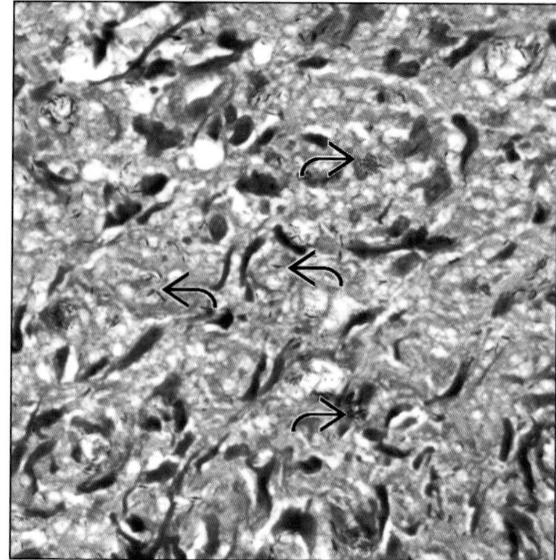

Abundant red staining M. lepra microorganisms, in clusters and as individual organisms ⇒, are present within the vacuolated histiocytes (lepra cells).

TERMINOLOGY

Abbreviations

- Lepromatous leprosy (LL)
- Tuberculoid leprosy (TL)

Synonyms

- Hansen disease

Definitions

- Infection caused by *Mycobacterium lepra* characterized by cutaneous, mucosal, and peripheral nerve involvement

ETIOLOGY/PATHOGENESIS

Infectious Agents

- *Mycobacterium lepra*
  - Low infectivity and exposure rarely results in infection
  - Believed to require cool host body temperature for survival
  - Affects cooler peripheral areas of the body, including digits, ears, nose, nasal cavity
- Sinonasal tract (mucosal) involvement fairly common and may be important in transmission of the disease
  - Nasal secretions contain high numbers of infectious bacilli
  - Initial site of infection may be nasal or oropharyngeal mucosa
  - Oral lesions are not uncommon
  - Less common sites of involvement of upper aerodigestive tract includes larynx

CLINICAL ISSUES

Site

- Patients with sinonasal tract involvement may present with
  - Mucopurulent rhinosinusitis, nosebleeds, and anosmia
    - Early lesions may appear plaque-like
    - Late lesions may be ulcerative and nodular and may result in collapse of bridge of nose
  - Due to involvement of peripheral nerves, pain and muscular atrophy as well as sensory loss occur frequently
    - Sensory loss begins in extremities and spreads to rest of body

Presentation

- 2 main clinical presentations occur based on immune reaction to the microorganism
  - **Lepromatous leprosy**
    - Also referred to as multibacillary leprosy
    - Develops in patients with reduced cell-mediated immune reaction
    - Disease is usually diffuse
    - Face is common site of involvement that may result in so-called "leonine facies" due to skin enlargement and facial distortion
    - Lepromin skin test is negative
    - Microorganisms are typically present in skin biopsy
  - **Tuberculoid leprosy**
    - Also referred to as paucicellular leprosy
    - Develops in patients with high immune reaction
    - Disease is usually localized

Treatment

- Surgical approaches
  - Reconstructive surgery may be required for cosmesis
- Drugs
  - Antibiotic therapy
    - Rifampin and dapsone for tuberculoid leprosy (6 month course)
    - Rifampin and dapsone and clofazimine for lepromatous leprosy (12 month course)

MYCOBACTERIA LEPRAE INFECTION

Key Facts

Terminology

- Infection caused by *M. lepra* characterized by cutaneous, mucosal, peripheral nerve involvement

Clinical Issues

- Peripheral nerve involvement results in pain and sensory loss
- Sinonasal tract involvement important in transmission of disease as numerous bacilli in nasal secretions

Microscopic Pathology

- **Lepromatous leprosy**
  - Absence of granulomatous inflammation
  - Presence of sheets of lymphocytes and vacuolated histiocytes (lepra cells)
  - Abundant microorganisms
- **Tuberculoid leprosy**
  - Noncaseating granulomatous inflammation
  - Paucity of microorganisms

MICROSCOPIC PATHOLOGY

Histologic Features

- 2 types of histopathologic processes can be seen
  - **Lepromatous leprosy**
    - Absence of granulomatous inflammation
    - Presence of sheets of lymphocytes and vacuolated histiocytes (lepra cells)
    - Abundant microorganisms by special stains
  - **Tuberculoid leprosy**
    - Well-formed granulomatous inflammation with admixture of histiocytes, multinucleated giant cells, and lymphocytes
    - Paucity of microorganisms by special stains
    - May approximate or surround peripheral nerves
  - **For both types**
    - Histopathologic process typically located in submucosa with intact surface epithelium
    - Pseudoepitheliomatous hyperplasia may be present

ANCILLARY TESTS

Histochemistry

- Fite stain (modified acid-fast bacilli)
  - Positive
    - Abundant organisms in lepromatous leprosy
    - Scarce to absent organisms in tuberculoid leprosy

PCR

- Available to assist in detecting presence of microorganisms

DIFFERENTIAL DIAGNOSIS

Mycobacterium Tuberculosis

- Characterized by caseating granulomatous inflammation
- Acid-fast bacilli may be identified by special stains

SELECTED REFERENCES

1. Bang PD et al: Evaluation of polymerase chain reaction-based detection of Mycobacterium leprae for the diagnosis of leprosy. J Dermatol. 36(5):269-76, 2009
2. Goulart IM et al: Leprosy: diagnostic and control challenges for a worldwide disease. Arch Dermatol Res. 300(6):269-90, 2008
3. Mahlberg MJ et al: Lepromatous leprosy. Dermatol Online J. 14(10):27, 2008
4. Bhat R et al: Otorhinolaryngologic manifestations of leprosy. Int J Dermatol. 46(6):600-6, 2007
5. de Freitas MR: Infectious neuropathy. Curr Opin Neurol. 20(5):548-52, 2007
6. Menger DJ et al: Reconstructive surgery of the leprosy nose: a new approach. J Plast Reconstr Aesthet Surg. 60(2):152-62, 2007

IMAGE GALLERY

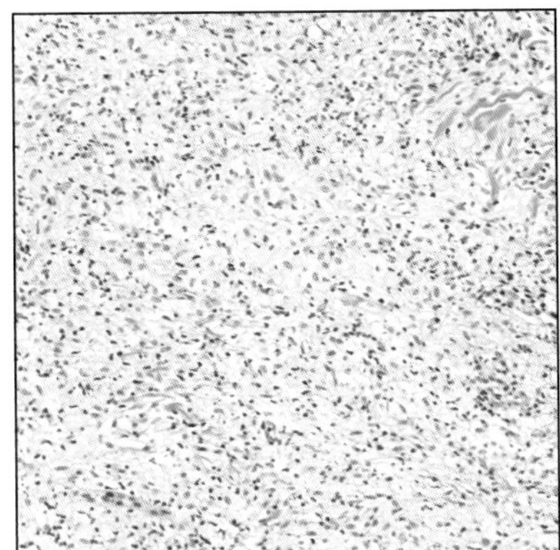

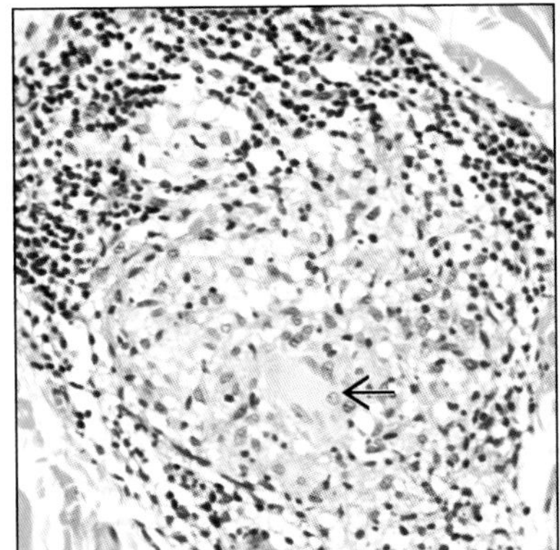

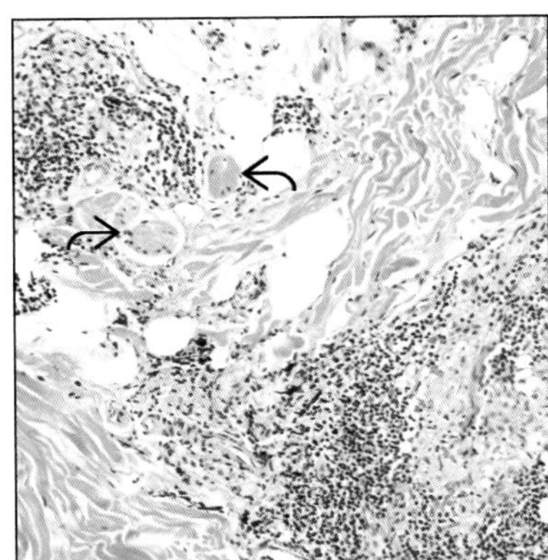

(Left) *A diffuse submucosal proliferation of vacuolated histiocytes (lepra cells) rather than well-formed granulomas characterizes lepromatous leprosy.* ***(Center)*** *Tuberculoid leprosy shows well-formed noncaseating granulomas comprised of epithelioid histiocytes and multinucleated giant cells ⇒. Microorganisms are sparse to absent.* ***(Right)*** *Granulomas of tuberculoid leprosy approximate small peripheral nerves ⇒; the latter were S100 protein positive (not shown).*

CHRONIC RHINOSINUSITIS

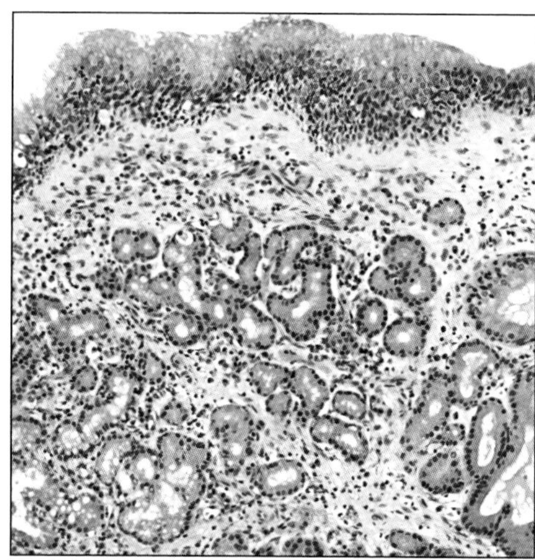

Nonspecific chronic sinusitis includes a mixed inflammatory cell infiltrate, including lymphocytes, plasma cells, and eosinophils with intact respiratory epithelium and seromucous glands.

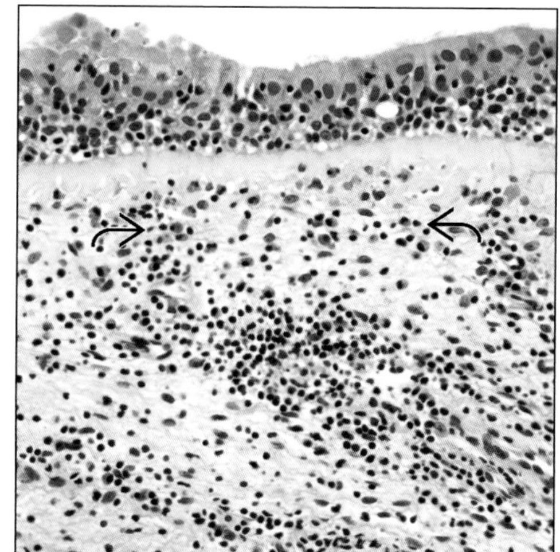

Chronic allergic rhinosinusitis shows submucosal edematous change and associated mixed inflammatory cell infiltrate, including numerous eosinophils ➔.

TERMINOLOGY

Synonyms

- Common cold
- Ozena (stench)
- Rhinitis sicca

Definitions

- Nonspecific or specific inflammation of sinonasal tract
  - May be isolated to nasal cavity (rhinitis)
  - Isolated to paranasal sinuses (sinusitis)
  - Involves both nasal cavity and paranasal sinuses (rhinosinusitis)

ETIOLOGY/PATHOGENESIS

Developmental Anomaly

- Structural or mechanical causes include
  - Deviated nasal septum, neoplasms, primary ciliary dyskinesia

Environmental Exposure

- **Allergic rhinosinusitis**
  - In adults, allergies most common cause
  - In children, viral upper respiratory infection most common cause followed by allergies
  - Caused by exposure to allergen in sensitized patient mediated via type I IgE immune reaction
    - Among more common allergens are pollens, animal dander, dust mites, mold
  - Allergic rhinosinusitis may predispose patients to recurrent or chronic sinusitis
  - May be familial

Infectious Agents

- **Infectious rhinosinusitis**
  - Caused by variety of microorganisms; most common are viruses and bacteria
  - Viral rhinosinusitis results in "common cold"
    - Symptoms include nasal congestion and watery nasal discharge
    - Common viruses implicated include rhinoviruses, influenza and parainfluenza viruses, adenoviruses, respiratory syncytial virus
    - Usually self-limiting disease course
  - Bacterial sinusitis
    - More common bacteria implicated include *Streptococcus pneumoniae*, *Hemophilias influenzae*, α-*hemolytic streptococci*

Other Causes

- Atrophic rhinosinusitis
  - Also referred to as "ozena" (stench) and "rhinitis sicca"
  - Caused by variety of factors, including the following
    - Chronic bacterial infection, nutritional deficiencies (e.g., vitamin A, iron)
    - Chronic exposure to irritants
    - Prior radiation or surgery
    - Endstage of chronic infections
    - Hypoestrogenemia
    - Autoimmune disease
- Aspirin intolerance
  - Also referred as Samter triad or syndrome: Includes aspirin intolerance, sinonasal polyps, asthma
- Nonallergic rhinosinusitis with eosinophilia (NARES) syndrome
  - May be precursor to aspirin intolerance syndrome
- Idiopathic
- Occupational or environmental exposure
- Systemic diseases
  - Cystic fibrosis, others
- Medication-induced
  - Referred to as rhinosinusitis medicamentosa
  - May be caused by topical or systemic medications (e.g., propranolol, oral contraceptives, reserpine), nasal sprays
- Pregnancy

CHRONIC RHINOSINUSITIS

Key Facts

Terminology
- Nonspecific or specific inflammation of sinonasal tract

Etiology/Pathogenesis
- Allergic rhinosinusitis
  - Most common cause in adults and 2nd most common cause (to viruses) in children
- Infectious rhinosinusitis
  - Caused by variety of microorganisms; most common include viruses and bacteria
- Atrophic rhinosinusitis
  - Caused by a variety of factors, including chronic bacterial infection, nutritional deficiencies, chronic exposure to irritants, prior radiation or surgery, endstage of chronic infections, autoimmune disease
- Aspirin intolerance
  - Referred to as Samter triad or syndrome: Includes aspirin intolerance, sinonasal polyps, asthma

Clinical Issues
- For all types of rhinosinusitis
  - Prognosis excellent with cure following appropriate therapy
  - Self-limiting disease
  - Atrophic rhinosinusitis may spontaneously arrest

Microscopic Pathology
- Submucosal mixed inflammatory cell infiltrate, including mature lymphocytes with variable admixture of plasma cells, eosinophils, histiocytes, and neutrophils

  - Thought to result from combined effects on nasal mucosa by pregnancy-related hormones, increased blood volume, and airway resistance

CLINICAL ISSUES

Epidemiology
- Incidence
  - Estimated 1 billion colds in USA annually
- Age
  - **Allergic, infectious, and nonspecific rhinosinusitis**
    - Occurs over wide age range from very young to very old
  - **Atrophic rhinosinusitis**
    - Begins in childhood often in 2nd decade of life at onset of puberty
  - **Aspirin intolerance**
    - Often begins in 3rd to 4th decades of life
- Gender
  - **Allergic, infectious, and nonspecific rhinosinusitis**
    - Equal gender distribution
  - **Atrophic rhinosinusitis**
    - Female > Male
  - **Aspirin intolerance**
    - Equal gender distribution

Presentation
- **Allergic rhinosinusitis**
  - In a sensitized patient, exposure results in allergic reaction, producing nasal congestion with rhinorrhea, sneezing, itching
    - Noninfected patient nasal secretions appear clear
    - Infected patient nasal secretions appear purulent
    - Reaction begins within minutes of exposure, peaking about 15 minutes later
- **Infectious rhinosinusitis**
  - Associated with pain localized over infected site, headaches are uncommon
  - Acute symptoms
    - Persistent and worsening symptoms longer than 7 days but less than 3 weeks
  - Subacute symptoms
    - 3 weeks to 3 months
  - Chronic symptoms
    - Lasting more than 3 months
    - Patients with resistant or refractory chronic sinusitis have increased incidence of *S. aureus*, anaerobic bacteria, gram-negative organisms
    - *Pseudomonas aeruginosa* commonly cultured organism in patients receiving multiple courses of antibiotics over extended periods
- **Nonspecific and atrophic rhinosinusitis**
  - Symptoms include nasal obstruction, headaches, nasal crusting, anosmia, epistaxis, halitosis, and foul-smelling nasal odor
- **Aspirin intolerance**
  - Within hours of aspirin ingestion, patients may experience bronchoconstriction and rhinorrhea
    - In some patients, may also follow ingestion of nonsteroidal anti-inflammatory medications
    - Symptoms may include nausea, vomiting, diarrhea with gastrointestinal cramping
    - Felt to be pharmacologic with interference in metabolism of arachidonic acid rather than allergic response

Endoscopic Findings
- **Allergic and nonspecific rhinosinusitis**
  - Sinonasal mucosa is pale to bluish
  - Inflammatory polyps may or may not be identified
- **Atrophic rhinosinusitis**
  - Characterized by atrophy of nasal mucosa, crust formation, and foul-smelling odor from nasal cavity
- **Aspirin intolerance**
  - Polyps can be identified and are usually bilateral
    - More severe symptoms with less improvement after surgery with significantly higher need for revision surgery

Laboratory Tests
- **Allergic rhinosinusitis**

CHRONIC RHINOSINUSITIS

- Gold standard for allergy testing is considered skin testing
  - Represents reaction between antigen and sensitized mast cells in skin causing wheal and flare skin response
  - Occasionally negative result in allergic rhinosinusitis patients due to local (nasal) synthesis of IgE with local (nasal) tissue less sensitive than distant (cutaneous) site
- **Infectious rhinosinusitis**
  - Microbiologic culturing for viral (e.g., H1N1) and bacterial pathogens
  - Drug sensitivity testing for bacterial infection

Treatment

- Surgical approaches
  - Surgery may be used in atrophic rhinosinusitis and aspirin intolerance, the latter for removal of polyps
- Drugs
  - **Allergic rhinosinusitis**
    - Antihistamines
    - Nasal cromolyn preparations (stabilizes mast cells against degranulation and release of inflammatory mediators)
    - Topical corticosteroids
    - Immunotherapy for documented IgE-mediated allergies
  - **Infectious rhinosinusitis**
    - Antibiotic therapy indicated for bacterial infection
  - **Atrophic rhinosinusitis**
    - Antibiotics and nutritional supplements (e.g., vitamin A, iron, estrogen)
  - **Aspirin intolerance**
    - Avoidance of instigating medications
    - Symptomatic relief
  - **Nonspecific rhinosinusitis**
    - Symptomatic relief

Prognosis

- For all types of rhinosinusitis, prognosis is excellent with cure following appropriate therapy

IMAGE FINDINGS

Radiographic Findings

- **Acute rhinosinusitis**
  - Air-fluid levels represent best diagnostic clue
- **Chronic rhinosinusitis**
  - Mucosal thickening or soft tissue opacification of nonexpanded sinus with thickening and sclerosis of sinus bony walls

MICROSCOPIC PATHOLOGY

Histologic Features

- **Allergic rhinosinusitis**
  - Submucosal edema with mixed inflammatory cell reaction dominated by presence of eosinophils
    - Neutrophils can be identified, especially in presence of secondary bacterial infection
  - Squamous metaplasia of surface epithelium may be present
- **Atrophic rhinosinusitis**
  - Squamous metaplasia of surface epithelium
  - Submucosal edema with nonspecific chronic inflammation, fibrosis
  - Atrophic changes of seromucous glands
  - Vascular dilatation
- **Aspirin intolerance**
  - Polyps histologically similar to sinonasal inflammatory polyps not occurring in aspirin-intolerant patients
- **Nonspecific chronic sinusitis**
  - Submucosal mixed inflammatory cell infiltrate, including mature lymphocytes with variable admixture of plasma cells, eosinophils, histiocytes, and neutrophils
    - Benign lymphoid aggregates may be present
  - Submucosal edematous change
  - Surface mucosa squamous metaplasia often (but not uniformly) present
  - Seromucous gland hyperplasia may be florid
  - Vascular proliferation may be seen
- In longstanding &/or recurrent/persistent disease, changes may include
  - Epithelial hyperplasia with papillary appearance (hyperplastic papillary sinusitis)

DIFFERENTIAL DIAGNOSIS

Adenocarcinoma

- Complex architectural growth patterns (e.g., back-to-back glands) composed of single-cell type

SELECTED REFERENCES

1. Kountakis SE: Relationship between clinical measures and histopathologic findings in chronic rhinosinusitis. Otolaryngol Head Neck Surg. 142(6):920-1; author reply 921, 2010
2. Ly TH et al: Diagnostic criteria for atrophic rhinosinusitis. Am J Med. 122(8):747-53, 2009
3. Babinski D et al: Rhinosinusitis in cystic fibrosis: not a simple story. Int J Pediatr Otorhinolaryngol. 72(5):619-24, 2008
4. Joe SA et al: Chronic rhinosinusitis and asthma. Otolaryngol Clin North Am. 41(2):297-309, vi, 2008
5. Mynatt RG et al: Squamous metaplasia and chronic rhinosinusitis: a clinicopathological study. Am J Rhinol. 22(6):602-5, 2008
6. Mafee MF et al: Imaging of rhinosinusitis and its complications: plain film, CT, and MRI. Clin Rev Allergy Immunol. 30(3):165-86, 2006
7. Meltzer EO et al: Allergic rhinitis, asthma, and rhinosinusitis: diseases of the integrated airway. J Manag Care Pharm. 10(4):310-7, 2004
8. Zeitz HJ: Bronchial asthma, nasal polyps, and aspirin sensitivity: Samter's syndrome. Clin Chest Med. 9(4):567-76, 1988

Diagrammatic, Imaging, and Variant Microscopic Features

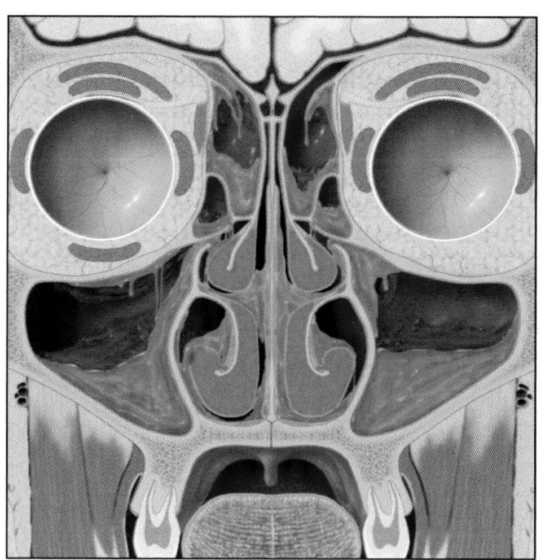

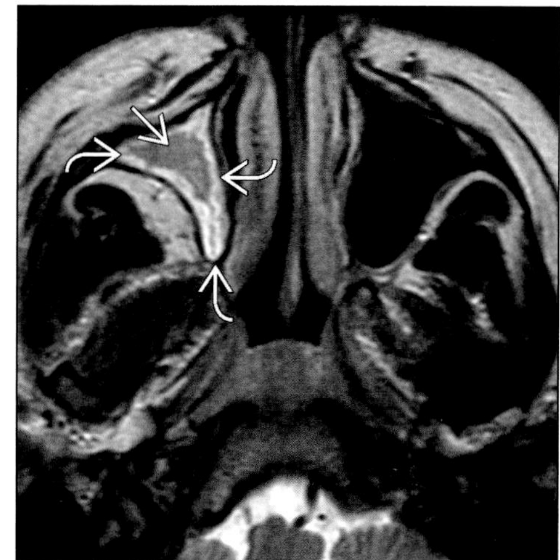

(Left) *Mucus accumulation in sinusitis results in variable accumulation with the nasal cavity and paranasal sinuses, which in turn results in clinical symptoms, including congestion, anosmia, and radiologic evidence of air-fluid levels and opacification.* ***(Right)*** *Axial T2 MR demonstrates an opacified, nonexpanded right maxillary sinus. The central secretions within the sinus are heterogeneous with low signal ➡, surrounded by hyperintense peripheral inflamed mucosa ➡.*

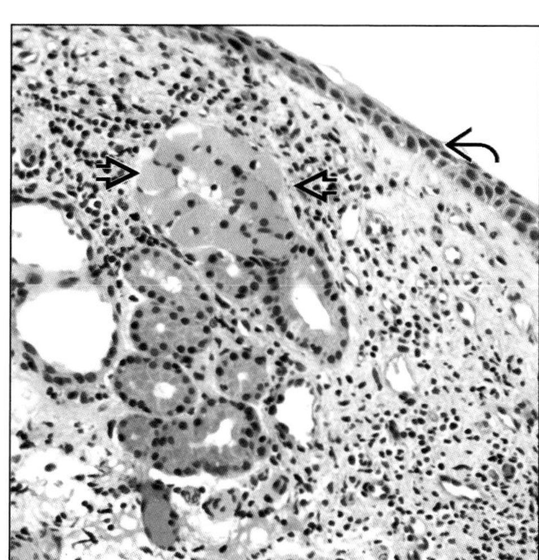

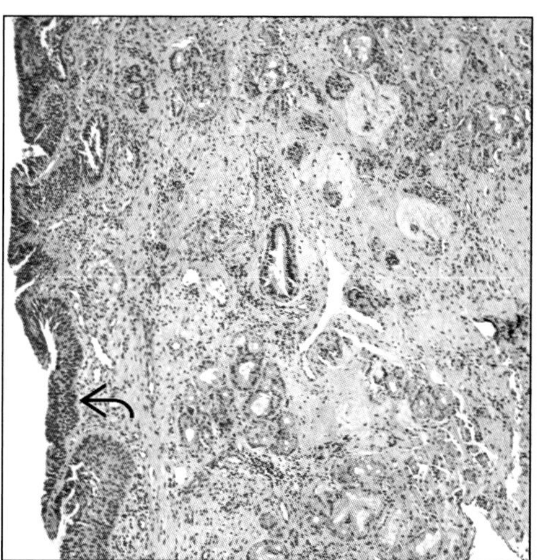

(Left) *Squamous metaplasia ➡ of the surface respiratory epithelium can be seen in all types of sinusitis. Although uncommon in association with (chronic) sinusitis, oncocytic metaplasia of seromucous glands ➡ may be seen.* ***(Right)*** *Atrophic rhinitis includes squamous metaplasia of surface epithelium ➡, atrophy of seromucous glands, nonspecific chronic inflammation, submucosal fibrosis, and submucosal edematous change.*

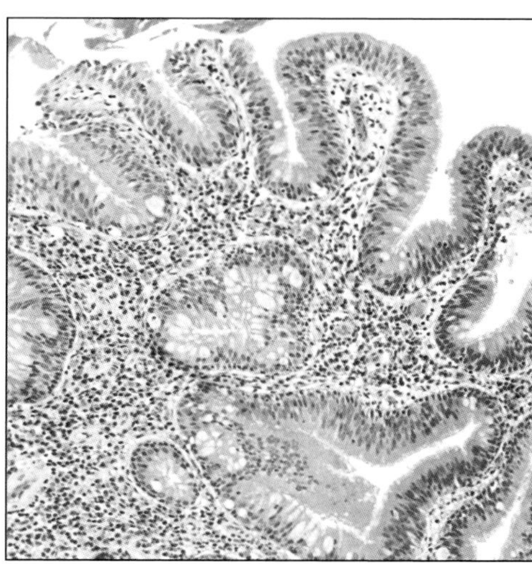

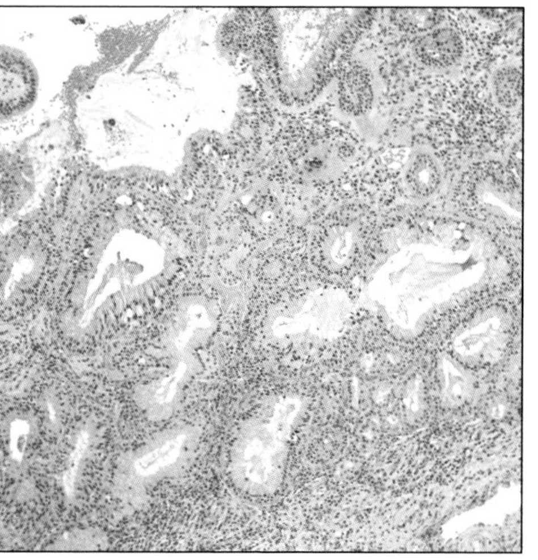

(Left) *In longstanding &/ or recurrent/persistent disease, changes may include epithelial hyperplasia with papillary appearance referred to as hyperplastic papillary sinusitis.* ***(Right)*** *In addition to surface epithelial changes, seromucous gland hyperplasia may be present and may be florid, raising concern for a possible diagnosis of a glandular neoplasm. In contrast to glandular neoplasms, the hyperplastic glands are widely separated, lacking the complex (back to back) growth patterns.*

WEGENER GRANULOMATOSIS

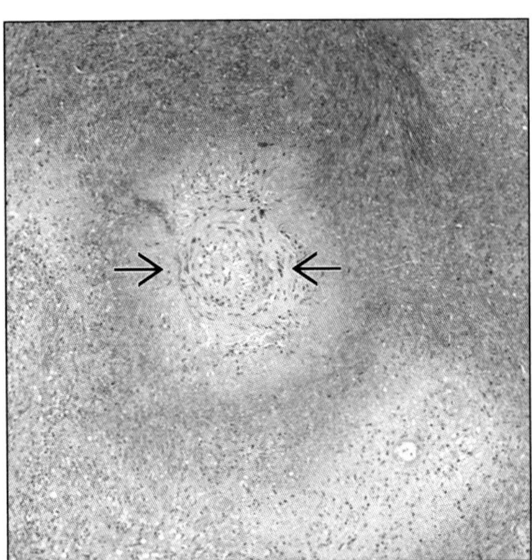

Ischemic-type necrosis with a basophilic smudgy appearance surrounds an ablated vascular space ➔. The necrosis should be deep within the tissue and not limited to the surface of the tissue.

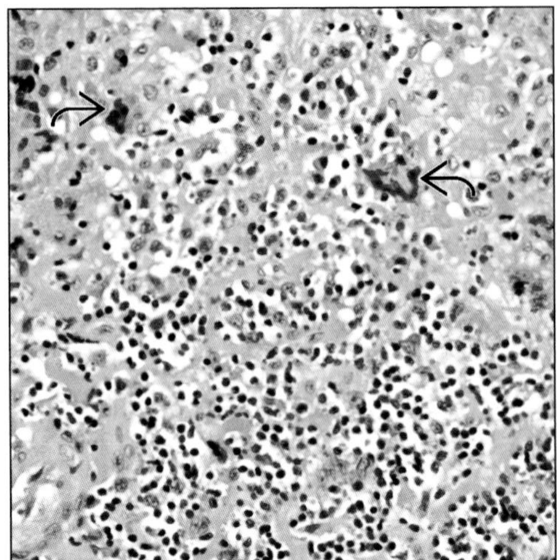

A mixed chronic inflammatory cell infiltrate is present, lacking atypia or malignant features. Scattered multinucleated giant cells are seen ➔, but well-formed granulomas are not identified.

TERMINOLOGY

Abbreviations

- Wegener granulomatosis (WG)

Definitions

- Nonneoplastic, idiopathic aseptic necrotizing disease characterized by vasculitis and destructive properties
  - Classic definition calls for involvement of head and neck region, lungs, and kidney
  - Majority of patients do not exhibit classic clinical triad simultaneously at time of initial presentation

ETIOLOGY/PATHOGENESIS

Idiopathic

- Although speculative, an infectious etiology (e.g., bacterial) either as cause or as cofactor in disease suggested based on
  - Reported beneficial effects of trimethoprim-sulfamethoxazole therapy on initial course of disease
  - Histologic features of disease similar to that found in infections diseases

CLINICAL ISSUES

Presentation

- May be systemic or localized
  - Extent of disease reflected in clinical manifestations such that limited or localized disease may be asymptomatic
    - Patients with systemic involvement always sick
- Disease may progress from localized to systemic involvement or may remain limited or even regress with treatment
- ELK classification includes
  - E = ear, nose, and throat involvement
  - L = lung involvement
  - K = kidney involvement
  - Patients with E or EL disease are considered to have limited form of WG
  - Patients with ELK disease correspond to systemic WG
- Localized upper aerodigestive tract (UADT) WG
  - Tends to affect men more than women
    - Exception in laryngeal WG seen predominantly in women
  - In UADT, most common site of occurrence is sinonasal region with nasal cavity > maxillary > ethmoid > frontal > sphenoid
  - Other sites of involvement include
    - Nasopharynx, larynx (subglottis), oral cavity, ear (external and middle ear including mastoid), and salivary glands
  - Symptoms vary according to site of involvement, including
    - Sinonasal tract: Sinusitis with or without purulent rhinorrhea, obstruction, pain, epistaxis, anosmia, headaches
    - Oral: Ulcerative lesion, gingivitis
    - Ear: Hearing loss, pain
    - Larynx: Dyspnea, hoarseness, voice changes
  - Involvement of larynx most often subglottic region
    - 8-25% of patients with WG will develop disease referable to larynx
    - Involvement of larynx seen more often in setting of preexisting disease elsewhere
    - Presentation with laryngeal WG rare event

Laboratory Tests

- Important adjunct evaluation includes
  - Elevated antineutrophil cytoplasmic antibody (ANCA)
  - Elevated proteinase 3 (PR3)
- Elevated ANCA
  - Reported specificity for diagnosis of WG from 85-98%

WEGENER GRANULOMATOSIS

Key Facts

Terminology

- Nonneoplastic, idiopathic, aseptic necrotizing disease characterized by vasculitis and destructive properties

Clinical Issues

- In UADT, most common site of occurrence is sinonasal region with nasal cavity > maxillary > ethmoid > frontal > sphenoid
- Important adjunct evaluation includes
  - Elevated antineutrophil cytoplasmic antibody (ANCA)
  - Elevated proteinase 3 (PR3)

Microscopic Pathology

- Classic triad includes vasculitis, granulomatous inflammation, tissue necrosis
- In practice, finding classic histologic triad in single biopsy or series of biopsies very uncommon
  - Seen in only 16% of biopsies from patients with proven WG
- Inflammatory cell infiltrate angiocentric and angioinvasive
- Ischemic- or geographic-type (multifocal necrobiosis) with basophilic smudgy appearance
- Well-formed granulomas not typical feature
  - Characterized by scattered or isolated multinucleated giant cells
- Polymorphous inflammatory infiltrate composed of lymphocytes, histiocytes, and plasma cells
- Microabscesses ± granuloma formation may be identified

  - ANCA reactivity seen in form of cytoplasmic (c-ANCA) vs. perinuclear (p-ANCA) staining
    - WG characteristically associated with c-ANCA and only infrequently with p-ANCA
    - c-ANCA of greater specificity than p-ANCA
  - Sensitivity of test varies with extent of disease
    - Patients with limited WG have 50-67% c-ANCA positivity
    - Patients with systemic WG have 60-100% positivity
    - Negative test does not rule out WG
  - May be identified in other vasculitides
    - Inflammatory bowel disease and hepatobiliary diseases
  - ANCA titers not elevated in infections or in lymphomas
  - ANCA titers follow the disease course
    - Titers revert to normal levels with remission and become elevated with recurrent or persistent disease
    - Decline in c-ANCA titer may lag behind clinical evidence of remission by up to 6-8 weeks
- Proteinase 3 (PR3)
  - PR3 is neutral serine proteinase present in azurophil granules of human polymorphonuclear leukocytes and monocyte lysosomal granules
  - Serves as major target antigen of ANCA with cytoplasmic staining pattern (c-ANCA) in WG
  - ANCA with specificity for PR3 characteristic for patients with WG
  - Patients with WG demonstrate significantly higher percentage of mPR3(+) neutrophils than healthy controls and patients with other inflammatory diseases
  - Detection of ANCA directed against proteinase 3 (PR3-ANCA) is highly specific for WG
  - ANCA positivity found only approximately 50% of patients with localized WG, whereas PR3-ANCA positivity seen in 95% of patients with generalized WG
  - Pathogenesis of vascular injury in WG ascribed to ANCA directed mainly against PR3
  - Interaction of ANCA with neutrophilic ANCA antigens necessary for the development of ANCA-associated diseases
    - ANCA bind to membrane-expressed PR3 and induce full-blown activation in primed neutrophils
  - In patients with WG, high expression of PR3 on surface of nonprimed neutrophils associated with increased incidence and rate of relapse
- ANCA-associated vasculitis (AAV) includes
  - WG, microscopic polyangiitis (MPA), and allergic granulomatous angiitis (AGA)
    - Major target antigens of ANCA-associated vasculitis include PR3 and myeloperoxidase (MPO)
    - PR3-ANCA is marker for WG; MPO-ANCA is related to MPA and AGA
  - ANCA appears to induce vasculitis by directly activating neutrophils
  - No immunoglobulins or complement components detected in vasculitis lesions
    - As such, AAV called pauci-immune vasculitis

Treatment

- Options, risks, complications
  - Once diagnosis and extent of disease is determined
    - Most patients receive combination of cyclophosphamide and prednisone for remission induction
  - Patients with limited disease treated with antibiotics (trimethoprim-sulfamethoxazole)
  - Rituximab therapy
    - Similar to daily cyclophosphamide treatment for induction of remission in severe ANCA-associated vasculitis
    - May be superior in relapsing disease
  - Patients with fulminating disease, especially with renal failure, treated with high doses of prednisone
    - Maintained until disease under control as evidenced by improved ESR, serum creatinine, or ANCA titer at which time cyclophosphamide therapy begun

        - Prednisone continued until cyclophosphamide takes effect; occurs approximately 2-3 weeks or following initiation of therapy

Prognosis

- Treatment with cyclophosphamide and prednisone results in 75% complete remission rate
    - Achieved although patients may experience one or more relapses from 3 months to 16 years after complete remission
    - Patients with WG who experience remission are not necessarily cured of disease
        - Remain at risk for recurrences throughout their life
- Limited WG responds well to cyclophosphamide &/or steroid therapy and has good prognosis
- Mortality rates of up to 28% have been reported
    - Major source of morbidity and mortality is renal or pulmonary insufficiency &/or complications of therapy (e.g., sepsis, drug-induced malignancies)
- Occasionally, spontaneous remissions may be seen with milder forms of disease when only one or a few organs are involved (but not kidneys)

MACROSCOPIC FEATURES

General Features

- Sinonasal area
    - Diffuse ulcerative and crusted lesions with tissue destruction
    - In advanced cases, septal perforation may be seen resulting in "saddle nose" deformity
- Oral cavity
    - Ulcerative, destructive lesions often seen along palate and alveolar region
- Larynx
    - Subglottic stenosis with associated ulcerative lesions

MICROSCOPIC PATHOLOGY

Histologic Features

- Histologic features of WG include classic triad of
    - Vasculitis, granulomatous inflammation, and tissue necrosis
        - In practice, finding classic histologic triad in a single or even series of biopsies very uncommon
        - Seen in only 16% of biopsies from patients with proven WG
        - Requiring presence of all features in a single biopsy in order to render diagnosis will result in "nondiagnostic" interpretation
        - Diagnosis can be suggested even when classic histologic changes not present in biopsy
        - Risk of underdiagnosing WG when all classic histologic components are lacking
        - Risk of overdiagnosing WG when excessive reliance placed on presence of minimal histologic changes
- **Vasculitis**
    - Involves small to medium-sized arteries
    - Difficult to definitively identify histologically and often absent
    - Angiocentric (surrounding vessels) and angioinvasive (invading through vessel wall) potentially results in thrombosis of involved blood vessel
    - Vasculitis not limited to WG seen in infectious diseases (e.g., mucormycosis, aspergillosis)
- **Necrosis**
    - Ischemic- or geographic-type (multifocal necrobiosis) with basophilic smudgy appearance
    - Necrotic foci should be within stromal connective tissues and not along surface or edge of tissue specimen
        - Surface or superficial ulceration considered nonspecific ulceration as seen in wide variety of lesions
- **Granulomatous inflammation**
    - Characterized by scattered or isolated multinucleated giant cells
    - Well-formed granulomas not typical feature of WG
- **Inflammatory cell infiltrate**
    - Polymorphous inflammatory infiltrate composed of lymphocytes, histiocytes, and plasma cells
    - Less often comprised of eosinophils and polymorphonuclear leukocytes
        - Eosinophils may be numerous on occasion
    - Microabscesses with or without granuloma formation may be identified
- Bacterial superinfection of diseased mucosa, particularly *Staphylococcus aureus*, may complicate clinical picture

ANCILLARY TESTS

Histochemistry

- Elastic stains
    - May assist in identification of vasculitis
    - Disruption of elastic membranes
- Staining for microorganisms negative
- Immunohistochemistry
    - Immunoreactivity present for B-cell (CD20) and T-cell (CD3) markers
        - Indicative of benign (polyclonal) cellular population

DIFFERENTIAL DIAGNOSIS

Infectious Diseases

- Fungal, mycobacterial, parasitic are identified by light microscopy &/or special stains

Cocaine Abuse

- Characterized by foreign body giant cell reaction, including polarizable material

Churg-Strauss Disease

- Also referred to as allergic granulomatosis and vasculitis
- Characterized by asthma, systemic vasculitis, tissue and peripheral eosinophilia, nasal manifestations

- These findings assist in differential diagnosis from WG
- Elevated ANCA levels reported in Churg-Strauss disease, so cannot be used to differentiate from WG
- Histology includes
  - Vasculitis of small to medium-sized vessels with transmural inflammatory cell infiltrate (angioinvasion)
  - Inflammatory infiltrate predominantly includes eosinophils
  - Granulomatous vasculitis may be seen characterized by multinucleated giant cells within vessel wall (seen in approximately 38% of cases)
  - Eosinophilic microabscesses unrelated to blood vessels may be present

NK-/T-cell Lymphoma, Nasal Type

- Cytologic characteristics of lymphoid infiltrate often permit distinction between WG and NK-/T-cell lymphoma, nasal type
  - Cytologic atypia to outright malignant cells characteristic of NK-/T-cell lymphoma, nasal type
  - Lymphoid infiltrates in WG lack appreciable degree of cytologic atypia
- Demonstration of monoclonality by immunohistochemistry or gene rearrangements by molecular analysis assists in recognition of lymphoma
- ANCA, PR3 negative
- Associated with Epstein-Barr virus (EBER[+])

Diffuse Large B-cell Lymphoma (DLBCL)

- Cytologic characteristics of lymphoid infiltrate often permit distinction between WG and DLBCL
  - Presence of malignant cells
  - Lymphoid infiltrate in WG lacks appreciable degree of cytologic atypia
- Demonstration of monoclonality by immunohistochemistry or gene rearrangements by molecular analysis assists in recognition of lymphoma
- ANCA, PR3 negative

Malignant Neoplasms

- Variety of nonhematolymphoid malignant neoplasms occur in sinonasal tract
  - Characterized by malignant neoplastic proliferation
  - WG characterized by mixed inflammatory cell infiltrate, absence of malignant cells

DIAGNOSTIC CHECKLIST

Clinically Relevant Pathologic Features

- Elevated ANCA, PR3 important adjunct studies

Pathologic Interpretation Pearls

- Triad of vasculitis, granulomatous inflammation, and tissue necrosis seen in only 16% of proven WG cases

SELECTED REFERENCES

1. Stone JH et al: Rituximab versus cyclophosphamide for ANCA-associated vasculitis. N Engl J Med. 363(3):221-32, 2010
2. Chen M et al: New advances in the pathogenesis of ANCA-associated vasculitides. Clin Exp Rheumatol. 27(1 Suppl 52):S108-14, 2009
3. Grindler D et al: Computed tomography findings in sinonasal Wegener's granulomatosis. Am J Rhinol Allergy. 23(5):497-501, 2009
4. Jayne D: Review article: Progress of treatment in ANCA-associated vasculitis. Nephrology (Carlton). 14(1):42-8, 2009
5. Oristrell J et al: Effectiveness of rituximab in severe Wegener's granulomatosis: report of two cases and review of the literature. Open Respir Med J. 3:94-9, 2009
6. Feng Z et al: Clinical relevance of anti-PR3 capture ELISA in diagnosing Wegener's granulomatosis. J Clin Lab Anal. 22(1):73-6, 2008
7. Srouji I et al: Rhinologic symptoms and quality-of-life in patients with Churg-Strauss syndrome vasculitis. Am J Rhinol. 22(4):406-9, 2008
8. Srouji IA et al: Patterns of presentation and diagnosis of patients with Wegener's granulomatosis: ENT aspects. J Laryngol Otol. 121(7):653-8, 2007
9. Lohrmann C et al: Sinonasal computed tomography in patients with Wegener's granulomatosis. J Comput Assist Tomogr. 30(1):122-5, 2006
10. Rodrigo JP et al: Idiopathic midline destructive disease: fact or fiction. Oral Oncol. 41(4):340-8, 2005
11. Benoudiba F et al: Sinonasal Wegener's granulomatosis: CT characteristics. Neuroradiology. 45(2):95-9, 2003
12. Rutgers A et al: The role of myeloperoxidase in the pathogenesis of systemic vasculitis. Clin Exp Rheumatol. 21(6 Suppl 32):S55-63, 2003
13. Kallenberg CG et al: New insights into the pathogenesis of antineutrophil cytoplasmic autoantibody-associated vasculitis. Autoimmun Rev. 1(1-2):61-6, 2002
14. Franssen CF et al: Antiproteinase 3- and antimyeloperoxidase-associated vasculitis. Kidney Int. 57(6):2195-206, 2000
15. Gross WL et al: Pathogenesis of Wegener's granulomatosis. Ann Med Interne (Paris). 149(5):280-6, 1998
16. McDonald TJ et al: Head and neck involvement in Wegener's granulomatosis (WG). Adv Exp Med Biol. 336:309-13, 1993
17. Bini P et al: Antineutrophil cytoplasmic autoantibodies in Wegener's granulomatosis recognize conformational epitope(s) on proteinase 3. J Immunol. 149(4):1409-15, 1992
18. Colby TV et al: Nasal biopsy in Wegener's granulomatosis. Hum Pathol. 22(2):101-4, 1991
19. Noorduyn LA et al: Sinonasal non-Hodgkin's lymphomas and Wegener's granulomatosis: a clinicopathological study. Virchows Arch A Pathol Anat Histopathol. 418(3):235-40, 1991
20. Devaney KO et al: Interpretation of head and neck biopsies in Wegener's granulomatosis. A pathologic study of 126 biopsies in 70 patients. Am J Surg Pathol. 14(6):555-64, 1990
21. Jennette JC et al: Antineutrophil cytoplasmic autoantibodies and associated diseases: a review. Am J Kidney Dis. 15(6):517-29, 1990
22. Specks U et al: Granulomatous vasculitis. Wegener's granulomatosis and Churg-Strauss syndrome. Rheum Dis Clin North Am. 16(2):377-97, 1990
23. McDonald TJ et al: Wegener's granulomatosis. Laryngoscope. 93(2):220-31, 1983
24. Olsen KD et al: Nasal manifestations of allergic granulomatosis and angiitis (Churg-Strauss syndrome). Otolaryngol Head Neck Surg. 88(1):85-9, 1980
25. DeRemee RA et al: Wegener's granulomatosis. Anatomic correlates, a proposed classification. Mayo Clin Proc. 51(12):777-81, 1976

WEGENER GRANULOMATOSIS

Differential Diagnosis of Sinonasal Tract WG

	WG	NK-/T-cell Lymphoma	DLBCL	AGV
Gender/age	M > F; 4th-5th decades	M > F; 6th decade	M > F; 7th decade	M > F; wide age range (3rd-6th decades)
Location	Localized upper aerodigestive tract WG most common in nasal cavity > paranasal sinuses	Generally limited to SNT region; extra-SNT represents higher stage tumor	Nasal cavity and one or more paranasal sinuses	Multisystem disease, including pulmonary, nasal, renal, skin, cardiac and nervous system
Presentation	SNT: Sinusitis with or without purulent rhinorrhea, obstruction, pain, epistaxis, anosmia, headaches	Destructive process of midfacial region; may include septal perforation, palate destruction, orbital swelling	Nonhealing ulcer, epistaxis, facial swelling, pain, cranial nerve manifestations	Asthma, allergic rhinitis, evidence of eosinophilia, serum and tissue (e.g., eosinophilic pneumonia, eosinophilic gastroenteritis, other)
Serology	ANCA, PR3 positive	ANCA, PR3 negative; no specific serologic marker(s)	ANCA, PR3 negative; no specific serologic marker(s)	ANCA levels may or may not be present; PR3 negative
Histology	Polymorphous (benign) cellular infiltrate, vasculitis (angiocentric, angioinvasive), ischemic-type necrosis, isolated multinucleated giant cells (not well-formed granulomas)	In forme fruste, overtly malignant cellular infiltrate with angiocentricity and angioinvasion, ischemic-type necrosis; no giant cells or granulomas	Diffuse dyscohesive cellular proliferation of medium to large cells with large round to oval vesicular (noncleaved) nuclei, prominent nucleoli, increased mitotic activity, and necrosis	Polymorphous (benign) cellular infiltrate predominantly eosinophils; vasculitis, which may be granulomatous vasculitis (multinucleated giant cells in wall of involved blood vessels); eosinophilic microabscesses
IHC/ molecular	Polymorphous and polyclonal; no gene rearrangement	CD56, CD2, cytoplasmic CD3e positive; T-cell markers (CD3, UCHL-1) positive; gene rearrangements	Leucocyte common antigen and B-cell markers (CD20, CD79) positive; gene rearrangements	Polymorphous and polyclonal; no gene rearrangement
EBV	Negative	Strong association	Negative to weak association	Negative
Treatment	Cyclophosphamide and prednisone	Radiotherapy for localized disease; chemotherapy for disseminated disease	Radiotherapy &/or chemotherapy	Systemic corticosteroids
Prognosis	Limited disease associated with good to excellent prognosis and occasional spontaneous remissions; mortality related to complications of renal and pulmonary involvement	Overall survival 30-50%; local recurrence/relapse and systemic failure common	Dependent on stage; survival rates 35-60%	62% 5-year survival; increased morbidity and mortality due to cardiac involvement resulting in congestive heart failure or myocardial infarction

WG = Wegener granulomatosis; DLBCL = diffuse large B-cell lymphoma; AGV = allergic granulomatosis and vasculitis (a.k.a. Churg-Strauss disease); SNT = sinonasal tract.

Microscopic, Clinical, and Radiographic Features

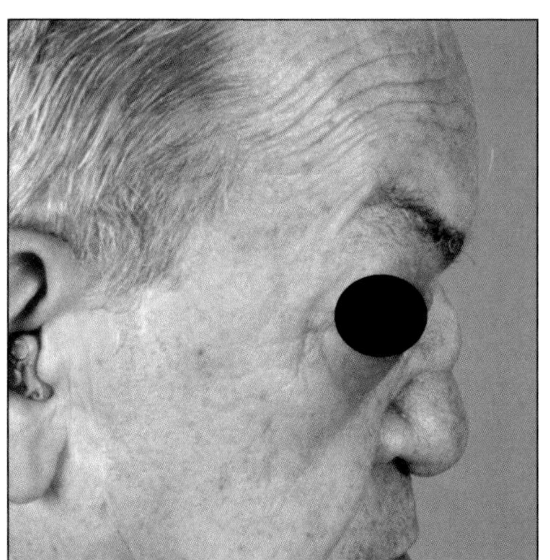

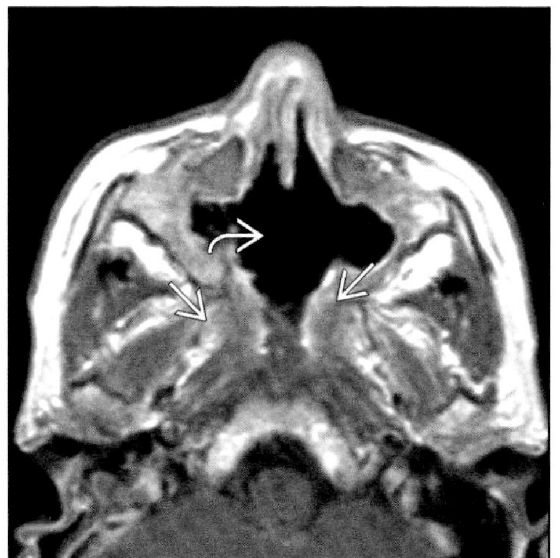

(Left) *Among the clinical findings that can be seen in association with Wegener granulomatosis is nasal septal destruction with saddle nose deformity.* ***(Right)*** *Axial T1WI C+ MR reveals enhancement of the nodular peripheral soft tissue within the maxillary sinuses with Wegener involvement extending into the nasopharynx ➡. A large septal perforation ➦ is present.*

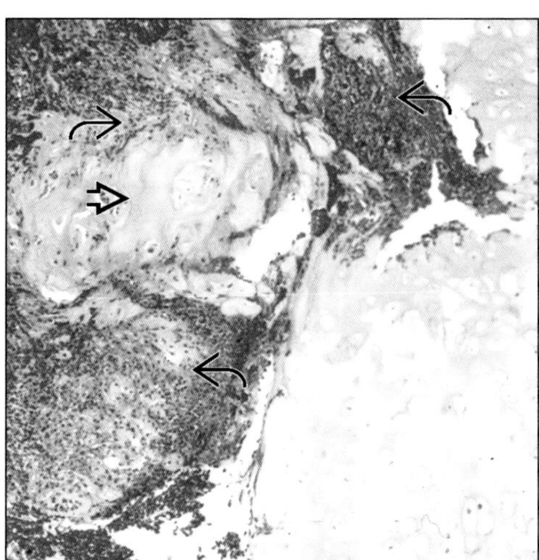

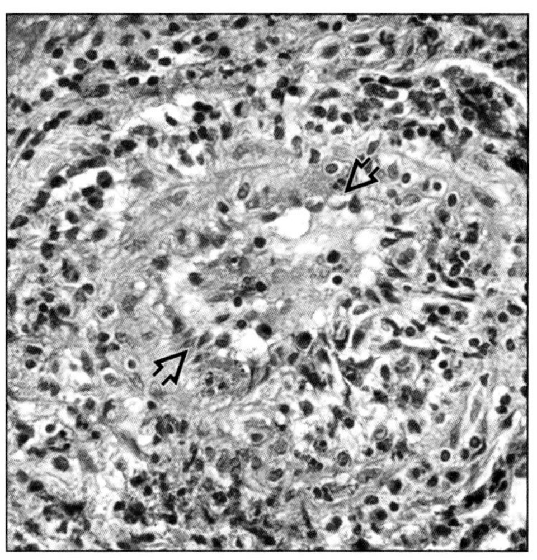

(Left) *Histologically, nasal septal destruction resulting in saddle nose deformity correlates to the presence of the inflammatory cell infiltrate ➦ extending into and throughout the septal elastic cartilage ⇨.* ***(Right)*** *Vasculitis includes inflammatory infiltrate concentrically surrounding a blood vessel (angiocentric) with (or without) invasion through the vessel wall (angioinvasion), resulting in near occlusion of the endothelial-lined lumen ⇨.*

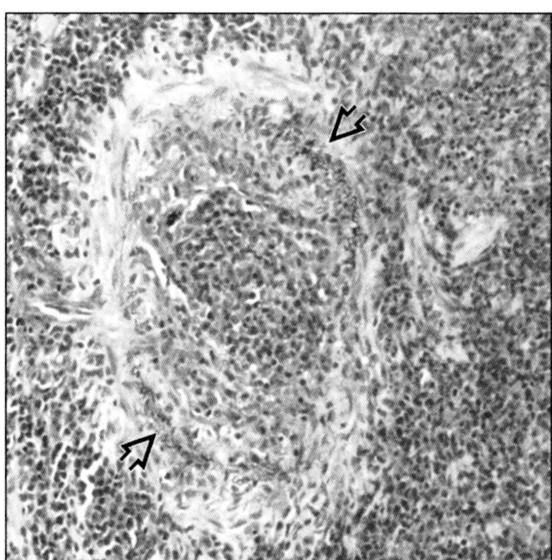

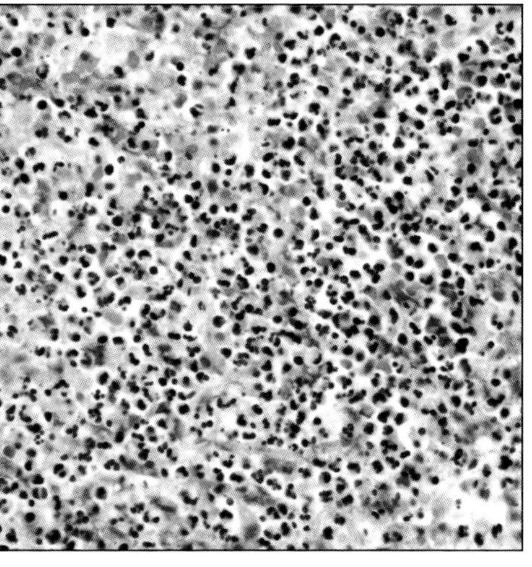

(Left) *Elastic stain shows disruption of the black staining external elastic membrane ⇨ by the angiocentric and angioinvasive inflammatory cell infiltrate. The inflammatory infiltrate completely obliterates the vessel lumen.* ***(Right)*** *Neutrophilic microabscess formation is another feature that can be seen in Wegener granulomatosis.*

EOSINOPHILIC ANGIOCENTRIC FIBROSIS

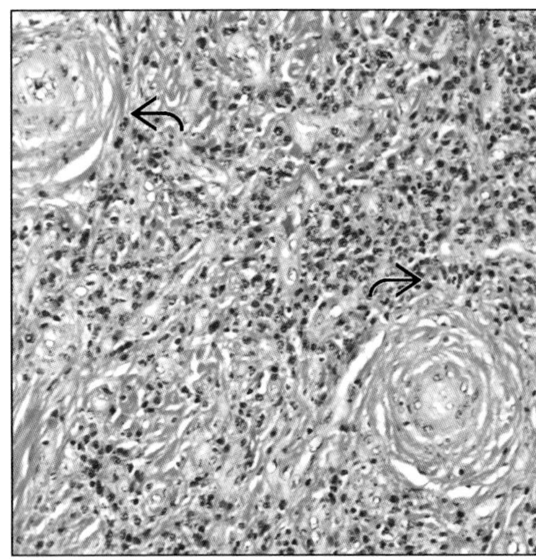

A mixed inflammatory cell infiltrate, including numerous eosinophils, is present and may be associated with small vessel walls ⮳ suggesting a small vessel angiitis.

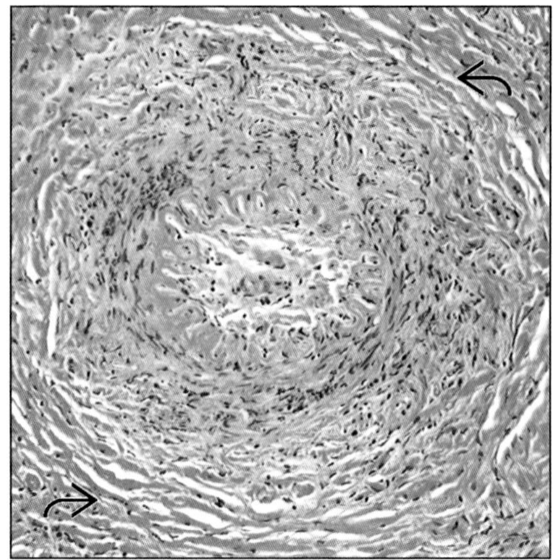

Prominent stromal fibrosis with layered "onion-skin-type" perivascular fibrosis ⮳ is a characteristic feature. Ischemic-type necrosis, granulomas, and multinucleated giant cells are absent.

TERMINOLOGY

Abbreviations

- Eosinophilic angiocentric fibrosis (EAF)

Definitions

- Rare, chronic, sclerosing, fibroinflammatory disorder of upper aerodigestive tract

ETIOLOGY/PATHOGENESIS

Idiopathic

- No known etiology; no known association with other (systemic or localized) diseases
- Postulated to represent mucosal variant of granuloma faciale due to
  - Histologic similarities of early nasal mucosal lesions to granuloma faciale
  - Concurrent occurrence of EAF and granuloma faciale in approximately 25% of cases

CLINICAL ISSUES

Epidemiology

- Incidence
  - Uncommon
- Age
  - Adults
- Gender
  - Female > > > Male
    - All reported cases occurred in women

Site

- Primarily involves nasal cavity (unilateral or bilateral)
  - Septum > lateral wall
  - Rarely extends to paranasal sinuses (usually maxillary sinus) or orbit
- Rarely involves subglottic region

Presentation

- Progressive airway (nasal) obstruction over several years
  - Some patients have associated allergies, including allergic rhinitis, chronic urticaria, sensitivity to penicillin
- Pain, epistaxis uncommon

Laboratory Tests

- Nonspecific
  - ANCA, PR3 levels not elevated
  - Erythrocyte sedimentation rate, urinalysis without abnormalities

Treatment

- Surgical approaches
  - Surgery may be required in patients with airway obstruction
- Drugs
  - Corticosteroids and antihistamines do not appear to be effective modes of treatment

Prognosis

- Disease progression stabilizes over time but typically not prior to development of airway obstruction

MICROSCOPIC PATHOLOGY

Histologic Features

- Early phase
  - Eosinophilic perivascular infiltrate in lamina propria
    - Eosinophils surround and extend into capillaries and venules (eosinophilic angiitis)
    - Plasma cells and mature lymphocytes may also be present
    - Thrombosis and ischemic-type necrosis are not identified
- Late phase

EOSINOPHILIC ANGIOCENTRIC FIBROSIS

Key Facts

Terminology
- Rare, chronic, sclerosing, fibroinflammatory disorder of upper aerodigestive tract

Etiology/Pathogenesis
- No known association with systemic or other localized disease(s)
- Postulated to represent mucosal variant of granuloma faciale

Clinical Issues
- Primarily involves nasal cavity
- Surgery may be required in patients with airway obstruction

Microscopic Pathology
- Early phase: Eosinophilic perivascular infiltrate in lamina propria with eosinophilic angiitis
- Late phase: Dense fibrosis with layered onion-skin-type perivascular fibrosis (angiocentric fibrosis)

  - Characteristic feature is presence of dense fibrosis with layered onion-skin-type perivascular fibrosis (angiocentric fibrosis)
  - Fibrosis is hypocellular, but areas of mixed inflammatory cells remain including eosinophils
- In both phases, no evidence of ischemic-type necrosis, granulomatous inflammation, or multinucleated giant cells

ANCILLARY TESTS

Histochemistry
- Special stains for microorganisms are negative

DIFFERENTIAL DIAGNOSIS

Infectious Disease
- Microorganisms identified

Wegener Granulomatosis
- Presence of ischemic-type necrosis, vasculitis, &/or multinucleated giant cells
- Elevated serologic ANCA, PR3 levels

Churg-Strauss Disease
- Characterized by asthma, systemic vasculitis, tissue and peripheral eosinophilia, nasal manifestations
- Vasculitis with transmural inflammation
  - Predominantly eosinophilic cell infiltrate
- Granulomatous vasculitis including multinucleated giant cells found within vessel wall

Fibromatosis
- Dense fibrosis lacking features of EAF

DIAGNOSTIC CHECKLIST

Pathologic Interpretation Pearls
- Believed to represent mucosal variant of granuloma faciale

SELECTED REFERENCES

1. Jain R et al: Sinonasal eosinophilic angiocentric fibrosis: a report of four cases and review of literature. Head Neck Pathol. 2(4):309-15, 2008
2. Narayan J et al: Eosinophilic angiocentric fibrosis and granuloma faciale: analysis of cellular infiltrate and review of literature. Ann Otol Rhinol Laryngol. 114(1 Pt 1):35-42, 2005
3. Pereira EM et al: Eosinophilic angiocentric fibrosis of the sinonasal tract: report on the clinicopathologic features of a case and review of the literature. Head Neck. 24(3):307-11, 2002
4. Thompson LD et al: Sinonasal tract eosinophilic angiocentric fibrosis. A report of three cases. Am J Clin Pathol. 115(2):243-8, 2001
5. Roberts PF et al: Eosinophilic angiocentric fibrosis of the upper respiratory tract: a mucosal variant of granuloma faciale? A report of three cases. Histopathology. 9(11):1217-25, 1985

IMAGE GALLERY

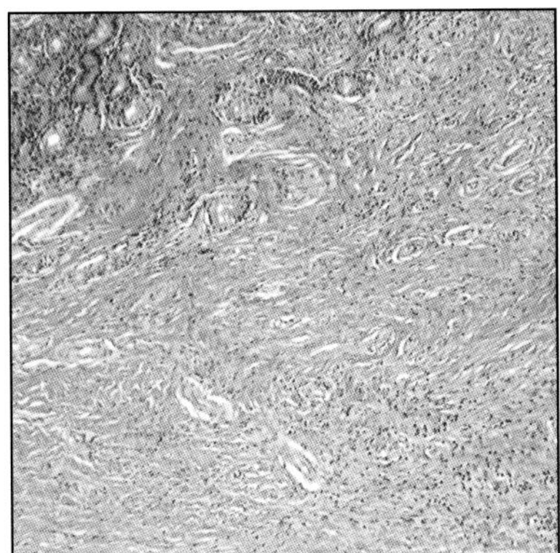

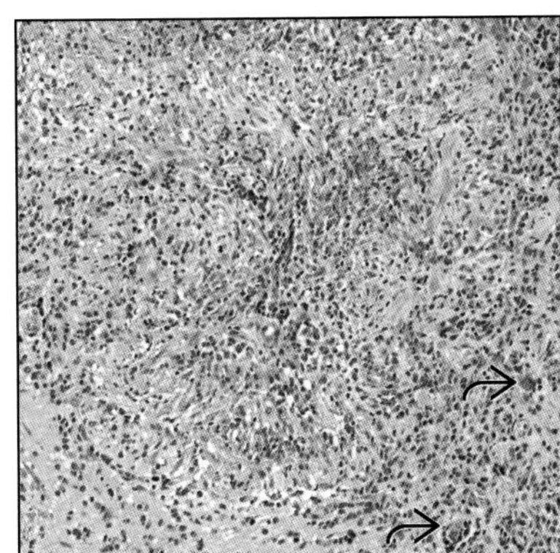

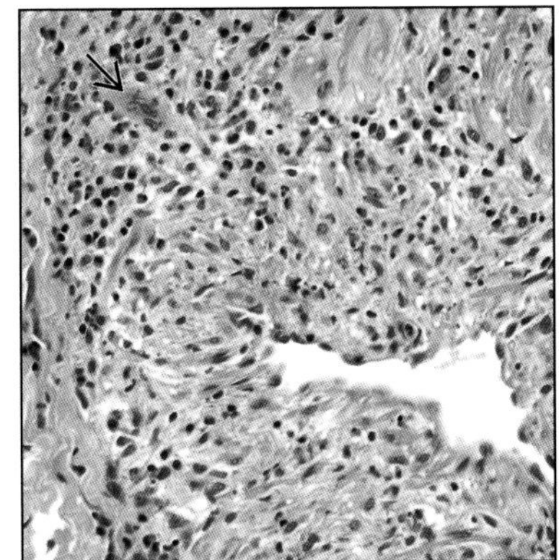

(Left) *Dense stromal fibrosis is a characteristic feature in eosinophilic angiocentric fibrosis.* ***(Center)*** *Histologic features of sinonasal Churg-Strauss disease include submucosal inflammatory cell infiltrate predominantly composed of eosinophils, as well as neutrophils, lymphocytes, plasma cells, and multinucleated giant cells ⇨.* ***(Right)*** *Churg-Strauss vasculitis with transmural inflammation is predominantly composed of eosinophils with neutrophils, lymphocytes, plasma cells, and a giant cell ⇨.*

SINONASAL INFLAMMATORY POLYP

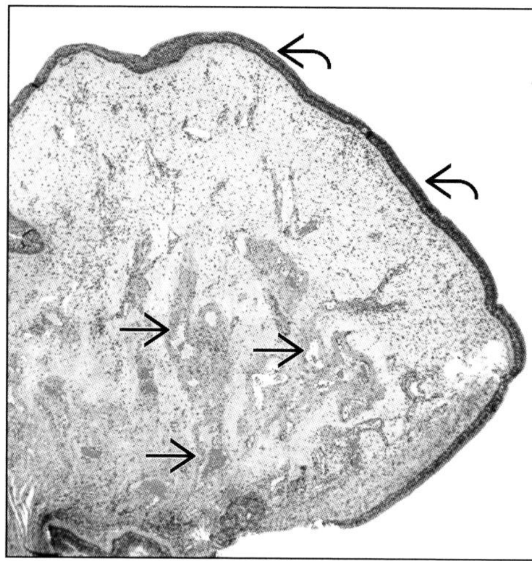

Polypoid mass is seen with intact surface (respiratory) epithelium ⇗ and underlying stroma characterized by edema, inflammatory infiltrate, increased vascularity ⇒, and absence of mucoserous glands.

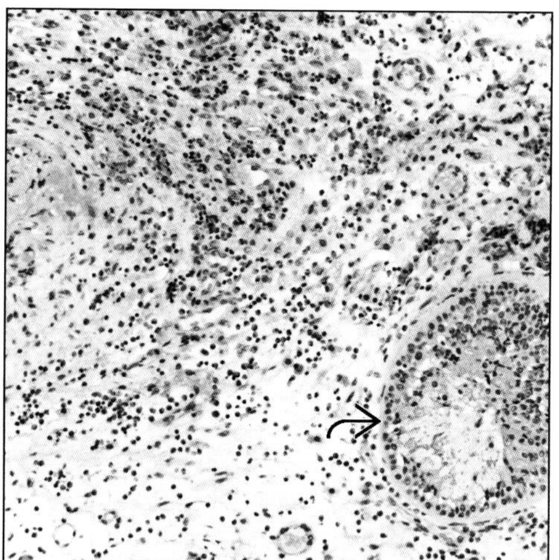

H&E shows edematous stroma with mixed chronic inflammatory cell infiltrate dominated by eosinophils, as well as mature lymphocytes, plasma cells, and neutrophils. A mucoserous gland is present ⇗.

TERMINOLOGY

Definitions

- Nonneoplastic inflammatory swellings of sinonasal mucosa

ETIOLOGY/PATHOGENESIS

Multifactorial

- Etiology linked to multiple factors including
  - Allergy (atopy)
  - Infections
  - Cystic fibrosis
  - Diabetes mellitus
  - Aspirin intolerance
  - Familial

CLINICAL ISSUES

Epidemiology

- Age
  - Occurs in all ages but commonly seen in adults over 20 years old
  - Rarely seen in children less than 5 years old
    - Exception in patients with cystic fibrosis who develop nasal polyps in 1st and 2nd decades of life
- Gender
  - Equal gender distribution

Site

- Most arise from lateral nasal wall or ethmoid recess
  - Normal physiologic parameters of lateral nasal cavity mucosa are such that prominent edema readily forms in mucosal lamina propria
    - Makes this site more susceptible to development of polyps
  - May be unilateral or bilateral, single or multiple
- Not infrequently, involvement of both nasal cavity and paranasal sinuses

Presentation

- Nasal obstruction, rhinorrhea, and headaches
- Samter triad
  - Nasal polyps, asthma, and aspirin intolerance
- Rarely, may be associated with bone erosion, destruction, blindness

Endoscopic Findings

- Mulberry turbinate
  - Clinical term referring to swollen nasal turbinate tissue
  - Formed as result of edema interspersed among thick vessel walls of normal turbinate vascularity
  - Appearance may clinically suggest pathologic process, such as vascular malformation

Treatment

- Options, risks, complications
  - Identification and treatment of possible etiologic factor(s) is initial approach in treatment
- Surgical approaches
  - Polypectomy
    - Medial maxillectomy (Caldwell-Luc procedure) including removal of stalk for antrochoanal polyps
- Drugs
  - Patients with cystic fibrosis may respond to medical therapy, but surgical resection may be required

Prognosis

- Approximately 50% of patients will have recurrence following surgery
  - Recurrence rates highest in patients with aspirin intolerance and asthma
- Development of functional endoscopic sinus surgery contributed to

SINONASAL INFLAMMATORY POLYP

Key Facts

Terminology
- Nonneoplastic inflammatory swellings of the sinonasal mucosa

Etiology/Pathogenesis
- Etiology linked to multiple factors

Clinical Issues
- Most arise from lateral nasal wall or from ethmoid recess
- Nasal obstruction, rhinorrhea, and headaches
- Polypectomy
- Approximately 50% of patients will have recurrence following surgery

Microscopic Pathology
- Surface ciliated respiratory epithelium typically intact; may show squamous metaplasia
- Markedly edematous stroma noteworthy for absence of mucoserous glands
- Mixed chronic inflammatory cell infiltrate predominantly composed of eosinophils, plasma cells, and lymphocytes
- Secondary changes may include
  - Surface ulceration
  - Fibrosis
  - Infarction
  - Granulation tissue
  - Atypical stromal cells
  - Granuloma formation
  - Deposition of amyloid-like stroma
  - Osseous &/or cartilaginous metaplasia

- Decreasing morbidity of sinonasal surgery and recurrence of nasal polyposis in patients with cystic fibrosis
- Improving sinonasal-related symptomatology for asthmatic patients

IMAGE FINDINGS

General Features
- Soft tissue densities, air-fluid levels, mucosal thickening, and opacification of paranasal sinuses
- When extensive, inflammatory polyps may expand and even destroy bone

MACROSCOPIC FEATURES

General Features
- Polyps are soft, fleshy, polypoid lesions with myxoid or mucoid appearance

Size
- Vary in size, ranging up to several centimeters in diameter

MICROSCOPIC PATHOLOGY

Histologic Features
- Surface ciliated respiratory epithelium typically intact
  - May show squamous metaplasia
  - Basement membrane may be thickened and eosinophilic in appearance
- Stroma
  - Markedly edematous; noteworthy for absence of mucoserous glands
  - Contains mixed chronic inflammatory cell infiltrate predominantly composed of eosinophils, plasma cells, and lymphocytes
    - Neutrophils may predominate in polyps of infectious origin
  - Bland-appearing fibroblasts and small to medium-sized blood vessels
    - Spaces containing watery-appearing fluid simulate appearance of lymphatic spaces, suggesting diagnosis of lymphangioma
    - Spaces lack endothelial cell lining
  - Prominent vascular component may be present
    - Variably termed angiomatous or angioectatic nasal polyps
    - May simulate appearance of neoplasm
- Secondary changes may include
  - Surface ulceration
  - Fibrosis
  - Infarction
  - Atypical stromal cells
    - Represent myofibroblasts
    - Often localized to areas of injury, especially around thrombosed vessels
  - Granulation tissue
  - Deposition of amyloid-like stroma
  - Osseous &/or cartilaginous metaplasia
  - Glandular hyperplasia
  - Causes for granuloma formation include
    - Ruptured mucous cysts
    - Cholesterol granulomas
    - Reaction to intranasal injections (steroids) or inhalants
  - Pseudogranulomas may be seen
    - Small patches of stromal nonedematous collagen with peripherally situated inflammatory cells

DIFFERENTIAL DIAGNOSIS

Infectious Diseases
- Identification of causative microorganism(s) by
  - Light microscopy
  - Special stains
- Absence of microorganisms in polyps

Schneiderian Papillomas
- Neoplastic epithelial proliferation characterized by

- Markedly thickened epithelial proliferation comprised of
  - Squamous, transitional, &/or columnar cells with admixed mucocytes (goblet cells)
- Intraepithelial mucous cysts
- Endophytic (inverted) &/or exophytic growth
- Oncocytic type characterized by
  - Multilayered epithelial proliferation composed of columnar cells with abundant eosinophilic and granular cytoplasm

Respiratory Epithelial Adenomatoid Hamartoma

- Histopathologic changes dominated by presence of glandular proliferation composed of
  - Widely-spaced, small to medium-sized glands separated by stromal tissue
- Glands can be seen in direct continuity with surface epithelium with invagination into submucosa
- Glands composed of multilayered ciliated respiratory epithelium with admixed mucin-secreting (goblet) cells
- Characteristic finding is presence of stromal hyalinization enveloping glands by thick, eosinophilic basement membrane
- Atrophic alterations may be present with glands lined by single layer of flattened to cuboidal epithelium

Nasopharyngeal Angiofibroma

- Neoplastic proliferation composed of variable admixture of
  - Slit-like vascular spaces lacking mural smooth muscle
  - Dense stromal fibrosis

Vascular and Lymphatic Neoplasm

- Lobular capillary hemangioma among more common sinonasal vascular neoplasms
  - Characterized by
    - Submucosal endothelial-lined vascular proliferation arranged in lobules or clusters
    - Composed of central capillaries and smaller ramifying tributaries
    - Central capillaries vary in caliber, as well as in shape; may include "staghorn" appearance
- Lymphangiomas rare in sinonasal tract

Heterotopic Central Nervous System Tissue/ Encephalocele

- Identification of central nervous system tissue by
  - Light microscopy
  - Glial fibrillary acidic protein immunostaining

Rhabdomyosarcoma (RMS)

- Atypical stromal cells may be confused with malignant cells (rhabdomyoblasts)
- Embryonal RMS most common type in sinonasal tract
- Diffusely cellular proliferation
- Variation in cellularity with alternating hyper- and hypocellular areas, latter often associated with myxoid stroma
- Cellular components consist of admixture of cell types including
  - Small undifferentiated (primitive-appearing) round or spindle-shaped cells with hyperchromatic nuclei and indistinct cytoplasm
  - Differentiated large round to oval cells with eosinophilic cytoplasm
  - Cross striations are rare in round cells but more apparent in spindle cell component
- Nuclear pleomorphism, increased mitotic activity, and necrosis are present
- Immunoreactivity for myogenic markers including
  - Desmin, myoglobin, myogenin

SELECTED REFERENCES

1. Ardehali MM et al: The comparison of histopathological characteristics of polyps in asthmatic and nonasthmatic patients. Otolaryngol Head Neck Surg. 140(5):748-51, 2009
2. Delagrand A et al: Nasal polyposis: is there an inheritance pattern? A single family study. Rhinology. 46(2):125-30, 2008
3. Sheahan P et al: Infarcted angiomatous nasal polyps. Eur Arch Otorhinolaryngol. 262(3):225-30, 2005
4. Yung MW et al: Nasal polyposis in children with cystic fibrosis: a long-term follow-up study. Ann Otol Rhinol Laryngol. 111(12 Pt 1):1081-6, 2002
5. Greisner WA 3rd et al: Hereditary factor for nasal polyps. Allergy Asthma Proc. 17(5):283-6, 1996
6. Holmberg K et al: Nasal polyps: medical or surgical management? Clin Exp Allergy. 26 Suppl 3:23-30, 1996
7. Drutman J et al: Sinonasal polyposis. Semin Ultrasound CT MR. 12(6):561-74, 1991
8. Levine HL: Functional endoscopic sinus surgery: evaluation, surgery, and follow-up of 250 patients. Laryngoscope. 100(1):79-84, 1990
9. Zeitz HJ: Bronchial asthma, nasal polyps, and aspirin sensitivity: Samter's syndrome. Clin Chest Med. 9(4):567-76, 1988
10. Som PM et al: CT appearance distinguishing benign nasal polyps from malignancies. J Comput Assist Tomogr. 11(1):129-33, 1987
11. Kindblom LG et al: Nasal polyps with atypical stroma cells: a pseudosarcomatous lesion. A light and electron-microscopic and immunohistochemical investigation with implications on the type and nature of the mesenchymal cells. Acta Pathol Microbiol Immunol Scand A. 92(1):65-72, 1984
12. Heffner DK: Problems in pediatric otorhinolaryngic pathology. I. Sinonasal and nasopharyngeal tumors and masses with myxoid features. Int J Pediatr Otorhinolaryngol. 5(1):77-91, 1983
13. Rejowski JE et al: Nasal polyps causing bone destruction and blindness. Otolaryngol Head Neck Surg. 90(4):505-6, 1982
14. Winestock DP et al: Benign nasal polyps causing bone destruction in the nasal cavity and paranasal sinuses. Laryngoscope. 88(4):675-9, 1978
15. Settipane GA et al: Nasal polyps in asthma and rhinitis. A review of 6,037 patients. J Allergy Clin Immunol. 59(1):17-21, 1977
16. Compagno J et al: Nasal polyposis with stromal atypia. Review of follow-up study of 14 cases. Arch Pathol Lab Med. 100(4):224-6, 1976
17. Wolff M: Granulomas in nasal mucous membranes following local steroid injections. Am J Clin Pathol. 62(6):775-82, 1974

Variant Microscopic Features

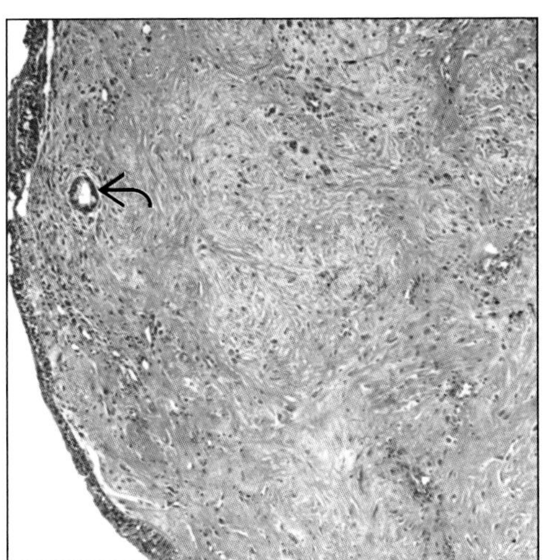

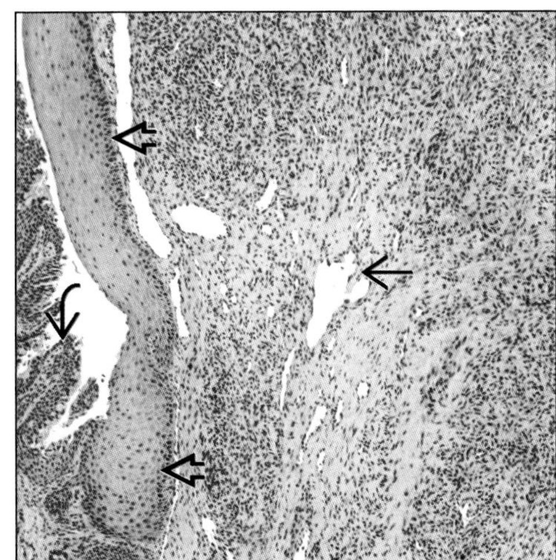

(Left) *A variety of reactive &/or degenerative changes can occur in inflammatory polyps, including submucosal dense fibrosis. Associated scattered inflammatory cells and an identifiable mucoserous gland ↪ are present.* ***(Right)*** *Additional reactive alterations in sinonasal polyps may include squamous metaplasia ⇨ of the respiratory epithelium ↪ and submucosal granulation tissue, including variably sized and shaped blood vessels →.*

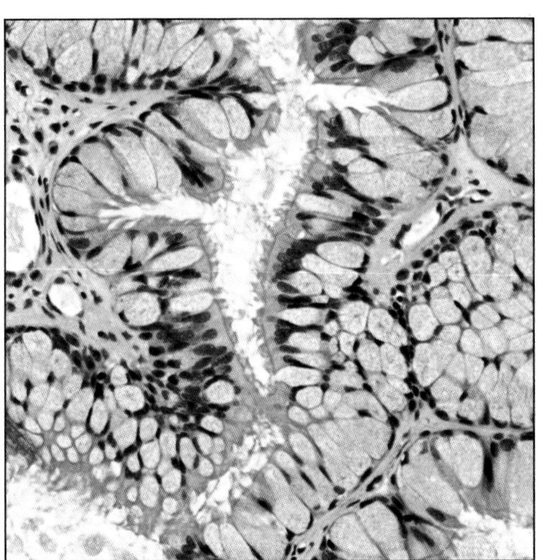

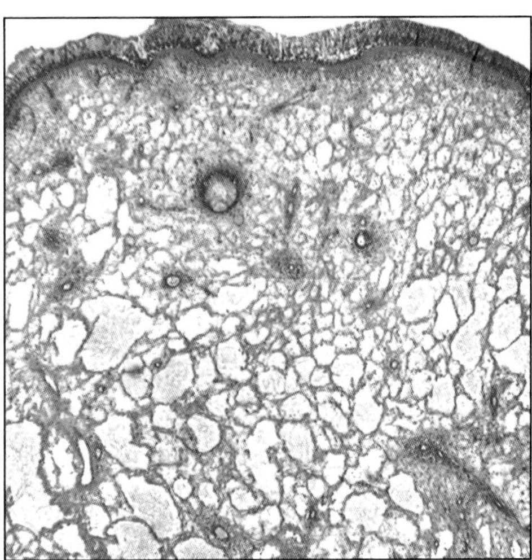

(Left) *Mucous gland hyperplasia may potentially create diagnostic concern for a glandular neoplasm. The background alterations typically seen in inflammatory polyps and the absence of complex (back-to-back) growth seen in glandular neoplasms allow for differentiation.* ***(Right)*** *Submucosal dilated spaces containing watery appearing fluid simulate lymphatic spaces, suggesting a diagnosis of lymphangioma. In contrast to lymphangioma, the spaces lack an endothelial lining.*

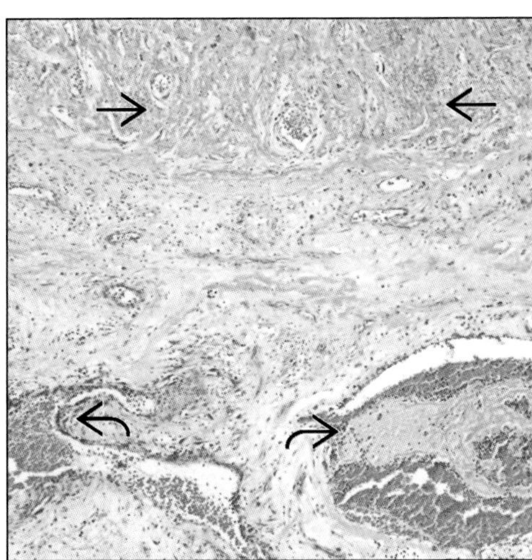

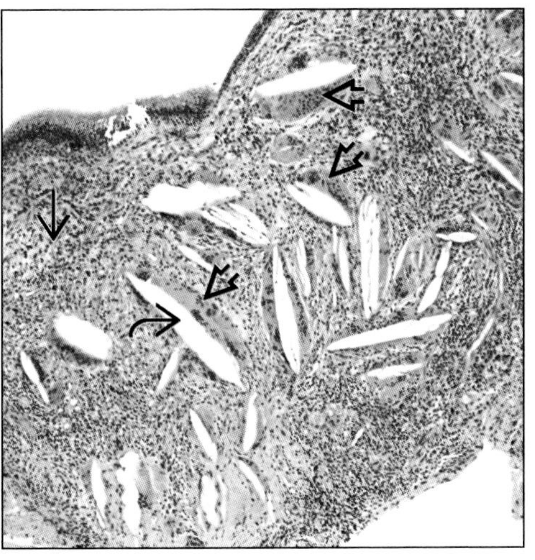

(Left) *Thrombosed blood vessels ↪ with hemorrhage → & infarction (not shown) can occur in traumatized sinonasal inflammatory polyps.* ***(Right)*** *Granulomas can be seen in polyps, including cholesterol granulomas comprised of clear needle-shaped spaces ↪ representing lipid from extravasated erythrocytes with associated multinucleated giant cells ⇨. Pigmented cells → represent hemosiderin deposition (iron positive, not shown), an indicator of past hemorrhage.*

ANTROCHOANAL POLYP

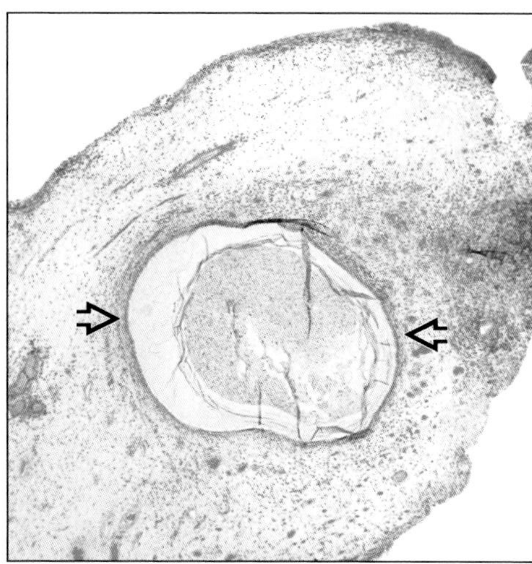

Polyp is shown with intact respiratory epithelium, edematous stroma with scattered inflammatory cells, and paucity of mucoserous glands, which may be dilated (ectatic) and filled with mucinous material ⇨.

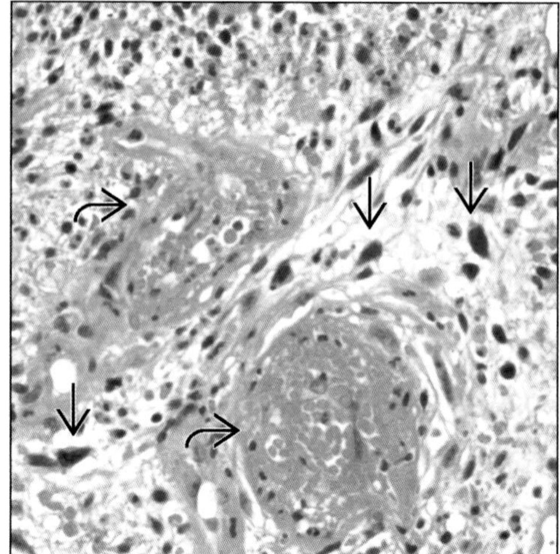

Due to torsion in its passage through the antrum, ACPs often have associated alterations that may include vascular thrombosis ↗ with nearby clusters of hyperchromatic atypical stromal cells →.

TERMINOLOGY

Abbreviations

- Antrochoanal polyp (ACP)
- Atypical stromal cell (ASC)

Definitions

- Clinically distinctive variant of sinonasal inflammatory polyp
  - Originates from within maxillary sinus (medial wall area) extending via stalk through ostium of maxillary sinus into nasal cavity

ETIOLOGY/PATHOGENESIS

Environmental Exposure

- Despite correlation in up to 40% of cases with history of allergies, felt to be of inflammatory etiology

CLINICAL ISSUES

Epidemiology

- Incidence
  - Represents approximately 3-6% of all sinonasal polyps
- Age
  - Occur in patients younger than those who present with nasal polyps
    - Primarily teenagers and young adults
- Gender
  - Male > Female

Site

- Maxillary sinus (medial wall area) and extending via a stalk through ostium of maxillary sinus into nasal cavity
- Posterior extension toward nasopharynx may result in obstruction of nasopharynx and clinical suspicion of primary nasopharyngeal tumor
- May extend ("hang") into oropharynx and be identifiable through open mouth

Presentation

- Generally presents as a single, unilateral polyp with nasal obstruction
- Often associated with bilateral maxillary sinusitis
- May be associated with more typical sinonasal polyps
- Rarely may coexist with sphenochoanal polyp
  - Sphenochoanal polyps originate from sphenoid sinus, extending
    - Through sphenoid ostium
    - Across sphenoethmoid recess
    - Into choana (boundary between nasal cavity and nasopharynx)

Treatment

- Surgical approaches
  - Complete surgical excision, including stalk, is treatment of choice

Prognosis

- Cured following complete surgical excision
- May recur if polyp, including stalk, is incompletely excised
  - High recurrence rate, especially in patients with history of allergies
  - Endoscopic removal (due to incomplete excision) may result in higher recurrence rate

MACROSCOPIC FEATURES

General Features

- Identical to other nasal polyps, except for presence of a stalk with attachment to maxillary sinus

ANTROCHOANAL POLYP

Key Facts

Terminology

- Clinically distinctive variant of sinonasal inflammatory polyp originating from within maxillary sinus and extending through ostium of maxillary sinus into nasal cavity

Clinical Issues

- Represents 3-6% of all sinonasal polyps
- Occur in patients younger in age than those who present with nasal polyps
- Complete surgical excision, including stalk, is curative

Microscopic Pathology

- Similar to sinonasal polyps except for relative absence of mucous glands
- Subject to secondary changes due to vascular compromise
  - Infarction, partial or complete
  - Presence of atypical stromal cells

MICROSCOPIC PATHOLOGY

Histologic Features

- Similar to sinonasal polyps except for relative lack of mucous glands and eosinophilic inflammatory infiltrate
- Subject to secondary changes resulting from chronic or subacute vascular compromise including
  - Presence of atypical stromal cells
    - Myofibroblastic origin and cellular component of wound healing
    - Bizarre-appearing cells with enlarged pleomorphic and hyperchromatic nuclei, indistinct to prominent nucleoli, eosinophilic to basophilic cytoplasm
    - Tend to cluster near areas of tissue injury (e.g., near thrombosed vascular spaces)
    - May be confused with malignant cells (e.g., rhabdomyoblasts)
    - Localization to limited areas of lesion coupled with absence of increased nuclear to cytoplasmic ratio, increased mitoses, or cross striations preclude diagnosis of malignancy
  - Infarction, partial or complete
    - Hemorrhage may be minimal or extensive
    - Associated reactive changes may include extensive neovascularization
    - Papillary endothelial hyperplasia may occur in conjunction with organizing thrombus
    - Presence of hemorrhage and reactive changes may result in bone erosion of lateral nasal cavity-medial maxillary sinus wall

ANCILLARY TESTS

Immunohistochemistry

- Atypical stromal cells
  - Vimentin and actins (smooth muscle, muscle specific) positive
  - Cytokeratin staining may be present
  - No immunoreactivity for desmin, myoglobin, myogenin

DIFFERENTIAL DIAGNOSIS

Rhabdomyosarcoma

- Atypical stromal cells may be confused with malignant cells (rhabdomyoblasts)
- In contrast to malignant cells, atypical stromal cells localized to areas around foci of injury

SELECTED REFERENCES

1. Yuca K et al: Evaluation and treatment of antrochoanal polyps. J Otolaryngol. 35(6):420-3, 2006
2. Batsakis JG et al: Choanal and angiomatous polyps of the sinonasal tract. Ann Otol Rhinol Laryngol. 101(7):623-5, 1992

IMAGE GALLERY

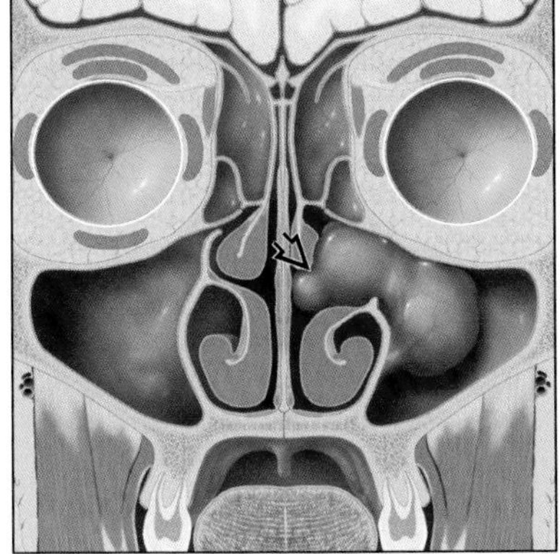
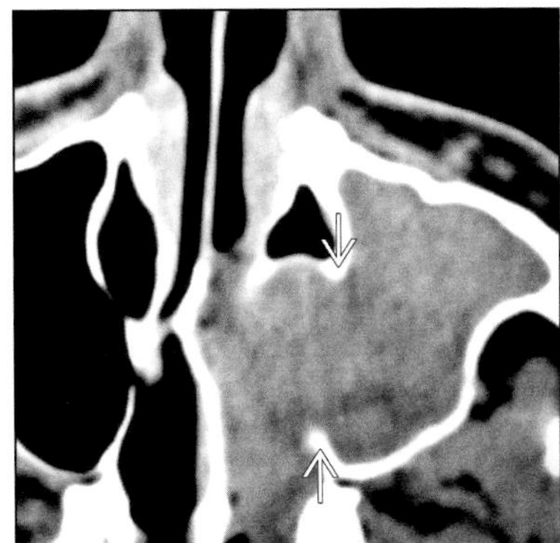
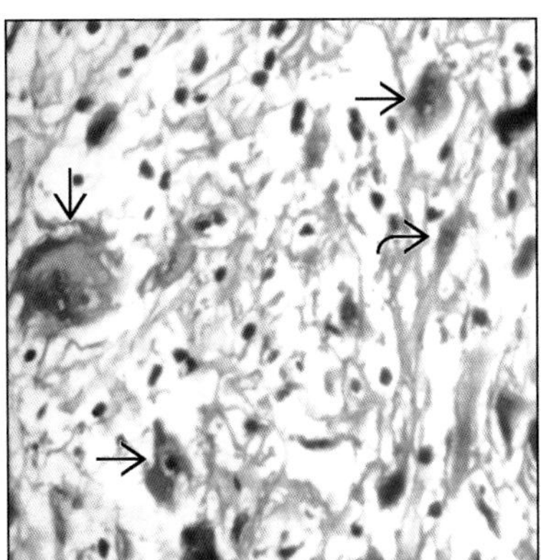

(Left) *This is a graphic depiction of ACP.* ***(Center)*** *Axial NECT shows antrochoanal polyp with somewhat heterogeneous increased density. This may be related to chronicity of polyp or fungal colonization. Widened secondary ostium is well seen.* ***(Right)*** *Despite their atypical appearance, ASCs have a low nuclear to cytoplasmic ratio, a fibrillar-appearing cytoplasm, and elongated appearance with axonal-like extensions lacking malignant cytomorphologic features.*

SINONASAL HAMARTOMA

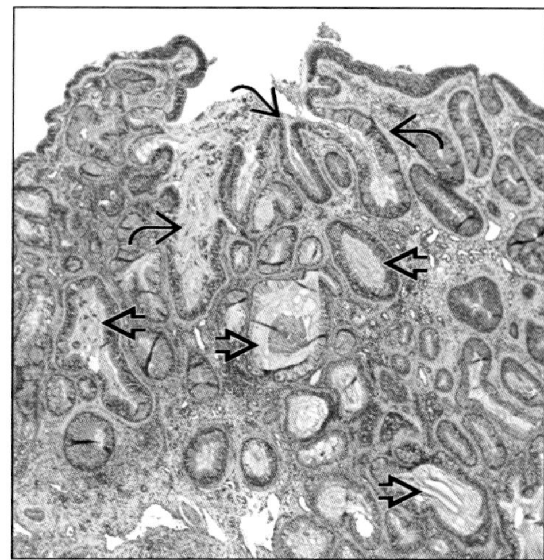

The histopathologic changes show a glandular proliferation composed of widely spaced, small to medium-sized glands ➾ separated by stromal tissue invaginating downward into the submucosa ➚.

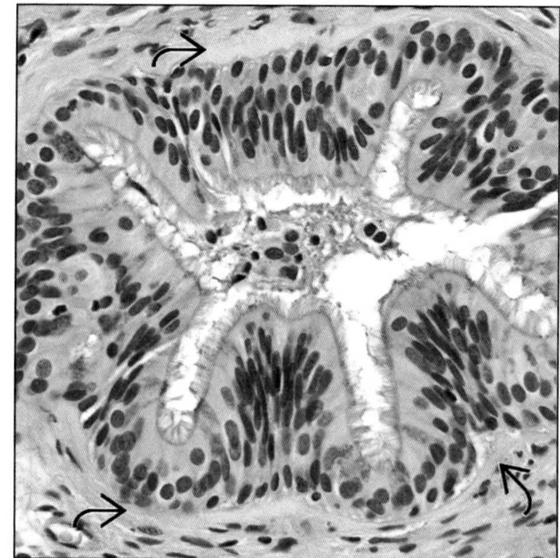

The glands are round to oval, composed of multilayered ciliated respiratory epithelium with characteristic envelopment of glands by a variably thickened, eosinophilic basement membrane ➚.

TERMINOLOGY

Abbreviations

- Respiratory epithelial adenomatoid (READ) hamartoma
- Chondro-osseous and respiratory epithelial (CORE) hamartomas
- Nasal chondromesenchymal hamartoma (NCH)

Synonyms

- Glandular hamartoma
- Seromucinous hamartoma
- Nasal hamartoma

Definitions

- **READ hamartoma**: Benign acquired nonneoplastic overgrowth of indigenous glands of sinonasal tract and nasopharynx
  - Arising from surface epithelium
  - Devoid of ectodermal, neuroectodermal, &/or mesodermal elements
- **CORE hamartoma**
  - Related to READ hamartoma but has additional feature of chondroid tissue
- NCH: Tumefactive process of sinonasal tract
  - Composed of admixture of chondroid and stromal elements with cystic features analogous to chest wall hamartoma
  - Histologic similarities to READ and CORE hamartomas; may be within spectrum of same lesion type

ETIOLOGY/PATHOGENESIS

Idiopathic

- No association with any specific etiologic agent

Developmental

- READ hamartomas arise in setting of inflammatory polyps
  - Raises possible developmental induction secondary to inflammatory process

CLINICAL ISSUES

Epidemiology

- Incidence
  - Rare lesions
- Age
  - **READ hamartoma**
    - Occurs in adult patients
    - Range from 3rd to 9th decades
    - Reported median in 6th decade
  - **CORE hamartoma**
    - Ranges from 11-73 years
  - NCH
    - Most of these lesions occur in newborns within 1st 3 months of life but may occur in 2nd decade of life
    - Occasionally in adults
- Gender
  - **READ hamartoma**
    - Equal gender distribution
  - **CORE hamartoma**
    - Equal gender distribution
  - NCH
    - Male > Female

Site

- Majority occur in nasal cavity, particularly posterior nasal septum
  - Involvement of other intranasal sites occurs less often and may be identified
    - Along lateral nasal wall, middle meatus, and inferior turbinate
- Other sites of involvement include nasopharynx, ethmoid sinus, and frontal sinus
- Majority of lesions are unilateral, but occasionally bilateral lesions may occur

SINONASAL HAMARTOMA

Key Facts

Terminology

- **READ hamartoma**: Benign acquired nonneoplastic overgrowth of indigenous glands of sinonasal tract and nasopharynx
- **CORE hamartoma**: Related to READ hamartoma but has additional feature of chondroid tissue
- **NCH**: Tumefactive process of sinonasal tract comprised of admixture of chondroid and stromal elements with cystic features analogous to chest wall hamartoma

Clinical Issues

- Conservative, but complete surgical excision treatment of choice
- Cured following surgical resection

Microscopic Pathology

- **READ hamartoma**
  - Changes dominated by presence of glandular proliferation enveloped by stromal hyalinization
- **CORE hamartoma**
  - Similar features to READ hamartomas but with intimate admixture of cartilaginous &/or osseous trabeculae
- **NCH**
  - Characterized by presence of nodules of cartilage varying in size, shape, and contour with varying differentiation
  - Chondromesenchymal elements are relatively cellular and "immature"

Presentation

- **READ hamartoma**
  - Clinical presentation may include one or more of the following symptoms
    - Nasal obstruction, nasal stuffiness, epistaxis, and chronic (recurrent) rhinosinusitis; associated complaints include allergies
    - Symptoms may occur over months to years
  - Nondestructive lesion
- **CORE hamartoma**
  - Polypoid mass lesion
- **NCH**
  - Respiratory difficulty and intranasal mass or facial swelling may be present
  - May erode into cranial cavity (through cribriform plate area), clinically simulating appearance of meningoencephalocele

Treatment

- Surgical approaches
  - Conservative, but complete surgical excision treatment of choice

Prognosis

- Cured following surgical resection

MACROSCOPIC FEATURES

General Features

- Typically polypoid or exophytic with rubbery consistency, tan-white to red-brown appearance

Size

- May measure up to 6 cm in greatest dimension

MICROSCOPIC PATHOLOGY

READ Hamartoma

- Changes dominated by presence of glandular proliferation composed of widely spaced, small to medium-sized glands separated by stromal tissue
  - In areas, glands are seen arising in direct continuity with surface epithelium, which invaginate downward into submucosa
  - Glands are round to oval, composed of multilayered ciliated respiratory epithelium often with admixed mucin-secreting (goblet) cells
  - Glandular dilatation distended with mucus can be seen
- Characteristic finding includes presence of stromal hyalinization with envelopment of glands by thick, eosinophilic basement membrane
- Atrophic glandular alterations may be present in which glands are lined by single layer of flattened to cuboidal-appearing epithelium
- Edematous or fibrous stroma containing mixed chronic inflammatory cell infiltrate
- Additional findings may include
  - Alterations of inflammatory sinonasal polyp(s)
  - Hyperplasia &/or squamous metaplasia of surface epithelium unrelated to adenomatoid proliferation
  - Osseous metaplasia
  - Rare association with
    - Schneiderian papilloma, inverted type
    - Solitary fibrous tumor

CORE Hamartoma

- Similar features to READ hamartomas but in addition
  - Intimately associated admixture of cartilaginous &/or osseous trabeculae
  - Spectrum of chondro-osseous differentiation can be found, including immature-appearing mesenchyme to well-developed bony trabeculae in myxoid to fibrous stroma
  - READ hamartoma components present but less prominent

NCH

- Characterized by presence of nodules of cartilage varying in size, shape, and contour
- Degree of differentiation varies with some nodules appearing similar to chondromyxomatous nodules

of chondromyxoid fibroma to nodules of well-differentiated cartilage
- Chondromesenchymal elements are relatively cellular and "immature"
- Loose spindle cell stroma or abrupt transition to hypocellular fibrous stroma are present at periphery of cartilaginous nodules
- Other findings include
  - Myxoid to spindle cell stroma
  - Fibroosseous proliferation with cellular stromal component
  - Ossicles or trabeculae of immature (woven) bone
  - Focal osteoclast-like giant cells in stroma
  - Erythrocyte-filled spaces resembling those of aneurysmal bone cyst
  - Mature adipose tissue can be present
  - Proliferating epithelial elements are not a prominent feature

ANCILLARY TESTS

Molecular Genetics

- Molecular profile of READ hamartoma
  - Reported to show a mean fractional allelic loss (FAL) of 31%
    - Considered unusually high for nonneoplastic entity
    - Suggests possibility that respiratory epithelial adenomatoid hamartoma may be benign neoplasm rather than hamartoma

DIFFERENTIAL DIAGNOSIS

Sinonasal Inflammatory Polyp

- Polypoid lesion characterized by stromal changes, including edema and mixed inflammatory cell infiltrate
- Typically lacks glandular proliferation as seen in READ hamartoma
  - Rarely may include seromucous gland hyperplasia
- Surface epithelial alterations may include squamous metaplasia

Schneiderian Papillomas

- Surface epithelial proliferation with endophytic (inverted) or exophytic growth
- Lacks glandular proliferation as seen in READ hamartoma

Nasopharyngeal Angiofibroma

- Neoplasm comprised of admixture of fibrous stromal component and benign endothelial-lined vascular component

Sinonasal Nonintestinal-Nonsalivary Adenocarcinoma

- Glandular neoplasm characterized by
  - Complex growth (back to back glands)
  - Glands lined by single cell type
  - Usually well-differentiated neoplasm lacking significant nuclear pleomorphism, increased mitoses, necrosis
  - Typically submucosal glandular proliferation lacking continuity to surface epithelium
  - Immunohistochemical staining of no diagnostic utility in differentiating adenocarcinoma from READ hamartoma
    - Myoepithelial cells as determined by p63 (or other basal cell markers) may be present or absent in benign sinonasal glandular lesions/neoplasms as well as in malignant glandular neoplasms
    - p63 and other myoepithelial markers cannot be used to discriminate between adenocarcinoma and hamartomas

SELECTED REFERENCES

1. Cao Z et al: Respiratory epithelial adenomatoid hamartoma of bilateral olfactory clefts associated with nasal polyposis: three cases report and literature review. Auris Nasus Larynx. 37(3):352-6, 2010
2. Seol JG et al: Respiratory epithelial adenomatoid hamartoma of the bilateral olfactory recesses: a neoplastic mimic? AJNR Am J Neuroradiol. 31(2):277-9, 2010
3. Weinreb I: Low grade glandular lesions of the sinonasal tract: a focused review. Head Neck Pathol. 4(1):77-83, 2010
4. Jo VY et al: Low-grade sinonasal adenocarcinomas: the association with and distinction from respiratory epithelial adenomatoid hamartomas and other glandular lesions. Am J Surg Pathol. 33(3):401-8, 2009
5. Perez-Ordoñez B: Hamartomas, papillomas and adenocarcinomas of the sinonasal tract and nasopharynx. J Clin Pathol. 62(12):1085-95, 2009
6. Weinreb I et al: Seromucinous hamartomas: a clinicopathological study of a sinonasal glandular lesion lacking myoepithelial cells. Histopathology. 54(2):205-13, 2009
7. Fitzhugh VA et al: Respiratory epithelial adenomatoid hamartoma: a review. Head Neck Pathol. 2(3):203-8, 2008
8. Ozolek JA et al: Basal/myoepithelial cells in chronic sinusitis, respiratory epithelial adenomatoid hamartoma, inverted papilloma, and intestinal-type and nonintestinal-type sinonasal adenocarcinoma: an immunohistochemical study. Arch Pathol Lab Med. 131(4):530-7, 2007
9. Sangoi AR et al: Respiratory epithelial adenomatoid hamartoma: diagnostic pitfalls with emphasis on differential diagnosis. Adv Anat Pathol. 14(1):11-6, 2007
10. Ozolek JA et al: Tumor suppressor gene alterations in respiratory epithelial adenomatoid hamartoma (REAH): comparison to sinonasal adenocarcinoma and inflamed sinonasal mucosa. Am J Surg Pathol. 30(12):1576-80, 2006
11. Roffman E et al: Respiratory epithelial adenomatoid hamartomas and chondroosseous respiratory epithelial hamartomas of the sinonasal tract: a case series and literature review. Am J Rhinol. 20(6):586-90, 2006
12. Metselaar RM et al: Respiratory epithelial adenomatoid hamartoma in the nasopharynx. J Laryngol Otol. 119(6):476-8, 2005
13. Delbrouck C et al: Respiratory epithelial adenomatoid hamartoma associated with nasal polyposis. Am J Otolaryngol. 25(4):282-4, 2004
14. Wenig BM et al: Respiratory epithelial adenomatoid hamartomas of the sinonasal tract and nasopharynx: a clinicopathologic study of 31 cases. Ann Otol Rhinol Laryngol. 104(8):639-45, 1995

Microscopic Features

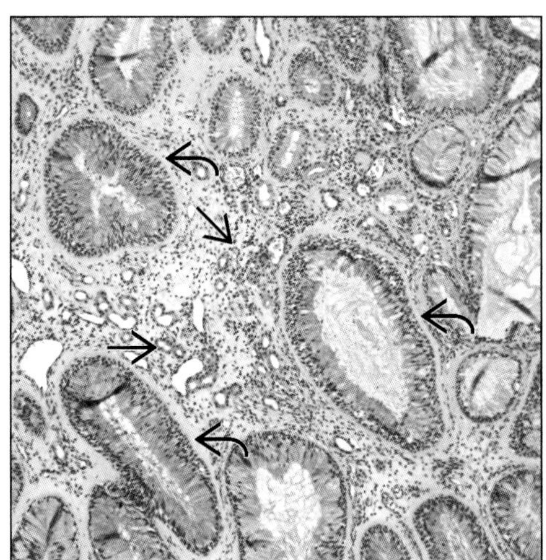

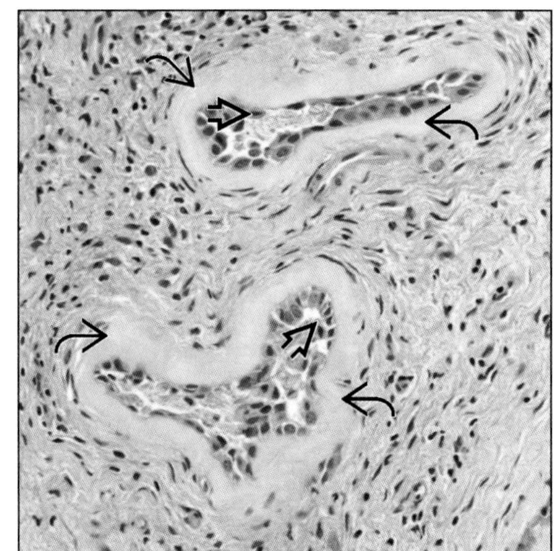

(Left) *The glands are round to oval, widely spaced, with variable amount of mucinous material & envelopment by eosinophilic basement membrane with fibrous to focally edematous stroma containing mixed chronic inflammatory cell infiltrate & scattered residual seromucinous glands.* ***(Right)*** *Atrophic glands include a single layer of flattened to cuboidal-appearing epithelium. Glands are enveloped by markedly thickened eosinophilic basement membranes.*

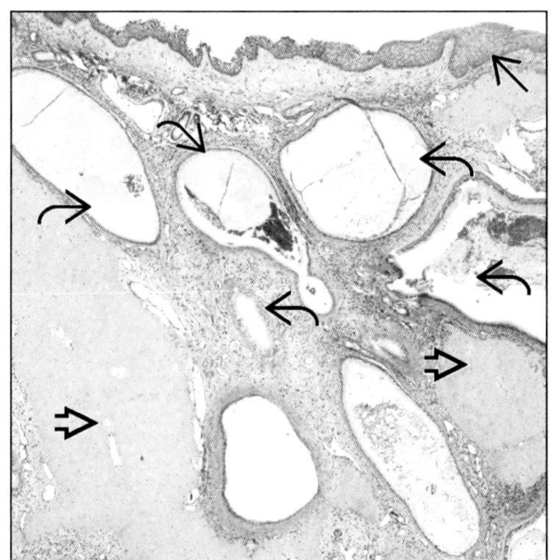

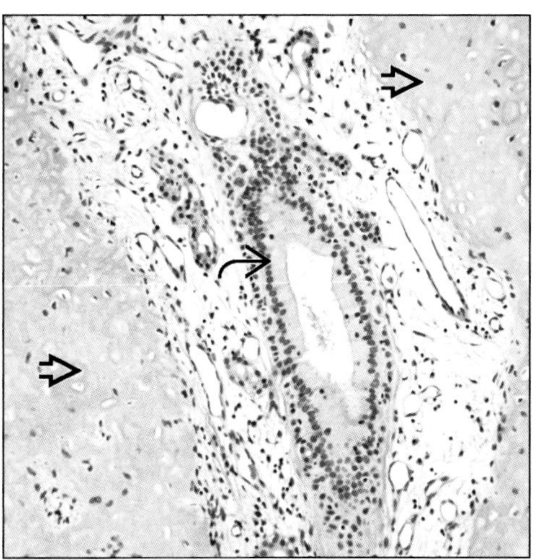

(Left) *CORE hamartoma includes a submucosal proliferation of glands that are less prominent compared to the READ hamartomas, as well as lightly eosinophilic-appearing cartilage. Note surface epithelial squamous metaplasia.* ***(Right)*** *At higher magnification, CORE hamartomas show an admixture of glands and cartilaginous nodules. A zonal-type phenomenon of the cartilage resembling endochondral ossification (not shown) may be present.*

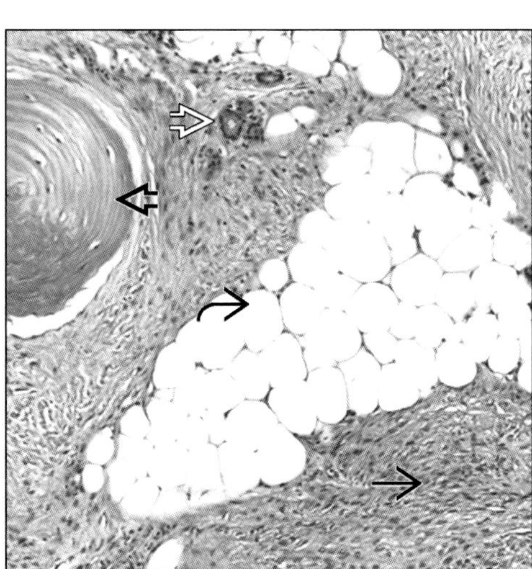

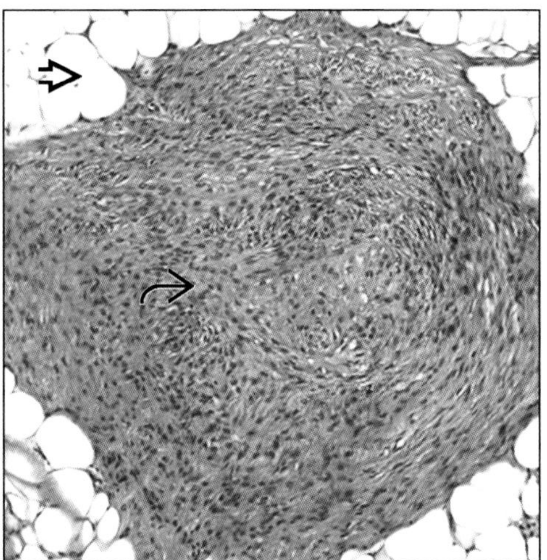

(Left) *NCH is shown composed of a submucosal proliferation of adipose tissue, bony trabeculae, and cellular nodules. Residual seromucous glands are present.* ***(Right)*** *Rounded myxochondroid-appearing cellular nodule composed of bland spindle-shaped cells is surrounded by adipose tissue. Additional findings (not shown) included cartilaginous nodules, bony trabeculae, and seromucous glands.*

MUCOCELE OF PARANASAL SINUS

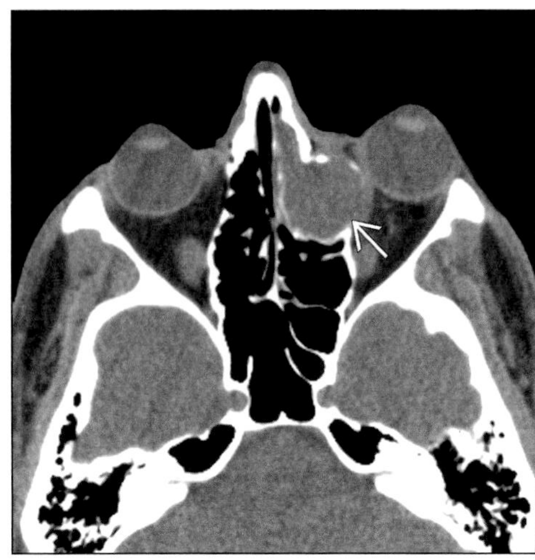

Axial NECT reveals a low-density, expansile, left ethmoid mucocele. The lamina papyracea is remodeled, and there is mass effect on the medial rectus muscle ➡.

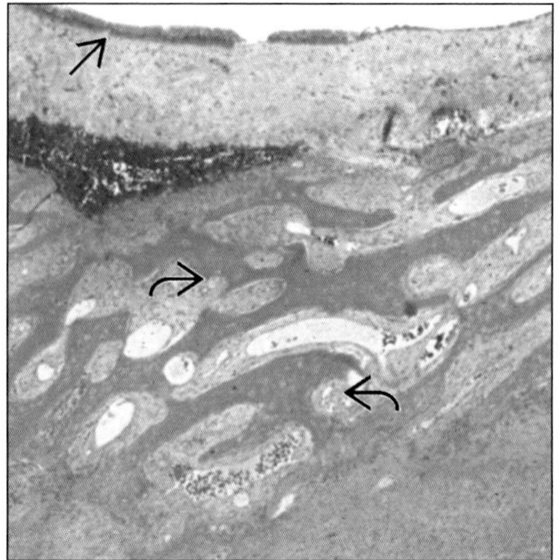

Histologic features associated with an internal mucocele include a respiratory epithelial-lined cyst ➡ lying near to the bony wall of the sinus ↗, as shown. The bone shows reactive changes.

TERMINOLOGY

Definitions

- Distinct clinicopathologic entity characterized by
  - Expansion of sinus cavity due to obstruction of outflow tract (ostium or duct) resulting in cystic lesion of paranasal sinus
  - Diagnosis requires correlation between clinical, radiographic, and pathologic findings, as histopathologic findings alone are nonspecific
  - Expansion of bony walls of sinus is sine qua non for paranasal sinus mucocele

ETIOLOGY/PATHOGENESIS

Developmental Anomaly

- Thought to occur as result of increase in pressure within a given sinus secondary to blockage of sinus outlet (ostium)
  - Most often result of inflammatory or allergic process
- Additional factors implicated include trauma, prior surgery, or neoplasm

CLINICAL ISSUES

Epidemiology

- Age
  - Occurs in all age groups
- Gender
  - Equal gender distribution

Site

- > 90% occur in frontal and ethmoid sinuses
  - Frontonasal duct relatively long and narrow, easily obstructed especially following surgery to this region
- Maxillary sinus uncommonly involved (5-10%)
- Sphenoid sinus involvement considered rare

Presentation

- Chronic process with signs and symptoms occurring over time rather than acutely
- Symptoms depend on site of involvement as well as direction, extent of expansion
  - Pain
  - Facial swelling or deformity
  - Proptosis, exophthalmos, diplopia
  - Rhinorrhea, nasal obstruction

Treatment

- Surgical approaches
  - Complete surgical excision is treatment of choice
    - Trend toward transnasal endoscopic management

Prognosis

- Excellent with long-term control
  - Near zero recurrence rates
- Complications may include superimposed infection (pyocele), meningitis, brain abscess

IMAGE FINDINGS

Radiographic Findings

- Opacification of involved sinus
- Erosion &/or destruction of sinus walls with loss of typical scalloped outline along mucoperiosteum
- Abnormal radiolucency due to loss of bone
- Sclerosis of adjacent bone
- Cavity manifests smoothly contoured, expanded wall with reactive bony thickening
- Radiographic picture can be highly characteristic based on
  - Strikingly rounded appearance, presence of homogeneous mucoid contents

MUCOCELE OF PARANASAL SINUS

Key Facts

Clinical Issues

- Distinct clinicopathologic entity characterized by
  - Expansion of sinus cavity due to obstruction resulting in cystic lesion of sinus
  - Expansion of sinus bony walls is sine qua non for paranasal sinus mucocele
- Thought to occur due to increase in sinus pressure secondary to blockage of sinus outlet, often as result of inflammatory or allergic process
- > 90% occur in frontal and ethmoid sinuses
- Complete surgical excision is treatment of choice

Macroscopic Features

- **Internal**: Herniation of cyst into submucosal tissue adjacent to bony wall of sinus
- **External**: Herniation of cyst through bony wall of sinus with extension into subcutaneous tissue or into cranial cavity

MACROSCOPIC FEATURES

General Features

- 2 types of mucoceles are identified
  - **Internal**
    - Herniation of cyst into submucosal tissue adjacent to bony wall of sinus
  - **External**
    - Herniation of cyst through bony wall of sinus with extension into subcutaneous tissue or into cranial cavity

MICROSCOPIC PATHOLOGY

Histologic Features

- Cysts lined by flattened, pseudostratified, ciliated, columnar epithelium
- In longstanding cases, squamous metaplasia may be present
  - Metaplastic changes uncommon
- Reactive bone formation lying in proximity to cyst epithelium
- Variable chronic inflammatory cell infiltrate may be present
- Additional changes may include
  - Fibrosis, granulation tissue, hemorrhage, cholesterol granuloma
  - Central nervous tissue can be seen if herniation into cranial cavity

DIFFERENTIAL DIAGNOSIS

Mucus Retention Cyst

- a.k.a. salivary mucocele
- Cystic lesion of minor salivary glands characterized by well-circumscribed, submucosal mucus-filled, epithelial-lined cyst

DIAGNOSTIC CHECKLIST

Pathologic Interpretation Pearls

- Diagnosis requires correlation between clinical, radiographic, and pathologic findings, as histopathologic findings alone are nonspecific

SELECTED REFERENCES

1. Socher JA et al: Diagnosis and treatment of isolated sphenoid sinus disease: a review of 109 cases. Acta Otolaryngol. 128(9):1004-10, 2008
2. Serrano E et al: Surgical management of paranasal sinus mucoceles: a long-term study of 60 cases. Otolaryngol Head Neck Surg. 131(1):133-40, 2004
3. Har-El G: Endoscopic management of 108 sinus mucoceles. Laryngoscope. 111(12):2131-4, 2001
4. Evans C: Aetiology and treatment of fronto-ethmoidal mucocele. J Laryngol Otol. 95(4):361-75, 1981
5. van Nostrand AW et al: Pathologic aspects of mucosal lesions of the maxillary sinus. Otolaryngol Clin North Am. 9(1):21-34, 1976

IMAGE GALLERY

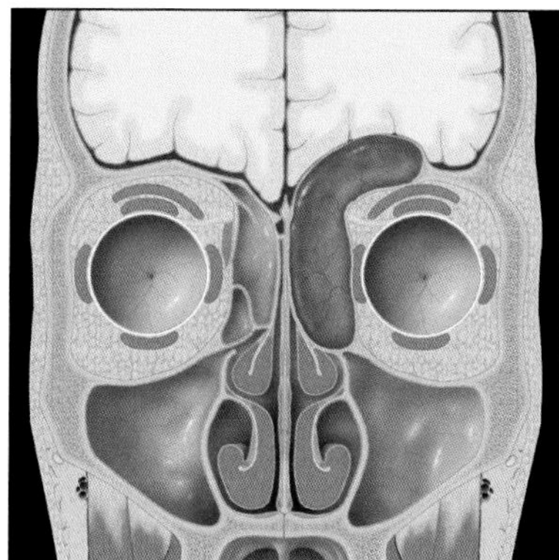

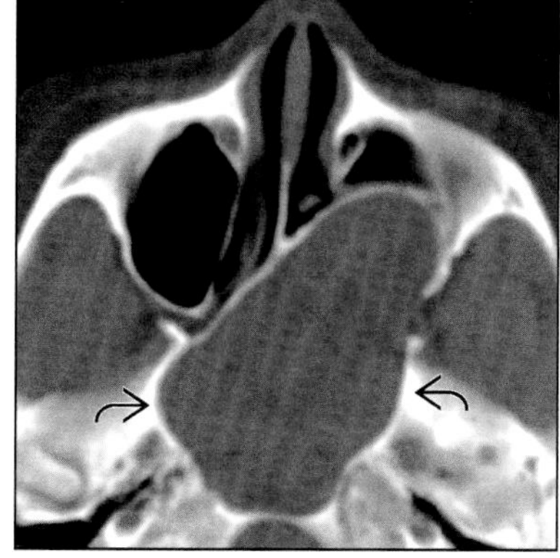

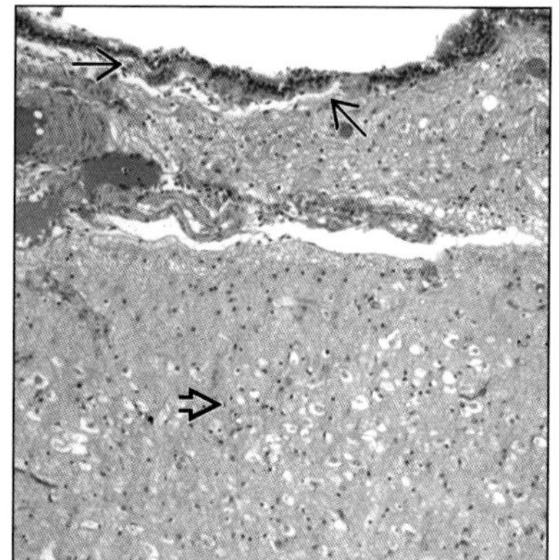

(Left) *Coronal graphic shows left anterior ethmoid mucocele extending into the left frontal sinus.* ***(Center)*** *Axial CT image demonstrates an airless and grossly expanded sphenoid sinus with smooth expansion of the bony walls ⇨ and areas of bone erosion, with extension into the medial and posterior orbit.* ***(Right)*** *External mucocele with herniation into the cranial cavity shows the respiratory epithelial-lined cyst ⇨ overlying central nervous system tissue ⇨.*

EXTRANODAL SINUS HISTIOCYTOSIS WITH MASSIVE LYMPHADENOPATHY

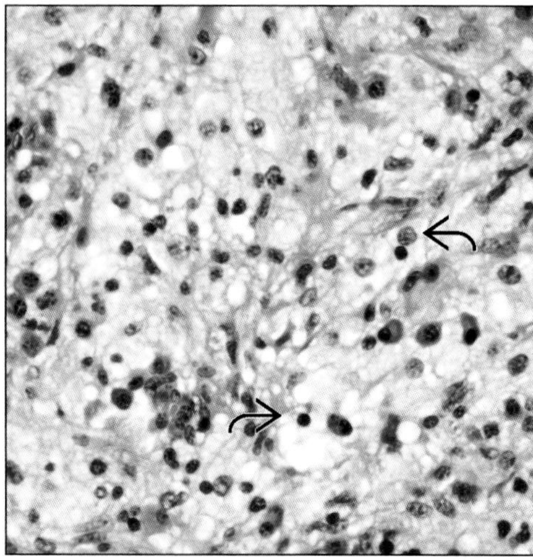

The histiocytic cells of SHML are composed of round nuclei with abundant clear to lightly eosinophilic cytoplasm that is seen occasionally engulfing mononuclear cells (emperipolesis) ➡.

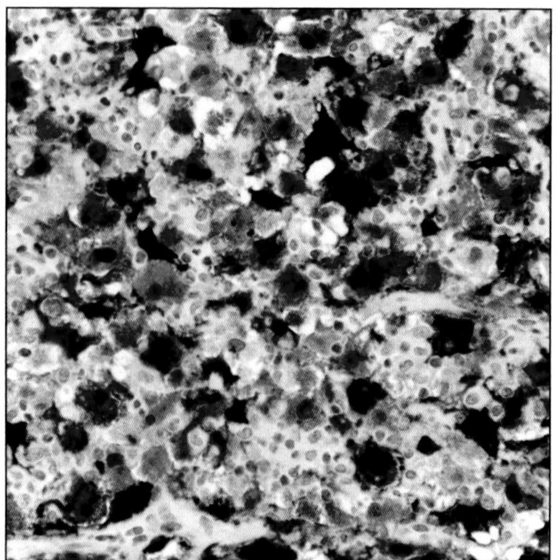

The histiocytes in SHML are diffusely immunoreactive for S100 protein but are CD1a and Langerin negative (not shown). The absence of CD1a and Langerin reactivity excludes Langerhans cell histiocytosis.

TERMINOLOGY

Abbreviations

- Extranodal sinus histiocytosis with massive lymphadenopathy (ESHML)
- Sinus histiocytosis with massive lymphadenopathy (SHML)

Synonyms

- Rosai-Dorfman disease
- Destombes-Rosai-Dorfman syndrome

Definitions

- Idiopathic histiocytic proliferative disorder characterized by lymph-node-based disease and indolent behavior
  - Extranodal manifestations occur with upper respiratory tract among more common sites of involvement

ETIOLOGY/PATHOGENESIS

Idiopathic

- Etiology remains obscure
- Infectious etiology has been suggested as cause, but infectious agent has never been isolated
  - Discrepancy in the literature relative to relationship to Epstein-Barr virus (EBV) and human herpes virus (HHV)
- Other considerations implicated but never substantiated, including
  - Immunodeficiency
  - Autoimmune disease
  - Neoplastic process

Immunophenotype

- Part of mononuclear phagocyte and immunoregulatory effector (M-PIRE) system belonging to macrophage/histiocytic family

CLINICAL ISSUES

Epidemiology

- Incidence
  - Uncommon disease
    - 40% of patients have extranodal disease with or without nodal involvement
- Age
  - Occurs over wide range
- Gender
  - Female > Male

Site

- SHML primarily nodal-based proliferation occurring as part of generalized process
- SHML may involve extranodal sites independent of lymph node status
- Head and neck region represents one of more common extranodal areas involved
  - Predilection for
    - Nasal cavity
    - Paranasal sinuses
  - All head and neck sites may be affected with or independent of nodal disease

Presentation

- Symptoms depend on site of occurrence
  - Sinonasal tract symptoms predominantly relate to nasal obstruction
  - Nonsinonasal tract related symptoms may include
    - Mass lesion
    - Pain, stridor, cranial nerve deficits
    - Proptosis, ptosis, decreased visual acuity
- Presentation often includes multiple concurrent sites of involvement
  - May occur without lymph node involvement

Laboratory Tests

- Hematologic and immunologic status generally intact

EXTRANODAL SINUS HISTIOCYTOSIS WITH MASSIVE LYMPHADENOPATHY

Key Facts

Terminology
- Idiopathic histiocytic proliferative disorder characterized by lymph-node-based disease
  - Extranodal manifestations occur with upper respiratory tract among more common sites of involvement

Etiology/Pathogenesis
- Etiology remains obscure

Clinical Issues
- Head and neck region represents one of more common extranodal areas involved
  - Predilection for sinonasal tract
- Considered indolent, self-limiting disease

Microscopic Pathology
- Submucosal lymphoid aggregates associated with pale-appearing areas composed of histiocytes and plasma cells
- Lymphoid aggregates composed of mature lymphocytes and histiocytic cells impart mottled appearance
- Histiocytes appear in clusters or nests
  - Lack atypical features
  - Characteristically demonstrate emperipolesis
  - Nuclei lack nuclear lobation, indentation, or longitudinal grooving

Ancillary Tests
- SHML cells are diffusely S100 protein positive but CD1a and Langerin (CD207) negative

- May be associated with polyclonal elevations in serum protein levels and raised erythrocyte sedimentation rates
- ANCA and proteinase 3 negative

Treatment
- Options, risks, complications
  - No ideal treatment
  - Treatment protocols mirror clinical manifestations
    - For airway compromise, treatment directed at alleviating the obstruction, requiring surgical intervention
    - In patients with extensive or progressive disease, more radical surgical intervention may be required
    - Surgical eradication may prove difficult in cases with involvement of craniofacial bones &/or cranial cavity
- Adjuvant therapy
  - Radiotherapy and chemotherapy utilized, but efficacy not proven

Prognosis
- Considered indolent, self-limiting disease
- Mortality related to SHML is rare
  - Severe morbidity and mortality attributed to **complications** of SHML
  - Extension of disease to vital structures (e.g., cranial cavity) may rarely result in death
- Unfavorable prognostic factors include
  - Disseminated nodal disease
  - Involvement of multiple extranodal organ systems
  - Deficiencies in hematologic &/or immunologic status

MACROSCOPIC FEATURES

General Features
- Mucosal thickening or polypoid, nodular, or exophytic growth with rubbery to firm consistency

MICROSCOPIC PATHOLOGY

Histologic Features
- Submucosal lymphoid aggregates associated with pale-appearing areas composed of histiocytes, plasma cells, and fibrosis
  - Lymphocytes and plasma cells are nondescript
  - Plasma cells include intracytoplasmic eosinophilic globules (Russell bodies)
- Lymphoid aggregates composed of mature lymphocytes and histiocytic cells impart mottled appearance
  - True germinal centers are not usually seen
- Histiocytic cells (so-called SHML cells) appear in clusters or cell nests
  - Uniform with mild pleomorphism, round to oval, vesicular to hyperchromatic nuclei, abundant amphophilic to eosinophilic, granular to foamy to clear-appearing cytoplasm
  - Nuclei lack
    - Nuclear lobation
    - Indentation
    - Longitudinal grooving
  - May be obscured by nonhistiocytic cell population (particularly plasma cells)
  - Characteristically demonstrate emperipolesis
    - Phagocytized cells (e.g., lymphocytes, plasma cells, erythrocytes, and polymorphonuclear leukocytes) engulfed within histiocytic cell cytoplasm
    - Tends to be less apparent as compared to nodal-based disease
- Well-formed granulomas and multinucleated giant cells not identified

ANCILLARY TESTS

Histochemistry
- Special stains for microorganisms negative
  - GMS
  - PAS

EXTRANODAL SINUS HISTIOCYTOSIS WITH MASSIVE LYMPHADENOPATHY

- AFB
- Others

Immunohistochemistry

- SHML cells
  - Diffusely S100 protein positive
  - Variably positive
    - CD68 (KP1)
    - CD163
    - HAM56 (CD64)
    - MAC387
    - Lysozyme
    - α-1-antichymotrypsin (ACT)
- SHML cells
  - CD1a negative
  - Langerin (CD207) negative
- Lymphocytes and plasma cells show polyclonal pattern of reactivity

DIFFERENTIAL DIAGNOSIS

Infectious (Granulomatous) Diseases

- e.g., rhinoscleroma, leprosy, others
- Absence of microorganisms

Langerhans Cell Histiocytosis

- Langerhans cells immunoreactive for
  - S100 protein
  - CD1a
  - Langerin (CD207)

Wegener Granulomatosis

- Active disease associated with elevations of serum ANCA and proteinase 3
- Histology includes
  - Ischemic-type necrosis
  - Vasculitis
  - Multinucleated giant cells
- Mixed inflammatory cell infiltrate but histiocytes not a prominent feature
- Absence of histologic features of SHML
- No immunoreactivity for S100 protein

Hematolymphoid Malignancy

- Monomorphic, monoclonal cell population in lymphoma allows for differentiation from SHML
  - Heterogeneous cell population, polyclonal immunoreactivity, S100 protein and CD68 reactivity in SHML allows for differentiation from hematolymphoid malignancy
- While rare, emperipolesis can be seen in association with B-cell lymphomas
- SHML on rare occasions has been identified in lymph nodes affected by malignant lymphoma
- Transformation of SHML to high-grade lymphoma reported

SELECTED REFERENCES

1. Belcadhi M et al: Rosai-Dorfman disease of the nasal cavities: A CO(2) laser excision. Am J Rhinol Allergy. 24(1):91-3, 2010
2. Walid MS et al: Ethmo-spheno-intracranial Rosai-Dorfman disease. Indian J Cancer. 47(1):80-1, 2010
3. Ensari S et al: Rosai-Dorfman disease presenting as laryngeal masses. Kulak Burun Bogaz Ihtis Derg. 18(2):110-4, 2008
4. La Barge DV 3rd et al: Sinus histiocytosis with massive lymphadenopathy (Rosai-Dorfman disease): imaging manifestations in the head and neck. AJR Am J Roentgenol. 191(6):W299-306, 2008
5. Kare M et al: Rosai Dorfman syndrome with sinonasal mucosa and intraocular involvement. J Assoc Physicians India. 55:448-50, 2007
6. Hagemann M et al: Nasal and paranasal sinus manifestation of Rosai-Dorfman disease. Rhinology. 43(3):229-32, 2005
7. Kaminsky J et al: Rosai-Dorfman disease involving the cranial base, paranasal sinuses and spinal cord. Clin Neuropathol. 24(4):194-200, 2005
8. Maeda Y et al: Rosai-Dorfman disease revealed in the upper airway: a case report and review of the literature. Auris Nasus Larynx. 31(3):279-82, 2004
9. Dodson KM et al: Rosai Dorfman disease presenting as synchronous nasal and intracranial masses. Am J Otolaryngol. 24(6):426-30, 2003
10. Ortonne N et al: Cutaneous Destombes-Rosai-Dorfman disease: absence of detection of HHV-6 and HHV-8 in skin. J Cutan Pathol. 29(2):113-8, 2002
11. Ku PK et al: Nasal manifestation of extranodal Rosai-Dorfman disease--diagnosis and management. J Laryngol Otol. 113(3):275-80, 1999
12. Luppi M et al: Expression of human herpesvirus-6 antigens in benign and malignant lymphoproliferative diseases. Am J Pathol. 153(3):815-23, 1998
13. Goodnight JW et al: Extranodal Rosai-Dorfman disease of the head and neck. Laryngoscope. 106(3 Pt 1):253-6, 1996
14. Tsang WY et al: The Rosai-Dorfman disease histiocytes are not infected by Epstein-Barr virus. Histopathology. 25(1):88-90, 1994
15. Wenig BM et al: Extranodal sinus histiocytosis with massive lymphadenopathy (Rosai-Dorfman disease) of the head and neck. Hum Pathol. 24(5):483-92, 1993
16. Paulli M et al: Immunophenotypic characterization of the cell infiltrate in five cases of sinus histiocytosis with massive lymphadenopathy (Rosai-Dorfman disease). Hum Pathol. 23(6):647-54, 1992
17. Eisen RN et al: Immunophenotypic characterization of sinus histiocytosis with massive lymphadenopathy (Rosai-Dorfman disease). Semin Diagn Pathol. 7(1):74-82, 1990
18. Foucar E et al: Sinus histiocytosis with massive lymphadenopathy (Rosai-Dorfman disease): review of the entity. Semin Diagn Pathol. 7(1):19-73, 1990
19. Komp DM: The treatment of sinus histiocytosis with massive lymphadenopathy (Rosai-Dorfman disease). Semin Diagn Pathol. 7(1):83-6, 1990
20. Foucar E et al: Immunologic abnormalities and their significance in sinus histiocytosis with massive lymphadenopathy. Am J Clin Pathol. 82(5):515-25, 1984
21. Foucar E et al: Sinus histiocytosis with massive lymphadenopathy. An analysis of 14 deaths occurring in a patient registry. Cancer. 54(9):1834-40, 1984
22. Rosai J et al: Sinus histiocytosis with massive lymphadenopathy: a pseudolymphomatous benign disorder. Analysis of 34 cases. Cancer. 30(5):1174-88, 1972
23. Rosai J et al: Sinus histiocytosis with massive lymphadenopathy. A newly recognized benign clinicopathological entity. Arch Pathol. 87(1):63-70, 1969

Imaging, Microscopic, and Immunohistochemical Features

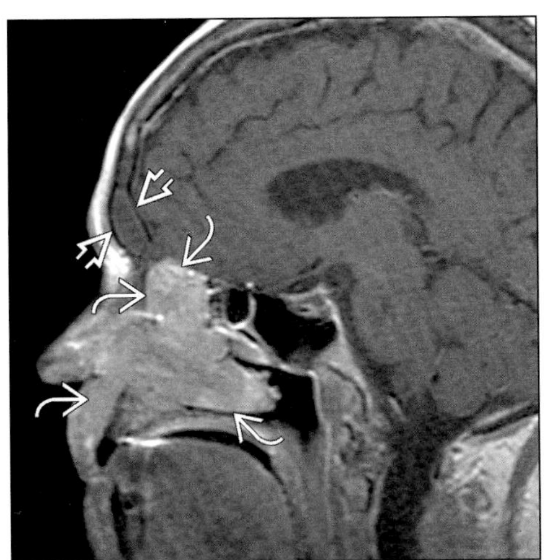

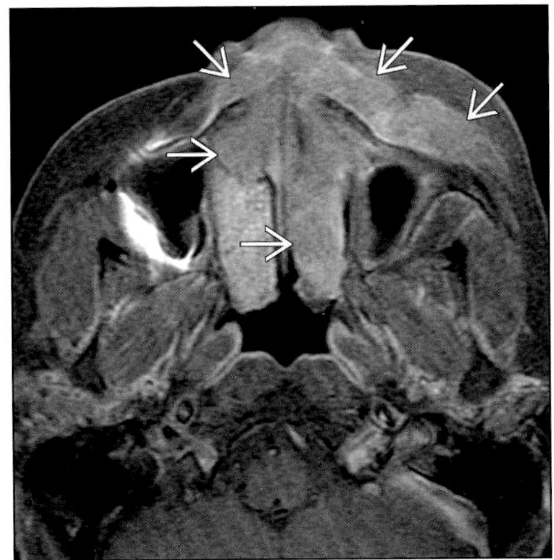

(Left) *This sagittal T1WI C+ MR shows enhancing foci of extranodal sinus histiocytosis ➡ with massive lymphadenopathy, obstructing the frontal recess and secretions trapped in the frontal sinus ➡.* ***(Right)*** *In this post-gadolinium fat-saturated axial image, the lesions ➡ enhance homogeneously but less strongly than the mucosa.*

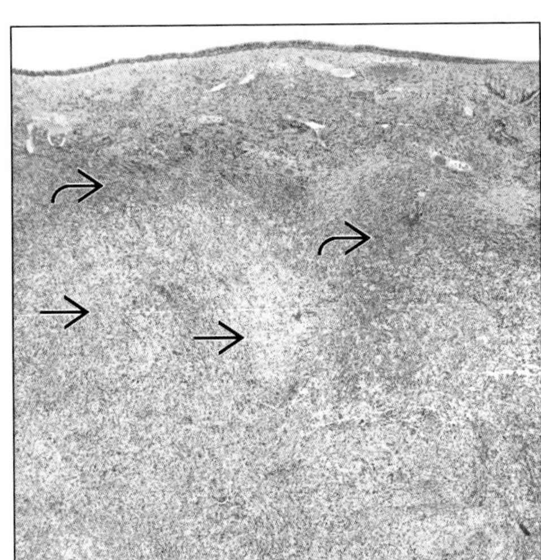

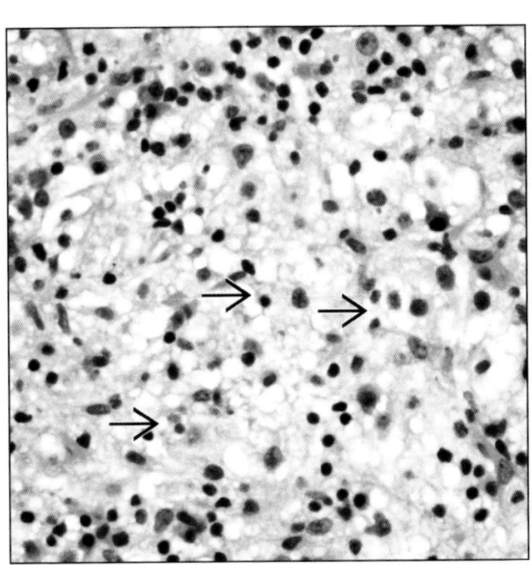

(Left) *Sinonasal tract ESHML shows the presence of a submucosal inflammatory cell infiltrate that includes lymphoid aggregates ➡ alternating with pale-appearing areas ➡, creating a mottled appearance.* ***(Right)*** *Readily identifiable histiocytic cells are composed of round nuclei lacking nuclear indentations with abundant lightly eosinophilic cytoplasm with ill-defined borders and scattered admixed mature lymphocytes and plasma cells; emperipolesis is present ➡.*

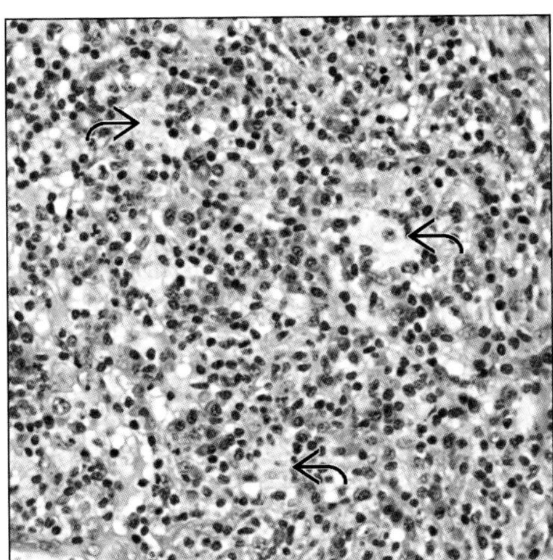

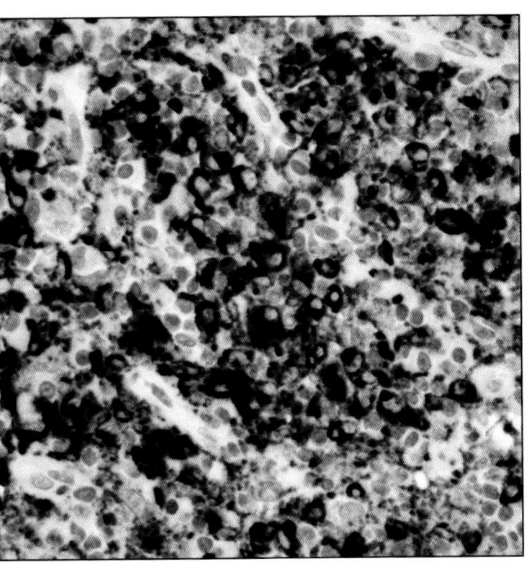

(Left) *The presence of a densely cellular mixed inflammatory cell infiltrate, including plasma cells and mature lymphocytes, may overrun and obscure the histiocytic cells ➡, potentially creating difficulties in recognizing them and in the diagnosis of (extranodal) sinus histiocytosis with massive lymphadenopathy.* ***(Right)*** *SHML cells are also reactive with histiocytic markers, including CD68, as well as with other markers, including CD163, HAM56, MAC387, and lysozyme (not shown).*

MYOSPHERULOSIS

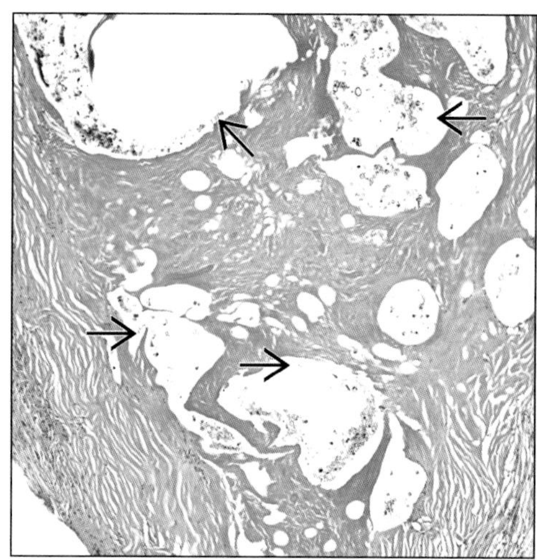

Myospherulosis shows irregularly shaped pseudocystic spaces ⇒ that are embedded in fibrotic tissue and contain round, sac-like structures ("parent bodies").

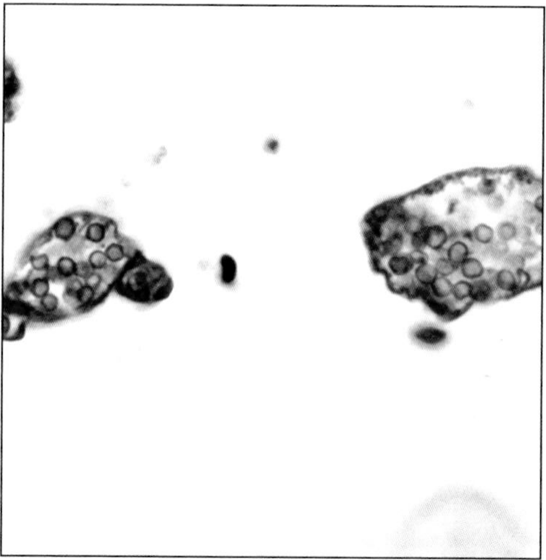

The "parent bodies" are brown staining and contain numerous spherules or endobodies resembling and potentially confused with microorganisms. Stains for microorganisms are negative.

TERMINOLOGY

Definitions

- Innocuous, iatrogenically induced pseudomycotic disease resulting from interaction of red blood cells and petrolatum-based ointments
  - Initially described in Africa where lesions primarily affected subcutaneous tissues or muscle resulting in the designation "myo"-spherulosis

ETIOLOGY/PATHOGENESIS

Iatrogenic

- History of surgery prior to the development of mass followed by packing of area with petrolatum-based ointment
- Results from injected or applied medicament acting as foreign substance
  - Origin of myospherules from red blood cells reacting with petrolatum or lanolin found in ointment utilized in "packing" nasal cavity following surgery
  - Emulsified fat may also induce formation of myospherules; thus, fat necrosis may result in myospherulosis
- Experimental studies show
  - Thin parent body wall of myospherulosis formed initially as result of physical emulsion phenomenon between lipid-containing materials and blood
  - Erythrocytes then enclosed in parent body
  - Parent body membrane gradually reinforced by deposition of plasma proteins, which are insoluble in ethanol
  - Erythrocytes become endobodies by deposition of their contents to membrane of parent body
  - Pores of endobodies formed in process of erythrocyte degeneration
  - Contents of erythrocytes (e.g., hemoglobin) attach to parent body completing myospherulosis

CLINICAL ISSUES

Site

- Nasal cavity and paranasal sinuses among more common sites of involvement
  - Other sites include
    - Ear
    - Soft tissues of extremities

Presentation

- In nose and paranasal sinuses, symptoms generally relate to mass lesion with or without airway obstruction
  - Local pain, tenderness may be present
  - May develop from 1 month to years after surgical procedure

Treatment

- Options, risks, complications
  - Prevention using non-petrolatum-based antibiotic substances
- Surgical approaches
  - Symptomatic treatment may include conservative surgical removal of fibrotic tissues

Prognosis

- Excellent

MICROSCOPIC PATHOLOGY

Histologic Features

- Pseudocysts or microcysts are embedded within fibrotic tissue creating "swiss cheese" appearance
  - Pseudocysts or microcysts measure up to 1 mm in diameter
    - Irregular contour containing round, sac-like structures called "parent bodies"
    - Parent bodies measure approximately 50 micrometers in diameter

MYOSPHERULOSIS

Key Facts

Terminology
- Innocuous, iatrogenically induced pseudomycotic disease

Clinical Issues
- Results from injected or applied medicament (petrolatum ointment) following surgery
- Nasal cavity and paranasal sinuses among more common sites
- Symptomatic treatment, which may include conservative surgical removal of fibrotic tissues

Microscopic Pathology
- Pseudocysts (microcysts) embedded within fibrotic tissue creating "swiss cheese" appearance
  - Pseudocysts contain parent bodies
  - Parent bodies contain dark brown endobodies
- Stains for microorganisms negative
- Characteristic spherules may be sparse or absent

    - Parent bodies contain numerous spherules or endobodies
  - Spherules or endobodies
    - Measure approximately 5 micrometers in diameter
    - Variable in size and shape with cup-shaped forms common
    - Usually dark brown
- Chronic inflammatory infiltrate usually present but may be sparse
  - Composed of
    - Lymphocytes
    - Histiocytes
    - Giant cells
    - Plasma cells
  - Occasional foreign body type multinucleated giant cells may be seen
- Characteristic spherules may be sparse or absent
- Diagnosis can be suggested even in absence of spherules given appropriate history, anatomic location, presence of fibrotic tissue with empty spaces

ANCILLARY TESTS

Histochemistry
- Stains for microorganisms (e.g., GMS, PAS, AFB, Warthin-Starry, others) negative

DIFFERENTIAL DIAGNOSIS

Fungal Infections
- Presence of microorganisms differentiate infectious disease from myospherulosis

DIAGNOSTIC CHECKLIST

Pathologic Interpretation Pearls
- Even in absence of spherules diagnosis suggested given
  - Appropriate history including
    - Prior surgery followed by packing of area with petrolatum-based ointment
  - Anatomic location
    - Nasal cavity and paranasal sinuses among more common sites of involvement
  - Histologic features
    - Presence of fibrotic tissue with empty spaces

SELECTED REFERENCES

1. Kakizaki H et al: Experimental study of the cause of myospherulosis. Am J Clin Pathol. 99(3):249-56, 1993
2. Wheeler TM et al: Myospherulosis: a preventable iatrogenic nasal and paranasal entity. Arch Otolaryngol. 106(5):272-4, 1980
3. Rosai J: The nature of myospherulosis of the upper respiratory tract. Am J Clin Pathol. 69(5):475-81, 1978
4. Kyriakos M. Myospherulosis of the paranasal sinuses et al: A possible iatrogenic disease. Am J Clin Pathol. 67(2):118-30, 1977

IMAGE GALLERY

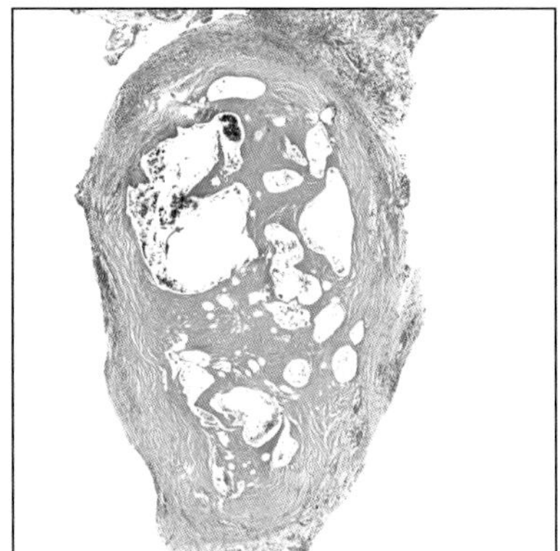

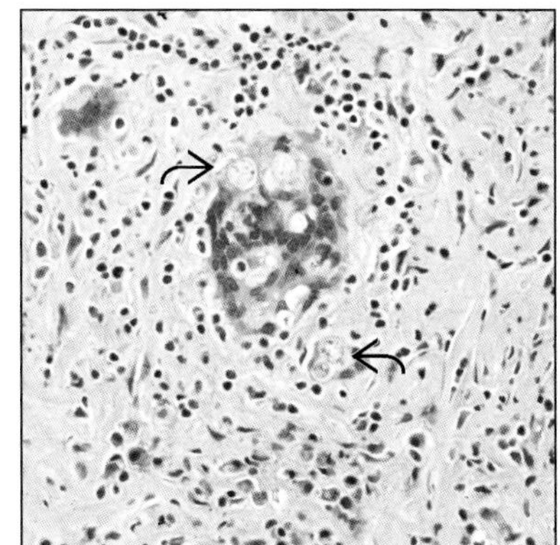

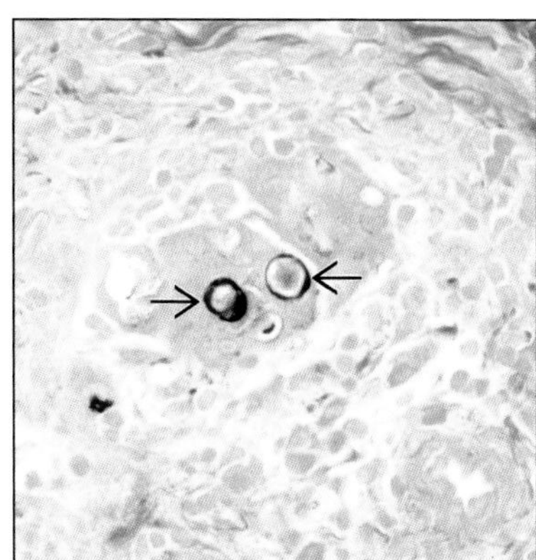

(Left) *Myospherulosis presents as a polypoid sinonasal mass. At low magnification, the lesion is densely fibrotic with irregularly shaped cysts.* ***(Center)*** *Sinonasal blastomycosis is characterized by microorganisms within submucosal multinucleated giant cells ⮫. The findings are dissimilar to myospherulosis, but endobodies in myospherulosis may be considered fungi.* ***(Right)*** *In contrast to the endospores in myospherulosis, fungal infections will stain positive ⮕ by histochemical staining (GMS).*

SINONASAL (SCHNEIDERIAN) PAPILLOMA

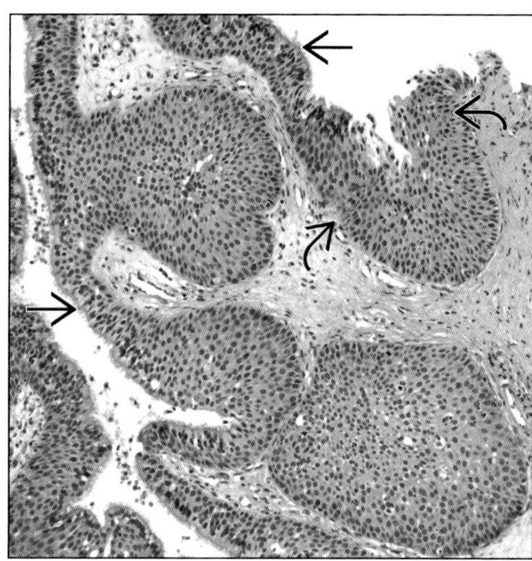

Endophytic or "inverted" growth pattern consists of thickened epithelial nests arising from the surface respiratory epithelium ➩ with downward growth. Surface squamous metaplasia is present ➦.

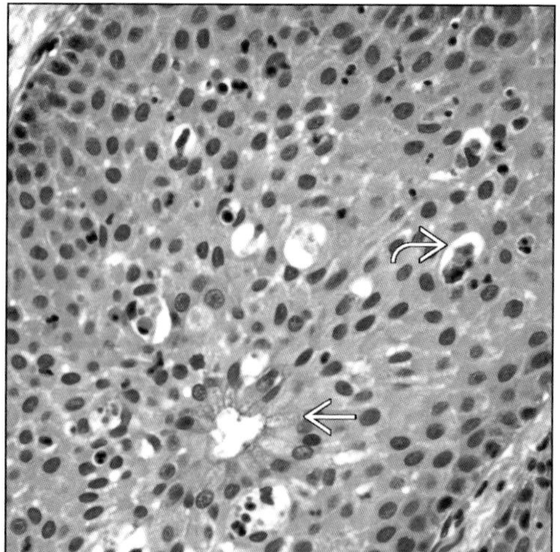

The epithelial proliferation is benign with an absence of cytologic atypia. Intraepithelial inflammatory cells, cysts ➦, and scattered mucocytes ➡ are features of Schneiderian papillomas.

TERMINOLOGY

Synonyms

- Sinonasal-type papillomas
- 3 morphologic types identified include
  - Inverted
  - Exophytic (fungiform, septal)
  - Oncocytic (cylindrical or columnar cell)

Definitions

- Group of benign epithelial neoplasms arising from sinonasal (Schneiderian) mucosa

ETIOLOGY/PATHOGENESIS

Infectious Agents

- Human papillomavirus (HPV)
  - Found in septal and inverted papillomas by in situ hybridization or polymerase chain reaction
  - Types 6/11 most common, less often 16/18, rarely other HPV types (e.g., HPV 57)
  - Cause and effect between presence of HPV and development of Schneiderian papillomas remains undetermined
  - Molecular biologic analysis to date on oncocytic papillomas has not identified presence of HPV
- Discrepant reports on presence of Epstein-Barr virus in Schneiderian papillomas

CLINICAL ISSUES

Epidemiology

- Incidence
  - Represent less than 5% of all sinonasal tract tumors
    - Literature supports septal type as most common, but in practical experience inverted type most common
    - Oncocytic type is least common
- Age
  - Occur over wide age range
    - Rare in children
  - **Inverted type**
    - Most common in 5th to 8th decades
  - **Exophytic type**
    - Tend to occur in younger age group
  - **Oncocytic type**
    - Tend to occur in older age range (> 50 years)
    - Uncommon under 4th decade of life

Site

- **Inverted type**
  - Occurs along lateral nasal wall (middle turbinate or ethmoid recesses)
    - Secondary extension may occur into maxillary and ethmoid sinuses
    - Less often extends/involves sphenoid and frontal sinuses
  - Less frequently may originate in paranasal sinus
  - May occur in paranasal sinus without involvement of nasal cavity
- **Exophytic type**
  - Almost invariably limited to nasal septum
- **Oncocytic type**
  - Most often occurs along lateral nasal wall
    - May originate within paranasal sinus (maxillary or ethmoid)
- Inverted and oncocytic types rarely occur on nasal septum
- Typically, Schneiderian papillomas are unilateral
  - Bilateral papillomas, particularly inverted type, may occur in up to 10%
  - In presence of bilateral disease
    - Clinical evaluation indicated to exclude extension from unilateral disease (i.e., septal perforation)
- Schneiderian-type papillomas may originate in nasopharynx or ear without connection to sinonasal tract

SINONASAL (SCHNEIDERIAN) PAPILLOMA

Key Facts

Terminology
- Group of benign epithelial neoplasms arising from sinonasal (Schneiderian) mucosa

Etiology/Pathogenesis
- Human papillomavirus (HPV)
  - Cause and effect between presence of HPV and development of Schneiderian papillomas remains undetermined

Clinical Issues
- Represent less than 5% of all sinonasal tract tumors
- Treatment for all types includes complete surgical excision, including adjacent uninvolved mucosa
  - Tumors recur if incompletely resected

Microscopic Pathology
- **Inverted type**
  - Endophytic or "inverted" growth pattern consisting of markedly thickened squamous epithelial proliferation growing downward
  - Thickened squamous epithelial proliferation with admixed mucocytes, intraepithelial mucous cysts
- **Exophytic type**
  - Exophytic (papillary) growth
  - Thickened squamous epithelial proliferation with admixed mucocytes, intraepithelial mucous cysts
- **Oncocytic type**
  - Exophytic &/or endophytic growth
  - Multilayered epithelial proliferation composed of columnar cells with abundant eosinophilic and granular cytoplasm
  - Admixed mucocytes (goblet cells) and intraepithelial mucous cysts

- Probably arise from misplaced ectodermal-derived epithelial rests from sinonasal tract

Presentation
- Symptoms vary according to site of occurrence
  - Airway obstruction, epistaxis, asymptomatic mass, pain

Treatment
- Surgical approaches
  - Treatment for all sinonasal papillomas includes complete surgical excision, including adjacent uninvolved mucosa
    - Growth and extension along mucosa results from induction of squamous metaplasia in adjacent sinonasal mucosa necessitating excision of adjacent mucosa
    - Adequate surgery includes lateral rhinotomy or medial maxillectomy with en bloc excision
- Adjuvant therapy
  - Chemo- and radiotherapy have not been shown to be of benefit
    - Radiation may prove beneficial in select population of patients with unresectable tumors due to locally advanced disease

Prognosis
- Good following complete surgical excision
- Complications
  - Tumors recur if incompletely resected
    - Recurrence probably represents persistence of disease rather than multicentricity of neoplasm
  - If left unchecked, capability of continued growth with extension along mucosal surface with invasion/ destruction of vital structures
- Malignant transformation
  - Incidence of malignant transformation varies per subtype
    - Inverted type ranges from 2-27%
    - Oncocytic type ranges from 4-17%
    - Exophytic type rarely, if ever
  - Majority of malignancies are keratinizing squamous cell carcinoma (SCC); less frequently nonkeratinizing SCC
  - Other carcinomas may occur, including
    - Verrucous carcinoma, mucoepidermoid carcinoma, small cell carcinoma, adenocarcinoma, and undifferentiated carcinoma
  - Carcinoma may occur synchronously or metachronously with papilloma
  - Carcinomatous foci may be limited or extensive, may show epithelial dysplasia/carcinoma in situ or invasive carcinoma
  - Evidence of preexisting papilloma
    - May be present with obvious transition from benign papilloma to overt carcinoma
    - May include predominantly benign tumor (papilloma) with limited foci of carcinoma
    - May predominantly include carcinoma with limited residual papilloma
    - May be no residual evidence of preexisting benign tumor; known to have prior papilloma only by history
  - No reliable histologic features predict which papillomas likely to become malignant
    - Moderate to severe epithelial dysplasia potential indicator of malignant transformation
    - Surface keratinization and dyskeratosis anecdotally considered possible predictors of malignant transformation
    - Any sinonasal papilloma showing moderate to severe dysplasia or surface keratinization should prompt histologic examination of all resected tissue
    - No correlation between number of recurrences and development of carcinoma
    - No correlation between presence of increased cellularity, pleomorphism, and mitotic activity and transformation to carcinoma
  - Treatment for malignant transformation includes surgery and radiotherapy
  - Prognosis for patients with malignant transformation varies

SINONASAL (SCHNEIDERIAN) PAPILLOMA

- Carcinoma only locally invasive associated with favorable prognosis following treatment
- Carcinoma extensively invasive with involvement of vital structures &/or metastatic disease associated with poor outcome
- Prognosis similar to de novo sinonasal squamous carcinoma

IMAGE FINDINGS

General Features

- Appearance varies with extent of disease
  - Soft tissue density seen early in disease
  - Opacification, mucosal thickening present with more extensive disease
  - Evidence of pressure erosion of bone may be seen

MACROSCOPIC FEATURES

General Features

- **Inverted type**
  - Large, bulky, translucent masses with red to gray color, varying from firm to friable in consistency
- **Exophytic type**
  - Papillary, exophytic, verrucoid lesion with pink to tan appearance, firm to rubbery consistency; often attached to mucosa by narrow or broad-based stalk
- **Oncocytic type**
  - Dark red to brown, papillary or polypoid lesions

MICROSCOPIC PATHOLOGY

Histologic Features

- **Inverted type**
  - Endophytic or "inverted" growth pattern consisting of markedly thickened squamous epithelial proliferation growing downward
  - Epithelium varies in cellularity composed of squamous, transitional, and columnar cells (all 3 may be present in a given lesion) with admixed mucocytes (goblet cells) and intraepithelial mucous cysts
    - Cells generally bland in appearance with uniform nuclei, no piling up, but pleomorphism and cytologic atypia may be present
    - Mitotic figures may be seen in basal and parabasal layers, but atypical mitotic figures are not identified
    - Epithelial cells may demonstrate extensive clear cell features indicative of abundant glycogen content
  - Mixed chronic inflammatory cell infiltrate characteristically seen within all layers of surface epithelium
  - Stromal component varies from myxoid to fibrous with admixed chronic inflammatory cells and variable vascularity
  - May occur simultaneously with nasal inflammatory polyps
  - Surface keratinization may be present
- **Exophytic type**
  - Papillary fronds composed of thick epithelium, which is predominantly squamous (epidermoid) and, less frequently, respiratory type
  - Mucocytes (goblet cells) and intraepithelial mucous cysts are present
  - Surface keratinization is uncommon
  - Stromal component is composed of delicate fibrovascular cores
- **Oncocytic type**
  - Exophytic &/or endophytic ("inverted") growth
  - Multilayered epithelial proliferation composed of columnar cells with abundant eosinophilic and granular cytoplasm
    - Nuclei vary from vesicular to hyperchromatic; nucleoli are usually indistinct
    - Outer surface of epithelial proliferation may demonstrate cilia
  - Intraepithelial mucin cysts, often containing polymorphonuclear leukocytes, are seen; cysts are not identified in submucosa
  - Stromal component varies from myxoid to fibrous with admixed chronic inflammatory cells and variable vascularity
  - May occur simultaneously with nasal inflammatory polyps

ANCILLARY TESTS

Histochemistry

- Mucicarmine
  - Intracytoplasmic mucin-positive material
- Periodic acid-Schiff with diastase
  - Diastase-resistant, PAS-positive material

Molecular Genetics

- Inverted papillomas shown to be monoclonal proliferations, but unlike squamous epithelial dysplasia, do not harbor key genetic alterations associated with malignant transformation
- *P53* gene mutation appears closely associated with malignant transformation in sinonasal papillomas

DIFFERENTIAL DIAGNOSIS

Sinonasal Inflammatory Polyps

- Often coexist with Schneiderian papillomas but lack epithelial proliferation with constituent cells of Schneiderian papillomas

Squamous Papilloma of Nasal Vestibular Skin

- Cutaneous lesion entirely comprised of squamous cells without identifiable intraepithelial mucocytes
- Staining for epithelial mucin (mucicarmine, DPAS) helpful in differential diagnosis

Verruca Vulgaris of Nasal Vestibular Skin

- Shows characteristic histopathologic findings including presence of prominent keratinization with verrucoid or papillomatous growth, keratohyaline granules, koilocytes and in turning of rete pegs, as well as absence of intraepithelial mucocytes

Sinonasal (Schneiderian) Papillomas

	Inverted Type	Exophytic Type	Oncocytic Type
Incidence	47-73%	20-50%	3-8%
Gender	M > F	M > F	M = F
Age	40-70 years	20-50 years	> 50 years
Location	Lateral nasal wall in region of middle turbinates; may extend into sinuses (maxillary or ethmoid)	Nasal septum	Lateral nasal wall and sinuses (maxillary or ethmoid)
Focality	Typically unilateral; rarely bilateral	Unilateral	Unilateral
Histology	Endophytic or "inverted" growth composed predominantly of squamous (epidermoid) cells with scattered admixed mucocytes and intraepithelial mucous cysts; mixed chronic inflammatory cell infiltrate characteristically seen within all layers of surface epithelium	Exophytic to papillary proliferation composed predominantly of squamous (epidermoid) epithelium with admixed mucocytes and intraepithelial mucous cysts; delicate fibrovascular cores	Multilayered epithelial proliferation composed of columnar cells with abundant eosinophilic and granular cytoplasm; outer surface of epithelial proliferation may demonstrate cilia; intraepithelial mucous cysts, often containing polymorphonuclear leukocytes
Association with HPV	~ 38% positive; HPV 6 and 11; less frequently HPV 16, 18; rarely HPV 57	~ 50% positive; HPV 6 and 11; less frequently HPV 16, 18; rarely HPV 57	Typically absent
Malignant transformation	2-27%; most common type is keratinizing SCC	Rare	4-17%; most common type is keratinizing SCC

HPV = human papillomavirus; SCC = squamous cell carcinoma.

Rhinosporidiosis

- Specific differential diagnosis with oncocytic-type papilloma
- Intraepithelial **and** submucosal cysts containing microorganisms

SELECTED REFERENCES

1. Giotakis E et al: Clinical outcomes of sinonasal inverted papilloma surgery. A retrospective study of 67 cases. B-ENT. 6(2):111-6, 2010
2. Shah AA et al: HPV DNA is associated with a subset of Schneiderian papillomas but does not correlate with p16(INK4a) immunoreactivity. Head Neck Pathol. 4(2):106-12, 2010
3. Guillemaud JP et al: Inverted papilloma of the sphenoid sinus: clinical presentation, management, and systematic review of the literature. Laryngoscope. 119(12):2466-71, 2009
4. Perez-Ordoñez B: Hamartomas, papillomas and adenocarcinomas of the sinonasal tract and nasopharynx. J Clin Pathol. 62(12):1085-95, 2009
5. Sham CL et al: Treatment results of sinonasal inverted papilloma: an 18-year study. Am J Rhinol Allergy. 23(2):203-11, 2009
6. Tanvetyanon T et al: Survival outcomes of squamous cell carcinoma arising from sinonasal inverted papilloma: report of 6 cases with systematic review and pooled analysis. Am J Otolaryngol. 30(1):38-43, 2009
7. Wu HH et al: Fascin over expression is associated with dysplastic changes in sinonasal inverted papillomas: a study of 47 cases. Head Neck Pathol. 3(3):212-6, 2009
8. Lawson W et al: The role of the human papillomavirus in the pathogenesis of Schneiderian inverted papillomas: an analytic overview of the evidence. Head Neck Pathol. 2(2):49-59, 2008
9. Oikawa K et al: Clinical and pathological analysis of recurrent inverted papilloma. Ann Otol Rhinol Laryngol. 116(4):297-303, 2007
10. Kaufman MR et al: Sinonasal papillomas: clinicopathologic review of 40 patients with inverted and oncocytic schneiderian papillomas. Laryngoscope. 112(8 Pt 1):1372-7, 2002
11. Kraft M et al: Significance of human papillomavirus in sinonasal papillomas. J Laryngol Otol. 115(9):709-14, 2001
12. Maitra A et al: Malignancies arising in oncocytic schneiderian papillomas: a report of 2 cases and review of the literature. Arch Pathol Lab Med. 125(10):1365-7, 2001
13. Califano J et al: Inverted sinonasal papilloma : a molecular genetic appraisal of its putative status as a precursor to squamous cell carcinoma. Am J Pathol. 156(1):333-7, 2000
14. Finkelstein SD et al: Malignant transformation in sinonasal papillomas is closely associated with aberrant p53 expression. Mol Diagn. 3(1):37-41, 1998
15. Mirza N et al: Identification of p53 and human papilloma virus in Schneiderian papillomas. Laryngoscope. 108(4 Pt 1):497-501, 1998
16. Gaffey MJ et al: Human papillomavirus and Epstein-Barr virus in sinonasal Schneiderian papillomas. An in situ hybridization and polymerase chain reaction study. Am J Clin Pathol. 106(4):475-82, 1996
17. Buchwald C et al: Human papillomavirus (HPV) in sinonasal papillomas: a study of 78 cases using in situ hybridization and polymerase chain reaction. Laryngoscope. 105(1):66-71, 1995
18. Buchwald C et al: Sinonasal papillomas: a report of 82 cases in Copenhagen County, including a longitudinal epidemiological and clinical study. Laryngoscope. 105(1):72-9, 1995
19. Lawson W et al: Inverted papilloma: a report of 112 cases. Laryngoscope. 105(3 Pt 1):282-8, 1995
20. Kapadia SB et al: Carcinoma ex oncocytic Schneiderian (cylindrical cell) papilloma. Am J Otolaryngol. 14(5):332-8, 1993
21. Barnes L et al: Oncocytic Schneiderian papilloma: a reappraisal of cylindrical cell papilloma of the sinonasal tract. Hum Pathol. 15(4):344-51, 1984
22. Heffner DK: Problems in pediatric otorhinolaryngic pathology. IV. Epithelial and lymphoid tumors of the sinonasal tract and nasopharynx. Int J Pediatr Otorhinolaryngol. 6(3):219-37, 1983

SINONASAL (SCHNEIDERIAN) PAPILLOMA

Imaging, Endoscopic, and Microscopic Features

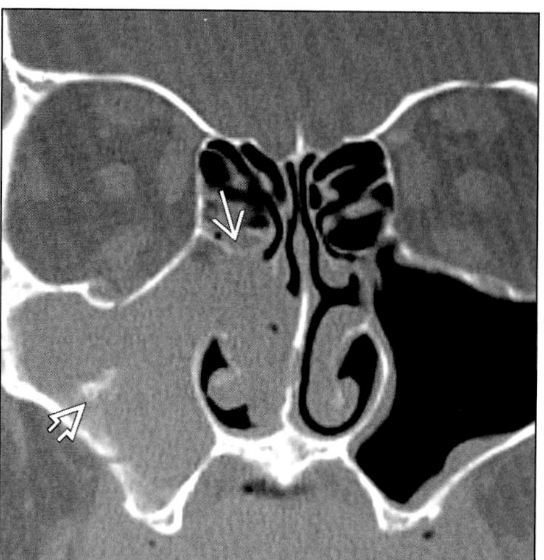

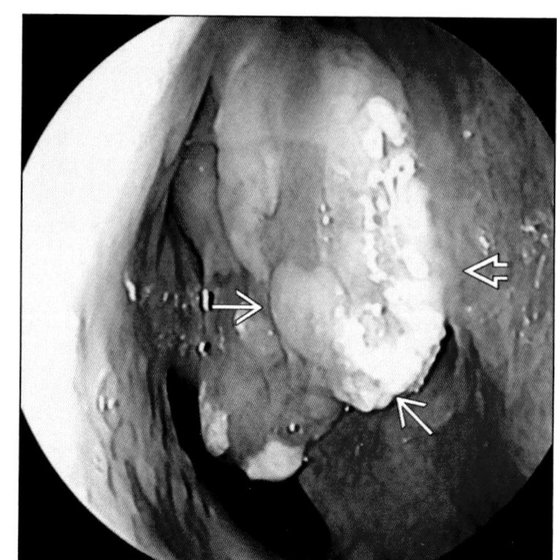

(Left) *Coronal bone CT shows a lobular inverted papilloma centered at the middle meatus ➡. The lesion enters the maxillary sinus via an enlarged infundibulum and is partially calcified ⇨.* ***(Right)*** *Endoscopic photograph during nasal endoscopy of an inverted papilloma shows a pale, lobular mass ➡ at the middle meatus. The lesion abuts the nasal septum ⇨ medially.*

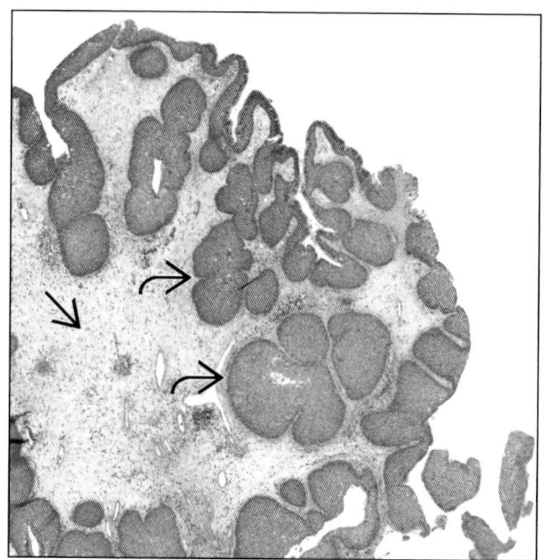

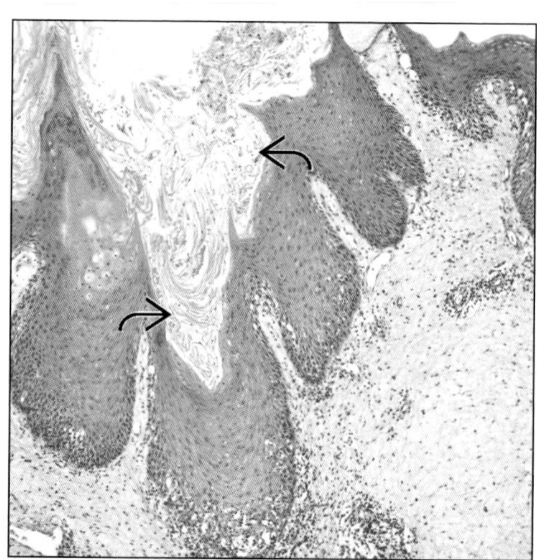

(Left) *Endophytic or "inverted" growth pattern of thickened epithelial nests ↪ arising from surface epithelium is characteristic of inverted-type papilloma. Stroma shows alterations similar to those seen in inflammatory polyps ➡.* ***(Right)*** *Sinonasal papillomas typically lack keratinization, and the presence of keratinization ↪ raises concern for the possibility of SCC (coexisting or development into a squamous cell carcinoma). With this occurrence, all of the tissue should be processed for histologic evaluation.*

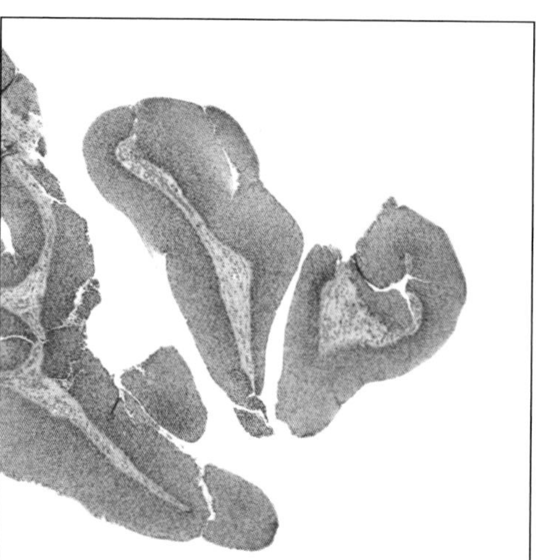

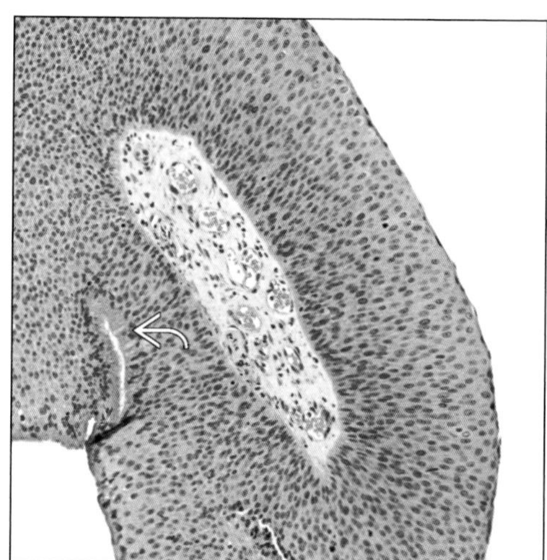

(Left) *Exophytic (fungiform) papilloma shows a papillary growth from the surface respiratory epithelium composed of a thickened nonkeratinized squamous (epidermoid) epithelium.* ***(Right)*** *At higher magnification the nonkeratinizing squamous epithelium shows cytomorphologic uniformity with cellular maturation, retention of cellular polarity, and absence of cytologic atypia. Focally, scattered mucocytes are present ↪.*

Microscopic Features

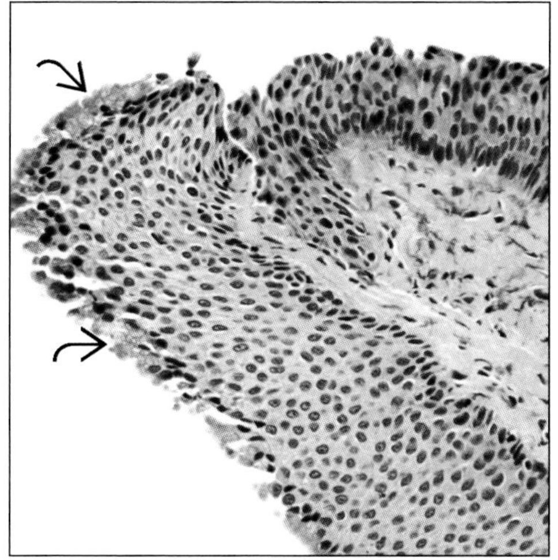

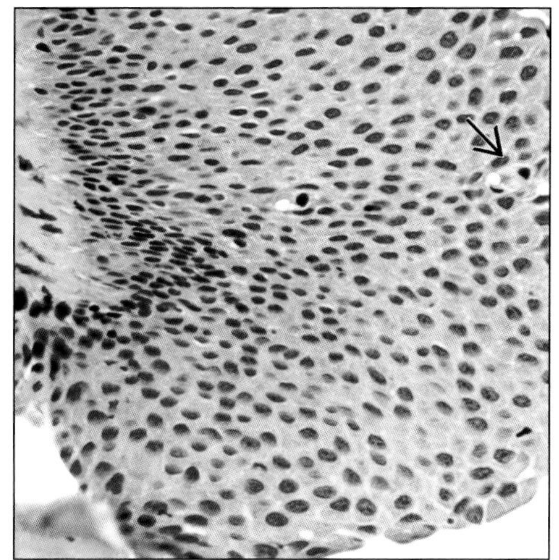

(Left) *Exophytic papilloma is the most superficial aspect retaining respiratory epithelial mucocytes* ⮫ *but is otherwise replaced by benign-appearing squamous (epidermoid) epithelium.* ***(Right)*** *An intraepithelial mucocyte is present* ⮕. *The identification of intraepithelial mucocytes assists in defining the papilloma as being of Schneiderian (mucosal) origin and not a squamous papilloma of cutaneous origin.*

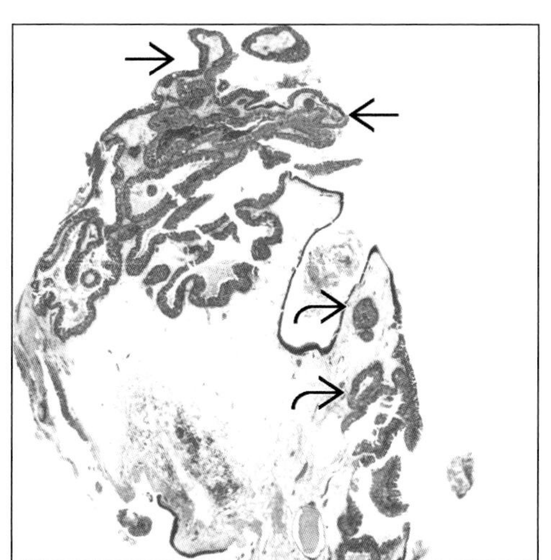

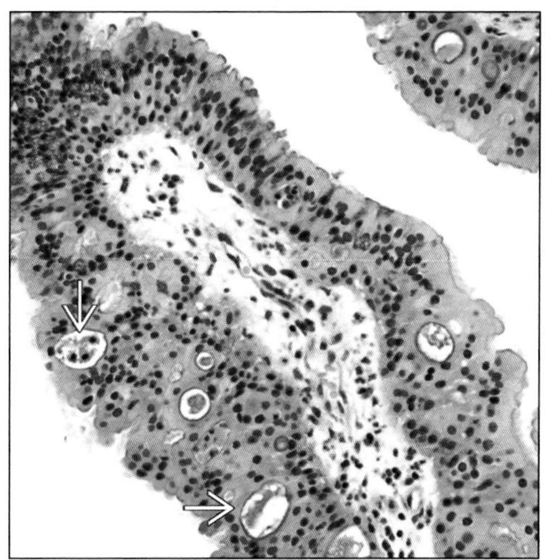

(Left) *Schneiderian papilloma, oncocytic type, shows an epithelial proliferation with exophytic/papillary* ⮕ *and focally endophytic* ⮫ *growth. The stroma shows edematous changes similar to that of sinonasal polyps.* ***(Right)*** *The lesion is characterized by a multilayered papillary epithelial proliferation with multiple intraepithelial mucin cysts* ⮕ *and a benign epithelial proliferation consisting of cells with prominent eosinophilic to granular-appearing cytoplasm (oncocytes).*

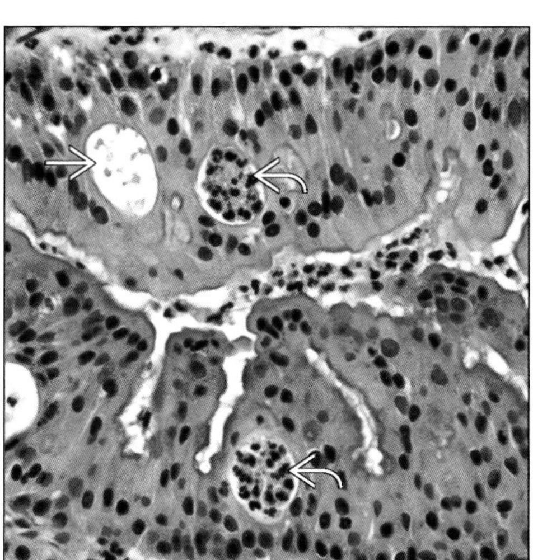

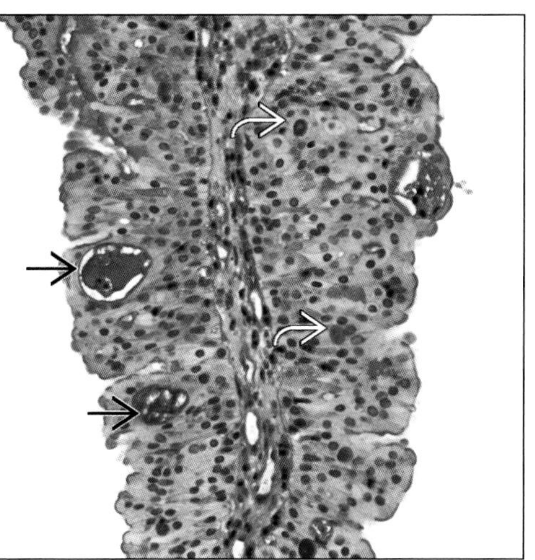

(Left) *The epithelium is multilayered, characterized by cells with prominent granular eosinophilic cytoplasm as well as the presence of intraepithelial mucin cysts containing amorphous pink material* ⮕ *&/or neutrophils* ⮫. ***(Right)*** *Histochemical staining shows the presence of intraluminal* ⮕ *and intracytoplasmic* ⮫ *diastase-resistant, PAS-positive material.*

PLEOMORPHIC ADENOMA

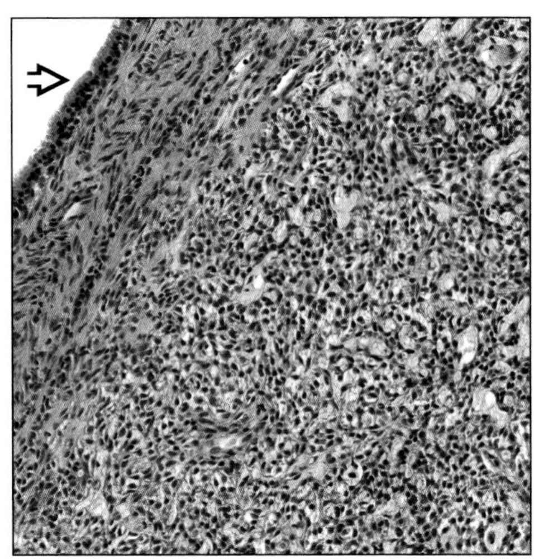

Hematoxylin & eosin shows an intact respiratory epithelium ⮚ overlying a cellular pleomorphic adenoma with a predominantly glandular pattern.

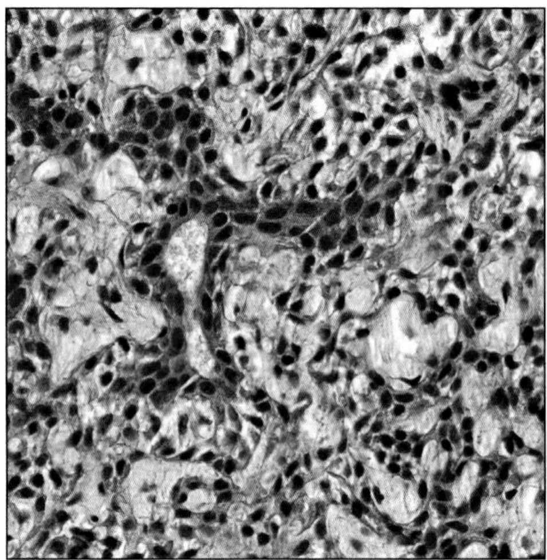

Hematoxylin & eosin shows myxoid matrix material with associated epithelial neoplasm. The epithelium shows gland-duct formation as well as ribbons and strips of epithelium.

TERMINOLOGY

Abbreviations

- Pleomorphic adenoma (PA)

Synonyms

- Benign mixed tumor (BMT), intranasal mixed tumor, nasal blastoma, mixed salivary tumor, chondroid syringoma

Definitions

- Benign, epithelial-derived neoplasm whose cells demonstrate both epithelial and mesenchymal differentiation

CLINICAL ISSUES

Epidemiology

- Incidence
  - Rare, although comprises ~ 25% of all sinonasal tract **glandular** neoplasms
- Age
  - Usually between 20 and 60 years (mean: 40 years)
- Gender
  - Slight Female > Male (1.1:1)

Site

- Mucosa of bony or cartilaginous nasal septum is most commonly affected
- Nasal turbinates next most common site affected, where it may extend into maxillary sinus(es)

Presentation

- Nonspecific signs and symptoms
  - Unilateral obstruction, mass, epistaxis
  - Congestion, difficulty breathing, discharge

Treatment

- Surgical approaches
  - Local, but complete, surgical excision to prevent recurrence/residual disease
    - Various surgical approaches: Endoscopic endonasal surgery, lateral rhinotomy, midfacial degloving, and transpalatal surgery

Prognosis

- Excellent
- Recurrences (< 8%) usually related to incomplete excision
- Rare, malignant transformation can be seen (usually adenoid cystic carcinoma)

IMAGE FINDINGS

Radiographic Findings

- Few studies, but MR shows mass with low signal intensity on T1-weighted images and heterogeneous, intermediate signal intensity on T2-weighted images
- Generally, bone "remodeling" or "resorption," but not bone "destruction"

MACROSCOPIC FEATURES

General Features

- Mucosa-covered, firm, pedunculated, polypoid or sessile, broad-based, fleshy mass
- Usually arising from septum

Size

- Usually small (range: 0.5-5 cm; mean: 2.5 cm)

MICROSCOPIC PATHOLOGY

Histologic Features

- Unencapsulated but usually circumscribed tumors
- Tumors are highly cellular and solid, with scant myxochondroid matrix

PLEOMORPHIC ADENOMA

Key Facts

Terminology
- Benign, epithelial-derived neoplasm whose cells demonstrate both epithelial and mesenchymal differentiation

Macroscopic Features
- Develop from mucosa of bony or cartilaginous nasal septum
- Mucosa-covered, firm, polypoid mass

Microscopic Pathology
- Unencapsulated, highly cellular tumors
- Myoepithelial cells with plasmacytoid appearance usually predominate
- Scant myxochondroid matrix material

Ancillary Tests
- Epithelial and myoepithelial reactions with keratins, GFAP, S100 protein, Actin-sm, p63

- Myoepithelial cells with plasmacytoid appearance usually predominate
- Epithelial elements revealed with admixture of well-formed, although rare tubuloductal structures
- Myoepithelial cells can be spindled, round, stellate, and polygonal
- Myxohyaline or cartilaginous stroma focally
- Cellular pleomorphism is limited
- Mitotic figures but not increased nor atypical
- Rarely, carcinoma ex-pleomorphic adenoma may develop

ANCILLARY TESTS

Immunohistochemistry
- Shows epithelial and myoepithelial expression: Keratins, GFAP, S100 protein, Actin-sm, calponin, p63

DIFFERENTIAL DIAGNOSIS

Basal Cell Adenoma
- Basal cells without plasmacytoid features; no myxoid matrix

Adenoid Cystic Carcinoma
- Infiltrative, destructive growth; cribriform; peg-shaped cells; increased mitotic activity

Polymorphous Low-Grade Adenocarcinoma
- Infiltrative; perineural invasion; vesicular nuclear chromatin; lacks chondroid matrix

Nonintestinal Sinonasal Adenocarcinoma
- Tubulo-glandular neoplasm; destructive growth; mitotic figures; pleomorphism

SELECTED REFERENCES

1. Baradaranfar MH et al: Endoscopic endonasal surgery for resection of benign sinonasal tumors: experience with 105 patients. Arch Iran Med. 9(3):244-9, 2006
2. Lee SL et al: Nasopharyngeal pleomorphic adenoma in the adult. Laryngoscope. 116(7):1281-3, 2006
3. Freeman SR et al: Carcinoma ex-pleomorphic adenoma of the nasal septum with adenoid cystic and squamous carcinomatous differentiation. Rhinology. 41(2):118-21, 2003
4. Hirai S et al: Pleomorphic adenoma in nasal cavity: immunohistochemical study of three cases. Auris Nasus Larynx. 29(3):291-5, 2002
5. Cho KJ et al: Carcinoma ex-pleomorphic adenoma of the nasal cavity: a report of two cases. J Laryngol Otol. 109(7):677-9, 1995
6. Nonomura N et al: Immunohistochemical study of pleomorphic adenoma of the nasal septum. Auris Nasus Larynx. 19(2):125-31, 1992
7. Compagno J et al: Intranasal mixed tumors (pleomorphic adenomas): a clinicopathologic study of 40 cases. Am J Clin Pathol. 68(2):213-8, 1977

IMAGE GALLERY

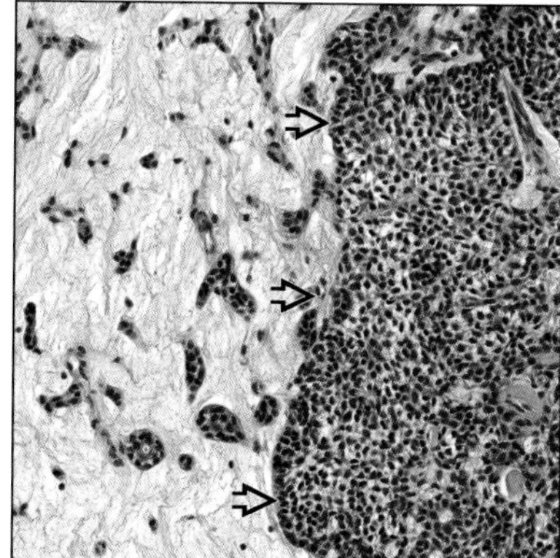
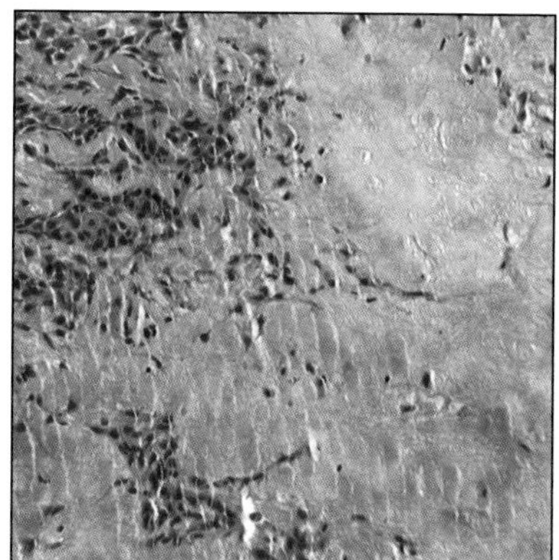
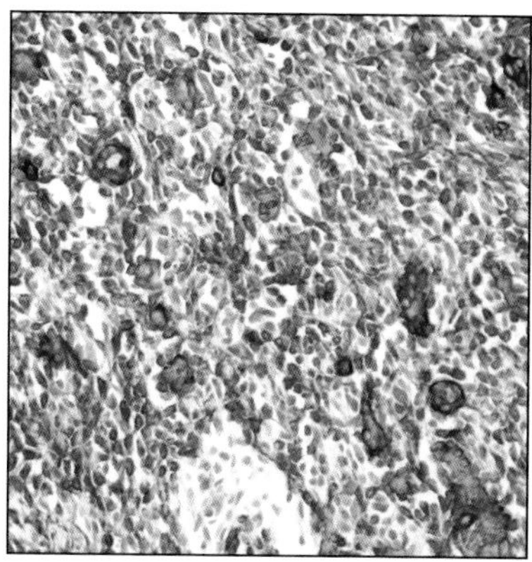

(Left) Hematoxylin & eosin demonstrates the abrupt juxtaposition between the cellular ⇒ and myxochondroid matrix compartments of this pleomorphic adenoma. *(Center)* Hematoxylin & eosin shows a predominantly myxochondroid matrix with only isolated glandular elements, an uncommon finding in minor salivary gland pleomorphic adenoma. *(Right)* CK-PAN highlights the epithelial glandular and spindle cell population seen in pleomorphic adenoma, in contrast to the myoepithelial differentiation highlighted by p63, actin-sm, &/or S100 protein.

ECTOPIC PITUITARY ADENOMA

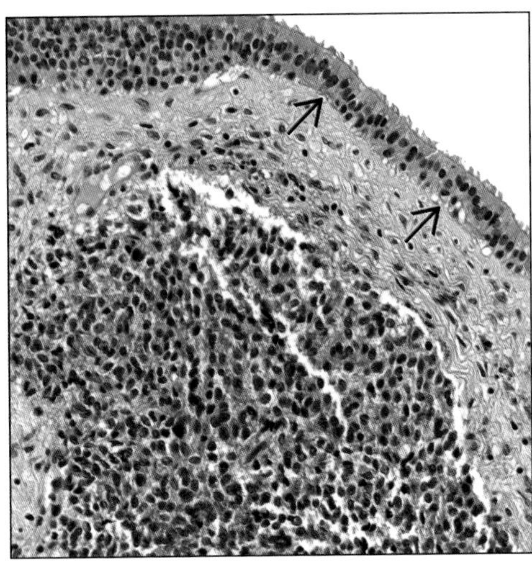

There is a submucosal location to this unencapsulated ectopic pituitary adenoma. The surface epithelium is intact → and uninvolved by the tumor, showing a well-developed Grenz zone of separation.

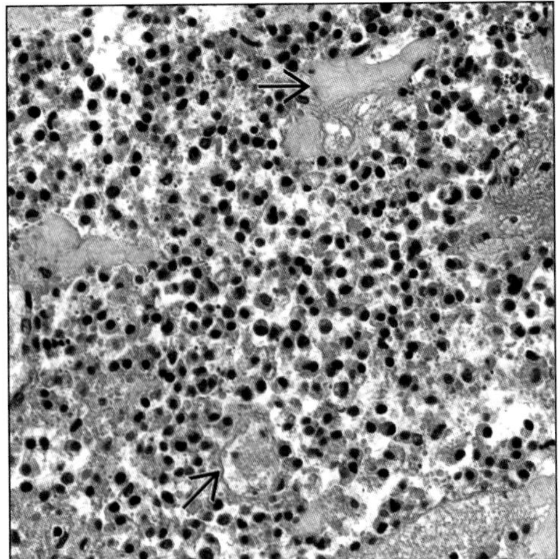

This very cellular tumor shows solid to vaguely trabecular architecture, separated by delicate fibrovascular septae →. The neoplastic population is monotonous, showing eccentrically located, round nuclei.

TERMINOLOGY

Definitions

- Benign pituitary gland neoplasm occurring separately from and without involvement of sella turcica (a normal anterior pituitary gland)
  - Direct extension from intrasellar neoplasm is much more common (seen in about 2% of pituitary tumors) and must be excluded

ETIOLOGY/PATHOGENESIS

Pathogenesis

- Anterior pituitary primordium appears at about 4 weeks of embryogenesis
- During 8th developmental week, pituitary divides into sellar and pharyngeal parts
  - Supradiaphragmatic attachment to pituitary stalk
  - Cephalic invagination of Rathke pouch (infrasellar)
- Migration into sphenoid or pharynx can be seen, often along craniopharyngeal canal
  - Ectopic pituitary adenomas are thought to be derived from these embryologic remnants along the migration path of Rathke pouch
  - Leptomeningeal locations are common but still intracranial
- Fully functional tissue in these ectopic locations is compatible with normal life
  - Pharyngeal pituitary begins hormone function at 17th-18th week, up to 8 weeks after sellar pituitary

CLINICAL ISSUES

Epidemiology

- Incidence
  - Pituitary adenomas account for 10-15% of intracranial neoplasms
  - Very rare in ectopic locations within upper aerodigestive tract
- Age
  - Wide range: 16-84 years
  - Mean: 50 years
- Gender
  - Female > Male (2:1)

Site

- Sphenoid sinus > > > cavernous sinus > 3rd ventricle > nasopharynx, nasal cavity, clivus > > petrous temporal bone
  - Must exclude "invasive sellar" tumors or direct extension from intracranial primary
  - Intact pituitary sellar is usually required

Presentation

- Space-occupying effects
  - Nasal obstruction or airway obstruction
  - Headaches
  - Bloody nasal discharge or epistaxis
  - Cerebrospinal fluid leakage (clear fluid)
  - Visual field defects (diplopia)
- Endocrine abnormalities seen in around 50% of patients
  - Cushing disease (adrenocorticotrophic hormone [ACTH]) most common
  - Acromegaly (growth hormone [GH])
  - Hyperthyroidism (thyroid-stimulating hormone [TSH])
  - Amenorrhea, hirsutism, impotence (prolactin [PRL])
  - Diagnosis unsuspected in functionally silent tumors
- Chronic sinusitis
- Rarely, cranial nerve(s) paralysis

Laboratory Tests

- All ectopic hormones can be measured serologically or via stimulation/suppression testing
  - ACTH, GH, TSH, prolactin, cortisol
  - Releasing hormones can also be measured

ECTOPIC PITUITARY ADENOMA

Key Facts

Terminology
- Benign pituitary gland neoplasm occurring separately from and without involvement of sella turcica (a normal anterior pituitary gland)

Clinical Issues
- Very rare in ectopic sinonasal tract locations
  - Sphenoid sinus > > > nasopharynx or nasal cavity
- Mean: 50 years
- Female > Male (2:1)
- Presents with space-occupying effects or endocrine abnormalities
- Complete surgical removal, followed by medical/ hormone manipulation

Image Findings
- Intrasphenoidal mass with erosion of sellar floor
- Early, intense, but heterogeneous enhancement

Microscopic Pathology
- Submucosal location of unencapsulated tumor
- Tumors arranged in many patterns
- Tumor groups separated by delicate fibrovascular septae
- Monotonous population of round to polygonal epithelial cells

Ancillary Tests
- Positive: Keratin, chromogranin-A &/or -B, synaptophysin, CD56, NSE, specific hormones

Top Differential Diagnoses
- Olfactory neuroblastoma, Ewing/PNET, neuroendocrine carcinoma, squamous cell carcinoma, lymphoma, meningioma

Treatment
- Surgical approaches
  - Surgery is treatment of choice but only if completely removed
    - Transnasal/transsphenoidal approach
- Drugs
  - Medical/hormonal manipulation
    - Dopamine-agonists (bromocriptine), somatostatin analogs (octreotide), corticosteroids (hydrocortisone, prednisone), thyroxine
- Radiation
  - Stereotactic radioablation, usually for larger or incompletely removed tumors
  - Conventional radiation therapy

Prognosis
- Excellent prognosis with control of endocrine abnormalities after complete surgical resection
  - Morbidity associated with hormonal manifestations and local invasion (bone or cranial cavity extension)
- Recurrence may develop in large tumors
- Malignant transformation is exceptionally rare
- Metastases are not reported

IMAGE FINDINGS

Radiographic Findings
- Thin section MR (with and without contrast) or CT yields best results
- Intrasphenoidal mass with erosion but usually not expansion of sellar floor
  - Sella may be involved by upward extension, although usually normal
- Usually show early, intense, but heterogeneous enhancement
- CT and MR define extent and location of tumor
- Diagnostic procedures usually suggest another type of neoplasm
  - Chordoma, nasopharyngeal carcinoma, or metastatic tumor

MR Findings
- T1WI: Rounded, isointense mass within sphenoid sinus; usually fills sinus; partially empty sella
  - Post contrast, mass will strongly enhance, although can be heterogeneous
- T2WI: Isointense mass within sphenoid
  - FLAIR technique results in hyperintense signal

CT Findings
- Variable attenuation, isodense with gray matter
- Rarely, hemorrhage and calcification can be seen
- Moderate, inhomogeneous enhancement with contrast

MACROSCOPIC FEATURES

General Features
- Polypoid and pedunculated mass
- Solitary mass
  - Exceedingly rare to have synchronous multifocal tumors

Size
- Mean: Usually 2 cm; range: 0.5-7.5 cm
- Tumor size does not seem to correlate with symptom severity

MICROSCOPIC PATHOLOGY

Histologic Features
- Submucosal location of unencapsulated tumor
  - Surface epithelium is intact and uninvolved
  - Minor mucoserous glands may be present
- Tumors arranged in many patterns
  - Solid, organoid, trabecular, glandular, festoons, ribbons, pseudorosettes
- Tumor groups separated by delicate fibrovascular septae
  - Extracellular stromal hyalinization may be seen
- Monotonous population of round to polygonal epithelial cells

- Round or oval nuclei with "salt and pepper," clumped chromatin
- Inconspicuous or small nucleoli
- Eosinophilic, amphophilic or clear, eccentrically located cytoplasm
- Most would be classified as chromophobe adenomas
- Isolated nuclear pleomorphism can be seen
- Mitoses and necrosis are rare

ANCILLARY TESTS

Immunohistochemistry

- **Positive**: Keratin, chromogranin-A, chromogranin-B, synaptophysin, CD56, NSE
  - Specific tumors (prolactin) are negative with chromogranin-A but positive with chromogranin-B
  - Hormone peptides: ACTH, prolactin most common (Golgi accentuation in some types)
  - Less common: GH, β-TSH, Pit-1, β-subunit and α-subunit of glycoprotein hormones, SF1, FSH, LH
  - May be mono-, pluri-, or nonhormonal adenoma

Electron Microscopy

- Intracytoplasmic neurosecretory granules
  - Number, size, shape, and type of granules dependent on tumor hormone production
- Often show prominent rough endoplastic reticulum, large Golgi apparatus

DIFFERENTIAL DIAGNOSIS

Olfactory Neuroblastoma

- Ethmoid sinus, destructive tumor, lobular architecture, syncytial architecture, neurofilament background, rosette formation, prominent nucleoli and mitoses in high-grade tumors
- **Positive**: Chromogranin, synaptophysin, CD56, S100 protein (sustentacular); usually **negative** with keratin and peptide markers

Ewing/PNET

- Small round blue cell tumor, sheets, tumor necrosis; finely distributed chromatin, mitoses
- **Positive**: FLI-1, CD99, SNF5, NSE, β-catenin (membrane); **negative**: Chromogranin, keratin (usually)

Neuroendocrine Carcinoma

- High-grade malignant neoplasm, syncytial architecture, "salt and pepper" nuclear chromatin, mitoses, necrosis
- **Positive**: Keratin, chromogranin, synaptophysin, CD56

Squamous Cell Carcinoma

- Epithelial proliferation of squamous cells, intercellular bridges, dyskeratosis, significant pleomorphism, mitoses
- **Positive**: Keratin; **negative**: Neuroendocrine and peptide markers

Lymphoma

- Depends on B- or T-cell type: Cleaved, irregular nuclei, diffuse, sheets, high nuclear to cytoplasmic ratio, coarse nuclear chromatin, prominent nucleoli, mitoses, necrosis
- **Positive**: Lymphoid markers; **negative**: Keratin, neuroendocrine markers

Meningioma

- Cellular tumors with whorled appearance, frequent calcifications, intranuclear cytoplasmic inclusions, coarse nuclear chromatin
- **Positive**: EMA, CK7; **negative**: Neuroendocrine and peptide markers

Mucosal Melanoma

- Dyscohesive epithelioid to spindled tumor cells, pigmented, intranuclear cytoplasmic inclusions, eccentric nuclei
- **Positive**: Melanoma markers (S100 protein, HMB-45, Melan-A, MITF); **negative**: Keratin, neuroendocrine markers

DIAGNOSTIC CHECKLIST

Pathologic Interpretation Pearls

- **Always** think of ectopic pituitary adenoma in sphenoid sinus tumor

SELECTED REFERENCES

1. Gondim JA et al: Acromegaly due to an ectopic pituitary adenoma in the sphenoid sinus. Acta Radiol. 45(6):689-91, 2004
2. Suzuki J et al: An aberrant ACTH-producing ectopic pituitary adenoma in the sphenoid sinus. Endocr J. 51(1):97-103, 2004
3. Wick MR et al: Ectopic neural and neuroendocrine neoplasms. Semin Diagn Pathol. 20(4):305-23, 2003
4. Matsuno A et al: Ectopic pituitary adenoma in the sphenoid sinus causing acromegaly associated with empty sella. ANZ J Surg. 71(8):495-8, 2001
5. Oruçkaptan HH et al: Pituitary adenomas: results of 684 surgically treated patients and review of the literature. Surg Neurol. 53(3):211-9, 2000
6. Hori A et al: Pharyngeal pituitary: development, malformation, and tumorigenesis. Acta Neuropathol. 98(3):262-72, 1999
7. Devaney K et al: Olfactory neuroblastoma and other round cell lesions of the sinonasal region. Mod Pathol. 9(6):658-63, 1996
8. Langford L et al: Pituitary gland involvement of the sinonasal tract. Ann Otol Rhinol Laryngol. 104(2):167-9, 1995
9. Tovi F et al: Ectopic pituitary adenoma of the sphenoid sinus: report of a case and review of the literature. Head Neck. 12(3):264-8, 1990
10. Melmed S et al: Ectopic pituitary and hypothalamic hormone syndromes. Endocrinol Metab Clin North Am. 16(3):805-21, 1987
11. Lloyd RV et al: Ectopic pituitary adenomas with normal anterior pituitary glands. Am J Surg Pathol. 10(8):546-52, 1986

Diagrammatic, Radiographic, and Microscopic Features

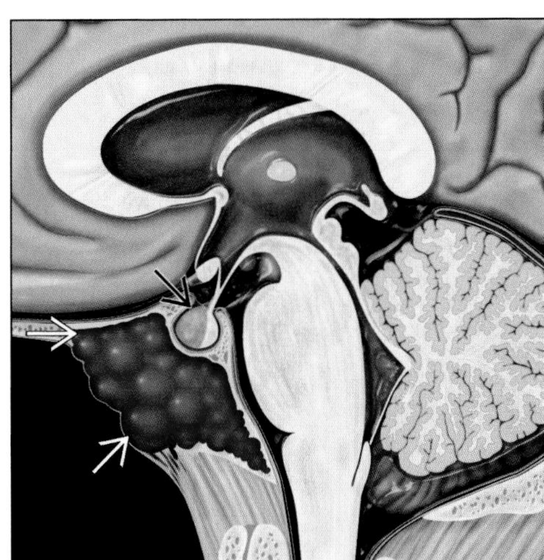

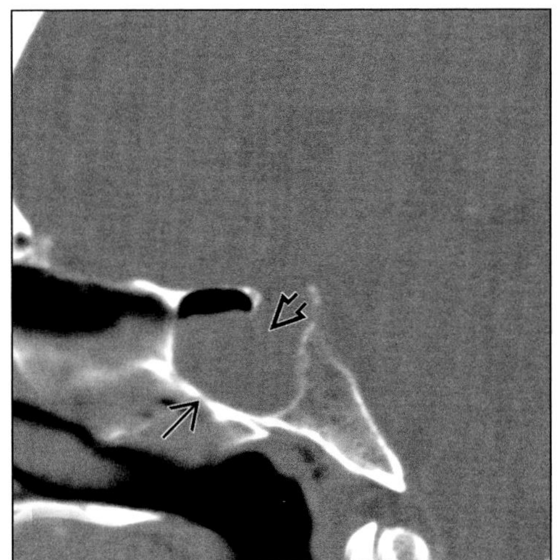

(Left) This is a diagrammatic representation of an ectopic pituitary adenoma. The sphenoid sinus is filled with tumor ➡, expanding into the nasopharynx, but there is a completely normal pituitary ➡, without any bony destruction. This is the appearance of many of these tumors. (Right) Sagittal bone CT shows an intrasphenoidal mass ➡ with erosion (but not expansion) of the sellar floor ➡. The sella is intact, a requirement for an "ectopic" location.

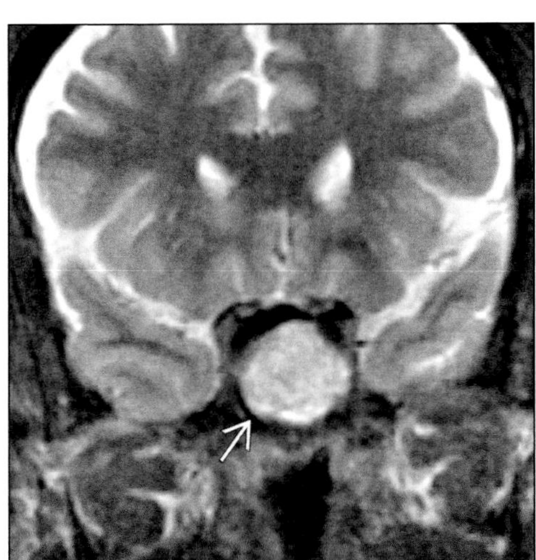

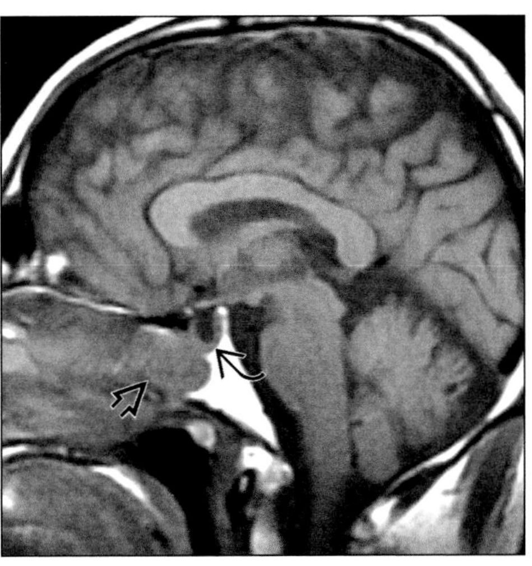

(Left) Coronal T2-weighted MR shows a hyperintense mass ➡ within the sphenoid sinus. This appearance does not confirm the diagnosis of ectopic pituitary adenoma, though it is part of the differential considerations for the anatomic site. (Right) Sagittal T1-weighted fat-suppressed MR shows a partially empty sella ➡ and a rounded, isointense mass in the sphenoid sinus ➡. While helping in confirming the diagnosis of a pituitary adenoma, the radiographic appearance is not diagnostic.

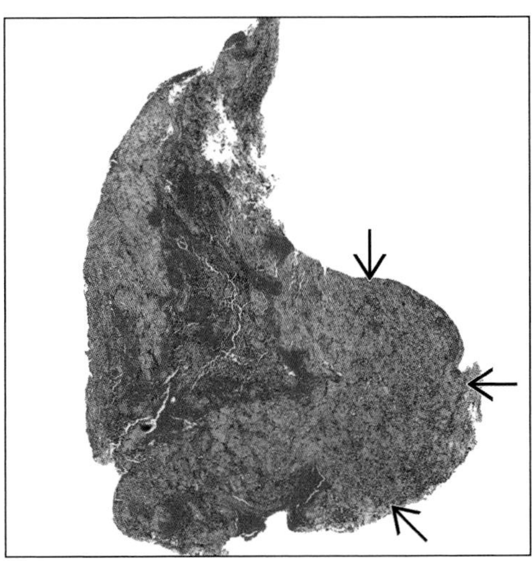

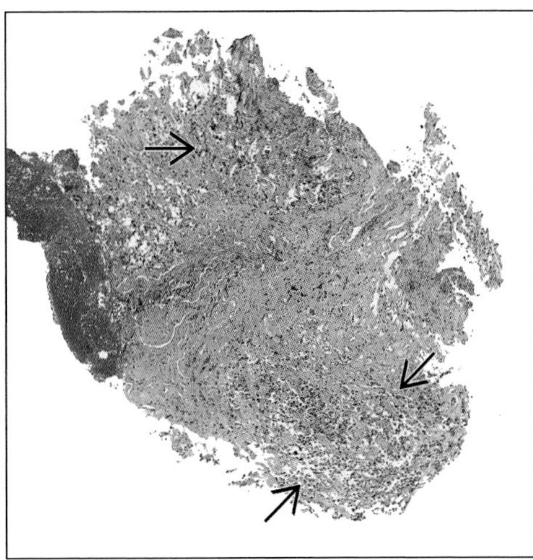

(Left) By macroscopic examination, the tumors tend to be polypoid or pedunculated masses. Most are solitary lesions. This tumor is < 1 cm. The surface epithelium is denuded, with a "small round blue cell" infiltrate ➡. (Right) In many cases, there are tissue fragments with fibrosis and blood, partially obscuring the true neoplasm ➡, which shows a ribbon-like or small cell "infiltrative pattern." The extracellular stromal hyalinization is prominent in this case.

ECTOPIC PITUITARY ADENOMA

Microscopic Features

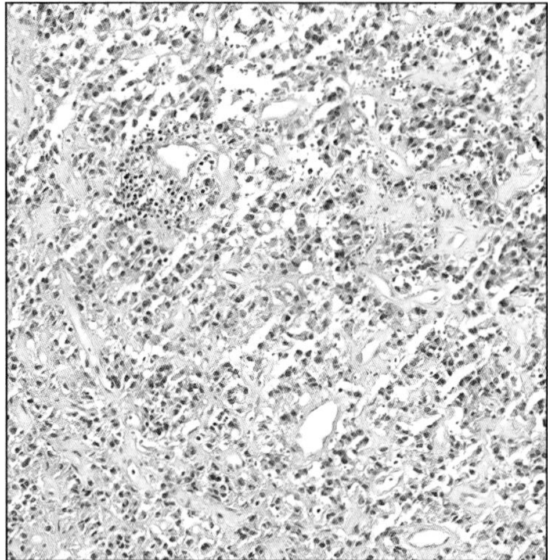

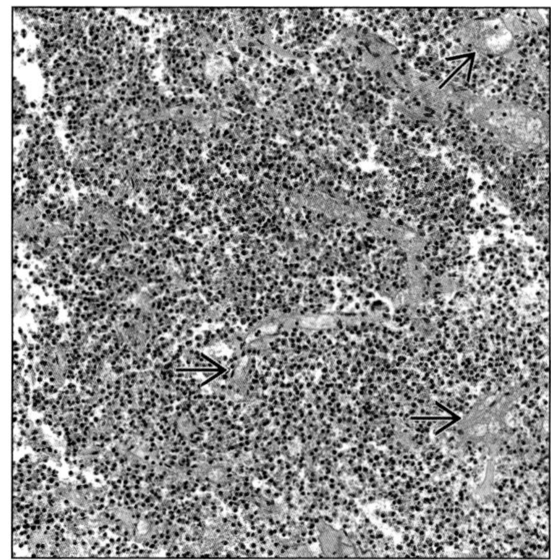

(Left) *There are usually a number of different patterns in the same tumor, with a glandular to ribbon-like appearance in this lesion. The neoplastic proliferation is a monotonous polygonal epithelial proliferation.* ***(Right)*** *A solid cellular tumor is seen in this field, although delicate fibrovascular septae ⇒ can be seen throughout. In many cases, a dilapidated or degenerated appearance can be seen.*

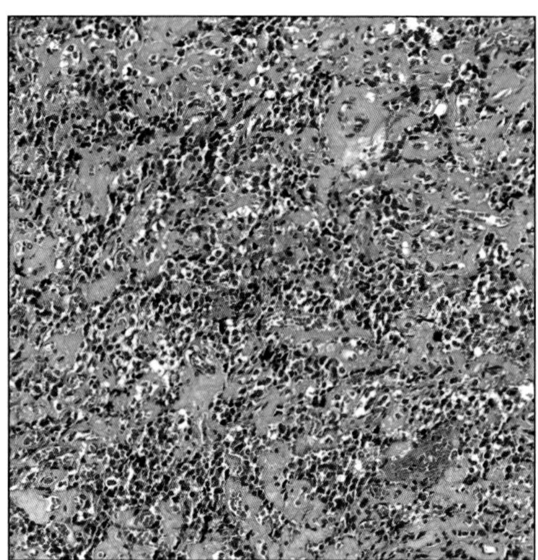

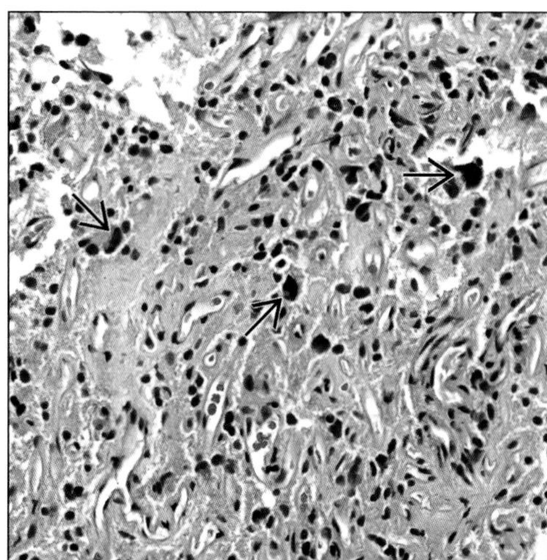

(Left) *An organoid neoplasm is separated by quite remarkable extracellular stromal hyalinization with blood. At this power, many "small round blue cell" tumors should be considered in the differential diagnosis.* ***(Right)*** *The heavy stromal hyalinization in this tumor has separated the neoplastic cells into small islands or single cells. The nuclei show hyperchromasia and pleomorphism ⇒, although the pleomorphism is not universally present.*

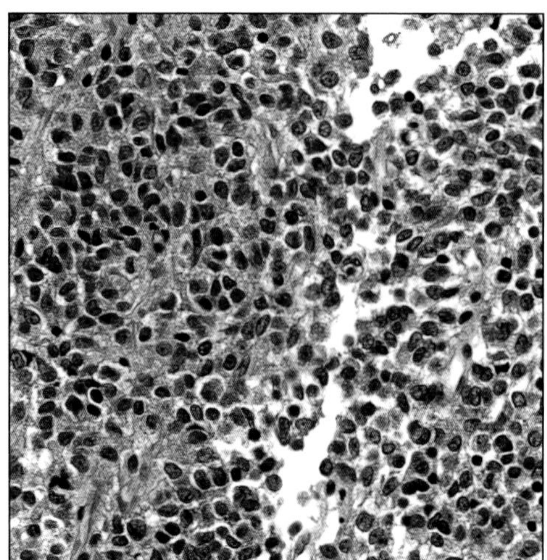

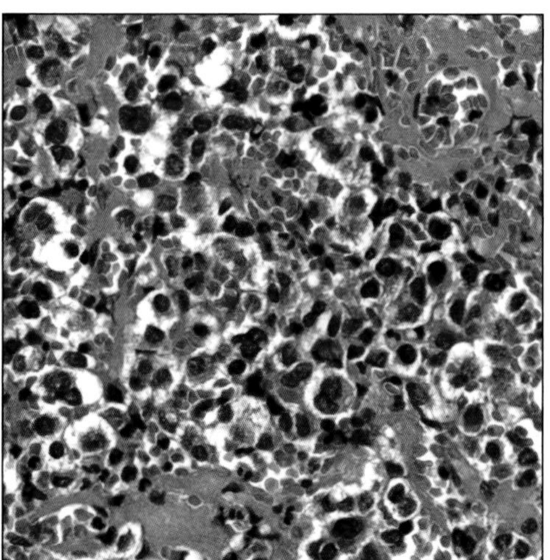

(Left) *There is a monotonous population of round to polygonal epithelial cells, showing round to oval nuclei with "salt and pepper" to slightly clumped chromatin. Nucleoli are inconspicuous. There is focal degeneration.* ***(Right)*** *These polygonal cells are arranged in a loose alveolar to festoon arrangement. The cells show focal binucleation, delicate, finely clumped chromatin, and isolated nucleoli. The cytoplasm is eosinophilic. There is a background of blood.*

Ancillary Techniques

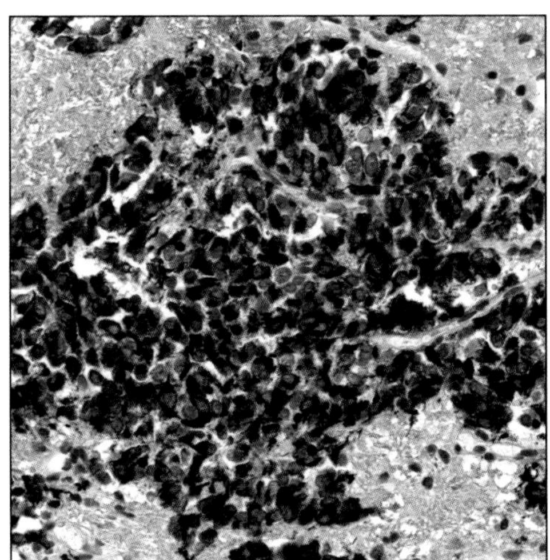

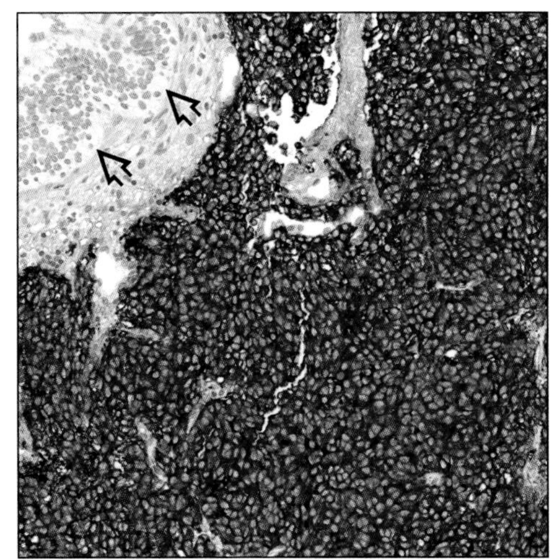

(Left) *A wide variety of immunohistochemistry markers can be used to confirm the diagnosis. The tumors will show keratin immunoreactivity, although a slightly "Golgi" pattern of deposition is noted in this tumor. There are often unique patterns of deposition based on specific hormone production.* ***(Right)*** *A number of different neuroendocrine markers will be positive, including CD56, chromogranin A or B, synaptophysin (shown), and NSE. Note the negative surface epithelium ⇨.*

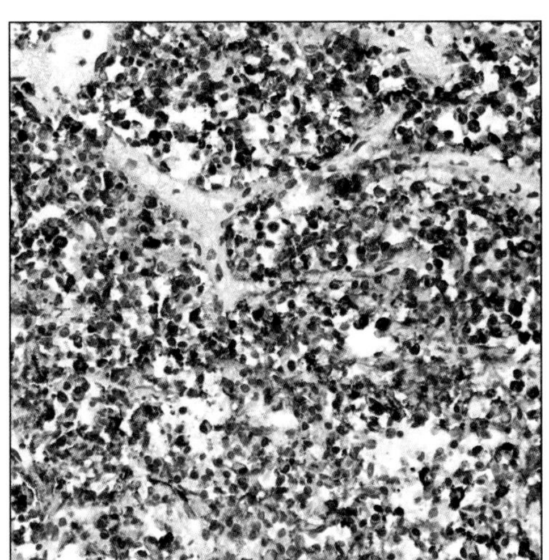

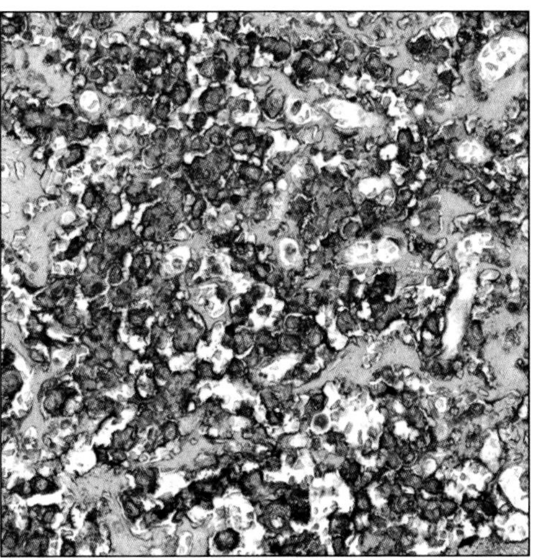

(Left) *This pituitary adenoma showed strong and diffuse cytoplasmic reaction with chromogranin A. Based on this finding, it is unlikely that prolactin was being produced. Sometimes no hormone is produced.* ***(Right)*** *If the type of tumor is uncertain, many lesions in the differential diagnosis do not react with specific peptides, which can also be secreted in the serum. This tumor shows a strong and diffuse cytoplasmic prolactin reaction.*

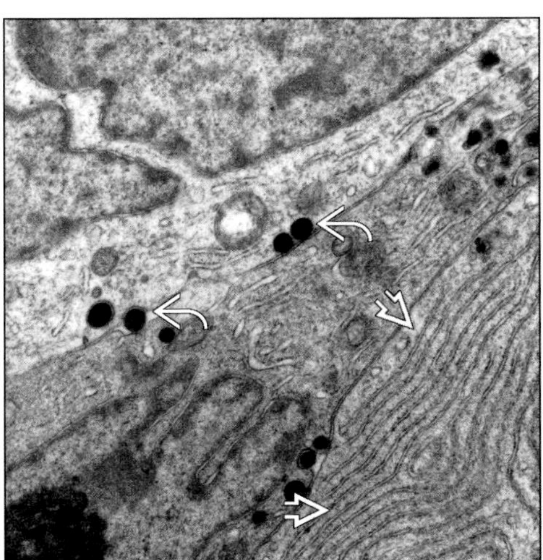

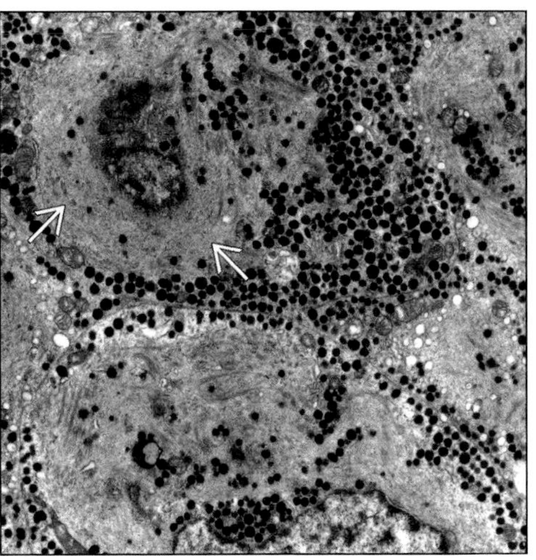

(Left) *A prolactin-secreting tumor cell is seen with large round cytoplasmic electron dense granules (200-300 nm in diameter), prominent rough endoplastic reticulum ➡, and misplaced lateral cell wall granule exocytosis ➡.* ***(Right)*** *In this functioning corticotroph cell adenoma (ACTH), densely granulated, the cytoplasm is densely populated with pleomorphic secretory granules ranging from 250-500 nm. Perinuclear bundles of intermediate filaments (Crooke change ➡) are diagnostic.*

MENINGIOMA

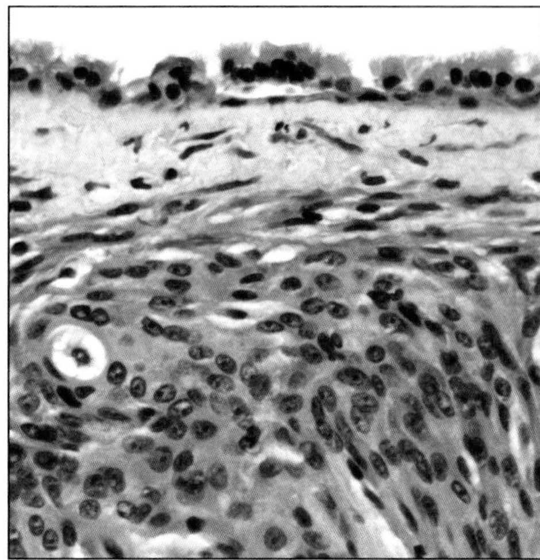

Hematoxylin & eosin shows an intact respiratory mucosa subtended by a syncytial neoplastic proliferation of meningothelial cells.

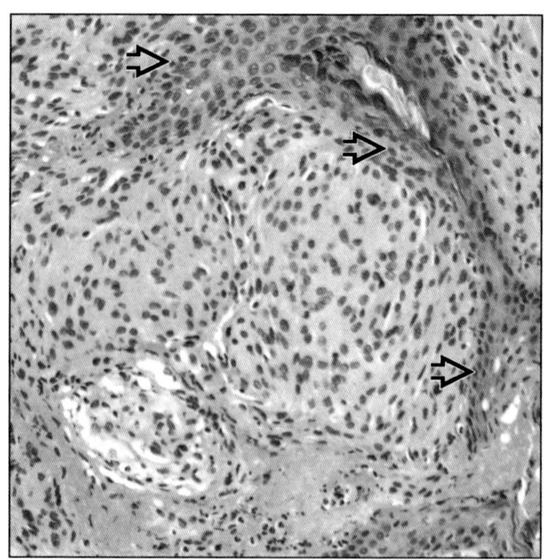

Hematoxylin & eosin shows a whorled pattern of meningothelial cells set adjacent to uninvolved surface squamous epithelium ⇨.

TERMINOLOGY

Definitions

- Benign neoplasm of meningothelial cells within nasal cavity, sinonasal tract, and nasopharynx

ETIOLOGY/PATHOGENESIS

Pathogenesis

- Arachnoid cells from arachnoid granulations or pacchionian bodies lining sheaths of nerves and vessels through skull foramina

CLINICAL ISSUES

Epidemiology

- Incidence
  - Approximately 0.2% of sinonasal tract and nasopharynx tumors
    - 20% of meningiomas have extracranial extension
- Age
  - Mean: 40-48 years old
  - Women older than men by over a decade
- Gender
  - Female > Male (1.2:1)

Site

- Mixed nasal cavity and paranasal sinuses (majority)
- Nasal cavity alone (~ 25%)
- Frontal sinus most commonly affected in isolation
- Majority are left sided

Presentation

- Mass, obstruction, discharge, and epistaxis
- Sinusitis, pain, headache, seizure activity
- Exophthalmos, periorbital edema, visual changes, ptosis

Treatment

- Surgical approaches
  - Excision (although difficult at times)

Prognosis

- Good outcome: 10-year survival (80%)
- Recurrences develop (usually < 5 years after primary)

IMAGE FINDINGS

Radiographic Findings

- Must exclude direct CNS extension from en plaque tumor
- Bony sclerosis with focal destruction of bony tissues
- Widening of suture lines and foramina at base of skull

MACROSCOPIC FEATURES

General Features

- Intact surface mucosa but infiltrative into bone
- Multiple fragments of grayish, white-tan, gritty, firm to rubbery masses
- Many are polypoid

Size

- Range: 1-8 cm, mean: 3.5 cm

MICROSCOPIC PATHOLOGY

Histologic Features

- Infiltrative growth of neoplastic cells, including soft tissue and bone
- Meningothelial (syncytial) lobules of neoplastic cells without distinct borders
- Whorled architecture
- Psammoma bodies or "pre-psammoma" bodies
- Epithelioid cells with round to regular nuclei and even nuclear chromatin

MENINGIOMA

Key Facts

Terminology
- Benign neoplasm of meningothelial cells

Clinical Issues
- Approximately 0.2% of sinonasal tract and nasopharynx tumors
- Female > Male (1.2:1)
  - Women older by over a decade
- Good outcome: 10-year survival (80%)

Image Findings
- Must exclude direct CNS extension

Microscopic Pathology
- Infiltrative growth of neoplastic cells, including soft tissue and bone
- Meningothelial (syncytial) lobules of neoplastic cells without distinct borders
- Whorled architecture, psammoma bodies
- Intranuclear cytoplasmic inclusions (invaginations)
- Histologic subtypes can be seen
  - Transitional, metaplastic, atypical

ANCILLARY TESTS

Immunohistochemistry
- Positive: EMA, keratin (pre-psammoma-body pattern), CAM5.2
- Weak positive: S100 protein
- Negative: Chromogranin, synaptophysin

DIFFERENTIAL DIAGNOSIS

Angiofibroma
- Males only; nasopharynx; collagenized stroma, stellate stromal cells, haphazard vessels (staghorn)

Aggressive Psammomatoid Ossifying Fibroma
- Young patients; abundant psammoma bodies; osteoclasts and osteoblasts; compact to storiform stroma

Olfactory Neuroblastoma
- Cribriform plate; lobular growth; small cells with scant cytoplasm; fibrillar background; rosette/pseudorosette formations

Melanoma
- Protean mimic; intranuclear cytoplasmic inclusions; prominent nucleoli; melanoma markers positive

Paraganglioma
- Rare in sinonasal tract; nested architecture, basophilic cytoplasm; S100 protein sustentacular and chromogranin paraganglia reaction

SELECTED REFERENCES

1. Dekker G et al: Meningioma presenting as an oropharyngeal mass--an unusual presentation. S Afr Med J. 97(5):342, 2007
2. Petrulionis M et al: Primary extracranial meningioma of the sinonasal tract. Acta Radiol. 46(4):415-8, 2005
3. Thompson LD et al: Extracranial sinonasal tract meningiomas: a clinicopathologic study of 30 cases with a review of the literature. Am J Surg Pathol. 24(5):640-50, 2000
4. Moulin G et al: Plaque-like meningioma involving the temporal bone, sinonasal cavities and both parapharyngeal spaces: CT and MRI. Neuroradiology. 36(8):629-31, 1994
5. Gabibov GA et al: Meningiomas of the anterior skull base expanding into the orbit, paranasal sinuses, nasopharynx, and oropharynx. J Craniofac Surg. 4(3):124-7; discussion 134, 1993
6. Perzin KH et al: Nonepithelial tumors of the nasal cavity, paranasal sinuses, and nasopharynx. A clinicopathologic study. XIII: Meningiomas. Cancer. 54(9):1860-9, 1984

IMAGE GALLERY

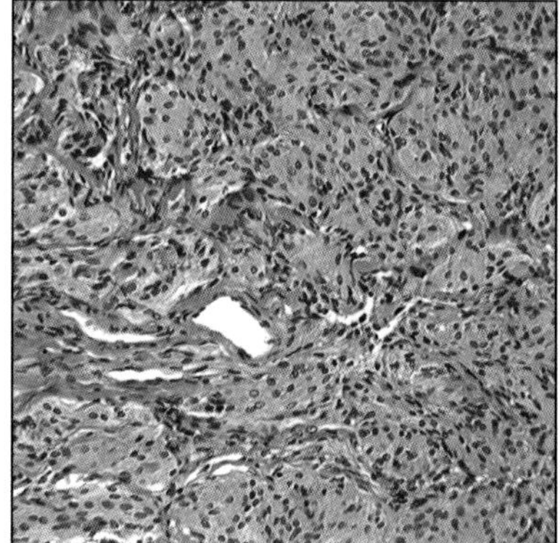

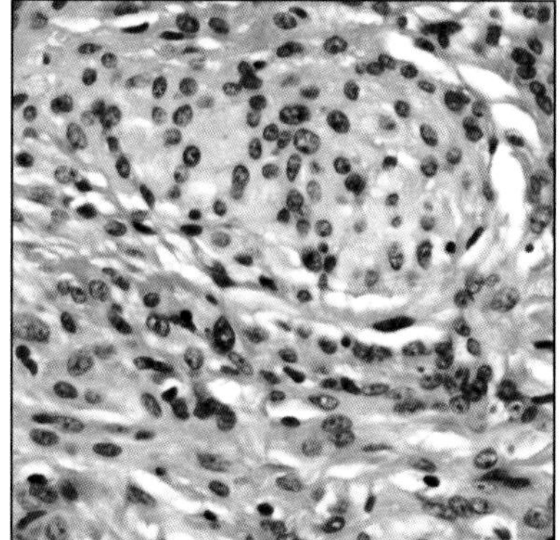

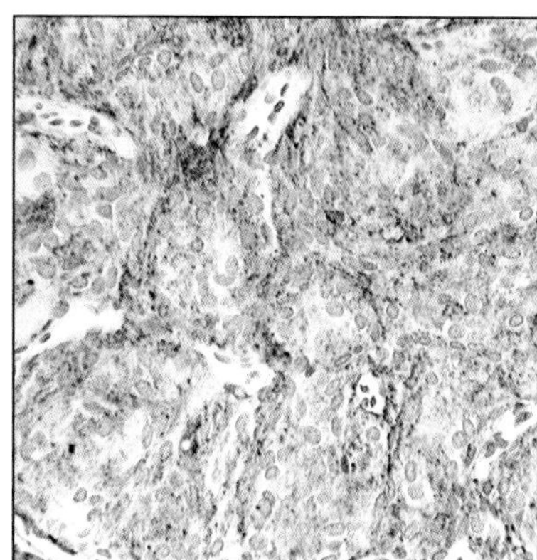

(Left) *Hematoxylin & eosin shows multiple small nests of meningothelial cells showing a slightly whorled appearance.* ***(Center)*** *Hematoxylin & eosin demonstrates a nest of cells without cell borders, showing nuclear hyperchromasia.* ***(Right)*** *EMA shows modest cytoplasmic reactivity.*

AMELOBLASTOMA

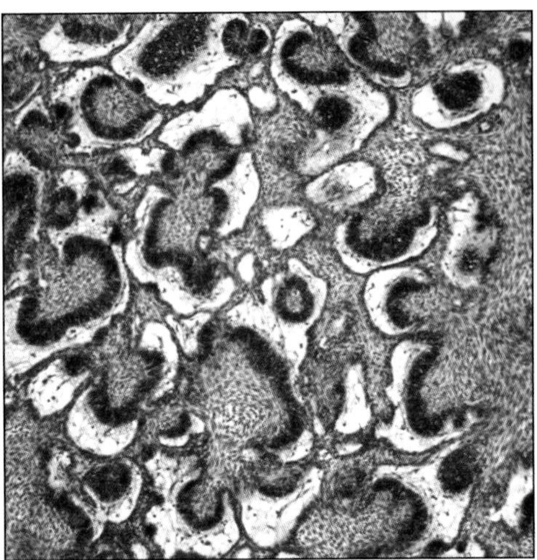

Hematoxylin & eosin shows the classic palisading of the nuclei with typical reverse polarity and sub-nuclear clearing. The stellate reticulum has a syncytial architecture. Edema is focally noted.

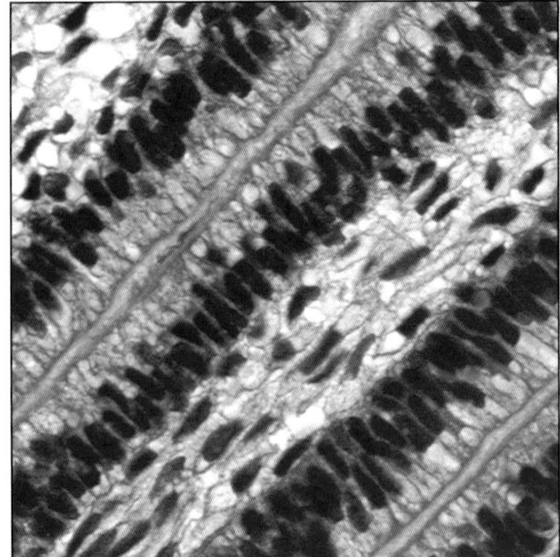

Note the prominent reverse polarity of the nuclei. The columnar nuclei are set within tall cells, illustrating the subnuclear vacuolization. The vacuoles are lined up against fibrovascular cores.

TERMINOLOGY

Definitions

- Locally aggressive, benign, epithelial odontogenic neoplasm arising from remnants of odontogenic epithelium

CLINICAL ISSUES

Epidemiology

- Incidence
  - Rare
- Age
  - Mean: 6th to 8th decades
    - Older than gnathic counterparts
- Gender
  - Male > Female (4:1)

Site

- Sinonasal cavity or maxillary sinus, with possible extension into other location
  - May present with combined involvement

Presentation

- Symptoms are nonspecific, including unilateral enlarging mass, sinusitis, nasal obstruction, epistaxis

Treatment

- Surgical approaches
  - Conservative surgery (polypectomy) or curettage to more aggressive surgery (radical maxillectomy), depending on patient status
  - Surgical excision with adequate margin is treatment of choice
- Radiation
  - Not used as first-line treatment

Prognosis

- Excellent, but long-term clinical follow-up is essential to manage potential recurrences
- Recurrence, usually within 1 year of initial surgery, occurs in up to 25%
- May die **with** but not **from** disease

IMAGE FINDINGS

General Features

- Multilocular, expansile lucency of bone
- Unilateral maxillary sinus opacification

MACROSCOPIC FEATURES

General Features

- Polypoid mass is most common
- Glistening, gray-white, pink, or yellow-tan
- Rubbery to granular
- Bone can be present

Size

- Range: 0.3 up to 9 cm

MICROSCOPIC PATHOLOGY

Histologic Features

- Blend of ameloblasts and epithelial cells trying to reduplicate enamel organ
- Intact overlying respiratory epithelium, possibly source of tumor
- Ameloblastic cells are palisaded about periphery of tumor nests in jigsaw-like configuration
- Basal cells arranged in anastomosing strands (plexiform pattern)
- Reverse polarity of basal columnar cells (a.k.a. "Vickers Gorlin change") with sub-nuclear vacuolization
  - Nuclei displaced away from basement membrane and are hyperchromatic
- Central, loosely arranged stellate reticulum, which can become cystic

AMELOBLASTOMA

Key Facts

Terminology
- Locally aggressive benign epithelial odontogenic neoplasm

Clinical Issues
- Older age (6th-8th decade) at presentation than gnathic counterparts
- Male > Female (4:1)
- Sinonasal cavity or maxillary sinus, with potential extension into adjacent areas
- Excellent, but requires long-term clinical follow-up to manage recurrences (up to 25%)

Microscopic Pathology
- Polypoid mass is most common
- Ameloblastic, basaloid columnar cells are palisaded about periphery of tumor nests showing reverse polarity (sub-nuclear vacuolization)
- Central, loosely arranged stellate reticulum
- Pleomorphism and mitoses are rare

  - Cells can be spindle-shaped, basaloid, granular, or show squamous differentiation
- Mitotic activity and cellular pleomorphism are rare
- Many histologic types: Plexiform, ameloblastic, and acanthomatous are most common in sinonasal tract

ANCILLARY TESTS

Cytogenetics
- Fos-oncogene and tumor-necrosis-factor-receptor-1 (*TNFRSF-1A*) are overexpressed
- Sonic hedgehog (*SHH*), cadherins 12 and 13 (CDH12 and 13), and transforming growth-factor-β1 (*TGF-β1*) are underexpressed

DIFFERENTIAL DIAGNOSIS

Basaloid Squamous Cell Carcinoma
- Basaloid peripheral palisade with abrupt squamous differentiation; may mimic acanthomatous pattern

Basal Cell Adenoma
- Small, basaloid cells with peripheral palisade; no subnuclear vacuolization; lacks stellate reticulum

Pleomorphic Adenoma
- Tubuloglandular structures; myoepithelial plasmacytoid cells; myxochondroid matrix

Adenoid Cystic Carcinoma
- Cribriform pattern; mucoid pseudoglandular structures; reduplicated basement membrane

Adenocarcinoma, Nonintestinal Type
- Glandular malignancy
- Lacks subnuclear vacuoles and stellate reticulum

SELECTED REFERENCES

1. Press SG: Odontogenic tumors of the maxillary sinus. Curr Opin Otolaryngol Head Neck Surg. 16(1):47-54, 2008
2. Bray D et al: Ameloblastoma: a rare nasal polyp. J Laryngol Otol. 121(1):72-5, 2007
3. Ereño C et al: Primary sinonasal ameloblastoma. APMIS. 113(2):148-50, 2005
4. Zwahlen RA et al: Maxillary ameloblastomas: a review of the literature and of a 15-year database. J Craniomaxillofac Surg. 30(5):273-9, 2002
5. Schafer DR et al: Primary ameloblastoma of the sinonasal tract: a clinicopathologic study of 24 cases. Cancer. 82(4):667-74, 1998
6. Wenig BL et al: An unusual cause of unilateral nasal obstruction: ameloblastoma. Otolaryngol Head Neck Surg. 93(3):426-32, 1985
7. Tsaknis PJ et al: The maxillary ameloblastoma: an analysis of 24 cases. J Oral Surg. 38(5):336-42, 1980
8. Vickers RA et al: Ameloblastoma: Delineation of early histopathologic features of neoplasia. Cancer. 26(3):699-710, 1970

IMAGE GALLERY

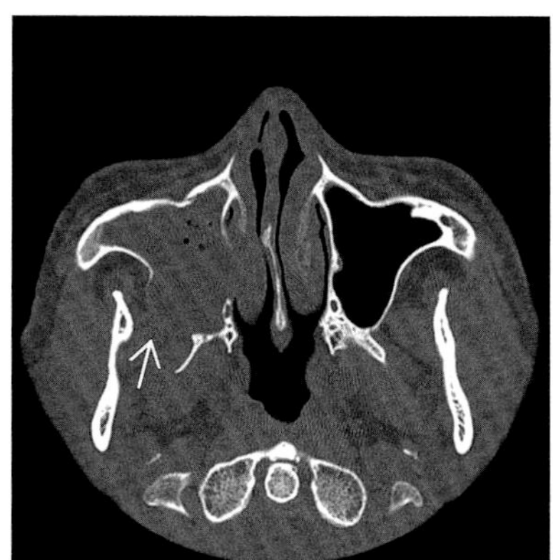
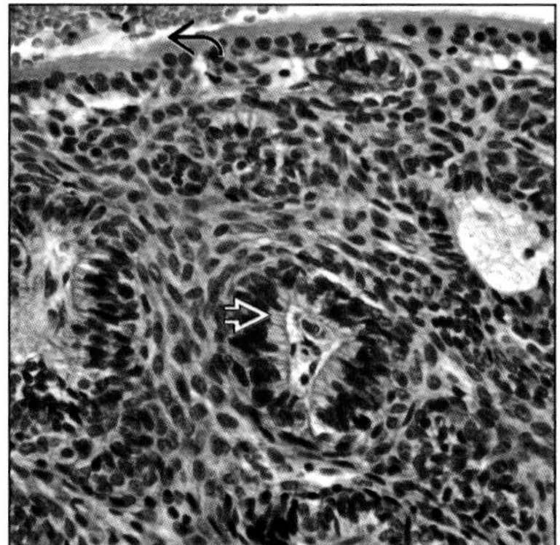
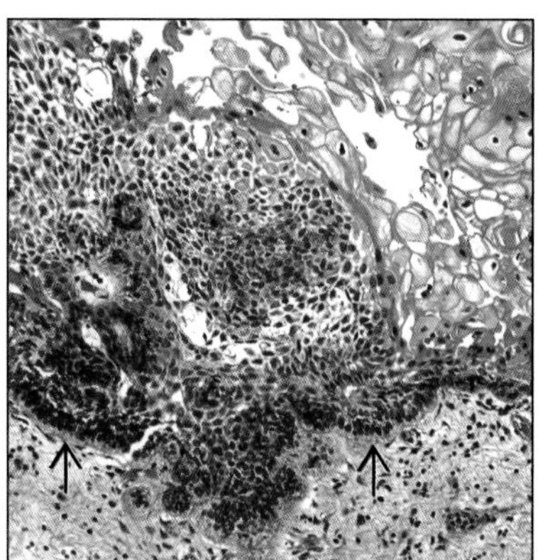

*(**Left**) Computed tomography scan demonstrates a cystic mass within the right maxillary sinus. Note the cystic foci with expanded cortical bone and focal remodeling and loss in the posterior portion ➡. (**Center**) Intact respiratory epithelium ↪ overlies the stellate reticulum with abrupt areas of columnar cells with reverse polarity and prominent subnuclear vacuoles ➡. (**Right**) Columnar cells with peripheral palisading ➡ are seen. Note the stellate reticulum with keratinization.*

LOBULAR CAPILLARY HEMANGIOMA (PYOGENIC GRANULOMA)

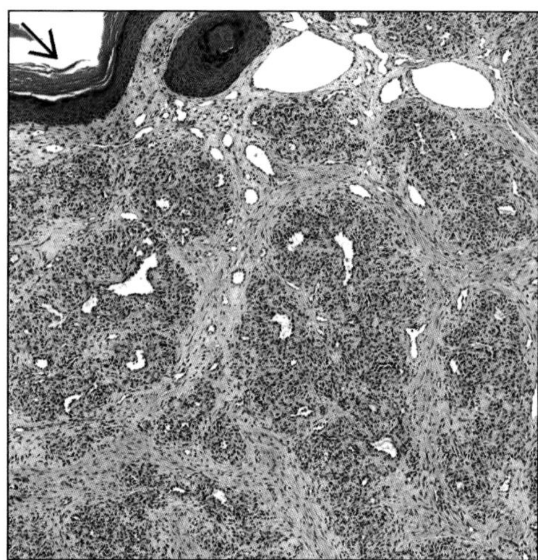

Part of the epithelial collarette ⇒ is identified overlying the circumscribed, lobular arrangement of capillaries. Each lobule shows a cluster of endothelial-lined capillaries with variable lumina. A central vessel is noted.

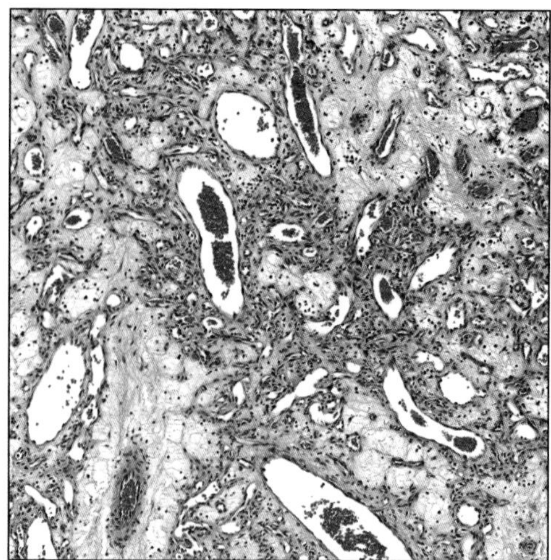

There is a lobular arrangement of capillaries lined by endothelial cells. A central vessel shows branching lumina. There is intimate association with spindled pericytes. Note small arteries and veins in the stroma.

TERMINOLOGY

Abbreviations

- Lobular capillary hemangioma (LCH)

Synonyms

- Pyogenic granuloma (PG)
  - While taxonomically inaccurate, PG is entrenched in medical literature
    - It is **not** purulent, infectious, or granulomatous
- Capillary hemangioma
- Epulis gravidarum

Definitions

- Benign overgrowth of capillary loops with obviously vascular phenotype

ETIOLOGY/PATHOGENESIS

Etiology

- Trauma or injury
  - Nose picking, nasal packing, cauterization, shaving/hair removal, nonspecific microtrauma
    - Nasal packing is commonly used for nasal bleeding and postoperative hemostasis
- Hormones
  - Increased in pregnancy or oral contraceptive use
    - Profound metabolic and endocrine changes in pregnancy seem to contribute to rapid growth

Familial Association

- Hemangioma(s) in sinonasal tract and multiple cutaneous hemangiomas
  - Consider Sturge-Weber or von Hippel-Lindau
- Kasabach-Merritt syndrome associated with cavernous hemangioma (vanishingly rare in sinonasal tract)

Pathogenesis

- Bicellular origin from endothelial and pericytic cells

CLINICAL ISSUES

Epidemiology

- Incidence
  - Mucosal hemangiomas account for about 10% of all head and neck hemangiomas
  - About 30% develop in nasal cavity
  - Account for approximately 25% of all nonepithelial tumors of sinonasal tract
- Age
  - Wide range: 1-65 years
  - Mean: 30 years
  - Peak: Adolescent males and reproductive females
  - Patients with an inherited syndrome tend to present at young age
- Gender
  - Female > Male (2:1)
  - Pediatric age (up to 18 years): Male > > Female
  - Reproductive years: Female > > Male
  - > 40 years: Equal gender distribution

Site

- Order of frequency in head and neck
  - Oral cavity (60%), nasal cavity (30%), paranasal sinuses (8%), and nasopharynx (2%)
    - Oral: Gingiva (75%), lips, tongue, buccal mucosa
    - Nasal cavity: Anterior nasal septum (Little's area; 60%), nasal vestibule, turbinate (tip)

Presentation

- Epistaxis is most common symptom (95%)
  - Spontaneous, intermittent, and unilateral bleeding
  - Bleed easily with minor trauma
- Nasal obstruction (35%) in larger tumors
- Rapidly growing, painless, hemorrhagic mass
- Symptoms usually present for short duration
  - Epistaxis is a dramatic symptom
  - Tumor tends to develop rapidly
- Sinus lesions present with sinusitis, proptosis, mass, anesthesia, pain

LOBULAR CAPILLARY HEMANGIOMA (PYOGENIC GRANULOMA)

Key Facts

Etiology/Pathogenesis
- Trauma or injury and hormones

Clinical Issues
- Mucosal hemangiomas represent ~ 10% of all head and neck hemangiomas
- Peak: Adolescent males and reproductive females
  - Pediatric age: Male > > Female
  - Reproductive years: Female > > Male
- Anterior nasal septum (Little's area; 60%)
- Epistaxis is most common symptom (95%)
- Rapidly growing, painless, hemorrhagic mass
- Biopsy should be **avoided** due to epistaxis
- Endoscopic resection is treatment of choice, removing a rim of normal tissue

Microscopic Pathology
- Polypoid, nodular, diffuse, or sessile mass
- Ulcerated surface with fibrinous exudate
- Collarette of epithelium around areas of ulceration
- Circumscribed, lobular arrangement of capillaries around central vessel
- Stroma is fibromyxoid to edematous, then hyalinized

Ancillary Tests
- Endothelial cells: CD31, CD34, FVIIIRAg, Ulex europaeus lectin, vimentin

Top Differential Diagnoses
- Sinonasal polyps, nasopharyngeal angiofibroma, glomangiopericytoma, angiosarcoma, granulation tissue

Endoscopic Findings
- Rhinoscopy shows well-defined, sessile or pedunculated, dark red-brown to purplish mass
- Ulcerated, friable surface with fibrinous exudate

Natural History
- May spontaneously involute after pregnancy

Treatment
- Options, risks, complications
  - Biopsy should be **avoided**, if possible, due to profound epistaxis
  - Preoperative radiology studies part of planning
    - Confirm nature and extent of lesion, avoiding biopsy and open procedures
  - Aplasia of nasal cartilages may cause disfigurement in young patients
  - Pregnancy related tumors will spontaneously involute after confinement
- Surgical approaches
  - Endoscopic resection is treatment of choice
    - Rim of normal mucosa/submucosa
    - Removal to epichondrium prevents recurrence
  - Preoperative embolization for large lesions

Prognosis
- Excellent long-term clinical outcome
  - Fatal exsanguination is reported
- Multiple recurrences (~ 20%) more common in children

IMAGE FINDINGS

Radiographic Findings
- Ultrasound &/or Doppler: Confirms anatomic site, extent, and vascular nature of process
- Computed tomography: Intensely enhancing mass within nasal cavity (septum)
- Magnetic resonance: Tumor with high signal intensity on T2-weighted images or after gadolinium injection
- Angiography (arteriography) identifies feeder vessel(s), useful in presurgical embolization

MACROSCOPIC FEATURES

General Features
- Polypoid (pedunculated), nodular, diffuse, or sessile mass (latter in children)
- Soft and compressible submucosal mass
- Ulcerated surface (40% of cases), partially covered by yellow to white fibrinous exudate
- Pink-red, blue to purple or gray-tan (depends on degree of congestion)
- Cavernous hemangiomas are spongy on sectioning

Size
- Range: 1-8 cm
- Mean: 1.5 cm

MICROSCOPIC PATHOLOGY

Histologic Features
- Polypoid, with high cellularity
- Surface ulceration with exudate and fibrin
  - Collarette of epithelium is seen on either side of ulcerated areas
  - Secondary, nonspecific changes can be present
    - Stromal edema, capillary dilation, inflammation, granulation tissue reaction
- Circumscribed, lobular arrangement of capillaries
  - Lobule has cluster of endothelial-lined capillaries
    - Lumina can be absent, slit-like to prominent
    - Endothelial cells range from plump to flattened
    - Immature to mature vessels
    - Bland nuclei with eosinophilic cytoplasm
  - Small capillaries and venules arranged around central vessel
    - May show branching lumina
  - Intimate association of spindled pericytes within perivascular spaces
  - Small arteries and veins may be present adjacent to lobules
- Surrounding stroma is fibromyxoid to edematous, but may be hyalinized, especially with chronicity

LOBULAR CAPILLARY HEMANGIOMA (PYOGENIC GRANULOMA)

- Mixed inflammatory cells and extravasated erythrocytes are usually present
  - Small lymphocytes, plasma cells, mast cells, neutrophils
  - Arranged on gradient: Greater at surface, less at center
- Mitotic figures easily identified, often increased
  - Atypical mitoses are absent

Subtypes

- Cavernous hemangioma
  - Very uncommon in nasal cavity
  - Most common in bones of paranasal sinuses and turbinates
  - Large, open, cystic, or cavernous spaces
  - Thin-walled spaces lined by bland endothelial cells
  - Scant connective tissue stroma
  - Hemorrhage with erythrocytes in spaces
  - Variably intense chronic inflammatory infiltrate in stroma
- Hemangiomatosis
  - Extensive, frequently involving bone and adjacent skin and sinuses
  - Vascular channels of variable size and shape
  - Flat endothelial cells
  - May contain fat

ANCILLARY TESTS

Histochemistry

- Reticulin: Highlights outline of endothelial cells
- Elastic: Identifies fibers in vascular walls

Immunohistochemistry

- Positive
  - Endothelial cells: CD31, CD34, FVIIIRAg, Ulex europaeus lectin, vimentin
    - Variably positive with estrogen and progesterone receptors
  - Perivascular cells: Smooth muscle and muscle-specific actins
  - Pericytes: Collagen IV and laminin (around endothelial cells)

Cytogenetics

- Clonal deletion (21)(q21.2q22.12) has been identified

DIFFERENTIAL DIAGNOSIS

Sinonasal Polyps

- Polyps may have haphazard vascular proliferation or become hemorrhagic
  - Vessels are dilated and patulous
- Usually have polypoid/pedunculated appearance
- Edematous to fibrotic stroma with limited mucoserous glands
- Eosinophils predominate

Angiofibroma (Nasopharyngeal)

- Develops exclusively in male patients and tends to involve nasopharynx to lateral nasal walls
- Variable vascular component from capillaries to muscle-walled vessels
- Hyalinized stroma with fine to coarse collagen deposition
- Spindle or stellate stromal cells with mast cells

Glomangiopericytoma

- Patternless to slightly fascicular arrangement of oval to spindled cells
- Richly vascularized tumor showing characteristic perivascular hyalinization
- Inflammatory infiltrate usually rich in mast cells and eosinophils

Angiosarcoma

- Widely infiltrative and destructive tumor
- Freely anastomosing vascular channels lined by atypical endothelial cells
- Increased mitotic figures and necrosis

Granulation Tissue

- More haphazard architecture
- Associated with significant inflammatory infiltrate
- Mitotic figures are common, but tumor necrosis is not present

Vascular Lesions

- Kaposi sarcoma, intravascular papillary endothelial hyperplasia, vascular malformation, bacillary angiomatosis, glomus tumor, lymphangioma, telangiectasia
  - All are exceedingly rare in sinonasal tract, showing features similar to other anatomic sites
  - Lobular architecture is not seen

SELECTED REFERENCES

1. Lee DG et al: CT features of lobular capillary hemangioma of the nasal cavity. AJNR Am J Neuroradiol. 31(4):749-54, 2010
2. Baradaranfar MH et al: Endoscopic endonasal surgery for resection of benign sinonasal tumors: experience with 105 patients. Arch Iran Med. 9(3):244-9, 2006
3. Puxeddu R et al: Lobular capillary hemangioma of the nasal cavity: A retrospective study on 40 patients. Am J Rhinol. 20(4):480-4, 2006
4. Truss L et al: Deletion (21)(q21.2q22.12) as a sole clonal cytogenetic abnormality in a lobular capillary hemangioma of the nasal cavity. Cancer Genet Cytogenet. 170(1):69-70, 2006
5. Sheen TS et al: Pyogenic granuloma--an uncommon complication of nasal packing. Am J Rhinol. 11(3):225-7, 1997
6. Lim IJ et al: 'Pregnancy tumour' of the nasal septum. Aust N Z J Obstet Gynaecol. 34(1):109-10, 1994
7. Kapadia SB et al: Pitfalls in the histopathologic diagnosis of pyogenic granuloma. Eur Arch Otorhinolaryngol. 249(4):195-200, 1992
8. Nichols GE et al: Lobular capillary hemangioma. An immunohistochemical study including steroid hormone receptor status. Am J Clin Pathol. 97(6):770-5, 1992
9. Mills SE et al: Lobular capillary hemangioma: the underlying lesion of pyogenic granuloma. A study of 73 cases from the oral and nasal mucous membranes. Am J Surg Pathol. 4(5):470-9, 1980

Imaging, Microscopic, and Immunohistochemical Features

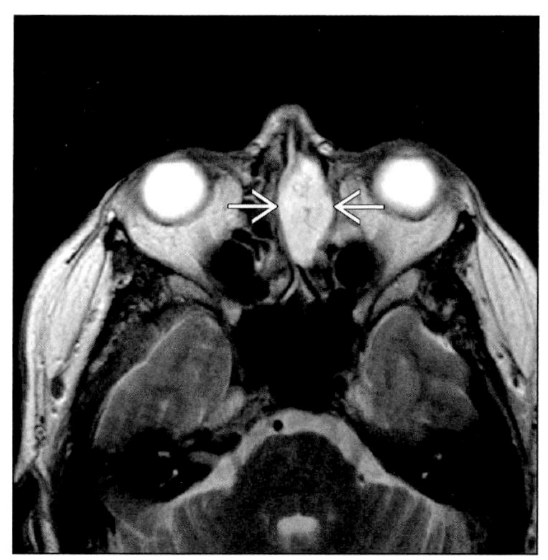

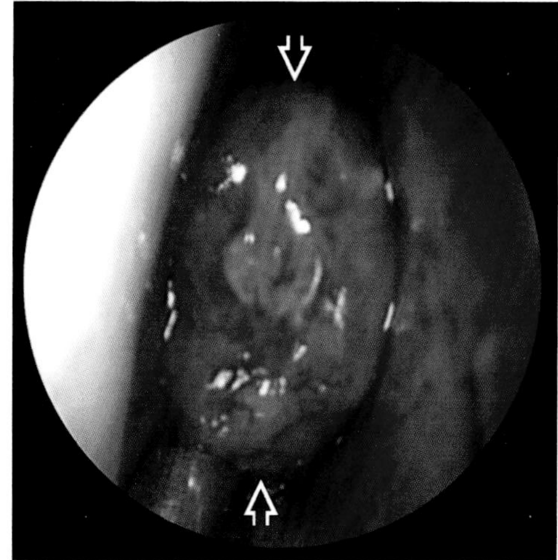

(Left) *There is an easily identified tumor in the nasal cavity ➡, showing a hyperintense mass compared with the surrounding tissues on a T2-weighted sequence. Gadolinium can also be used.* ***(Right)*** *Rhinoscopy shows a well-defined polypoid or pedunculated reddish mass within the nasal cavity ➡. The surface shows erythema and ulceration, with a friable surface containing a fibrinous exudate. (Courtesy G.G. Calzada, MD.)*

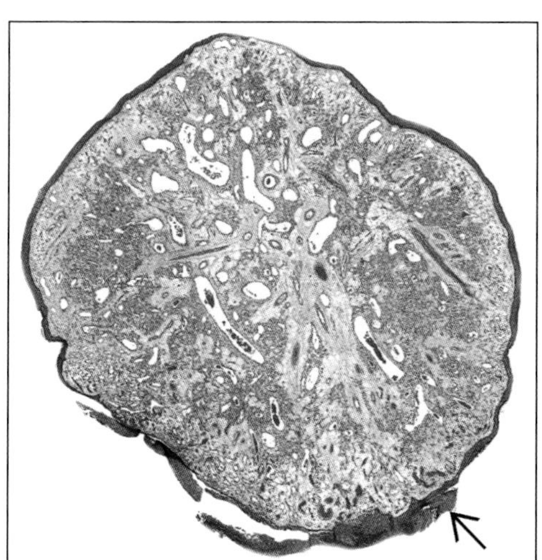

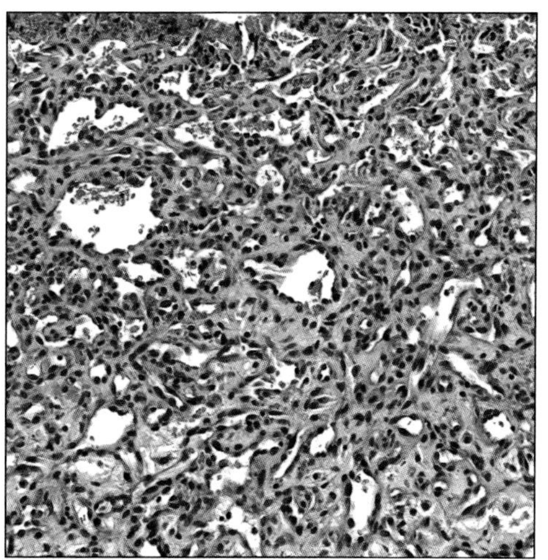

(Left) *LCH tend to be very polypoid (pedunculated), nodular masses. The surfaces are frequently ulcerated ➡. A vague lobularity can be easily identified even at this magnification.* ***(Right)*** *There is a more haphazard arrangement to the endothelial cells lining the variably sized vessels. The vessels are mature to immature with bland endothelial cells. Intimate association of spindled pericytes is also noted. The stroma is slightly fibrous.*

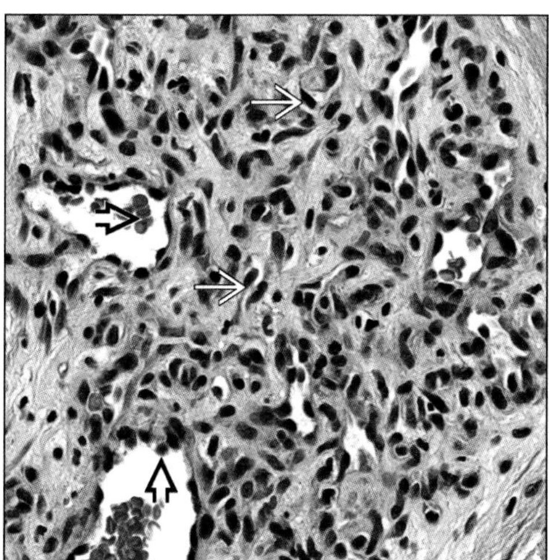

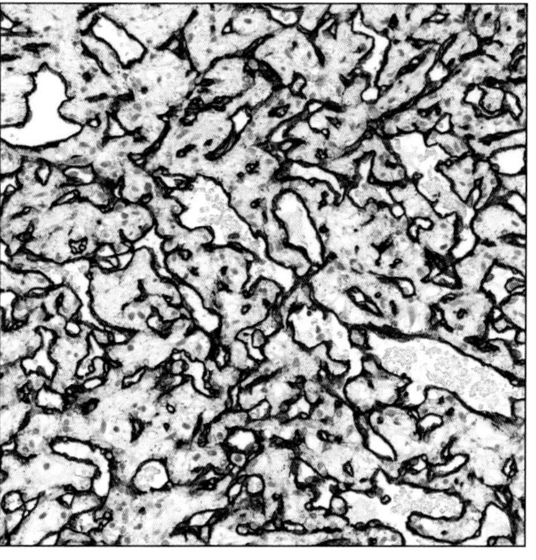

(Left) *This high-power image highlights the well-circumscribed, lobular arrangement of capillaries. The lobule has clusters of endothelial-lined capillaries with lumina that are prominent ➡ to slit-like ➡. The cells are bland.* ***(Right)*** *The endothelial cells can be highlighted by CD34 (shown), along with CD31, FVIIIRAg, and vimentin. The perivascular cells are highlighted by actins, with collagen IV and laminin surrounding them.*

SCHWANNOMA/NEUROFIBROMA

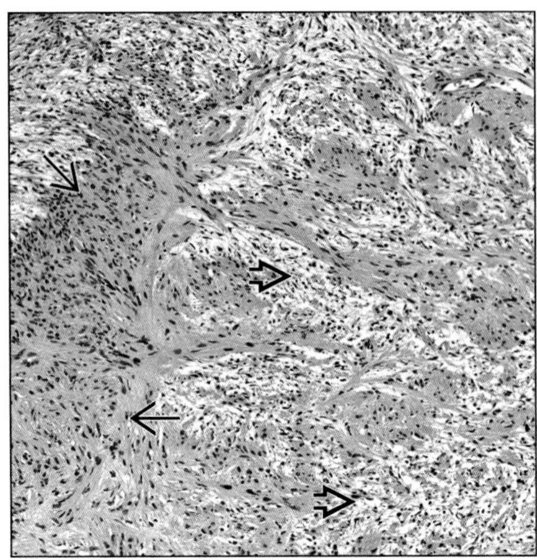

There is a juxtaposition and blending of cellular Antoni A areas ➔ with hypocellular Antoni B areas ⇨. The nuclei have palisading. Note the areas of myxoid-type change.

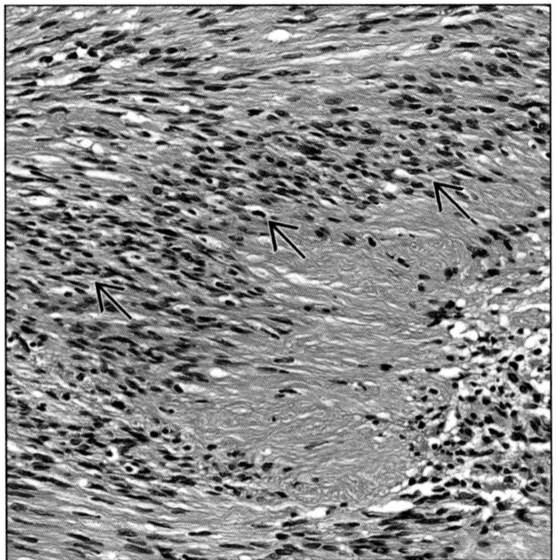

This Antoni A area shows elongated nuclei stacked in neat rows ➔ (palisade resembling a fortification) with Schwann cell cytoplasm in the center. This Verocay body is characteristic of schwannoma.

TERMINOLOGY

Synonyms

- Neurilemmoma
- Benign peripheral nerve sheath tumor

Definitions

- **Schwannoma**: Benign peripheral nerve sheath tumor showing differentiated Schwann cells
- **Neurofibroma**: Schwann cell tumor with perineurial hybrid cells and intraneural fibroblasts

ETIOLOGY/PATHOGENESIS

Genetic Factors

- Association with neurofibromatosis type 2 (NF2) is limited
- Schwannomatosis: Multiple schwannomas but not affecting hearing or vestibular nerves

CLINICAL ISSUES

Epidemiology

- Incidence
  - Very rare in sinonasal tract
    - < 4% of all schwannomas involve sinonasal tract
  - Neurofibromas are very rare in sinonasal tract
- Age
  - Mean: 5th-6th decades
    - Younger in patients with NF2
- Gender
  - Equal gender distribution

Site

- Ethmoid and maxillary sinuses
  - Involve branches of 5th (trigeminal) cranial nerve or autonomic nervous system
    - Ophthalmic or maxillary branches of 5th nerve
- Less frequently: Nasal cavity, sphenoid and frontal sinuses
- Tend to develop along midline
- Rarely, expands into orbit, nasopharynx, pterygomaxillary fossa, cranial cavity

Presentation

- Nonspecific symptoms
  - Obstruction, swelling/mass, rhinorrhea, epistaxis, anosmia, headache, pain, dysphagia, facial or orbital swelling

Treatment

- Surgical approaches
  - Complete excision is treatment of choice

Prognosis

- Benign tumor with very low recurrence potential
- Malignant transformation is exceptional (although seen in setting of NF1)

IMAGE FINDINGS

Radiographic Findings

- Best study: T1WI MR with contrast and fat suppression, especially images showing branches of 5th cranial nerve
- Sharply and smoothly marginated soft tissue mass

MR Findings

- T1WI: Iso- to **hypointense** mass; hyperintense if hemorrhagic
- T2WI: Iso- to **hyperintense** mass, depending on cellularity and degenerative changes

MACROSCOPIC FEATURES

General Features

- Well-delineated but nonencapsulated polypoid mass
- Globular, firm to rubbery, yellow-tan mass

SCHWANNOMA/NEUROFIBROMA

Key Facts

Terminology

- **Schwannoma**: Benign peripheral nerve sheath tumor showing differentiated Schwann cells
- **Neurofibroma**: Schwann cell tumor with perineurial hybrid cells and intraneural fibroblasts

Clinical Issues

- < 4% of all schwannomas involve sinonasal tract
- Mean: 5th-6th decades
- Ethmoid and maxillary sinuses
- Complete excision is treatment of choice

Image Findings

- Sharply and smoothly marginated soft tissue mass

Macroscopic Features

- Well-delineated, polypoid, globular, firm to rubbery, yellow-tan mass

Microscopic Pathology

- Submucosal mass with intact surface epithelium
- Cellular Antoni A areas blended with hypocellular Antoni B areas
  - Verocay bodies are palisaded nuclear aggregates
- Fusiform cells with fibrillar cytoplasm surrounding spindled, wavy/buckled nuclei
- Medium-sized ectatic vessels with marked hyalinization and sometimes thrombosis

Ancillary Tests

- **S100 protein**: Strong, diffuse, nuclear and cytoplasmic

Top Differential Diagnoses

- Meningioma, leiomyoma, malignant peripheral nerve sheath tumor

---

- Cut surfaces are myxoid and cystic, frequently with hemorrhage

Size

- Range: Up to 7 cm

MICROSCOPIC PATHOLOGY

Schwannoma

- Submucosal mass with intact surface epithelium
- Cellular Antoni A areas blended with hypocellular Antoni B areas
  - Verocay bodies are palisaded nuclear aggregates
- Hypocellular Antoni B areas with microcystic degeneration
  - Loose reticular pattern can be seen
  - Degenerative changes may be quite prominent (histiocytes, cyst formation, hemorrhage)
- Fusiform cells with fibrillar cytoplasm
- Spindled, wavy/buckled nuclei
- Pleomorphism is limited to absent
- Medium-sized ectatic vessels with marked hyalinization and sometimes thrombosis
- Mitoses are rare
- Glandular variant is rare in this location

Neurofibroma

- Paucicellular submucosal mass
- Spindled cells with wavy, dark-staining nuclei and scanty cytoplasm
- Background of wavy collagen fibers, myxoid stroma, and mast cells

ANCILLARY TESTS

Immunohistochemistry

- Positive
  - S100 protein strong, diffuse, nuclear & cytoplasmic
  - Vimentin
  - CD34 focally present in slender cells in Antoni B
  - GFAP and NSE may have focal reaction
- Negative: Neurofilament, keratin, desmin

Molecular Genetics

- Sinonasal schwannoma/neurofibroma are generally not associated with NF1 or NF2

Electron Microscopy

- Schwann cells: Thin, interdigitating cytoplasmic processes, covered by a discrete, continuous basal lamina wrapping long spacing collagen (Luse body)

DIFFERENTIAL DIAGNOSIS

Meningioma

- Whorled architecture, psammoma bodies, intranuclear cytoplasmic inclusions, EMA-positive immunoreactivity

Leiomyoma

- Spindled cells, cigar-shaped nuclei, perinuclear clearing, short fascicles; actin immunoreactivity

Malignant Peripheral Nerve Sheath Tumor

- Greater degree of pleomorphism, necrosis, increased mitoses, destructive growth, S100 protein is often decreased or limited
- Includes **Triton** tumor, if rhabdomyoblasts are present

SELECTED REFERENCES

1. Mey KH et al: Sinonasal schwannoma--a clinicopathological analysis of five rare cases. Rhinology. 44(1):46-52, 2006
2. Buob D et al: Schwannoma of the sinonasal tract: a clinicopathologic and immunohistochemical study of 5 cases. Arch Pathol Lab Med. 127(9):1196-9, 2003
3. Kardon DE et al: Sinonasal mucosal malignant melanoma: report of an unusual case mimicking schwannoma. Ann Diagn Pathol. 4(5):303-7, 2000
4. Hasegawa SL et al: Schwannomas of the sinonasal tract and nasopharynx. Mod Pathol. 10(8):777-84, 1997
5. Heffner DK et al: Sinonasal fibrosarcomas, malignant schwannomas, and "Triton" tumors. A clinicopathologic study of 67 cases. Cancer. 70(5):1089-101, 1992

SCHWANNOMA/NEUROFIBROMA

Radiographic and Microscopic Features

*(**Left**) Axial T1WI MR shows a mass ➔ that is hypointense relative to brain and appears sharply marginated from adjacent tissues. Note smooth remodeling of the posterior wall of the right maxillary sinus ➔. This "nondestructive" pattern is characteristic of a benign tumor. (**Right**) Axial T1WI MR with contrast and fat suppression shows the typical appearance of a hemorrhagic masticator space schwannoma. The mass enhances homogeneously and intensely ➔.*

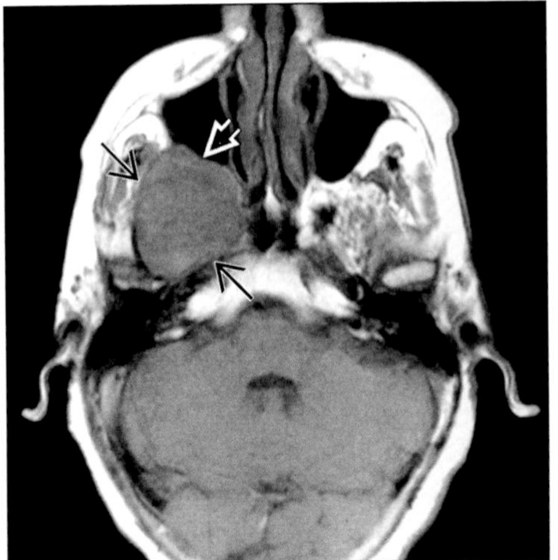

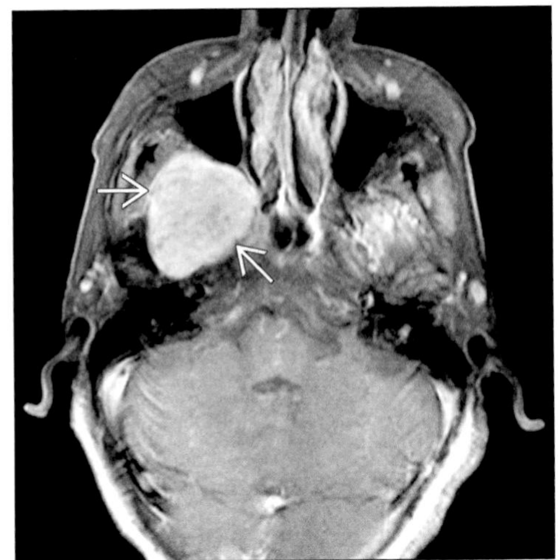

*(**Left**) This polypoid tumor shows a submucosal mass with an intact surface epithelium. Obviously, the exact tumor type cannot be determined from this magnification, although hyper- and hypocellular areas can be seen. (**Right**) The surface epithelium is intact ➔, with a submucosal proliferation of spindled neoplastic cells. They are arranged in long, sweeping fascicles, which expand into the subepithelial stroma.*

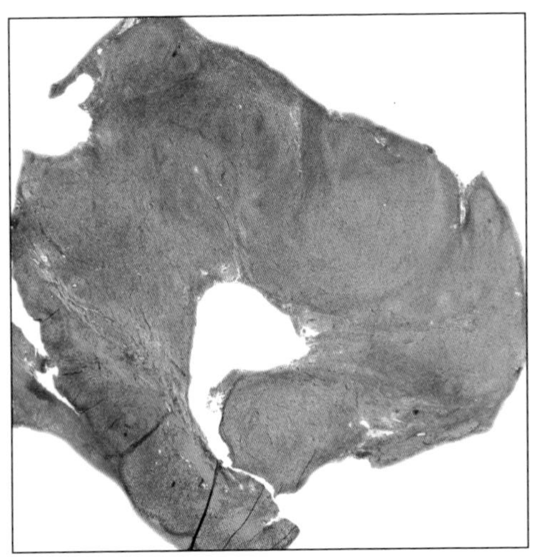

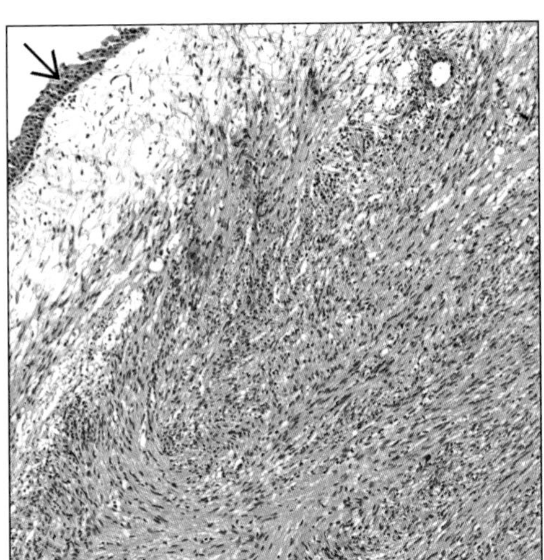

*(**Left**) The cellularity of tumors can be quite variable. In this field, the tumor is overall hypocellular, although areas of increased cellularity are still present. This is a typical schwannoma. (**Right**) This is a cellular Antoni A area, showing palisading and lined up nuclei. The cytoplasm is eosinophilic and fibrillar, surrounding spindled, buckled nuclei. There is no cytologic atypia.*

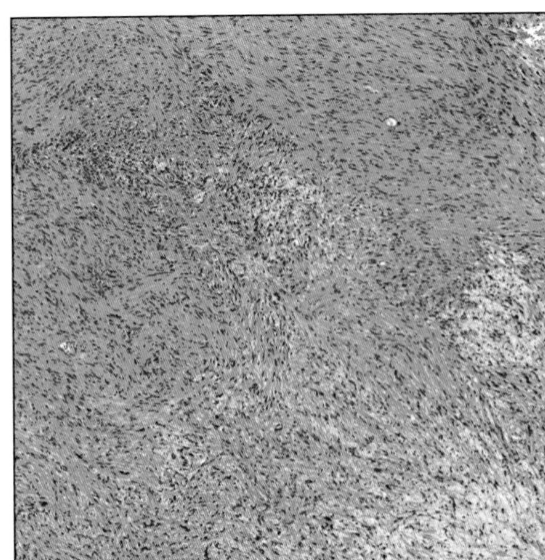

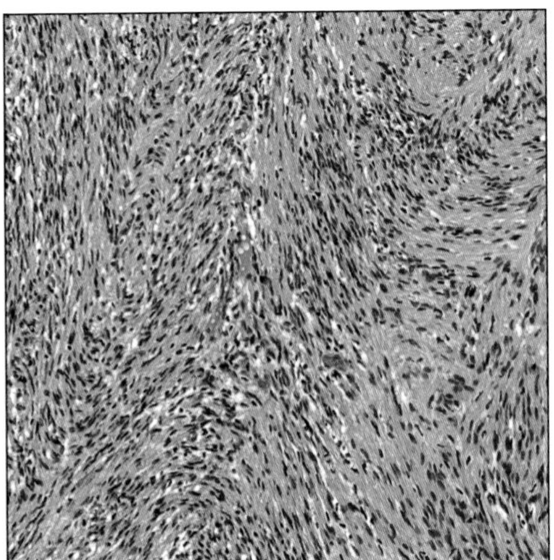

Microscopic and Immunohistochemical Features

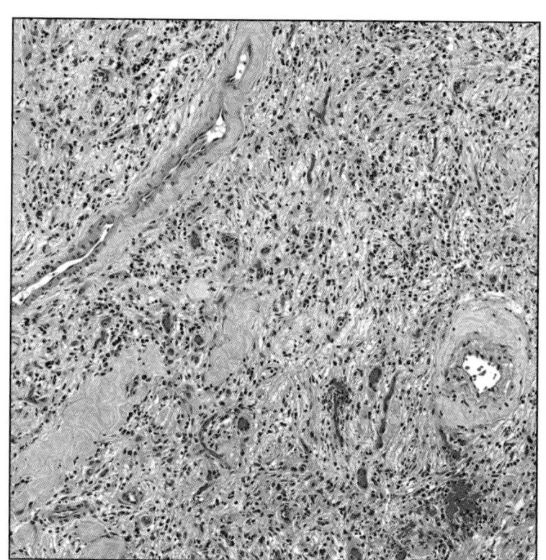

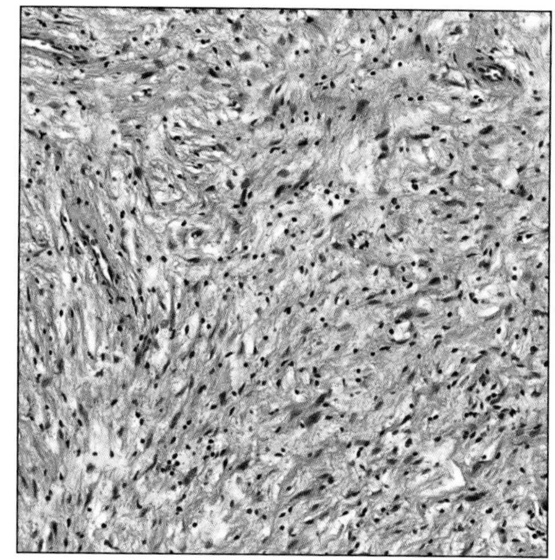

(Left) *This is a hypocellular Antoni B area in which there are well-developed, medium-sized ectatic vessels with marked hyalinization of the wall.* ***(Right)*** *In some hypocellular areas, a more loose stroma is appreciated. However, the fusiform cells with fibrillar cytoplasm are still present throughout. There is limited to absent nuclear pleomorphism. Cystic spaces, although not visible here, can be seen in some tumors.*

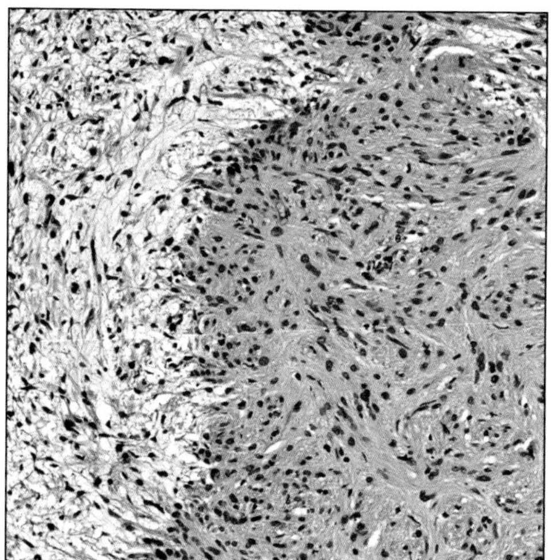

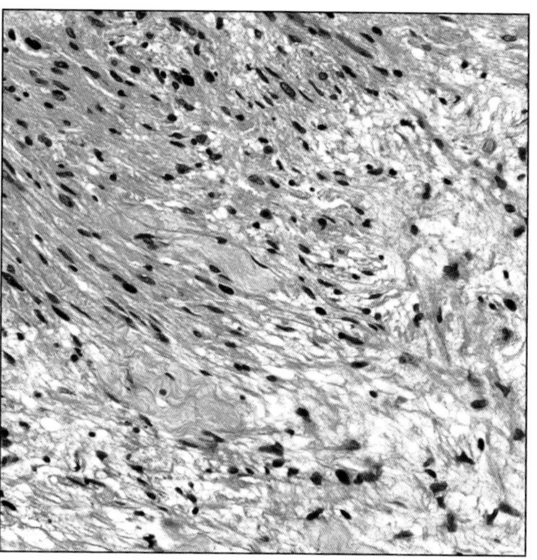

(Left) *The separation between a cellular Antoni A and hypocellular Antoni B area can sometimes be quite abrupt. In this example, the hypocellular area still has many nuclei, but it does not have the same number as the Antoni A areas, nor are palisades present.* ***(Right)*** *The fusiform, spindled neoplastic cells have a fibrillar cytoplasm surrounding hyperchromatic buckled or wavy nuclei. This zone blends into an area of lesser cellularity (Antoni B).*

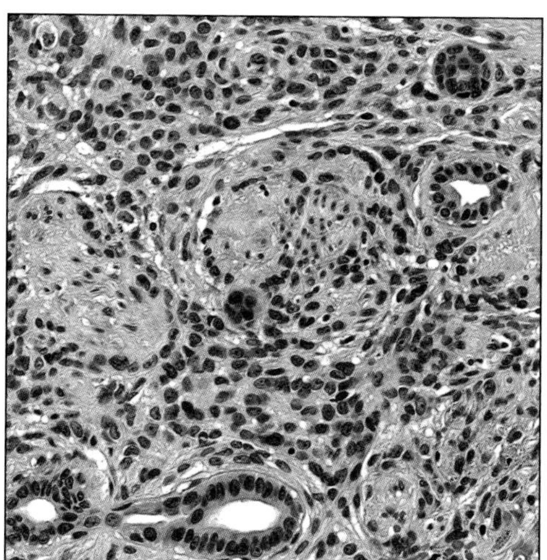

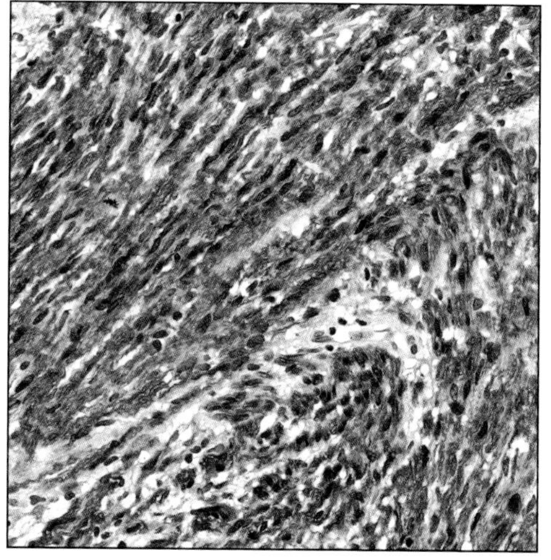

(Left) *A glandular variant is very rare, composed of glandular profiles set intimately within the spindle cell, fusiform Antoni A area. Separation of native serous gland entrapment from glands that are part of the tumor is challenging.* ***(Right)*** *The neoplastic cells of a schwannoma are strongly and diffusely positive in both the nucleus and cytoplasm with S100 protein. A similar strong reaction can be seen in the cytoplasm with vimentin.*

LEIOMYOMA & SMOOTH MUSCLE TUMORS OF UNCERTAIN MALIGNANT POTENTIAL

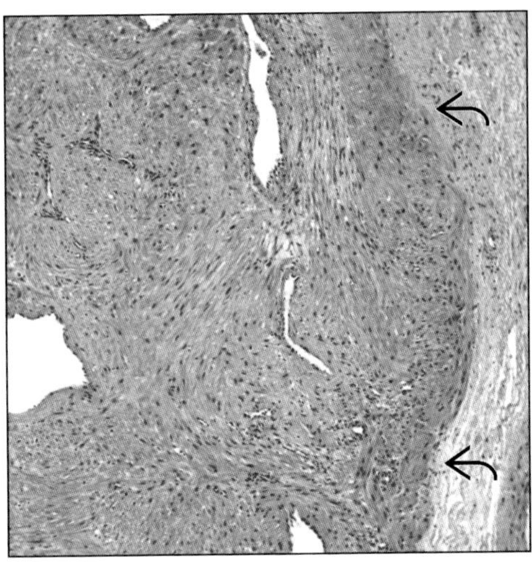

Circumscribed to delineated ➢ spindle cell proliferation shows fascicular growth composed of interlacing bundles with associated prominent vascular spaces.

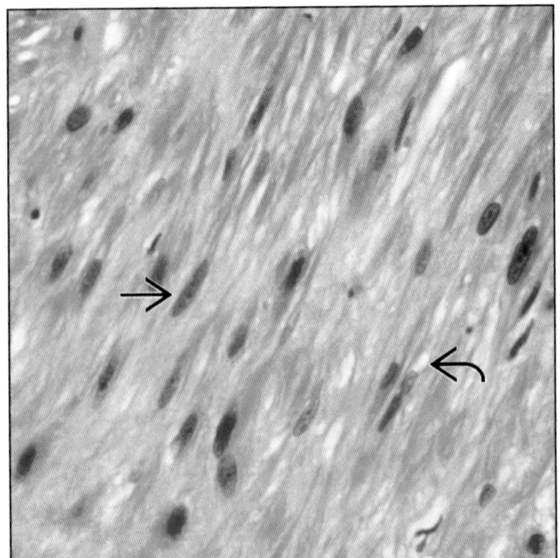

The cellular component consists of cells with blunt-ended or cigar-shaped nuclei ➔, abundant eosinophilic cytoplasm, and perinuclear vacuolization ➢.

TERMINOLOGY

Abbreviations

- Smooth muscle tumor of uncertain malignant potential (SMTUMP)

Synonyms

- Vascular leiomyoma

Definitions

- Benign tumor of smooth muscle

ETIOLOGY/PATHOGENESIS

Idiopathic

- No known etiologic factors

CLINICAL ISSUES

Epidemiology

- Incidence
  - One of least common mesenchymal tumors in head and neck mucosal sites
    - Relative paucity of smooth muscle in region other than related to blood vessels
    - Thought to originate from smooth muscle within vascular structures (vascular leiomyoma)
- Age
  - All ages but generally tumor of adult life
    - Peak incidence in 6th decade
- Gender
  - Male > Female

Site

- Most common sites of occurrence in head and neck include
  - Skin
  - Oral cavity (lips, tongue, and palate)
  - Sinonasal tract
    - Most often involves turbinates

Presentation

- Painless mass, nasal obstruction
- Other symptoms include dysphagia, voice changes, pain

Treatment

- Surgical approaches
  - Complete surgical excision is curative

Prognosis

- Excellent
- Rarely recur

IMAGE FINDINGS

Radiographic Findings

- CT, MR show well-defined, homogeneous, expansile mass without bony erosion

MACROSCOPIC FEATURES

General Features

- Solitary, well-demarcated, sessile, tan-white submucosal lesion
- On cut section, appears homogeneous with whorled appearance

Size

- Usually measures < 3 cm in diameter
- May attain larger sizes

MICROSCOPIC PATHOLOGY

Histologic Features

- Localized to submucosa, appears delineated, characterized by presence of interlacing bundles or fascicles of cells

LEIOMYOMA & SMOOTH MUSCLE TUMORS OF UNCERTAIN MALIGNANT POTENTIAL

Key Facts

Clinical Issues
- Benign tumor of smooth muscle
- One of least common mesenchymal tumors in head and neck mucosal sites
- Presentation includes painless mass, nasal obstruction
- Thought to originate from smooth muscle within vascular structures (vascular leiomyoma)

Macroscopic Features
- On cut section, appears homogeneous with whorled appearance

Microscopic Pathology
- Interlacing bundles or fascicles of cells
- Blunt-ended or cigar-shaped nuclei, abundant eosinophilic cytoplasm
- **Cellular leiomyoma**
  - Increase in cells but lacking significant pleomorphism, mitotic activity, necrosis
- **Smooth muscle tumor of uncertain malignant potential**
  - Similar clinical features to leiomyoma
  - Increased cellularity
  - Moderate nuclear pleomorphism
  - Presence of no more than 4 mitoses per 10 HPF
  - Locally infiltrative growth may occur

Ancillary Tests
- Actins, vimentin, desmin positive

Top Differential Diagnoses
- Benign peripheral nerve sheath tumor, solitary fibrous tumor, leiomyosarcoma

  - Blunt-ended or cigar-shaped nuclei with abundant eosinophilic cytoplasm
  - Nuclei may appear epithelioid
- Nuclear palisading, perinuclear vacuolization may be seen
- No significant pleomorphism, mitotic activity, necrosis
- Neoplastic cells seen in intimate association with vascular spaces
- Degenerative-type changes may include stromal fibrosis, mucinous or myxoid alterations
- **Cellular leiomyoma**
  - Characterized by absolute increase in cells lacking significant pleomorphism, mitotic activity, necrosis
- **Smooth muscle tumor of uncertain malignant potential**
  - Similar clinical features to leiomyoma
  - Histologically characterized by
    - Increased cellularity
    - Moderate nuclear pleomorphism
    - Presence of no more than 4 mitoses per 10 HPF
    - Locally infiltrative growth may occur

ANCILLARY TESTS

Histochemistry
- Masson trichrome
  - Cytoplasmic myofibrils appear red
- Phosphotungstic acid-hematoxylin
  - Cytoplasmic myofibrils appear blue

Immunohistochemistry
- Actins (smooth muscle and muscle specific), vimentin, desmin positive
- S100 protein, CD34, CD31 negative
- Low proliferation rate (< 5%) by MIB-1 (Ki-67) staining

Electron Microscopy
- Myofilaments, pinocytotic vesicles, investing basal laminae

DIFFERENTIAL DIAGNOSIS

Benign Peripheral Nerve Sheath Tumors
- Presence of diffuse S100 protein reactivity
- Absent immunoreactivity for actins

Solitary Fibrous Tumor
- Characterized stromal collagenization ("ropey" collagen)
- Perivascular hyalinization, pericytic-type vasculature
- Presence of CD34 immunoreactivity

Leiomyosarcoma
- Increased cellularity with nuclear pleomorphism
- Increased mitotic activity (≥ 5 per HPF)
- Infiltrative growth

SELECTED REFERENCES

1. Yang BT et al: Leiomyoma of the sinonasal cavity: CT and MRI findings. Clin Radiol. 64(12):1203-9, 2009
2. Farah-Klibi F et al: Sinonasal leiomyoma: an exceptional localization. Tunis Med. 86(8):752-4, 2008
3. Agarwal AK et al: Sinonasal leiomyoma: report of 2 cases. Ear Nose Throat J. 84(4):224, 226-30, 2005
4. Bel Haj Salah M et al: Leiomyoma of the nasal cavity. A case report. Pathologica. 97(6):376-7, 2005
5. Huang HY et al: Sinonasal smooth muscle cell tumors: a clinicopathologic and immunohistochemical analysis of 12 cases with emphasis on the low-grade end of the spectrum. Arch Pathol Lab Med. 127(3):297-304, 2003
6. Bloom DC et al: Leiomyoma of the nasal septum. Rhinology. 39(4):233-5, 2001
7. Trott MS et al: Sinonasal leiomyomas. Otolaryngol Head Neck Surg. 111(5):660-4, 1994
8. Fu YS et al: Nonepithelial tumors of the nasal cavity, paranasal sinuses, and nasopharynx: a clinicopathologic study. IV. Smooth muscle tumors (leiomyoma, leiomyosarcoma). Cancer. 35(5):1300-8, 1975

LEIOMYOMA & SMOOTH MUSCLE TUMORS OF UNCERTAIN MALIGNANT POTENTIAL

Gross, Microscopic, and Immunohistochemical Features

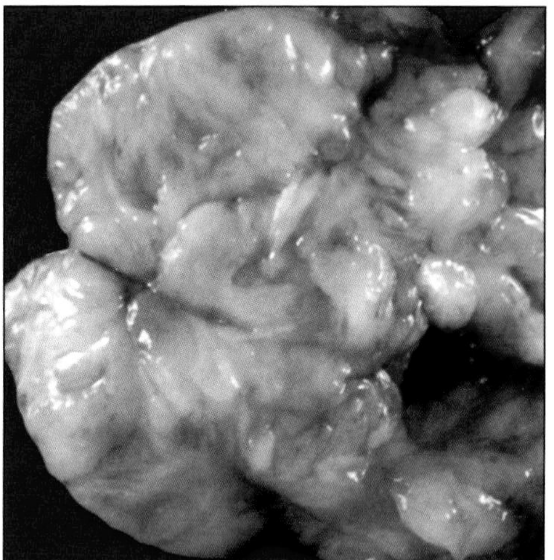

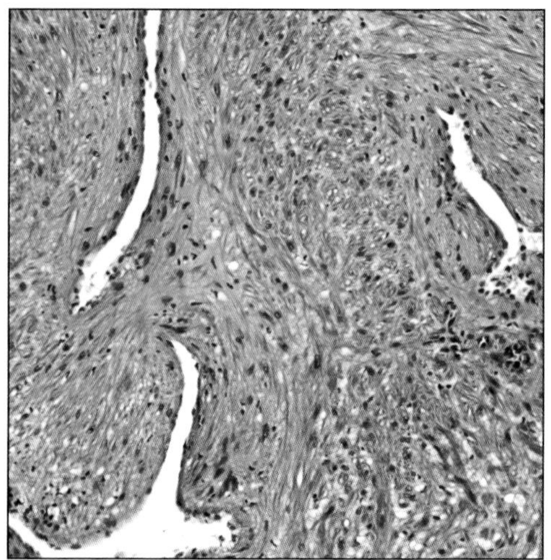

*(**Left**) On cut section, the resected sinonasal leiomyoma shows characteristic macroscopic findings, including a tan-white color and whorled appearance. Histologically, this lesion was noteworthy for the presence of increased cellularity. (**Right**) The neoplastic cells lie in continuity with endothelial-lined blood vessels, supporting the theory that the origin of sinonasal (and other mucosal-based) leiomyomas originate from smooth muscle cells of vascular walls conferring the designation of vascular leiomyoma.*

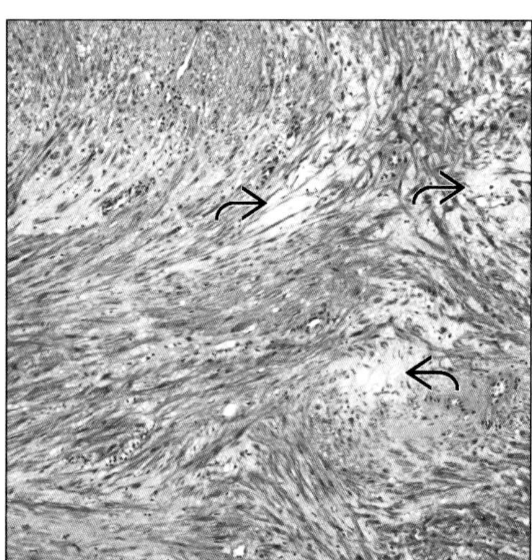

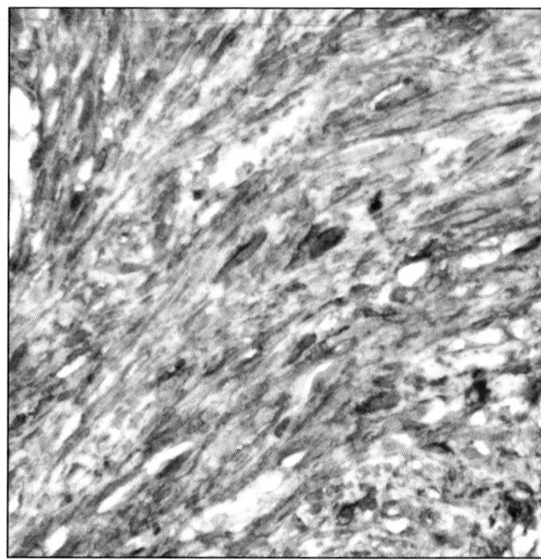

*(**Left**) The neoplastic proliferation shows fascicular growth composed of interlacing cellular bundles. Interspersed between the fascicles are mucinous foci ⮫ representing associated degenerative changes. (**Right**) The myogenic nature of the lesional cells is confirmed by the presence of diffuse and strong reactivity for smooth muscle actin (SMA).*

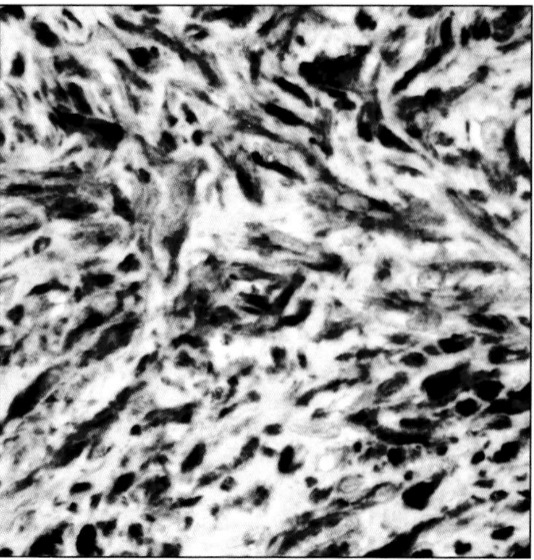

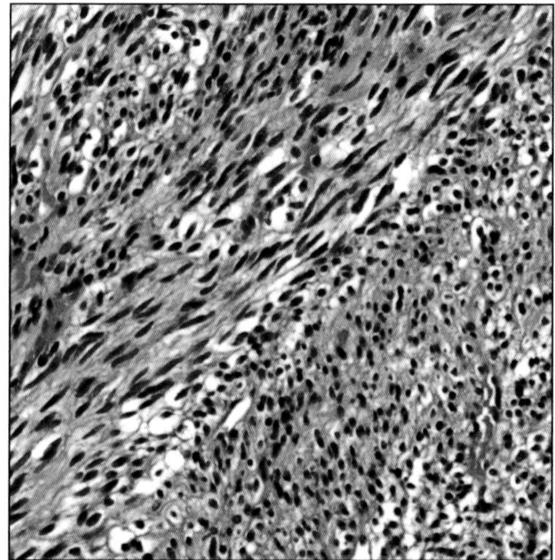

*(**Left**) In addition to actin staining, lesional cells are diffusely reactive for desmin. Light microscopic features coupled with immunoreactivity for myogenic markers allows differentiation from benign peripheral nerve sheath tumors (e.g., schwannoma) and solitary fibrous tumor. (**Right**) In comparison to "conventional" leiomyomas, cellular leiomyomas show increased cellularity. Like "conventional" leiomyomas, there is fascicular growth composed of interlacing bundles of neoplastic cells.*

Microscopic and Immunohistochemical Features

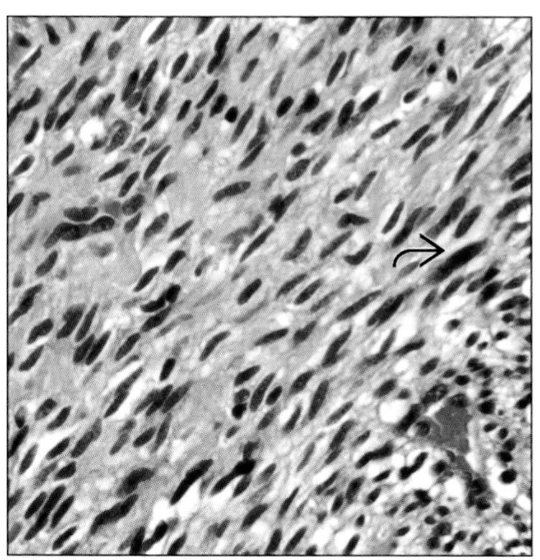
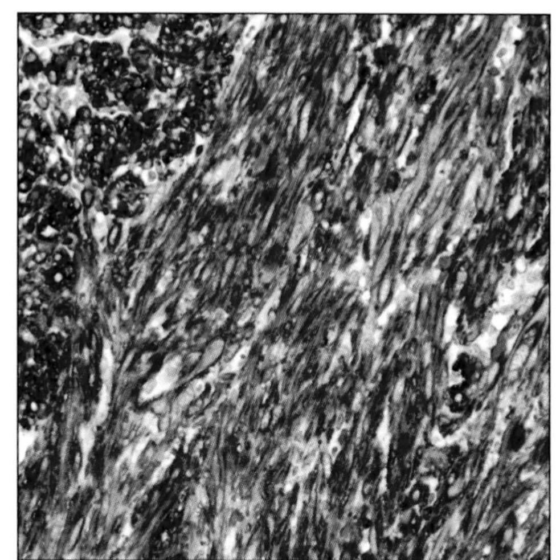

***(Left)** In spite of increased cellularity, there is no significant evidence of nuclear pleomorphism and no increase in mitotic activity. Scattered enlarged hyperchromatic nuclei are seen ➢. **(Right)** There is diffuse and strong immunoreactivity for smooth muscle actin. Other than the increased cellularity, the overall findings are those of a leiomyoma, albeit a cellular one, without evidence to support a diagnosis of a leiomyosarcoma.*

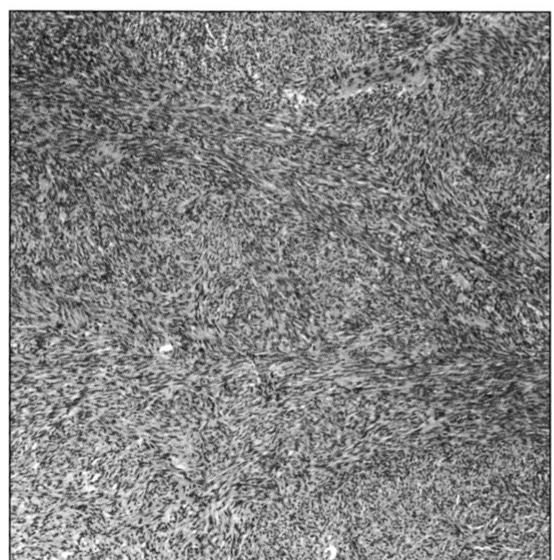
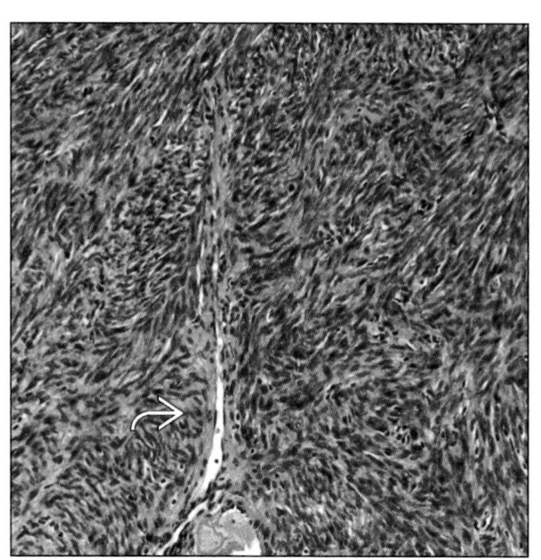

***(Left)** Sinonasal smooth muscle tumor of uncertain malignant potential (SMTUMP) shows fascicular to storiform growth with marked increase in cellularity. This tumor was located in the submucosa and revealed focally infiltrative growth (not shown). **(Right)** Similar to sinonasal leiomyomas, SMTUMPs of the sinonasal tract likely arise from the smooth muscle in the wall of blood vessels, accounting for the intimate association of the neoplasm with sinonasal vessels ➢.*

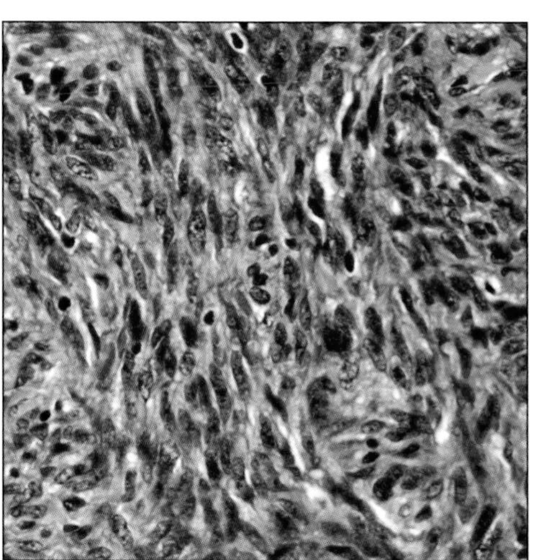
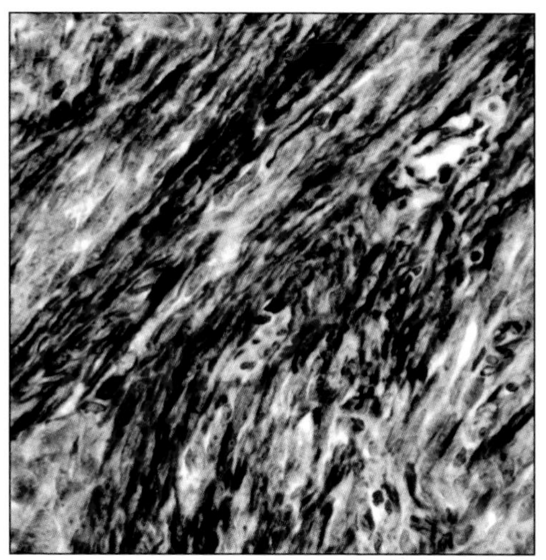

***(Left)** In contrast to cellular leiomyomas, the cellular component of SMTUMP reveals moderate nuclear pleomorphism and increased mitotic activity (not shown), the latter not greater than 4 mitoses per 10 HPF. **(Right)** SMTUMP shows diffuse and strong immunoreactivity for smooth muscle actin. SMTUMP may show locally infiltrative growth, but the absence of significant increase in mitotic activity (≥ 4 mitoses per 10 HPF) allows differentiation from leiomyosarcoma.*

FIBROMATOSIS/DESMOID-TYPE FIBROMATOSIS

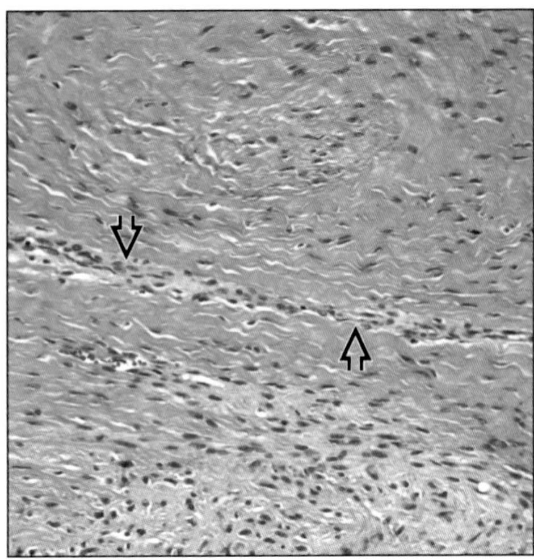

Hematoxylin & eosin shows a parallel arrangement of elongated blood vessels ⊳ to the bland spindle cell population. There is a slight variation in cellularity.

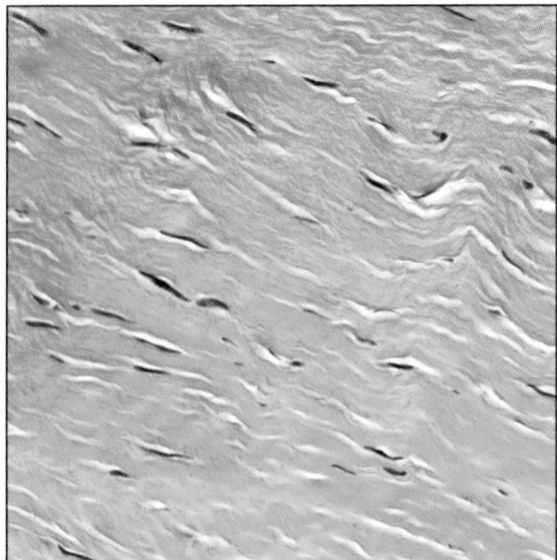

Hematoxylin & eosin shows broad fascicles of bland-looking spindle cells arranged in the same direction. Note the very heavy collagen deposition. There are usually no mitotic figures or pleomorphism.

TERMINOLOGY

Synonyms

- Desmoid tumor
- Extraabdominal desmoid
- Extraabdominal fibromatosis
- Aggressive fibromatosis
- Juvenile desmoid-type fibromatosis
- Infantile fibromatosis
- Desmoma

Definitions

- Locally aggressive, intermediate type of nonmetastasizing, well-differentiated, unencapsulated myofibroblastic tissue proliferations with a tendency for local invasion and recurrence
  - Intermediate between benign fibrous lesions and fibrosarcoma

ETIOLOGY/PATHOGENESIS

Environmental Exposure

- Hyperestrogenism during pregnancy, trauma, and surgery have been suggested

CLINICAL ISSUES

Epidemiology

- Incidence
  - Uncommon, although approximately 15% of fibromatoses occur in head and neck
- Age
  - All ages affected, though more frequent in young people
    - Mean: 29 years
- Gender
  - Male > Female (2:1)

Site

- Maxillary sinus and turbinates
- Nasal cavity, other paranasal sinuses, and nasopharynx are rarely affected

Presentation

- Nonspecific signs and symptoms
  - Nasal obstruction, epistaxis, mass, facial pain, tooth displacement
- Bilateral disease in about 25%

Treatment

- Surgical approaches
  - Local but complete surgical excision

Prognosis

- Excellent without morbidity of other anatomic sites
- Recurrence/residual disease in about 20% of patients
  - Parapharyngeal tumors may spread to oropharynx, subglottic area, pharynx, and can laterally displace sternocleidomastoid muscle
- No metastases for sinonasal and nasopharynx lesions

IMAGE FINDINGS

General Features

- CT and MR are useful in delineating tumor extent

MACROSCOPIC FEATURES

General Features

- Tan-white, glistening, and rubbery firm mass
- Often infiltrative, although it may be polypoid
- May be multicentric, especially in setting of Gardner syndrome

Size

- Usually small, although nasopharyngeal tumors are larger (up to 7 cm)

FIBROMATOSIS/DESMOID-TYPE FIBROMATOSIS

Key Facts

Terminology
- Locally aggressive, well-differentiated, unencapsulated myofibroblastic tissue proliferations

Clinical Issues
- Male > Female (2:1)
- Young people more frequently afflicted (mean: 29 years old)
- Maxillary sinus and turbinates
- Local but complete surgical excision helps decrease recurrence (20%)

Microscopic Pathology
- Infiltrative growth with low to moderate cellularity
- Broad fascicles of bland-looking myofibroblastic spindle cells arranged in uniform direction with parallel blood vessels
- Vimentin and actins positive

MICROSCOPIC PATHOLOGY

Histologic Features
- Infiltrative growth with low to moderate cellularity
- Broad fascicles of bland-looking spindle cells
- Cells arranged in uniform direction
- Elongated blood vessels are frequently observed running parallel to each other
- Spindle cells have myofibroblastic appearance, with low nuclear to cytoplasmic ratio and uniformly bland ovoid nuclei with indistinct nucleoli
- Mitotic figures are infrequent and never atypical
- Matrix is collagenized to focally myxoid; keloid-like collagen may be present

ANCILLARY TESTS

Immunohistochemistry
- Vimentin and actins positive, desmin focally positive

DIFFERENTIAL DIAGNOSIS

Ossifying Fibroma
- Bony or calcified spicules within cellular stroma

Solitary Fibrous Tumor
- "Wavy" spindle nuclei with "ropy" collagen
- CD34 and Bcl-2 immunoreactive

Hypertrophic Scar
- Heavy collagen deposition with scant cellularity
- No purposeful vessels

Juvenile Ossifying Fibroma (Psammomatous)
- Psammomatoid ossicles of calcification
- No heavy collagen deposition; swirled growth

Glomangiopericytoma
- Cellular with patternless appearance
- Perivascular hyalinization; mast cells and eosinophils

Chondromyxoid Fibroma
- Myxoid or chondroid matrix; fibrous connective tissue

SELECTED REFERENCES

1. Neri HA et al: Ethmoidal desmoid tumor in a pediatric patient. Otolaryngol Head Neck Surg. 136(1):137-8, 2007
2. Eller R et al: Common fibro-osseous lesions of the paranasal sinuses. Otolaryngol Clin North Am. 39(3):585-600, x, 2006
3. Mannan AA et al: Infantile fibromatosis of the nose and paranasal sinuses: report of a rare case and brief review of the literature. Ear Nose Throat J. 83(7):481-4, 2004
4. Gnepp DR et al: Desmoid fibromatosis of the sinonasal tract and nasopharynx. A clinicopathologic study of 25 cases. Cancer. 78(12):2572-9, 1996
5. el-Sayed Y: Fibromatosis of the head and neck. J Laryngol Otol. 106(5):459-62, 1992
6. West CB Jr et al: Nonsurgical treatment of aggressive fibromatosis in the head and neck. Otolaryngol Head Neck Surg. 101(3):338-43, 1989

IMAGE GALLERY

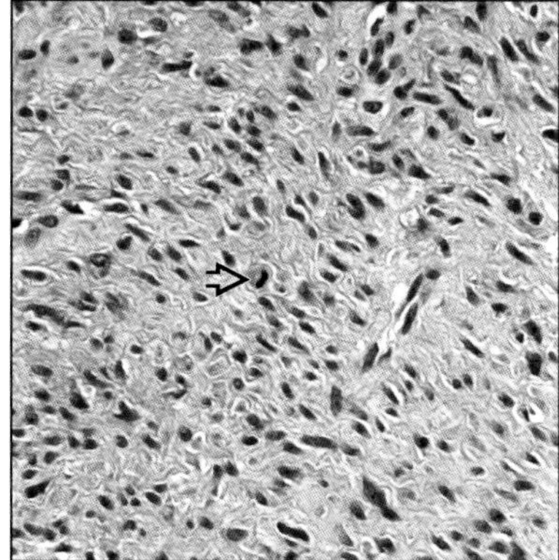

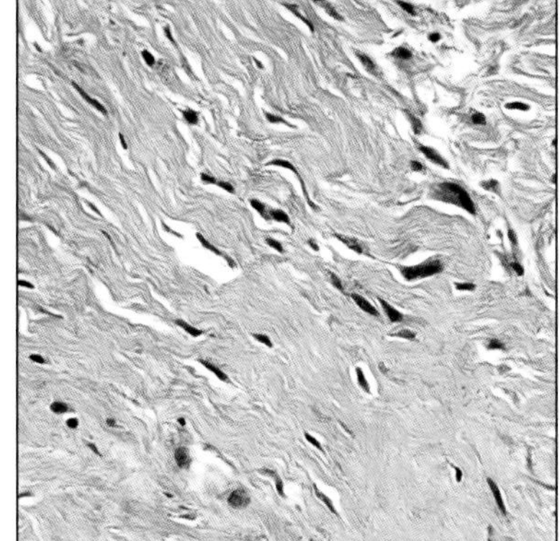

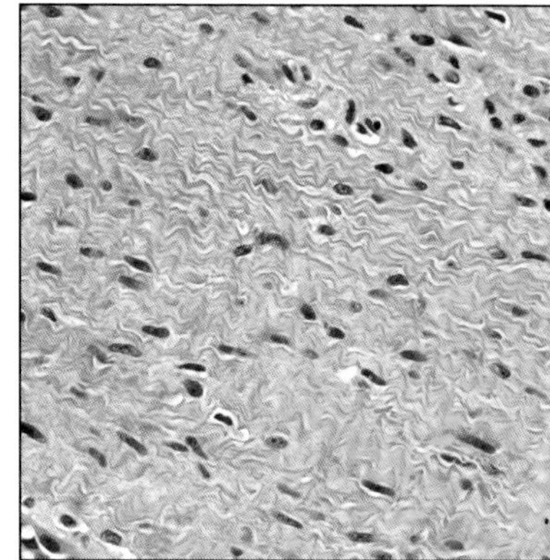

(Left) *The spindle cells have a myofibroblastic appearance, with low nuclear to cytoplasmic ratio and uniformly bland ovoid nuclei. Note the single mitotic figure ⮚, an uncommon finding (it is not atypical).* ***(Center)*** *Bland spindle cells in a heavily collagenized stroma are shown.* ***(Right)*** *Hematoxylin & eosin shows a spindled population set in a collagenized background. The cells are bland cytologically with no nucleoli and even nuclear chromatin distribution.*

SOLITARY FIBROUS TUMOR

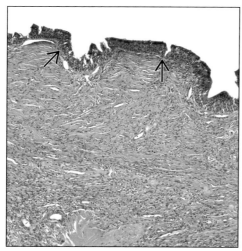

The respiratory epithelium is intact ➔, subtended by a cellular proliferation of a patternless spindle cell population with associated collagen deposition. Small vessels are noted.

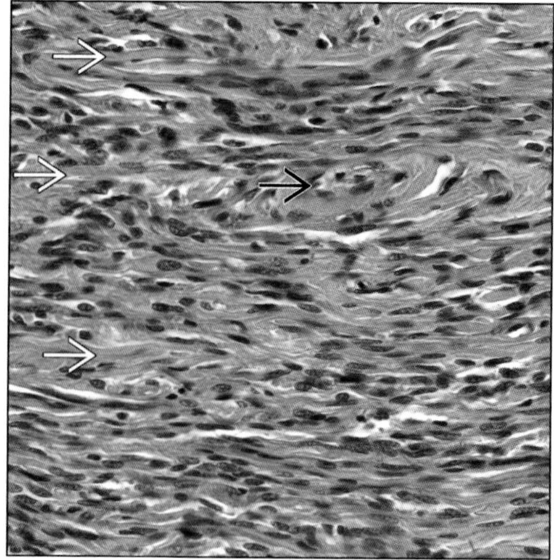

Hematoxylin & eosin shows a spindle cell proliferation arranged in a patternless growth of hypercellular areas with isolated blood vessels ➔. Note the "ropy" eosinophilic ➔ collagen deposition.

TERMINOLOGY

Abbreviations

- Solitary fibrous tumor (SFT)

Synonyms

- Extrapleural solitary fibrous tumor
- Fibrous mesothelioma
- Hemangiopericytoma
  - SFT to hemangiopericytoma is considered morphologic continuum
  - However, this is not the same as **glomangiopericytoma**, considered a unique tumor entity in sinonasal tract

Definitions

- Mesenchymal tumor of probable fibroblastic type identical to pleural SFTs
  - Previously called hemangiopericytoma (although not in sinonasal tract)

CLINICAL ISSUES

Epidemiology

- Incidence
  - Very rare (< 50 reported cases)
  - Comprise < 0.1% of all neoplasms of sinonasal tract
- Age
  - Median: 50 years old
  - Range: 20-80 years old
  - Rare in children and adolescents
- Gender
  - Equal gender distribution

Site

- Anywhere in sinonasal tract
  - Orbit (direct extension from meninges) > maxillary sinus > sphenoid-ethmoid sinuses > nasal cavity (direct extension from sinuses) > oral cavity > nasopharynx

Presentation

- Painless, unilateral, slow-growing mass
- Obstructive symptoms
- Epistaxis and rhinorrhea
- Nonspecific findings are common (headaches)
- Paraneoplastic syndrome (hypoglycemia due to secretion of insulin-like growth factor) has been reported

Treatment

- Surgical approaches
  - Complete but conservative local excision yields best patient outcome
    - Endoscopic sinus surgery can work well (monobloc excision)
    - Clear surgical margins reduces recurrence risk

Prognosis

- Overall, excellent long-term prognosis
- Although most cases are benign, behavior is unpredictable and often not predicated on histologic parameters
  - Therefore, long-term clinical follow-up is advocated
- Infrequently, recurrences will develop (< 10%)
- Rare cases (< 2%) may have malignant behavior
  - Based on increased tumor size, atypical mitotic figures, necrosis
  - If metastases develop, lungs, bone, and liver are most frequently affected

IMAGE FINDINGS

General Features

- Most tumors are well delineated
- Computed tomography images show well-circumscribed tumors that strongly enhance with contrast
- Most tumors are hypointense on T2-weighted MR images but may be isointense

SOLITARY FIBROUS TUMOR

Key Facts

Terminology

- Mesenchymal tumor of probable fibroblastic type identical to pleural SFTs

Clinical Issues

- Median age: 50 years old
- Painless, unilateral, slow-growing mass with obstructive symptoms
- Complete but conservative local excision yields best patient outcome
- Excellent long-term prognosis

Macroscopic Features

- Usually polypoid and firm
- Multinodular, whitish cut surface, although myxoid and hemorrhagic areas can be observed

Microscopic Pathology

- Requires combination of architectural, cytomorphologic, and immunophenotypic features as diagnosis of exclusion
- Proliferation of bland, blunt spindle-shaped cells in patternless growth of alternating hypo- and hypercellular areas
- Cells are separated by thick bands of "ropy" keloidal collagen bundles

Ancillary Tests

- CD34, Bcl-2, and CD99 immunoreactive

Top Differential Diagnoses

- Sinonasal glomangiopericytoma
- Fibrosarcoma and schwannoma

- Tumors show enhancement with gadolinium contrast on T1-weighted images
- Reactive remodeling of bone may be seen

MACROSCOPIC FEATURES

General Features

- Usually polypoid and firm
- Well circumscribed but partially encapsulated
- Multinodular, whitish cut surface, although myxoid and hemorrhagic areas can be observed
- Malignant tumors tend to be locally infiltrative and may have necrosis

Size

- Mean: 2.5 cm
  - Size may be constrained due to anatomic confines
- Range: 1-6 cm

MICROSCOPIC PATHOLOGY

Histologic Features

- Diagnosis rests on combination of architectural, cytomorphologic, and immunophenotypic features
- Separated into benign and malignant forms
- Diagnosis of exclusion in many instances
  - Tumors lack features characteristic of other primary tumors of region
- Nonencapsulated mass below intact, uninvolved respiratory epithelium
- Patternless growth of variably cellular, alternating hypo- and hypercellular areas
  - Hemangiopericytoma-like vascular pattern can be seen
- Proliferation of bland, blunt, spindle-shaped cells, often syncytial in appearance
- Round to spindle-shaped cells with indistinct borders can be seen
- Cells are separated by thick bands of "ropy" keloidal or hyalinized collagen bundles
- Neoplastic cells are intersected by thin-walled vascular spaces
  - Vessels are sometimes patulous or hemangiopericytoma-like
- Myxoid change, areas of fibrosis, and interstitial mast cells may be present
- Mitoses are uncommon
- Fat deposition and giant cells are exceedingly uncommon in sinonasal tract cases
- Malignant SFT is very rare
  - Infiltrative borders, high cellularity, pleomorphism, tumor necrosis, increased mitotic figures

Margins

- Positive margins tend to be associated with recurrences

ANCILLARY TESTS

Immunohistochemistry

- Characteristically, CD34, Bcl-2, and CD99 immunoreactive

Flow Cytometry

- Most tumors are diploid, but seldom evaluated

Cytogenetics

- Cytogenetics are heterogeneous, but abnormalities tend to increase in larger tumors (uncommon in sinonasal tract)

Electron Microscopy

- Primitive myofibroblastic or fibroblast-like cells
- Ultrastructural features are usually nonspecific in SFT

DIFFERENTIAL DIAGNOSIS

Sinonasal Glomangiopericytoma

- Formerly, **sinonasal type hemangiopericytoma**
- Ovoid cells in syncytium
- Vessels are prominent, often patulous, and seen throughout
- Perivascular hyalinization nearly pathognomonic

SOLITARY FIBROUS TUMOR

Immunohistochemistry

Antibody	Reactivity	Staining Pattern	Comment
CD34	Positive	Cytoplasmic	Strong and diffuse in neoplastic cells
Bcl-2	Positive	Cytoplasmic	Strong in most neoplastic cells
CD99	Positive	Cytoplasmic	Many tumor cells will be positive
Vimentin	Positive	Cytoplasmic	Strong and diffuse in neoplastic cells
Actin-sm	Positive	Cytoplasmic	Weak, < 25% of cells reactive
Actin-HHF-35	Positive	Cytoplasmic	Isolated, rare cells may be positive
EMA	Positive	Cell membrane & cytoplasm	Weak, < 25% of cells reactive
GFAP	Positive	Cytoplasmic	Isolated, rare cells may be positive
Ki-67	Positive	Nuclear	< 3-5% of nuclei
CK-PAN	Negative		
S100	Negative		
HBME-1	Negative		

- Eosinophils, mast cells, and extravasated erythrocytes
- Strong SMA and MSA immunoreactivity
- Negative with CD34, Bcl-2, and CD99

Fibrosarcoma

- Highly cellular
- Tumor cells arranged in short, interlacing fascicles
- Mitotic figures are easily identified
- Strongly and diffusely positive with only vimentin

Schwannoma

- Alternating hyper- and hypocellular areas with palisading
  - Antoni A areas are more common in sinonasal tumors
- Wavy nuclei with elongated nuclear extensions
- Lacks keloid-like collagen deposition
- Vascular hyalinization can be seen, usually in Antoni B areas
- Strongly and diffusely immunoreactive with S100 protein
- Negative with CD34, Bcl-2, and SMA

Synovial Sarcoma

- Frequently biphasic tumor
- Highly cellular, arranged in short interlacing fascicles
- Glandular profiles may be seen in biphasic type
- Strong epithelial immunoreactivity (EMA, keratin)
- Characteristic and unique cytogenetics: t(X;18)(p11.2; q11.2) translocation resulting in *SYT-SSX* fusion transcript

Fibrous Histiocytoma

- Haphazard, storiform proliferation of fibroblastic cells with histiocytes

Leiomyoma

- Rare in sinonasal tract
- Cellular tumors with short interlacing fascicles of blunt spindled cells with spindle nuclei
- Positive with SMA, MSA, and desmin
- Negative with CD34

SELECTED REFERENCES

1. Kodama S et al: Solitary fibrous tumor in the maxillary sinus treated by endoscopic medial maxillectomy. Auris Nasus Larynx. 36(1):100-3, 2009
2. Furze AD et al: Pathology case quiz 2. Solitary fibrous tumor of the nasal cavity and ethmoid sinus with intracranial extension. Arch Otolaryngol Head Neck Surg. 134(3):334, 336-7, 2008
3. Smith LM et al: Solitary fibrous tumor of the maxillary sinus. Ear Nose Throat J. 86(7):382-3, 2007
4. Zeitler DM et al: Malignant solitary fibrous tumor of the nasal cavity. Skull Base. 17(4):239-46, 2007
5. Eloy PH et al: Endonasal endoscopic resection of an ethmoidal solitary fibrous tumor. Eur Arch Otorhinolaryngol. 263(9):833-7, 2006
6. Ganly I et al: Solitary fibrous tumors of the head and neck: a clinicopathologic and radiologic review. Arch Otolaryngol Head Neck Surg. 132(5):517-25, 2006
7. Morales-Cadena M et al: Solitary fibrous tumor of the nasal cavity and paranasal sinuses. Otolaryngol Head Neck Surg. 135(6):980-2, 2006
8. Abe T et al: Solitary fibrous tumor arising in the sphenoethmoidal recess: a case report and review of the literature. Auris Nasus Larynx. 32(3):285-9, 2005
9. Alobid I et al: Solitary fibrous tumour of the nasal cavity and paranasal sinuses. Acta Otolaryngol. 123(1):71-4, 2003
10. Cassarino DS et al: Widely invasive solitary fibrous tumor of the sphenoid sinus, cavernous sinus, and pituitary fossa. Ann Diagn Pathol. 7(3):169-73, 2003
11. Konstantinidis I et al: A rare case of solitary fibrous tumor of the nasal cavity. Auris Nasus Larynx. 30(3):303-5, 2003
12. Kessler A et al: Solitary fibrous tumor of the nasal cavity. Otolaryngol Head Neck Surg. 121(6):826-8, 1999
13. Kohmura T et al: Solitary fibrous tumor of the paranasal sinuses. Eur Arch Otorhinolaryngol. 256(5):233-6, 1999
14. Kim TA et al: Solitary fibrous tumor of the paranasal sinuses: CT and MR appearance. AJNR Am J Neuroradiol. 17(9):1767-72, 1996
15. Fukunaga M et al: Solitary fibrous tumor of the nasal cavity and orbit. Pathol Int. 45(12):952-7, 1995
16. Batsakis JG et al: Solitary fibrous tumor. Ann Otol Rhinol Laryngol. 102(1 Pt 1):74-6, 1993
17. Witkin GB et al: Solitary fibrous tumor of the upper respiratory tract. A report of six cases. Am J Surg Pathol. 15(9):842-8, 1991
18. Zukerberg LR et al: Solitary fibrous tumor of the nasal cavity and paranasal sinuses. Am J Surg Pathol. 15(2):126-30, 1991

Microscopic and Immunohistochemical Features

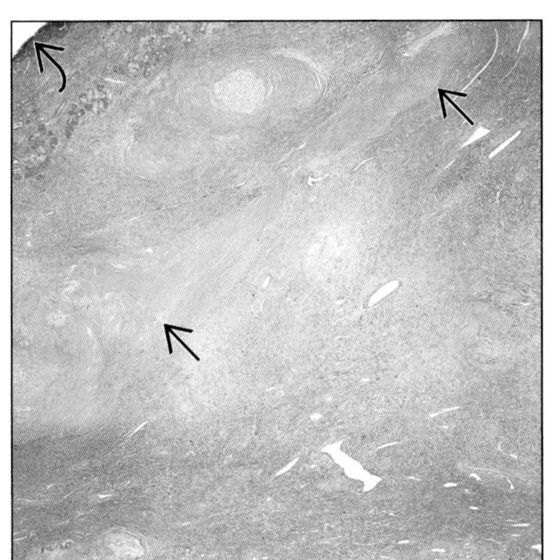

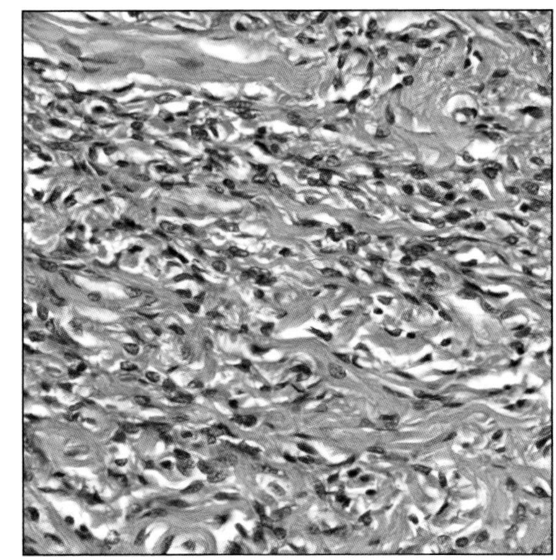

(Left) *There is intact surface epithelium ⮫ overlying the mesenchymal neoplasm. Collagen is deposited, although in this case, a heavier deposition → is noted due to previous biopsy site changes. There is a syncytium of cells without a specific pattern.* ***(Right)*** *Cells are separated by thick bands of "ropy" keloidal collagen bundles, brightly eosinophilic with hematoxylin and eosin stain. There is a "waviness" to the proliferation, with elongated, blunt spindle-shaped nuclei.*

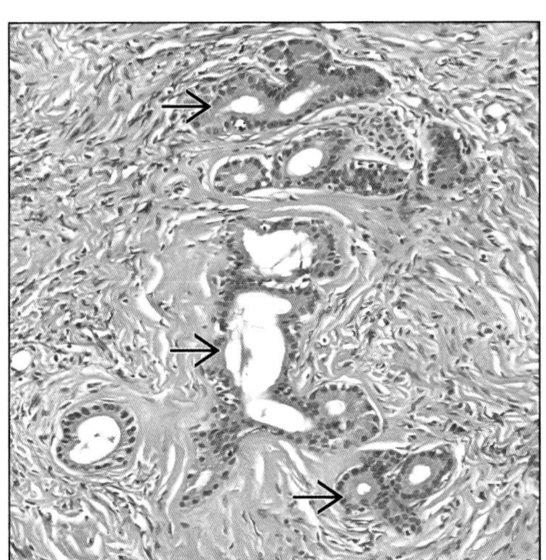

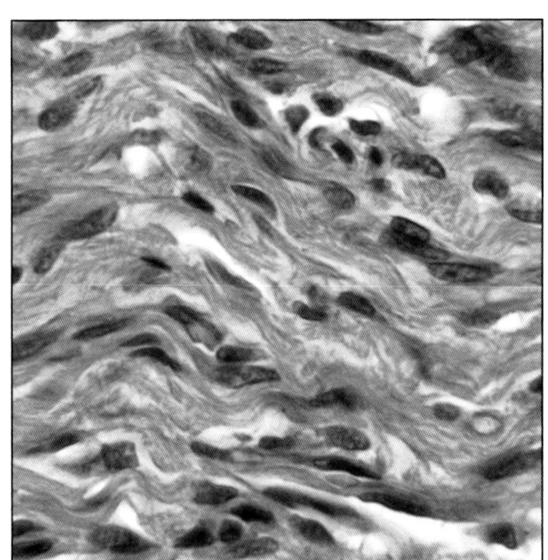

(Left) *Hematoxylin & eosin demonstrates entrapment of the minor mucoserous glands →. The proliferation surrounds these glands but does not destroy them. There is a haphazard distribution to the proliferation, with heavy keloid-like collagen deposition.* ***(Right)*** *This high magnification shows bland spindle cells with slightly wavy, spindle-shaped nuclei. There is wiry, keloid-like collagen deposition. There are isolated inflammatory cells.*

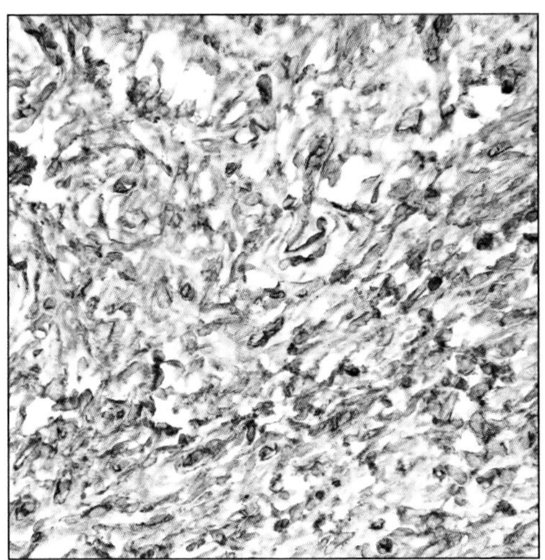

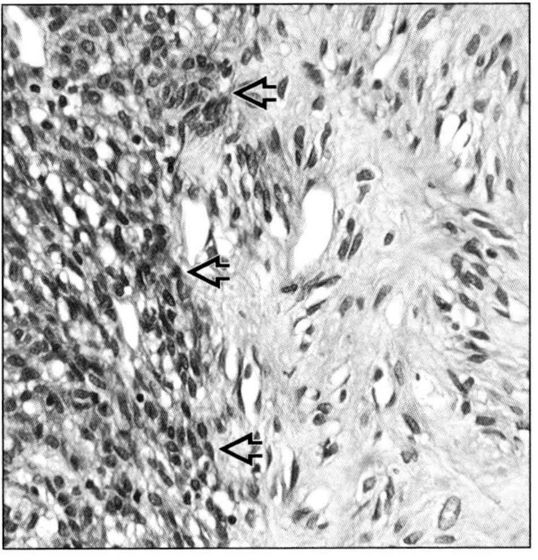

(Left) *CD34 shows strong and diffuse positive immunoreactivity with nearly all of the spindle cells in a solitary fibrous tumor. Bcl-2 and CD99 will often give the same type of reaction.* ***(Right)*** *This is an example of a collision tumor. The left side highlights the findings of a glomangiopericytoma ⇨ with a high cellularity and a lack of collagen deposition, while the right side shows the characteristic findings of a solitary fibrous tumor. Collision tumors are rare.*

MYXOMA/FIBROMYXOMA

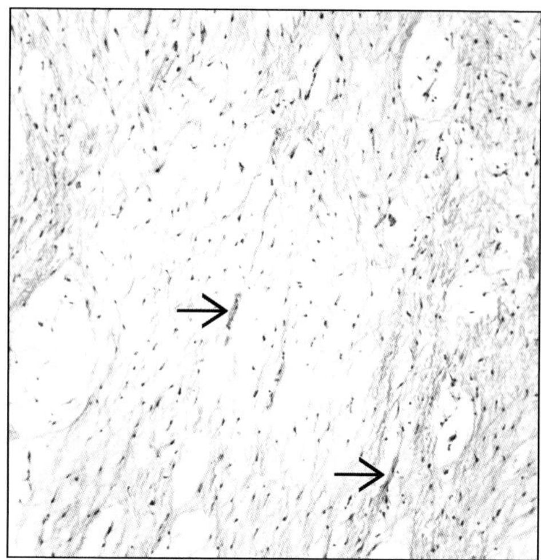

Sinonasal myxoma is seen with predominant myxoid stroma and a relatively hypocellular spindle-shaped cellular proliferation. The vascular component is scant but identifiable ⇨.

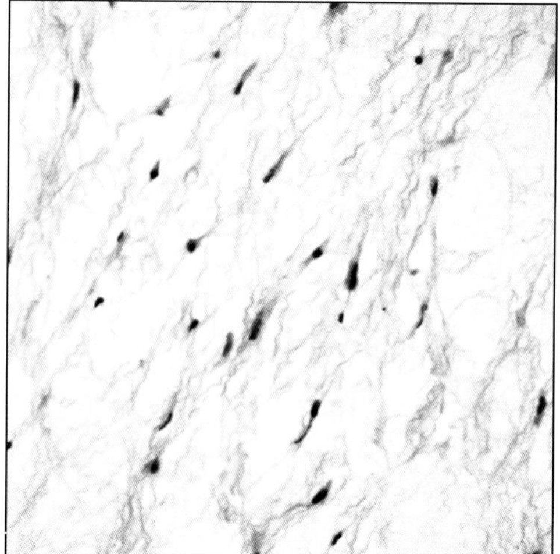

Loosely cellular proliferation consisting of spindle-shaped or stellate-appearing cells in a mucinous or myxomatous stroma lacking significant nuclear pleomorphism and presence of arborizing vessels is shown.

TERMINOLOGY

Definitions

- Benign neoplasm of uncertain histogenesis characterized by bland-appearing spindle to stellate cells set in a myxoid to fibromyxoid stroma
  - 2 forms identified in head and neck
    - Facial skeletal-derived
    - Soft tissue derived

ETIOLOGY/PATHOGENESIS

Idiopathic

- No known etiologic factors

Developmental

- Localization to jaw bones suggests origin from primordial odontogenic mesenchyme or osteogenic embryonic connective tissue
- Sinonasal tract tumors appear to be of osseous derivation

CLINICAL ISSUES

Epidemiology

- Incidence
  - Rare
- Age
  - Occurs over wide age range
    - Most frequent in 2nd and 3rd decades of life
- Gender
  - Equal gender distribution

Site

- **Facial skeleton derived**
- Gnathic sites
  - More common than extragnathic sites
  - Mandible > maxilla
    - Mandible most common in posterior and condylar regions
    - Maxilla most common in zygomatic process and alveolar bone
- Extragnathic tumors
  - Primarily involve sinonasal tract
    - Maxillary sinus (antrum) most often involved with secondary extension into nasal cavity
    - Extension to orbit and cranial cavity may occur
- **Soft tissue derived**
  - In head and neck
    - Common sites include paraoral soft tissues, pharynx, larynx, parotid gland, tonsil/ear
    - Myxomas of ear associated with Carney complex
  - Association between soft tissue myxomas and fibrous dysplasia noted
    - Referred as Mazabraud syndrome
    - Multiple myxomas present
    - Tend to be intramuscular
    - Majority have polyostotic fibrous dysplasia
    - Patients may suffer from Albright syndrome

Presentation

- Painless swelling of affected area

Treatment

- Surgical approaches
  - Wide local excision treatment of choice

Prognosis

- Slow growing, usually follows benign course
  - Potential for local recurrence with destructive growth following inadequate excision
- Presence of metastasis should seriously question benign diagnosis; probably represents sarcoma

MACROSCOPIC FEATURES

General Features

- Delineated but unencapsulated

MYXOMA/FIBROMYXOMA

Key Facts

Terminology

- Benign neoplasm of uncertain histogenesis characterized by bland appearing spindle to stellate cells set in a myxoid to fibromyxoid stroma

Clinical Issues

- Gnathic sites more common than extragnathic sites
  - Mandible > maxilla
- Extragnathic tumors primarily involve sinonasal tract
- Slow-growing, usually follows benign course
- Locally recur following inadequate excision
  - May show invasive growth

Microscopic Pathology

- Scant, loosely cellular proliferation consisting of spindle-shaped or stellate-appearing cells embedded in abundant mucinous stroma
- Vascular component present but limited in extent
  - Absence of delicate vascular capillary vasculature

- Multinodular, rubbery to firm
- Tan-yellow with gelatinous appearance

MICROSCOPIC PATHOLOGY

Histologic Features

- Histology is same, irrespective of site/setting of occurrence
  - Scant, loosely cellular proliferation of spindle-shaped or stellate-appearing cells embedded in abundant mucinous stroma
  - Small, hyperchromatic nuclei
  - Cellular pleomorphism, mitotic figures, and necrosis are absent
  - Amount of collagenous fibrillary stroma may vary
    - Depending on extent, may confer term fibromyxoma
  - Periphery appears circumscribed, but local infiltration may be present
- Vascular component present but limited in extent
  - Absence of delicate vascular capillary vasculature
- Intraoral lesions may include odontogenic epithelium
- Paucity of inflammatory cells

ANCILLARY TESTS

Histochemistry

- Mucinous stroma stains positive for acid mucopolysaccharides
- In general, special stains are of limited diagnostic utility

DIFFERENTIAL DIAGNOSIS

Sinonasal Inflammatory Polyps

- Abundant mixed inflammatory cells
- Edematous rather than mucinous stromal changes

Sarcomas with Myxoid Component

- Increased cellularity, pleomorphism, presence of delicate arborizing vasculature

DIAGNOSTIC CHECKLIST

Clinically Relevant Pathologic Features

- Metastatic distribution
  - Presence of metastasis even with "benign" histology likely indicative of sarcoma

SELECTED REFERENCES

1. Andrews T et al: Myxomas of the head and neck. Am J Otolaryngol. 21(3):184-9, 2000
2. Evans HL: Low-grade fibromyxoid sarcoma. A report of 12 cases. Am J Surg Pathol. 17(6):595-600, 1993
3. Heffner DK: Sinonasal myxomas and fibromyxomas in children. Ear Nose Throat J. 72(5):365-8, 1993
4. Fu YS et al: Non-epithelial tumors of the nasal cavity, paranasal sinuses and nasopharynx: a clinico-pathologic study. VII. Myxomas. Cancer. 39(1):195-203, 1977

IMAGE GALLERY

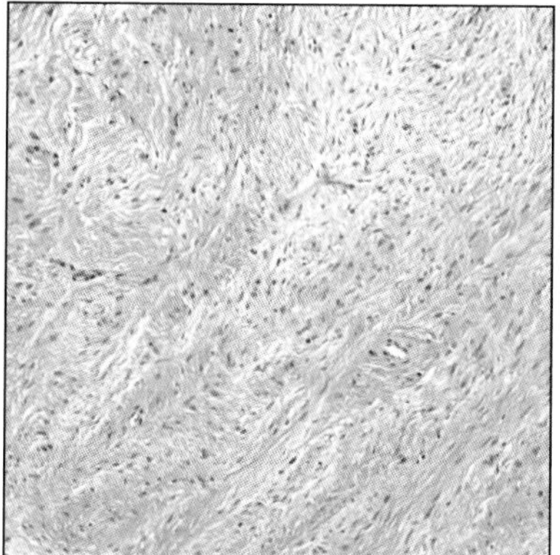

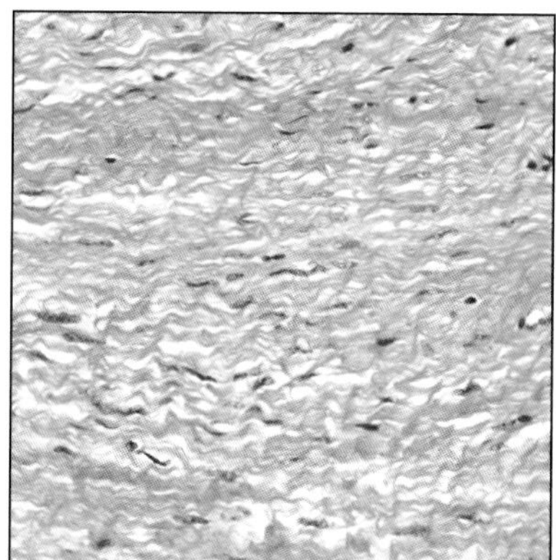

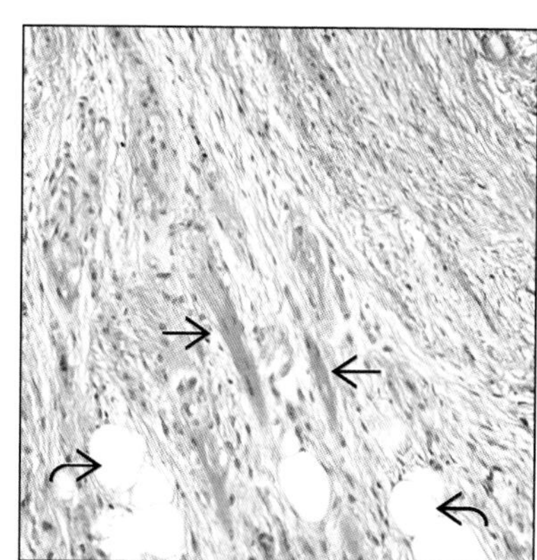

(Left) *A greater degree of fibrous to fibromxyomatous stroma confers the designation of fibromyxoma.* ***(Center)*** *There is a slight increase in cellularity; however, the spindle-shaped cells are bland and embedded in a fibrous or fibromyxomatous stroma.* ***(Right)*** *Lesional cells may infiltrate into soft tissue (skeletal muscle →, fat ↗) at the periphery of the lesion, creating difficulties in assuring complete surgical resection, potentially resulting in local recurrent tumor.*

GLOMANGIOPERICYTOMA (SINONASAL-TYPE HEMANGIOPERICYTOMA)

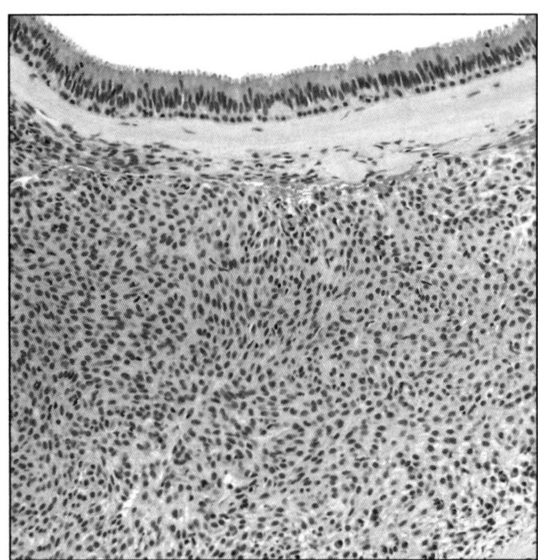

Hematoxylin & eosin shows an intact, uninvolved respiratory epithelium subtended by a thick band of fibrosis. Below this is a patternless, bland, cellular proliferation.

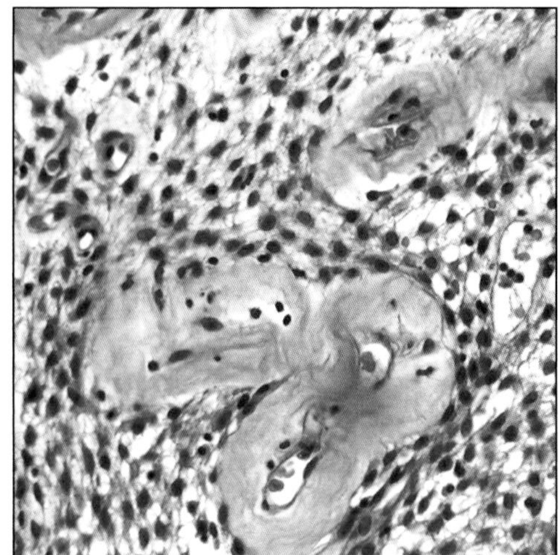

The strong, heavy, perivascular (peritheliomatous) hyalinization is quite characteristic for this tumor in the setting of a monotonous proliferation. The neoplasm is bland and arranged in a syncytium.

TERMINOLOGY

Abbreviations

- Sinonasal-type hemangiopericytoma (SNTHPC)

Synonyms

- Sinonasal hemangiopericytoma-like tumor
- Glomus tumor
- Hemangiopericytoma
- Solitary fibrous tumor (inaccurate in sinonasal site)
- Intranasal myopericytoma

Definitions

- Soft tissue tumor showing perivascular myoid differentiation defined by glomus (myoid) and hemangiopericytoma (pericyte) features within same lesion

ETIOLOGY/PATHOGENESIS

Myopericyte

- May arise from plentiful pericytes associated with vessels of nasal cavity

CLINICAL ISSUES

Epidemiology

- Incidence
  - Rare, comprising < 0.5% of sinonasal primary neoplasms
- Age
  - Broad range at presentation (5-90 years old)
  - Mean: 7th decade
  - Age at presentation does not affect prognosis
- Gender
  - Female > Male (1.2:1)
  - No difference in outcome based on gender

Site

- Nasal cavity is usually affected in isolation
  - Turbinate and septum are occasionally affected in isolation
- Maxillary and ethmoid sinuses may also be affected in conjunction with nasal cavity
- Bilateral tumors are uncommon (approximately 5%)

Presentation

- Nasal obstruction
- Epistaxis
- Mass, polyps
- Difficulty breathing
- Sinusitis
- Headache, congestion, pain
- Discharge
- Changes in smell
- Symptoms usually present for < 1 year
- Rare association with osteomalacia

Treatment

- Options, risks, complications
  - Surgery is treatment of choice, although radiation has been used in nonsurgical candidates
  - Chemotherapy is not used
- Surgical approaches
  - Polypectomy or wide surgical excision
  - Complete surgical extirpation decreases risk of recurrence (residual or recrudescence)

Prognosis

- Excellent long-term survival (5-year survival ~ 90%)
- Recurrences may develop (~ 18%)
  - Multiple recurrences may be seen
- Recurrences are associated with
  - Long duration of symptoms
  - Bone invasion
  - Severe nuclear pleomorphism
- Long-term clinical follow-up advocated as recurrences may develop late

GLOMANGIOPERICYTOMA (SINONASAL-TYPE HEMANGIOPERICYTOMA)

Key Facts

Terminology
- Soft tissue tumor showing perivascular myoid differentiation

Clinical Issues
- Nasal cavity is usually affected in isolation
- Present with nasal obstruction and epistaxis
- Excellent long-term outcome with surgery alone, although recurrences develop

Macroscopic Features
- Tends to be polypoid mass about 3 cm

Microscopic Pathology
- Peritheliomatous (perivascular) hyalinization is characteristic
- Cellular, diffuse, syncytial arrangement
- Surface epithelium usually intact (respiratory type or metaplastic squamous mucosa)
- Many patterns of growth, often within same tumor
- Ramifying, branching pattern of vessels
- Mixture of inflammatory cells in background
  - Eosinophils, mast cells, and lymphocytes, although first two predominate
- Extravasated erythrocytes

Ancillary Tests
- Shows myoid phenotype (actins positive)
- Lacks vascular markers (CD34, CD31, FVIIIRAg)

Top Differential Diagnoses
- Lobular capillary hemangioma
- Solitary fibrous tumor
- Nasopharyngeal angiofibroma

IMAGE FINDINGS

CT Findings
- Nasal cavity opacification by polypoid mass accompanied by bone erosion or sclerosis
- Destructive mass of nasal cavity and paranasal sinuses
- No cribriform plate involvement
- Angiograms show tumor blush
- Nonspecific sinusitis frequently concurrent

MACROSCOPIC FEATURES

General Features
- Tends to be polypoid
- Beefy red to grayish pink
- Soft, edematous, and fleshy
- Frequently associated with hemorrhage

Size
- Range: 0.8-8 cm
- Mean: 3.1 cm
  - Tumors in females often larger than in males (mean: 3.3 cm vs. 2.8 cm)
- Size does not correlate with recurrence

MICROSCOPIC PATHOLOGY

Histologic Features
- Surface epithelium usually intact (respiratory type or metaplastic squamous mucosa)
- Subepithelial proliferation separated from surface (Grenz zone)
- Proliferation effaces normal architecture, although entrapped minor mucoserous glands can be seen
- Bone remodeling or compression may occur but not direct invasion
- Cellular, diffuse, syncytial arrangement
- Many patterns of growth, often within same tumor
  - May be be fascicular (short not long fascicles), storiform, solid, whorled, meningothelial, reticulated, palisaded, peritheliomatous
- Spindled, epithelioid or rounded cells with indistinct cell borders
- Clear to amphophilic to slightly eosinophilic cytoplasm
- Absent to mild pleomorphism
- Oval to spindle nuclei with coarse nuclear chromatin
- Mitotic figures uncommon (< 1/10 HPFs)
- Atypical mitotic figures absent
- Ramifying, branching pattern of thin-walled vessels
  - "Staghorn" or antler-like vessels
- Peritheliomatous (perivascular) hyalinization is characteristic
- Extravasated erythrocytes
- Mixture of inflammatory cells in background
  - Eosinophils, mast cells, and lymphocytes, though the first two predominate
- Tumor giant cells can be seen but are uncommon
- Fatty (lipomatous) change rare
- Hematopoiesis very rare
- Other tumors (solitary fibrous tumor, fibrosarcoma, respiratory epithelial adenomatoid hamartoma) and reactive changes (sinonasal polyps) can be seen
- Rare cases may show profound pleomorphism, increased mitotic activity, and necrosis
  - These tumors are considered to be "malignant"

ANCILLARY TESTS

Histochemistry
- May-Grünwald Giemsa highlights mast cells

Immunohistochemistry
- Shows myoid phenotype (actins positive)
- Lacks vascular markers in neoplastic cells (only background vessels will be positive)

DIFFERENTIAL DIAGNOSIS

Lobular Capillary Hemangioma
- Lobular growth around central vessel
- Granulation tissue with ulcerated surface

GLOMANGIOPERICYTOMA (SINONASAL-TYPE HEMANGIOPERICYTOMA)

Immunohistochemistry

Antibody	Reactivity	Staining Pattern	Comment
Vimentin	Positive	Cytoplasmic	100% of tumor cells
Actin-sm	Positive	Cytoplasmic	Majority of tumor cells positive
Actin-HHF-35	Positive	Cytoplasmic	Majority of tumor cells positive
FXIIIA	Positive	Cytoplasmic	Focal, granular immunoreactivity
Laminin	Positive	Stromal matrix	Adjacent to neoplastic cells
CD34	Positive	Cytoplasmic	< 5% of cases
S100	Positive	Nuclear & cytoplasmic	< 3% of cases
CD68	Positive	Cytoplasmic	< 2% of cases
GFAP	Positive	Cytoplasmic	< 1% of cases
Bcl-2	Positive	Nuclear	< 1% of cases
CD117	Positive	Cytoplasmic	Only in mast cells
Ki-67	Positive	Nuclear	Usually < 5% of nuclei
CD31	Negative		
FVIIIRAg	Negative		
Desmin	Negative		
CK-PAN	Negative		
EMA	Negative		
NSE	Negative		

- Rich inflammatory infiltrate
- Lacks perivascular hyalinization

Solitary Fibrous Tumor
- Spindle cell tumor with thin-walled vascular proliferation
- Heavy ropy-keloid-like collagen deposition
- Lacks inflammatory cells
- Strong and diffuse CD34, Bcl-2, and CD99 immunoreactivity

Nasopharyngeal Angiofibroma
- Nasopharynx origin
- Heavy stromal hyalinization around variably sized vessels with possible smooth muscle walls
- Lacks elastic fibers and increased mast cells
- Lacks myoid phenotype

Fibrosarcoma
- Cellular tumor with short, interlacing fascicles of elongated spindle cells with tapered spindle nuclei
- Lacks vascular background
- Has increased mitoses
- Vimentin positive only

Meningioma
- Whorled pattern of growth comprised of meningothelial or epithelioid cells
- Intranuclear cytoplasmic inclusions
- Psammoma bodies
- EMA immunoreactivity

Peripheral Nerve Sheath Tumor
- a.k.a. schwannoma or neurilemmoma
- Palisaded growth of spindle cells
- Arranged in Antoni A and Antoni B areas
- Perivascular hyalinization
- Myxoid change
- Verocay bodies
- Strong S100 protein immunoreactivity

SELECTED REFERENCES

1. Beech TJ et al: A haemangiopericytoma of the ethmoid sinus causing oncogenic osteomalacia: a case report and review of the literature. Int J Oral Maxillofac Surg. 36(10):956-8, 2007
2. Wilson T et al: Intranasal myopericytoma. A tumour with perivascular myoid differentiation: the changing nomenclature for haemangiopericytoma. J Laryngol Otol. 121(8):786-9, 2007
3. Kuo FY et al: Sinonasal hemangiopericytoma-like tumor with true pericytic myoid differentiation: a clinicopathologic and immunohistochemical study of five cases. Head Neck. 27(2):124-9, 2005
4. Folpe AL et al: Most osteomalacia-associated mesenchymal tumors are a single histopathologic entity: an analysis of 32 cases and a comprehensive review of the literature. Am J Surg Pathol. 28(1):1-30, 2004
5. Thompson LD: Sinonasal tract glomangiopericytoma (hemangiopericytoma). Ear Nose Throat J. 83(12):807, 2004
6. Thompson LD et al: Sinonasal-type hemangiopericytoma: a clinicopathologic and immunophenotypic analysis of 104 cases showing perivascular myoid differentiation. Am J Surg Pathol. 27(6):737-49, 2003
7. Tse LL et al: Sinonasal haemangiopericytoma-like tumour: a sinonasal glomus tumour or a haemangiopericytoma? Histopathology. 40(6):510-7, 2002
8. Watanabe K et al: True hemangiopericytoma of the nasal cavity. Arch Pathol Lab Med. 125(5):686-90, 2001
9. Weber W et al: Haemangiopericytoma of the nasal cavity. Neuroradiology. 43(2):183-6, 2001
10. Marianowski R et al: Nasal haemangiopericytoma: report of two cases with literature review. J Laryngol Otol. 113(3):199-206, 1999

Microscopic and Immunohistochemical Features

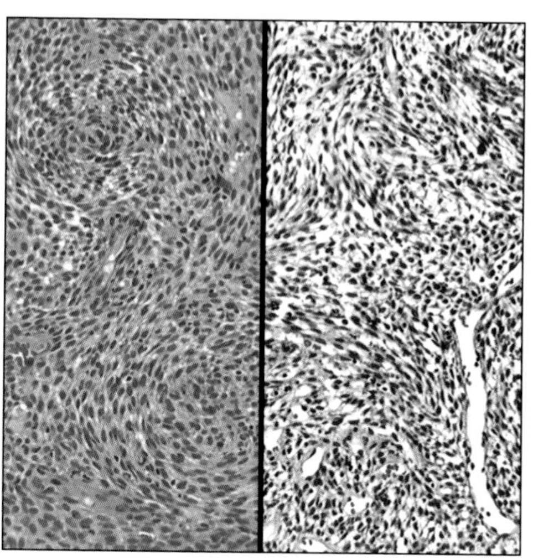

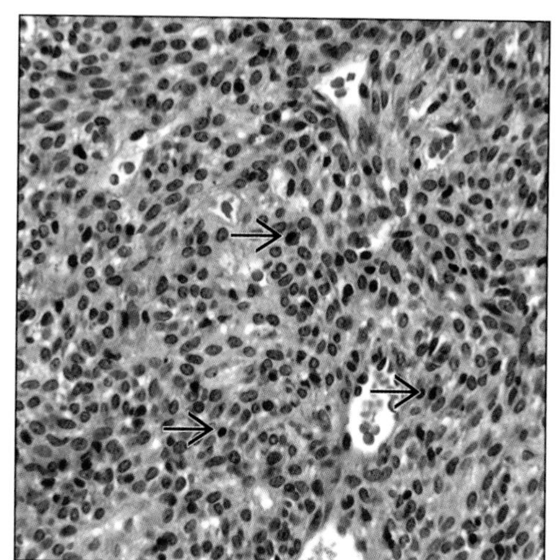

(Left) *A variety of different patterns can be seen. The left side demonstrates a whorled appearance with a richly vascularized stroma. The right side shows patulous, open vessels with extravasated erythrocytes.* ***(Right)*** *There is no specific pattern to this proliferation although the vessels are easily identified between the lesional cells. Mast cells →, eosinophils, and extravasated erythrocytes are quite characteristic for the tumor.*

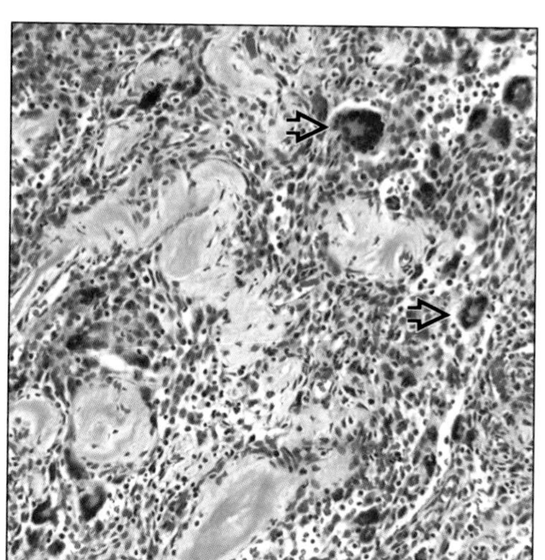

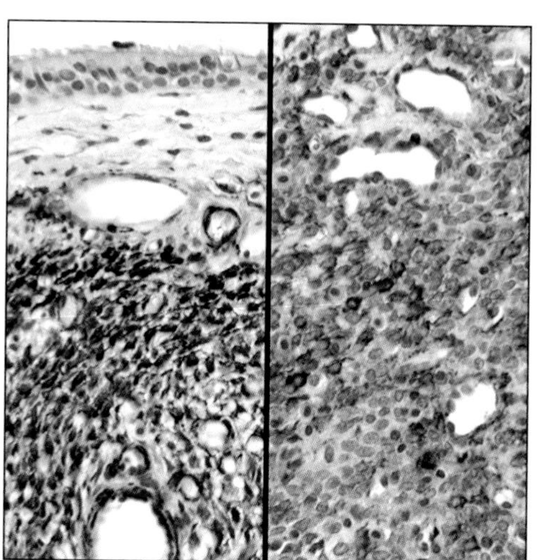

(Left) *Occasionally, tumor multinucleated giant cells ⇒ will be seen within the proliferation. These cells have an identical immunohistochemistry to the rest of the tumor cells, confirming their neoplastic nature. Note the peritheliomatous hyalinization.* ***(Right)*** *Actins will be strongly and diffusely immunoreactive in the neoplastic cells, although there can be some variation to the intensity of the staining. A smooth muscle actin (left) or a muscle specific actin (right).*

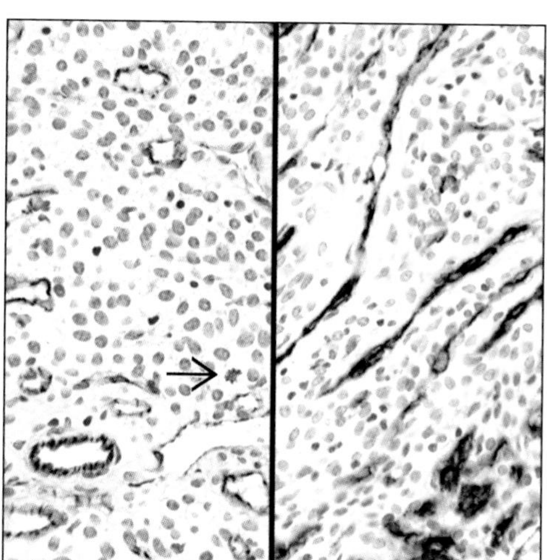

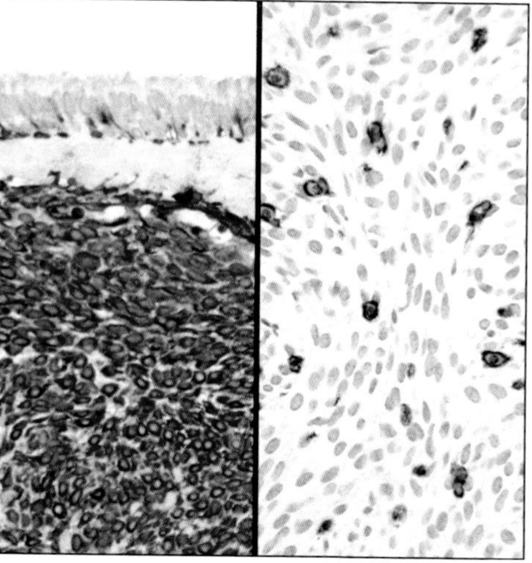

(Left) *Vascular markers are not positive in the neoplastic cells, although CD31 (left), CD34, and FVIIIRAg (right) are positive in the endothelial cells within the vessels. Note a mitotic figure →, occasionally seen.* ***(Right)*** *Vimentin (left) is strongly and diffusely immunoreactive. CD117 (right) is not required for the diagnosis, but it is a well-known marker for mast cells, and so the mast cells within the tumor will be immunoreactive.*

SQUAMOUS CELL CARCINOMA

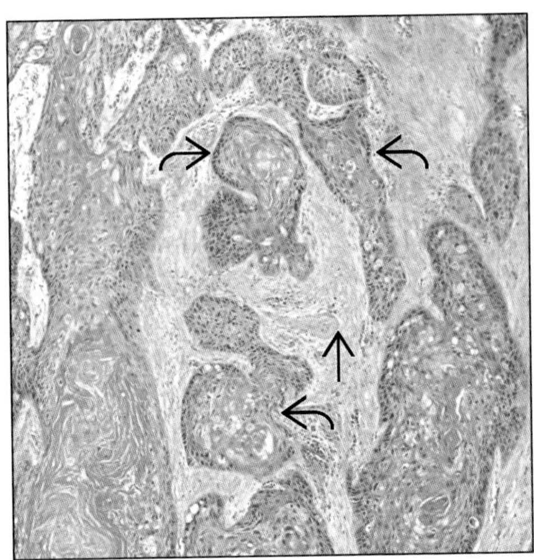

Sinonasal invasive keratinizing well-differentiated squamous cell carcinoma shows cohesive nests and cords of carcinoma ⮫ with an associated desmoplastic stroma →.

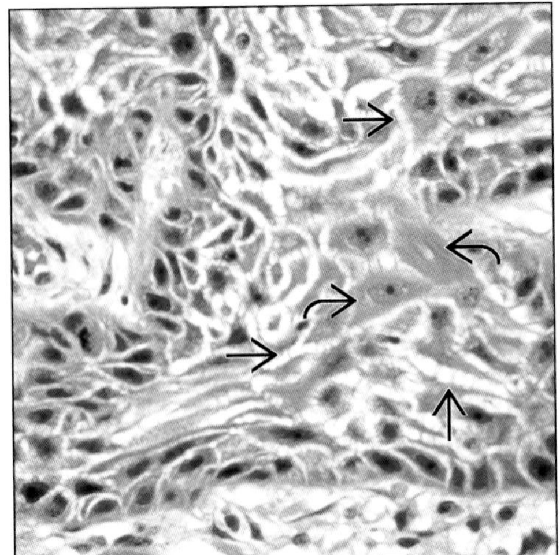

Nests of invasive well-differentiated squamous cell carcinoma show readily identifiable keratinization ⮫ and intercellular bridges → indicative of a better differentiated carcinoma.

TERMINOLOGY

Abbreviations

- Squamous cell carcinoma (SCC)

Synonyms

- For keratinizing squamous cell carcinoma
  - Sinonasal carcinoma
  - Epidermoid carcinoma
- For nonkeratinizing squamous cell carcinoma
  - Transitional carcinoma
  - Respiratory epithelial carcinoma
  - Ringertz carcinoma
  - Cylindrical cell carcinoma

Definitions

- Malignant epithelial neoplasm arising from surface epithelium with squamous cell differentiation
  - 2 histologic subtypes
    - Keratinizing SCC
    - Nonkeratinizing SCC
  - Variants of SCC occur (discussed elsewhere) including
    - Verrucous carcinoma
    - Papillary SCC
    - Spindle cell squamous carcinoma
    - Basaloid SCC
    - Adenosquamous carcinoma

ETIOLOGY/PATHOGENESIS

Environmental Exposure

- Associated risk factors include
  - Nickel exposure
  - Exposure to textile dust
  - Tobacco smoking
  - Prior Thorotrast use

Developmental

- May develop from sinonasal (schneiderian) papilloma
  - Majority transform to keratinizing SCC
  - Majority arise in association with inverted-type sinonasal papilloma
  - Human papillomavirus (HPV) may be found
    - Direct cause and effect not definitively found

CLINICAL ISSUES

Epidemiology

- Incidence
  - Represents approximately 3% of head and neck malignant neoplasms
  - Represents < 1% of all malignant neoplasms
  - Most common malignant epithelial neoplasm of sinonasal tract
- Age
  - Most frequent in 6th and 7th decades of life
    - 95% of cases arise in patients older than 40 years
- Gender
  - Male > Female

Site

- In decreasing order of frequency, sites of occurrence include
  - Antrum of maxillary sinus > nasal cavity > ethmoid sinus > sphenoid and frontal sinuses
  - Maxillary sinus
    - No lateralization
  - Nasal cavity
    - Primarily lateral wall
    - No lateralization
    - 10% bilateral although may represent extension from one side via septal perforation
  - Nasal septum
    - Most arise from anterior rather than posterior septum
  - Nasal vestibule SCC cutaneous (not mucosal) derived

SQUAMOUS CELL CARCINOMA

Key Facts

Terminology
- Malignant epithelial neoplasm arising from surface epithelium with squamous cell differentiation

Etiology/Pathogenesis
- Associated risk factors include
  - Nickel exposure, exposure to textile dust, tobacco smoking, prior Thorotrast use
- May develop from sinonasal (schneiderian) papilloma; majority transform to keratinizing SCC

Clinical Issues
- Represents approximately 3% of head and neck malignant neoplasms
- Sites in decreasing order of frequency
  - Maxillary sinus antrum > nasal cavity > ethmoid sinus > sphenoid, frontal sinuses

Microscopic Pathology
- Divided into keratinizing and nonkeratinizing subtypes
- **Keratinizing squamous cell carcinoma**
  - Most common type representing 80-85% of all cases
  - Divided into well-, moderately, poorly differentiated carcinomas
- **Nonkeratinizing squamous cell carcinoma**
  - Represents approximately 15-20% of all cases
  - Often shows downward (inverted or endophytic) growth with broad interconnecting bands or nests of neoplastic epithelium
  - Composed of elongated cells with cylindrical or columnar appearance

Presentation
- Maxillary sinus
  - Early symptoms often confused with sinusitis resulting in delay in diagnosis
  - With progression of disease, grouped in 5 categories
    - Nasal: Nasal obstruction, persistent purulent rhinorrhea, nonhealing sore/ulcer, epistaxis, mass
    - Oral: Referred pain including to upper premolar, molar teeth, ulceration, loosening of teeth, fistula
    - Facial: Swelling, asymmetry
    - Ocular: Eyelid swelling, proptosis/exophthalmos
    - Neurologic: Numbness, paraesthesia, pain, cranial neuropathy
- Nasal cavity
  - Unilateral obstruction, nonhealing sore, rhinorrhea, epistaxis
  - Mass
  - Pain in minority of cases

Treatment
- Options, risks, complications
  - Complete surgical resection plus adjuvant radiotherapy
- Surgical approaches
  - Surgical advances permit complex tumor removal and reconstruction surrounding these structures
    - Results in functional, cosmetic improvements

Prognosis
- **Keratinizing SCC**
- Maxillary sinus
  - Poor prognosis
    - Often presents with advanced clinical stage
    - Clinical stage of greater prognostic import than histologic type
  - 30-45% local recurrence
  - Metastatic disease uncommon if tumor confined to involved sinus, but over disease course
    - 25-30% locoregional nodal spread
    - 10-20% distant spread
  - Poorer prognosis related to
    - Higher clinical stage disease involving more than one anatomic area
    - Recurrent tumor following initial curative therapy
    - Regional lymph node metastasis
    - Presence of facial numbness/swelling, orbital-related symptoms, oral cavity involvement, skin involvement
- Nasal cavity
  - Generally > 50% 5-year survival
  - Approximately 20% local recurrence
  - Approximately 30% develop locoregional nodal spread
  - Approximately 20% distant spread
  - Spread may occur to paranasal sinuses, orbit, oral cavity, skin, cranial cavity
  - Patients at greater risk for 2nd primary malignancy
    - Other mucosal site in upper aerodigestive tract
    - Sites other than head and neck (e.g., lung, gastrointestinal tract, breast)
- Nasal septum
  - 60-80% 5-year survival
  - Approximately 11% local recurrence
  - Approximately 25% develop locoregional nodal spread
  - Approximately 15% develop distant spread
  - Poor prognosis related to
    - Tumors larger than 2 cm
    - Lymph node metastasis
- Nasal vestibule
  - 65-87% 5-year survival
  - Approximately 24% local recurrence
  - Approximately 18% develop locoregional nodal spread
  - < 5% distant spread
  - Poor prognosis related to
    - Tumors larger than 1.5 cm
    - Involvement of ≥ 2 sites in vestibule
    - Local recurrence
    - Lymph node metastasis especially at presentation
    - Spread to cartilage, bone, upper lip, columella
- **Nonkeratinizing SCC**
  - Better prognosis than keratinizing SCC

SQUAMOUS CELL CARCINOMA

- Tend to be locally aggressive
  - Approximately 10% metastasize to regional lymph nodes or distant sites

IMAGE FINDINGS

Radiographic Findings

- Indispensable in determining extent of disease
- In advanced disease
  - Involved sinus filled by tumor
  - Destruction of bony walls
  - Extension into adjacent structures
    - Oral cavity, skin, infratemporal fossa, periorbital soft tissue, orbit

MACROSCOPIC FEATURES

General Features

- Polypoid, papillary, fungating or inverted growth patterns
- May be well circumscribed with expansile growth and limited invasion
- May be overtly invasive with destructive growth, necrotic with friable, hemorrhagic appearance

MICROSCOPIC PATHOLOGY

Histologic Features

- Divided into keratinizing and nonkeratinizing subtypes
- **Keratinizing squamous cell carcinoma**
  - Most common type representing 80-85% of all cases
  - Stromal invasion includes
    - Cohesive nests or cords
    - Isolated invasive malignant cells
    - Desmoplasia present, including collagen deposition with/without associated inflammatory cell reaction
  - Dysplasia of adjacent or overlying surface epithelium may be seen
    - If present, may vary from mild to moderate to severe dysplasia
- **Grading keratinizing SCC**
  - Divided into well, moderately, and poorly differentiated carcinomas
  - Well- to moderately differentiated carcinomas show
    - Readily apparent keratinization, keratin pearl formation, individual cell keratinization
    - Intercellular bridges
    - Mild to moderate nuclear atypia with enlarged, hyperchromatic nuclei
    - Dyskeratosis (abnormal keratinization)
    - Low mitotic activity
  - Poorly differentiated carcinomas show
    - Less keratinization
    - Greater nuclear atypia
    - Increased mitotic activity, atypical mitoses
    - Evidence of keratinization usually focally present
- **Nonkeratinizing squamous cell carcinoma**
  - Represents approximately 15-20% of all cases
  - May have papillary or exophytic growth pattern
  - Often shows downward (inverted or endophytic) growth with broad interconnecting bands or nests of neoplastic epithelium
    - Tumor nests may appear rounded, with smooth borders, or delineated by basement membrane-like material
    - May not be interpreted as invasive but rather as papilloma with severe dysplasia
    - Growth pattern similar to bladder cancers resulting in prior (obsolete) terminology of transitional-type carcinoma
  - Composed of elongated cells with cylindrical or columnar appearance
    - Oriented perpendicular to surface
    - Generally lack evidence of keratinization
    - Keratin may be present focally but does not represent significant component
  - Generally hypercellular neoplasm characterized by
    - Nuclear pleomorphism, hyperchromasia
    - Increased nuclear:cytoplasmic ratio
    - Loss of cell polarity
    - Increased mitotic activity, including atypical forms
  - Dysplasia of surface epithelium may be seen
    - May vary from mild to moderate to severe

ANCILLARY TESTS

Immunohistochemistry

- Positive for epithelial markers (e.g., cytokeratins)
  - Not typically required for diagnosis
- Nonkeratinizing SCC reported to be p16 positive
  - Unlike oropharyngeal nonkeratinizing carcinoma, no specific cause and effect with HPV
- Epstein-Barr virus (EBV) negative

DIFFERENTIAL DIAGNOSIS

Schneiderian Papillomas

- Differential diagnosis primarily with inverted-type papilloma
- Histologically characterized by
  - Epithelial proliferation primarily composed of squamous cells with admixed mucocytes
  - Intraepithelial mucous cysts present
  - Endophytic or "inverted" growth pattern
    - Downward growth into underlying stroma
  - Epithelial cells generally bland in appearance with uniform nuclei
    - Cytologic atypia may be present
    - Mitotic figures may be seen in basal and parabasal layers, but atypical mitotic figures not seen
  - Mixed chronic inflammatory cell infiltrate characteristically seen within all layers of surface epithelium
- In contrast to carcinomas
  - Lack malignant cytomorphology
  - Absence of invasive growth lacking
    - Cohesive nests or cords
    - Isolated invasive malignant cells

- Associated desmoplasia
- Absence of broad interconnecting cords as evidence in nonkeratinizing SCC

Oropharyngeal Nonkeratinizing Carcinoma

- Represents tonsil and base of tongue carcinomas
- Oropharyngeal nonkeratinizing carcinomas (in contrast to sinonasal nonkeratinizing carcinoma)
  - Invade as tumor nests often with associated central (comedo-type) necrosis
  - May invade as individual malignant cells or small nests with
    - Associated lymphoid infiltrate
    - May invade without desmoplastic response
  - Frequently metastasize to cervical neck
    - Unilateral or bilateral
  - Metastatic disease may occur in absence of known primary carcinoma
    - Primary carcinoma may be small &/or located in crypt epithelium; makes clinical detection difficult
    - PET scan helpful in locating primary tumor
  - Strong association with HPV16
    - p16 immunoreactivity &/or identification by PCR or in situ hybridization
    - Presence of p16 shown to be reliable predictor of oropharyngeal origin (i.e., tonsils and base of tongue)
    - Presence of p16 correlates to presence of HPV16 (HPV-associated SCC)
  - As compared to HPV-negative head & neck SCC (HNSCC), HPV-positive HNSCC
    - Frequently occur in patients with no known risk factors for HNSCC
    - Associated with better outcome (better overall- and disease-specific survival)
    - Tend to be radioresponsive

NUT Midline Carcinoma

- Carcinomas originating from midline epithelial structures with balanced chromosomal translocation t(15;19) resulting in *BRD4-NUT* oncogene
- Predominantly but not exclusively occur in sites above diaphragm, including
  - Sinonasal tract, nasopharynx
  - Orbit
  - Supraglottic larynx (epiglottis)
  - Trachea, thymus, mediastinum, lung
- Female > Male
- Predominantly affects children, young adults
  - Occurs in older adults
- Poorly differentiated or undifferentiated carcinoma with squamous differentiation
  - Squamous differentiation > 80% of cases
  - With or without keratinization
- Immunohistochemistry
  - Cytokeratins positive
  - CD34 positive
- Cytogenetics and molecular genetics
  - Unique chromosomal translocation disease identifier
  - t(15;19) results in novel fusion oncogene *BRD4-NUT*
  - Some patients harbor *NUT* with *BRD4* gene break point (*BRD4-NUT* fusion)
  - Some patients harbor *NUT* without *BRD4* gene break point (*NUT* variant)
- Highly lethal despite intensive therapies
  - *NUT* variant carcinomas may have less fulminant clinical course than *BRD4-NUT* fusions
- Tends to disseminate widely

SELECTED REFERENCES

1. Agger A et al: Squamous cell carcinoma of the nasal vestibule 1993-2002: a nationwide retrospective study from DAHANCA. Head Neck. 31(12):1593-9, 2009
2. Haack H et al: Diagnosis of NUT midline carcinoma using a NUT-specific monoclonal antibody. Am J Surg Pathol. 33(7):984-91, 2009
3. Stelow EB et al: Carcinomas of the upper aerodigestive tract with rearrangement of the nuclear protein of the testis (NUT) gene (NUT midline carcinomas). Adv Anat Pathol. 16(2):92-6, 2009
4. Allen MW et al: Long-term radiotherapy outcomes for nasal cavity and septal cancers. Int J Radiat Oncol Biol Phys. 71(2):401-6, 2008
5. Dowley A et al: Squamous cell carcinoma of the nasal vestibule: a 20-year case series and literature review. J Laryngol Otol. 122(10):1019-23, 2008
6. Stelow EB et al: NUT rearrangement in undifferentiated carcinomas of the upper aerodigestive tract. Am J Surg Pathol. 32(6):828-34, 2008
7. Fasunla AJ et al: Sinonasal malignancies: a 10-year review in a tertiary health institution. J Natl Med Assoc. 99(12):1407-10, 2007
8. Hoppe BS et al: Treatment of nasal cavity and paranasal sinus cancer with modern radiotherapy techniques in the postoperative setting--the MSKCC experience. Int J Radiat Oncol Biol Phys. 67(3):691-702, 2007
9. El-Mofty SK et al: Prevalence of high-risk human papillomavirus DNA in nonkeratinizing (cylindrical cell) carcinoma of the sinonasal tract: a distinct clinicopathologic and molecular disease entity. Am J Surg Pathol. 29(10):1367-72, 2005
10. Bhattacharyya N: Cancer of the nasal cavity: survival and factors influencing prognosis. Arch Otolaryngol Head Neck Surg. 128(9):1079-83, 2002
11. Dulguerov P et al: Nasal and paranasal sinus carcinoma: are we making progress? A series of 220 patients and a systematic review. Cancer. 92(12):3012-29, 2001
12. Paulino AF et al: Epstein-Barr virus in squamous carcinoma of the anterior nasal cavity. Ann Diagn Pathol. 4(1):7-10, 2000
13. Hermans R et al: Squamous cell carcinoma of the sinonasal cavities. Semin Ultrasound CT MR. 20(3):150-61, 1999
14. Tufano RP et al: Malignant tumors of the nose and paranasal sinuses: hospital of the University of Pennsylvania experience 1990-1997. Am J Rhinol. 13(2):117-23, 1999
15. Harbo G et al: Cancer of the nasal cavity and paranasal sinuses. A clinico-pathological study of 277 patients. Acta Oncol. 36(1):45-50, 1997
16. Taxy JB: Squamous carcinoma of the nasal vestibule: an analysis of five cases and literature review. Am J Clin Pathol. 107(6):698-703, 1997
17. Haraguchi H et al: Malignant tumors of the nasal cavity: review of a 60-case series. Jpn J Clin Oncol. 25(5):188-94, 1995
18. Spiro JD et al: Squamous carcinoma of the nasal cavity and paranasal sinuses. Am J Surg. 158(4):328-32, 1989

SQUAMOUS CELL CARCINOMA

Imaging and Microscopic Features

*(**Left**) Axial T1 C+ MR with fat saturation shows an anterior maxillary sinus SCC. V2 perineural tumor ➔ enters pterygopalatine fossa ➢. Note Vidian canal involvement ➔. (**Right**) A rather large peripheral nerve ➔ is completely surrounded by invasive squamous cell carcinoma ➢. This finding correlates to a clinical presentation that includes complaints of pain. Typically, pain associated with a head and neck mass is indicative of a malignancy until proven otherwise.*

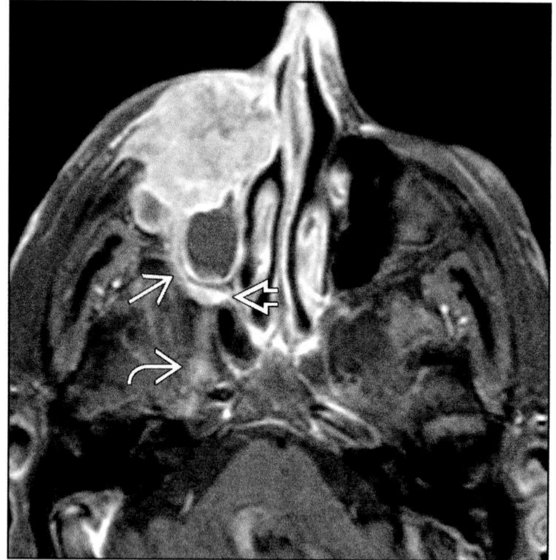

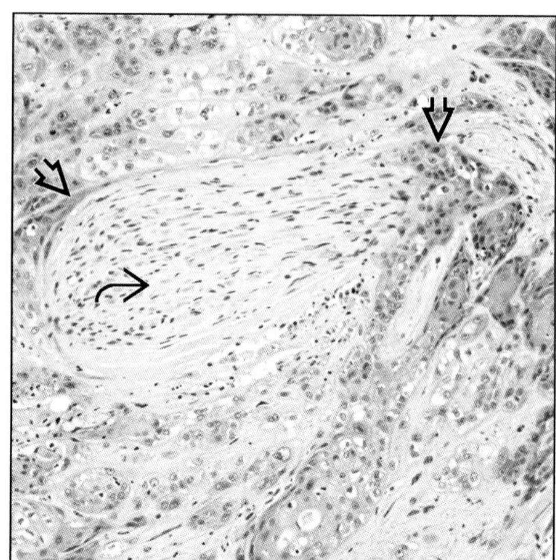

*(**Left**) Coronal bone CT demonstrates aggressive maxillary antral squamous cell carcinoma associated with marked bony destruction ➔ and extension into the nasal cavity and superior alveolus ➢. (**Right**) A resection specimen showed a widely infiltrative squamous cell carcinoma including neurotropism (not shown), angioinvasion (not shown), and invasion into bone. Nests of poorly differentiated squamous cell carcinoma ➢ invade into bone ➔.*

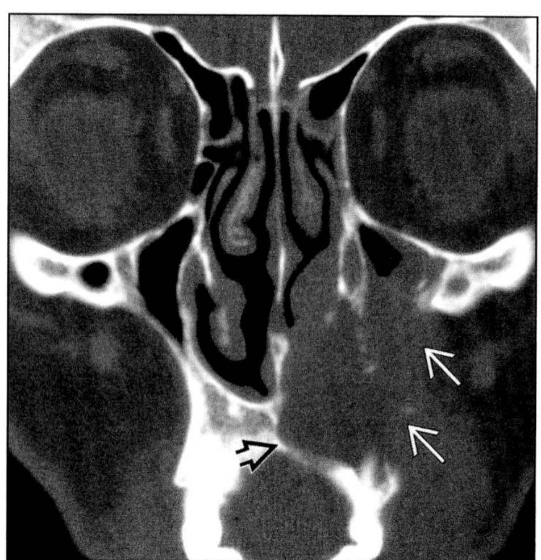

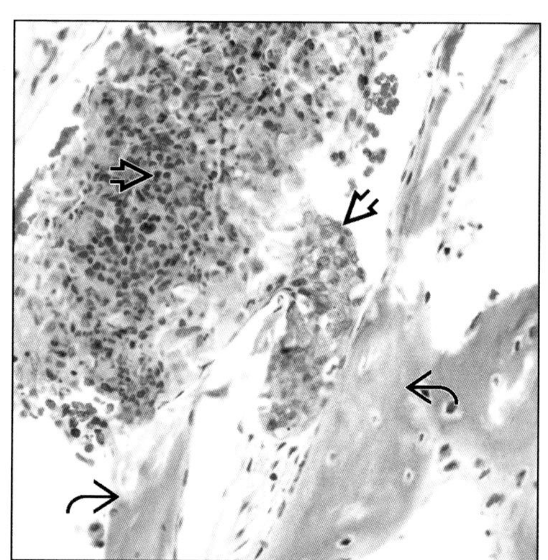

*(**Left**) Moderately differentiated keratinizing squamous cell carcinoma shows greater nuclear pleomorphism and less differentiation than well-differentiated carcinomas but still retains readily identifiable keratinization ➢ and intercellular bridges ➔. (**Right**) Poorly differentiated squamous cell carcinoma retains less identifiable evidence of squamous differentiation, but the nested growth and limited but identifiable keratinized cells ➔ support this diagnosis.*

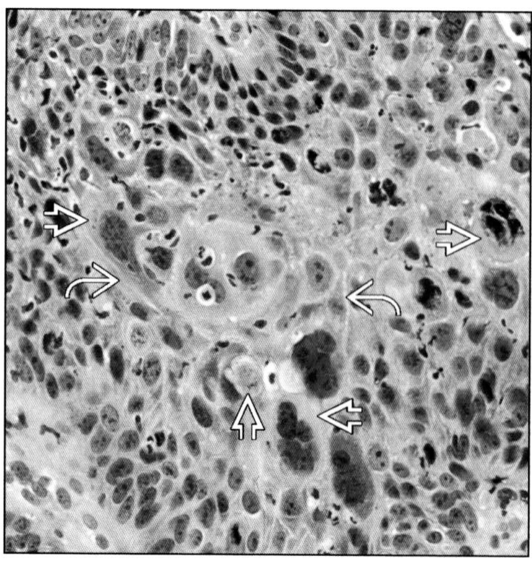

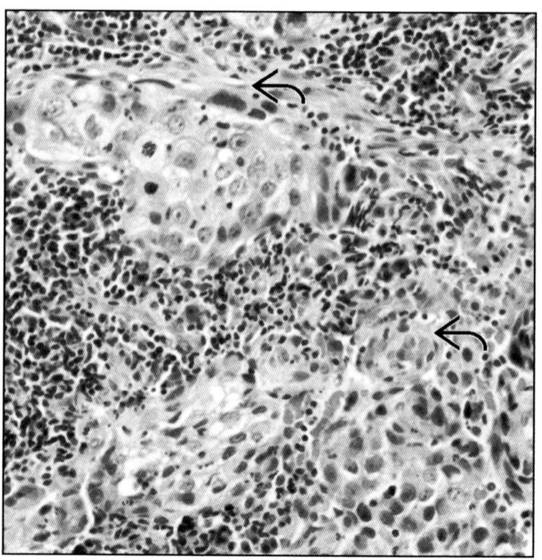

SQUAMOUS CELL CARCINOMA

Microscopic Features

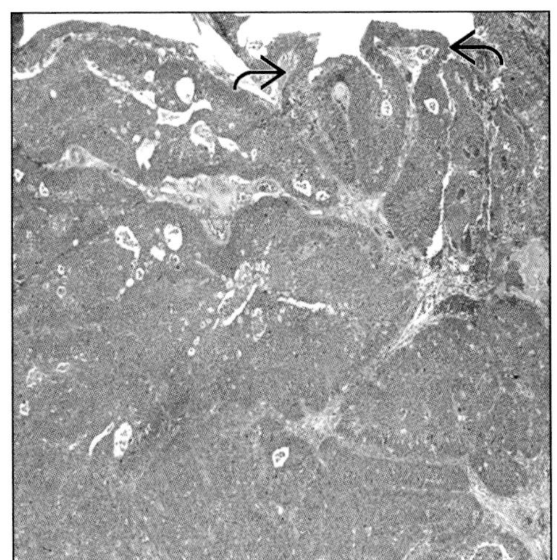

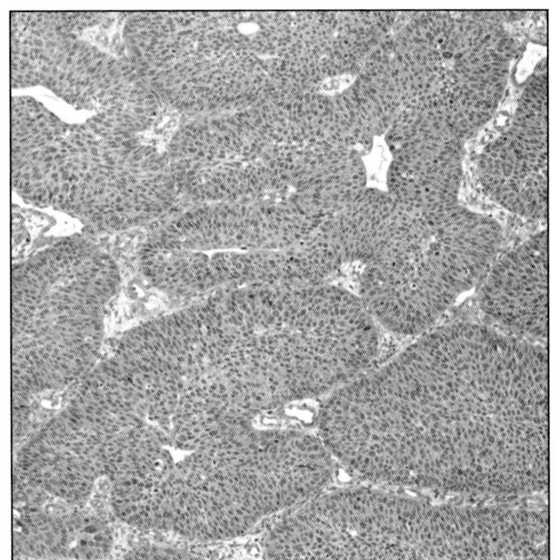

(Left) *Nonkeratinizing squamous cell carcinoma originates from the surface epithelium and invades into the submucosa as broad interconnecting bands of neoplastic epithelium growing down ("inverted") into the stroma.* ***(Right)*** *The pattern of growth includes interconnecting/ramifying bands of the neoplastic epithelium, which is a hallmark feature of sinonasal nonkeratinizing carcinoma and starkly contrasts the absence of such growth in sinonasal (schneiderian) papillomas.*

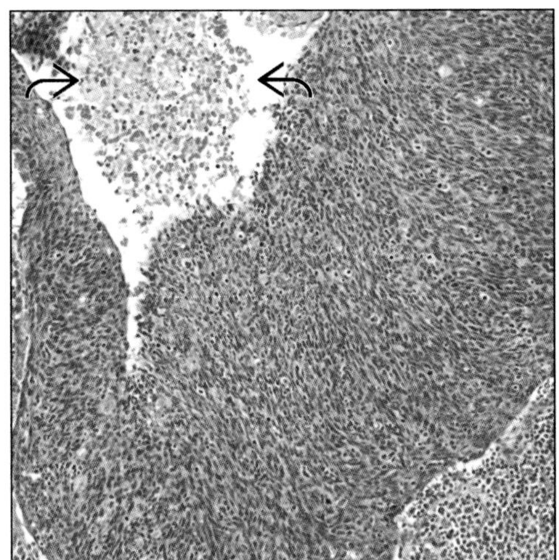

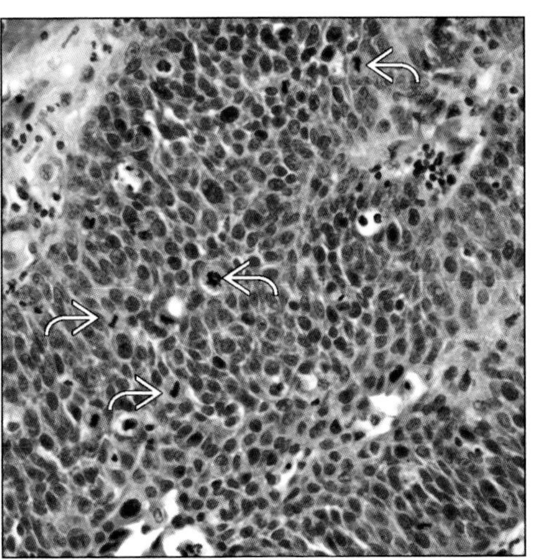

(Left) *The neoplastic epithelium is nonkeratinizing and may show cystic change.* ***(Right)*** *Nonkeratinizing squamous carcinoma shows nuclear pleomorphism, hyperchromasia, loss of cellular polarity, increased nuclear:cytoplasmic ratio, and increased mitotic activity. The diagnosis of nonkeratinizing carcinoma can be made even in the presence of focal keratinization (not shown) as long as the majority of the neoplasm shows diagnostic features of nonkeratinizing carcinoma.*

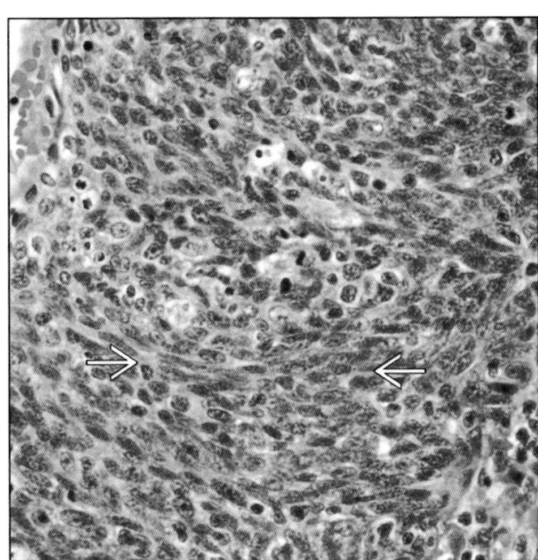

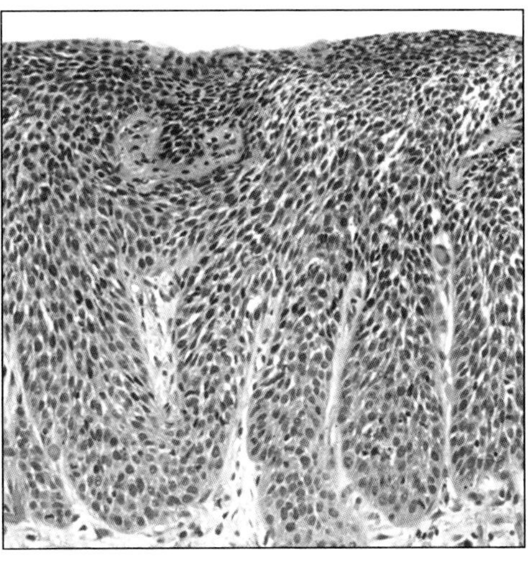

(Left) *Areas of nonkeratinizing carcinoma may include a spindle-shaped cell population.* ***(Right)*** *Carcinoma in situ may be present. The light microscopic features of sinonasal nonkeratinizing carcinoma may be similar to oropharyngeal (tonsil, base of tongue) nonkeratinizing carcinomas. The latter are consistently p16 positive, whereas sinonasal nonkeratinizing carcinomas have not been shown to be highly correlated with HPV.*

SINONASAL UNDIFFERENTIATED CARCINOMA

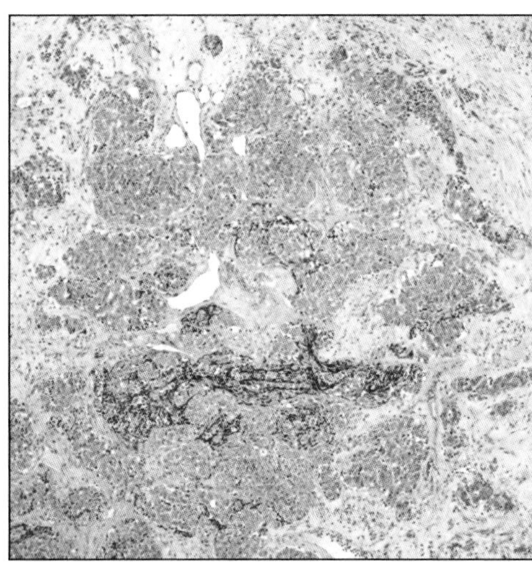

Invasive neoplasm shows lobular and trabecular growth, a consistent but not pathognomonic feature seen in SNUCs. Similar growth characteristics occur in other high-grade SNT malignant neoplasms.

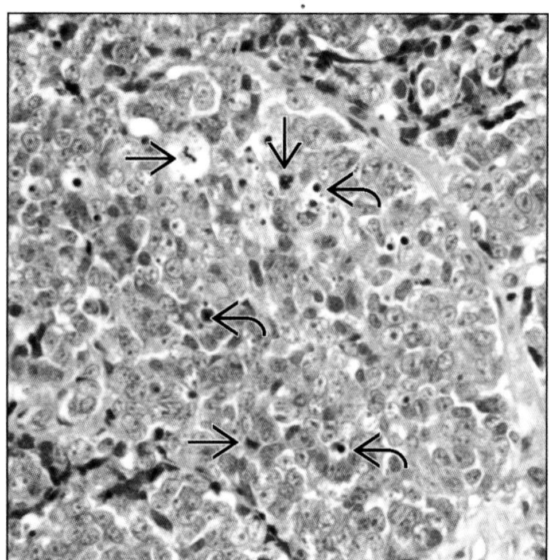

Undifferentiated (nasopharyngeal-like) malignant cells show vesicular nuclei, small to prominent nucleoli, and ill-defined cell membranes. Mitoses ➔ and individual cell necrosis ➔ are present.

TERMINOLOGY

Abbreviations

- Sinonasal undifferentiated carcinoma (SNUC)
- Sinonasal tract (SNT)

Definitions

- Original definition considered SNUC a high-grade malignant epithelial neoplasm of nasal cavity and paranasal sinuses
  - Uncertain histogenesis
  - ± neuroendocrine differentiation
  - Without evidence of squamous or glandular differentiation
- More currently, SNUC defined as highly aggressive and clinicopathologically distinctive carcinoma
  - Uncertain histogenesis
  - Typically presenting with locally extensive disease
  - Composed of pleomorphic tumor cells with frequent necrosis
  - Should be differentiated from lymphoepithelial (and other) carcinomas or olfactory neuroblastoma

ETIOLOGY/PATHOGENESIS

Idiopathic

- No known etiologic agents
- SNUCs typically negative for Epstein-Barr virus (EBV)
  - Reports of EBV RNA identified in Asian and Italian patients with SNUC but not in other western patients with SNUC
- Some cases reported to develop following radiation therapy for nasopharyngeal carcinoma
- Although no specific etiology linked to development of SNUC, cigarette smoking and nickel exposure identified in patients with SNUC
- Deletion of retinoblastoma gene implicated in development of SNUC

CLINICAL ISSUES

Epidemiology

- Incidence
  - Uncommon tumor
    - Recognized with greater frequency
- Age
  - Occurs over wide age range, including
    - 3rd to 9th decades of life
    - Median: 6th decade at presentation
- Gender
  - Male > Female

Site

- Extensively infiltrative at presentation and involving multiple sites including
  - Nasal cavity
  - One or more paranasal sinuses
  - Orbit, skull base, brain

Presentation

- Multiple symptoms including
  - Nasal obstruction, epistaxis, proptosis, visual disturbances (e.g., diplopia)
  - Facial pain
  - Symptoms of cranial nerve involvement
- Characteristically, clinical symptoms develop over relatively short duration (weeks to months)
  - Rapid onset not typically seen in association with other SNT malignant neoplasms
  - Rapid clinical onset represents a helpful, although not pathognomonic, diagnostic finding

Treatment

- Options, risks, complications
  - Uncertainty remains in optimal management for SNUC including
    - Sequencing of various therapeutic modalities, optimal chemotherapy agent and dosing, optimal radiation dose and target

SINONASAL UNDIFFERENTIATED CARCINOMA

Key Facts

Terminology
- SNUC currently defined as highly aggressive and clinicopathologically distinctive carcinoma
  - Uncertain histogenesis
  - Typically presents with locally extensive disease
  - Composed of pleomorphic tumor cells with frequent necrosis
  - Should be differentiated from lymphoepithelial (and other) carcinomas or olfactory neuroblastoma

Clinical Issues
- Extensively infiltrative at presentation involving multiple sites
- Characteristically, symptoms develop over relatively short duration (weeks to months)

Microscopic Pathology
- Hypercellular proliferation with varied growth, including trabecular, sheet-like, ribbon-like, solid, lobular and organoid
- Histologically high-grade undifferentiated neoplastic proliferation with
  - Increased mitotic activity, including atypical mitoses
  - Prominent tumor necrosis (confluent areas and individual cells)
  - Lymph-vascular invasion, neurotropism

Ancillary Tests
- Consistently immunoreactive with cytokeratins

    - Significant improvements in outcomes owing to use of multimodality approaches to management
    - For patients who are medically inoperable, definitive chemoradiation used
    - Resectable or potentially resectable tumors receive neoadjuvant chemoradiation followed by surgical resection

Prognosis
- Highly aggressive neoplasm that is neither completely eradicated by surgery nor responsive to radiation treatment
- Mean survival of 4 months with no disease-free patients reported
- Extent of resection most reliable predictor of tumor control
- Improved survival following treatment with chemotherapy (cyclophosphamide, doxorubicin, and vincristine), followed by radiotherapy and then radical surgery
- Local recurrence common
  - Represents major cause of morbidity and mortality
- Metastatic disease occurs to bone, brain, liver, cervical lymph nodes

IMAGE FINDINGS

Radiographic Findings
- CT and MR often demonstrates large (sinonasal) mass typically with local invasive growth extending beyond its bony confines with involvement of orbital &/or cranial bones
- Intracranial extension may occur

MACROSCOPIC FEATURES

General Features
- Tend to be fungating with poorly defined margins
  - With invasion into adjacent structures &/ or anatomic compartments, including bone destruction

Size
- Typically measure > 4 cm in greatest dimension

MICROSCOPIC PATHOLOGY

Histiologic Features
- Characterized by hypercellular proliferation with varied growth, including
  - Lobular (organoid), trabecular, solid, sheet-like, ribbon-like
- Surface involvement in form of dysplasia/carcinoma in situ usually not present
  - May be present
  - Often ulceration is present precluding evidence of surface epithelial derivation
- Cellular infiltrate consists of
  - Polygonal cells of medium to large size
  - Round to oval, hyperchromatic to vesicular nuclei
  - Inconspicuous to prominent nucleoli
  - Varying amount of eosinophilic appearing cytoplasm with poorly defined cell membranes, although distinct cell borders may be present
  - Cells with clear cytoplasm may be present
- Additional findings include
  - High nuclear to cytoplasmic ratio
  - Increased mitotic activity, including atypical mitoses
  - Prominent tumor necrosis (confluent areas and individual cells), apoptosis
  - Lymph-vascular invasion, neurotropism often present
- 3 cell types described including
  - "**Western**" **type** characterized by
    - Cells with round to oval hyperchromatic nuclei
    - Inconspicuous to small nucleoli
    - Limited pink to amphophilic cytoplasm
  - **Cells similar to nasopharyngeal undifferentiated carcinoma** including
    - Large vesicular nuclei, prominent nucleoli, associated (nonneoplastic) lymphocytic infiltrate
    - Reported predominantly in (but not exclusive to) Asian patients

SINONASAL UNDIFFERENTIATED CARCINOMA

- **Large cell type** with features similar to large cell carcinoma of lung
    - Large cells with pleomorphic nuclei, prominent eosinophilic nucleoli
    - Reported predominantly in (but not exclusive to) Asian patients
- 3 cell types described can be seen to variable extent in single tumor
- Neurofibrillary material and neural rosettes not identified
- Squamous or glandular differentiation should not be present
- Rare examples may show squamous cell differentiation, but in this setting strict criteria required for diagnosis
    - Clinical parameters are those typically associated with SNUC (i.e., rapid onset)
    - Squamous foci (keratinization and intercellular bridges) extremely limited in extent
    - Occurs in neoplasm where dominant histologic features are those of SNUC
    - **Note**: Presence of undifferentiated carcinoma with abrupt keratinization may represent *NUT* carcinoma

ANCILLARY TESTS

Histochemistry

- Noncontributory to diagnosis of SNUC
- Stains for epithelial mucin negative

DIFFERENTIAL DIAGNOSIS

Olfactory Neuroblastoma (High Grade)

- Neuron-specific enolase
    - Most consistently positive marker
    - Diffuse, strong staining
- S100 protein (characteristic peripheral or sustentacular cell-like pattern)
- Neuroendocrine markers (chromogranin, synaptophysin, CD57, CD56) variably positive
- Typically cytokeratin negative
    - Very focal positive staining can be seen
    - Lacks diffuse staining seen in SNUC
    - Rare olfactory carcinoma may show more diffuse cytokeratin staining

Small Cell Undifferentiated Neuroendocrine Carcinoma (SCUNC)

- Consistently immunoreactive for neuroendocrine markers (chromogranin, synaptophysin, CD57)
    - SNUCs variably reactive and often nonreactive for neuroendocrine markers

Nasopharyngeal Carcinoma (NPC), Nonkeratinizing Undifferentiated

- Clinical, radiologic evaluation critical in determining location of tumor
- Presence of Epstein-Barr virus (EBV)
    - SNUCs lack EBV staining
- Purported differential cytokeratin staining from SNUC
    - NPC: CK5/6, CK13 positive
    - SNUC: CK5/6, CK13 negative

Sinonasal Lymphoepithelial Carcinoma

- Rare tumor with overlapping morphology with SNUC
- Radioresponsive with favorable outcomes
- Presence of Epstein-Barr virus (EBV)
    - SNUCs lack EBV staining

Mucosal Malignant Melanoma (MMM)

- S100 protein, HMB-45, Melan-A, tyrosinase positive
- Cytokeratin negative

NK-/T-cell Lymphoma, Nasal Type

- Hematolymphoid markers (CD45, CD3, CD56, others) positive
- Cytokeratin negative (< 5% positive)
- p63, a marker of epithelial and myoepithelial cells, may be positive

Rhabdomyosarcoma (RMS)

- Desmin, muscle specific actin, myoglobin, myogenin positive
- Cytokeratin negative (< 5% positive)
- CD56 and CD57 may be positive

Squamous Cell Carcinoma (SCC), Keratinizing

- Presence of squamous differentiation (keratinization, intercellular bridges)
- Intraepithelial dysplasia
- Purported differential cytokeratin staining from SNUC
    - SCC: CK5/6, CK13, CK14 positive
    - SNUC: CK5/6, CK13, CK14 negative

Squamous Cell Carcinoma, Nonkeratinizing (NKSCC)

- Tumor grows in broad interconnecting, ramifying cords
- May be p16 positive
- Purported differential cytokeratin staining from SNUC
    - NKSCC: CK5/6, CK13, CK14 positive; CK7 negative
    - SNUC: CK5/6, CK13, CK14 negative; CK7 positive

PNET/Ewing Sarcoma

- FLI-1 (nuclear) and CD99 (O13) positive
- Epithelial markers negative to very focally positive
- Defining translocation t(11;22)(q24;q12)

NUT Midline Carcinoma

- Poorly differentiated or undifferentiated carcinoma with squamous differentiation
    - Squamous differentiation > 80% of cases
- Unique chromosomal translocation sole identifier of this disease
    - t(15;19) results in novel fusion oncogene *BRD4-NUT*

DIAGNOSTIC CHECKLIST

Clinically Relevant Pathologic Features

- Symptom time frame
    - Characteristically, symptoms develop over short duration (weeks to months)

SNUC: Differential Diagnosis Based on Immunohistochemical Staining

IHC	SNUC	ONB	SCUNC	MMM	NK/T	RMS
CK	+	-	+	-	-	-
p63	±	-	±	-	±	-
CK5/6	+	-	-	-	-	-
CHR	±	+	+	-	-	-
SYN	±	+	+	-	-	-
CD57	-	+	+	-	-	±
NSE	- (may be focally +)	+	+	±	-	-
S100 protein	- (may be focally +)	+ (peripheral pattern)	+ (lacks peripheral pattern)	+ (diffuse)	-	-
VIM	-	±	±	+ (diffuse)	±	+
Melanocytic markers	-	-	-	+	-	-
CD45RB	-	-	-	-	+	-
CD56	±	+	+	-	+	±
Muscle markers	-	-	-	-	-	+
EBER	-	-	-	-	+	-

SNUC = sinonasal undifferentiated carcinoma; ONB = olfactory neuroblastoma; SCUNC = small cell undifferentiated neuroendocrine carcinoma; NK/T = angiocentric NK-/T-cell lymphoma; RMS = rhabdomyosarcoma; CK = cytokeratin (AE1/AE3, CAM5.2); CHR = chromogranin; SYN = synaptophysin; NSE = neuron-specific enolase; VIM = vimentin; LCA = leucocyte common antigen (CD45RB); EBER = Epstein-Barr encoded RNA (in situ hybridization). Melanocytic markers include HMB-45, Melan-A, and tyrosinase; muscle markers are desmin, myoglobin, and myogenin.

- Rapid onset not typical with other sinonasal malignant neoplasms
- Rapid clinical onset represents helpful diagnostic finding

SELECTED REFERENCES

1. Menon S et al: Sinonasal malignancies with neuroendocrine differentiation: case series and review of literature. Indian J Pathol Microbiol. 53(1):28-34, 2010
2. Cordes B et al: Molecular and phenotypic analysis of poorly differentiated sinonasal neoplasms: an integrated approach for early diagnosis and classification. Hum Pathol. 40(3):283-92, 2009
3. Wenig BM: Undifferentiated malignant neoplasms of the sinonasal tract. Arch Pathol Lab Med. 133(5):699-712, 2009
4. Schmidt ER et al: Diagnosis and treatment of sinonasal undifferentiated carcinoma: report of a case and review of the literature. J Oral Maxillofac Surg. 66(7):1505-10, 2008
5. Stelow EB et al: NUT rearrangement in undifferentiated carcinomas of the upper aerodigestive tract. Am J Surg Pathol. 32(6):828-34, 2008
6. Weinreb I et al: Non-small cell neuroendocrine carcinoma of the sinonasal tract and nasopharynx. Report of 2 cases and review of the literature. Head Neck Pathol. 1(1):21-6, 2007
7. Mendenhall WM et al: Sinonasal undifferentiated carcinoma. Am J Clin Oncol. 29(1):27-31, 2006
8. Ejaz A et al: Sinonasal undifferentiated carcinoma: clinical and pathologic features and a discussion on classification, cellular differentiation, and differential diagnosis. Adv Anat Pathol. 12(3):134-43, 2005
9. Enepekides DJ: Sinonasal undifferentiated carcinoma: an update. Curr Opin Otolaryngol Head Neck Surg. 13(4):222-5, 2005
10. Iezzoni JC et al: "Undifferentiated" small round cell tumors of the sinonasal tract: differential diagnosis update. Am J Clin Pathol. 124 Suppl:S110-21, 2005
11. Kim BS et al: Sinonasal undifferentiated carcinoma: case series and literature review. Am J Otolaryngol. 25(3):162-6, 2004
12. Kramer D et al: Sinonasal undifferentiated carcinoma: case series and systematic review of the literature. J Otolaryngol. 33(1):32-6, 2004
13. Franchi A et al: Sinonasal undifferentiated carcinoma, nasopharyngeal-type undifferentiated carcinoma, and keratinizing and nonkeratinizing squamous cell carcinoma express different cytokeratin patterns. Am J Surg Pathol. 26(12):1597-604, 2002
14. Jeng YM et al: Sinonasal undifferentiated carcinoma and nasopharyngeal-type undifferentiated carcinoma: two clinically, biologically, and histopathologically distinct entities. Am J Surg Pathol. 26(3):371-6, 2002
15. Musy PY et al: Sinonasal undifferentiated carcinoma: the search for a better outcome. Laryngoscope. 112(8 Pt 1):1450-5, 2002
16. Cerilli LA et al: Sinonasal undifferentiated carcinoma: immunohistochemical profile and lack of EBV association. Am J Surg Pathol. 25(2):156-63, 2001
17. Smullen JL et al: Sinonasal undifferentiated carcinoma: a review of the literature. J La State Med Soc. 153(10):487-90, 2001
18. Houston GD et al: Sinonasal undifferentiated carcinoma: a distinctive clinicopathologic entity. Adv Anat Pathol. 6(6):317-23, 1999
19. Phillips CD et al: Sinonasal undifferentiated carcinoma: CT and MR imaging of an uncommon neoplasm of the nasal cavity. Radiology. 202(2):477-80, 1997
20. Mills SE et al: "Undifferentiated" neoplasms of the sinonasal region: differential diagnosis based on clinical, light microscopic, immunohistochemical, and ultrastructural features. Semin Diagn Pathol. 6(4):316-28, 1989
21. Levine PA et al: Sinonasal undifferentiated carcinoma: a distinctive and highly aggressive neoplasm. Laryngoscope. 97(8 Pt 1):905-8, 1987
22. Frierson HF Jr et al: Sinonasal undifferentiated carcinoma. An aggressive neoplasm derived from schneiderian epithelium and distinct from olfactory neuroblastoma. Am J Surg Pathol. 10(11):771-9, 1986

Imaging and Microscopic Features

*(**Left**) Axial NECT demonstrates a large mass in the left maxillary antrum with marked bone destruction and extension into the nasal cavity ➔, masticator space ➔, and soft tissues of the cheek. Foci of air are seen within the necrotic portion of this rapidly growing lesion. (**Right**) Coronal T1 C+ FS MR shows a thick, nodular enhancing rim at the periphery of the mass with central necrosis. There is aggressive invasion of the orbit ➔.*

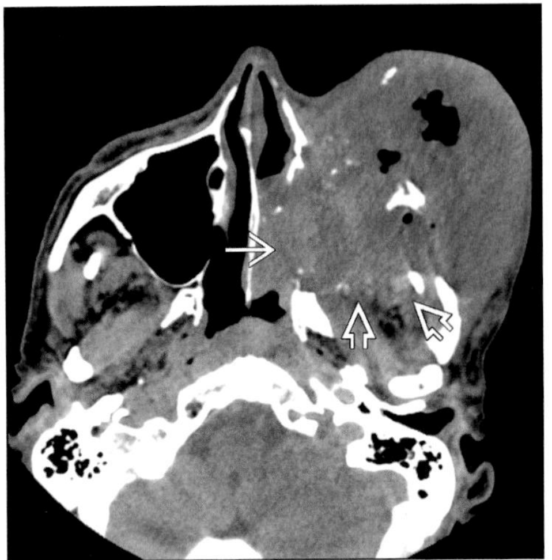

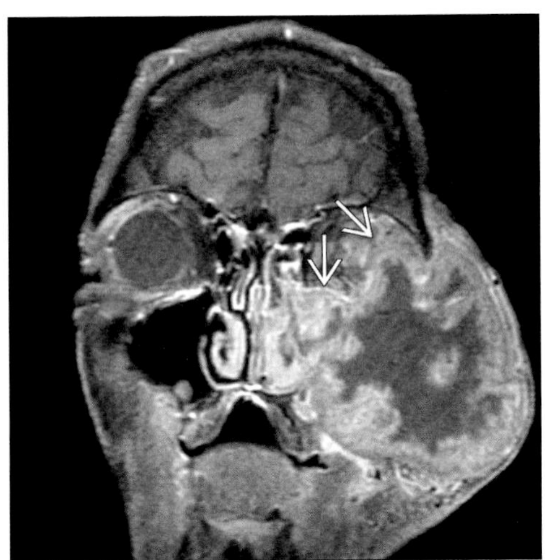

*(**Left**) Histologic features of the "Western" type SNUC include cells with round to oval hyperchromatic nuclei, inconspicuous to small nucleoli, and limited pink to amphophilic appearing cytoplasm. (**Right**) Undifferentiated malignant cellular proliferation is similar to large cell carcinoma of the lung, including large polygonal cells with pleomorphic nuclei, prominent eosinophilic nucleoli, and a moderate amount of eosinophilic cytoplasm. Mitoses, including atypical forms ➔, are seen.*

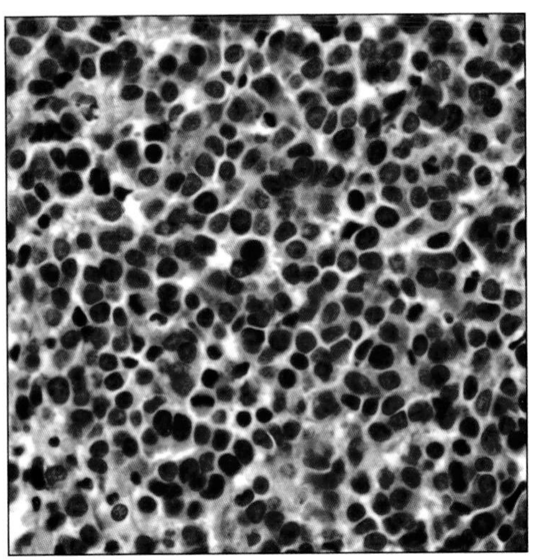

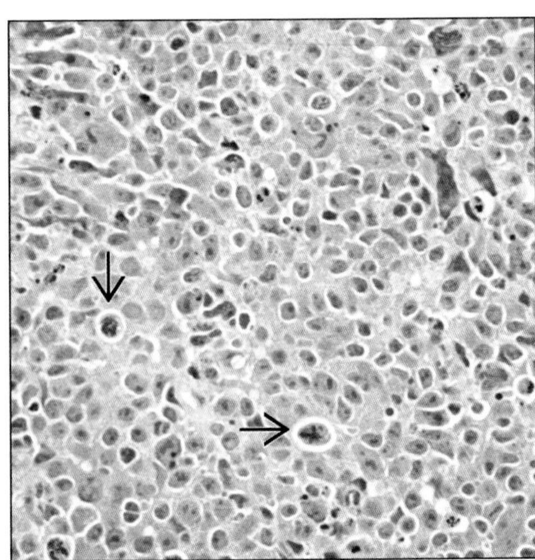

*(**Left**) Transitional area includes nonneoplastic surface epithelium (showing squamous metaplasia ➔) to carcinoma ➔. Typically, it is uncommon to find intraepithelial neoplasia in SNUCs. Such a finding lends support that SNUC originates from the sinonasal surface epithelium. Submucosal invasive carcinoma with lobular growth is present ➔. (**Right**) In addition to individual cell necrosis, SNUCs typically include confluent areas of tumor necrosis ➔.*

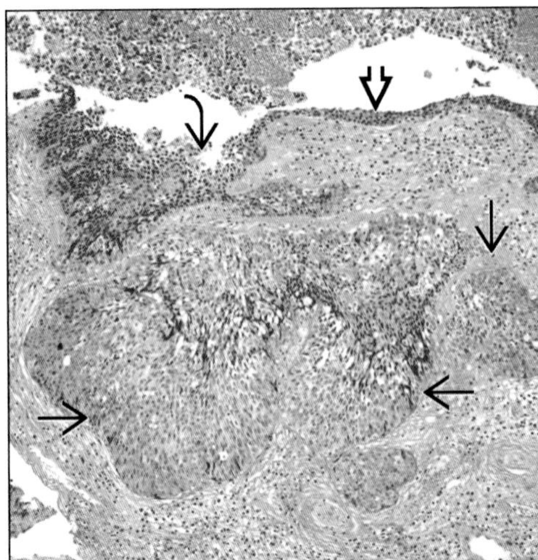

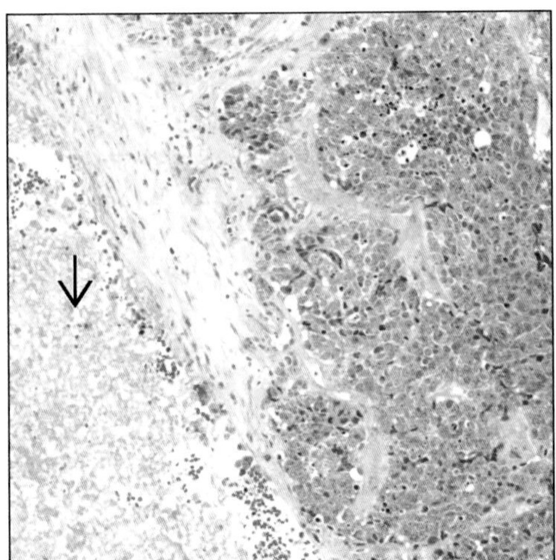

Immunohistochemical Features and Differential Diagnosis

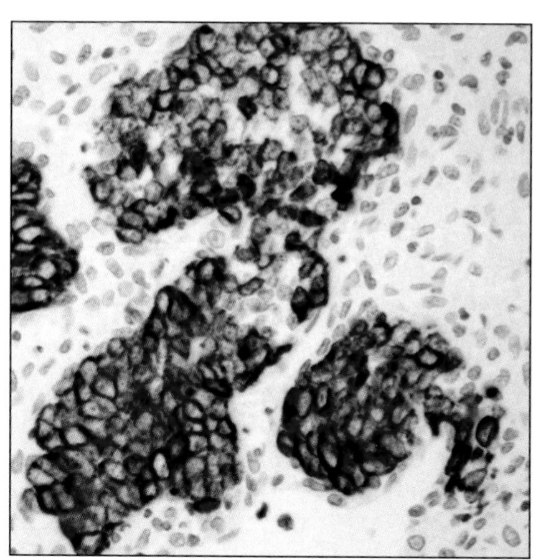

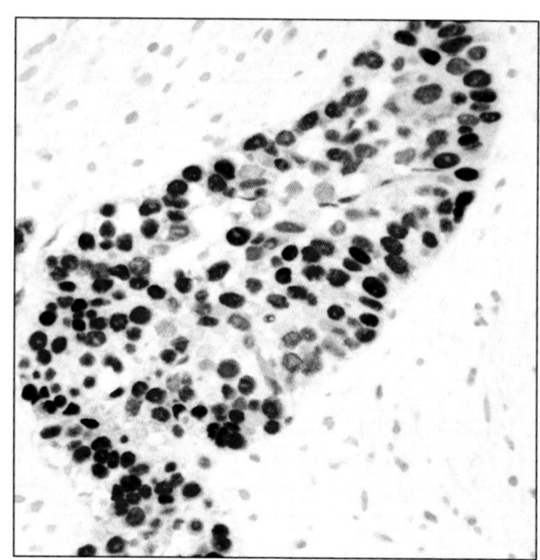

(Left) *IHC antigenic profile of SNUCs invariably includes cytokeratin reactivity.* **(Right)** *p63 immunoreactivity, a marker of squamous cell differentiation, varies from case to case and even within the same case. Diffuse (nuclear) p63 reactivity is present, but adjacent areas of tumor were p63 negative. The combination of intraepithelial neoplasia and cytokeratin and p63 reactivity in the absence of reactivity for other markers support a surface epithelial origin.*

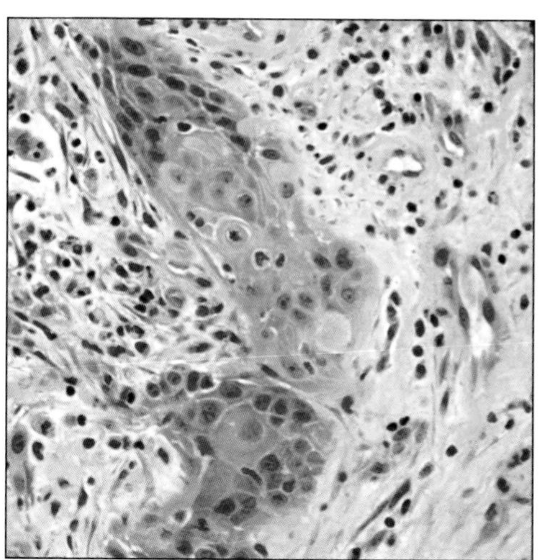

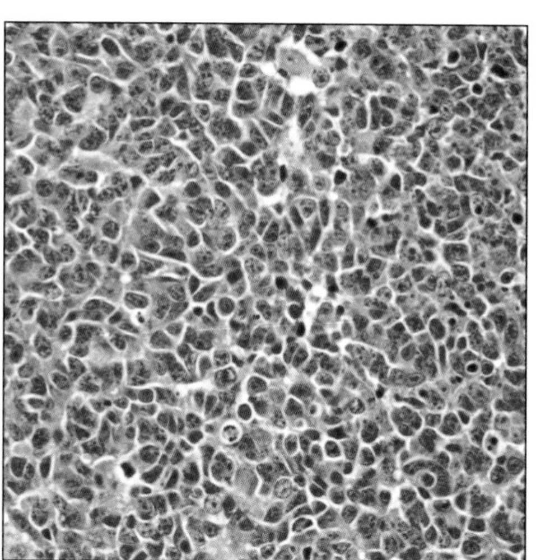

(Left) *Rarely foci of squamous differentiation may be seen in SNUCs. However, the clinical parameters typical for SNUC (rapid onset) with evidence of aggressive growth must be present. If not, alternative diagnostic considerations may include squamous cell carcinoma or variant thereof and NUT midline carcinoma. The latter would require the presence of t(15;19).* **(Right)** *High-grade olfactory neuroblastoma (ONB) shares overlapping histologic features with SNUC.*

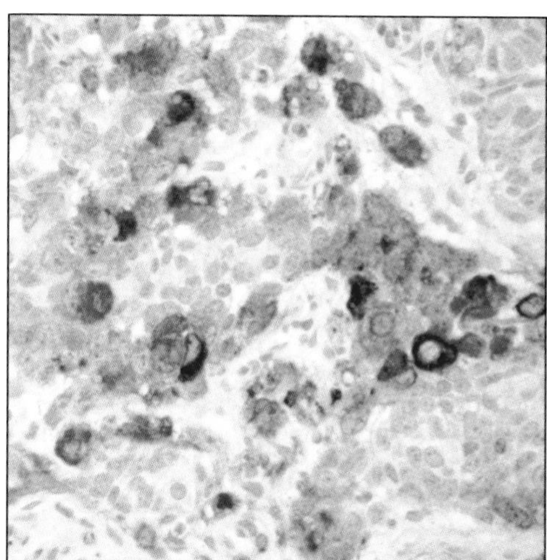

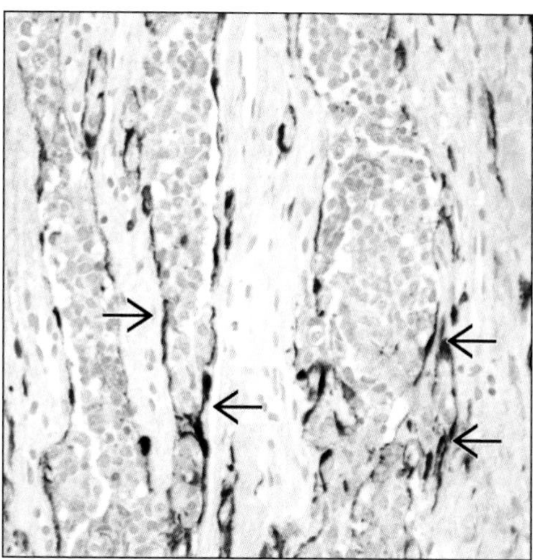

(Left) *Differentiating SNUC from ONB requires immunohistochemical staining. ONBs are consistently reactive for NSE and are consistently negative for cytokeratins (or show extremely limited [focal and weak] cytokeratin staining). SNUCs are uniformly cytokeratin reactive (diffuse and strong) but may show limited NSE reactivity.* **(Right)** *ONBs show characteristic peripheral S100 protein staining ⇒, a finding not seen with SNUC or other high-grade SNT malignancies.*

LYMPHOEPITHELIAL CARCINOMA

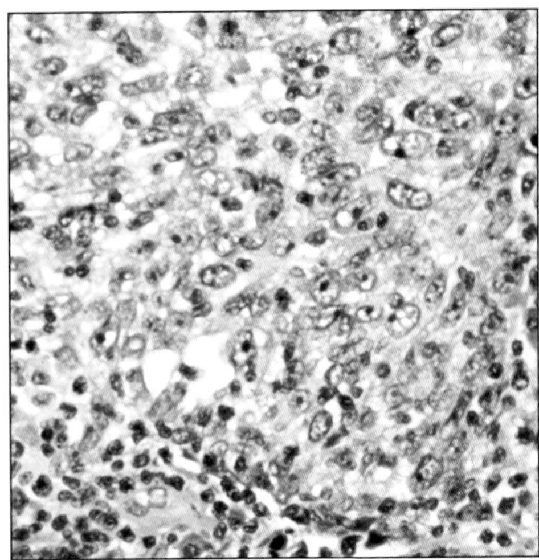

Sinonasal lymphoepithelial carcinoma (LEC) includes cells with identical morphology to its nasopharyngeal counterpart including enlarged vesicular nuclei and prominent eosinophilic nucleoli.

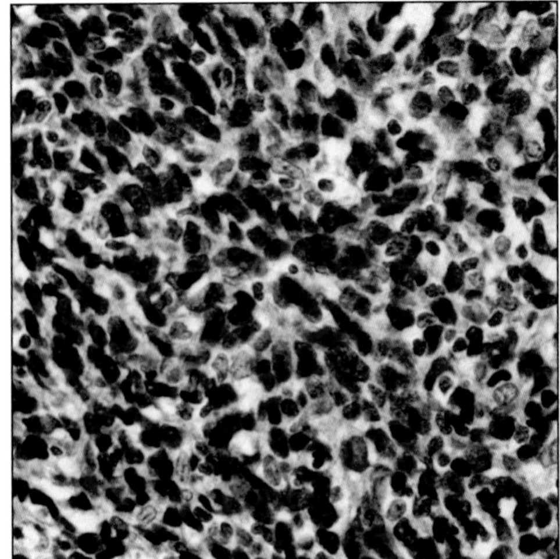

The presence of EBER (along with cytokeratin staining) represents supportive diagnostic features for LEC and assist in differentiating it from other sinonasal-type carcinomas.

TERMINOLOGY

Abbreviations

- Lymphoepithelial carcinoma (LEC)

Synonyms

- Lymphoepithelial-like carcinoma
- Nasopharyngeal-type undifferentiated carcinoma
- Undifferentiated carcinoma
- Undifferentiated carcinoma with lymphoid stroma

Definitions

- Undifferentiated carcinoma of the sinonasal tract that is morphologically similar to counterpart in nasopharynx

ETIOLOGY/PATHOGENESIS

Infectious Agents

- Strong association with Epstein-Barr virus (EBV)
  - Almost all sinonasal LECs associated with EBV
  - Only minority of LECs of larynx, hypopharynx are EBV positive

CLINICAL ISSUES

Epidemiology

- Incidence
  - Rare sinonasal tract carcinoma
- Age
  - 5th to 7th decades of life
    - Range: 31-75 years
- Gender
  - Male > Female (3:1)

Site

- More common in nasal cavity than paranasal sinuses
  - May rarely originate in other upper aerodigestive mucosal sites
    - Salivary glands (parotid)
    - Larynx
    - Hypopharynx

Presentation

- Nasal obstruction, blood-tinged rhinorrhea, epistaxis
- Proptosis, visual disturbances, cranial nerve dysfunction may be present

Treatment

- Radiation
  - Represents treatment of choice

Prognosis

- Favorable owing to good response to radiotherapy
  - 61% disease-free survival reported (median follow-up: 48 months)

MICROSCOPIC PATHOLOGY

Histologic Features

- Neoplastic cells
  - Enlarged round nuclei, prominent eosinophilic nucleoli, dispersed (vesicular) nuclear chromatin, scant eosinophilic to amphophilic cytoplasm
  - Absent keratinization
  - Intraepithelial dysplasia, spindle-shaped cells may be present
- Prominent nonneoplastic lymphoid component composed of mature lymphocytes and plasma cells present
  - May be abundant or relatively absent
  - When abundant, may obscure neoplastic cells
- May demonstrate syncytial growth with cohesive cells or diffuse noncohesive cellular infiltrate
  - Stromal desmoplastic response typically absent
- Mitoses, necrosis infrequently present

LYMPHOEPITHELIAL CARCINOMA

Key Facts

Terminology
- Undifferentiated carcinoma of sinonasal tract that is morphologically similar to counterpart in nasopharynx

Etiology/Pathogenesis
- Strong association with Epstein-Barr virus (EBV)

Clinical Issues
- Rare sinonasal tract carcinoma
- More common in nasal cavity than paranasal sinuses
- Favorable prognosis owing to good response to radiotherapy

Microscopic Pathology
- Enlarged round nuclei, prominent eosinophilic nucleoli, dispersed (vesicular) nuclear chromatin
- Absent keratinization
- Prominent nonneoplastic lymphoid component
- Cytokeratin positive, EBV encoded RNA (EBER)(+)

ANCILLARY TESTS

Immunohistochemistry
- Cytokeratin positive (AE1/AE3, CAM5.2)
  - CK5/6, CK13 positive
- EBV encoded RNA (EBER) positive
- NSE, neuroendocrine markers negative

DIFFERENTIAL DIAGNOSIS

Sinonasal Undifferentiated Carcinoma (SNUC)
- May share light microscopic & immunohistochemical (i.e., cytokeratins) features with LEC
- Differentiation based on clinical presentation, light microscopy, association with EBV
  - Rapid clinical onset and growth of tumor typical for SNUC, not LEC
  - SNUC characterized by increased mitotic activity, atypical mitoses, necrosis
  - SNUC not associated with EBV
  - Purported differential cytokeratin staining from LEC
    - SNUC: CK5/6, CK13 negative
    - LEC: CK5/6, CK13 positive

Nasopharyngeal Undifferentiated Carcinoma
- Identical histologic, immunohistochemical features, shared strong EBV association
- Imperative to exclude sinonasal involvement from nasopharyngeal primary tumor
  - Detailed clinical/radiologic evaluation indicated to determine origin of neoplasm

Mucosal Malignant Melanoma
- Presence of S100 protein and melanocytic markers (HMB-45, Melan-A, tyrosinase)
- Absence of epithelial markers (cytokeratins)

Non-Hodgkin Lymphoma
- Presence of hematolymphoid markers (CD45RB), lineage (B-, T-cell) specific markers, CD56
- Absence of epithelial markers (cytokeratins)

SELECTED REFERENCES

1. Hajiioannou JK et al: Nasopharyngeal-type undifferentiated carcinoma (lymphoepithelioma) of paranasal sinuses: Rare case and literature review. J Otolaryngol. 35(2):147-51, 2006
2. Franchi A et al: Sinonasal undifferentiated carcinoma, nasopharyngeal-type undifferentiated carcinoma, and keratinizing and nonkeratinizing squamous cell carcinoma express different cytokeratin patterns. Am J Surg Pathol. 26(12):1597-604, 2002
3. Jeng YM et al: Sinonasal undifferentiated carcinoma and nasopharyngeal-type undifferentiated carcinoma: two clinically, biologically, and histopathologically distinct entities. Am J Surg Pathol. 26(3):371-6, 2002
4. Zong Y et al: Epstein-Barr virus infection of sinonasal lymphoepithelial carcinoma in Guangzhou. Chin Med J (Engl). 114(2):132-6, 2001

IMAGE GALLERY

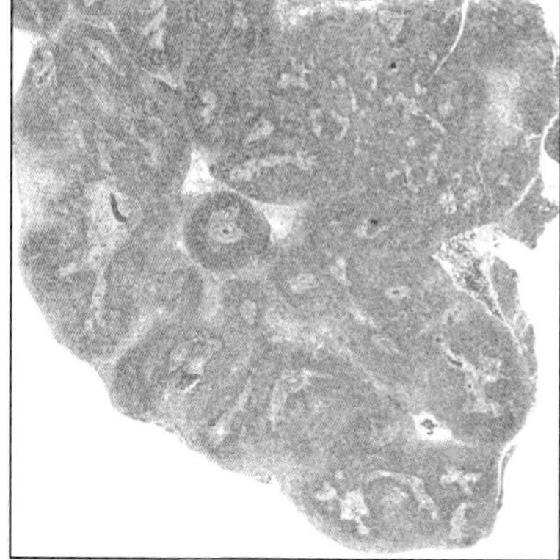

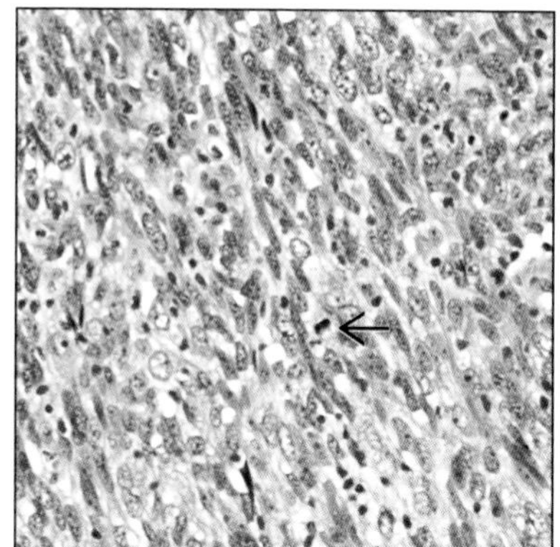

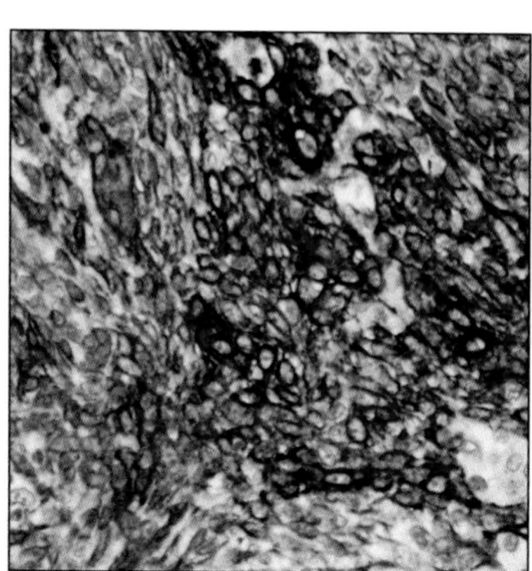

(Left) *Sinonasal LEC shows polypoid appearance with interconnecting cords of tumor representing histologic features more commonly seen in the sinonasal nonkeratinizing carcinoma. The latter, while cytokeratin positive, is negative for EBER.* ***(Center)*** *Spindle-shaped neoplastic cells are seen. Scattered mitotic figures are present ➡.* ***(Right)*** *Cytokeratin immunoreactivity confirms the presence of a carcinoma and, in conjunction with EBER staining, supports a diagnosis of LEC.*

SINONASAL ADENOCARCINOMA, INTESTINAL TYPE

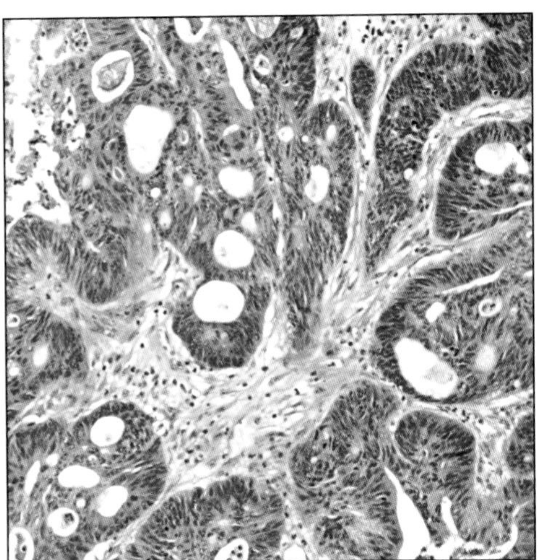

In this sinonasal tract intestinal-type adenocarcinoma, colonic type, a prevalence of tubuloglandular architecture, virtually identical to primary colonic adenocarcinoma, is shown.

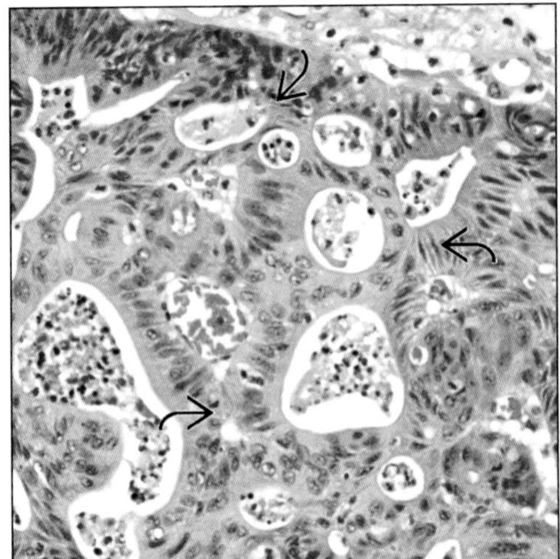

The colonic type shows complex glandular growth with back to back glands ➚. The histologic, histochemical, and immunohistochemical findings are identical to colonic adenocarcinoma.

TERMINOLOGY

Abbreviations

- Intestinal-type adenocarcinoma (ITAC)

Synonyms

- Colonic-type adenocarcinoma
- Enteric-type adenocarcinoma

Definitions

- Malignant epithelial glandular tumors of sinonasal tract (SNT) that histologically resemble intestinal adenocarcinoma

ETIOLOGY/PATHOGENESIS

Environmental Exposure

- Exposure to hardwood dust, leather, and softwood
  - Increased incidences in
    - Woodworkers
    - Workers in shoe and furniture industries
  - May occur sporadically without environmental exposure

CLINICAL ISSUES

Epidemiology

- Incidence
  - Adenocarcinomas (all types) comprise 10-20% of sinonasal tract malignant neoplasms
    - ITACs are rare
- Age
  - Occurs over wide range
    - Most common in 5th to 7th decades of life
- Gender
  - ITAC associated with environmental exposure
    - Male > Female
  - ITAC not associated with environmental exposure
    - Female > Male

Site

- May arise anywhere in SNT but in decreasing order of frequency
  - Ethmoid sinus > nasal cavity (inferior and middle turbinates) > maxillary sinus

Presentation

- Early symptoms
  - Nonspecific, varying from nasal stuffiness to obstruction
  - May be associated with epistaxis
- Due to delay in diagnosis, tumors may reach large size with extensive invasion at time of presentation
  - Advanced tumors present with pain, cranial nerve deficits, visual disturbances, and exophthalmos

Treatment

- Surgical approaches
  - Complete surgical resection with radiation
    - Depending on extent of neoplasm, surgery varies from local excision to more radical procedures (maxillectomy, ethmoidectomy, and additional exenterations)
  - Neck dissection not indicated
- Radiation
  - Radiotherapy may be utilized for extensive disease &/or for higher grade neoplasms

Prognosis

- All ITACs considered as potentially aggressive, lethal tumors
- 5-year cumulative survival rate is around 40%, with most deaths occurring within 3 years
- Generally are locally aggressive tumors with frequent local failure (approximately 50%)
- Metastasis to cervical lymph nodes and spread to distant sites are infrequent, occurring in approximately 10% and 20%, respectively

SINONASAL ADENOCARCINOMA, INTESTINAL TYPE

Key Facts

Terminology
- Malignant epithelial glandular tumors of sinonasal tract that histologically resemble intestinal adenocarcinoma

Etiology/Pathogenesis
- Exposure to hardwood dust, leather, and softwood
  - Increased incidences in woodworkers, workers in shoe and furniture industries
  - May occur sporadically without environmental exposure

Clinical Issues
- May arise anywhere in SNT but in decreasing order of frequency
  - Ethmoid sinus > nasal cavity (inferior and middle turbinates) > maxillary sinus
- Complete surgical resection with radiation
- All ITACs considered potentially aggressive, lethal
- 5-year cumulative survival rate is around 40%, with most deaths occurring within 3 years

Microscopic Pathology
- Barnes classification
  - Papillary
  - Colonic
  - Solid
  - Mucinous
  - Mixed

Ancillary Tests
- Reactive for gastrointestinal type markers
  - CK20, CDX-2, villin, mucin-related antigens (MUCs)

- Death results from uncontrollable local or regional disease with extension and invasion of vital structures &/or metastatic disease
- Most patients present with advanced local disease, so clinical staging generally has no relevant prognostic significance
- Histologic subtype identified as indicative of clinical behavior
  - Papillary type (grade I) behave more indolently than other histologic variants
- No difference in behavior between ITAC occurring in occupational exposed individuals and sporadically occurring ITACs

IMAGE FINDINGS

Radiographic Findings
- Essential in determining extent of disease and planning surgery
- Early lesions
  - Soft tissue mass
  - Absent to minimal bone destruction
- More advance lesions associated with
  - Osteodestruction
  - Invasion of contiguous anatomic structures/ compartments
    - e.g., orbit, cranial cavity

MICROSCOPIC PATHOLOGY

Histologic Features
- 2 histologic classifications proposed
  - Barnes vs. Kleinsasser and Schroeder
    - Either classification is acceptable, but for simplicity Barnes classification is preferred
  - Barnes classification
    - Papillary
    - Colonic
    - Solid
    - Mucinous
    - Mixed
  - Kleinsasser and Schroeder classification
    - Papillary tubular cylinder (PTCC) types I-III (I = well differentiated, II = moderately differentiated, III = poorly differentiated)
    - Alveolar goblet type
    - Signet ring type
    - Transitional type
- **Papillary type**
  - Represents approximately 18% of cases
  - Shows predominance of papillary architecture with occasional tubular glands, minimal cytologic atypia, rare mitotic figures
- **Colonic type**
  - Represents approximately 40% of cases
  - Prevalence of tubuloglandular architecture, rare papillae, with increased nuclear pleomorphism and mitotic activity
- **Solid type**
  - Represents approximately 20% of cases
  - Loss of differentiation characterized by solid and trabecular growth with isolated tubule formation
  - Marked increase in smaller cuboidal cells with nuclear pleomorphism, round vesicular nuclei, prominent nucleoli, and increased mitotic figures
- **Mucinous type**
  - Uncommon type
  - One pattern shows
    - Solid clusters of cells, individual glands, signet ring cells, short papillary fronds with or without fibrovascular cores
    - Mucin predominantly intracellular, and mucomyxoid matrix may be present
  - Another pattern shows
    - Presence of large, well-formed glands distended by mucus and extracellular mucin pools
    - Pools of extracellular mucin separated by thin connective tissue septa creating alveolar-type pattern
    - Predominantly cuboidal or goblet tumor cells present in single layers at periphery of mucus lakes

SINONASAL ADENOCARCINOMA, INTESTINAL TYPE

- Mucus extravasation elicits inflammatory response that may include multinucleated giant cells
- Tumors where mucus component predominates (> 50%) are similar to their gastrointestinal counterparts and may be classified as mucinous adenocarcinomas

- Papillary and colonic types are most common histologic types, whether occurring in association with environmental exposure or sporadically
- Irrespective of histologic type, ITACs histologically simulate normal intestinal mucosa and may include
  - Villi, Paneth cells, enterochromaffin cells, and muscularis mucosa
- In rare instances, lesion is composed of well-formed villi lined by columnar cells resembling resorptive cells
  - In such cases, bundles of smooth muscle cells resembling muscularis mucosae may also be identified under villi
- **Mixed type**
  - Rare type
  - Composed of admixture of 2 or more of the previously defined patterns

ANCILLARY TESTS

Histochemistry

- Mucicarmine
  - Intracytoplasmic and intraluminal positive
- PAS with diastase
  - Diastase-resistant, PAS-positive intracytoplasmic and intraluminal material

Immunohistochemistry

- Reactive for gastrointestinal type markers
  - CK20 positivity (up to 86% of cases)
  - CDX-2 is nuclear transcription factor involved in differentiation of intestinal epithelial cells and diffusely expressed in intestinal adenocarcinomas reactive in ITACs
  - Expression of villin also present
  - Mucin-related antigens (MUCs) include MUC2(+), MUC5(+)
- Strongly reactive with pancytokeratins
- Variable CK7 reactivity (43-93% of cases)
- Variably positive for other epithelial markers including
  - Epithelial membrane antigen, B72.3, Ber-EP4, BRST-1, Leu-M1, and human milk fat globule (HMFG-2)
  - Variable CEA staining
- Neoplastic cells may express variety of hormone peptides including
  - Serotonin, cholecystokinin, gastrin, somatostatin, leu-enkephalin
- Chromogranin, synaptophysin, CD56 positivity can be identified
  - Rare examples of mixed ITAC-small cell neuroendocrine carcinoma reported
- Epidermal growth factor receptor (EGFR) protein expression and *EGFR* gene copy gains reported
  - Frequency of EGFR overexpression significantly higher in woodworkers than in leatherworkers or those with no known occupational history
  - High levels of EGFR often associated with either gene amplification or chromosome 7 polysomy
- p53 immunoreactivity can be identified
- Increased proliferation rate by Ki-67 (MIB-1) staining

Cytogenetics

- Chromosomal gains and losses identified by comparative genomic hybridization (CGH)
  - Gains at 5p15, 20q13, and 8q24
  - Losses at 4q31-qter, 18q12-22, 8p12-pter, and 5q11-qter
  - Microsatellite instability (MSI) not detected

Molecular Genetics

- Discrepant molecular findings including
  - *K-ras* mutations from 0-20%
  - *H-ras* mutations from 0-25%
  - *P53* mutations from 14-44%

DIFFERENTIAL DIAGNOSIS

Metastatic Adenocarcinoma of Gastrointestinal Origin

- Rare occurrence to sinonasal tract
- Clinical history critical and mandatory in excluding a metastasis to sinonasal tract from primary gastrointestinal tract (GIT) neoplasm
- Histology, histochemistry, and immunohistochemistry of ITAC essentially identical to GIT adenocarcinomas

Sinonasal Nonintestinal-Nonsalivary Adenocarcinoma

- Morphologic features differ from ITACs
- Lack immunoreactivity for gastrointestinal-type markers
  - e.g., CK20, CDX-2, villin, mucins

Salivary Gland Adenocarcinomas

- Most common type in SNT is adenoid cystic carcinoma
- Less common types include
  - Acinic cell adenocarcinoma
  - Mucoepidermoid carcinoma
- Overall histology of salivary gland carcinomas differ from SNT ITACs

Nasopharyngeal Low-Grade Papillary Adenocarcinoma

- Localization to nasopharynx most often along lateral wall
- Immunoreactive for thyroid transcription factor 1 (TTF-1)
- Lack immunoreactivity for gastrointestinal-type markers

Papillary Sinusitis

- Comprised of ciliated respiratory epithelium with simple papillae lacking complex growth
- Absence of dysplastic epithelial changes
- Absence of infiltrative growth

SINONASAL ADENOCARCINOMA, INTESTINAL TYPE

Sinonasal Tract ITACs Classification

Barnes	Kleinsasser & Schroeder	Percentage of Cases	3-Year Cumulative Survival
Papillary type	Papillary tubular cylinder cell I	18%	82%
Colonic type	Papillary tubular cylinder cell II	40%	54%
Solid type	Papillary tubular cylinder cell III	20%	36%
Mucinous type	Alveolar goblet	Uncommon	48%
	Signet ring	Uncommon	0%
Mixed type	Transitional	Rare	71%

SELECTED REFERENCES

1. Mayr SI et al: Characterization of initial clinical symptoms and risk factors for sinonasal adenocarcinomas: results of a case-control study. Int Arch Occup Environ Health. 83(6):631-8, 2010
2. Stelow EB et al: Adenocarcinoma of the upper aerodigestive tract. Adv Anat Pathol. 17(4):262-9, 2010
3. Thompson LD: Intestinal-type sinonasal adenocarcinoma. Ear Nose Throat J. 89(1):16-8, 2010
4. Hermsen MA et al: Genome-wide analysis of genetic changes in intestinal-type sinonasal adenocarcinoma. Head Neck. 31(3):290-7, 2009
5. Jain R et al: Composite intestinal-type adenocarcinoma and small cell carcinoma of sinonasal tract. J Clin Pathol. 62(7):634-7, 2009
6. Llorente JL et al: Genetic and clinical aspects of wood dust related intestinal-type sinonasal adenocarcinoma: a review. Eur Arch Otorhinolaryngol. 266(1):1-7, 2009
7. Martínez JG et al: Microsatellite instability analysis of sinonasal carcinomas. Otolaryngol Head Neck Surg. 140(1):55-60, 2009
8. Perez-Ordoñez B: Hamartomas, papillomas and adenocarcinomas of the sinonasal tract and nasopharynx. J Clin Pathol. 62(12):1085-95, 2009
9. Castillo C et al: Signet-ring cell adenocarcinoma of sinonasal tract: an immunohistochemical study of the mucins profile. Arch Pathol Lab Med. 131(6):961-4, 2007
10. Ozolek JA et al: Basal/myoepithelial cells in chronic sinusitis, respiratory epithelial adenomatoid hamartoma, inverted papilloma, and intestinal-type and nonintestinal-type sinonasal adenocarcinoma: an immunohistochemical study. Arch Pathol Lab Med. 131(4):530-7, 2007
11. Luna MA: Sinonasal tubulopapillary low-grade adenocarcinoma: a specific diagnosis or just another seromucous adenocarcinoma? Adv Anat Pathol. 12(3):109-15, 2005
12. Yom SS et al: Genetic analysis of sinonasal adenocarcinoma phenotypes: distinct alterations of histogenetic significance. Mod Pathol. 18(3):315-9, 2005
13. Ariza M et al: Comparative genomic hybridization in primary sinonasal adenocarcinomas. Cancer. 100(2):335-41, 2004
14. Cathro HP et al: Immunophenotypic differences between intestinal-type and low-grade papillary sinonasal adenocarcinomas: an immunohistochemical study of 22 cases utilizing CDX2 and MUC2. Am J Surg Pathol. 28(8):1026-32, 2004
15. Franchi A et al: CDX-2, cytokeratin 7 and cytokeratin 20 immunohistochemical expression in the differential diagnosis of primary adenocarcinomas of the sinonasal tract. Virchows Arch. 445(1):63-7, 2004
16. Kennedy MT et al: Expression pattern of CK7, CK20, CDX-2, and villin in intestinal-type sinonasal adenocarcinoma. J Clin Pathol. 57(9):932-7, 2004
17. Perez-Ordonez B et al: Expression of mismatch repair proteins, beta catenin, and E cadherin in intestinal-type sinonasal adenocarcinoma. J Clin Pathol. 57(10):1080-3, 2004
18. Bashir AA et al: Sinonasal adenocarcinoma: immunohistochemical marking and expression of oncoproteins. Head Neck. 25(9):763-71, 2003
19. Sklar EM et al: Sinonasal intestinal-type adenocarcinoma involvement of the paranasal sinuses. AJNR Am J Neuroradiol. 24(6):1152-5, 2003
20. Franchi A et al: Clinical relevance of the histological classification of sinonasal intestinal-type adenocarcinomas. Hum Pathol. 30(10):1140-5, 1999
21. Gallo O et al: Prognostic significance of c-erbB-2 oncoprotein expression in intestinal-type adenocarcinoma of the sinonasal tract. Head Neck. 20(3):224-31, 1998
22. Saber AT et al: K-ras mutations in sinonasal adenocarcinomas in patients occupationally exposed to wood or leather dust. Cancer Lett. 126(1):59-65, 1998
23. Franchi A et al: Prognostic implications of Sialosyl-Tn antigen expression in sinonasal intestinal-type adenocarcinoma. Eur J Cancer B Oral Oncol. 32B(2):123-7, 1996
24. Van den Oever R: Occupational exposure to dust and sinonasal cancer. An analysis of 386 cases reported to the N.C.C.S.F. Cancer Registry. Acta Otorhinolaryngol Belg. 50(1):19-24, 1996
25. Leung SY et al: Epstein-Barr virus is present in a wide histological spectrum of sinonasal carcinomas. Am J Surg Pathol. 19(9):994-1001, 1995
26. McKinney CD et al: Sinonasal intestinal-type adenocarcinoma: immunohistochemical profile and comparison with colonic adenocarcinoma. Mod Pathol. 8(4):421-6, 1995
27. Urso C et al: Intestinal-type adenocarcinoma of the sinonasal tract: a clinicopathologic study of 18 cases. Tumori. 79(3):205-10, 1993
28. Franquemont DW et al: Histologic classification of sinonasal intestinal-type adenocarcinoma. Am J Surg Pathol. 15(4):368-75, 1991
29. López JI et al: Intestinal-type adenocarcinoma of the nasal cavity and paranasal sinuses. A clinicopathologic study of 6 cases. Tumori. 76(3):250-4, 1990
30. Alessi DM et al: Nonsalivary sinonasal adenocarcinoma. Arch Otolaryngol Head Neck Surg. 114(9):996-9, 1988
31. Hayes RB et al: Wood-related occupations, wood dust exposure, and sinonasal cancer. Am J Epidemiol. 124(4):569-77, 1986
32. Mills SE et al: Aggressive sinonasal lesion resembling normal intestinal mucosa. Am J Surg Pathol. 6(8):803-9, 1982

SINONASAL ADENOCARCINOMA, INTESTINAL TYPE

Imaging and Microscopic Features

*(**Left**) Axial CECT shows a heterogeneous mass ➡ with cystic foci, which arises in the anterior ethmoid sinuses, a frequent location for sinonasal adenocarcinomas associated with environmental exposures. The mass shows extensive local invasion, including into the nasal soft tissues ↗. (**Right**) Axial CT demonstrates a destructive lesion in the right sinonasal cavities with erosion of the medial antral wall ➡ and spread into the pterygopalatine fossa ⇨.*

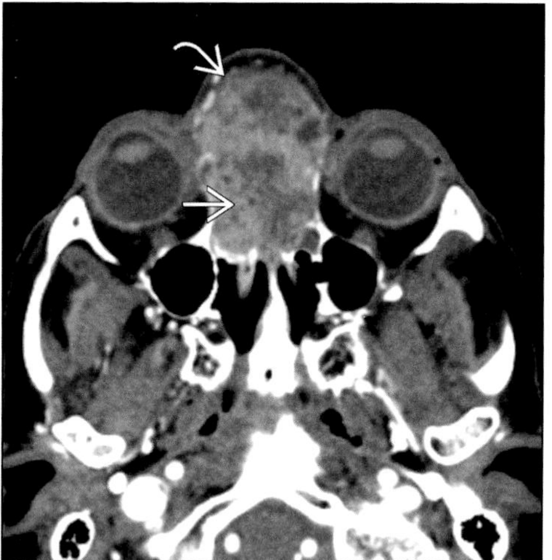

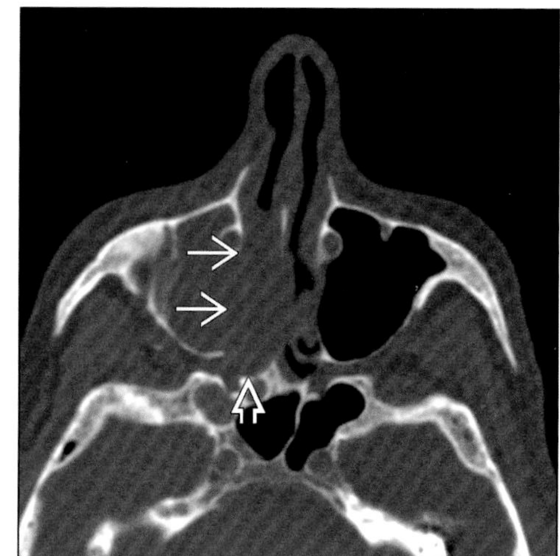

*(**Left**) Sinonasal intestinal-type adenocarcinoma, papillary type, arises in the submucosa and is characterized by the presence of papillary architecture ↗ as well as glandular and cystic growth patterns. (**Right**) Prominent papillary architecture ↗ is seen with fibrovascular cores ⇨. These findings recapitulate the histologic features of primary intestinal adenocarcinoma.*

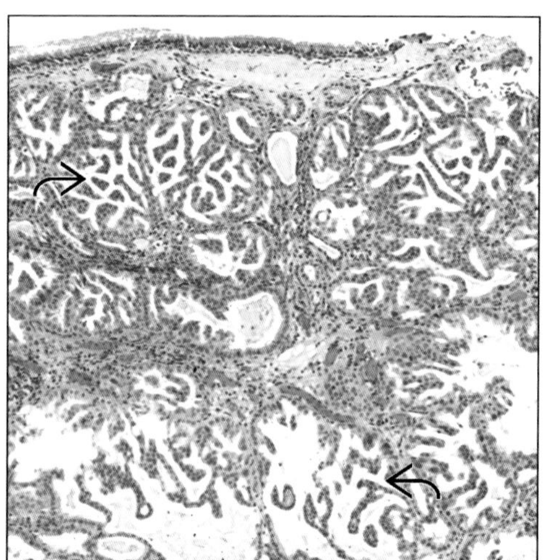

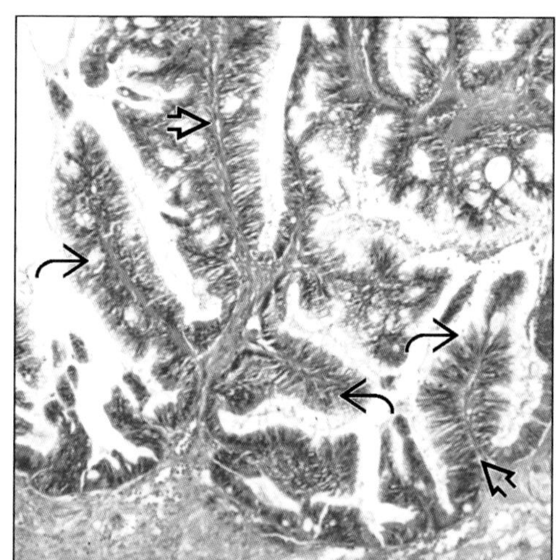

*(**Left**) Sinonasal adenocarcinoma, mucinous type, shows abundant extracellular mucin pools ↗ as well as scattered glandular epithelial structures ⇨. (**Right**) Scattered malignant neoplastic cells ↗, including cells with intracellular mucin ⇨, lie within copious extracellular mucinous pools ➡. The extent of the extracellular mucinous material defines the extent of the tumor even if epithelial structures are not uniformly seen.*

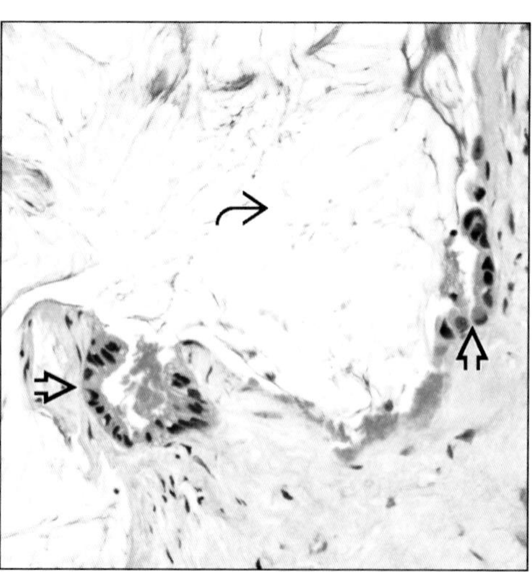

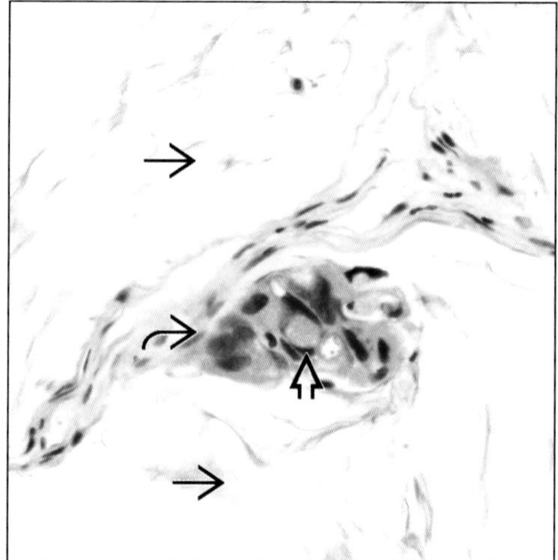

Microscopic and Immunohistochemical Features

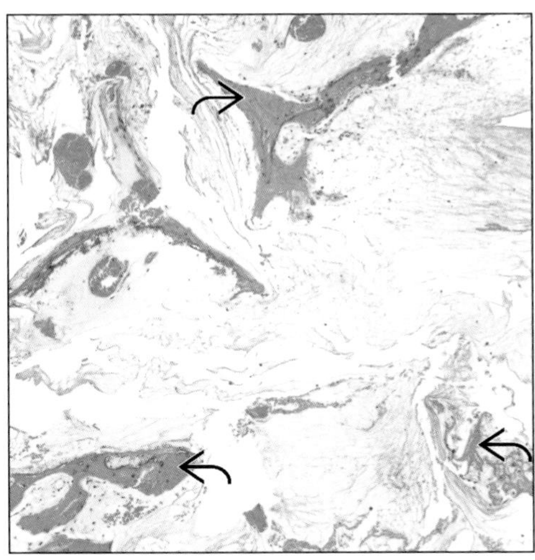

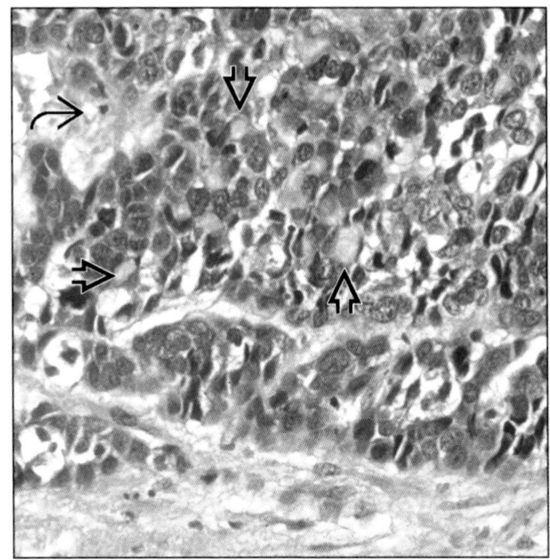

(Left) All types of sinonasal intestinal-type adenocarcinomas, irrespective of their histology, including mucinous type, are capable of aggressive growth with extensive invasion of bone ⮫. (Right) The solid type of sinonasal intestinal adenocarcinoma shows a loss of differentiation characterized by solid growth with attempts at tubule formation ⮫, scattered goblet cells ⇨, and nuclear pleomorphism.

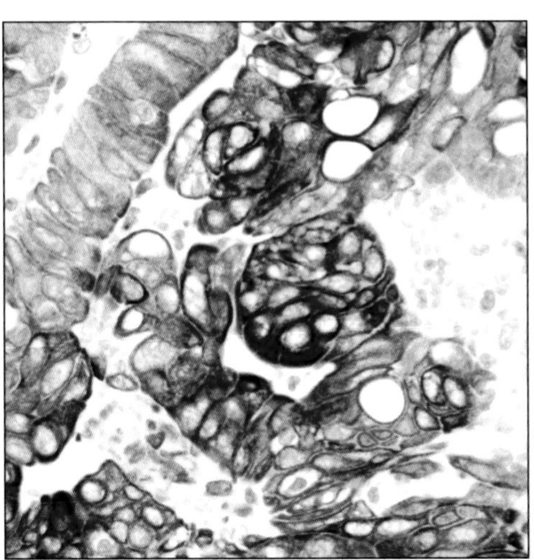

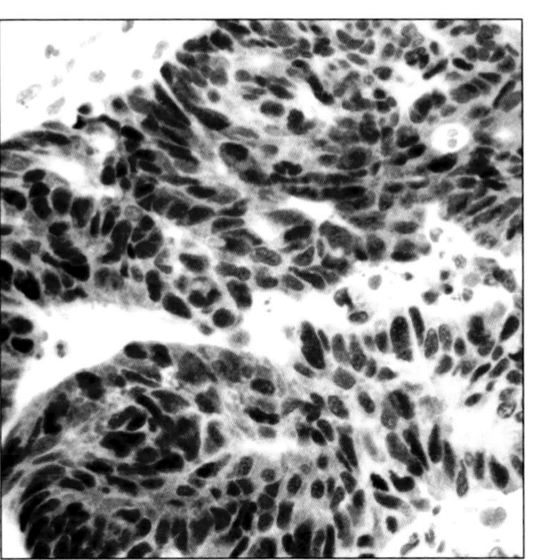

(Left) Immunohistochemical staining of sinonasal intestinal-type adenocarcinoma is similar to that of primary colonic adenocarcinomas, including the presence of diffuse CK20 immunoreactivity. (Right) Diffuse and strong (nuclear) immunoreactivity is present for CDX-2, which is a nuclear transcription factor involved in the differentiation of intestinal epithelial cells and diffusely expressed in primary intestinal adenocarcinomas.

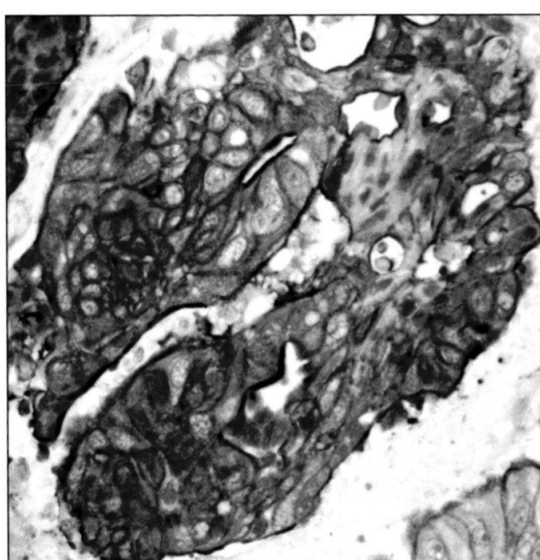

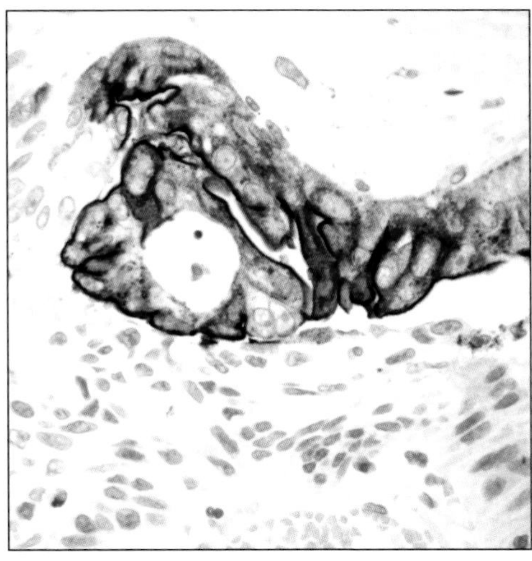

(Left) In addition to CK20 and CDX-2, the immunoreactivity of sinonasal ITACs may also include villin. (Right) Mucin-related antigens (MUCs), including MUC2, are also present in sinonasal ITACs. On the basis of light microscopy, histochemical and immunohistochemical staining, there is no difference between primary colonic adenocarcinoma and ITACs. Clinical history is important in trying to differentiate between ITAC and a metastasis.

SINONASAL NONINTESTINAL-NONSALIVARY ADENOCARCINOMA

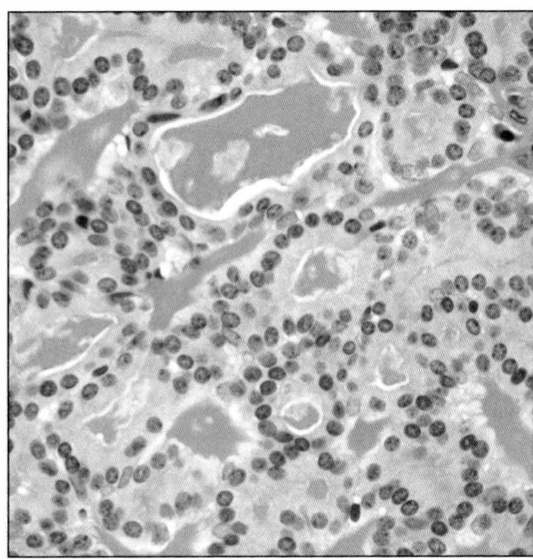

Low-grade adenocarcinoma shows back to back glandular growth with glands lined by a single layer of nonciliated, cuboidal cells with uniform, round nuclei lacking pleomorphism and mitotic activity.

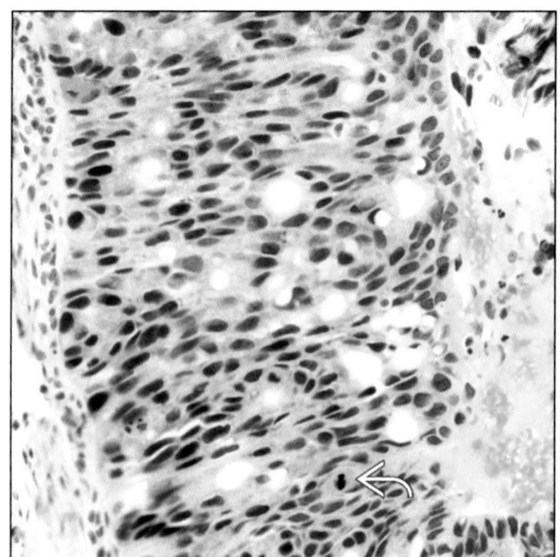

High-grade adenocarcinoma with cribriform (gland in gland) growth characterized by cells with nuclear hyperchromasia, pleomorphism, and increased mitotic activity ➡.

TERMINOLOGY

Abbreviations

- Sinonasal tract (SNT)

Synonyms

- Seromucinous adenocarcinoma
- Nonenteric adenocarcinoma
- Sinonasal tubulopapillary low-grade adenocarcinoma

Definitions

- SNT adenocarcinomas that are neither "intestinal" type nor (minor) salivary gland adenocarcinomas
  - Divided into 2 histologic types
    - Low grade
    - High grade

ETIOLOGY/PATHOGENESIS

Idiopathic

- No known occupational or environmental factors

CLINICAL ISSUES

Epidemiology

- Incidence
  - Adenocarcinomas (all types) comprise 10-20% of sinonasal tract malignant neoplasms
    - Nonintestinal, nonsalivary gland sinonasal adenocarcinomas are rare
- Age
  - **Low grade**
    - Predominantly in adults with mean age at presentation approximately 55-65 years
    - Occurs over wide age range from 9-89 years
  - **High grade**
    - Predominantly in adults with mean age at presentation of 59 years
    - Occurs over wide age range from 15-80 years
- Gender
  - **Low grade**
    - Male > Female
  - **High grade**
    - Male > > > Female

Site

- **Low grade**
  - May occur at any site but predilect to nasal cavity and ethmoid sinus
    - Ethmoid sinus involvement occurs to a lesser extent as compared with "intestinal" type adenocarcinoma
- **High grade**
  - May occur at any site but predilect to maxillary sinus

Presentation

- **Low grade**
  - Nasal obstruction
  - Epistaxis
- **High grade**
  - Nasal obstruction
  - Epistaxis
  - Pain and facial deformity (e.g., proptosis)
  - Duration of symptoms range from 2 weeks to 5 years with median duration of 2.5 months

Treatment

- Surgical approaches
  - Complete surgical excision is treatment of choice
    - Generally via lateral rhinotomy
    - Depending on extent and histology of neoplasm, surgery varies from local excision to more radical procedures (e.g., maxillectomy, ethmoidectomy, and additional exenterations)
- Adjuvant therapy
  - Radiotherapy may be utilized for extensive disease or for higher grade neoplasms

SINONASAL NONINTESTINAL-NONSALIVARY ADENOCARCINOMA

Key Facts

Terminology

- SNT adenocarcinomas that are neither "intestinal" type nor (minor) salivary gland adenocarcinomas

Clinical Issues

- **Low grade**
  - Predilect to nasal cavity and ethmoid sinus
  - Excellent prognosis
- **High grade**
  - Predilect to maxillary sinus
  - 20% 3-year survival rate

Microscopic Pathology

- **Low grade**
  - Numerous uniform small glands or acini with back to back growth pattern without intervening stroma
  - Cells are uniform with round nuclei and eosinophilic to clear- to oncocytic-appearing cytoplasm
  - Glands lined by single layer of nonciliated, cuboidal to columnar cells
- **High grade**
  - May show glandular and papillary growth patterns but less as compared to low-grade adenocarcinomas
  - Moderate to marked nuclear pleomorphism
  - Increased mitotic activity, including atypical forms

Ancillary Tests

- Nonreactive for intestinal type markers including CK20, CDX-2, villin, mucins

Prognosis

- **Low grade**
  - Excellent prognosis
    - 20-30% local recurrence usually within 4 years of surgery
    - Rarely metastasizes (locoregional, distant)
    - Death due to disease rare
- **High grade**
  - 30% distant metastases
  - 20% 3-year survival rate

MICROSCOPIC PATHOLOGY

Histologic Features

- **Low grade**
  - Submucosal unencapsulated glandular &/or papillary growth
  - May be circumscribed
  - Numerous uniform small glands or acini with back to back growth pattern without intervening stroma
  - Occasionally, large irregular cystic spaces seen
  - Glands lined by single layer of nonciliated, cuboidal to columnar cells
    - Cells are uniform with round nuclei and eosinophilic to clear- to oncocytic-appearing cytoplasm
    - Nuclei often localized to basal aspect of cell or may demonstrate stratification with loss of nuclear polarity
  - Cellular pleomorphism is mild to moderate
    - Occasional mitotic figures seen, but atypical mitoses and necrosis are absent
  - Invasive growth may be present
- **High grade**
  - Submucosal invasive tumor predominantly with solid or sheet-like growth
    - May show glandular and papillary growth patterns but less as compared to low-grade adenocarcinomas
  - Characterized by presence of
    - Moderate to marked nuclear pleomorphism
    - Increased mitotic activity, including atypical forms
    - Necrosis
  - Invasive growth may include
    - Effacement of normal architecture
    - Angioinvasion
    - Neurotropism
    - Invasion of soft tissues and bone

ANCILLARY TESTS

Histochemistry

- Mucicarmine
  - Intraluminal staining
  - Intracytoplasmic staining may be identified
- Periodic acid-Schiff with diastase
  - Intraluminal staining
  - Intracytoplasmic staining may be identified

Immunohistochemistry

- Reactive for pancytokeratin and other keratins
- Cytokeratin 7 positive
- Nonreactive for intestinal type markers, including CK20, CDX-2, villin, mucins
- May be S100 protein positive
- Negative for myoepithelial markers
  - e.g., p63, calponin
- Typically nonreactive for neuroendocrine markers
  - e.g., chromogranin, synaptophysin, CD56

DIFFERENTIAL DIAGNOSIS

Intestinal-type Adenocarcinoma

- Morphologic features differ from nonintestinal, nonsalivary gland type adenocarcinomas
- Immunoreactivity for gastrointestinal type markers
  - CK20
  - CDX-2
  - Villin
  - Mucins

SINONASAL NONINTESTINAL-NONSALIVARY ADENOCARCINOMA

Hamartomas

- Surface epithelial-derivation
- Widely separated glands enveloped by thickened basement membrane lacking complex growth
- Glands lined by ciliated epithelium with nuclear stratification

Sinonasal (Schneiderian) Papilloma

- Surface epithelial derivation
- Histology characterized by
  - Proliferation of epidermoid cells &/or respiratory epithelium including admixture of mucocytes
  - Presence of
    - Intraepithelial cysts
    - Microabscesses
    - Mixed inflammatory cells

Salivary Gland Neoplasms

- Adenomas
  - Pleomorphic adenoma and myoepithelial-predominant pleomorphic adenoma most common in SNT
  - Overall histologic findings as well as presence of myoepithelial cells differ from SNT nonintestinal, nonsalivary gland adenocarcinomas
    - Myoepithelial differentiation seen by light microscopy and immunostaining (i.e., p63, calponin)
- Carcinomas
  - Most common type in SNT is adenoid cystic carcinoma
  - Less common types include
    - Acinic cell adenocarcinoma
    - Mucoepidermoid carcinoma
  - Overall histology of salivary gland carcinomas differ from SNT nonintestinal, nonsalivary gland adenocarcinomas

Metastatic Adenocarcinoma

- Rare occurrence to SNT
- Most common types include
  - Renal (clear) cell carcinoma
  - Prostatic adenocarcinoma
  - Breast adenocarcinoma
  - Melanoma
- Immunohistochemical staining assists in differential diagnosis
  - Renal cell carcinoma
    - CD10, renal cell carcinoma marker positive
  - Prostatic adenocarcinoma
    - Prostate specific antigen, prostate specific acid phosphatase positive
  - Breast adenocarcinoma
    - BRST-2, mammoglobin positive
  - Melanoma
    - S100 protein, HMB-45, Melan-A, tyrosinase, vimentin positive

SELECTED REFERENCES

1. Mayr SI et al: Characterization of initial clinical symptoms and risk factors for sinonasal adenocarcinomas: results of a case-control study. Int Arch Occup Environ Health. 83(6):631-8, 2010
2. Stelow EB et al: Adenocarcinoma of the upper aerodigestive tract. Adv Anat Pathol. 17(4):262-9, 2010
3. Jardeleza C et al: Surgical outcomes of endoscopic management of adenocarcinoma of the sinonasal cavity. Rhinology. 47(4):354-61, 2009
4. Jo VY et al: Low-grade sinonasal adenocarcinomas: the association with and distinction from respiratory epithelial adenomatoid hamartomas and other glandular lesions. Am J Surg Pathol. 33(3):401-8, 2009
5. Perez-Ordoñez B: Hamartomas, papillomas and adenocarcinomas of the sinonasal tract and nasopharynx. J Clin Pathol. 62(12):1085-95, 2009
6. Tripodi D et al: Gene expression profiling in sinonasal adenocarcinoma. BMC Med Genomics. 2:65, 2009
7. Ozolek JA et al: Basal/myoepithelial cells in chronic sinusitis, respiratory epithelial adenomatoid hamartoma, inverted papilloma, and intestinal-type and nonintestinal-type sinonasal adenocarcinoma: an immunohistochemical study. Arch Pathol Lab Med. 131(4):530-7, 2007
8. Day TA et al: Management of paranasal sinus malignancy. Curr Treat Options Oncol. 6(1):3-18, 2005
9. Orvidas LJ et al: Adenocarcinoma of the nose and paranasal sinuses: a retrospective study of diagnosis, histologic characteristics, and outcomes in 24 patients. Head Neck. 27(5):370-5, 2005
10. Yom SS et al: Genetic analysis of sinonasal adenocarcinoma phenotypes: distinct alterations of histogenetic significance. Mod Pathol. 18(3):315-9, 2005
11. Cathro HP et al: Immunophenotypic differences between intestinal-type and low-grade papillary sinonasal adenocarcinomas: an immunohistochemical study of 22 cases utilizing CDX2 and MUC2. Am J Surg Pathol. 28(8):1026-32, 2004
12. Licitra L et al: Head and neck tumors other than squamous cell carcinoma. Curr Opin Oncol. 16(3):236-41, 2004
13. Choi HR et al: Sinonasal adenocarcinoma: evidence for histogenetic divergence of the enteric and nonenteric phenotypes. Hum Pathol. 34(11):1101-7, 2003
14. Neto AG et al: Sinonasal tract seromucous adenocarcinomas: a report of 12 cases. Ann Diagn Pathol. 7(3):154-9, 2003
15. Skalova A et al: Sinonasal tubulopapillary low-grade adenocarcinoma. Histopathological, immunohistochemical and ultrastructural features of poorly recognised entity. Virchows Arch. 443(2):152-8, 2003
16. Lee CF et al: Sinonasal adenocarcinoma: clinical study of nine cases in Taiwan. Acta Otolaryngol. 122(8):887-91, 2002
17. Rice DH: Endonasal approaches for sinonasal and nasopharyngeal tumors. Otolaryngol Clin North Am. 34(6):1087-93, viii, 2001
18. Alessi DM et al: Nonsalivary sinonasal adenocarcinoma. Arch Otolaryngol Head Neck Surg. 114(9):996-9, 1988
19. Heffner DK et al: Low-grade adenocarcinoma of the nasal cavity and paranasal sinuses. Cancer. 50(2):312-22, 1982

Microscopic Features

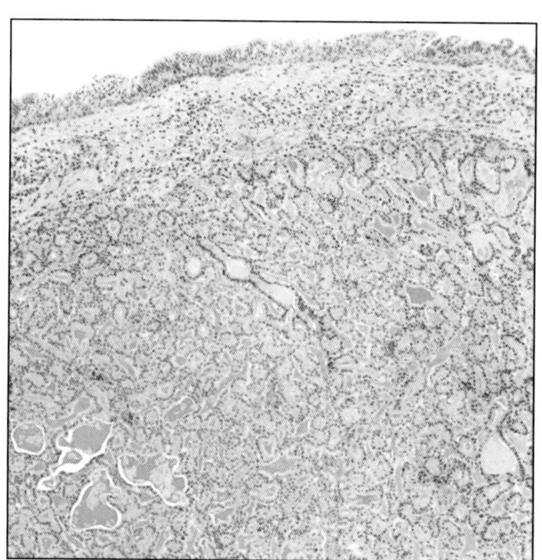

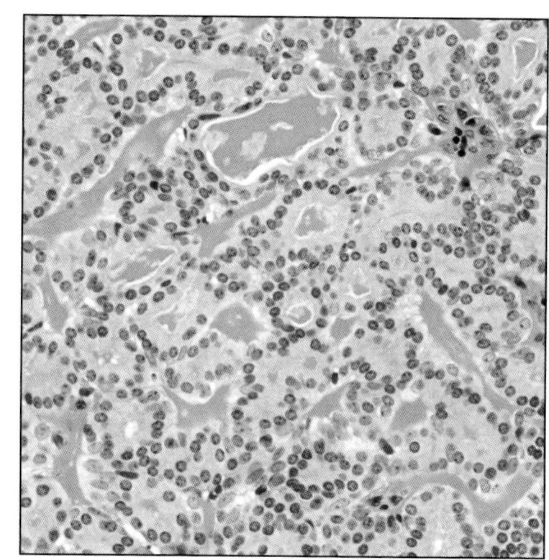

(Left) *A submucosal, circumscribed but unencapsulated tumor with complex glandular growth is seen.* ***(Right)*** *The presence of complex growth, including back to back glands without intervening stroma and the presence of glands lined by a single cell layer, is diagnostic for low-grade adenocarcinoma even in the absence of nuclear pleomorphism, mitotic activity, &/or invasive growth. There are no benign neoplasms in the sinonasal tract that have these overall morphologic findings.*

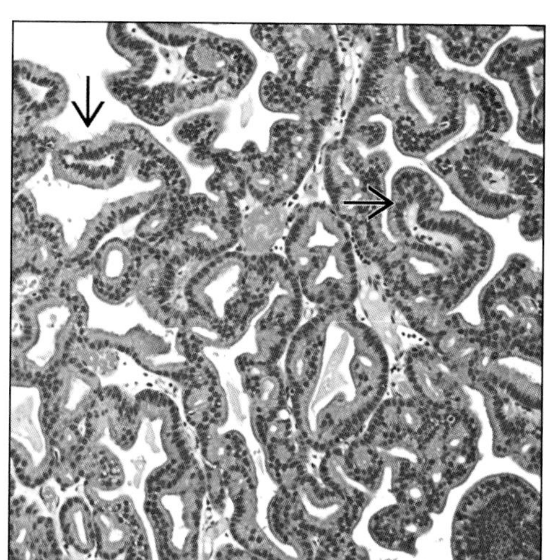

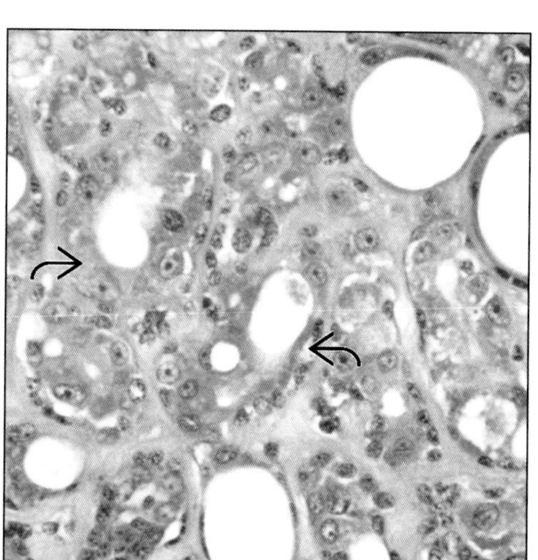

(Left) *Sinonasal low-grade adenocarcinoma shows complex glandular growth as well as papillary architecture ⇒.* ***(Right)*** *Sinonasal low-grade adenocarcinoma comprised of oncocytic cells is characterized by brightly eosinophilic granular-appearing cytoplasm ⇒ with enlarged vesicular nuclei and prominent nucleoli. In spite of the enlarged nuclei, the features are those of low-grade adenocarcinoma, including absence of significant nuclear pleomorphism and scarce to absent mitoses.*

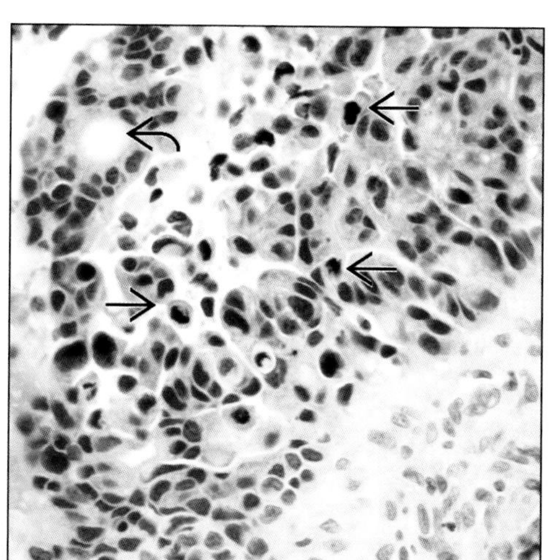

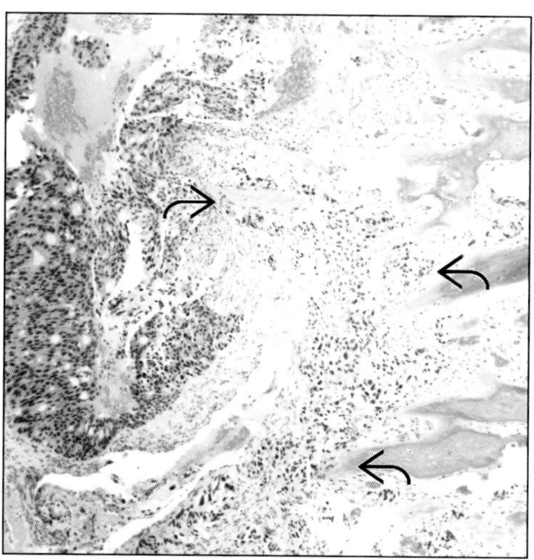

(Left) *Sinonasal high-grade adenocarcinoma shows focal glandular differentiation ⇒ but is predominantly solid with hyperchromatic and pleomorphic nuclei and increased mitotic activity ⇒. The light microscopic and immunohistochemical features of this neoplasm contrast to that of intestinal-type adenocarcinomas and salivary gland carcinomas.* ***(Right)*** *Sinonasal high-grade adenocarcinomas are often extensively infiltrative at presentation and may include invasion into bone ⇒.*

OLFACTORY NEUROBLASTOMA

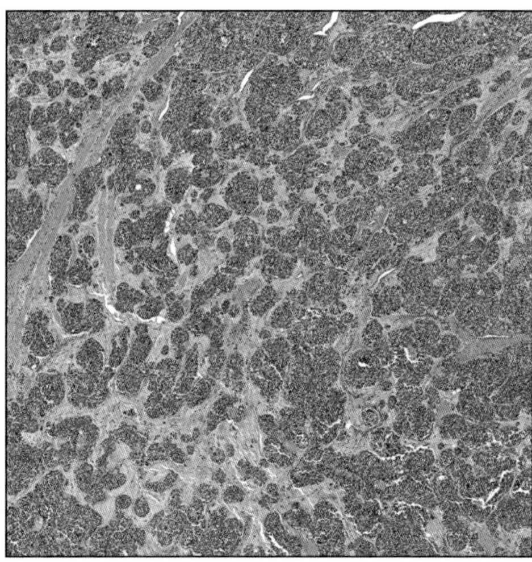

This low-power H&E shows the well-developed lobular architecture of the primitive neuroblastoma cells that is so characteristic for olfactory neuroblastoma (ONB). There are richly vascularized fibrovascular septa.

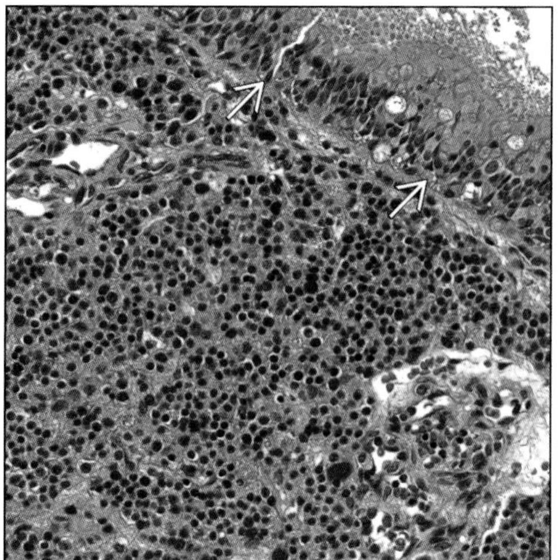

An intact respiratory epithelial surface ➡ overlies the neoplastic proliferation of "small round blue cells." There is a moderate degree of variability in this grade 2 ONB.

TERMINOLOGY

Abbreviations

- Olfactory neuroblastoma (ONB)

Synonyms

- Esthesioneuroblastoma (ENB)
- Olfactory placode tumor
- Esthesioneurocytoma
- Esthesioneuroepithelioma
- Esthesioneuroma

Definitions

- Malignant neoplasm arising from specialized sensory neuroepithelial (neuroectodermal) olfactory cells normally found in upper part of nasal cavity, specifically cribriform plate of ethmoid sinus

ETIOLOGY/PATHOGENESIS

Proposed Origin

- Arise from specialized sensory neuroepithelial olfactory cells (bipolar neurons) of olfactory membrane
- Normally identified in
  - Jacobson organ (vomeronasal organ)
  - Sphenopalatine ganglion (pterygoid gland)
  - Ectodermal olfactory placode
  - Ganglion of Loci (nervus terminalis)
  - Autonomic ganglia of nasal mucosa
  - Olfactory neuroepithelium
    - Cribriform plate
    - Upper 1/3 to 1/2 of nasal septum
    - Superomedial surface of superior turbinate (concha)
    - Upper nasopharynx
- Olfactory epithelium contains 3 cell types (also present in tumor)
  - Basal cells (stem cell compartment, thought to give rise to tumor)
  - Olfactory neurosensory cells
  - Supporting sustentacular cells

CLINICAL ISSUES

Epidemiology

- Incidence
  - Represents ~ 2-3% of all sinonasal tract tumors
  - ~ 0.4/1,000,000 population/year
- Age
  - Range: 2-94 years
  - Bimodal peak: 2nd and 6th decades
- Gender
  - Male > Female (1.2:1)

Site

- Nearly always involves cribriform plate of ethmoid sinus
- Much less common: Superior nasal concha, upper part of septum, roof of nose

Presentation

- Unilateral nasal obstruction (70%)
- Epistaxis (50%)
- Other symptoms include
  - Headaches, pain, excessive lacrimation, rhinorrhea, visual disturbances
  - Anosmia: < 5% of patients, even though tumor involves olfactory epithelium
- Symptoms are nonspecific, so usually present for some time
- Rarely, may produce ectopic adrenocorticotrophic hormone (ACTH) or antidiuretic hormone secretion (vasopressin)

Treatment

- Options, risks, complications
  - Due to tumor vascularity, biopsy is discouraged

OLFACTORY NEUROBLASTOMA

Key Facts

Terminology
- Malignant neoplasm arising from specialized sensory neuroepithelial (neuroectodermal) olfactory cells

Clinical Issues
- Bimodal age peak: 2nd and 6th decades
- Unilateral nasal obstruction (70%), epistaxis (50%)
  - Anosmia: < 5% of patients
- Involves cribriform plate of ethmoid sinus
- Complete craniofacial resection with follow-up radiation is standard treatment
- Overall survival: 70% 5-year (stage and grade dependent)

Microscopic Pathology
- Lobular arrangement of primitive neuroblastoma cells is characteristic
- **Small round blue cells**
  - Arranged in a syncytium, with a tangle of neuronal processes
  - **Pseudorosettes**: Neoplastic cells palisaded around finely fibrillary neural matrix
  - **True rosettes**: True tight annular formation by neoplastic cells

Ancillary Tests
- Positive: Neuroendocrine markers; S100 protein sustentacular cells; rarely, keratin

Top Differential Diagnoses
- Sinonasal undifferentiated carcinoma, neuroendocrine carcinoma, *NUT* midline carcinoma, extranodal NK-/T-cell lymphoma nasal-type, rhabdomyosarcoma, PNET/Ewing sarcoma

---

  - Consider combination surgery and radiation for best outcome
  - Meningitis, CSF leak (liquorrhea), and dermatitis are potential complications
- Surgical approaches
  - Complete craniofacial resection, including removal of cribriform plate, is treatment of choice
    - Endoscopic-assisted endonasal and anterior craniotomy resection (bi-cranial-facial approach; trephination)
    - Endoscopic surgery vs. open techniques tend to have better survival rate
    - Larger tumors tend to be managed by open technique
    - Patients with clear margins do better than those with positive margins
  - Neck dissection recommended if clinically suspicious
- Drugs
  - Chemotherapy is reserved for large, high-grade, unresectable, disseminated, &/or salvage
    - High-dose chemotherapy with cisplatin and etoposide (adjuvant did better)
- Radiation
  - Full-course radiotherapy post surgery
  - Patients managed with radiation **alone** have worse outcome
  - Proton-beam therapy may yield better dose distribution
  - Elective neck irradiation may be of value
- Autologous bone marrow transplantation
  - Limited cases have shown promise

Prognosis
- Overall survival: 70% 5-year survival (stage and grade dependent)
  - Low grade: 80% 5-year survival
  - High grade: 25% 5-year survival
  - Most patients present with Kadish stage C disease
  - Best outcome with combination surgery and radiotherapy (~ 85% 5-year survival)
- Most tumors show local invasion (orbit, cranial cavity)
- Local recurrence: Up to 30% (range: 15-70%)
  - Tend to develop within 1st 2 years after presentation
- 35% of patients develop metastatic disease
  - Cervical lymph nodes (up to 25%): Poor prognosis, < 30% 5-year survival
  - Distant metastases (10%): Parotid glands, lung, bone, liver, skin, and spinal cord
- **Negative** prognostic indicators include
  - High-grade tumor (Hyams grade 3 or 4)
  - Cervical or distant metastasis
  - Female
  - Age: < 20 or > 50 years at presentation
  - Extensive intracranial spread
  - Tumor recurrence
  - High proliferation index
  - Polyploidy/aneuploidy

IMAGE FINDINGS

General Features
- Best diagnostic clue
  - Classic appearance: Dumbbell-shaped mass with upper portion in intracranial fossa & lower portion in upper nasal cavity
    - "Waist" at level of cribriform plate
  - Presence of peripheral tumor cysts at intracranial tumor margin is highly suggestive of diagnosis of ONB
  - Radiographic findings dependent on tumor size and symptom duration
    - Small: Unilateral nasal mass centered on superior nasal wall
    - Large: Anterior cranial fossa, maxillary sinuses, orbit

MR Findings
- T1WI
  - Hypointense to intermediate signal intensity mass compared to brain
  - Areas of hemorrhage/necrosis are hypointense
- T1WI with gadolinium contrast
  - Avid homogeneous tumor enhancement

OLFACTORY NEUROBLASTOMA

- Enhancement heterogeneous in areas of necrosis
- T2WI
  - Intermediate to hyperintense compared to brain
  - Areas of cystic degeneration are hyperintense

CT Findings

- Bone CT (no contrast)
  - Bone erosion/remodeling of lamina papyracea, cribriform plate, &/or fovea ethmoidalis
  - Speckled calcifications within tumor matrix frequently present
- Contrast enhanced
  - Homogeneously enhancing mass
  - Nonenhancing areas suggest necrosis

MACROSCOPIC FEATURES

General Features

- Glistening, unilateral, mucosal-covered, soft, polypoid mass
- Red-gray, with gray-tan to pink cut surface
- Mimics other sinonasal tract primary malignancies

Size

- Range: < 1 cm to huge mass filling nasal cavity and intracranial regions
  - Possible extension into adjacent paranasal sinuses and nasopharynx

MICROSCOPIC PATHOLOGY

Histologic Features

- Histologic appearance varies based on degree of differentiation
- Lobular arrangement of primitive neuroblastoma cells is characteristic (irrespective of grade)
  - Lobule of cells surrounded by richly vascularized stroma creating fibrovascular septa
  - Sustentacular supporting cells line the lobule (S100 protein highlighted)
- Surface epithelium is intact
  - "**In situ**" tumor within respiratory epithelium is rarely identified
- Neoplastic cells are classic "**small round blue cells**," slightly larger than mature lymphocytes
  - High nuclear to cytoplasmic ratio
  - Small, uniform nuclei with delicate, "salt and pepper" chromatin distribution
  - Nucleoli are small to absent
- Cells arranged in syncytium, with a tangle of neuronal processes
  - Centrally located neurofibrillary material creates pseudorosette (Homer Wright type)
- Nuclear pleomorphism, mitoses, and necrosis
  - Absent or limited in low-grade lesions (grade 1 or 2)
  - Present in high-grade lesions (grade 3 or 4)
- 2 types of rosettes are recognized
  - **Pseudorosettes** (Homer Wright type)
    - Neoplastic cells palisading or cuffing around finely fibrillary, delicate edematous neural matrix material
    - Up to 30% of cases
    - Seen in grade 1 and 2 tumors
  - **True rosettes** (of Flexner-Wintersteiner)
    - Gland-like, tight annular formation by neoplastic cells creating duct-like space with nonciliated columnar cells
    - About 5% of cases
    - Seen in grade 3 and 4 tumors
  - Peritheliomatous "rosettes" are not considered of diagnostic utility
- Calcification (psammomatous or concretion) may be seen
  - Decrease in frequency as grade increases
- Rarely present
  - Vascular invasion
  - Ganglion cells
  - Melanin-containing cells
  - Rhabdomyoblastic cells
- Tumors are separated into 4 grades
  - Overall grade based on degree of differentiation, presence of neural stroma, mitotic figures, and necrosis

ANCILLARY TESTS

Histochemistry

- Silver stains highlight neurosecretory granules
  - Bodian, Churukian-Schenck, Grimelius

Immunohistochemistry

- Positive: Neuroendocrine markers; S100 protein sustentacular cells
  - Rare reaction with low molecular weight cytokeratin (CAM5.2)
- Negative: Desmin, myogenin, CD45RB, CD99

Flow Cytometry

- High rate of polyploidy and aneuploidy, related to adverse prognosis

Cytogenetics

- Chromosomal alterations of 19, 8q, 15q, 22q, 4q
- Deletion of chromosome 11 and gains of 1p associated with increased risk of metastases and worse prognosis
- RT-PCR of human achaete-scute homologue (*hASH1*) expression may be specific marker of ONB
- **No** *EWS/FLI1* gene fusion

Electron Microscopy

- Membrane-bound dense core **neurosecretory granules** present in cytoplasm and nerve processes
  - Granule diameter: 50-250 μm
- Fibrillary stroma corresponds to immature nerve processes
  - Nerve processes may contain neurotubules and neurofilaments
    - Occasionally, Schwann-like cells can be seen
- Flexner-Wintersteiner rosette lining cells may have apical cilia or microvilli and olfactory vesicles

DIFFERENTIAL DIAGNOSIS

Sinonasal Undifferentiated Carcinoma (SNUC)

- High-grade, usually widely destructive neoplasm
- Extensive coagulative necrosis and vascular invasion
- Strong and diffuse keratin immunoreactivity; may show limited neuroendocrine markers

Neuroendocrine Carcinoma

- High-grade tumors with extensive necrosis, high mitoses, and apoptosis
- Punctate paranuclear keratin immunoreactivity; may show TTF-1 positive

NUT Midline Carcinoma

- Poorly differentiated, high-grade carcinoma, often with squamous differentiation, usually in young patients, vast majority in midline, with t(15;19)(q14;p13)
- Requires identification of nuclear protein in testis (*NUT*) gene on chromosome 15q14 (FISH or RT-PCR techniques)
  - Balanced translocation: *BRD4* (19p13.1) with *NUT* (15q14), creating fusion gene *BRD4-NUT*
- Frequently also show CD34 expression

Extranodal NK-/T-cell Lymphoma, Nasal Type

- High-grade tumors with extensive vascular invasion and coagulative necrosis
- **Positive**: NK- or T-cell markers; **negative** with neuroendocrine markers, S100 protein, keratin

Rhabdomyosarcoma

- Often in same bimodal age distribution; similar radiographic, gross, and clinical findings
- Rhabdomyoblastic differentiation with strap cells and eccentric, eosinophilic cytoplasm
- **Positive**: Muscle markers; keratin and CD56 can be positive in 5-10% of cases

Malignant Melanoma

- Wide variety of architectural patterns and wide variety of morphologic appearances
- Polygonal cells, eosinophilic, plasmacytoid cytoplasm, intranuclear cytoplasmic inclusions and pigment
- **Positive**: S100 protein, HMB-45, Melan-A, MIFT; **negative**: Neuroendocrine markers

PNET/Ewing Sarcoma

- Characteristic "small round blue cell" tumor, showing coagulative necrosis
- Diffuse, sheet-like cells with indistinct cell borders, uniform small cells with finely dispersed chromatin distribution and small nucleoli
- **Positive**: FLI-1, CD99, NSE; sometimes synaptophysin; **negative**: Chromogranin, GFAP
- FISH for t(11;22)(q24;q12)

Pituitary Adenoma

- Sphenoid sinus mass, ribbons, festoons, lobular architecture, polygonal cells, lacking pleomorphism and mitoses
- **Positive**: Neuroendocrine and peptide markers, keratin

Extramedullary Plasmacytoma

- Plasmacytoid cells with "clockface" nuclear chromatin distribution, Hof-zone in cytoplasm
- **Positive**: CD138, CD79a, κ or λ restricted
- **Negative**: Epithelial or neuroendocrine markers

Metastatic Neuroblastoma

- Histologically identical, but has *myc* amplification

GRADING

Hyams Grading

- **Grade 1**: Majority of tumors; lobular, syncytial, neurofibrillary matrix, vesicular chromatin, no mitoses or necrosis
- **Grade 2**: Less neurofibrillary matrix, scattered mitoses
- **Grade 3**: More pleomorphic cells, Flexner-Wintersteiner rosettes, possible necrosis
- **Grade 4**: Least number of tumors; anaplastic, high mitoses, necrosis

STAGING

Kadish Staging

- **A**: Tumor confined to nasal cavity (18%)
- **B**: Tumor involves nasal cavity plus one or more paranasal sinuses (32%)
- **C**: Extension of tumor beyond sinonasal cavities (50%)

SELECTED REFERENCES

1. Ozsahin M et al: Outcome and prognostic factors in olfactory neuroblastoma: a rare cancer network study. Int J Radiat Oncol Biol Phys. 78(4):992-7, 2010
2. Bragg TM et al: Clinicopathological review: esthesioneuroblastoma. Neurosurgery. 64(4):764-70; discussion 770, 2009
3. Devaiah AK et al: Treatment of esthesioneuroblastoma: a 16-year meta-analysis of 361 patients. Laryngoscope. 119(7):1412-6, 2009
4. Faragalla H et al: Olfactory neuroblastoma: a review and update. Adv Anat Pathol. 16(5):322-31, 2009
5. Folbe A et al: Endoscopic endonasal resection of esthesioneuroblastoma: a multicenter study. Am J Rhinol Allergy. 2009 Jan-Feb;23(1):91-4. Erratum in: Am J Rhinol Allergy. 23(2):238, 2009
6. Thompson LD: Olfactory neuroblastoma. Head Neck Pathol. 3(3):252-9, 2009
7. Wenig BM: Undifferentiated malignant neoplasms of the sinonasal tract. Arch Pathol Lab Med. 133(5):699-712, 2009
8. Bachar G et al: Esthesioneuroblastoma: The Princess Margaret Hospital experience. Head Neck. 30(12):1607-14, 2008
9. Wang SL et al: Absence of Epstein-Barr virus in olfactory neuroblastoma. Pathology. 39(6):565-6, 2007
10. Sugita Y et al: Olfactory neuroepithelioma: an immunohistochemical and ultrastructural study. Neuropathology. 26(5):400-8, 2006

OLFACTORY NEUROBLASTOMA

Immunohistochemistry

Antibody	Reactivity	Staining Pattern	Comment
EpCAM/BER-EP4/ CD326	Positive	Cytoplasmic	Nearly all neoplastic cells
Chromogranin-A	Positive	Cytoplasmic	Majority of tumor cells
Synaptophysin	Positive	Cytoplasmic	Majority of tumor cells
CD56	Positive	Cell membrane & cytoplasm	Nearly all neoplastic cells
NSE	Positive	Cytoplasmic	Nearly all neoplastic cells
NFP	Positive	Cytoplasmic	Accentuates neural matrix
β-tubulin	Positive	Cytoplasmic	Most tumor cells
S100	Positive	Nuclear & cytoplasmic	Accentuates peripheral sustentacular cells
GFAP	Positive	Cytoplasmic	Highlights peripheral sustentacular cells
CK8/18/CAM5.2	Positive	Cytoplasmic	Only about 5% of tumors
Ki-67	Positive	Nuclear	Proliferation index ranges from 5-50%
EBER	Negative		
CD99	Negative		
Desmin	Negative		
Myogenin	Negative		
CD45RB	Negative		

Histologic Grading (Hyams's Criteria)

Microscopic Features	Grade 1	Grade 2	Grade 3	Grade 4
Architecture	Lobular	Lobular	± lobular	± lobular
Pleomorphism	Absent to slight	Present	Prominent	Marked
Neurofibrillary matrix	Prominent	Present	May be present	Limited
Rosettes	Homer Wright pseudorosettes	Homer Wright pseudorosettes	Flexner-Wintersteiner rosettes	Flexner-Wintersteiner rosettes
Mitoses	Absent	Present	Prominent	Marked
Necrosis	Absent	Absent	Present	Prominent
Glands	May be present	May be present	Usually limited	Focally present
Calcifications	Variable	Variable	Absent	Absent

Hyams VJ et al. Tumors of the Upper Respiratory Tract and Ear. Armed Forces Institute of Pathology Fascicles. 2nd series. Washington: American Registry of Pathology Press, Armed Forces Institute of Pathology, 1988.

Kadish Staging System

Stage	Criteria	Outcome
Stage A	Tumor confined to nasal cavity	5-year survival: > 90%
Stage B	Tumor involves nasal cavity plus one or more paranasal sinuses	5-year survival: ~ 70%
Stage C	Extension of tumor beyond sinonasal cavities	5-year survival: < 50%

Kadish S et al: Olfactory neuroblastoma. A clinical analysis of 17 cases. Cancer. 37(3):1571-6, 1976.

11. Iezzoni JC et al: "Undifferentiated" small round cell tumors of the sinonasal tract: differential diagnosis update. Am J Clin Pathol. 124 Suppl:S110-21, 2005
12. Klepin HD et al: Esthesioneuroblastoma. Curr Treat Options Oncol. 6(6):509-18, 2005
13. Theilgaard SA et al: Esthesioneuroblastoma: a Danish demographic study of 40 patients registered between 1978 and 2000. Acta Otolaryngol. 123(3):433-9, 2003
14. Ingeholm P et al: Esthesioneuroblastoma: a Danish clinicopathological study of 40 consecutive cases. APMIS. 110(9):639-45, 2002
15. Rinaldo A et al: Esthesioneuroblastoma and cervical lymph node metastases: clinical and therapeutic implications. Acta Otolaryngol. 122(2):215-21, 2002
16. Dulguerov P et al: Esthesioneuroblastoma: a meta-analysis and review. Lancet Oncol. 2(11):683-90, 2001
17. Resto VA et al: Esthesioneuroblastoma: the Johns Hopkins experience. Head Neck. 22(6):550-8, 2000
18. Broich G et al: Esthesioneuroblastoma: a general review of the cases published since the discovery of the tumour in 1924. Anticancer Res. 17(4A):2683-706, 1997
19. Hirose T et al: Olfactory neuroblastoma. An immunohistochemical, ultrastructural, and flow cytometric study. Cancer. 76(1):4-19, 1995
20. Frierson HF Jr et al: Olfactory neuroblastoma. Additional immunohistochemical characterization. Am J Clin Pathol. 94(5):547-53, 1990

Imaging, Gross, and Microscopic Features

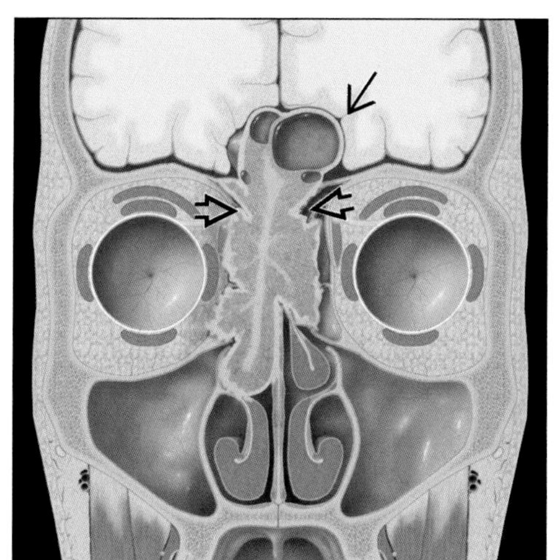

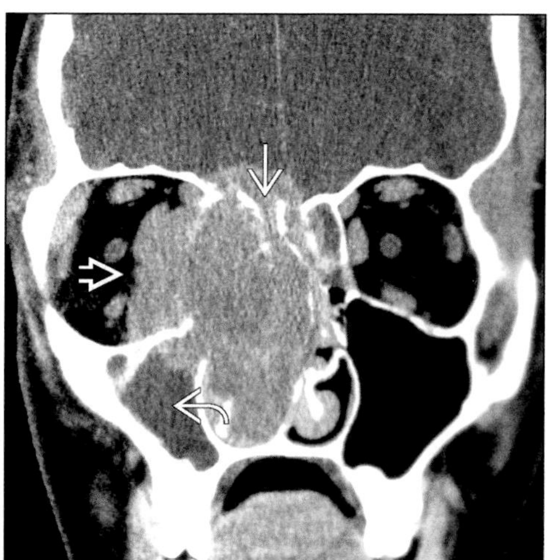

(Left) *Coronal graphic of invasive ONB shows the lesion centered high in the nasal cavity, invading the anterior cranial fossa through the cribriform plate ⇨. Note characteristic intracranial cysts →, a helpful radiographic finding for this tumor.* ***(Right)*** *Coronal CECT demonstrates right nasal cavity ONB with destruction of the cribriform plate → and lamina papyracea ⇨. Note low-density obstructed maxillary secretions ↷.*

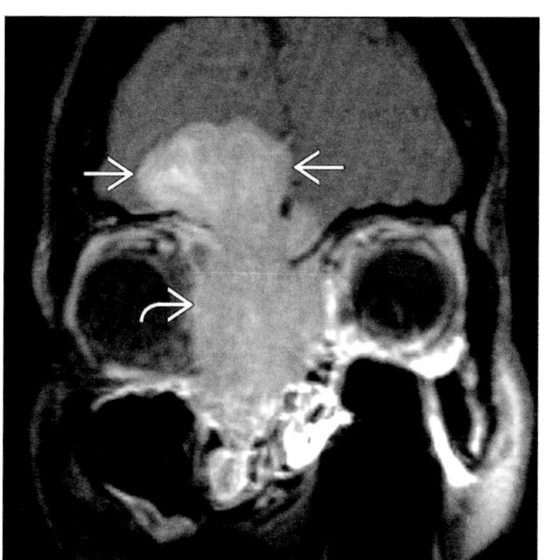

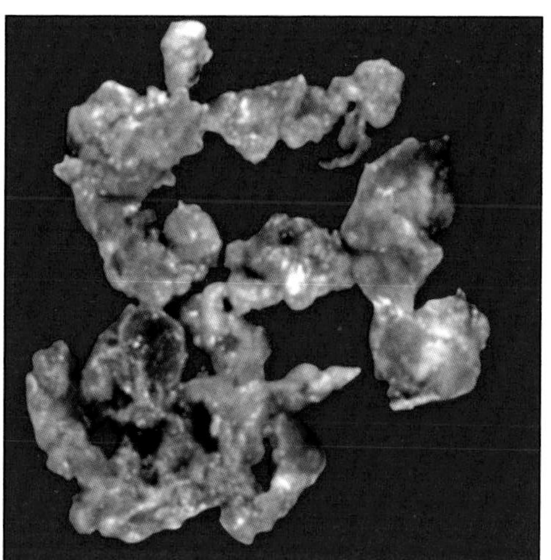

(Left) *Coronal T1-weighted contrast-enhanced MR image shows slightly heterogeneous enhancement throughout the large mass, destroying the cribriform plate and expanding into the frontal lobe →. Extension into the right orbit ↷ is also apparent.* ***(Right)*** *Multiple polypoid fragments of mucosal-covered soft tissue show a red to red-tan appearance, suggesting the rich vascularity of the tumor.*

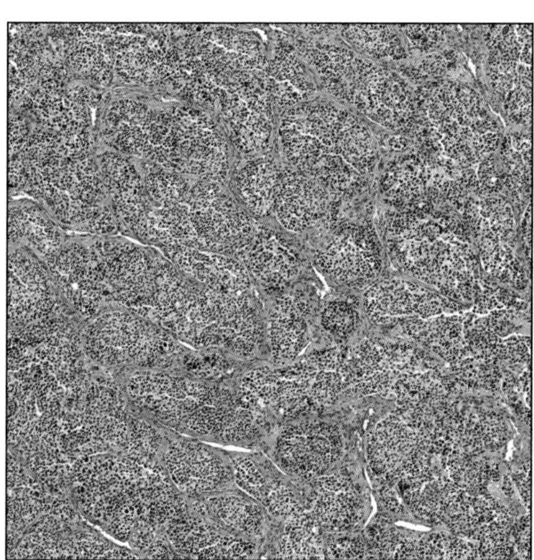

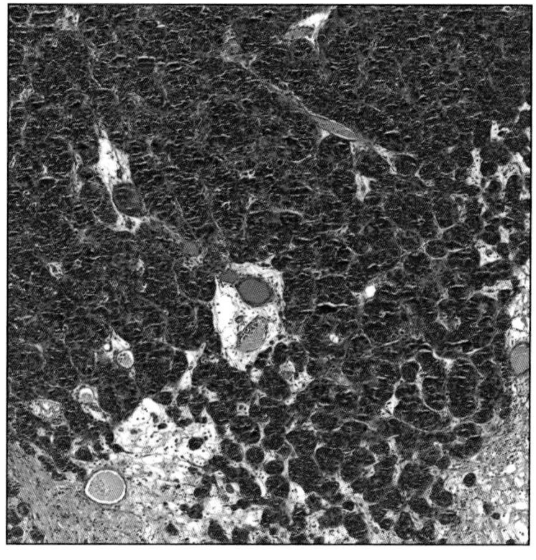

(Left) *Many fibrovascular septa dissect and surround the tumor lobules. The lobular architecture is present to a variable degree in all ONB no matter what histologic grade.* ***(Right)*** *There are multiple small, tight lobules of tumor set within an edematous to richly vascularized stroma. This lobular architecture is quite characteristic of ONB and is a histologic feature at low power that can be quite helpful in confirming the diagnosis.*

OLFACTORY NEUROBLASTOMA

Microscopic Features

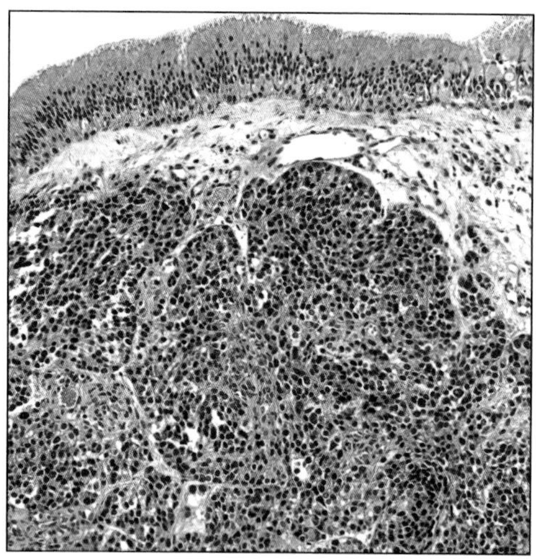
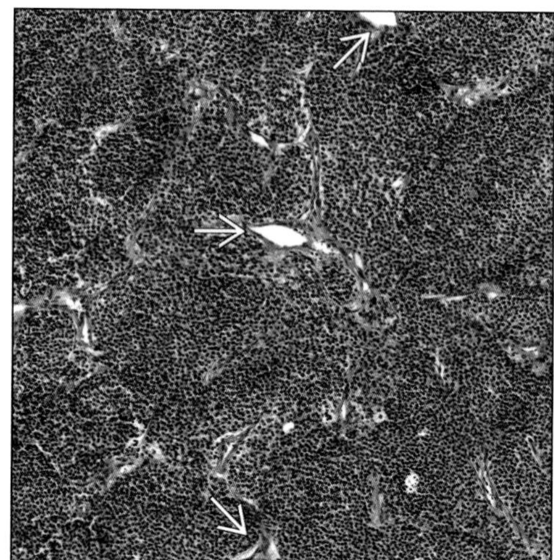

(Left) *The respiratory epithelium is intact, separated by fibrous connective tissue from the lobular neoplastic infiltrate in the stroma. There is limited pleomorphism, with a fibrillary matrix noted between the syncytium of cells.* ***(Right)*** *The tumors are quite cellular, showing lobules of primitive neuroblastoma-like cells that have a very high nuclear to cytoplasmic ratio and are arranged in a syncytium. A few vessels ➔ can be easily identified even at this low magnification.*

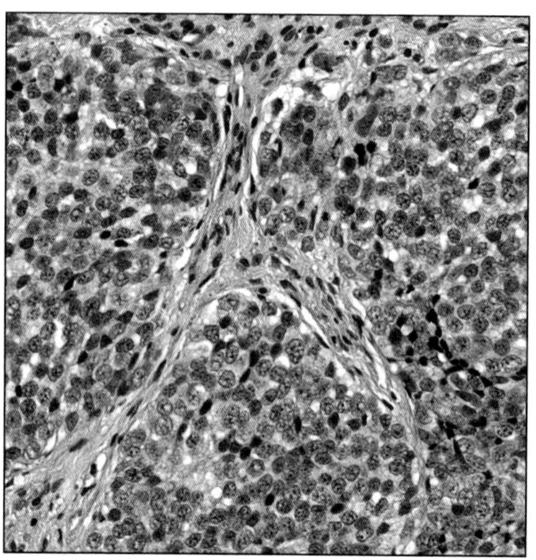
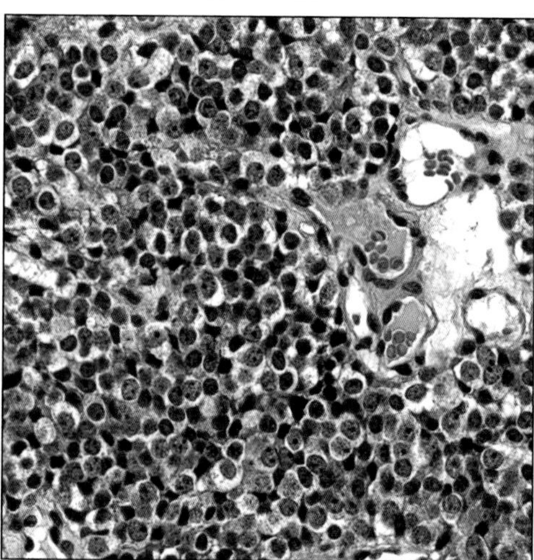

(Left) *This grade 1 tumor shows classic "salt and pepper" nuclear chromatin without any cellular variability. The fibrovascular septa separate the neoplastic cells into lobules. Neuronal matrix material is noted within the lobules.* ***(Right)*** *The neoplastic cells show the "small round blue cell" pattern so characteristic of neuroblastoma. The nuclei are monotonous, with evenly distributed chromatin. The vascularized stroma is noted.*

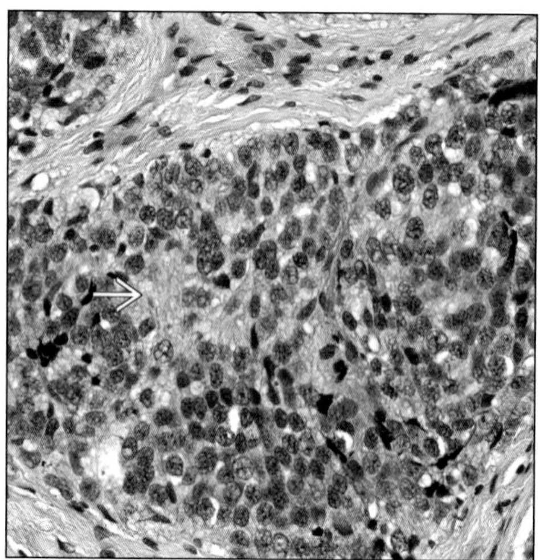
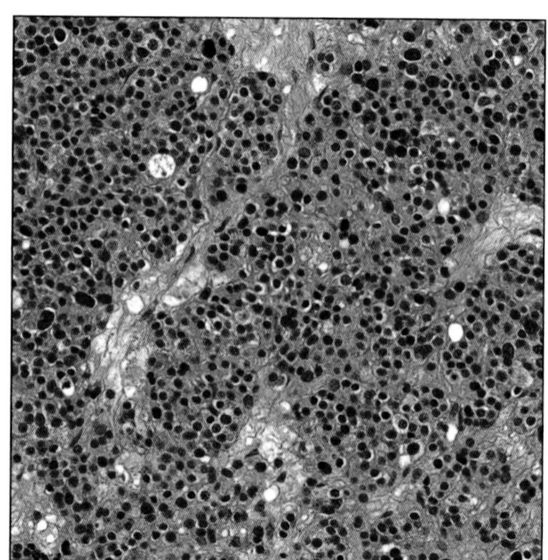

(Left) *The neoplastic cells are arranged in a syncytium, lacking any well-defined cell borders. There is a high nuclear to cytoplasmic ratio. Nucleoli are focally identified in cells that show delicate, "salt and pepper" nuclear chromatin distribution. Note the Homer Wright rosette ➔, a finding seen in up to 30% of grade 2 tumors.* ***(Right)*** *There is a greater degree of nuclear pleomorphism and variability in this grade 2 tumor, showing nuclear hyperchromasia. Mitoses and necrosis are absent.*

Microscopic Features

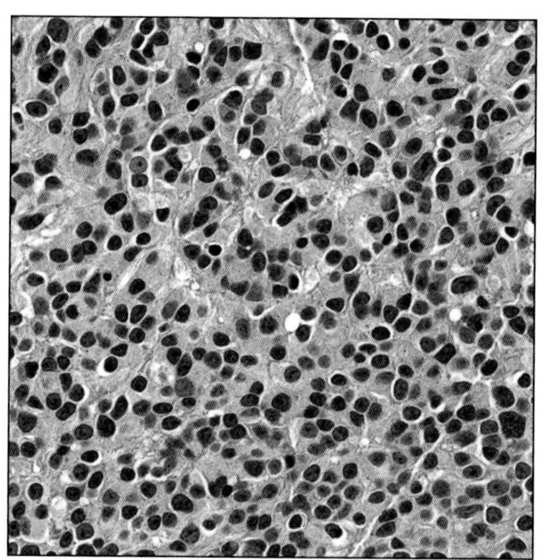

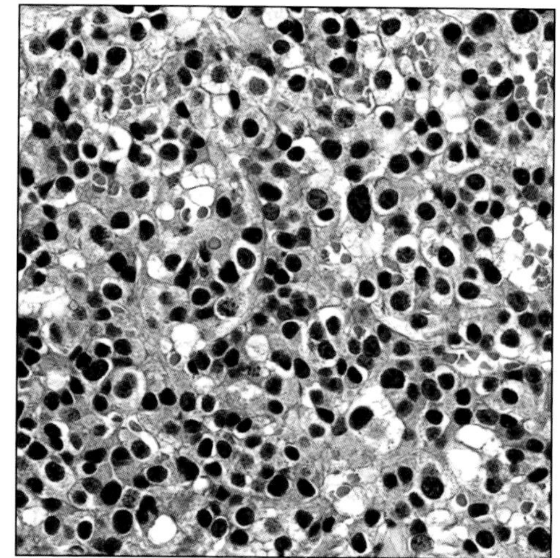

(Left) Within a lobule, the neoplastic cells have a high nuclear to cytoplasmic ratio, nuclear hyperchromasia, and a suggestion of pseudorosettes. This tumor shows a syncytial architecture. **(Right)** There is slightly more variability among the nuclei of this tumor, with marked nuclear hyperchromasia. This is an example of a grade 3 tumor. Other histologic features were present elsewhere in the sample.

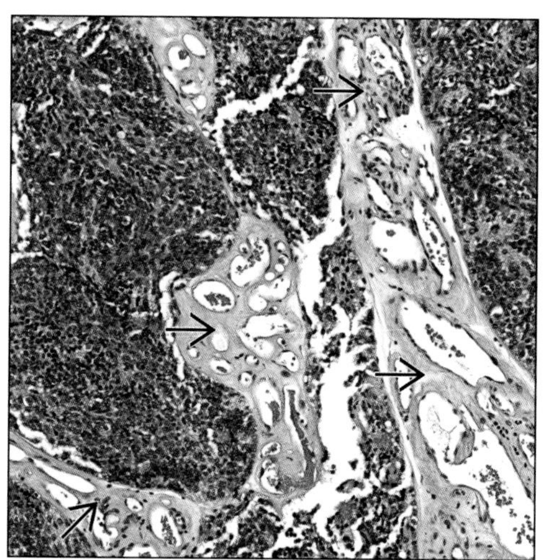

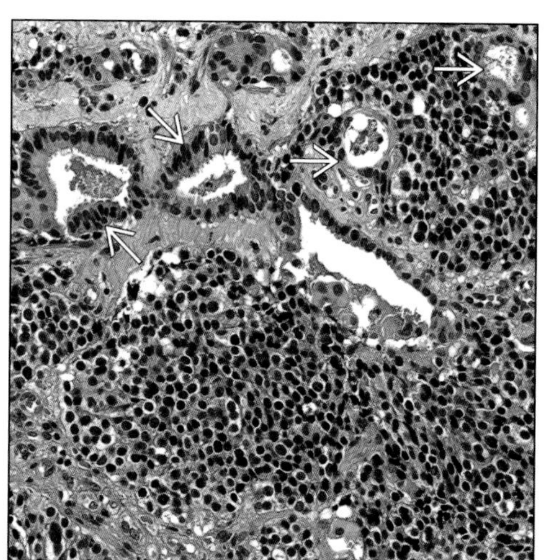

(Left) ONB are very vascular tumors, with a richly vascularized fibrovascular stroma and septa ⇨. This tumor would bleed quite profusely if it were biopsied; hence biopsies are discouraged. **(Right)** Native, residual minor mucoserous glands ➡ can be surrounded or invaded by the neoplastic proliferation. It is important to separate these structures from true rosettes (Flexner-Wintersteiner), which are only identified in high-grade tumors.

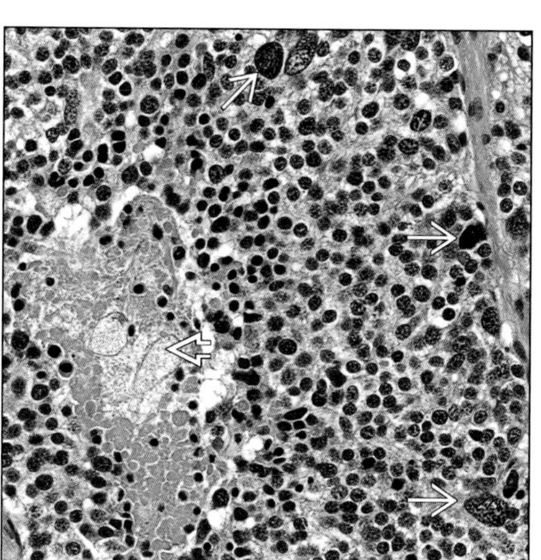

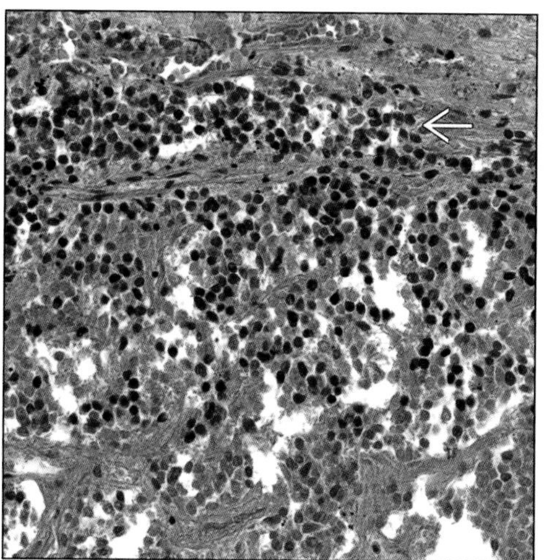

(Left) A grade 3 ONB will show nuclear pleomorphism ➡ and tumor necrosis ⇨, along with increased mitoses. There is a greater degree of nuclear hyperchromasia. **(Right)** There are still areas of viable tumor at the periphery of this lobule ➡, otherwise showing coagulative-type necrosis of the tumor. This is a pattern of growth that would be seen in a grade 3 or 4 ONB.

Microscopic Features

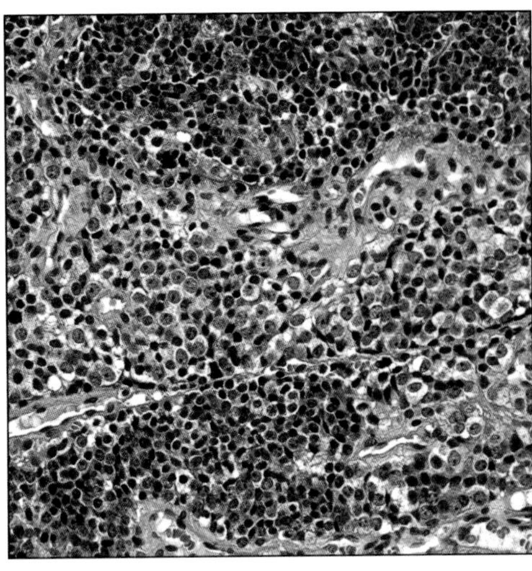

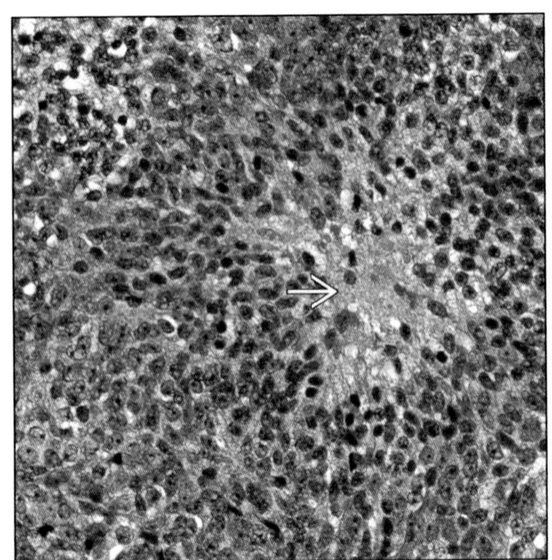

*(**Left**) It is not uncommon in a single tumor to have a number of different appearances, in which the cells become slightly larger (center) than the remaining cells, a finding seen more commonly in higher grade tumors. (**Right**) A pseudorosette (Homer Wright type) shows a peripheral palisade of neoplastic cells cuffing a finely fibrillary neural matrix material in the center ➡. This pseudorosette is seen in up to 30% of grade 1 and 2 tumors.*

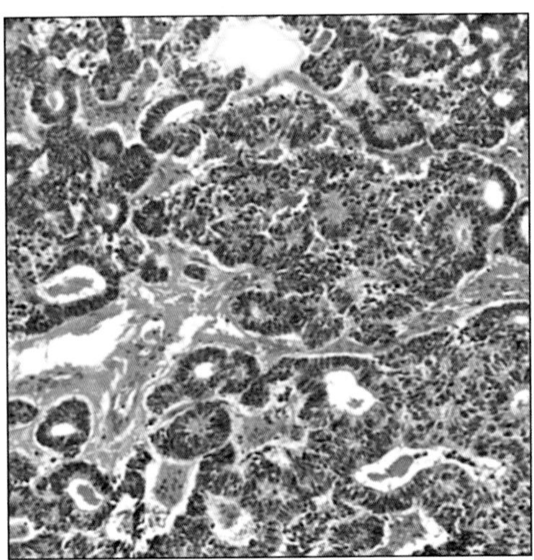

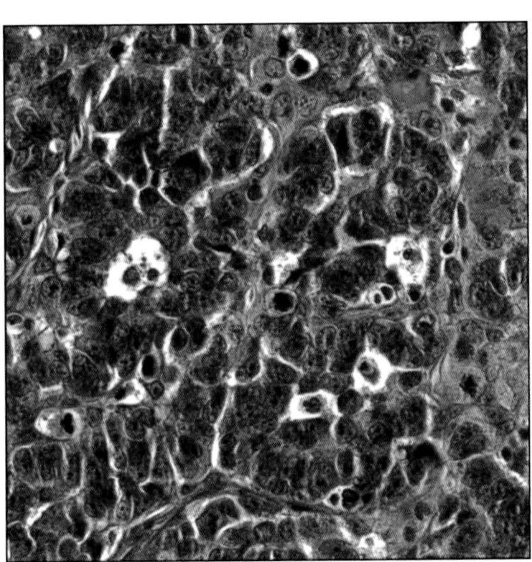

*(**Left**) True rosettes (of Flexner-Wintersteiner) have gland-like, tight annular formations with concretions in the lumen. The cells lining these duct-like spaces are nonciliated columnar cells. These rosettes are present in ~ 5% of grade 3 or 4 tumors. (**Right**) This grade 3 tumor shows a number of gland-like structures, but a true lumen with the cells arranged around the periphery is not present in this case. There is significant nuclear pleomorphism and prominent nucleoli.*

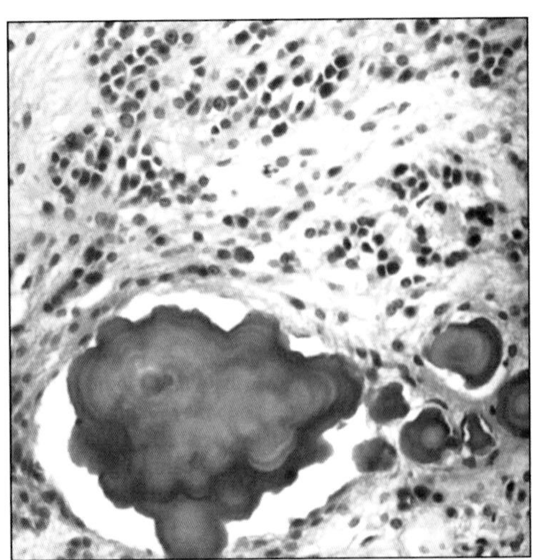

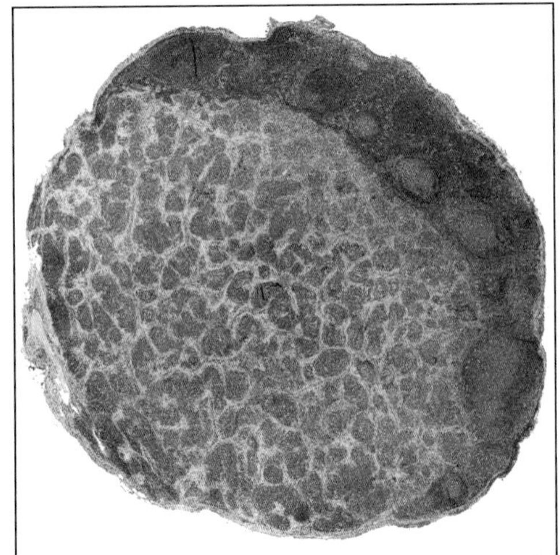

*(**Left**) Calcifications can be seen in ONB, although they tend to be seen more frequently in lower grade tumors. Multiple psammomatoid calcifications are seen in this grade 1 tumor. (**Right**) Cervical lymph node metastases are seen in up to 25% of patients. In this case, nearly 7/8 of the lymph node is replaced by the neoplasm. The metastatic foci recapitulate the primary, maintaining a lobular architecture and a richly vascularized stroma.*

Ancillary Techniques

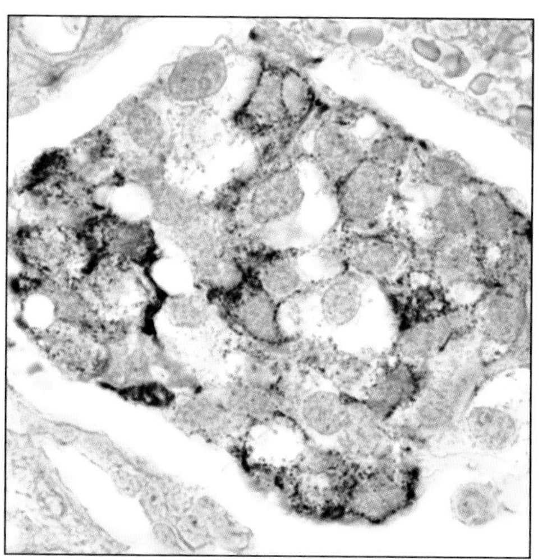

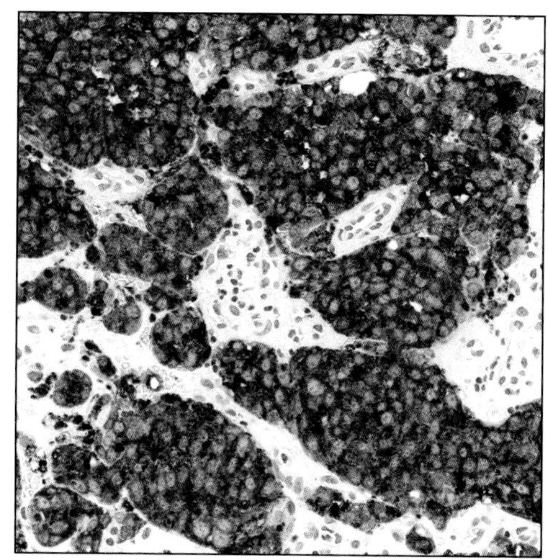

(Left) *The neurosecretory granules can be highlighted in the neoplastic cells by applying silver stains, with the Grimelius stain illustrated. (Stain courtesy L. Grimelius, MD.)* ***(Right)*** *A wide variety of neuroendocrine markers can be applied to highlight the neoplastic cells. Synaptophysin often gives a very strong, heavy chromogen deposition in the neoplastic cells, as illustrated here. There is a slight granularity to the staining pattern.*

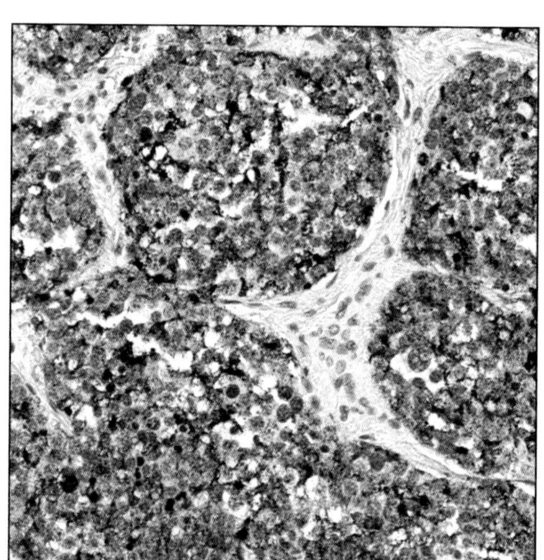

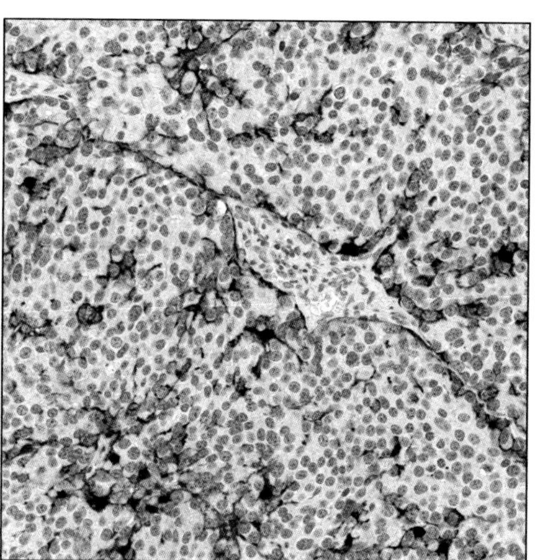

(Left) *Chromogranin yields a very strong, diffuse, cytoplasmic reaction in ONB. While chromogranin-A or -B can be used, A tends to give a more consistent result.* ***(Right)*** *The sustentacular cells at the periphery of the lobule are strongly highlighted with S100 protein, yielding a nuclear and cytoplasmic reaction. This pattern of reactivity supports the notion that the various cellular components of olfactory epithelium are all present in the tumor (basal, neurosensory, sustentacular cells).*

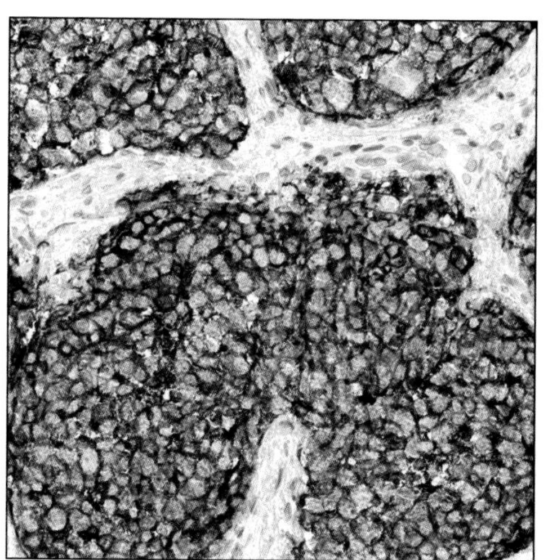

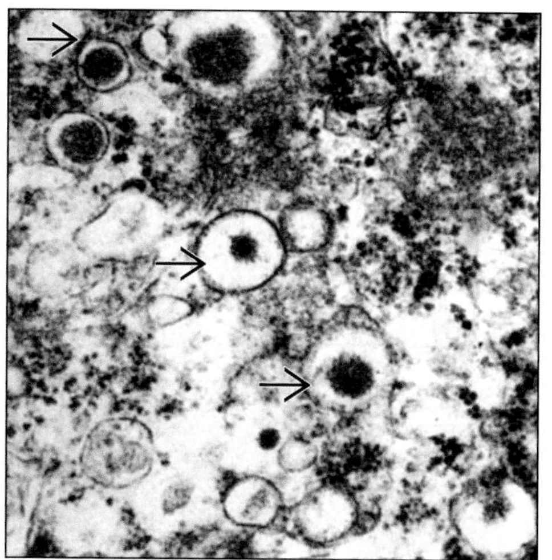

(Left) *CD56 yields a very strong and diffuse membranous and cytoplasmic reaction in the ONB cells. It is important to remember that CD56 is also reactive in rhabdomyosarcoma and NK-/T-cell lymphoma nasal-type tumors that are included in the differential diagnosis.* ***(Right)*** *A poorly differentiated olfactory neuroblastoma shows distinct halos ⇒ around the dense core granules in the neuroendocrine cells by ultrastructural examination.*

MALIGNANT MUCOSAL MELANOMA

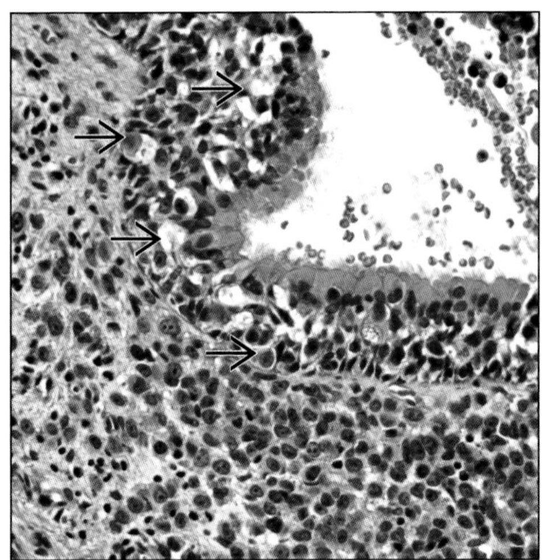

Atypical junctional melanocytes are noted within the respiratory epithelium, arranged in a pagetoid spread ➔. The tumor cells are also present within the stroma.

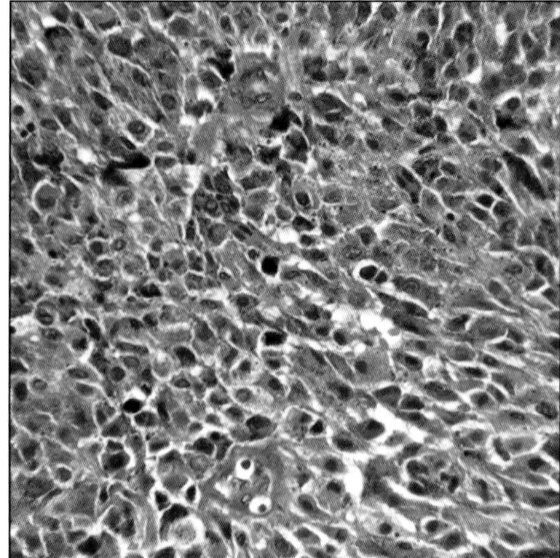

Hematoxylin & eosin shows a spindled to polygonal population of highly atypical, pigmented neoplastic cells. These changes are characteristic for a pigmented melanoma.

TERMINOLOGY

Abbreviations

- Malignant mucosal melanoma (MMM)
- Sinonasal tract and nasopharynx mucosal malignant melanoma (STMMM)

Definitions

- Neural crest-derived neoplasms originating from melanocytes and demonstrating melanocytic differentiation

ETIOLOGY/PATHOGENESIS

Environmental Exposure

- Formalin
- Possibly radiation
- UV exposure

CLINICAL ISSUES

Epidemiology

- Incidence
  - Rare
    - Represents < 1% of all melanomas
    - < 5% of all sinonasal tract neoplasms
    - 15-20% of all skin melanomas occur in head and neck
    - STMMM represent < 4% of all head and neck melanomas
- Age
  - Wide range, usually in 5th to 8th decades
- Gender
  - Equal gender distribution
- Ethnicity
  - Increased incidence in Japanese patients

Site

- About 15-20% of melanomas arise in head and neck
  - 80% are cutaneous in origin
  - Ocular origin account for majority of remaining MMM
  - Sinonasal tract is next most common site
- Anterior nasal septum > maxillary sinus

Presentation

- Nasal obstruction
- Epistaxis or nasal discharge
  - Melanorrhea: Black-flecked (melanin) discharge
- Polyp
- Pain is uncommon

Treatment

- Options, risks, complications
  - Metastatic melanoma to sinonasal tract can develop but is vanishingly rare
  - Breslow thickness and Clark level are not used in sinonasal tract
- Surgical approaches
  - Wide local excision is treatment of choice
- Radiation
  - Can be used after surgery
    - In most cases, it is palliative

Prognosis

- Poor overall
- 5-year survival (17-47%)
- Recurrences are common
- Poor prognosis associated with
  - Obstruction as presenting symptom
  - Nasopharynx or "mixed site" of involvement
  - Tumor ≥ 3 cm
  - Undifferentiated histology
  - High mitotic count
  - Recurrence
  - Stage of tumor
- Matrix metalloproteinases (MMPs) (proteolytic enzymes required for extracellular matrix degradation) expression may be associated with patient outcome

MALIGNANT MUCOSAL MELANOMA

Key Facts

Terminology
- Neural crest-derived neoplasms originating from melanocytes and demonstrating melanocytic differentiation

Clinical Issues
- Anterior nasal septum > maxillary sinus
- Overall prognosis is poor

Macroscopic Features
- Most are polypoid

Microscopic Pathology
- Protean histology, mimic of many other primary tumor types
- Junctional activity and epidermal migration (Pagetoid spread) help to confirm primary tumor
- Many patterns of growth
- Variety of cell types can be seen
- Prominent, irregular, brightly eosinophilic, enlarged nucleoli
- Intranuclear cytoplasmic inclusions usually present
- Melanin-containing tumor cells can be seen

Ancillary Tests
- Positive: S100 protein, HMB-45, Melan-A, microphthalmia transcription factor, tyrosinase, vimentin

Top Differential Diagnoses
- Olfactory neuroblastoma
- Sinonasal undifferentiated carcinoma
- Melanotic neuroectodermal tumor of infancy
- Rhabdomyosarcoma
- Lymphoma

  - Decreased *MMP2* expression associated with greater overall survival
  - Positive *MMP14* expression associated with poor survival

IMAGE FINDINGS

Radiographic Findings
- Usually identifies extent of tumor and bone invasion
- Positron emission tomography (PET) tends to show posterior nasal cavity and sinus tumors better than anterior nasal tumors
- Locoregional and metastatic disease can be detected

MACROSCOPIC FEATURES

General Features
- Most are polypoid
- White to gray, brown, or black
- Surface ulceration/erosion is common

Size
- Range up to 6 cm
- Mean: 2-3 cm

MICROSCOPIC PATHOLOGY

Histologic Features
- Protean histology, mimic of many other primary tumor types
- Junctional activity and epidermal migration (Pagetoid spread) help to confirm primary tumor
- Surface ulceration is common, obscuring "in situ" component
- Bone or soft tissue invasion is common
- Many patterns of growth
  - Peritheliomatous: Distinctive and unique for STMMM
  - Epithelioid
  - Solid
  - Organoid
  - Sheets
  - Nests
  - Fascicles and interlacing bundles
  - Storiform
  - Meningothelial
  - Hemangiopericytoma-like
  - Papillary
- Variety of cell types can be seen
  - Undifferentiated
  - Epithelioid, polygonal
  - Small cell
  - Plasmacytoid
  - Rhabdoid
  - Giant cell
- Vesicular nuclei although sometimes hyperchromatic
- Prominent, irregular, brightly eosinophilic, enlarged nucleoli
- Intranuclear cytoplasmic inclusions usually present
- Melanin-containing tumor cells can be seen
- Tumor cell necrosis is common
- Mitotic figures, including atypical forms, usually easily found and increased
- Inflammation may be present but not of consequence
- Desmoplastic type fibrosis can be seen, but is not common
- Perineural invasion, when present, is poor prognostic indicator
- Tumor depth of invasion (Clark) impossible to accurately assess
- Tumor thickness (Breslow) not meaningful in sinonasal tract

Lymphatic/Vascular Invasion
- Usually present but difficult to assess

Margins
- Difficult to assess, as samples are frequently fragmented and removed piecemeal

MALIGNANT MUCOSAL MELANOMA

ANCILLARY TESTS

Histochemistry

- Fontana-Masson
  - Reactivity: Positive
  - Staining pattern
    - Melanin bleach will confirm melanin in cytoplasm

Immunohistochemistry

- Positive: S100 protein, HMB-45, Melan-A, microphthalmia transcription factor, tyrosinase, vimentin
- p16 expression is lost in most MMM (74%)

Cytogenetics

- Comparative genomic hybridization (CGH) shows chromosome arm 1q is gained in nearly all tumors studied
- Gains of 6p (93%) and 8q (57%) are also identified

Electron Microscopy

- Premelanosomes and melanosomes confirms melanocytic origin

DIFFERENTIAL DIAGNOSIS

Olfactory Neuroblastoma

- Lobular architecture
- Fibrillary matrix material associated with rosettes and pseudorosettes
- CD56, chromogranin, synaptophysin, and sustentacular S100 protein reaction

Sinonasal Undifferentiated Carcinoma

- Small cells with high nuclear to cytoplasmic ratio
- Necrosis, destructive growth, and vascular invasion
- Strong, diffuse keratin immunoreactivity

Melanotic Neuroectodermal Tumor of Infancy

- Tumor of neonatal period, affecting gnathic bones
- Biphasic tumor with small and large cells, with pigment easily identified

Rhabdomyosarcoma

- Tends to develop in younger patients (although not alveolar type)
- Nests, alveolar patterns are similar
- Strap and rhabdoid patterns are helpful
- Cross striations can confirm diagnosis
- Immunoreactive with desmin, MYOD1, myogenin, SMA, MSA, CD56

Leiomyosarcoma

- Fascicular architecture, frequently associated with necrosis and high mitotic index
- Perinuclear vacuoles and cigar-shaped nuclei are rare in melanoma
- Muscle markers positive, while nonreactive with melanoma markers

Plasmacytoma

- Hematologic neoplasm giving sheet-like pattern of plasmacytoid cells
- "Hof" zone, paranuclear clearing, and rounded nuclei with clock face-like chromatin distribution
- CD138, CD79a, κ or λ, and other hematologic markers will be positive

Metastatic Melanoma

- While theoretic consideration, junctional/Pagetoid spread helps to exclude this possibility
- Clinical and radiographic examinations are the only way to make definitive separation

Mesenchymal Chondrosarcoma

- Small, undifferentiated cell appearance, but if enough sections are taken, cartilaginous features can be seen
- S100 protein will be positive (chondrocytic tumors are positive), but HMB-45, tyrosinase, Melan-A will not react

SELECTED REFERENCES

1. Wenig BM: Undifferentiated malignant neoplasms of the sinonasal tract. Arch Pathol Lab Med. 133(5):699-712, 2009
2. Bachar G et al: Mucosal melanomas of the head and neck: experience of the Princess Margaret Hospital. Head Neck. 30(10):1325-31, 2008
3. Dauer EH et al: Sinonasal melanoma: a clinicopathologic review of 61 cases. Otolaryngol Head Neck Surg. 138(3):347-52, 2008
4. Kim DK et al: Ki67 antigen as a predictive factor for prognosis of sinonasal mucosal melanoma. Clin Exp Otorhinolaryngol. 1(4):206-10, 2008
5. Kondratiev S et al: Expression and prognostic role of MMP2, MMP9, MMP13, and MMP14 matrix metalloproteinases in sinonasal and oral malignant melanomas. Hum Pathol. 39(3):337-43, 2008
6. McLean N et al: Primary mucosal melanoma of the head and neck. Comparison of clinical presentation and histopathologic features of oral and sinonasal melanoma. Oral Oncol. 44(11):1039-46, 2008
7. Cheng YF et al: Toward a better understanding of sinonasal mucosal melanoma: clinical review of 23 cases. J Chin Med Assoc. 70(1):24-9, 2007
8. Martin JM et al: Outcomes in sinonasal mucosal melanoma. ANZ J Surg. 74(10):838-42, 2004
9. Prasad ML et al: Clinicopathologic differences in malignant melanoma arising in oral squamous and sinonasal respiratory mucosa of the upper aerodigestive tract. Arch Pathol Lab Med. 127(8):997-1002, 2003
10. Thompson LD et al: Sinonasal tract and nasopharyngeal melanomas: a clinicopathologic study of 115 cases with a proposed staging system. Am J Surg Pathol. 27(5):594-611, 2003
11. van Dijk M et al: Distinct chromosomal aberrations in sinonasal mucosal melanoma as detected by comparative genomic hybridization. Genes Chromosomes Cancer. 36(2):151-8, 2003
12. Patel SG et al: Primary mucosal malignant melanoma of the head and neck. Head Neck. 24(3):247-57, 2002
13. Kardon DE et al: Sinonasal mucosal malignant melanoma: report of an unusual case mimicking schwannoma. Ann Diagn Pathol. 4(5):303-7, 2000
14. Regauer S et al: Primary mucosal melanomas of the nasal cavity and paranasal sinuses. A clinicopathological analysis of 14 cases. APMIS. 106(3):403-10, 1998

MALIGNANT MUCOSAL MELANOMA

Immunohistochemistry

Antibody	Reactivity	Staining Pattern	Comment
S100	Positive	Nuclear & cytoplasmic	Diffuse and strong stain usually; identified in about 90% of cases
HMB-45	Positive	Cytoplasmic	Variably reactive in most cases (~ 75%)
Tyrosinase	Positive	Cytoplasmic	Variably reactive in most cases (~ 75%)
melan-A103	Positive	Cytoplasmic	Variably reactive in majority of cases (~ 66%)
MITF	Positive	Nuclear	Positive in majority of cases (~ 55%)
NSE	Positive	Cytoplasmic	Positive in < 50% of tumor cells, often focal
CD117	Positive	Cytoplasmic	Positive in ~ 33% of cases
CD99	Positive	Cytoplasmic	Positive in ~ 25% of cases
Vimentin	Positive	Cytoplasmic	All tumor cells
CD56	Positive	Cell membrane & cytoplasm	~ 7% of cases
Synaptophysin	Positive	Cytoplasmic	Nonspecific, in ~ 10% of cases
EMA	Positive	Cytoplasmic	< 5% of tumor cells
Chromogranin-A	Negative		
CD45RB	Negative		
CK-PAN	Negative		
GFAP	Negative		
CD45RB	Negative		
Actin-HHF-35	Negative		
Actin-sm	Negative		
Desmin	Negative		
MYOD1	Negative		

Proposed Staging for Sinonasal Tract Melanomas

Classification	Description
Primary Tumor	
T1	Single anatomic site
T2	2 or more anatomic sites
Regional Lymph Nodes	
N0	No lymph node involvement
N1	Any lymph node metastases
Distant Metastasis	
M0	No distant metastases
M1	Distant metastasis
Stage Grouping	
I	T1 N0 M0
II	T2 N0 M0
III	Any T, N1, M0
IV	Any T, Any N, M1

MALIGNANT MUCOSAL MELANOMA

Radiographic and Microscopic Features

__(Left)__ This MR image (T2-weighted axial) demonstrates high signal within the maxillary sinus, focally associated with fluid in the posterior portion ➡. This lesion was a maxillary sinus malignant melanoma, without associated involvement of the nasal cavity. __(Right)__ The nasal septum cartilage ⇨ is being destroyed by the infiltrative neoplasm. The tumor forms a thick, sheet-like distribution. No pattern of growth can be seen at this magnification, although ulceration is present.

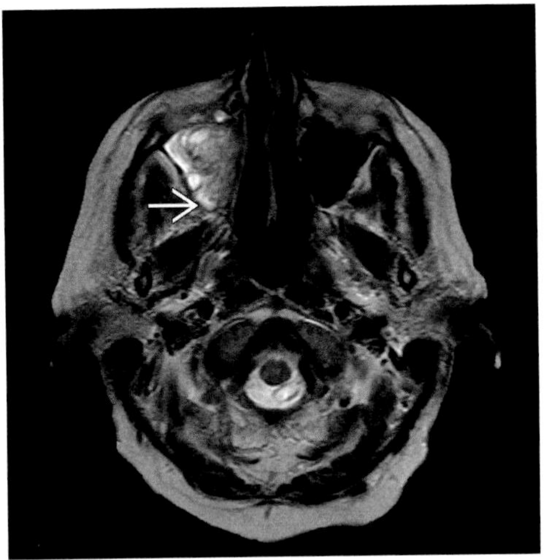

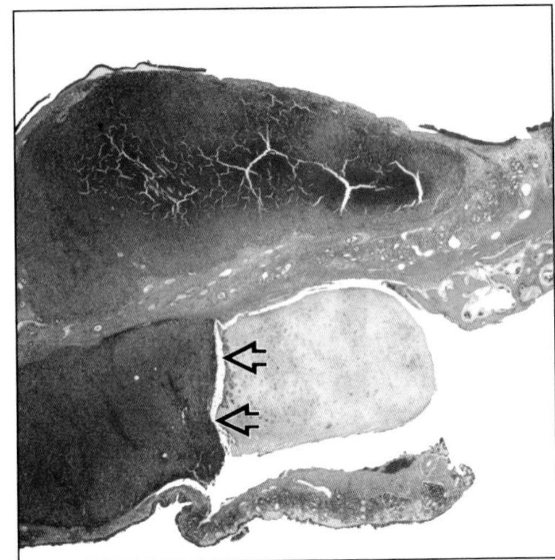

__(Left)__ Isolated junctional neoplastic cells are noted ⇨ in this MMM. The neoplastic cells in the stroma show pleomorphism and a plasmacytoid appearance. Pigment is easily identified. __(Right)__ This "peritheliomatous" or perivascular ➡ distribution of the neoplastic cells is quite characteristic for a melanoma. It is thought to represent viable tumor cells remaining around vessels. This pattern can be seen in other tumors but not to the same frequency as it is in melanoma.

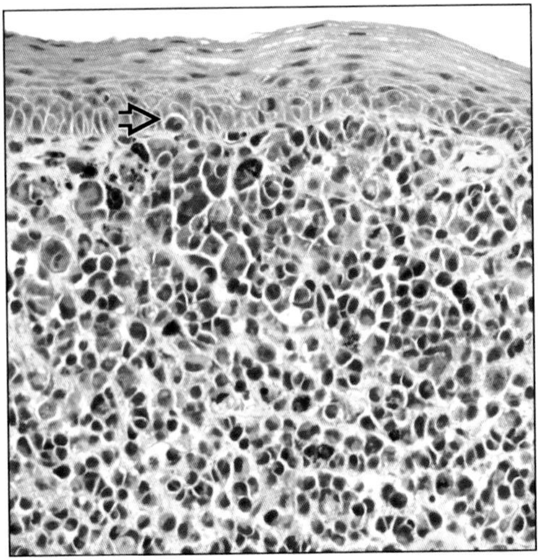

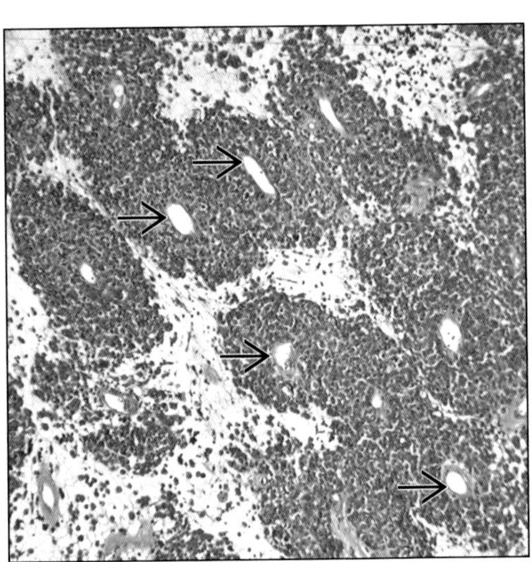

__(Left)__ MMM can be arranged in a number of different architectures, with a fascicular architecture seen here. The spindle cells are arranged in short, intersecting fascicles. The cells are somewhat syncytial in appearance. __(Right)__ It is not uncommon to have an "undifferentiated" or "small round blue cell" appearance to MMM. There is a slightly plasmacytoid appearance to the cells. Note the very prominent nucleoli. Mitotic figures are noted, but pigment is absent.

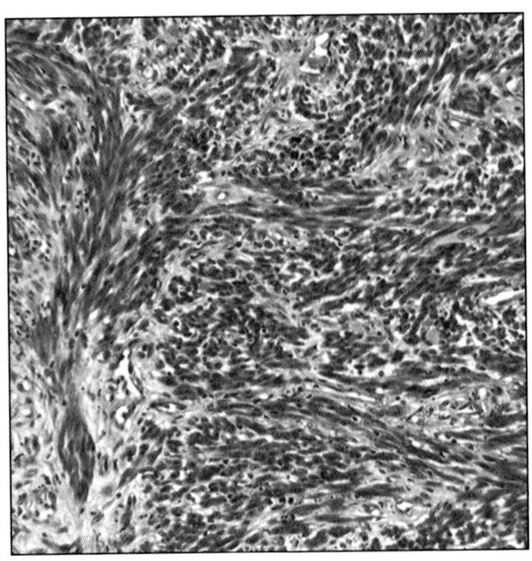

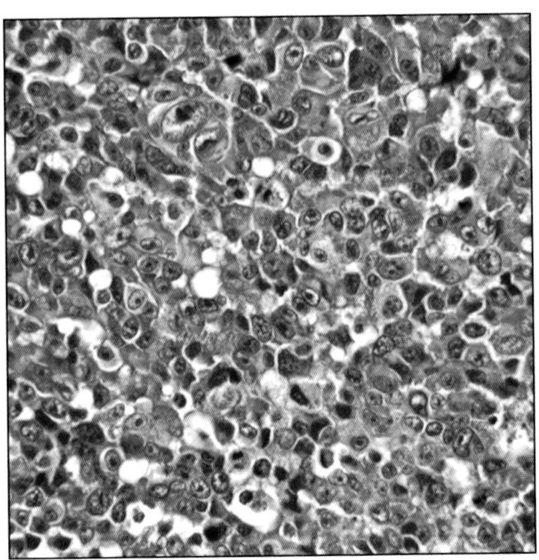

Microscopic and Immunohistochemical Features

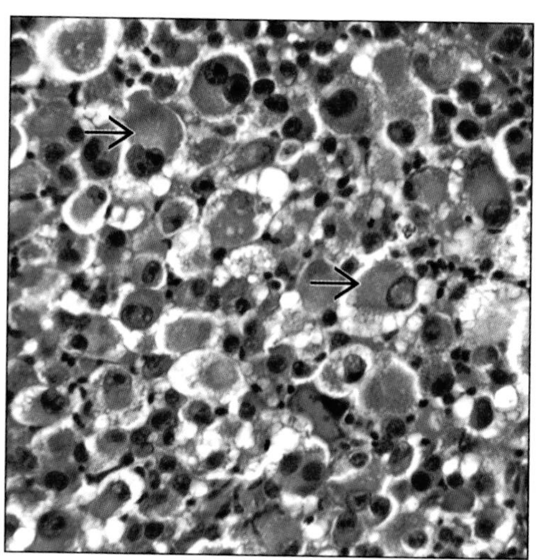

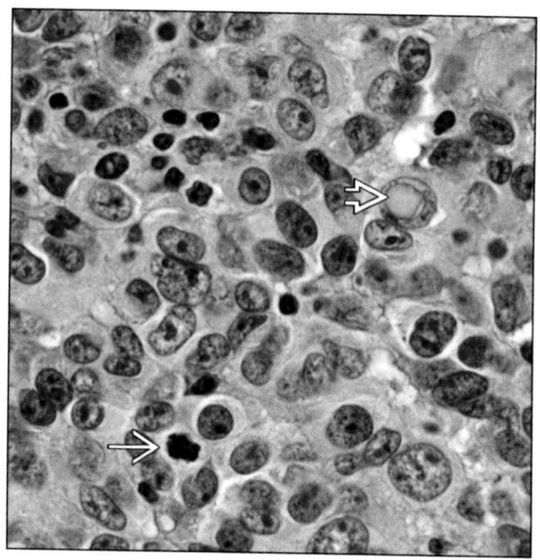

(Left) *This tumor shows a very pronounced plasmacytoid appearance, including a "Hof zone" adjacent to the nucleus ➔. There are intranuclear cytoplasmic inclusions as well as binucleation in this MMM.* **(Right)** *Pleomorphic polygonal cells comprise this melanoma. There is remarkable variability between cells. Prominent, eosinophilic nucleoli are noted, along with intranuclear cytoplasmic inclusions ➔. Mitotic figures are also noted ➔.*

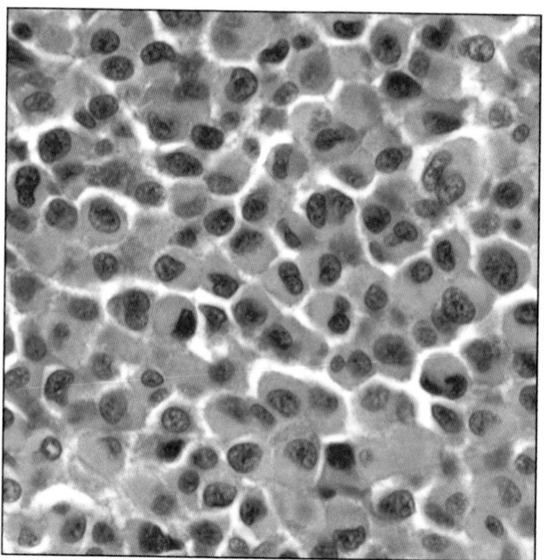

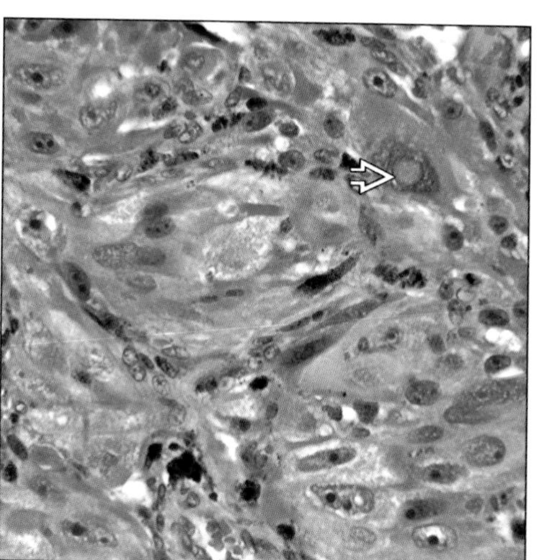

(Left) *A rhabdoid appearance with darkly opacified, eosinophilic cytoplasm is the dominant pattern in this MMM. Nucleoli are not as enlarged. Mitotic figures, necrosis, and pigment are not appreciated.* **(Right)** *It is not uncommon to have a variable architecture and cellular morphology in a single tumor. Here a polygonal and spindled cell population shows melanin pigment, prominent nucleoli, and intranuclear cytoplasmic inclusions ➔.*

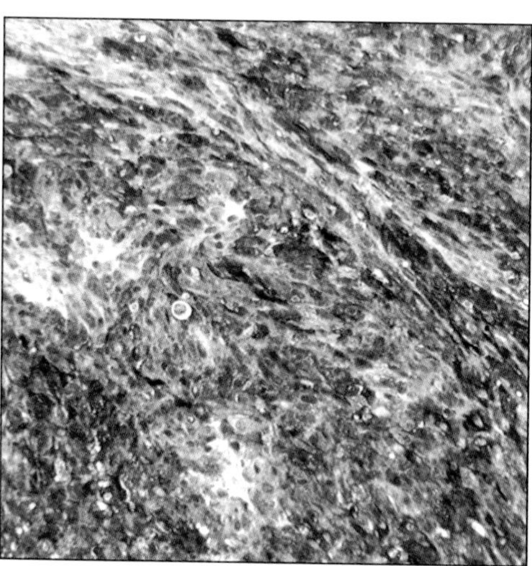

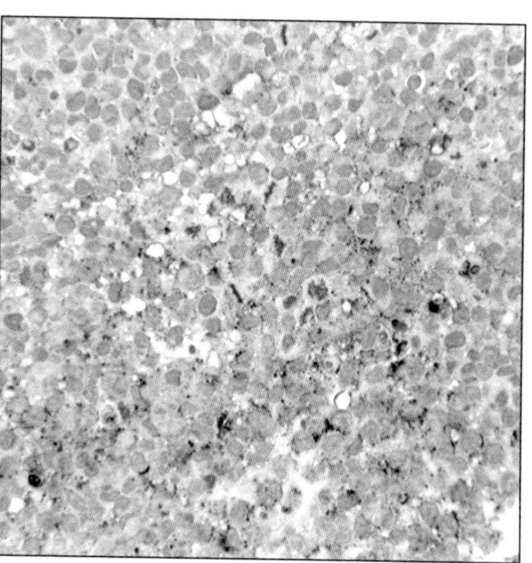

(Left) *Positive S100 protein is immunoreactive in this spindled cell melanoma. There is both cytoplasmic and nuclear reactivity with this marker that highlights nearly all of the cells.* **(Right)** *Positive HMB-45 in this "small round blue cell" pattern demonstrates some of the variability that can be seen both within a tumor as well as between tumors. The intensity of the staining as well as the number of cells, which are positive, can be quite variable.*

EWING SARCOMA

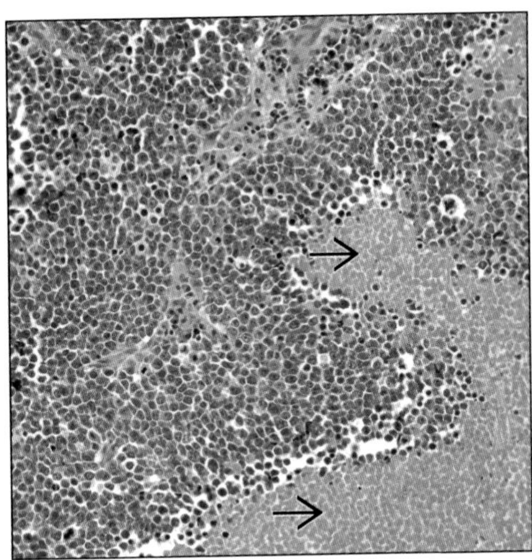

There is a very cellular tumor arranged in a diffuse sheet-like pattern. Note isolated fibrous connective tissue septae. Areas of coagulative and geographic necrosis are seen ⇒. There is often peritheliomatous tumor sparing.

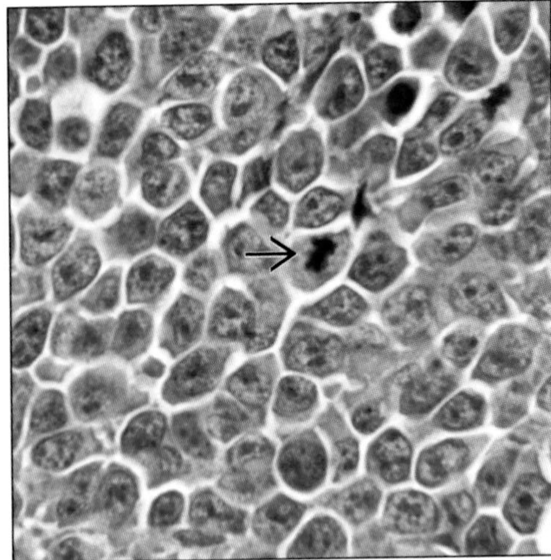

A relatively uniform population of medium cells shows a high nuclear to cytoplasmic ratio. The nuclei are round to slightly irregular with dispersed, fine chromatin distribution and small nucleoli. Note mitotic figures ⇒.

TERMINOLOGY

Abbreviations

- Ewing sarcoma (EWS)
- Primitive neuroectodermal tumor (PNET)

Synonyms

- PNET encompasses many tumors
  - Medulloblastoma, medulloepithelioma, olfactory neuroblastoma, retinoblastoma, pineoblastoma, ependymoblastoma, neuroblastoma

Definitions

- High-grade malignant tumor composed of primitive small, round tumor cells of undifferentiated or neuroectodermal phenotype analogous to pluripotential periventricular germinal matrix cells
  - EWS and PNET considered on morphologic spectrum, with both expressing similar genetic alterations
  - **Extraskeletal** tumors only considered

ETIOLOGY/PATHOGENESIS

Familial

- Sinonasal EWS/PNET has been reported in association with retinoblastoma

Pathogenesis

- Pluripotential fetal neuroectodermal cell is considered the progenitor
- Common neural crest origin with variable neural differentiation

CLINICAL ISSUES

Epidemiology

- Incidence
  - Exceedingly rare
    - Worldwide overall tumor incidence: 2/1,000,000 children
  - Approximately 20% of EWS/PNET occur in head and neck
    - About 20% of these cases develop in sinonasal tract
- Age
  - Predominantly a tumor of children and young adults
    - ~ 80% of tumors develop in < 20 year olds
    - Median: 12 years
  - Older adults uncommonly affected
- Gender
  - Slight male predilection
- Ethnicity
  - Blacks are rarely affected

Site

- Most common sites in sinonasal tract
  - Maxillary sinus > nasal fossa > > turbinates

Presentation

- Patients present with pain, mass, and obstruction
  - Bone pain specifically

Laboratory Tests

- Elevated serum LDH helps in managing recurrence

Treatment

- Options, risks, complications
  - Multimodality therapy (chemotherapy, radiation, and surgery) achieves best outcome
  - High-dose myeloablative radiochemotherapy with autologous bone marrow or peripheral blood stem cell rescue is aggressive alternative
- Surgical approaches
  - Wide excision after chemotherapy
- Adjuvant therapy
  - Generally, neoadjuvant chemotherapy
- Drugs
  - Multiple chemotherapeutic agents in combination

Key Facts

Terminology
- High-grade malignant tumor composed of primitive small, round tumor cells of undifferentiated or neuroectodermal phenotype

Clinical Issues
- Approximately 20% of EWS occur in head and neck
- ~ 80% of tumors develop in < 20 year olds
- Slight male predilection
- Maxillary sinus > nasal fossa > > turbinates
- Multimodality therapy (chemotherapy, radiation, and surgery) achieves best outcome
  - Overall, 60-70% 5-year survival
  - ~ 30% have metastases at presentation

Microscopic Pathology
- Diffuse, densely cellular tumor
- Coagulative necrosis with high mitotic index
- Uniform, small to medium round cells with scant, vacuolated cytoplasm
- Nuclei are round with dispersed fine chromatin distribution and small nucleoli

Ancillary Tests
- PAS with diastase identifies glycogen
- FLI-1 nuclear stain is nearly always positive
- FISH or RT-PCR for t(11;22)(q24;q12) (*EWS/FLI1*)

Top Differential Diagnoses
- Olfactory neuroblastoma, lymphoma, rhabdomyosarcoma, *NUT* midline carcinoma
- Pituitary adenoma, mesenchymal chondrosarcoma, osteosarcoma (small cell type), sinonasal undifferentiated carcinoma, mucosal melanoma

    - Vincristine, doxorubicin, cyclophosphamide, and dactinomycin; ifosfamide and etoposide may be used
  - Fenretinide shows promise
- Radiation
  - Used as adjuvant therapy for local disease control

Prognosis
- Overall, 60-70% 5-year survival
  - Aided by excellent radiographic studies and multimodality therapy
- Head and neck tumors have much better prognosis than tumors in other anatomic sites
- Size and stage are most important prognostic factors
  - Tumors with *EWS/FLI1* fusion have better prognosis than less common fusion types
- Intranasal tumors frequently spread into paranasal sinuses
- Up to 30% of patient have metastases at presentation
- Common sites of spread
  - Lungs, bone marrow, bone, brain, and lymph nodes
  - Isolated lung metastases may have better outcome
- Unfavorable prognosis dictated by
  - Tumor > 8 cm
  - Elevated WBC and sedimentation rate
  - Filigree microscopic pattern
  - No response to chemotherapy prior to resection

IMAGE FINDINGS

Radiographic Findings
- Destructive osteolytic lesion with bony erosion
- Periosteal reaction ("onion skin") frequently seen
  - Not as common in sinonasal tract tumors as in appendicular skeleton

MACROSCOPIC FEATURES

General Features
- Tumors are frequently multilobular and polypoid
- Gray-white and glistening cut surface
- Surface mucosal ulceration and hemorrhage
- Bone erosion is common

Size
- Range: Up to 6 cm
  - Sinonasal tract EWS/PNET tend to be smaller than other anatomic sites
  - This is probably due to anatomic confines of sinonasal tract vs. pelvis and long bones

MICROSCOPIC PATHOLOGY

Histologic Features
- Diffuse, densely cellular tumor
- Sheets and large nests of cells with indistinct cell borders
- Coagulative and geographic necrosis is easy to identify
  - Peritheliomatous tumor sparing
- Uniform, small to medium-sized round cells
- High nuclear to cytoplasmic ratio
- Nuclei are round with dispersed fine chromatin distribution and small nucleoli
- Scant, vacuolated cytoplasm
- Mitotic figures are increased
- Uncommonly, true rosettes and pseudorosettes may be seen (10% of cases)
  - Interpreted to be neural differentiation

Atypical
- Lobular architecture
- Increased extracellular matrix
- Alveolar pattern
- Increased mitoses (> 2/HPF)
- Pleomorphism
- Increased spindle cells (often at tumor margin)
- Lack of glycogen in cytoplasm (PAS stain)

ANCILLARY TESTS

Cytology
- Cellular smears with undifferentiated cells

EWING SARCOMA

- Focal clusters but predominantly single cells
  - Round tumor cells with high nuclear to cytoplasmic ratio
  - Small cells with scant cytoplasm
  - Pale cytoplasm with cytoplasmic vacuoles
    - Irregular, "punched out" cytoplasmic vacuoles due to glycogen
  - Nuclei with fine to smudged chromatin and small, basophilic nucleoli
  - Naked nuclei focally showing crush artifacts (but **not** typically nuclear molding)
- Mitoses and necrosis uncommon
- **Absence** of lymphoglandular bodies, cellular dyscohesion, rosettes, eosinophilic fibrillar material, and plasmacytoid cells
- Cytochemistry, immunocytochemistry, electron microscopy, cytogenetics, chromosomal analysis, &/ or molecular techniques can help differentiate among small round cell tumors

Histochemistry

- Diastase-sensitive PAS-positive intracytoplasmic material identifies glycogen

Immunohistochemistry

- CD99 (MIC2, O13, HBA-71, p30/32, 12E7) is nearly always positive
  - CD99 represents the monoclonal antibody to *EWS/FLI1* fusion product

Cytogenetics

- Translocation between chromosomes 11 and 22
  - Fusion of *EWS* gene on chromosome 22 to *FLI1* gene of chromosome 11
  - *FLI1*: Friend leukemia integration 1 transcription factor
- Other translocation partners can also be seen: t(21;22)(q22;q12)

In Situ Hybridization

- Dual-color break-apart probe fluorescence in situ hybridization (FISH) analysis will confirm translocation
  - Detected in about 95% of cases

Molecular Genetics

- Reverse transcriptase-polymerase chain reaction (RT-PCR) detects *EWS/FLI1* fusion product and can be performed on paraffin-embedded tissue
  - Chromosomal translocation: t(11;22)(q24;q12) or t(21;22)(q22;q12)
    - Many chimeric *EWS/FLI1* transcripts, representing different combinations of exons from *EWS* and *FLI1*
    - *ERG*, *ETV1*, *E1A-F*, *FEV* may be translocation partners
  - *EWS* is proto-oncogene: Present in native cells, but when activated, becomes oncogene
  - *EWS* gene amino-terminal domain (22q12) fuses with carboxy-terminal domain of *FLI1* (11q24) to create chimeric protein

Electron Microscopy

- Interdigitating cellular processes (neurite-like), filaments, and microtubules
- Dense core neurosecretory granules rarely identified
- Abundant intracellular glycogen
- Primitive cell-cell junctions resembling poorly formed desmosomes

DIFFERENTIAL DIAGNOSIS

Olfactory Neuroblastoma

- Specific anatomic site of involvement (ethmoid sinus, cribriform plate)
- Lobular architecture, with neural matrix, rosettes (true and pseudorosettes)
- In low-grade lesions, mitotic figures and necrosis are absent
- Chromogranin, CD56, synaptophysin positive, with sustentacular S100 protein reactivity
- Keratin can be seen, along with NSE; CD99 negative

Lymphoma

- Dispersed population without molding or cohesive groups
- Positive with lymphoid markers: CD45RB, CD20, CD3, CD56, based on specific tumor type

Rhabdomyosarcoma

- Small blue round cell phenotype can show significant overlap
- Slightly plasmacytoid appearance, with eosinophilic perinuclear cytoplasm condensation, strap cells
- Also rich in glycogen
- Myogenic immunohistochemistry: Desmin, MYOD1, myogenin, MYF4, myoglobin, actin

Mesenchymal Chondrosarcoma

- Hemangiopericytoma-like vascular pattern
- Small round blue cell morphology for most of tumor
- Must submit many sections to see areas of chondroid differentiation
- S100 protein may help with separation

Osteosarcoma, Small Cell Type

- Uncommon tumor type in sinonasal tract
- Lacy, osteoid matrix present

Pituitary Adenoma

- Sphenoid sinus usually affected
- Bland cytology, with sheet-like to lobular architecture
- Various neuroendocrine markers positive but CD99 absent
- Molecular studies are negative

Mucosal Malignant Melanoma

- Frequently show mucosal origin (in situ)
- Pleomorphic population, plasmacytoid and spindled cell appearance, intranuclear cytoplasmic inclusions, pigmentation, peritheliomatous distribution
- Strong S100 protein, HMB-45, Melan-A immunoreactivity

EWING SARCOMA

Immunohistochemistry

Antibody	Reactivity	Staining Pattern	Comment
CD99	Positive	Cytoplasmic	Nearly all tumor cells with membrane accentuation
FLI-1	Positive	Nuclear	Most tumor cells
SNF5	Positive	Nuclear	All tumor cells
p14	Positive	Nuclear	Nearly all tumor cells
Rb	Positive	Nuclear	Nearly all tumor cells
Vimentin	Positive	Cytoplasmic	Most tumor cells
NSE	Positive	Cytoplasmic	Usually more frequently seen in PNET than Ewing
β-catenin-cytoplasm	Positive	Cell membrane & cytoplasm	Majority of tumor cells
PGP9.5	Positive	Cytoplasmic	Most tumor cells
Claudin-1	Positive	Cytoplasmic	Approximately 50% of cases
CD117	Positive	Cytoplasmic	About 25% of cases
Synaptophysin	Positive	Cytoplasmic	About 20% of cases
S100	Positive	Nuclear & cytoplasmic	About 20% of cases
CK-PAN	Positive	Cytoplasmic	Only about 15% of cells
Myogenin	Negative		
WT1	Negative		
Chromogranin-A	Negative		
GFAP	Negative		

Sinonasal Undifferentiated Carcinoma

- Old age at initial presentation, with midline destruction
- Significant destruction, vascular invasion, bone invasion, perineural invasion
- Strong, diffuse keratin immunoreactivity

NUT Midline Carcinoma

- Poorly differentiated carcinoma presenting in patients of young age (< 30 years)
- Majority are midline, although sinonasal tract is not frequent location
- Specific molecular alteration required for diagnosis (rearrangement of nuclear protein in testis [*NUT*] gene on chromosome 15q14 [detected by FISH])

Melanotic Neuroectodermal Tumor of Infancy

- Pigmented tumor of maxilla presenting during neonatal or early childhood
- Large, pigmented epithelioid cells associated with smaller, blue round cells
- Set in heavy background stromal reaction
- HMB-45 and S100 protein positive

STAGING

Same as Rhabdomyosarcoma

- Staging is according to Clinical Groups of the Intergroup Rhabdomyosarcoma Study

SELECTED REFERENCES

1. Cordes B et al: Molecular and phenotypic analysis of poorly differentiated sinonasal neoplasms: an integrated approach for early diagnosis and classification. Hum Pathol. 40(3):283-92, 2009
2. Franchi A et al: Pediatric sinonasal neuroendocrine carcinoma after treatment of retinoblastoma. Hum Pathol. 40(5):750-5, 2009
3. Wenig BM: Undifferentiated malignant neoplasms of the sinonasal tract. Arch Pathol Lab Med. 133(5):699-712, 2009
4. Rischin D et al: Sinonasal malignancies of neuroendocrine origin. Hematol Oncol Clin North Am. 22(6):1297-316, xi, 2008
5. Iezzoni JC et al: "Undifferentiated" small round cell tumors of the sinonasal tract: differential diagnosis update. Am J Clin Pathol. 124 Suppl:S110-21, 2005
6. Mills SE: Neuroectodermal neoplasms of the head and neck with emphasis on neuroendocrine carcinomas. Mod Pathol. 15(3):264-78, 2002
7. Tsai EC et al: Tumors of the skull base in children: review of tumor types and management strategies. Neurosurg Focus. 12(5):e1, 2002
8. Cope JU et al: Ewing sarcoma and sinonasal neuroectodermal tumors as second malignant tumors after retinoblastoma and other neoplasms. Med Pediatr Oncol. 36(2):290-4, 2001
9. Parham DM: Neuroectodermal and neuroendocrine tumors principally seen in children. Am J Clin Pathol. 115 Suppl:S113-28, 2001
10. Toda T et al: Primitive neuroectodermal tumor in sinonasal region. Auris Nasus Larynx. 26(1):83-90, 1999
11. Klein EA et al: Sinonasal primitive neuroectodermal tumor arising in a long-term survivor of heritable unilateral retinoblastoma. Cancer. 70(2):423-31, 1992
12. Frierson HF Jr et al: Unusual sinonasal small-cell neoplasms following radiotherapy for bilateral retinoblastomas. Am J Surg Pathol. 13(11):947-54, 1989

EWING SARCOMA

Radiographic, Gross, and Microscopic Features

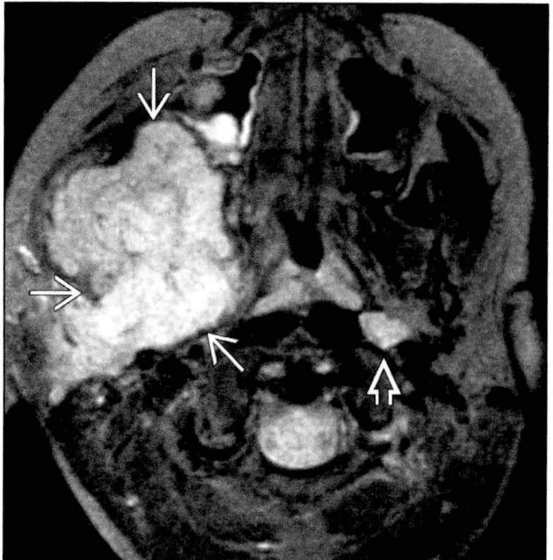

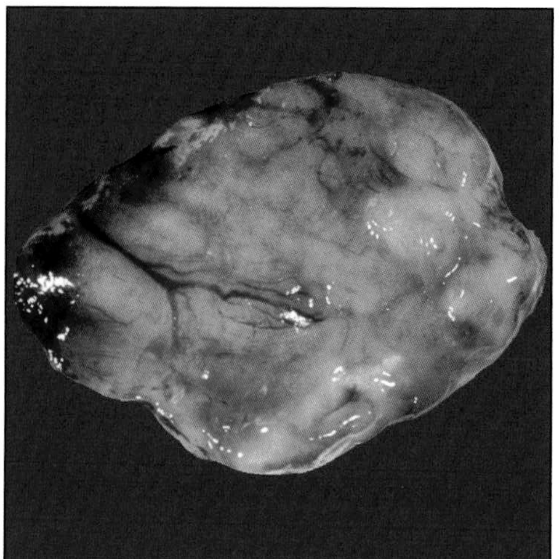

(Left) *Axial T2-weighted fat-suppressed MR shows a markedly hyperintense but heterogeneous tumor ➡. A prominent left retropharyngeal node ➡ is incidentally noted. This appearance supports the diagnosis of a tumor but is not specific for Ewing.* ***(Right)*** *This is a polypoid, multilobular tumor removed from the nasal cavity of a 28-year-old man. The surface is intact, although showing areas of erosion and subepithelial hemorrhage. Necrosis is seen as yellow streaks.*

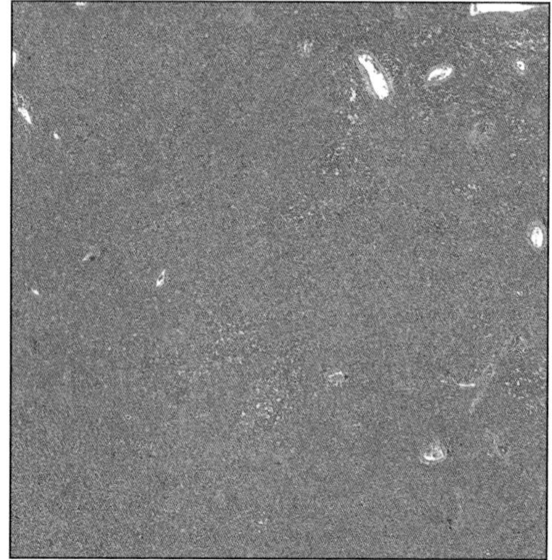

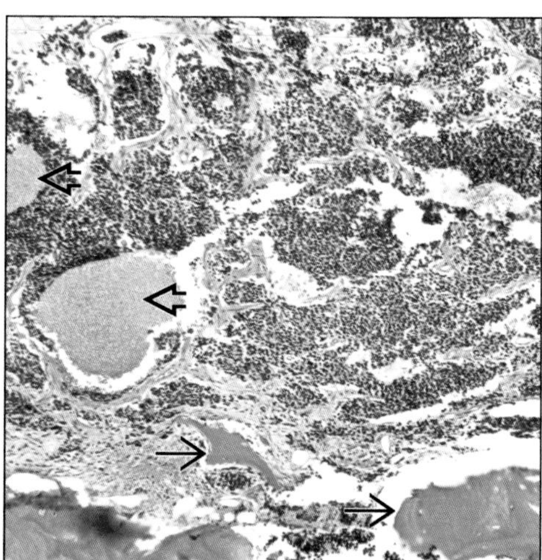

(Left) *The tumors are usually extremely cellular, with a dense, solid to sheet-like distribution of cells. A delicate vascularity is noted, but overall this is a solid population of cells.* ***(Right)*** *Areas of bone invasion are often easy to see ➡. There is a "small round blue cell" population, associated with areas of necrosis ➡ and hemorrhage. This pattern on low power is not specific for Ewing sarcoma but can be seen in a variety of different sinonasal tract tumors.*

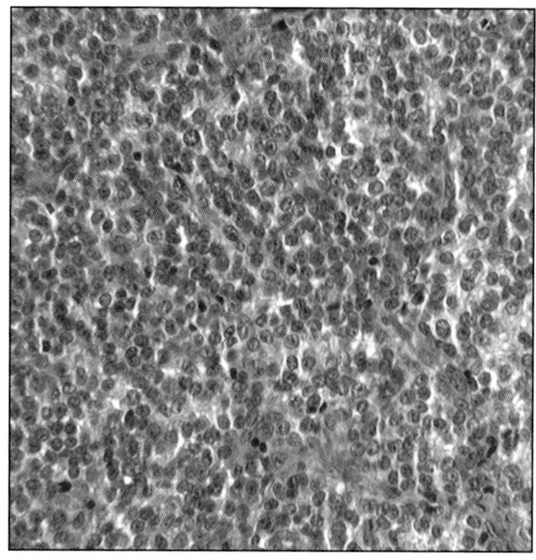

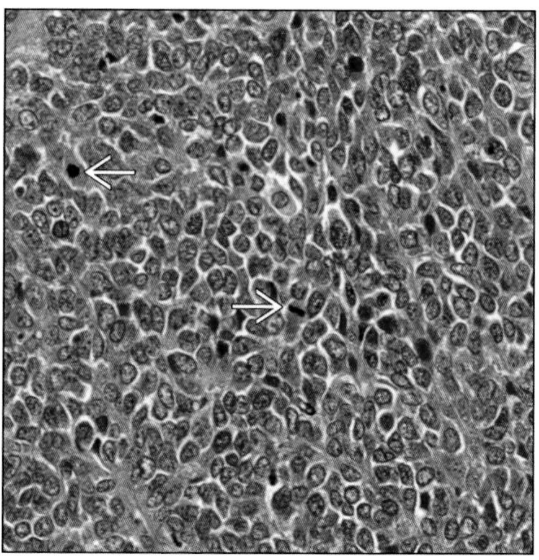

(Left) *There is a vaguely lobular appearance to this monotonous tumor cell population. The cells have round nuclei with delicate nuclear chromatin distribution. Nucleoli are small and inconspicuous. A background vascularity is noted.* ***(Right)*** *There is no unique pattern to this sheet of neoplastic cells. The cells have a high nuclear to cytoplasmic ratio, but the cells are small. The nuclear chromatin is evenly distributed. A number of mitotic figures are seen ➡.*

Microscopic Features and Ancillary Techniques

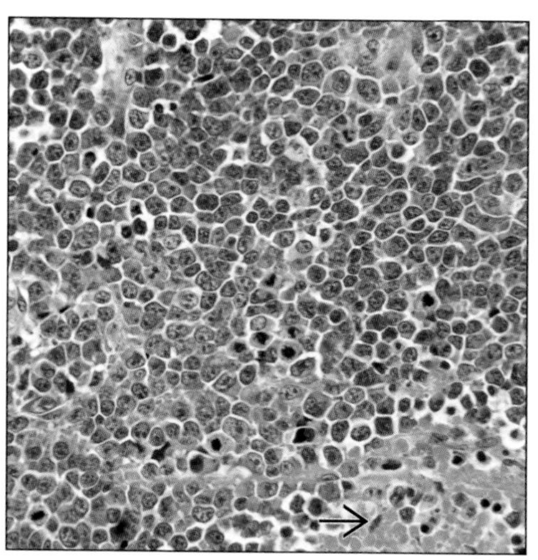

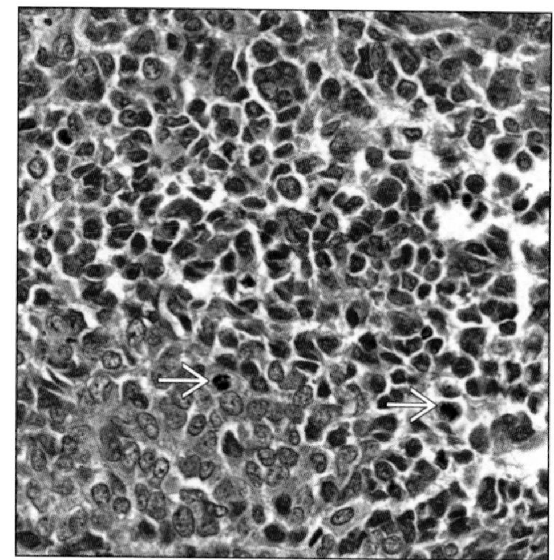

(Left) *The cells do not really show distinct cell borders but are arranged in a syncytium. There are areas of coagulative necrosis → and a number of apoptotic bodies and mitotic figures.* ***(Right)*** *This tumor is beginning to undergo degeneration with a number of apoptotic bodies. Mitoses are also easily identified throughout the tumor →, a feature that can aid in the diagnostic separation of Ewing sarcoma from other tumor types.*

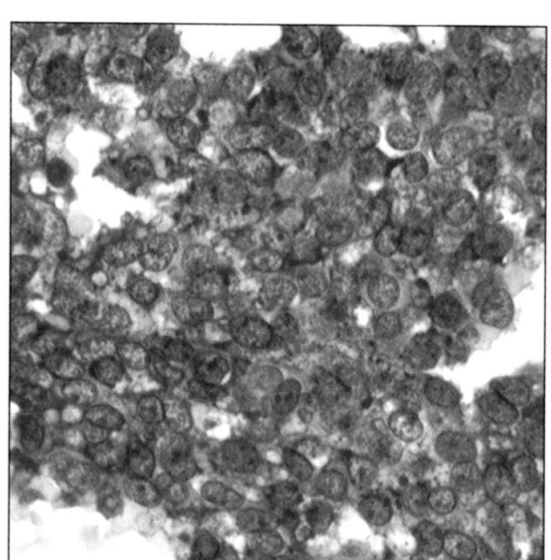

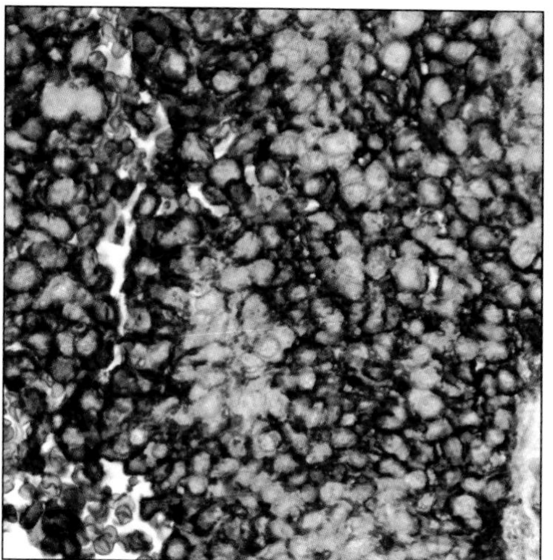

(Left) *This PAS stain without digestion shows a very strong cytoplasmic pink glycogenation. Glycogen (dissolved with diastase) is quite helpful in the diagnosis, although rhabdomyosarcoma also shows glycogen in the cytoplasm.* ***(Right)*** *There is a strong, diffuse, cytoplasmic reaction with CD99. This type of pattern is not as frequently seen in other tumor types. CD99 is an antibody to the fusion protein between EWS and FLI1.*

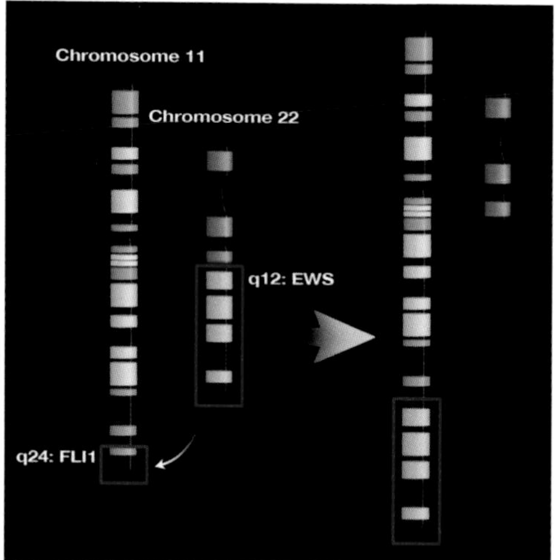

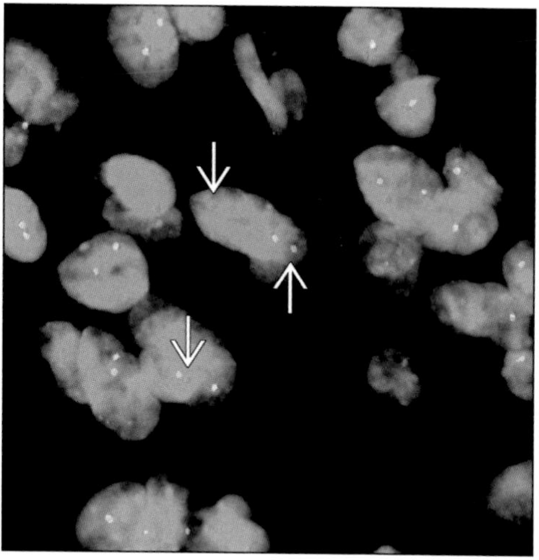

(Left) *The characteristic t(11;22)(q24;q12) translocation between the carboxy-terminal domain of FLI1 (11q24) and the EWS gene amino-terminal domain (22q12) creates a fusion product.* ***(Right)*** *A probe that spans the known breakpoints of the EWS gene on chromosome 22 (introns 7-10) is labeled with spectrum green and orange (3' and 5' respectively). With rearrangement, discrete separate red → and green signals are seen instead of the fused yellow signal. (Courtesy A. Nguyen.)*

TERATOCARCINOSARCOMA

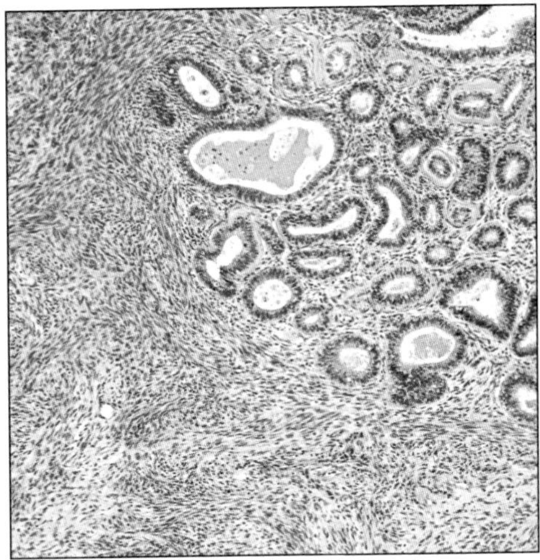

The heterogeneous nature of the neoplasm shows intermingled features of adenocarcinoma and spindled cell sarcoma in this field. Fibrosarcoma is a frequent tumor type.

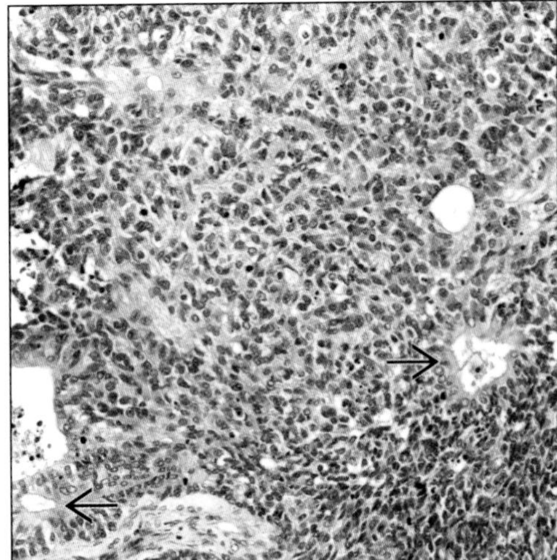

This field shows intermingled features of carcinoma, with immature spindled elements (sarcoma) and areas of blastemal tissue (teratoma). There are a number of rosettes ⇒ within this field.

TERMINOLOGY

Abbreviations

- Sinonasal teratocarcinosarcoma (SNTCS)

Synonyms

- Malignant teratoma
- Blastoma
- Teratocarcinoma
- Teratoid carcinosarcoma
- Mixed olfactory neuroblastoma-craniopharyngioma

Definitions

- Complex malignant sinonasal neoplasm with immature and malignant endodermal, mesodermal, and neuroepithelial elements resembling immature teratoma
- By definition, germ cell tumor is absent (embryonal carcinoma, choriocarcinoma, seminoma)

ETIOLOGY/PATHOGENESIS

Pathogenesis

- Probably arises from primitive cell in olfactory membrane that possess capacity to show multilineage differentiation
- Some consider it a germ cell tumor

CLINICAL ISSUES

Epidemiology

- Incidence
  - Extremely rare
- Age
  - Median: 60 years
  - Range: 18-79 years
- Gender
  - Male > > > Female

Site

- Most common high in nasal cavity, ethmoid and maxillary sinuses
- Frequently involves more than 1 paranasal sinus

Presentation

- Most common symptoms: Nasal obstruction and epistaxis
- Symptoms are of short duration
  - Mean: < 4 months
- May also experience
  - Nasal discharge
  - Frontal headaches
  - Sinusitis

Laboratory Tests

- Vasopressin may be ectopically or inappropriately elevated (ADH)

Treatment

- Options, risks, complications
  - Aggressive multimodality therapy (combination of surgery, radiation therapy, and chemotherapy) yields best outcome
    - 40% of patients survive disease-free > 3 years, although 60% of patients die in that time
- Surgical approaches
  - Complete surgical eradication by craniofacial resection, open surgery, or endoscopic resection
- Drugs
  - Combined with radiation and surgery in most cases
- Radiation
  - Postoperatively

Prognosis

- Guarded prognosis with highly aggressive clinical behavior
  - 60% of patients are dead within 3 years
    - Mean: 1.7 years
  - Most common cause of treatment failure is local recurrence

TERATOCARCINOSARCOMA

Key Facts

Terminology

- Complex malignant sinonasal neoplasm with immature and malignant endodermal, mesodermal, and neuroepithelial elements resembling immature teratoma

Clinical Issues

- Median: 60 years
- Male > > > Female
- Most common high in nasal cavity, ethmoid and maxillary sinuses
- Most common symptoms: Nasal obstruction and epistaxis
- Aggressive multimodality therapy (combination of surgery, radiation therapy, and chemotherapy) yields best outcome
- Guarded prognosis with highly aggressive clinical behavior

Microscopic Pathology

- Heterogeneous neoplasm with **intermingled** features of carcinoma, sarcoma, and immature teratoma
  - **Carcinoma** can be squamous or adenocarcinoma
  - **Sarcoma** composed of cartilage, bone, or muscle in varying degrees of maturation
  - **Neural** elements show primitive neuroepithelial tissue, blastomatous cells, neurofibrillary matrix, and prominent rosettes

Top Differential Diagnoses

- Olfactory neuroblastoma, rhabdomyosarcoma, sinonasal undifferentiated carcinoma, adenocarcinoma, germ cell tumor

---

  - 40% of patients respond to multimodality therapy
    - Mean survival: 6 years
- Rapid recurrences are very common (up to 70%) usually in < 2 years
  - Local paranasal sinus disease, intracranial or orbital extension
- Metastatic disease
  - Cervical metastases in ~ 30%
  - Distant metastases to lung are uncommon

IMAGE FINDINGS

Radiographic Findings

- Aggressive, poorly marginated, large, soft tissue density mass with bone destruction and invasion across fascial planes
- Best studies: Bone CT and T1WI MR with contrast
  - MR: Soft tissue and neural involvement
  - CT: Bone destruction

MACROSCOPIC FEATURES

General Features

- Large, bulky, polypoid, friable masses
- Soft, fleshy with necrosis

Size

- Mean: > 4 cm

MICROSCOPIC PATHOLOGY

Histologic Features

- Heterogeneous neoplasm with **intermingled** features of carcinoma, sarcoma, and immature teratoma
  - By definition, germ cell tumor is absent (embryonal carcinoma, choriocarcinoma, seminoma)
- Benign and malignant, immature epithelial, mesenchymal, and neural elements topographically mixed, with transition between elements
  - **Carcinoma** can be squamous or adenocarcinoma
    - Keratinizing or nonkeratinizing squamous epithelium, occasionally cystic
    - Clear cell immature squamous epithelium
    - Pseudostratified columnar, ciliated epithelium
    - Glandular structures with cuboidal or columnar cells, with or without mucus production
  - **Sarcoma** composed of cartilage, bone, or muscle in varying degrees of maturation
    - Spindled, immature mesenchymal cells in matrix (myxoid, mucinous)
    - Cartilage, bone, skeletal or smooth muscle in embryonal form
    - Fibrosarcoma pattern
  - **Neural** elements show primitive neuroepithelial tissue, blastomatous cells, neurofibrillary matrix, and prominent rosettes
    - Neuronal maturation is rarely seen post chemotherapy

ANCILLARY TESTS

Immunohistochemistry

- Highlights the various constituent elements
- **Positive**
  - Epithelial
    - Cytokeratins, EMA
  - Spindle cell
    - Vimentin, GFAP, calponin, desmin, myoglobin, myogenin, actins
  - Neuroepithelial/blastema
    - Neuron specific enolase, CD56, chromogranin, synaptophysin, CD99, S100 protein; rarely AFP
- **Negative**
  - β human chorionic gonadotrophin
  - Neurofilament protein
  - CD45RB

Molecular Genetics

- Trisomy 12 and 1p deletion have been identified

Electron Microscopy

- **Primitive** cells

  - Neural processes, parallel microtubules, dense core granules
- **Spindle** cells
  - Actin filaments, skeletal muscle differentiation
- **Epithelial** cells
  - Desmosomes, intermediate filaments, microvilli, tonofilaments

DIFFERENTIAL DIAGNOSIS

Olfactory Neuroblastoma

- Ethmoid sinus and cribriform plate involvement
- Lobular architecture
- Neurofibrillary matrix, pseudorosettes, and rosettes
- Monotonous "small round blue cell" neoplasm
- Positive with neuroendocrine markers
- Negative with mesenchymal and epithelial markers (isolated keratin-positive cells can be seen)

Rhabdomyosarcoma

- Embryonal or alveolar types most common in sinonasal tract
- Lacks epithelial and neuroendocrine differentiation (neural tissue)
- Positive: Myogenic markers, but also positive with CD56 and keratin (5%)

Sinonasal Undifferentiated Carcinoma

- Poorly differentiated epithelial neoplasm, showing destructive midline growth, extensive necrosis, and vascular invasion
- May have rosettes but tends to lack mesenchyma or teratoma-like appearance
- Strong keratin expression, lacking other markers

Adenocarcinoma

- Epithelial elements only
- Arranged in distinctive pattern
  - High- or low-grade sinonasal adenocarcinoma
  - Salivary gland-type adenocarcinomas (all variants)
- Lacks neural, blastemal, and sarcomatoid elements

Germ Cell Tumor

- Distinct features of embryonal, yolk sac, and seminoma are not identified in teratocarcinosarcoma
- Unique immunohistochemistry profile helps with separation

DIAGNOSTIC CHECKLIST

Pathologic Interpretation Pearls

- Highly malignant tumor with carcinoma, sarcoma, and teratoma (blastema/primitive) intermingled

SELECTED REFERENCES

1. Budrukkar A et al: Management and clinical outcome of sinonasal teratocarcinosarcoma: single institution experience. J Laryngol Otol. 124(7):739-43, 2010
2. Nguyen BD: Sinonasal teratocarcinosarcoma: MRI and F18-FDG-PET/CT imaging. Ear Nose Throat J. 89(3):106-8, 2010
3. Su YY et al: Sinonasal teratocarcinosarcoma. Am J Otolaryngol. 31(4):300-3, 2010
4. Kane SV et al: Chemotherapy-induced neuronal maturation in sinonasal teratocarcinosarcoma--a unique observation. Head Neck Pathol. 3(1):31-6, 2009
5. Salem F et al: Teratocarcinosarcoma of the nasal cavity and paranasal sinuses: report of 3 cases with assessment for chromosome 12p status. Hum Pathol. 39(4):605-9, 2008
6. Smith SL et al: Sinonasal teratocarcinosarcoma of the head and neck: a report of 10 patients treated at a single institution and comparison with reported series. Arch Otolaryngol Head Neck Surg. 134(6):592-5, 2008
7. Vranic S et al: Hamartomas, teratomas and teratocarcinosarcomas of the head and neck: Report of 3 new cases with clinico-pathologic correlation, cytogenetic analysis, and review of the literature. BMC Ear Nose Throat Disord. 8:8, 2008
8. Wei S et al: Sinonasal teratocarcinosarcoma: report of a case with review of literature and treatment outcome. Ann Diagn Pathol. 12(6):415-25, 2008
9. Carrizo F et al: Pharyngeal teratocarcinosarcoma: review of the literature and report of two cases. Ann Diagn Pathol. 10(6):339-42, 2006
10. Shimazaki H et al: Sinonasal teratocarcinosarcoma: ultrastructural and immunohistochemical evidence of neuroectodermal origin. Ultrastruct Pathol. 24(2):115-22, 2000
11. Pai SA et al: Teratocarcinosarcoma of the paranasal sinuses: a clinicopathologic and immunohistochemical study. Hum Pathol. 29(7):718-22, 1998
12. Heffner DK et al: Teratocarcinosarcoma (malignant teratoma?) of the nasal cavity and paranasal sinuses A clinicopathologic study of 20 cases. Cancer. 53(10):2140-54, 1984

Radiographic and Microscopic Features

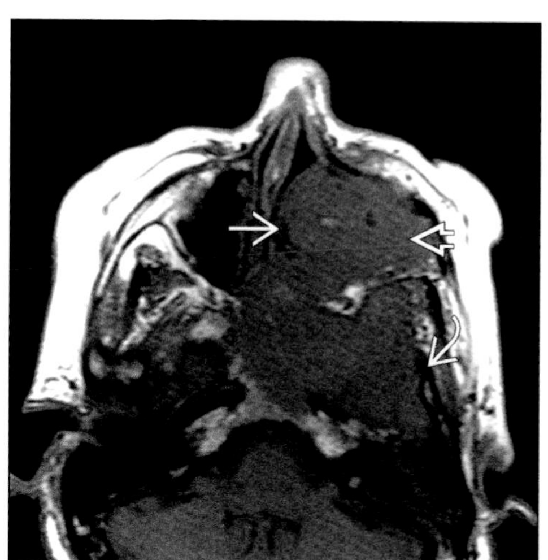

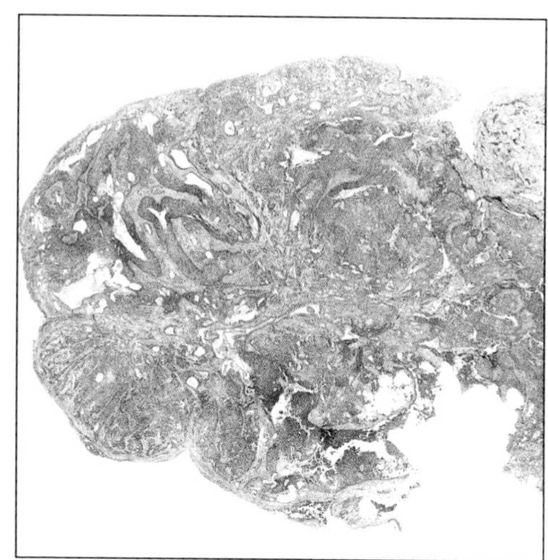

(Left) *Axial T1WI MR demonstrates a heterogeneous soft tissue mass, which extensively involves the sinonasal cavities and central skull base. The mass fills the maxillary sinus ➡, ipsilateral nasal cavity ➡, and nasopharynx ➡.* ***(Right)*** *A polypoid mass shows a number of different components within the tumor, all intermingled: Carcinoma, sarcoma, and neural blastema-type tissue.*

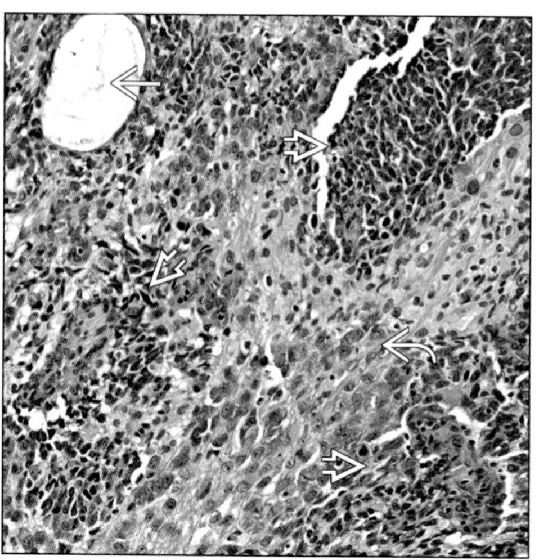

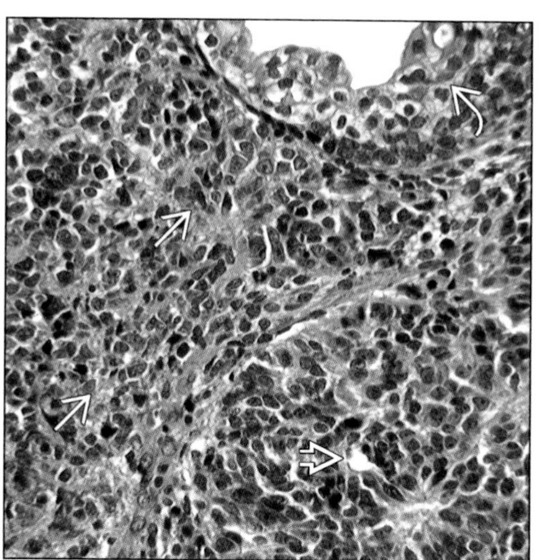

(Left) *A glandular space ➡ is immediately surrounded by areas of sarcoma ➡, showing slightly rhabdoid features. The neural elements show blastomatous cells ➡.* ***(Right)*** *On high power, the immature squamous ➡ element is juxtaposed to immature mesenchymal tissue ➡, which is juxtaposed to immature neural tissue, the latter showing a rosette ➡. Note the blending between these elements as they form the tumor.*

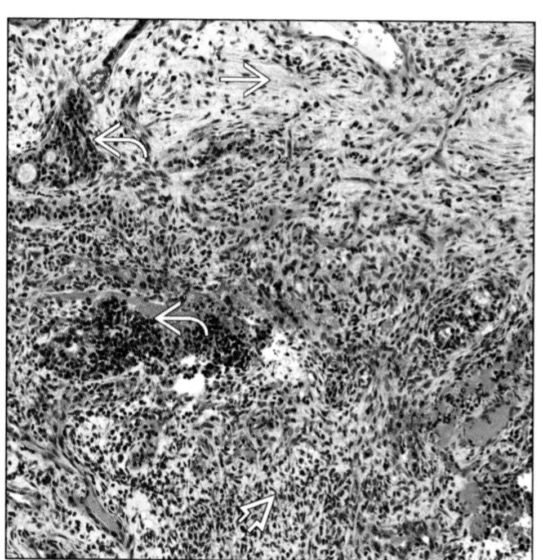

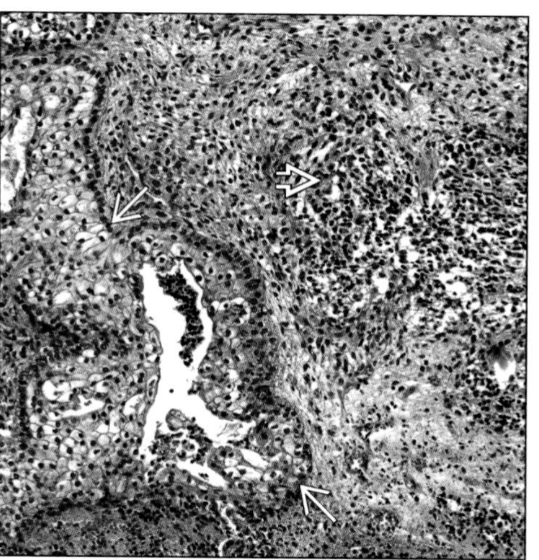

(Left) *In this field, the immature mesenchymal tissue has a myxoid appearance ➡ that blends into more fibrous areas ➡. Teratoid areas are identified by the immature neural elements with rosettes ➡.* ***(Right)*** *Squamous cell carcinoma ➡ with well-developed cell borders is surrounded by a cellular immature mesenchyma. The mesenchyma blends into an immature neural matrix ➡. There is no sharp line of demarcation between each of these elements.*

FIBROSARCOMA

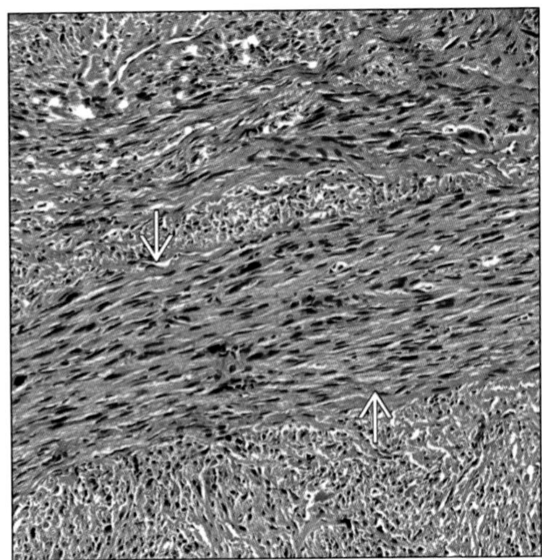

Unencapsulated tumor demonstrates a moderate to high cellularity, with fascicles showing acute angles. One of the fascicles is perpendicular to the others ➡. There is focal pleomorphism.

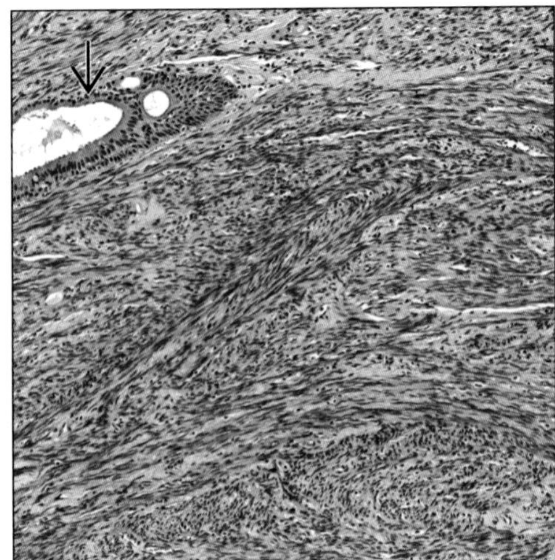

The surface epithelium ➡ is frequently entrapped or invaginated into the neoplastic proliferation. The spindled cell proliferation is present throughout the rest of the resection.

TERMINOLOGY

Synonyms

- Fibromyxosarcoma

Definitions

- Malignant neoplasm with only fibroblastic &/or myofibroblastic differentiation
  - Tumors must lack additional histologic or immunophenotypic differentiation features

ETIOLOGY/PATHOGENESIS

Etiology

- Isolated patients with documented radiation exposure

CLINICAL ISSUES

Epidemiology

- Incidence
  - Uncommon sinonasal tract tumor
    - 2nd most common sinonasal tract nonepithelial malignancy (lymphoma is 1st)
    - ~ 3% of sinonasal **malignancies**
- Age
  - Peak: 5th to 6th decades
- Gender
  - Female > Male (3:2)

Site

- One or more paranasal sinuses (maxillary, ethmoid)
  - Nasal cavity alone is much less common

Presentation

- Nasal obstruction and epistaxis most common
- Pain, sinusitis, nasal discharge, swelling less common
- Symptoms usually of short duration
- Anosmia and proptosis very rare

Treatment

- Surgical approaches
  - En bloc resection yields best long-term outcome
- Radiation
  - Adjuvant radiation after surgical extirpation

Prognosis

- Generally good, with 75% 5-year survival
  - Better prognosis for low-grade tumors (majority of patients have low-grade tumors)
- May result in death due to local infiltration or by distant metastasis
  - Recurrences are high (up to 60%) especially in incompletely excised tumors
  - Recurrences precede distant metastases
  - Distant metastases in ~ 15%: Lung and bones most common (rarely lymph nodes)
- Poor prognosis associated with
  - Males, large tumors, tumor stage, high-grade tumors (including high mitotic index, high cellularity), incompletely excised tumors (positive margins)

IMAGE FINDINGS

Radiographic Findings

- Aggressive, poorly marginated soft tissue mass with bone destruction and fascial plane destruction
- Best study: Thin section bone CT combined with MR T1WI with contrast

MACROSCOPIC FEATURES

General Features

- Smooth, nodular, fungating, ulcerated, fleshy mass
- Firm, homogeneous, circumscribed cut surface
- Necrosis and hemorrhage in higher grade tumors

Size

- Range: 2-8 cm

FIBROSARCOMA

Key Facts

Terminology
- Malignant neoplasm with only fibroblastic &/or myofibroblastic differentiation

Clinical Issues
- Uncommon sinonasal tract tumor
- Peak age: 5th-6th decades
- Female > Male (3:2)
- One or more paranasal sinuses (maxillary, ethmoid)
- Present with nasal obstruction and epistaxis
- Recurrences high especially in incompletely excised tumors
- En bloc resection yields best long-term outcome
- Prognosis generally good with 75% 5-year survival

Microscopic Pathology
- Unencapsulated, often with bone invasion
- Surface epithelial invagination common (~ 1/3)
- Spindled tumor cells arranged in short, compact fascicles at acute angles
- "Herringbone" or "chevron" pattern
- Fusiform cells with centrally placed, hyperchromatic, needle-like nuclei with tapering cytoplasm

Ancillary Tests
- Positive: Strong, diffuse vimentin

Top Differential Diagnoses
- Fibromatosis (desmoid type), synovial sarcoma, solitary fibrous tumor, spindle cell squamous cell carcinoma, spindle cell melanoma, peripheral nerve sheath tumor

MICROSCOPIC PATHOLOGY

Histologic Features
- Unencapsulated, circumscribed, often with bone invasion
  - Calcification (**not** osteosarcoma) is seen at periphery
- Surface epithelial invagination common (~ 1/3)
  - Surface ulceration occasionally present
  - Epithelial entrapment must not be mistaken for part of tumor (inverted papilloma, synovial sarcoma)
- Cellularity is variable but usually high
- Spindled tumor cells arranged in short, compact fascicles at acute angles
  - "Herringbone" or "chevron" pattern
  - Storiform pattern is usually absent
  - Vague fasciculated pattern can be seen
- Fusiform cells with centrally placed, hyperchromatic, needle-like nuclei with tapering cytoplasm
  - Mild pleomorphism, small nucleoli, clumped heterochromatin
  - Syncytial appearance is common
- Mitotic figures: Low in low-grade tumors
  - Increased to high in high-grade tumors
- Bizarre, pleomorphic cells are usually absent
- Stroma shows vascularity with delicate collagen fibrils to dense, keloid-like deposition
  - Myxoid and edematous change can be seen
- **Low grade**
  - Vast majority of tumor; moderate cellularity, limited pleomorphism, few mitoses, no necrosis
- **High grade**
  - Nuclear pleomorphism, high mitotic activity, scant collagenous stroma, necrosis, and hemorrhage

ANCILLARY TESTS

Immunohistochemistry
- **Positive**: Strong, diffuse cytoplasmic vimentin
  - Rarely, weak, focal actin

DIFFERENTIAL DIAGNOSIS

Fibromatosis (Desmoid Type)
- Mature fibroblasts without atypia in rich collagenous matrix

Solitary Fibrous Tumor
- Plump fibroblasts in mature collagenous stroma, sometimes with vessels, lacking mitoses
- Strong, diffuse CD34, Bcl-2, and vimentin reactions

Spindle Cell Squamous Cell Carcinoma
- Epithelial malignancy with spindled &/or epithelioid morphology with epithelial immunohistochemistry (although absent in up to 30%)

Melanoma (Spindle Cell Type)
- S100 protein, HMB-45, Melan-A, tyrosinase positive

Malignant Peripheral Nerve Sheath Tumor (MPNST)
- Low- and high-grade tumors show variable S100 protein staining
- Malignant "triton" tumor is an MPNST with S100 protein staining and rhabdomyoblastic differentiation

Undifferentiated Pleomorphic Sarcoma
- Pleomorphism, high-grade nuclear appearance, high mitotic index, necrosis

SELECTED REFERENCES

1. Heffner DK et al: Sinonasal fibrosarcomas, malignant schwannomas, and "Triton" tumors. A clinicopathologic study of 67 cases. Cancer. 70(5):1089-101, 1992
2. Fu YS et al: Nonepithelial tumors of the nasal cavity, paranasal sinuses, and nasopharynx. A clinicopathologic study. VI. Fibrous tissue tumors (fibroma, fibromatosis, fibrosarcoma). Cancer. 37(6):2912-28, 1976

FIBROSARCOMA

Imaging and Microscopic Features

(Left) Contrast-enhanced CT shows a large hypodense mass ➡ filling the left masticator space with extensive bone remodeling and erosion ➡. This soft tissue mass is not specific for a sarcoma, although clearly worrisome for malignancy. *(Right)* There are numerous areas of surface epithelial invagination. The entrapment of the epithelium may morphologically mimic an inverted papilloma, respiratory epithelial adenomatoid hamartoma, or synovial sarcoma. However, the epithelium lacks atypia.

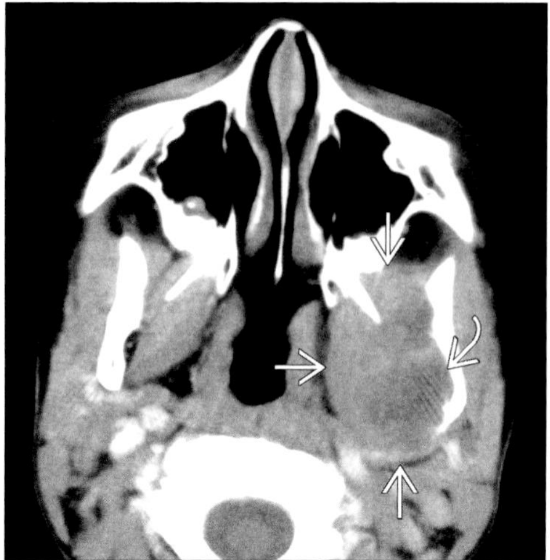

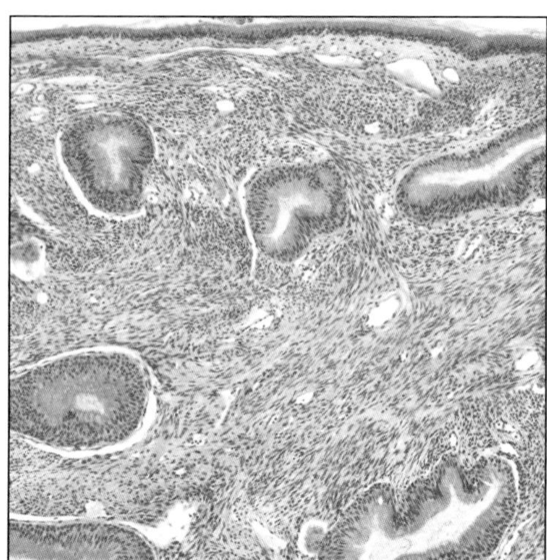

(Left) The surface epithelium ➡ is separated from the neoplastic proliferation by a Grenz zone of fibrosis. The tumor shows areas of collagenized stroma, but the pattern of growth is difficult to detect from this high-power field. *(Right)* This low-power view of a fibrosarcoma shows acute angle intersection of fascicles of spindled cells. Fibrosarcomas are usually quite cellular tumors, although there is usually a lack of significant pleomorphism.

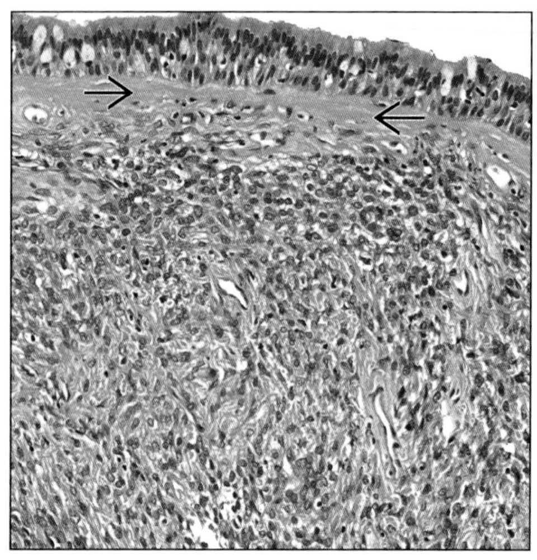

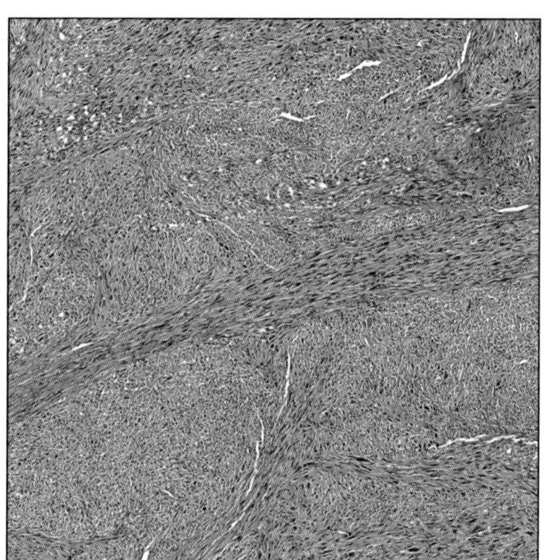

(Left) Occasional areas of degeneration ➡, with histiocytes, may be seen in a fibrosarcoma. The tumor is quite cellular with coarse nuclear chromatin distribution in the cells that have a syncytial architecture. *(Right)* There are short, abrupt, right angle intersections to these fascicles of a fibrosarcoma. Note the elongated and tapered cells with hyperchromatic fusiform nuclei. This degree of cellularity is characteristic for a fibrosarcoma.

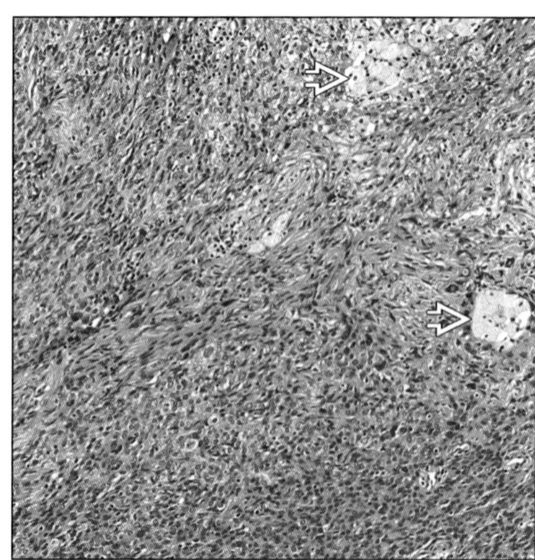

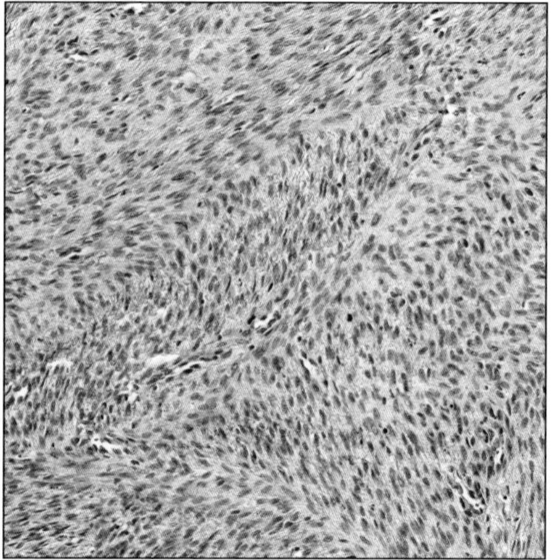

Microscopic Features

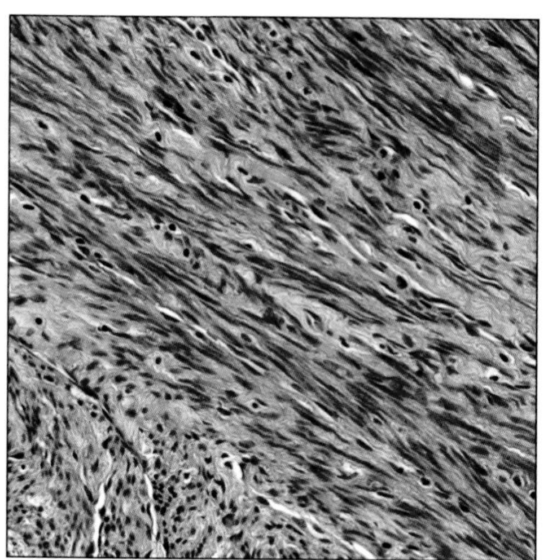

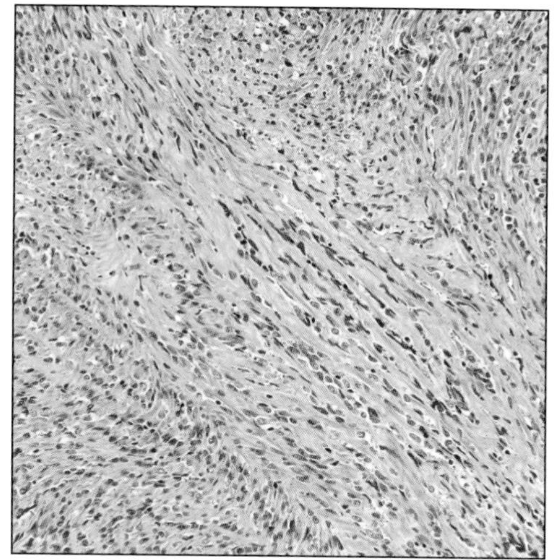

(Left) *Fusiform cells are arranged in a compact fascicle. The syncytial cells show centrally placed, hyperchromatic, needle-like nuclei with tapering cytoplasm. There is limited to absent pleomorphism.* ***(Right)*** *The elongated spindled cells are set in a variable stroma. In this case, there are delicate collagen fibrils aggregated to form dense, almost keloid-like bundles of brightly eosinophilic collagen. Collagen formation is seen in nearly all tumors.*

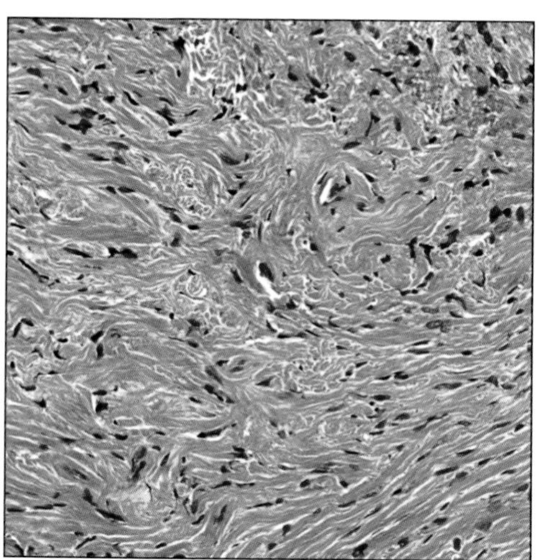

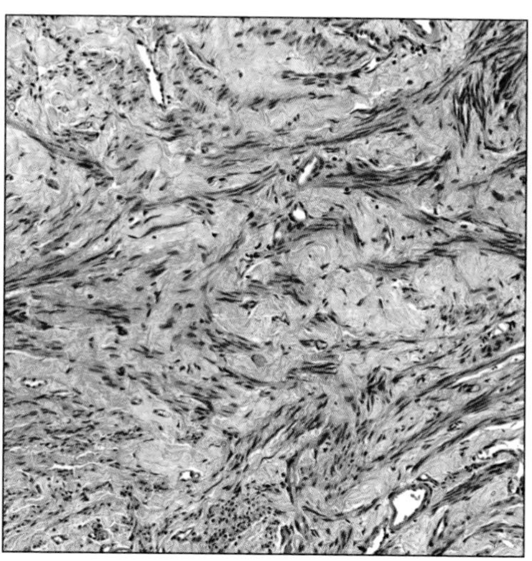

(Left) *A minority of fibrosarcoma cases will show an exceedingly heavy, keloid-like collagen deposition with only a limited cellularity. In this field, there are single, isolated, atypical spindled cells. Note that in this field there is a vague storiform appearance, a finding not present in the remaining tumor.* ***(Right)*** *The tumors are usually variably cellular, and this is an example from a hypocellular and low-grade tumor. The cellularity is still beyond that of a reactive lesion.*

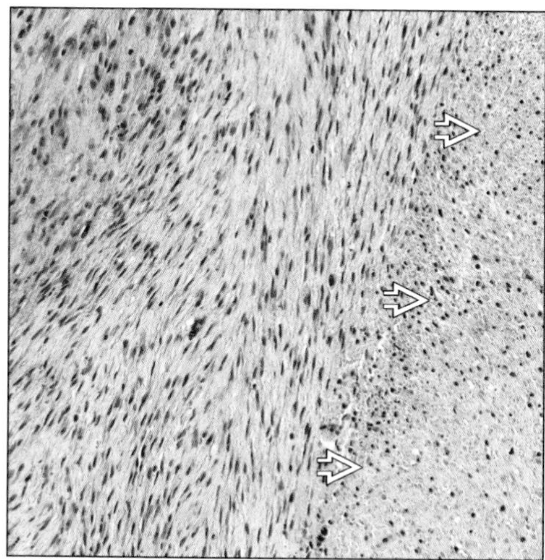

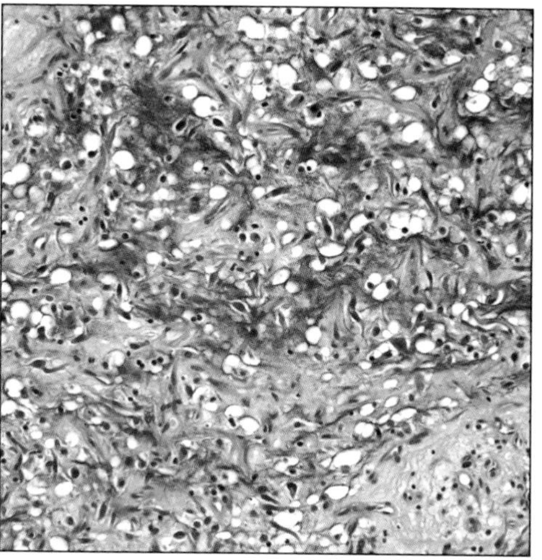

(Left) *The presence of genuine, comedo-type or coagulative necrosis ➡ is an uncommon finding. When this is present, it dictates placing the tumor in the high-grade category.* ***(Right)*** *A fibromyxosarcoma has a myxoid stroma in the background of the neoplastic proliferation. In this tumor type, it is not uncommon for the short, compact fascicle pattern to be lost. There can be slight atypia; however, there is usually not profound nuclear pleomorphism.*

LEIOMYOSARCOMA

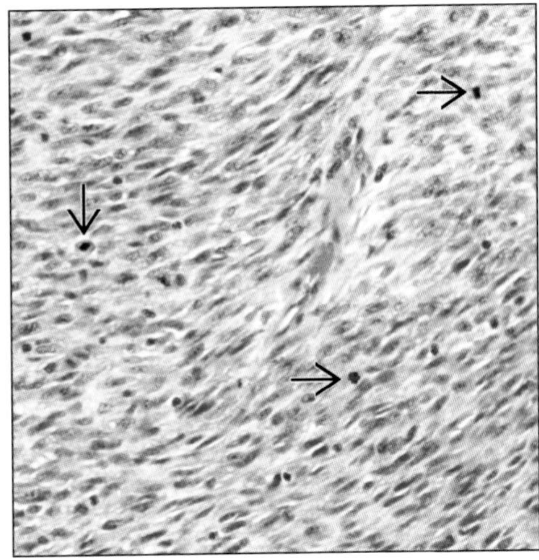

Sinonasal spindle-shaped cellular proliferation is shown with nuclear pleomorphism and increased mitotic activity →. The overall mitotic count was ≥ 4 mitoses per 10 high-power fields.

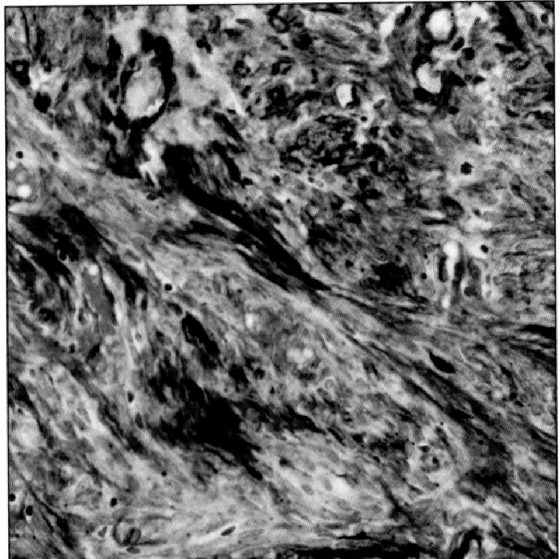

The presence of smooth muscle actin staining supports the light microscopic features in leiomyosarcoma (LMS). As head and neck LMS is rare, differentiation is required from other spindle cell neoplasms.

TERMINOLOGY

Abbreviations

- Leiomyosarcoma (LMS)

Definitions

- Malignant tumor of smooth muscle

ETIOLOGY/PATHOGENESIS

Environmental Exposure

- May develop following irradiation or cyclophosphamide exposure

Infectious Agents

- Link between LMS and Epstein-Barr virus (EBV) identified
- Occurs in immunocompromised patients

Histogenesis

- Appears to arise from vascular structures
  - Due to relative lack of smooth muscle in head and neck region
  - Other than relationship to vascular walls, histology similar to non-vascular-derived LMS

CLINICAL ISSUES

Epidemiology

- Incidence
  - Approximately 4% arise in head and neck
  - Increased incidence in immunocompromised patients
    - Post-transplantation (e.g., kidney, heart, liver)
    - AIDS
    - Epstein-Barr virus (EBV) found in these tumors, termed EBV smooth muscle tumors (EBVSMT)
    - Clonal EBV DNA and EBV surface receptor protein
    - Different episomal DNA clones found in separate tumors in same patient; suggests multifocal tumor rather than metastatic disease
- Age
  - **Non-immunocompromise-associated LMS**
    - Occurs in wide age range
    - Most common in 6th decade
  - **Immunocompromise-associated LMS**
    - Tends to occur in children or young adults
- Gender
  - Equal gender distribution

Site

- **Non-immunocompromise-associated LMS**
  - Most common sites
    - Oral cavity (buccal mucosa, gingiva, tongue, floor of mouth)
    - Sinonasal tract
    - Skin and subcutaneous tissue
  - Less common sites
    - Larynx
    - Trachea
    - Neck
    - Hypopharynx
    - Orbit
    - External auditory canal
- **Immunocompromise-associated LMS**
  - Tend to occur in relationship to viscera (e.g., GI tract, lung)
  - May be multifocal

Presentation

- Nasal obstruction
- Pain
- Epistaxis
- Painless mass
- Ulceration

Treatment

- Surgical approaches
  - Radical surgical excision

LEIOMYOSARCOMA

Key Facts

Terminology
- LMS: Malignant tumor of smooth muscle

Etiology/Pathogenesis
- May develop following irradiation or cyclophosphamide exposure
- Appears to arise from vascular structures
- Link between LMS and Epstein-Barr virus (EBV) identified
  - Occurs in immunocompromised patients

Clinical Issues
- Approximately 4% arise in head and neck
- Increased incidence in immunocompromised patients

Microscopic Pathology
- Interlacing fascicular to storiform bundles of spindle-shaped cells
  - Typically intersect at right angles
- Neoplastic cells are elongated (spindle) with centrally located, blunt-ended, cigar-shaped nuclei and eosinophilic cytoplasm
- Perinuclear vacuole or clear halo may be seen, giving nucleus an indented or concave contour
- Variable degree of cellular anaplasia with nuclear pleomorphism, nuclear hyperchromasia, and increased mitotic activity (typical and atypical forms)
- Actins (smooth muscle and muscle specific) positive
- Criteria for malignancy
  - Tumors with 1-4 mitoses per 10 HPF considered potentially malignant especially in conjunction with nuclear atypia and necrosis
  - > 4 mitoses per 10 HPF is malignant

    - Treatment of choice
- Radiation and chemotherapy are of questionable utility

Prognosis
- Dependent on site and extent of tumor
- Not necessarily contingent on histology
  - Nasal cavity
    - Good prognosis
    - Cured following complete removal
  - Both nasal cavity and paranasal sinuses
    - Aggressive neoplasm associated with increased recurrence (70% of patients)
    - Increased mortality rates (45% of patients with death occurring within 2 years of diagnosis)
- Local recurrence frequent
  - Usually associated with extensive, uncontrollable local infiltration
- Metastases (hematogenous) infrequent early but can occur late in disease course
- Cutaneous leiomyosarcoma
  - Dermal based
    - Tend to be small (< 2 cm)
    - Tend to be histologically low grade
    - May recur but do not metastasize, even histologically higher grade tumors
    - Favorable prognosis
  - Subcutaneous tumors
    - Up to 40% may metastasize
    - Metastasis most often to lungs; nodal metastasis uncommon
    - Prognosis comparable to that of soft tissue leiomyosarcomas
  - Wide surgical resection indicated
- EBVSMT may disseminate and be lethal

IMAGE FINDINGS

General Features
- Soft tissue density
- Sinus opacification
- Bone erosion &/or invasion

MACROSCOPIC FEATURES

General Features
- Circumscribed but not encapsulated
- Tan-white to pink-red
- Rubbery to firm
- Polypoid or sessile lesion
- Ulceration, hemorrhage, necrosis, and invasion of adjacent structures often identifiable

Size
- Usually > 5 cm in diameter

MICROSCOPIC PATHOLOGY

Histologic Features
- Interlacing fascicular to storiform bundles of spindle-shaped cells
  - Typically intersect at right angles
- Neoplastic cells are elongated (spindle) with centrally located, blunt-ended, cigar-shaped nuclei and eosinophilic cytoplasm
  - Perinuclear vacuole or clear halo may be seen, giving nucleus an indented or concave contour
- Variable degree of cellular anaplasia with nuclear pleomorphism, nuclear hyperchromasia, and increased mitotic activity (typical and atypical forms)
  - Marked nuclear pleomorphism may be present
- Nuclear palisading may be prominent
  - May suggest diagnosis of peripheral nerve sheath tumor
- Other cell types
  - Multinucleated giant cells commonly seen
  - Epithelioid cells may predominate, conferring designation "epithelioid LMS"
- Stroma tends to be richly vascular with close apposition of tumor to vascular structures
  - Myxomatous stromal changes may be prominent, conferring designation "myxoid LMS"
- Infiltrative
  - Usually indicative of malignancy

LEIOMYOSARCOMA

  - Limited infiltrative growth can be seen in smooth muscle tumors of uncertain malignant potential

Epithelioid LMS

- Predominantly composed of epithelioid cells with round to oval nuclei
- Clear or vacuolated-appearing cytoplasm may be prominent
- Transitional areas from epithelioid to spindle-shaped areas

Myxoid LMS

- Extensive myxoid change may create gelatinous appearance
- Prominent myxoid stroma rich in hyaluronic acid is present between spindled neoplastic cells
- Overall appearance relatively hypocellular
  - In presence of low mitotic rate, overall histology may not be suggestive of malignant neoplasm
- Even mitotic rates ≤ 2 mitotic figures should prompt consideration for malignancy

Inflammatory Leiomyosarcoma

- Characterized by presence of prominent inflammatory cell infiltrate
  - Including xanthoma cells, lymphocytes, and occasionally neutrophils
  - Not associated with systemic (constitutional) symptoms

Granular Cell LMS

- Rare LMS variant characterized by cells with granular eosinophilic cytoplasm

Criteria for Malignancy

- Tumors with 1-4 mitoses per 10 HPF considered potentially malignant
  - Especially in conjunction with nuclear atypia and necrosis
- > 4 mitoses per 10 HPF is malignant
- If tumors have no/very few mitoses and absence of nuclear atypia, then tumor is likely benign
  - Even in presence of increased cellularity
  - Even in presence of focal infiltrative growth
  - Especially if significant hyalinization or calcification

ANCILLARY TESTS

Histochemistry

- Masson trichrome
  - Deep red, longitudinal lines
- PTAH
  - Purple
- Glycogen demonstrable as diastase-sensitive, PAS-positive material

Immunohistochemistry

- Actins (smooth muscle and muscle specific) positive
- Variable desmin reactivity present but usually positive
- No immunoreactivity for
  - Epithelial markers (e.g., cytokeratins)
    - Cytokeratin expression may occur, usually perinuclear localization, usually seen in association with desmin reactivity
  - Melanocytic markers, markers of skeletal muscle, vascular endothelial markers
- S100 protein may be positive

Electron Microscopy

- Entire cell membrane enveloped by
  - Deeply indented nuclei
  - Numerous well-oriented filaments (6-8 nm)
  - Pinocytotic vesicles
  - Intercellular connections
  - Basal lamina

DIFFERENTIAL DIAGNOSIS

Leiomyoma

- Even if cellular, lacks significant pleomorphism and mitotic activity

Smooth Muscle Tumor of Uncertain Malignant Potential

- Shows moderate nuclear pleomorphism but not more than 4 mitoses per 10 HPF

Spindle Cell Squamous Carcinoma

- Presence of squamous cell carcinoma (i.e., dysplasia, invasive differentiated carcinoma)
- Immunoreactivity for epithelial markers (cytokeratins, p63) seen in majority of cases

Malignant Peripheral Nerve Sheath Tumor (MPNST)

- Overlapping features but typically only S100 protein immunoreactive, lacking actin staining

Fibrosarcoma/Undifferentiated Pleomorphic Sarcoma

- Diagnosis of exclusion lacking immunoreactivity associated with LMS

Rhabdomyosarcoma

- Consistent immunoreactivity for markers of skeletal muscle differentiation including
  - Desmin, muscle specific actin, myoglobin, MYOD1, myogenin

SELECTED REFERENCES

1. Ulrich CT et al: Sinonasal leiomyosarcoma: review of literature and case report. Laryngoscope. 115(12):2242-8, 2005
2. Hsu JL et al: Epstein-barr virus-associated malignancies: epidemiologic patterns and etiologic implications. Crit Rev Oncol Hematol. 34(1):27-53, 2000
3. McClain KL et al: Association of Epstein-Barr virus with leiomyosarcomas in children with AIDS. N Engl J Med. 332(1):12-8, 1995
4. Kuruvilla A et al: Leiomyosarcoma of the sinonasal tract. A clinicopathologic study of nine cases. Arch Otolaryngol Head Neck Surg. 116(11):1278-86, 1990

Variant Microscopic and Immunohistochemical Features

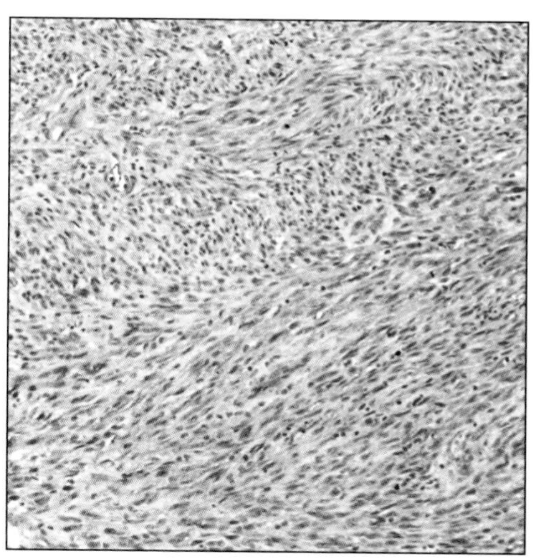

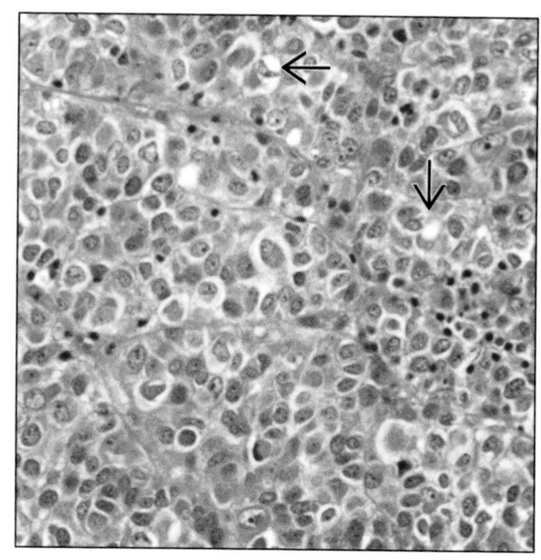

(Left) *Sinonasal submucosal cellular infiltrate shows fascicular growth composed of interlacing bundles of neoplastic cells intersecting at right angles. This overall appearance suggests a possible diagnosis of a smooth muscle neoplasm.* ***(Right)*** *Epithelioid LMS is composed of epithelioid cells with round to oval nuclei and eosinophilic to vacuolated ➔ appearing cytoplasm. There were foci transitioning from spindled to epithelial cells, as well as smooth muscle actin staining (not shown).*

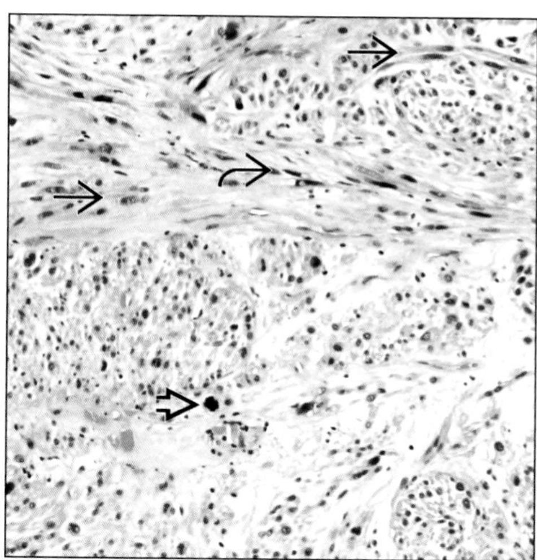

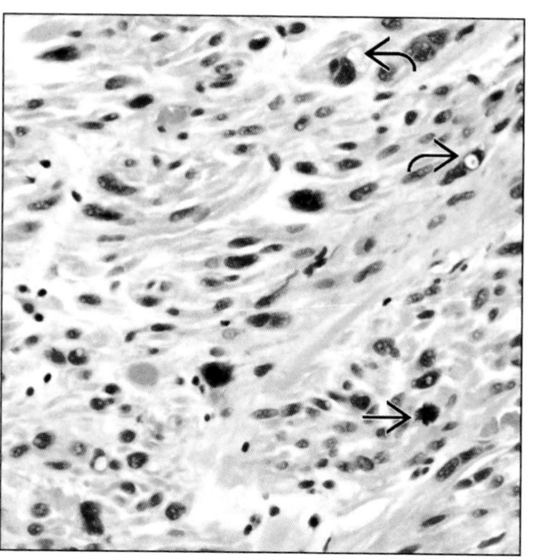

(Left) *Myxoid LMS shows fascicular growth and the presence of prominent myxoid stroma. The neoplastic cells are elongated with blunt-ended nuclei ➔, eosinophilic cytoplasm, and occasional perinuclear vacuoles ➚. Note mitotic figure ➔.* ***(Right)*** *Myxoid LMS shows pleomorphic and hyperchromatic nuclei, eosinophilic cytoplasm, cytoplasmic vacuoles ➚, & increased mitotic activity ➔. Neoplastic cells were immunoreactive for smooth muscle actin (not shown).*

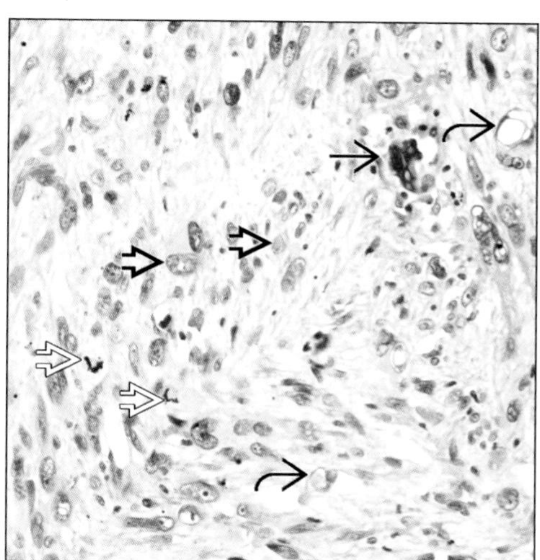

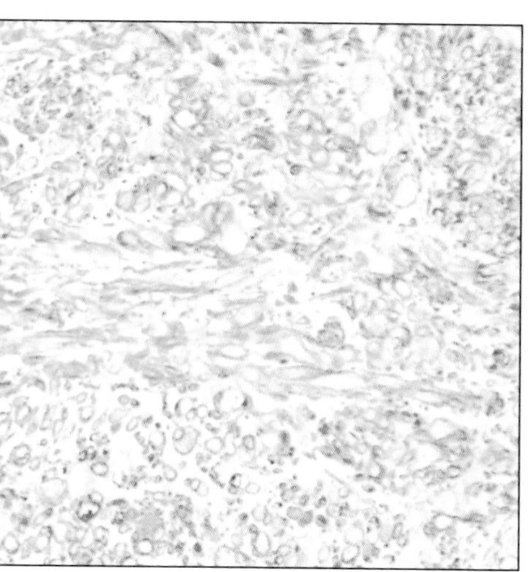

(Left) *LMS shows markedly pleomorphic nuclei including a multinucleated cell ➔, eosinophilic intranuclear inclusions ➔, vacuolated cells ➚, and increased mitotic activity ➔. The histologic features suggest a tumor of possible smooth muscle origin but require immunohistochemical staining for the diagnosis.* ***(Right)*** *Smooth muscle actin immunoreactivity with absence of reactivity for other markers (e.g., epithelial, melanocytic, other sarcomas) is confirmatory of LMS.*

MALIGNANT PERIPHERAL NERVE SHEATH TUMOR

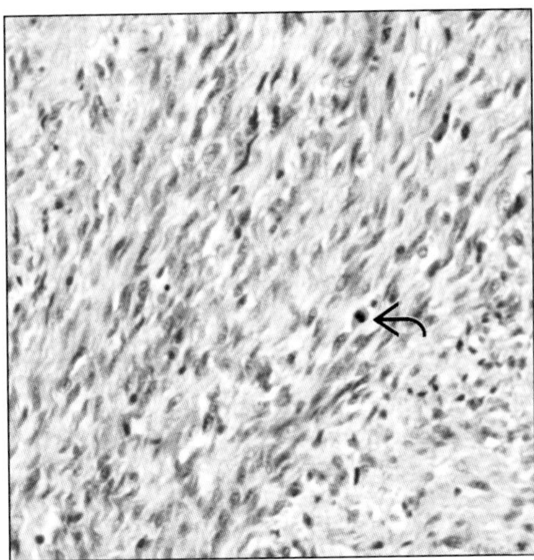

Low-grade MPNST shows fascicular growth with "wavy" appearing nuclei. As compared to benign schwannomas, there is increased cellularity with nuclear pleomorphism and increased mitotic activity ➚.

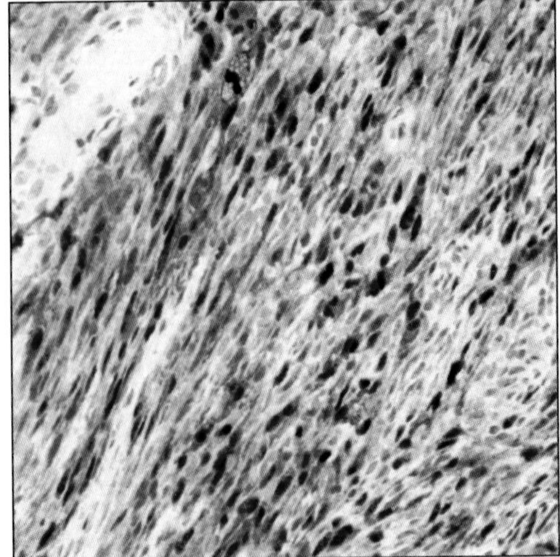

In low-grade MPNSTs, S100 protein staining tends to be diffuse and strong, similar to that in benign schwannomas. Differentiation is based on cellularity, atypia, mitotic activity, and infiltrative growth.

TERMINOLOGY

Abbreviations

- Malignant peripheral nerve sheath tumor (MPNST)

Synonyms

- Malignant schwannoma
- Neurogenic sarcoma
- Neurofibrosarcoma

Definitions

- Malignant tumor of peripheral nerves or having differentiation along the lines of various elements of nerve sheath
  - Occurs de novo (sporadic) or in association with neurofibromatosis type 1 (NF1)

ETIOLOGY/PATHOGENESIS

Neurofibromatosis

- Occurs in setting of NF1

Idiopathic

- De novo (sporadic) MPNST

Post Irradiation

- Infrequently may occur in areas previously irradiated

CLINICAL ISSUES

Epidemiology

- Incidence
  - Accounts for approximately 5-10% of all soft tissue sarcomas
    - Most commonly occurs in lower extremity
  - Up to 20% may occur in head and neck
  - Approximately 25-50% of all MPNST occur in association with NF1
  - Estimated risk of patients with NF1 developing MPNST varies (4-50%)
    - Occurrence typically follows latent period of 10-20 years
- Age
  - **De novo MPNST**
    - Occurs over wide age range, but most frequently in 5th decade
  - **MPNST associated with NF1**
    - Primarily seen in 3rd-4th decades of life
- Gender
  - **De novo MPNST**
    - No gender predilection or slightly more common in females
  - **MPNST associated with NF1**
    - No gender predilection or slightly more common in females

Site

- Most common site of involvement is neck
  - Less frequently, other sites of involvement include sinonasal tract, nasopharynx, oral cavity

Presentation

- Neck symptoms include
  - Mass with associated pain, paresthesia, weakness
- Sinonasal tract, nasopharynx, oral cavity symptoms include
  - Mass lesion, pain, epistaxis, and nasal obstruction

Treatment

- Surgical approaches
  - Complete surgical excision is treatment of choice
    - Most MPNSTs are high-grade malignancies necessitating wide en bloc resection and postoperative radiotherapy
- Adjuvant therapy
  - Chemotherapy utilized for inoperable tumors and disseminated tumors

MALIGNANT PERIPHERAL NERVE SHEATH TUMOR

Key Facts

Terminology

- Malignant tumor of peripheral nerves or having differentiation along the lines of various elements of nerve sheath
- Occurs de novo (sporadic) or in association with NF1

Clinical Issues

- Accounts for approximately 5-10% of all soft tissue sarcomas
- Up to 20% may occur in head and neck
- Approximately 25-50% of all MPNST occur in association with NF1
- Most common site of involvement is neck
  - Less frequently, other sites of involvement include sinonasal tract, nasopharynx, oral cavity

Microscopic Pathology

- Cells have elongated nuclei with irregular contour, tapered ends
- Nuclei appear wavy or buckled in profile and asymmetrically oval en face
- Nuclear palisading may be seen
- In sinonasal cavity, MPNST can occur in setting of inflammatory polyp
- Divided into low- and high-grade tumors depending on degree of cellularity, pleomorphism, mitotic activity, and necrosis

Ancillary Tests

- S100 protein reactivity seen in 50-90% of tumors with extent and intensity of reactivity dependent on histologic grade of tumor

Prognosis

- Survival rates differ for de novo vs. NF1-associated MPNST
  - De novo 5-year survival rate: ~ 50%
  - NF1-associated 5-year survival rate: 15-30%
- Additional adverse prognostic findings include
  - Larger tumor size (greater than 5 cm)
  - Positive surgical margins
  - Radiation-induced sarcoma
- Local recurrence common; reported in up to 50% of patients

MACROSCOPIC FEATURES

General Features

- Fusiform-shaped mass with fleshy, tan-white appearance
- Attachment to nerve may be identified

Size

- Usually measures more than 5 cm in diameter

MICROSCOPIC PATHOLOGY

Histologic Features

- Unencapsulated hypercellular proliferation composed of spindle-shaped cells
  - Cells arranged in fascicular growth with long sweeping (herringbone-like) fascicles that swirl or interdigitate with one another
    - Less common growth patterns may include nodules or whorled arrangement of neoplastic cells
    - Hypocellular areas with myxoid stroma can be seen alternating with areas of greater cellularity
  - Cells have elongated nuclei with irregular contour, tapered ends
    - Nuclei appear wavy or buckled in profile and asymmetrically oval en face
    - Indistinct cytoplasm
  - Nuclear palisading may be seen
    - Typically is present in minority of cases (less than 10%)
    - When present, tends to be focally identified within a given tumor
  - Other findings include
    - Hyaline bands and nodules resembling giant rosettes when seen in cross section
    - Perineural and intraneural spread of tumor
    - Proliferation of tumor in subendothelial zones of blood vessels creates appearance of tumor cells herniating into lumen
  - Heterologous elements can be identified in up to 15% of cases
    - Most common elements include mature cartilage and bone
    - Tend to be more commonly seen in association with MPNST than other sarcomas
  - In sinonasal cavity, MPNST can occur in setting of inflammatory polyp
    - Often low grade
    - Appears as nondescript spindle cell proliferation in and around benign glandular proliferation
    - S100 protein reactivity invaluable in confirming diagnosis

Histologic Variants

- **MPNST with rhabdomyosarcoma (malignant Triton tumor)**
  - Approximately 60% associated with NF1
  - Rhabdomyoblasts identified scattered throughout tumor; numbers vary from case to case
- **MPNST with glands (glandular malignant schwannoma)**
  - 75% associated with NF1
  - Contains gland formation
    - Most often benign appearing; rarely, glands histologically malignant
    - Composed of well-differentiated, nonciliated cuboidal or columnar cells with clear cytoplasm
    - Goblet cells may be present
    - Intra- and intercellular mucin may be present
    - Rarely, squamous differentiation may be present

MALIGNANT PERIPHERAL NERVE SHEATH TUMOR

- Immunoreactivity for cytokeratin, CEA, EMA, CK20, neuroendocrine markers (chromogranin, somatostatin, Leu-7, calcitonin)
- Ultrastructurally glands have features of intestinal epithelium with microvilli

- **Epithelioid MPNST**
  - Unusual variant not associated with NF1
  - May be located in superficial (superficial epithelioid MPNST) or deep soft tissues
  - Predominantly or exclusively composed of cells with polygonal epithelioid appearance
    - Large round nuclei with prominent eosinophilic nucleoli
    - May include tumors with clear cells or rhabdoid cells
    - Diffuse and intense S100 protein staining
    - Typically negative for epithelial markers and melanocytic markers
- **MPNST with angiosarcoma**
  - Rare
  - Most develop in association with NF1
  - Tends to occur in younger patients
  - Poor prognosis

Grading

- Divided into low- and high-grade tumors depending on degree of cellularity, pleomorphism, mitotic activity, and necrosis
- **Low-grade MPNST**
  - Cellular with mild to focally moderate nuclear pleomorphism, increased mitotic figures (as compared to schwannomas)
  - Mitoses may be few in number
  - Atypical mitoses not usually present
  - Necrosis not usually present
  - Infiltrative growth focally present
    - May represent sole parameter separating cellular (atypical) schwannoma from low-grade MPNST
- **High-grade MPNST**
  - Hypercellular with markedly pleomorphic cells, hyperchromatic nuclei, increased mitotic activity, atypical mitoses, necrosis
  - Infiltrative growth

ANCILLARY TESTS

Immunohistochemistry

- S100 protein reactivity seen in 50-90% of tumors with extent and intensity of reactivity dependent on grade of tumor
  - **Low-grade MPNST**
    - S100 protein positivity present but, in contrast to schwannoma and neurofibroma, is less diffusely/intensely positive
  - **High-grade MPNST**
    - S100 protein may be focally positive with even less immunoreactivity than low-grade tumors
    - May be S100 protein negative
- Other markers that may be positive include Leu-7 (CD57), glial fibrillary acidic protein, TLE1 (~ 10%)
- Epithelial, neuroendocrine, melanocytic, hematolymphoid markers typically negative

Molecular Genetics

- MPNST associated with NF1 have
  - Germline inactivation of *NF1*
  - Progression of neurofibroma to MPNST associated with chromosomal translocation including
    - 17q, 7p, 5p, 8q, 12q representing most common translocations
    - Accumulation of additional mutations of multiple genes, including *INK4A/ARF* and *P53* with resulting abnormalities of respective signal cascades

DIFFERENTIAL DIAGNOSIS

Synovial Sarcoma (SS)

- Shares overlapping histologic features with MPNST
  - SS immunoreactive for epithelial markers (EMA, CK7, CK19), S100 protein (30%), CD99, TLE1
  - Presence of SS18 (SYT) gene rearrangement

Fibrosarcoma

- More uniform fascicular growth pattern
- Cells resemble fibroblasts with symmetric fusiform appearance
- Absence of neural differentiation

Leiomyosarcoma (LMS)

- Overlapping features with MPNST; some distinguishing features include
  - Presence of blunt-ended, cigar-shaped nuclei, juxtanuclear vacuoles
  - Presence of myogenic markers (actins, desmin, caldesmon)

Malignant Melanoma

- Distinguished on basis of immunohistochemical findings
  - Melanomas reactive for melanocytic markers, including HMB-45, Melan-A, tyrosinase

SELECTED REFERENCES

1. Gottfried ON et al: Neurofibromatosis Type 1 and tumorigenesis: molecular mechanisms and therapeutic implications. Neurosurg Focus. 28(1):E8, 2010
2. Minovi A et al: Malignant peripheral nerve sheath tumors of the head and neck: management of 10 cases and literature review. Head Neck. 29(5):439-45, 2007
3. Heffner DK et al: Sinonasal fibrosarcomas, malignant schwannomas, and "Triton" tumors. A clinicopathologic study of 67 cases. Cancer. 70(5):1089-101, 1992
4. Laskin WB et al: Epithelioid variant of malignant peripheral nerve sheath tumor (malignant epithelioid schwannoma). Am J Surg Pathol. 15(12):1136-45, 1991
5. Ducatman BS et al: Malignant peripheral nerve sheath tumors. A clinicopathologic study of 120 cases. Cancer. 57(10):2006-21, 1986
6. Ducatman BS et al: Postirradiation neurofibrosarcoma. Cancer. 51(6):1028-33, 1983

Microscopic and Immunohistochemical Features

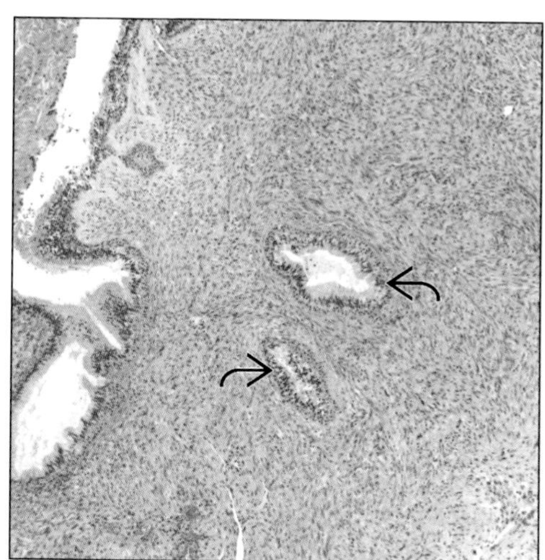

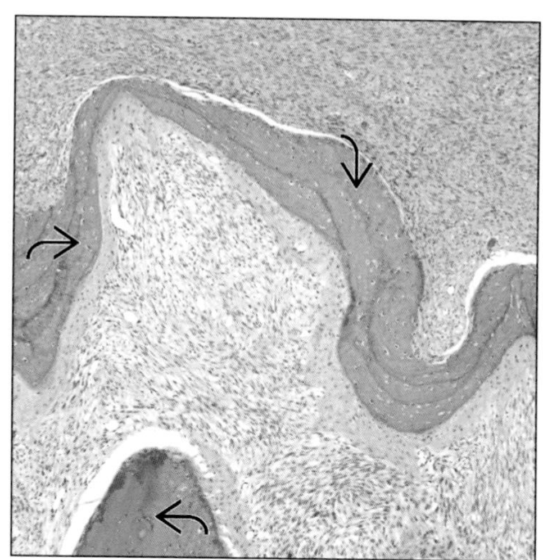

(Left) *Unlike their soft tissue counterparts, mucosal-based peripheral nerve sheath tumors of the head and neck are all unencapsulated. In the sinonasal tract, whether benign or malignant, these tumors tend to meander in and around normal structures, such as mucoserous glands ⮫.* ***(Right)*** *In contrast to benign peripheral nerve sheath tumors of the sinonasal tract, malignant peripheral nerve sheath tumors may also show invasive growth, including into and around bone ⮫.*

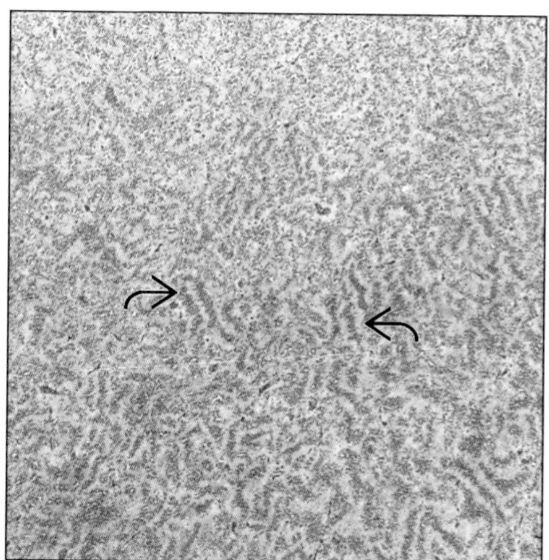

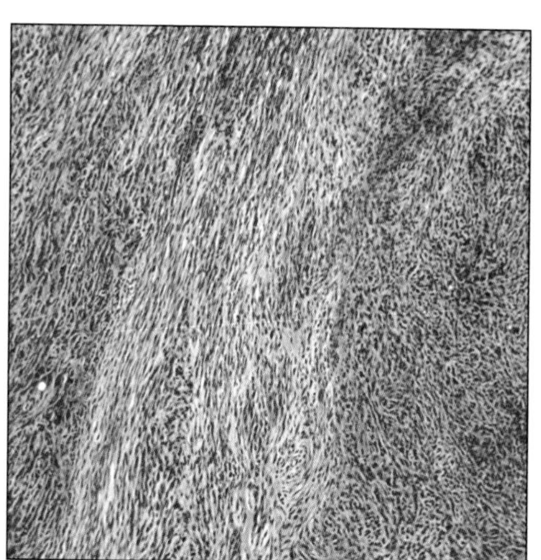

(Left) *Nuclear palisading with parallel arrangement of the neoplastic cells ⮫ is a feature that can be seen in both benign and malignant peripheral nerve sheath tumors (and in other tumor types). In addition to the nuclear palisading, low-grade MPNSTs show nuclear atypia, increased mitotic activity, and may have infiltrative growth.* ***(Right)*** *High-grade MPNST shows hypercellularity often with less conspicuous but still identifiable fascicular growth as compared to low-grade MPNSTs.*

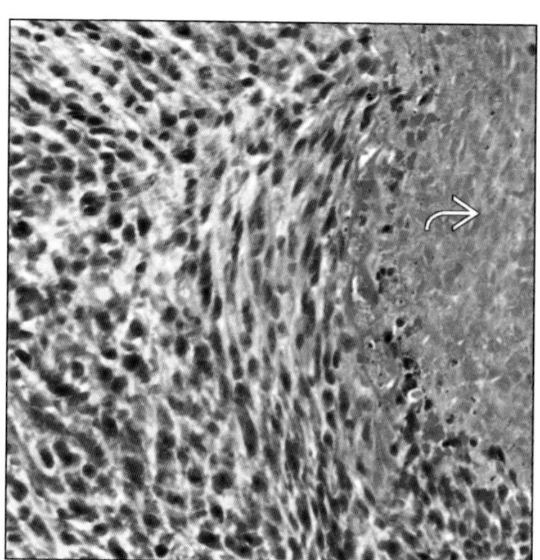

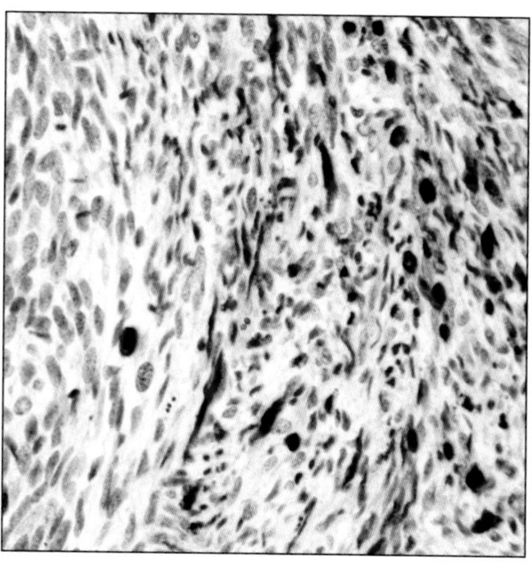

(Left) *High-grade MPNST shows increased cellularity, nuclear pleomorphism, necrosis ⮫, and increased mitotic activity (not shown). The overall features are not diagnostic for a neurogenic neoplasm & could represent any high-grade malignant neoplasm. Transitional areas from foci more diagnostic of a peripheral nerve sheath tumor (not shown), as well as focal S100 protein staining, supported the diagnosis.* ***(Right)*** *S100 protein staining supports the diagnosis of a high-grade MPNST.*

MALIGNANT FIBROUS HISTIOCYTOMA/UNDIFFERENTIATED PLEOMORPHIC SARCOMA

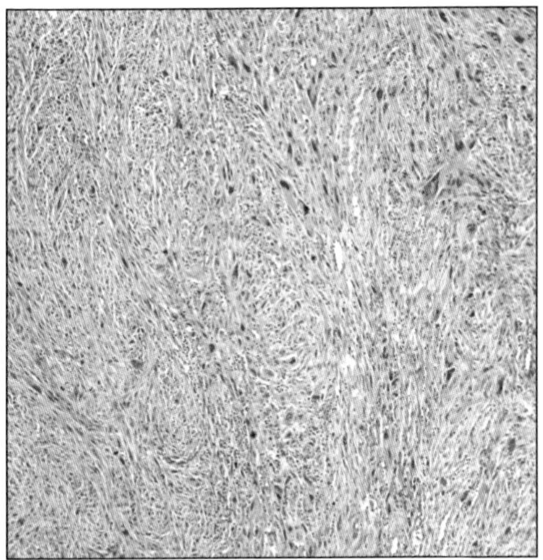

Sinonasal malignant fibrous histiocytoma (MFH), pleomorphic-storiform type, shows a densely cellular infiltrate with fascicular and storiform growth patterns. These growth characteristics are not unique to MFH.

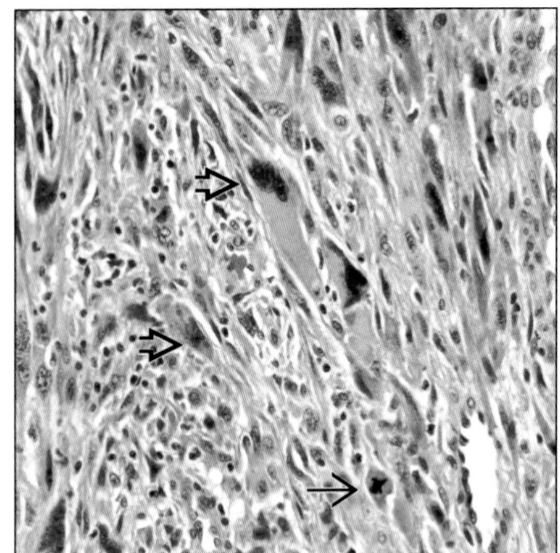

MFH shows spindle-shaped cells with marked nuclear pleomorphism and hyperchromasia ⇨. There is increased mitotic activity, including typical and atypical forms →.

TERMINOLOGY

Abbreviations

- Malignant fibrous histiocytoma (MFH)

Definitions

- High-grade pleomorphic malignant mesenchymal neoplasm
  - Diagnosis made by excluding another more specific sarcoma or nonsarcomatous neoplasm

ETIOLOGY/PATHOGENESIS

Idiopathic

- Majority occur de novo

Post Radiation

- Represents most common post-irradiation sarcoma
- To qualify as post-irradiation sarcoma
  - Must develop in radiation field
  - Latency period of at least 3 years between irradiation and development of malignancy
  - Histologic confirmation
  - Documentation that region of sarcoma was normal prior to irradiation

CLINICAL ISSUES

Epidemiology

- Incidence
  - Once considered one of the more common soft tissue sarcomas of late adult life
    - With more advanced diagnostic techniques (e.g., immunohistochemistry) classification into another class of sarcomas decreased incidence
  - Uncommon neoplasm in head and neck
    - Approximately 3% occur in head and neck
- Age
  - Occurs over wide range
    - Most commonly seen in adults
- Gender
  - Male > Female

Site

- Sinonasal tract most common site of occurrence
  - Maxillary sinus > ethmoid sinus and nasal cavity
  - Rare occurrence in frontal and sphenoid sinuses
- Neck 2nd most common site of occurrence
- Rare in other head and neck sites

Presentation

- Mass with or without associated pain, nasal obstruction, epistaxis, facial asymmetry, proptosis

Treatment

- Surgical approaches
  - Complete surgical excision is treatment of choice
  - Lymph node metastasis occurs in less than 15% of cases
    - Unless clinically suspect for nodal disease, neck dissection of limited value
- Adjuvant therapy
  - Chemotherapy used in presence of metastasis
- Radiation
  - Radiotherapy may be used for tumors with positive surgical margins or close surgical margins

Prognosis

- 5-year overall, disease-free, and disease-specific survival rates reported as 55%, 44%, and 69%, respectively
- Recurrence rate: ~ 27% reported
- Metastatic rate: ~ 35% reported
  - Occurs to lung > lymph nodes > liver and bone
- Prognosis dependent on
  - Depth of tumor
    - Deep soft tissue tumors more likely to metastasize compared to tumors of subcutis
  - Size of tumor

MALIGNANT FIBROUS HISTIOCYTOMA/UNDIFFERENTIATED PLEOMORPHIC SARCOMA

Key Facts

Terminology
- High grade, pleomorphic, malignant, mesenchymal
  - Diagnosis is one of excluding another more specific sarcoma or nonsarcomatous neoplasm

Etiology/Pathogenesis
- Majority occur de novo
- Represents most common post-irradiation sarcoma

Clinical Issues
- Approximately 3% occur in head and neck
- Sinonasal tract most common site of occurrence
  - Neck 2nd most common site of occurrence
- Recurrence rate: ~ 27% reported
- Metastatic rate: ~ 35% reported

Microscopic Pathology
- Histologic variants include
  - Storiform-pleomorphic
  - Myxoid
  - Giant cell
  - Inflammatory (xanthomatous)
- Storiform-pleomorphic type most common histologic variant in sinonasal tract
  - Fascicular and storiform growth patterns
  - Marked nuclear pleomorphism, increased mitotic activity, including typical and atypical forms
  - Multinucleated giant cells
- Heterologous elements, including bone and cartilage, may be present in any histologic subtype

Ancillary Tests
- No specific immunoreactivity

    - Smaller tumors (less than 2.5 cm) less likely to metastasize compared to larger tumors
  - Prior radiation exposure
    - Reported 5-year disease-free survival rates of post-irradiated MFH of 0%
  - Positive margins
    - Associated with worse survival
  - Inflammatory cell component
    - Tumors with increased numbers of inflammatory cells less likely to metastasize compared to tumors lacking significant inflammatory cell infiltrate
  - Myxoid component
    - Tumors with prominent myxoid component less likely to metastasize compared to tumors lacking significant myxoid component

MACROSCOPIC FEATURES

General Features
- Nodular or multinodular appearing tan-white to gray lesion
- Necrosis and hemorrhage may be apparent
- Myxoid variant appears translucent or gelatinous

MICROSCOPIC PATHOLOGY

Histologic Features
- Histologic variants include
  - Storiform-pleomorphic
  - Myxoid
  - Giant cell
  - Inflammatory (xanthomatous)
- Most are histologically high grade
- Heterologous elements, including bone and cartilage, may be present in any histologic subtype
- **Storiform-pleomorphic type**
  - Most common histologic variant in sinonasal tract
  - Fascicular and storiform growth patterns
    - Storiform growth characterized by formation of short fascicles in "pinwheel" or "cartwheel" configuration
  - Hypercellular neoplasm consisting of spindle-shaped to epithelioid-appearing cells
  - Marked nuclear pleomorphism, increased mitotic activity, including typical and atypical forms
  - Multinucleated giant cells
  - Bizarre giant cells with multiple hyperchromatic nuclei identified
  - Necrosis commonly seen
  - Variable amount of chronic inflammatory cells, xanthoma (foam) cells
  - Granulomas may be identified
  - Stromal findings include variable fibrosis, hyalinization, myxoid change, and vascularity
- **Myxoid MFH type**
  - Diagnosis requires that at least 50% of tumor has myxoid stroma
  - Myxoid foci are hypocellular but contain spindle-shaped and epithelioid malignant cells arranged in storiform or fascicular growth
  - Cells are spindled to round with moderate to marked atypia
  - Cells may show features suggestive of lipoblasts, including vacuolated cytoplasm with indentation of nuclei
  - Characteristic stromal vasculature, including delicate vessels arranged in curvilinear fashion
- **Giant cell MFH type**
  - Nodular or multinodular growth but also diffuse growth without nodularity
  - Characterized by presence of multinucleated giant cells containing numerous (up to 100) round to oval nuclei with vesicular chromatin, identifiable nucleoli, and eosinophilic cytoplasm
    - Multinucleated giant cells admixed with mononuclear cells and spindle-shaped cells
    - Diagnosis requires that multinucleated giant cells and mononuclear cells represent over 50% of tumor
- **Inflammatory MFH type**
  - Admixture of histiocytic-appearing cells, xanthomatous cells, and inflammatory cells
  - Inflammatory cells include neutrophils

MALIGNANT FIBROUS HISTIOCYTOMA/UNDIFFERENTIATED PLEOMORPHIC SARCOMA

- Typically not associated with necrosis
- May be intense, obscuring neoplastic cells
- Patients may have constitutional symptoms, including fever and peripheral granulocytosis

ANCILLARY TESTS

Immunohistochemistry

- No specific immunoreactivity
  - Vimentin positive
  - Actin may be focally positive
  - Absence of
    - Epithelial markers
    - Melanocytic markers
    - Myogenic markers
    - Hematolymphoid markers

DIFFERENTIAL DIAGNOSIS

Other Pleomorphic Sarcomas

- Examples include
  - Liposarcoma
  - Leiomyosarcoma
  - Rhabdomyosarcoma
- Targeted panel of immunohistochemical stains
- Identification of diagnostic cells
  - e.g., lipoblasts, rhabdomyoblasts
- Dedifferentiated liposarcoma shares similar histologic features to MFH
  - Differentiation achieved by evaluating for lipogenic tumor markers including
    - Peroxisome proliferator-activated receptor γ (PPAR-γ), CDK4, p16, and MDM2
    - High sensitivity for malignant lipomatous tumors

Spindle Cell Squamous Carcinoma

- Typically superficially located, not deep-seated
- Often associated with differentiated squamous cell carcinoma in form of
  - Intraepithelial dysplasia
  - Invasive differentiated squamous cell carcinoma
  - Immunoreactivity for epithelial markers, including cytokeratins, p63
    - Significant percentage keratin, p63 negative
    - Consistently vimentin reactive with variable desmin and actin immunoreactivity

DIAGNOSTIC CHECKLIST

Pathologic Interpretation Pearls

- Diagnosis is one of excluding another more specific sarcoma or nonsarcomatous malignant neoplasm
  - Requires targeted panel of immunostains
  - May require molecular genetic testing

SELECTED REFERENCES

1. Alaggio R et al: Undifferentiated high-grade pleomorphic sarcomas in children: a clinicopathologic study of 10 cases and review of literature. Pediatr Dev Pathol. 13(3):209-17, 2010
2. Clark DW et al: Malignant fibrous histiocytoma of the head and neck region. Head Neck. Epub ahead of print, 2010
3. Chung L et al: Overlapping features between dedifferentiated liposarcoma and undifferentiated high-grade pleomorphic sarcoma. Am J Surg Pathol. 33(11):1594-600, 2009
4. Matushansky I et al: MFH classification: differentiating undifferentiated pleomorphic sarcoma in the 21st Century. Expert Rev Anticancer Ther. 9(8):1135-44, 2009
5. Wang CP et al: Malignant fibrous histiocytoma of the sinonasal tract. Head Neck. 31(1):85-93, 2009
6. Franco Gutiérrez V et al: Radiation-induced sarcomas of the head and neck. J Craniofac Surg. 19(5):1287-91, 2008
7. Nascimento AF et al: Diagnosis and management of pleomorphic sarcomas (so-called "MFH") in adults. J Surg Oncol. 97(4):330-9, 2008
8. Dei Tos AP: Classification of pleomorphic sarcomas: where are we now? Histopathology. 48(1):51-62, 2006
9. Fletcher CD: The evolving classification of soft tissue tumours: an update based on the new WHO classification. Histopathology. 48(1):3-12, 2006
10. Sabesan T et al: Malignant fibrous histiocytoma: outcome of tumours in the head and neck compared with those in the trunk and extremities. Br J Oral Maxillofac Surg. 44(3):209-12, 2006
11. Sturgis EM et al: Sarcomas of the head and neck region. Curr Opin Oncol. 15(3):239-52, 2003
12. Iguchi Y et al: Malignant fibrous histiocytoma of the nasal cavity and paranasal sinuses: review of the last 30 years. Acta Otolaryngol Suppl. (547):75-8, 2002
13. Rodrigo JP et al: Malignant fibrous histiocytoma of the nasal cavity and paranasal sinuses. Am J Rhinol. 14(6):427-31, 2000
14. Patel SG et al: Radiation induced sarcoma of the head and neck. Head Neck. 21(4):346-54, 1999
15. Ko JY et al: Radiation-induced malignant fibrous histiocytoma in patients with nasopharyngeal carcinoma. Arch Otolaryngol Head Neck Surg. 122(5):535-8, 1996
16. Wanebo HJ et al: Head and neck sarcoma: report of the Head and Neck Sarcoma Registry. Society of Head and Neck Surgeons Committee on Research. Head Neck. 14(1):1-7, 1992
17. Barnes L et al: Malignant fibrous histiocytoma of the head and neck. A report of 12 cases. Arch Otolaryngol Head Neck Surg. 114(10):1149-56, 1988
18. Heffner DK: Problems in pediatric otorhinolaryngic pathology. I. Sinonasal and nasopharyngeal tumors and masses with myxoid features. Int J Pediatr Otorhinolaryngol. 5(1):77-91, 1983
19. Perzin KH et al: Non-epithelial tumors of the nasal cavity, paranasal sinuses and nasopharynx: a clinico-pathologic study XI. fibrous histiocytomas. Cancer. 45(10):2616-26, 1980

Microscopic Features

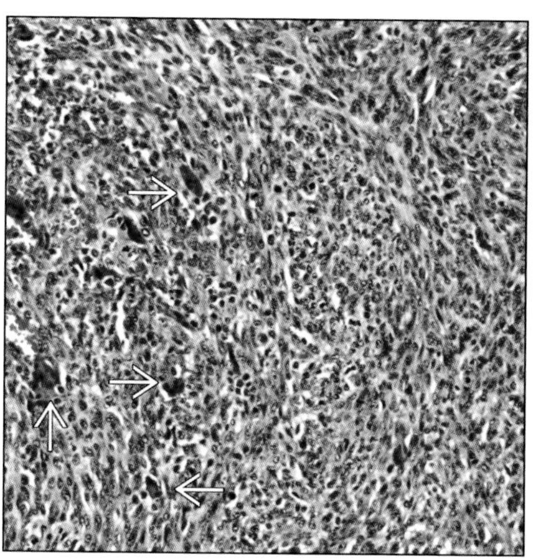

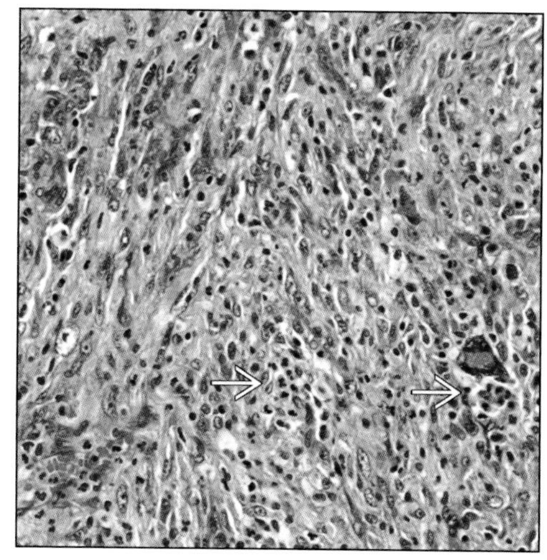

(Left) *MFH, pleomorphic-storiform type, shows the presence of scattered multinucleated giant cells ➔. The diagnosis of MFH is one of exclusion; only after other (more common) types of undifferentiated malignant neoplasms are excluded can the diagnosis of MFH be proffered.* ***(Right)*** *MFH may include a variable number of inflammatory cells typically including mature lymphocytes and plasma cells, but increased numbers of neutrophils ➔ may be seen in a minority of cases.*

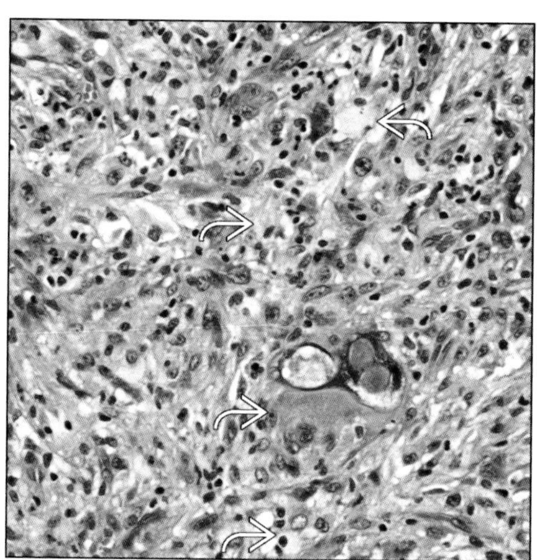

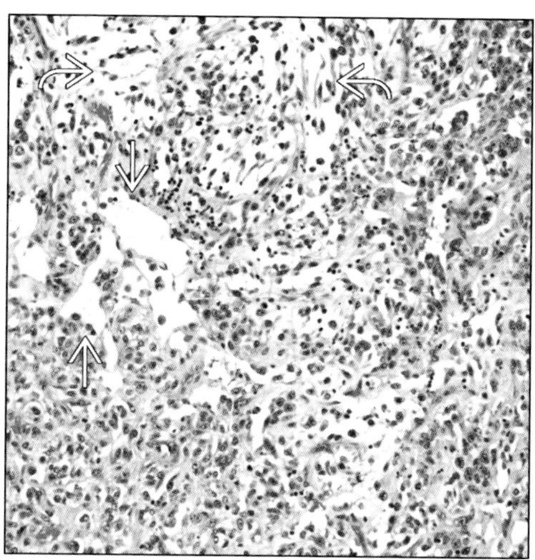

(Left) *MFH shows a mixed inflammatory cell infiltrate, including lymphocytes, plasma cells, eosinophils, and neutrophils as well as xanthoma cells ➔. Such findings, in particular the presence of xanthoma cells, correlate to the designation of the inflammatory type of MFH.* ***(Right)*** *The vascular pattern in MFH may include vessels with a "staghorn" or hemangiopericytoma-like configuration ➔. In addition, focal myxoid stroma may be present ➔.*

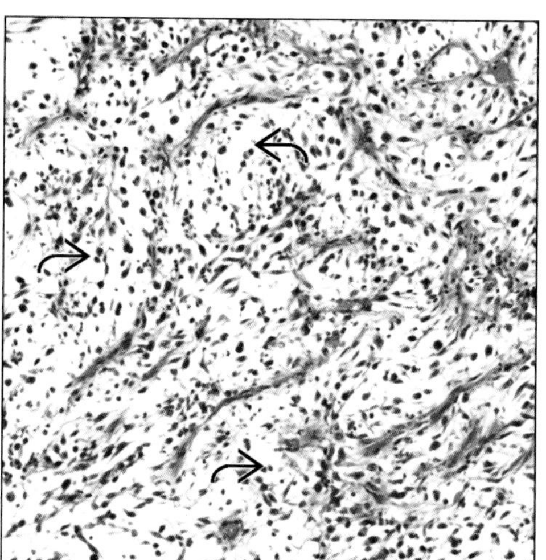

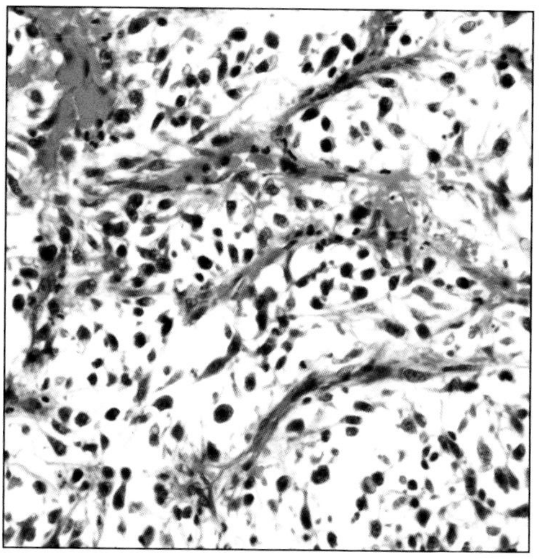

(Left) *A diagnosis of myxoid MFH requires that at least 50% of the tumor show myxoid stroma ➔. The degree of cellularity may vary from relatively paucicellular to hypercellular. The vascular component, composed of an intricate plexiform pattern, is noteworthy.* ***(Right)*** *The neoplastic and inflammatory cells condense along the arcing vessels. The intricate plexiform pattern seen in myxoid MFH is also a feature seen in other sarcomas, in particular myxoid liposarcoma.*

MESENCHYMAL CHONDROSARCOMA

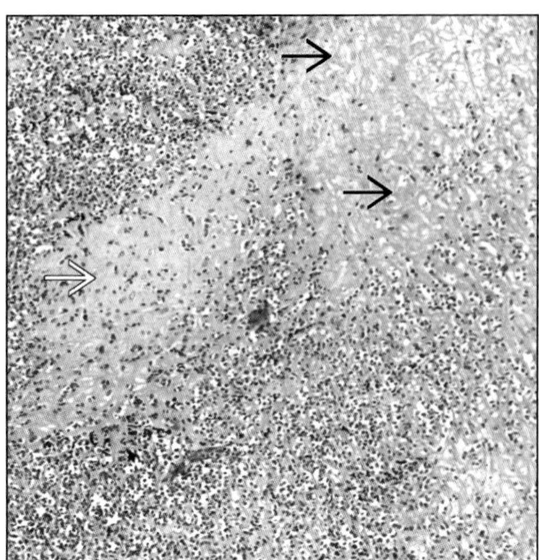

Low-power view reveals an island of cartilage ➡ in a sea of small cells with associated necrosis ⇨. The mix of cartilage and small blue cells is a clue to this diagnosis.

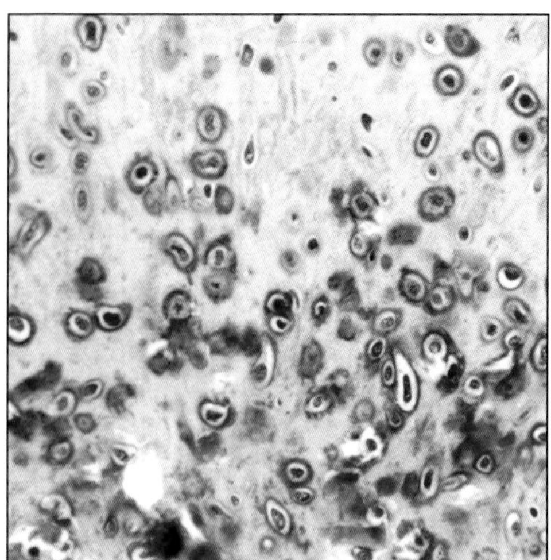

High-power view demonstrates cartilage with an increase in cellularity and mild atypia. This finding indicates a low-grade cartilage lesion, a finding commonly seen in this tumor type.

TERMINOLOGY

Definitions

- Malignant mesenchymal tumor with cartilaginous differentiation
  - Biphasic tumors with 2 separate cell populations

CLINICAL ISSUES

Epidemiology

- Incidence
  - Rare
    - < 1% of head and neck chondrosarcomas
- Age
  - Affects all ages
  - Usually seen in 2nd and 3rd decades of life
- Gender
  - Equal gender distribution

Site

- Most often in maxilla or mandible
  - May occur in sinonasal tract and orbit

Presentation

- Nonspecific symptoms
  - Mass, teeth displacement, nasal obstruction, epistaxis
- Usually no history of radiation exposure

Treatment

- Options, risks, complications
  - Moderate to high risk of recurrence
    - Due to anatomy and difficulty obtaining adequate margins
- Surgical approaches
  - Radical surgical resection is preferred treatment
- Adjuvant therapy
  - No benefit in cartilaginous tumors
- Radiation
  - No benefit in cartilaginous tumors

Prognosis

- Varies from complete tumor response and long-term survival to rapid local tumor progression
- When metastases are present, usually widespread to lungs and bones
  - Demise in months
- Overall survival guarded
  - 5-year survival (55%)
  - 10-year survival (27%)

IMAGE FINDINGS

Radiographic Findings

- No radiographic findings that are pathognomonic for chondrosarcoma

MR Findings

- Noncalcified portions demonstrate signal intensity lower than or equal to gray matter on T1-weighted images
- Isointense to gray matter on T2-weighted images
- T1-weighted images after gadolinium contrast show inhomogeneous enhancement in calcified and uncalcified areas

CT Findings

- CT shows moderate contrast enhancement and well-defined mass with multiple areas of fine and coarse calcification
- Dynamic CT reveals delayed contrast enhancement

Bone Scan

- Bone scan will be "hot" (positive)

MACROSCOPIC FEATURES

General Features

- Similar to conventional chondrosarcoma
- Fleshy areas indicating small cell-spindle component

MESENCHYMAL CHONDROSARCOMA

Key Facts

Terminology
- Malignant mesenchymal tumor with cartilaginous differentiation

Clinical Issues
- 2nd and 3rd decades, usually gnathic bones
- Radical surgical resection is treatment of choice
- Variable prognosis: Long-term survival or rapid local tumor progression

Microscopic Pathology
- Mesenchymal chondrosarcoma has 3 characteristic components
  - Dense population of anaplastic small cells; arranged in solid sheets or in hemangiopericytoma-like pattern; chondroid matrix in abrupt islands

Top Differential Diagnoses
- Small cell tumors when cartilage is not seen

Sections to Be Submitted
- Must submit **all** tissue to document cartilage

Size
- 2-10 cm

MICROSCOPIC PATHOLOGY

Histologic Features
- 3 characteristic components
  - Dense population of anaplastic small cells
  - Arranged in solid sheets or in hemangiopericytoma-like pattern
  - Chondroid matrix in abrupt islands

ANCILLARY TESTS

Immunohistochemistry
- Small cells positive for CD99
- Negative for S100 protein, distinctly different from most chondrocytic chondrosarcomas

DIFFERENTIAL DIAGNOSIS

Small Cell Neoplasms
- When cartilaginous component is absent (not sampled) small cell neoplasms are considered
- Hemangiopericytoma
- Synovial sarcoma
- Ewing sarcoma/PNET
- Olfactory neuroblastoma
- Rhabdomyosarcoma
- Small cell osteosarcoma
- Anaplastic carcinoma (especially "oat cell" carcinoma)
- Leukemic deposits (granulocytic sarcoma) and malignant lymphoma

SELECTED REFERENCES

1. Pellitteri PK et al: Mesenchymal chondrosarcoma of the head and neck. Oral Oncol. 43(10):970-5, 2007
2. Lee SY et al: Chondrosarcoma of the head and neck. Yonsei Med J. 46(2):228-32, 2005
3. Knott PD et al: Mesenchymal chondrosarcoma of the sinonasal tract: a clinicopathological study of 13 cases with a review of the literature. Laryngoscope. 113(5):783-90, 2003
4. Chidambaram A et al: Mesenchymal chondrosarcoma of the maxilla. J Laryngol Otol. 114(7):536-9, 2000
5. Patel SC et al: Sarcomas of the head and neck. Top Magn Reson Imaging. 10(6):362-75, 1999
6. Skoog L et al: Fine-needle aspiration cytology and immunocytochemistry of soft-tissue tumors and osteo/chondrosarcomas of the head and neck. Diagn Cytopathol. 20(3):131-6, 1999
7. Granter SR et al: CD99 reactivity in mesenchymal chondrosarcoma. Hum Pathol. 27(12):1273-6, 1996
8. Takahashi K et al: Mesenchymal chondrosarcoma of the jaw--report of a case and review of 41 cases in the literature. Head Neck. 15(5):459-64, 1993
9. Bloch DM et al: Mesenchymal chondrosarcomas of the head and neck. J Laryngol Otol. 93(4):405-12, 1979

IMAGE GALLERY

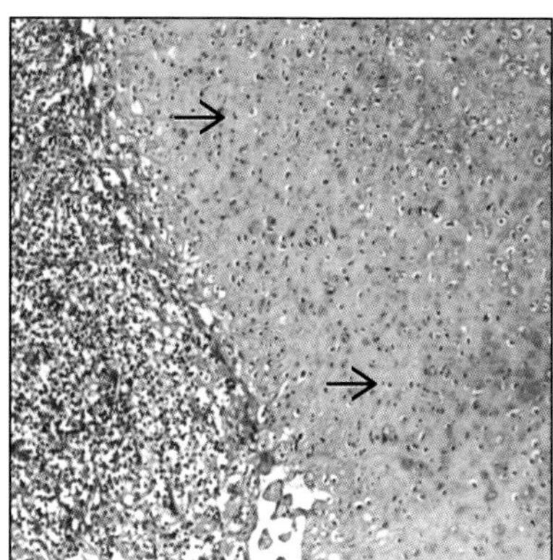

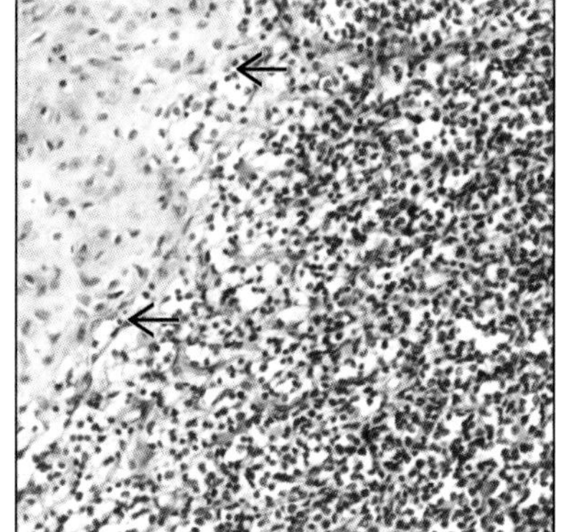

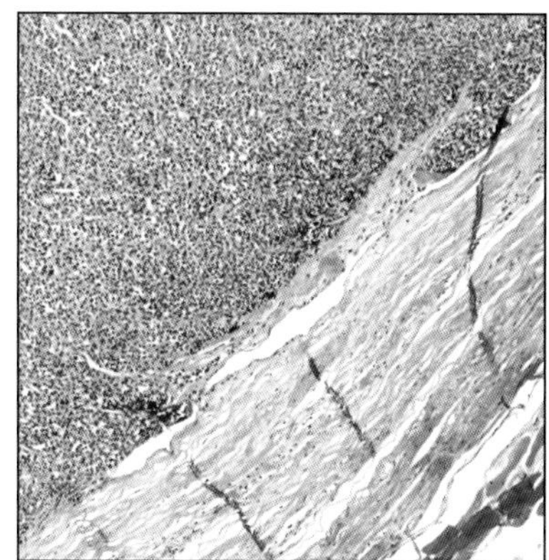

(Left) *Medium-power view shows the interface between the cartilaginous ⇒ and noncartilaginous components. The interface can often show an eosinophilic quality to the cartilage matrix, which can mimic osteoid. The cartilage is usually sharply demarcated from the surrounding tissue.* ***(Center)*** *High-power view shows "small round blue cells" in nests and sheets, juxtaposed to the cartilage ⇒.* ***(Right)*** *There is a fibrous capsule surrounding this tumor. No cartilage is seen.*

ANGIOSARCOMA

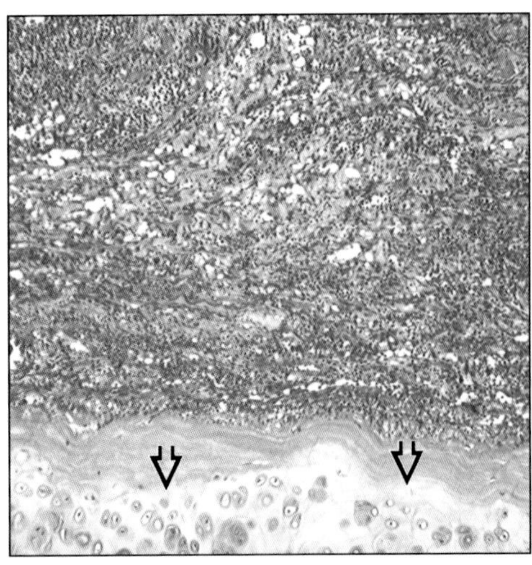

Hematoxylin & eosin shows a highly cellular vascular neoplasm with extravasated erythrocytes adjacent to septal cartilage ⇨.

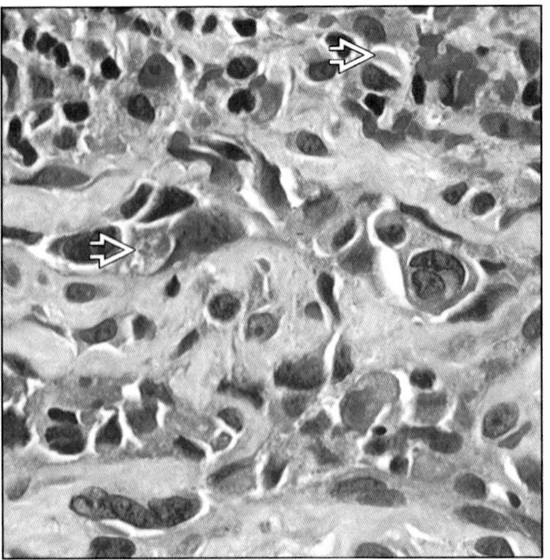

Hematoxylin & eosin shows highly pleomorphic cells projecting into slit-like lumens. A neolumen formation is present ➡.

TERMINOLOGY

Synonyms

- Epithelioid hemangioendothelioma
- Malignant hemangioendothelioma
- Malignant angioendothelioma
- Lymphangiosarcoma
- Hemangiosarcoma
- Hemangioblastoma

Definitions

- High-grade malignant vascular neoplasm

ETIOLOGY/PATHOGENESIS

Radiation

- May result in tumor development after long latent period

Environmental Exposure

- Chemicals have not been reported to result in tumor development

CLINICAL ISSUES

Epidemiology

- Incidence
  - Rare, < 0.1% of all sinonasal tract malignancies
  - ~ 50% of all angiosarcomas develop in head and neck
    - Most common in skin (scalp) and superficial soft tissues
- Age
  - Mean: 47 years
  - Range: 8-82 years
  - Females tend to be younger than males at presentation
- Gender
  - Male > Female (2:1)

Site

- Nasal cavity alone
  - May involve paranasal sinuses
- Paranasal sinuses alone

Presentation

- Epistaxis is most common symptom
- Nasal discharge
- Nasal obstruction
- Not syndrome associated (Kasabach-Merritt specifically)

Treatment

- Options, risks, complications
  - Best outcome achieved with combination of surgery, radiation, and chemotherapy
- Surgical approaches
  - Wide surgical excision
- Adjuvant therapy
  - Multiagent chemotherapy
- Radiation
  - Postoperative radiation

Prognosis

- Generally poor
  - ~ 60% die from disease in approximately 2 years
  - Better prognosis than skin or soft tissue sarcomas, perhaps due to earlier detection
- Recurrences are common, up to 40%
- Female patients have worse prognosis (increased percentage of patients die from disease), although overall length of survival is identical to male patients
- Older patients have worse prognosis than younger patients
- Larger tumors or tumors from maxillary sinuses tend to have poorer prognosis
- Metastatic disease identified in lung, liver, spleen, and bone marrow
- Patients with specific etiologic factor (radiation) seem to have shorter survival

ANGIOSARCOMA

Key Facts

Terminology
- High-grade malignant vascular neoplasm

Clinical Issues
- Epistaxis is most common symptom
- Not syndrome associated (Kasabach-Merritt specifically)

Macroscopic Features
- Nodular, polypoid masses

Microscopic Pathology
- Ulcerated surface epithelium (usually respiratory type)
- Necrosis and hemorrhage prominent
- Freely anastomosing vascular channels
- Tortuous, irregular, small to large, and cleft-like spaces
- Atypical, enlarged, spindled to epithelioid endothelial cells line channels
- Intracytoplasmic vacuoles or neolumen
- Extravasated erythrocytes are noted throughout
- Increased mitotic figures, including atypical forms
- Extracellular eosinophilic hyaline globules are absent

Ancillary Tests
- Positive with a variety of vascular markers
  - CD31, CD34, FVIIIRAg

Top Differential Diagnoses
- Granulation tissue
- Lobular capillary hemangioma
- Juvenile nasopharyngeal angiofibroma
- Epithelioid hemangioma
- Kaposi sarcoma

IMAGE FINDINGS

General Features
- Radiolucent or radiopaque density associated with destructive growth in soft tissue, cartilage, &/or bone
- CT determines extent of tumor (contrast-enhanced mass)
- Magnetic resonance image (MR) shows bright mass on T2-weighted images
- Angiography identifies extent of tumor and shows feeder vessel(s), allowing for presurgical angiographic embolization, if desired

MACROSCOPIC FEATURES

General Features
- Nodular, polypoid masses
- Soft, friable
- Red to purple
- Hemorrhagic with clots and necrosis

Size
- Range: 0.7-8 cm
- Mean: 4 cm
- Tumors in female patients tend to be larger (6 cm vs. 3 cm)
- Paranasal sinus tumors tend to be larger than nasal cavity tumors (6.8 cm vs. 2.2 cm)

MICROSCOPIC PATHOLOGY

Histologic Features
- Ulcerated surface epithelium (usually respiratory type)
- Necrosis and hemorrhage prominent
- Infiltrative neoplasm into surrounding soft and hard tissues
- Extravasated erythrocytes are noted throughout
- Freely anastomosing vascular channels
  - Tortuous, irregular, small to large, and cleft-like spaces
- Atypical, enlarged, spindled to epithelioid endothelial cells line channels
  - Endothelial cells may be single, multi-layered or papillary, tufted
- Intracytoplasmic vacuoles or neolumen
  - Frequently contain erythrocytes
- Nuclear chromatin is heavy, coarse, with irregular nuclear contours
- Increased mitotic figures, including atypical forms
- Extracellular eosinophilic hyaline globules are absent
- Inflammatory cells are present but may depend on ulceration and reaction

ANCILLARY TESTS

Immunohistochemistry
- Positive with a variety of vascular markers

DIFFERENTIAL DIAGNOSIS

Granulation Tissue
- Proliferation of vessels arranged perpendicular to surface with plump endothelial cells
- Ulcerated surface is common
- Mixed inflammatory infiltrate, with prominent histiocytes
- No cytologic atypia, freely anastomosing vessels, or atypical mitotic figures

Lobular Capillary Hemangioma
- Pyogenic granuloma (misnomer, since it is not infection or granulomatous)
- Polypoid mass with surface ulceration and fibrinoid necrosis
- Lobular architecture with central perpendicular vessels with surrounding capillaries
- Plump endothelial cells with bland nuclei
- Mitotic activity is usually brisk
- Edematous to fibrotic stroma with hemosiderin-laden macrophages
- Variable inflammatory infiltrate

ANGIOSARCOMA

Immunohistochemistry

Antibody	Reactivity	Staining Pattern	Comment
CD34	Positive	Cytoplasmic	> 98% of neoplastic cells
CD31	Positive	Cytoplasmic	> 95% of neoplastic cells
FVIIIRAg	Positive	Cytoplasmic	> 90% of neoplastic cells
Actin-sm	Positive	Cytoplasmic	Adjacent to vascular spaces
Ki-67	Positive	Nuclear	> 10% of cells
EMA	Positive	Cell membrane	Variably reactive
CK-PAN	Negative		
S100	Negative		
Actin-HHF-35	Equivocal	Cytoplasmic	Variably reactive

Juvenile Nasopharyngeal Angiofibroma

- Arises in nasopharynx (pterygoid region) in young male patients exclusively
- Cellular and richly vascularized mesenchymal neoplasm
- Background fibrous connective tissue stroma with many variable-sized, disorganized vessels of varying thickness with patchy muscle content
- Plump endothelial cells without atypia
- Elastic tissue is lacking in vessel walls
- Mast cells are common

Epithelioid Hemangioma

- Also called "angiolymphoid hyperplasia with eosinophilia" or "histiocytoid hemangioma"
- Extranodal proliferation of vessels associated with heavy nodular to diffuse lymphocytic infiltrate with eosinophils
- Enlarged nonatypical endothelial cells protruding into lumen in cobblestone or hobnail type fashion, often occluding vessel lumen
- Cytoplasmic vacuoles may be seen

Glomangiopericytoma

- Diffuse syncytial growth of closely packed round to oval cells
- Arranged in short interlacing fascicles, which are richly vascularized
- Capillary to large patulous spaces that may have ramifying "staghorn" configuration
- Prominent peritheliomatous hyalinization
- Extravasated erythrocytes, mast cells, and eosinophils
- Positive with actins but not with vascular markers (CD34, CD31, or FVIIIRAg)

Kaposi Sarcoma

- Plaque-tumor stage shows sieve-like vasoformative pattern
- Slightly atypical spindled tumor cells
- Eosinophilic, glassy-hyaline intra- and extracellular globules (PAS positive)
- HHV8 is usually positive, helping to confirm diagnosis

Thrombosed Vessel

- Recanalization of thrombosed vessels (Masson vegetant endothelial hyperplasia or intravascular papillary endothelial hyperplasia)
- Vessel wall usually easy to identify
- No atypia of endothelial cells as they line papillary projections within organizing spaces

SELECTED REFERENCES

1. Heffner DK: Sinonasal angiosarcoma? Not likely (a brief description of infarcted nasal polyps). Ann Diagn Pathol. 14(4):233-4, 2010
2. Wang ZH et al: Sinonasal intravascular papillary endothelial hyperplasia successfully treated by endoscopic excision: a case report and review of the literature. Auris Nasus Larynx. 36(3):363-6, 2009
3. Nelson BL et al: Sinonasal tract angiosarcoma: a clinicopathologic and immunophenotypic study of 10 cases with a review of the literature. Head Neck Pathol. 1(1):1-12, 2007
4. Fukushima K et al: A case of angiosarcoma of the nasal cavity successfully treated with recombinant interleukin-2. Otolaryngol Head Neck Surg. 134(5):886-7, 2006
5. Ordoñez-Escalante KG et al: [Nasal cavity angiosarcoma: a case report and literature review.] Gac Med Mex. 142(2):155-8, 2006
6. Yang C et al: [Clinical analysis of 48 cases sarcoma in nasal cavity and sinuses.] Lin Chuang Er Bi Yan Hou Ke Za Zhi. 18(10):597-8, 2004
7. Di Girolamo A et al: Epithelioid haemangioendothelioma arising in the nasal cavity. J Laryngol Otol. 117(1):75-7, 2003
8. Wong KF et al: Sinonasal angiosarcoma with marrow involvement at presentation mimicking malignant lymphoma: cytogenetic analysis using multiple techniques. Cancer Genet Cytogenet. 129(1):64-8, 2001
9. Alameda F et al: Reactive vascular lesion of nasal septum simulating angiosarcoma in a cocaine abuser. Hum Pathol. 31(2):239-41, 2000
10. Velegrakis GA et al: Angiosarcoma of the maxillary sinus. J Laryngol Otol. 114(5):381-4, 2000
11. Kimura Y et al: Angiosarcoma of the nasal cavity. J Laryngol Otol. 106(4):368-9, 1992
12. Solomons NB et al: Haemangiosarcoma of the maxillary antrum. J Laryngol Otol. 104(10):831-4, 1990
13. Kurien M et al: Angiosarcoma of the nasal cavity and maxillary antrum. J Laryngol Otol. 103(9):874-6, 1989
14. Heffner DK: Problems in pediatric otorhinolaryngic pathology. II. Vascular tumors and lesions of the sinonasal tract and nasopharynx. Int J Pediatr Otorhinolaryngol. 5(2):125-38, 1983
15. Bankaci M et al: Angiosarcoma of the maxillary sinus: literature review and case report. Head Neck Surg. 1(3):274-80, 1979

Microscopic and Immunohistochemical Features

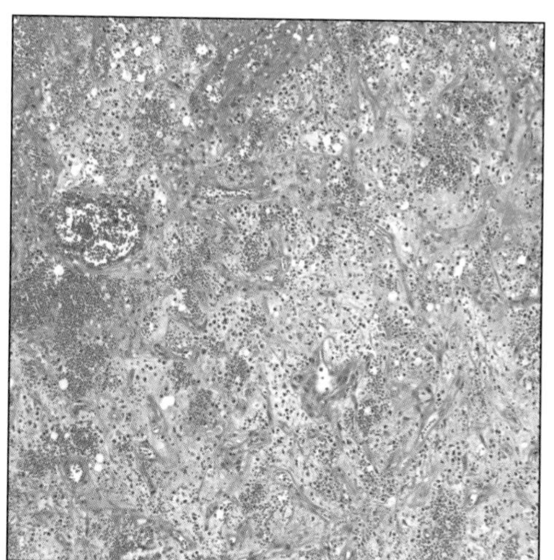

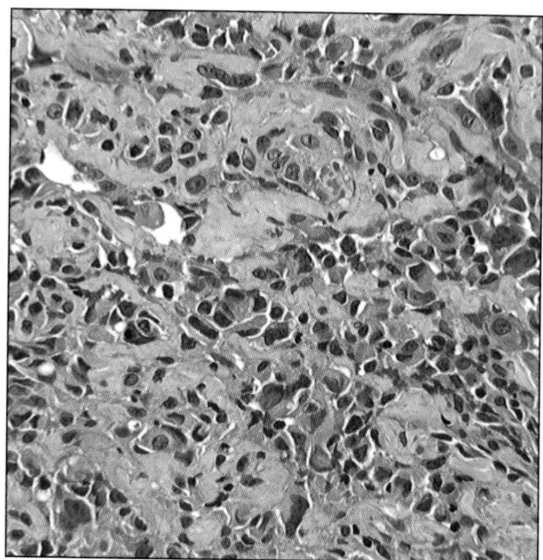

(Left) *Hematoxylin & eosin shows hemorrhagic and degenerated material within a vascular neoplasm.* ***(Right)*** *Hematoxylin & eosin shows a cellular pleomorphic population arranged in a haphazard distribution, lining the irregular vascular channels with extravasated erythrocytes.*

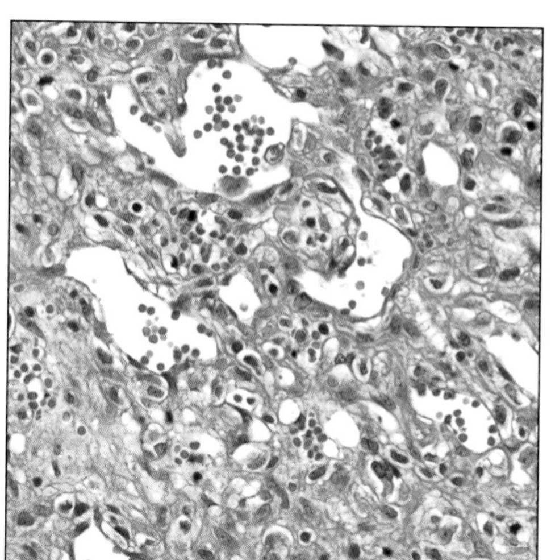

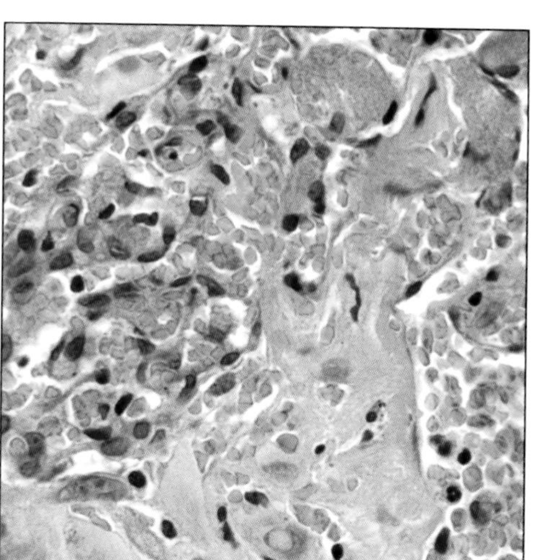

(Left) *Hematoxylin & eosin shows variable-sized vascular channels associated with a neoplastic proliferation of atypical endothelial cells. Erythrocytes are noted throughout.* ***(Right)*** *Hematoxylin & eosin shows a hobnail or tufted pattern of endothelial cells projecting into vascular spaces filled with erythrocytes.*

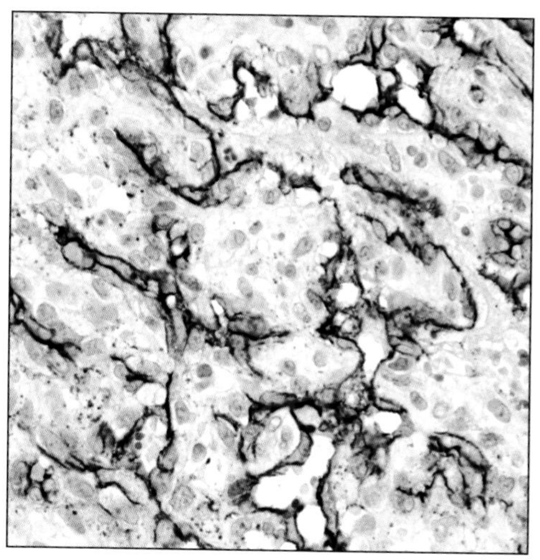

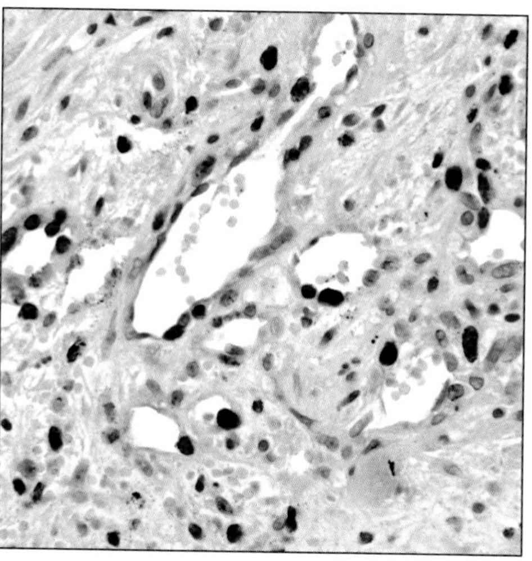

(Left) *CD34 shows strong reactivity in the cytoplasm of the endothelial cells arranged in an anastomosing pattern.* ***(Right)*** *Ki-67 shows a positive reaction within the nuclei of the endothelial cells in the stroma, as well as lining the vascular spaces.*

EXTRANODAL NK-/T-CELL LYMPHOMA, NASAL TYPE

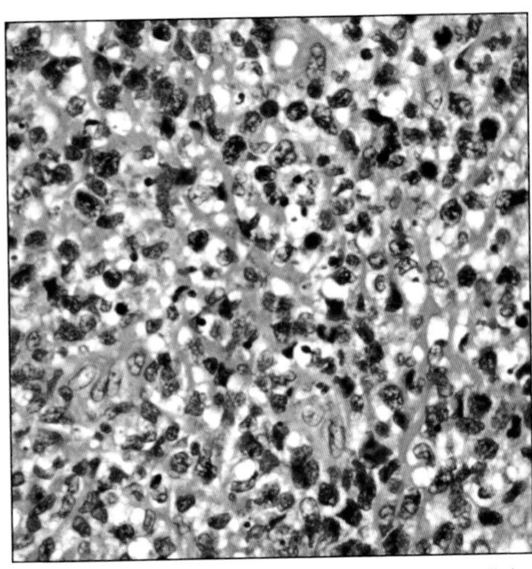

Dyscohesive undifferentiated malignant cellular proliferation is comprised of medium to large cells with round to oval nuclei, vesicular to hyperchromatic chromatin, and eosinophilic to clear cytoplasm.

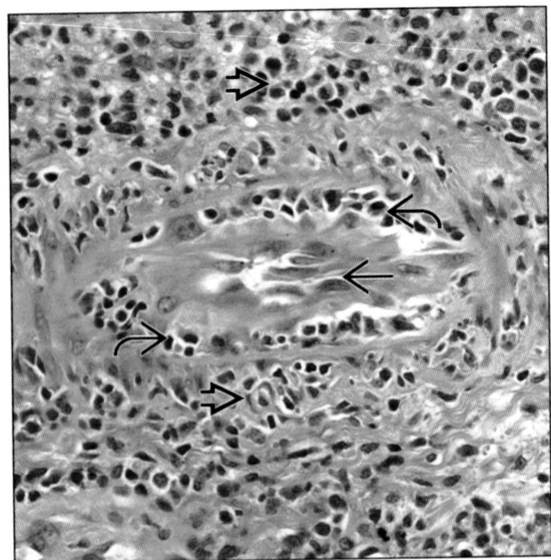

The neoplastic cells surround (angiocentric) ⇨ and invade (angioinvasive) ➔ an endothelial cell-lined ➔ vascular space. Vascular obliteration causes ischemic-type necrosis (not shown).

TERMINOLOGY

Synonyms

- Angiocentric immunoproliferative lesions; peripheral T-cell lymphoma
- Angiocentric NK-/T-cell lymphoma of nasal type
- Polymorphic reticulosis
- Lethal midline granuloma
- Midline malignant reticulosis
- Idiopathic midline destructive disease
- Stewart granuloma
- World Health Organization classifies NK-cell tumors into 3 types
  - Extranodal NK-/T-cell lymphomas, nasal type
  - Extranodal NK-/T-cell lymphomas, nonnasal type
  - NK-cell leukemias

Definitions

- Polymorphic neoplastic infiltrate with
  - Angioinvasion &/or angiodestruction
  - CD2(+), CD3(-), cCD3ε(+), CD56(+) phenotype
  - Strong association with Epstein-Barr virus (EBV)

ETIOLOGY/PATHOGENESIS

Infectious Agents

- Strongly associated with EBV
  - > 95% of cases
- Clonal EBV infection is almost invariably present

Immunosuppression

- Occurs with increased frequency in setting of immune suppression, especially after organ transplantation

CLINICAL ISSUES

Epidemiology

- Incidence
  - Prevalent in Asia and South America
  - Rare in Western countries
  - Peripheral T-cell lymphomas uncommon, accounting for 10-15% of all non-Hodgkin lymphomas
- Age
  - Disease of adults with median age in 6th decade of life
  - Closely related entity seen mainly in children is hydroa vacciniforme-like lymphoma
    - Also EBV positive
- Gender
  - Male > Female
- Ethnicity
  - Most common in Asians
  - Reported with significant frequency in South and Central America and Mexico
    - In these populations, primarily occurs in individuals of Native American origin
    - Findings suggest racial predisposition
  - Although uncommon, occurs in Western populations in Caucasians

Site

- Most commonly affects nasal cavity

Presentation

- Destructive process of mid-facial region with
  - Nasal septal destruction
  - Palatal destruction/perforation
  - Orbital swelling
  - Obstructive symptoms related to a mass
- Clinical features of major importance in defining NK-/T-cell lymphoma
- Small percentage of cases present with hematophagocytic syndrome with pancytopenia
- Hyper-IgE syndrome (Job syndrome)
  - Rare primary immunodeficiency associated with increased risk for malignancies
    - Includes extranodal natural killer/T-cell lymphoma

EXTRANODAL NK-/T-CELL LYMPHOMA, NASAL TYPE

Key Facts

Terminology

- Polymorphic neoplastic infiltrate with
  - Angioinvasion &/or angiodestruction
  - CD2(+), CD3(-), cCD3ε(+), CD56(+) phenotype
  - Strong association with EBV

Clinical Issues

- Most commonly affects nasal cavity
- Destructive process of mid-facial region
- First-line radiotherapy most important key to successful treatment
  - Early radiation is advocated for localized NK-/T-cell lymphoma, nasal type
  - Effectiveness of radiotherapy evident in limited disease but questionable in extensive disease
- Despite early stage of disease at presentation, overall survival is poor

Microscopic Pathology

- Polymorphic neoplastic infiltrate with angioinvasive and angiodestructive pattern
- Broad cytologic spectrum
  - Nuclear pleomorphism, irregular and elongated nuclei, prominent nucleoli, eosinophilic to clear cytoplasm
- Angiocentric and angiodestructive pattern
- Presence of geographic ("ischemic type") necrosis

Ancillary Tests

- Most common immunophenotype: CD2(+), surface CD3(-), cytoplasmic CD3(+), CD56(+)
- In situ hybridization for EBV-encoded RNA (EBER)

Laboratory Tests

- Serum EBV-DNA copy number useful as specific tumor marker
  - May be predictive prognostic factor

Treatment

- Options, risks, complications
  - Most nasal NK-cell lymphomas present with stage I/II disease
  - Based on currently available data, treatment of nasal NK-/T-cell lymphoma consists of radiotherapy with or without multiagent chemotherapy
- Adjuvant therapy
  - Many stage I/II patients treated with radiotherapy fail systemically, implying that concomitant chemotherapy may be needed
  - Chemotherapy is indicated for advanced nasal NK-cell lymphoma and nonnasal and aggressive subtypes
    - NK-/T-cell lymphoma is resistant to anthracycline-based chemotherapy
    - Nonanthracycline combination chemotherapy (e.g., ifosfamide, methotrexate, etoposide, and prednisolone) has activity against NK-/T-cell lymphoma either as first-line or as second-line treatment
    - Treatment results are unsatisfactory
  - High-dose chemotherapy with hematopoietic stem cell transplantation may be beneficial to selected patients
  - Therapeutic approaches to advanced stage or relapsed and refractory disease not well established
- Radiation
  - First-line radiotherapy most important key to successful treatment
    - Early radiation is advocated for localized nasal-type NK/T-cell lymphoma
    - Effectiveness of radiotherapy evident in limited disease but questionable in extensive disease

Prognosis

- Despite early stage of disease at presentation, overall survival is poor
- No apparent differences in survival between radiotherapy alone or in combination with chemotherapy
- 5-year survival rates
  - Approximately 70% for limited I(E)
  - Approximately 41% for extended I(E)
- 10-year survival rates
  - Approximately 57% for limited I(E)
  - Approximately 36% for extended I(E)
- Poor prognostic factors include
  - Bulky disease
  - Advanced stage
  - Multiple extranodal sites of involvement
  - Older age

IMAGE FINDINGS

Radiographic Findings

- Locally destructive disease typically presenting with obliteration of nasal passages and maxillary sinuses
- Involvement of adjacent anatomic structures (e.g., alveolar bone, hard palate, orbits, nasopharynx) associated with extensive soft tissue masses present in majority of cases

MICROSCOPIC PATHOLOGY

Histologic Features

- Polymorphic neoplastic infiltrate with angioinvasive and angiodestructive pattern
- Broad cytologic spectrum
- Usually (but not always) cytologically atypical cells are present
  - Vary from small and medium-sized cells to large, hyperchromatic cells with

EXTRANODAL NK-/T-CELL LYMPHOMA, NASAL TYPE

        - Nuclear pleomorphism, irregular and elongated nuclei, prominent nucleoli, eosinophilic to clear cytoplasm
- Early phase of disease may not include overtly malignant appearing cells
    - Infiltrate appears nonspecific including admixture of chronic inflammatory cells
    - "Disconnect" between destructive clinical process and absence of overtly malignant infiltrate
    - Presence of EBV even in absence of malignant cellular process supportive of diagnosis
        - EBV-positive cells are typically absent in nasal cavity mucosa &/or in inflammatory sinonasal diseases
- Increased mitotic activity, including atypical mitoses, often present
- Epitheliotropism and pseudoepitheliomatous hyperplasia may be present
- Associated prominent admixed inflammatory cell infiltrate may be present
    - Polymorphous inflammatory cell infiltrate may obscure atypical cells
    - Benign inflammatory cell infiltrate includes lymphocytes, plasma cells, histiocytes, and eosinophils
    - Multinucleated giant cells and granulomas absent
- Angiocentric and angiodestructive pattern
    - Atypical cells invade and destroy blood vessels
        - Tumor cells around and within vascular spaces with infiltration and destruction of vessel wall
        - Perivascular localization alone insufficient for designation of angiocentricity
        - Vascular invasion and destruction responsible for designation "angiocentric lymphoma"
- Presence of geographic ("ischemic-type") necrosis characterized by
    - Tissue destruction with bluish or "gritty" appearance
    - Necrosis is virtually constant (but not pathognomonic) feature
    - Zonal pattern of distribution suggests vascular pathogenesis

ANCILLARY TESTS

Histochemistry

- Elastic stains may be useful in identification of angiocentric/angioinvasive growth
    - Disruption of elastic membrane with permeation of vessel wall by neoplastic cells
- Stains for microorganisms are negative

Immunohistochemistry

- NK-cell lineage most common immunophenotype seen in approximately 65-75% of cases
    - CD2(+), surface CD3(-), cytoplasmic CD3ε(+), CD56(+), CD94(+)
    - Expression of cytotoxic markers
        - TIA, granzyme B (GZM-B), perforin
- T-cell lineage in approximately 25-35% of cases
    - CD2(+), cytoplasmic CD3ε(+), CD5(+), CD8 (±), CD56(-/+), cytotoxic markers(+)
- CD45RB (leucocyte common antigen) positive
- In situ hybridization (ISH) for EBV-encoded RNA (EBER)
- Tumors CD56 negative may still be classified as NK/T-cell lymphomas if express
    - T-cell markers
    - Cytotoxic markers
    - EBV positive
- May be p63 positive
- Vimentin positive
- Negative for epithelial markers (cytokeratins), melanocytic markers, neuroendocrine markers, mesenchymal myogenic markers

Cytogenetics

- Loss of chromosomes 6q, 11q, 13q, and 17p are recurrent aberrations

Molecular Genetics

- Clonal Epstein-Barr virus (EBV) infection almost invariably present (> 95% of cases)
- T-cell receptor (TCR) gene rearrangement
    - Present in T-cell tumors
        - T-cell receptor gene is germline
    - NK-cell tumors do not carry *TCR* gene rearrangements

DIFFERENTIAL DIAGNOSIS

Nonspecific Chronic Sinusitis

- Innocuous clinical symptoms lacking destructive nature of NK-/T-cell lymphoma, nasal type
- EBV negative

Wegener Granulomatosis

- Mixed inflammatory infiltrate, scattered multinucleated giant cells, vasculitis
- Elevated antineutrophil cytoplasmic antibodies (ANCA), proteinase 3 (PR3)
- EBV negative

Sinonasal B-cell Lymphoma

- Most often diffuse large B-cell lymphoma
    - Submucosal diffuse cellular infiltrate of monotonous population of large cells
- Less commonly shows angiocentricity and angioinvasion compared to NK-/T-cell lymphoma, nasal type
- Immunophenotype is B-cell, including
    - CD20(+), CD79a(+), CD3(-)
- Molecular evaluation shows
    - Monoclonal *IgH* gene rearrangements
- EBV negative

Carcinomas

- Immunoreactive for cytokeratins
- Nonreactive for hematolymphoid markers
- EBV negative

Olfactory Neuroblastoma, High Grade

- Immunoreactive for neuron-specific enolase, neuroendocrine markers, S100 protein including peripheral sustentacular cell-type pattern
- EBV negative

Mucosal Malignant Melanoma
- Immunoreactive for vimentin, melanocytic markers (S100 protein, HMB-45, Melan-A, tyrosinase)
- EBV negative

Small Cell Undifferentiated Neuroendocrine Carcinoma
- Immunoreactive for cytokeratins, neuroendocrine markers (chromogranin, synaptophysin, CD57)
- CD56 positive
- EBV negative

Rhabdomyosarcoma
- Immunoreactive for desmin, myoglobin, myogenin, and vimentin
- EBV negative

Primitive (Peripheral) Neuroectodermal Tumor/Extraosseous Ewing Sarcoma
- Immunoreactive for FLI-1, CD99; variable reactivity for neuroendocrine markers, neuron-specific enolase, epithelial markers
- EBV negative

DIAGNOSTIC CHECKLIST

Clinically Relevant Pathologic Features
- Clinical features are of major importance in defining NK-/T-cell lymphoma

Pathologic Interpretation Pearls
- Presence of EBV confirmatory of diagnosis even in situation where cellular infiltrate not overly malignant
  - EBV-positive cells typically absent in nasal cavity mucosa or in inflammatory diseases of nasal cavity

SELECTED REFERENCES

1. Chang CH et al: Hyper-IgE syndrome with Epstein-Barr virus associated extranodal NK/T cell lymphoma of skin. Kaohsiung J Med Sci. 26(4):206-10, 2010
2. Chen SW et al: Upper aerodigestive tract lymphoma in Taiwan. J Clin Pathol. 63(10):888-93, 2010
3. Huang YH et al: Nasopharyngeal Extranodal NK/T-Cell Lymphoma, Nasal Type: Retrospective Study of 18 Consecutive Cases in Guangzhou, China. Int J Surg Pathol. Epub ahead of print, 2010
4. Watanabe K et al: A unique case of nasal NK/T cell lymphoma with frequent remission and relapse showing different histological features during 12 years of follow up. J Clin Exp Hematop. 50(1):65-9, 2010
5. Greer JP et al: Natural killer-cell neoplasms. Curr Hematol Malig Rep. 4(4):245-52, 2009
6. Harabuchi Y et al: Nasal natural killer (NK)/T-cell lymphoma: clinical, histological, virological, and genetic features. Int J Clin Oncol. 14(3):181-90, 2009
7. Kim TM et al: Extranodal NK / T-cell lymphoma, nasal type: new staging system and treatment strategies. Cancer Sci. 100(12):2242-8, 2009
8. Kohrt H et al: Extranodal natural killer/T-cell lymphoma: current concepts in biology and treatment. Leuk Lymphoma. 50(11):1773-84, 2009
9. Zeglaoui I et al: Nasal NK/T-cell lymphoma in the paediatric population. Two case reports. B-ENT. 5(2):119-23, 2009
10. Bourne TD et al: p63 Expression in olfactory neuroblastoma and other small cell tumors of the sinonasal tract. Am J Clin Pathol. 130(2):213-8, 2008
11. Brodkin DE et al: Nasal-type NK/T-cell lymphoma presenting as hemophagocytic syndrome in an 11-year-old Mexican boy. J Pediatr Hematol Oncol. 30(12):938-40, 2008
12. Liang X et al: Natural killer cell neoplasms. Cancer. 112(7):1425-36, 2008
13. Li YX et al: Radiotherapy as primary treatment for stage IE and IIE nasal natural killer/T-cell lymphoma. J Clin Oncol. 2006 Jan 1;24(1):181-9. Erratum in: J Clin Oncol. 24(18):2973, 2006
14. Kim K et al: Treatment outcome of angiocentric T-cell and NK/T-cell lymphoma, nasal type: radiotherapy versus chemoradiotherapy. Jpn J Clin Oncol. 35(1):1-5, 2005
15. Nakashima Y et al: Genome-wide array-based comparative genomic hybridization of natural killer cell lymphoma/leukemia: different genomic alteration patterns of aggressive NK-cell leukemia and extranodal Nk/T-cell lymphoma, nasal type. Genes Chromosomes Cancer. 44(3):247-55, 2005
16. Nava VE et al: The pathology of NK-cell lymphomas and leukemias. Adv Anat Pathol. 12(1):27-34, 2005
17. Ng SB et al: Nasal-type extranodal natural killer/T-cell lymphomas: a clinicopathologic and genotypic study of 42 cases in Singapore. Mod Pathol. 17(9):1097-107, 2004
18. Cheung MM et al: Natural killer cell neoplasms: a distinctive group of highly aggressive lymphomas/leukemias. Semin Hematol. 40(3):221-32, 2003
19. Cheung MM et al: Early stage nasal NK/T-cell lymphoma: clinical outcome, prognostic factors, and the effect of treatment modality. Int J Radiat Oncol Biol Phys. 54(1):182-90, 2002
20. Hu W et al: Multivariate prognostic analysis of stage I(E) primary non-Hodgkin's lymphomas of the nasal cavity. Am J Clin Oncol. 24(3):286-9, 2001
21. Ooi GC et al: Nasal T-cell/natural killer cell lymphoma: CT and MR imaging features of a new clinicopathologic entity. AJR Am J Roentgenol. 174(4):1141-5, 2000
22. Siu LL et al: Consistent patterns of allelic loss in natural killer cell lymphoma. Am J Pathol. 157(6):1803-9, 2000
23. Jaffe ES et al: Extranodal peripheral T-cell and NK-cell neoplasms. Am J Clin Pathol. 111(1 Suppl 1):S46-55, 1999
24. Yoon TY et al: Nasal-type T/natural killer cell angiocentric lymphoma, Epstein-Barr virus-associated, and showing clonal T-cell receptor gamma gene rearrangement. Br J Dermatol. 140(3):505-8, 1999
25. Cheung MM et al: Primary non-Hodgkin's lymphoma of the nose and nasopharynx: clinical features, tumor immunophenotype, and treatment outcome in 113 patients. J Clin Oncol. 16(1):70-7, 1998
26. Jaffe ES et al: Report of the Workshop on Nasal and Related Extranodal Angiocentric T/Natural Killer Cell Lymphomas. Definitions, differential diagnosis, and epidemiology. Am J Surg Pathol. 20(1):103-11, 1996
27. Jaffe ES: Classification of natural killer (NK) cell and NK-like T-cell malignancies. Blood. 87(4):1207-10, 1996
28. Abbondanzo SL et al: Non-Hodgkin's lymphoma of the sinonasal tract. A clinicopathologic and immunophenotypic study of 120 cases. Cancer. 75(6):1281-91, 1995
29. Heffner DK: Idiopathic midline destructive disease. Ann Otol Rhinol Laryngol. 104(3):258, 1995

EXTRANODAL NK-/T-CELL LYMPHOMA, NASAL TYPE

Clinical, Imaging, and Microscopic Features

*(**Left**) Clinically, NK-/T-cell lymphoma is a destructive process of mid-facial region that may include facial deformities due to destruction of bony walls between adjacent anatomic sites. (**Right**) CT scan shows a destructive nasal cavity mass with almost completely opacified maxillary sinus and thickening of mucosa in the nasopharynx. This patient was shown to have extranodal NK-/T-cell lymphoma, nasal type.*

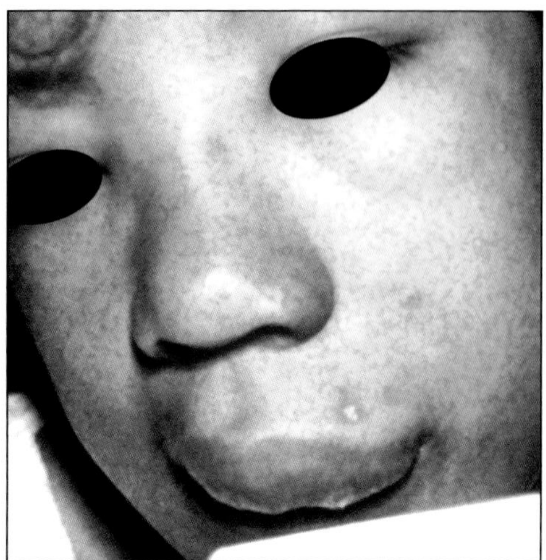

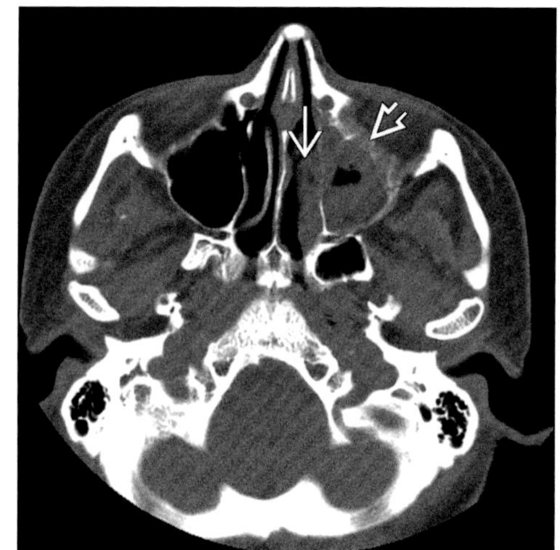

*(**Left**) At low magnification, ischemic-type ("geographic") necrosis is present lying adjacent to area of viable tumor and an obliterated vascular space. (**Right**) Diffuse cellular proliferation comprised of cells with varying size and shape, including cells with elongated convoluted appearing nuclei, vesicular to hyperchromatic chromatin, inconspicuous to prominent nucleoli, and indistinct eosinophilic to clear cytoplasm. Note scattered mitotic figures.*

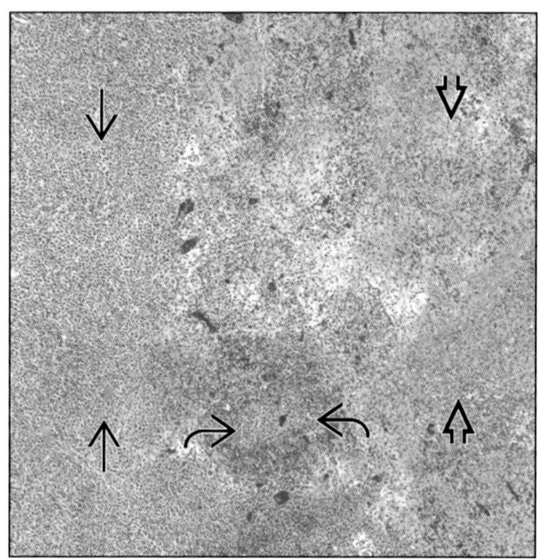

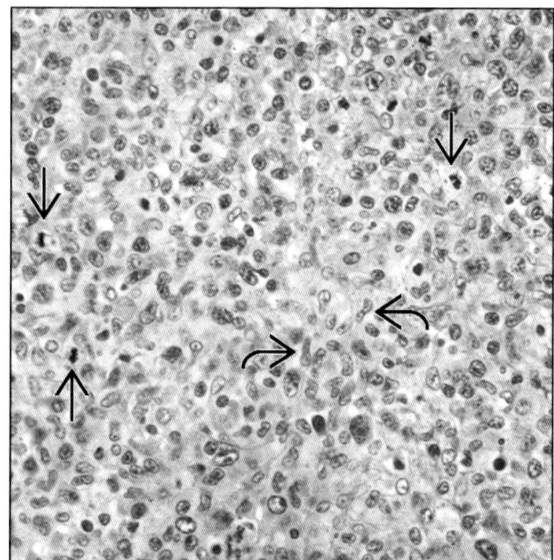

*(**Left**) The neoplastic cells surround (angiocentric) and invade (angioinvasion) vascular spaces with near obliteration of the endothelial cell-lined vascular lumen with thrombus-like effects. The results of the vascular compromise will be ischemic-type necrosis (not shown). (**Right**) Vasculitis can be difficult to identify and elastic stain may assist in showing disruption of elastic membranes due to tumor invasion through the wall with plugging of the vessel lumen.*

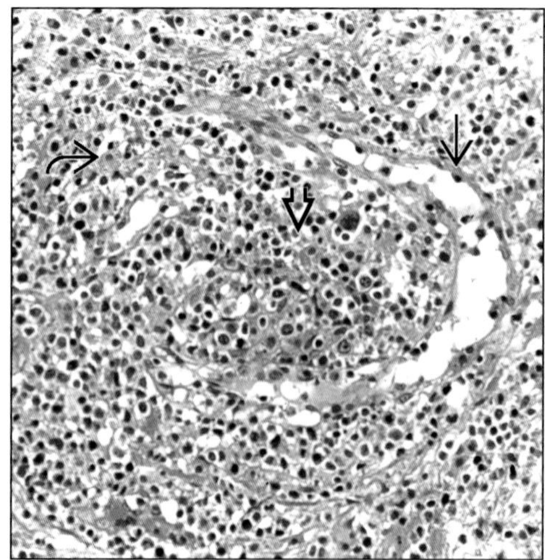

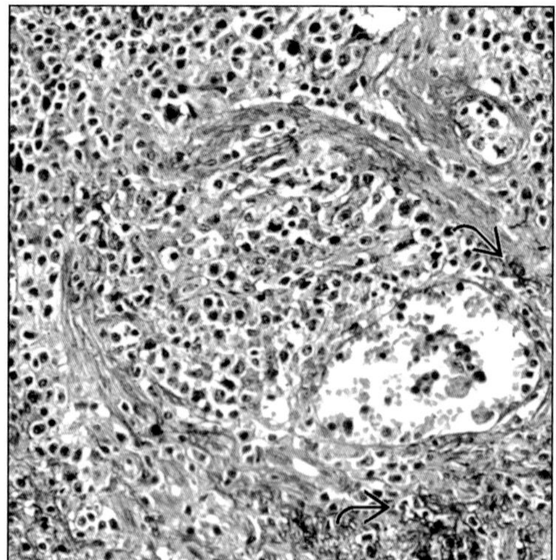

Microscopic and Immunohistochemical Features

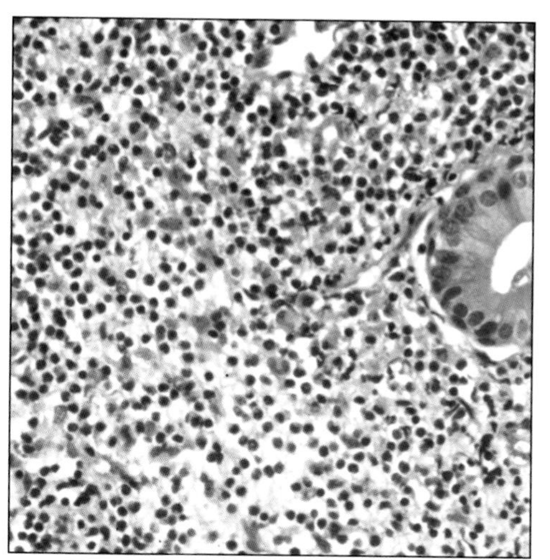

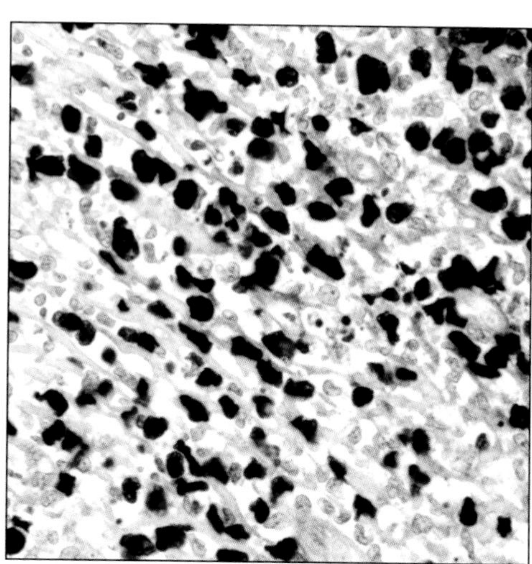

(Left) *In spite of aggressive clinical behavior, histology may show a polymorphous cell population lacking malignant cytomorphologic features with a polyclonal phenotype and absence of TCR gene rearrangements weighing against a malignant diagnosis. In this case, EBV staining would support a diagnosis of NK-/T-cell lymphoma.* ***(Right)*** *Diffuse EBER reactivity is present. Relative to SNT undifferentiated malignancies, EBER is uniquely identified in NK-/T-cell lymphoma.*

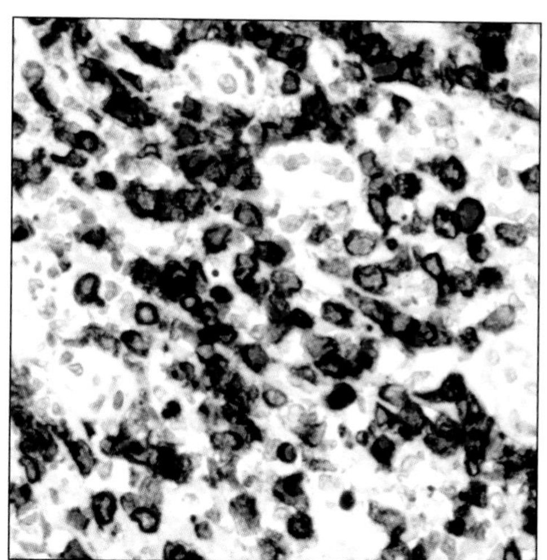

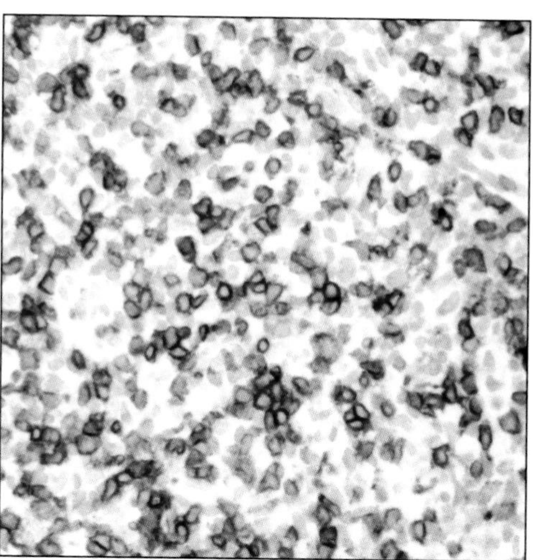

(Left) *IHC antigenic profile of NK-/T-cell lymphoma includes reactivity for hematolymphoid markers (e.g., CD45RB or leucocyte common antigen [not shown]), as well as CD2 positive staining.* ***(Right)*** *Diffuse CD3 (cytoplasmic not surface) positive neoplastic cells are present. NK-cell lineage is the most common immunophenotype, seen in approximately 65-75% of cases, and characterized by CD2(+), cytoplasmic CD3ϵ(+), CD56(+), and expression of cytotoxic markers.*

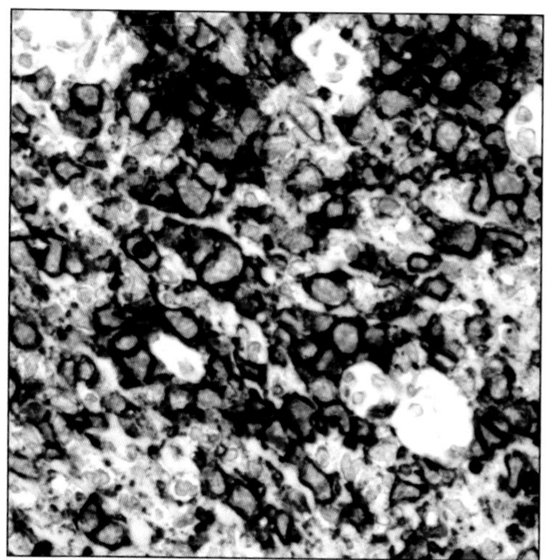

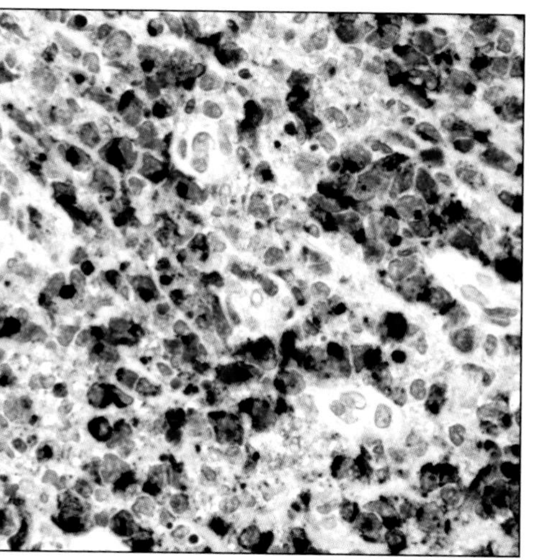

(Left) *The neoplastic cells are diffusely immunoreactive for CD56.* ***(Right)*** *The neoplastic cells are diffusely immunoreactive for the cytotoxic granule marker TIA1. Given overlapping of light microscopic features shared among sinonasal undifferentiated malignant neoplasms, especially in limited biopsy material, a broad immunohistochemical antigenic panel is required in the diagnosis and differential diagnosis of these neoplasms, including but not limited to NK-/T-cell lymphoma.*

METASTATIC/SECONDARY TUMORS

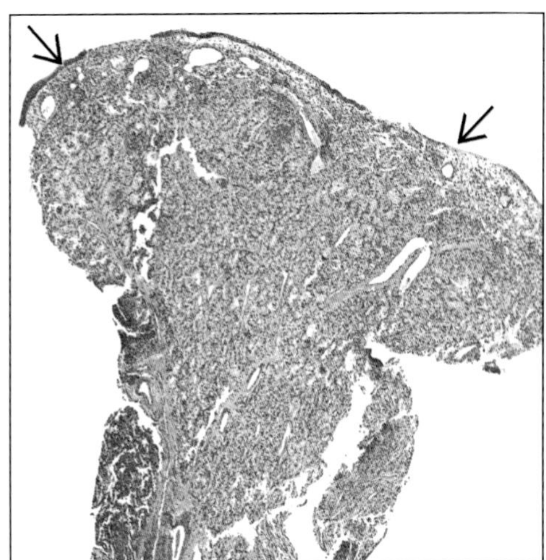

This "polyp" shows an intact squamous mucosa ➔ but has a very cellular epithelial neoplasm in the stroma. This is a metastatic renal cell carcinoma, showing some vascularity.

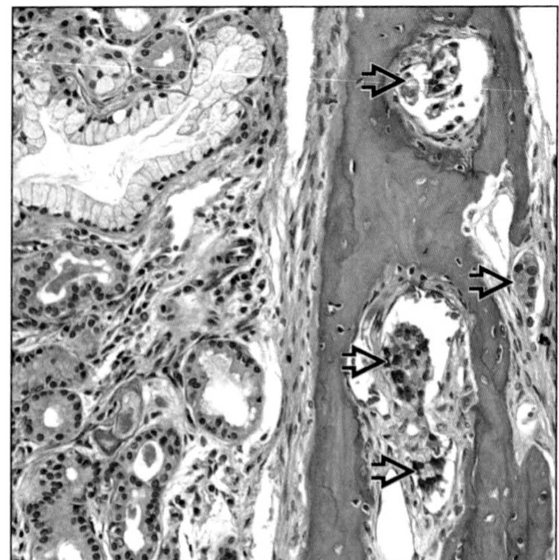

A metastatic prostate adenocarcinoma is identified within the bony fragments of this curettage sample. The native minor mucoserous glands are quite different from the intra-bony metastases ➲.

TERMINOLOGY

Definitions

- Tumors secondarily involving nasal cavity and paranasal sinuses that originate from, but are not in continuity with, primary malignancies of other sites
  - Lymphomas and leukemias are excluded by definition

CLINICAL ISSUES

Epidemiology

- Incidence
  - Uncommon
    - < 0.5% of all malignancies of nasal cavity and paranasal sinuses
- Age
  - Older ages, correlated with increased malignancies of other anatomic sites
    - In review of 82 cases, median age was 57 years
- Gender
  - Male > Female (3:2)

Site

- Maxillary sinus (33%)
- Sphenoid sinus (22%)
- Multiple sinuses (22%)
- Ethmoid sinus (14%)
- Frontal sinus (9%)
- Limited to nasal cavity (10-15%)

Presentation

- Identical to primary tumors
- Nasal obstruction
- Epistaxis
  - Especially metastatic renal and thyroid carcinomas
- Headache
- Facial pain
- Visual disturbances
- Exophthalmos
- Cranial nerve deficits

Treatment

- Options, risks, complications
  - Metastasis may be 1st manifestation of occult carcinoma
  - Rarely, metastatic disease to sinonasal tract may be the only, isolated metastasis
    - Most commonly with renal cell carcinoma
- Surgical approaches
  - Excision is performed for symptomatic relief

Prognosis

- Matches underlying disease but usually part of disseminated disease
- Prognosis is usually grave
  - Also depends on whether sinonasal metastasis is isolated or part of widespread disseminated disease
    - Localized metastasis, treated aggressively, can yield survival of 2-3 years
  - Renal cell carcinoma may be exception, associated with good prognosis with isolated metastatic foci

MACROSCOPIC FEATURES

General Features

- Metastases may be solitary or multifocal
- Polyp can be seen
- Surface epithelium is usually intact
- Often a subepithelial (submucosal) mass

Size

- Variable
  - Lesions of sinuses tend to be larger than nasal cavity

METASTATIC/SECONDARY TUMORS

Key Facts

Terminology

- Tumors secondarily involving nasal cavity and paranasal sinuses that originate from primary malignancies of other sites

Clinical Issues

- < 0.5% of all malignancies of nasal cavity and paranasal sinuses
- Male > Female (3:2)
- Maxillary sinus (33%), sphenoid sinus (22%), multiple sinuses (22%)

Microscopic Pathology

- Specific tumor type dictates histology
- Most common tumors are carcinomas
  - Kidney (40%)
  - Lung (9%)
  - Breast and thyroid (8% each)
  - Prostate (7%)

MICROSCOPIC PATHOLOGY

Histologic Features

- Metastases to sinonasal tract are hematogenous
  - Look in patulous vessels for tumor thrombi
- Specific tumor type dictates histology
- Most common tumors are carcinomas (adenocarcinomas)
  - Kidney (40%)
  - Lung (9%)
  - Breast (8%)
  - Thyroid (8%)
  - Prostate (7%)
  - Miscellaneous (28%)
- Clear cell primary salivary gland-type tumors may be difficult to separate from metastases
- Melanoma may invade from overlying skin

ANCILLARY TESTS

Immunohistochemistry

- Prudent and judicious target studies will help with separation from primary tumors

DIFFERENTIAL DIAGNOSIS

Primary Tumor

- Primary, poorly differentiated tumors may need to be separated from metastatic tumors
  - Separation can usually be achieved by history, radiographic studies, and immunohistochemistry
  - Salivary gland-type primaries are more common than metastatic tumors

Direct Extension

- Oral cavity primaries (squamous cell carcinoma, melanoma, salivary gland-type adenocarcinomas) may directly extend into nasal cavity or paranasal sinuses
  - Clinical and radiographic evaluation helps
- Gnathic tumors (multiple myeloma, ameloblastoma, odontogenic tumors) may expand into paranasal sinuses and should be considered in differential of an unusual tumor
- Brain (pituitary adenoma, chordoma, meningioma) may extend into these spaces, mimicking primary tumors

SELECTED REFERENCES

1. Barnes L: Metastases to the head and neck: an overview. Head Neck Pathol. 3(3):217-24, 2009
2. Prescher A et al: [Metastases to the paranasal sinuses: case report and review of the literature.] Laryngorhinootologie. 80(10):583-94, 2001
3. Kent SE et al: Metastases of malignant disease of the nasal cavity and paranasal sinuses. J Laryngol Otol. 98(5):471-4, 1984
4. Bernstein JM et al: Metastatic tumors to the maxilla, nose, and paranasal sinuses. Laryngoscope. 76(4):621-50, 1966

IMAGE GALLERY

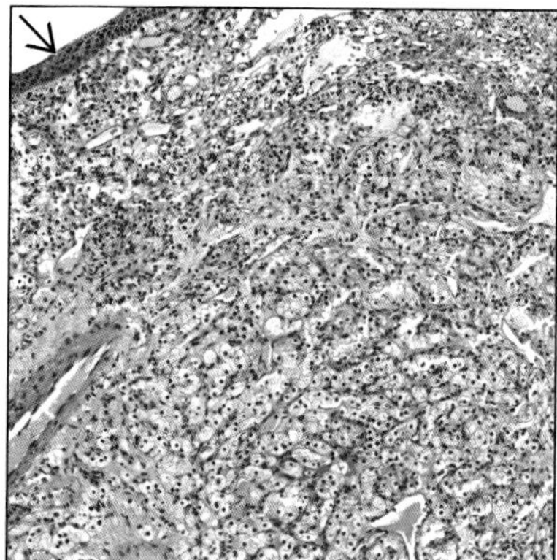

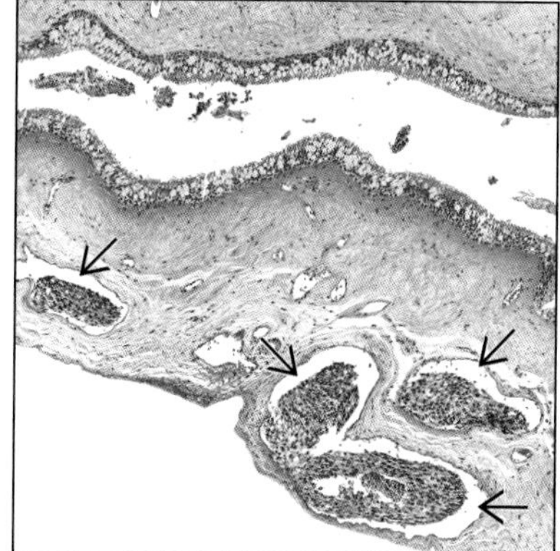

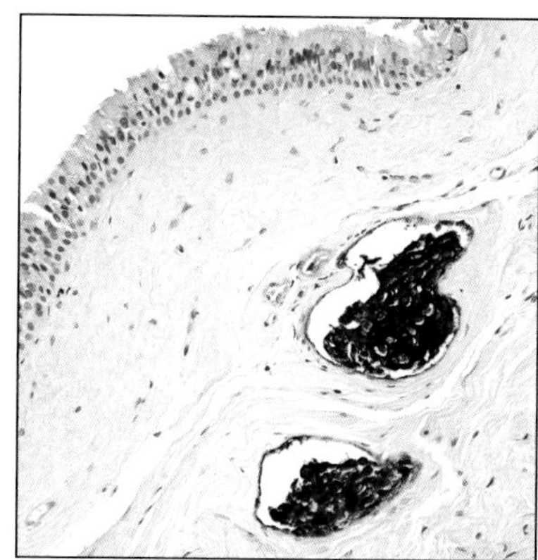

(Left) *The intact respiratory epithelium ⇒ overlies the very cellular neoplastic proliferation of a metastatic renal cell carcinoma. The alveolar pattern is associated with extravasated erythrocytes.* ***(Center)*** *Metastases frequently occupy dilated vascular spaces ⇒. While the type of malignancy is difficult to determine at this power, the intravascular distribution is obvious.* ***(Right)*** *A PSA stain helps to confirm the presence of metastatic prostate carcinoma.*

PROTOCOL FOR THE EXAMINATION OF NASAL CAVITY AND PARANASAL SINUS SPECIMENS

Nasal Cavity and Paranasal Sinuses

Incisional Biopsy, Excisional Biopsy, Resection

Specimen (select all that apply)

___ Nasal cavity
  ___ Septum
  ___ Floor
  ___ Lateral wall
  ___ Vestibule
___ Paranasal sinus(es), maxillary
___ Paranasal sinus(es), ethmoid
___ Paranasal sinus(es), frontal
___ Paranasal sinus(es), sphenoid
___ Other (specify): ____________________________
___ Not specified

Received

___ Fresh
___ In formalin
___ Other (specify): ____________________________

Procedure (select all that apply)

___ Incisional biopsy
___ Excisional biopsy
___ Resection (specify type)
  ___ Partial maxillectomy
  ___ Radical maxillectomy
___ Neck (lymph node) dissection (specify): ____________________________
___ Other (specify): ____________________________
___ Not specified

**Specimen Integrity*

*___ Intact
*___ Fragmented

Specimen size

Greatest dimensions: _________ x _________ x _________ cm
*Additional dimensions (if more than 1 part): _________ x _________ x _________ cm

Specimen Laterality

___ Right
___ Left
___ Bilateral
___ Midline
___ Not specified

Tumor Site (select all that apply)

___ Nasal cavity
  ___ Septum
  ___ Floor
  ___ Lateral wall
  ___ Vestibule
___ Paranasal sinus(es), maxillary
___ Paranasal sinus(es), ethmoid
___ Paranasal sinus(es), frontal
___ Paranasal sinus(es), sphenoid
___ Other (specify): ____________________________
___ Not specified

PROTOCOL FOR THE EXAMINATION OF NASAL CAVITY AND PARANASAL SINUS SPECIMENS

Tumor Focality

___ Single focus

___ Bilateral

___ Multifocal (specify): ___

Tumor Size

Greatest dimension: ___ cm

*Additional dimensions: ___ x ___ cm

___ Cannot be determined

**Tumor Description (select all that apply)*

*Gross subtype

*___ Polypoid

*___ Exophytic

*___ Endophytic

*___ Ulcerated

*___ Sessile

*___ Other (specify): ___

**Macroscopic Extent of Tumor*

*Specify: ___

Histologic Type (select all that apply)

___ Squamous cell carcinoma, conventional

  ___ Keratinizing

  ___ Nonkeratinizing (formerly cylindrical cell, transitional cell)

___ Variants of squamous cell carcinoma

  ___ Acantholytic squamous cell carcinoma

  ___ Adenosquamous carcinoma

  ___ Basaloid squamous cell carcinoma

  ___ Papillary squamous cell carcinoma

  ___ Spindle cell squamous cell carcinoma

  ___ Verrucous carcinoma

___ Giant cell carcinoma

___ Lymphoepithelial carcinoma (non-nasopharyngeal)

___ Sinonasal undifferentiated carcinoma (SNUC)

___ Adenocarcinoma, nonsalivary gland type

  ___ Intestinal type

    ___ Papillary type

    ___ Colonic type

    ___ Solid type

    ___ Mucinous type

    ___ Mixed type

  ___ Nonintestinal type

    ___ Low grade

    ___ Intermediate grade

    ___ High grade

___ Carcinomas of minor salivary glands

  ___ Acinic cell carcinoma

  ___ Adenoid cystic carcinoma

  ___ Adenocarcinoma, not otherwise specified (NOS)

    ___ Low grade

    ___ Intermediate grade

    ___ High grade

  ___ Carcinoma ex-pleomorphic adenoma (malignant mixed tumor)

  ___ Clear cell adenocarcinoma

  ___ Epithelial-myoepithelial carcinoma

PROTOCOL FOR THE EXAMINATION OF NASAL CAVITY AND PARANASAL SINUS SPECIMENS

____ Mucoepidermoid carcinoma

____ Low grade

____ Intermediate grade

____ High grade

____ Myoepithelial carcinoma (malignant myoepithelioma)

____ Oncocytic carcinoma

____ Polymorphous low-grade adenocarcinoma

____ Salivary duct carcinoma

____ Other (specify): ________________________

____ Neuroendocrine carcinoma

____ Typical carcinoid tumor (well-differentiated neuroendocrine carcinoma)

____ Atypical carcinoid tumor (moderately differentiated neuroendocrine carcinoma)

____ Small cell carcinoma (poorly differentiated neuroendocrine carcinoma)

____ Combined (or composite) small cell carcinoma, neuroendocrine type

____ Mucosal malignant melanoma

____ Other (specify): ________________________

____ Carcinoma, type cannot be determined

Histologic Grade

____ Not applicable

____ GX: Cannot be assessed

____ G1: Well differentiated

____ G2: Moderately differentiated

____ G3: Poorly differentiated

____ Other (specify): ________________________

**Microscopic Tumor Extension*

*Specify: ________________________

Margins (select all that apply)

____ Cannot be assessed

____ Margins uninvolved by invasive carcinoma

Distance from closest margin: ________ mm or ________ cm

Specify margin(s) per origination, if possible: ________________________

____ Margins uninvolved by carcinoma in situ (includes moderate and severe dysplasia†)

Distance from closest margin: ________ mm or ________ cm

Specify margin(s), per orientation, if possible: ________________________

____ Margins involved by carcinoma in situ (includes moderate and severe dysplasia†)

Specify margin(s), per orientation, if possible: ________________________

____ Not applicable

**Treatment Effect (applicable to carcinomas treated with neoadjuvant therapy)*

*____ Not identified

*____ Present (specify): ________________________

*____ Indeterminate

Lymph-Vascular Invasion

____ Not identified

____ Present

____ Indeterminate

Perineural Invasion

____ Not identified

____ Present

____ Indeterminate

Lymph Nodes, Extranodal Extension

____ Not identified

____ Present

___ Indeterminate

Pathologic Staging (pTNM)

TNM descriptors (required only if applicable) (select all that apply)

___ m (multiple primary tumors)

___ r (recurrent)

___ y (post-treatment)

Primary tumor (pT)

___ pTX: Cannot be assessed

___ pT0: No evidence of primary tumor

___ pTis: Carcinoma in situ

For all carcinomas excluding mucosal malignant melanoma

Primary tumor (pT): Maxillary sinus

___ pT1: Tumor limited to maxillary sinus mucosa with no erosion or destruction of bone

___ pT2: Tumor causing bone erosion or destruction including extension into hard palate &/or middle nasal meatus

except invasion to posterior wall of maxillary sinus and pterygoid plates

___ pT3: Tumor invades any of the following

Bone of posterior wall of maxillary sinus, subcutaneous tissues, floor or medial wall of orbit, pterygoid fossa, ethmoid sinuses

___ pT4a: Moderately advanced local disease

Tumor invades anterior orbital contents, skin of cheek, pterygoid plates, infratemporal fossa, cribriform plate, sphenoid or frontal sinuses

___ pT4b: Very advanced local disease; tumor invades any of the following

Orbital apex, dura, brain, middle cranial fossa, cranial nerves other than maxillary division of trigeminal nerve (V_2), nasopharynx, or clivus

Primary tumor (pT): Nasal cavity and ethmoid sinus

___ pT1: Tumor restricted to any 1 subsite, ± bone invasion

___ pT2: Tumor invading 2 subsites in a single region

or extending to involve an adjacent region within nasoethmoidal complex, ± bone invasion

___ pT3: Tumor extends to invade medial wall or floor of orbit, maxillary sinus, palate, or cribriform plate

___ pT4a: Moderately advanced local disease; tumor invades any of the following

Anterior orbital contents, skin of nose or cheek, minimal extension to anterior cranial fossa, pterygoid plates, sphenoid or frontal sinuses

___ pT4b: Very advanced local disease; tumor invades any of the following

Orbital apex, dura, brain, middle cranial fossa, cranial nerves other than maxillary division of trigeminal nerve (V_2), nasopharynx, or clivus

Regional lymph nodes (pN)††

___ pNX: Cannot be assessed

___ pN0: No regional lymph node metastasis

___ pN1: Metastasis in a single ipsilateral lymph node, ≤ 3 cm in greatest dimension

___ pN2: Metastasis in a single ipsilateral lymph node > 3 cm but ≤ 6 cm in greatest dimension

or in multiple ipsilateral lymph nodes, none > 6 cm in greatest dimension

or in bilateral or contralateral nodes, none > 6 cm in greatest dimension

___ pN2a: Metastasis in single ipsilateral lymph node, > 3 cm but ≤ 6 cm in greatest dimension

___ pN2b: Metastasis in multiple ipsilateral lymph nodes, none > 6 cm in greatest dimension

___ pN2c: Metastasis in midlateral or contralateral lymph nodes, none > 6 cm in greatest dimension

___ pN3: Metastasis in lymph node > 6 cm in greatest dimension

Specify: Number of lymph nodes examined: ________

Number of positive lymph nodes: ________

*Size of largest positive lymph node: ________

*Size of associated metastatic focus: ________

*Position of involved node (level): ________

Distant metastasis (pM)

___ Not applicable

___ pM1: Distant metastasis

*Specify site(s) if known: ____________________

PROTOCOL FOR THE EXAMINATION OF NASAL CAVITY AND PARANASAL SINUS SPECIMENS

*Source of pathologic metastatic specimen (specify): ____________________

For mucosal malignant melanoma

Primary tumor (pT)

___ pT3: Mucosal disease

___ pT4a: Moderately advanced disease; tumor involving deep soft tissue, cartilage, bone, or overlying skin

___ pT4b: Very advanced disease

Tumor involving brain, dura, skull base, lower cranial nerves (IX, X, XI, XII), masticator space, carotid artery, prevertebral space, or mediastinal structures

Regional lymph nodes (pN)

___ pNX: Regional lymph nodes cannot be assessed

___ pN0: No regional lymph node metastases

___ pN1: Regional lymph node metastases present

Distant metastasis (pM)

___ Not applicable

___ pM1: Distant metastasis present

*Specify site(s), if known: ____________________

*Source of pathologic metastatic specimen (specify): ____________________

*Additional Pathologic Findings (select all that apply)

*___ None identified

*___ Carcinoma in situ

*___ Epithelial dysplasia

*Specify: ____________________

*___ Inflammation (specify type): ____________________

*___ Squamous metaplasia

*___ Epithelial hyperplasia

*___ Colonization

*___ Fungal

*___ Bacterial

*___ Other (specify): ____________________

*Ancillary Studies

*Specify type(s): ____________________

*Specify result(s): ____________________

*Clinical History (select all that apply)

*___ Neoadjuvant therapy

*___ Yes (specify type): ____________________

*___ No

*___ Indeterminate

*___ Other (specify): ____________________

**Data elements with asterisks are not required. However, these elements may be clinically important but are not yet validated or regularly used in patient management. †Applicable only to squamous cell carcinoma and histologic variants. ††Metastases at level VII are considered regional lymph node metastases. Midline nodes are considered ipsilateral nodes. Adapted with permission from College of American Pathologists, "Protocol for the Examination of Specimens from Patients with Carcinoma of the Nasal Cavity and Paranasal Sinuses." Web posting date October 2009, www.cap.org.*

Stage Groupings: For All Cancers Except Mucosal Malignant Melanoma

Stage	T	N	M
0	Tis	N0	M0
I	T1	N0	M0
II	T2	N0	M0
III	T1	N1	M0
	T2	N1	M0
	T3	N0, N1	M0
IVA	T1, T2, T3	N2	M0
	T4a	N0, N1, N2	M0
IVB	T4b	Any N	M0
	Any T	N3	M0
IVC	Any T	Any N	M1

Adapted from 7th edition AJCC Staging Forms.

Stage Groupings: For Mucosal Malignant Melanoma

Stage	T	N	M
III	T3	N0	M0
IVA	T4a	N0	M0
	T3-T4a	N1	M0
IVB	T4b	Any N	M0
IVC	Any T	Any N	M1

Adapted from 7th edition AJCC Staging Forms.

PROTOCOL FOR THE EXAMINATION OF NASAL CAVITY AND PARANASAL SINUS SPECIMENS

Anatomic and Tumor Staging Graphics

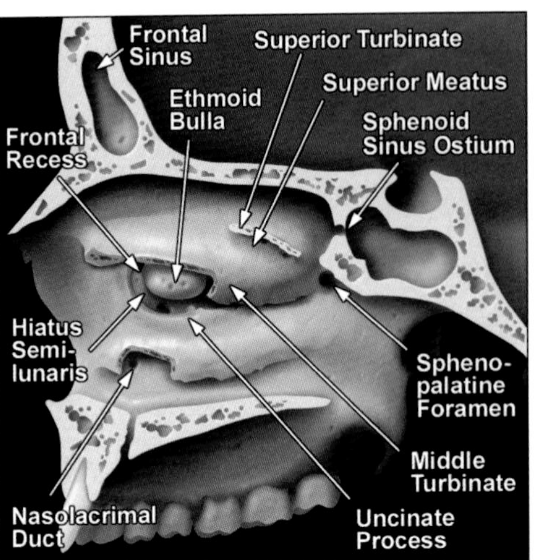

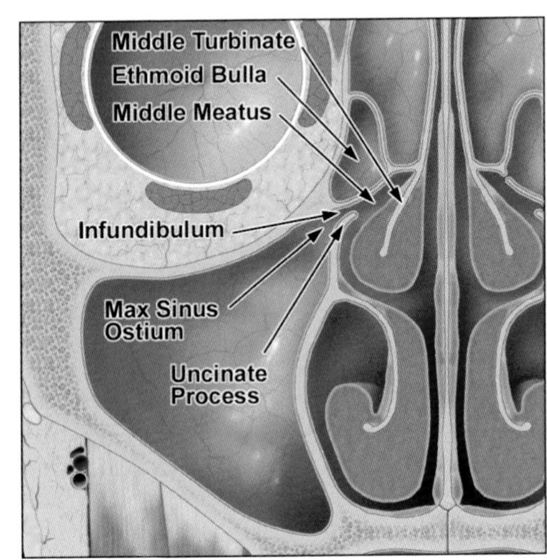

*(**Left**) Sagittal graphic demonstrates the specific anatomic sites within the nasal cavity and paranasal sinus that are useful in accurately classifying tumors of these sites. (**Right**) Coronal graphic demonstrates the anatomic separations of the maxillary sinus from the nasal cavity. The ethmoid sinus and orbit are shown. These anatomic drawings are useful in accurately classifying tumor stage.*

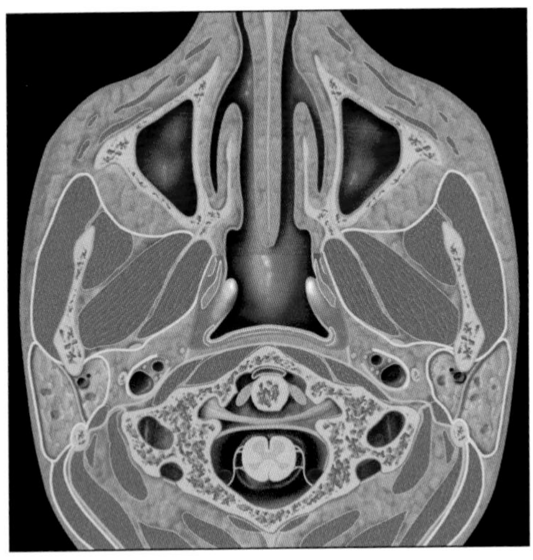

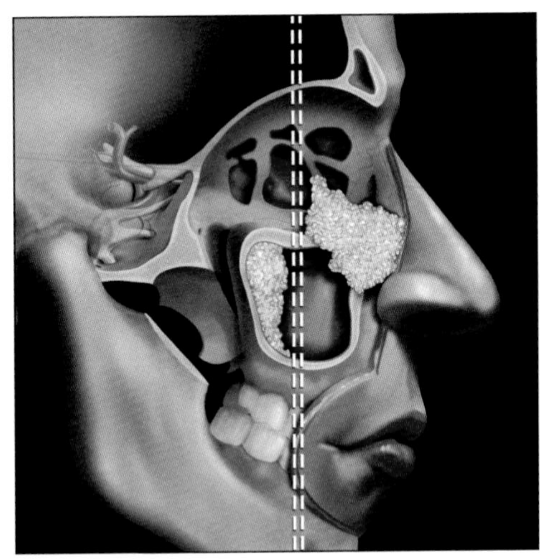

*(**Left**) Axial graphic demonstrates the mucosal surface (purple) of the nasopharynx, while also demonstrating the regions of the maxillary sinus and nasal cavity. (**Right**) Mid-sagittal graphic demonstrates a tumor that involves the maxillary sinus and nasal cavity and expands into the ethmoid sinus. This type of multifocal carcinoma showing origin in the nasal cavity and extension into the ethmoid complex, with bone invasion and maxillary sinus involvement, would be a pT3 tumor.*

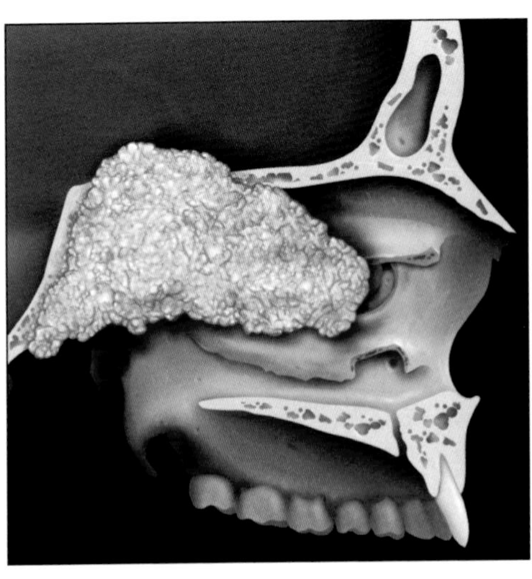

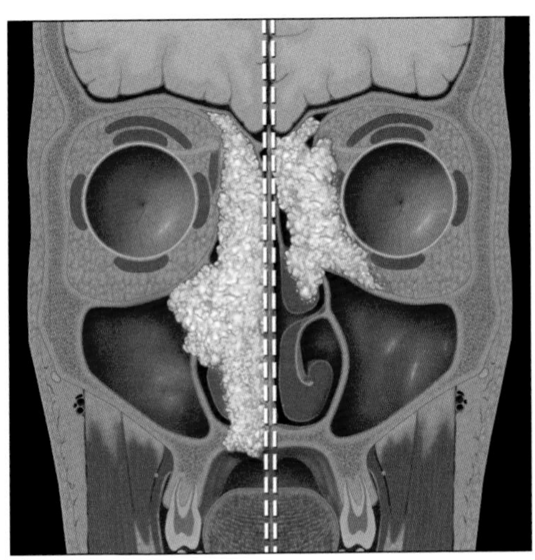

*(**Left**) Sagittal graphic demonstrates a large tumor involving the nasal cavity, sphenoid sinus with base of skull invasion and expansion into the nasopharynx. A tumor of this type would be considered a pT4a since there is only limited cranial fossa involvement. (**Right**) Coronal graphic shows tumor involving both nasal cavities, with expansion into the ethmoid, frontal, and maxillary sinuses as well as anterior orbital content invasion (subcutaneous tissue). This tumor would be considered pT4a.*

Pharynx (Nasal, Oro-, Hypo-)

Congenital/Genetic/Hereditary

Infectious

Reactive

Benign Neoplasm

Malignant Neoplasm

Staging and Grading, Pharynx

DERMOID CYST

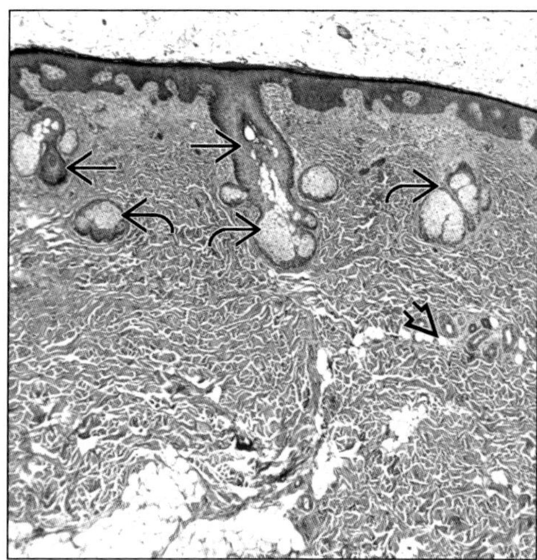

The cyst is lined by stratified squamous epithelium with cutaneous adnexal structures in the fibroconnective tissue wall, including hair follicles ➙, sebaceous glands ➙, and eccrine glands ➙.

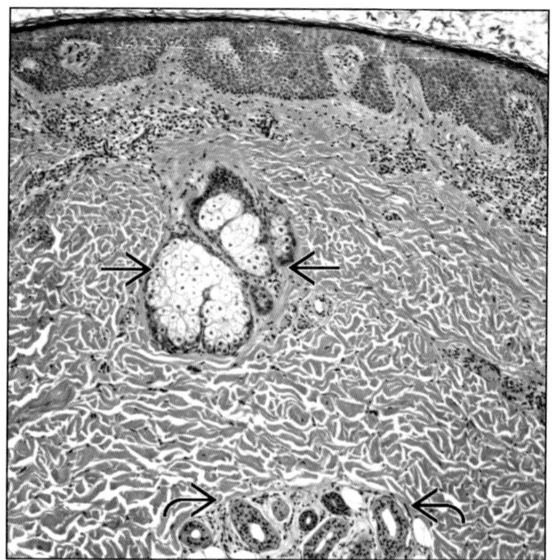

Higher magnification of the cyst wall showing the adnexal structures, including sebaceous glands ➙ and eccrine glands ➙.

TERMINOLOGY

Definitions

- Benign, developmental cystic anomaly originating from ectoderm and mesoderm, but not endoderm

CLINICAL ISSUES

Epidemiology

- Incidence
  - Head & neck
    - Common site of cyst occurrence
    - Accounts for approximately 34% of all dermoid cysts
- Age
  - Most common in 1st decade of life
    - May occur over wide age range
- Gender
  - Equal gender distribution

Site

- Predominantly subcutaneous lesion in head and neck, but may occur in other (mucosal) sites
  - Common noncutaneous sites of occurrence
    - Orbit
    - Oral cavity
    - Nasal cavity
  - Less common sites of occurrence
    - Mandible and maxilla
    - Middle ear
    - Neck (midline or near midline)
    - Upper neck
    - Near thyroid cartilage

Presentation

- Slow-growing mass lesion not associated with pain

Treatment

- Surgical approaches
  - Simple surgical excision is treatment of choice

Prognosis

- Cured following surgical resection

MACROSCOPIC FEATURES

General Features

- Thin-walled cysts containing gray-white friable material
- Internal aspect of cyst has smooth lining

Size

- Range: A few mm to 12 cm in greatest dimension

MICROSCOPIC PATHOLOGY

Histologic Features

- Lined by stratified squamous epithelium with cutaneous adnexal structures in fibroconnective tissue wall
  - Adnexal structures may include
    - Hair shafts
    - Sebaceous glands
    - Eccrine glands
    - Apocrine glands
- Cyst content may include keratin or sebaceous material
- May rupture, resulting in florid foreign body giant cell reaction

DIFFERENTIAL DIAGNOSIS

Teratoma

- Represent true neoplasm comprised of tissues from all 3 germ layers

Epidermal Inclusion Cyst

- Lined by stratified squamous epithelium with keratin-filled cyst lacking adnexal structures

Key Facts

Terminology

- Benign, developmental cystic anomaly originating from ectoderm and mesoderm, but not endoderm

Clinical Issues

- May occur over wide age range but most common in 1st decade of life
- Predominantly subcutaneous lesion in head and neck but may occur in other (mucosal) sites
- Cured following surgical resection

Microscopic Pathology

- Lined by stratified squamous epithelium with cutaneous adnexal structures in fibroconnective tissue wall
- Cyst content may include keratin or sebaceous material
- May rupture, resulting in florid foreign body giant cell reaction

Trichilemmal (Sebaceous) Cyst

- Lined by stratified squamous epithelium showing trichilemmal keratinization with individual cells increasing in bulk and vertical diameter toward luminal aspect
  - Occurs without formation of keratohyaline granules
  - Abrupt change from epithelium to eosinophilic keratin in lumen
  - Resembles external root sheath in region of follicular isthmus

SELECTED REFERENCES

1. Al-Khateeb TH et al: Cutaneous cysts of the head and neck. J Oral Maxillofac Surg. 67(1):52-7, 2009
2. Papadogeorgakis N et al: Surgical management of a large median dermoid cyst of the neck causing airway obstruction. A case report. Oral Maxillofac Surg. 13(3):181-4, 2009
3. Handa U et al: Epidermal inclusion cyst: cytomorphological features and differential diagnosis. Diagn Cytopathol. 36(12):861-3, 2008
4. Rosa PA et al: Congenital neck masses. Oral Maxillofac Surg Clin North Am. 20(3):339-52, 2008
5. Naujoks C et al: Dermoid cyst of the parotid gland--a case report and brief review of the literature. Int J Oral Maxillofac Surg. 36(9):861-3, 2007
6. Golden BA et al: Cutaneous cysts of the head and neck. J Oral Maxillofac Surg. 63(11):1613-9, 2005
7. Pryor SG et al: Pediatric dermoid cysts of the head and neck. Otolaryngol Head Neck Surg. 132(6):938-42, 2005
8. Longo F et al: Midline (dermoid) cysts of the floor of the mouth: report of 16 cases and review of surgical techniques. Plast Reconstr Surg. 112(6):1560-5, 2003
9. Torske KR et al: Dermoid cyst of the maxillary sinus. Ann Diagn Pathol. 5(3):172-6, 2001
10. Coppit GL 3rd et al: Nasopharyngeal teratomas and dermoids: a review of the literature and case series. Int J Pediatr Otorhinolaryngol. 52(3):219-27, 2000
11. Rosen D et al: Dermoid cyst of the lateral neck: a case report and literature review. Ear Nose Throat J. 77(2):125, 129-32, 1998
12. Kayhan FT et al: A nasopharyngeal dermoid causing neonatal airway obstruction. Int J Pediatr Otorhinolaryngol. 40(2-3):195-201, 1997
13. Heffner DK et al: Pharyngeal dermoids ("hairy polyps") as accessory auricles. Ann Otol Rhinol Laryngol. 105(10):819-24, 1996
14. Smirniotopoulos JG et al: Teratomas, dermoids, and epidermoids of the head and neck. Radiographics. 15(6):1437-55, 1995
15. Black EE et al: Dermoid cyst of the floor of the mouth. Oral Surg Oral Med Oral Pathol. 75(5):556-8, 1993
16. Ward RF et al: Teratomas of the head and neck. Otolaryngol Clin North Am. 22(3):621-9, 1989
17. Holt GR et al: Dermoids and teratomas of the head and neck. Ear Nose Throat J. 58(12):520-31, 1979
18. McAvoy JM et al: Dermoid cysts of the head and neck in children. Arch Otolaryngol. 102(9):529-31, 1976
19. Brownstein MH et al: Subcutaneous dermoid cysts. Arch Dermatol. 107(2):237-9, 1973
20. Taylor BW et al: Dermoids of the head and neck. Minn Med. 49(10):1535-40, 1966

IMAGE GALLERY

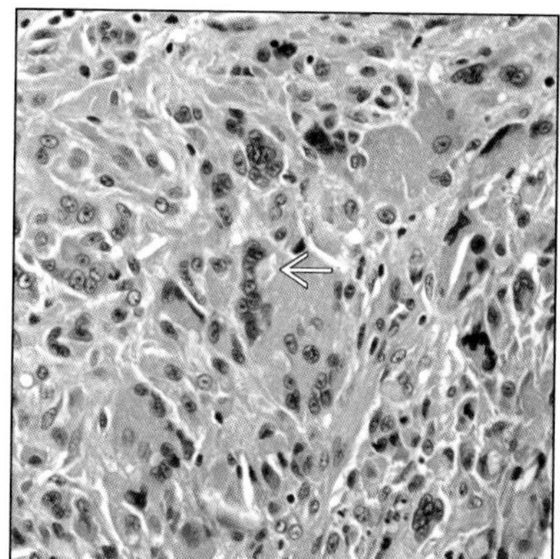

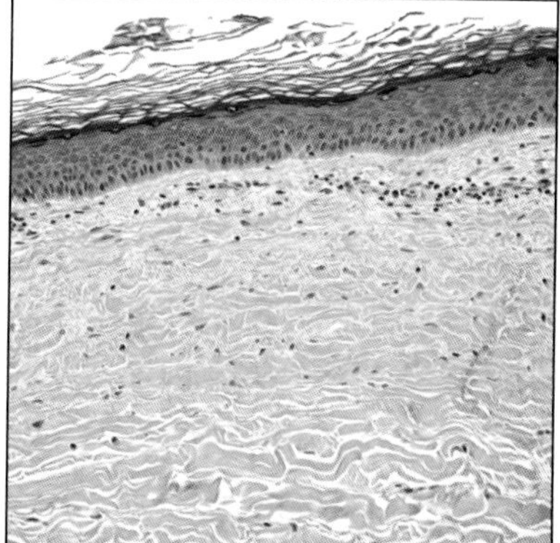

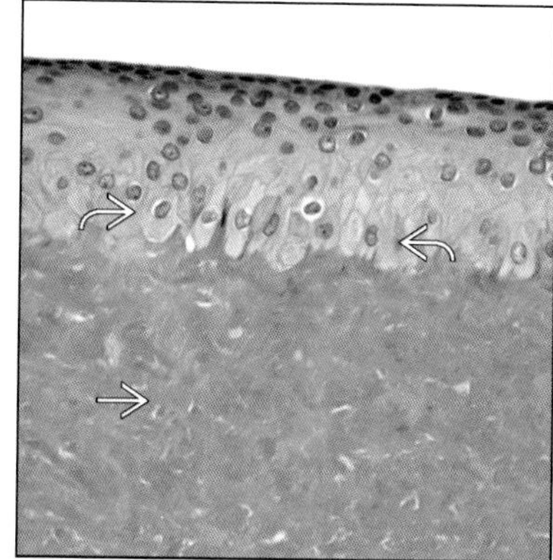

(Left) Rupture of the cyst may result in a foreign body giant cell reaction, including numerous multinucleated giant cells focally with keratin debris ➡. *(Center)* Epidermal inclusion cysts are lined by keratinizing stratified squamous epithelium, but they lack cutaneous adnexal structures in their fibroconnective tissue walls. *(Right)* Trichilemmal cyst is lined by stratified squamous epithelium with trichilemmal keratinization ➡ and abrupt change to keratin in the lumen ➡.

RATHKE CLEFT CYST

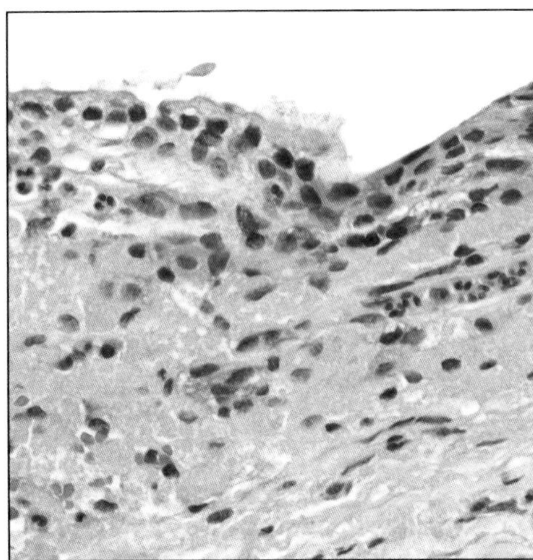

Hematoxylin & eosin shows a ciliated cuboidal to columnar epithelium lining a cystic space. There is fibrosis immediately below. There is no cytologic atypia and pituitary cells are not present.

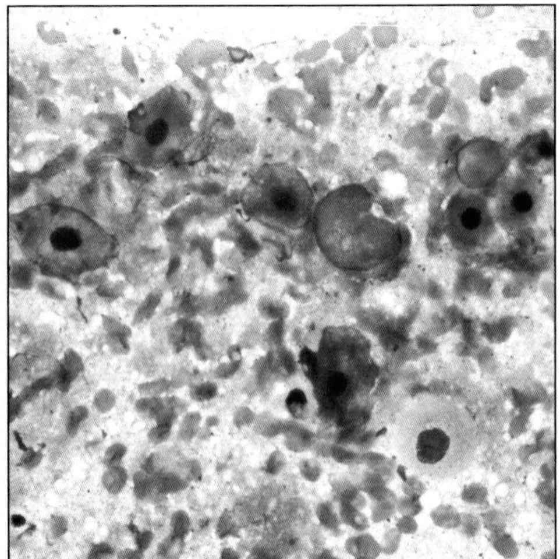

Nucleated squames are shown in a background of blood. This finding can be seen in an epidermoid cyst as well as in a Rathke cleft cyst. Additional clinical and radiographic correlation would be required.

TERMINOLOGY

Abbreviations

- Rathke cleft cyst (RCC)

Definitions

- Cystic tumor located in sellar region filled with fluid, comprised of ciliated epithelium and metaplastic squamous epithelium

ETIOLOGY/PATHOGENESIS

Developmental Anomaly

- Abnormal proliferation of Rathke pouch epithelium

CLINICAL ISSUES

Epidemiology

- Incidence
  - Uncommon in clinical practice, but common incidental autopsy finding
- Age
  - Wide range, but peak in 4th to 5th decades
- Gender
  - Female > Male (1.3:1)

Site

- Intra- or suprasellar

Presentation

- Most commonly presents with headache
- Visual impairment (pressure on optic chiasm/apparatus)
- Pituitary-hypothalamic endocrine disturbance frequently identified
  - Hyperprolactinemia, growth hormone excess, amenorrhea; diabetes insipidus can be seen
  - Pituitary apoplexy is rare

Treatment

- Options, risks, complications
  - Cysts can be followed radiographically (MR) if asymptomatic and nonenlarging (i.e., incidental lesions)
  - Persistent pituitary or visual dysfunction requires management
    - Surgical complication includes diabetes insipidus
  - Packing sella may result in predisposition to recurrent cyst formation
- Surgical approaches
  - Transsphenoidal (transnasal) or transcranial sella surgery
- Drugs
  - Instillation of sclerosing agent (absolute alcohol) to treat residual cyst lining

Prognosis

- Persistence or recurrences develop in about 1/3 of patients
  - Extent of cyst removal and presence of squamous metaplasia in cyst wall increase likelihood of recurrence
  - Follow-up imaging is recommended for at least 10 years as recurrences may take time to develop

IMAGE FINDINGS

MR Findings

- Variable intensity of cystic material in RCC makes radiographic images overlap with other entities
- Suprasellar or intrasellar mass with ovoid shape, small tumor volume, cystic characteristics, no calcifications, and no or thin cyst wall enhancement are more common in RCC
- Enhancement on MR imaging coincides with displacement of pituitary gland, giving posterior ledge sign
- Cyst wall lacks enhancement with gadolinium

RATHKE CLEFT CYST

Key Facts

Etiology/Pathogenesis
- Abnormal proliferation of Rathke pouch epithelium

Clinical Issues
- Intra- or suprasellar lesion
- Presents with headache, visual impairment, endocrine disturbances
- Cysts can be followed if asymptomatic and nonenlarging
- Persistence/recurrence in about 1/3 of patients
- Diabetes insipidus may be a complication

Microscopic Pathology
- Cyst contents are clear to yellow, mucoid to hemorrhagic
- Cyst lined by tall, ciliated, pseudostratified columnar epithelium
- Squamous metaplasia and stratified squamous epithelium
- Inflammatory cells present

MACROSCOPIC FEATURES

General Features
- Cyst contents intraoperatively are clear (CSF-like) to yellow, mucoid to hemorrhagic

Size
- Range: 0.5-4 cm, mean: 2 cm

MICROSCOPIC PATHOLOGY

Histologic Features
- Cyst filled with mucinous and squamous debris
- Lining of tall, ciliated, pseudostratified columnar epithelium
- Squamous metaplasia and stratified squamous epithelium seen
- Inflammatory cells can be seen, including acute and chronic cells
- Isolated glands may be seen
- Concurrent pituitary adenoma can be demonstrated

ANCILLARY TESTS

Cytology
- Clinicoradiologic features and anatomic site used in conjunction with cytology
- Aspirates show single and aggregates of keratinizing squamous cells, anucleate squames, and hemosiderin-laden macrophages

Immunohistochemistry
- Positive with LMW keratins: CK8 and CK20
- Negative for nuclear accumulation of β-catenin

DIFFERENTIAL DIAGNOSIS

Craniopharyngioma
- Tends to be larger
- Has calcifications, keratinaceous debris, multinucleated giant cells, basaloid epithelium
- Negative with CK8 and CK20

Epidermoid Cyst
- Pituitary tissue immediately adjacent to squamous epithelium, prominent keratohyaline granules

Metastatic Squamous Cell Carcinoma
- Remarkably atypical epithelial cells, background of necroinflammatory debris

SELECTED REFERENCES

1. Aho CJ et al: Surgical outcomes in 118 patients with Rathke cleft cysts. J Neurosurg. 102(2):189-93, 2005
2. Parwani AV et al: Keratinized squamous cells in fine needle aspiration of the brain. Cytopathologic correlates and differential diagnosis. Acta Cytol. 47(3):325-31, 2003
3. Kleinschmidt-DeMasters BK et al: The pathologic, surgical, and MR spectrum of Rathke cleft cysts. Surg Neurol. 44(1):19-26; discussion 26-7, 1995

IMAGE GALLERY

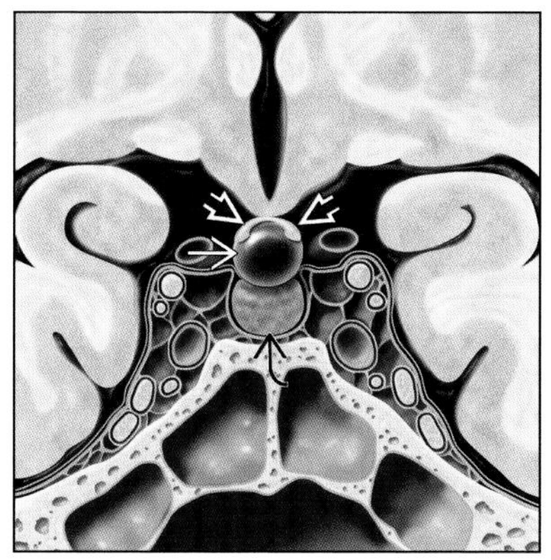

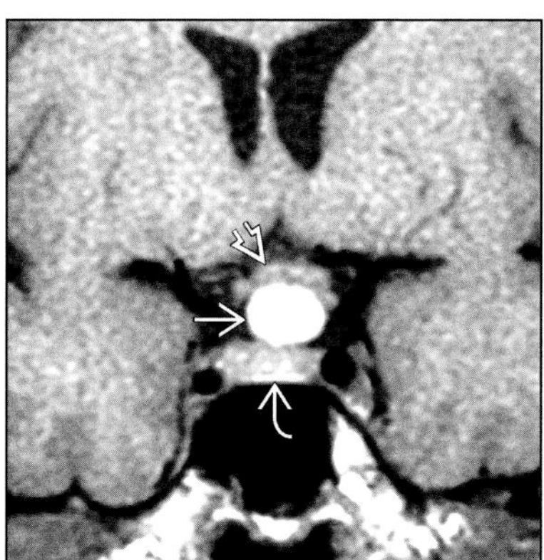

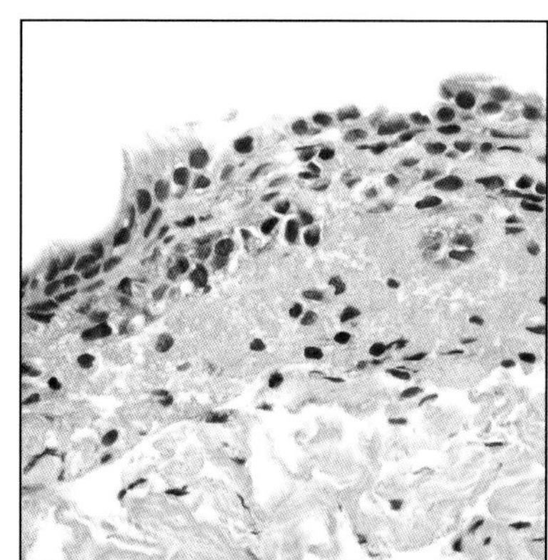

*(**Left**) Coronal graphic shows a typical suprasellar Rathke cyst ➡ interposed between pituitary gland ➡ & optic chiasm ➡. Note optic chiasm is bowed upward by cyst mass effect. (**Center**) Coronal T1 MR shows a classic Rathke cyst ➡ that elevates & drapes the optic chiasm ➡. Pituitary gland ➡ is normal. 50% of Rathke cysts are high signal (bright) on T1 MR imaging, while the other 50% are low signal (dark). (**Right**) Delicate cilia is seen on the surface of cuboidal cells. There are no contents in the lumen of this cyst. There is fibrosis below the epithelium.*

TORNWALDT CYST

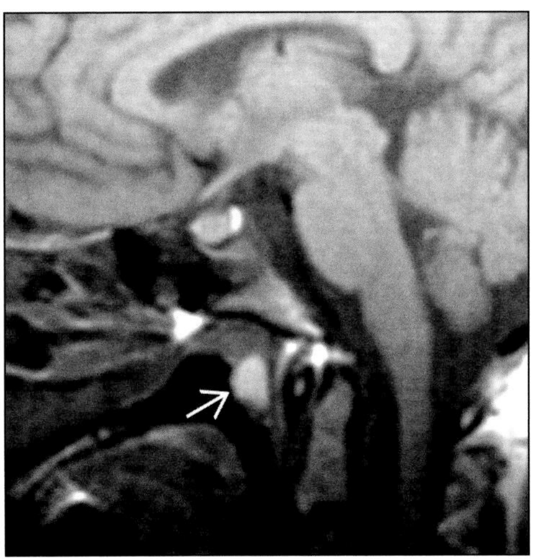

Sagittal T1WI MR shows a high signal Tornwaldt cyst ➡ in the superficial nasopharyngeal soft tissues. The high signal is the result of high protein content in the cyst fluid.

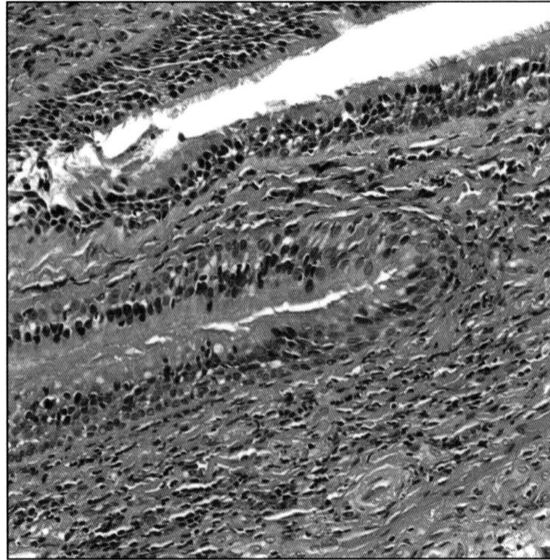

Hematoxylin & eosin shows a respiratory epithelial-lined cystic cavity. This is a common finding in a Tornwaldt cyst, and it requires a clinical &/or radiographic correlation.

TERMINOLOGY

Synonyms

- Thornwaldt, Thornwald, Tornwald, Tornwaldt cyst
- Thornwaldt disease

Definitions

- Expansion of a virtual space in nasopharynx midline into a mucosal cyst at a point where embryonic notochord and nasopharyngeal ectoderm meet
  - Initially small diverticulum retracts and expands into a cyst with time
    - Especially under the influence of inflammation, which obliterates cyst opening (mouth)
  - Notochord gives rise to vertebrae
    - Cysts are close to vertebrae

ETIOLOGY/PATHOGENESIS

Developmental Anomaly

- Pharyngeal bursa (Tornwaldt bursa) is persistent communication between roof of nasopharynx and notochord
  - Formed within space between notochord and pharyngeal ectoderm
  - If the opening that drains bursa into nasopharynx becomes obstructed, Tornwaldt cyst develops
  - Around 10th week of embryonic development, pouch forms by adhesion of pharyngeal ectoderm to notochord at most cranial end of notochord

Mechanical Injury

- Adenoidectomy may cause injury of pharyngeal duct orifice, with subsequent inflammation resulting in cyst development

CLINICAL ISSUES

Epidemiology

- Incidence
  - Identified in up to 5% of healthy adults
    - Detected during radiographic evaluation for different reasons
    - Large study identified 0.06% (32 of 53,013 CTs and MRs performed)
- Age
  - Peak incidence at 30-55 years
- Gender
  - Equal gender distribution

Site

- Posterior-superior nasopharynx midline

Presentation

- Most cases are asymptomatic, radiographically detected
  - Symptoms can be induced by mechanical stimuli
- Upper respiratory tract infection type symptoms
  - Inflammation or abscess of cyst may yield symptoms
- Long symptom duration; cyst forms gradually as fluid accumulates following duct obliteration
- Periodic, purulent, foul-tasting discharge of fluid into mouth, or postnasal drip
- Nasal obstruction, obstructive sleep apnea
- Halitosis
- Ear fullness, ear ache, ear discomfort (eustachian tube dysfunction)
- Clearing of throat
- Occipital pain/headaches, neck pain
- Dizziness and vertigo

Treatment

- Options, risks, complications
  - Asymptomatic patients can be followed with serial images (stable size)
  - Complications may include middle ear effusion

TORNWALDT CYST

Key Facts

Terminology
- Expansion of virtual space in nasopharynx midline into a cyst where embryonic notochord and nasopharyngeal ectoderm meet

Clinical Issues
- Peak incidence: 30-55 years of age
- Posterior-superior nasopharynx midline
- Most cases are asymptomatic, radiographically detected
- Symptoms include foul-tasting discharge, headaches, halitosis, and ear symptoms

Image Findings
- ≥ 7 mm mass between longus capitis muscles, without soft tissue inflammatory changes

Microscopic Pathology
- Cyst lined by respiratory epithelium

- Surgical approaches
  - Marsupialization
  - Complete excision (endoscopic or transpalatal)

IMAGE FINDINGS

MR Findings
- MR is exam of choice
  - Up to 5% of brain MR exams reveal incidental Tornwaldt cysts
- High signal intensity on both T1- and T2-weighted images due to protein &/or hemorrhage within cyst
- Mass between longus capitis muscles, ≥ 7 mm in diameter, without soft tissue inflammatory changes or concurrent bone involvement
  - Fat-saturated axial T1-weighted, pre- and post-contrast images are optimal
  - Adhesion to cervical vertebrae is noted

MICROSCOPIC PATHOLOGY

Histologic Features
- Cyst up to 3 cm (mean: 0.6 cm)
- Well-circumscribed rounded cyst immediately deep to mucosa
- Cyst lined by respiratory epithelium
- Fluid with variable proteinaceous and inflammatory debris

DIFFERENTIAL DIAGNOSIS

Nasopharyngeal Teratoma
- Sessile-polypoid mass; cranial deformities (anencephaly, hemicrania, palate fissures); mature glial tissue mixed with skin, hair, bone, and teeth

Branchial Cleft Cyst
- Usually paired lateral masses with inflammation adjacent to epithelium

Encephalocele/Meningocele
- Brain or meninges within cystic space; no epithelium

SELECTED REFERENCES

1. Christmas DA Jr et al: Endoscopic view of obstructing nasopharyngeal cysts (Tornwaldt's cysts). Ear Nose Throat J. 86(10):591-2, 2007
2. Magliulo G et al: Tornwaldt's cyst and magnetic resonance imaging. Ann Otol Rhinol Laryngol. 110(9):895-6, 2001
3. Ikushima I et al: MR imaging of Tornwaldt's cysts. AJR Am J Roentgenol. 172(6):1663-5, 1999
4. Miyahara H et al: Tornwaldt's disease. Acta Otolaryngol Suppl. 517:36-9, 1994
5. Weissman JL: Thornwaldt cysts. Am J Otolaryngol. 13(6):381-5, 1992
6. Kwok P et al: Tornwaldt's cyst: clinical and radiological aspects. J Otolaryngol. 16(2):104-7, 1987
7. Miller RH et al: Tornwaldt's bursa. Clin Otolaryngol Allied Sci. 10(1):21-5, 1985

IMAGE GALLERY

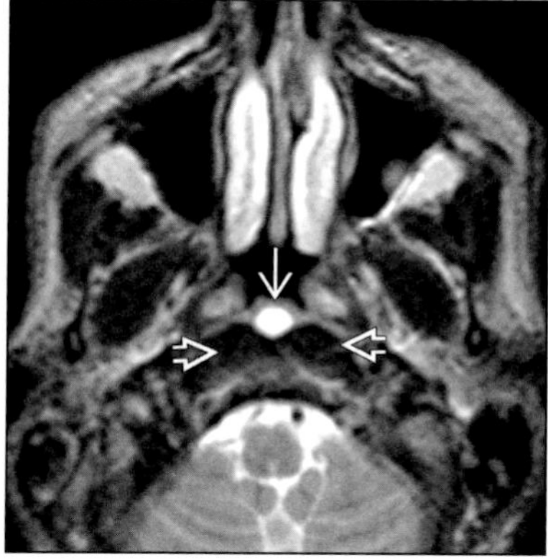
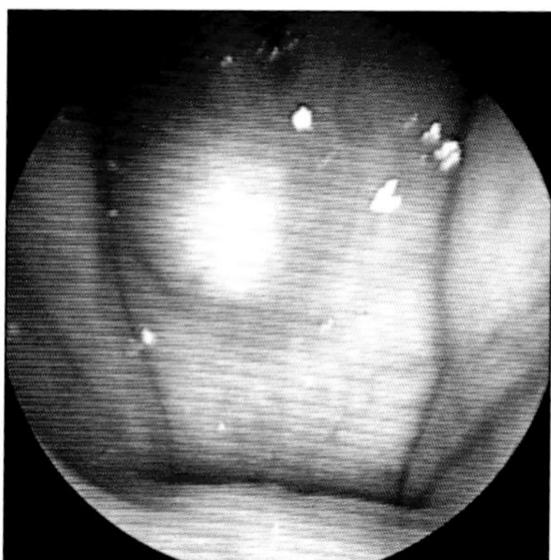
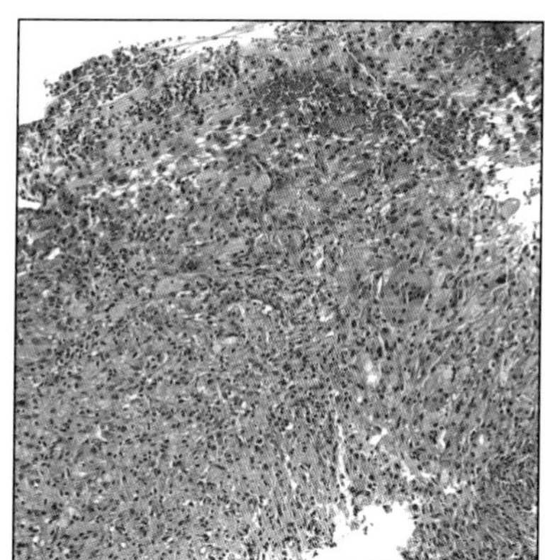

*(**Left**) Axial T2-weighted MR shows a well-circumscribed, oval, high signal cyst in the posterior midline nasopharynx wall ➡. Note the lesion is anterior to the prevertebral muscles ⇨. (**Center**) Endoscopic photograph shows a nodule on the nasopharynx mucosa. There is a yellow, bulging nodule in the nasopharynx. (Courtesy D. Cua, MD.) (**Right**) A foreign body giant cell-type reaction is seen with inflammatory cells and histiocytes due to cyst rupture.*

TANGIER DISEASE

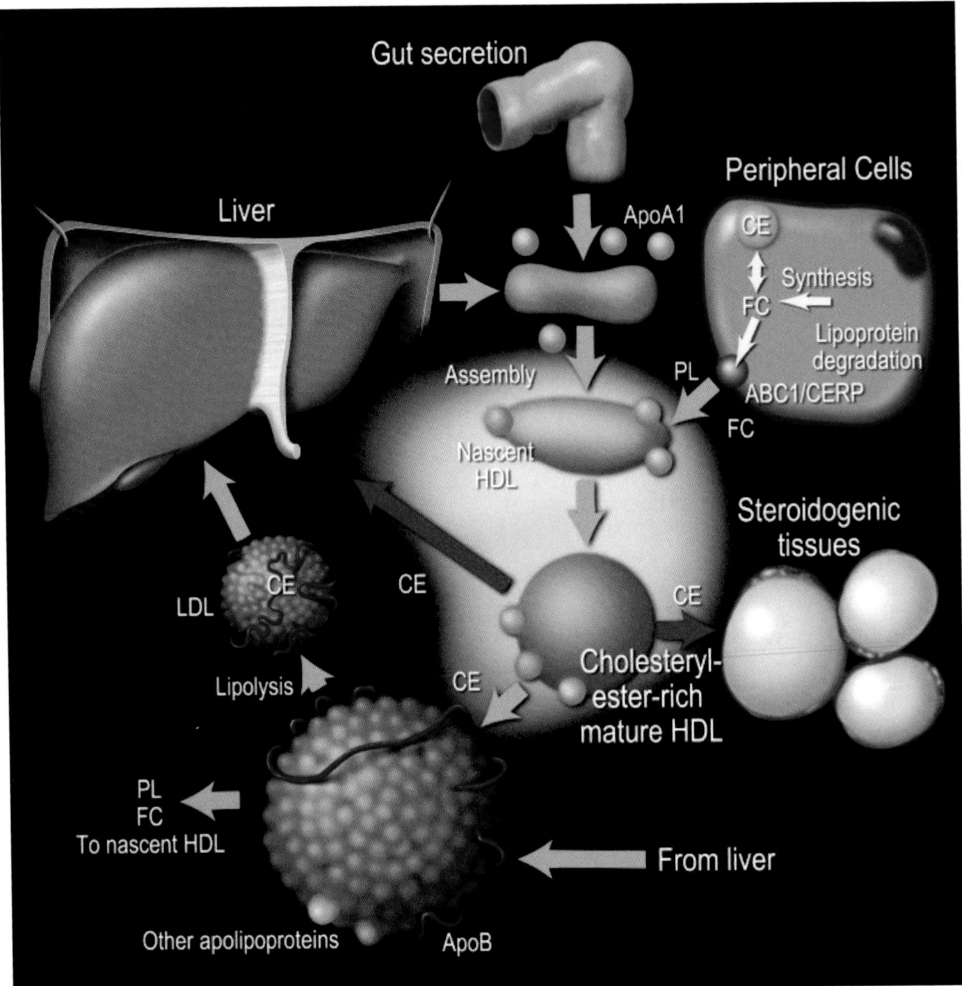

CERP is necessary for bulk transfer of free cholesterol (FC) and phospholipids out of cells. ApoA1 and HDL act as acceptors for cholesterol. The FC is esterified (cholesteryl ester, CE) and transferred to LDL and to cells by SRB1. TD patients have defects in CERP, with ApoA1 rapidly cleared from the circulation and degraded (defects of TD are light green).

TERMINOLOGY

Definitions

- Severe high-density lipoprotein (HDL) deficiency syndrome characterized by accumulation of cholesterol in tissue macrophages with prevalent atherosclerosis (α-lipoprotein deficiency)

ETIOLOGY/PATHOGENESIS

Developmental Anomaly

- Autosomal-recessive inherited disorder
  - Defect in chromosome 9q31
  - May be due to different metabolic errors or common metabolic error subject to genetic influences
- HDLs play a central role in transporting cholesterol from peripheral tissues to liver for elimination
- Defect of HDL-mediated cholesterol transport favors cholesterol deposition in arterial walls
- Caused by mutations in cell membrane protein adenosine triphosphate (ATP)-binding cassette transporter A1 (*ABCA1*) and cholesterol-efflux regulatory protein (*CERP*) pathways

CLINICAL ISSUES

Epidemiology

- Incidence
  - Rare, autosomal-recessive inherited disorder
  - Affected families identified on Tangier Island, VA, in Chesapeake Bay
    - Also in Missouri, Kentucky, and Europe
- Age
  - All ages, but usually < 40 years at initial presentation
  - Childhood deposition of cholesterol esters yields grotesquely enlarged tonsils and adenoids
- Gender
  - Equal gender distribution

TANGIER DISEASE

Key Facts

Terminology
- Severe HDL deficiency syndrome characterized by accumulation of cholesterol in tissue macrophages and prevalent atherosclerosis

Etiology/Pathogenesis
- Autosomal-recessive inherited disorder, mutation in *ABCA1* and *CERP* pathways

Clinical Issues
- Affected families live on Tangier Island, Virginia
- Massive accumulation of cholesterol esters in macrophages

Microscopic Pathology
- Bright orange-yellow tonsils and adenoids
- Prominent accumulation of foamy histiocytes (xanthoma cells) in clusters

Site
- Massive, abnormal accumulation of cholesterol esters in macrophages in many tissues
- Accumulation is most conspicuous in tonsils
- Also occurs in nerves and vessels

Presentation
- Presentation is related to abnormal storage of cholesteryl esters
- Abnormal accumulation in tonsils, lymph nodes, spleen, liver, and bone marrow
- Peripheral neuropathy
  - Multiple different nerves may be affected
  - Slowly progressive neuropathy
  - Prominent peripheral nerve demyelination and remyelination may be seen
- Atherosclerosis
- Corneal infiltrates may affect vision

Laboratory Tests
- Depends on homozygous or heterozygous state
- Heterozygotes have low concentrations of HDL
- Homozygotes
  - Severe deficiency or absence of HDL-C in plasma
    - One of A proteins is reduced to < 1% of normal
  - LDL levels tend to be reduced
- Normal or elevated triglyceride levels

Prognosis
- Premature vascular disease may develop and give heart disease at very early age

MACROSCOPIC FEATURES

General Features
- Bright orange-yellow tonsils and adenoids
- Large, lobulated, and hyperplastic tonsils and adenoids

MICROSCOPIC PATHOLOGY

Histologic Features
- Prominent accumulation of foamy histiocytes (xanthoma cells) in clusters
- In parafollicular or interfollicular zones
- Histiocytes contain lipid droplets (cholesterol esters) and occasionally crystalline material
- Must exclude infectious etiology

DIFFERENTIAL DIAGNOSIS

Klebsiella Rhinoscleromatis
- Foamy histiocytes are filled with infectious organisms

SELECTED REFERENCES

1. Kolovou GD et al: Tangier disease four decades of research: a reflection of the importance of HDL. Curr Med Chem. 13(7):771-82, 2006
2. Nofer JR et al: Tangier disease: still more questions than answers. Cell Mol Life Sci. 62(19-20):2150-60, 2005
3. Nelson BL et al: Tonsil with Tangier disease. Ear Nose Throat J. 82(3):178, 2003

IMAGE GALLERY

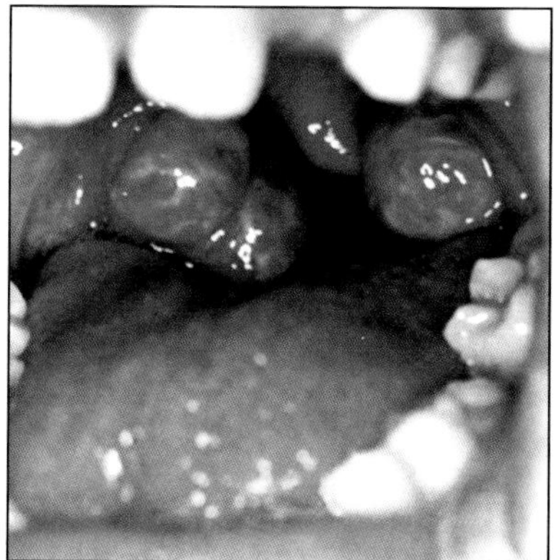

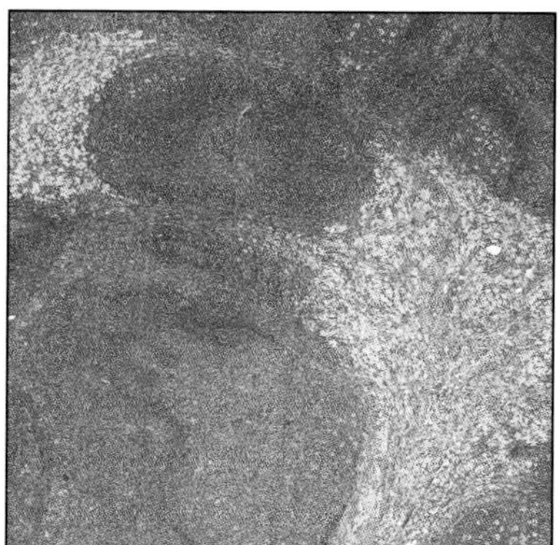

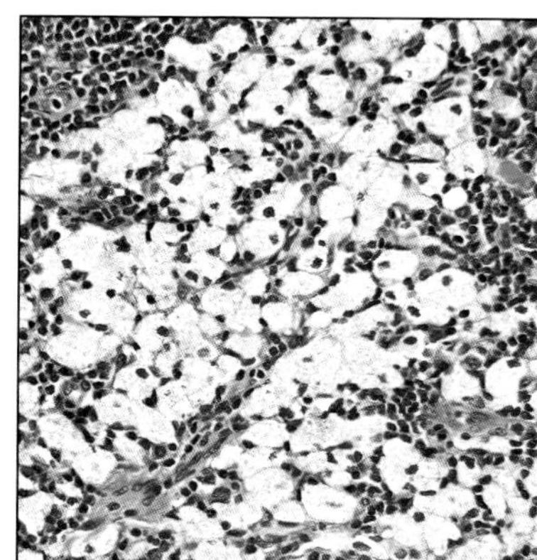

(Left) *Gross photograph of the enlarged tonsils shows a slightly orange appearance. (National Library of Medicine: Jiménez Díaz Memorial Lecture, Madrid, 1974.)* ***(Center)*** *There is a parafollicular accumulation of pale-staining, foamy histiocytes.* ***(Right)*** *Hematoxylin and eosin stained material shows histiocytes filled with clear esters. Organisms are not identified (using other histochemistries).*

INFECTIOUS MONONUCLEOSIS

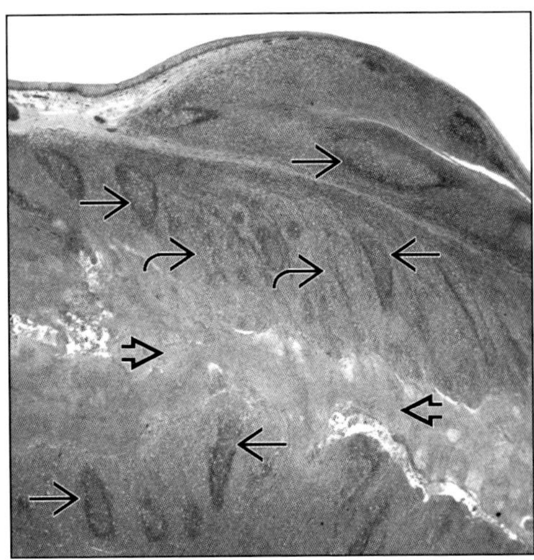

Excised tonsil shows distortion and partial effacement of tonsillar architecture with preservation of germinal centers ➔ with interfollicular (cellular) expansion ➔ and foci of necrosis ➔.

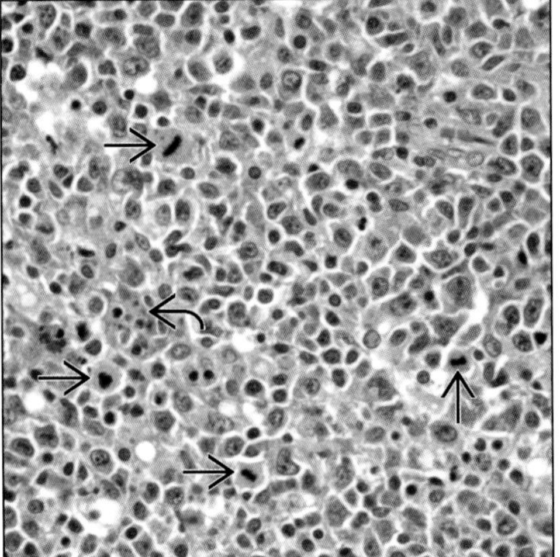

Cellular components of the interfollicular area show marked nuclear atypia with increased mitotic activity ➔ and individual cell necrosis ➔, findings worrisome for a lymphoma.

TERMINOLOGY

Abbreviations

- Infectious mononucleosis (IM)

Definitions

- Systemic, benign, self-limiting infectious lymphoproliferative disease primarily caused by, but not limited to, Epstein-Barr virus (EBV) infection

ETIOLOGY/PATHOGENESIS

Infectious Agents

- EBV estimated to cause 80-95% of IM cases
- EBV
  - Enveloped icosahedral herpesvirus with double-stranded linear DNA
  - Strongly tropic for B lymphocytes
    - Also tropic for T lymphocytes
  - Associated with
    - Oral hairy leukoplakia
    - NK-/T-cell lymphoma, nasal type
    - Burkitt lymphoma
    - Hodgkin lymphoma
    - Nasopharyngeal-type nonkeratinizing carcinomas (differentiated and undifferentiated)
  - Virus penetrates nasopharyngeal epithelium and infects B lymphocytes
  - EBV-infected B-cells proliferate and elicit humoral and cellular immune responses
- Other microorganisms associated with mononucleosis-like syndromes include
  - Cytomegalovirus (CMV)
  - *Toxoplasma gondii*
  - Rubella
  - Hepatitis A virus
  - Adenoviruses

CLINICAL ISSUES

Epidemiology

- Age
  - May occur in all age groups, but primarily affects adolescents and young adults
- Gender
  - Equal gender distribution

Site

- Tonsils

Presentation

- Acute pharyngotonsillitis with patients experiencing sore throat, fever, and malaise
  - Pharyngotonsillitis often severe and may be exudative
  - Pharyngitis characterized by marked swollen and enlarged tonsils covered by dirty gray exudates
- Lymphadenopathy and hepatosplenomegaly with chemical evidence of hepatitis may represent systemic manifestations of disease
  - Lymphadenopathy commonly affects posterior cervical lymph nodes, but both anterior and posterior nodes may be involved
  - Tender lymphadenopathy
- Prodromal period of 2-5 days with malaise and fatigue frequently occurs prior to onset of full syndrome

Laboratory Tests

- Absolute lymphocytosis with > 50% lymphocytes in total leukocyte population of > 5,000/mm^3
- Prominent atypical lymphocytes (Downey cells) often > 10% of total leukocyte count
  - Atypical lymphocytes in peripheral blood thought to represent mostly activated T-lymphocyte populations in response to B-cell infection
- Mild to moderate elevations of liver enzymes, including aspartate and alanine aminotransferase

INFECTIOUS MONONUCLEOSIS

Key Facts

Terminology
- Systemic, benign, self-limiting infectious lymphoproliferative disease primarily caused by, but not limited to, Epstein-Barr virus (EBV) infection

Etiology/Pathogenesis
- EBV estimated to cause 80-95% of IM cases

Clinical Issues
- May occur in all age groups, but primarily affects adolescents and young adults
- Acute pharyngotonsillitis with patients experiencing sore throat, fever, and malaise
- Prodromal period of 2-5 days with malaise and fatigue frequently occurs prior to onset of full syndrome
- Absolute lymphocytosis with > 50% lymphocytes in total leukocyte population of > 5,000/mm^3
- Prominent atypical lymphocytes (Downey cells) often > 10% of total leukocyte count
- Therapy is supportive, including rest and fluid intake

Microscopic Pathology
- Distortion &/or partial effacement of nodal/tonsillar architecture with
  - Reactive follicular hyperplasia characterized by enlarged and irregularly shaped germinal centers
- Expansion of interfollicular areas with polymorphous proliferation of
  - Small lymphocytes, transformed lymphocytes, immunoblasts, plasma cells, and Reed-Sternberg-like cells

- Diagnosis confirmed by demonstration of serum antibodies to
  - Horse red cells (positive monospot test)
  - Sheep erythrocytes (positive Paul-Bunnell heterophile antibody test)
- Non-EBV infectious agents causing IM not associated with positive heterophile antibody test and monospot test
- Patients consistently heterophile antibody or monospot negative; serodiagnosis is invaluable and includes
  - Appreciable serum response to EBV viral capsid antigen (VCA) with both IgM and IgG antibodies at time of clinical presentation
    - IgM antibodies to VCA disappear within 2-3 months following infection
    - IgG antibodies to VCA persist for life, indicative of chronic carrier state
  - At presentation or shortly thereafter, many infected patients will develop antibodies to early antigen complex (EA)
    - Antibodies to EA disappear within 2-6 months following infection
  - During early phase of primary infection, antibodies to EBV nuclear antigens (EBNA) are usually not demonstrable
    - Anti-EBNA antibodies persist for life, indicative of chronic carrier state

Treatment
- Options, risks, complications
  - Therapy is supportive, including rest and fluid intake

Prognosis
- Favorable clinical course, often with resolution of symptoms over a period of several months
- Rarely, serious and potentially fatal complications may develop and include
  - Airway obstruction and splenic rupture, the latter secondary to splenic involvement with massive splenomegaly

MICROSCOPIC PATHOLOGY

Histologic Features
- Distortion &/or partial effacement of nodal/tonsillar architecture with reactive follicular hyperplasia
  - Characterized by enlarged and irregularly shaped germinal centers
- Expansion of interfollicular areas with polymorphous proliferation of
  - Small lymphocytes
  - Transformed lymphocytes
  - Immunoblasts
  - Plasma cells
  - Reed-Sternberg-like cells
  - Presence of immunoblasts may result in mottled appearance
- Lymphocytic and immunoblastic proliferations often display marked cytologic atypia with
  - One or more prominent nucleoli
  - Increased mitotic activity
  - Phagocytosis
- Immunoblasts may
  - Cluster or form sheets effacing portions of tissue, simulating malignant lymphoma
  - Occasionally be binucleate, simulating appearance of Reed-Sternberg cells of Hodgkin lymphoma
- Necrosis may be seen
  - Usually focal
  - Characterized by individual cell necrosis, although larger confluent zones may be present
- Vascular proliferation with prominent endothelial cells always present

ANCILLARY TESTS

Histochemistry
- Stains for microorganisms are negative

Immunohistochemistry
- B-cell and T-cell reactivity without im
  for CD15 (Leu M1)

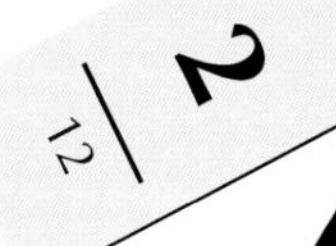

- Immunoblasts may be CD30(+)
- Immunoreactivity can be seen for
  - EBV latent membrane protein
  - In situ hybridization for Epstein-Barr encoded RNA (EBER)

Cytogenetics

- Absence of gene rearrangements

Molecular Genetics

- PCR analysis detects virus
  - Generation of proteins containing EBV-encoded polypeptide sequences
  - Represent more reliable and sensitive means for detecting presence of virus than serodiagnosis

DIFFERENTIAL DIAGNOSIS

HIV Infection

- Morphologic features of acute & chronic phases of HIV tonsils not present in IM
  - Florid follicular hyperplasia
  - Follicle lysis
  - Attenuation to loss of mantle lymphocytes
  - Giant cells localized to surface &/or crypt epithelium
- Presence of immunoreactivity for HIV p24

Lymphoma

- Diffuse large cell B-cell lymphoma and anaplastic CD30(+) large cell lymphoma
  - Typically includes effacement of architecture with loss of germinal centers
  - Monoclonality by immunohistochemistry
  - Presence of gene rearrangements

Hodgkin Lymphoma

- Primary Hodgkin lymphoma of tonsils &/or mucosal sites of upper aerodigestive tract exceedingly rare
- Hodgkin lymphoma involving tonsils &/or mucosal sites of upper aerodigestive tract usually secondary to primary nodal-based disease

SELECTED REFERENCES

1. Gulley ML et al: Laboratory assays for Epstein-Barr virus-related disease. J Mol Diagn. 10(4):279-92, 2008
2. Rezk SA et al: Epstein-Barr virus-associated lymphoproliferative disorders. Hum Pathol. 38(9):1293-304, 2007
3. Kutok JL et al: Spectrum of Epstein-Barr virus-associated diseases. Annu Rev Pathol. 1:375-404, 2006
4. Kojima M et al: Lymph node lesion in infectious mononucleosis showing geographic necrosis containing cytologically atypically B-cells. A case report. Pathol Res Pract. 200(1):53-7, 2004
5. Vetsika EK et al: Infectious mononucleosis and Epstein-Barr virus. Expert Rev Mol Med. 6(23):1-16, 2004
6. Taylor GH: Cytomegalovirus. Am Fam Physician. 67(3):519-24, 2003
7. Kojima M et al: Lymph node infarction associated with infectious mononucleosis: report of a case resembling lymph node infarction associated with malignant lymphoma. Int J Surg Pathol. 10(3):223-6, 2002
8. Chan SC et al: The management of severe infectious mononucleosis tonsillitis and upper airway obstruction. J Laryngol Otol. 115(12):973-7, 2001
9. Beazley DM et al: Toxoplasmosis. Semin Perinatol. 22(4):332-8, 1998
10. Peter J et al: Infectious mononucleosis. Pediatr Rev. 19(8):276-9, 1998
11. Kapadia SB et al: Hodgkin's disease of Waldeyer's ring. Clinical and histoimmunophenotypic findings and association with Epstein-Barr virus in 16 cases. Am J Surg Pathol. 19(12):1431-9, 1995
12. Bailey RE: Diagnosis and treatment of infectious mononucleosis. Am Fam Physician. 49(4):879-88, 1994
13. Strickler JG et al: Infectious mononucleosis in lymphoid tissue. Histopathology, in situ hybridization, and differential diagnosis. Arch Pathol Lab Med. 117(3):269-78, 1993
14. Gaffey MJ et al: Association of Epstein-Barr virus with human neoplasia. Pathol Annu. 27 Pt 1:55-74, 1992
15. Isaacson PG et al: Epstein-Barr virus latent membrane protein expression by Hodgkin and Reed-Sternberg-like cells in acute infectious mononucleosis. J Pathol. 167(3):267-71, 1992
16. Abbondanzo SL et al: Acute infectious mononucleosis. CD30 (Ki-1) antigen expression and histologic correlations. Am J Clin Pathol. 93(5):698-702, 1990
17. Childs CC et al: Infectious mononucleosis. The spectrum of morphologic changes simulating lymphoma in lymph nodes and tonsils. Am J Surg Pathol. 11(2):122-32, 1987

Microscopic and Immunohistochemical Features

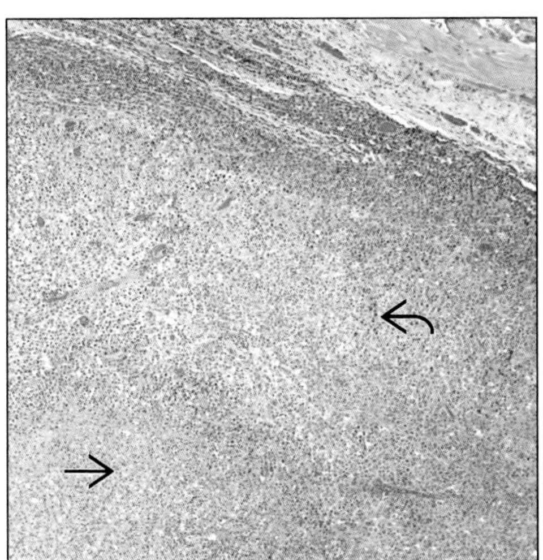
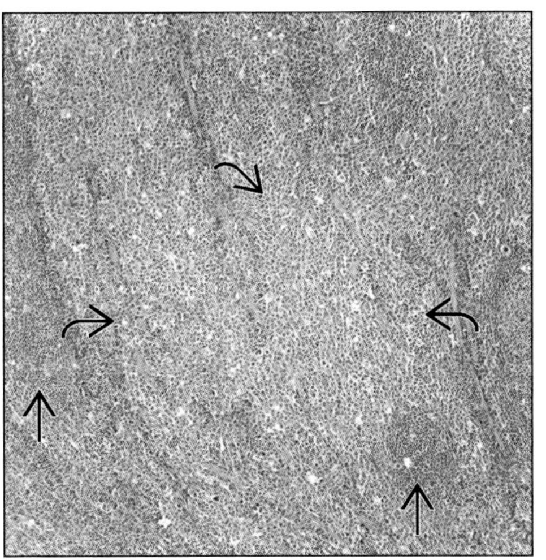

(Left) *Juxtaposition of diffuse cellular proliferation ↷ and area of confluent necrosis → is shown.* ***(Right)*** *There is preservation of germinal centers → with distortion of the tonsillar architecture due to marked interfollicular (cellular) expansion ↷. The overall light microscopic features, including necrosis and especially the presence of a markedly atypical cellular infiltrate, raise concern for a diagnosis of lymphoma.*

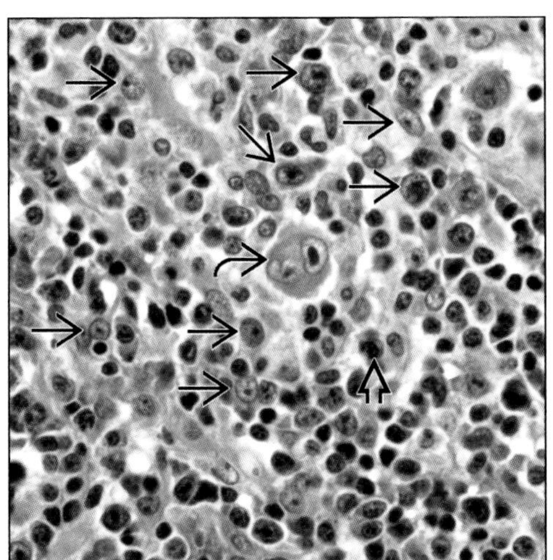
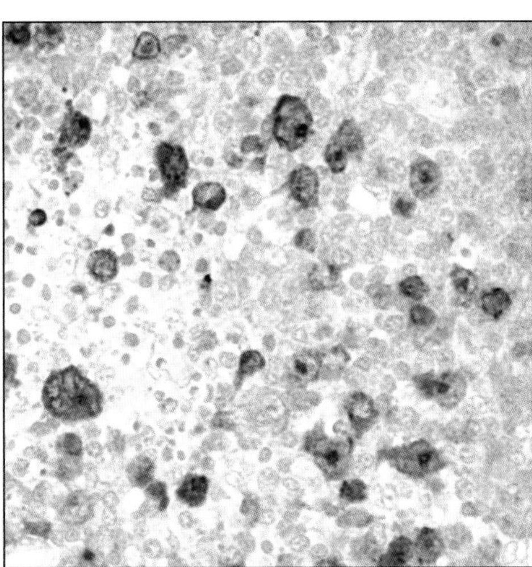

(Left) *The interfollicular area includes a proliferation of numerous immunoblasts →, as well as lymphocytes, plasma cells ⇨, and Reed-Sternberg-like cells ↷. Out of context, at higher magnification the cytomorphologic features certainly suggest a possible diagnosis of a lymphoma.* ***(Right)*** *Epstein-Barr virus (EBV) is the cause in the majority of cases of infectious mononucleosis as shown by the presence of immunoreactivity for EBV latent membrane protein.*

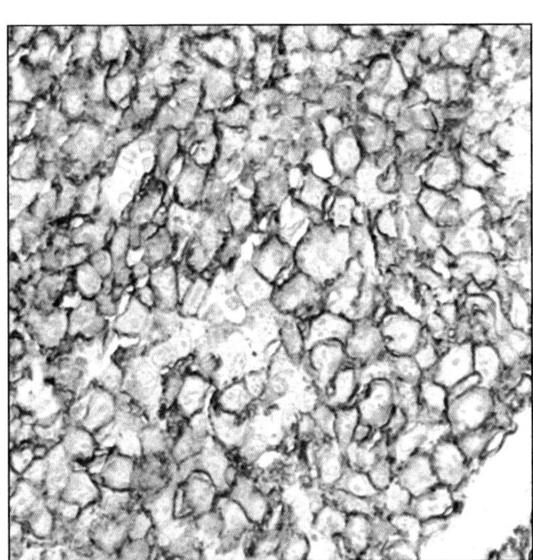
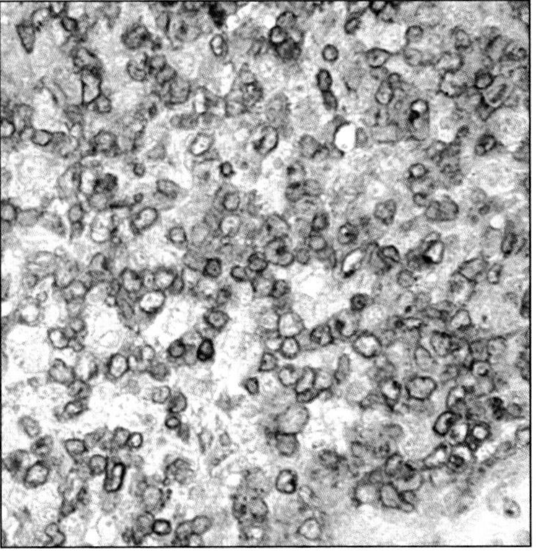

(Left) *Immunoreactivity is present for the B-cell marker CD20.* ***(Right)*** *Immunoreactivity for the T-cell marker CD3 is shown. Immunoreactivity for B- and T-cell markers, even in the presence of a markedly atypical cellular proliferation with increased mitotic activity and necrosis, would support a benign lymphoid cell proliferation rather than a lymphoma. A diagnosis of IM is established in a patient with typical clinical presentations and appropriate laboratory findings.*

HIV INFECTION OF TONSILS AND ADENOIDS

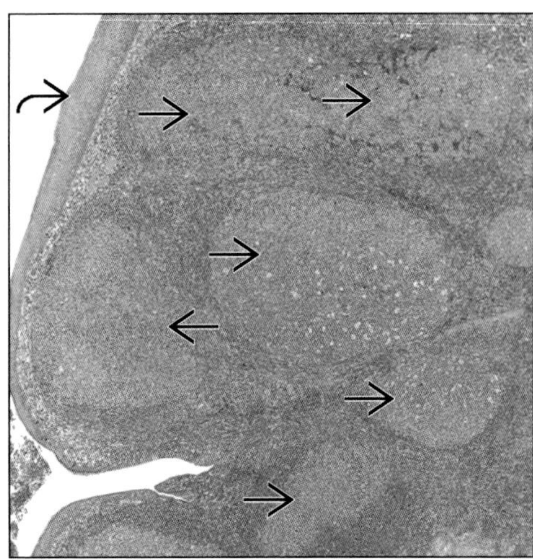

Early HIV infection of the tonsil includes florid follicular hyperplasia characterized by enlarged and irregularly shaped germinal centers ➔, some approximating the surface epithelium ➚.

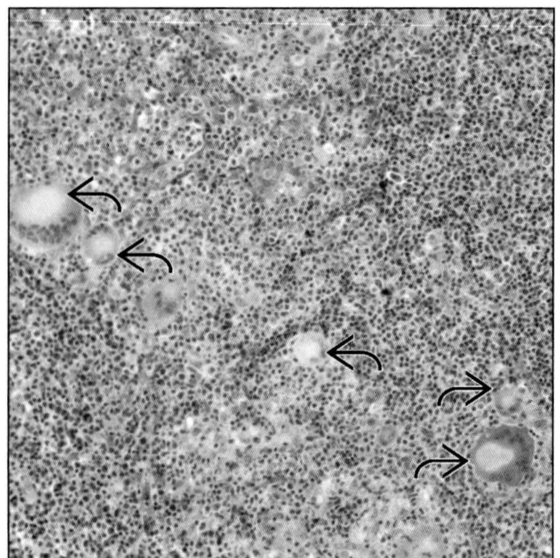

In conjunction with the florid follicular hyperplasia, the presence of multinucleated giant cells ➚, characteristically localized to the epithelium (not shown), is a feature of HIV infection.

TERMINOLOGY

Definitions

- Primary HIV infection of extranodal tissues of Waldeyer ring
  - Occurs in association with known systemic disease
  - May represent initial manifestation of HIV infection in patients not known to be HIV infected

ETIOLOGY/PATHOGENESIS

Infectious Agents

- HIV infection
  - Leads to destruction of cellular immunity leading to immunosuppression rendering host susceptible to opportunistic infections and tumors, a hallmark of AIDS
  - Belongs to human retrovirus of lentivirus genus
  - Preferentially infects CD4(+) (helper) T-cell lymphocytes and other cells of immune system that bear both CD4 receptor and 1 of 2 chemokine receptors (CCR-5 and CXCR-4) on their surface
    - Also includes dendritic cells and macrophages
  - Transmission occurs through
    - Blood
    - Sexual contact (bodily fluids)
    - Maternofetal routes

CLINICAL ISSUES

Epidemiology

- Incidence
  - More than 30 million persons are infected with HIV-1 worldwide
  - Majority of early cases in western countries reported in men who have sex with men (homosexual and bisexual)
    - Remains major risk group (53%)
    - But highest increased incidence in intravenous drug users (36%) and women (18%) in USA
  - Most cases in Africa and Asia heterosexually transmitted
- Age
  - Occurs most frequently in 3rd-5th decades of life (median age 4th decade)
    - May occur in pediatric age groups
- Gender
  - Male > Female

Site

- Nasopharyngeal tonsil (adenoids) and palatine tonsils

Presentation

- Clinical presentation varies, including
  - Nasal congestion
  - Airway obstruction
  - Sore throat (pharyngitis)
  - Otitis media unresponsive to antibiotic therapy
  - Otalgia, facial weakness, fever
  - Nasopharyngeal or tonsillar mass
    - Usually bilateral tonsillar or adenoidal enlargement but may be unilateral
    - Large ulcers may be present
    - Concurrent cervical adenopathy may be present
    - May raise concern for neoplastic (hematolymphoid or epithelial) proliferation

Laboratory Tests

- Serologic evaluation confirmatory for HIV infection

Treatment

- Options, risks, complications
  - Antiretroviral chemotherapy
    - Typically includes 3 or 4 medications taken in combination
    - Approach known as highly active antiretroviral therapy (HAART)
- Surgical approaches

HIV INFECTION OF TONSILS AND ADENOIDS

Key Facts

Terminology
- Primary HIV infection of tonsils &/or adenoids
  - Occurs in association with known systemic disease
  - May represent initial manifestation of HIV infection in patients not known to be HIV infected

Etiology/Pathogenesis
- HIV-1 belongs to human retrovirus of lentivirus genus
- Preferentially infects CD4(+) (helper) T-cell lymphocytes

Clinical Issues
- Nasopharyngeal or tonsillar mass usually bilateral but may be unilateral
- Concurrent cervical adenopathy may be present
- Use of antiretroviral chemotherapy may significantly prolong life and disease-free interval

Microscopic Pathology
- Acute &/or chronic stage
  - Florid follicular hyperplasia, follicle lysis with areas of follicular involution
  - Monocytoid B-cell hyperplasia
  - Multinucleated giant cells cluster adjacent to &/or within surface epithelium/crypt epithelium
- Advanced stage
  - Loss of normal lymphoid cell population replaced by benign plasma cell infiltrate, increased vascularity, absence of multinucleated giant cells

Ancillary Tests
- Reactivity for HIV core antigen p24 (gag protein)

  - Presence of mass may raise concern for neoplastic proliferation prompting surgical removal of adenoids or tonsils

Prognosis
- Early management with antiretroviral chemotherapy may significantly prolong life and disease-free interval

MICROSCOPIC PATHOLOGY

Histologic Features
- Histomorphologic changes represent continuum varying according to duration and progression of disease
- Acute &/or chronic stage
  - Florid follicular hyperplasia with and without follicular fragmentation
  - Follicle lysis with areas of follicular involution
  - Monocytoid B-cell hyperplasia
  - Paracortical and interfollicular zone expansion with immunoblasts and plasma cells
  - Interfollicular clusters of high endothelial venules
  - Intrafollicular hemorrhage
  - Multinucleated giant cells (MGC)
    - Characteristically cluster adjacent to or within adenoidal surface epithelium or tonsillar crypt epithelium
- Advanced stage
  - Features correlate with lymphoid obliteration seen in terminal stages of HIV infection or AIDS
  - Effacement of nodal architecture
  - Loss of normal lymphoid cell population replaced by benign plasma cell infiltrate
  - Presence of increased vascularity
  - MGC characteristically seen in early and chronic stages of disease are not identified in more advanced stages

ANCILLARY TESTS

Histochemistry
- Special stains for microorganisms (other than HIV) negative

Immunohistochemistry
- Reactivity for HIV core antigen p24 (gag protein)
  - Indicator of active HIV infection consistently identified in early and chronic stages of disease
  - Anti-HIV p24 reactivity
    - Within follicular dendritic cell (FDC) network of germinal centers
    - Scattered interfollicular lymphocytes
    - Multinucleated giant cells
    - Intraepithelial cells of crypt epithelium
  - HIV p24(+) intraepithelial multinucleated giant cells are S100 protein (dendritic cell marker) positive
    - Morphologic appearance correlates with appearance of dendritic cells (DC)
- Reactivity with B-cell (CD20) and T-cell markers or subsets (CD45RO, CD3, OPD4)
  - Seen within germinal centers and interfollicular regions, as well as in scattered intraepithelial cells
- Advanced stages of disease
  - Relative absence of lymphoid cell markers (CD45RB, CD3, or OPD4)
  - Plasma cell infiltrate shows reactivity with κ and λ light chains indicative of benign proliferation
- Absent immunoreactivity for
  - Epstein-Barr virus-latent membrane protein (EBV-LMP)
  - In situ hybridization for Epstein-Barr encoded RNA (EBER)
  - Herpes simplex virus (HSV)
  - Cytomegalovirus (CMV)
- Surface and crypt epithelia reactive for epithelial markers (cytokeratins, others)

Molecular Genetics
- In situ hybridization for HIV RNA seen in
  - Follicular dendritic cell network

HIV INFECTION OF TONSILS AND ADENOIDS

- Multinucleated giant cells
- Mature lymphocytes localized to
  - Germinal centers
  - Interfollicular zones
  - Within surface &/or crypt epithelia

Electron Microscopy

- Transmission
  - Presence of abundant HIV particles associated with complex follicular dendritic cell network

DIFFERENTIAL DIAGNOSIS

Infectious Diseases (Other than HIV)

- May be characterized by granulomatous inflammation
  - With or without caseating necrosis
    - Mycobacterial diseases
    - Fungal infections
    - Sarcoidosis
- May be characterized by intranuclear inclusions
  - Cytomegalovirus (CMV)
  - Herpes simplex virus (HSV)
- Histochemical &/or immunohistochemical stains may confirm presence of another infectious agent
  - Acid-fast bacilli for mycobacterial disease
  - Immunoreactivity for CMV or HSV

Infectious Mononucleosis (IM)

- IM lacks constellation of histologic features present in HIV infection
- Marked cytologic atypia of cells in IM absent in HIV
- Serologic markers associated with IM

Non-Hodgkin Lymphoma

- Effacement of architecture with loss of germinal centers
- Most commonly large B-cell lymphomas
  - Sheet-like proliferation of dyscohesive cells with
    - Enlarged vesicular nuclei
    - Prominent eosinophilic nucleoli
  - Expression of B-cell antigens (i.e., CD20)
    - T-cell markers(-)
  - Absence of HIV p24 immunoreactivity
  - Monoclonality may be demonstrated by flow cytometry immunophenotyping as light chain restriction
  - Presence of gene rearrangements

SELECTED REFERENCES

1. Orenstein JM: Hyperplastic lymphoid tissue in HIV/AIDS: an electron microscopic study. Ultrastruct Pathol. 32(4):161-9, 2008
2. Orenstein JM: The macrophage in HIV infection. Immunobiology. 204(5):598-602, 2001
3. Blauvelt A et al: HIV-infected human Langerhans cells transmit infection to human lymphoid tissue ex vivo. AIDS. 14(6):647-51, 2000
4. Dargent JL et al: HIV-associated multinucleated giant cells in lymphoid tissue of the Waldeyer's ring: a detailed study. Mod Pathol. 13(12):1293-9, 2000
5. Kapadia SB et al: HIV-associated Waldeyer's ring lymphoid hyperplasias: characterization of multinucleated giant cells and the role of Epstein-Barr virus. Hum Pathol. 30(11):1383-8, 1999
6. Orenstein JM et al: The macrophage origin of the HIV-expressing multinucleated giant cells in hyperplastic tonsils and adenoids. Ultrastruct Pathol. 23(2):79-91, 1999
7. Pope M: Mucosal dendritic cells and immunodeficiency viruses. J Infect Dis. 179 Suppl 3:S427-30, 1999
8. Vicandi B et al: HIV-1 (p24)-positive multinucleated giant cells in HIV-associated lymphoepithelial lesion of the parotid gland. A report of two cases. Acta Cytol. 43(2):247-51, 1999
9. Orenstein JM: The Warthin-Finkeldey-type giant cell in HIV infection, what is it? Ultrastruct Pathol. 22(4):293-303, 1998
10. Frankel SS et al: Active replication of HIV-1 at the lymphoepithelial surface of the tonsil. Am J Pathol. 151(1):89-96, 1997
11. Frankel SS et al: Replication of HIV-1 in dendritic cell-derived syncytia at the mucosal surface of the adenoid. Science. 272(5258):115-7, 1996
12. Wenig BM et al: Lymphoid changes of the nasopharyngeal and palatine tonsils that are indicative of human immunodeficiency virus infection. A clinicopathologic study of 12 cases. Am J Surg Pathol. 20(5):572-87, 1996
13. Heath SL et al: Follicular dendritic cells and human immunodeficiency virus infectivity. Nature. 377(6551):740-4, 1995
14. Schuurman HJ et al: Follicular dendritic cells and infection by human immunodeficiency virus type 1--a crucial target cell and virus reservoir. Curr Top Microbiol Immunol. 201:161-88, 1995
15. Sprenger R et al: Follicular dendritic cells productively infected with immunodeficiency viruses transmit infection to T cells. Med Microbiol Immunol. 184(3):129-34, 1995
16. Steinman RM: Dendritic cells: clinical aspects. Res Immunol. 140(9):911-8; discussion 918-26, 1989

Microscopic Features and Ancillary Techniques

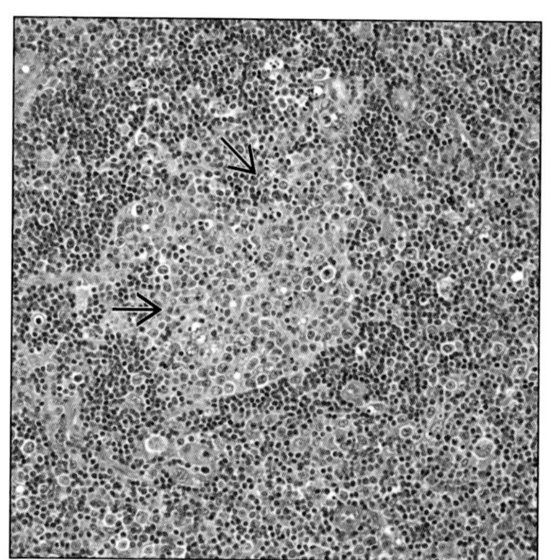

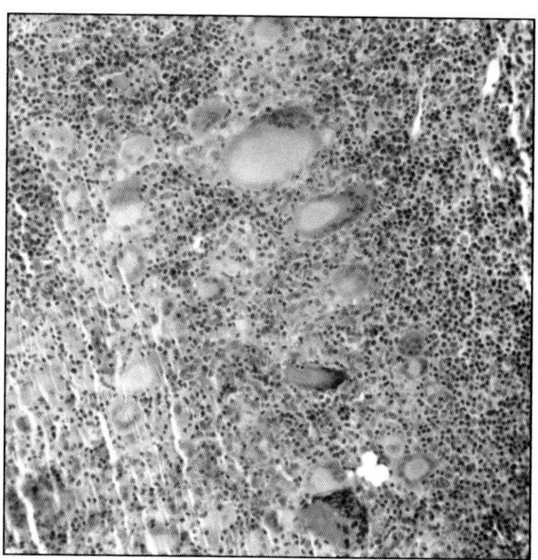

(Left) *Higher magnification of a lymphoid follicle in the early to chronic phase of infection shows attenuated to partially absent mantle cell lymphocytes and follicle lysis, characteristic infiltration of the follicle by small lymphocytes, creating a "moth eaten" appearance.* ***(Right)*** *Warthin-Finkeldey-like multinucleated giant cells (MGC) may or may not be present in a given case, but they are a rather consistent feature including cases with readily identifiable clusters of MGC.*

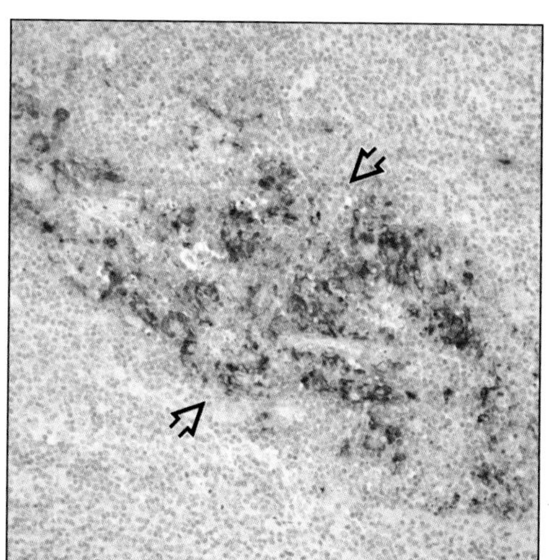

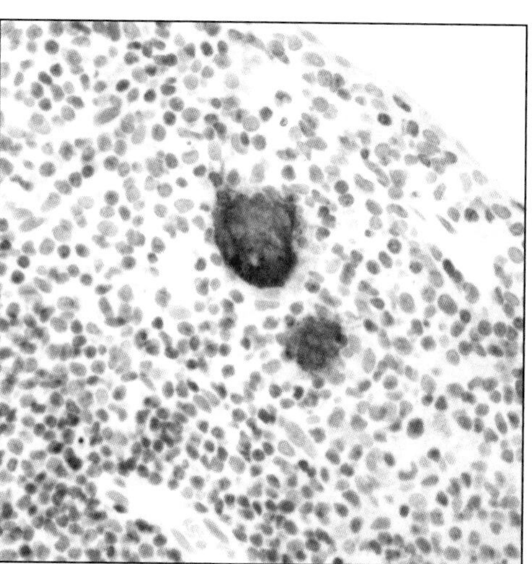

(Left) *The constellation of light microscopic features suggest the possible presence of HIV infection, but confirmation is required. To this end, aside from serologic confirmation of HIV infection, the presence of HIV p24 immunoreactivity in follicular dendritic cells is confirmatory of the diagnosis.* ***(Right)*** *In addition to the follicles, p24 immunoreactivity is also present in the multinucleated giant cells. These cells are also S100 protein positive.*

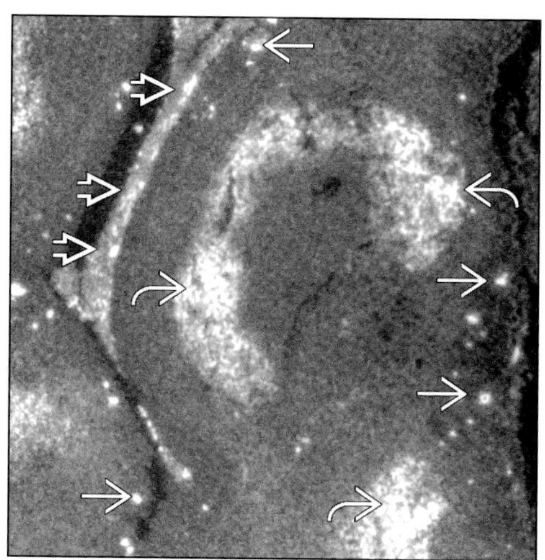

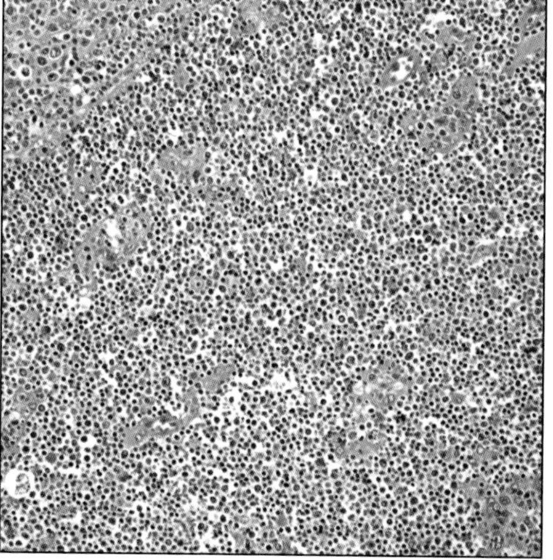

(Left) *In situ hybridization for HIV-1 RNA using antisense riboprobe, darkfield microscopy shows signal in enlarged and irregularly shaped germinal centers and in scattered multinucleated giant cells in interfollicular locations and within the epithelial layer.* ***(Right)*** *In more advanced stages, the findings include effacement of lymphoid architecture, loss of normal lymphoid cell population with replacement by a benign plasma cell infiltrate, and increased vascularity.*

HAIRY POLYP

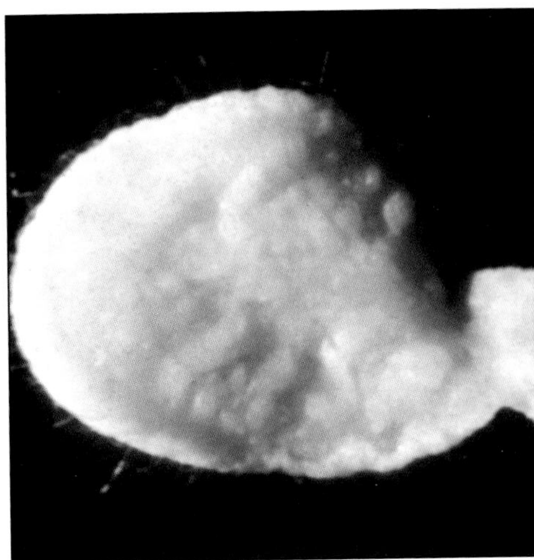

Hairy polyp is also known as a nasopharyngeal dermoid. This lesion occurred in a neonate with airway obstruction and appears as a polypoid solid mass with identifiable hairs on the surface.

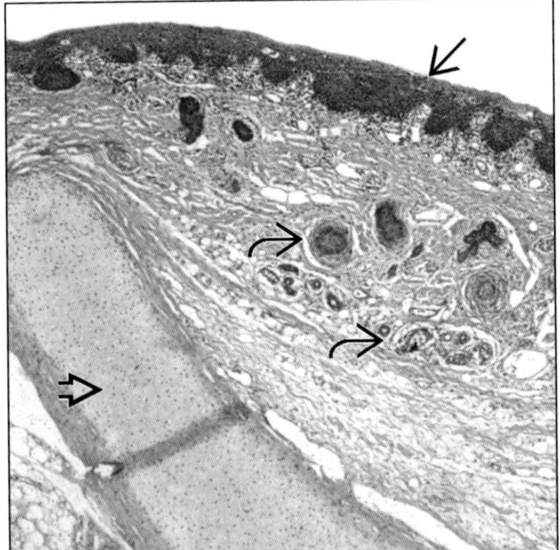

The histology of hairy polyp includes a combination of ectodermal and mesodermal tissues, such as keratinizing squamous epithelium ➔, adnexal structures ➔, and cartilage ➔.

TERMINOLOGY

Synonyms

- Nasopharyngeal dermoid or teratoid lesion

Definitions

- Developmental (congenital) anomaly predominantly composed of ectodermal and mesodermal tissue but lacking endodermal-derived tissues

ETIOLOGY/PATHOGENESIS

Developmental Anomaly

- Proposed classification includes
  - 1st branchial arch origin
    - Presence of skin, including hair follicles and sebaceous glands and identification of elastic cartilage
    - Findings identical to those of congenital accessory auricles akin to accessory tragus, which is of 1st branchial arch origin
  - Choristoma
    - Suggested by presence of skin, tissue type not normally found in nasopharynx
  - Teratoma
    - On basis of histologic features, some authorities feel these lesions best classified as subset of benign teratoma
    - Absence of endodermal-derived structures and presence of limited heterogeneity of tissue types argue against inclusion as benign teratoma

CLINICAL ISSUES

Epidemiology

- Age
  - Occurs in newborns or infants
- Gender
  - Equal gender distribution

Site

- Nasopharynx

Presentation

- Difficulties in breathing, swallowing, or sucking

Treatment

- Surgical approaches
  - Simple surgical excision is treatment of choice

Prognosis

- Cured following surgical resection

MACROSCOPIC FEATURES

General Features

- Polypoid, predominantly solid but partially cystic lesions
- May be pedunculated or sessile

MICROSCOPIC PATHOLOGY

Histologic Features

- Combination of various ectodermal and mesodermal tissues including
  - Ectodermal structures
    - Skin (keratinizing squamous epithelium)
    - Cutaneous adnexa
  - Mesodermal structures
    - Cartilage, bone
    - Muscle (striated or smooth)
    - Fibrous tissue
    - Mature adipose tissue
    - Vascular tissue
- Polypoid lesions covered by
  - Skin with identification of hair follicles and sebaceous glands within submucosa and identification of elastic cartilage

HAIRY POLYP

Key Facts

Terminology
- Developmental (congenital) anomaly predominantly composed of ectodermal and mesodermal tissue

Etiology/Pathogenesis
- Presence of skin suggests classification as choristoma
- Possibly of 1st branchial arch origin

Clinical Issues
- Occurs in newborns or infants
- Difficulties in breathing, swallowing, or sucking
- Cured following surgical resection

Microscopic Pathology
- Combination of various ectodermal and mesodermal tissues including
  - Skin (keratinizing squamous epithelium) and cutaneous adnexa
  - Cartilage, bone, muscle, fibrous tissue, mature adipose tissue, vascular tissue

  - These histologic findings suggest branchial cleft origin representing congenital accessory auricles akin to accessory tragus

DIFFERENTIAL DIAGNOSIS

Teratoma
- Represents true neoplasm composed of tissues from all 3 germ layers
- Presence of endodermal-derived tissue and presence of wide variety of tissue types usually seen in teratoma will allow for distinguishing these lesions

Epidermal Inclusion Cyst
- Lined by stratified squamous epithelium with keratin-filled cyst
- Lacks adnexal structures in cyst wall

SELECTED REFERENCES

1. Russo E et al: Dermoid of the nasopharynx: an unusual finding in an older child. Ear Nose Throat J. 89(4):162-3, 2010
2. Gambino M et al: Two unusual cases of pharyngeal hairy polyp causing intermittent neonatal airway obstruction. Int J Oral Maxillofac Surg. 37(8):761-2, 2008
3. Roh JL: Transoral endoscopic resection of a nasopharyngeal hairy polyp. Int J Pediatr Otorhinolaryngol. 68(8):1087-90, 2004
4. Burns BV et al: 'Hairy polyp' of the pharynx in association with an ipsilateral branchial sinus: evidence that the 'hairy polyp' is a second branchial arch malformation. J Laryngol Otol. 115(2):145-8, 2001
5. Coppit GL 3rd et al: Nasopharyngeal teratomas and dermoids: a review of the literature and case series. Int J Pediatr Otorhinolaryngol. 52(3):219-27, 2000
6. Kayhan FT et al: A nasopharyngeal dermoid causing neonatal airway obstruction. Int J Pediatr Otorhinolaryngol. 40(2-3):195-201, 1997
7. Heffner DK et al: Pharyngeal dermoids ("hairy polyps") as accessory auricles. Ann Otol Rhinol Laryngol. 105(10):819-24, 1996
8. Kelly A et al: Hairy polyp of the oropharynx: case report and literature review. J Pediatr Surg. 31(5):704-6, 1996
9. Olivares-Pakzad BA et al: Oropharyngeal hairy polyp with meningothelial elements. Oral Surg Oral Med Oral Pathol Oral Radiol Endod. 79(4):462-8, 1995
10. Nicklaus PJ et al: Hairy polyp of the eustachian tube. J Otolaryngol. 20(4):254-7, 1991
11. Aughton DJ et al: Nasopharyngeal teratoma ('hairy polyp'), Dandy-Walker malformation, diaphragmatic hernia, and other anomalies in a female infant. J Med Genet. 27(12):788-90, 1990
12. Kochanski SC et al: Neonatal nasopharyngeal hairy polyp: CT and MR appearance. J Comput Assist Tomogr. 14(6):1000-1, 1990
13. Resta L et al: The s.c. 'hairy polyp' or 'dermoid' of the nasopharynx. (An unusual observation in older age). J Laryngol Otol. 98(10):1043-6, 1984
14. Heffner DK. Problems in pediatric otorhinolaryngic pathology et al: Teratoid and neural tumors of the nose, sinonasal tract, and nasopharynx. Int J Pediatr Otorhinolaryngol. 6(1):1-21, 1983

IMAGE GALLERY

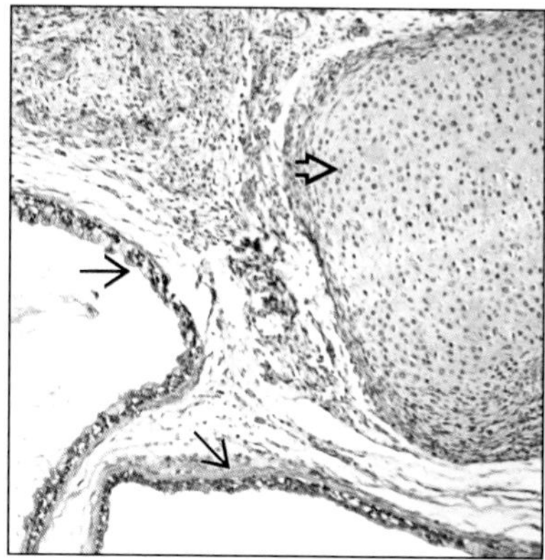

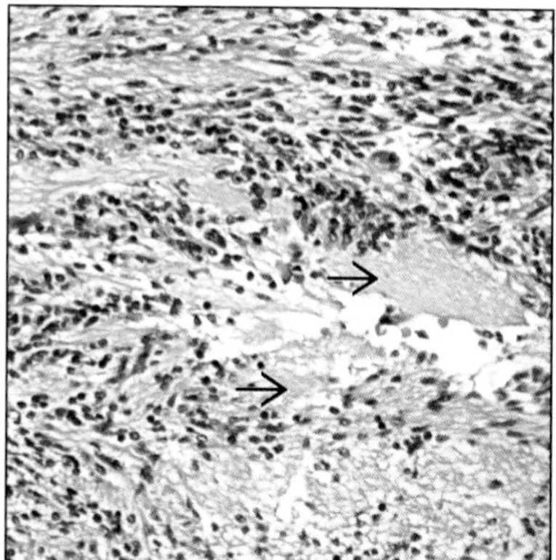

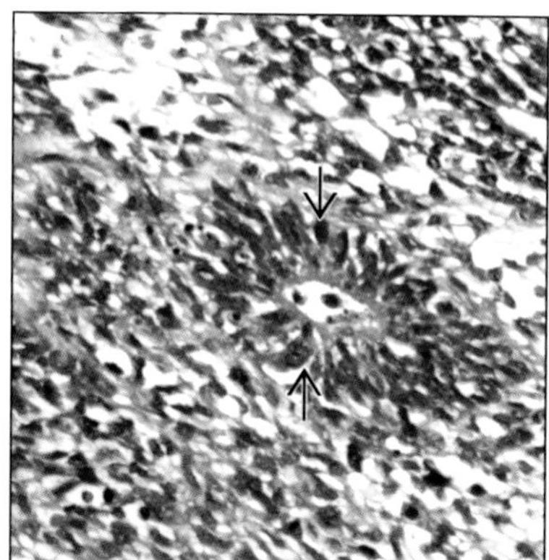

(Left) *Histologically, teratomas include elements from all germ cell layers, including epithelial, mesenchymal structures, and central nervous system tissue. Epithelial-lined glands* ⇒ *and immature cartilage* ⇒ *are present.* ***(Center)*** *In addition to epithelial and mesenchymal tissues, teratomas may also show central nervous system tissue, including neurofibrillary matrix* ⇒*.* ***(Right)*** *The central nervous system tissue in teratomas may show true neural rosettes* ⇒*.*

NASOPHARYNGEAL ANGIOFIBROMA

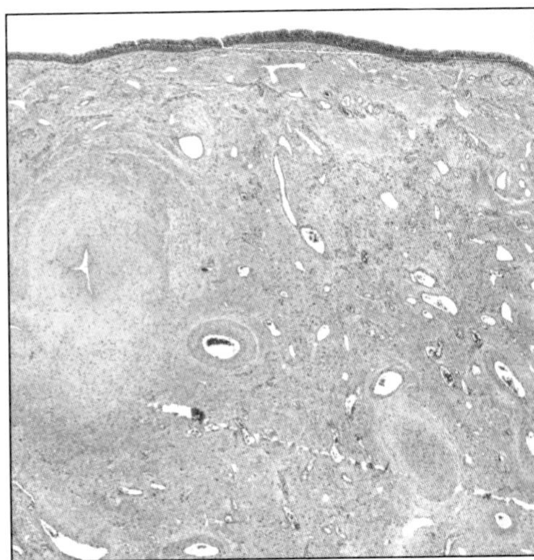

Hematoxylin & eosin shows an intact surface with a wide variety of vessels set within a fibrous stroma. Some of the vessels have smooth muscle and others do not. Patulous and compressed vessels are noted.

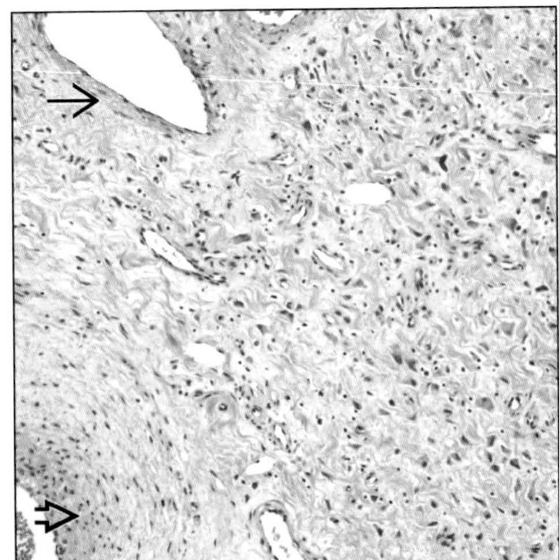

Hematoxylin & eosin shows smooth-muscle-walled vessels ⇨ adjacent to vessels without smooth muscle →, along with numerous capillaries within a fibrous stroma.

TERMINOLOGY

Abbreviations

- Juvenile angiofibroma (JNA)
- Angiofibroma (AF)

Synonyms

- Angiomyofibroblastoma-like tumor
- Angiofibroma
- Fibroangioma
- Fibroma

Definitions

- Benign, highly cellular and richly vascularized mesenchymal neoplasm arising in nasopharynx in males

ETIOLOGY/PATHOGENESIS

Hormonal

- Testosterone-dependent puberty-induced growth can be blocked with estrogen &/or progesterone therapy

Genetic

- Reported association with familial adenomatous polyposis

CLINICAL ISSUES

Epidemiology

- Incidence
  - < 1% of all nasopharyngeal tumors
  - < 0.1% of all head and neck neoplasms
- Age
  - < 20 years old
    - Adolescents to young men
    - Peak in 2nd decade of life
- Gender
  - Males exclusively
  - If diagnosed in female, studies of sex chromosomes required to confirm gender
- Ethnicity
  - Higher frequency in fair-skinned, red-haired patients
    - Develops throughout the world

Site

- Nasopharynx usually affected
- Pterygoid region usually affected
- May expand to involve surrounding structures (30% of cases)
  - Anterior: Nasal cavity and maxillary sinus via roof of nasopharynx
  - Lateral: Temporal and infratemporal fossae via pterygomaxillary fissure, resulting in cheek or intraoral buccal mass
  - Posterior: Middle cranial fossa
  - Superior: Pterygopalatine fossa and orbit via inferior and superior orbital fissures resulting in proptosis
  - Medial: Contralateral side

Presentation

- Nasal obstruction
- Recurrent, spontaneous epistaxis
- Nasal discharge
- Facial deformity (proptosis), exophthalmia, diplopia
- Rhinolalia, sinusitis
- Otitis media, tinnitus, deafness
- Headaches
- Rarely, anosmia or pain
- Increased frequency in red-haired, fair-skinned boys
  - Predicated on Caucasian population
- Symptoms present for 12-24 months (nonspecific presentation)

Treatment

- Options, risks, complications
  - Benign tumor can show aggressive local growth
  - Biopsy is contraindicated due to potential exsanguination
  - Potential for facial deformity if allowed to grow

Key Facts

Terminology
- Benign, highly cellular and richly vascularized mesenchymal neoplasm arising in nasopharynx in males

Clinical Issues
- Recurrent, spontaneous epistaxis
- Nasopharynx is nearly always affected
- Patients < 20 years old
- Males exclusively
- Recurrences in ~ 20% of patients
- Range up to 22 cm in size

Image Findings
- Anterior bowing of posterior wall of maxillary sinus with posterior displacement of pterygoid plates (Holman-Miller sign)
- Angiography identifies feeding vessel(s) and allows for presurgical embolization
- Tumor blush is characteristic

Microscopic Pathology
- Submucosal proliferation of vascular component within fibrous stroma
- Many variably sized, disorganized vessels
- Fibrous stroma consists of plump spindle, angular, or stellate-shaped cells
- Variable amounts of fine and coarse collagen fibers
- Elastic tissue is not identified within stroma

Top Differential Diagnoses
- Lobular capillary hemangioma
- Inflammatory polyp
- Antrochoanal polyp

- Surgical approaches
  - Surgery is treatment of choice
  - Definitive resection is frequently associated with significant morbidity
- Drugs
  - Preoperative hormone therapy
    - Not as popular as other modalities
    - Giving estrogens to pubertal males is undesirable
- Radiation
  - Used to manage large, intracranial, or recurrent tumors
- Angiography
  - Selective angiography allows embolization with sclerosing agent or cryotherapy

Prognosis
- Good
- May have fatal exsanguination if incorrectly managed
- Recurrences in ~ 20% of patients
  - Usually develop within 2 years of diagnosis
  - Commonly extends intracranially

IMAGE FINDINGS

General Features
- Best diagnostic clue
  - Anterior bowing of posterior wall of maxillary sinus with posterior displacement of pterygoid plates (Holman-Miller sign)
- Location
  - Nasopharynx with extension into surrounding structures
- Angiography identifies feeding vessel(s) and allows for presurgical embolization
  - Tumor blush is characteristic

CT Findings
- Allows for accurate determination of size and extent
- Enhancement is different from adjacent muscle, accentuated with contrast
- Bony margins may be eroded

MACROSCOPIC FEATURES

General Features
- Polypoid mass with multinodular contour
- Red, gray-tan cut surface

Size
- Mean: 4 cm
- Range: Up to 22 cm

MICROSCOPIC PATHOLOGY

Histologic Features
- Submucosal proliferation of vascular component within fibrous stroma
- Many variably sized disorganized vessels
  - Varying thickness of vessel wall with patchy muscle content
  - Vessels are mostly thin-walled, slit-like ("staghorn")
  - Range from capillary size to large, dilated, patulous vessels
- Focal, pad-like, smooth muscle thickenings within vessel walls
- Endothelial cells may be plump but are usually attenuated
- Fibrous stroma consists of plump spindle, angular, or stellate-shaped cells
- Variable amounts of fine and coarse collagen fibers
- Myxoid degeneration is common (especially in embolized specimens)
  - May see foreign material within vessels in embolized cases
- As stroma increases, vascular compression results in virtually nonexistent lumina
- Elastic tissue is not identified within stroma
- Stromal cells may be angulated, multinucleated, and pleomorphic
- Mitotic figures are sparse
- Mast cells may be seen
- Hormone treated cases show increased collagenization of stroma with fewer, but thicker-walled vessels

NASOPHARYNGEAL ANGIOFIBROMA

Immunohistochemistry

Antibody	Reactivity	Staining Pattern	Comment
Vimentin	Positive	Cytoplasmic	All elements of tumor
Actin-sm	Positive	Cytoplasmic	Smooth muscle of vessel walls highlighted
Actin-HHF-35	Positive	Cytoplasmic	Smooth muscle of vessel walls highlighted
Desmin	Positive	Cytoplasmic	Only within larger vessel walls
Androgen receptor	Positive	Nuclear	Stromal cells and endothelial cell nuclei
ER	Positive	Nuclear	Variably reactive, mostly in vascular nuclei
PR	Positive	Nuclear	Variably reactive, mostly in vascular nuclei
FVIIIRAg	Positive	Cytoplasmic	Endothelial cells only
CD34	Positive	Cytoplasmic	Endothelial cells only
CD31	Positive	Cytoplasmic	Endothelial cells only
PDGF-B	Positive	Cytoplasmic	
IGF-2	Positive	Cytoplasmic	
S100	Positive	Nuclear & cytoplasmic	Highlights entrapped nerves but not tumor cells

Staging for Nasopharyngeal Angiofibroma

Stage	Radiographic, Clinical, or Pathologic Finding
I	Tumor limited to nasopharynx with no bone destruction
II	Tumor invading nasal cavity, maxillary, ethmoid, and sphenoid sinus with no bone destruction
III	Tumor invading pterygo-palatine fossa, infratemporal fossa, orbit, and parasellar region
IV	Tumor with massive invasion of cranial cavity, cavernous sinus, optic chiasm, or pituitary fossa

- Sarcomatous transformation is exceedingly uncommon event
  - Develops following massive doses of radiation

ANCILLARY TESTS

Histochemistry

- Reticulin shows positive black staining around stromal cells and blood vessels
- Elastic van Gieson highlights elastic tissue within vessel walls

Immunohistochemistry

- Vessels are highlighted within myofibroblastic stroma

DIFFERENTIAL DIAGNOSIS

Lobular Capillary Hemangioma

- Lesion is ulcerated; arises from different anatomic site; has granulation-type tissue and lots of inflammation; vessels are more organized

Inflammatory Polyp

- Especially if there are atypical stromal cells; usually more edematous; lacks rich vascular investment

Antrochoanal Polyp

- Arises from different location; heavy stromal fibrosis, but usually lacks characteristic vascular pattern of JNA

SELECTED REFERENCES

1. Bleier BS et al: Current management of juvenile nasopharyngeal angiofibroma: a tertiary center experience 1999-2007. Am J Rhinol Allergy. 23(3):328-30, 2009
2. Carrillo JF et al: Juvenile nasopharyngeal angiofibroma: clinical factors associated with recurrence, and proposal of a staging system. J Surg Oncol. 98(2):75-80, 2008
3. Coutinho-Camillo CM et al: Genetic alterations in juvenile nasopharyngeal angiofibromas. Head Neck. 30(3):390-400, 2008
4. Glad H et al: Juvenile nasopharyngeal angiofibromas in Denmark 1981-2003: diagnosis, incidence, and treatment. Acta Otolaryngol. 127(3):292-9, 2007
5. Tyagi I et al: Staging and surgical approaches in large juvenile angiofibroma--study of 95 cases. Int J Pediatr Otorhinolaryngol. 70(9):1619-27, 2006
6. Thompson LDR et al: Tumours of the Nasopharynx: Nasopharyngeal angiofibroma. Barnes EL et al: Pathology and Genetics of Head and Neck Tumours. World Health Organization Classification of Tumours. Lyon, France: IARC Press. 102-3, 2005
7. Fletcher CD: Distinctive soft tissue tumors of the head and neck. Mod Pathol. 15(3):324-30, 2002
8. Lee JT et al: The role of radiation in the treatment of advanced juvenile angiofibroma. Laryngoscope. 112(7 Pt 1):1213-20, 2002
9. Coffin CM et al: Fibroblastic-myofibroblastic tumors in children and adolescents: a clinicopathologic study of 108 examples in 103 patients. Pediatr Pathol. 11(4):569-88, 1991
10. Makek MS et al: Malignant transformation of a nasopharyngeal angiofibroma. Laryngoscope. 99(10 Pt 1):1088-92, 1989

Radiographic and Microscopic Features

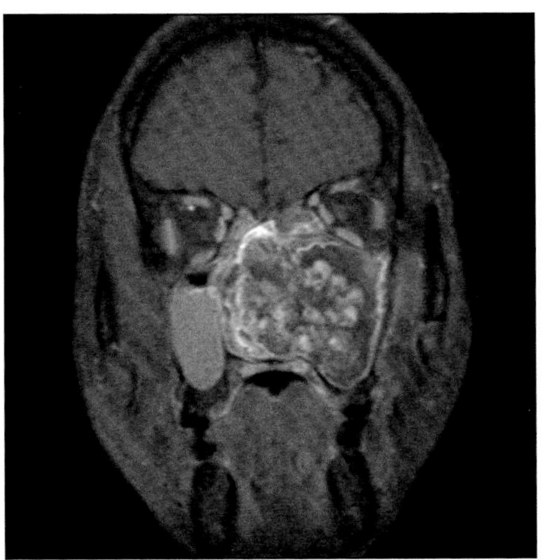

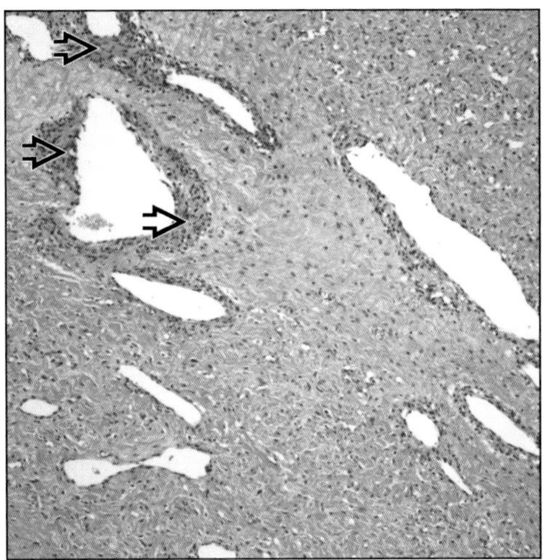

(Left) *MR shows intracranial extension of a large, destructive, hyperintense mass in the nasopharynx. The bone has been remodeled and pushed aside. Note the fluid collection in the sinuses as a postobstructive phenomenon.* ***(Right)*** *Hematoxylin & eosin shows numerous vessels of various calibers, some with smooth muscle ⇨ set in a heavily collagenized stroma. The stroma shows hypocellularity.*

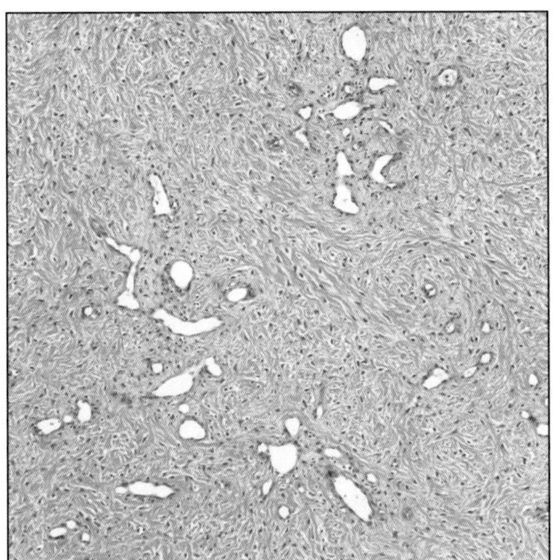

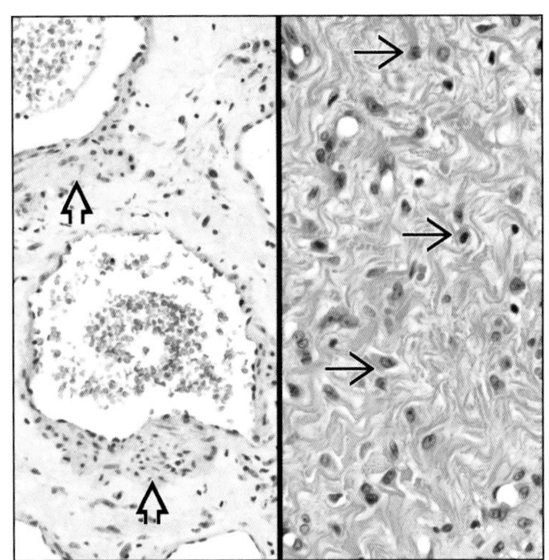

(Left) *Hematoxylin & eosin shows increased collagen deposition, often seen in lesions of a long duration. Note how the vessels are compressed and narrowed to a nearly slit-like configuration.* ***(Right)*** *Hematoxylin & eosin shows a "pad" of smooth muscle within the vessel wall ⇨. The vessel contains erythrocytes. Note the increased number of mast cells → in the stroma, which has wavy collagen deposition.*

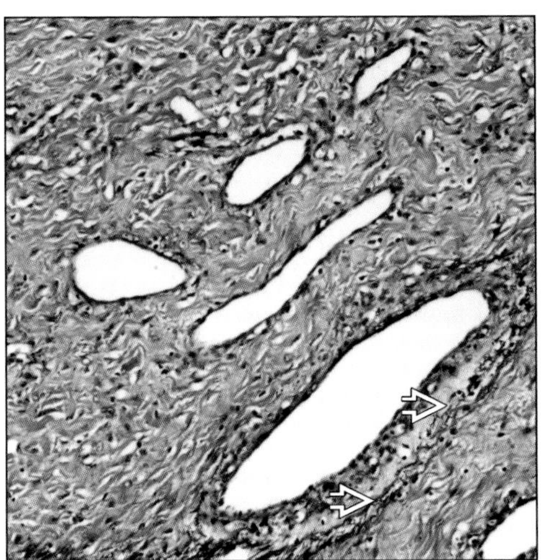

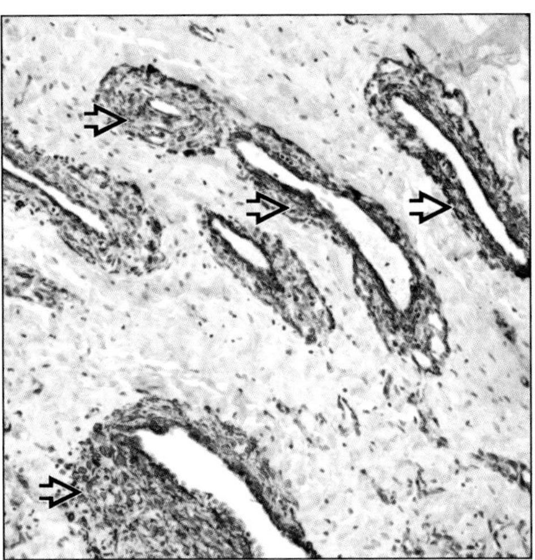

(Left) *Elastic von Gieson shows elastic tissue (black deposition as short to wavy fragments) in the larger vessel ➡ but not in the smaller vessels. This results in profuse epistaxis, as the vessels are unable to contract and staunch bleeding.* ***(Right)*** *Muscle specific actin highlights the muscle walls around vessels ⇨. The variable intensity of the reaction helps to demonstrate the variable amounts of smooth muscle associated with the vessels.*

NASOPHARYNGEAL CARCINOMA, NONKERATINIZING TYPES

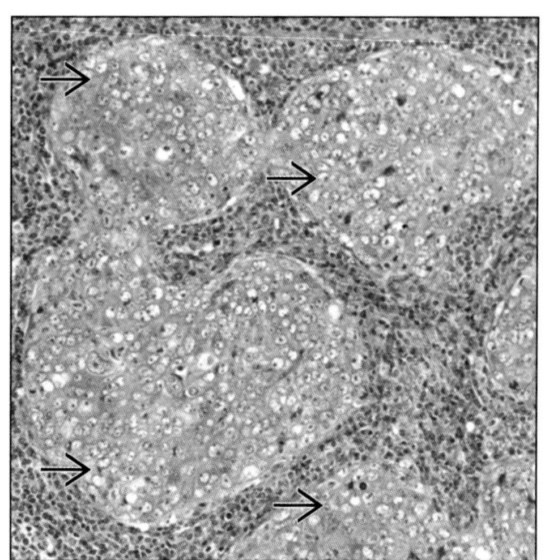

Nonkeratinizing undifferentiated nasopharyngeal carcinoma is characterized by tumor nests ➔ demarcated from surrounding stroma, the latter lacking a desmoplastic reaction.

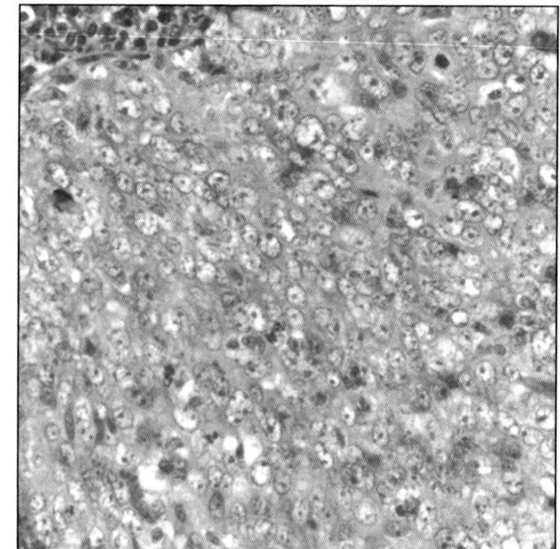

The neoplastic nests are composed of enlarged oval to round nuclei with vesicular chromatin, prominent eosinophilic nucleoli, scant cytoplasm, and indistinct cell margins creating a syncytial appearance.

TERMINOLOGY

Abbreviations

- Nasopharyngeal carcinoma (NPC)

Synonyms

- Lymphoepithelioma, Rigaud and Schmincke types of lymphoepithelioma; transitional carcinoma
  - Lymphoepithelioma is a misnomer
    - Tumor entirely of epithelial origin with secondary associated benign lymphoid component
  - Designations Rigaud and Schmincke refer to syncytial vs. individual cell growth patterns, respectively, with no biologic import

Definitions

- Type of squamous cell carcinoma originating from nasopharyngeal mucosa with evidence of squamous differentiation
- World Health Organization classification of NPC
  - I. Keratinizing
  - II. Nonkeratinizing
    - Differentiated
    - Undifferentiated
- Prior designations of WHO no longer used including
  - Types I (squamous cell carcinoma), II (nonkeratinizing carcinoma), III (undifferentiated carcinoma)

ETIOLOGY/PATHOGENESIS

Infectious Agents

- Strong association with Epstein-Barr virus (EBV)
  - Both nonkeratinizing differentiated and undifferentiated types linked to EBV
  - Strong association indicates probable oncogenic role of EBV in development of NPC
  - EBV early initiating event in development of NPC
    - EBV found in preinvasive (precursor) nasopharyngeal lesions
    - Clonal EBV-DNA identified, suggesting preinvasive lesions arose from single EBV-infected cell progressing to invasive cancer
- Role of human papillomavirus (HPV) uncertain

Environmental Exposure

- Purported risk factors include
  - High dietary levels of nitrosamines in preserved food in high incidence regions implicated as carcinogen
  - Cigarette smoking
  - Occupational exposure to chemical fumes, smoke, formaldehyde
  - Prior radiation exposure

Genetic and Geographic Factors

- Increased incidence of NPC in China (especially in south: Kwantung province) and Taiwan
- Incidence among Chinese people decreases after emigration to low-incidence areas but still remains higher than in non-Chinese populations

CLINICAL ISSUES

Epidemiology

- Incidence
  - In China, NPC accounts for 18% of all cancers, and 1 in 40 men develop NPC before age 72 years
  - NPC, nonkeratinizing differentiated
    - Least common, representing < 15% of cases
  - NPC, nonkeratinizing undifferentiated
    - Most common, representing > 60% of cases
- Age
  - Most common in 4th-6th decades
  - Nonkeratinizing undifferentiated may occur in pediatric patients
    - Less than 20% occur in pediatric age groups
    - Pediatric NPC most common in northern and central Africa, accounting for 10-20% of all cases

NASOPHARYNGEAL CARCINOMA, NONKERATINIZING TYPES

Key Facts

Terminology
- Type of squamous cell carcinoma originating from nasopharyngeal mucosa showing evidence of squamous differentiation

Etiology/Pathogenesis
- Strong association with Epstein-Barr virus (EBV)
- Role of human papillomavirus (HPV) uncertain

Clinical Issues
- Asymptomatic cervical neck mass typically localized to posterior cervical triangle or superior jugular nodal chain
- Supervoltage radiotherapy (6,500-7,000+ rads) considered treatment of choice for all NPC histologic subtypes
- Overall 5-year survival approximately 65%

Microscopic Pathology
- Nonkeratinizing differentiated type composed of stratified cells with pleomorphic, hyperchromatic nuclei showing little to absent keratinization
- Nonkeratinizing undifferentiated type composed of cells with enlarged vesicular nuclei, prominent eosinophilic nucleoli

Ancillary Tests
- Detection of EBV
  - By polymerase chain reaction (PCR) or in situ hybridization (ISH) found in 75-100% of NPCs, nonkeratinizing types
  - Nonreactive for p16

    - Approximately 2% of NPC in China occurs in children
- Gender
  - Male > Female
- Ethnicity
  - Endemic populations include Chinese, southeast Asians, north Africans, natives of Arctic region

Site
- Lateral wall (fossa of Rosenmüller) > superior posterior wall

Presentation
- Presence of asymptomatic cervical neck mass typically localized to posterior cervical triangle or superior jugular nodal chain commonly present
- Additional signs and symptoms include
  - Nasal obstruction, nasal discharge, epistaxis, pain, serous otitis media, otalgia, hearing loss, headache
- Signs and symptoms in early stages often subtle and nonspecific resulting in delay in diagnosis
  - Presentation often at more advanced clinical stage
- Up to 25% of patients may experience cranial nerve involvement
  - Considered adverse prognostic finding
  - Cranial nerves involved may include
    - III, IV, ophthalmic branch of V, 3rd division of V (through parapharyngeal space in proximity to lateral nasopharyngeal wall), VI, IX-XII

Laboratory Tests
- Positive serology against EBV in 90% of patients reported
  - Elevated titers of IgA antibodies (vs. viral capsid antigen [VCA]) and IgG antibodies (vs. early antigen [EA])
    - Detection rates range up to 93%
    - Elevated titers used as marker to screen populations in high-risk areas and as potential indicator of disease relapse
  - Quantitative PCR testing for elevated circulating EBV-DNA in plasma and serum reported sensitivity rates of up to 96%
  - Newer antibody tests based on recombinant EBV antigens (e.g., EBV nuclear antigens [EBNA], membrane antigen [MA], others) utilized in diagnosis
  - Expression of EBV nuclear antigen-1 (EBNA-1), latent membrane protein-1 (LMP-1), EBV encoded RNA (EBER)

Treatment
- Options, risks, complications
  - Due to anatomic constraints imposed by nasopharynx and tendency of NPCs to present with advanced stage, supervoltage radiotherapy is treatment of choice
- Surgical approaches
  - Surgical intervention reserved for patients who fail radiation therapy
- Adjuvant therapy
  - Chemotherapy integrated with radiation (RT) in advanced stage disease
- Radiation
  - Supervoltage radiotherapy (6,500-7,000+ rads) considered treatment of choice for all NPC histologic subtypes
    - Given to nasopharynx and neck using megavoltage radiation with median dose of 70 Gy

Prognosis
- Overall 5-year survival (approximately 75%)
- Clinical stage at presentation represents most important prognostic factor
  - 5-year disease-specific survival (DSS) for
    - Stage I (98%)
    - Stage IIA-B (95%)
    - Stage III (86%)
    - Stage IVA-B (73%)
- Long-term outcomes in patients treated with induction chemotherapy and radiotherapy (CRT) vs. radiotherapy alone (RT) show
  - Modest but significant decrease in relapse and improvement in disease-specific survival in advanced stage NPC

NASOPHARYNGEAL CARCINOMA, NONKERATINIZING TYPES

        - Includes addition of cisplatin-based induction chemotherapy (cisplatin, bleomycin, fluorouracil or cisplatin, and epirubicin) to RT
    - No substantive improvement in overall survival reported
- Factors affecting prognosis may include
    - Better prognosis associated with lower clinical stage, younger patient age, female gender
    - Worse prognosis with higher stage tumors, older patients, male gender
    - Frequently metastasizes to regional lymph nodes
        - Presence of lymph node metastasis decreases survival by approximately 10-20%
    - Large percentage of NPCs, particularly undifferentiated type, metastasize to sites below clavicle, including lungs, bone (ribs and spine), liver
        - Associated with worse prognosis
    - Poorer prognosis seen in patients with HLA-Aw33-C3-B58/DR3 haplotype, while patients with A2-Cw11-Bw46/DR9 haplotype have longer survival
    - Prominent tumor angiogenesis and c-erb-B22 expression suggested as indicators of poor prognosis
- Risk of developing synchronous or metachronous 2nd primary malignancy approximately 4%
    - 2nd malignancies tend to occur in upper aerodigestive tract

IMAGE FINDINGS

Radiographic Findings

- Important diagnostic aid in assessing extent of disease and presence of metastatic disease
- Positron emission tomography and computed tomography (PET/CT) is used in detection of locoregional and distant spread of tumor

MR Findings

- Preferred study for detection of invasion into soft tissues, intracranial extension, and invasion into bone

MACROSCOPIC FEATURES

General Features

- Varies to include
    - No visible mass
    - Mucosal bulge with overlying intact epithelium
    - Demonstrable mass with extensive involvement of surface epithelium
    - Frankly infiltrative mass

MICROSCOPIC PATHOLOGY

Histologic Features

- Nonkeratinizing differentiated
    - Growth includes presence of interconnecting cords or trabeculae
        - Cystic change with associated necrosis commonly present
        - Often metastases to lymph nodes include cystic change with central necrosis
    - Stratified cells with pleomorphic, hyperchromatic nuclei showing little to absent keratinization
        - Well-defined cell borders and vague intercellular bridges may be present
        - Keratinized cells may be identified
    - Sharp delineation from surrounding stroma
    - Increased mitotic activity, including atypical mitoses
    - Typically, absence of desmoplastic stromal response to invasive growth
- Nonkeratinizing undifferentiated
    - Variable growth including cohesive or nested cell nests (syncytial pattern) to diffuse cellular infiltrate composed of dyscohesive cells
    - Neoplastic cells characterized by
        - Enlarged round nuclei with vesicular chromatin, prominent eosinophilic nucleoli, scant eosinophilic to amphophilic cytoplasm, indistinct borders
        - Keratinization is typically absent but in any case may be focally present
    - Mitoses can be seen but typically not prominently present
    - Prominent nonneoplastic lymphoid component composed of
        - Mature lymphocytes and plasma cells
        - May overrun and obscure invasive carcinoma
    - Infiltrative growth generally does not produce host desmoplastic response
        - Absence of desmoplasia in conjunction with prominent benign lymphocytic infiltrate obscuring lesional cells may make diagnosis problematic
        - Absence of desmoplastic response may also be present in association with nodal metastasis
- Uncommon to identify precursor lesion (i.e., intraepithelial dysplasia &/or carcinoma in situ)
    - Intraepithelial dysplasia can be seen in surface or crypt epithelium
    - Most cases of invasive carcinoma occur without identifying intraepithelial dysplasia/carcinoma in situ
    - NPC originates from nasopharyngeal surface &/ or crypt epithelium even in absence of identifying intraepithelial dysplasia &/or carcinoma in situ
- Approximately 25% of NPCs show more than 1 histologic type
    - Classification in "mixed" tumors according to dominant cell component
- Histologic distinction among NPC, nonkeratinizing types may not always be clear
    - Overlapping histology may be present in any given tumor

ANCILLARY TESTS

Immunohistochemistry

- Strong immunoreactivity for cytokeratins
    - Pan-cytokeratins and high molecular weight cytokeratins strongly positive
    - Weak immunoreactivity is present for low molecular weight cytokeratins
    - Typically negative for cytokeratin 7, cytokeratin 20

Clinicopathologic Comparison of Nasopharyngeal Carcinoma

	Keratinizing	NK, Differentiated	NK, Undifferentiated
Incidence	Approximately 25%	Approximately 15%	Approximately 60%
Gender/age	M > F; 4th-6th decades; rare < 40 years of age	M > F; 4th-6th decades	M > F; 4th-6th decades; may occur in children
Histology	Keratinization, intercellular bridges; conventional squamous carcinoma graded as well-, moderately, or poorly differentiated; desmoplastic response to invasion	Little to absent keratinization, growth pattern interconnecting cords; typically, limited to absent desmoplastic response to invasion	Absence of keratinization, syncytial growth, cohesive or noncohesive cells with round nuclei, prominent eosinophilic nucleoli, scant cytoplasm; prominent nonneoplastic lymphoid component; typically, absent desmoplastic response to invasion
Association with EBV	Weak association	Strong association	Strong association
Treatment	Supervoltage radiotherapy (6,500-7,000+ rads)	Supervoltage radiotherapy (6,500-7,000+ rads)	Supervoltage radiotherapy (6,500-7,000+ rads)
Prognosis	5-year survival (20-40%)	5-year survival (~ 75%)	5-year survival (~ 75%)

NK = nonkeratinizing.

- Positive for EBV
  - Immunoreactivity for EBV
  - In situ hybridization for Epstein-Barr encoded RNA (EBER)
- Negative for p16

Molecular Genetics

- Detection of EBV by polymerase chain reaction (PCR) or in situ hybridization (ISH) found in 75-100% of NPCs, nonkeratinizing types
  - Not true in keratinizing subtype, in which detection of EBV genomes is variable
  - Presence of EBV in keratinizing subtype generally limited to scattered dysplastic intraepithelial cells
- Development of NPC likely involves cumulative genetic and epigenetic changes in background of predisposed genetic and environmental factors

DIFFERENTIAL DIAGNOSIS

Oropharyngeal Nonkeratinizing Carcinoma

- Tonsillar and base of tongue carcinomas may share histomorphologic features with NPC, differentiated and undifferentiated types
  - Such tumors are p16(+) and EBER(-)
  - Nodal metastatic p16(+), EBER(-) carcinomas may originate from occult primary oropharyngeal carcinomas
  - Work-up for nodal metastatic carcinomas with features of NPC, differentiated and undifferentiated, should include staining for EBER **and** p16

Diffuse Large B-cell Lymphoma

- Positive for hematolymphoid markers including CD45 (leucocyte common antigen) and B-cell markers
- Negative for cytokeratins and EBV

Mucosal Malignant Melanoma

- Positive for S100 protein, melanoma markers (HMB-45, Melan-A, tyrosinase)
- Negative for cytokeratins and EBV

Rhabdomyosarcoma

- Positive for myogenic markers (desmin, myoglobin, myogenin)
- Negative for cytokeratins and EBV

SELECTED REFERENCES

1. Caponigro F et al: Treatment approaches to nasopharyngeal carcinoma: a review. Anticancer Drugs. 21(5):471-7, 2010
2. Singhi AD et al: Lymphoepithelial-like carcinoma of the oropharynx: a morphologic variant of HPV-related head and neck carcinoma. Am J Surg Pathol. 34(6):800-5, 2010
3. Afqir S et al: Nasopharyngeal carcinoma in adolescents: a retrospective review of 42 patients. Eur Arch Otorhinolaryngol. 266(11):1767-73, 2009
4. Liu T et al: FDG-PET, CT, MRI for diagnosis of local residual or recurrent nasopharyngeal carcinoma, which one is the best? A systematic review. Radiother Oncol. 85(3):327-35, 2007
5. Tao Q et al: Nasopharyngeal carcinoma: molecular pathogenesis and therapeutic developments. Expert Rev Mol Med. 9(12):1-24, 2007
6. Thompson LD: Update on nasopharyngeal carcinoma. Head Neck Pathol. 1(1):81-6, 2007
7. Brennan B: Nasopharyngeal carcinoma. Orphanet J Rare Dis. 1:23, 2006
8. Mirzamani N et al: Detection of EBV and HPV in nasopharyngeal carcinoma by in situ hybridization. Exp Mol Pathol. 81(3):231-4, 2006
9. Wei WI et al: Nasopharyngeal carcinoma. Lancet. 365(9476):2041-54, 2005
10. Licitra L et al: Cancer of the nasopharynx. Crit Rev Oncol Hematol. 45(2):199-213, 2003
11. Ensley JF et al: Locally advanced nasopharyngeal cancer. Curr Treat Options Oncol. 2(1):15-23, 2001
12. Erkal HS et al: Nasopharyngeal carcinomas: analysis of patient, tumor and treatment characteristics determining outcome. Radiother Oncol. 61(3):247-56, 2001
13. Wenig BM: Nasopharyngeal carcinoma. Ann Diagn Pathol. 3(6):374-85, 1999

NASOPHARYNGEAL CARCINOMA, NONKERATINIZING TYPES

Microscopic and Immunohistochemical Features

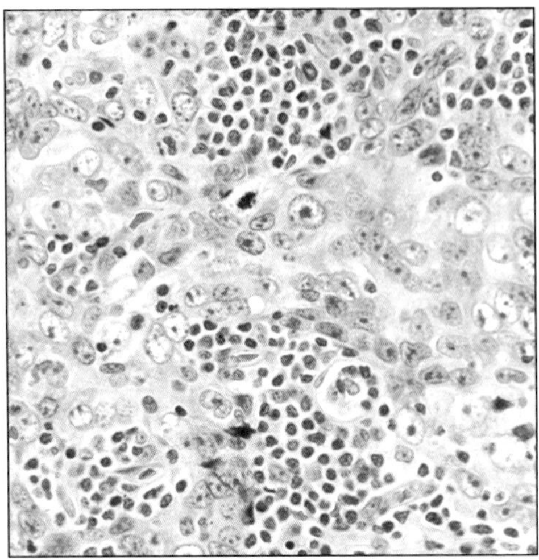

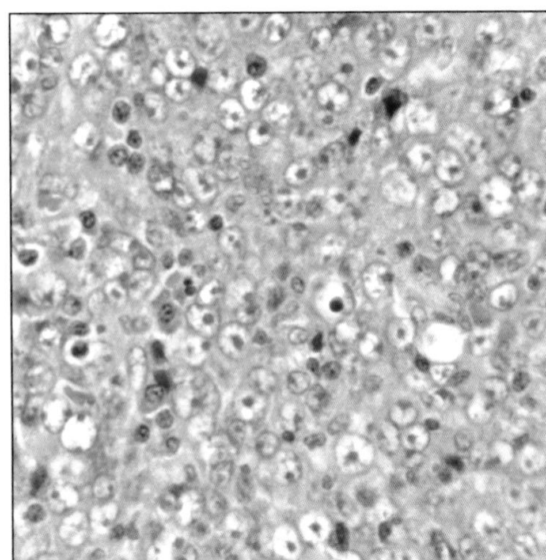

(Left) *A benign lymphocytic cell infiltrate is often present in association with the neoplastic cells of NPC, nonkeratinizing undifferentiated type. In spite of the invasive growth, there is an absence of desmoplasia.* ***(Right)*** *NPC, nonkeratinizing undifferentiated type, shows a diffuse pattern of growth composed of dyscohesive cells with enlarged vesicular chromatin and prominent nucleoli. These overall features raise concern for a possible misdiagnosis of large B-cell lymphoma.*

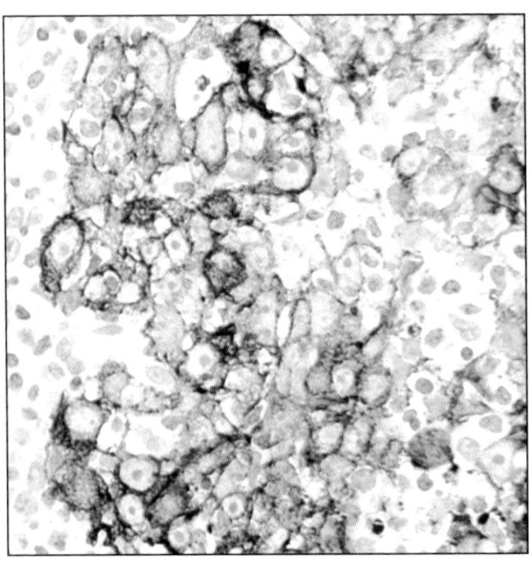

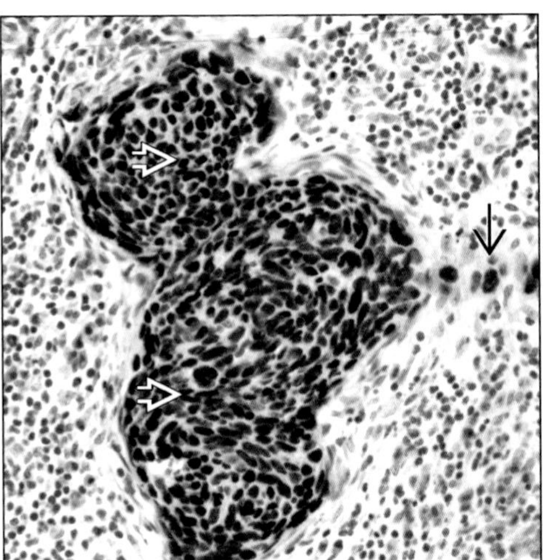

(Left) *Although similarities in the appearance of the neoplastic cells make them difficult to distinguish, the presence of cytokeratin immunoreactivity confirms the diagnosis of carcinoma and allows for differentiation from diffuse large B-cell lymphoma.* ***(Right)*** *NPC, nonkeratinizing undifferentiated type is strongly associated with EBV, as indicated by the presence of nuclear labeling of tumor cells (in nests ➡ and individual cells →) by in situ hybridization for EBER.*

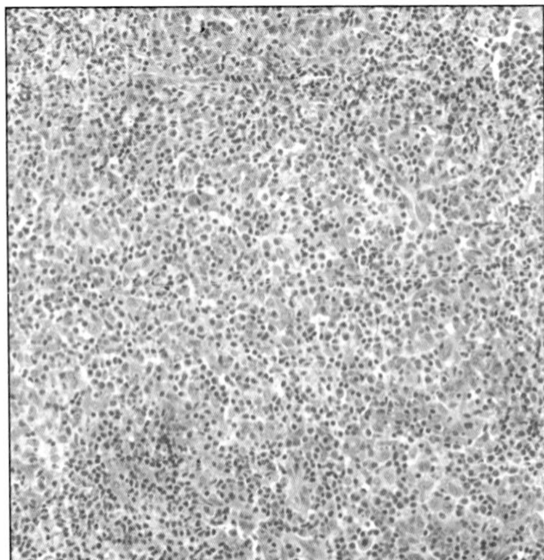

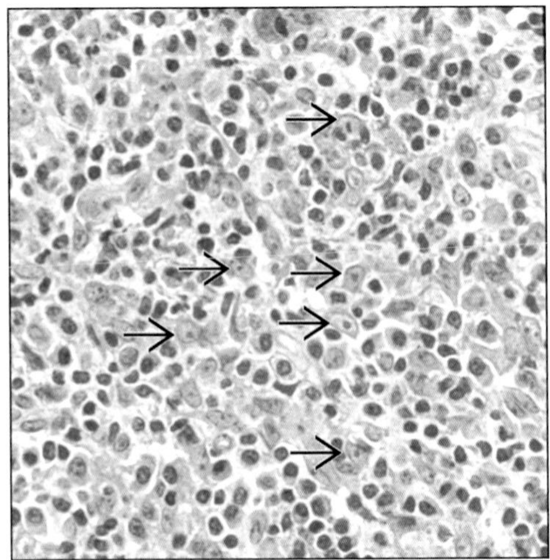

(Left) *At low magnification, there is no suggestion that an invasive carcinoma is present in this NPC, nonkeratinizing undifferentiated, due to the absence of a host desmoplastic response to invasive NPC. Instead, the impression may be that of a mixed reactive inflammatory cell proliferation.* ***(Right)*** *At higher magnification, the neoplastic cells are seen → but may be easily overlooked and viewed as part of a reactive inflammatory cell infiltrate, given the absence of associated desmoplasia.*

Microscopic and Immunohistochemical Features

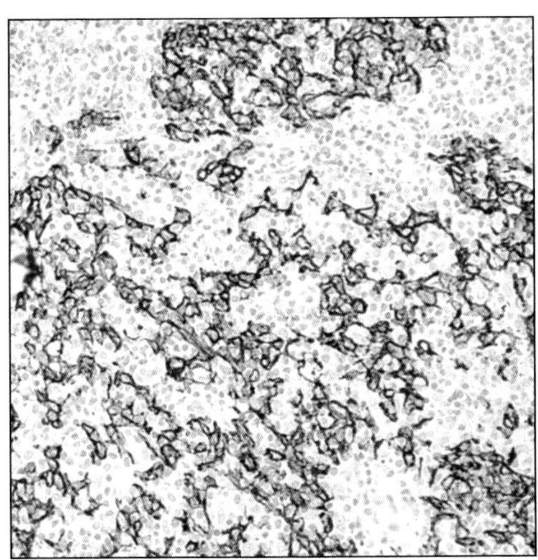

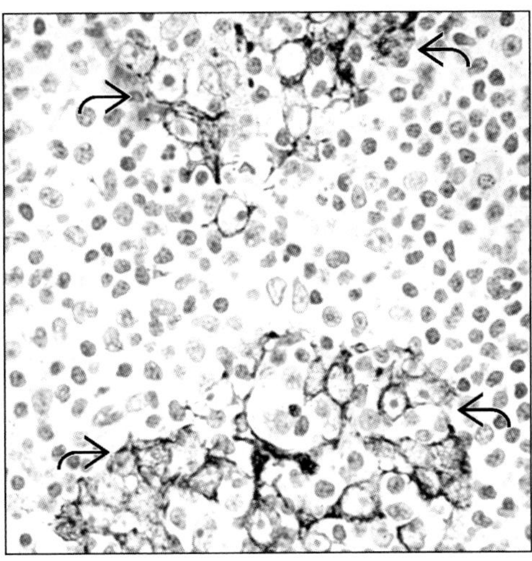

(Left) *Cytokeratin staining highlights the irregular clusters of carcinoma cells, as well as the extent of the invasive carcinoma. The extent of the invasive carcinoma as demonstrated by the cytokeratin staining may not be appreciated by light microscopic evaluation.* ***(Right)*** *At high magnification, cytokeratin reactivity delineates the carcinoma cells demonstrating a meshwork pattern of staining* ⮫*. The neoplastic epithelial cells would be nonreactive for hematolymphoid markers.*

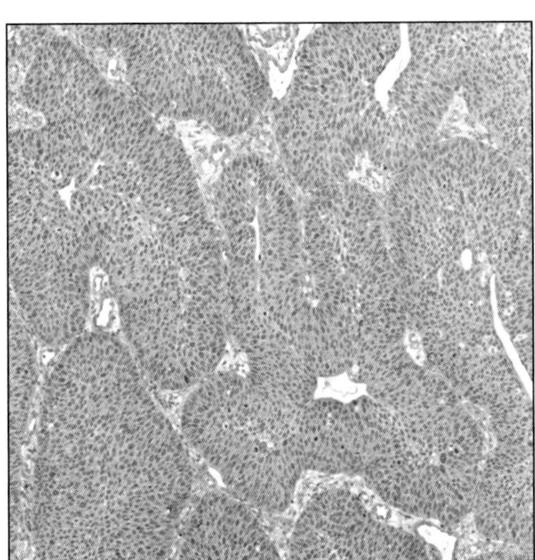

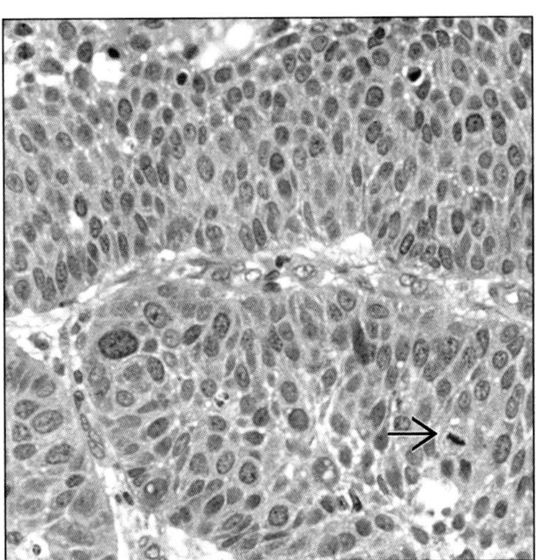

(Left) *Nasopharyngeal carcinoma, nonkeratinizing differentiated type, is characterized by broad interconnecting cords and trabeculae of infiltrative carcinoma. This pattern of growth is indicative of an infiltrative neoplasm.* ***(Right)*** *At higher magnification, the neoplastic cells of NPC, nonkeratinizing differentiated type, are stratified with nuclear pleomorphism, increased nuclear to cytoplasmic ratio, and increased mitotic activity* ⇨*.*

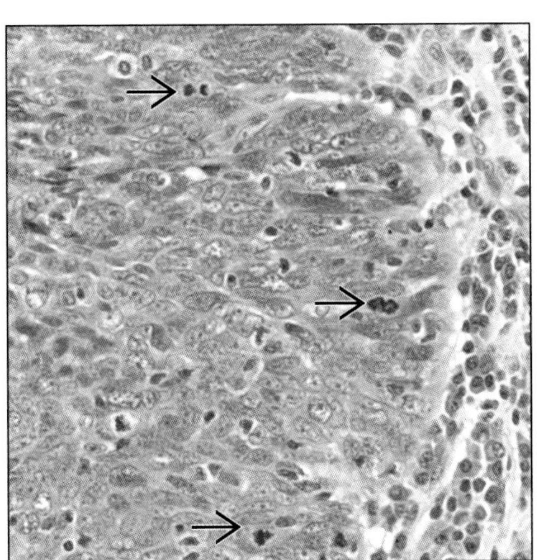

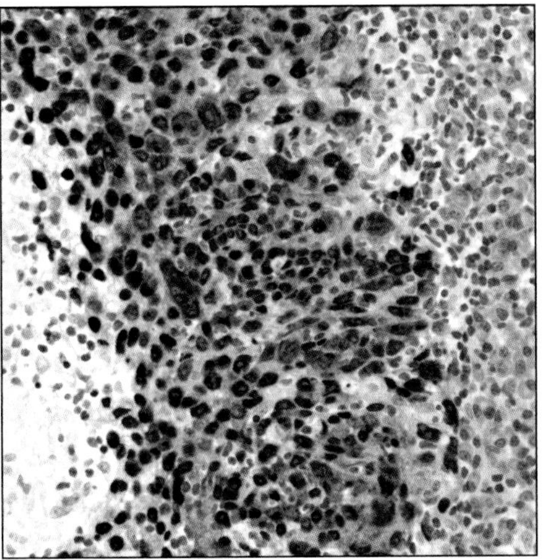

(Left) *NPC, nonkeratinizing differentiated type, shows nuclear stratification with nuclear pleomorphism, increased mitotic figures* ⇨*, absent keratinization, and absent intercellular bridges.* ***(Right)*** *NPC, nonkeratinizing differentiated type is strongly associated with EBV. Note the presence of in situ hybridization for EBER nuclear labeling in the neoplastic cells.*

NASOPHARYNGEAL CARCINOMA, NONKERATINIZING TYPES

Microscopic and Immunohistochemical Features

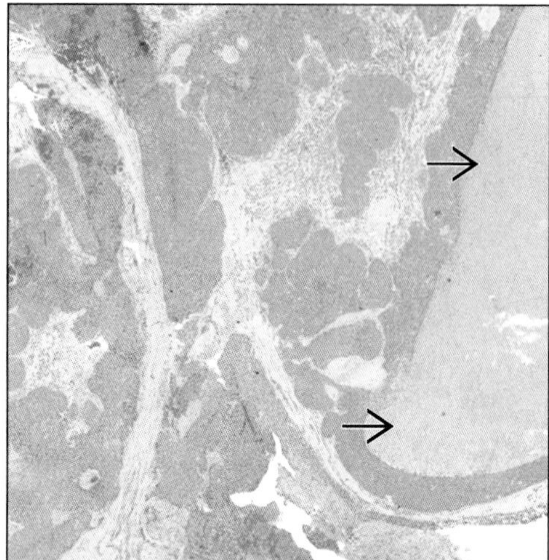

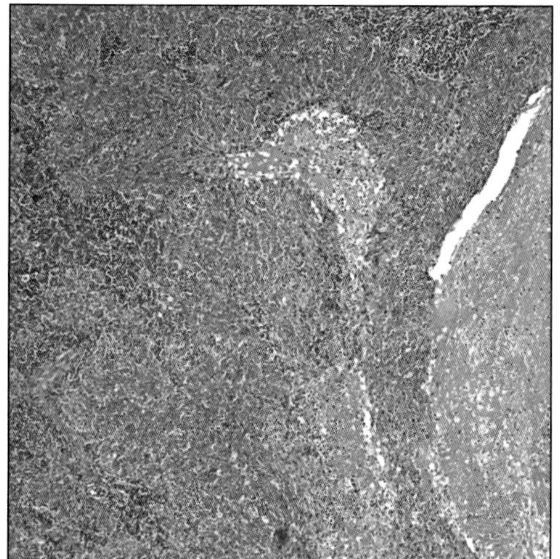

(Left) *NPC, nonkeratinizing differentiated type, shows cystic degeneration characterized by large cyst filled with necrotic material* → *. This cystic appearance with associated necrosis is the pattern that can be seen when this carcinoma metastasizes to cervical lymph nodes (i.e., cystic metastatic nonkeratinizing carcinoma).* ***(Right)*** *Nodal metastasis from a NPC, nonkeratinizing undifferentiated type, shows cystic degeneration and absent desmoplastic reaction.*

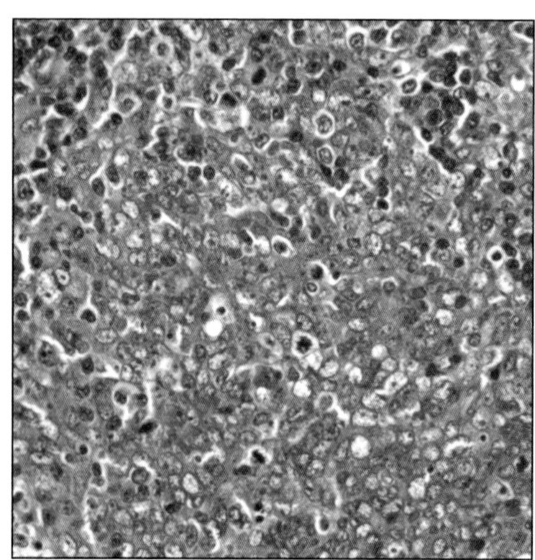

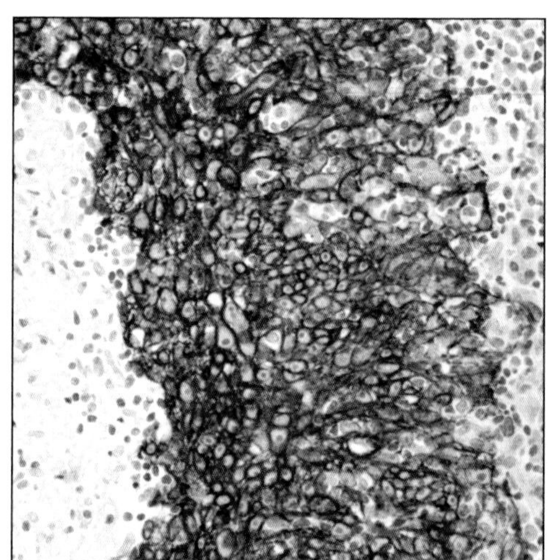

(Left) *At higher magnification, the cells of metastatic NPC, nonkeratinizing undifferentiated type, include dyscohesive cells with enlarged vesicular chromatin and prominent nucleoli. These findings may erroneously suggest a diagnosis of diffuse large B-cell lymphoma.* ***(Right)*** *Given similarities in the appearance of the neoplastic cells, the presence of cytokeratin immunoreactivity confirms the diagnosis of carcinoma and allows for differentiation from diffuse large B-cell lymphoma.*

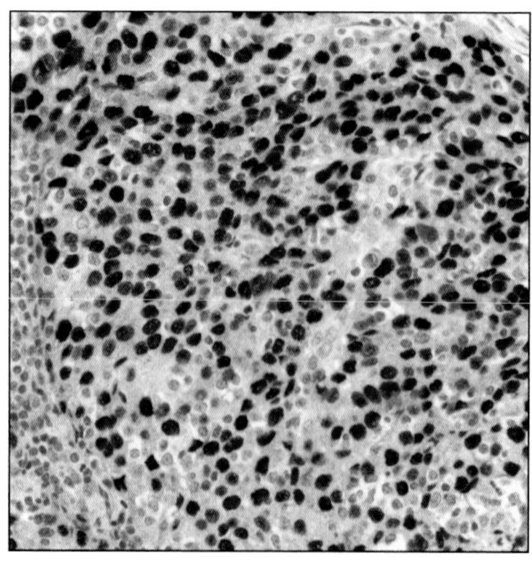

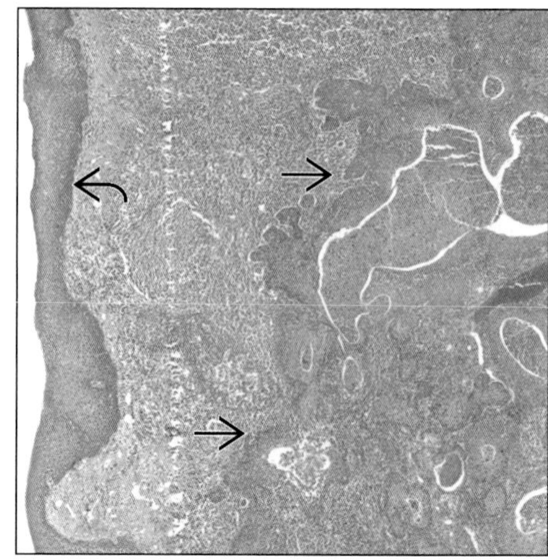

(Left) *Metastatic NPC, nonkeratinizing undifferentiated type, demonstrates the presence of in situ hybridization for EBER nuclear labeling.* ***(Right)*** *NPC, nonkeratinizing differentiated, may originate in the crypt epithelium* → *within the depth of the submucosa while the surface epithelium* ↶ *is uninvolved by dysplasia &/ or carcinoma. The carcinoma shows cystic change and associated necrosis and may metastasize to cervical lymph nodes as an occult primary carcinoma.*

Differential Diagnosis

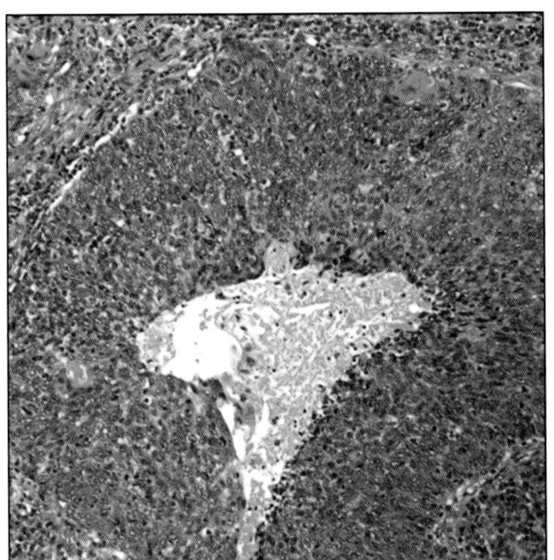

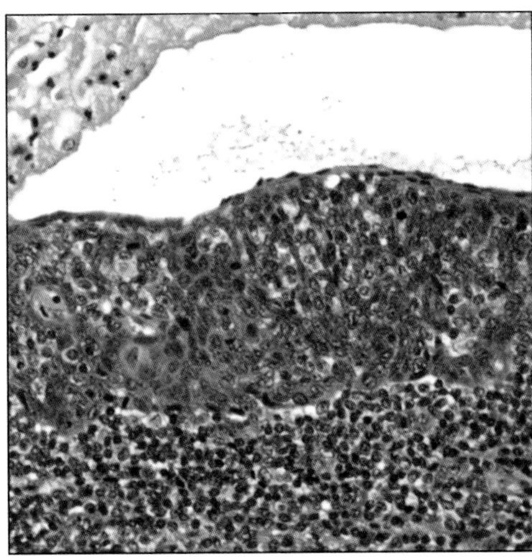

(Left) *Oropharyngeal (i.e., tonsil, base of tongue) nonkeratinizing cystic carcinoma with associated necrosis is histologically similar to NPC, nonkeratinizing differentiated type.* ***(Right)*** *At higher magnification, the neoplastic cells of oropharyngeal (i.e., tonsil, base of tongue) nonkeratinizing carcinoma, including nuclear stratification and minimal to absent keratinization, is histologically similar to NPC, nonkeratinizing differentiated type.*

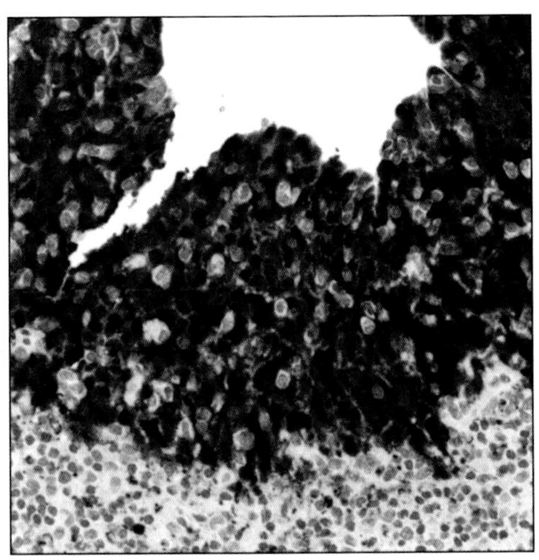

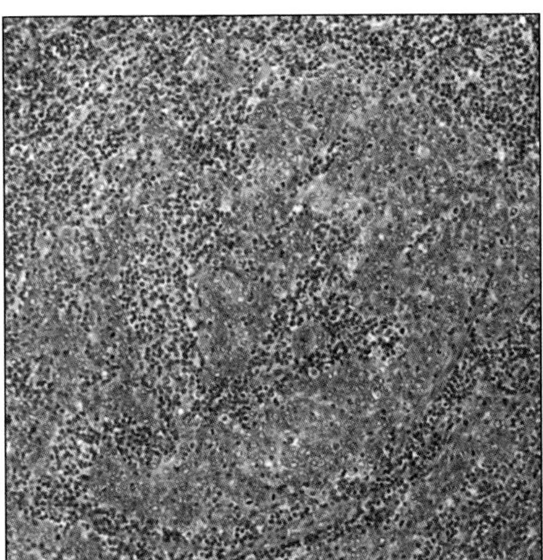

(Left) *In contrast to the strong association of NPC, nonkeratinizing types to EBV, the histologically similar appearing oropharyngeal nonkeratinizing carcinoma is associated with HPV by p16 nuclear and cytoplasmic staining, as seen here.* ***(Right)*** *Oropharyngeal (i.e., tonsil, base of tongue) nonkeratinizing carcinoma may also show similar histologic features to NPC, nonkeratinizing undifferentiated type, including associated lymphocytic cell infiltrate and absence of desmoplasia.*

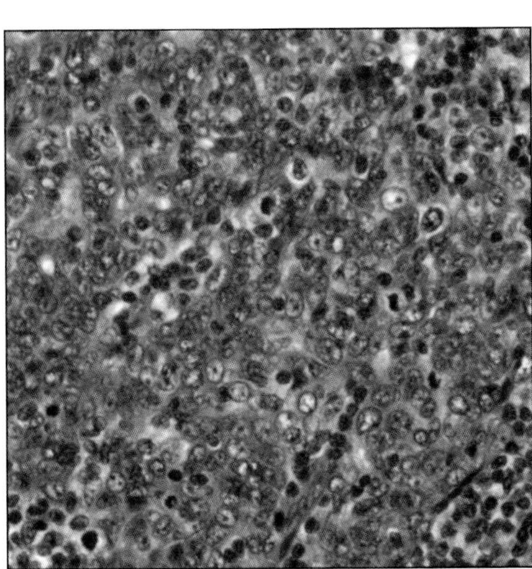

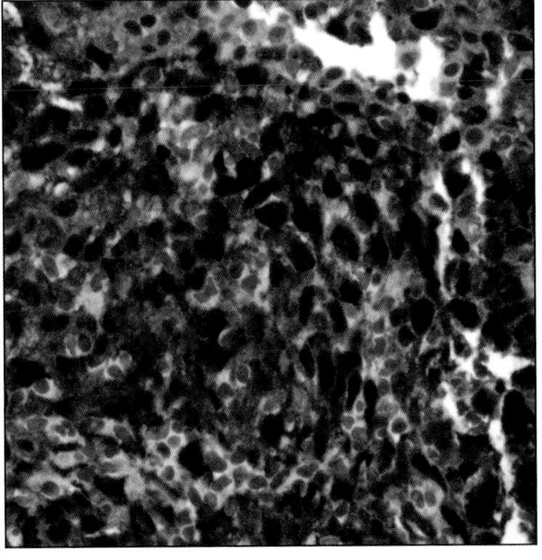

(Left) *The neoplastic cells of oropharyngeal nonkeratinizing carcinoma, including enlarged nuclei with prominent eosinophilic nucleoli, are similar to those of NPC, nonkeratinizing undifferentiated type.* ***(Right)*** *Oropharyngeal nonkeratinizing carcinoma shows strong p16 staining. This carcinoma may metastasize as an occult primary, suggesting possible nasopharyngeal origin. The presence of p16 staining strongly correlates to a primary oropharyngeal carcinoma.*

NASOPHARYNGEAL CARCINOMA, KERATINIZING TYPE

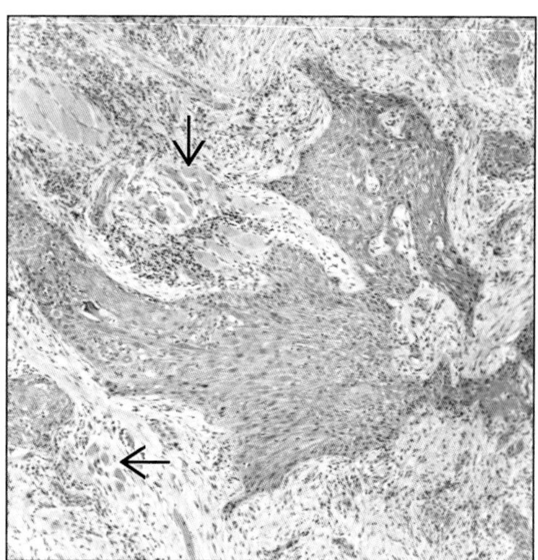

Nasopharyngeal invasive keratinizing squamous cell carcinoma invades into the submucosa with associated desmoplastic stromal reaction and invasion into skeletal muscle ➔.

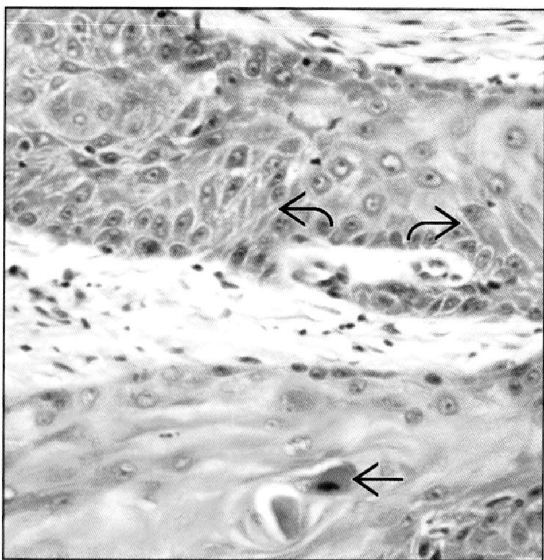

Well-differentiated keratinizing squamous cell carcinoma is characterized by the presence of limited (mild) cytologic atypia, cells with identifiable keratinization ➔, and intercellular bridges ➔.

TERMINOLOGY

Abbreviations

- Nasopharyngeal carcinoma (NPC)

Definitions

- Type of squamous cell carcinoma originating from nasopharyngeal mucosa showing evidence of squamous differentiation
- World Health Organization classification of NPC
  - Keratinizing
  - Nonkeratinizing
    - Differentiated
    - Undifferentiated
- Prior numerical designations of WHO types 1 (squamous cell carcinoma), 2 (nonkeratinizing carcinoma), and 3 (undifferentiated carcinoma) no longer used

ETIOLOGY/PATHOGENESIS

Environmental Exposure

- Purported risk factors include
  - High dietary levels of nitrosamines in preserved food in high incidence regions implicated as carcinogen
  - Cigarette smoking
  - Occupational exposure to chemical fumes, smoke, formaldehyde
  - Prior radiation exposure
- NPC, keratinizing type, not considered to be associated with Epstein-Barr virus (EBV)
  - NPC, nonkeratinizing types associated with EBV

CLINICAL ISSUES

Epidemiology

- Incidence
  - Represents approximately 25% of all NPC
- Age
  - Most common in 4th-6th decades
    - Rarely occurs in patients under 40 years of age
- Gender
  - Male > Female
- Ethnicity
  - Endemic populations include Chinese, southeast Asians, north Africans, natives of Arctic region

Site

- Lateral wall > superior posterior wall

Presentation

- Nasal obstruction, nasal discharge, epistaxis, pain, serous otitis media, otalgia, hearing loss, headache
- Cranial nerve involvement may be present in more advanced disease

Treatment

- Surgical approaches
  - Surgical intervention reserved for patients who fail radiation therapy
- Adjuvant therapy
  - Chemotherapy integrated with radiation in advanced stage disease
- Radiation
  - Supervoltage radiotherapy (6,500 to > 7,000 rads) considered treatment of choice for all NPC histologic subtypes

Prognosis

- Overall 5-year survival: 20-40%
  - Higher incidence of locally advanced tumor but lower incidence of lymphatic &/or distant spread
  - Poorer 5-year survival rate due to higher incidence of deaths secondary to local uncontrollable disease

NASOPHARYNGEAL CARCINOMA, KERATINIZING TYPE

Key Facts

Terminology
- Type of squamous cell carcinoma originating from nasopharyngeal mucosa showing evidence of squamous differentiation

Etiology/Pathogenesis
- Not considered associated with Epstein-Barr virus

Clinical Issues
- Represents approximately 25% of all NPC
- Supervoltage radiotherapy treatment of choice
- Overall 5-year survival: 20-40%

Microscopic Pathology
- Infiltrative carcinoma characterized by presence of keratinization and intercellular bridges
- Graded as well-, moderately, or poorly differentiated

IMAGE FINDINGS

Radiographic Findings
- Represents important diagnostic aid in assessing extent of disease and presence of metastatic disease
- MR preferred study for detection of invasion into soft tissues, intracranial extension, and invasion into bone

MICROSCOPIC PATHOLOGY

Histologic Features
- Infiltrative carcinoma characterized by presence of keratinization and intercellular bridges
  - Graded as well-, moderately, or poorly differentiated
- Desmoplastic stroma present in response to invasive carcinoma
- Relative absence of associated lymphoid cell infiltrate

ANCILLARY TESTS

Immunohistochemistry
- Consistent strong staining for cytokeratins, p63

Molecular Genetics
- Molecular studies for EBV
  - Positive in endemic areas, generally negative in nonendemic areas

DIFFERENTIAL DIAGNOSIS

Reactive Epithelial Hyperplasia
- May show reactive atypia but lack
  - Significant dysplastic epithelial changes
  - Invasive nests of tumor
  - Associated desmoplasia

SELECTED REFERENCES

1. Mirzamani N et al: Detection of EBV and HPV in nasopharyngeal carcinoma by in situ hybridization. Exp Mol Pathol. 81(3):231-4, 2006
2. Licitra L et al: Cancer of the nasopharynx. Crit Rev Oncol Hematol. 45(2):199-213, 2003
3. Ensley JF et al: Locally advanced nasopharyngeal cancer. Curr Treat Options Oncol. 2(1):15-23, 2001
4. Wenig BM: Nasopharyngeal carcinoma. Ann Diagn Pathol. 3(6):374-85, 1999
5. Marks JE et al: The National Cancer Data Base report on the relationship of race and national origin to the histology of nasopharyngeal carcinoma. Cancer. 83(3):582-8, 1998
6. Zhang JX et al: Epstein-Barr virus expression within keratinizing nasopharyngeal carcinoma. J Med Virol. 55(3):227-33, 1998
7. Nicholls JM et al: The association of squamous cell carcinomas of the nasopharynx with Epstein-Barr virus shows geographical variation reminiscent of Burkitt's lymphoma. J Pathol. 183(2):164-8, 1997

IMAGE GALLERY

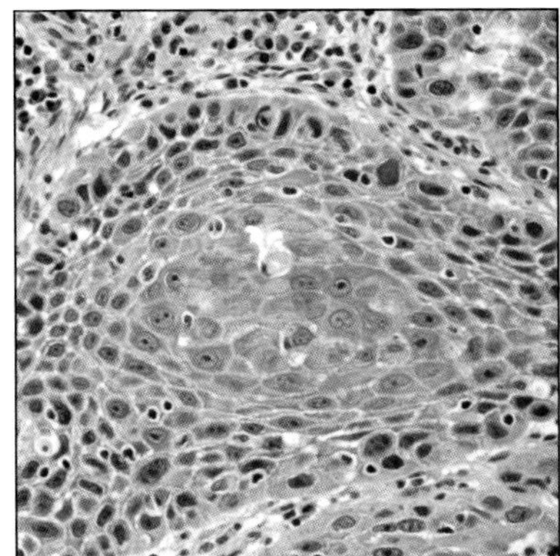

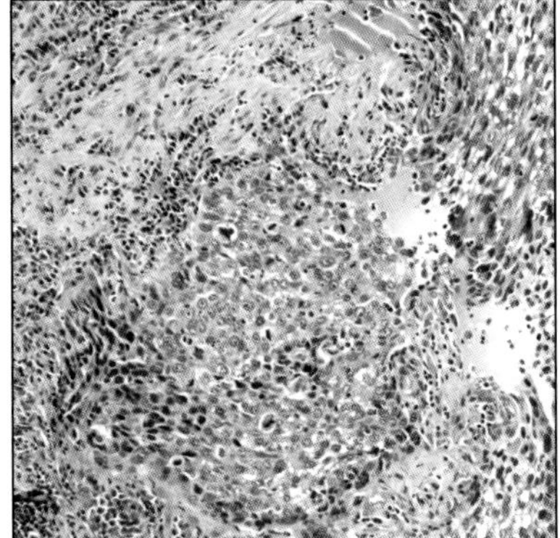

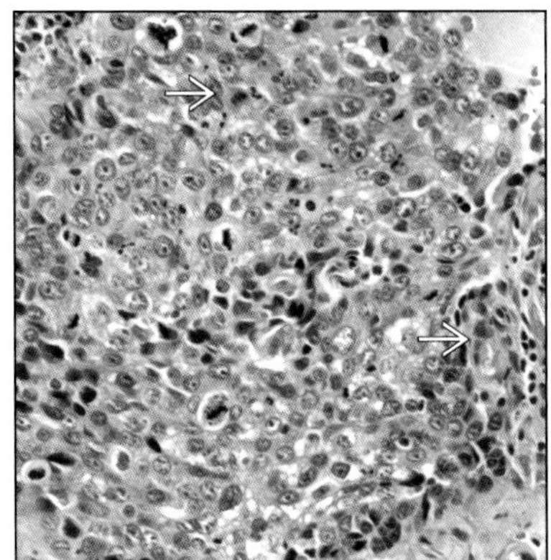

*(**Left**) Nasopharyngeal invasive moderately differentiated keratinizing squamous cell carcinoma with greater nuclear pleomorphism than well-differentiated carcinoma is shown. (**Center**) Nasopharyngeal invasive poorly differentiated squamous cell carcinoma with associated desmoplasia is shown. (**Right**) At higher magnification, there is less evidence of squamous differentiation compared to better differentiated carcinomas although keratinization is present ➡, indicative of squamous carcinoma.*

NASOPHARYNGEAL CARCINOMA, BASALOID SQUAMOUS CELL CARCINOMA

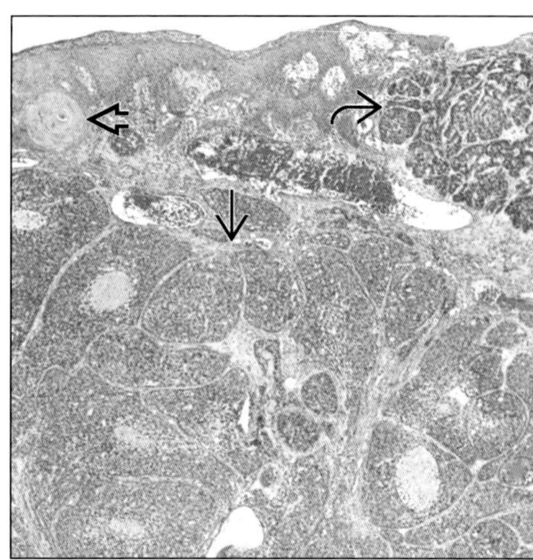

Basaloid squamous cell carcinoma is an infiltrative basaloid cell neoplasm with varied growth, including lobular ➔ and trabecular ➔ patterns; abrupt squamous differentiation is present ➔.

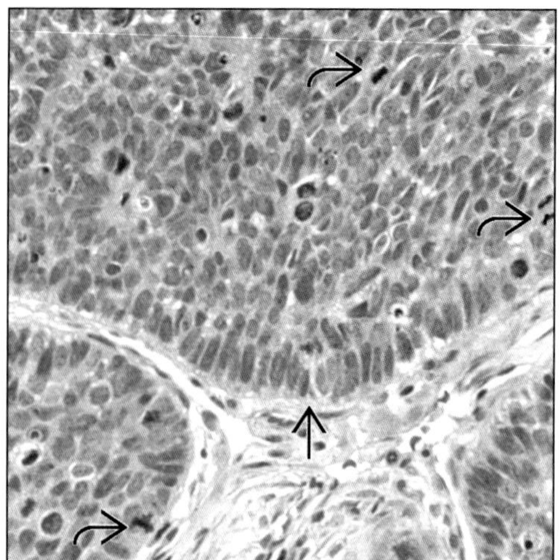

The basaloid cells show marked nuclear pleomorphism, hyperchromasia, and increased mitotic activity ➔. Peripheral nuclear palisading is present ➔, but retraction artifact is not identified.

TERMINOLOGY

Abbreviations

- Basaloid squamous cell carcinoma (BSCC)

Definitions

- High-grade variant of squamous cell carcinoma histologically characterized by invasive neoplasm composed predominantly of basaloid pleomorphic cells and variable squamous component

ETIOLOGY/PATHOGENESIS

Alcohol and Tobacco

- Etiologic factors of BSCC occurring in more common sites include excessive alcohol &/or tobacco use

Infectious Agents

- Confusion in literature relative to association with Epstein-Barr virus (EBV)
  - Asian patients reported EBV(+) while non-Asians reported EBV(-)
    - Likely not EBV associated; presence of EBV endemic to Asian population
  - BSCC are typically not associated with human papillomavirus (HPV)

CLINICAL ISSUES

Epidemiology

- Incidence
  - Uncommon type of primary nasopharyngeal carcinoma
  - May occur in any mucosal site of upper aerodigestive tract, but majority predilect to hypopharynx (piriform sinus), larynx (supraglottis), and palatine tonsil
- Age
  - Occurs over wide age range from 3rd to 8th decades of life (mean: 55 years)
- Gender
  - Male > Female

Presentation

- Symptoms depend on site of occurrence and relative to laryngeal tumors include
  - Hoarseness, dysphagia, pain, or neck mass

Treatment

- Options, risks, complications
  - Radical surgical excision
  - Due to early regional lymph node as well as distant visceral metastases, radical neck dissection, and supplemental radio- and chemotherapy may be included in initial management protocol

Prognosis

- Nasopharyngeal BSCCs appear to have lower clinical aggressiveness compared to BSCC of other head and neck sites
  - Of 6 cases reported
    - 4 clinical stage T3 or T4
    - 2 with nodal metastasis
    - None with distant metastasis
    - 3 with no evidence of disease at 34-52 months
    - 3 alive with disease from 19-46 months
- BSCCs of more common head and neck sites are aggressive, high-grade tumors with increased tendency to be multifocal, deeply invasive, and metastatic
  - Metastases occur via lymphatics and blood vessels with sites of predilection, including regional and distant lymph nodes, lung, bone, skin, and brain
  - Metastases include both basaloid and squamous cell components
  - Rapidly fatal associated with high mortality rates within 1st year following diagnosis

NASOPHARYNGEAL CARCINOMA, BASALOID SQUAMOUS CELL CARCINOMA

Key Facts

Terminology
- High-grade variant of squamous cell carcinoma histologically characterized by invasive neoplasm composed predominantly of basaloid pleomorphic cells and variable squamous component

Clinical Issues
- Uncommon type of primary nasopharyngeal carcinoma
- Nasopharyngeal BSCCs appear to have lower clinical aggressiveness compared to BSCC of other head and neck sites

Microscopic Pathology
- Invasive neoplasm predominantly composed of basaloid cells with associated squamous component
- Varied growth patterns, including lobular (with or without comedonecrosis), solid, trabecular
- Basaloid cell component is predominant cell type characterized by pleomorphic, hyperchromatic nuclei with increased mitotic activity
- Squamous cell component typically represents minor component and may include keratinization, invasive squamous cell carcinoma
- Intraepithelial dysplasia and carcinoma in situ may be present

Ancillary Tests
- Immunoreactivity consistently present for cytokeratins
- Neuroendocrine markers usually negative but occasionally may be positive

MACROSCOPIC FEATURES

General Features
- Firm to hard, tan-white mass often with associated central necrosis
- Infrequently may be exophytic in appearance

Size
- May reach large size, measuring up to 6 cm in greatest dimension

MICROSCOPIC PATHOLOGY

Histologic Features
- Invasive neoplasm predominantly composed of basaloid cells with associated squamous component
  - Varied growth patterns, including solid, lobular, cribriform, cords, trabeculae, and gland-like or cystic
  - Tends to be deeply invasive at presentation, including neurotropism and lymph-vascular invasion
    - Shallow biopsies may belie depth and extent of invasion
- Basaloid cell component
  - Predominant cell type
  - May be seen in direct continuity with surface epithelium
  - Pleomorphic, hyperchromatic nuclei, scanty cytoplasm and variably sized but identifiable nucleoli
  - Peripheral nuclear palisading may be present
  - Increased mitotic activity, including atypical mitoses
  - Necrosis commonly seen, including
    - Comedonecrosis seen in center of neoplastic lobules
    - Individual cell necrosis
  - Intercellular deposition of hyalin or mucohyalin material can be seen
    - Similar in appearance to reduplicated basement membrane material seen in some salivary gland tumors
  - Additional findings may include
    - Cells with clear appearing cytoplasm may be seen either focally or more extensively
    - Spindle cell component may be identified but usually very focal, not predominate cell type
    - Infrequently, true neural-type rosettes may be present
    - Calcifications may be present
- Squamous cell component
  - Typically, represents minor component
    - May only be focally present
    - In biopsies, squamous cell component may be absent
  - Includes intraepithelial dysplasia (moderate to severe dysplasia) &/or invasive squamous cell carcinoma with or without foci of abrupt keratinization
  - Continuity with surface epithelium may be present

ANCILLARY TESTS

Histochemistry
- Diastase-sensitive, periodic acid-Schiff(+) intracytoplasmic material indicative of glycogen may be present especially in cells with clear cytoplasm

Immunohistochemistry
- Immunoreactivity consistently present for epithelial markers, including cytokeratins (AE1/3, CAM5.2, others), EMA, and CEA
- Neuroendocrine markers, including chromogranin, synaptophysin, CD56 usually negative but occasionally may be positive (synaptophysin > chromogranin)
- Likely EBV(-) although discrepant results reported
- p16(-)
  - Oropharyngeal (tonsil, base of tongue) BSCC may be p16(+)
  - Nonoropharyngeal BSCCs mostly p16(-)
- Variable expression seen for vimentin, NSE, S100 protein, actin

Differential Diagnosis of Basaloid Squamous Cell Carcinoma

	BSCC	AdCC	SCUNC
Age/gender	6th-7th decades; M > F	5th-7th decades; equal gender distribution except for submandibular tumors, which predilect to females	6th-7th decades; M > F
Location	Predilects to hypopharynx (piriform sinus), larynx (supraglottis), and oropharynx (palatine tonsil)	Major and minor salivary glands	Uncommon in head and neck; supraglottic larynx most common site
Surface involvement	Present in the form of intraepithelial dysplasia	Absent	Absent
Squamous component	Present but is the minor component and may only be found focally	Absent	May be present; limited in extent when found
Neurotropism	Present	Present	Present
Immunohistochemistry	Immunoreactive for cytokeratins; neuroendocrine markers (chromogranin, synaptophysin, others) usually negative but occasionally may be positive	Immunoreactivity for cytokeratins, p63, S100 protein, calponin, actins, and vimentin; negative for neuroendocrine markers	Positive for cytokeratins; immunoreactive for neuroendocrine markers (chromogranin, synaptophysin, CD56, CD57, TTF-1); calcitonin rarely is positive
HPV association	No	No	No
Treatment	Surgery, radiotherapy, chemotherapy	Surgery, radiotherapy	Systemic chemotherapy and therapeutic irradiation
Prognosis	Dependent on clinical stage but overall considered to be poor; nasopharyngeal-based BSCC appears to be less biologically aggressive than other head and neck BSCCs	Short-term prognosis is good but long-term prognosis is poor; survival rates include 5-year (71-89%), 10-year (29-71%), 15-year (29-55%)	Poor: 2-year survival (16%), 5-year survival (5%)

BSCC = basaloid squamous cell carcinoma of all head and neck sites; AdCC = adenoid cystic carcinoma; SCUNC = small cell undifferentiated neuroendocrine carcinoma.

- Melanocytic markers (HMB-45, Melan-A, tyrosinase) and hematolymphoid markers negative

Electron Microscopy

- Cell groups with numerous and prominent tonofilament bundles, increased desmosomes, epithelial pearls, loose stellate granules, or replicated basal lamina within cystic spaces
- Absence of glandular differentiation

DIFFERENTIAL DIAGNOSIS

Oropharyngeal Nonkeratinizing Carcinoma

- HPV-associated carcinoma distinct from BSCC
- In situ and invasive carcinoma characterized by broad interconnecting cords of tumor often with cystic change and central necrosis
- Cells are nonkeratinizing characterized by pleomorphic basaloid-appearing nuclei with increased mitotic activity
- Limited foci of squamous cell differentiation (keratinization) may be seen
- Immunoreactivity for p16

Adenoid Cystic Carcinoma

- Characterized by isomorphic hyperchromatic basaloid cells lacking pleomorphism, mitotic activity, and necrosis
- Squamous differentiation not feature of AdCC
- Immunohistochemical staining not helpful in differential diagnosis

Small Cell Undifferentiated Neuroendocrine Carcinoma

- Consistent immunoreactivity for neuroendocrine markers (chromogranin, synaptophysin, CD56, CD57, TTF-1)

SELECTED REFERENCES

1. Begum S et al: Basaloid squamous cell carcinoma of the head and neck is a mixed variant that can be further resolved by HPV status. Am J Surg Pathol. 32(7):1044-50, 2008
2. Muller E et al: The basaloid squamous cell carcinoma of the nasopharynx. Rhinology. 38(4):208-11, 2000
3. Paulino AF et al: Basaloid squamous cell carcinoma of the head and neck. Laryngoscope. 110(9):1479-82, 2000
4. Barnes L et al: Basaloid squamous cell carcinoma of the head and neck: clinicopathological features and differential diagnosis. Ann Otol Rhinol Laryngol. 105(1):75-82, 1996
5. Wan SK et al: Basaloid-squamous carcinoma of the nasopharynx. An Epstein-Barr virus-associated neoplasm compared with morphologically identical tumors occurring in other sites. Cancer. 76(10):1689-93, 1995
6. Raslan WF et al: Basaloid squamous cell carcinoma of the head and neck: a clinicopathologic and flow cytometric study of 10 new cases with review of the English literature. Am J Otolaryngol. 15(3):204-11, 1994
7. Klijanienko J et al: Basaloid squamous carcinoma of the head and neck. Immunohistochemical comparison with adenoid cystic carcinoma and squamous cell carcinoma. Arch Otolaryngol Head Neck Surg. 119(8):887-90, 1993
8. Banks ER et al: Basaloid squamous cell carcinoma of the head and neck. A clinicopathologic and immunohistochemical study of 40 cases. Am J Surg Pathol. 16(10):939-46, 1992

Microscopic Features

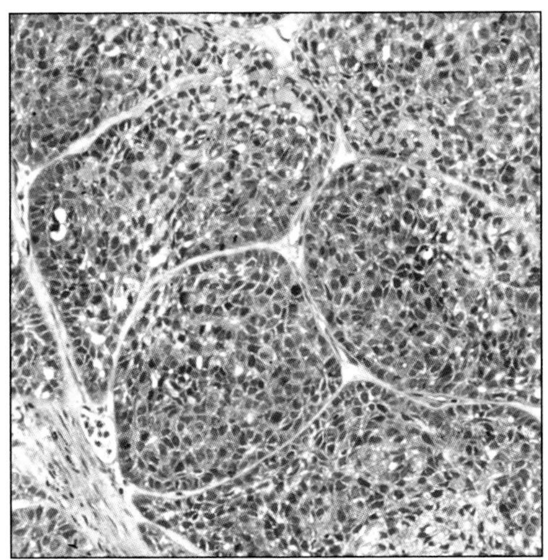

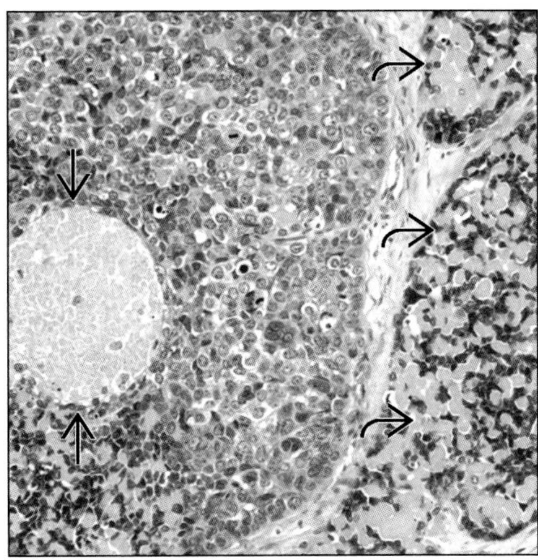

(Left) *Infiltrative nests or lobules show a jigsaw-puzzle-like configuration predominantly composed of malignant basaloid cells showing marked nuclear pleomorphism; squamous differentiated foci are not identified.* ***(Right)*** *Infiltrative nest or lobule with comedo-type necrosis* → *and adjacent area show reduplicated basement membrane-like material reminiscent of salivary gland tumors* ↪*. Basaloid cells predominate without squamous differentiation.*

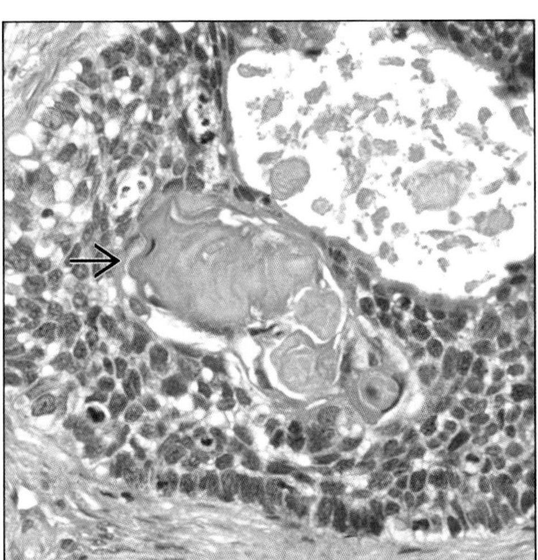

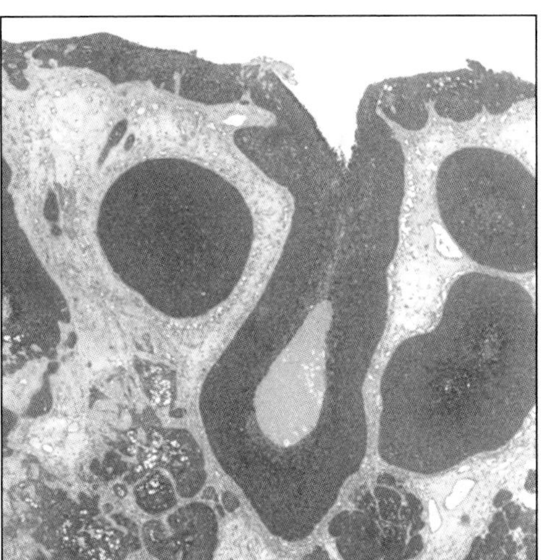

(Left) *The squamous differentiated component of BSCC represents the minor component and may be represented by presence of focal areas of abrupt keratinization* → *to larger confluent foci of keratinization or invasive keratinizing squamous cell carcinoma (not shown).* ***(Right)*** *In addition to keratinization or invasive squamous cell carcinoma, there may be intraepithelial dysplasia or carcinoma in situ, a feature supporting origin from surface epithelium.*

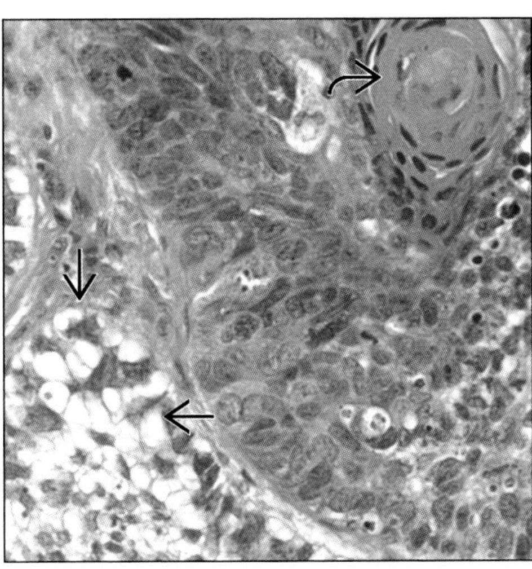

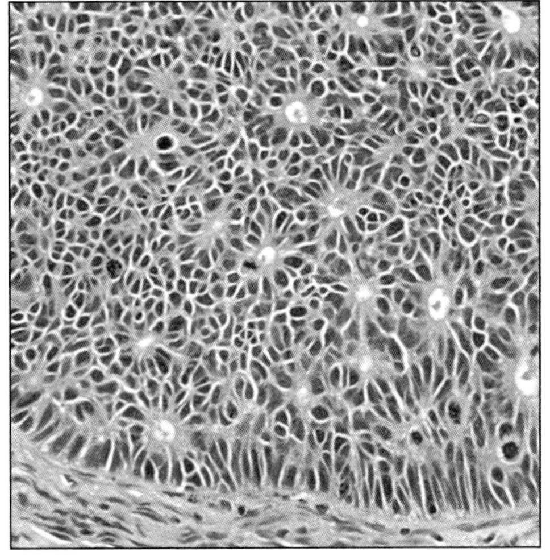

(Left) *Additional cell types that can be seen in BSCC are clear cells* → *that by special stain contain glycogen (not shown). Note the prominent malignant basaloid cells as well as a focus of abrupt keratinization* ↪*.* ***(Right)*** *Neural-type rosettes can be seen in BSCC raising concern for a possible diagnosis of small cell undifferentiated neuroendocrine carcinoma (SCUNC). BSCC typically lacks immunostaining for neuroendocrine markers, assisting in differentiating it from SCUNC.*

NASOPHARYNGEAL PAPILLARY ADENOCARCINOMA

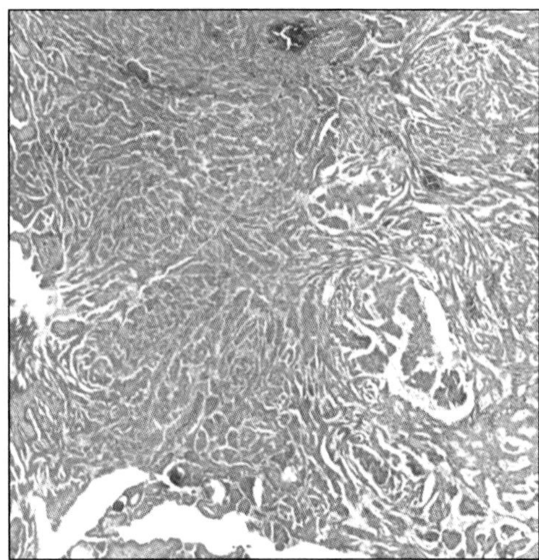

Infiltrating tumor with complex glandular and papillary growth is characteristically seen in NPPA. Such an appearance even at low magnification suggests a malignant neoplasm.

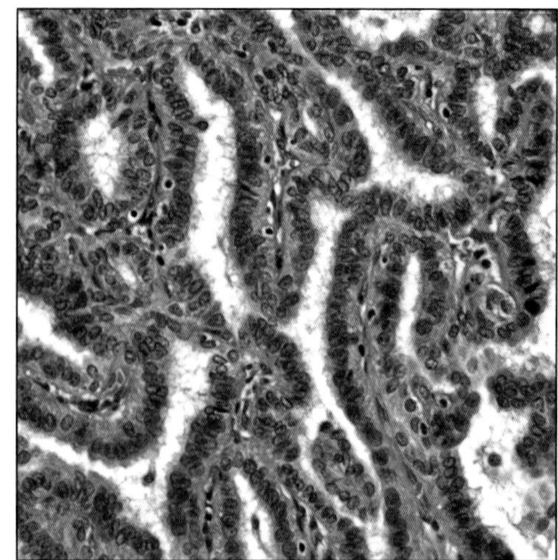

Papillary growth and fibrovascular cores are seen composed of pseudostratified columnar to cuboidal cells with enlarged nuclei that are crowded or overlap and have dispersed to clear-appearing chromatin.

TERMINOLOGY

Abbreviations

- Nasopharyngeal papillary adenocarcinoma (NPPA)

Definitions

- Surface epithelial-derived malignant tumor with adenocarcinomatous differentiation and indolent biologic behavior
  - Light microscopic findings and immunohistochemical findings support derivation of this neoplasm from surface epithelium rather than from subjacent minor salivary glands

ETIOLOGY/PATHOGENESIS

Idiopathic

- No known etiologic factors
- No association with infectious agents (e.g., Epstein-Barr virus, human papillomavirus, others)
- Rare case identified in association with Turner syndrome but no known link to other diseases/ syndromes

CLINICAL ISSUES

Epidemiology

- Incidence
  - Rare primary tumor of nasopharynx
- Age
  - Occurs over wide age range from 2nd-7th decades of life (median: 37 years)
- Gender
  - Equal gender distribution

Site

- May occur anywhere in nasopharynx but is most common in posterior and lateral nasopharyngeal walls and roof

Presentation

- Nasal obstruction most common symptom
  - Occasional association to otitis media with or without associated hearing deficits and postnasal drip

Treatment

- Options, risks, complications
  - Complete surgical excision via transpalatal approach is treatment of choice
- Radiation
  - Radiotherapy (pre- and postoperative) not warranted

Prognosis

- Cured by surgical resection
- Slow-growing tumor with potential to recur if incompletely excised
- Metastatic disease does not occur

MACROSCOPIC FEATURES

General Features

- Exophytic, soft to gritty mass with papillary, nodular, and cauliflower-like appearance

Size

- Varies from few millimeters to 3 cm or greater

MICROSCOPIC PATHOLOGY

Histologic Features

- Unencapsulated and infiltrative tumor composed of papillary and glandular growth patterns
  - Papillary structures are complex with arborization and hyalinized fibrovascular cores
  - Complex glandular pattern characterized by back-to-back and cribriform growth

NASOPHARYNGEAL PAPILLARY ADENOCARCINOMA

Key Facts

Terminology

- Surface epithelial-derived malignant tumor with adenocarcinomatous differentiation and indolent biologic behavior

Clinical Issues

- Occurs 2nd-7th decades (median: 37 years)
- Most common in posterior and lateral nasopharyngeal walls and roof
- Nasal obstruction most common symptom
- Complete surgical excision treatment of choice

Microscopic Pathology

- Unencapsulated and infiltrative tumor composed of papillary and glandular growth patterns
- Round to oval nuclei with vesicular to optically clear chromatin
- Psammoma bodies can be identified
- Thyroid transcription factor 1 (TTF-1) positive, thyroglobulin negative

---

  - Transition from normal nasopharyngeal surface epithelium to neoplastic proliferation present supporting surface epithelial derivation
- Cells vary in appearance from pseudostratified columnar to cuboidal
  - Nuclei are round to oval with vesicular to optically clear-appearing chromatin pattern
  - Mild to moderate nuclear pleomorphism may be present
  - Nuclear crowding and overlapping with loss of basal polarity
  - Nuclear (pseudo)inclusions not typically seen
  - Psammoma bodies can be identified
- Mitoses and prominent nucleoli not commonly identified
- Necrosis may be present

ANCILLARY TESTS

Histochemistry

- Epithelial mucin material present
  - Intracytoplasmic and intraluminal mucicarmine positive material
  - Intracytoplasmic diastase-resistant, PAS-positive material

Immunohistochemistry

- Diffuse and intense reactivity with cytokeratins and epithelial membrane antigen (EMA)
- Thyroid transcription factor 1 (TTF-1) positivity
- Carcinoembryonic antigen (CEA) focally reactive
- Negative for thyroglobulin, S100 protein, or glial fibrillary acidic protein (GFAP)

DIFFERENTIAL DIAGNOSIS

Papilloma (Surface Epithelial or Minor Salivary Gland Origin)

- Exophytic lesion lacking complex (back to back) growth and infiltrative pattern of NPPA

Minor Salivary Gland Neoplasms

- Differentiation based on surface epithelial origin, complex papillary growth, cytomorphologic features, immunohistochemical findings (i.e., TTF-1 reactivity)

Metastatic Thyroid Papillary Carcinoma

- Both tumor types are TTF-1 positive but thyroglobulin only positive in thyroid papillary carcinoma

SELECTED REFERENCES

1. Fu CH et al: Primary thyroid-like papillary adenocarcinoma of the nasopharynx. Auris Nasus Larynx. 35(4):579-82, 2008
2. Pineda-Daboin K et al: Nasopharyngeal adenocarcinomas: a clinicopathologic study of 44 cases including immunohistochemical features of 18 papillary phenotypes. Ann Diagn Pathol. 10(4):215-21, 2006
3. Wenig BM et al: Nasopharyngeal papillary adenocarcinoma. A clinicopathologic study of a low-grade carcinoma. Am J Surg Pathol. 12(12):946-53, 1988

IMAGE GALLERY

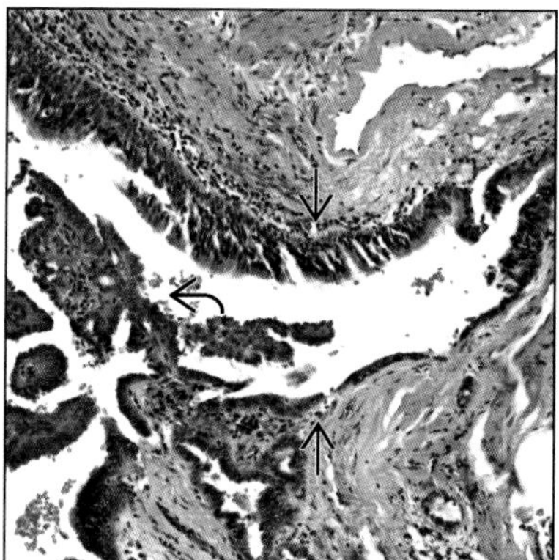

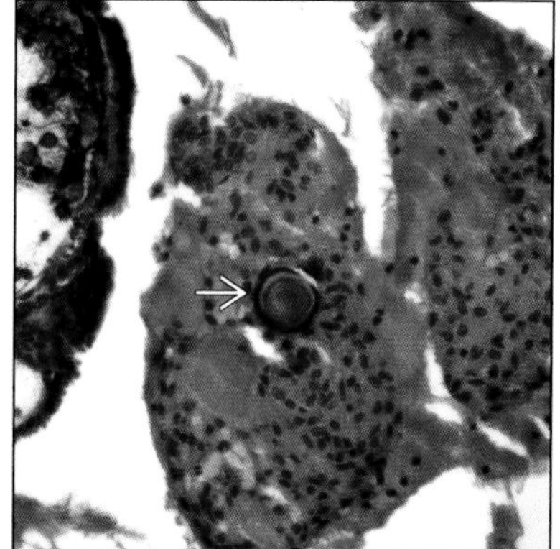

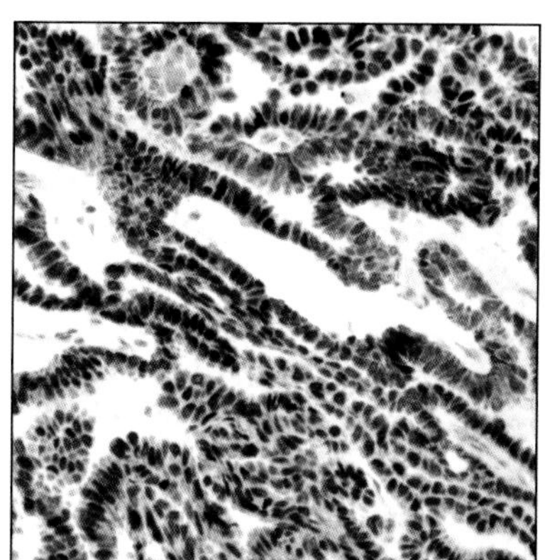

*(**Left**) The presence of transitional areas from normal surface epithelium ⇨ to the neoplastic proliferation ⇨ confirms origin from the nasopharyngeal surface epithelium. (**Center**) Psammoma bodies ➡ can be seen that, in addition to papillary growth and nuclear features, are reminiscent of thyroid papillary carcinoma. (**Right**) Thyroid transcription factor 1 immunoreactivity (nuclear staining) is consistently present, but thyroglobulin staining is absent (not shown).*

DIFFUSE LARGE B-CELL LYMPHOMA

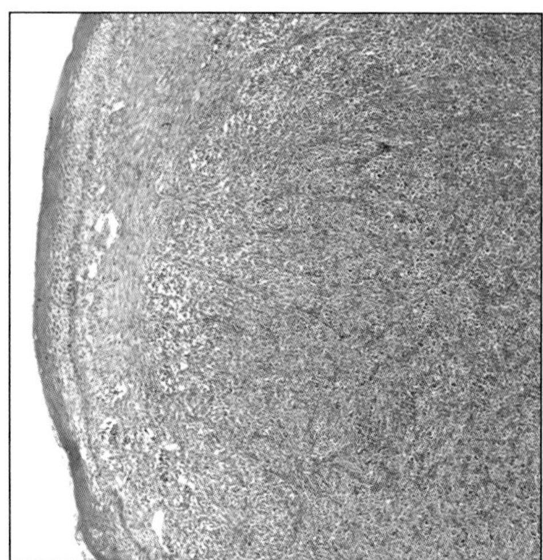

Diffuse large B-cell lymphoma of the nasopharynx shows effacement of the normal architecture by a submucosal diffuse cellular proliferation.

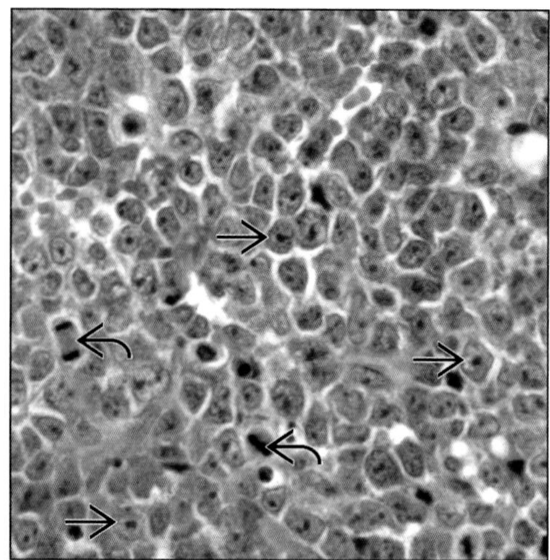

At higher power the neoplastic cells are large with vesicular chromatin, prominent eosinophilic nucleoli →, and increased mitotic activity ↶.

TERMINOLOGY

Abbreviations

- Diffuse large B-cell lymphoma (DLBCL)

Definitions

- Primary malignant hematolymphoid neoplasm with bulk of disease occurring in Waldeyer ring
  - Group of extranodal lymphoid tissues, including palatine tonsils, nasopharyngeal tonsils (adenoids), base of tongue/lingual tonsils
- Any non-Hodgkin lymphoma (NHL) type can occur, but DLBCL most common, representing > 50% of Waldeyer NHLs

ETIOLOGY/PATHOGENESIS

Idiopathic

- Minority of patients have underlying/associated immunodeficiency condition that may predispose to NHL
  - Post-transplantation, HIV/AIDS
- Weak association of NHL, especially diffuse large B-cell lymphoma, with Epstein-Barr virus

CLINICAL ISSUES

Epidemiology

- Incidence
  - Waldeyer NHLs represent approximately
    - 5-10% of NHLs in western countries
    - 20-25% of NHLs in Asian countries
    - 16% of all head and neck NHLs
    - 50% of all primary extranodal lymphomas in head and neck
  - Oropharyngeal (and oral cavity) NHLs account for 13% of all primary extranodal NHLs
    - Approximately 70% occur in tonsils
  - Nasopharyngeal NHLs account for 2.5% of all extranodal NHLs
- Age
  - Wide age range but most common in 6th-8th decades of life
    - Patients with underlying immunodeficiency condition usually are younger
- Gender
  - Male > Female

Site

- Tonsils > nasopharynx > base of tongue

Presentation

- Most common symptoms include dysphagia, odynophagia, swelling or lump in throat, decreased hearing, pain, and sore throat
  - Majority are unilateral (80-90% of cases)
  - Cervical adenopathy present in approximately 65% of patients
  - Systemic symptoms (e.g., fever, night sweats, other) not common
  - Multifocality may be present

Treatment

- Options, risks, complications
  - Treatment options include surgical excision, radiotherapy, and chemotherapy
- Surgical approaches
  - Surgical resection may be needed for symptomatic relief
- Adjuvant therapy
  - Treatment primarily includes radiotherapy &/or chemotherapy

Prognosis

- Majority (80%) of NHL of Waldeyer tonsillar ring have localized disease/low clinical stage (i.e., stage IE, IIE)
- For B-cell lymphomas, including DLBCL, prognosis is dependent on clinical stage

DIFFUSE LARGE B-CELL LYMPHOMA

Key Facts

Terminology

- Primary malignant hematolymphoid neoplasm with bulk of disease occurring in Waldeyer ring
- DLBCL represents more than 50% of all NHLs of Waldeyer ring

Etiology/Pathogenesis

- No known etiology in majority of patients
- Weak association of NHL, especially diffuse large B-cell lymphoma, with Epstein-Barr virus

Clinical Issues

- Most common in tonsils > nasopharynx > base of tongue
- Majority are unilateral (80-90% of cases)
- Treatment primarily by radiotherapy &/or chemotherapy
- Majority (80%) localized disease/low clinical stage
- Overall 5-year survival approximately 65%

Microscopic Pathology

- Diffuse submucosal dyscohesive cellular infiltrate with effacement of normal architecture, including absence/loss of germinal centers
- Pleomorphic cells with large round to oval vesicular nuclei and prominent eosinophilic nucleoli

Ancillary Tests

- CD45RB, CD20, CD79a, Bcl-6, CD10 positive; T-cell markers negative; may be p63 positive
- Absence of epithelial, melanocytic, neuroendocrine, and myogenic markers
- Clonal rearrangement of immunoglobulin heavy and light chains genes

- Overall 5-year survival (for all treatment modalities) is approximately 65%
- Relapse occurs in 30-45% of patients
  - May be localized to cervical lymph nodes
  - May involve non-H&N sites, primarily gastrointestinal tract (GIT) in up to 20% of patients
  - GIT involvement may occur at presentation or prior to involvement of Waldeyer ring, necessitating clinical evaluation of these sites
  - Less commonly may involve other sites, such as bone marrow, liver, or spleen
- Factors associated with adverse prognosis include
  - Advanced clinical stage (e.g., number of extranodal sites)
  - Higher histologic grade
  - Aberrant T-cell antigen expression
  - High proliferative (i.e., Ki-67) index
  - Poor performance status
  - Tumor bulk
  - B symptoms, including fever, drenching night sweats, loss of > 10% original weight within 6 months

MACROSCOPIC FEATURES

General Features

- Often large exophytic submucosal mass with or without surface ulceration

MICROSCOPIC PATHOLOGY

Histologic Features

- Diffuse submucosal dyscohesive cellular infiltrate with effacement of normal architecture, including absence/loss of germinal centers
  - Residual germinal centers may be identified due to incomplete involvement by lymphoma
- Medium to large cells with
  - Large round to oval vesicular (noncleaved) pleomorphic nuclei
  - Membrane-bound small nucleoli or single centrally located prominent eosinophilic nucleolus
- Nuclear lobulation may be present
- Increased mitotic activity, including atypical forms
- Confluent necrosis and apoptotic figures seen
- Surface epithelium may be intact or ulcerated; crypt epithelium usually intact

ANCILLARY TESTS

Immunohistochemistry

- Waldeyer ring NHLs are predominantly follicular center cell-derived, which are positively reactive with pan B-cell markers and negatively reactive with T-cell markers
  - Leukocyte common antigen (LCA or CD45) and pan B-cell markers, including CD20(+) and CD79a(+)
  - Expression of CD10 (30-60%), Bcl-6 (60-90%)
  - High proliferation rate (Ki-67 or MIB-1), may be greater than 90%
  - p63(+); vimentin(+)
  - Absence of epithelial, melanocytic, neuroendocrine, and myogenic markers
  - Negative for Epstein-Barr virus testing (immunohistochemistry, in situ hybridization, others)

Cytogenetics

- Clonal rearrangement of immunoglobulin heavy and light chains genes
- Translocation of *BCL2* gene, t(14;18) occurs in 20-30% of cases
  - t(14;18) is hallmark of follicular lymphoma
- Abnormalities of 3q27 region involving candidate proto-oncogene *BCL6* in up to 30% of cases

DIFFERENTIAL DIAGNOSIS

Reactive Lymphoid (Follicular) Hyperplasia

- Admixture of cellular infiltrate including mature lymphocytes, plasma cells, histiocytes, others

DIFFUSE LARGE B-CELL LYMPHOMA

Ann Arbor and AJCC Staging System for Lymphomas

Stage	Definition	Treatment	5-Year Survival
I	Involvement of a single lymphatic site (i.e., nodal region, Waldeyer ring, thymus, or spleen) (I); or localized involvement of a single extralymphatic organ or site in the absence of any lymph node involvement (IE)	Radiotherapy (4,500-5,000 rads)	50%
II	Involvement of ≥ 2 lymph node regions on the same side of the diaphragm (II); or localized involvement of a single extralymphatic organ or site in association with regional lymph node involvement with or without involvement of other lymph node regions on the same side of the diaphragm (IIE)	Radiotherapy (4,500-5,000 rads)	25%
III	Involvement of lymph node regions on both sides of the diaphragm (III), which also may be accompanied by extralymphatic extension in association with adjacent lymph node involvement (IIIE) or by the involvement of the spleen (IIIS) or both (IIIE,S)	Total lymphoid radiation; chemotherapy if the spleen is involved	17%
IV	Diffuse or disseminated involvement of ≥ 1 extralymphatic organ, with or without associated lymph node involvement; or isolated extralymphatic organ involvement in the absence of adjacent regional lymph node involvement, but in conjunction with disease in distant site(s)	Chemotherapy	Very poor

Each stage should be classified as either A or B according to the absence or presence of defined constitutional symptoms: Fever (> 38°C), drenching night sweats, and unexplained loss of more than 10% original weight within 6 months.

- Retention (rather than effacement) of normal architecture including germinal centers
- Polyclonal staining including reactivity for both B-cell and T-cell markers

Infectious Mononucleosis

- Histology may suggest DLBCL, but findings that allow for differentiation include
  - Younger patients
  - Preservation of germinal centers
  - Presence of B- and T-cell markers
  - Presence of serologic confirmation
  - Absence of gene rearrangement

Nasopharyngeal Carcinoma, Nonkeratinizing

- Presence of immunoreactivity for cytokeratins and in situ hybridization for Epstein-Barr virus
- Absence of immunoreactivity for hematolymphoid markers

Mucosal Malignant Melanoma

- Presence of immunoreactivity for S100 protein and melanocytic markers (e.g., HMB-45, Melan-A, tyrosinase)
- Absence of immunoreactivity for hematolymphoid markers

Rhabdomyosarcoma

- Presence of immunoreactivity for myogenic markers (desmin, myoglobin, myogenin)
- Absence of immunoreactivity for hematolymphoid markers

SELECTED REFERENCES

1. Aanaes K et al: Improved prognosis for localized malignant lymphomas of the head and neck. Acta Otolaryngol. 130(5):626-31, 2010
2. Laskar S et al: Non-Hodgkin lymphoma of the Waldeyer's ring: clinicopathologic and therapeutic issues. Leuk Lymphoma. 49(12):2263-71, 2008
3. Hedvat CV et al: Expression of p63 in diffuse large B-cell lymphoma. Appl Immunohistochem Mol Morphol. 13(3):237-42, 2005
4. Mohammadianpanah M et al: Treatment results of tonsillar lymphoma: a 10-year experience. Ann Hematol. 84(4):223-6, 2005
5. Vega F et al: Extranodal lymphomas of the head and neck. Ann Diagn Pathol. 9(6):340-50, 2005
6. Krol AD et al: Waldeyer's ring lymphomas: a clinical study from the Comprehensive Cancer Center West population based NHL registry. Leuk Lymphoma. 42(5):1005-13, 2001
7. Hanna E et al: Extranodal lymphomas of the head and neck. A 20-year experience. Arch Otolaryngol Head Neck Surg. 123(12):1318-23, 1997
8. Economopoulos T et al: Primary extranodal non-Hodgkin's lymphoma in adults: clinicopathological and survival characteristics. Leuk Lymphoma. 21(1-2):131-6, 1996
9. Economopoulos T et al: Primary extranodal non-Hodgkin's lymphoma of the head and neck. Oncology. 49(6):484-8, 1992
10. Goldwein JW et al: Prognostic factors in patients with early stage non-Hodgkin's lymphomas of the head and neck treated with definitive irradiation. Int J Radiat Oncol Biol Phys. 20(1):45-51, 1991
11. Burton GV et al: Extranodal head and neck lymphoma. Prognosis and patterns of recurrence. Arch Otolaryngol Head Neck Surg. 116(1):69-73, 1990
12. Shima N et al: Extranodal non-Hodgkin's lymphoma of the head and neck. A clinicopathologic study in the Kyoto-Nara area of Japan. Cancer. 66(6):1190-7, 1990
13. Shirato H et al: Early stage head and neck non-Hodgkin's lymphoma. The effect of tumor burden on prognosis. Cancer. 58(10):2312-9, 1986
14. Saul SH et al: Primary lymphoma of Waldeyer's ring. Clinicopathologic study of 68 cases. Cancer. 56(1):157-66, 1985

Microscopic and Immunohistochemical Features

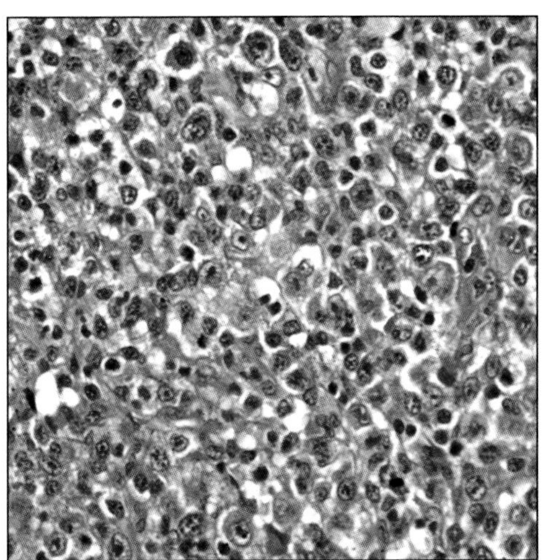

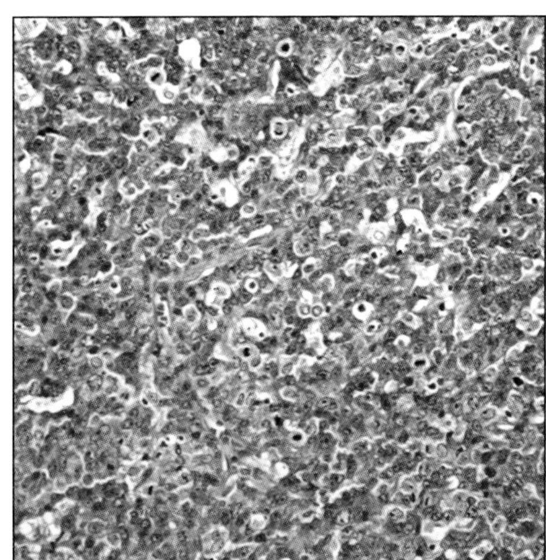

(Left) *In the majority of examples of DLBCL, the light microscopic appearance is that of a diffuse malignant cellular proliferation in which the neoplastic cells lack cohesive growth. This pattern is not unique to lymphomas but would suggest a hematolymphoid lesion.* ***(Right)*** *In a minority of examples of DLBCL, the neoplastic infiltrate may show cohesive pattern of growth, a feature more commonly seen in other types of malignant neoplasms including but not limited to carcinomas.*

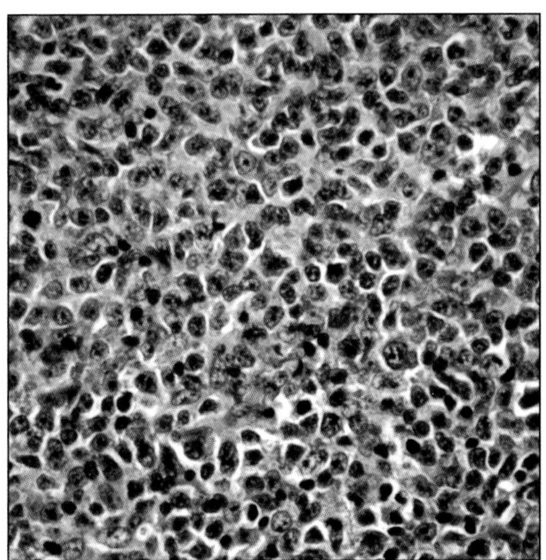

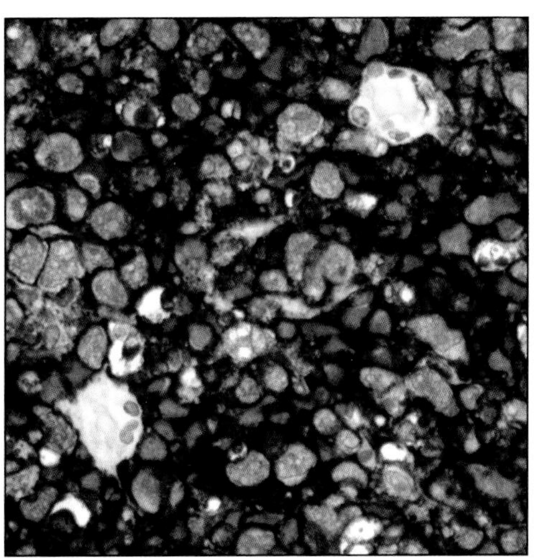

(Left) *Irrespective of the growth pattern, DLBCL is characterized by a diffuse population of malignant cells showing nuclear pleomorphism with enlarged vesicular chromatin and prominent eosinophilic nucleoli. While these features suggest a hematolymphoid lesion, the differential diagnosis includes other tumor types necessitating immunohistochemical staining to confirm the diagnosis of a lymphoma.* ***(Right)*** *DLBCL shows diffuse CD20 immunoreactivity, a marker of B-cells.*

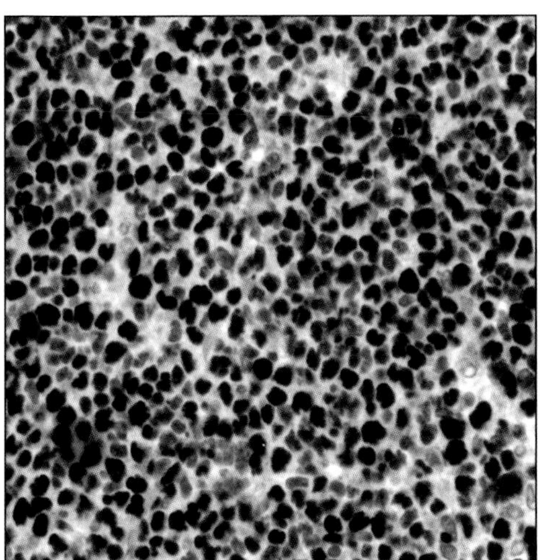

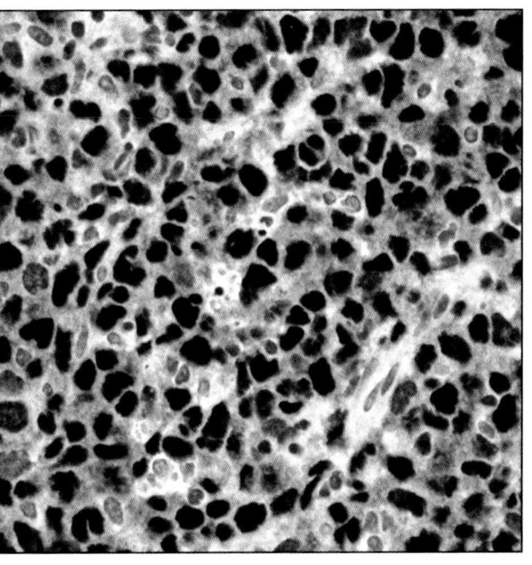

(Left) *Positive bcl-6 (nuclear staining) supports the diagnosis of DLBCL and is present in 60-90% of cases.* ***(Right)*** *p63 (nuclear) staining is seen in malignant lymphomas, including DLBCL. In limited tissue sampling, the presence of p63 may suggest an epithelial malignancy, as p63 is expressed in squamous and myoepithelial cells. However, the absence of markers specific for another tumor type (epithelial, melanocytic, others) should prompt consideration of a lymphoma.*

PROTOCOL FOR THE EXAMINATION OF PHARYNX SPECIMENS

Pharynx (Nasopharynx, Oropharynx, Hypopharynx)

Excisional Biopsy, Resection

Specimen (select all that apply)

___ Nasopharynx
___ Oropharynx
___ Hypopharynx
___ Other (specify): ___________________________
___ Not specified

Received

___ Fresh
___ In formalin
___ Other (specify): ___________________________

Procedure (select all that apply)

___ Incisional biopsy
___ Excisional biopsy
___ Resection
 ___ Tonsillectomy
 ___ Laryngopharyngectomy
 ___ Other (specify): ___________________________
___ Neck (lymph node) dissection (specify): ___________________________
___ Other (specify): ___________________________
___ Not specified

****Specimen Integrity***

*___ Intact
*___ Fragmented

Specimen Size

Greatest dimensions: _________ x _________ x _________ cm
*Additional dimensions (if more than 1 part): _________ x _________ x _________ cm

Specimen Laterality

___ Left
___ Right
___ Bilateral
___ Midline
___ Not specified

Tumor Site (select all that apply)

___ **Nasopharynx**
 ___ Nasopharyngeal tonsils (adenoids)
___ **Oropharynx**
 ___ Palatine tonsil
 ___ Base of tongue, including lingual tonsil
 ___ Soft palate
 ___ Uvula
 ___ Pharyngeal wall (posterior)
___ **Hypopharynx**
 ___ Piriform sinus
 ___ Postcricoid
 ___ Pharyngeal wall (posterior &/or lateral)
 ___ Other
___ Other (specify): ___________________________
___ Not specified

PROTOCOL FOR THE EXAMINATION OF PHARYNX SPECIMENS

Tumor Laterality

___ Left
___ Right
___ Bilateral
___ Midline
___ Not specified

Tumor Focality

___ Single focus
___ Bilateral
___ Multifocal (specify): ______________________

Tumor Size

Greatest dimension: _______ cm
*Additional dimensions: _______ x _______ cm
___ Cannot be determined

****Tumor Description (select all that apply)***

*Gross subtype
*___ Polypoid
*___ Exophytic
*___ Endophytic
*___ Ulcerated
*___ Sessile
*___ Other (specify): ______________________

****Macroscopic Extent of Tumor***

*Specify: ______________________

Histologic Type (select all that apply)

___ **Carcinomas of nasopharynx**
  ___ Keratinizing squamous cell carcinoma
  ___ Nonkeratinizing carcinoma
    ___ Differentiated carcinoma
    ___ Undifferentiated carcinoma
  ___ Basaloid squamous cell carcinoma
___ **Carcinomas of oropharynx and hypopharynx**
  ___ Squamous cell carcinoma, conventional
    ___ Variants of squamous cell carcinoma
      ___ Acantholytic squamous cell carcinoma
      ___ Adenosquamous carcinoma
      ___ Basaloid squamous cell carcinoma
      ___ Papillary squamous cell carcinoma
      ___ Spindle cell squamous carcinoma
      ___ Verrucous carcinoma
  ___ Lymphoepithelial carcinoma (non-nasopharyngeal)
___ **Adenocarcinomas (non-salivary gland type)**
  ___ Nasopharyngeal papillary adenocarcinoma
  ___ Adenocarcinoma, not otherwise specified (NOS)
    ___ Low grade
    ___ Intermediate grade
    ___ High grade
  ___ Other (specify): ______________________
___ **Carcinomas of minor salivary glands**
  ___ Acinic cell carcinoma
  ___ Adenoid cystic carcinoma
  ___ Adenocarcinoma, not otherwise specified (NOS)

____ Low grade
____ Intermediate grade
____ High grade
____ Basal cell adenocarcinoma
____ Carcinoma ex-pleomorphic adenoma (malignant mixed tumor)
____ Carcinoma, type cannot be determined
____ Clear cell adenocarcinoma
____ Cystadenocarcinoma
____ Epithelial-myoepithelial carcinoma
____ Mucoepidermoid carcinoma
____ Low grade
____ Intermediate grade
____ High grade
____ Mucinous adenocarcinoma (colloid carcinoma)
____ Myoepithelial carcinoma (malignant myoepithelioma)
____ Oncocytic carcinoma
____ Polymorphous low-grade adenocarcinoma
____ Salivary duct carcinoma
____ Other (specify): __________________________
____ **Neuroendocrine carcinoma**
____ Typical carcinoid tumor (well-differentiated neuroendocrine carcinoma)
____ Atypical carcinoid tumor (moderately differentiated neuroendocrine carcinoma)
____ Small cell carcinoma (poorly differentiated neuroendocrine carcinoma)
____ Combined (or composite) small cell carcinoma, neuroendocrine type
____ Mucosal malignant melanoma
____ Other carcinoma (specify): __________________________
____ Carcinoma, type cannot be determined

Histologic Grade

____ Not applicable
____ GX: Cannot be assessed
____ G1: Well differentiated
____ G2: Moderately differentiated
____ G3: Poorly differentiated
____ Other (specify): __________________________

**Microscopic Tumor Extension*

*____ Specify: __________________________

Margins (select all that apply)

____ Cannot be assessed
____ Margins uninvolved by invasive carcinoma
Distance from closest margin: ________ mm or ________ cm
Specify margin(s), per orientation, if possible: __________________________
____ Margins involved by invasive carcinoma
Specify margin(s), per orientation, if possible: __________________________
____ Margins uninvolved by carcinoma in situ (includes moderate and severe dysplasia)
Distance from closest margin: ________ mm or ________ cm
Specify margin(s), per orientation, if possible: __________________________
____ Margins involved by carcinoma in situ (includes moderate and severe dysplasia)
Specify margin(s), per orientation, if possible: __________________________
____ Not applicable
Applicable only to squamous cell carcinoma and histologic variants

**Treatment Effect (applicable to carcinomas treated with neoadjuvant therapy)*

*____ Not identified
*____ Present (specify): __________________________

*___ Indeterminate

Lymph-Vascular Invasion

___ Not identified

___ Present

___ Indeterminate

Perineural Invasion

___ Not identified

___ Present

___ Indeterminate

Lymph Nodes, Extranodal Extension

___ Not identified

___ Present

___ Indeterminate

Pathologic Staging (pTNM)

TNM descriptors (required only if applicable) (select all that apply)

___ m (multiple primary tumors)

___ r (recurrent)

___ y (post-treatment)

Primary tumor (pT)

___ pTX: Cannot be assessed

___ pT0: No evidence of primary tumor

___ pTis: Carcinoma in situ

For all carcinomas (excluding mucosal malignant melanoma)

Primary tumor (pT): Nasopharynx†

___ pT1: Tumor confined to nasopharynx, or tumor extends to oropharynx &/or nasal cavity without parapharyngeal extension

___ pT2: Tumor with parapharyngeal extension

___ pT3: Tumor invades bony structures of skull base &/or paranasal sinuses

___ pT4: Tumor with intracranial extension &/or involvement of cranial nerves, hypopharynx, orbit or with extension to infratemporal fossa/masticator space

Parapharyngeal extension denotes posterolateral infiltration of tumor

Primary tumor (pT): Oropharynx†

___ pT1: Tumor ≤ 2 cm in greatest dimension

___ pT2: Tumor > 2 cm but ≤ 4 cm in greatest dimension

___ pT3: Tumor > 4 cm in greatest dimension or extension to lingual surface of epiglottis

___ pT4a: Moderately advanced local disease

Tumor invades larynx, deep/extrinsic muscle of tongue, medial pterygoid muscles, hard palate, or mandible

___ pT4b: Very advanced local disease

Tumor invades lateral pterygoid muscle, pterygoid plates, lateral nasopharynx, or skull base, or encases carotid artery

Note: Mucosal extension to lingual surface of epiglottis from primary tumors of the base of the tongue and vallecula does not constitute invasion of larynx

Primary tumor (pT): Hypopharynx†

___ pT1: Tumor limited to 1 subsite of hypopharynx &/or ≤ 2 cm in greatest dimension

___ pT2: Tumor invades > 1 subsite of hypopharynx or an adjacent site or measures > 2 but ≤ 4 cm in greatest dimension without fixation of hemilarynx

___ pT3: Tumor measures > 4 cm in greatest dimension **or** with fixation of hemilarynx or extension to esophagus

___ pT4a: Moderately advanced local disease

Tumor invades thyroid/cricoid cartilage, hyoid bone, thyroid gland, or central compartment soft tissue

___ pT4b: Very advanced local disease

Tumor invades prevertebral fascia, encases carotid artery, or involves mediastinal structures

Note: Central compartment soft tissue includes prelaryngeal strap muscles and subcutaneous fat

Regional lymph nodes (pN)

___ pNX: Cannot be assessed

___ pN0: No regional lymph node metastasis

PROTOCOL FOR THE EXAMINATION OF PHARYNX SPECIMENS

Regional lymph nodes (pN): Nasopharynx†

___ pN1: Unilateral metastasis in lymph node(s), ≤ 6 cm in greatest dimension, above supraclavicular fossa

___ pN2: Bilateral metastasis in lymph node(s), ≤ 6 cm in greatest dimension, above supraclavicular fossa

___ pN3: Metastasis in a lymph node > 6 cm &/or to supraclavicular fossa

___ pN3a: > 6 cm in dimension

___ pN3b: Extension to supraclavicular fossa

Specify: Number examined: _________

Number involved: _________

*Size (greatest dimension) of largest positive lymph node: _________

Metastases at level VII are considered regional lymph node metastases. Midline nodes are considered ipsilateral nodes

Supraclavicular zone or fossa is relevant to staging of nasopharyngeal carcinoma and is the triangular region defined by 3 points

1: Superior margin of sternal end of clavicle

2: Superior margin of lateral end of clavicle

3: Point where neck meets shoulder. Note that this would include caudal portions of levels IV and VB. All cases with lymph nodes (whole or in part) in fossa are considered N3b

Regional lymph nodes (pN): Oropharynx and hypopharynx†

___ pN1: Metastasis in single ipsilateral lymph node, ≤ 3 cm in greatest dimension

___ pN2: Metastasis in single ipsilateral lymph node, > 3 cm but ≤ 6 cm in greatest dimension

or in multiple ipsilateral lymph nodes, none > 6 cm in greatest dimension

or in bilateral or contralateral lymph nodes, none > 6 cm in greatest dimension

___ pN2a: Metastasis in single ipsilateral lymph node, > 3 cm but ≤ 6 cm in greatest dimension

___ pN2b: Metastasis in multiple ipsilateral lymph nodes, none > 6 cm in greatest dimension

___ pN2c: Metastasis in bilateral or contralateral lymph nodes, none > 6 cm in greatest dimension

___ pN3: Metastasis in lymph node > 6 cm in greatest dimension

Specify: Number examined: _________

Number involved: _________

*Size (greatest dimension) of largest positive lymph node: _________

Note: Metastases at level VII are considered regional lymph node metastases. Midline nodes are considered ipsilateral nodes

Distant metastasis (pM)

___ Not applicable

___ pM1: Distant metastasis

*Specify site(s), if known: ___________________________

For mucosal malignant melanoma

Primary tumor (pT)†

___ pT3: Mucosal disease

___ pT4a: Moderately advanced disease

Tumor involving deep soft tissue, cartilage, bone, or overlying skin

___ pT4b: Very advanced disease

Tumor involving brain, dura, skull base, lower cranial nerves (IX, X, XI, XII), masticator space, carotid artery, prevertebral space, or mediastinal structures

Regional lymph nodes (pN)†

___ pNX: Regional lymph nodes cannot be assessed

___ pN0: No regional lymph node metastases

___ pN1: Regional lymph node metastases present

Distant metastasis (pM)†

___ Not applicable

___ pM1: Distant metastasis present

*Specify site(s), if known: ___________________________

*Source of pathologic metastatic specimen† (specify): ___________________________

*Additional Pathologic Findings (select all that apply)

*___ None identified

*___ Keratinizing dysplasia

*___ Mild

*____ Moderate
*____ Severe (carcinoma in situ)
*____Nonkeratinizing dysplasia
*____ Mild
*____ Moderate
*____ Severe (carcinoma in situ)
*____Inflammation (specify type): __________________________
*____Squamous metaplasia
*____Epithelial hyperplasia
*____Colonization
*____ Fungal
*____ Bacterial
*____Other (specify): __________________________

Ancillary Studies (select all that apply)

____ Human papillomavirus-associated carcinoma (p16 immunoreactivity, in situ hybridization, other)
____ Present
____ Negative
____ Epstein-Barr virus (Epstein-Barr virus encoded RNA [EBER], other)
____ Present
____ Negative
____ Other (specify): __________________________
____ Not specified

****Clinical History (select all that apply)***

*____Neoadjuvant therapy
*____ Yes (specify type): __________________________
*____ No
*____ Indeterminate
*____Other (specify): __________________________

**Data elements with asterisks are not required. However, these elements may be clinically important but are not yet validated or regularly used in patient management. †These phrases include clinical findings required for AJCC staging. This clinical information may be unknown to the pathologist. It is included here only for the sake of completeness. Adapted with permission from College of American Pathologists, "Protocol for the Examination of Specimens from Patients with Carcinomas of the Pharynx." Web posting date October 2009, www.cap.org. Protocol applies to all invasive carcinomas of the pharynx (nasopharynx, oropharynx, hypopharynx) including the base of tongue, tonsils, soft palate, and uvula. Mucosal malignant melanoma is included. Lymphomas and sarcomas are not included.*

PROTOCOL FOR THE EXAMINATION OF PHARYNX SPECIMENS

Anatomic Stage/Prognostic Groups: Nasopharynx

Group	T	N	M
0	Tis	N0	M0
I	T1	N0	M0
II	T1	N1	M0
	T2	N0	M0
	T2	N1	M0
III	T1	N2	M0
	T2	N2	M0
	T3	N0	M0
	T3	N1	M0
	T3	N2	M0
IVA	T4	N0	M0
	T4	N1	M0
	T4	N2	M0
IVB	Any T	N3	M0
IVC	Any T	Any N	M1

Adapted from 7th edition AJCC Staging Forms.

Anatomic Stage/Prognostic Groups: Oropharynx, Hypopharynx

Group	T	N	M
0	Tis	N0	M0
I	T1	N0	M0
II	T2	N0	M0
	T2	N0, N1	M0
III	T3	N0,N1	M0
IVA	T1, T2, T3	N2	M0
	T4a	N0, N1, N2	M0
IVB	T4b	Any N	M0
	Any T	N3	M0
IVC	Any T	Any N	M1

Adapted from 7th edition AJCC Staging Forms.

General Notes, Staging

Note	Description
m suffix	Indicates presence of multiple primary tumors in a single site and is recorded in parentheses: pT(m)NM
y prefix	Indicates cases in which classification is performed during or following initial multimodality therapy. The cTNM or pTNM category is identified by a "y" prefix. ycTNM or ypTNM categorizes the extent of tumor actually present at the time of that examination. The "y" categorization is not an estimate of tumor prior to multimodality therapy
r prefix	Indicates a recurrent tumor when staged after a disease-free interval and is identified by the "r" prefix: rTNM
a prefix	Designates the stage determined at autopsy: aTNM
Surgical margins	Data field recorded by registrars describing the surgical margins of the resected primary site specimen as determined only by the pathology report
Neoadjuvant treatment	Radiation therapy or systemic therapy (consisting of chemotherapy, hormone therapy, or immunotherapy) administered prior to a definitive surgical procedure. If the surgical procedure is not performed, the administered therapy no longer meets the definition of neoadjuvant therapy

Adapted from 7th edition AJCC Staging Forms.

Anatomic and Tumor Staging Graphics

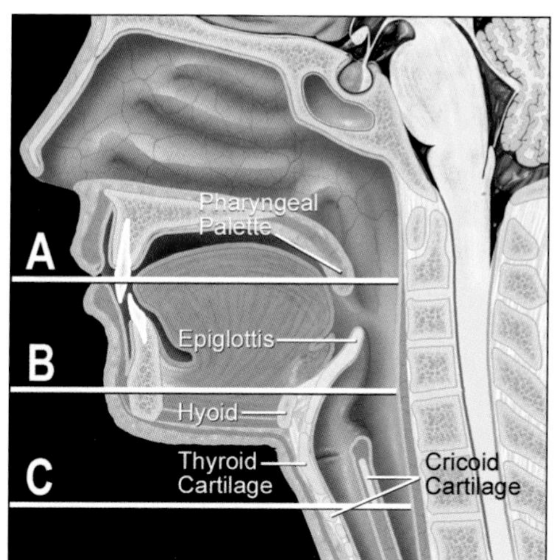

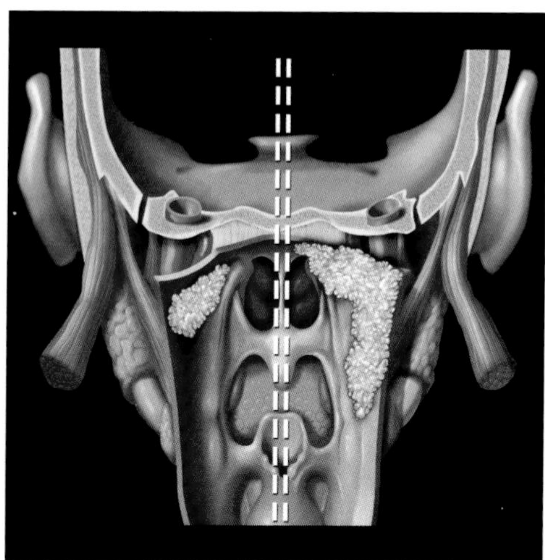

(Left) *The pharynx is divided into naso- (A), oro- (B), and hypopharynx (C), using the junction between the hard and soft palate as the start of the nasopharynx, the inferior surface of the soft palate, uvula, base of tongue, tonsils and tonsillar pillars within the oropharynx, and the hypopharynx extending from the superior border of the hyoid bone to the inferior border of the cricoid cartilage.* ***(Right)*** *Graphic shows bilateral nasopharyngeal tumors with parapharyngeal extension (pT2).*

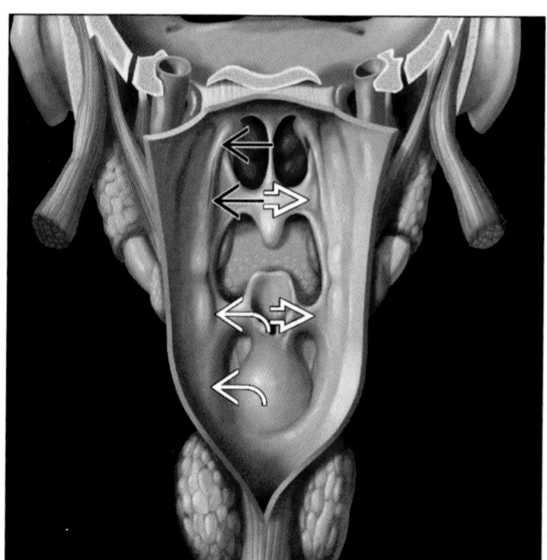

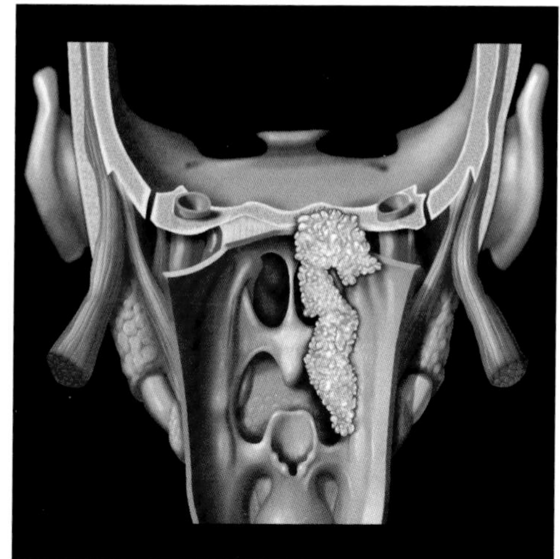

(Left) *This splayed open posterior view of the pharynx highlights the anatomic divisions from a different perspective. Note nasopharynx →, oropharynx ➡, and hypopharynx ➡. These separations are important due to metastatic potential of each anatomic site.* ***(Right)*** *This tumor involves the nasopharynx and oropharynx and expands into the posterior nasal cavity, with parapharyngeal extension and involvement of the bony structures of the skull base (pT3).*

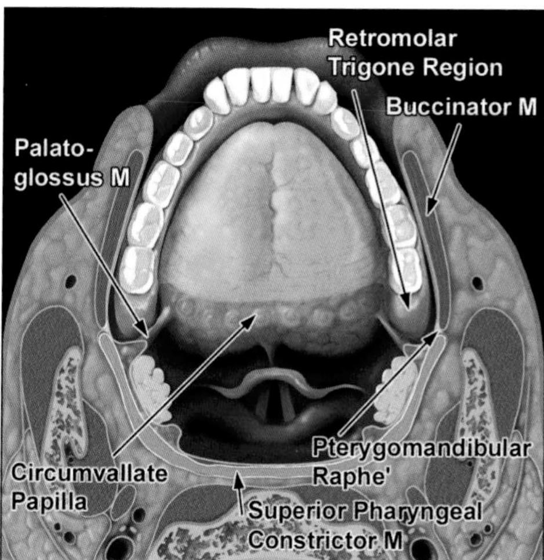

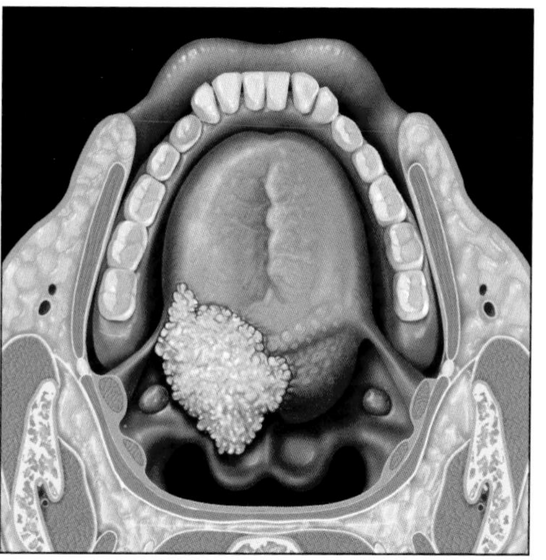

(Left) *The oropharynx (highlighted in purple) includes the base of the tongue (posterior 1/3), vallecula, tonsil, tonsillar fossa and pillars, inferior surface of the soft palate and the uvula, and the posterior wall of the pharynx. Other anatomic landmarks are highlighted as points of reference.* ***(Right)*** *This oropharyngeal carcinoma measures 4.8 cm, with extension to the lingual surface of the epiglottis and middle 1/3 of the tongue. This tumor is in the pT3 category.*

PROTOCOL FOR THE EXAMINATION OF PHARYNX SPECIMENS

Anatomic and Tumor Staging Graphics

(Left) Coronal view from the posterior demonstrates the very intimate relationship between all of the structures of the oropharynx and the hypopharynx as it joins with the larynx. Each of the anatomic landmarks shown (hyoid and cricoid especially) help to divide the hypopharynx from the oropharynx. ***(Right)*** This hypopharynx carcinoma is 5.1 cm, showing expansion into the central compartment soft tissue. There is no artery involvement. This tumor would be placed in pT4a.

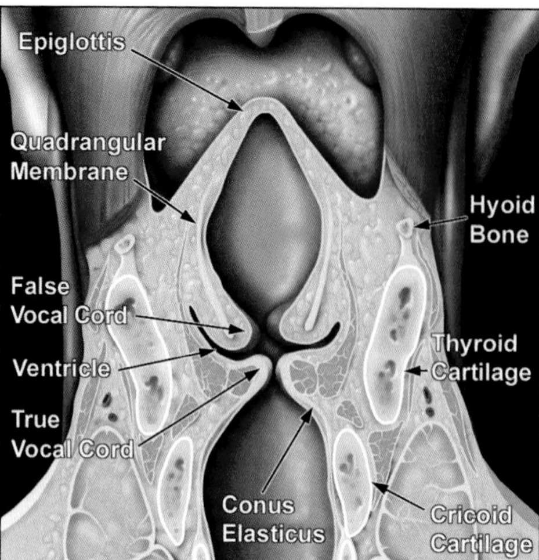

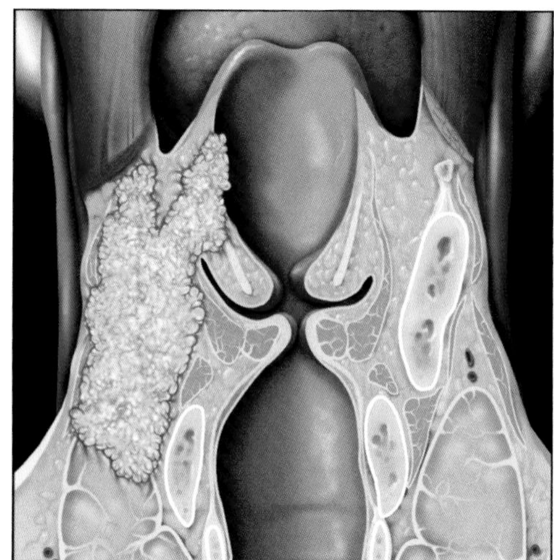

(Left) Axial anatomic view of the hypopharynx identifies the various anatomic compartments, as well as the bones and neurovascular bundles of the region. ***(Right)*** Graphic shows a bilateral hypopharyngeal carcinoma expanding to involve the superior border of the larynx and the esophagus. This is a pT3 tumor, as there is no advanced local disease.

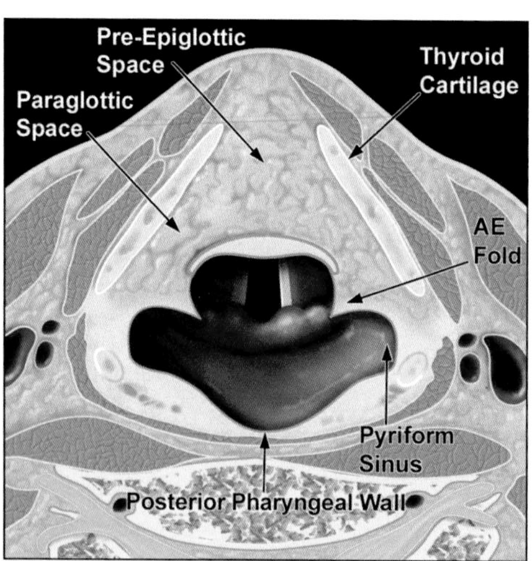

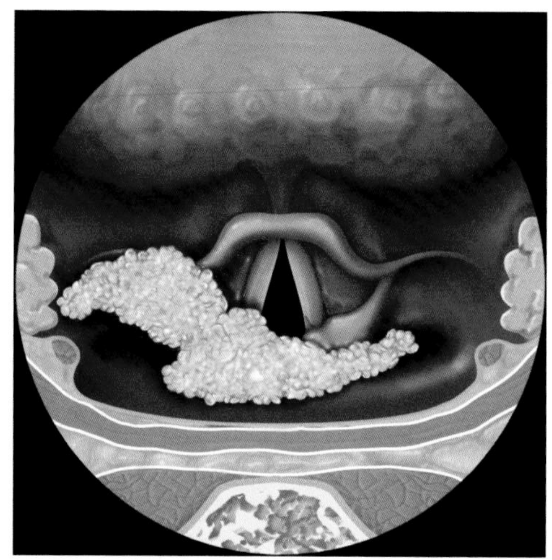

(Left) All tumors of the pharynx (naso-/oro-/ hypopharynx) will frequently show metastases to the various lymph nodes in the cervical chains. They are separated into ipsilateral, contralateral, and bilateral, as well as anatomic compartments using the internal jugular vein (upper, middle, and lower 1/3) and sternocleidomastoid muscle (anterior). The posterior triangle is behind the SCM. ***(Right)*** This hypopharyngeal tumor shows level III and IV lymph node metastases (pN2b).

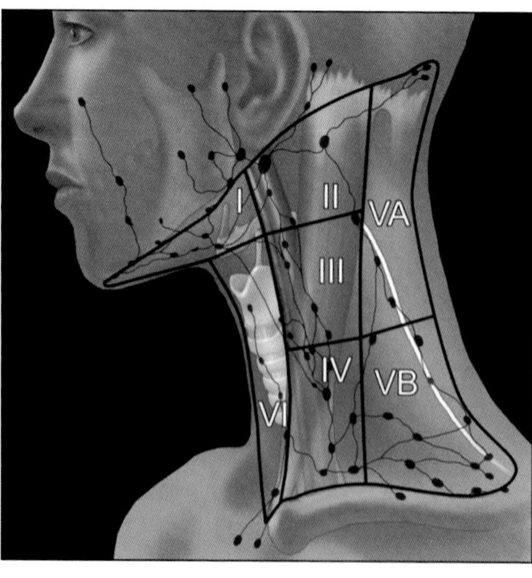

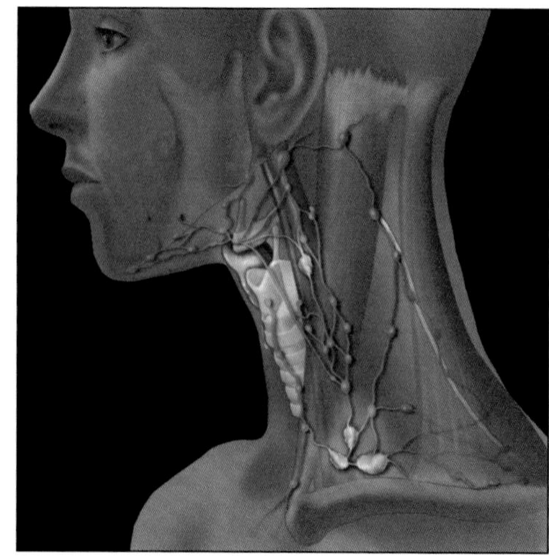

Larynx and Trachea

LARYNGOCELE AND LARYNGEAL CYSTS

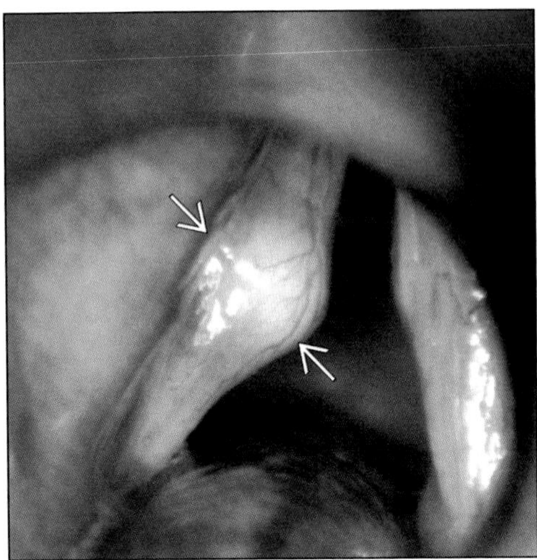

This endoscopic view demonstrates a nodule within the middle portion of the left vocal cord ➔. The histologic type of the cyst cannot be determined from this appearance.

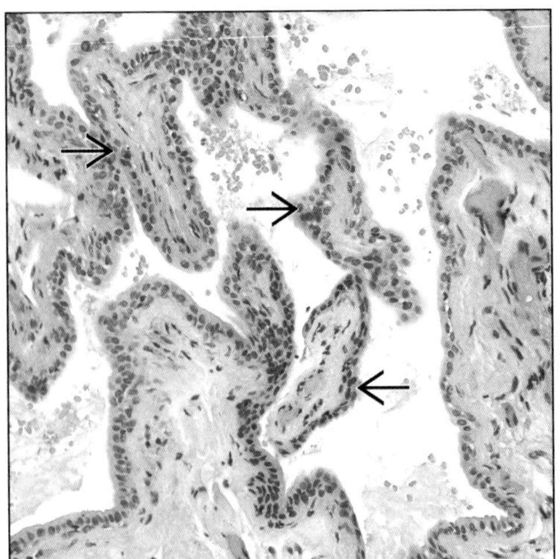

Hematoxylin & eosin shows multiple papillary projections into the lumen of this ductal cyst ➔, lined by a double-layered ductal epithelium. There is no cytologic atypia.

TERMINOLOGY

Synonyms

- Saccular, ductal, oncocytic, or tonsillar cysts

Definitions

- Laryngocele (L)
- Laryngeal cysts (LC)
- Saccular cyst (SC)
- Ductal cyst (DC)
- Oncocytic cyst (OC)
- Tonsillar cyst (TC)
- Dilatation of air-filled saccule (appendix of ventricle) communicating with laryngeal lumen (L)
- Obstruction of intramucosal ducts of seromucinous glands (DC) or laryngeal saccule without communication with laryngeal lumen (SC)

ETIOLOGY/PATHOGENESIS

Developmental Anomaly

- Congenital appearance of laryngocele

Environmental Exposure

- Repeated increases of intralaryngeal pressure in adults
- Tumors
- Infection or trauma

CLINICAL ISSUES

Epidemiology

- Incidence
  - Rare (1 in 2,500,000 for laryngocele)
  - 5% of benign laryngeal lesions
    - DC are 75% and SC are 25% of all LC
- Age
  - All ages, but most common between 50 and 60 years
- Gender
  - Male > Female (L)
  - Equal gender distribution (LC)

Site

- Unilateral, internal L in laryngeal lumen (30%), external L in neck through thyrohyoid membrane (26%), mixed L with both locations (44%)
- Larynx lumen between true and false cords (SC)
- Vocal cords, ventricle of Morgagni, ventricular folds, aryepiglottic folds, and pharyngeal side of epiglottis, solitary or multiple (DC)
- Ventricle of Morgagni, ventricular folds (OC)
- Epiglottis (TC)

Presentation

- Hoarseness, cough, dyspnea, dysphagia, and foreign body sensation in internal and mixed L
- Fluctuating lateral neck mass in external L, asymptomatic L in 12% of cases
- Hoarseness, respiratory and feeding problems, foreign body sensation, and asymptomatic LC

Treatment

- Endoscopic or external surgery in symptomatic L
- Conservative treatment of LC by aspiration, marsupialization, endoscopic removal

Prognosis

- Excellent, although rarely airway obstruction and infection (laryngopyocele) or recurrences (incompletely excised LC)
- Relationship between L and laryngeal squamous cell carcinoma in up to 29% of cases

IMAGE FINDINGS

CT Findings

- Circumscribed, air-/fluid-filled cystic, intra- &/or extralaryngeal lesion, with possible communication

LARYNGOCELE AND LARYNGEAL CYSTS

Key Facts

Terminology
- Laryngocele is defined as air-filled saccule communicating with laryngeal lumen
- Laryngeal cysts are designed with regard to pathogenesis (DC, SC) or typical histologic features (OC)

Clinical Issues
- All age groups, most common over 50 years
- Specific anatomic sites depending on L or LC
- Fluctuating lateral neck mass in external and mixed L

Microscopic Pathology
- Normal histologic structures of laryngeal saccule; respiratory epithelium or double-layered ductal epithelium (± oncocytes)

Top Differential Diagnoses
- Different types of cyst, including saccular cyst, branchiogenic cyst, dermoid cyst, laryngocele, teratoma

MACROSCOPIC FEATURES

General Features
- Type of LC defines gross appearance, with internal, external, or mixed appearance
- Communicating (L) or noncommunicating (LC) with laryngeal lumen
- Air-filled (L), mucus, or keratin-filled

Size
- 0.5-7.5 cm (LC)

MICROSCOPIC PATHOLOGY

Histologic Features
- Laryngocele
  - Respiratory or columnar epithelium, with focal squamous or oncocytic metaplasia
  - Fibrous wall with focal chronic mononuclear inflammatory cells
- Saccular cyst
  - Ciliated respiratory epithelium with increased number of goblet cells and partially or completely metaplastic squamous or oncocytic epithelium
  - Fibrous wall with focal lymphocytic infiltrates
- Ductal cyst
  - Double-layered cylindrical, cuboidal, or flattened ductal epithelium with squamous or oncocytic metaplasia
  - Fibrous wall, focal lymphocytic infiltrates
- Oncocytic cyst
  - Folded cystic wall with papillary infolding, double-layered epithelium
  - Columnar eosinophilic cells with granular cytoplasm encircling cystic lumina, with outer layer of small basal cells
- Tonsillar cyst
  - Cystic formation resembling tonsillar crypt with squamous epithelium, keratin-filled lumen, and lymphoid tissue in wall

DIFFERENTIAL DIAGNOSIS

Different Types of Cysts
- Separation between saccular, branchiogenic, dermoid, laryngocele, & teratoma based on histology

SELECTED REFERENCES

1. Pennings RJ et al: Giant laryngoceles: a cause of upper airway obstruction. Eur Arch Otorhinolaryngol. 258(3):137-40, 2001
2. Arens C et al: Clinical and morphological aspects of laryngeal cysts. Eur Arch Otorhinolaryngol. 254(9-10):430-6, 1997
3. Celin SE et al: The association of laryngoceles with squamous cell carcinoma of the larynx. Laryngoscope. 101(5):529-36, 1991
4. Newman BH et al: Laryngeal cysts in adults: a clinicopathologic study of 20 cases. Am J Clin Pathol. 81(6):715-20, 1984

IMAGE GALLERY

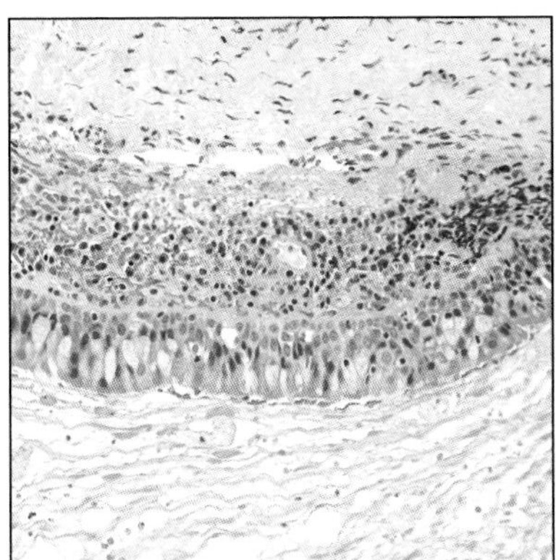

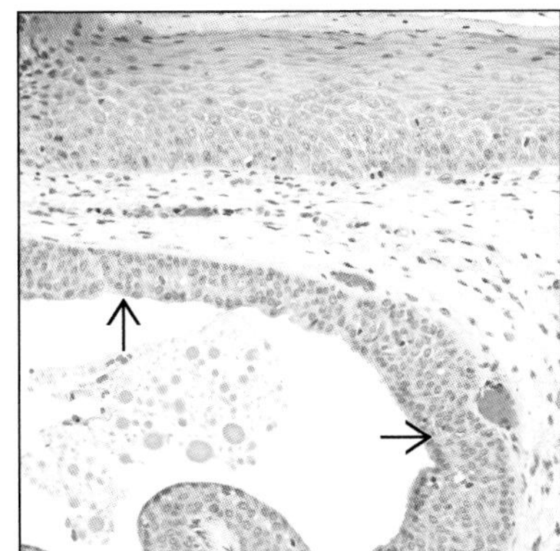

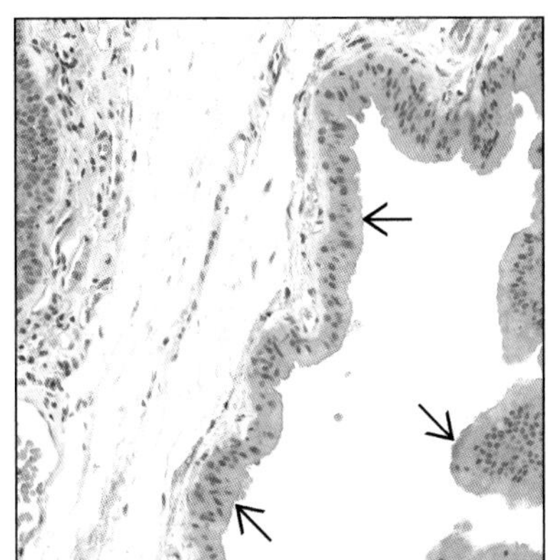

*(**Left**) A saccular cyst is seen with distended saccule filled with mucinous material. The cystic wall is lined by respiratory-type epithelium with mucinous cells. (**Center**) A distended duct is lined by a metaplastic squamous epithelium ⇒ in this ductal cyst. Beneath the epithelium, there is an edematous fibrous stroma. (**Right**) The inner layer of this oncocytic cyst is composed of cylindrical eosinophilic oncocytic cells ⇒, with an outer layer lined by basal cells.*

TRACHEOPATHIA OSTEOPLASTICA

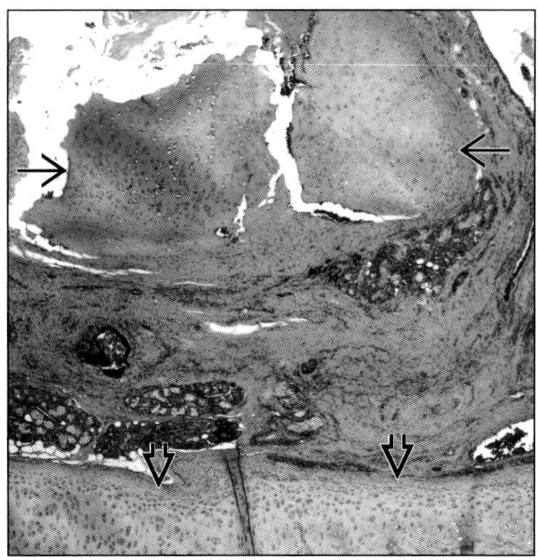

Hematoxylin & eosin shows cartilage rings ⇨ with a number of nodules of cartilage immediate below the surface mucosa →. The minor mucoserous glands are noted in the stroma.

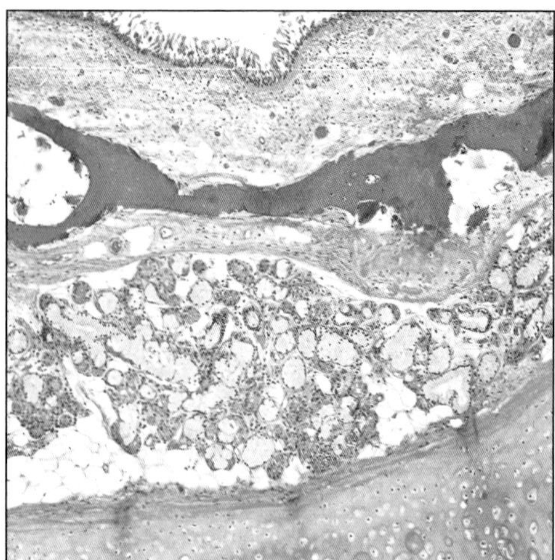

Hematoxylin & eosin shows calcification and bone formation below an intact respiratory-type epithelium. The minor mucoserous glands and fat separate this bone from the underlying cartilage ring.

TERMINOLOGY

Abbreviations

- Tracheopathia osteoplastica (TPO)

Synonyms

- Tracheopathia osteochondroplastica
- Osteochondroplastic tracheopathy
- Tracheopathia chondro-osteoplastica

Definitions

- Segmental degenerative disorder of tracheobronchial tree characterized by multiple submucosal cartilaginous and osseous nodules of various sizes narrowing upper respiratory tract

ETIOLOGY/PATHOGENESIS

Infectious

- Persistent purulent tracheitis followed by calcium deposition, resulting in bone and cartilage forming around accumulations

Degenerative

- Nodules develop as eccondroses of tracheal cartilage rings

CLINICAL ISSUES

Epidemiology

- Incidence
  - Rare disease in clinical practice
    - Identified at autopsy > clinical practice
- Age
  - Mean: > 50 years; range: 11-71 years
  - Females older than males by about a decade
- Gender
  - Male > Female

Site

- Tracheobronchial tree, usually in subglottic space
  - Posterior membranous portion of tracheobronchial tree is spared

Presentation

- Most patients are asymptomatic (90%)
- If symptomatic, signs and symptoms are nonspecific, overlapping with asthma
- Stridor, dyspnea, and shortness of breath
- Chronic, recurrent cough, hoarseness, wheezing
- Hemoptysis or expectoration
- May result in difficult intubation
- Rarely involves entire trachea with progression to airway obstruction
- Associated with atrophic rhinitis or pharyngitis in some cases

Endoscopic Findings

- Bronchoscopy considered diagnostic
- Submucosal projections into laryngotracheal lumen

Treatment

- Options, risks, complications
  - Localized disease may not require treatment
  - Significant narrowing may require laser removal and dilatation
- Surgical approaches
  - Endoscopic CO_2 laser or complete linear tracheoplasty
    - While stents (silicone tubes) are difficult to insert, they can yield extended opening of larynx/trachea

Prognosis

- Disease tends to be slowly progressive
- Meticulous tracheobronchial hygiene is imperative for long-term clinical management
- With little morbidity or mortality, correct diagnosis prevents unnecessary operation

TRACHEOPATHIA OSTEOPLASTICA

Key Facts

Terminology
- Segmental degenerative disorder characterized by multiple submucosal osteocartilaginous nodules of various sizes narrowing upper respiratory tract

Clinical Issues
- Male > Female; mean age: > 50 years
- Most patients are asymptomatic (90%)
- Bronchoscopy considered diagnostic

Image Findings
- Submucosal projections into laryngotracheal lumen
- Beaded or scalloped, nodular, submucosal calcified opacities of tracheal cartilages
- Posterior membranous portion of tracheobronchial tree is spared

Microscopic Pathology
- Metaplastic or heterotopic cartilage and bone in submucosa

IMAGE FINDINGS

Radiographic Findings
- X-ray or CT may show calcified soft tissue masses in the trachea or larynx
- Beaded or scalloped, nodular, submucosal calcified opacities of tracheobronchial cartilages

MACROSCOPIC FEATURES

General Features
- Bronchoscopy shows submucosal firm nodules

Size
- Usually < 3-4 mm nodules studding cartilage rings

MICROSCOPIC PATHOLOGY

Histologic Features
- Metaplastic or heterotopic cartilage and bone in submucosa
- Shows continuity with inner surface of tracheal cartilage
- Bone may protrude into mucosa
- Overlying mucosa is intact and may appear normal or metaplastic
- Irregular bony spicules have thin walls surrounding fatty marrow
- Residua of inflammation (tracheitis) may be seen
- Small biopsies and lack of radiographic/bronchoscopic information make diagnosis difficult

DIFFERENTIAL DIAGNOSIS

Diffuse Tracheal Stenosis
- Endstage of multiple different diseases, lacking calcification or ossification, usually measures 2-4 cm, results in airway compromise, producing concentric or eccentric narrowing

Relapsing Polychondritis
- Mixed inflammation with destruction of cartilage from outside in; systemic disorder

Tracheobronchomegaly and Tracheomalacia
- Both disorders present with softening, flexibility, or dilatation of trachea

SELECTED REFERENCES

1. Penner CR et al: Tracheopathia osteoplastica. Ear Nose Throat J. 82(6):427, 2003
2. Tibesar RJ et al: Tracheopathia osteoplastica: effective long-term management. Otolaryngol Head Neck Surg. 129(3):303-4, 2003
3. Young RH et al: Tracheopathia osteoplastica: clinical, radiologic, and pathological correlations. J Thorac Cardiovasc Surg. 79(4):537-41, 1980
4. Härmä RA et al: Tracheopathia chondro-osteoplastica. A clinical study of thirty cases. Acta Otolaryngol. 84(1-2):118-23, 1977

IMAGE GALLERY

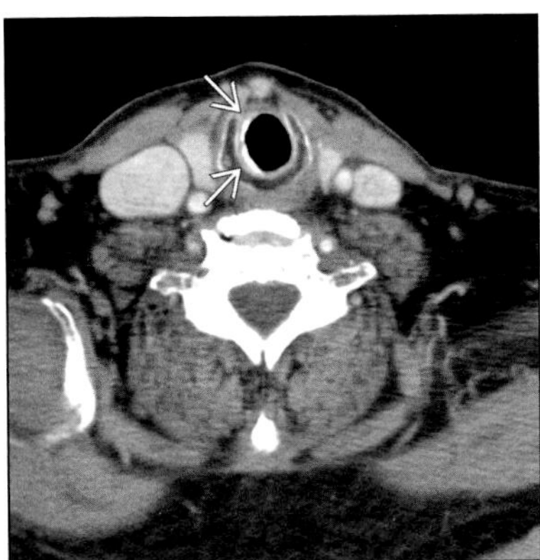

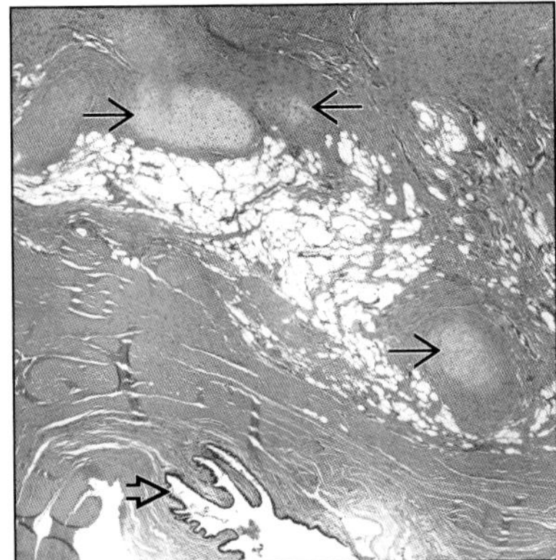

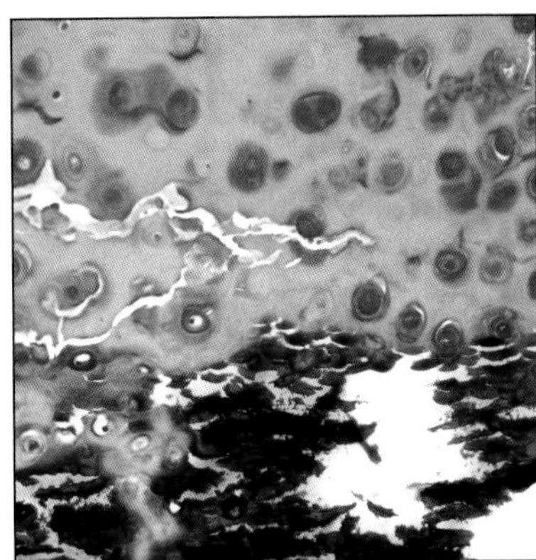

(Left) *Axial CECT shows diffuse calcified subglottic submucosa ➔. TPO can be thin and non-nodular or focal with discrete ossification.* ***(Center)*** *The respiratory-type epithelium ⇨ is subtended by fibrosis. Within the fibrosis are a number of nodules of benign, mature cartilage ➔.* ***(Right)*** *A nodule of cartilage associated with calcification is shown. The "osteoplastica" component may be calcification, bony spicules, or mature lamellar bone, dependent on length of time with disease and stage.*

LARYNGITIS: VIRAL, BACTERIAL, FUNGAL

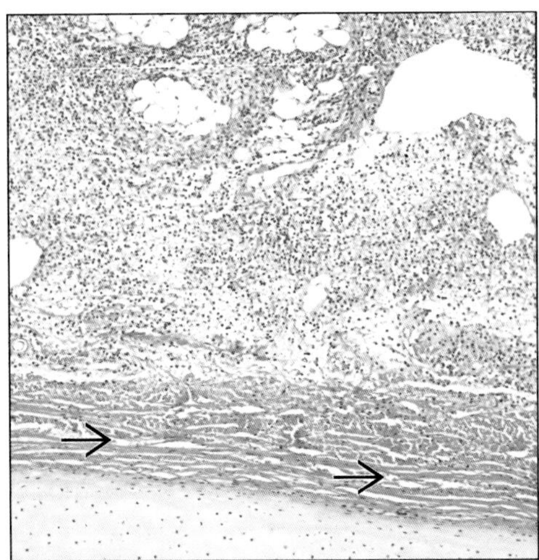

The surface epithelium is lost. There is a mixed inflammatory infiltrate associated with fat and edema fluid. There is some fibrosis immediately associated with the cartilage ➔.

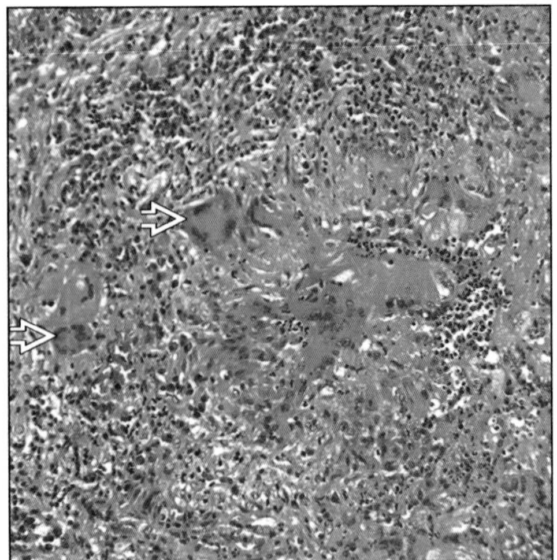

There are caseating granulomas associated with mixed inflammatory cells in the background. There are isolated giant cells ⊳. This is from a case of tuberculosis laryngitis.

TERMINOLOGY

Synonyms

- Different terms based on specific anatomic site affected
  - Laryngotracheobronchitis, pharyngitis, laryngitis, croup, epiglottitis

Definitions

- Laryngitis can be infectious or inflammatory, acute or chronic
  - Antecedent events may predispose to laryngitis, which tends to be multifactorial

ETIOLOGY/PATHOGENESIS

Infectious

- Many viruses, bacteria, and fungi can cause laryngitis
  - Parainfluenza virus type 1 (croup)
- Different etiologies may be present synchronously

Trauma/Mechanical

- Foreign bodies getting caught
- Ulceration by foreign body predisposes to laryngitis

Neoplasm

- Tumors can cause ulceration

Iatrogenic

- Surgery (vascular compromise)
- Feeding tube, tracheostomy tube (especially when inserted during airway emergencies)
- Post-radiation
- Environmental exposures to noxious substances

CLINICAL ISSUES

Epidemiology

- Incidence
  - Common (6%), with seasonal and age variability
  - Laryngitis usually a clinical diagnosis
- Age
  - Same organism causes different clinical disease based on age
    - Bronchiolitis in infant
    - Croup in older child
    - Pharyngitis in young adult
    - Subclinical syndrome in middle-aged adult
  - Croup: usually < 6 years
  - Herpes: Very young, very old, pregnant, or immunocompromised patients

Presentation

- Thorough history, including occupation and vocal demands, may guide further evaluation
- Clinical manifestations depend on age, sex, nutritional and immunity status
- Croup: Hoarseness, barking cough, inspiratory stridor (noisy, labored breathing)
- Epiglottitis: Tripod sign, fever, stridor, sore throat, odynophagia, shortness of breath, drooling
- Immunocompromised patients: Herpes simplex or fungal laryngitis
  - AIDS, cancer, leukemia/lymphoma, corticosteroids, diabetes mellitus, pulmonary disease, organ transplantation
- Cord function may be compromised

Endoscopic Findings

- Direct laryngoscopy to evaluate airway

Laboratory Tests

- Extensive laboratory investigation for specific infectious agent is not warranted, except in extreme or unique cases
  - Serologic pre- and postinfection titers may document infectious agent (complement fixation; precipitant tests)

LARYNGITIS: VIRAL, BACTERIAL, FUNGAL

Key Facts

Terminology
- Different terms based on specific anatomic site affected
- Laryngitis can be infectious or inflammatory, acute or chronic

Clinical Issues
- Same organism causes different clinical disease based on age
- Clinical manifestations depend on age, sex, nutritional and immunity status
- Croup: Hoarseness, barking cough, inspiratory stridor (noisy, labored breathing)
- Epiglottitis: Tripod sign, fever, stridor, sore throat, odynophagia, shortness of breath, drooling
- Generally, supportive measures to control symptoms
  - Culture sensitivities dictate type and duration of antimicrobial regimen

Microscopic Pathology
- Nonspecific inflammatory cells and edema fluid
- Surface epithelial erosion or ulceration
- Hyperkeratosis commonly associated with intraepithelial neutrophils
- Pseudoepitheliomatous hyperplasia associated with fungal infections

Top Differential Diagnoses
- Gastroesophageal reflux disease
- Squamous cell carcinoma (SCC)
- Wegener granulomatosis
- Relapsing polychondritis

Treatment
- Drugs
  - Culture sensitivities dictate type and duration of antimicrobial regimen
    - In practice, infrequently performed
  - Single dose corticosteroids and bronchodilators reduce croup severity and duration
  - Nebulized epinephrine in patients with severe croup
  - Antifungal therapy if fungal organisms
- Generally, supportive measures to control symptoms
  - Humidified air, analgesics

Prognosis
- Excellent for self-limited viral illnesses
- Rarely, intubation to maintain airway
  - Avoid repeated intubation attempts
- Rarely, death results from complications

MACROSCOPIC FEATURES

General Features
- Mucus membranes are erythematous and swollen
- Exudate can be seen

MICROSCOPIC PATHOLOGY

Histologic Features
- Nonspecific inflammatory cells and edema fluid
- Surface epithelial erosion or ulceration
- Hyperkeratosis commonly associated with intraepithelial neutrophils
- Secondary bacterial colonies within exudate
- Pseudoepitheliomatous hyperplasia associated with fungal infections
- Multinucleated giant cells with opacified, "ground-glass" nuclei (herpes simplex) or prominent Cowdry-A-type inclusion (CMV)
- Atrophy or hyperplasia associated with nonspecific inflammatory infiltrate in chronic laryngitis cases

ANCILLARY TESTS

Histochemistry
- Specific histochemistry stains highlight organisms
  - Gram, acid-fast, fluoro, GMS, PAS/light green

Immunohistochemistry
- Selectively: HSV, CMV

DIFFERENTIAL DIAGNOSIS

Gastroesophageal Reflux Disease
- Fibrinoid necrosis; granulation tissue, organized

Squamous Cell Carcinoma (SCC)
- Pseudoepitheliomatous hyperplasia in fungal infection can mimic SCC

Wegener Granulomatosis
- Biocollagenolysis; blue-granular geographic necrosis; foreign body giant cells; vasculitis, ↑ ANCA titers

Relapsing Polychondritis
- Cartilage destroyed by mixed inflammation; no granuloma; auto-antibodies

SELECTED REFERENCES

1. Tulunay OE: Laryngitis--diagnosis and management. Otolaryngol Clin North Am. 41(2):437-51, ix, 2008
2. Thompson L: Herpes simplex virus laryngitis. Ear Nose Throat J. 85(5):304, 2006
3. Cherry JD: State of the evidence for standard-of-care treatments for croup: are we where we need to be? Pediatr Infect Dis J. 24(11 Suppl):S198-202, discussion S201, 2005
4. Leung AK et al: Viral croup: a current perspective. J Pediatr Health Care. 18(6):297-301, 2004
5. Mehanna HM et al: Fungal laryngitis in immunocompetent patients. J Laryngol Otol. 118(5):379-81, 2004
6. Sack JL et al: Identifying acute epiglottitis in adults. High degree of awareness, close monitoring are key. Postgrad Med. 112(1):81-2, 85-6, 2002

LARYNGITIS: VIRAL, BACTERIAL, FUNGAL

Microscopic Features

(Left) The surface epithelium is heavily spongiotic with degenerated bullae ➔. Inflammatory cells are arranged within the surface epithelium and within the stroma below. This acute laryngitis shows predominantly acute inflammatory cells. Biopsy is seldom performed in this setting. *(Right)* There is a heavy inflammatory infiltrate filling the subepithelial space of this case of acute laryngitis (viral). There is a suggestion of abscess formation in this disorder.

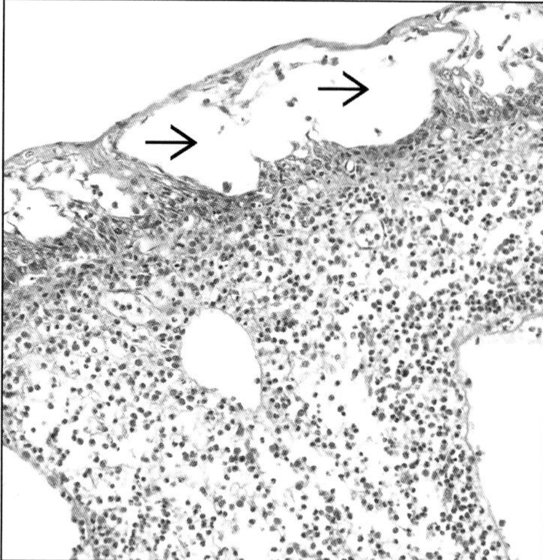

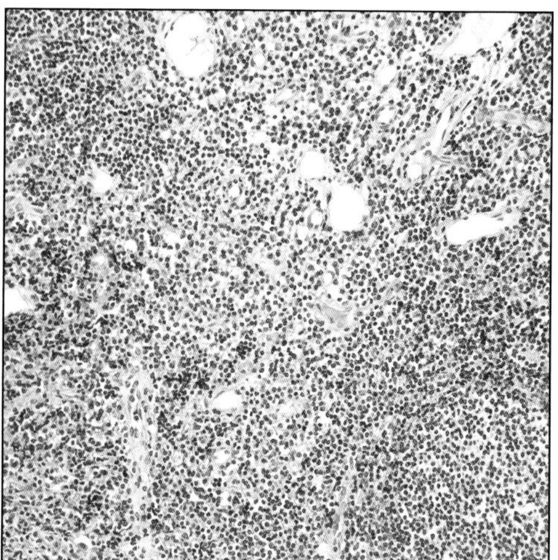

(Left) The surface epithelium is metaplastic, subtended by a band of heavy chronic inflammatory cells. This is from a case of chronic laryngitis in a patient with a long exposure to noxious fumes in the workplace. *(Right)* This case of acute viral laryngitis was associated with a secondary bacterial infection in a patient with a history of squamous cell carcinoma and radiation therapy. Bacterial colonies ➔ are frequently seen as a concurrent finding in erosions/ ulcerations.

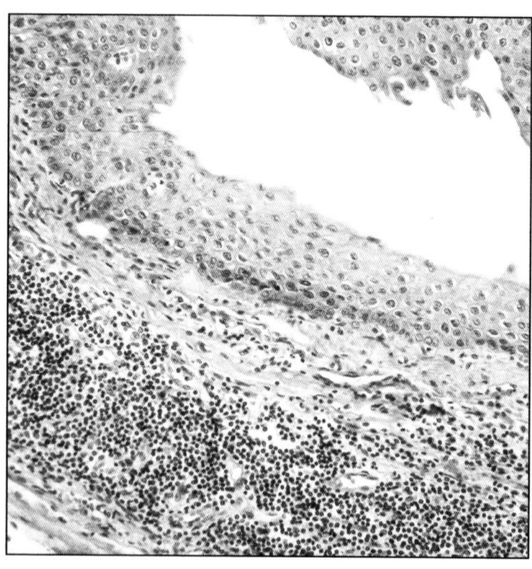

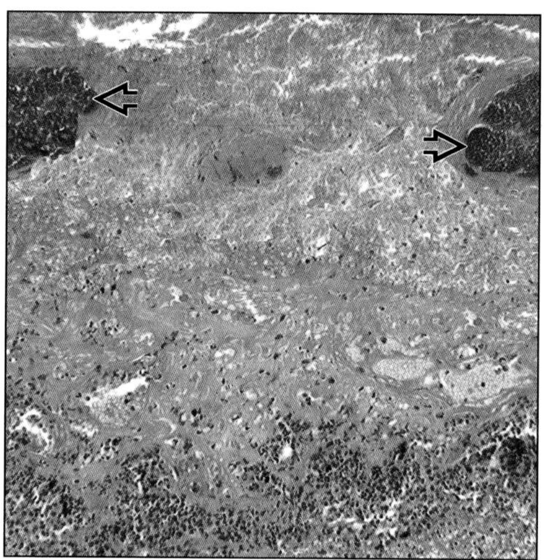

(Left) There is a heavy inflammatory infiltrate composed of acute and chronic inflammatory cells. Within this background, a number of multinucleated giant cells ➔ can be seen, part of a herpes simplex infection. This type of giant cell is pathognomonic for herpes infections. *(Right)* The characteristic multinucleated giant cells of herpes simplex infection ➔ are shown. Note the nuclear overlapping and the powdery, smudged nuclear chromatin within the giant cells.

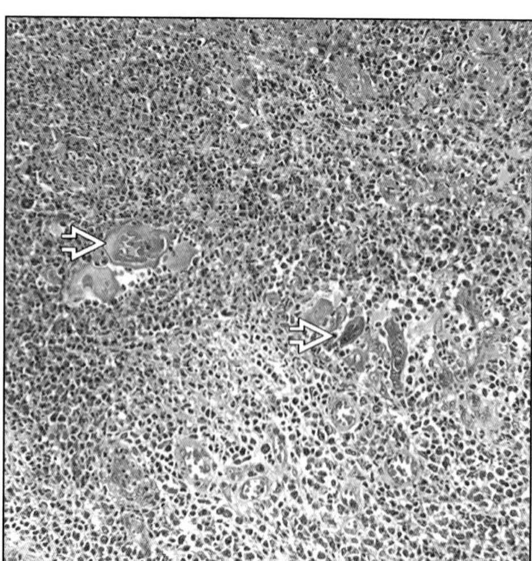

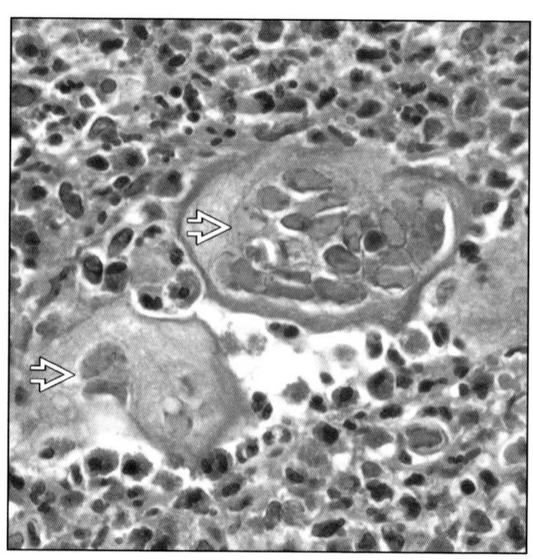

Microscopic and Histochemical Features

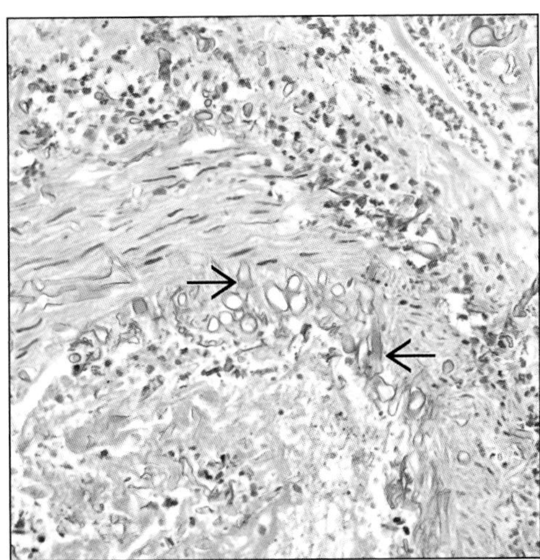

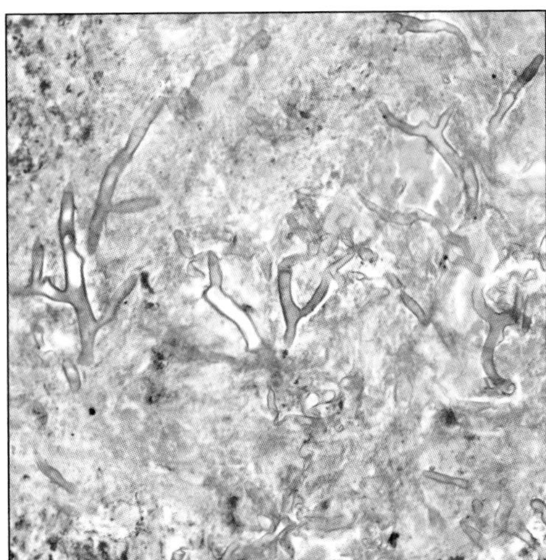

(Left) *Fungal infections can involve the surface epithelium or present as deep fungal infections. This deep fungal infection shows numerous fungal hyphae within a vessel wall* →. ***(Right)*** *Fungal hyphae are haphazardly identified within the necrotic debris and inflammatory exudate of this example of a fungal laryngitis. Antifungal therapy is required for this type of "invasive" laryngitis.*

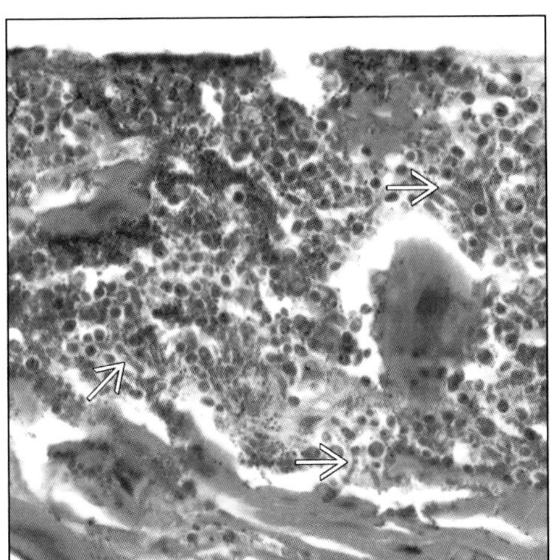

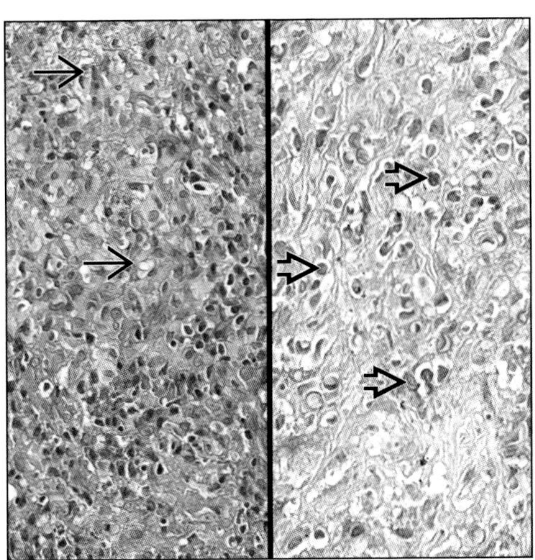

(Left) *The keratin is filled with fungal spores, although well-developed fungal hyphae* ➡ *are noted throughout. It is required to see fungal hyphae attached to the keratin to qualify as a legitimate fungal infection.* ***(Right)*** *The tissue shows a heavy granulomatous type inflammation. Cleared spaces can be seen* → *but organisms are not easily identified. However, with a mucicarmine stain, the cryptococcal organisms* ⇨ *are highlighted in magenta, present throughout the sample.*

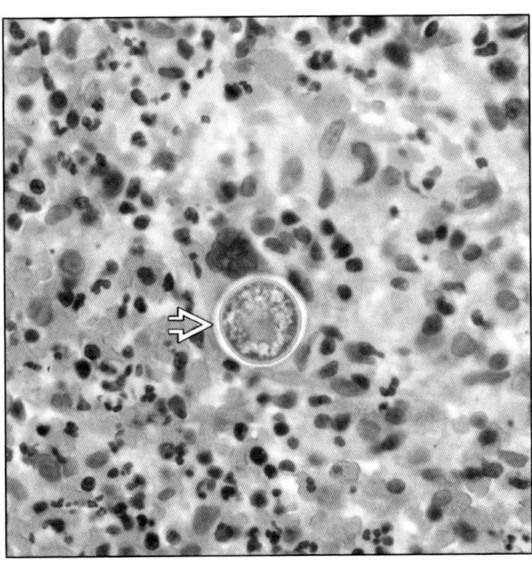

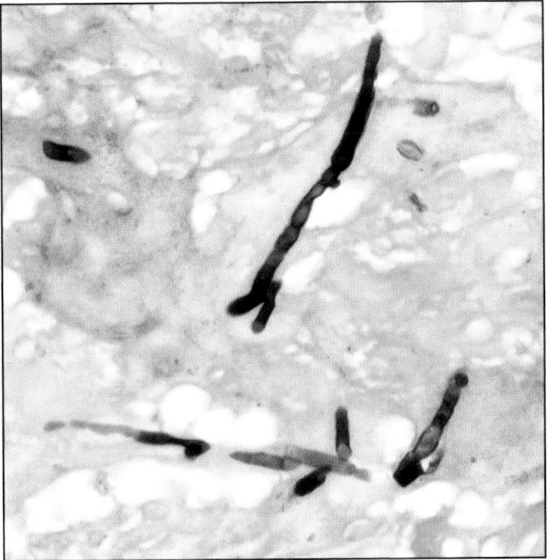

(Left) *Coccidiomycosis infection of the larynx can be seen as part of systemic disease. The spherule* ➡ *filled with endospores is characteristic for this type of fungal organism. Note the mixed inflammatory infiltrate & background giant cell formation.* ***(Right)*** *A silver impregnation stain highlights numerous fungal hyphae in this example of fungal laryngitis. This type of finding requires antifungal chemotherapy agents (amphotericin B or azoles).*

VOCAL CORD NODULES AND POLYPS

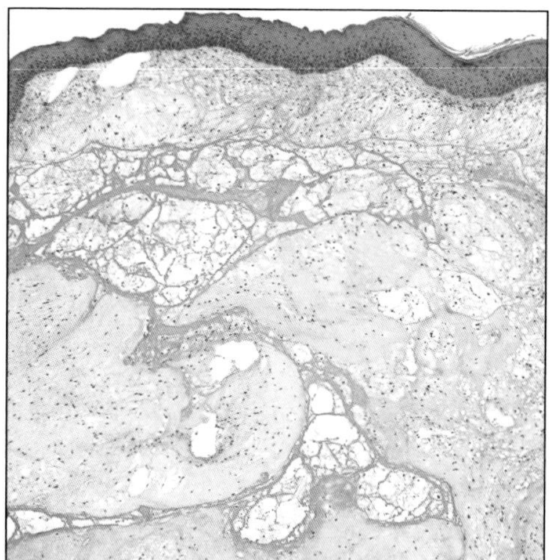

The overlying squamous mucosa is intact. There is an edematous stroma with fibrinous degeneration of the stroma. Hyaline deposition is noted. Inflammatory cells are present.

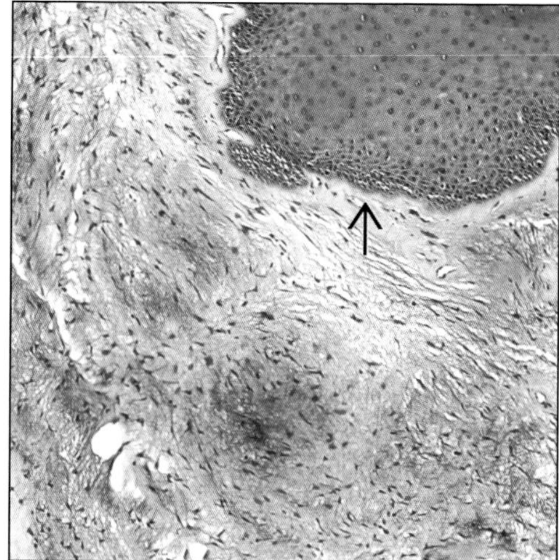

A metaplastic squamous mucosa ⇒ overlies a myxoid stroma. The predominant pattern in a polyp may be an intermediate cellularity in a bluish myxoid-mucinous stroma.

TERMINOLOGY

Synonyms

- Nodule
- Polyp

Definitions

- Reactive changes of laryngeal mucosa and adjacent stroma, which results in benign polypoid or nodular growth

ETIOLOGY/PATHOGENESIS

Multifactorial

- Laryngeal trauma may result from vocal abuse, accidents, or surgery
  - Excessive and improper use of voice
  - Iatrogenic or functional lesions
- Infection
- Hypothyroidism
- Smoking

Pathogenesis

- Personality traits, specifically extroversion, associated with development of vocal cord polyps and nodules

CLINICAL ISSUES

Epidemiology

- Incidence
  - Infrequent
    - Approximately 1.5% of population has hoarseness
    - Polyp/nodule is one of the most frequent significant causes of hoarseness
    - Approximately 2.5% of children have nodules (prevalence)
- Age
  - Variable between nodule or polyp
  - Nodule
    - Usually young to middle-aged patients
    - Uncommon in children
  - Polyp: Any age group
- Gender
  - Nodule
    - Female > Male in young patients
    - Boys > Girls (~ 2:1) in children (7-16 years old)
  - Polyp: Equal gender distribution

Site

- Nodule
  - Anterior to middle 3rd of true vocal cord
  - Nearly always bilateral
- Polyp
  - Aryepiglottic fold, ventricular space, vocal fold, Reinke space
  - > 90% unilateral

Presentation

- Behavior-induced vocal changes
  - Affects speaking voice of nonprofessionals and professionals
    - Professional voice users
    - Singers, actors, public speakers, lecturers, coaches
  - Excessive (overuse) and improper (abuse) use of voice
  - Stressing or straining of voice
- Disease-related vocal cord disease
  - Infection
  - Hypothyroidism
  - Smoking association
- Hoarseness
- Phonation changes

Endoscopic Findings

- Laryngoscopic and stroboscopic findings can be combined in reaching diagnosis
- Nodules more frequently bilateral, sometimes showing hemorrhage
- Polyps appear as protuberances, erythematous, and edematous

VOCAL CORD NODULES AND POLYPS

Key Facts

Terminology
- Reactive changes of laryngeal mucosa and adjacent stroma, which results in benign polypoid or nodular growth

Clinical Issues
- Excessive and improper use of voice
- Patients present with hoarseness and phonation changes
- Nodule: Nearly always bilateral < 0.3 cm nodule on anterior to middle 1/3 of vocal cord
- Polyp: > 90% unilateral, ventricular or Reinke space, > 0.3 cm raspberry-like mass
- Voice therapy is first-line treatment
  - Surgery for refractory cases

Microscopic Pathology
- Shows arc of development (histologic features based on phase at time of biopsy)
- Edema, proteinaceous subepithelial deposition
- Loose myxoid matrix associated with hemorrhage and vascularized stroma
- Dilated vessels (telangiectasia) associated with granulation tissue and hemorrhage/fibrin
- Myxoid, pale blue-pink material
- Fibrous connective tissue deposition

Top Differential Diagnoses
- Amyloidosis, contact ulcer, ligneous conjunctivitis
- Myxoma, spindle cell squamous cell carcinoma, granular cell tumor

- Use of ultrasonography and virtual laryngoscopy may be of benefit
  - Spectrophotometric analysis of hemoglobin concentration in various disease conditions may help clinical assessment
    - Lower hemoglobin concentrations in polyps

Treatment
- Options, risks, complications
  - Among professional voice users, voice problems have significant personal negative impact
    - Ability to work, overall sense of well-being, sense of self
- Surgical approaches
  - Little evidence for surgical intervention as first-line therapy
    - If needed, either CO_2 laser &/or microdissection are equivalent modalities
- Management strategies include voice re-education, drug therapy, and surgery
- Voice therapy is first-line treatment
  - Good vocal function is required by more than 1/3 of labor force to fulfill their job requirements
  - Behavior modification
  - General vocal hygiene is beneficial
  - If there is no improvement with initial speech and language therapy, referral to specialist voice clinic (speech pathologist) should be considered
- Treatment of hypothyroidism can be beneficial

Prognosis
- Excellent, usually without any long-term follow-up required
- Recurrences if inciting factor is not identified and removed or managed

MACROSCOPIC FEATURES

General Features
- Nodule
  - Bilateral, affecting opposing surfaces of vocal cords
  - Usually middle to anterior 1/3 of vocal cord
  - Range from edematous, gelatinous, hemorrhagic, firm or fixed
- Polyp
  - Single
  - Soft, rubbery mass
  - Translucent to red
  - Sessile
  - Raspberry-like to pedunculated

Size
- Nodule: Usually < 0.3 cm
- Polyp: Usually > 0.3 cm
  - Can be up to a few centimeters

MICROSCOPIC PATHOLOGY

Histologic Features
- No definitive histological distinction between laryngeal nodules and polyp
  - While distinctive clinically, interchangeable terms histologically
- Arc of development
  - Edema and proteinaceous material deposited in interstitium and subepithelial tissue
  - Loose myxoid matrix associated with hemorrhage within vascularized stroma
    - Inflammation is usually sparse to absent
  - Dilated vessels (telangiectasia) associated with granulation tissue and hemorrhage/fibrin
  - Myxoid, pale blue-pink material may predominate
  - Fibrous connective tissue deposition
    - Fibrin-type material adjacent to vascular spaces
    - May become completely collagenized/fibrotic at end stage
    - Only isolated fibroblasts present
- Polyps divided into 4 main histologic subtypes depending on stage of development at time of biopsy and dominant histologic pattern
  - Edematous
  - Vascular
  - Myxoid
  - Hyaline or fibrous

VOCAL CORD NODULES AND POLYPS

  - Not uncommon to have overlap or mixture of these features
- Surface epithelium
  - Metaplastic
  - Atrophic
  - Keratotic
  - Hyperplastic
  - Not atypical or pleomorphic
- Crystals rarely identified in some polyps

DIFFERENTIAL DIAGNOSIS

Amyloidosis

- False vocal cord most common
- Acellular, extracellular, eosinophilic, matrix material
- Perivascular and periglandular accentuation
- Positive with Congo red &/or cresyl violet
- May show light chain restriction (uncommon)
  - κ or λ restricted

Myxoma

- Uncommon mass lesion
- Hypocellular myxoid lesion with stellate spindle cells
- Usually clear to very light blue matrix
- Difficult to separate from myxoid polyp in some cases

Spindle Cell Squamous Cell Carcinoma

- Polypoid mass with surface ulceration or denudation
- Epithelium can be identified (usually in crypts or base of polyp)
- Cellular stroma
- Comprised of atypical spindled cells with pleomorphism and nuclear hyperchromasia
- Mitotic figures can be seen, including atypical forms
- May be positive with keratin (approximately 70% of cases) immunohistochemistry
- Proliferation markers tend to be increased

Contact Ulcer

- Bilateral, posterior larynx
- Opposing surfaces of true vocal cords
- Polypoid mass
- Surface ulceration with fibrinoid necrosis
- Granulation tissue with vessels arranged perpendicular to surface
- Inflammation with hemosiderin-laden macrophages
- Mitotic figures can be seen (vessels or fibroblasts)

Granular Cell Tumor

- Pseudoepitheliomatous hyperplasia of epithelium
  - Overlying neoplastic cells only
- Large polygonal cells with abundant, granular, eosinophilic cytoplasm
- Frequently associated with nerves
- Strong S100 protein immunoreactivity

Ligneous Conjunctivitis

- Uncommon in larynx
- Firm, clotted fibrin-rich matrix material deposition
- Hard, subepithelial nodule

SELECTED REFERENCES

1. Syed I et al: Hoarse voice in adults: an evidence-based approach to the 12 minute consultation. Clin Otolaryngol. 34(1):54-8, 2009
2. Altman KW: Vocal fold masses. Otolaryngol Clin North Am. 40(5):1091-108, viii, 2007
3. Franco RA et al: Common diagnoses and treatments in professional voice users. Otolaryngol Clin North Am. 40(5):1025-61, vii, 2007
4. Akif Kiliç M et al: The prevalence of vocal fold nodules in school age children. Int J Pediatr Otorhinolaryngol. 68(4):409-12, 2004
5. Wallis L et al: Vocal fold nodule vs. vocal fold polyp: answer from surgical pathologist and voice pathologist point of view. J Voice. 18(1):125-9, 2004
6. Johns MM: Update on the etiology, diagnosis, and treatment of vocal fold nodules, polyps, and cysts. Curr Opin Otolaryngol Head Neck Surg. 11(6):456-61, 2003
7. Marcotullio D et al: Exudative laryngeal diseases of Reinke's space: a clinicohistopathological framing. J Otolaryngol. 31(6):376-80, 2002
8. Thompson LD: Diagnostically challenging lesions in head and neck pathology. Eur Arch Otorhinolaryngol. 254(8):357-66, 1997
9. Milutinović Z et al: Functional trauma of the vocal folds: classification and management strategies. Folia Phoniatr Logop. 48(2):78-85, 1996
10. Yamaguchi M et al: Mucosal blood volume and oxygen saturation in the human vocal fold. Acta Otolaryngol. 110(3-4):300-8, 1990

Endoscopic and Microscopic Features

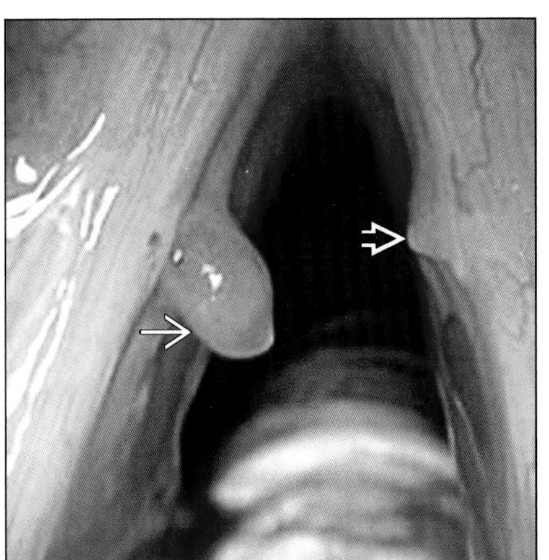

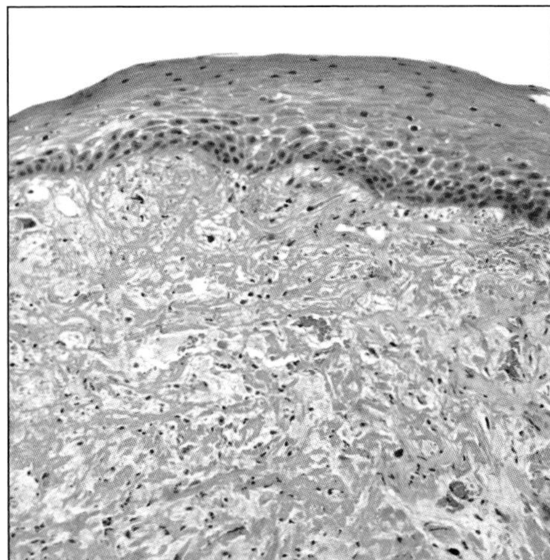

(Left) *A polypoid projection from the vocal cord ➡ is noted. There is a slight nodularity on the contralateral vocal cord ➡, suggesting "bilateral" disease.* ***(Right)*** *There is a mixed fibrous connective tissue stroma with myxoid material between the fibrosis. This is a common finding in the arc of development seen in a polyp/nodule.*

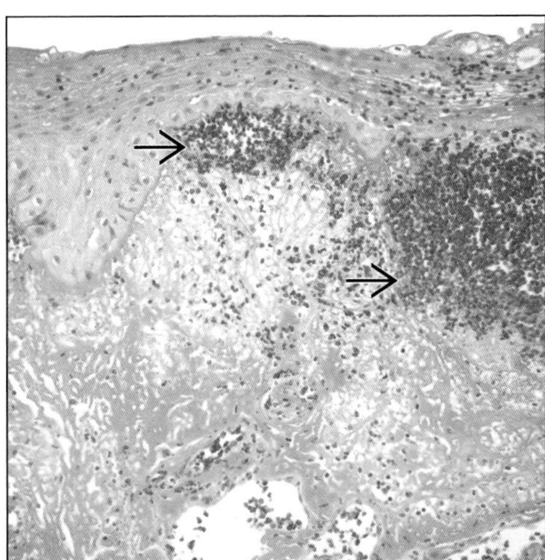

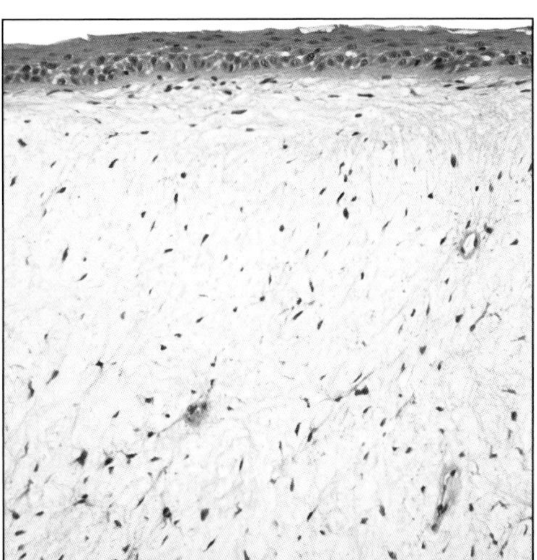

(Left) *Early in the development of a polyp, there is edema and hemorrhage into the stroma ➡ below an intact or possibly ulcerated epithelium. Fibrinous material is noted in the stroma as organization of the hemorrhage is suggested.* ***(Right)*** *The stroma is hypocellular in this polyp, although there is a very edematous to myxomatous stroma. There are a few isolated spindled cells in the stroma, but they are not atypical. Mitotic figures are absent.*

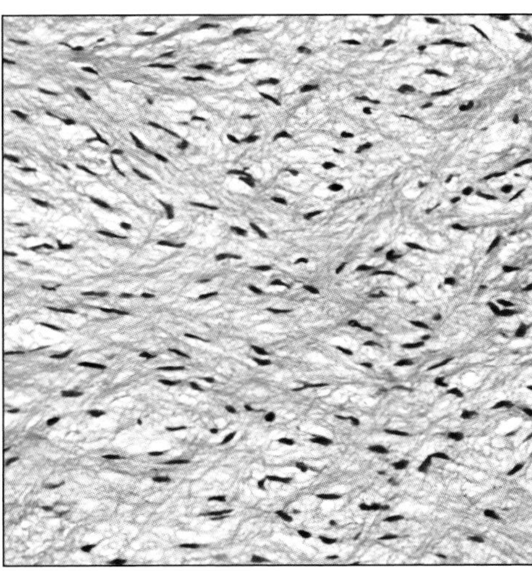

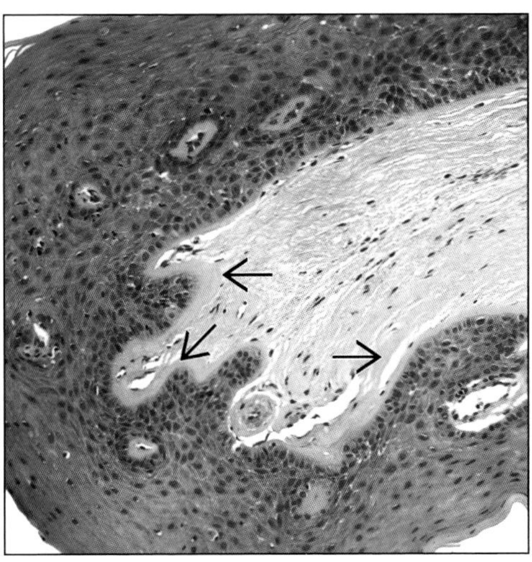

(Left) *As the arc of development for a polyp continues, there is a mingling of myxoid matrix with the fibrous connective tissue stroma. Note the bland spindle fibroblastic cells.* ***(Right)*** *The end stage of a polyp/nodule shows heavy subepithelial fibrosis ➡, sometimes creating an accentuated basement membrane material. The epithelium may be hyperplastic, with keratosis. However, cellular atypia is absent.*

REACTIVE EPITHELIAL CHANGES

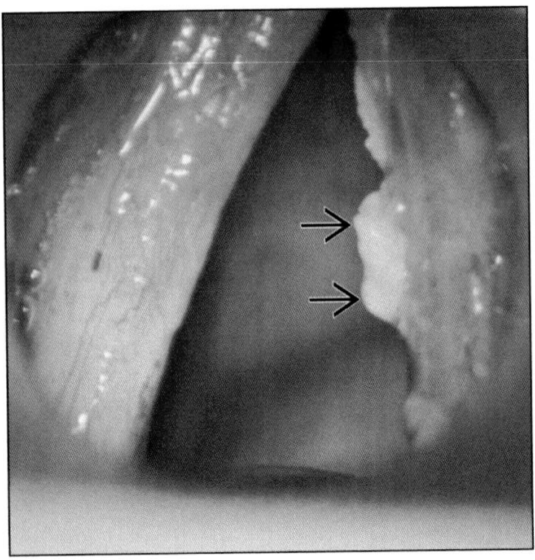

Endoscopic view shows a well-circumscribed, uneven, exophytic white plaque (leukoplakia) ⇒ on the right vocal cord. This clinical appearance encompasses a wide variety of histologic changes.

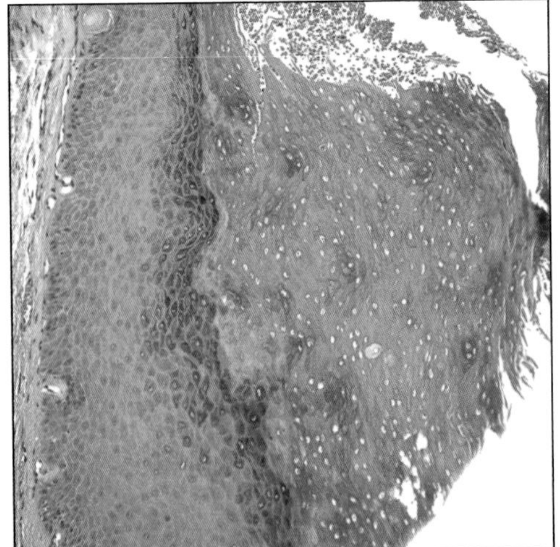

Hematoxylin & eosin shows hyperplastic squamous epithelium with keratohyaline layer and exuberant layer of keratin termed keratosis. Parakeratosis is not appreciated. There is no cytologic atypia.

TERMINOLOGY

Synonyms

- Leukoplakia
- Keratosis without atypia
- Pseudoepitheliomatous hyperplasia
- Teflonoma

Definitions

- Keratosis
  - Keratin layer on surface of squamous epithelium, often accompanied by granular cell layer
- Pseudoepitheliomatous hyperplasia (PEH)
  - Extensive hyperplasia of prickle cell layer of squamous epithelium without cytologic atypia
  - Has irregular epithelial projections into underlying stroma mimicking squamous cell carcinoma
- Radiation change (RC)
  - Long-lasting or life persistent morphologic changes caused by radiotherapy
  - Affects surface epithelium, minor salivary glands, fibrous tissue, vessels, and cartilages
- Teflon granuloma (TG)
  - Foreign body granuloma caused by overinjection or too superficial or too deep injection of Teflon paste
    - Teflon is used to treat paralyzed vocal cord

ETIOLOGY/PATHOGENESIS

Environmental Exposure

- Keratosis: Smoking, air pollution, chronic irritation
- PEH: Chronic irritation, smoking
- RC: Radiation therapy of larynx, usually for carcinoma, but may be part of head and neck radiation for a different reason
- TG: Injection of Teflon paste
  - Tetrafluoroethylene and glycerin

Infectious Agents

- Various bacteria and fungi can cause PEH
  - Mycobacteria, *Blastomyces dermatitidis*, *Cryptococcus*

Tumor

- Granular cell tumor is frequently associated with PEH

CLINICAL ISSUES

Site

- Specific anatomic site for certain types of reactive changes
  - True vocal folds/cords: Keratosis, PEH, and Teflon granuloma
  - True vocal folds in relation to tuberculosis
  - Posterior true vocal folds, false cords, and subglottis: Granular cell tumor and PEH
  - Any location as a complication of radiation

Presentation

- Hoarseness
- Cough
- Foreign body sensation
- Airway obstruction
- Dysphagia

Endoscopic Findings

- Raised, flat, or sometimes ulcerated
- Leukoplakia
- Erythroplakia
- Findings are usually nonspecific and can significantly overlap with carcinoma

Natural History

- Most reactive conditions resolve spontaneously
  - Depends if etiologic agent is removed

Treatment

- Options, risks, complications
  - Most lesions resolve on their own

REACTIVE EPITHELIAL CHANGES

Key Facts

Terminology
- Keratosis: Exuberant keratin layer
- Pseudoepitheliomatous hyperplasia: Epithelial hyperplasia without atypia but with irregular projections
- Radiation: Atrophic epithelium, fibrosis, bizarre fibroblasts, glandular atrophy
- Teflon granuloma: Foreign body reaction around Teflon particles

Macroscopic Features
- Keratosis: Elevated white plaque of vocal cord
- PEH: Polypoid thickening with smooth, whitish surface
- Radiation: Atrophic mucosa, glottic stenosis, cartilage necrosis or osteonecrosis
- TG: Firm polypoid lesion (up to 2 cm)

Microscopic Pathology
- Keratosis
  - Thickened keratotic layer, hyperplastic spinous layer, no dysplastic changes
- Pseudoepitheliomatous hyperplasia
  - Hyperplastic squamous epithelium, irregular epithelial projections, no atypia
- Radiation change
  - Acute stage: Acute necrotizing inflammation
  - Chronic stage: Atrophic epithelium and minor salivary glands, fibrosis, plump endothelial cells, bizarre fibroblasts, intimal proliferation

Top Differential Diagnoses
- Invasive squamous cell carcinoma
- Gouty tophus

  - No prospective features that suggest reactive vs. carcinoma
- Surgical approaches
  - Endoscopic removal provides a diagnosis, rather than necessarily the treatment

Prognosis
- Excellent, when truly a reactive lesion
- No risk of malignant transformation if atypia or dysplasia is absent

MACROSCOPIC FEATURES

General Features
- Keratosis: Usually well-circumscribed, slightly elevated white plaque of vocal cord
- PEH: Thickening or polypoid lesion with smooth, whitish surface
- Radiation changes
  - Early: Edema, mucositis, ulceration, blood
  - Late: Atrophic or hyperplastic mucosa, fibrosis, glottic stenosis, osteonecrosis
- TG: Well-circumscribed, firm polypoid lesion (~ 2 cm)

MICROSCOPIC PATHOLOGY

Histologic Features
- Keratosis is variably thickened keratotic layer ± nuclei; granular layer may be present; irregularly hyperplastic spinous layer; possible chronic inflammation
- PEH shows hyperplastic epithelium without atypia, well-defined basement membrane with irregular epithelial projections into stroma
  - Exclude granular cell tumor or infection
  - Special studies to exclude infectious agent
  - TB fluorostain, acid-fast, PAS/light green, GMS
- Radiation changes have stages
  - Acute stage: Acute necrotizing inflammation
  - Chronic stage: Surface ulceration, squamous atypia, atrophic epithelium, and minor salivary glands
  - Ductal squamous metaplasia, endothelial cell hypertrophy, bizarre fibroblasts in dense fibrosis, bizarre skeletal muscle changes
  - Rarely, chondronecrosis or osteonecrosis
- TG: Teflon, polarizable, birefringent foreign material with foreign body giant cell reaction in fibrous stroma (arc of development)

DIFFERENTIAL DIAGNOSIS

Squamous Cell Carcinoma (SCC)
- Pseudoepitheliomatous hyperplasia can mimic invasive carcinoma
- Invasive growth of atypical epithelial cells
- Increased mitotic figures, including atypical forms

Dysplasia or Carcinoma
- Radiation change or PEH may overestimate grade of dysplasia or invasive SCC

Gouty Tophus
- Amorphous crystals, enveloped by giant cells and histiocytes
- Needle-shaped crystals on unstained sections

SELECTED REFERENCES

1. Hamdan AL et al: Vocal changes following radiotherapy to the head and neck for non-laryngeal tumors. Eur Arch Otorhinolaryngol. 266(9):1435-9, 2009
2. Thompson LD: Diagnostically challenging lesions in head and neck pathology. Eur Arch Otorhinolaryngol. 254(8):357-66, 1997
3. Wenig BM et al: Teflonomas of the larynx and neck. Hum Pathol. 21(6):617-23, 1990
4. Dedo HH et al: Histologic evaluation of Teflon granulomas of human vocal cords. A light and electron microscopic study. Acta Otolaryngol. 93(5-6):475-84, 1982
5. Hellquist H et al: Hyperplasia, keratosis, dysplasia and carcinoma in situ of the vocal cords--a follow-up study. Clin Otolaryngol Allied Sci. 7(1):11-27, 1982

REACTIVE EPITHELIAL CHANGES

Microscopic Features

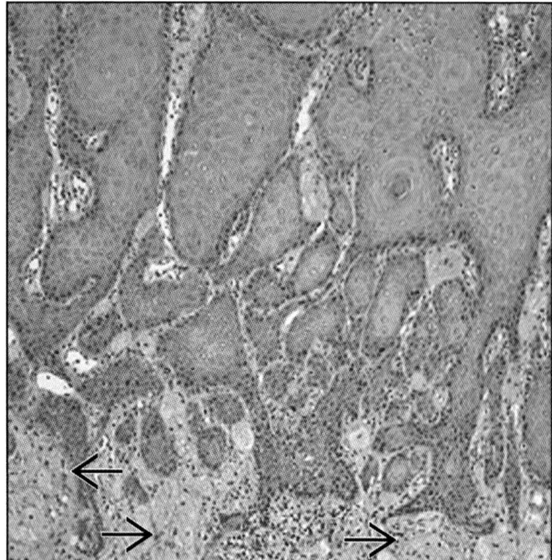

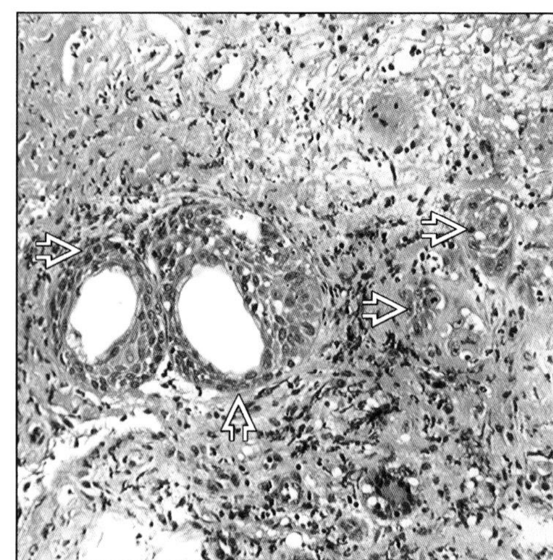

(Left) *Hematoxylin & eosin shows irregular epithelial projections of pseudoepitheliomatous hyperplasia expanding into underlying stroma. Note well-formed nests with a defined basement membrane. There is a granular cell tumor in the stroma ⇒.* ***(Right)*** *At high power, a loss of the surface epithelium with associated fibrinoid material is shown. The glandular epithelium is lost, but the architecture is maintained. The minor mucoserous glands show metaplastic squamous epithelium ⇨.*

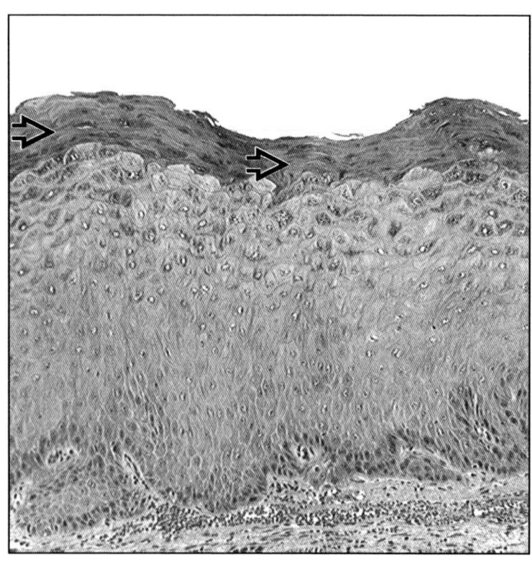

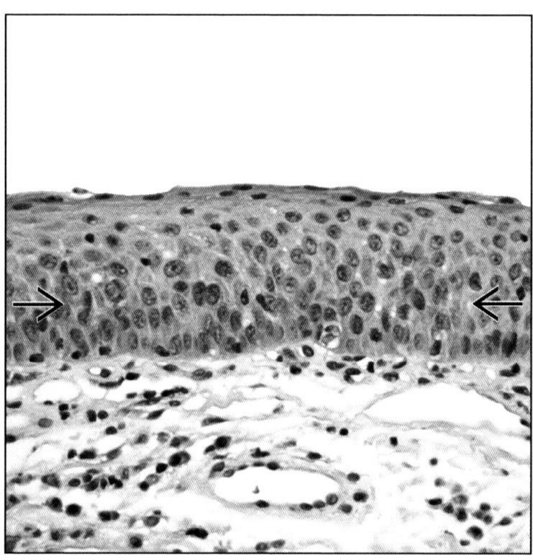

(Left) *The squamous epithelium is thickened, showing a prominent granular cell layer and keratosis ⇨. There is associated parakeratosis in this case too.* ***(Right)*** *The basal zone of the epithelium is thickened in this example of basal cell hyperplasia ⇒. Basal hyperplasia is quite frequently identified at the transition from 1 epithelium to another and should not be confused for dysplasia. There is a lack of atypia.*

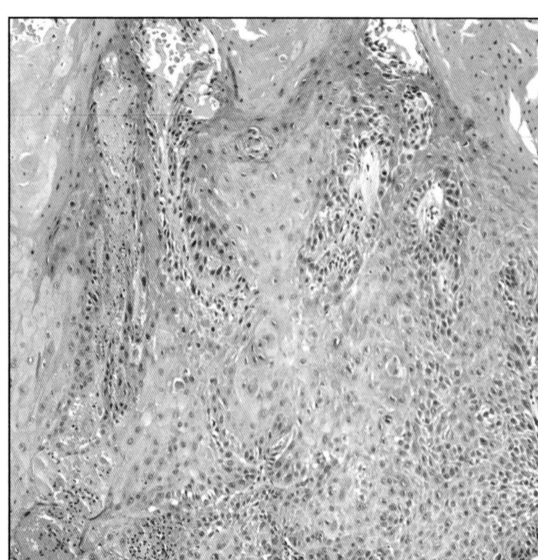

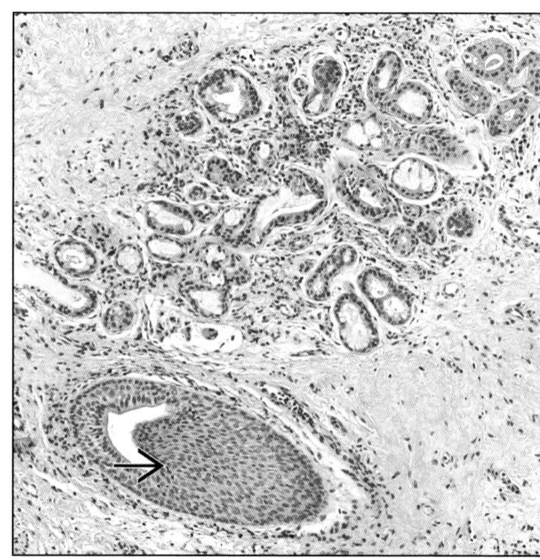

(Left) *Verrucous hyperplasia is difficult to diagnose accurately. There is abundant keratin, projections of epithelium, and a lack of cytologic atypia. However, verrucous squamous cell carcinoma can have these same features, especially if the biopsy is superficial.* ***(Right)*** *Radiation-induced changes of minor salivary glands in the stroma of a larynx biopsy show acinar atrophy, increased intercalated ducts, and squamous metaplasia of the duct ⇒. Note the background fibrosis.*

Microscopic Features

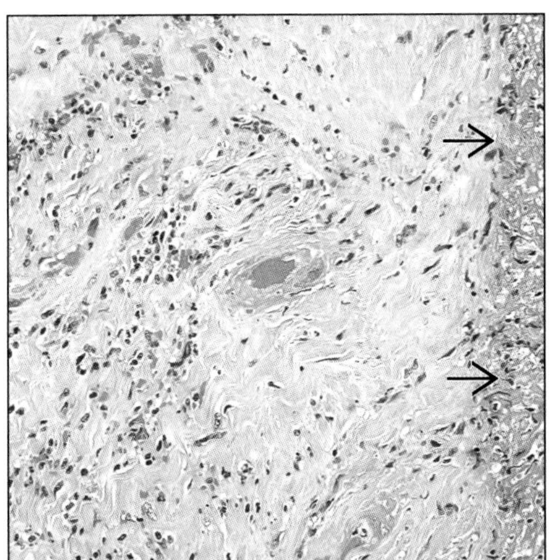

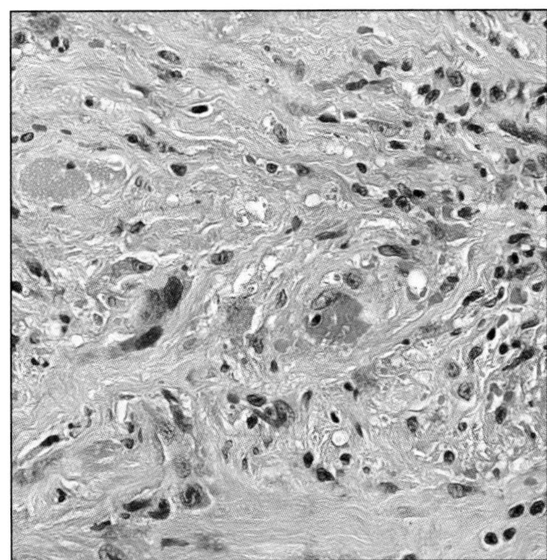

(Left) *Hematoxylin & eosin shows radiation-induced changes of laryngeal mucosa with surface necrosis ⇨, increased fibrosis, and mixed cell type inflammatory infiltration.* ***(Right)*** *Hematoxylin & eosin shows radiation-induced changes as fibrosis, mixed cell type inflammatory reaction, and pleomorphic-appearing fibroblasts with hyperchromatic atypical nuclei. However, the nuclear to cytoplasmic ratio is maintained.*

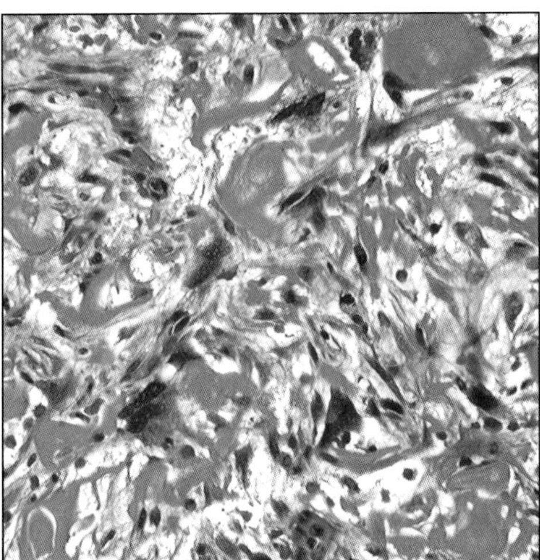

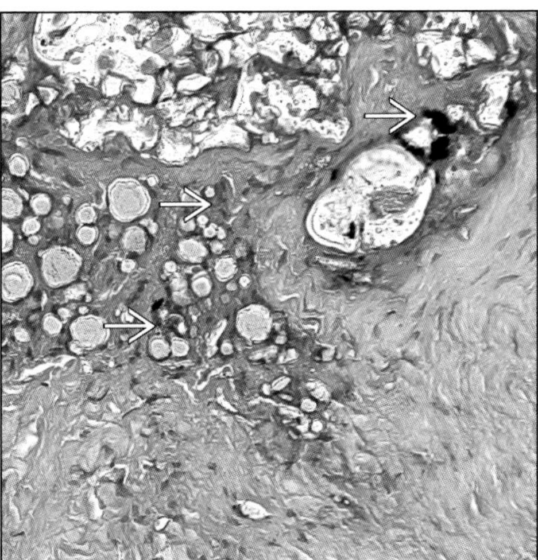

(Left) *There are remarkably atypical fibroblastic cells present in the stroma of this larynx biopsy taken from a patient previously managed with radiation. Note the intense fibrosis. There is a "stellate" appearance to the fibroblasts. Mitotic figures are usually absent.* ***(Right)*** *Hematoxylin & eosin shows Teflon particles surrounded by multinucleated giant cells ➡. Teflon particles of oval and rounded shape have clear centers and darker borders. Teflon is used infrequently today.*

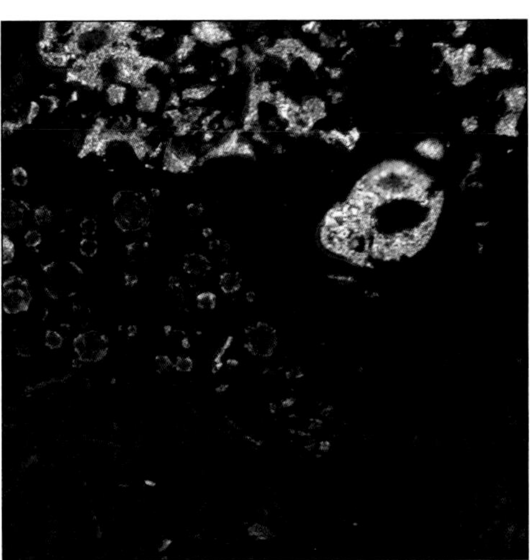

(Left) *The Teflon particles appear quite prominent and polarizable under polarized light. Talc may polarize but would appear differently on H&E stained material. The crystals of gout are sheaf-like, and are not arranged in this fashion.* ***(Right)*** *The smaller particles of Teflon are frequently not identified on H&E stained material, but are embedded within background fibrosis, only highlighted when performing an evaluation with polarized light.*

CONTACT ULCER

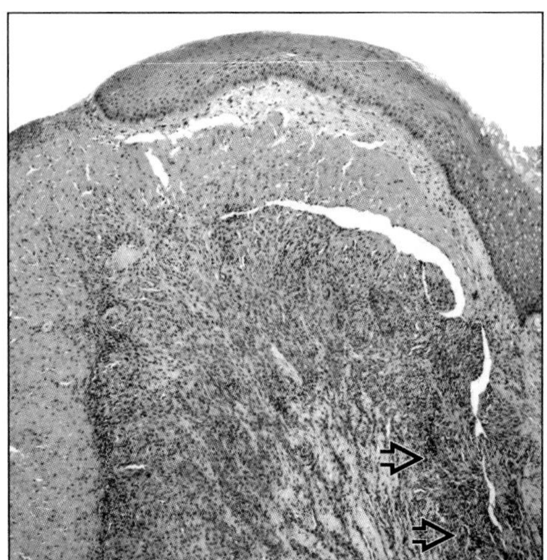

Hematoxylin & eosin shows fibrinoid necrosis, ulceration, and perpendicular vessels with granulation tissue and hemosiderin-laden macrophages ➾.

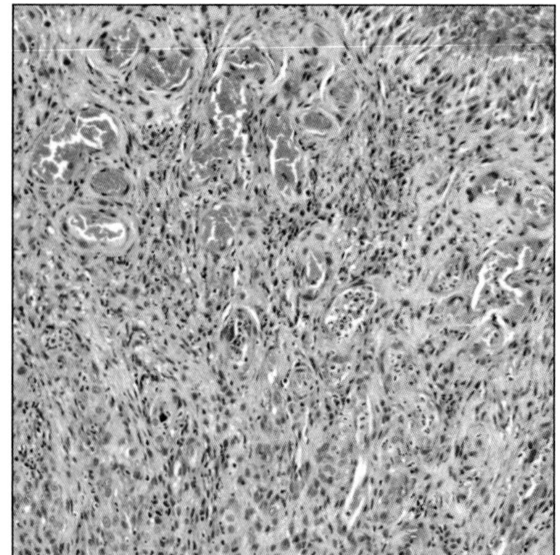

Hematoxylin & eosin shows granulation-type tissue with plump endothelial cells and mixed inflammation.

TERMINOLOGY

Synonyms

- Pyogenic granuloma
- Vocal process granuloma
- Intubation granuloma
- Peptic granuloma

Definitions

- Benign reactive epithelial response to injury

ETIOLOGY/PATHOGENESIS

Environmental Exposure

- Gastroesophageal reflux disease (GERD)
- Intubation complication, especially when incorrect endotracheal (ET) tube is used emergently
  - More common in females than males
- Vocal abuse

CLINICAL ISSUES

Epidemiology

- Incidence
  - Frequent
  - Increased incidence in GERD
- Age
  - Usually adults
- Gender
  - Male > Female (except post-intubation)

Site

- Posterior larynx (true vocal cord, posterior commissure)

Presentation

- Hoarseness, cough, sore throat, vocal abuse/misuse, chronic throat clearing
- Heartburn as part of gastroesophageal reflux disease (gastrolaryngeal reflux)

Treatment

- Options, risks, complications
  - Remove inciting factor
    - Aggressive acid-suppressive therapy to control gastroesophageal reflux disease
    - Discontinue habitual coughing or throat clearing, shouting
    - Vocal rehabilitation (especially in singers)
- Surgical approaches
  - Excision

Prognosis

- Excellent

MACROSCOPIC FEATURES

General Features

- Bilateral, polypoid masses affecting posterior larynx
  - Results in "kissing ulcer" on contralateral cord

Size

- Up to 3 cm

MICROSCOPIC PATHOLOGY

Histologic Features

- Surface ulceration
- Significant fibrinoid necrosis at surface
- Exuberant granulation tissue
- Vessels in granulation tissue are often perpendicular to surface
- Endothelial cells are plump and reactive but not atypical
- Rich investment with lymphocytes, plasma cells, neutrophils, and histiocytes
- Hemosiderin-laden macrophages (especially at base)

CONTACT ULCER

Key Facts

Terminology
- Benign reactive epithelial response to injury

Etiology/Pathogenesis
- Gastroesophageal reflux disease (GERD)

Clinical Issues
- Posterior larynx
- Bilateral, polypoid, beefy red masses
- Remove inciting factor

Macroscopic Features
- Bilateral, polypoid masses, resulting in "kissing ulcer" on contralateral cord

Microscopic Pathology
- Surface ulceration with fibrinoid necrosis
  - Necrosis present immediately below surface when healing (clue to diagnosis)
- Surface regeneration or re-epithelialization with time

  - Increased in frequency with prolonged clinical history
- Surface bacterial overgrowth can be seen
- Surface regeneration or re-epithelialization with time
  - Fibrinoid necrosis is still present immediately below surface (clue to diagnosis)
  - Epithelial hyperplasia with reactive atypia
  - Prominent fibrosis in stroma with time

DIFFERENTIAL DIAGNOSIS

Vascular Tumors
- Very rare in larynx
- Kaposi sarcoma and angiosarcoma rare
  - Show significant pleomorphism, freely anastomosing vessels, atypical mitotic figures, and hyaline, eosinophilic globules (in Kaposi)

Inflammatory Conditions
- Wegener granulomatosis: Geographic, biocollagenolytic, blue granular necrosis, vasculitis, and rare granulomas
- Special stains can be used to exclude infectious agent

Spindle Cell "Sarcomatoid" Squamous Cell Carcinoma
- Atypical spindle cell population with increased mitotic figures, including atypical forms

SELECTED REFERENCES

1. Qadeer MA et al: Correlation between symptoms and laryngeal signs in laryngopharyngeal reflux. Laryngoscope. 115(11):1947-52, 2005
2. Thompson L: Larynx contact ulcer. Ear Nose Throat J. 84(6):340, 2005
3. Thompson LD: Diagnostically challenging lesions in head and neck pathology. Eur Arch Otorhinolaryngol. 254(8):357-66, 1997
4. Toohill RJ et al: Role of refluxed acid in pathogenesis of laryngeal disorders. Am J Med. 103(5A):100S-106S, 1997
5. Shin T et al: Contact granulomas of the larynx. Eur Arch Otorhinolaryngol. 251(2):67-71, 1994
6. Benjamin B et al: Vocal granuloma, including sclerosis of the arytenoid cartilage: radiographic findings. Ann Otol Rhinol Laryngol. 102(10):756-60, 1993
7. Olson NR: Laryngopharyngeal manifestations of gastroesophageal reflux disease. Otolaryngol Clin North Am. 24(5):1201-13, 1991
8. Wenig BM et al: Contact ulcers of the larynx. A reacquaintance with the pathology of an often underdiagnosed entity. Arch Pathol Lab Med. 114(8):825-8, 1990
9. Miko TL: Peptic (contact ulcer) granuloma of the larynx. J Clin Pathol. 42(8):800-4, 1989
10. Ward PH et al: Contact ulcers and granulomas of the larynx: new insights into their etiology as a basis for more rational treatment. Otolaryngol Head Neck Surg. 88(3):262-9, 1980

IMAGE GALLERY

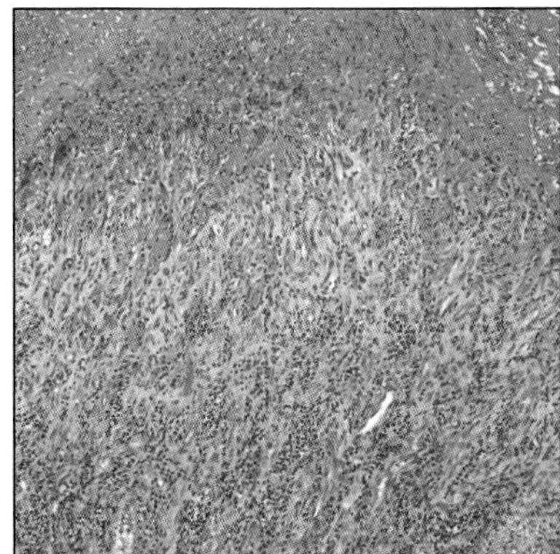

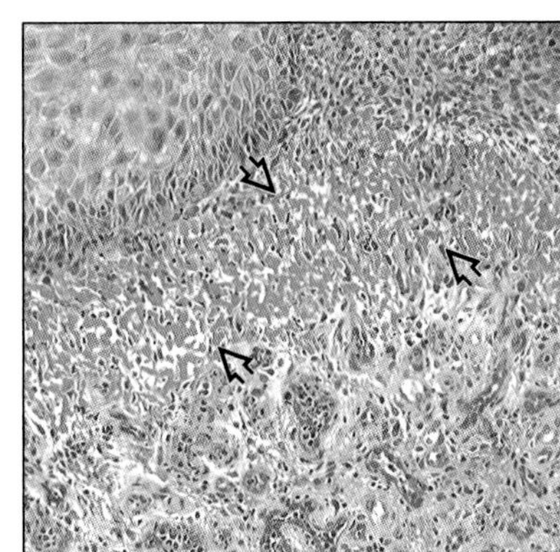

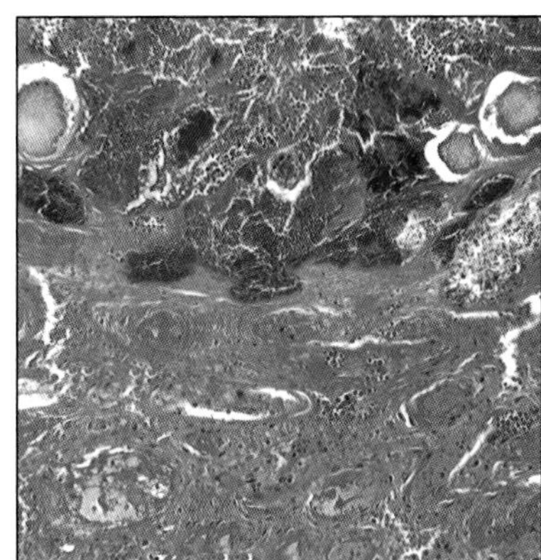

(Left) Hematoxylin & eosin shows surface ulceration and replacement with fibrinoid necrosis. Note the perpendicular arrangement of the vessels to the surface. Inflammation is easily identified throughout. *(Center)* Hematoxylin & eosin shows surface re-epithelialization over the granulation tissue but still with fibrinoid necrosis between the layers ⮚. *(Right)* Hematoxylin & eosin shows fibrinoid exudate with mixed inflammation and numerous bacterial colonies on the surface.

SQUAMOUS PAPILLOMA

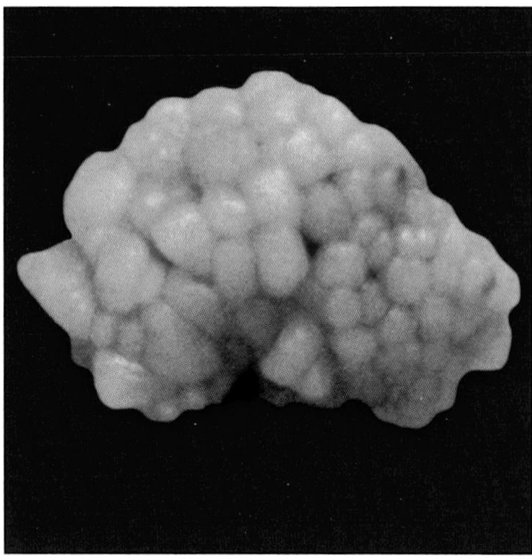

A gross photograph shows a sessile growth with finely lobulated surface. This pattern matches the histologic features of multiple bulbous projections of epithelium. There is no ulceration.

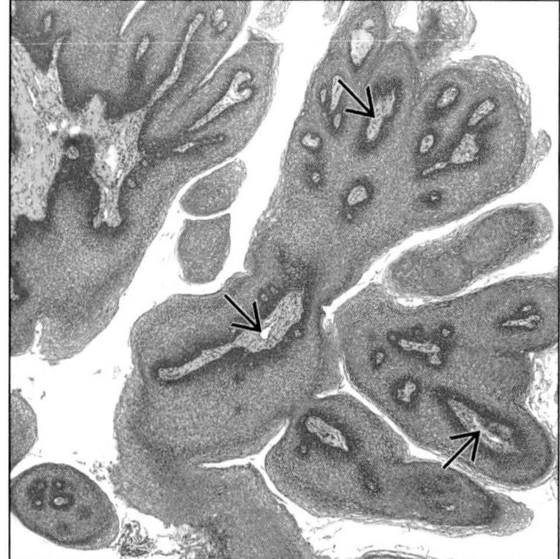

A laryngeal biopsy of an exophytic gross lesion demonstrates multiple, papillary branching projections of squamous epithelium surrounding delicate fibrovascular stromal cores ⇒. There is no atypia.

TERMINOLOGY

Abbreviations

- Squamous papilloma (SP)

Synonyms

- Recurrent respiratory papillomatosis
- Laryngeal papillomatosis
- Juvenile-onset papillomatosis
- Adult-onset papillomatosis
- Aggressive papillomatosis

Definitions

- Benign epithelial tumor arranged in exophytic fashion of branching fronds, showing fibrovascular tissue covered by squamous epithelium, causally related to human papillomavirus (HPV) infection

ETIOLOGY/PATHOGENESIS

Infectious Agents

- HPV infection
  - Genotypes 6 or 11
  - Rarely genotypes 16, 18, 31, 33, 35, 39
- Different modes of infection based on age at presentation
  - Children
    - Perinatal transmission from infected mother to child
  - Adults
    - Sexual transmission, reactivation of perinatally acquired infection

Pathogenesis

- HPV in basal cells of squamous epithelium through microtraumatized spots
- Viral replication in spinous layer associated with disturbance of epithelial maturation
- Separated into juvenile and adult groups with unified biological entity, but with differences in clinical course

CLINICAL ISSUES

Epidemiology

- Incidence
  - 0.4-4.3 per million persons annually
- Age
  - 1st peak: Before 5 years
  - 2nd peak: 20-40 years
- Gender
  - Children
    - Equal gender distribution
  - Adults
    - Male > Female (3:2)

Site

- True and false vocal cords, subglottis and ventricles most often
  - Not uncommon to have multiple squamous papillomas in endolarynx
- Rarely extralaryngeal spread to trachea, bronchi, hypopharynx &/or oropharynx

Presentation

- Presentation is different based on age at initial presentation
- Children
  - Dysphonia
  - Hoarseness
  - Stridor
  - Less frequently, chronic cough and life-threatening events
  - Tend to have more aggressive course
    - Multiple papillomas
    - More frequent recurrences
    - Extralaryngeal spread in 30%
- Adults
  - Dysphonia
  - Hoarseness
  - Tend to have less aggressive course
    - May have multiple squamous papillomas

SQUAMOUS PAPILLOMA

Key Facts

Etiology/Pathogenesis
- Multiple benign papillary tumors related to HPV infection

Clinical Issues
- Endolarynx, rarely spread to trachea, bronchi, hypopharynx, and oropharynx
- Presentation varies based on age
  - Children: Usually before 5 years
  - Adults: Usually between 20 to 40 years
  - Male > Female (3:2) in adults
- Treated with multiple surgeries
  - CO_2 laser can be used
- Can be treated with antiviral drugs

Macroscopic Features
- Usually involves true and false vocal cords
- Subglottis and ventricles involved less frequently

Microscopic Pathology
- Papillary branching projections of squamous epithelium overlying fibrovascular stroma
- Basal-parabasal cell hyperplasia
- Koilocytes in upper part of epithelium
- Atypical epithelium rarely appeared

Ancillary Tests
- HPV detection: Immunohistochemistry, ISH, PCR

Top Differential Diagnoses
- Adult solitary keratinizing squamous papilloma
- Verrucous carcinoma
- Papillary squamous cell carcinoma

    - Recurrences are less common
    - Extralaryngeal spread in 16%

Endoscopic Findings
- Papillary to exophytic lesion(s)
- One or more tumors may be identified

Treatment
- Surgical approaches
  - Surgical excision
  - Endolaryngeal procedure by CO_2 laser
- Adjuvant therapy
  - Antiviral drugs
    - Cidofovir

Prognosis
- Unpredictable biologic behavior
- Presence of HPV in apparently normal mucosa acts as virus reservoir and cause of recurrence
- Neonatal squamous papilloma
  - Negative prognostic factor
  - Associated with greater need for tracheostomy
  - Increased likelihood of mortality
  - High proliferation index and aneuploidy may correlate with increased risk of recurrence
- HPV genotypes 11 and 16
  - Associated with more aggressive clinical coarse
  - Increased frequency of recurrences
- Malignant transformation
  - Tends to develop in patients with history of heavy smoking
  - Identified in 14% of patients with history of previous irradiation
  - Identified in 2% of patients who have not been irradiated
  - Pediatrics: Malignancies develop preferentially in tracheobronchial locations
  - Adults: Malignancies develop preferentially in larynx
- Overall mortality rate 4-14%
  - Death causally related to
    - Asphyxia
    - Pulmonary involvement
    - Carcinomatous transformation

MACROSCOPIC FEATURES

General Features
- Frequently multiple lesions
- Pedunculated or sessile
- Exophytic branching
- Frequently in clusters
- Pink to reddish
- Lobular surface

Size
- Wide range
- Generally < 1 cm in greatest dimension

MICROSCOPIC PATHOLOGY

Histologic Features
- Finger-like projections
- Thin fibrovascular cores
- Core lined or covered by squamous epithelium
- Basal and parabasal hyperplasia
  - Usually to mid-portion of squamous epithelium
  - Mitotic activity in this basal/parabasal zone may be increased
- Clusters of koilocytes in upper part of epithelium
  - Crenated, hyperchromatic nucleus
  - Perinuclear halo or clearing
  - Prominent intercellular borders
- Cellular and nuclear atypia is uncommon
- Architectural disturbance of epithelium is very rare
- Increased mitoses throughout whole epithelium is rare

ANCILLARY TESTS

Immunohistochemistry
- HPV-positive staining
  - p16 can be used as surrogate marker
  - Will not give specific serotype if p16 is used

- High Ki-67 proliferative index is associated with increased risk of disease recurrence in pediatric patients

Flow Cytometry

- Detection of DNA aneuploidy seems to predict increased risk of disease recurrence in pediatric patients

In Situ Hybridization

- Nuclear HPV signals in koilocytes

PCR

- Most sensitive method for HPV detection, including different HPV genotypes
- Not used frequently in daily practice (research setting)

DIFFERENTIAL DIAGNOSIS

Solitary Keratinizing Squamous Papilloma

- Develops in adults
- Prominent surface keratinization
- Keratohyaline granules present
- Lack of koilocytes
- Frequently atypical hyperplastic epithelium

Verrucous Carcinoma

- Larger macroscopic lesion
- Prominent superficial keratin layer (hyperkeratosis)
  - Church-spire type hyperkeratosis
- Broad, pushing border of infiltration at epithelial-stromal junction
- Parakeratotic crypting
- Usually a nonmitotically active lesion
  - Mitoses may be seen in basal/parabasal zone
- Shows maturation toward surface
- Lack of koilocytes

Papillary Squamous Cell Carcinoma

- Broad-based to delicate fronds of fibrovascular stroma covered with atypical epithelium
- Very cellular tumor
- Lack of maturation toward surface
- Remarkable cellular pleomorphism
- Increased mitotic figures, identified throughout epithelium
- Atypical mitotic figures
- Invasion into stroma may or may not be present

Verruca Vulgaris

- Very uncommon in larynx
- Lack of branching of fibrovascular cores
- Prominent surface keratinization
- Prominent keratohyaline granules

REPORTING CONSIDERATIONS

Key Elements to Report

- When premalignant changes (dysplasia) are present, they should be documented

SELECTED REFERENCES

1. Broekema FI et al: Side-effects of cidofovir in the treatment of recurrent respiratory papillomatosis. Eur Arch Otorhinolaryngol. 265(8):871-9, 2008
2. Derkay CS et al: Recurrent respiratory papillomatosis: a review. Laryngoscope. 118(7):1236-47, 2008
3. Stamataki S et al: Juvenile recurrent respiratory papillomatosis: still a mystery disease with difficult management. Head Neck. 29(2):155-62, 2007
4. Gerein V et al: Incidence, age at onset, and potential reasons of malignant transformation in recurrent respiratory papillomatosis patients: 20 years experience. Otolaryngol Head Neck Surg. 132(3):392-4, 2005
5. Shehab N et al: Cidofovir for the treatment of recurrent respiratory papillomatosis: a review of the literature. Pharmacotherapy. 25(7):977-89, 2005
6. Wiatrak BJ: Overview of recurrent respiratory papillomatosis. Curr Opin Otolaryngol Head Neck Surg. 11(6):433-41, 2003
7. Aaltonen LM et al: Human papillomavirus in larynx. Laryngoscope. 112(4):700-7, 2002
8. Derkay CS: Recurrent respiratory papillomatosis. Laryngoscope. 111(1):57-69, 2001
9. Bauman NM et al: Recurrent respiratory papillomatosis. Pediatr Clin North Am. 43(6):1385-401, 1996
10. Mahnke CG et al: Recurrent laryngeal papillomatosis. Retrospective analysis of 95 patients and review of the literature. Otolaryngol Pol. 50(6):567-78, 1996
11. Gale N et al: Laryngeal papillomatosis: molecular, histopathological, and clinical evaluation. Virchows Arch. 425(3):291-5, 1994
12. Gaylis B et al: Recurrent respiratory papillomatosis: progression to invasion and malignancy. Am J Otolaryngol. 12(2):104-12, 1991

SQUAMOUS PAPILLOMA

Microscopic Features with Differential Considerations

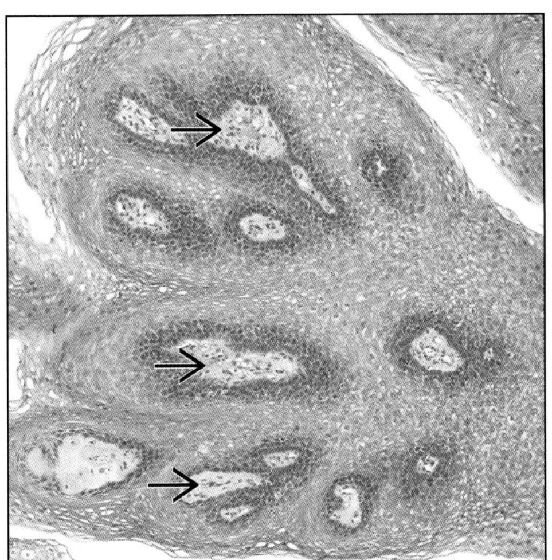

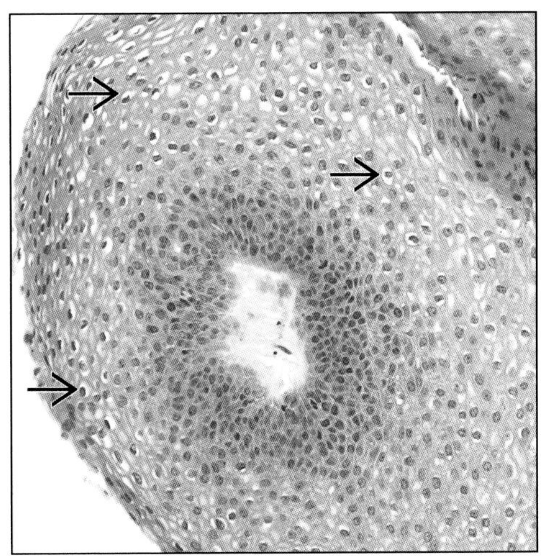

(Left) *Hematoxylin & eosin shows branching of papillary projections consisting of mainly hyperplastic squamous epithelium and thin fronds of fibrovascular tissue* ⇒*. The epithelium shows maturation toward the surface, where koilocytic atypia can be seen.* ***(Right)*** *The papillary frond is sectioned tangentially (perpendicular to the fibrovascular core). There are many koilocytes* ⇒ *identified at the surface, the most common location to document their presence.*

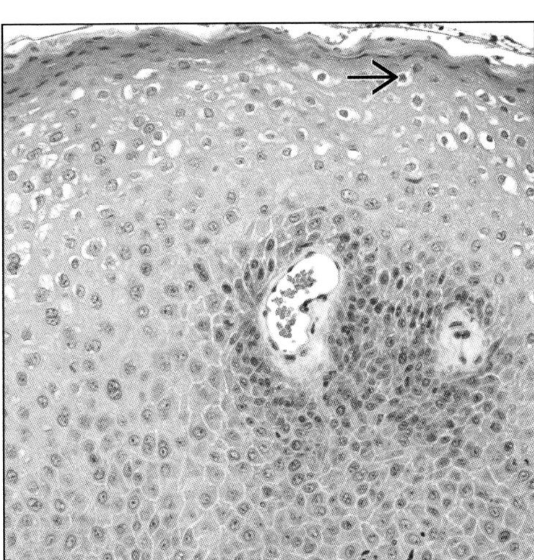

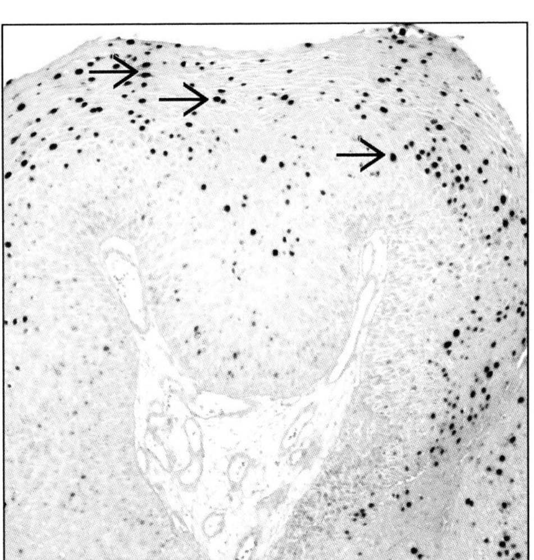

(Left) *The squamous epithelium of the papillary projection displays numerous koilocytes on the surface* ⇒ *of the epithelial projection. There is also slight parakeratosis on the surface. This degree of cytologic atypia is well within the spectrum of squamous papilloma.* ***(Right)*** *In situ hybridization for HPV genotypes 6 and 11 shows multiple positive signals* ⇒ *in the upper part of the squamous epithelium. In general, ISH is not required to confirm the diagnosis.*

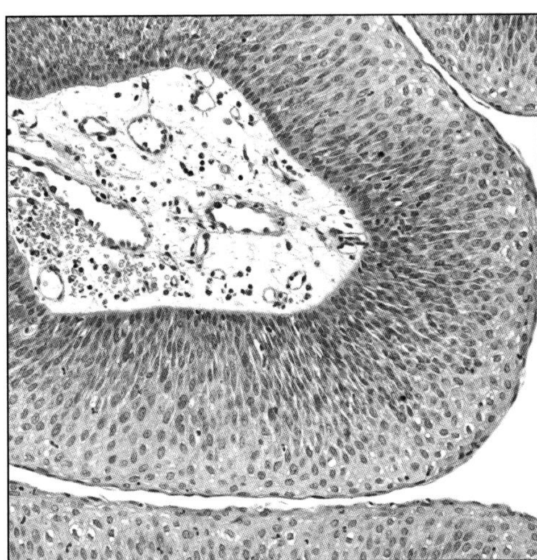

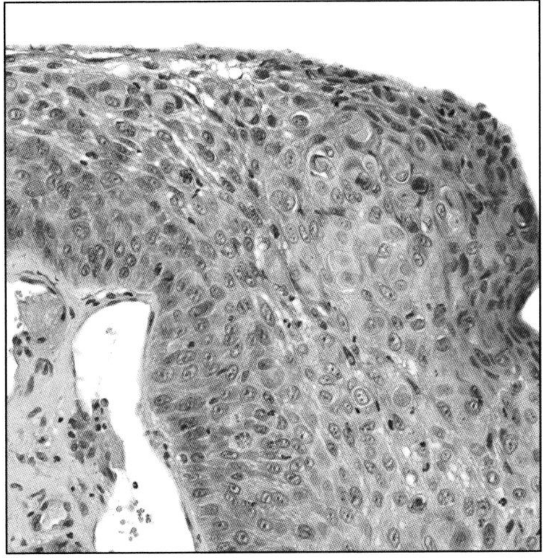

(Left) *This squamous papilloma shows an increased amount of cytologic atypia, in which there is mild dysplasia (basal-parabasal cell hyperplasia). The reproducibility of this degree of cytologic atypia is limited, with high intra- and interobserver variability. This lesion shows maturation toward the surface.* ***(Right)*** *Epithelial abnormalities are identified throughout the epithelial thickness, a finding of severe dysplasia. There is limited surface maturation. Mitoses are increased.*

GRANULAR CELL TUMOR

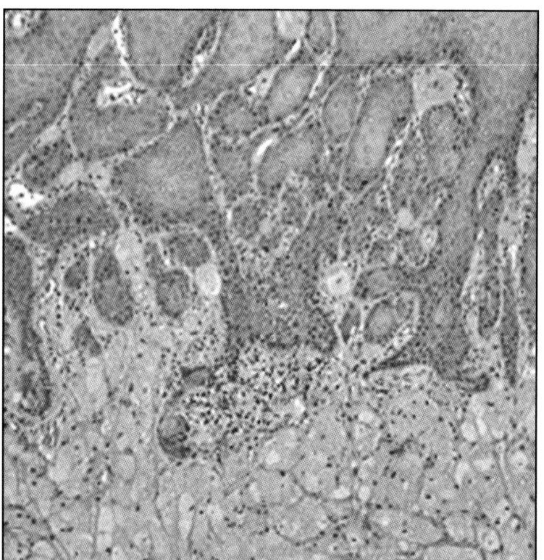

Hematoxylin & eosin shows pseudoepitheliomatous hyperplasia, which overlies a granular cell tumor. It is usually limited to the tumor proliferation but simulates invasive squamous cell carcinoma.

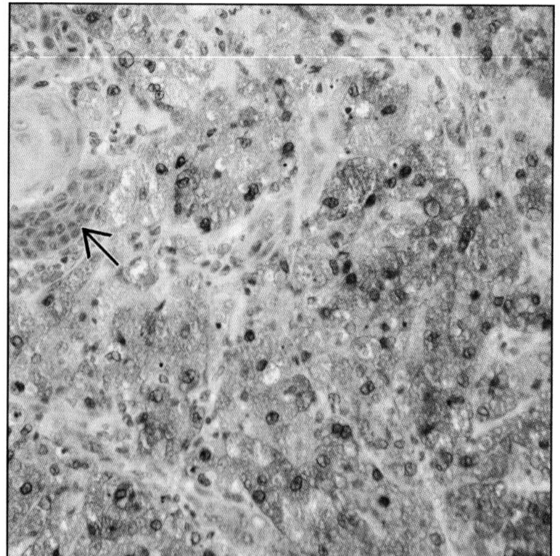

The neoplastic cells of a granular cell tumor show strong and diffuse nuclear and cytoplasmic reactivity for S100 protein. The surface epithelium ⇨ is negative.

TERMINOLOGY

Abbreviations

- Granular cell tumor (GCT)

Synonyms

- Myoblastoma
- Granular cell myoblastoma
- Schwann cell tumor
- Laryngeal xanthoma
- Abrikossoff tumor

Definitions

- Benign tumor of Schwann cell origin, composed of polygonal to spindle cells with abundant granular cytoplasm due to increased number of lysosomes

CLINICAL ISSUES

Epidemiology

- Incidence
  - Frequent tumor, larynx is involved in about 10% of cases
    - Most frequent sites are skin, tongue, breast, & larynx
- Age
  - Broad age range: 4-70 years
  - Mean: 34 years
    - Uncommon in children
- Gender
  - Female > Male (2:1)

Site

- Posterior 1/3 of true vocal cord is most common location
  - Anywhere in larynx

Presentation

- Hoarseness
- Airway obstruction

Treatment

- Surgical approaches
  - Complete but conservative surgery

Prognosis

- Excellent prognosis with low recurrence rate
  - Recurrences in up to 10%

MACROSCOPIC FEATURES

General Features

- Firm, polypoid or sessile tumor
- Rarely cystic
- Usually covered by intact mucosa
- Grayish-yellow cut surface
- Multiple GCTs may develop

Size

- Usually < 2 cm

MICROSCOPIC PATHOLOGY

Histologic Features

- Poorly circumscribed tumor
- Syncytial pattern is often present
- Composed of large, rounded, polygonal or elongated cells with ill-defined borders
  - Syncytium is common
- Small hyperchromatic to vesicular nuclei, centrally located
- Cytoplasm is eosinophilic, abundant, coarsely granular
- Pseudoepitheliomatous hyperplasia of surface epithelium
  - Usually limited to extent of granular cell tumor
  - Mimics invasive squamous cell carcinoma
- Abundant desmoplasia, especially in old GCT
- Perineural growth
  - Not significant, since nerves are entrapped within proliferation

GRANULAR CELL TUMOR

Key Facts

Terminology
- Benign tumor of Schwann cell origin

Clinical Issues
- Young patients, predominantly female (F:M = 2:1)
- Most frequent sites include skin, tongue, and larynx
- Complete excision yields excellent prognosis

Macroscopic Features
- Firm, polypoid tumor, with intact mucosa

Microscopic Pathology
- Pseudoepitheliomatous hyperplasia of surface epithelium
- Ill-defined borders, poorly circumscribed tumor
- Large polygonal cells with granular cytoplasm
- Positive for S100 protein

Top Differential Diagnoses
- Squamous cell carcinoma, adult rhabdomyoma, paraganglioma, malignant granular cell tumor

- Cellular atypia, mitoses, and necrosis uncommon
  - If these features are present, it raises suspicion for malignant GCT

ANCILLARY TESTS

Histochemistry
- PAS-positive, diastase-resistant cytoplasmic granules (not glycogen)

Immunohistochemistry
- Strong and diffuse positivity
  - S100 protein, vimentin, NSE, and MBP
- Negative
  - Cytokeratin and muscle markers

Electron Microscopy
- Transmission
  - Characteristic intracytoplasmic abundance of lysosomes, in various stages of fragmentation

DIFFERENTIAL DIAGNOSIS

Squamous Cell Carcinoma
- Lack of pleomorphism and nuclear atypia of epithelial cells in GCT
- Lack of increased mitotic activity in overlying epithelium of GCT

Adult Rhabdomyoma
- Well-delineated cell borders
- Large, granular, vacuolated cells with abundance of glycogen and cross striation
- Immunohistochemical positivity for skeletal muscle markers

Paraganglioma
- Organoid pattern (zellballen)
- Chief cells positive for neuroendocrine markers (chromogranin and synaptophysin)

Malignant Variant of GCT
- Cellular and nuclear atypia, necrosis, increased mitoses

SELECTED REFERENCES

1. Thompson LD: Laryngeal granular cell tumor. Ear Nose Throat J. 88(3):824-5, 2009
2. Arevalo C et al: Laryngeal granular cell tumor. J Voice. 22(3):339-42, 2008
3. Scala WA et al: Granular cell tumor of the larynx in children: a case report. Braz J Otorhinolaryngol. 74(5):780-5, 2008
4. Lassaletta L et al: Immunoreactivity in granular cell tumours of the larynx. Auris Nasus Larynx. 26(3):305-10, 1999
5. Kamal SA et al: Granular cell tumour of the larynx. J Laryngol Otol. 112(1):83-5, 1998
6. Brandwein M et al: Atypical granular cell tumor of the larynx: an unusually aggressive tumor clinically and microscopically. Head Neck. 12(2):154-9, 1990
7. Compagno J et al: Benign granular cell tumors of the larynx: a review of 36 cases with clinicopathologic data. Ann Otol Rhinol Laryngol. 84(3 Pt 1):308-14, 1975

IMAGE GALLERY

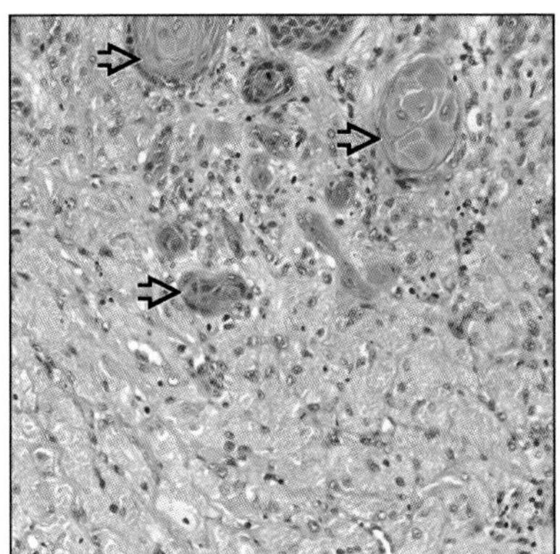

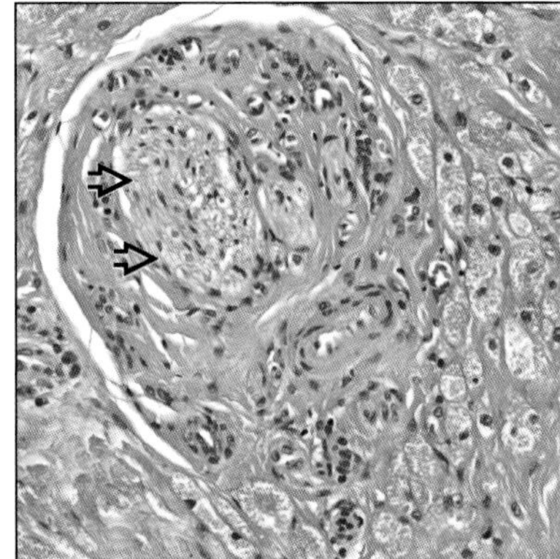

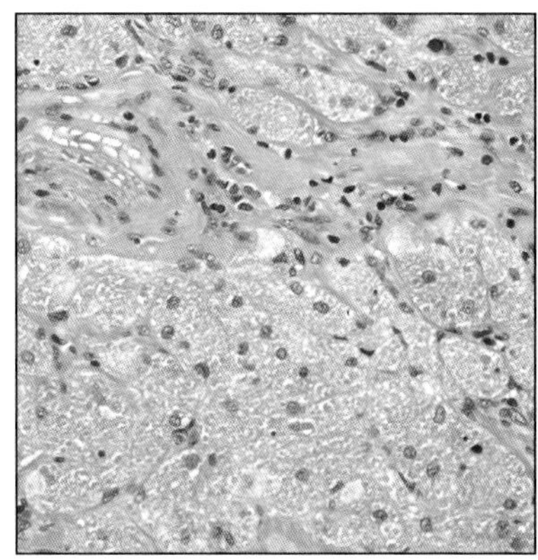

*(**Left**) The overlying surface pseudoepitheliomatous hyperplasia ➾ is seen to blend imperceptibly with the granular cell proliferation. This is a characteristic finding. (**Center**) There is desmoplasia and perineural growth of granular cells. A peripheral nerve ➾ is entrapped within the neoplastic proliferation. (**Right**) The neoplastic cells are arranged in a characteristic syncytial appearance. Note the pale granular cytoplasm surrounding vesicular nuclei.*

AMYLOID (AMYLOIDOMA)

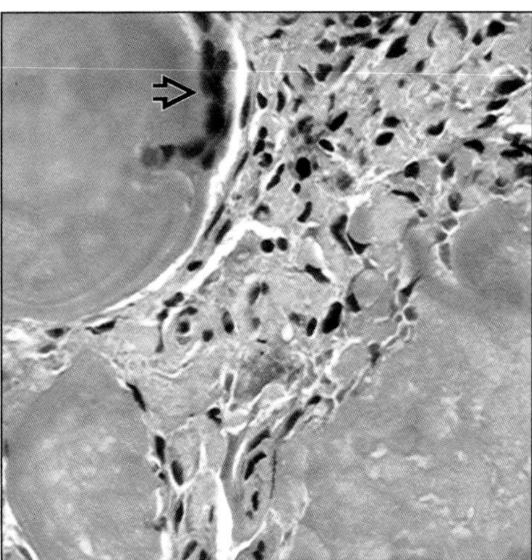

H&E shows acellular, eosinophilic, extracellular matrix material with giant cells ➡. There are a few inflammatory cells in the interstitium. This is quite characteristic of amyloid deposition.

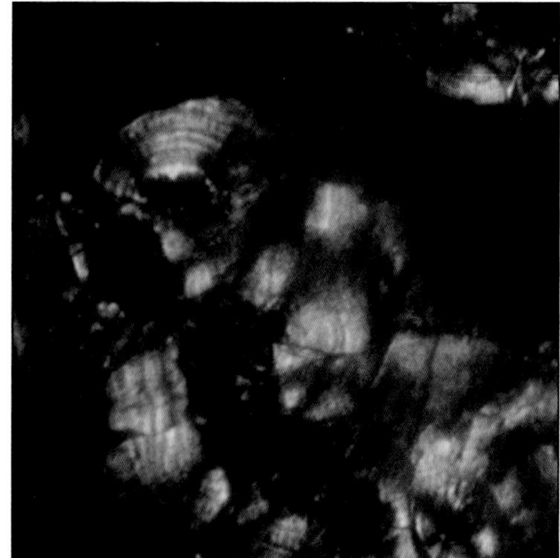

Positive Congo red stain shows "apple-green" birefringence of amyloid when viewed under polarized light. Note the "rings," which can be highlighted by this technique.

TERMINOLOGY

Synonyms

- Amyloidoma

Definitions

- Benign accumulation of extracellular, acellular, eosinophilic, insoluble protein

ETIOLOGY/PATHOGENESIS

Tumor Associated

- Part of mucosa-associated lymphoid tissue (MALT) or neuroendocrine tumor product

CLINICAL ISSUES

Epidemiology

- Incidence
  - < 1% of all laryngeal neoplasms
- Age
  - Most common in adults
- Gender
  - Equal gender distribution

Site

- False vocal cord most commonly affected
- Multifocal disease elsewhere in upper aerodigestive tract in up to 15% of patients

Presentation

- Hoarseness
- Voice changes

Laboratory Tests

- Quantitative immunoglobulin assay
- Serologic rheumatoid factor tests
- Serum &/or urine electrophoresis to exclude monoclonal gammopathy (Bence-Jones proteins)

Treatment

- Surgical approaches
  - Excision

Prognosis

- Good, but depends on localized vs. systemic and primary vs. secondary disease
- Multiple myeloma may have deposits in larynx as part of systemic disease

MACROSCOPIC FEATURES

General Features

- Cut surface shows starch-like, waxy, translucent material below surface

Size

- Up to 4 cm, though usually less

MICROSCOPIC PATHOLOGY

Histologic Features

- Subepithelial, extracellular, acellular, eosinophilic, homogeneous deposits
- Peritheliomatous and periglandular predilection
- Foreign body giant cell reaction
- Lymphoplasmacytic infiltrate
  - May be monoclonal if part of MALT origin

ANCILLARY TESTS

Histochemistry

- Congo red: Apple-green birefringence with polarized light
- Crystal violet: Metachromatic reaction

AMYLOID (AMYLOIDOMA)

Key Facts

Clinical Issues
- Outcome dependent on localized vs. systemic, and primary vs. secondary disease
- Multifocal disease in upper aerodigestive tract in up to 15% of patients

Macroscopic Features
- Starch-like, waxy, translucent material below surface
- False vocal cord is most commonly affected

Microscopic Pathology
- Extracellular, eosinophilic, homogeneous deposits
- Peritheliomatous and periglandular predilection

Ancillary Tests
- Occasional light chain restriction in plasma cells
- Congo red: Apple-green with polarized light

Top Differential Diagnoses
- MALT, vocal cord polyp, neuroendocrine carcinoma

Immunohistochemistry
- Plasma cell light chain restriction (κ or λ) in some cases
- Amyloid P positive
- Mixed population of CD3 and CD20 positive cells in reactive lymphoid tissue

Electron Microscopy
- Interlacing meshwork of nonbranching fibrils
- β-pleated sheets

DIFFERENTIAL DIAGNOSIS

Mucosa-associated Lymphoid Tissue
- Extranodal marginal zone B-cell lymphoma can be associated with amyloid
- Light chain restriction

Vocal Cord Polyp
- Hyalinized polyps do not have inflammatory infiltrate or matrix deposition

Ligneous Conjunctivitis
- May be systemic disorder, but negative amyloid stains

Lipoid Proteinosis
- Negative amyloid stains

Tumor Associated
- Larynx neuroendocrine tumors
  - May produce amyloid, but without serum calcitonin elevation
- Medullary thyroid carcinoma
  - Direct invasion from thyroid gland with elevated serum calcitonin levels

SELECTED REFERENCES

1. Penner CR et al: Head and neck amyloidosis: a clinicopathologic study of 15 cases. Oral Oncol. 42(4):421-9, 2006
2. Bartels H et al: Laryngeal amyloidosis: localized versus systemic disease and update on diagnosis and therapy. Ann Otol Rhinol Laryngol. 113(9):741-8, 2004
3. Piazza C et al: Endoscopic management of laryngo-tracheobronchial amyloidosis: a series of 32 patients. Eur Arch Otorhinolaryngol. 260(7):349-54, 2003
4. Thompson LD et al: Amyloidosis of the larynx: a clinicopathologic study of 11 cases. Mod Pathol. 13(5):528-35, 2000
5. Lewis JE et al: Laryngeal amyloidosis: a clinicopathologic and immunohistochemical review. Otolaryngol Head Neck Surg. 106(4):372-7, 1992
6. Hellquist H et al: Amyloidosis of the larynx. Acta Otolaryngol. 88(5-6):443-50, 1979
7. Michaels L et al: Amyloid in localised deposits and plasmacytomas of the respiratory tract. J Pathol. 128(1):29-38, 1979
8. Barnes EL Jr et al: Laryngeal amyloidosis: clinicopathologic study of seven cases. Ann Otol Rhinol Laryngol. 86(6 Pt 1):856-63, 1977

IMAGE GALLERY

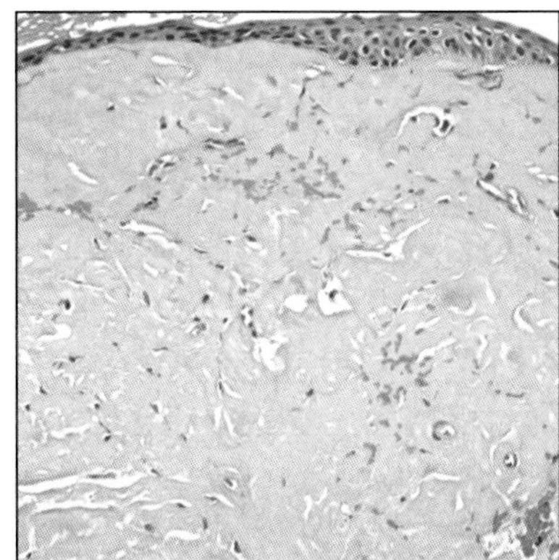

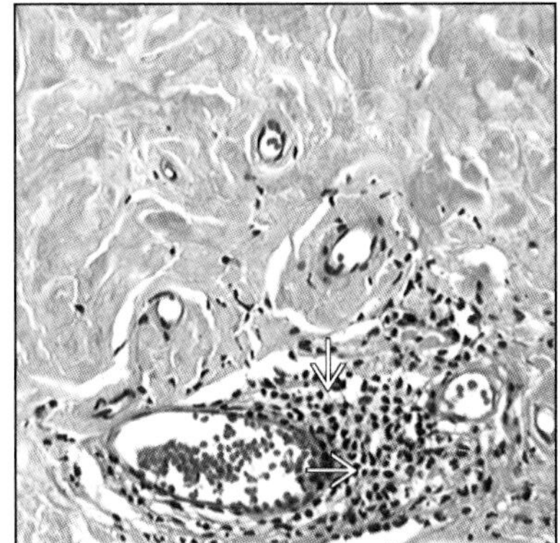

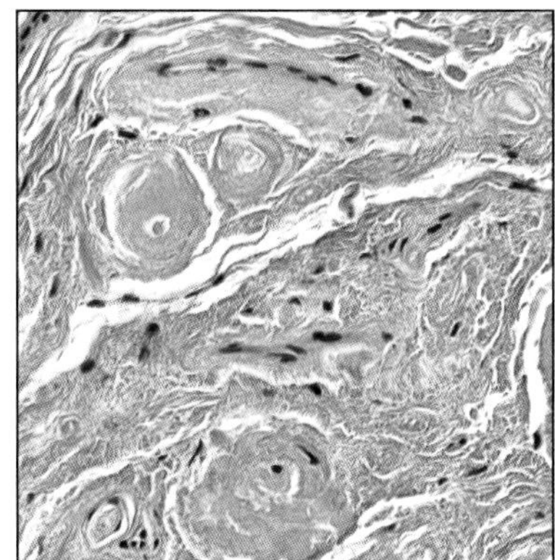

(Left) The surface epithelium is thinned and attenuated. There is a heavy deposition of acellular, eosinophilic, waxy extracellular matrix, destroying the subepithelial connective tissue. (Center) A slight perivascular accentuation of amyloid with a sprinkling of inflammatory cells (predominantly plasma cells and lymphocytes) ➡ is noted in this example of amyloid. (Right) The perivascular proclivity for amyloid deposition is highlighted in this image.

ADULT RHABDOMYOMA

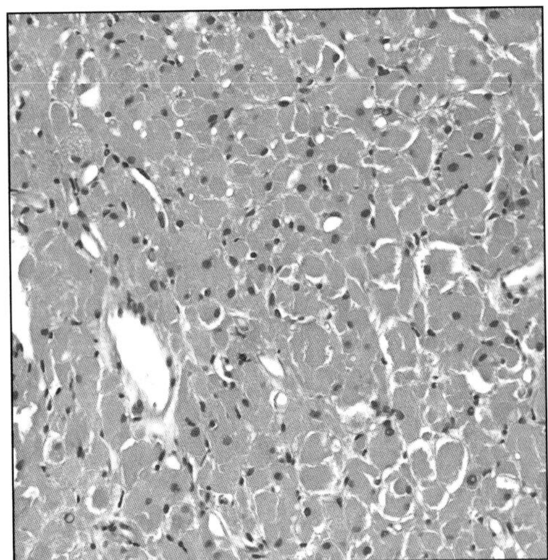

There is a diffuse growth pattern of polygonal cells with abundant eosinophilic cytoplasm and small rounded nuclei. Note the delicate fibrovascular stroma between the neoplastic cells.

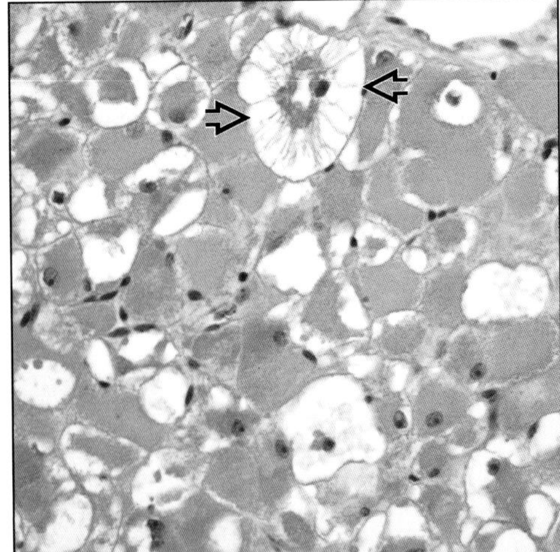

The characteristic polygonal cells have eosinophilic, vacuolated, granular cytoplasm. The small, hyperchromatic nuclei are mainly peripherally located. Note the spiderweb-like cell ⇨.

TERMINOLOGY

Abbreviations

- Adult rhabdomyoma (AR)

Definitions

- Benign tumor of skeletal muscle differentiation
- Tumors separated into cardiac and extracardiac types
  - Extracardiac divided into adult (70% in head & neck), fetal, and genital types

ETIOLOGY/PATHOGENESIS

Pathogenesis

- Arise from unsegmented mesoderm from 3rd and 4th branchial arches (not from myotomes)

CLINICAL ISSUES

Epidemiology

- Incidence
  - Very uncommon tumor
- Age
  - Mean: 6th decade; range: 16-82 years
- Gender
  - Male > > Female (3-4:1)

Site

- Larynx (supraglottic, glottis) and hypopharynx
  - Neck is most common soft tissue site

Presentation

- Dysphagia, dyspnea, hoarseness

Treatment

- Complete surgical excision

Prognosis

- Excellent long-term prognosis
  - Larynx tumors lack local aggressiveness or malignant potential
- Recurrences may develop (up to 40%) if incompletely excised

MACROSCOPIC FEATURES

General Features

- Rounded, lobulated, well-circumscribed, unencapsulated submucosal tumor
- Solitary, but may be multinodular
- Tan to grayish-red brown

Size

- Median: 3 cm; range: 1.5-8 cm

MICROSCOPIC PATHOLOGY

Histologic Features

- Sheets, nests, or lobules
- Closely packed, large polygonal cells separated by delicate fibrovascular stroma
- Abundant eosinophilic, granular &/or vacuolated cytoplasm (due to glycogen)
  - Vacuolation creates spiderweb-like appearance due to radially oriented strands of cytoplasm separating vacuoles
- Small, rounded, centrally or peripherally located nuclei
- Cytoplasmic cross striations
- Crystalline-like cytoplasmic structures called jackstraw inclusions (rod-like)

ANCILLARY TESTS

Histochemistry

- PAS-positive, diastase-resistant glycogen granules
- PTAH highlights cross striations and crystals

ADULT RHABDOMYOMA

Key Facts

Terminology
- Benign extracardiac tumor of skeletal muscle origin

Clinical Issues
- Rare tumors predominating in middle-aged men (Male > > Female [3-4:1])

Macroscopic Features
- Rounded, lobulated, well-circumscribed submucosal tumor

Microscopic Pathology
- Large polygonal cells with abundant eosinophilic, granular, vacuolated cytoplasm
- "Spiderweb" appearance to cytoplasm

Ancillary Tests
- Desmin, actin, and myoglobin

Top Differential Diagnoses
- Granular cell tumor, paraganglioma, oncocytoma

Immunohistochemistry

Antibody	Reactivity	Staining Pattern	Comment
Desmin	Positive	Cytoplasmic	Skeletal muscle cells
Actin-HHF-35	Positive	Cytoplasmic	Skeletal muscle cells
Myoglobin	Positive	Cytoplasmic	Skeletal muscle cells
CK-PAN	Negative		
CD68	Negative		
Actin-sm	Equivocal	Cytoplasmic	Skeletal muscle cells
S100	Equivocal	Nuclear & cytoplasmic	Skeletal muscle cells

Immunohistochemistry
- Positive for skeletal muscle markers

Molecular Genetics
- Reciprocal translocation of chromosome 15 and 17
- Variety of changes in 10q

Electron Microscopy
- Alternating thick and thin myofilaments
- Condensation of rudimentary myofibrils (hypertrophied Z bands)
- Variable amount of glycogen and mitochondria

DIFFERENTIAL DIAGNOSIS

Granular Cell Tumor
- Pseudoepitheliomatous hyperplasia; indistinct cellular borders, lacking vacuolization; S100 protein positive

Paraganglioma
- Organoid pattern; positive for neuroendocrine markers and sustentacular S100 protein

Oncocytoma
- Lacking vacuolization and cross striations

SELECTED REFERENCES

1. Brys AK et al: Rhabdomyoma of the larynx: case report and clinical and pathologic review. Ear Nose Throat J. 84(7):437-40, 2005
2. Johansen EC et al: Rhabdomyoma of the larynx: a review of the literature with a summary of previously described cases of rhabdomyoma of the larynx and a report of a new case. J Laryngol Otol. 109(2):147-53, 1995
3. Kapadia SB et al: Adult rhabdomyoma of the head and neck: a clinicopathologic and immunophenotypic study. Hum Pathol. 24(6):608-17, 1993

IMAGE GALLERY

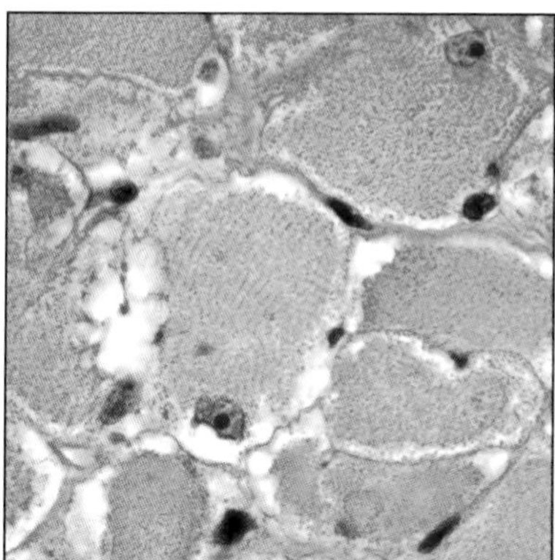

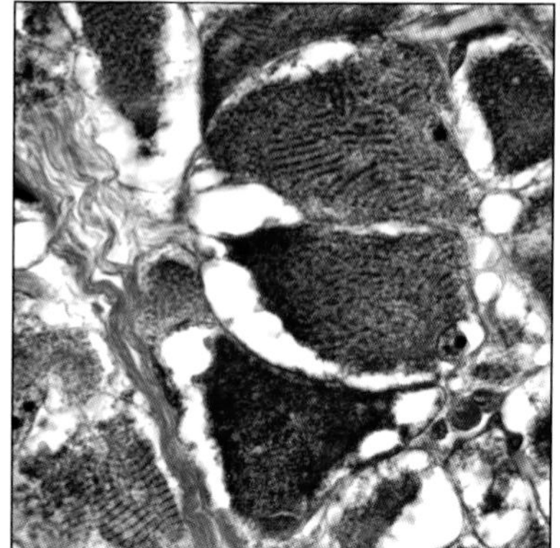

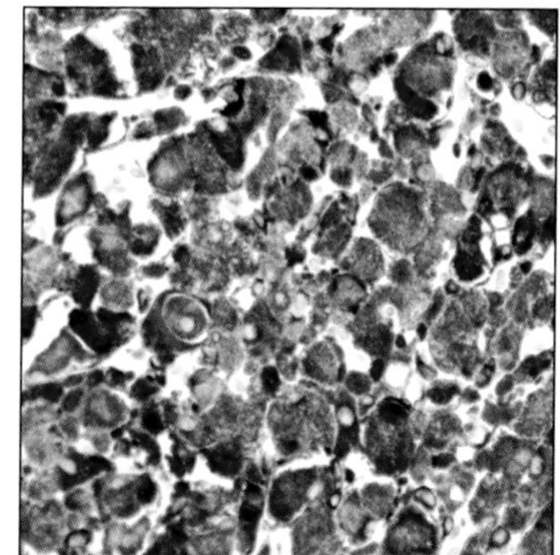

(Left) *Hematoxylin & eosin at high power demonstrates the characteristic cross striations that can be seen in the cytoplasm of the neoplastic cells. The nuclei are vesicular with a single, prominent nucleolus.* ***(Center)*** *PTAH stain highlights the cross striations within the cytoplasm of the muscle cells, creating a fingerprint-like appearance within the cytoplasm.* ***(Right)*** *Desmin stain demonstrates strong and diffuse cytoplasmic reactivity, characteristic for rhabdomyoma.*

CHONDROMA

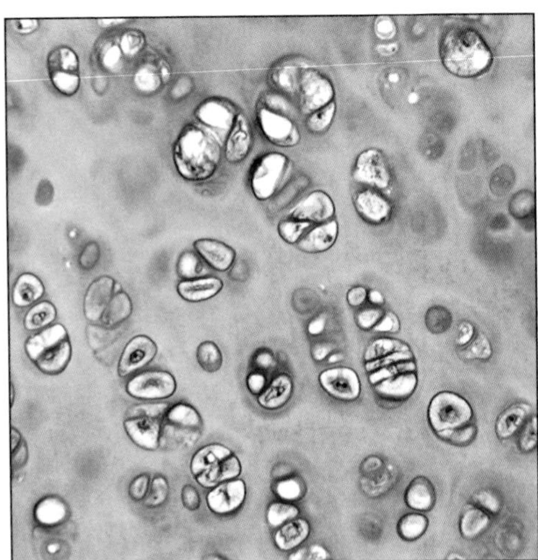

There is increased cellularity but no disarray, binucleation, or atypia. This case would be difficult to separate from a low-grade chondrosarcoma without radiographic and macroscopic correlation.

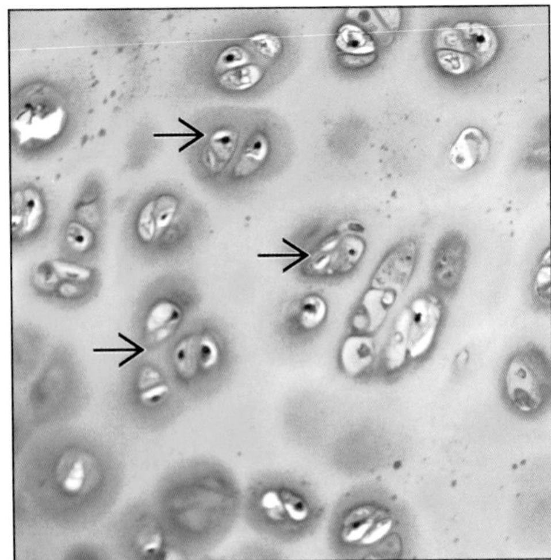

Hematoxylin & eosin shows slightly increased cellularity ➙, but no cytologic atypia, binucleation, or cluster disarray. The cellular features in this case are characteristic of a chondroma.

TERMINOLOGY

Synonyms

- Osteochondroma

Definitions

- Benign mesenchymal neoplasm of cartilaginous supporting structures of larynx

ETIOLOGY/PATHOGENESIS

Pathogenesis

- Endochondral ossification of laryngeal hyaline cartilages at points of mechanical stress/tension (muscle insertion points)
- With ischemic change, malignant transformation is more likely to develop

CLINICAL ISSUES

Epidemiology

- Incidence
  - Rare: < 1% of laryngeal tumors
    - Chondrosarcomas > > > chondroma (17:1)
- Age
  - Mean: 5th decade (approximately 10 years younger than chondrosarcoma)
- Gender
  - Male > Female (2-3:1)

Site

- Anterior surface of posterior lamina of cricoid cartilage
  - Thyroid, arytenoid, and epiglottic cartilages infrequently affected

Presentation

- Slowly progressive obstruction
- Subglottic tumors: Dyspnea, hoarseness, and stridor
- Supraglottic tumors: Hoarseness, dyspnea, dysphagia, and odynophagia
- Neck mass (thyroid cartilage specifically)

Endoscopic Findings

- Posterior larynx, endolaryngeal firm projection into laryngeal space

Treatment

- Options, risks, complications
  - Adequate sampling to exclude chondrosarcoma
  - If cricoid ring is destroyed, laryngeal stabilization is required
- Surgical approaches
  - Complete but conservative resection (includes endoscopic laser)

Prognosis

- Excellent, although recurrence may develop
  - May be that original lesion was underdiagnosed chondrosarcoma
  - Up to 10% recurrence; develops many years after resection (mean: 9 years)
- Transformation to chondrosarcoma (about 7%)
- Concurrent chondrosarcomas (up to 60%), especially if ischemic change in chondroma
- Very important to adequately sample tumors and follow patients

IMAGE FINDINGS

General Features

- CT accurately demonstrates size, extent of tumor, and whether "destructive" growth is present
  - Hypodense, well-circumscribed mass with regular margins centered in cartilage
  - Minimal calcifications are present
- MR better for tumor to soft tissue relationship and extent of tumor than CT

CHONDROMA

Key Facts

Etiology/Pathogenesis
- Ischemic change associated with malignant transformation

Clinical Issues
- Present approximately 10 years earlier than chondrosarcoma (5th decade)
- Male > Female (2-3:1)
- Anterior surface of posterior lamina of cricoid

Macroscopic Features
- Adequate sampling to exclude chondrosarcoma
- Firm, glassy, blue-white cut surface
- By definition, < 2 cm in diameter

Microscopic Pathology
- Hyaline cartilage with low cellularity
- Evenly distributed, well-defined, lobular pattern
- Individual, bland chondrocytes within lacunae

MACROSCOPIC FEATURES

General Features
- Firm, glassy, blue-white cut surface

Size
- By definition, < 2 cm in diameter

MICROSCOPIC PATHOLOGY

Histologic Features
- Usually intact epithelium
- Hyaline cartilage with low cellularity
- Evenly distributed, well defined, lobular pattern
- Individual, bland chondrocytes within lacunae
- Cells with single, uniform, small hyperchromatic nuclei surrounded by clear to eosinophilic cytoplasm
- Exceptionally, double-nucleated chondrocytes
- Calcification and ossification may be seen

ANCILLARY TESTS

Cytology
- Normal-appearing chondrocytes in fibrillar matrix

DIFFERENTIAL DIAGNOSIS

Chondrosarcoma
- On biopsy, differentation may be impossible
- In biopsy cases, use "cartilaginous lesion without definitive evidence of malignancy, requiring examination of complete lesion" as diagnosis
- Bone destruction or invasion
- Increased cellularity, loss of organization, lobular disarray, increased pleomorphism, multinucleation

Chondrometaplasia
- Ill-defined, submucosal, elastic-rich cartilage nodule affecting vocal cord, without cartilaginous connection

Tracheopathia Osteochondroplastica
- Multiple submucosal nodules, attached to cartilage

Pleomorphic Adenoma
- Epithelial/myoepithelial components blended with myxochondroid stroma

SELECTED REFERENCES

1. Franco RA Jr et al: Laryngeal chondroma. J Voice. 16(1):92-5, 2002
2. Thompson LD et al: Chondrosarcoma of the larynx: a clinicopathologic study of 111 cases with a review of the literature. Am J Surg Pathol. 26(7):836-51, 2002
3. Bielecki I et al: [Laryngeal chondromas: review of the literature and report of three cases.] Otolaryngol Pol. 55(3):331-4, 2001
4. Chiu LD et al: Laryngeal chondroma: a benign process with long-term clinical implications. Ear Nose Throat J. 75(8):540-2, 544-9, 1996
5. Jones SR et al: Benign neoplasms of the larynx. Otolaryngol Clin North Am. 17(1):151-78, 1984

IMAGE GALLERY

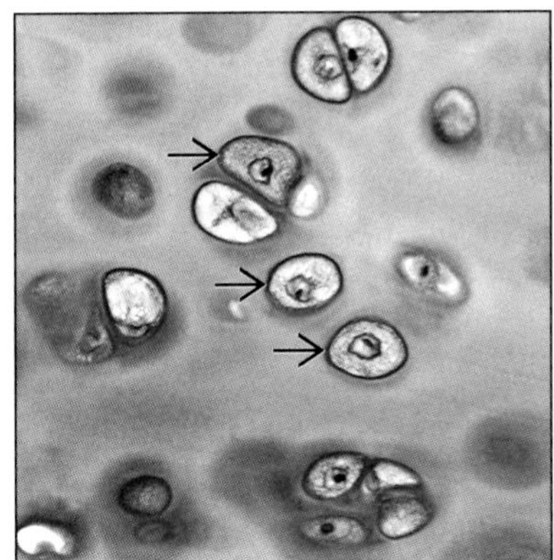

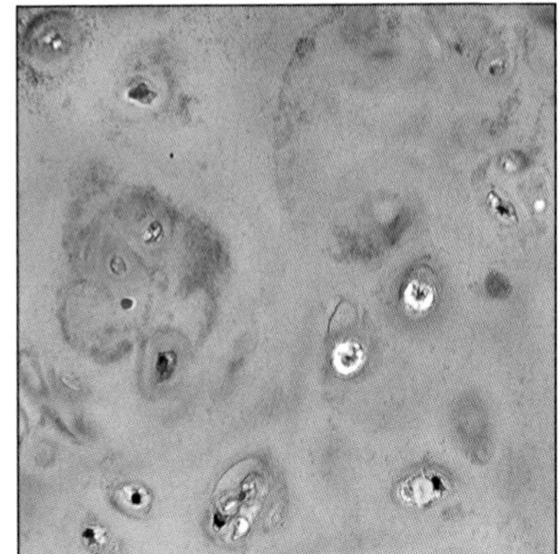

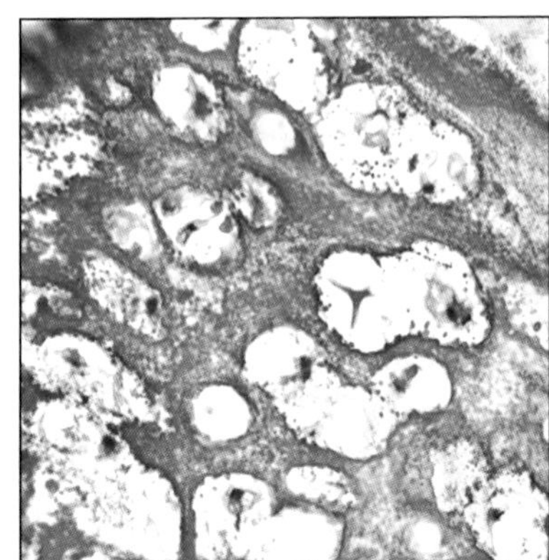

(Left) *Note the relative paucity of cells, each lacunae containing only a single cell ⇒, with a normal-appearing nucleus. There is no clustering or disorganization.* ***(Center)*** *This tumor shows only slightly increased cellularity and were this lesion not clinically and radiographically identifiable, it may fall within normal cartilage limits.* ***(Right)*** *This chondroma shows ischemic change, with blue, granular material in the cytoplasm of the cell and in the adjacent matrix.*

INFLAMMATORY MYOFIBROBLASTIC TUMOR

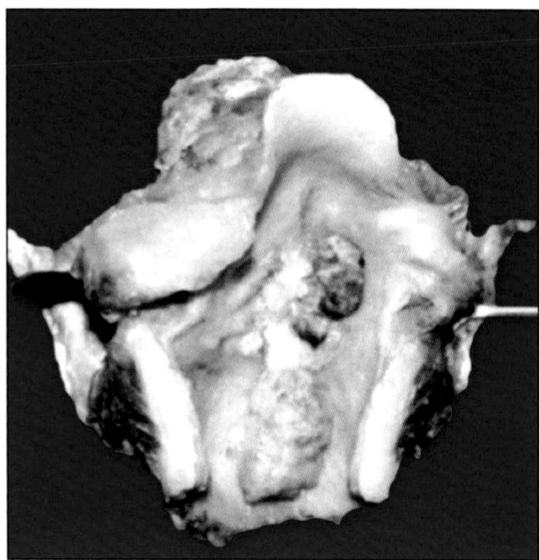

Laryngeal IMT appears as a polypoid and nodular lesion. Conservative surgical excision is usually curative, but this patient's lesion recurred multiple times, necessitating a laryngectomy.

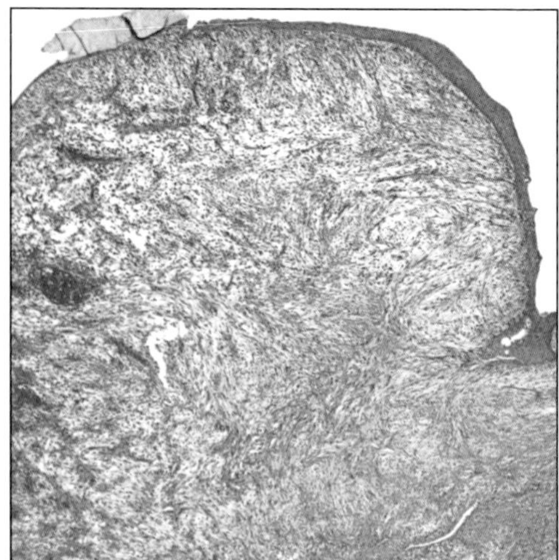

Laryngeal IMT appears as a polypoid lesion with an intact surface epithelium and a submucosal loosely cellular proliferation with storiform to fascicular growth and edematous myxoid stroma.

TERMINOLOGY

Abbreviations

- Inflammatory myofibroblastic tumor (IMT)

Synonyms

- Inflammatory (myofibroblastic) pseudotumor
- Plasma cell granuloma
- Plasma cell pseudotumor
- Pseudosarcomatous (myofibroblastic) lesion/tumor

Definitions

- Distinctive lesion composed predominantly of myofibroblastic cells with variable admixture of chronic inflammatory cells and extracellular collagen

ETIOLOGY/PATHOGENESIS

Etiology

- Unknown for IMTs in general, upper aerodigestive tract lesions in particular
- Cases associated with
  - Tobacco smoking
  - Prior history of traumatic intubation
  - Development nearly a decade after kidney transplantation
  - HHV-8 DNA sequences and overexpression of interleukin 6 and cyclin-D1 recently reported in IMTs
  - Epstein-Barr virus
    - Identified in inflammatory pseudotumors by in situ hybridization

CLINICAL ISSUES

Epidemiology

- Age
  - Upper aerodigestive tract IMT
    - Wide age range, including pediatric population but more common in adult populations
  - Laryngeal IMT
    - Median age: 59 years
- Gender
  - Laryngeal IMT
    - Male > Female

Site

- Upper aerodigestive tract IMTs rare
  - Larynx most common
    - True vocal cord (glottis) most common > supraglottis, subglottis
  - Nonlaryngeal sites include oral cavity, tonsil, parapharyngeal space, sinonasal tract, salivary glands, and trachea

Presentation

- Laryngeal IMTs
  - Hoarseness, stridor, dysphonia, foreign body sensation in throat
    - Duration of symptoms range from days to months
- Upper aerodigestive tract IMTs
  - Painless mass (± ulceration), nasal obstruction, epistaxis, headache, dysphagia
- Soft tissue and visceral IMTs
  - Constitutional &/or systemic signs and symptoms (not usually component of upper aerodigestive tract IMTs)
    - Fever, weight loss, pain, malaise, anemia, thrombocytosis, polyclonal hyperglobulinemia, elevated erythrocyte sedimentation rate

Treatment

- Surgical approaches
  - Conservative surgical resection, including local excision by laser removal or via laryngoscopic techniques
- Drugs

INFLAMMATORY MYOFIBROBLASTIC TUMOR

Key Facts

Terminology

- Distinctive lesion composed predominantly of myofibroblastic cells with variable admixture of inflammatory cells, including mature lymphocytes, histiocytes, plasma cells, eosinophils, and extracellular collagen

Clinical Issues

- True vocal cord (glottis) most common
- Conservative resection usually curative

Microscopic Pathology

- Spindle-shaped or stellate, enlarged round to oblong nuclei, inapparent to prominent eosinophilic nucleoli and abundant basophilic fibrillar-appearing cytoplasm
- Epithelioid or histiocytoid myofibroblasts with round to oval nuclei, prominent nuclei, and abundant basophilic fibrillar-appearing cytoplasm
- Axonal (spider-like) cells with elongated nuclei, inapparent nucleoli, and long cytoplasmic extensions creating bipolar to multipolar (tadpole-like) cells
- Intranuclear inclusions may be seen

Ancillary Tests

- Strong diffuse cytoplasmic immunoreactivity for vimentin
- Smooth muscle actin and muscle specific actin present, varying from focal to diffuse
- Cytoplasmic reactivity for ALK1 can be seen
- ALK1 reactivity also present in the intranuclear inclusions

  - Corticosteroid and nonsteroidal anti-inflammatory agents have been used, resulting in regression in some patients

Prognosis

- Conservative resection usually curative
- Rarely, tumors recur following surgical resection
  - Recurrence rate of approximately 25% reported for extrapulmonary IMTs
  - Rare examples of extrapulmonary (non-head and neck) IMTs metastasize
- Some evidence that nuclear atypia, ganglion-like cells, expression of TP53 and DNA aneuploidy may portend more aggressive behavior

MACROSCOPIC FEATURES

General Features

- Polypoid, pedunculated, or nodular firm lesion with smooth appearance and fleshy to firm consistency
- IMTs of upper aerodigestive tract usually present as solitary lesions

Size

- 0.4-3 cm in greatest dimension

MICROSCOPIC PATHOLOGY

Histologic Features

- Polypoid and unencapsulated submucosal loosely cellular proliferation of spindle-shaped to stellate cells
- Cellular proliferation loosely arranged with storiform to fascicular growth patterns and edematous myxoid to fibromyxoid stroma, prominent vascularity, and variable inflammatory cell infiltrate
  - Mature lymphocytes, histiocytes, plasma cells, eosinophils, and scattered polymorphonuclear leukocytes

Myofibroblasts

- Spindle-shaped or stellate, enlarged round to oblong nuclei, inapparent to prominent eosinophilic nucleoli and abundant basophilic fibrillar-appearing cytoplasm
- Myofibroblasts may also appear
  - Epithelioid or histiocytoid with round to oval nuclei, prominent nucleoli, and abundant basophilic fibrillar-appearing cytoplasm
  - Axonal (spider-like) cells with elongated nuclei, inapparent nucleoli, and long cytoplasmic extensions creating cells with bipolar to multipolar appearance (tadpole-like)
- In all examples, low nuclear to cytoplasmic ratio
- Intranuclear inclusions may be seen
- Increased mitotic figures are common and may be numerous but atypical mitoses not usually seen
- Marked nuclear pleomorphism and necrosis not present

Stroma

- Varies from edematous myxoid background to fibromyxoid and more fibrous stroma
- Fibrillar-appearing stroma resembling neurofibrillary matrix may rarely be seen
- Vascular component varies, including widely dilated medium-sized vascular channels to narrow, slit-like blood vessels
  - Can be obscured by myofibroblasts and inflammatory cells
- Vascular thrombosis not present

Surface Epithelium

- May be intact and unremarkable to ulcerated and hyperplastic in appearance
- Myofibroblastic proliferation approximates surface epithelium
  - There is usually separation between myofibroblasts and surface epithelium
- Reactive epithelial atypia may be seen
  - Significant epithelial dysplasia (i.e., moderate to severe dysplasia), carcinoma in situ, and invasive squamous carcinoma not present

INFLAMMATORY MYOFIBROBLASTIC TUMOR

ANCILLARY TESTS

Immunohistochemistry

- Strong diffuse cytoplasmic immunoreactivity for vimentin
- Variable immunoreactivity for smooth muscle actin, muscle specific actin, calponin, and caldesmon
- Desmin immunoreactivity may be seen
- Cytoplasmic reactivity for anaplastic lymphoma kinase (ALK) can be seen
    - Positive in < 50% of cases
    - ALK1 reactivity also present in intranuclear inclusions
- Cytokeratin, S100 protein, HMB-45, myoglobin, myogenin, MYOD1, CD34, CD117 (c-kit) usually negative

Molecular Genetics

- Anaplastic lymphoma kinase (*ALK*) gene rearrangements and expression seen in IMTs
    - IMTs of children and young adults often have clonal cytogenetic rearrangements activating *ALK* receptor kinase gene in chromosome band 2p23
        - Such rearrangements are uncommon in adults > 40 years of age with IMT
- Gene rearrangements and protein activation restricted to myofibroblastic component of IMTs
    - Inflammatory cell component lacks gene rearrangements or expression of ALK protein
- Fusion of *ALK* to Ran-binding protein 2 (*RANBP2*) gene in IMTs expand spectrum of *ALK* abnormalities seen in IMT further confirming clonal, neoplastic nature of IMTs

Electron Microscopy

- Transmission
    - Myofibroblastic and fibroblastic differentiation with cytoplasmic organelles, including
        - Well-developed, prominent rough endoplasmic reticulum and Golgi complexes
        - Bundles of microfilaments arranged in parallel along long axis of cells with focal densities ("stress fibers")
        - Fragmented basal lamina, pinocytotic vesicles, and fibronexus junctions
        - Fibronexus junctions represent foci on the cell surface where intracellular myofilaments and extracellular fibronectin filaments converge

DIFFERENTIAL DIAGNOSIS

Contact Ulcer

- Unilateral or bilateral mass often localized to posterior vocal cord
- Myofibroblasts present but usually sparse as 1 component of a mixed chronic inflammatory cell reaction in background of granulation tissue

Spindle Cell Squamous Carcinoma

- Histologically high-grade variant of squamous cell carcinoma
- Usually densely cellular composed of malignant spindle-shaped &/or pleomorphic cell population with increased mitotic figures and atypical mitoses
- Intraepithelial dysplasia (moderate to severe) &/or invasive differentiated squamous cell carcinoma may be present
    - Surface ulceration is common and differentiated squamous cell component may not be present
- Cytokeratin immunoreactivity present in > 70% of cases

Low-Grade Myofibrosarcoma

- Cytologically, more cellular uniformity but greater cellularity and nuclear pleomorphism than IMT
- More widely infiltrative growth than IMT
- ALK negative

SELECTED REFERENCES

1. Chabbi AG et al: Inflammatory myofibroblastic tumor of the larynx: A case report. Tunis Med. 88(12):942-4, 2010
2. Völker HU et al: Laryngeal inflammatory myofibroblastic tumors: Different clinical appearance and histomorphologic presentation of one entity. Head Neck. 32(11):1573-8, 2010
3. Biron VL et al: Inflammatory pseudotumours of the larynx: three cases and a review of the literature. J Otolaryngol Head Neck Surg. 37(2):E32-8, 2008
4. Qiu X et al: Inflammatory myofibroblastic tumor and low-grade myofibroblastic sarcoma: a comparative study of clinicopathologic features and further observations on the immunohistochemical profile of myofibroblasts. Hum Pathol. 39(6):846-56, 2008
5. Coffin CM et al: Inflammatory myofibroblastic tumor: comparison of clinicopathologic, histologic, and immunohistochemical features including ALK expression in atypical and aggressive cases. Am J Surg Pathol. 31(4):509-20, 2007
6. Tavora F et al: Absence of human herpesvirus-8 in pulmonary inflammatory myofibroblastic tumor: immunohistochemical and molecular analysis of 20 cases. Mod Pathol. 20(9):995-9, 2007
7. Cessna MH et al: Expression of ALK1 and p80 in inflammatory myofibroblastic tumor and its mesenchymal mimics: a study of 135 cases. Mod Pathol. 15(9):931-8, 2002
8. Coffin CM et al: ALK1 and p80 expression and chromosomal rearrangements involving 2p23 in inflammatory myofibroblastic tumor. Mod Pathol. 14(6):569-76, 2001
9. Cook JR et al: Anaplastic lymphoma kinase (ALK) expression in the inflammatory myofibroblastic tumor: a comparative immunohistochemical study. Am J Surg Pathol. 25(11):1364-71, 2001
10. Coffin CM et al: Inflammatory myofibroblastic tumor, inflammatory fibrosarcoma, and related lesions: an historical review with differential diagnostic considerations. Semin Diagn Pathol. 15(2):102-10, 1998
11. Coffin CM et al: Extrapulmonary inflammatory myofibroblastic tumor (inflammatory pseudotumor). A clinicopathologic and immunohistochemical study of 84 cases. Am J Surg Pathol. 19(8):859-72, 1995
12. Wenig BM et al: Inflammatory myofibroblastic tumor of the larynx. A clinicopathologic study of eight cases simulating a malignant spindle cell neoplasm. Cancer. 76(11):2217-29, 1995

Microscopic and Immunohistochemical Features

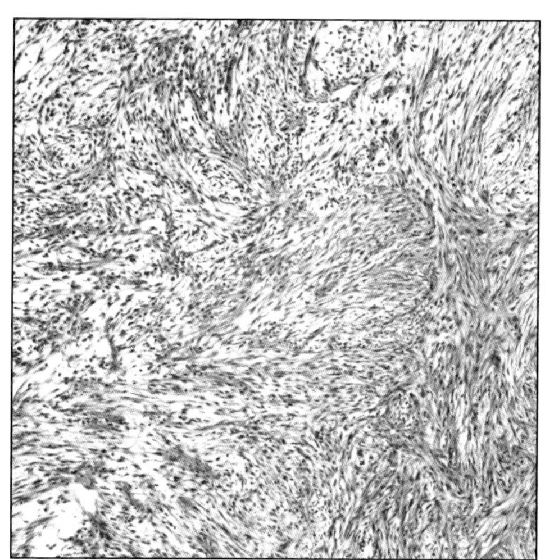

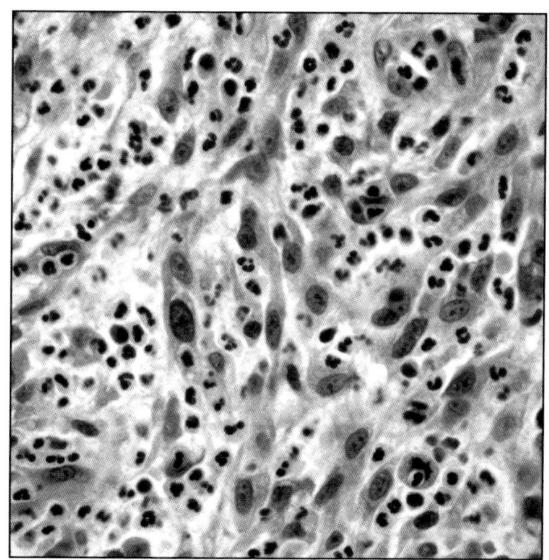

(Left) *Histologic similarities to nodular fasciitis are seen, including loosely arranged spindle cell proliferation with storiform to fascicular growth and myxoid stroma.* ***(Right)*** *Myofibroblasts vary in appearance from case to case and in the same case. Here, the myofibroblasts include spindle-shaped to stellate cells with round to oblong nuclei, inapparent to prominent eosinophilic nucleoli, and ample basophilic fibrillar cytoplasm; background inflammatory cell infiltrate is present.*

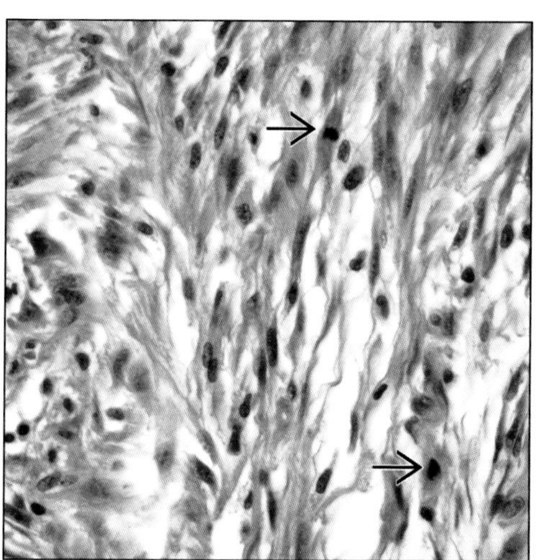

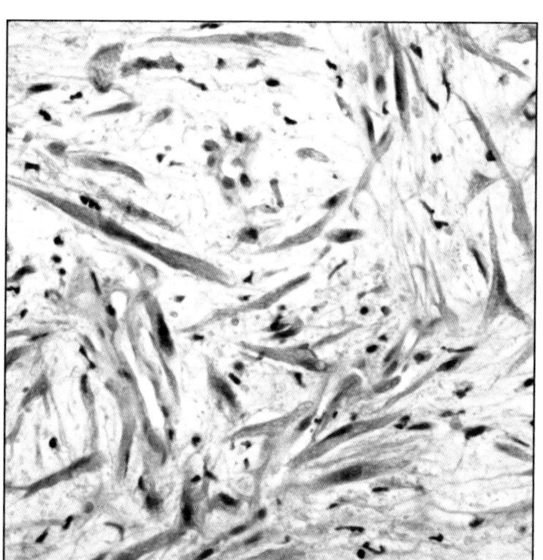

(Left) *Myofibroblasts are predominantly spindle-shaped in this image with elongated nuclei and abundant eosinophilic to basophilic cytoplasm. Note mitotic figures* ⇒*.* ***(Right)*** *Myofibroblasts appear axonal (spider-like) with long cytoplasmic extensions, creating cells with bipolar to multipolar (tadpole-like) appearance. A variable admixed inflammatory cell infiltrate is present. Inflammatory cell component may vary considerably from case to case in IMTs.*

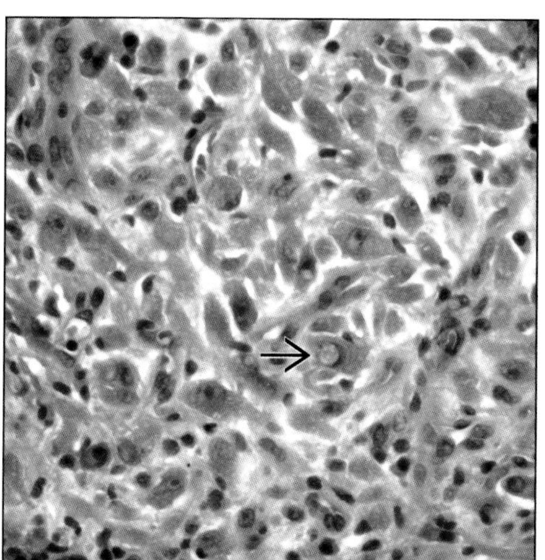

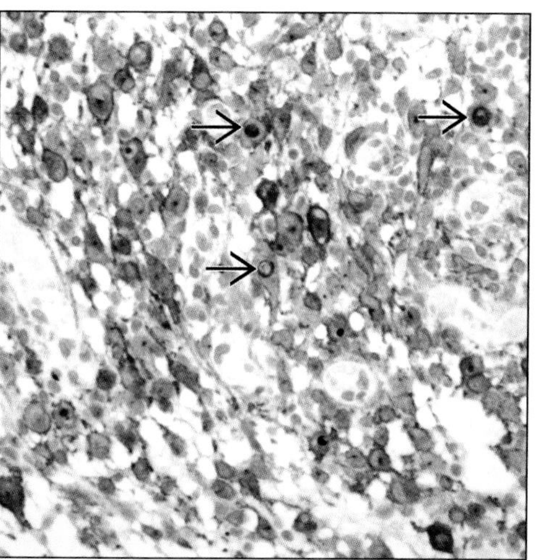

(Left) *In this image, the myofibroblasts are epithelioid in appearance with round to oval nuclei, prominent eosinophilic nucleoli, and abundant basophilic to eosinophilic appearing-fibrillar cytoplasm. In addition, an intranuclear inclusion* ⇒ *is present.* ***(Right)*** *Immunoreactivity for ALK1 is a helpful diagnostic finding in IMTs. The lesional cells show the presence of intracytoplasmic ALK staining; the intranuclear inclusions* ⇒ *are also immunoreactive for ALK1.*

PARAGANGLIOMA

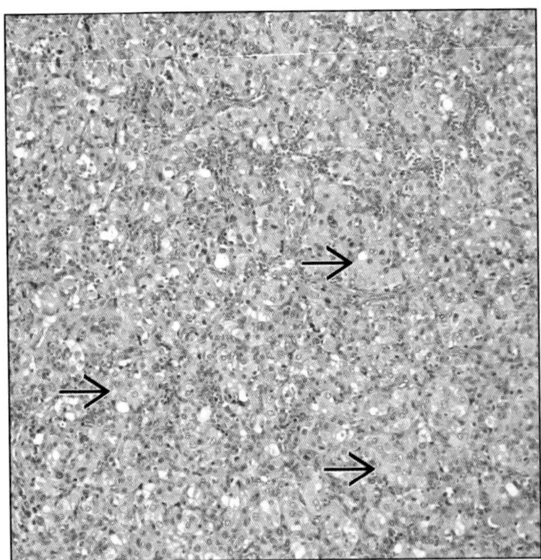

Hematoxylin & eosin shows the characteristic alveolar pattern (zellballen) of paraganglioma. Small nests of cells ⇒ are surrounded by a fibrovascular, richly vascularized stroma.

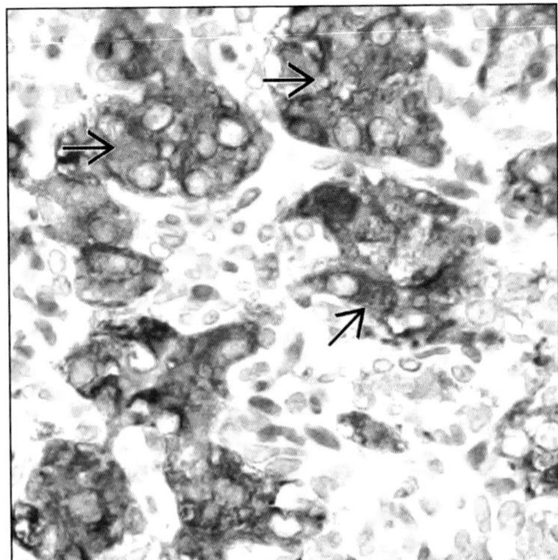

Synaptophysin shows strong and diffuse immunoreactivity of the chief cells ⇒. There is no reactivity of the supporting sustentacular cells (which would stain with S100 protein).

TERMINOLOGY

Synonyms

- Chemodectoma
- Neuroendocrine tumor
- Nonchromaffin paraganglioma

Definitions

- Neuroendocrine tumor arising from either superior or inferior laryngeal paraganglia, composed of chief and sustentacular cells arranged in organoid pattern

CLINICAL ISSUES

Epidemiology

- Incidence
    - Very rare laryngeal tumor
- Age
    - Mean: 47 years
    - Range: 5-83 years
- Gender
    - Female > Male (3:1)

Site

- Supraglottis (82%)
- Subglottis (15%)
- Glottis (3%)
- Rarely multicentric

Presentation

- Hoarseness is major symptom
- Dysphagia, dyspnea, stridor, sore throat

Treatment

- Surgical approaches
    - Excision with external approach
        - Intraoperative bleeding may be significant

Prognosis

- Excellent
- ~ 20% of patients may develop local recurrences
    - 1-16 years after excision

IMAGE FINDINGS

General Features

- Preoperative angiogram is rarely used

MACROSCOPIC FEATURES

General Features

- Rounded submucosal mass
- Cut surface is homogeneous or nodular
- Pink to tan and dark red

Size

- Range: 0.5-6 cm

MICROSCOPIC PATHOLOGY

Histologic Features

- Nests of tumor cells are surrounded by highly vascular fibrous tissue
- 2 cell types
    - Chief and sustentacular cells form alveolar (**zellballen**) pattern
- Chief cells have eosinophilic, finely granular cytoplasm, and centrally located nuclei
    - Cellular pleomorphism may be present but is prognostically unimportant
- Sustentacular cells are inconspicuous spindle-shaped at periphery of cell balls
- Rare mitoses

DIFFERENTIAL DIAGNOSIS

Neuroendocrine Tumors

- Both typical and atypical carcinoid

PARAGANGLIOMA

Key Facts

Terminology

- Benign tumor arising from laryngeal paraganglia

Clinical Issues

- Sporadic predominantly supraglottic tumor
- Female > Male (3:1)
- Surgery yields excellent prognosis

Microscopic Pathology

- Rounded, submucosal tumor
- Clustered, alveolar (zellballen) pattern
- Chief cells with granular cytoplasm
- Highly vascular fibrous stroma

Ancillary Tests

- Neuroendocrine markers and S100 protein positive

Top Differential Diagnoses

- Typical & atypical carcinoid, melanoma, metastatic renal cell carcinoma, medullary thyroid carcinoma

Immunohistochemistry

Antibody	Reactivity	Staining Pattern	Comment
Chromogranin-A	Positive	Cytoplasmic	Chief, paraganglia cells
Synaptophysin	Positive	Cytoplasmic	Chief, paraganglia cells
CD56	Positive	Cell membrane	Chief, paraganglia cells
NSE	Positive	Cytoplasmic	Chief, paraganglia cells
S100	Positive	Nuclear & cytoplasmic	Sustentacular cells
GFAP	Positive	Cytoplasmic	Sustentacular cells
CK-PAN	Negative		

- Organoid, trabecular, or glandular patterns
- Positive: **Both** neuroendocrine and epithelial markers

Melanoma

- Multiple patterns of growth
- Positive: S100 protein, HMB-45, Melan-A

Metastatic Renal Cell Carcinoma

- Organoid pattern
- Positive: Keratin, vimentin, CD10, pax-2, renal cell carcinoma marker
- Negative: Chromogranin, S100 protein

Medullary Thyroid Carcinoma

- Multiple patterns with amyloid
- Positive: Calcitonin, TTF-1, CEA-m

SELECTED REFERENCES

1. Ferlito A et al: Neuroendocrine neoplasms of the larynx: advances in identification, understanding, and management. Oral Oncol. 42(8):770-88, 2006
2. Myssiorek D et al: Laryngeal and sinonasal paragangliomas. Otolaryngol Clin North Am. 34(5):971-82, vii, 2001
3. Peterson KL et al: Subglottic paraganglioma. Head Neck. 19(1):54-6, 1997
4. Ferlito A et al: Laryngeal paraganglioma versus atypical carcinoid tumor. Ann Otol Rhinol Laryngol. 104(1):78-83, 1995
5. Ferlito A et al: Identification, classification, treatment, and prognosis of laryngeal paraganglioma. Review of the literature and eight new cases. Ann Otol Rhinol Laryngol. 103(7):525-36, 1994
6. Barnes L: Paraganglioma of the larynx. A critical review of the literature. ORL J Otorhinolaryngol Relat Spec. 53(4):220-34, 1991

IMAGE GALLERY

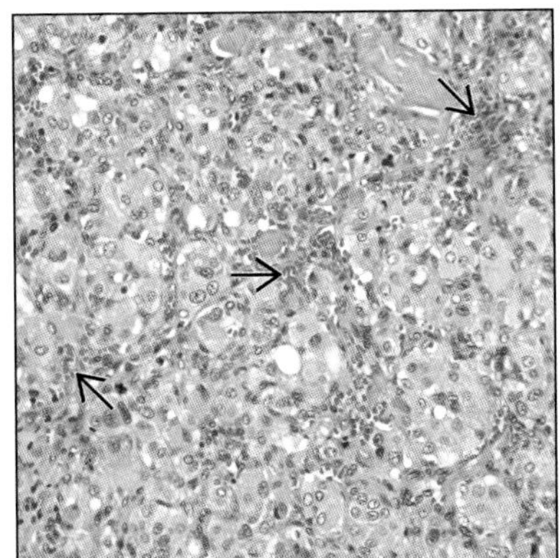

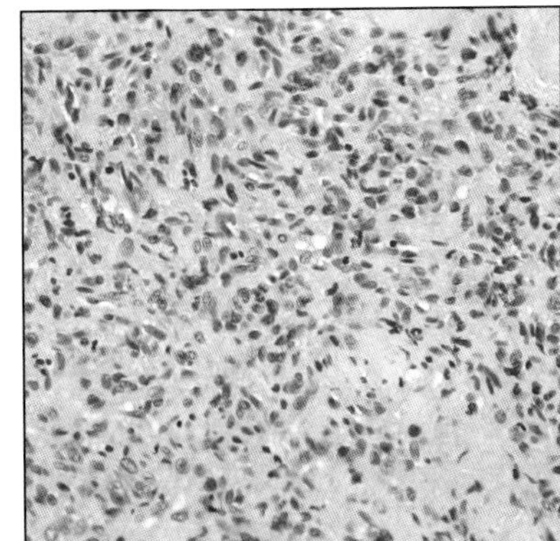

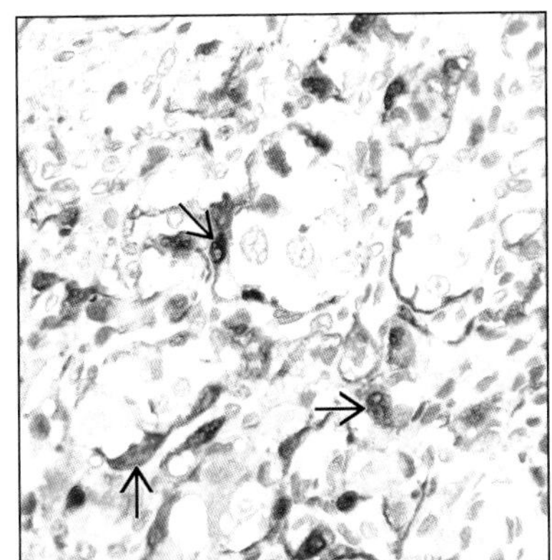

*(**Left**) Hematoxylin & eosin shows paraganglioma with the characteristic pattern of small islands of cells separated by thin fibrovascular stroma. Extravasated erythrocytes are noted ⇒. (**Center**) Hematoxylin & eosin shows a region of paraganglioma where the characteristic nested or alveolar pattern is not well recognized. This case would be more difficult to diagnose. (**Right**) S100 protein positive supporting, sustentacular cells ⇒ are shown surrounding the negative chief cells.*

KERATINIZING DYSPLASIA AND CARCINOMA IN SITU

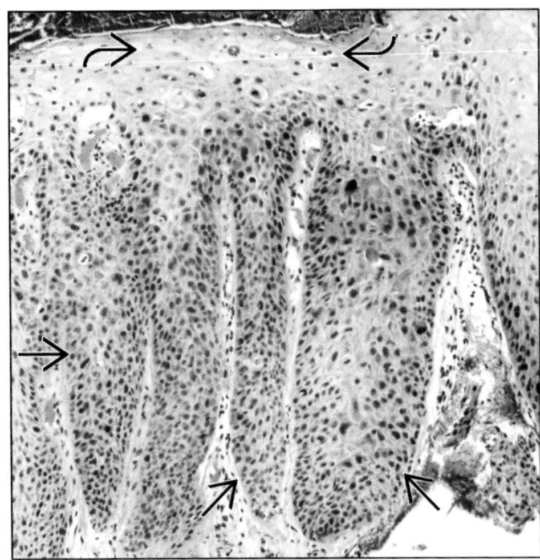

Keratinizing severe dysplasia shows widened and downwardly growing rete ⇒ and marked dysplastic cellular changes, albeit limited to the basal zone with surface epithelial maturation ⇒.

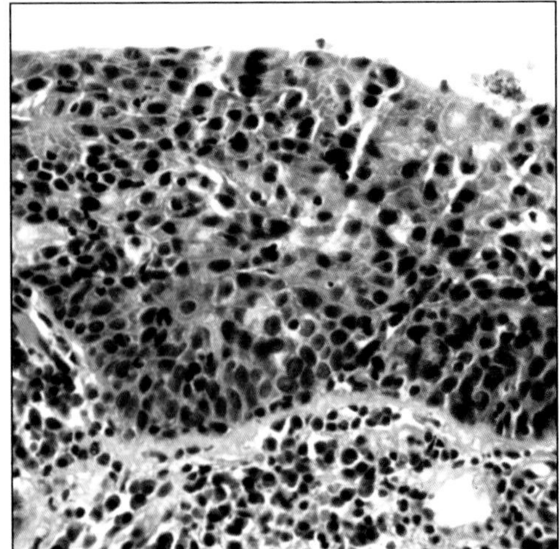

Severe (nonkeratinizing) dysplasia representing "classic" carcinoma in situ shows full thickness dysplasia of surface epithelium without invasion beyond the basement membrane.

TERMINOLOGY

Abbreviations

- Carcinoma in situ (CIS)

Synonyms

- Keratosis with atypia
- Dysplasia (mild, moderate, severe)
- Squamous intraepithelial lesion (SIL) or neoplasia (SIN)
- Laryngeal intraepithelial neoplasia (LIN)
- Simple hyperplasia
- Basal/parabasal hyperplasia
- Atypical hyperplasia

Definitions

- **Keratinizing dysplasia**
  - Potentially reversible (qualitative) alteration in malignant direction in appearance of epithelial cells with increased likelihood to progress to squamous cell carcinoma
- **Carcinoma in situ (CIS)**
  - "Classically" defined as malignant alteration characterized by cellular dysplasia involving entire thickness of surface epithelium without violation of basement membrane
  - Considered irreversible process that will progress to invasive carcinoma if left untreated
  - Dysplasia may extend into mucoserous glands but is still considered an in situ lesion

ETIOLOGY/PATHOGENESIS

Environmental Exposure

- Tobacco smoking (most common) and excess alcohol use
  - Alcohol potentiates the effect of tobacco smoking
  - Risk of developing dysplastic lesions increases with duration of smoking &/or alcohol use

Infectious Agents

- Role of human papillomavirus (HPV) in development of these lesions remains unproven
  - Prevalence of HPV in premalignant epithelial lesions reported in approximately 12% of cases
  - DNA reported in 12-25% of normal (clinically and histologically) larynges
  - Increasing evidence linking HPV to certain head and neck squamous cell carcinomas
    - Uncertainty remains whether HPV plays any direct role in development of upper aerodigestive tract premalignant epithelial dysplasias

CLINICAL ISSUES

Epidemiology

- Incidence
  - Carcinoma in situ
    - Represents 1-13% of all laryngeal carcinomas
- Age
  - **Keratinizing dysplasia**
    - Generally limited to adult population with mean age at diagnosis in 6th-7th decade of life
  - **Carcinoma in situ**
    - Wide age range but most common in 7th decade of life
- Gender
  - Male > Female

Site

- **Keratinizing dysplasia**
  - May occur anywhere in larynx but mainly identified along true vocal cord
    - Typically is unilateral but may be bilateral in up to 30% of cases
- **Carcinoma in situ**
  - Can occur anywhere in larynx but most often involves anterior 1/3 of one or both true vocal cords
    - May involve entire cord

KERATINIZING DYSPLASIA AND CARCINOMA IN SITU

Key Facts

Terminology

- **Keratinizing dysplasia**
  - Potentially reversible (qualitative) alteration in malignant direction in appearance of epithelial cells with increased likelihood to progress to squamous cell carcinoma
- **Carcinoma in situ (CIS)**
  - "Classically" defined as malignant alteration characterized by cellular dysplasia involving entire thickness of surface epithelium without violation of basement membrane
  - Considered irreversible process that will progress to invasive carcinoma if left untreated

Microscopic Pathology

- **"Classic" or nonkeratinizing dysplasia**
  - Uncommon in upper aerodigestive tract, especially in laryngeal glottis and oral cavity
- **Keratinizing dysplasia**
  - Most common type of dysplasia in upper aerodigestive tract
  - Similar grading as nonkeratinizing dysplasia (i.e., mild, moderate, and severe) depending on degree and extent of cellular and maturation alterations
  - Definition of keratinizing severe dysplasia, especially laryngeal and oral cavity, broader, more heterogeneous, and less reproducible than nonkeratinizing dysplasias
  - Invasive carcinoma may develop in epithelium showing dysplasia limited only to basal zone (i.e., absence of full thickness dysplasia)

    - May be bilateral
    - Frequently associated with invasive squamous cell carcinoma either lying adjacent to or remote from one another
    - May exist as isolated lesion unrelated to invasive carcinoma
    - Multifocal areas can occur

Presentation

- Hoarseness or voice changes most common

Natural History

- Risk of progression to invasive carcinoma
  - Circumstantial evidence supports the idea that preinvasive dysplasias are potentially reversible following cessation or removal of instigating factor, such as tobacco use
  - Mild and moderate dysplasias felt to be potentially reversible alterations
  - Determining whether mild to moderate dysplasia is reactive or neoplastic not always achievable
  - Clinically abnormal lesions falling under the designation reactive atypias or hyperplastic lesions represent
    - Reversible changes that rarely, if ever, progress to carcinoma
    - Reactive atypias or hyperplastic lesions managed conservatively
  - Problem of predicting malignant potential of dysplastic lesion greatest in moderate dysplasia
    - Impossible to differentiate moderately dysplastic lesions that are reversible from moderate dysplasias representing earliest form of malignant transformation
    - Diagnosis of moderate dysplasia should warrant vigilant patient follow-up
    - Recurrence or persistence may be indicative of malignant transformation
  - Keratotic epithelium without dysplasia carries very low risk of developing invasive carcinoma with reported incidences of 1-5%
  - Keratotic epithelium with dysplasia associated with increased risk for progression or development of premalignant or overtly carcinomatous changes, varying from 11-18%
  - Risk of malignant transformation in keratosis with dysplasia represents increase of 3-5x compared to carcinoma arising in keratotic lesions without dysplasia
  - Risk for progression to invasive carcinoma in keratosis with atypia varies depending on degree of atypia/dysplasia
    - Mild dysplasia: Approximately 6%
    - Moderate dysplasia: Approximately 23%
    - Severe dysplasia: Approximately 28%
    - Average latency period from diagnosis of keratosis with atypia to invasive carcinoma is 3.8 years
  - No statistical difference in risk to progression to invasive carcinoma in upper aerodigestive tract moderate dysplasia and severe dysplasia
    - Based on similar risk to invasive carcinoma
    - Classification akin to Bethesda system used for uterine cervix being considered to include 2 categories for upper aerodigestive tract dysplasia
    - Low-grade squamous intraepithelial neoplasia (i.e., mild dysplasia)
    - High-grade squamous intraepithelial neoplasia (i.e., moderate and severe dysplasia)
  - Important to note that diagnosis of severe keratinizing dysplasia/CIS associated with
    - Multifocal lesions, including other foci of keratinizing severe dysplasia &/or invasive carcinoma
    - Frequently occurs adjacent to or near synchronous foci of invasive carcinoma
    - Requires clinical evaluation of entire upper aerodigestive tract to exclude possible presence of additional foci of dysplasia or carcinoma
  - Wide variation in the literature relative to incidence of laryngeal CIS progressing to invasive carcinoma
    - Discrepant statistics reflects inconsistencies in diagnosis of CIS, which is a notoriously subjective diagnosis

KERATINIZING DYSPLASIA AND CARCINOMA IN SITU

- Collated incidence of laryngeal CIS progressing to invasive carcinoma is 23-27%
- Latent period of 3-5 years from diagnosis of CIS to invasive carcinoma

Treatment

- Options, risks, complications
  - Cessation of contributing risk factors
    - Mild and moderate dysplasias potentially reversible alterations
    - Circumstantial evidence supports the notion that preinvasive dysplasias are potentially reversible following cessation or removal of instigating factor, such as tobacco use
- Surgical approaches
  - **Keratinizing dysplasia**
    - Excisional biopsy by vocal cord stripping or by forceps is treatment of choice
  - **Carcinoma in situ**
    - Treatment is not standardized; includes vocal cord stripping, laser ablation, cordectomy, hemilaryngectomy, radiation, or combination of procedures

Prognosis

- **Keratinizing dysplasia**
  - Excellent cure rates but recurrent or persistent disease varies from 15-30% following initial therapy
- **Carcinoma in situ**
  - High cure rate (approximately 75%) but vigilant follow-up, including periodic laryngoscopic examinations indicated
  - Treatment failures result from
    - Extensive &/or multifocal disease
    - Associated undetected invasive squamous carcinoma
    - Extension of CIS to subjacent mucoserous glands harboring residual disease following mucosal stripping, which may in turn be the nidus for subsequent invasive carcinoma

MACROSCOPIC FEATURES

General Features

- **Keratinizing dysplasia**
  - Localized, circumscribed flat or papillary area with white (leukoplakic), red (erythroplakic), or gray appearance
- **Carcinoma in situ**
  - Circumscribed or diffuse lesion with white, red, or gray color and smooth to granular appearance

MICROSCOPIC PATHOLOGY

Histologic Features

- Histomorphologic changes separated into cellular abnormalities and maturation abnormalities and include proliferation of immature or "uncommitted" cells
  - Cellular abnormalities
    - Nuclear pleomorphism (i.e., variations in size and shape of nuclei)
    - Nuclear hyperchromasia with irregularities in nuclear contour
    - Increased mitotic activity, especially away from basal zone involving mid and upper (superficial) portions of surface epithelium; may include atypical forms
    - Prominent nucleoli (not unique to dysplasia and may be seen in reactive or reparative process)
  - Maturation abnormalities
    - Loss of maturation with increased cellularity in superficial epithelium
    - Normally in mature squamous epithelium there is decrease in cellularity from basal zone toward keratinizing layers (referred to as maturation)
    - Crowding of cells with loss of polarity
    - Increase in nuclear size relative to cytoplasm (increased nuclear-to-cytoplasmic ratio)
    - Abnormal keratosis (dyskeratosis)
  - Dysplastic process begins in basal and parabasal area
- **Grading dysplasia**
  - Mild dysplasia (grade I)
    - Dysplasia limited to lower portions or inner 1/3 of epithelium (basal zone dysplasia)
  - Moderate dysplasia (grade II)
    - Dysplasia involves up to 2/3 of thickness of epithelium
  - Severe dysplasia (grade III)
    - Dysplasia involves from 2/3 to almost complete thickness of epithelium
    - For all intents and purposes, synonymous with carcinoma in situ
- **"Classic" or nonkeratinizing dysplasia**
  - Uncommon in upper aerodigestive tract, especially in laryngeal glottis and oral cavity
  - Absent surface keratosis
  - Increasing gradations of dysplasia include
    - Mild dysplasia (grade I)
    - Moderate dysplasia (grade II)
    - Severe dysplasia (grade III) representing full thickness replacement of squamous epithelium by atypical, small, immature basaloid cells and synonymous with carcinoma in situ
  - Grading scheme is reproducible and clinically useful
- **Keratinizing dysplasia**
  - Most common type of dysplasia in upper aerodigestive tract
  - Keratinizing dysplasias include surface keratinization with maturation but cellular (and often architectural) abnormalities
    - Surface maturation retained with only partial replacement of epithelium by dysplastic cells from which invasive carcinoma may develop
    - Similar grading as nonkeratinizing dysplasia (i.e., mild, moderate, and severe) depending on degree and extent of cellular and maturation alterations
    - Criteria for evaluating keratinizing dysplasias are less defined than nonkeratinizing dysplasia and diagnosis of keratinizing severe dysplasia remains controversial
    - Definition of keratinizing severe dysplasia, especially laryngeal and oral cavity, broader,

more heterogeneous and less reproducible than nonkeratinizing dysplasias
    - Keratinizing dysplastic epithelium often hyperplastic with elongated and irregular-appearing rete pegs extending downward into submucosa
    - Keratinizing severe dysplasia includes epithelial alterations so severe that there would be high probability for progression to invasive carcinoma if left untreated
    - Prior statement, while true, represents major source of subjectivity in evaluating these lesions as well as reason for lack of diagnostic reproducibility
  - Histopathologic interpretation and grading of keratinizing dysplasias of upper aerodigestive tract are imprecise and subjective
    - Confusion and misunderstandings occur between clinician and pathologist that may result in inappropriate patient management
- **Carcinoma in situ**
  - Dysplastic process involves entire thickness of squamous epithelium without violation of basement membrane
  - Uncommon in upper aerodigestive tract and, when identified, typically seen in nonkeratinizing epithelia
  - Squamous epithelium may or may not be thickened
  - Alterations include
    - Loss of cellular maturation and polarity
    - Increase in nuclear to cytoplasmic ratio
    - Nuclear pleomorphism with hyperchromasia and irregular nuclear contours
    - Presence of mitoses in all layers of mucosa, including normal and abnormal forms
    - Dyskeratosis may be present
    - Extension to mucoserous glands still represents CIS
  - Use of CIS as classically defined (i.e., full thickness dysplasia) in keratinizing dysplasias is inappropriate as full thickness dysplasia is uncommon
    - More appropriate designation is severe keratinizing dysplasia
    - Such lesions capable of progressing to invasive carcinoma in absence of full thickness epithelial dysplasia

DIFFERENTIAL DIAGNOSIS

Reactive Epithelial Changes

- May include keratosis with thickened epithelium, elongated rete pegs but absent dysplastic epithelium
- Discerning reactive from dysplastic cellular changes can be problematic

Transitional Epithelium

- Normal epithelium lying at transition between respiratory-type epithelium of supra- and subglottis and squamous epithelium of glottis
- On biopsy, may present diagnostic challenge with dysplastic epithelium
- Characterized by increased cellularity with lack of maturation but absence of nuclear pleomorphism, mitotic activity

Infectious Disease

- Presence of neutrophilic infiltrate along surface &/or within epithelium may indicate presence of fungi
- Special stains for fungi, including periodic acid-Schiff &/or Grocott methenamine silver indicated
  - Fungal forms (spores &/or hyphae) limited to superficial aspect of epithelium represents colonization
  - Fungal forms within depth of epithelium represents infestation and requires antifungal therapy
  - Fungal infestation may cause clinical and histopathologic lesion simulating squamous epithelial lesion

Microinvasive Carcinoma

- Diagnosis reserved for examples showing definitive evidence of dissociated squamous cells at epithelial-to-stromal interface with superficial invasion of lamina propria

SELECTED REFERENCES

1. Baumann JL et al: Human papillomavirus in early laryngeal carcinoma. Laryngoscope. 119(8):1531-7, 2009
2. Eversole LR: Dysplasia of the upper aerodigestive tract squamous epithelium. Head Neck Pathol. 3(1):63-8, 2009
3. Gale N et al: Current review on squamous intraepithelial lesions of the larynx. Histopathology. 54(6):639-56, 2009
4. Sadri M et al: Management of laryngeal dysplasia: a review. Eur Arch Otorhinolaryngol. 263(9):843-52, 2006
5. Wenig BM: Squamous cell carcinoma of the upper aerodigestive tract: precursors and problematic variants. Mod Pathol. 15(3):229-54, 2002
6. Gale N et al: The Ljubljana classification: a practical strategy for the diagnosis of laryngeal precancerous lesions. Adv Anat Pathol. 7(4):240-51, 2000
7. Blackwell KE et al: Laryngeal dysplasia: epidemiology and treatment outcome. Ann Otol Rhinol Laryngol. 104(8):596-602, 1995
8. Bouquot JE et al: Laryngeal precancer: a review of the literature, commentary, and comparison with oral leukoplakia. Head Neck. 13(6):488-97, 1991
9. Stenersen TC et al: Carcinoma in situ of the larynx: an evaluation of its natural clinical course. Clin Otolaryngol Allied Sci. 16(4):358-63, 1991
10. Crissman JD et al: Dysplasia, in situ carcinoma, and progression to invasive squamous cell carcinoma of the upper aerodigestive tract. Am J Surg Pathol. 13 Suppl 1:5-16, 1989
11. Crissman JD et al: Carcinoma in situ and microinvasive squamous carcinoma of the laryngeal glottis. Arch Otolaryngol Head Neck Surg. 114(3):299-307, 1988
12. Crissman JD et al: Preinvasive lesions of the upper aerodigestive tract: histologic definitions and clinical implications (a symposium). Pathol Annu. 22 Pt 1:311-52, 1987
13. Gillis TM et al: Natural history and management of keratosis, atypia, carcinoma-in situ, and microinvasive cancer of the larynx. Am J Surg. 146(4):512-6, 1983
14. Hellquist H et al: Hyperplasia, keratosis, dysplasia and carcinoma in situ of the vocal cords--a follow-up study. Clin Otolaryngol Allied Sci. 7(1):11-27, 1982

KERATINIZING DYSPLASIA AND CARCINOMA IN SITU

Classification Schemes for Epithelial Precursor Lesions

WHO Classification*	SIN	Ljubljana Classification
Mild dysplasia	SIN 1	Basal/parabasal cell hyperplasia
Moderate dysplasia	SIN 2	Atypical hyperplasia
Severe dysplasia**	SIN 3	Atypical hyperplasia
CIS	SIN 3	CIS

*CIS = carcinoma in situ. *Recommended classification scheme; **For all intents and purposes, severe dysplasia and CIS represent the same lesion.*

Histomorphologic Changes of Dysplasia

Cellular Abnormalities	Maturation Abnormalities
Nuclear pleomorphism with abnormal variation of nuclear size (anisonucleosis) and cell size (anisocytosis)	Loss of maturation
Nuclear hyperchromasia	Loss of cellular polarity
Increased mitotic activity, especially away from basal zone	Increased nuclear to cytoplasmic ratio
Atypical mitoses	Abnormal keratosis (dyskeratosis)
Prominent nucleoli	

In conjunction with cellular and maturation abnormalities, alterations in the architectural appearance, including elongated and irregular-appearing rete pegs, may factor in to the determination of the extent of dysplasia.

Upper Aerodigestive Tract Intraepithelial Dysplasia

Proposed 2-Tier Classification

Low-grade squamous intraepithelial lesion encompassing mild dysplasia

High-grade squamous intraepithelial lesion encompassing moderate and severe dysplasia*

**The risk of progression to invasive carcinoma relative to upper aerodigestive tract moderate dysplasia (approximately 23%) and severe dysplasia (approximately 28%) is not statistically significant. As such, consideration is being given to group moderate and severe dysplasia under a single category of high-grade squamous intraepithelial neoplasia akin to the Bethesda classification for uterine cervical dysplasias.*

KERATINIZING DYSPLASIA AND CARCINOMA IN SITU

Microscopic Features

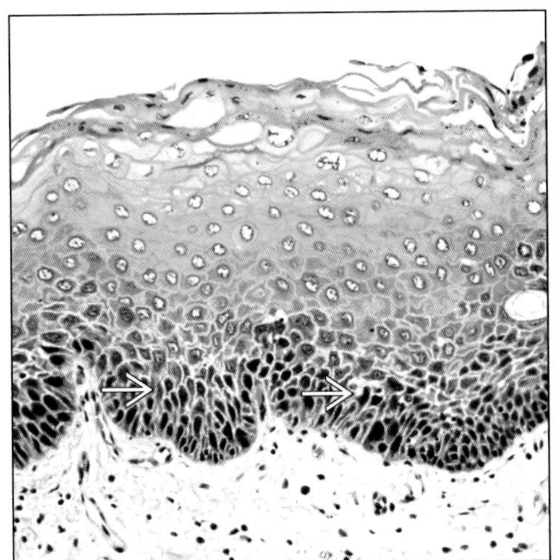

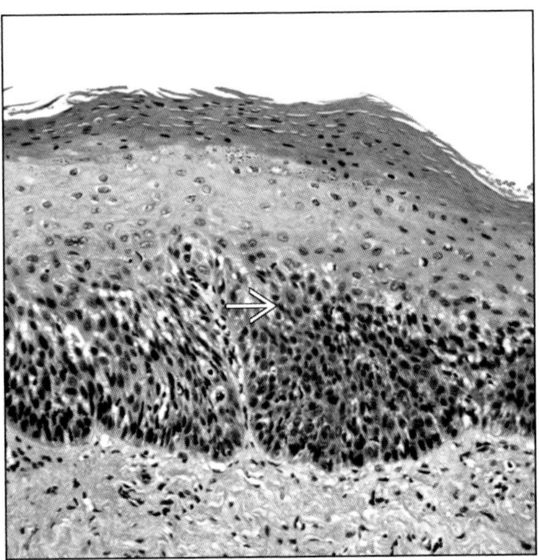

*(**Left**) Keratosis with mild dysplasia shows dysplastic epithelium ➡ that is limited to the basal zone (lower 1/3 of the thickness of the surface epithelium) with only slight elongation of the rete pegs. (**Right**) Keratosis is shown with moderate dysplasia in which the dysplastic epithelium ➡ involves 2/3 of the thickness of the surface epithelium. In addition, the rete pegs are slightly elongated but not extending downward into the submucosa.*

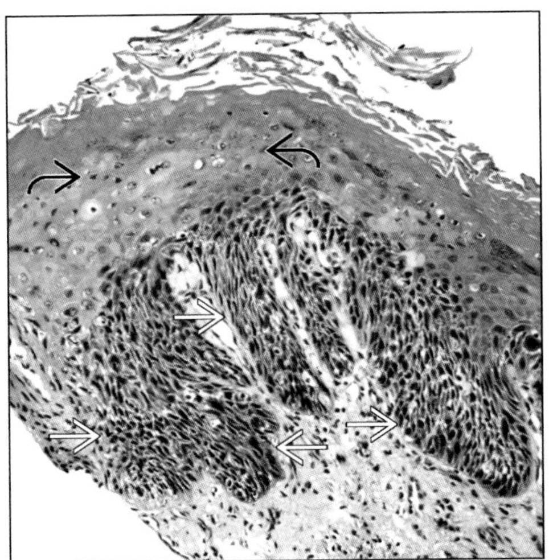

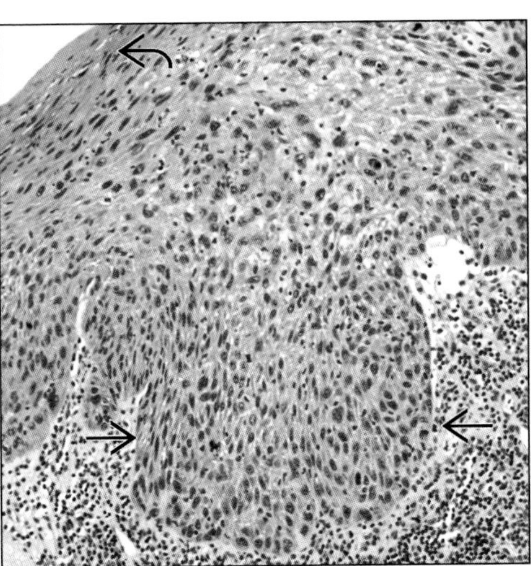

*(**Left**) Keratinizing severe dysplasia shows dysplastic alterations limited to the basal zone ➡ with surface maturation ↗. (**Right**) Keratinizing severe dysplasia shows dysplastic alterations limited to the basal zone ➡ with surface maturation ↗. These findings fall short of classically defined carcinoma in situ (full thickness dysplasia), but the architectural and cytomorphologic changes warrant a diagnosis of keratinizing severe dysplasia.*

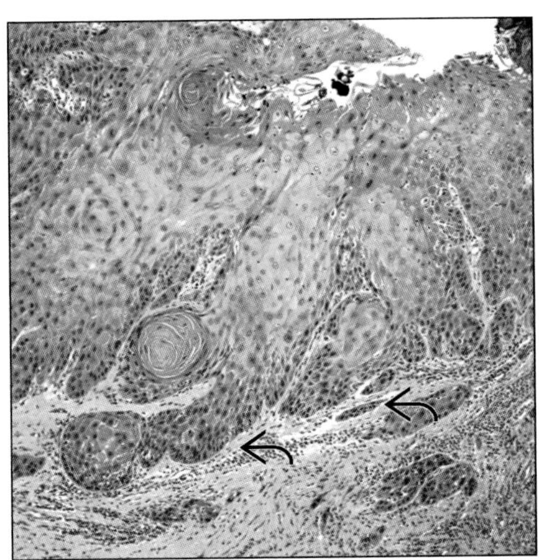

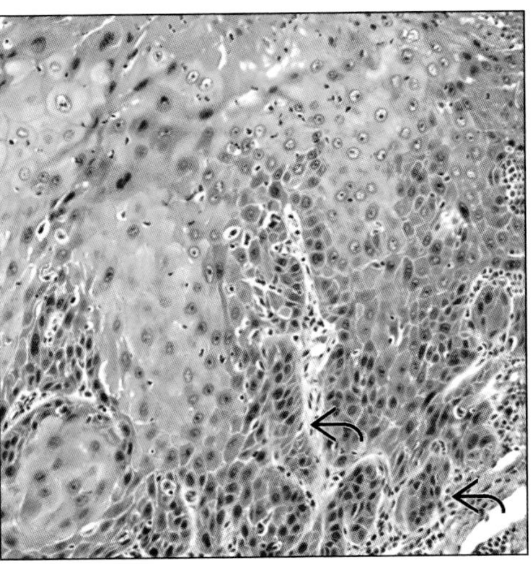

*(**Left**) Invasive squamous carcinoma ↗ is seen arising from keratinizing dysplasia in which the dysplasia is limited to the lower zone in the absence of full thickness dysplasia. Such an occurrence is the reason that the grading of keratinizing severe dysplasia is problematic, lacking reproducibility. (**Right**) Invasive squamous carcinoma ↗ develops from dysplasia limited to the lower 1/3 of the surface epithelium in the absence of full thickness dysplasia.*

KERATINIZING DYSPLASIA AND CARCINOMA IN SITU

Microscopic Features

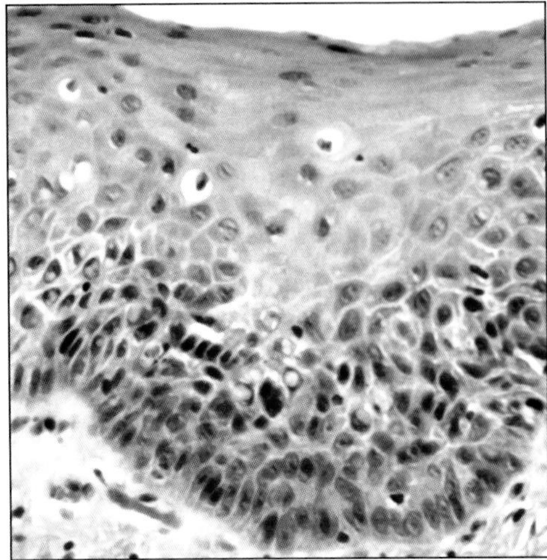

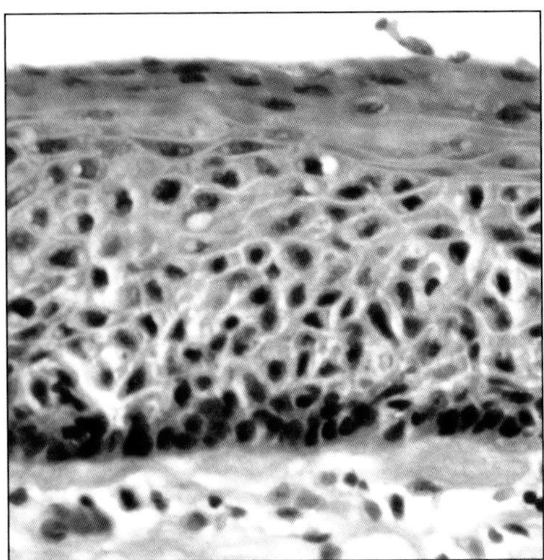

(Left) Laryngeal nonkeratinizing mild dysplasia is characterized by the dysplastic changes limited to the lower 1/3 of the surface epithelium. The grading in nonkeratinizing dysplastic lesions is similar to that of the uterine cervix and is more reproducible than keratinizing dysplasia. *(Right)* Laryngeal nonkeratinizing moderate dysplasia is characterized by the dysplastic changes involving 2/3 of the surface epithelium.

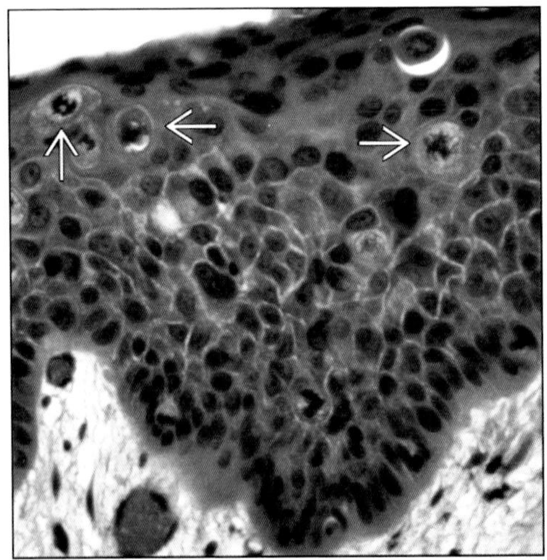

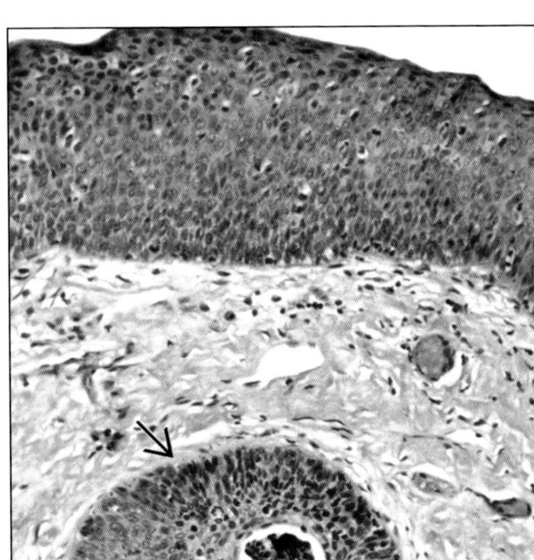

(Left) Nonkeratinizing severe dysplasia shows dysplastic changes involving the entire surface epithelium without violation of the basement membrane. Note the numerous mitotic figures ➔, including atypical forms well above the basal zone. These changes are synonymous with carcinoma in situ. *(Right)* Laryngeal nonkeratinizing severe dysplasia is shown with extension of the dysplasia to mucoserous gland ➔, a finding that still constitutes in situ changes and not invasive carcinoma.

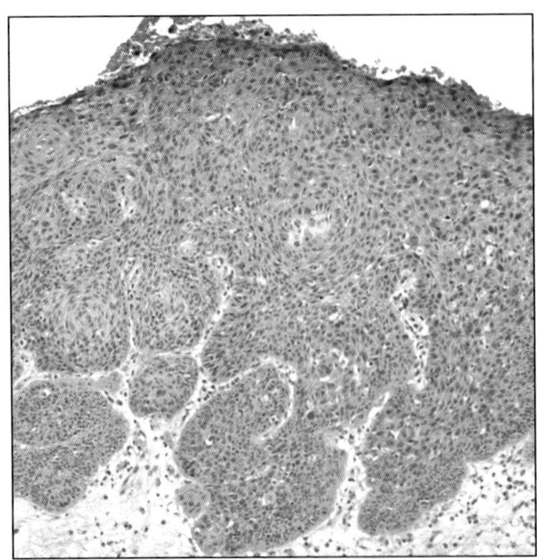

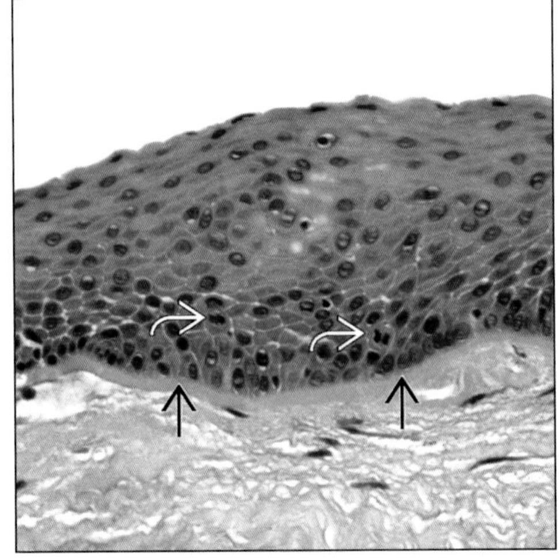

(Left) Invasive carcinoma developing from nonkeratinizing severe dysplasia conforms to classic carcinoma in situ. Such a finding is much less common than the development of invasive carcinoma from keratinizing dysplasia lacking full thickness dysplasia of the surface epithelium. *(Right)* Normal true vocal cord shows nonkeratinizing squamous epithelium characterized by cellular maturation. Normally, mitotic figures ➔ can be seen in the basal zone ➔ (proliferation zone).

Differential Diagnosis

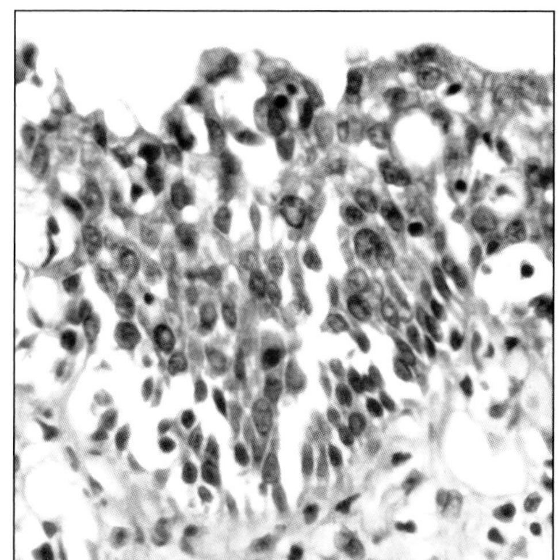

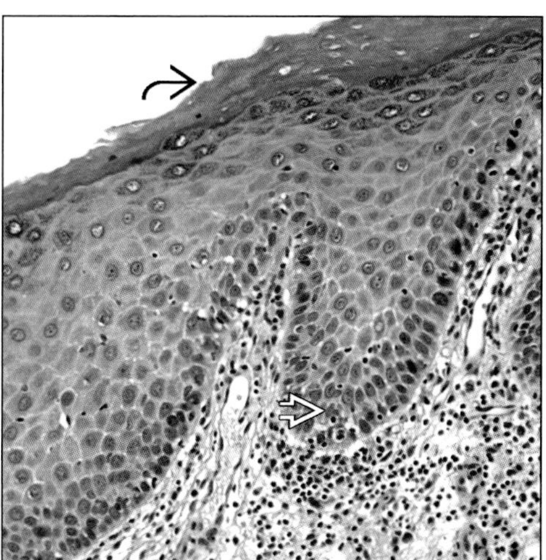

(Left) *Transitional-type epithelium predominantly composed of basaloid or immature squamous cells may be misdiagnosed as carcinoma in situ, but cells have vesicular nuclei, smooth nuclear contours, absence of significant pleomorphism, and absence of mitoses away from the basement membrane.* ***(Right)*** *Abnormal vocal cord epithelium shows surface keratinization ⮫, epithelial hyperplasia, and elongated rete pegs ➡ but absence of dysplasia. Clinically, this is a leukoplakic lesion.*

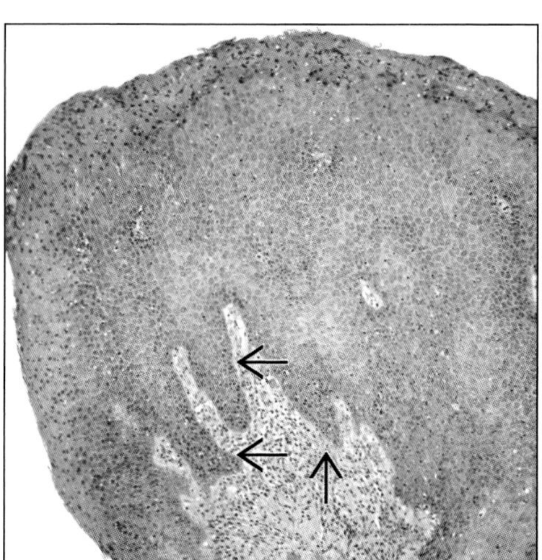

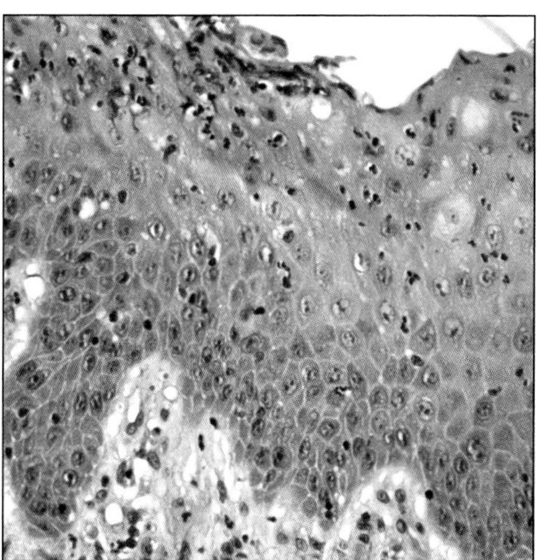

(Left) *Laryngeal leukoplakic lesion that was clinically suspicious for a carcinoma is shown. At low magnification there is a keratotic epithelial proliferation with downward extension of the rete pegs ➔ raising concern for a possible diagnosis of keratinizing dysplasia &/ or carcinoma.* ***(Right)*** *At higher magnification, there is reactive epithelial atypia but absent dysplasia and a neutrophilic infiltrate along the surface epithelium as well as throughout the epithelial layers.*

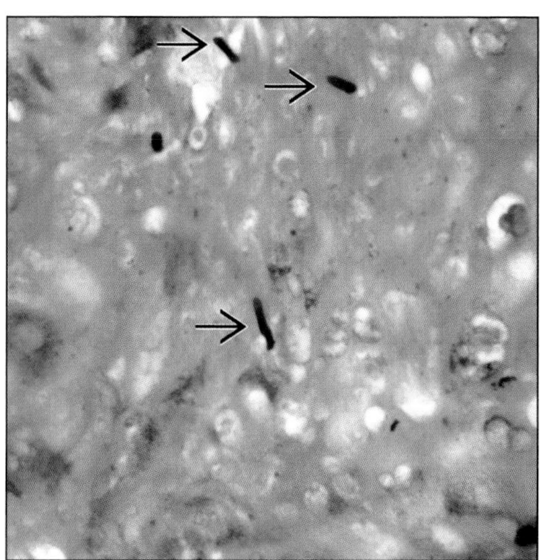

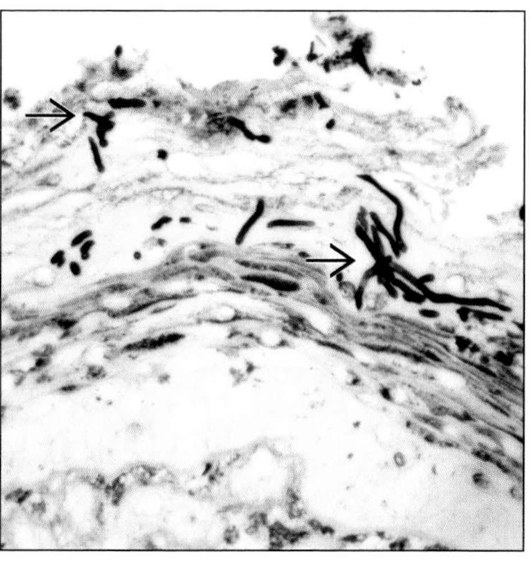

(Left) *Histochemical (GMS) staining shows the presence of fungal hyphae ➔ within the depth of the epithelium indicative of fungal infestation, the likely cause of the keratosis and irregular epithelial hyperplasia.* ***(Right)*** *In contrast to fungal infestation, fungal colonization shows the fungal forms ➔ limited to the surface &/or superficial aspects of the squamous epithelium but not in the depths of the surface epithelium.*

CONVENTIONAL SQUAMOUS CELL CARCINOMA

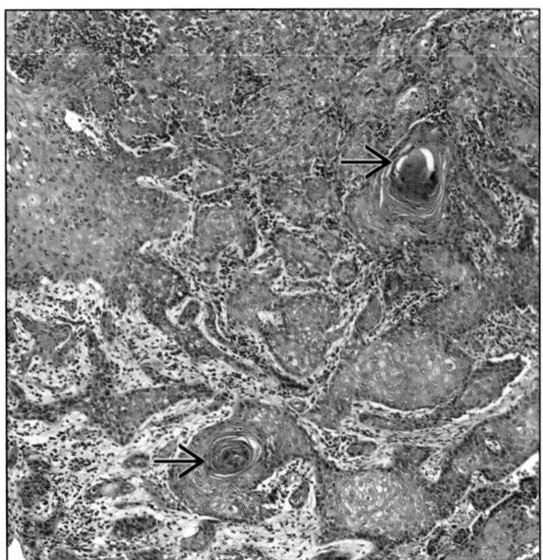

The characteristic features of squamous cell carcinoma include an infiltration into the stroma, abnormal keratinization →, irregular nests of squamous epithelium, and cellular pleomorphism.

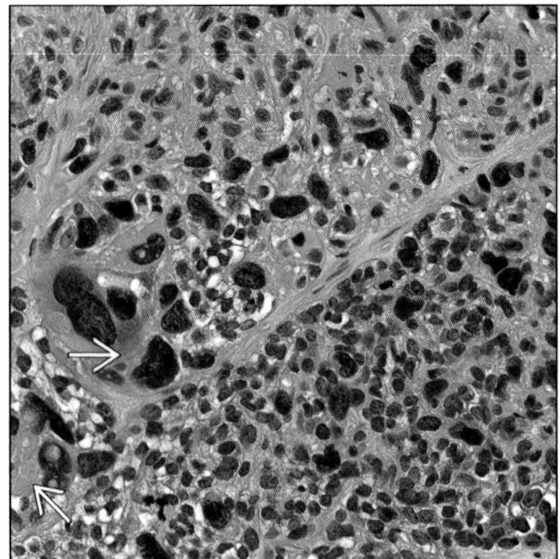

There are many cases where the degree of cytologic atypia can be quite profound. There is cytoplasmic opacification →, a feature highlighting squamous differentiation. There are bands of fibrosis.

TERMINOLOGY

Abbreviations

- Squamous cell carcinoma (SCC)

Synonyms

- Epidermoid carcinoma

Definitions

- Malignant neoplasm characterized by squamous cell differentiation

ETIOLOGY/PATHOGENESIS

Developmental Anomaly

- Genetic predisposition is uncommon, but immune deficiency and old age play a role
  - Lynch II syndrome, Bloom syndrome, Fanconi anemia, xeroderma pigmentosum, ataxia telangiectasia, and Li-Fraumeni syndrome are all associated with SCC

Environmental Exposure

- Tobacco (cigarette, cigar, pipe, smokeless) use
- Alcohol consumption
  - Independent of tobacco, but multiplicative if both are used
  - Maté drinking is a suggested risk factor
- Gastroesophageal reflux or laryngo-pharyngeal reflux (chronic inflammation as a mutagen)
- Radiation exposure (therapeutic and environmental)
- Occupational factors/exposures may play a role
- Protective effect by high intake of fruits and vegetables

Infectious Agents

- Human papilloma virus (HPV), HHV-8, Epstein-Barr virus may have a minor causative role (association vs. effect?)

Precursor Lesions

- SCC originates from squamous mucosa or metaplastic squamous mucosa
- Leukoplakia clinically: 50% show no dysplasia histologically
- Epithelium goes through arc of development to invasive carcinoma
  - Reactive/keratosis: 1-5% of patients develop SCC
  - Mild dysplasia: 6% of patients develop SCC
  - Moderate/severe dysplasia/CIS: 28% of patients develop SCC

Multifactorial

- All factors probably interact in multistep process

CLINICAL ISSUES

Epidemiology

- Incidence
  - About 1% of all cancers
    - 90% of head and neck cancers
  - > 95% of laryngeal malignancies
    - 10/100,000 men
    - 1/100,000 women
  - Slightly more common in urban than rural areas
  - Incidence is on the rise, presumably related to increases in tobacco and alcohol consumption
- Age
  - All ages affected
  - Mean: 6th to 7th decades
    - Children are rarely affected
- Gender
  - Male > > > Female (6:1)
- Ethnicity
  - Highest in European, South American, and USA blacks
  - Lowest in southeast Asians and central Africans

CONVENTIONAL SQUAMOUS CELL CARCINOMA

Key Facts

Etiology/Pathogenesis
- Tobacco & alcohol, gastroesophageal reflux

Clinical Issues
- Accounts for > 95% of laryngeal malignancies
- Affects men in 6th to 7th decades
- Supraglottic & glottic regions most commonly affected
- Treatment includes surgery &/or radiation
- TNM classification (site, size, and stage) correlates significantly with disease-free and overall survival
  - Resection margins, lymph-vascular and perineural invasion, lymph node metastases, and extracapsular lymph node spread

Microscopic Pathology
- Histologic categories: In situ or invasive
  - Expansive vs. jagged, single cell infiltration
- Grade: Well, moderately, or poorly differentiated
  - Disorganized growth, loss of polarity, loss of maturation
  - Increased nuclear to cytoplasmic ratio, nuclear chromatin irregularities, prominent nucleoli
  - Increased mitoses, atypical mitoses
  - Desmoplastic stroma, inflammatory infiltrate
- Dyskeratosis, paradoxical pearl formation
- Margins must be reported

Top Differential Diagnoses
- Pseudoepitheliomatous hyperplasia, radiation changes, variants of SCC, squamous papilloma, necrotizing sialometaplasia

Site
- Supraglottic and glottic regions are most common
- Geographic differences
  - In Europe (France, Spain, Italy, Finland, the Netherlands): Supraglottic SCC predominates
  - In USA, England, and Sweden: Glottic SCC predominates
  - In Japan: No differences noted

Presentation
- Glottic tumors: Hoarseness is earliest symptom
- Supraglottic &/or hypopharyngeal tumors: Dysphagia, changes in phonation, foreign body sensation in throat, and odynophagia
- Subglottic tumors: Dyspnea and stridor most common
- Tracheal tumors: Dyspnea, stridor (wheezing), cough, and hemoptysis most common
- Neck mass (lymph nodes) more common in transglottic tumors

Endoscopic Findings
- Imaging studies should always precede endoscopy
  - Endoscopy may cause edema and decrease accuracy of image studies
- Evaluate extent of disease, document synchronous primaries (seen in up to 10% of patients), and obtain a biopsy
- Well-defined, exophytic, polypoid, flat, or endophytic mass
- Rolled, raised borders vs. abrupt, irregular borders
- Leukoplakia, erythroplakia, tan
- Ulceration may be present

Laboratory Tests
- Hepatic function (evaluation for possible metastatic disease)

Treatment
- Options, risks, complications
  - Treatment goals include cure, voice sparing (preservation), optimal swallowing, and minimal xerostomia
    - Larynx functions include phonation, respiration, deglutition, air humidification, and contributes to taste and smell
  - Clinical stage and site play important role in patient management
  - Important factors: Pathologic diagnosis, local tumor extent, regional lymph node status, and distant metastasis
  - Stomal recurrence is infrequent complication (subglottic and postcricoid tumors)
  - Treatment options include surgery &/or radiation
- Surgical approaches
  - Surgical removal of tumor
    - Transoral laser microsurgery, vocal cord stripping, limited resection, open partial laryngectomy, total laryngectomy, &/or neck dissection
    - Movement toward noninvasive, nondestructive management
- Adjuvant therapy
  - Neoadjuvant chemotherapy rarely employed to maintain larynx function
- Radiation
  - Radiotherapy: Definitive and postoperative
  - External beam radiation, including brachytherapy

Prognosis
- TNM classification (site, size, and stage) correlates most closely and significantly with disease-free status and overall survival
  - **T1**: 90% 5-year survival rate
  - **T4**: < 50% 5-year survival rate
  - **Glottic**: 80-85% 5-year survival rate
  - **Supraglottic**: 65-75% 5-year survival rate
  - **Subglottic**: 40% 5-year survival rate
  - **Tracheal**: 50% 5-year survival rate
- Resection margins
  - Negative resection margins associated with decreased recurrence and improved survival
  - Exact distance difficult to determine: Generally > 3-5 mm considered adequate
- Lymph-vascular invasion

CONVENTIONAL SQUAMOUS CELL CARCINOMA

- Vessel invasion associated with increased lymph node &/or distant metastases
  - Associated with recurrence and poor survival
- Perineural invasion
  - Intra- and perineural invasion associated with increased local recurrence and regional lymph node metastases
  - Associated with decreased survival
- Regional lymph node metastases are relatively common
- Extracapsular spread in lymph node metastases
  - Presence of lymph node metastasis is **single most adverse prognostic factor**
  - Carcinoma penetrating lymph node capsule and infiltrating extracapsular tissue
    - Extracapsular spread is divided into macroscopic and microscopic
    - **Macroscopic**: Identified by naked eye (matted lymph nodes)
    - **Microscopic**: Only identified histologically
  - Extracapsular extension in lymph nodes is strongly associated with both regional recurrence and distant metastases, both associated with decreased survival
- Proliferation fraction
  - Higher proliferation index (MIB-1/Ki-67) strongly correlates with poorly differentiated tumors and lymph node metastases
  - It is **not** an independent prognostic factor
- Hematogenous metastases are uncommon, usually late in disease
  - Distant spread: Lung, followed by liver and bone
- Up to 25% mortality (site and stage dependent)
- If "limited" interventions fail, then delayed, salvage, partial or total laryngectomy can still achieve a good outcome
- Additional prognostic factors include age, comorbidity (concurrent diseases), and performance status
- Prognostic markers
  - *EGFR* (epidermal growth factor receptor) and cyclin-D1 overexpression associated with worse clinical outcome
    - *EGFR* status is only useful for patients treated by induction chemotherapy followed by exclusive radiotherapy and not with laryngectomy
  - *CCND1* amplification is associated with poor prognosis
  - Simultaneous *CDK4* and *CCND1* overexpression is associated with poor prognosis
  - *CDKN2A* mutations are associated with poor prognosis (in advanced tumors)

IMAGE FINDINGS

General Features

- Computed tomography (CT), magnetic resonance imaging (MR), and PET (positron emission tomography) document extent and location of disease
  - Studies highlight submucosal invasion patterns
  - Demonstrate preepiglottic space, paraglottic space, and laryngeal cartilages extension
    - These parameters are helpful in staging the tumor
- Imaging studies of lung and bones may help to document metastatic disease

MACROSCOPIC FEATURES

General Features

- Supraglottis, glottis, and subglottis are embryologically distinct and separately compartmentalized
  - Lymphatic drainage is unique for each location
  - Glottic tumors: Tend to be smaller (have earlier clinical presentation)
  - Supraglottic tumors: Reach larger size before clinical presentation
- Erythematous to white to tan
- Flat, well-defined, raised edge, polypoid, exophytic, verrucous or endophytic, and ulcerated
- Firm to friable on palpation

Size

- Minute mucosal thickening to large masses filling lumen
- Mean: ~ 2 cm

MICROSCOPIC PATHOLOGY

Histologic Features

- SCC is generally divided into a number of categories
  - Histologic categories: In situ, superficially invasive, or deeply invasive
  - Histologic grade: Well, moderately, or poorly differentiated
  - Keratinization: Present or absent
- Surface epithelium confined by basement membrane: In situ tumor
- Invasion manifested by extension through and disruption of basement membrane: Superficially vs. deeply invasive tumor
  - Invasion may be seen without atypical surface epithelium
  - Broad (expansive) infiltration: Large tumor islands with well-defined pushing margins
  - Jagged, scattered, irregular cords or individual/single cell infiltration with poorly defined margin
  - Type of border of infiltration associated with prognosis (jagged is worse)
- Variable degrees of squamous differentiation
  - Disorganized growth
  - Loss of polarity and lack of maturation
  - Dyskeratosis and keratin pearl formation, especially at base (paradoxical keratinization)
  - Intercellular bridges easily identified
  - Increased nuclear to cytoplasmic ratio
  - Nuclear chromatin irregularities (coarse, hyperchromatic)
  - Prominent eosinophilic nucleoli
  - Increased mitotic figures
  - Atypical mitoses
- Inflammatory infiltrate (usually lymphocytes, plasma cells) present at tumor to stroma junction
- Dense, desmoplastic fibrous stroma

- Deposition of extracellular matrix and proliferation of fibroblasts
- Perineural and vascular invasion should be documented when present
  - Correlates with management &/or outcome
- Keratinizing-type SCC is seen more frequently than nonkeratinizing or poorly differentiated types
- Mitotic figures and necrosis increase as grade increases
- May spread directly to contiguous structures
  - Supraglottic: Piriform sinus, base of tongue, thyroid cartilage
  - Glottic: Opposite true vocal cord, supraglottis and subglottis, thyroid cartilage, and neck soft tissue
  - Subglottic: Thyroid gland, hypopharynx, cervical esophagus, and tracheal wall
  - Transglottic: Crosses ventricles, involving supraglottis and glottis

Lymphatic/Vascular Invasion

- Prognostic factor, associated with worse prognosis

Margins

- Must be reported
- Shrinkage (up to 50%) after removal must be taken into consideration
- Assessed by frozen section vs. permanent sections
  - Post-removal (artifactual) shrinkage
  - Margin status affects recurrence and patient outcome
  - Larynx functional preservation
  - Bone margins difficult to assess

Lymph Nodes

- Must be reported
- Especially if extracapsular lymph node extension by tumor (worse prognosis)

ANCILLARY TESTS

Cytology

- Not usually performed on primary larynx tumor
- May be used in lymph node assessment

Frozen Sections

- 5 areas result in possible errors
  - Inaccurate communication
    - Must have clear, open, levelheaded, and direct communication
    - Physical presence in operating room or gross laboratory, by surgeon &/or pathologist respectively, achieves best result
  - Indications for intraoperative assessment
    - Submit only a portion of tissue when specimen adequacy is assessed to allocate tissue for special procedures (cultures, molecular studies, ultrastructural examination, flow cytometry)
    - Different definitive therapy would be performed
    - Numerous previous attempts at diagnosis have been unsuccessful
    - Assessing surgical margins
    - **Never** performed for intellectual or academic curiosity, gamesmanship, family reassurance, financial gain, or rote examination
    - Should be avoided for primary diagnosis
  - Inadequate sampling (by surgeon or pathologist)
    - Proper orientation is extremely important
    - Use of sutures or tissue pen to orient specimen margins is crucial
    - Take multiple sections from main specimen
  - Incorrect interpretation
    - Epithelial lesions, such as hyperplasia, pseudoepitheliomatous hyperplasia, radiation changes, and SCC (verrucous and spindle cell types) can be misinterpreted
    - Mesenchymal and inflammatory lesions need deep tissue samples
    - Lack of clinical history (previous radiation, chemotherapy, &/or surgery) may result in error
    - While a personal bias, it is better to err on the side of benignancy and delay definitive therapy rather than perform radical surgery for benign disease
  - Technical difficulties
    - Specimens must be received fresh (not in formalin), kept moist with sterile, saline-soaked gauze
    - Calcified and fatty tissues cannot be easily cut
    - Small samples may be exhausted in preparation of frozen section
    - Cryostat difficulties to poor staining quality can result in technical problems
- SCC expresses epithelial markers, such as cytokeratins
- Specific keratin subtypes may relate to histologic grade, degree of keratinization, and likelihood of metastases

Cytogenetics

- Cytogenetics and comparative genomic hybridization (CGH) show +3q21-29 and -3p most commonly
- *CCND1* (at 11q13) is amplified and overexpressed; expression is lower in metastatic tumors
  - Gene expression silencing of *CDH1* by promoter hypermethylation is more frequent in metastatic tumors
- *MMP13* expression and *MMP14* overexpression are associated with advanced tumors
- *EGFR* may be amplified but it is not overexpressed
- *P53* mutations are early event in SCC but not a prognostic marker
- Losses at 8p, 9q, and 13 are more frequent in metastatic than in primary tumors
- Molecular margins are not yet determined in routine daily practice

Electron Microscopy

- SCC exhibits desmosomes, hemidesmosomes, and attached tonofilaments

DIFFERENTIAL DIAGNOSIS

Pseudoepitheliomatous Hyperplasia (PEH)

- Benign reactive proliferation of elongated, rounded, bulbous epithelial projections, associated with infections and granular cell tumor
- Cellular atypia or nuclear pleomorphism is absent

CONVENTIONAL SQUAMOUS CELL CARCINOMA

Immunohistochemistry

Antibody	Reactivity	Staining Pattern	Comment
AE1/AE3	Positive	Cytoplasmic	Nearly all tumor cells
CK1	Positive	Cytoplasmic	In most carcinomas
CK-HMW-NOS	Positive	Cytoplasmic	**Low-grade** tumors tend to express HMW keratins
CK-LMW-NOS	Positive	Cytoplasmic	**High-grade** tumors tend to express LMW keratins
CK8/18/CAM5.2	Positive	Cytoplasmic	**High-grade** tumors tend to show expression
CK5/6	Positive	Cytoplasmic	May highlight the membranes
CK10	Positive	Cytoplasmic	Positive in most carcinomas
p63	Positive	Nuclear	**High-grade** tumors tend to show reaction
p16	Positive	Nuclear & cytoplasmic	Rarely positive
CK7	Positive	Cytoplasmic	Most tumors of the larynx
EMA	Positive	Cytoplasmic	Variably reactive but usually limited or weak
p53	Positive	Nuclear & cytoplasmic	About 75% of tumors; correlated with lymph node metastases
EGFR	Positive	Cell membrane & cytoplasm	Upregulation (expression) may be useful in chemotherapy regimen choice
CK20	Negative		

Squamous Cell Carcinoma Grading

Grade	Features
Grade 1 (well differentiated)	Resembles normal squamous epithelium but shows invasion
Grade 2 (moderately differentiated)	Easily identified nuclear pleomorphism, loss of polarity, disorganization, increased mitotic activity, usually less keratinization
Grade 3 (poorly differentiated)	Immature cells predominate, high nuclear to cytoplasmic ratio, limited keratinization, numerous typical and atypical mitoses

Radiation Changes

- Epithelial, endothelial, and stromal cells affected
- Profound nuclear pleomorphism, but enlarged cells have low nuclear to cytoplasmic ratio
- Glands may become atrophic; vessels may be hyperplastic; stroma contains isolated atypical cells

Variants of Squamous Cell Carcinoma

- Basaloid SCC has peripheral palisade, small, basaloid cells, comedonecrosis, only focal keratinization
- Verrucous SCC shows papillary projections and bulbous invaginations, lacking cytological atypia

Squamous Papilloma

- No disorganized growth, no invasion, and lacks pleomorphism

Necrotizing Sialometaplasia

- Lobular architecture maintained, associated necrosis, variable cytologic atypia, mucocytes can be seen
- Must have biopsy of sufficient size

STAGING

TNM System (AJCC and UICC)

- Stage is one of most important prognostic considerations
- Most patients present with pT1 or pT2 tumors

SELECTED REFERENCES

1. Gale N et al: Current review on squamous intraepithelial lesions of the larynx. Histopathology. 54(6):639-56, 2009
2. Lefebvre JL et al: Larynx preservation clinical trial design: key issues and recommendations--a consensus panel summary. Head Neck. 31(4):429-41, 2009
3. Becker M et al: Imaging of the larynx and hypopharynx. Eur J Radiol. 66(3):460-79, 2008
4. Chang AR et al: Expression of epidermal growth factor receptor and cyclin D1 in pretreatment biopsies as a predictive factor of radiotherapy efficacy in early glottic cancer. Head Neck. 30(7):852-7, 2008
5. Chu EA et al: Laryngeal cancer: diagnosis and preoperative work-up. Otolaryngol Clin North Am. 41(4):673-95, v, 2008
6. Isenberg JS et al: Institutional and comprehensive review of laryngeal leukoplakia. Ann Otol Rhinol Laryngol. 117(1):74-9, 2008
7. Galli J et al: Laryngeal carcinoma and laryngo-pharyngeal reflux disease. Acta Otorhinolaryngol Ital. 26(5):260-3, 2006
8. Heffner DK: Infinitesimals, quantum mechanics, and exiguous carcinomas: how to possibly save a patient's larynx. Ann Diagn Pathol. 7(3):187-94, 2003
9. Koren R et al: The spectrum of laryngeal neoplasia: the pathologist's view. Pathol Res Pract. 198(11):709-15, 2002
10. Kau RJ et al: Diagnostic procedures for detection of lymph node metastases in cancer of the larynx. ORL J Otorhinolaryngol Relat Spec. 62(4):199-203, 2000
11. Batsakis JG: Surgical excision margins: a pathologist's perspective. Adv Anat Pathol. 6(3):140-8, 1999

Diagrammatic, Gross, and Microscopic Features

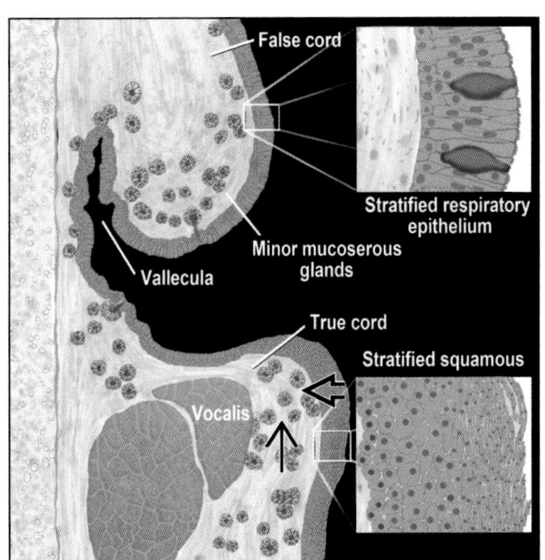

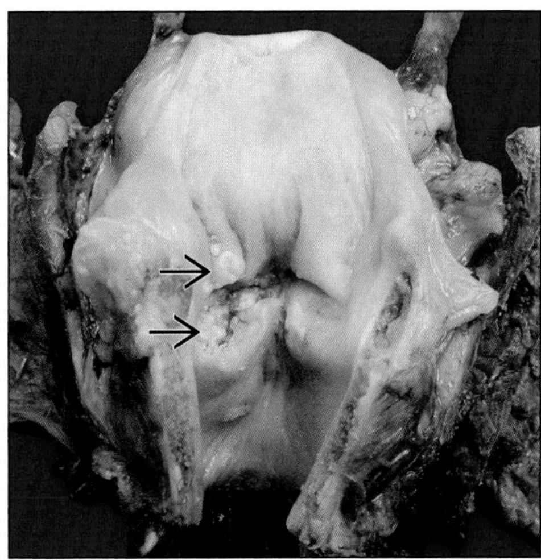

*(**Left**) This graphic shows the normal histology of the larynx, with a transition from pseudostratified respiratory to squamous type epithelium. Reinke space ⇨ is adjacent to the conus elasticus →, which overlies the vocalis muscle. (**Right**) This laryngectomy specimen demonstrates a transglottic → tumor. The exophytic tumor involves the vocal cords, subglottic and supraglottic spaces. The specimen has been opened in the midline posteriorly. (Courtesy J.C. Fowler, MPAS, PA-C.)*

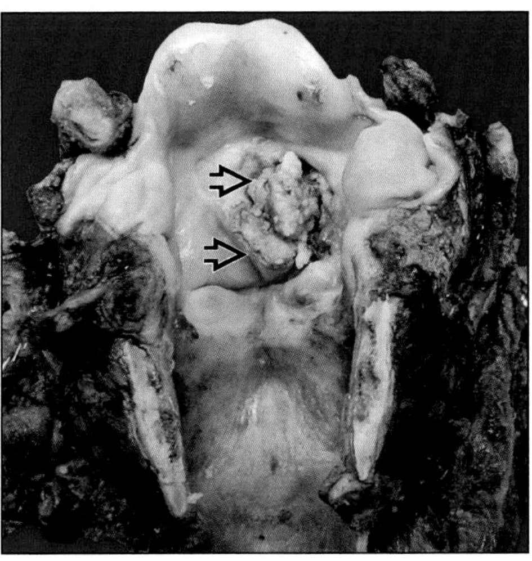

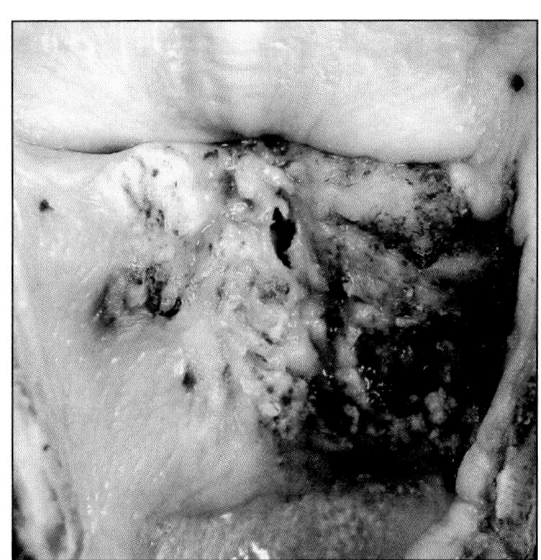

*(**Left**) The squamous cell carcinoma is within the supraglottis ⇨. The tumor is exophytic, although showing multiple projections of tissue into the laryngeal lumen. There is no involvement of the true vocal cord. (Courtesy J.C. Fowler, MPAS, PA-C.) (**Right**) This tumor only involves the subglottic space. This is an uncommon occurrence. There is significant ulceration and tissue destruction. The tumor has an irregular border. (Courtesy J.C. Fowler, MPAS, PA-C.)*

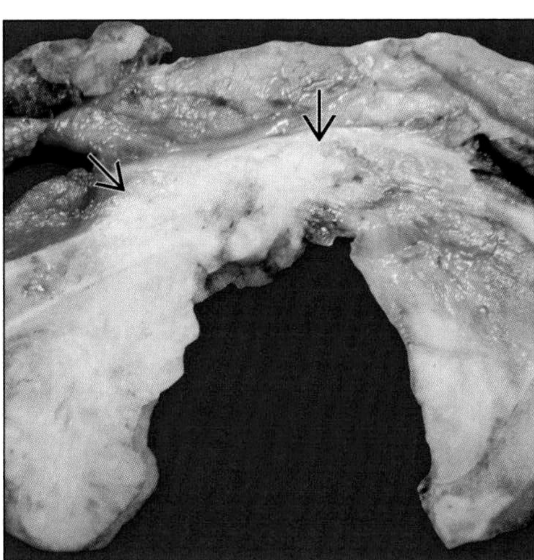

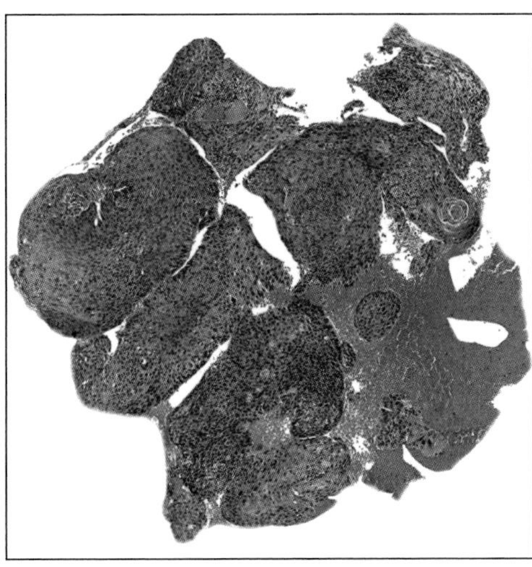

*(**Left**) Cross section through a laryngectomy specimen demonstrates tumor that invades into and destroys the cartilage →. The tumor appears white and is firm to palpation. (Courtesy J.C. Fowler, MPAS, PA-C.) (**Right**) Many biopsies contain multiple fragments of tissue. There is very scant stroma-tumor interface in this specimen. Note the atypical epithelial proliferation. However, even though this may be diagnostic of SCC in situ, invasion requires inclusion of the stroma in the sample.*

CONVENTIONAL SQUAMOUS CELL CARCINOMA

Microscopic Features

(Left) *Invasive squamous cell carcinoma shows broad, tongue-like projections of the epithelium into the underlying stroma. This pattern of infiltration has a better prognosis than the more "jagged" or irregular pattern.* ***(Right)*** *The invasive pattern in this tumor is of individual cells and small nests within a desmoplastic-type stroma. Cytologic atypia is easily identified. The sheet-like pattern can sometimes obscure the invasive nature of the lesion.*

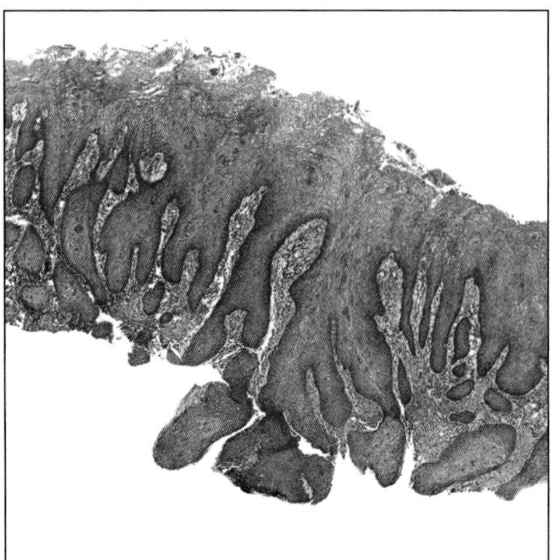

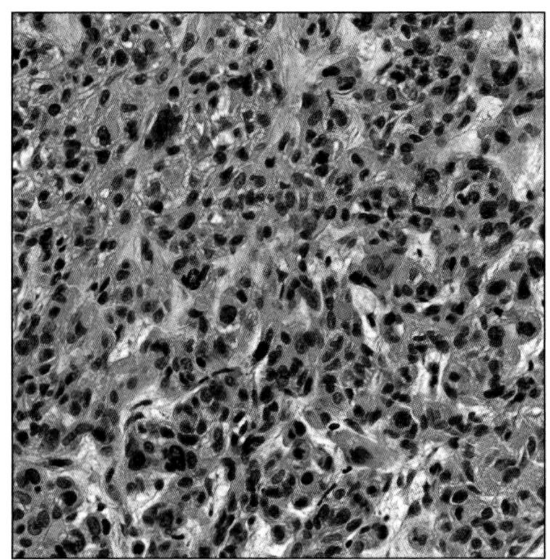

(Left) *Well-differentiated squamous cell carcinoma shows easily recognized squamous epithelium, invading into the stroma in a destructive pattern. Note the inflammatory infiltrate ➔.* ***(Right)*** *This poorly differentiated squamous cell carcinoma still shows isolated cells with keratinization ➔. Note the "inky-black" atypical nuclei. There is uninvolved minor mucoserous glands ➔, a finding that is frequently present in supraglottic tumors.*

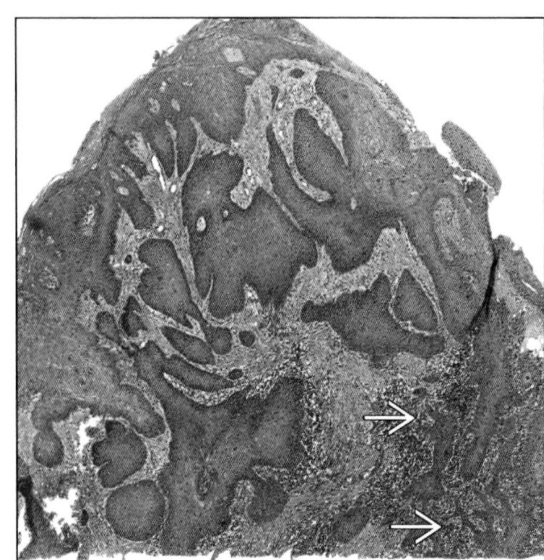

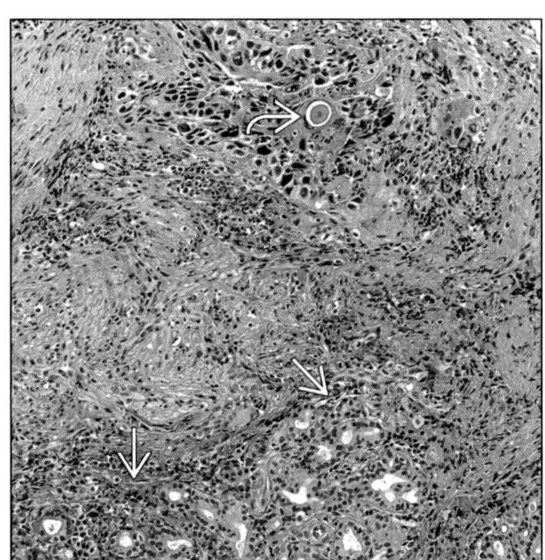

(Left) *Desmoplastic stroma has a slightly different tinctural quality than fibrosis or degenerative change. There are fibroblasts present within the stroma. Note the isolated small nests and strands of squamous epithelium ➔.* ***(Right)*** *It is not uncommon to have a SCC that does not show involvement of the surface epithelium. There is a grenz ➔ zone between the mucosa and the tumor. Note the remarkable pleomorphism ➔ in this poorly differentiated squamous cell carcinoma.*

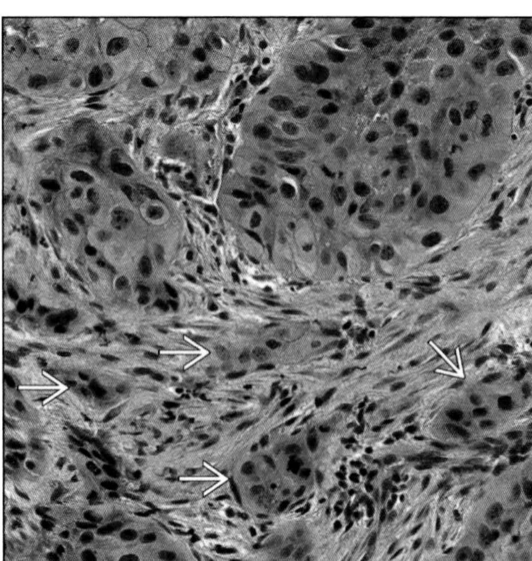

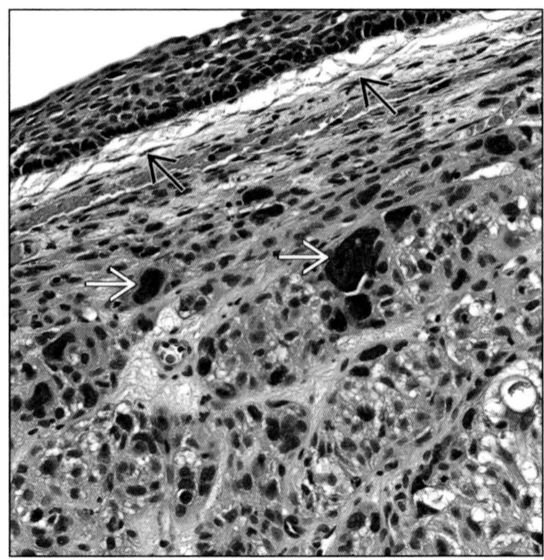

Microscopic and Immunohistochemical Features

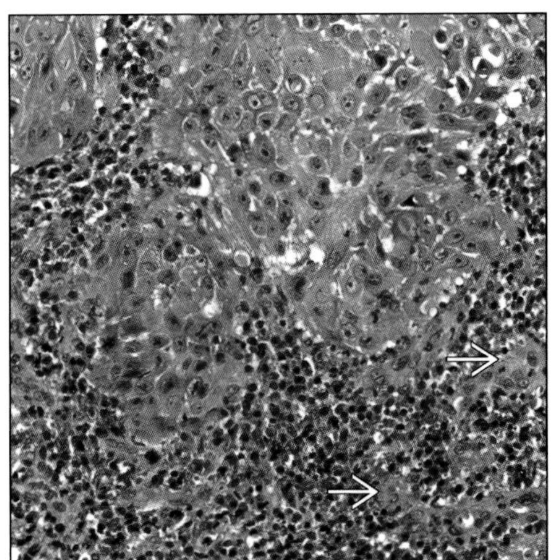

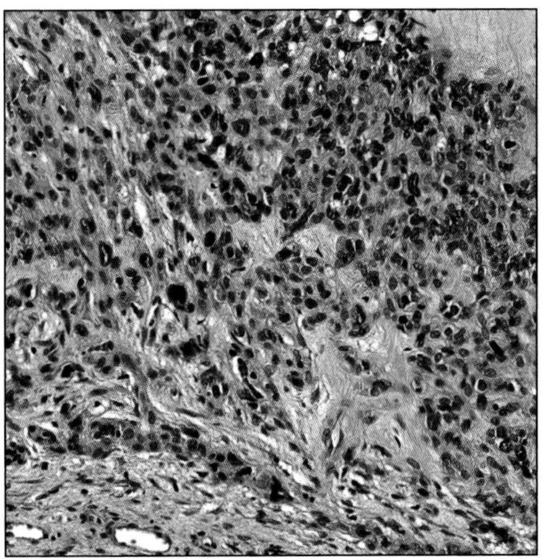

(Left) *The "blending" of the tumor cells with the inflammatory infiltrate can sometimes make the assessment of invasion challenging. In this case, the individual cells* ➡ *and cellular pleomorphism help to support the diagnosis of carcinoma.* ***(Right)*** *The basal region of a SCC can be subtle to assess, especially if there has been tangential sectioning. The strips, ribbons, and streams of epithelial cells in the slightly bluish, desmoplastic stroma can help with the diagnosis of invasion.*

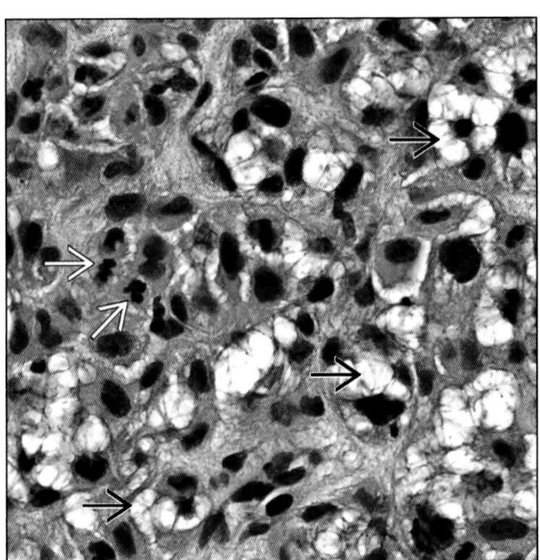

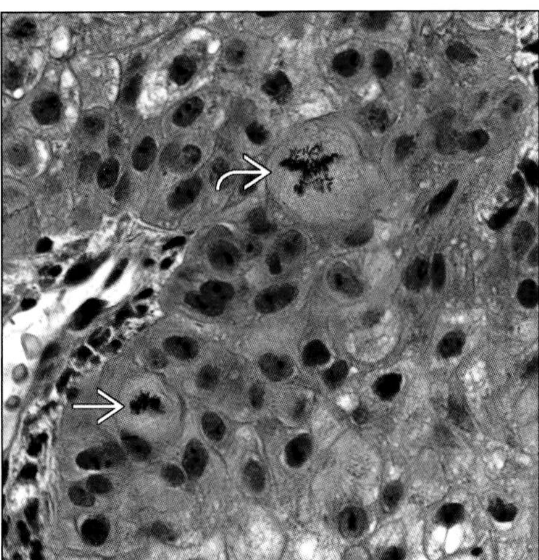

(Left) *Squamous differentiation can be confirmed when there are intercellular bridges* ⇨ *(retraction artifact between adjacent cells). Many times these will appear as "ladders" or "strands" between cells. Note the mitoses* ➡*.* ***(Right)*** *Increased mitotic figures are usually easy to identify in SCC* ➡*. Atypical mitoses* ➦ *help to confirm the diagnosis of a malignancy, although atypical mitoses can be seen in a variety of different malignancies.*

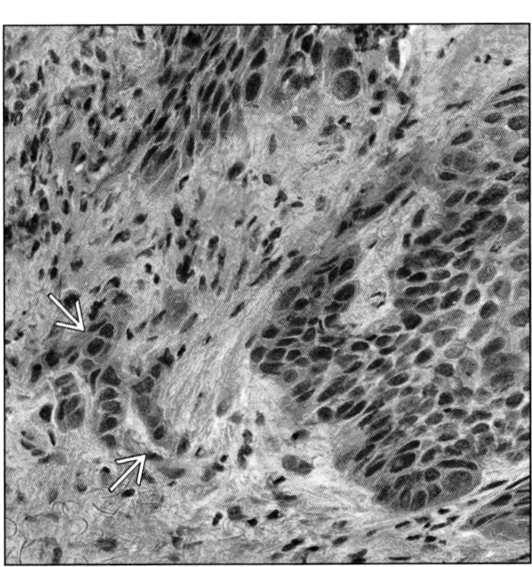

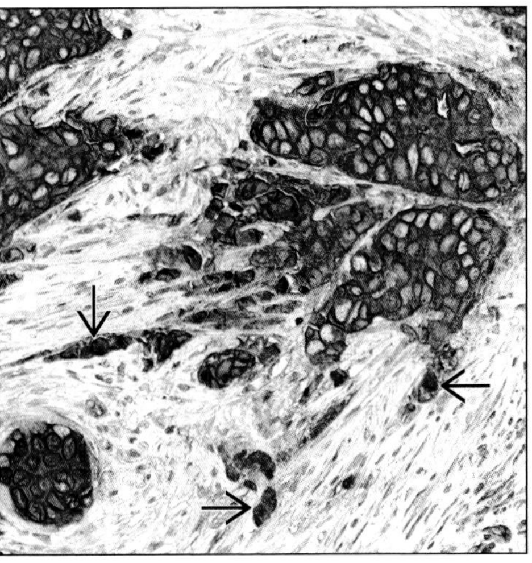

(Left) *Frozen section shows an irregular and invasive neoplasm* ➡ *in which the squamous differentiation can be seen. This would be interpreted as a positive margin if present in the frozen margin section. There is atypia beyond what would be expected in a benign condition.* ***(Right)*** *Immunohistochemistry is seldom necessary to confirm squamous differentiation. CK5/6 stain highlights the epithelial cells within the desmoplastic stroma* ⇨*. Other keratins may have similar results.*

VERRUCOUS SQUAMOUS CELL CARCINOMA

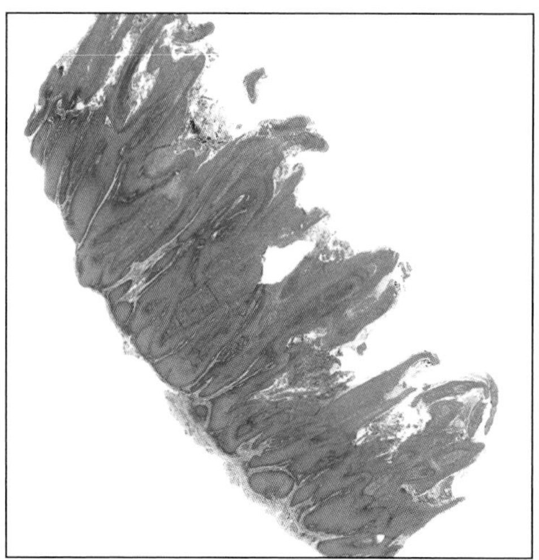

A low-power view shows a highly differentiated, exophytic, warty squamous neoplasm with pushing borders. There are papillary projections associated with extensive keratosis. This is an adequate biopsy.

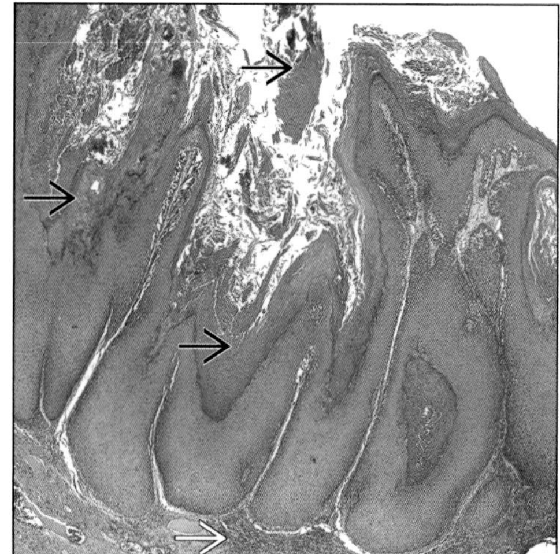

Broadly implanted, blunt-based, club-shaped papillae show maturation toward the surface. There is significant keratosis ⇒, with a dense lymphoplasmacytic inflammatory basal response ➡.

TERMINOLOGY

Abbreviations

- Verrucous squamous cell carcinoma (VSCC)

Synonyms

- Ackerman tumor
- Verrucous acanthosis

Definitions

- Highly differentiated, low-grade squamous cell carcinoma variant characterized by exophytic, warty neoplasm with pushing borders and cytologically bland, amitotic squamous epithelium

ETIOLOGY/PATHOGENESIS

Environmental Exposure

- Strong association with tobacco and alcohol abuse

Infectious Agents

- Human papillomavirus (HPV) genotypes 16 and 18 (rarely 6 and 11) are identified in some VSCC

CLINICAL ISSUES

Epidemiology

- Incidence
  - Comprises up to 4% of all laryngeal SCC
- Age
  - Mean: 6th and 7th decades
- Gender
  - Male > Female (4:1)
    - In oral cavity, Female > Male (3:2)

Site

- Larynx is 2nd most common site of VSCC
  - Oral cavity is most commonly affected (56%), then larynx (35%), sinonasal tract, and nasopharynx
  - Accounts for 15-35% of all VSCC
- Glottis, specifically anterior true vocal cords
  - Supraglottis, subglottis, hypopharynx, and trachea uncommonly affected

Presentation

- Long-lasting hoarseness is most common symptom
- Other symptoms include airway obstruction, weight loss, dysphagia, and throat pain
- Enlarged lymph nodes are common, but they are reactive rather than neoplastic

Endoscopic Findings

- "Benign" papilloma-like appearance makes initial diagnosis difficult and may delay treatment
- Broad-based, fungating, firm mass
- May have extensive surrounding leukoplakia
- Surface ulceration uncommon

Treatment

- Options, risks, complications
  - Voice preservation strategies are encouraged
  - Even though neck lymph nodes appear enlarged, they are reactive, not representing metastatic disease
    - No neck dissection indicated
  - Surgery alone seems to yield best outcome
  - Radiotherapy
    - Theoretic risk of post-radiation anaplastic transformation
    - Rarely, post-radiation neoplasm may develop
- Surgical approaches
  - Early (T1 or T2) tumors treated by local excision
    - Endoscopic resection (carbon dioxide [CO_2] laser) or extended laser cordectomy
  - More aggressive procedures for extensive or recurrent tumors
    - Partial or total laryngectomy
- Adjuvant therapy
  - Rarely, chemotherapy and concomitant radiation for nonsurgical candidates
- Radiation

VERRUCOUS SQUAMOUS CELL CARCINOMA

Key Facts

Terminology
- Highly differentiated, low-grade SCC variant characterized by exophytic growth with pushing borders and cytologically bland, amitotic squamous epithelium

Etiology/Pathogenesis
- Strong association with tobacco and alcohol abuse, occasionally with HPV

Clinical Issues
- Affects glottis, specifically anterior true vocal cords
- Surgery alone seems to yield best outcome
- ~ 20% recurrence/persistence rate overall (treatment dependent)
- Pure VSCC does **not** metastasize

Macroscopic Features
- Warty, exophytic, papillary or fungating tumor
- Biopsy large enough to include deep margin and sufficient amount to make an accurate diagnosis

Microscopic Pathology
- Multiple filiform, finger-like projections of well-differentiated squamous epithelium, maturing to surface
- Abundant keratosis (ortho- and parakeratosis), "church spire" keratosis, with parakeratotic crypting
- Broad pushing border of infiltration with dense inflammatory response

Top Differential Diagnoses
- Verrucous hyperplasia, exophytic/papillary SCC, squamous papilloma, verruca vulgaris

  - While not entirely radioresistant, significantly less radiosensitive than ordinary SCC
  - Radiation allows for functional preservation
  - Useful for tumors that cannot be resected
  - Approximately 30-35% recurrence/persistence rate
    - Surgical salvage of radiation failures still effective
  - Survival is lower if treated with radiation only

Prognosis
- Slow, locally aggressive neoplasm
- Pure VSCC does **not** metastasize
  - Considering superficial, nondestructive invasion, there is very slight metastatic capacity
- Overall 5-year survival: 85-95%
  - Similar to age- and sex-matched controls
    - Only about 5% of patients die from VSCC (disease-specific survival)
  - Survival lower with radiation only (65%)
- Most tumors present at pT1 or pT2 (stage I or II)
  - Although controversial, T stage, clinical stage, and type of surgery fail to predict survival
- For localized disease, surgery alone yields better outcome than irradiation alone
- ~ 20% recurrence/persistence rate overall (treatment dependent)
  - If extensive surrounding leukoplakia, may have increased recurrence
- When VSCC coexists with **conventional** SCC, treatment is identical to invasive, conventional SCC

MACROSCOPIC FEATURES

General Features
- Sharply circumscribed, broadly implanted
- Warty, exophytic, papillary or fungating tumor
- Bulky, firm to hard; tan to white mass

Sections to Be Submitted
- Large enough to include the deep margin and sufficient amount to make an accurate diagnosis
  - If biopsy is small, superficial, or fragmented, state: **Verrucous lesion, defer to adequate sample**
- Must have perpendicular orientation (not tangential) to render definitive diagnosis

Size
- Large, up to 8 cm

MICROSCOPIC PATHOLOGY

Histologic Features
- VSCC is highly differentiated type of SCC
- Squamous epithelium lacks cytologic criteria of malignancy
  - Very well-differentiated squamous epithelium
  - Cells are typically larger than those seen in conventional SCC
  - Maturation toward surface
  - If dysplasia is present, it is focal and limited to basal zone
- Surface contains papillary fronds
  - Multiple filiform, finger-like projections of well-differentiated squamous epithelium
  - Thickened, club-shaped papillae with thin fibrovascular cores
  - Papillae may show surface ulceration
- Abundant keratosis (ortho- and parakeratosis)
  - Thick, keratinized layer covering epithelium
  - "Church spire" keratosis
  - Parakeratotic crypting (collections of parakeratotic cells with debris)
  - Intraepithelial microabscesses can be identified
  - Extravasated keratin may elicit foreign body giant-cell stromal reaction
- Broad pushing border of infiltration
  - Blunt, intrastromal invaginated folds
  - Bulbous coalescing rete ridges
  - Downward dipping of epithelium creates "cup" or "arms" around periphery
    - This interface is excellent location for biopsy
  - Associated with dense lymphoplasmacytic inflammatory response
- Limited mitotic figures, if present at all
  - Limited to basal zone if found, and not atypical

VERRUCOUS SQUAMOUS CELL CARCINOMA

- Surrounding epithelium may show changes of hyperplasia (progression to carcinoma)
- Hybrid tumors seen in about 10% of VSCC
  - Conventional SCC and concurrent VSCC
  - If hybrid tumor is present, SCC **must** be diagnosis, as it predicts management and outcome

ANCILLARY TESTS

Frozen Sections

- Must be adequate sample size, including deep stroma, perpendicularly sectioned
  - Almost unavoidable tangential sectioning, curled, piecemeal or fragmented biopsy material
- Must know clinical size and appearance

Immunohistochemistry

- p53 overexpression can be seen (~ 40%)

Cytogenetics

- Specific LOH patterns not present in hyperplasia

PCR

- HPV types 6, 11, 16, and 18 are variably detected

DIFFERENTIAL DIAGNOSIS

Verrucous Hyperplasia

- Considered on developmental spectrum
  - Size and extent of hyperplasia may help
  - One of most difficult and problematic lesions to diagnose
  - Requires pathologist and clinician to communicate, with pathologist thoroughly explaining all that is present histologically
- Hyperplastic squamous epithelium, regularly spaced, verrucous projections, hyperkeratosis, sharply defined stromal interface
- Close patient follow-up recommended to exclude recurrence or progression

Exophytic/Papillary SCC

- Significant pleomorphism or atypia, mitotic figures, atypical mitoses, invasion

Hybrid VSCC and SCC

- Concurrent cytologically malignant epithelium (conventional SCC)
- Irregular-shaped invasive islands or individual cells
- When present, SCC "trumps" VSCC, as it determines management and prognosis

Squamous Papilloma

- Papillomas have thin, well-formed papillary fronds
- Limited keratinization
- Koilocytic atypia usually present

Pseudoepitheliomatous Hyperplasia

- Nonatypical inverted epithelial proliferation, with bulbous rete extensions into stroma
- Lacks exophytic/papillary growth, and usually is not large lesion clinically
- Associated with infection or granular cell tumor

Verruca Vulgaris

- Uncommon larynx lesion, characterized by layers of parakeratotic squamous cells with prominent keratohyaline granules and sharply defined acanthotic rete ridges

DIAGNOSTIC CHECKLIST

Clinically Relevant Pathologic Features

- Close cooperation and communication between laryngologist and pathologist
  - Histologically benign, but broadly implanted, fungating clinical mass suggests malignancy
- Must have adequate biopsy to include stroma

STAGING

Cautions

- Presumed clinically positive lymph nodes **fail** to demonstrate histologic metastatic disease

Low Stage

- Approximately 75% are pT1 tumors at presentation

SELECTED REFERENCES

1. Huang SH et al: Truths and myths about radiotherapy for verrucous carcinoma of larynx. Int J Radiat Oncol Biol Phys. 73(4):1110-5, 2009
2. Güvenç MG et al: Detection of HHV-8 and HPV in laryngeal carcinoma. Auris Nasus Larynx. 35(3):357-62, 2008
3. Strojan P et al: Verrucous carcinoma of the larynx: determining the best treatment option. Eur J Surg Oncol. 32(9):984-8, 2006
4. McCaffrey TV et al: Verrucous carcinoma of the larynx. Ann Otol Rhinol Laryngol. 107(5 Pt 1):391-5, 1998
5. Orvidas LJ et al: Verrucous carcinoma of the larynx: a review of 53 patients. Head Neck. 20(3):197-203, 1998
6. Damm M et al: CO2 laser surgery for verrucous carcinoma of the larynx. Lasers Surg Med. 21(2):117-23, 1997
7. Thompson LD: Diagnostically challenging lesions in head and neck pathology. Eur Arch Otorhinolaryngol. 254(8):357-66, 1997
8. López-Amado M et al: Human papillomavirus and p53 oncoprotein in verrucous carcinoma of the larynx. J Laryngol Otol. 110(8):742-7, 1996
9. Lundgren JA et al: Verrucous carcinoma (Ackerman's tumor) of the larynx: diagnostic and therapeutic considerations. Head Neck Surg. 9(1):19-26, 1986
10. Ferlito A: Diagnosis and treatment of verrucous squamous cell carcinoma of the larynx: a critical review. Ann Otol Rhinol Laryngol. 94(6 Pt 1):575-9, 1985
11. Batsakis JG et al: The pathology of head and neck tumors: verrucous carcinoma, Part 15. Head Neck Surg. 5(1):29-38, 1982
12. Fechner RE et al: Verruca vulgaris of the larynx: a distinctive lesion of probable viral origin confused with verrucous carcinoma. Am J Surg Pathol. 6(4):357-62, 1982
13. Ferlito A et al: Ackerman's tumor (verrucous carcinoma) of the larynx: a clinicopathologic study of 77 cases. Cancer. 46(7):1617-30, 1980

Microscopic Features

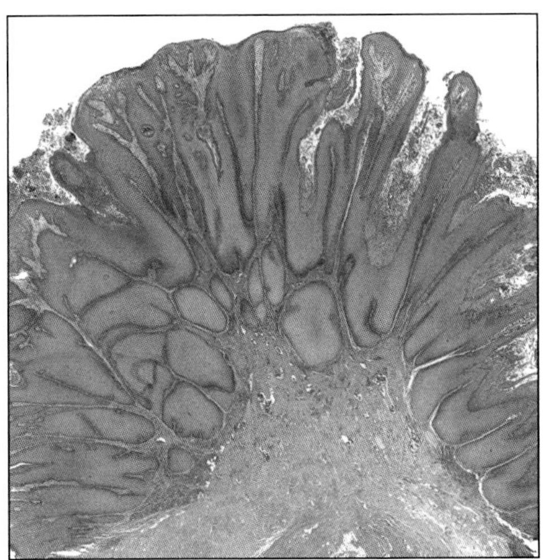

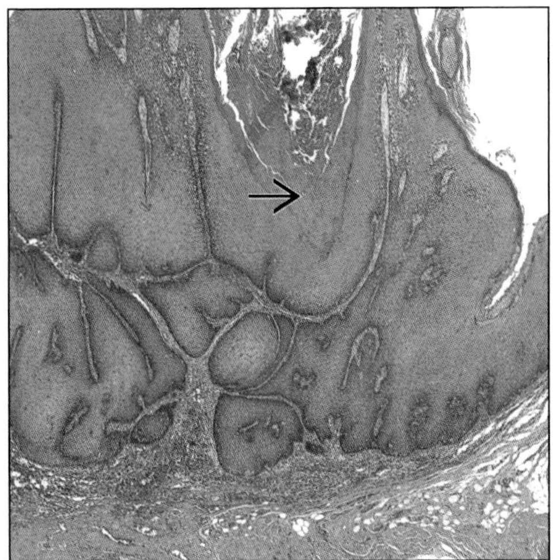

(Left) There is a broad, pushing border of infiltration with thickened, bulbous coalescing rete ridges. Keratosis lines papillary projections. An inflammatory infiltrate is present at the sharply defined stroma-epithelial interface. (Right) There is a very well-defined, broadly implanted epithelial proliferation. The rete are thickened, bulbous, and club-shaped. The epithelium shows maturation toward the surface. Parakeratotic crypting ⇒ is noted.

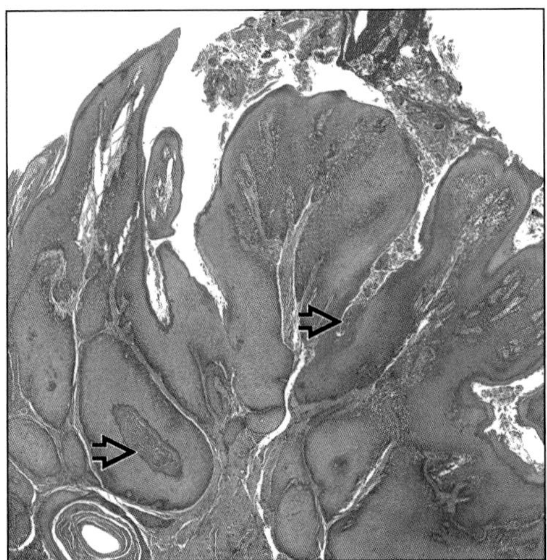

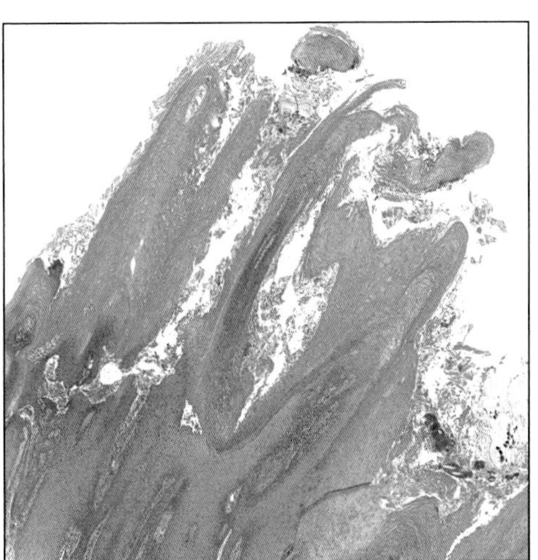

(Left) Multiple filiform and finger-like projections comprised of well-differentiated squamous epithelium make up this VSCC. There are thin fibrovascular cores. Parakeratotic crypting is noted ⇨. (Right) These delicate papillae are associated with "church spire" keratosis. Ortho- &/ or parakeratosis can be seen. This illustration only shows the surface tips of papillae. If this were all that was available, it would be an inadequate biopsy.

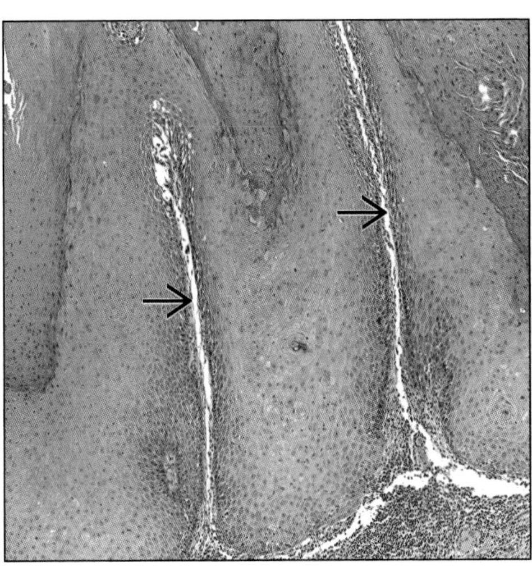

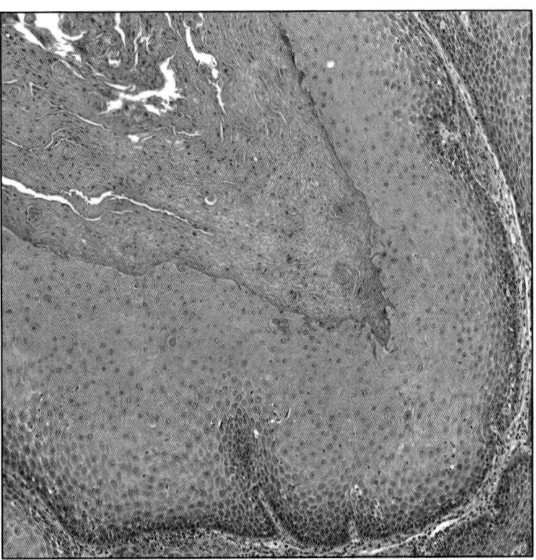

(Left) There is maturation toward the surface in these papillary projections, showing delicate fibrovascular cores ⇒. There is extensive keratinization, showing parakeratosis in this sample. (Right) This is a cytologically bland, nonmitotically active, maturing squamous epithelium. It shows a "bulbous" pushing border. Keratinization is present, filling the space between papillary projections. This is a characteristic high-power appearance for VSCC.

SPINDLE CELL "SARCOMATOID" SQUAMOUS CELL CARCINOMA

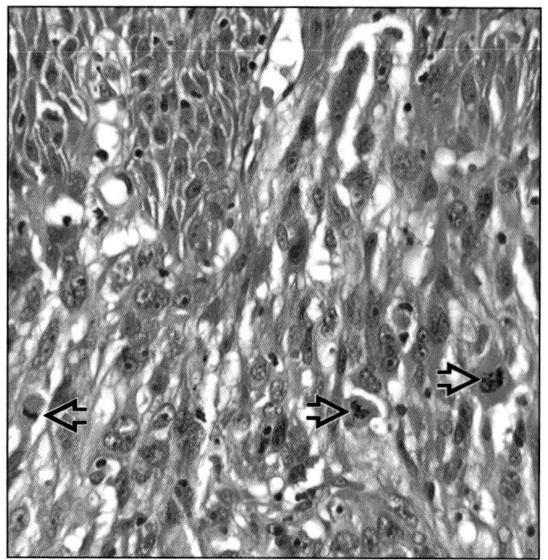

Hematoxylin & eosin shows surface epithelium transforming into a spindle cell population that blends with the surface epithelium. There are a remarkable number of mitotic figures ➪.

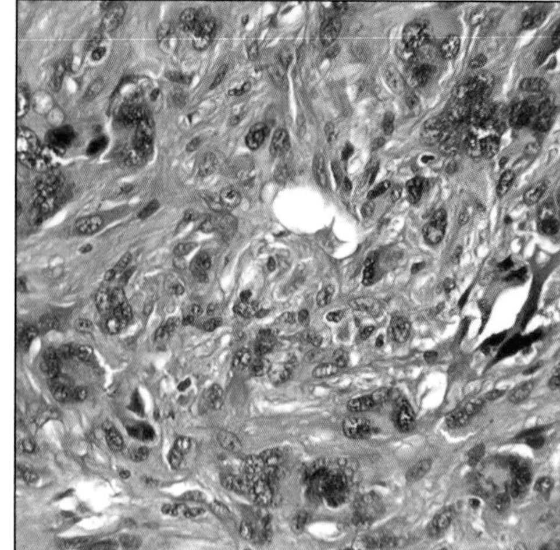

Hematoxylin & eosin shows significant pleomorphism within a spindled population. Stromal fibrosis is noted. Mitotic figures are not appreciated in this field but are generally easy to find.

TERMINOLOGY

Abbreviations

- Spindle cell "sarcomatoid" squamous cell carcinoma (SCSCC)

Synonyms

- Carcinosarcoma
- Pseudosarcoma
- Pseudocarcinoma
- Pseudocarcinosarcoma
- Pseudosarcomatous carcinoma
- Spindle cell carcinoma
- Spindle cell variant of squamous carcinoma
- Squamous cell carcinoma with pseudosarcoma
- Lane tumor
- Carcinoma with pseudosarcoma
- Pleomorphic carcinoma
- Metaplastic carcinoma

Definitions

- Squamous cell carcinoma with biphasic appearance yielding spindle cell transformation

ETIOLOGY/PATHOGENESIS

Environmental Exposure

- Strong smoking association
- Strong alcohol association
- Radiation exposure occasionally reported (~ 10%)

CLINICAL ISSUES

Epidemiology

- Incidence
  - ~ 2-3% of all laryngeal tumors
- Age
  - Mean: 65 years
  - Wide range: 30-95 years
- Gender
  - Male > > > > Female (12:1)

Site

- Glottic (true vocal cord, anterior commissure, posterior commissure) (~ 70%)
- Supraglottic (15%)
- Transglottic (12%)
- Subglottic (2%)

Presentation

- Polypoid mass
- Hoarseness
- Changes in voice
- Airway obstruction, shortness of breath, dyspnea
- Sore throat
- Dysphagia
- Cough and stridor

Endoscopic Findings

- Polypoid, ulcerated mass, often attached by pedicle arising from vocal cords

Treatment

- Options, risks, complications
  - "Polypectomy" may be curative in many cases
  - ~ 85% of patients identified at low-stage disease
- Surgical approaches
  - Wide local excision
  - May require additional surgery if polypectomy was not definitive
- Radiation
  - Postoperative, limited field radiation similar to grade and stage-matched squamous cell carcinoma patients (majority receive radiation)

Prognosis

- 5-year disease-free overall survival (~ 80%)
- Prognosis is worse
  - High-stage disease
  - Nonglottic tumors

SPINDLE CELL "SARCOMATOID" SQUAMOUS CELL CARCINOMA

Key Facts

Terminology

- Squamous cell carcinoma with biphasic appearance yielding spindle cell transformation

Clinical Issues

- Male > > > > Female (12:1)
- Glottic (true vocal cord, anterior commissure, posterior commissure) (~ 70%)
- Polypoid mass
- 5-year disease-free overall survival (~ 80%)
- Glottic tumors have better prognosis than nonglottic tumors
- Previous history of radiation decreases prognosis
- Epithelial negative tumors behave better than positive tumors

Macroscopic Features

- Polyp in vast majority of cases (> 98%)
- Almost always ulcerated surface

Microscopic Pathology

- Polypoid mass with surface ulceration
- Imperceptible blending between squamous and spindle cells
- Hypocellular lesions are very difficult to diagnose
- Mitotic figures found, including atypical forms
- Pleomorphism seen, although isolated atypical cells are common

Ancillary Tests

- Epithelial immunoreactivity is absent in up to 30% of cases

---

  - Larger tumors
  - Fixed vocal cords
  - Previous history of radiation
  - Presence of necrosis by histology
  - Epithelial positive immunoreactivity
- ~ 20% metastatic rate to regional lymph nodes
  - Usually identified in nonglottic tumors

MACROSCOPIC FEATURES

General Features

- Polypoid, pedunculated, exophytic tumor
  - Vast majority of cases (> 98%)
- Almost always ulcerated surface

Sections to Be Submitted

- Include junction of polyp with stalk
  - Most likely location for epithelium to be identified in ulcerated lesion

Size

- Mean: < 2 cm
- Range: 0.2 cm up to 8.5 cm

MICROSCOPIC PATHOLOGY

Histologic Features

- Polypoid mass with surface ulceration and fibrinoid necrosis
- Areas of classic squamous cell carcinoma (surface or deep within lesion) can usually be identified, although limited
- Imperceptible blending between squamous and spindle cells
- Storiform, solid, and fascicular architecture
- Low to intermediate cellularity most common
  - Hypocellular lesions are very difficult to diagnose
- Tumor necrosis is usually absent
- Mitotic figures are easily identified, including atypical forms
  - Mean: 12 mitoses/10 HPF
- Mild to moderate nuclear pleomorphism, although isolated atypical cells are common
- Tumor giant cells and multinucleated cells are seen
- Desmoplastic, stromal fibrosis is seen in ~ 1/2 of cases
- Benign or malignant bone or cartilage within spindle cell population
- Myxoid changes or acute inflammatory cells can be seen

ANCILLARY TESTS

Immunohistochemistry

- Epithelial immunoreactivity absent in up to 30% of cases

DIFFERENTIAL DIAGNOSIS

Contact Ulcer

- Bilateral ulcerated polyps
- Lacks cytologic atypia
- Mitotic figures can be seen

Fibrosarcoma

- Herringbone arrangement
- Spindle cells
- Arises from soft tissues of neck rather than endoluminal tissues of larynx

Synovial Sarcoma

- Young age at presentation
- Epithelial and spindle cell tumor
- Epithelial markers positive (EMA, keratin)
- Specific molecular alterations [t(X,18)]

Mucosal Melanoma

- Spindle cell melanoma
- Surface origin
- Positive melanocytic marker immunoreactivity

Nodular Fasciitis

- Pseudosarcomatous proliferation of soft tissues adjacent to larynx

SPINDLE CELL "SARCOMATOID" SQUAMOUS CELL CARCINOMA

Immunohistochemistry

Antibody	Reactivity	Staining Pattern	Comment
CK-PAN	Positive	Cytoplasmic	Approximately 70% of cases
Vimentin	Positive	Cytoplasmic	Present in nearly 100% of cases
EMA	Positive	Cytoplasmic	Up to 20% of cases
CK1	Positive	Cytoplasmic	Up to 40% of cases
CK5/6	Positive	Cytoplasmic	About 7% of cases
CK7	Positive	Cytoplasmic	About 5% of cases
CK14	Positive	Cytoplasmic	About 15% of cases
CK18	Positive	Cytoplasmic	About 25% of cases
CK17	Positive	Cytoplasmic	About 15% of cases
34B312	Positive	Cytoplasmic	About 10% of cases
Actin-sm	Positive	Cytoplasmic	About 30% of cases
Actin-HHF-35	Positive	Cytoplasmic	About 15% of cases
S100	Positive	Nuclear & cytoplasmic	About 5% of cases
p63	Positive	Nuclear	About 5% of cases
CK4	Negative		
CK10	Negative		
CK20	Negative		
CK8/18/CAM5.2	Negative		
HMB-45	Negative		

- Myxoid stroma, storiform spindle cell population
- Extravasated erythrocytes, keloid-like collagen, giant cells, mitotic figures
- Actin-sm, MSA, desmin, and myofibroblastic markers positive (keratin negative)

DIAGNOSTIC CHECKLIST

Pathologic Interpretation Pearls

- Nearly always polypoid projections into lumen
- Ulcerated surface with fibrinoid necrosis
- Spindle cell cellularity can be variable
- Do not rely on epithelial marker reactivity for diagnosis

STAGING

TNM

- Most are T1 and T2 lesions (> 85%)
- Survival depends on stage and tumor location

SELECTED REFERENCES

1. Marioni G et al: Squamous cell carcinoma of the larynx with osteosarcoma-like stromal metaplasia. Acta Otolaryngol. 124(7):870-3, 2004
2. Thompson LD et al: Spindle cell (sarcomatoid) carcinomas of the larynx: a clinicopathologic study of 187 cases. Am J Surg Pathol. 26(2):153-70, 2002
3. Ballo MT et al: Radiation therapy for early stage (T1-T2) sarcomatoid carcinoma of true vocal cords: outcomes and patterns of failure. Laryngoscope. 108(5):760-3, 1998
4. Lewis JE et al: Spindle cell carcinoma of the larynx: review of 26 cases including DNA content and immunohistochemistry. Hum Pathol. 28(6):664-73, 1997
5. Olsen KD et al: Spindle cell carcinoma of the larynx and hypopharynx. Otolaryngol Head Neck Surg. 116(1):47-52, 1997
6. Thompson LD: Diagnostically challenging lesions in head and neck pathology. Eur Arch Otorhinolaryngol. 254(8):357-66, 1997
7. Cassidy M et al: Pseudosarcoma of the larynx: the value of ploidy analysis. J Laryngol Otol. 108(6):525-8, 1994
8. Klijanienko J et al: True carcinosarcoma of the larynx. J Laryngol Otol. 106(1):58-60, 1992
9. Avagnina A et al: [Spindle cell carcinomas. Immunohistochemical analysis of 15 cases] Medicina (B Aires). 50(4):325-9, 1990
10. Hellquist H et al: Spindle cell carcinoma of the larynx. APMIS. 97(12):1103-13, 1989
11. Slootweg PJ et al: Spindle-cell carcinoma of the oral cavity and larynx. Immunohistochemical aspects. J Craniomaxillofac Surg. 17(5):234-6, 1989
12. Toda S et al: Polypoid squamous cell carcinoma of the larynx. An immunohistochemical study for ras p21 and cytokeratin. Pathol Res Pract. 185(6):860-6, 1989
13. Recher G: Spindle cell squamous carcinoma of the larynx. Clinico-pathological study of seven cases. J Laryngol Otol. 99(9):871-9, 1985
14. Lambert PR et al: Pseudosarcoma of the larynx: a comprehensive analysis. Arch Otolaryngol. 106(11):700-8, 1980
15. Kleinsasser OK et al: [Sarcomalike patterns in laryngeal carcinoma (pseudosarcoma, carcinosarcoma, spindle-cell-carcinoma, pleomorphic carcioma (author's transl)] Laryngol Rhinol Otol (Stuttg). 57(3):225-34, 1978
16. Hyams VJ: Spindle cell carcinoma of the larynx. Can J Otolaryngol. 4(2):307-13, 1975

Clinical and Microscopic Features

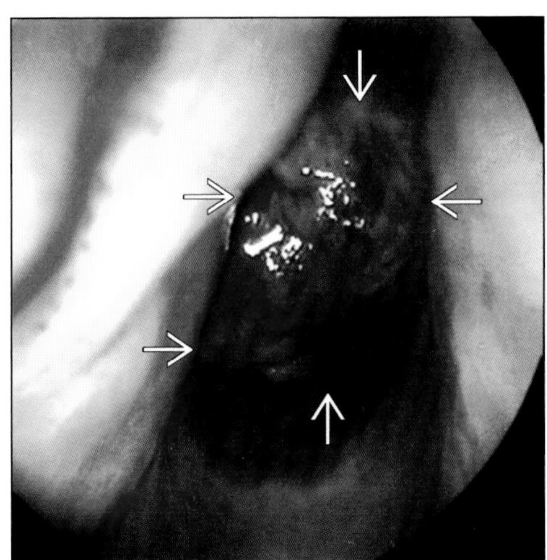

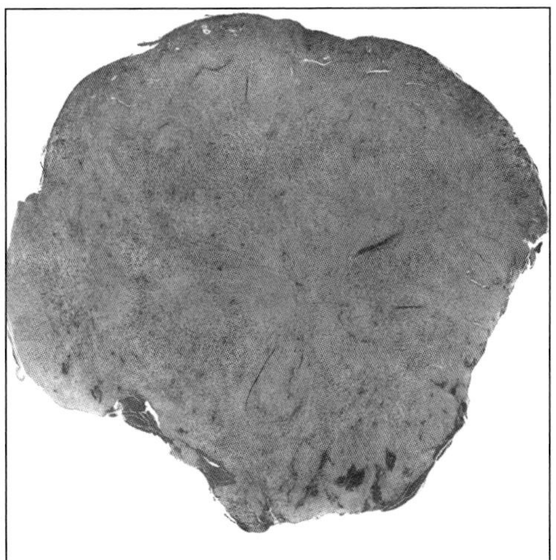

(Left) *Clinical photograph shows a polypoid tumor mass ➡ nearly completely occluding the endolaryngeal lumen. This may result in a "ball-valve" phenomenon, with alteration of the patient's position resulting in complete airway obstruction.* ***(Right)*** *Hematoxylin & eosin shows a polypoid mass with surface ulceration. The stalk leads into an area of central collagen deposition, frequently seen as a degenerative phenomenon.*

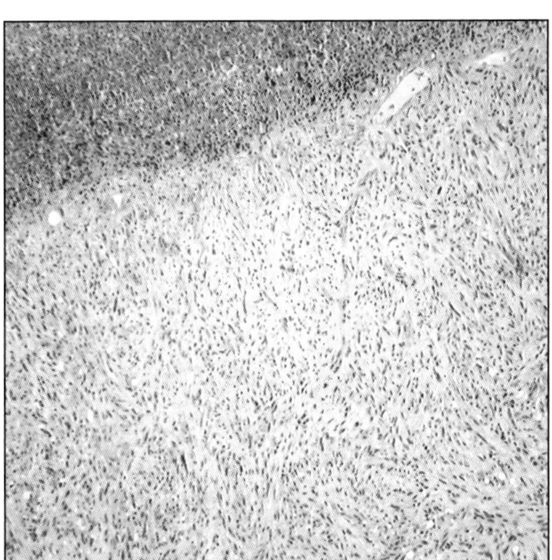

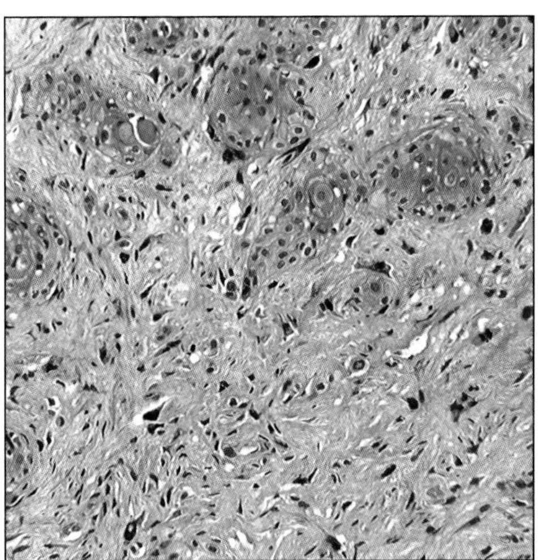

(Left) *Hematoxylin & eosin shows surface ulceration with fibrinoid necrosis subtended by an atypical spindle cell population. The cellularity is quite high and lacks a vascular proliferation.* ***(Right)*** *Hematoxylin & eosin shows abrupt juxtaposition of squamous cell carcinoma with the spindle cell stroma. The stroma contains many remarkably atypical fusiform to stellate cells.*

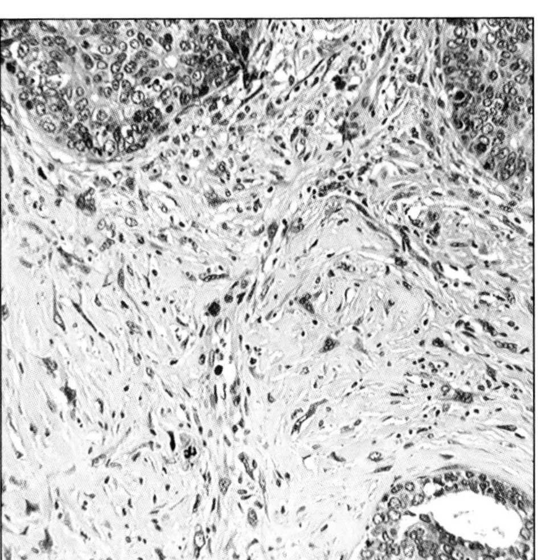

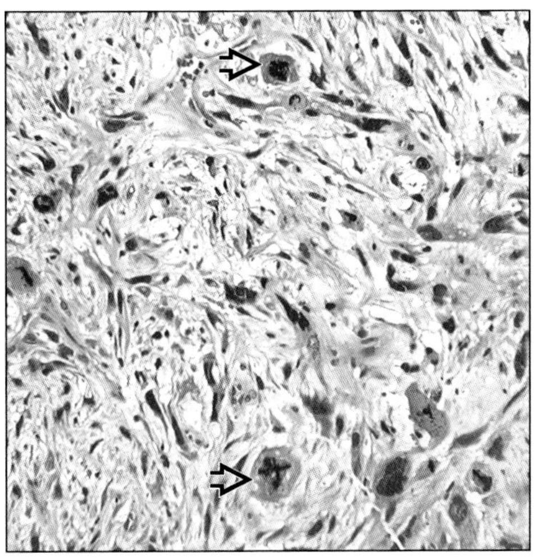

(Left) *Hematoxylin & eosin shows remarkably atypical squamous epithelium with an atypical spindle cell population within the collagenized stroma. The cellularity of the spindled population is variable and ranges from hypercellular to hypocellular.* ***(Right)*** *Hematoxylin & eosin shows a haphazard to storiform arrangement of remarkably atypical spindled to stellate cells with atypical mitotic figures ⇨. The cytoplasm is opacified.*

SPINDLE CELL "SARCOMATOID" SQUAMOUS CELL CARCINOMA

Microscopic Features

(Left) *Hematoxylin & eosin shows short interlacing fascicles in a pseudo-herringbone fashion. The cells are spindled with elongated nuclei.* ***(Right)*** *Hematoxylin & eosin shows a storiform, haphazard arrangement of interlacing spindle cells. The spindle cells tend to have a high nuclear to cytoplasmic ratio and pleomorphism.*

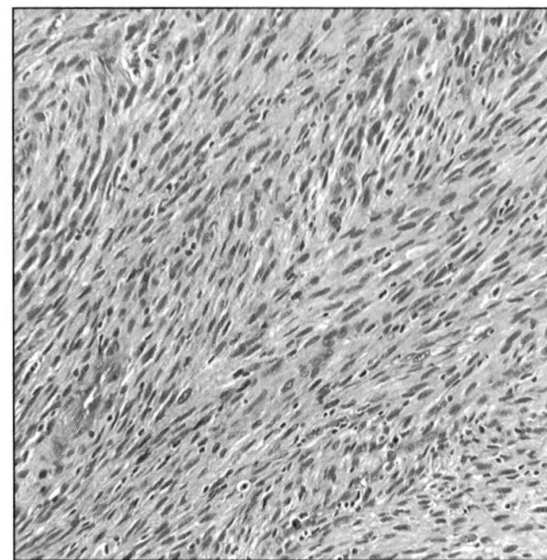

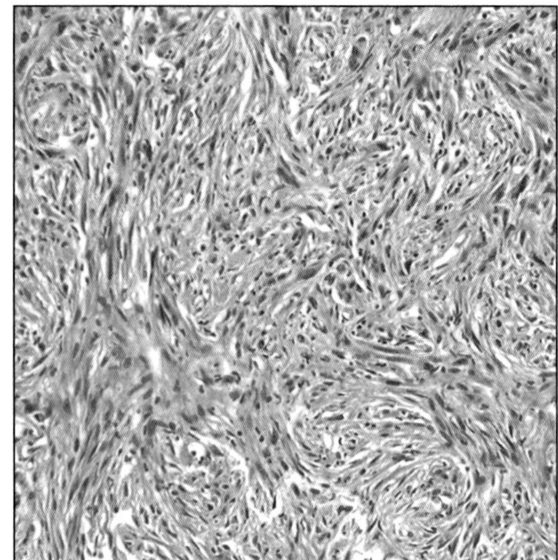

(Left) *Hematoxylin & eosin shows hypocellular and hypercellular areas within this spindle cell carcinoma. The heavy collagen deposition can be a mimic for other benign and reactive lesions of the larynx.* ***(Right)*** *Hematoxylin & eosin shows spindle cells with eosinophilic intracytoplasmic globules ⇨. The globules are nonspecific but are not seen in many other laryngeal lesions. Mitotic figures are also noted →.*

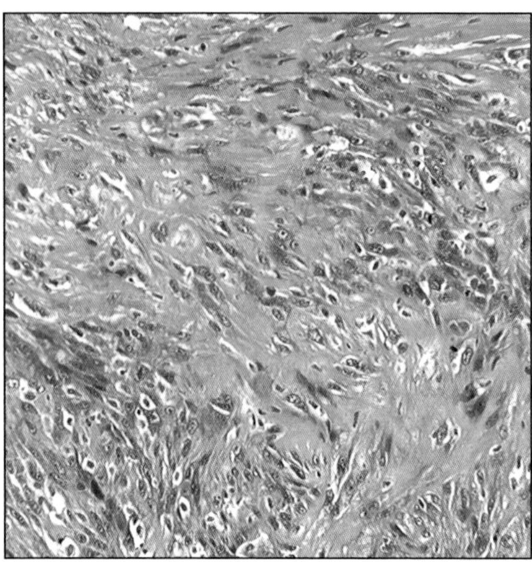

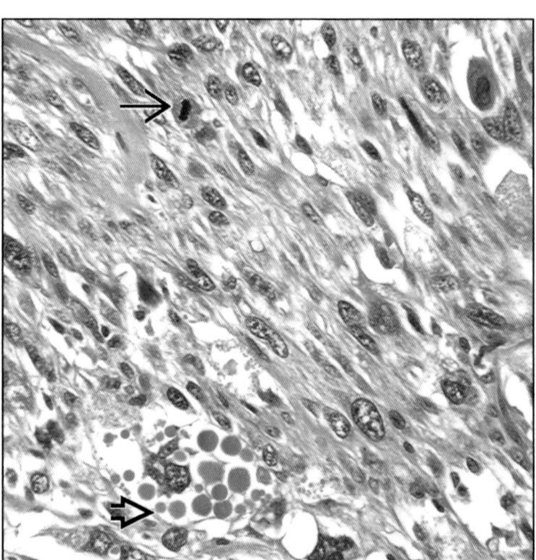

(Left) *Hematoxylin & eosin shows a spindle cell population adjacent to areas of necrosis →. There are areas of hypocellularity immediately adjacent to the regions of necrosis. This type of tumor necrosis is not seen in benign tumors of the larynx.* ***(Right)*** *Hematoxylin & eosin shows a hypocellular tumor with single, highly pleomorphic neoplastic cells. The cells are usually set in a heavily collagenized stroma. Vessels can be seen but are usually small capillaries.*

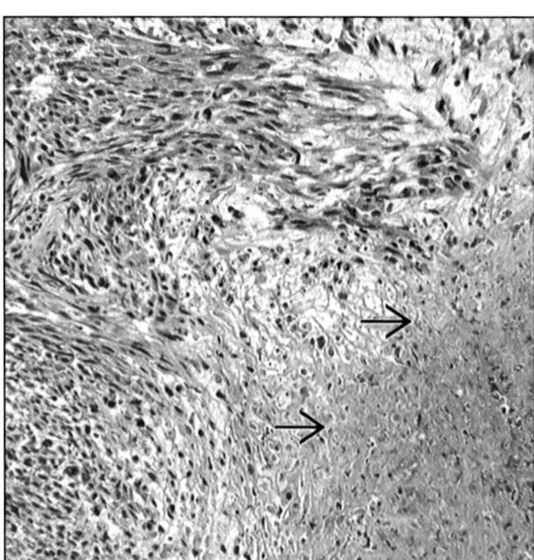

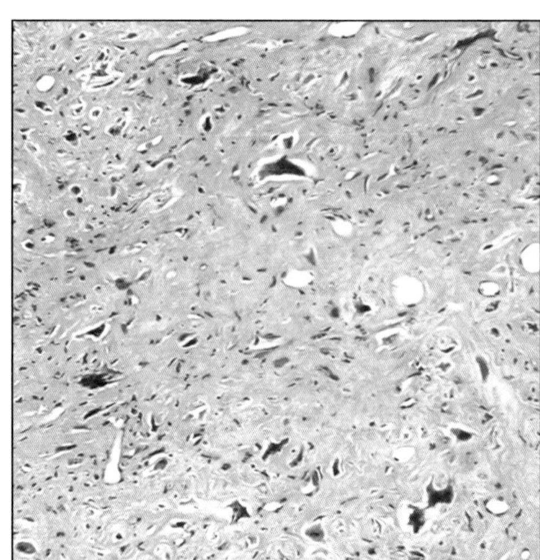

Microscopic and Immunohistochemical Features

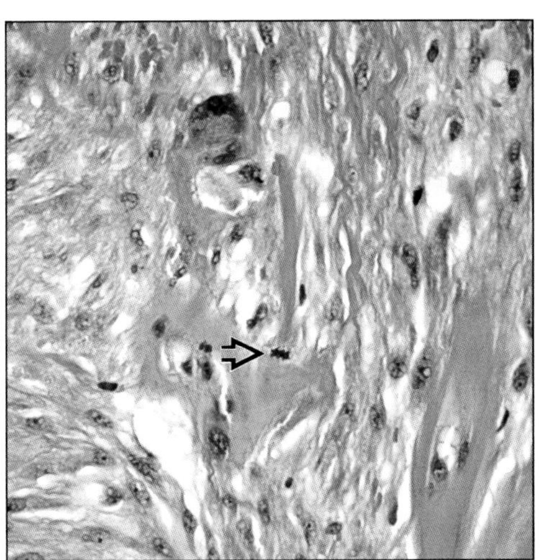

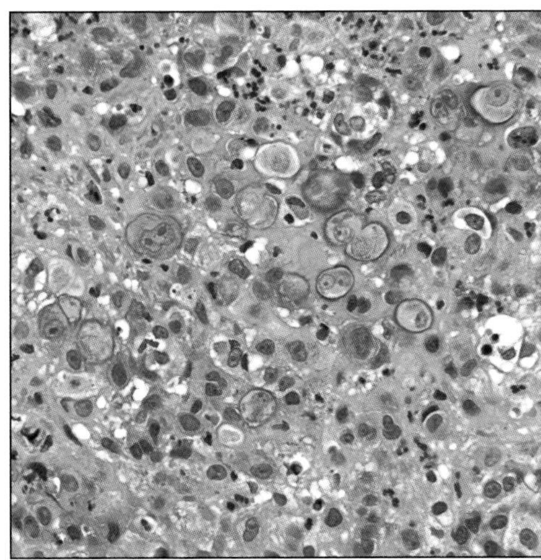

(Left) *Hematoxylin & eosin shows heavy stromal fibrosis separating atypical spindle cells with mitotic figures ⇨. The hypocellular appearance can mimic benign reactive lesions, and is one of the difficulties with this diagnosis.* ***(Right)*** *Hematoxylin & eosin shows cartilaginous differentiation within this spindle cell carcinoma. The cartilage can be malignant (chondrosarcoma) or benign (cartilage). This case shows a chondrosarcoma, separate topographically from the larynx cartilages.*

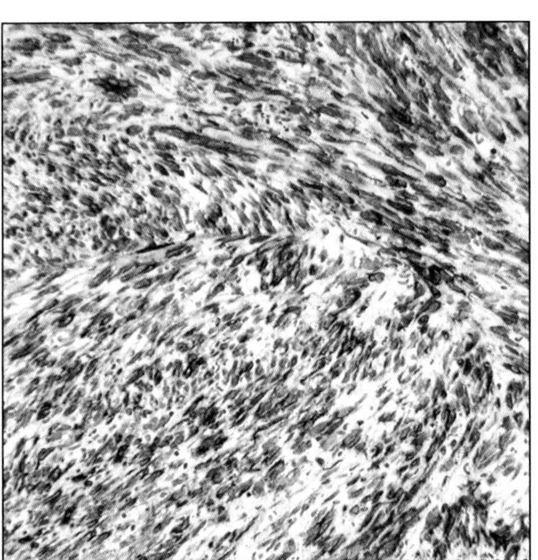

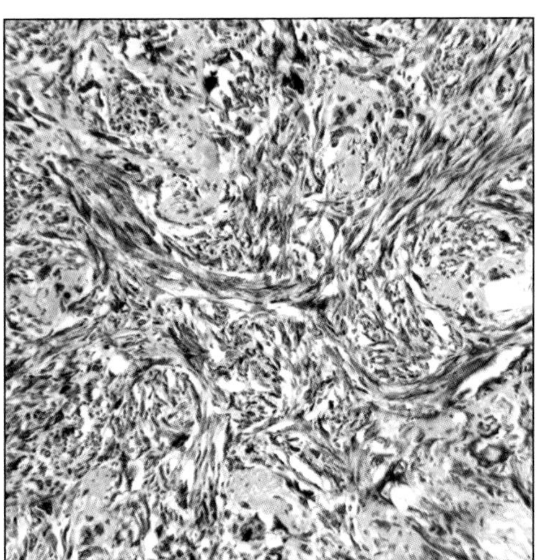

(Left) *CK-PAN shows strong and diffuse cytoplasmic immunoreactivity of the spindled neoplastic cells. The spindle shape is accentuated by this study.* ***(Right)*** *CK18 shows strong and diffuse immunoreactivity within the spindled cells. The vessels and collagen do not stain.*

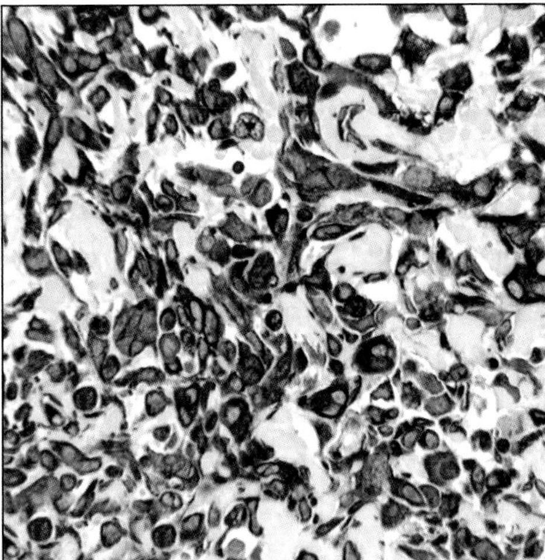

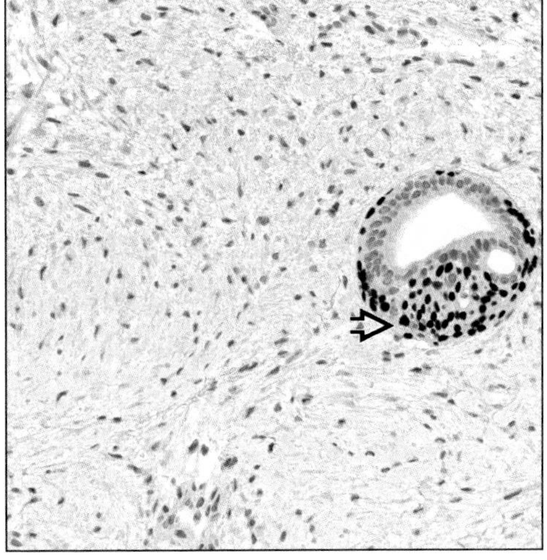

(Left) *Vimentin shows heavy and diffuse cytoplastic immunoreactivity within the atypical spindle and polygonal population. Vimentin can be used to test the tumor tissue antigenicity also but does not help to separate between tumor types of the larynx.* ***(Right)*** *p63 shows a basal proliferation of positive epithelial cells ⇨, while the spindle cell population is negative. If SCSCC, the spindle cell population may be p63 positive, but it is not a common occurrence.*

BASALOID SQUAMOUS CELL CARCINOMA

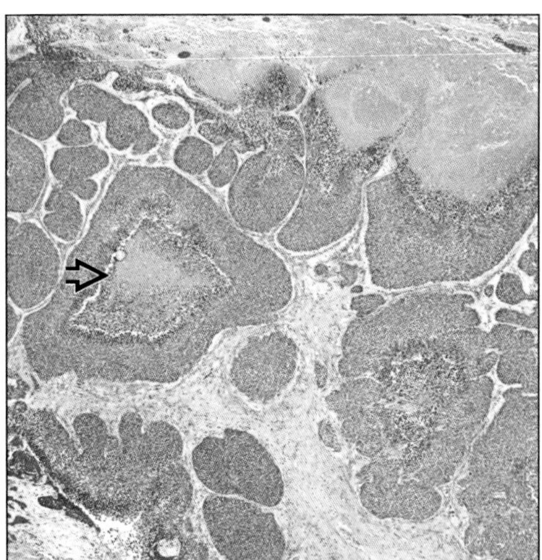

Hematoxylin & eosin shows lobules of basaloid cells with areas of central comedonecrosis ➯.

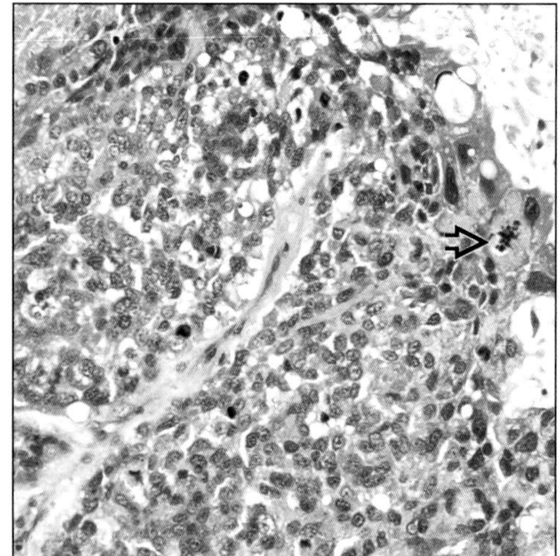

Hematoxylin & eosin shows basaloid cells with abrupt areas of remarkably atypical squamous epithelium, including atypical mitotic figures ➯.

TERMINOLOGY

Abbreviations

- Squamous cell carcinoma (SCC)
- Basaloid squamous cell carcinoma (BSCC)

Definitions

- Distinct variant of SCC showing predominantly basaloid cells with associated squamous differentiation (keratinization, dysplasia, in situ, or invasive tumor)

ETIOLOGY/PATHOGENESIS

Environmental Exposure

- High frequency of tobacco and alcohol use

Stem Cell

- Pluripotent stem cell with divergent differentiation

CLINICAL ISSUES

Epidemiology

- Incidence
  - Rare tumor
- Age
  - Mean: 6th to 7th decade
- Gender
  - Male > > Female

Site

- Piriform sinus (hypopharynx)
- Supraglottic or transglottic (larynx)

Presentation

- Dysphagia
- Pain
- Cough
- Hemoptysis
- Neck mass (less common)
- Frequently shows multifocal disease

Treatment

- Surgical approaches
  - Radical surgery (laryngectomy), with radical neck dissection
- Adjuvant therapy
  - Chemotherapy should be contemplated
- Radiation
  - Postoperative radiation

Prognosis

- Regional and distant metastases are common
- Significantly higher stage at presentation than other forms of SCC
- Appears biologically more aggressive, although stage-dependent
  - Majority of patients die of disease in < 3 years

MACROSCOPIC FEATURES

General Features

- Hard, white-tan mass associated with central necrosis

Size

- Up to 6 cm

MICROSCOPIC PATHOLOGY

Histologic Features

- Basaloid neoplasm arranged in many patterns, but smooth contoured lobules predominate
  - Solid, lobular, cords, cribriform, cystic, glandular
- Peripherally palisaded cells
- High nuclear to cytoplasmic ratio with vesicular-round nuclei
- High mitotic index
- Comedonecrosis within tumor lobules

BASALOID SQUAMOUS CELL CARCINOMA

Key Facts

Terminology
- Variant of SCC showing predominantly basaloid cells with associated squamous differentiation (keratinization, dysplasia, in situ, or invasive tumor)

Clinical Issues
- Male > > Female
- Mean: 6th to 7th decades
- Supraglottic or transglottic (larynx)
- Regional and distant metastases are common

Macroscopic Features
- Hard, white-tan mass associated with central necrosis

Microscopic Pathology
- Basaloid neoplasm arranged in many patterns
- Peripherally palisaded cells
- Comedonecrosis within tumor lobules
- Squamous differentiation, usually limited in degree
- High mitotic index
- High nuclear to cytoplasmic ratio

- Occasional mucohyaline type material may be seen in cystic spaces
- Squamous differentiation, usually limited in degree
  - Dysplastic surface epithelium, abrupt keratinization, keratin pearl formation, SCC in situ, invasive SCC
- Rosettes may be seen; ~ 5% may have spindle component

ANCILLARY TESTS

Immunohistochemistry
- Positive
  - AE1/AE3, 34βE12, CAM5.2, EMA, CK5/6
  - p63, p53, CEA, and MIB-1 (Ki-67 > 50%)
- Negative
  - Chromogranin, synaptophysin, p27Kip1, HPV, and EBV

DIFFERENTIAL DIAGNOSIS

Squamous Cell Carcinoma
- Superficial, shallow biopsies may miss basaloid component

Adenoid Cystic Carcinoma
- Prominent cribriform pattern, angulated nuclei, no nucleoli, lacks squamous differentiation, positive for S100 protein

Atypical Carcinoid, Small Cell Carcinoma
- Nuclear molding, lacks cysts and peripheral palisading, no squamous cell component
- Positive with neuroendocrine markers and TTF-1

SELECTED REFERENCES

1. Khaldi L et al: Basaloid squamous carcinoma of the larynx. A potential diagnostic pitfall. Ann Diagn Pathol. 10(5):297-300, 2006
2. Erisen LM et al: Basaloid squamous cell carcinoma of the larynx: a report of four new cases. Laryngoscope. 114(7):1179-83, 2004
3. Kleist B et al: Different risk factors in basaloid and common squamous head and neck cancer. Laryngoscope. 114(6):1063-8, 2004
4. Bahar G et al: Basaloid squamous carcinoma of the larynx. Am J Otolaryngol. 24(3):204-8, 2003
5. Paulino AF et al: Basaloid squamous cell carcinoma of the head and neck. Laryngoscope. 110(9):1479-82, 2000
6. Wieneke JA et al: Basaloid squamous cell carcinoma of the sinonasal tract. Cancer. 85(4):841-54, 1999
7. Morice WG et al: Distinction of basaloid squamous cell carcinoma from adenoid cystic and small cell undifferentiated carcinoma by immunohistochemistry. Hum Pathol. 29(6):609-12, 1998
8. Ferlito A et al: Basaloid squamous cell carcinoma of the larynx and hypopharynx. Ann Otol Rhinol Laryngol. 106(12):1024-35, 1997
9. Ereño C et al: Basaloid-squamous cell carcinoma of the larynx and hypopharynx. A clinicopathologic study of 7 cases. Pathol Res Pract. 190(2):186-93, 1994

IMAGE GALLERY

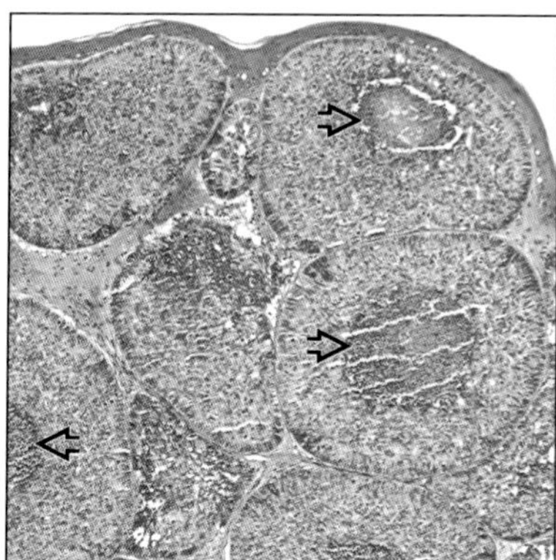
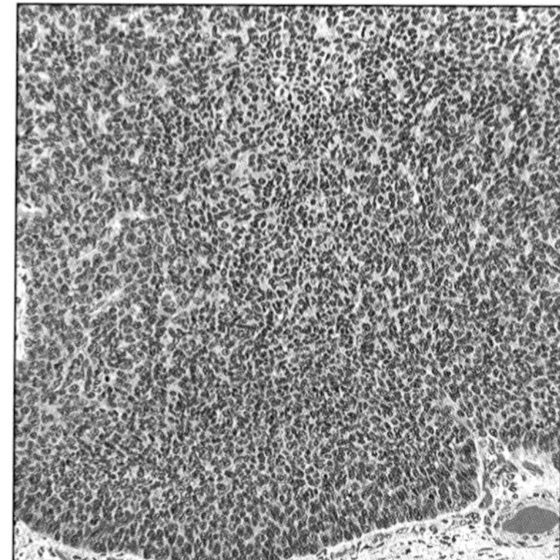
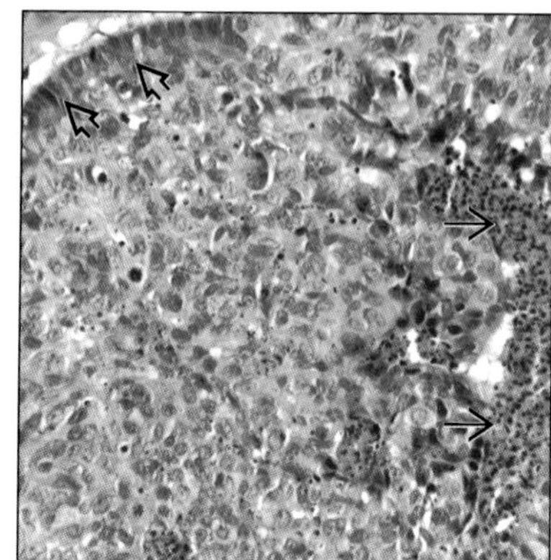

(Left) *Hematoxylin & eosin shows intact surface mucosa. The basaloid proliferation demonstrates peripheral palisading of the cells, with central comedonecrosis ⇨.* ***(Center)*** *Hematoxylin & eosin shows peripheral palisading in a sheet-like growth of basaloid cells.* ***(Right)*** *Hematoxylin & eosin demonstrates focal palisading ⇨ and necrosis → of basaloid cells with a high nuclear to cytoplasmic ratio and vesicular nuclear chromatin distribution.*

EXOPHYTIC AND PAPILLARY SQUAMOUS CELL CARCINOMA

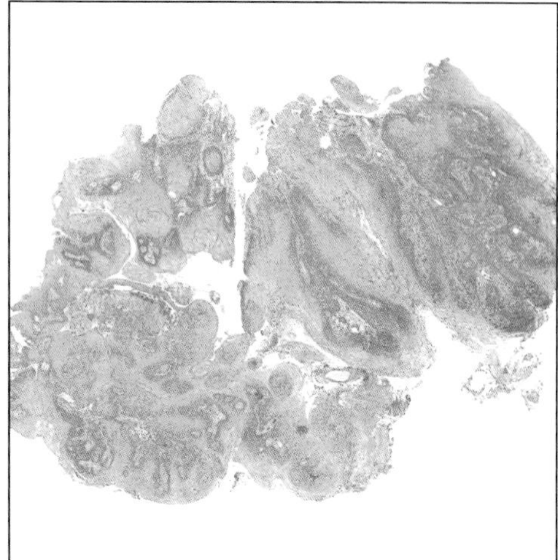

Papillary SCC are frequently sectioned tangentially, creating an "end-on" appearance. However, more than 70% of the proliferation is papillary, with delicate fibrovascular cores.

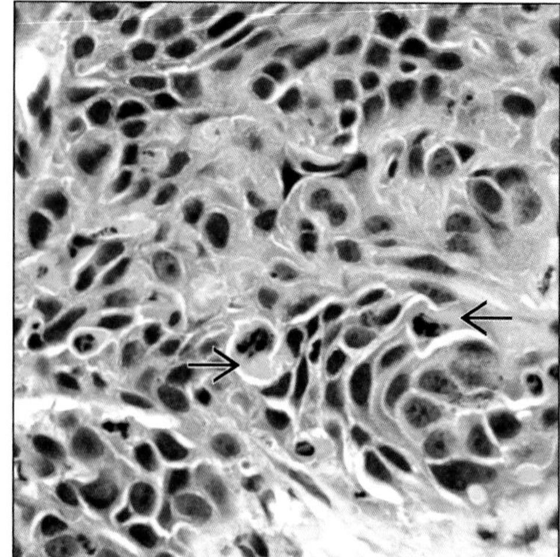

This high-power view shows a highly atypical squamous epithelium with dyskeratosis ⇒, architectural disarray, lack of polarization, along with nuclear hyperchromasia and pleomorphism.

TERMINOLOGY

Abbreviations

- Exophytic squamous cell carcinoma (ESCC)
- Papillary squamous cell carcinoma (PSCC)

Definitions

- ESCC is characterized by broad, cauliflower-like projections of malignant squamous epithelium
- PSCC is characterized by delicate, stalk-like papillary growth of malignant squamous epithelium

ETIOLOGY/PATHOGENESIS

Environmental Exposure

- Tobacco use (smoking)
- Alcohol abuse
- HPV is suggested etiologic factor in ~ 15-20% of cases
  - Types 6 or 16 (by ISH) most frequently

Malignant Transformation

- May evolve from preexisting squamous papilloma or papillary hyperplasia

CLINICAL ISSUES

Epidemiology

- Incidence
  - Uncommon variant of SCC
- Age
  - Mean: 6th and 7th decades
- Gender
  - Male > > Female (4:1)

Site

- Supraglottis > > glottis > > subglottis

Presentation

- Hoarseness and airway obstruction
- Other symptoms include dysphagia, sore throat, cough, hemoptysis
- Multifocality (synchronous or metachronous) commonly identified

Treatment

- Surgical approaches
  - Complete excision
    - Excisional biopsy, vocal cord stripping
    - Laryngectomy reserved for recalcitrant cases
- Radiation
  - Postoperative radiation therapy is employed for most patients

Prognosis

- PSCC has better prognosis than SCC (NOS)
  - Better prognosis is probably related to limited invasion
- ESCC has better prognosis than SCC (NOS), site and stage matched
  - More aggressive than PSCC
- Recurrences develop
  - Approximately 1/3 of patients
    - Recurrences are often multiple
  - Conservative treatment initially, then more aggressive management
- Most tumors present at low tumor stage (T1 or T2)
- Regional lymph node metastases are uncommon
  - Especially seen in stage T3 and T4 tumors
- Distant metastases are rare
  - Lung, liver, and bone
- *P53* inversely related to HPV prevalence and associated with worse prognosis

MACROSCOPIC FEATURES

General Features

- Polypoid, exophytic, bulky, papillary, or fungiform tumors
  - Arising from broad base or narrow, thin pedicle

EXOPHYTIC AND PAPILLARY SQUAMOUS CELL CARCINOMA

Key Facts

Terminology
- ESCC is characterized by broad, cauliflower-like projections of malignant squamous epithelium
- PSCC is characterized by delicate, stalk-like papillary growth of malignant squamous epithelium

Etiology/Pathogenesis
- Tobacco (smoking) and alcohol abuse
- HPV present in 15-20% of cases (types 6 or 16)

Clinical Issues
- Male > > Female (4:1)
- Supraglottis > > glottis > > subglottis
- Multifocality (synchronous or metachronous) commonly identified
- Most tumors present at low tumor stage (T1 or T2)
- Recurrences develop

Microscopic Pathology
- SCC demonstrating dominant (> 70%) exophytic or papillary architecture
- Exophytic pattern
  - Broad-based, bulbous exophytic growth, with rounded projections
- Papillary pattern
  - Multiple, thin, delicate, filiform projections with fibrovascular core
- Stromal invasion can be found

Top Differential Diagnoses
- Verrucous squamous cell carcinoma
- Carcinoma in situ
- Papillary hyperplasia
- Squamous papilloma

- Soft to firm, frequently friable

Size
- Exophytic SCC: Mean = 1.5 cm
- Papillary SCC: Mean = 1 cm

MICROSCOPIC PATHOLOGY

Histologic Features
- Neoplastic squamous epithelial proliferation demonstrating dominant (> 70%) exophytic or papillary architecture
- Exophytic pattern
  - Broad-based, bulbous exophytic growth
  - Projections are rounded and cauliflower-like
  - Tangential sectioning yields a number of central fibrovascular cores with lobular periphery
- Papillary pattern
  - Multiple, thin, delicate, filiform, finger-like papillary projections
  - Papillae contain delicate fibrovascular core surrounded by neoplastic epithelium
  - Tangential sectioning yields "bunch of celery" cut across the stalk
- Patterns may overlap and coexist
  - When overlapping, ESCC is default
- Unequivocal cytomorphologic evidence of malignancy
  - Both types usually have limited surface keratosis
  - Architectural distortion with loss of cellular polarity
  - Nuclear enlargement, increased nuclear to cytoplasmic ratio, prominent nucleoli
  - Frequently an immature, basaloid phenotype
  - Numerous mitotic figures, including atypical forms
  - Focal necrosis can be found
- Stromal invasion can be found
  - Cohesive nests or single cell infiltration
  - Associated with chronic inflammatory infiltrate
  - May require serial sections or reorientation to demonstrate invasion
  - Invasion is usually superficial, lacking perineural, vascular, or chondro-osseous invasion
- "Koilocytic atypia" is frequently noted
  - Hyperchromatic, crenated nucleus surrounded by clear halo with prominent cell border

DIFFERENTIAL DIAGNOSIS

Verrucous Squamous Cell Carcinoma
- Broad, pushing border of infiltration
- Parakeratotic crypting, "church spire" keratosis
- Maturation, limited pleomorphism, and limited mitotic figures

Carcinoma In Situ
- Atypical epithelial proliferation without forming appreciable clinical lesion
- Invasion may be difficult to assess, especially in tangentially sectioned tumors
  - If questionable, large tumor weighs heavily toward invasive carcinoma

Papillary Hyperplasia
- Lacks fibrovascular cores; devoid of pleomorphism; no atypical mitoses

Squamous Papilloma
- Noncomplex papillae; lacks pleomorphism, invasion, necrosis, atypical mitoses

SELECTED REFERENCES

1. Cobo F et al: Review article: relationship of human papillomavirus with papillary squamous cell carcinoma of the upper aerodigestive tract: a review. Int J Surg Pathol. 16(2):127-36, 2008
2. Suarez PA et al: Papillary squamous cell carcinomas of the upper aerodigestive tract: a clinicopathologic and molecular study. Head Neck. 22(4):360-8, 2000
3. Thompson LD et al: Exophytic and papillary squamous cell carcinomas of the larynx: A clinicopathologic series of 104 cases. Otolaryngol Head Neck Surg. 120(5):718-24, 1999
4. Ishiyama A et al: Papillary squamous neoplasms of the head and neck. Laryngoscope. 104(12):1446-52, 1994
5. Crissman JD et al: Squamous papillary neoplasia of the adult upper aerodigestive tract. Hum Pathol. 19(12):1387-96, 1988

EXOPHYTIC AND PAPILLARY SQUAMOUS CELL CARCINOMA

Microscopic Features

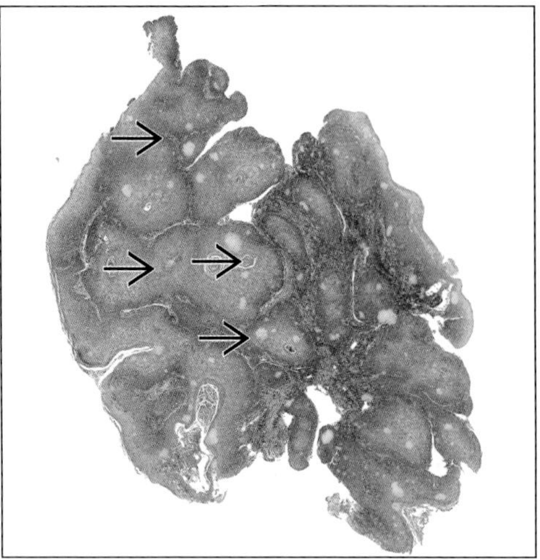

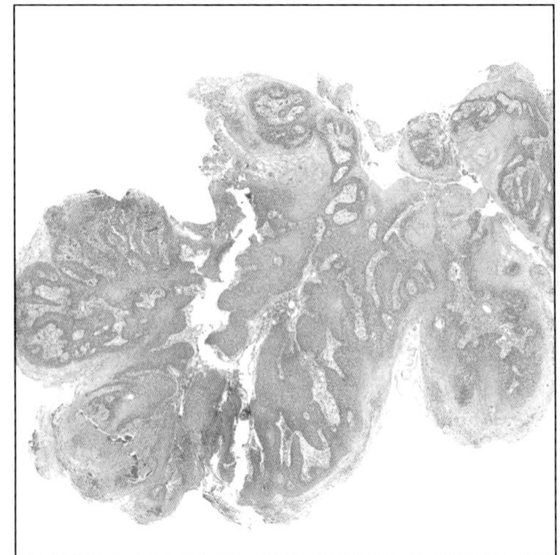

(Left) The outer contour of this carcinoma shows a cauliflower-like appearance, although numerous fibrovascular cores → are easily identified within the tumor. This is characteristic for an exophytic pattern SCC. (Right) Multiple, delicate, filiform papillary projections are crowded together in this papillary SCC. Tangentially, sections still demonstrate numerous projections toward the periphery of the tumor. Fibrovascular cores are thin.

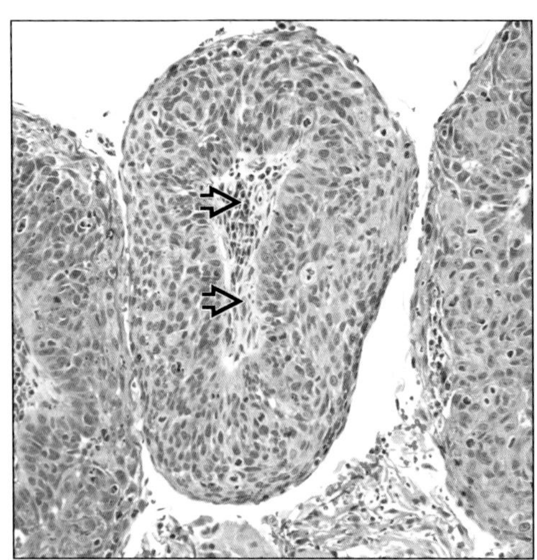

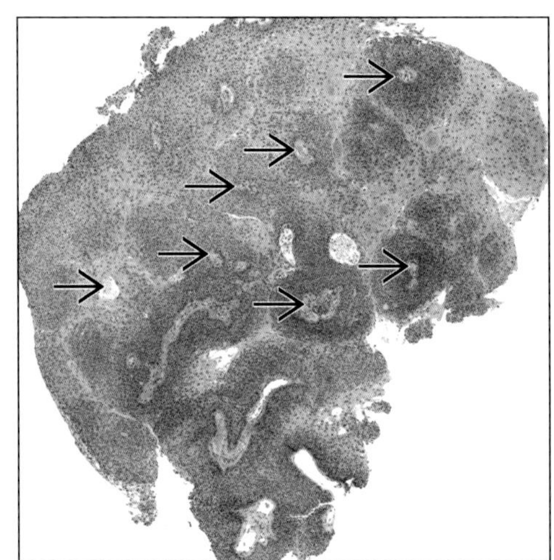

(Left) A papillary projection shows a central fibrovascular core → that is surrounded by a highly atypical squamous proliferation in this papillary SCC. There is loss of maturation, focal surface keratosis, and increased mitotic figures. (Right) An exophytic SCC shows a smooth exterior. However, multiple fibrovascular cores → are noted extending toward the surface of this neoplasm. This needs to be the dominant pattern in order to diagnose this variant of SCC.

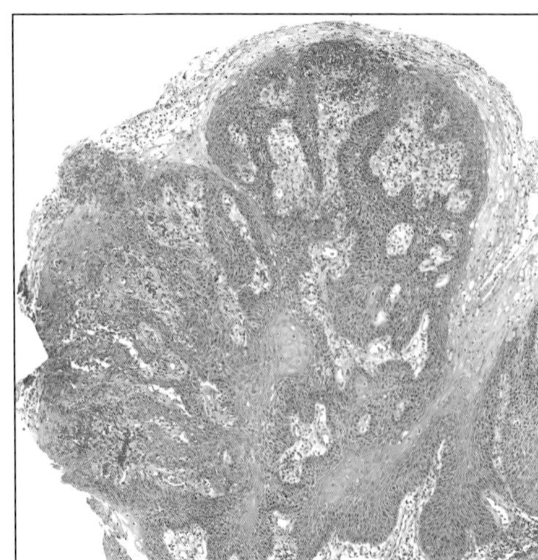

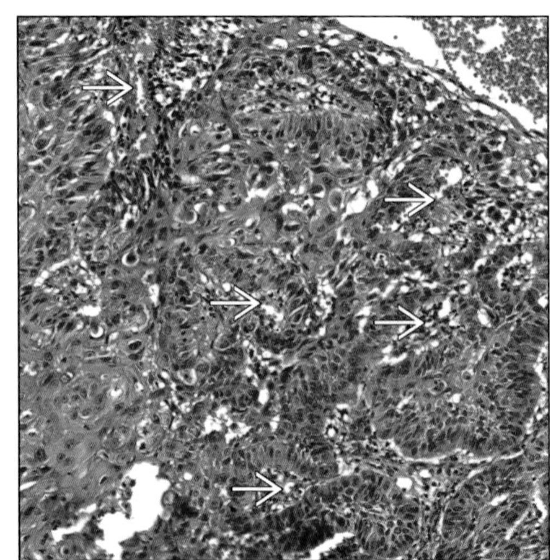

(Left) The surface epithelium is denuded in this papillary SCC. Note the parallel arrangement of the epithelial fingers as they extend through the sample. Inflammation is present at the epithelial to stromal interface. (Right) There are numerous delicate papillary projections surrounding fibrovascular cores in this papillary SCC →. The epithelium shows significant pleomorphism, dyskeratosis, lack of maturation, and mitotic figures. However, "invasion" is difficult to prove.

Microscopic Features

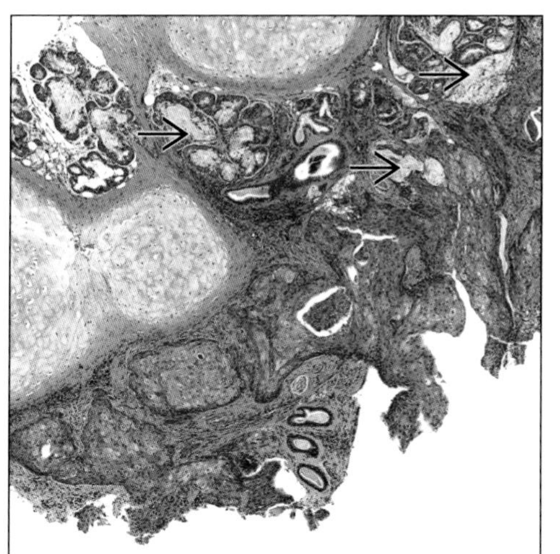

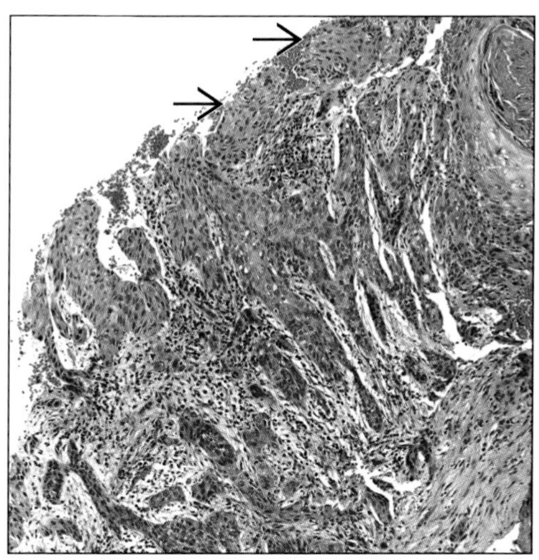

*(**Left**) In other areas of this tumor, an exophytic pattern was identified. However, invasion was present in this part of the sample, showing extension down to the cartilage. Note the minor mucoserous glands ⇒, focally surrounded by the neoplastic proliferation. (**Right**) At the surface of this papillary SCC, the epithelium shows nests and finger-like projections of the neoplastic epithelium into the stroma. These areas qualify for invasion. Note the surface ulceration ⇒.*

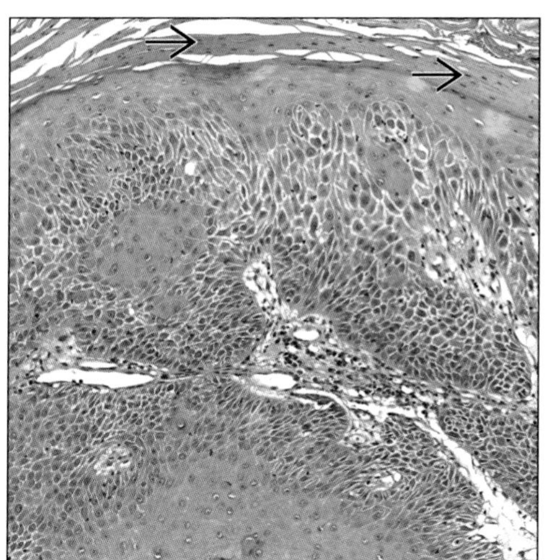

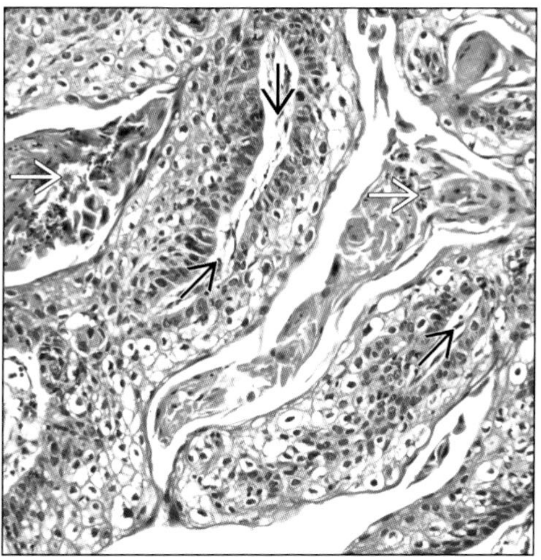

*(**Left**) The bulbous projections of the exophytic SCC show the "surface" epithelium on either side of this broad projection. There is parakeratosis ⇒ and keratosis. There is a suggestion of maturation toward the surface of this tumor. (**Right**) Multiple delicate, finger-like or filiform papillary projections comprise this papillary SCC. There is keratosis and keratin debris ➡ between the papillae. The fibrovascular cores are delicate and thin ⇒.*

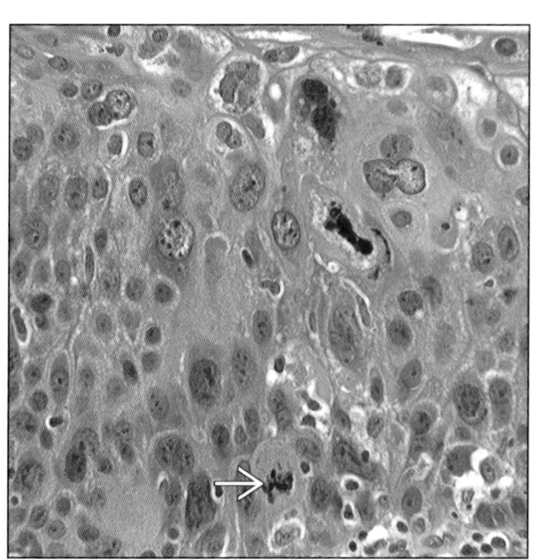

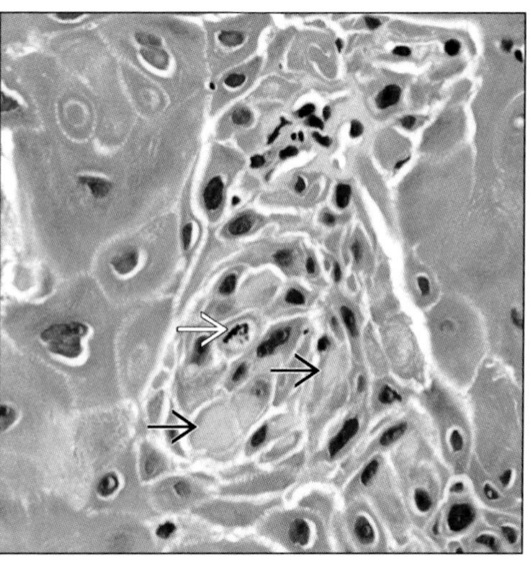

*(**Left**) The cytomorphonuclear features of carcinoma are usually easily recognized. There is an atypical mitotic figure ➡, lack of maturation toward the surface, profound nuclear pleomorphism, and increased nuclear to cytoplasmic ratio. Dyskeratosis is also present. (**Right**) The abnormal keratinization is seen on either side of the central part of the papillary projection. There is dyskeratosis ⇒ and a mitotic figure ➡ in this papillary SCC. Pleomorphism is moderate.*

ADENOSQUAMOUS CARCINOMA

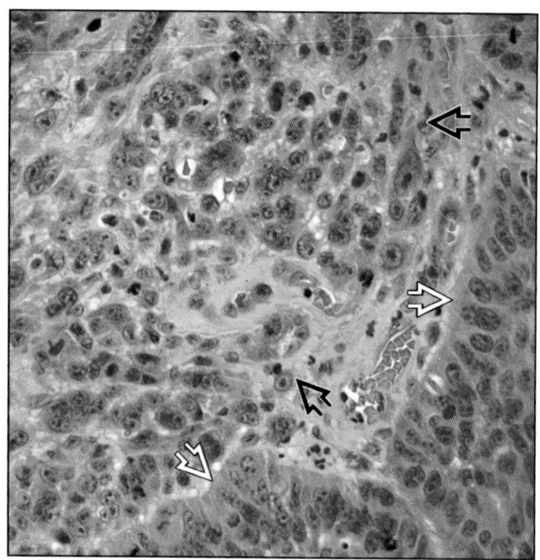

Two different carcinoma types are seen. The adenocarcinoma ⇨ shows a sheet to glandular profile of cells with prominent nucleoli. The squamous cell carcinoma ➡ shows a "pavement" appearance.

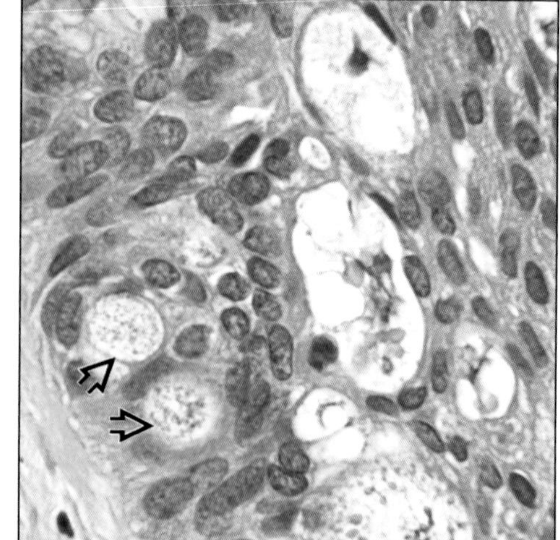

The squamous epithelial component is in direct approximation of the adenocarcinoma portion of this tumor. Note the mucin production ⇨, confirming the adenocarcinoma portion of the tumor.

TERMINOLOGY

Abbreviations

- Adenosquamous carcinoma (ASC)
- Squamous cell carcinoma (SCC)

Definitions

- Tumor that demonstrates admixture of biphasic components of true adenocarcinoma and squamous cell carcinoma

ETIOLOGY/PATHOGENESIS

Environmental Exposure

- Cigarette smoking and alcohol consumption have been implicated
- Role of gastroesophageal reflux is not as well established

Pathogenesis

- Adenosquamous carcinoma originates from basal cells of surface epithelium that are capable of divergent differentiation

CLINICAL ISSUES

Epidemiology

- Incidence
  - While > 90% of all head and neck mucosal malignancies are squamous cell carcinoma, < 1% of these tumors are adenosquamous carcinoma
- Age
  - Usually older age at initial presentation
  - Mean: 6th to 7th decades
- Gender
  - Male > Female (1.2:1)

Site

- Any region of larynx, with hypopharynx occasionally affected

Presentation

- Hoarseness
- Sore throat
- Dysphagia
- Hemoptysis
- Neck lymph node metastases in up to 75% of patients at presentation

Treatment

- Surgical approaches
  - Aggressive surgery required
  - Neck dissection may be warranted even without clinical disease
- Radiation
  - Radiation combined with surgery can yield a benefit

Prognosis

- Poor prognosis; significantly worse than conventional squamous cell carcinoma
- 5-year survival: 15-25%
  - 2-year survival: 55%
- Majority of patients present with lymph node metastases
  - Mean: 65%
- Most patients present with high-stage disease
  - Stage is predictive of outcome
  - Multivariant analysis between stage and tumor type is unavailable
- Distant metastases develop in about 25% of patients
  - Most commonly to lungs

MACROSCOPIC FEATURES

General Features

- Exophytic mass
- Polypoid mass

ADENOSQUAMOUS CARCINOMA

Key Facts

Terminology
- Tumor that demonstrates admixture of biphasic components of true adenocarcinoma and squamous cell carcinoma

Clinical Issues
- Rare, < 1% of SCC
- Lymph node metastases at presentation (up to 75%)
- Aggressive surgery required, including neck dissection
- Poor prognosis (5-year survival: 15-25%)

Macroscopic Features
- Exophytic, polypoid mass to indurated submucosal nodule, often with ulceration, ~ 1 cm

Microscopic Pathology
- Biphasic appearance of separate or blended tumors, showing areas of transition
- SCC component can be in situ or invasive
- Adenocarcinoma identified away from surface
- Tubular, alveolar, or glandular
- Mucin (intraluminal or intracellular) can be seen, but not required
- Undifferentiated or "intermediate" transitional cells can be seen, often with clear cytoplasm
- Metastases may display both components

Ancillary Tests
- Adenocarcinoma usually CK7 positive
- SCC is CK5/6 and p63 positive

Top Differential Diagnoses
- Mucoepidermoid carcinoma, acantholytic SCC, basaloid SCC
- Necrotizing sialometaplasia

- Poorly defined indurated submucosal nodule
- Ulceration is frequent

Size
- Mean: ~ 1 cm
  - Can be up to 5 cm in maximum dimension

MICROSCOPIC PATHOLOGY

Histologic Features
- Admixture of both true adenocarcinoma and squamous cell carcinoma
  - Biphasic appearance
- Can be distinct, separate tumors in close proximity, but many are blended, intermixed, and commingled, showing areas of transition
- Squamous cell carcinoma component can be in situ or invasive
  - Tumors can be well to poorly differentiated
  - Squamous differentiation confirmed
    - Pavemented growth
    - Intercellular bridges
    - Keratin pearl formation
    - Dyskeratosis
    - Individual cell keratinization
- Adenocarcinoma tends to develop deep in tumor (away from surface)
  - Tubular structures that give rise to "glands within glands," alveolar to glandular
    - Adenocarcinoma cells can be basaloid
    - Separation from basaloid squamous cell carcinoma can be arbitrary
  - Mucin production is typically present (intraluminal or intracellular), but not required
    - Rarely, signet ring cells may be present
- Undifferentiated or "intermediate" transitional cells can be seen, often with clear cytoplasm
- Both components may have
  - Necrosis
  - Increased mitotic figures
  - Infiltration into surrounding tissues, including perineural invasion
- Tends to have sparse inflammatory cell infiltrate
- Desmoplastic stromal response is usually minimal to absent
- Metastases may display both components although one usually predominates

ANCILLARY TESTS

Histochemistry
- Mucicarmine
  - Reactivity: Positive
  - Staining pattern
    - In adenocarcinoma component only

Immunohistochemistry
- Generally, positive in both components with high molecular weight cytokeratins
- Glandular component expresses
  - CEA
  - Low molecular weight cytokeratins
    - Specifically, CK7 is positive
    - CK20 is negative
- Squamous cell component usually expresses
  - CK5/6
  - p63

Flow Cytometry
- High prevalence of aneuploidy has been demonstrated

Electron Microscopy
- Features of both squamous and glandular differentiation are present

DIFFERENTIAL DIAGNOSIS

Mucoepidermoid Carcinoma (MEC)
- MEC has much better prognosis than adenosquamous carcinoma
- Does not have surface component
  - Lacks dysplasia or carcinoma in situ
- MEC lacks true "squamous cell" differentiation, showing intermediate cells

ADENOSQUAMOUS CARCINOMA

- No true adenocarcinoma adjacent to squamous cell carcinoma in MEC
- True "mucocytes" (squashed, eccentric nucleus) rare in adenosquamous carcinoma
- Separation may be impossible in some cases
  - Some view adenosquamous cell carcinoma as high-grade MEC

Acantholytic (Adenoid) SCC

- Acantholysis or dilapidated appearance can mimic adenocarcinoma
- Mucin in true glandular spaces is not seen in acantholytic squamous cell carcinoma

Basaloid SCC

- Dominant pattern of growth is basaloid cells
- Peripheral nuclear palisading usually present
- Squamous differentiation
  - May have isolated keratinization
  - Squamous metaplasia without atypia
  - Can have squamous cell carcinoma
- No intra- and extracellular mucin

Necrotizing Sialometaplasia

- Squamous cell carcinoma can extend down gland-duct units, entrapping minor mucoserous glands
  - Glandular component appears benign
- Preservation of lobular, gland architecture (especially on low power)
- Areas of necrosis or inflammation are common
- Cellular atypia may be present, but frank pleomorphism is absent

Adenocarcinoma with Squamous Metaplasia

- Absence of malignant appearance to squamous component
- Usually isolated and minor component of tumor

Concurrent Tumors

- Requires identification of contemporaneous tumors that are temporally separated

SELECTED REFERENCES

1. Passon P et al: Long-surviving case of adenosquamous carcinoma of the larynx: case report and review of literature. Acta Otorhinolaryngol Ital. 25(5):301-3, 2005
2. Alos L et al: Adenosquamous carcinoma of the head and neck: criteria for diagnosis in a study of 12 cases. Histopathology. 44(6):570-9, 2004
3. Thompson LDR: Squamous cell carcinoma variants of the head and neck. Curr Diag Pathol. (9):384-396, 2003
4. Keelawat S et al: Adenosquamous carcinoma of the upper aerodigestive tract: a clinicopathologic study of 12 cases and review of the literature. Am J Otolaryngol. 23(3):160-8, 2002
5. Ferlito A et al: Mucosal adenoid squamous cell carcinoma of the head and neck. Ann Otol Rhinol Laryngol. 105(5):409-13, 1996
6. Fujino K et al: Adenosquamous carcinoma of the larynx. Am J Otolaryngol. 16(2):115-8, 1995
7. Snow RT et al: Mucoepidermoid carcinoma of the larynx. J Am Osteopath Assoc. 91(2):182-4, 187-9, 1991
8. Batsakis JG et al: Basaloid-squamous carcinomas of the upper aerodigestive tracts. Ann Otol Rhinol Laryngol. 98(11):919-20, 1989
9. Damiani JM et al: Mucoepidermoid-adenosquamous carcinoma of the larynx and hypopharynx: a report of 21 cases and a review of the literature. Otolaryngol Head Neck Surg. 89(2):235-43, 1981
10. Ferlito A et al: Mucoepidermoid carcinoma of the larynx. A clinicopathological study of 11 cases with review of the literature. ORL J Otorhinolaryngol Relat Spec. 43(5):280-99, 1981

ADENOSQUAMOUS CARCINOMA

Microscopic and Histochemical Features

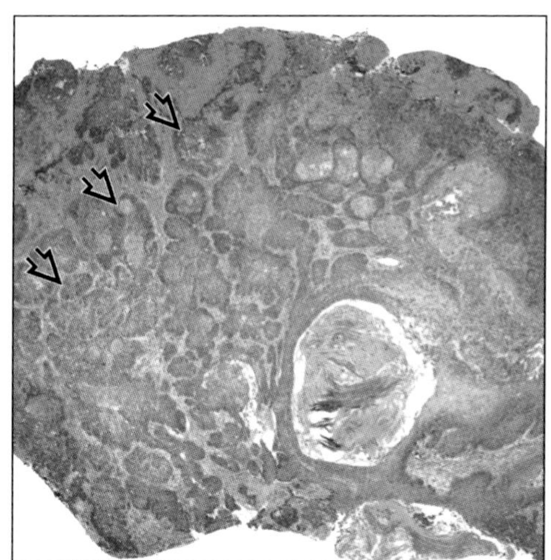
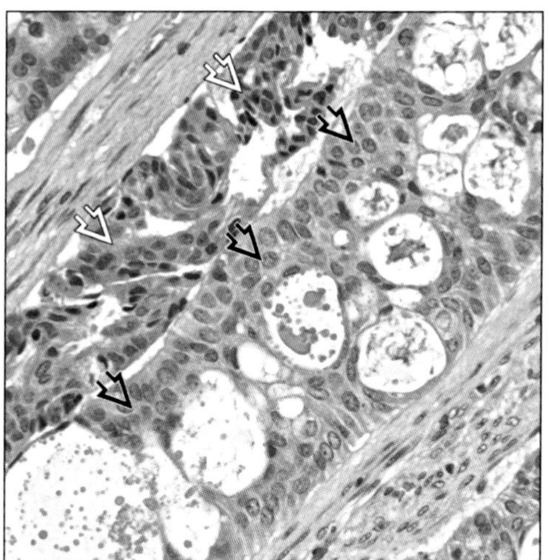

(Left) *This low-power view of a larynx tumor demonstrates a mixture of squamous cell carcinoma and adenocarcinoma in the same biopsy. The squamous cell carcinoma is more toward the surface, while the adenocarcinoma* ⇨ *is deeper in the biopsy.* ***(Right)*** *The remarkable proximity of adenosquamous carcinoma is evident in this biopsy. The adenocarcinoma shows mucinous material* ⇨*, while the squamous cell component shows dyskeratosis and opaque cytoplasm* ➡*.*

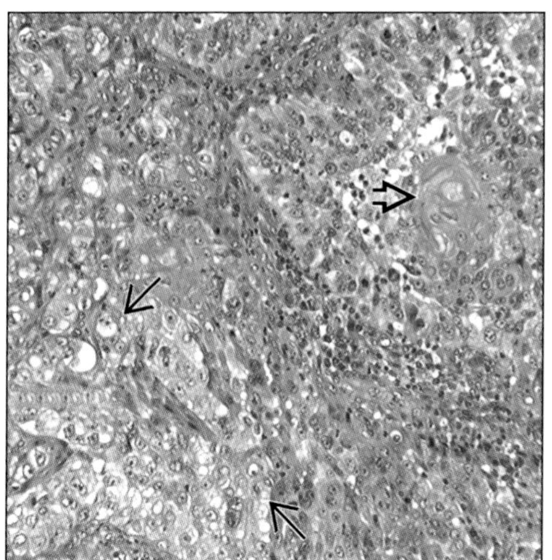
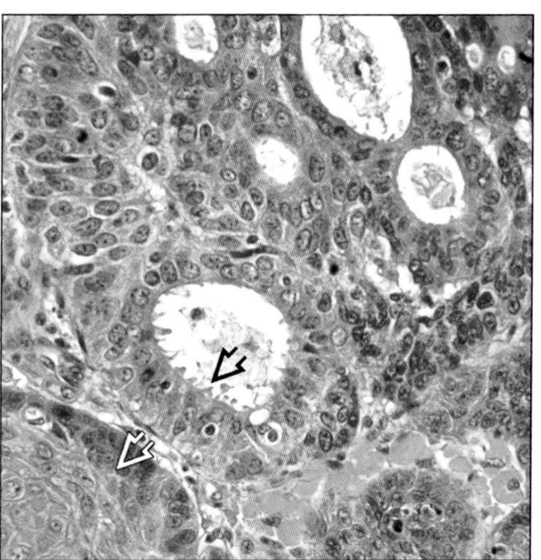

(Left) *There is a remarkable blending of the tumors in this example, with an intermediate or "undifferentiated" component in between. The squamous elements are highlighted by the keratin pearl formation* ⇨*, while the more "undifferentiated" component has clearing of the cytoplasm* →*.* ***(Right)*** *The adenocarcinoma shows well-formed glands with blebs on the surface* ⇨*, along with inspissated material. An area of squamous carcinoma is noted* ➡*.*

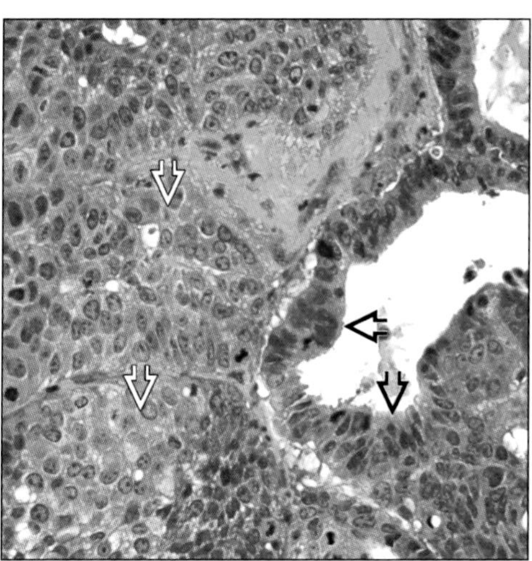
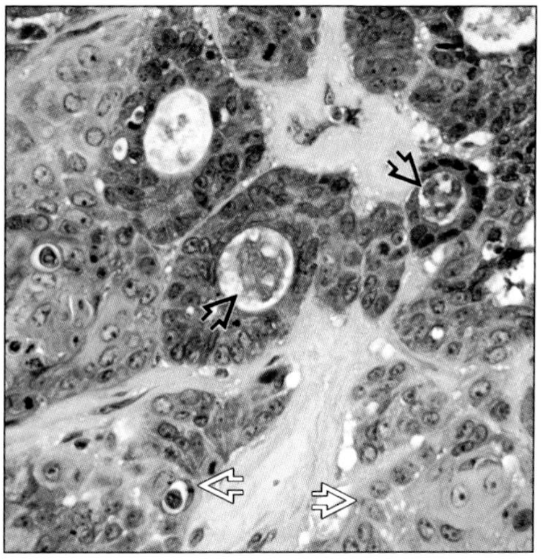

(Left) *There is such a blending of the tumors that it is difficult to accurately separate the squamous and adenocarcinoma components. The adenocarcinoma has a lumen* ⇨*, but the squamous cell carcinoma has a clear to transitional cell component blended in with it* ➡*.* ***(Right)*** *The mucicarmine stain highlights mucinous material within the lumen of a number of the islands of adenocarcinoma* ⇨*, while no reaction is noted in the squamous epithelium* ➡*.*

NEUROENDOCRINE CARCINOMA

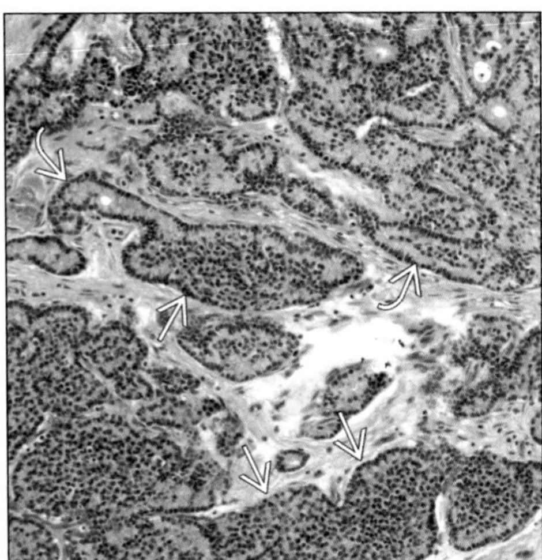

Laryngeal carcinoid tumor ➔ with a submucosal cellular neoplasm ➔ shows trabecular, solid, and organoid growth patterns.

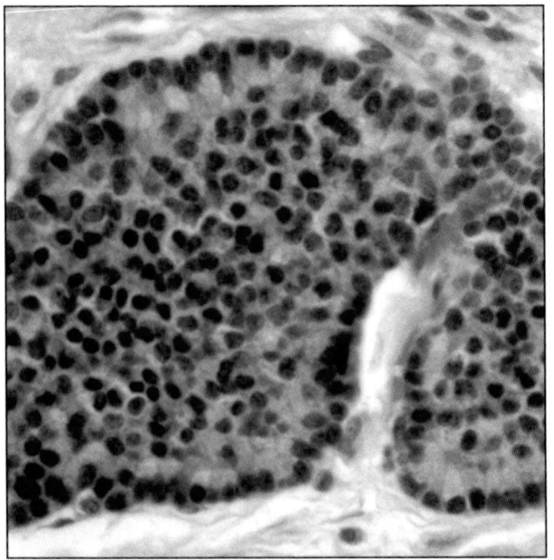

The tumor is composed of uniform cells with centrally located round nuclei and dispersed nuclear chromatin lacking nuclear pleomorphism, mitoses, or necrosis.

TERMINOLOGY

Abbreviations

- Neuroendocrine carcinoma (NEC)

Synonyms

- Classification of (laryngeal) neuroendocrine carcinomas of head and neck includes
  - Carcinoid tumor or well-differentiated neuroendocrine tumor (WDNEC)
  - Atypical carcinoid or moderately differentiated neuroendocrine carcinoma (MDNEC)
  - Small cell undifferentiated neuroendocrine carcinoma (SCUNC) or poorly differentiated neuroendocrine carcinoma (PDNEC)
    - "Oat" cell carcinoma

Definitions

- Heterogeneous group of malignant neoplasms characterized by presence of epithelial and neuroendocrine differentiation with prognosis predicated on tumor type

ETIOLOGY/PATHOGENESIS

Environmental Exposure

- Atypical carcinoid and SCUNC
  - History of cigarette smoking
- Carcinoid tumor
  - Generally not associated with smoking history

CLINICAL ISSUES

Epidemiology

- Incidence
  - In general, NECs are uncommon in head and neck
  - May be identified in virtually all sites of head and neck
    - More common sites include larynx > sinonasal cavity, salivary glands
  - Significant overlap in demographics and clinical features for all subtypes of laryngeal NECs
- Age
  - Generally in 6th and 7th decades of life
- Gender
  - Male > Female

Site

- Larynx is most common site of occurrence
  - Supraglottic larynx most common single site of occurrence
  - Glottis and subglottis occasionally
- Frequency of tumor type in larynx
  - Atypical carcinoid (MDNEC) > small cell carcinoma (PDNEC) > carcinoid tumor (WDNEC)

Presentation

- Hoarseness
  - Most common complaint
- Paraneoplastic syndrome
  - Rarely occurs in association with carcinoid tumor and atypical carcinoid
  - Occasionally may occur in association with small cell carcinoma and may include
    - Cushing syndrome, Lambert-Eaton syndrome, Schwartz-Bartter syndrome

Treatment

- Surgical approaches
  - **Carcinoid tumor**
    - Conservative complete resection
    - Neck dissection not indicated given low incidence of nodal metastasis at presentation
  - **Atypical carcinoid**
    - Depending on site of occurrence surgery may include partial or total laryngectomy
    - High incidence of cervical node metastasis necessitates neck dissection even in clinically N0 necks

NEUROENDOCRINE CARCINOMA

Key Facts

Terminology
- Heterogeneous group of malignant neoplasms characterized by presence of epithelial and neuroendocrine differentiation with prognosis predicated on tumor type

Clinical Issues
- Larynx is most common site of occurrence
  - Supraglottic larynx most common single site of occurrence
- Atypical carcinoid (MDNEC) > small cell carcinoma (PDNEC) > carcinoid tumor (WDNEC)
- Carcinoid tumor (WDNEC) indolent with excellent behavior generally cured following surgical resection
- Atypical carcinoid tumor (MDNEC) 5-year survival: 48%, 10-year survival: 30%
- Small cell undifferentiated neuroendocrine carcinoma has poor prognosis (2-year survival: 16%, 5-year survival: 5%)

Microscopic Pathology
- All NECs are submucosal tumors showing variety of growth patterns, including organoid, trabecular, ribbons, cribriform or solid growth ± fibrovascular stroma

Ancillary Tests
- All NECs variably immunoreactive for cytokeratins (AE1/AE3, CAM5.2, others) and neuroendocrine markers (chromogranin, synaptophysin, CD56, CD57, TTF-1, others)
- Atypical carcinoid (primary and metastatic) calcitonin immunoreactive in > 80%

- Adjuvant therapy
  - For SCUNC, primary mode of therapy includes systemic chemotherapy and radiation
  - Adjunctive radiation and chemotherapy used for atypical carcinoid tumor but of questionable utility

Prognosis
- **Carcinoid tumor (WDNEC)**
  - Indolent biology with excellent behavior generally cured following surgical resection
  - May metastasize in approximately 1/3 of patients
    - Metastases may occur late in disease course to liver and bone
- **Atypical carcinoid tumor (MDNEC)**
  - Prognosis is dependent on extent of disease at presentation
    - Tumor confined to larynx 62% tumor-free over median of 3.9 years
    - Overall 5-year survival: 48%
    - Overall 10-year survival: 30%
  - Often metastasizes, and presence of metastatic disease (either at presentation or developing subsequently) is ominous sign with death at intervals ranging from 1-6 years
    - Cervical lymph nodes (43% of patients)
    - Lungs, bone, liver (44% of patients)
    - Skin and subcutaneous tissue (22% of patients)
    - Death results from metastatic disease
- **Small cell undifferentiated neuroendocrine carcinoma (SCUNC)**
  - Poor
    - 2-year survival: 16%
    - 5-year survival: 5%
  - Metastases are common
    - Regional lymph nodes in majority of patients (60-90%)
    - Liver, lung, bone, and brain

MACROSCOPIC FEATURES

General Features
- **Carcinoid tumor**
  - Submucosal nodular or polypoid mass with tan-white appearance, varying in size from a few millimeters up to 3 cm in diameter
  - Surface ulceration generally absent
- **Atypical carcinoid**
  - Submucosal nodular or polypoid mass with tan-white appearance, varying in size from a few millimeters up to 4 cm in diameter
  - Surface ulceration may be present
- **SCUNC**
  - Submucosal mass usually with surface ulceration

MICROSCOPIC PATHOLOGY

Histologic Features
- **Carcinoid tumor**
  - Submucosal tumor arranged in organoid, trabecular, ribbons, or solid growth pattern with fibrovascular stroma
  - Uniform cells, centrally located round nuclei, vesicular chromatin, and eosinophilic cytoplasm
    - Low nuclear to cytoplasmic ratio
    - Stippled ("salt and pepper") nuclear chromatin pattern
  - Absence of pleomorphism, mitoses, necrosis
  - Glands &/or squamous differentiation can be seen
  - Surface ulceration uncommon
  - Vascular, lymphatic, and perineural invasion absent
- **Atypical carcinoid**
  - Submucosal tumor in organoid, trabecular, ribbons, cribriform, or solid growth pattern with prominent fibrovascular stroma
    - Infiltrative growth when present may include neurotropism and lymphovascular invasion
  - Hypercellular with mild to marked nuclear pleomorphism, round to oval nuclei, stippled to vesicular chromatin, and eosinophilic to clear to oncocytic cytoplasm
    - Nuclei can be centrally or eccentrically (plasmacytoid) located
    - Nucleoli may be prominent

NEUROENDOCRINE CARCINOMA

  - Mitoses uncommon but can be seen, including atypical forms
  - Necrosis may be focally identified
  - Glands, squamous differentiation, and neural-type rosettes can be identified
  - Surface ulceration may be prominent
- SCUNC
  - Submucosal tumor arranged in solid nests, sheets, or ribbons with absence of fibrovascular stromal component
  - Hypercellular with hyperchromatic, pleomorphic, oval to spindle-shaped nuclei, increased nuclear to cytoplasmic ratio, nondescript cytoplasm, and indistinct cell borders
    - Stippled ("salt and pepper") nuclear chromatin with absent to inconspicuous nucleoli
    - "Crush" artifact frequent
    - Abundant mitoses, including atypical forms
    - Confluent foci of necrosis and individual cell necrosis common
    - Nuclear molding identified
  - Glands, squamous differentiation, and neural-type rosettes can be identified
  - May occur in association with squamous cell carcinoma and less often with adenocarcinoma
    - Referred to as combined or composite tumors
  - Surface ulceration present
  - Neurotropism and lymphovascular invasion common
  - Large cell type of neuroendocrine carcinoma akin to lung large cell neuroendocrine carcinoma reported in larynx

ANCILLARY TESTS

Immunohistochemistry

- All NECs immunoreactive for
  - Cytokeratins (AE1/AE3, CAM5.2, others), epithelial membrane antigen
  - Neuroendocrine markers (chromogranin, synaptophysin, CD56, CD57, others)
  - Neuron specific enolase (NSE)
- Atypical carcinoid (primary and metastatic) calcitonin immunoreactive in > 80%

Electron Microscopy

- Transmission
  - Neurosecretory granules, cellular junctional complexes, inter- and intracellular lumina

DIFFERENTIAL DIAGNOSIS

Laryngeal Paraganglioma

- Absent cytokeratin immunoreactivity
- Characteristic S100 protein immunoreactivity along periphery of cell nests (sustentacular cell-like pattern)

Thyroid Medullary Carcinoma

- Thyroid-based mass
- Overlapping light microscopic and immunohistochemical findings with atypical carcinoid
  - Serum calcitonin levels almost invariably elevated in thyroid medullary carcinoma and almost always within normal limits in atypical carcinoid

Malignant Melanoma

- Presence of S100 protein and melanocytic immunomarkers (HMB-45, Melan-A, tyrosinase)
- Absent cytokeratin and neuroendocrine marker immunoreactivity

Malignant Lymphoma

- Presence of hematolymphoid immunomarkers
- Absent cytokeratin and neuroendocrine marker immunoreactivity

DIAGNOSTIC CHECKLIST

Pathologic Interpretation Pearls

- All NECs show stippled ("salt and pepper") chromatin with differentiation among types predicated on degree of nuclear pleomorphism, extent of mitotic activity, and presence of necrosis

SELECTED REFERENCES

1. Davies-Husband CR et al: Primary, combined, atypical carcinoid and squamous cell carcinoma of the larynx: a new variety of composite tumour. J Laryngol Otol. 124(2):226-9, 2010
2. Ferlito A et al: Neuroendocrine neoplasms of the larynx: an overview. Head Neck. 31(12):1634-46, 2009
3. Gillenwater A et al: Moderately differentiated neuroendocrine carcinoma (atypical carcinoid) of the larynx: a clinically aggressive tumor. Laryngoscope. 115(7):1191-5, 2005
4. Greene L et al: Large cell neuroendocrine carcinoma of the larynx: a case report and a review of the classification of this neoplasm. J Clin Pathol. 58(6):658-61, 2005
5. Jaiswal VR et al: Primary combined squamous and small cell carcinoma of the larynx: a case report and review of the literature. Arch Pathol Lab Med. 128(11):1279-82, 2004
6. Mills SE: Neuroectodermal neoplasms of the head and neck with emphasis on neuroendocrine carcinomas. Mod Pathol. 15(3):264-78, 2002
7. Wenig BM: Neuroendocrine tumors of the larynx. Head Neck. 14(4):332-4, 1992
8. el-Naggar AK et al: Carcinoid tumor of the larynx. A critical review of the literature. ORL J Otorhinolaryngol Relat Spec. 53(4):188-93, 1991
9. Gnepp DR: Small cell neuroendocrine carcinoma of the larynx. A critical review of the literature. ORL J Otorhinolaryngol Relat Spec. 53(4):210-9, 1991
10. Woodruff JM et al: Atypical carcinoid tumor of the larynx. A critical review of the literature. ORL J Otorhinolaryngol Relat Spec. 53(4):194-209, 1991
11. Wenig BM et al: The spectrum of neuroendocrine carcinomas of the larynx. Semin Diagn Pathol. 6(4):329-50, 1989
12. Wenig BM et al: Moderately differentiated neuroendocrine carcinoma of the larynx. A clinicopathologic study of 54 cases. Cancer. 62(12):2658-76, 1988
13. Woodruff JM et al: Neuroendocrine carcinomas of the larynx. A study of two types, one of which mimics thyroid medullary carcinoma. Am J Surg Pathol. 9(11):771-90, 1985
14. Mills SE et al: Small cell undifferentiated carcinoma of the larynx. Report of two patients and review of 13 additional cases. Cancer. 51(1):116-20, 1983

NEUROENDOCRINE CARCINOMA

Clinical Features of Laryngeal Neuroendocrine Neoplasms (LNEC)

	Laryngeal Paraganglioma	Carcinoid Tumor	Atypical Carcinoid	Small Cell Neuroendocrine Carcinoma
Frequency	Rare	Least common LNEC	Most common LNEC	2nd most common LNEC
Age/gender	5th decade; F > M	7th decade (on avg.); M > F	7th decade (on avg.); M > F	6th-7th decade; M > F
Risk factor(s)	None known	None known	Smoking	Smoking
Site	Supraglottis; aryepiglottic fold and false vocal cord			
Symptoms	Hoarseness; dysphagia, dyspnea, stridor	Hoarseness	Hoarseness	Hoarseness
Paraneoplastic syndrome	Exceptional; may be multicentric occurring in association with other head & neck paragangliomas	Rare	Rare	Occasional
Treatment	Surgery is curative	Surgery	Surgery; adjuvant radiotherapy and chemotherapy used but of questionable utility	Systemic chemotherapy and therapeutic irradiation
Metastasis	None	Approximately 33% have distant metastases (liver and bone)	Metastasis common to cervical lymph nodes, lung, bone, liver, skin	Metastasis frequent (even at presentation) to regional lymph nodes and to liver, lung, bone, and brain
Prognosis	Excellent	Indolent biology with excellent behavior	Fully malignant neoplasm; tumor confined to larynx: 3.9-y survival (62%), 5-y survival (48%), 10-y survival (30%)	Poor: 2-y survival (16%), 5-y survival (5%)

Pathology of Laryngeal Neuroendocrine Neoplasms

	Laryngeal Paraganglioma	Carcinoid Tumor	Atypical Carcinoid	Small Cell Neuroendocrine Carcinoma
Histology	Cell nest or "zellballen" pattern separated by prominent fibrovascular tissue	Submucosal tumor with organoid or trabecular growth pattern and fibrovascular stroma	Submucosal tumor with organoid, trabecular, cribriform or solid growth and fibrovascular stroma	Submucosal tumor with solid nests, sheets or ribbons and absence of a fibrovascular stroma
	Chief cells are predominant cell type	Neoplastic cells are uniform with "salt and pepper" nuclear chromatin	Neoplastic cells retain "salt and pepper" chromatin	Hypercellular tumor with "salt and pepper" nuclear chromatin; "crush" artifact frequently present
	Sustentacular cells lie at periphery of cells nests but are difficult, if not impossible, to identify by light microscopy	Absence of pleomorphism, mitoses, necrosis	Mild to marked nuclear pleomorphism and increased mitotic activity are present; necrosis uncommon	Confluent foci of necrosis and individual cell necrosis seen; abundant mitoses, including atypical forms
Invasiveness	Absent	Typically absent	Present; may include neurotropism and lymphovascular invasion	Present; commonly includes neurotropism and lymphovascular invasion
Histochemistry	Reticulin staining delineates cell nest growth pattern; tumor cells are argyrophilic (Churukian-Schenck[+]); argentaffin (Fontana), mucicarmine and periodic acid-Schiff stains are negative	Presence of epithelial mucin: Diastase-resistant, PAS(+); argyrophilic	Presence of epithelial mucin: Diastase-resistant, PAS(+) and occasionally mucicarmine(+); argyrophilic; rarely, argentaffin(+)	Epithelial mucin usually absent but may be present; argyrophilia rarely present
IHC	Chief cells: CHR, SYN, NSE, NFP positive; sustentacular cells: S100 protein(+); CK(-)	Positive for CK, CHR, SYN, CD56, CD57, NSE, EMA, CEA, TTF-1; may be positive for calcitonin, serotonin, somatostatin, bombesin	Positive for CK, CHR, SYN, CD56, CD57, calcitonin (> 80%); also positive for NSE, NFP, EMA, CEA, TTF-1	Positive CK, CHR, SYN, CD56, CD57; also positive for NSE, NFP, EMA, CEA, TTF-1; calcitonin rarely is positive

IHC = immunohistochemistry; CEA = carcinoembryonic antigen; CHR =chromogranin; CK = cytokeratins; EMA = epithelial membrane antigen; NFP = neurofibrillary protein; NSE = neuron specific enolase; SYN = synaptophysin; TTF-1 = thyroid transcription factor 1.

NEUROENDOCRINE CARCINOMA

Microscopic and Immunohistochemical Features

*(**Left**) At high magnification, cytomorphologic features of carcinoid include uniform round to oval nuclei with characteristic dispersed ("salt and pepper") nuclear chromatin and absence of nuclear pleomorphism, mitotic activity, and necrosis. (**Right**) Lesional cells are diffusely immunoreactive for cytokeratin (CAM5.2). The extent of cytokeratin reactivity varies from case to case and even within the same case such that cytokeratin staining may be diffusely present or only focally seen.*

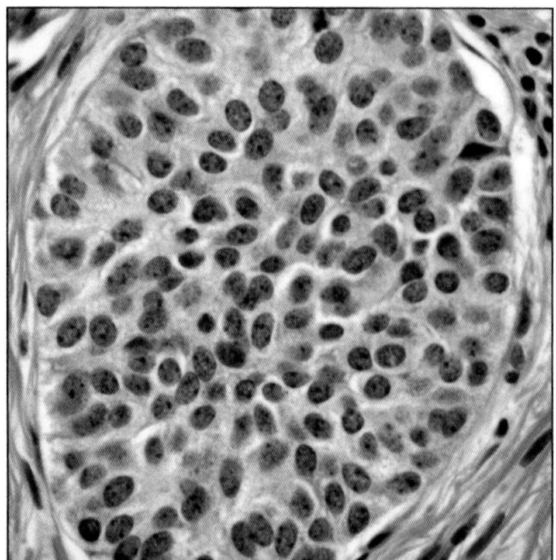

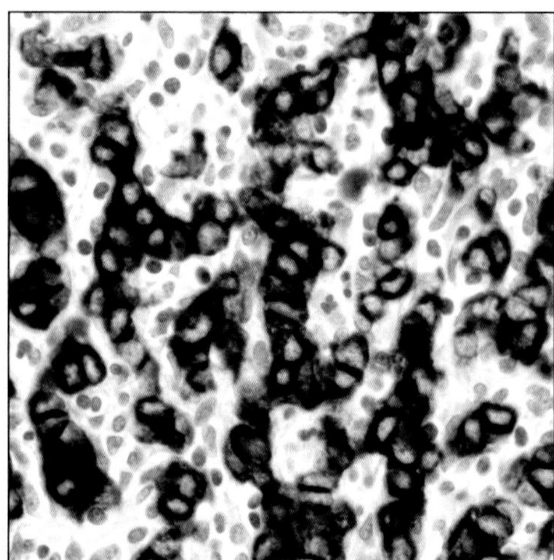

*(**Left**) In addition to epithelial markers, carcinoid tumors also include diffuse immunoreactivity for chromogranin. (**Right**) Lesional cells are diffusely immunoreactive for synaptophysin. Light microscopic features, including character of nuclear chromatin pattern, absence of significant pleomorphism & mitotic activity, coupled with the presence of immunostaining for epithelial markers & neuroendocrine markers, points to a neuroendocrine-type neoplasm (i.e., carcinoid tumor).*

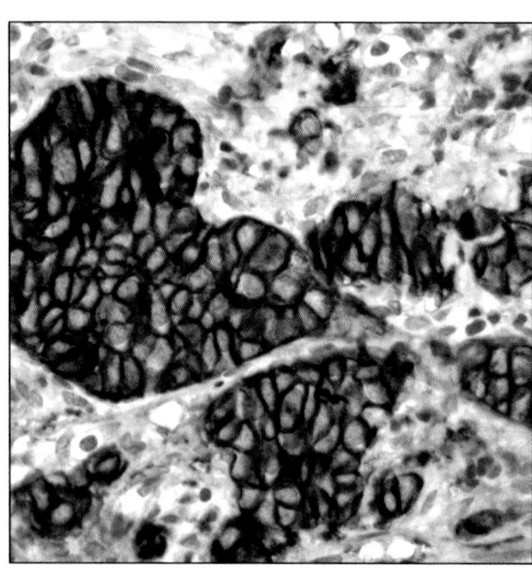

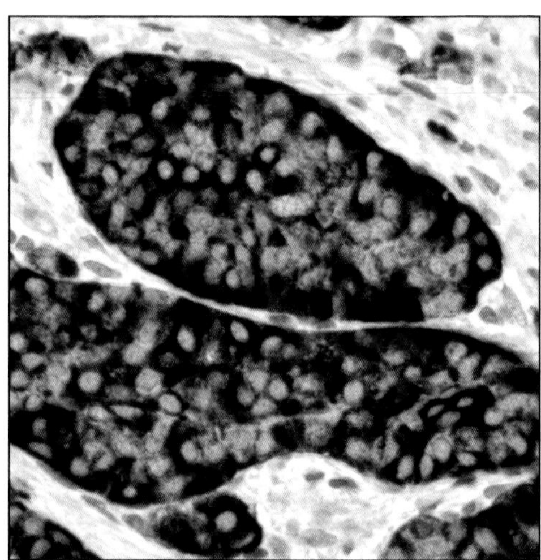

*(**Left**) Atypical carcinoid appears as a submucosal cellular infiltrate with organoid growth and fibrovascular stroma. (**Right**) At high magnification, the cell nest pattern is present composed of cells with round to oval nuclei, dispersed ("salt and pepper") nuclear chromatin, inconspicuous to small nucleoli and eosinophilic cytoplasm; variable but identifiable nuclear pleomorphism is present, but there is an absence of mitotic figures and necrosis.*

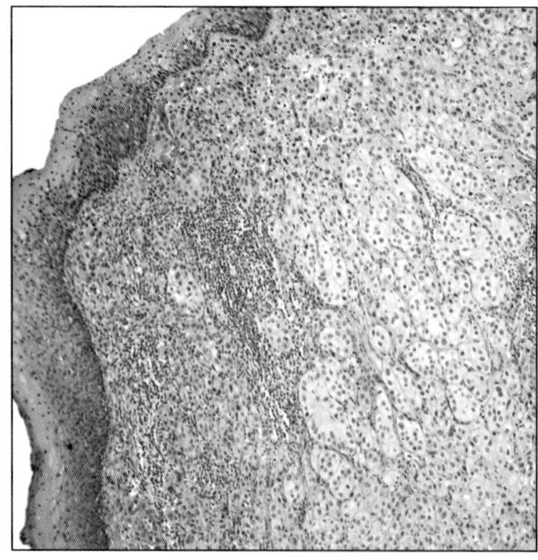

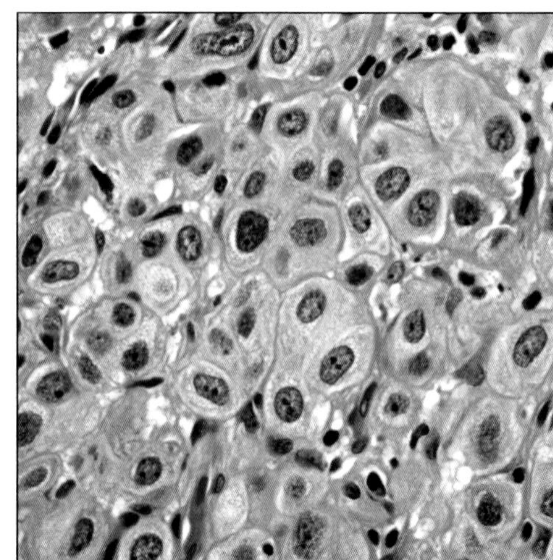

Microscopic and Immunohistochemical Features

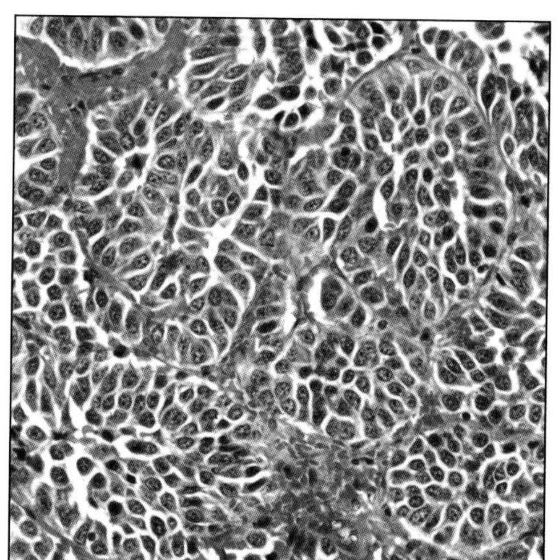

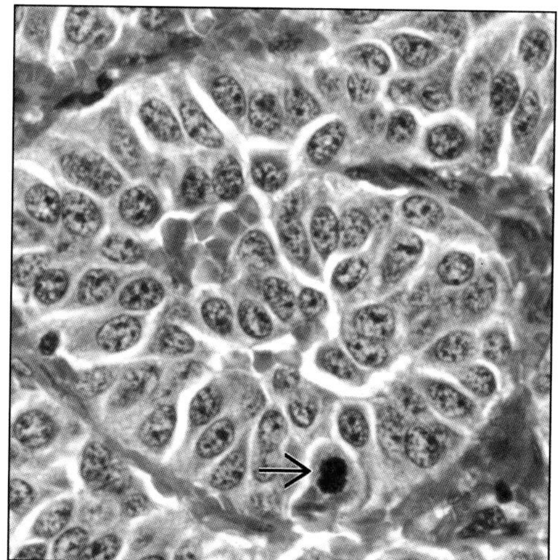

(Left) *Atypical carcinoid shows organoid (cell nest) growth with fibrovascular stroma.* ***(Right)*** *Cell nest comprised of cells with round to oval nuclei, dispersed ("salt and pepper") nuclear chromatin, inconspicuous to small nucleoli, and basophilic to eosinophilic cytoplasm is shown. Nuclear pleomorphism is present, and there is a mitotic figure ⊡. The greater nuclear pleomorphism and presence of mitotic figures separates carcinoids from atypical carcinoids.*

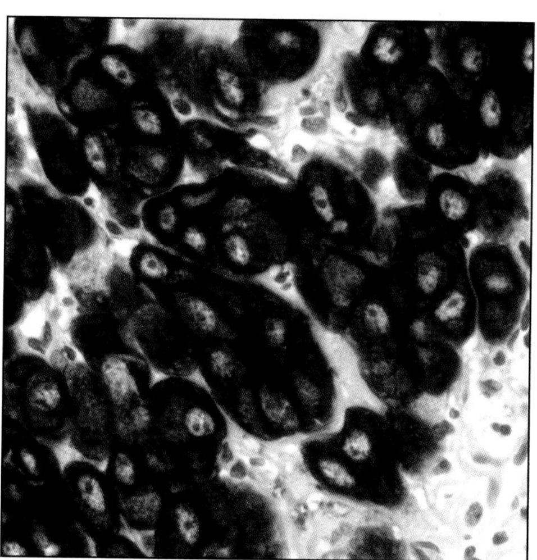

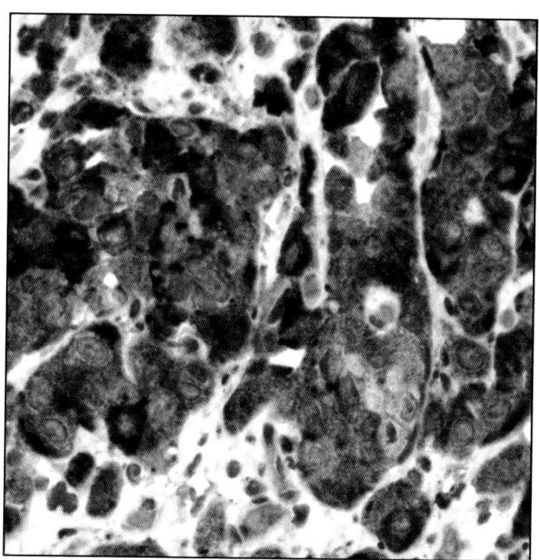

(Left) *Atypical carcinoid shows diffuse immunoreactivity for CAM 5.2.* ***(Right)*** *Atypical carcinoid shows immunoreactivity for synaptophysin. Similar to carcinoid tumors, the combination of the light microscopic features, including dispersed chromatin coupled with the presence of immunoreactivity for cytokeratins and neuroendocrine markers, points to a possible diagnosis of a neuroendocrine carcinoma.*

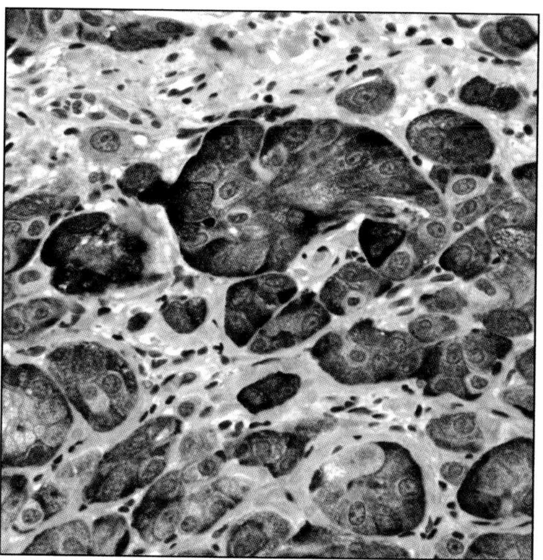

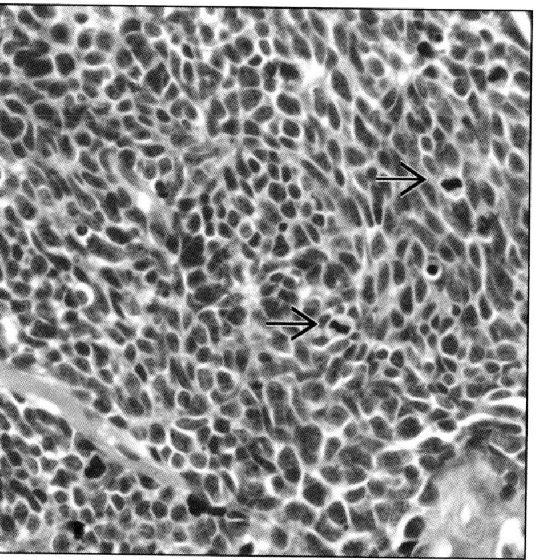

(Left) *Immunoreactivity for calcitonin can be seen in a majority of atypical carcinoids. In contrast to thyroid medullary carcinoma, levels of serum calcitonin are not elevated.* ***(Right)*** *Laryngeal small cell undifferentiated neuroendocrine carcinoma is characterized by a hypercellular proliferation with solid growth comprised of hyperchromatic nuclei with dispersed ("salt and pepper") nuclear chromatin, nuclear molding, inconspicuous nucleoli, and increased mitotic activity ⊡.*

NEUROENDOCRINE CARCINOMA

Microscopic and Immunohistochemical Features

*(**Left**) In this image of laryngeal small cell undifferentiated neuroendocrine carcinoma, the neoplastic cells have more spindle-shaped-appearing nuclei characterized by stippled ("salt and pepper") appearing chromatin, inconspicuous to small nucleoli, increased mitotic activity ⇒, and individual cell necrosis ⇗. (**Right**) In this laryngeal small cell undifferentiated neuroendocrine carcinoma, a confluent area of necrosis ⇒ is seen adjacent to the small round cell malignant infiltrate.*

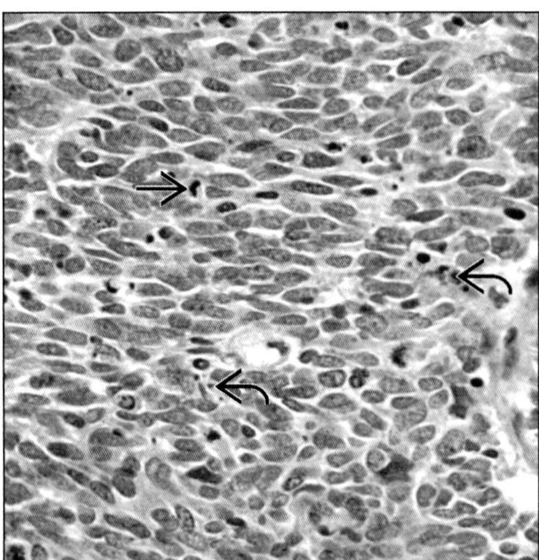

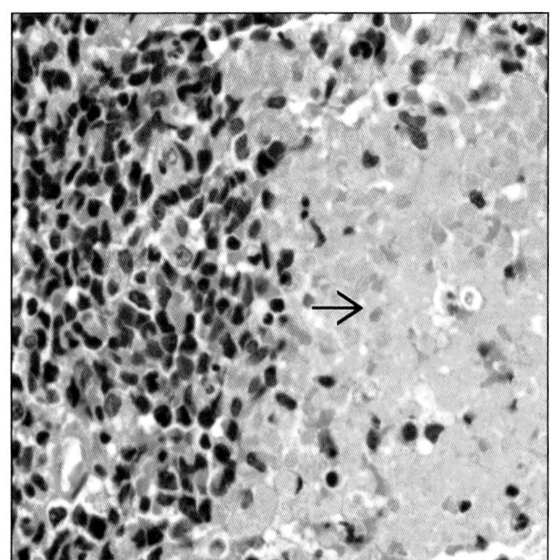

*(**Left**) In this example of a laryngeal small cell undifferentiated neuroendocrine carcinoma, neural-type rosettes ⇒ are present. Rosettes are not unique to neuroendocrine carcinomas and can be seen in other tumor types, including olfactory neuroblastoma and basaloid squamous cell carcinoma. (**Right**) Diffuse immunoreactivity is present for CAM5.2.*

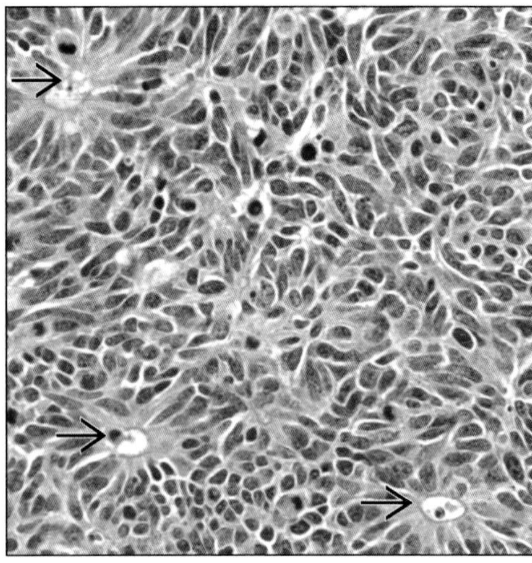

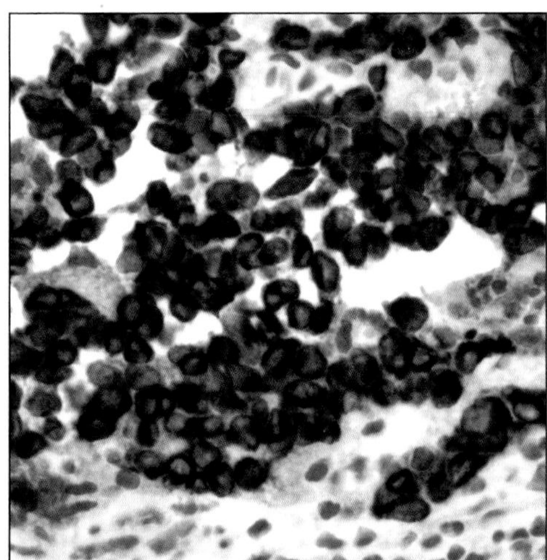

*(**Left**) Immunoreactivity is present for chromogranin. (**Right**) Immunoreactivity is present for synaptophysin. Similar to the carcinoids and atypical carcinoids, the combination of the light microscopic features and immunoreactivity for epithelial and neuroendocrine markers assist in the diagnosis. The nuclear pleomorphism, increased mitotic activity, and necrosis differentiates small cell neuroendocrine carcinoma from carcinoid and atypical carcinoid.*

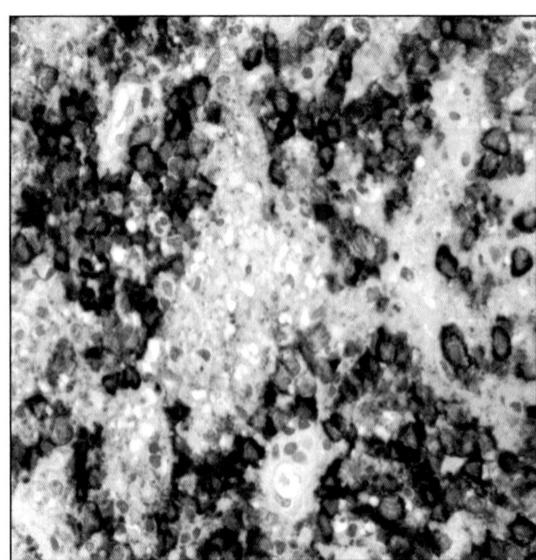

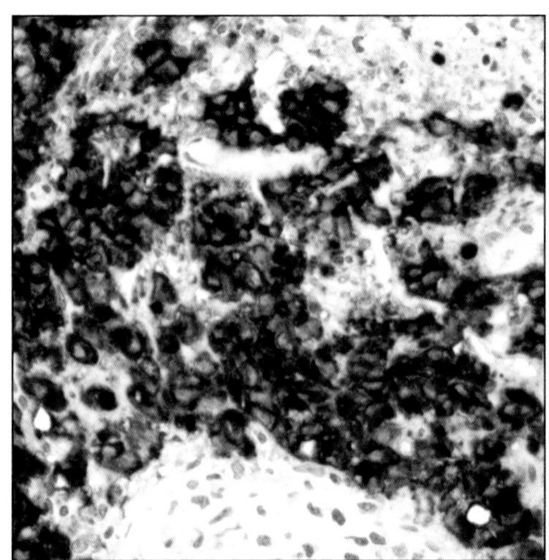

Microscopic and Immunohistochemical Features

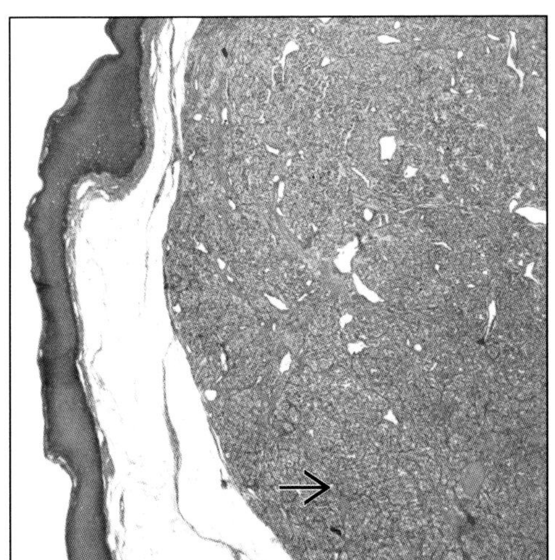

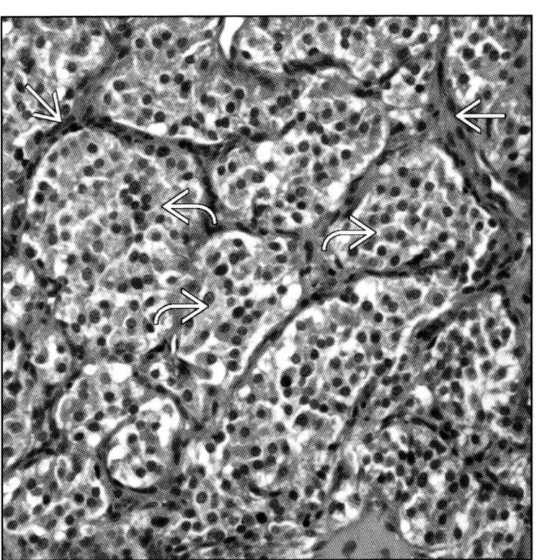

(Left) *Laryngeal paraganglioma shows the presence of a cellular submucosal neoplasm with organoid growth* ⇒ *and prominent vascularity, including variably sized blood vessels.* ***(Right)*** *Classic cell nest (zellballen) growth pattern* ⇒ *with nests separated by fibrovascular stroma* ⇒ *is a characteristic feature of paragangliomas of all sites. Similar architectural features are seen in neuroendocrine carcinomas, especially carcinoid and atypical carcinoid tumors.*

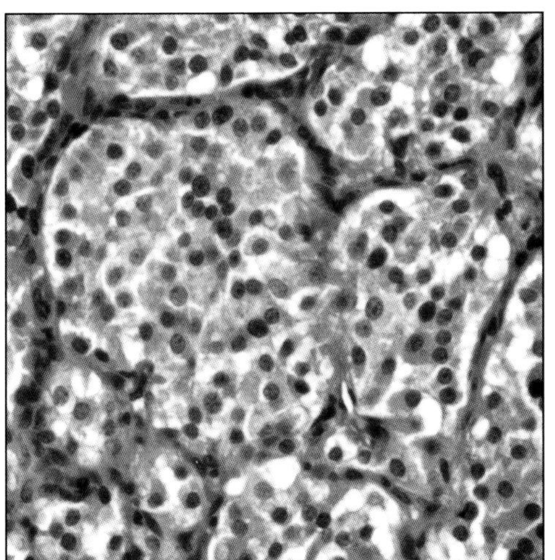

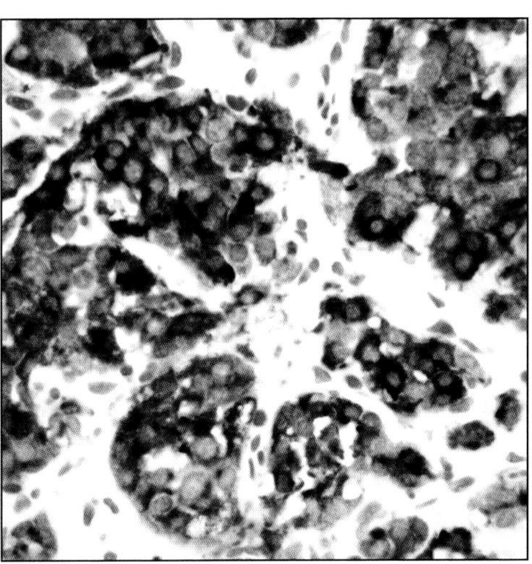

(Left) *Paragangliomas are predominantly composed of chief cells, which are round or oval with uniform nuclei, dispersed chromatin pattern, and abundant eosinophilic, granular, or vacuolated cytoplasm. The sustentacular cells are difficult to identify by light microscopy as they have similar features (i.e., spindle-shaped, basophilic cells) as cells within the fibrovascular cores.* ***(Right)*** *The chief cells of paragangliomas are diffusely immunoreactive with chromogranin.*

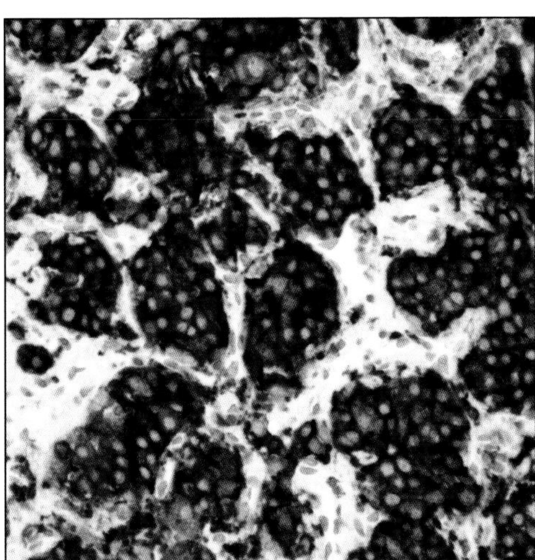

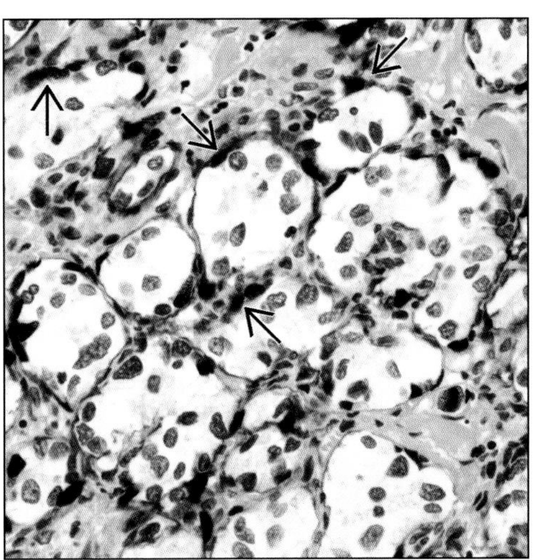

(Left) *In addition to chromogranin, chief cells of paragangliomas are diffusely immunoreactive with synaptophysin. Carcinoid tumors may share overlapping light microscopic and IHC features with paragangliomas but will be immunoreactive for epithelial markers (e.g., cytokeratins), a finding not expected to be seen in paragangliomas.* ***(Right)*** *S100 protein staining in paragangliomas typically is limited to the peripherally located sustentacular cells* ⇒.

CHONDROSARCOMA

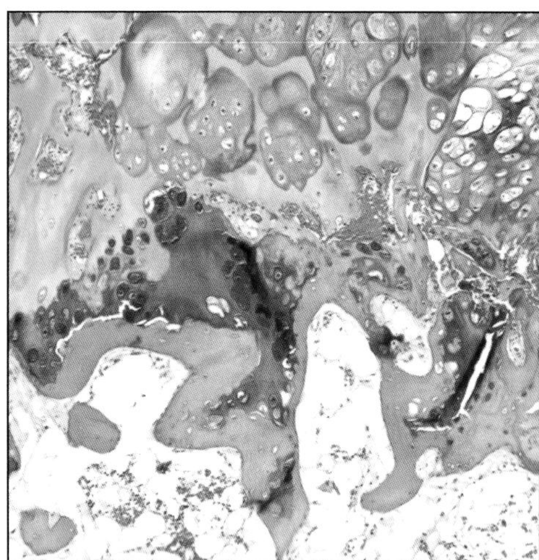

Hematoxylin & eosin shows neoplastic cartilage in the upper field infiltrating bone and native cartilage. There is cluster disarray.

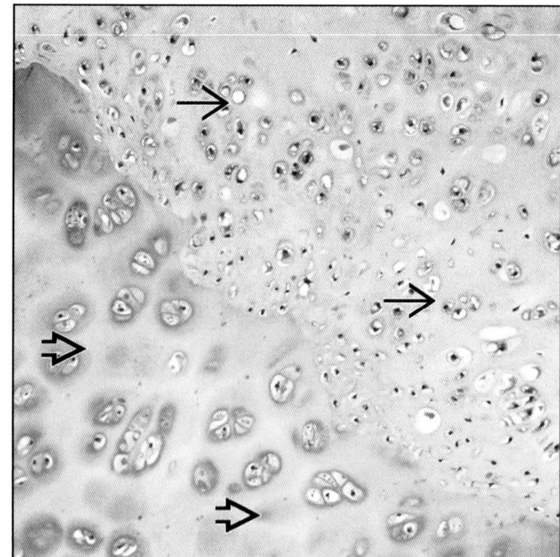

Hematoxylin & eosin shows normal cartilage ⇨ immediately juxtaposed to the increased cellularity of low-grade chondrosarcoma →. A difference in cell size and lacunar distribution is noted.

TERMINOLOGY

Definitions

- Malignant neoplasm forming neoplastic cartilage

ETIOLOGY/PATHOGENESIS

Disordered Ossification

- Ossification of laryngeal hyaline cartilages at points of mechanical stress/tension (muscle insertion points)

Ischemic Change

- Ischemic change in chondromas related to mechanical trauma predisposes to malignant transformation

Continuum with Chondroma

- Usually develop a decade earlier, suggesting arc of development (continuum)

CLINICAL ISSUES

Epidemiology

- Incidence
  - Represents 1% of all laryngeal primary malignancies but 75% of laryngeal sarcomas
- Age
  - Mean: 60-65 years
  - Range: 25-91 years
- Gender
  - Male > > Female (4:1)

Site

- Cricoid cartilage (85%)
- Does not develop in elastic cartilages (i.e., epiglottis)

Presentation

- Difficulty breathing due to progressive narrowing by endolaryngeal growth
- Hoarseness, dyspnea, dysphagia, stridor
- Mass for thyroid cartilage neoplasms specifically
- Symptoms present for long duration (> 2 years)

Treatment

- Options, risks, complications
  - Requires long-term follow-up, often with repeated "limited" surgeries to maintain phonation
- Surgical approaches
  - Complete but conservative laryngeal function-preserving surgery
    - Multiple surgeries over many years for recurrences
    - Voice-preserving surgeries give best long-term quality of life (tracheal autotransplantation and rib interposition)

Prognosis

- Excellent, > 95% 10-year survival
- Recurrences develop in up to 40% of patients, but metastatic disease is rare
- Tumor grade does not alter prognosis
- Histologic subtype does not change outcome, but myxoid tumors may be more likely to recur

IMAGE FINDINGS

CT Findings

- Ill-defined, invasive, destructive, hypodense mass
- Fine, punctate to coarse (popcorn) calcifications

MACROSCOPIC FEATURES

General Features

- Inner, posterior, midline lamina of cricoid
- Crunchy, hard, lobular mass
- Glistening, blue-gray, semitranslucent myxoid-mucoid cut surface
- Dedifferentiated tumors have fleshy areas

CHONDROSARCOMA

Key Facts

Etiology/Pathogenesis
- Disordered ossification of laryngeal cartilages at points of mechanical stress/tension (muscle insertion points)

Clinical Issues
- Cricoid cartilage (85%)
- Does not develop in elastic cartilages (i.e., epiglottis)
- Male > > Female (4:1)
- Mean: 60-65 years
- Conservative laryngeal-function preserving surgery
- Grade does not alter prognosis
- Metastatic disease is vanishingly rare

Image Findings
- Fine, punctate stippled to coarse (popcorn) calcifications within mass

Macroscopic Features
- Inner, posterior lamina (midline) of cricoid cartilage most commonly affected

Microscopic Pathology
- Bone invasion and destruction
- Increased cellularity in comparison to normal cartilage
- Loss of normal architecture and lacunar distribution (cluster disarray)
- Tumors separated into 3 grades
- 3 tumor subtypes: Myxoid, mesenchymal, dedifferentiated

Top Differential Diagnoses
- Chondroma
- Spindle cell (sarcomatoid) squamous cell carcinoma

Size
- Mean: 3.5 cm
- Range: Up to 12 cm

MICROSCOPIC PATHOLOGY

Histologic Features
- Bone invasion and destruction
- Basophilic cartilaginous matrix in comparison to eosinophilic normal cartilage
- Cellular tumors with loss of normal architecture and lacunar distribution (cluster disarray)
- Nuclear atypia with bi- and multinucleation of cells with increased nuclear to cytoplasmic ratio
- Ischemic change (blue, granular cytoplasm) can be seen in background
- Mitotic figures and necrosis rarely present (only in high-grade tumors)
- Tumors separated into 3 grades
- 3 tumor subtypes
  - Myxoid chondrosarcoma (grade II)
  - Mesenchymal chondrosarcoma (grade III)
  - Dedifferentiated chondrosarcoma (grade III)

DIFFERENTIAL DIAGNOSIS

Chondroma
- Small lesion (< 2 cm), very uncommon, showing slightly increased cellularity over normal

Spindle Cell "Sarcomatoid" Squamous Cell Carcinoma
- Metaplastic/malignant cartilage may develop, but tumor is polypoid, associated with spindle cell proliferation
- Keratin immunoreactive in 70% of cases

Chondrometaplasia
- Multifocal elastic cartilage nodules within vocal cord, blending with surrounding tissue (no mass)

GRADING

Low Grade
- Mildly increased cellularity, mild pleomorphism

Intermediate Grade
- Moderate cellularity, moderate pleomorphism, less cartilaginous matrix

High Grade
- High cellularity, severe pleomorphism, increased mitoses, necrosis

SELECTED REFERENCES

1. Delaere P et al: Organ preservation surgery for advanced unilateral glottic and subglottic cancer. Laryngoscope. 117(10):1764-9, 2007
2. Sauter A et al: Chondrosarcoma of the larynx and review of the literature. Anticancer Res. 27(4C):2925-9, 2007
3. Baatenburg de Jong RJ et al: Chondroma and chondrosarcoma of the larynx. Curr Opin Otolaryngol Head Neck Surg. 12(2):98-105, 2004
4. Casiraghi O et al: Chondroid tumors of the larynx: a clinicopathologic study of 19 cases, including two dedifferentiated chondrosarcomas. Ann Diagn Pathol. 8(4):189-97, 2004
5. Garcia RE et al: Dedifferentiated chondrosarcomas of the larynx: a report of two cases and review of the literature. Laryngoscope. 112(6):1015-8, 2002
6. Thompson LD et al: Chondrosarcoma of the larynx: a clinicopathologic study of 111 cases with a review of the literature. Am J Surg Pathol. 26(7):836-51, 2002
7. Rinaldo A et al: Laryngeal chondrosarcoma: a 24-year experience at the Royal National Throat, Nose and Ear Hospital. Acta Otolaryngol. 120(6):680-8, 2000
8. Kozelsky TF et al: Laryngeal chondrosarcomas: the Mayo Clinic experience. J Surg Oncol. 65(4):269-73, 1997
9. Lewis JE et al: Cartilaginous tumors of the larynx: clinicopathologic review of 47 cases. Ann Otol Rhinol Laryngol. 106(2):94-100, 1997
10. Devaney KO et al: Cartilaginous tumors of the larynx. Ann Otol Rhinol Laryngol. 104(3):251-5, 1995

CHONDROSARCOMA

Radiographic, Gross, and Microscopic Features

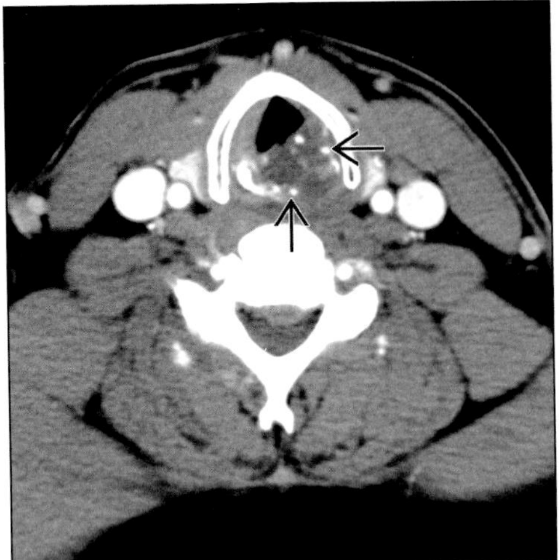

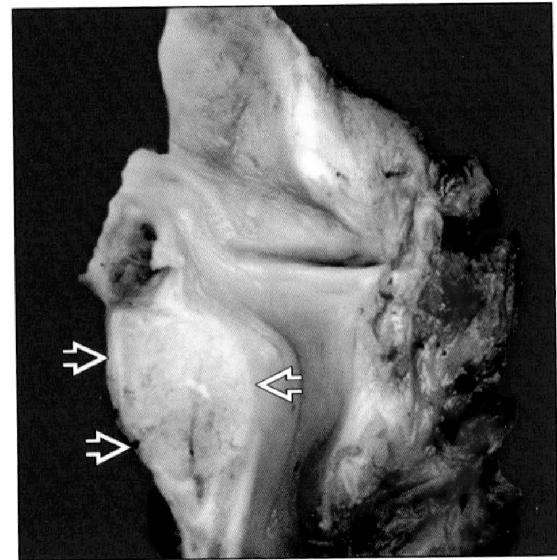

(Left) *Radiologic image shows destruction of the posterior lamina of the cricoid cartilage by a neoplastic proliferation. Note the speckled calcifications ➔.* ***(Right)*** *Gross photograph shows a neoplastic proliferation within the cricoid cartilage ➔.*

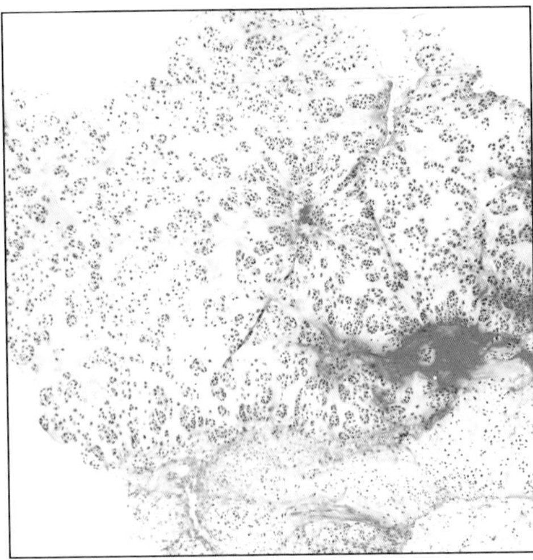

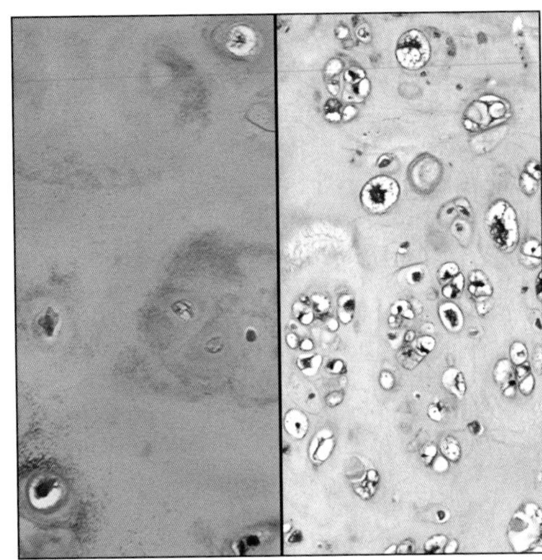

(Left) *Hematoxylin & eosin shows a highly cellular neoplastic cartilaginous neoplasm.* ***(Right)*** *Hematoxylin & eosin shows normal cartilage (left) with neoplastic cartilage (right) taken at the same magnification. This shows an increased number of lacunar spaces and increased nuclear to cytoplasmic ratio.*

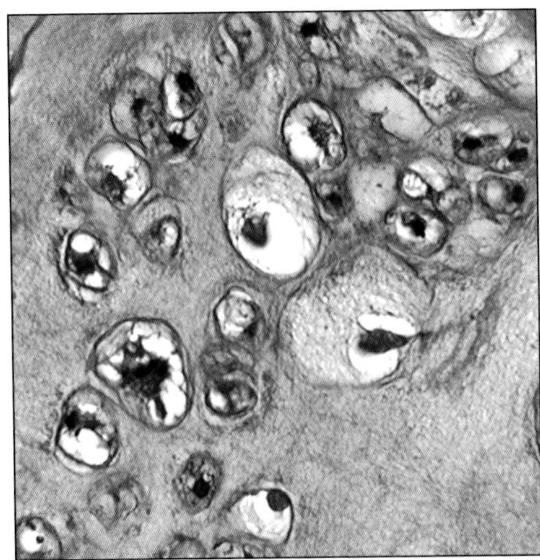

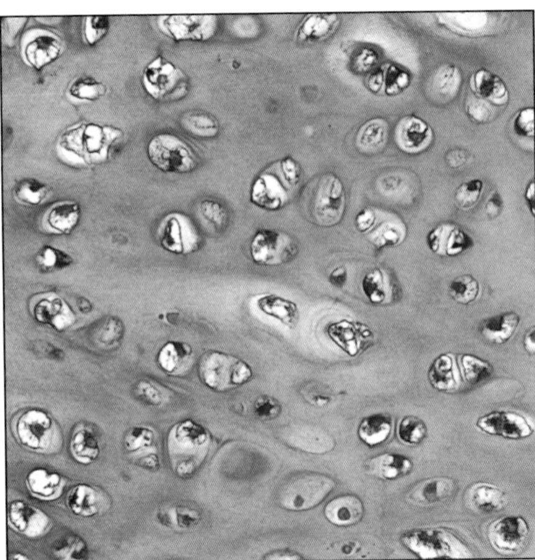

(Left) *Hematoxylin & eosin shows atypical nuclei within enlarged lacunar spaces in this grade I chondrosarcoma.* ***(Right)*** *Hematoxylin & eosin shows lacunar disarray and increased cellularity in this grade I chondrosarcoma.*

Microscopic Features

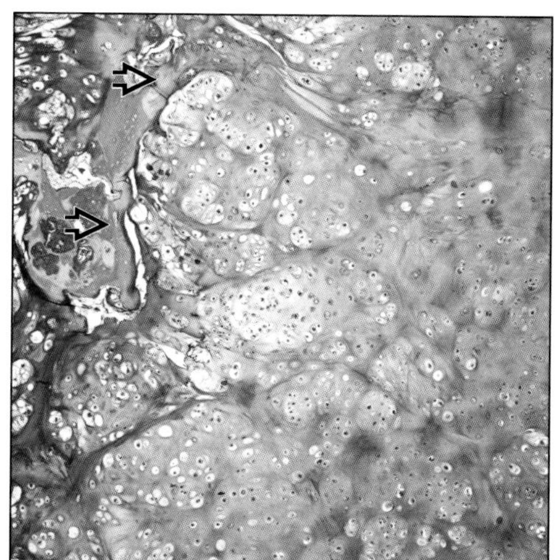

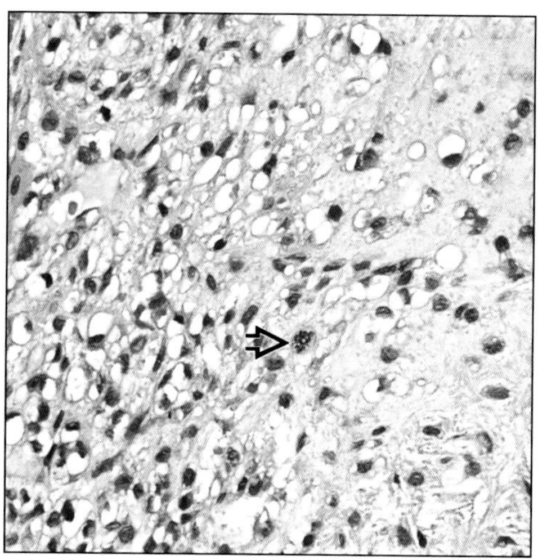

*(**Left**) Hematoxylin & eosin shows an increased cellularity within a cartilaginous neoplasm that destroys bone ➲ in this grade I chondrosarcoma. (**Right**) Hematoxylin & eosin shows increased cellularity and a single mitotic figure ➲ in this grade II chondrosarcoma.*

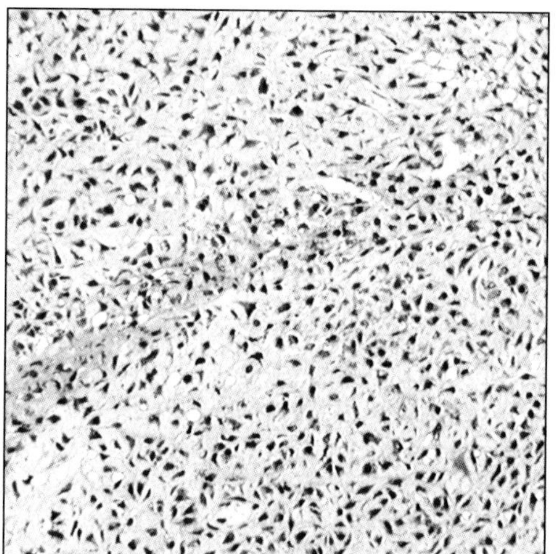

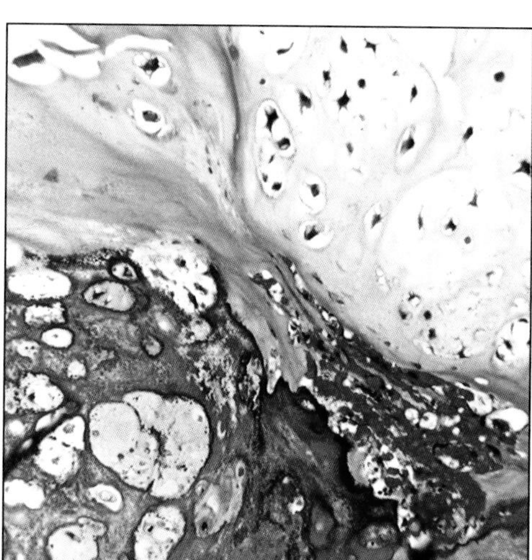

*(**Left**) Hematoxylin & eosin shows remarkably increased cellularity and lacunar space disorganization in this grade III chondrosarcoma. (**Right**) Hematoxylin & eosin shows ischemic change in a chondroma (bottom left) immediately adjacent to a chondrosarcoma (right upper).*

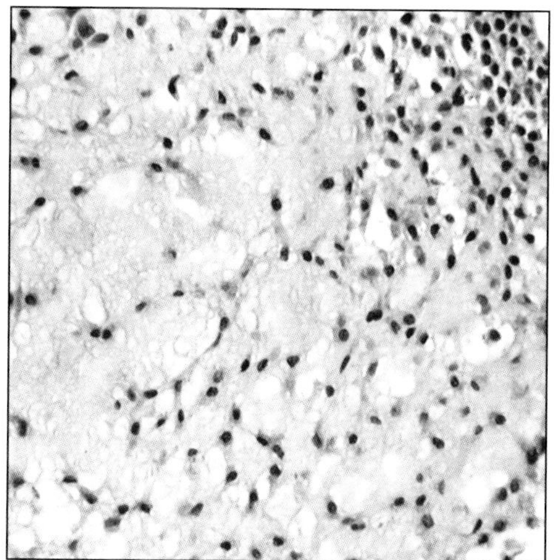

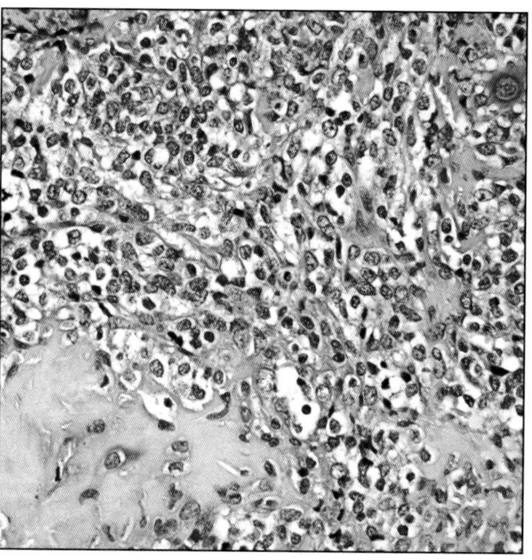

*(**Left**) Hematoxylin & eosin shows the "string of beads" or "string of pearls" pattern diagnostic for a myxoid chondrosarcoma. (**Right**) Hematoxylin & eosin shows a "small round blue cell" population with associated cartilage, diagnostic of mesenchymal chondrosarcoma. This is different from dedifferentiated chondrosarcoma, which shows a spindle cell population (sarcoma).*

METASTATIC/SECONDARY TUMORS

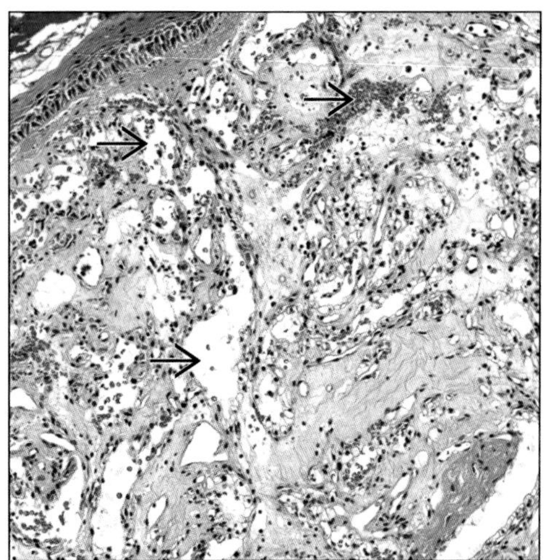

Hematoxylin & eosin shows an intact squamous mucosa overlying the richly vascularized metastatic clear cell renal cell carcinoma. Note the vascularized neoplastic spaces ⇒.

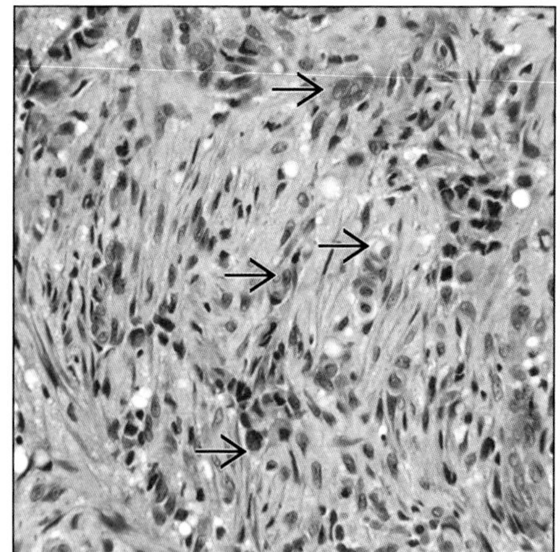

There is an infiltration by neoplastic adenocarcinoma cells in a single file ⇒. The primary tumor was identified in the breast. There is a heavy fibroblastic stroma separating the tumor cells.

TERMINOLOGY

Definitions

- Tumors secondarily involving larynx or hypopharynx that originate from, but are not in continuity with, primary malignancies of other sites
  - Lymphomas and leukemias are excluded by definition

CLINICAL ISSUES

Epidemiology

- Incidence
  - Uncommon
    - < 0.2% of all malignancies of larynx
- Age
  - Older ages, correlated with increased malignancies of other anatomic sites
- Gender
  - Male > Female (2:1)

Site

- Mucosa-submucosa
  - Supraglottis most common (40%)
  - Subglottis (20%)
  - Glottis (10%)
- Cartilages
  - Usually areas that have undergone endochondral ossification
- Multifocal sites within larynx are common
  - Approximately 35% of cases

Presentation

- Hoarseness
- Voice changes
- Difficulty breathing
- Stridor

Treatment

- Options, risks, complications
  - Rarely, metastatic disease to larynx may be the only, isolated metastasis
    - Most commonly with renal cell carcinoma
- Surgical approaches
  - Excision is performed for symptomatic relief

Prognosis

- Matches underlying disease but usually part of disseminated disease
- Prognosis is usually grave
  - However, renal cell carcinoma may be exception, associated with good prognosis with isolated metastatic foci

MACROSCOPIC FEATURES

General Features

- Submucosal mass
- Surface epithelium usually intact

MICROSCOPIC PATHOLOGY

Histologic Features

- Specific tumor type dictates histology
- Most common tumors are melanomas or carcinomas
  - Melanoma (40%)
  - Kidney (13%)
  - Breast (9%)
  - Lung (8%)
  - Prostate (7%)
  - Gastrointestinal tract (colon and stomach) (6%)
- Of carcinomas, adenocarcinomas are most frequent, a tumor type that is uncommon as a primary larynx tumor
- Mesenchymal tumors rarely metastasize to larynx
  - Leiomyosarcoma is most common of mesenchymal lesions to metastasize

METASTATIC/SECONDARY TUMORS

Key Facts

Terminology

- Tumors that secondarily involve larynx or hypopharynx that originate from, but are not in continuity with, primary malignancies of other sites
  - Lymphomas and leukemias are excluded by definition

Clinical Issues

- Uncommon (< 0.2% of all malignancies of larynx)
- Male > Female (2:1)
- Supraglottis most common (40%)
- Prognosis is usually grave

Microscopic Pathology

- Specific tumor type dictates histology
- Most common tumors are melanomas or carcinomas
  - Melanoma (40%)
  - Kidney (13%)
  - Breast (9%)
  - Lung (8%)

DIFFERENTIAL DIAGNOSIS

Primary Tumor

- Primary poorly differentiated tumors may need to be separated from metastatic tumors
  - Separation can usually be achieved by history, radiographic studies, and immunohistochemistry
  - Primary adenocarcinomas of larynx are rare
  - Salivary gland tumor-type primaries are more frequent

Direct Extension

- Thyroid gland tumors (especially medullary carcinoma) must be separated from primary and metastatic lesions
  - Frequently radiographic correlation is required, as immunohistochemistry is insufficient
    - Primary atypical carcinoid tumors of larynx are usually calcitonin immunoreactive
    - Serum calcitonin levels usually positive in thyroid gland tumors and negative in primary larynx carcinoma
- Squamous cell carcinoma of esophagus may extend into larynx
- Hematologic neoplasms (lymphoma and plasmacytoma/multiple myeloma) may mimic primary tumors
  - Clinical, radiographic, or laboratory investigation will usually resolve this question

SELECTED REFERENCES

1. Ferlito A et al: Primary and secondary small cell neuroendocrine carcinoma of the larynx: a review. Head Neck. 30(4):518-24, 2008
2. Ramanathan Y et al: Laryngeal metastasis from a rectal carcinoma. Ear Nose Throat J. 86(11):685-6, 2007
3. Marioni G et al: Laryngeal metastasis from sigmoid colon adenocarcinoma followed by peristomal recurrence. Acta Otolaryngol. 126(6):661-3, 2006
4. Abbas A et al: Leiomyosarcoma of the larynx: A case report. Ear Nose Throat J. 84(7):435-6, 440, 2005
5. Sano D et al: A case of metastatic colon adenocarcinoma in the larynx. Acta Otolaryngol. 125(2):220-2, 2005
6. Prescher A et al: Laryngeal prostatic cancer metastases: an underestimated route of metastases? Laryngoscope. 112(8 Pt 1):1467-73, 2002
7. Nicolai P et al: Metastatic neoplasms to the larynx: report of three cases. Laryngoscope. 106(7):851-5, 1996
8. Bernáldez R et al: Pulmonary carcinoma metastatic to the larynx. J Laryngol Otol. 108(10):898-901, 1994
9. Marlowe SD et al: Metastatic hypernephroma to the larynx: an unusual presentation. Neuroradiology. 35(3):242-3, 1993
10. Batsakis JG et al: Metastases to the larynx. Head Neck Surg. 7(6):458-60, 1985
11. Ritchie WW et al: Uterine carcinoma metastatic to the larynx. Laryngoscope. 95(1):97-8, 1985
12. Coakley JF et al: Metastasis to the larynx from a prostatic carcinoma. A case report. J Laryngol Otol. 98(8):839-42, 1984
13. Abemayor E et al: Metastatic cancer to the larynx. Diagnosis and management. Cancer. 52(10):1944-8, 1983

IMAGE GALLERY

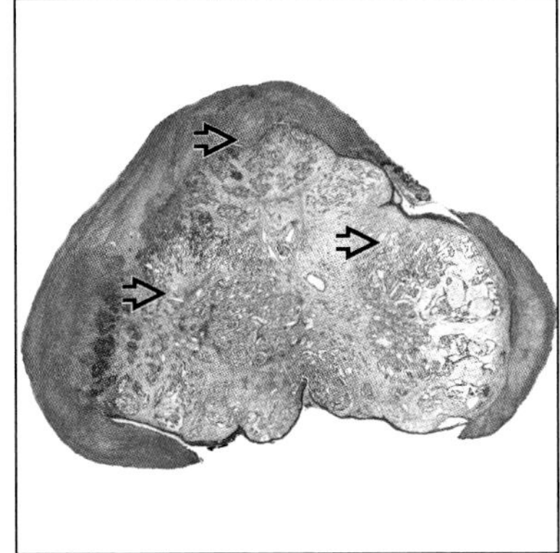

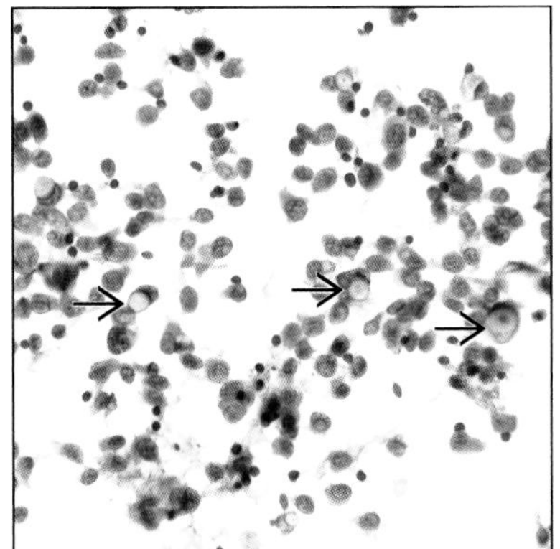

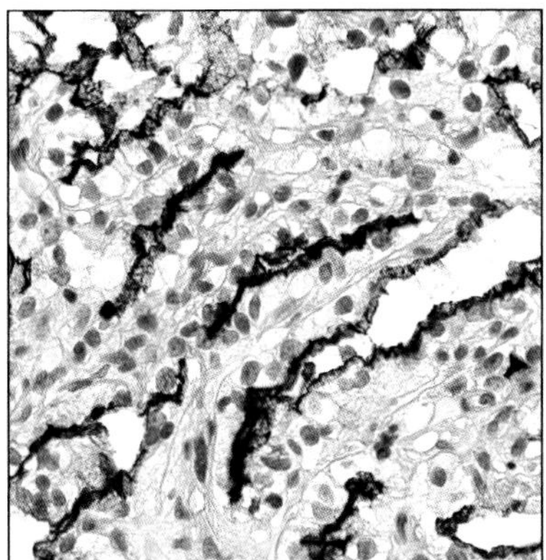

(Left) *Hematoxylin & eosin reveals a polypoid mass showing ulceration. The neoplastic proliferation is seen filling the stroma of the polyp ⇨. This is a metastatic renal cell carcinoma with vascularized stroma.* ***(Center)*** *Papanicolaou stain of a cellular smear shows mucin vacuoles → in the cytoplasm of metastatic breast carcinoma to the larynx.* ***(Right)*** *CD10 shows strong membrane reactivity, helping to confirm the diagnosis of metastatic renal cell carcinoma.*

PROTOCOL FOR THE EXAMINATION OF LARYNX SPECIMENS

Larynx (Supraglottis, Glottis, Subglottis)

Incisional Biopsy, Excisional Biopsy, Resection

Specimen (select all that apply)

___ Larynx, supraglottis
___ Larynx, glottis
___ Larynx, subglottis
___ Other (specify): ______________________
___ Not specified

Received

___ Fresh
___ In formalin
___ Other (specify): ______________________

Procedure (select all that apply)

___ Incisional biopsy
___ Excisional biopsy
___ Resection
  ___ Stripping (glottis)
  ___ Transoral laser excision (glottis)
  ___ Supraglottic laryngectomy
  ___ Vertical hemilaryngectomy (specify side): _______
  ___ Partial laryngectomy (specify type): _______
  ___ Total laryngectomy
___ Neck (lymph node dissection) (specify): ______________________
___ Other (specify): ______________________

**Specimen Integrity*

*___Intact
*___Fragmented

Laryngectomy

___ Open
___ Unopened

Specimen Size

Greatest dimensions: _______ x _______ x _______ cm
*Additional dimensions (if more than 1 part): _______ x _______ x _______ cm

Tumor Laterality (select all that apply)

___ Right
___ Left
___ Bilateral
  Transglottic
  ___ Yes
  ___ No
___ Midline
___ Not specified

Tumor Site (select all that apply)

___ Larynx, supraglottis
  ___ Epiglottis
    ___ Lingual aspect
    ___ Laryngeal aspect
  ___ Aryepiglottic folds
  ___ Arytenoid(s)
  ___ False vocal cord
  ___ Ventricle

___ Larynx, glottis
  ___ True vocal cord
  ___ Anterior commissure
  ___ Posterior commissure
___ Larynx, subglottis
___ Other (specify): ____________________________
___ Not specified

Tumor Focality

___ Single focus
___ Bilateral
___ Multifocal (specify): ____________________________
___ Not specified

Tumor Size

Greatest dimension: __________ cm
*Additional dimensions: __________ x __________ cm
___ Cannot be determined

Tumor Description (select all that apply)

*Gross subtype
  *___ Polypoid
  *___ Exophytic
  *___ Endophytic
  *___ Ulcerated
  *___ Sessile
  *___ Other (specify): ____________________________

*Macroscopic Extent of Tumor

*Specify: ____________________________

Histologic Type (select all that apply)

___ Squamous cell carcinoma, conventional
___ Variants of squamous cell carcinoma
  ___ Acantholytic squamous cell carcinoma
  ___ Adenosquamous carcinoma
  ___ Basaloid squamous cell carcinoma
  ___ Papillary squamous cell carcinoma
  ___ Spindle cell squamous cell carcinoma
  ___ Verrucous carcinoma
___ Giant cell carcinoma
___ Lymphoepithelial carcinoma (non-nasopharyngeal)
___ Neuroendocrine carcinoma
  ___ Typical carcinoid tumor (well-differentiated neuroendocrine carcinoma)
  ___ Atypical carcinoid tumor (moderately differentiated neuroendocrine carcinoma)
  ___ Small cell carcinoma, neuroendocrine type (poorly differentiated neuroendocrine carcinoma)
  ___ Combined (or composite) small cell carcinoma, neuroendocrine type
___ Mucosal malignant melanoma
___ Carcinomas of minor salivary glands
  ___ Adenoid cystic carcinoma
  ___ Mucoepidermoid carcinoma
    ___ Low grade
    ___ Intermediate grade
    ___ High grade
  ___ Other (specify): ____________________________
___ Other carcinoma (specify): ____________________________
___ Carcinoma, type cannot be determined

PROTOCOL FOR THE EXAMINATION OF LARYNX SPECIMENS

Histologic Grade

___ Not applicable
___ GX: Cannot be assessed
___ G1: Well differentiated
___ G2: Moderately differentiated
___ G3: Poorly differentiated
___ Other (specify): ___________________________

****Microscopic Tumor Extension***

*Specify: ___________________________

Margins (select all that apply)

___ Cannot be assessed
___ Margins uninvolved by invasive carcinoma
Distance from closest margin: _________ mm or _________ cm
Specify margin(s), per orientation, if possible: ___________________________
___ Margins involved by invasive carcinoma
Specify margin(s), per orientation, if possible: ___________________________
___ Margins uninvolved by carcinoma in situ (includes moderate and severe dysplasia)†
Distance from closest margin: _________ mm or _________ cm
Specify margin(s), per orientation, if possible: ___________________________
___ Margins involved by carcinoma in situ (includes moderate and severe dysplasia)†
Specify margin(s), per orientation, if possible: ___________________________
___ Not applicable

****Treatment Effect (applicable to carcinomas treated with neoadjuvant therapy)***

*___Not identified
*___Present (specify): ___________________________
*___Indeterminate

Lymph-Vascular Invasion

___ Not identified
___ Present
___ Indeterminate

Perineural Invasion

___ Not identified
___ Present
___ Indeterminate

Lymph Nodes, Extranodal Extension

___ Not identified
___ Present
___ Indeterminate

Pathologic Staging (pTNM)

TNM descriptors (required only if applicable) (select all that apply)
___ m (multiple primary tumors)
___ r (recurrent)
___ y (post-treatment)

Primary tumor (pT)
___ pTX: Cannot be assessed
___ pT0: No evidence of primary tumor
___ pTis: Carcinoma in situ

For All Carcinomas Excluding Mucosal Malignant Melanoma

Primary tumor (pT): Supraglottis
___ pT1: Tumor limited to 1 subsite of supraglottis **with normal vocal cord mobility**
___ pT2: Tumor invades > 1 adjacent subsite of supraglottis or glottis or region outside supraglottis

(e.g., mucosa of base of tongue, vallecula, medial wall of pyriform sinus) **without fixation of larynx**

___ pT3: Tumor limited to larynx **with vocal cord fixation** &/or invades any of the following

Postcricoid area, preepiglottic space, paraglottic space, &/or inner cortex of thyroid cartilage

___ pT4a: Moderately advanced local disease; tumor invades through thyroid cartilage &/or invades tissues beyond larynx

(e.g., trachea, soft tissues of neck including deep extrinsic muscle of tongue, strap muscles, thyroid, or esophagus)

___ pT4b: Very advanced local disease; tumor invades prevertebral space, encases carotid artery, or invades mediastinal structures

Primary tumor (pT): Glottis

___ PT1: Tumor limited to vocal cord(s) (may involve anterior or posterior commissure) **with normal mobility**

___ pT1a: Tumor limited to 1 vocal cord

___ pT1b: Tumor involves both vocal cords

___ pT2: Tumor extends to supraglottis &/or subglottis **&/or with impaired vocal cord mobility**

___ pT3: Tumor limited to larynx **with vocal cord fixation** &/or invades paraglottic space &/or minor thyroid cartilage erosion

(e.g., inner cortex)

___ pT4a: Moderately advanced local disease; tumor invades through outer cortex of thyroid cartilage &/or invades tissues beyond larynx

(e.g., trachea, soft tissues of neck including deep extrinsic muscle of tongue, strap muscles, thyroid, or esophagus)

___ pT4b: Very advanced local disease; tumor invades prevertebral space, encases carotid artery, or invades mediastinal structures

Primary tumor (pT): Subglottis

___ pT1: Tumor limited to subglottis

___ pT2: Tumor extends to vocal cord(s) **with normal or impaired mobility**

___ pT3: Tumor limited to larynx **with vocal cord fixation**

___ pT4a: Moderately advanced local disease; tumor invades cricoid or thyroid cartilage &/or invades tissues beyond the larynx

(e.g., trachea, soft tissues of neck including deep extrinsic muscles of the tongue, strap muscles, thyroid, or esophagus)

___ pT4b: Very advanced local disease; tumor invades prevertebral space, encases carotid artery, or invades mediastinal structures

Regional lymph nodes (pN)††

___ pNX: Cannot be assessed

___ pN0: No regional lymph node metastasis

___ pN1: Metastasis in single ipsilateral lymph node, ≤ 3 cm in greatest dimension

___ pN2: Metastasis in single ipsilateral lymph node, > 3 cm but ≤ 6 cm in greatest dimension, or in multiple ipsilateral lymph nodes, none > 6 cm in greatest dimension, or in bilateral or contralateral lymph nodes, none > 6 cm in greatest dimension

___ pN2a: Metastasis in single ipsilateral lymph node, > 3 cm but ≤ 6 cm in greatest dimension

___ pN2b: Metastasis in multiple ipsilateral lymph nodes, none > 6 cm in greatest dimension

___ pN2c: Metastasis in bilateral or contralateral lymph nodes, none more than 6 cm in greatest dimension

___ pN3: Metastasis in lymph node > 6 cm in greatest dimension

Specify: Number examined: ________

Number involved: ________

*Size (greatest dimension) of largest positive lymph node: ________

Distant metastasis (pM)

___ Not applicable

___ pM1: Distant metastasis

*Specify site(s), if known: ________________________

*Source of pathologic metastatic specimen (specify): ________________________

For Mucosal Malignant Melanoma

Primary tumor (pT)

___ pT3: Mucosal disease

___ pT4a: Moderately advanced disease; tumor involving deep soft tissue, cartilage, bone, or overlying skin

___ pT4b: Very advanced disease; tumor invading brain, dura, skull base, lower cranial nerves (IX, X, XI, XII), masticator space, carotid artery, prevertebral space, or mediastinal structures

Regional lymph nodes (pN)

___ pNX: Regional lymph nodes cannot be assessed

___ pN0: No regional lymph node metastases

___ pN1: Regional lymph node metastases present

Distant metastasis (pM)

___ Not applicable

___ pM1: Distant metastasis present

PROTOCOL FOR THE EXAMINATION OF LARYNX SPECIMENS

*Specify site(s), if known: ___________________________

*Source of pathologic metastatic specimen (specify): ___________________________

*Additional Pathologic Findings (select all that apply)

*____None identified

*____Keratinizing dysplasia

*____ Mild

*____ Moderate

*____ Severe (carcinoma in situ)

*____Nonkeratinizing dysplasia

*____ Mild

*____ Moderate

*____ Severe (carcinoma in situ)

*____Inflammation (specify type): ___________________________

*____Squamous metaplasia

*____Epithelial hyperplasia

*____Colonization

*____ Fungal

*____ Bacterial

*____Other (specify): ___________________________

*Ancillary Studies

*Specify type(s): ___________________________

*Specify result(s): ___________________________

*Clinical History (select all that apply)

*____Neoadjuvant therapy

*____ Yes (specify type): ___________________________

*____ No

*____ Indeterminate

*____Other (specify): ___________________________

*Data elements with asterisks are not required. However, these elements may be clinically important but are not yet validated or regularly used in patient management. †Applicable only to squamous cell carcinoma and histologic variants. ††Superior mediastinal lymph nodes are considered regional lymph nodes (level VII). Midline nodes are considered ipsilateral nodes. Adapted with permission from College of American Pathologists, "Protocol for the Examination of Specimens from Patients with Carcinomas of the Larynx." Web posting date October 2009, www.cap.org.

Anatomic Stage/Prognostic Groups; Stage Groupings: Supraglottis, Glottis, and Subglottis: For All Cancers Except Mucosal Malignant Melanoma

Stage	T	N	M
Stage 0	Tis	N0	M0
Stage I	T1	N0	M0
Stage II	T2	N0	M0
Stage III	T1	N1	M0
	T2	N1	M0
	T3	N0, N1	M0
Stage IVA	T1, T2, T3	N2	M0
	T4a	N0, N1, N2	M0
Stage IVB	T4b	Any N	M0
	Any T	N3	M0
Stage IVC	Any T	Any N	M1

Adapted from 7th edition AJCC Staging Forms.

Anatomic Stage/Prognostic Groups; Stage Groupings: For Mucosal Malignant Melanoma

Stage	T	N	M
Stage III	T3	N0	M0
Stage IVA	T4a	N0	M0
	T3-T4a	N1	M0
Stage IVB	T4b	Any N	M0
Stage IVC	Any T	Any N	M1

Adapted from 7th edition AJCC Staging Forms.

PROTOCOL FOR THE EXAMINATION OF LARYNX SPECIMENS

Anatomic and Tumor Staging Graphics

(Left) Basic anatomic landmarks of the larynx are used in accurate classification and separation of specific tumors into location and stage. The vocal cords are used to separate tumors into supraglottic, glottic, and subglottic regions, one of the most useful staging parameters. Extension into cartilage or across membranes also changes the tumor stage. *(Right)* A large supraglottic tumor fills the laryngeal side of the epiglottis, with expansion into the thyrohyoid membrane.

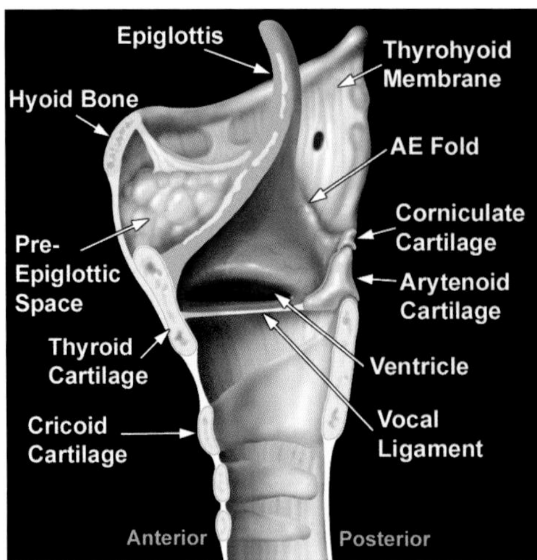

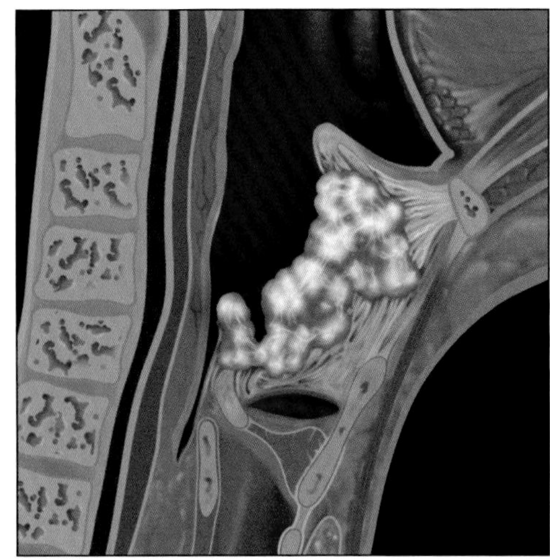

(Left) Coronal graphic of the larynx at the midcord level demonstrates the anatomic compartments and specific barriers, which would be important in documentation of the primary tumor. The supraglottic, glottic, and subglottic regions would be used in tumor staging. *(Right)* Coronal graphic shows a transglottic squamous cell carcinoma, involving the true ➔ and false ➔ vocal cord (transglottic), with expansion into the thyroid cartilage and paraglottic space.

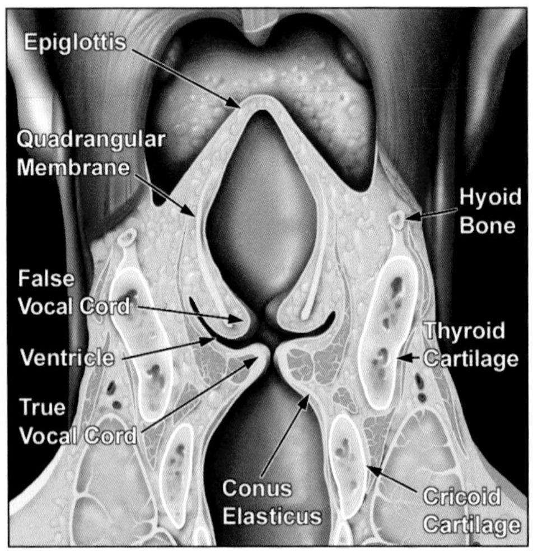

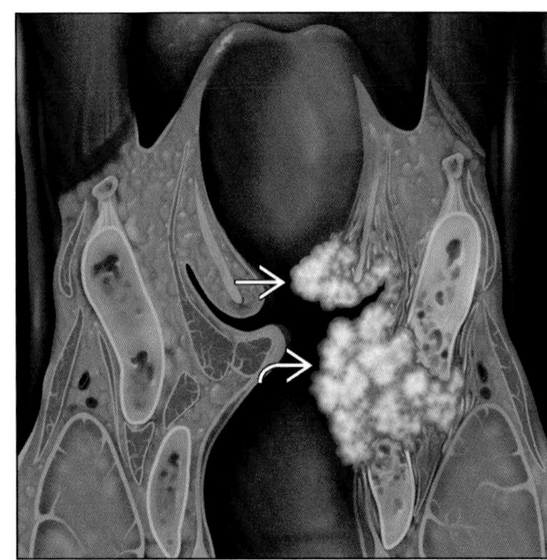

(Left) Axial graphic demonstrates the various compartments and barriers of the larynx. These parameters are important in the staging of tumors of the larynx. The natural barriers can contain the tumor or, with invasion, suggest the specific pathway of metastatic spread. *(Right)* Laryngoscopic graphic shows the glottis with a large tumor within the glottic space, replacing the vocal cord.

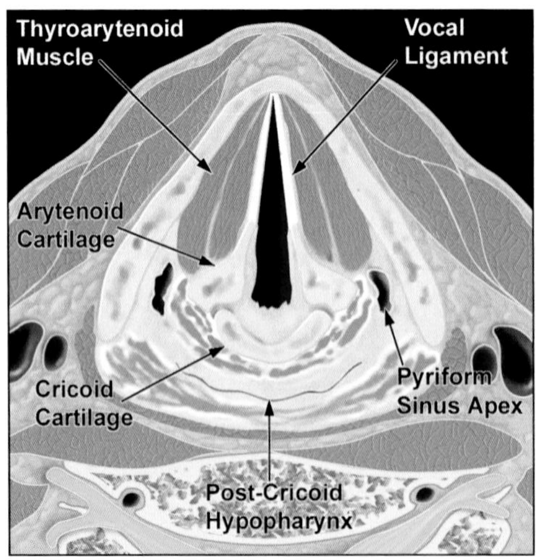

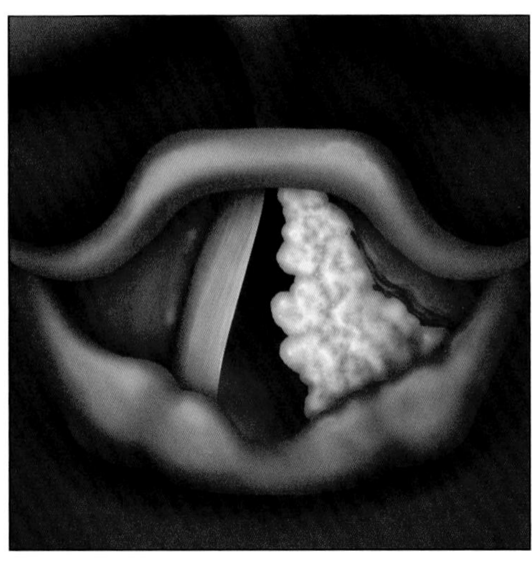

Oral Cavity

Congenital/Genetic/Hereditary

Infectious

Inflammatory-Immune Dysfunction

Reactive

Nonneoplastic Lesions

Benign Neoplasm

Malignant Neoplasm

Staging and Grading, Lip and Oral Cavity

ECTOPIC (LINGUAL) THYROID

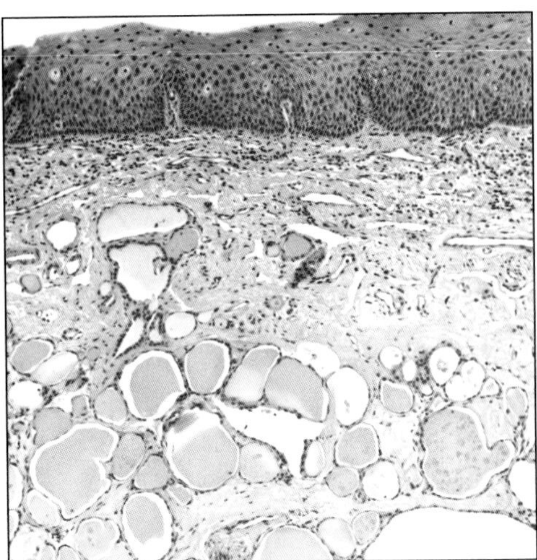

H&E shows ectopic lingual thyroid. Normal stratified squamous epithelium overlies benign, unencapsulated thyroid follicles, which interdigitate between the surrounding connective tissue and muscle.

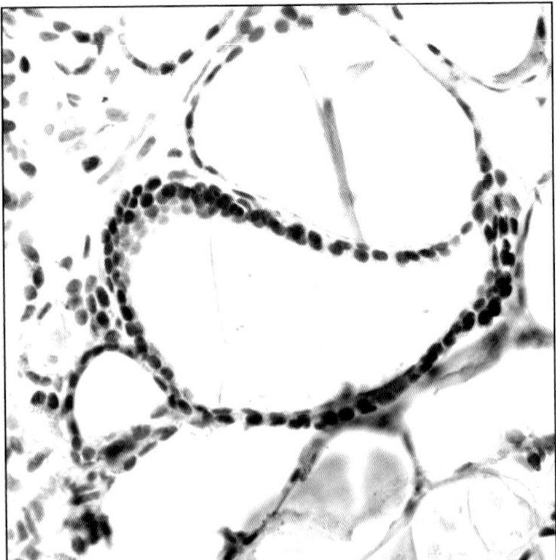

TTF-1 immunohistochemistry demonstrates strong nuclear staining of the follicular cells, although immunohistochemistry is seldom necessary to confirm the thyroid origin of the cells.

TERMINOLOGY

Definitions

- Developmental anomaly due to failure of thyroid gland to descend to normal prelaryngeal site during embryologic development

ETIOLOGY/PATHOGENESIS

Developmental Anomaly

- During embryogenesis, thyroid tissue descends from foramen cecum located at midline dorsal tongue along thyroglossal tract
- Ectopic thyroid tissue can be found anywhere along course of thyroglossal tract
  - > 90% occur in tongue
    - Mostly occur between foramen cecum and epiglottis
    - Rarely seen anterior to foramen cecum

Pathogenesis

- Cause of thyroid descent failure is unknown
  - Conflicting reports on possible role of maternal thyroid blocking immunoglobulins in development of congenital thyroid disease

CLINICAL ISSUES

Epidemiology

- Incidence
  - Uncommon, reported incidence of 1 in 100,000
- Age
  - Seen in all ages (mean: 44 years)
- Gender
  - Female > Male (range up to 7:1)

Site

- Posterior 2/3 of midline dorsal tongue

Presentation

- Dysphagia most common symptom
- Dyspnea may result if thyroid grows
- Foreign body or globus sensation
- Dysphonia
- Sleep apnea
- Possible bleeding
- 1/3 of patients with lingual thyroid are hypothyroid
  - In > 75% of patients with lingual thyroid, it is **only** functioning thyroid

Treatment

- Options, risks, complications
  - Preoperative work-up includes Tc-99m pertechnetate scanning or radioiodine studies
    - Will identify normal thyroid gland, if present
    - Will identify any other possible ectopic thyroid
  - Incisional biopsies may cause necrosis or sloughing of lingual thyroid
  - Fine needle aspiration can confirm diagnosis of ectopic thyroid
- Surgical approaches
  - Surgical excision for symptomatic patients
    - Intraoral approach or pharyngotomy
    - Autotransplantation into neck muscles of patients without normal thyroid has been suggested
- Radiation
  - ^{131}Iodine will shrink mass
    - Useful in nonsurgical candidates
    - Therapy not selective and can affect normal thyroid tissue in normal location, if present
- Suppression therapy
  - Thyroxin will reduce size, thereby relieving symptoms

Prognosis

- Excellent
- Rare reports of malignant transformation (< 1%)

ECTOPIC (LINGUAL) THYROID

Key Facts

Terminology
- Developmental anomaly due to failure of thyroid gland to descend to normal prelaryngeal site during embryologic development

Etiology/Pathogenesis
- During embryogenesis, thyroid tissue descends from foramen cecum located at midline dorsal tongue along thyroglossal tract

Clinical Issues
- Uncommon (incidence of 1 in 100,000)
- Seen in all ages (mean: 44 years)

Microscopic Pathology
- Normal-appearing thyroid tissue
- Unencapsulated

Top Differential Diagnoses
- Microscopic findings are pathognomonic

MICROSCOPIC PATHOLOGY

Histologic Features
- Normal-appearing thyroid tissue
  - Variably sized follicles lined by cuboidal epithelium
  - Lumen containing proteinaceous colloid material
- Unencapsulated
- Thyroid tissue in submucosa, possibly extending into tongue skeletal muscle
- May be nodular and hypercellular (goiter clinically)

ANCILLARY TESTS

Immunohistochemistry
- Positive cytoplasmic staining with thyroglobulin, low molecular weight cytokeratin, and epithelial membrane antigen
- Positive nuclear staining with TTF-1

DIFFERENTIAL DIAGNOSIS

Clinical DDx
- Vascular anomaly
  - Lymphangioma
  - Hemangioma
- Abscess
- Hyperplastic lingual tonsil

Pathologic DDx
- Microscopic findings are pathognomonic
- Exclude papillary carcinoma (rare)

DIAGNOSTIC CHECKLIST

Clinically Relevant Pathologic Features
- Nodular hyperemic mass at base of tongue

Pathologic Interpretation Pearls
- Normal-appearing thyroid follicles, usually unencapsulated

SELECTED REFERENCES

1. Iglesias P et al: Iodine 131 and lingual thyroid. J Clin Endocrinol Metab. 93(11):4198-9, 2008
2. Rahbar R et al: Lingual thyroid in children: a rare clinical entity. Laryngoscope. 118(7):1174-9, 2008
3. Kang HC: Lingual thyroid: marked response to suppression therapy. Thyroid. 14(5):401-2, 2004
4. Abdallah-Matta MP et al: Lingual thyroid and hyperthyroidism: a new case and review of the literature. J Endocrinol Invest. 25(3):264-7, 2002
5. Basaria S et al: Ectopic lingual thyroid masquerading as thyroid cancer metastases. J Clin Endocrinol Metab. 86(1):392-5, 2001
6. Massine RE et al: Lingual thyroid carcinoma: a case report and review of the literature. Thyroid. 11(12):1191-6, 2001
7. Kalan A et al: Lingual thyroid gland: clinical evaluation and comprehensive management. Ear Nose Throat J. 78(5):340-1, 345-9, 1999
8. Rojananin S et al: Transposition of the lingual thyroid: A new alternative technique. Head Neck. 21(5):480-3, 1999

IMAGE GALLERY

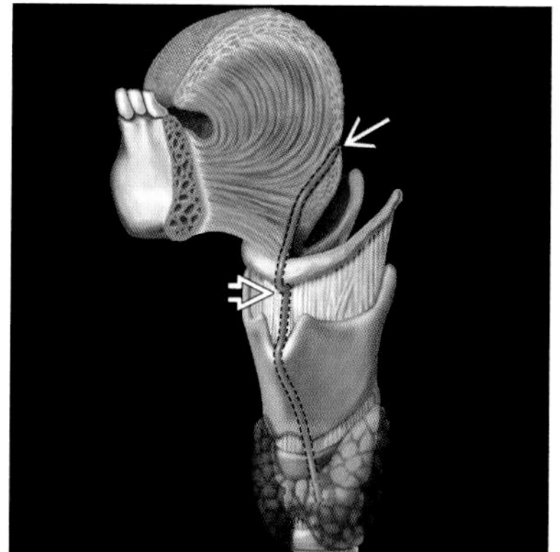

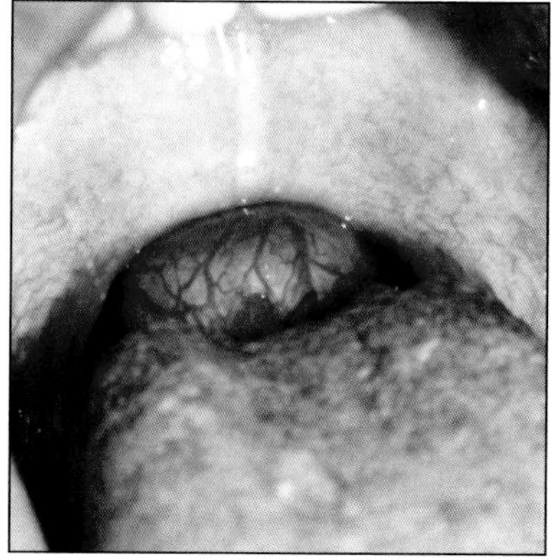

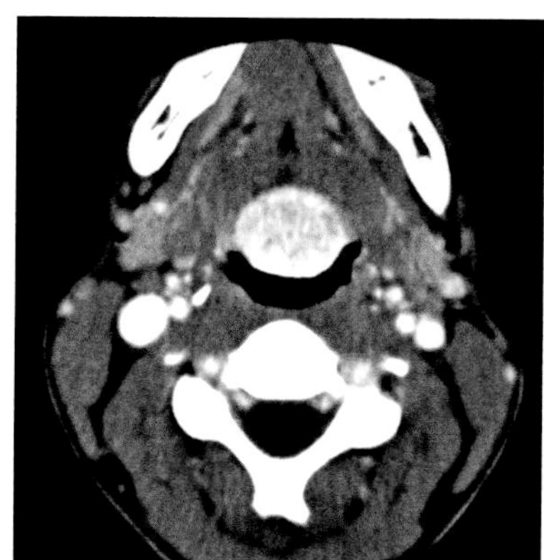

(Left) *The path of descent ⮕ of the thyroid gland from the foramen cecum ⮕ to the normal location in the neck can be arrested. Lingual thyroid involves the tongue base.* ***(Center)*** *Clinical photograph shows a lingual thyroid that presents as a smooth, sessile, hyperemic mass on the dorsal tongue just posterior to the circumvallate papillae.* ***(Right)*** *Axial CT of a lingual thyroid with IV contrast shows a large, well-defined mass with distinct margins localized at the tongue base.*

WHITE SPONGE NEVUS

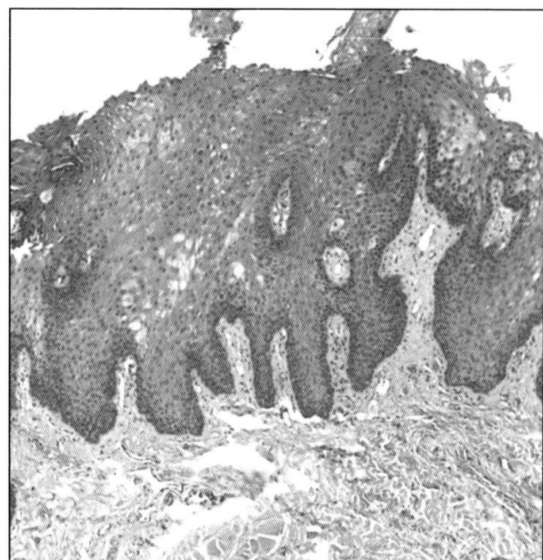

Low-power photomicrograph of a white sponge nevus shows prominent parakeratosis, acanthosis, and spongiosis with blunting of the large rete. Inflammation is not usually present.

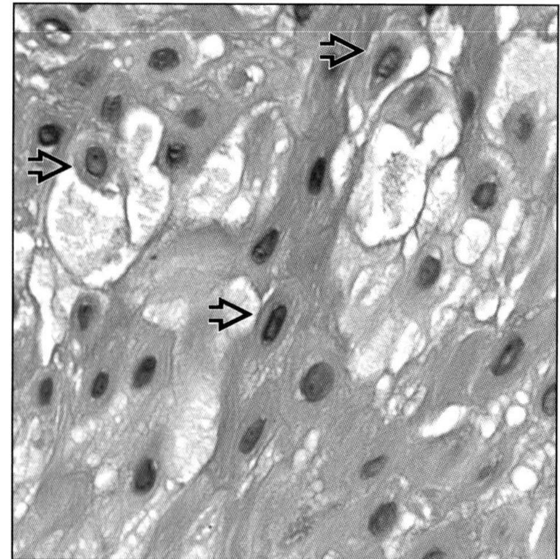

High-power photomicrograph of a white sponge nevus from the spinous layer reveals prominent vacuolation and perinuclear eosinophilic condensation ⮚.

TERMINOLOGY

Abbreviations

- White sponge nevus (WSN)

Synonyms

- Cannon disease
- Familial white folded mucosal dysplasia
- Hereditary leukokeratosis

Definitions

- Rare autosomal dominant genodermatosis exhibiting marked leukokeratosis

ETIOLOGY/PATHOGENESIS

Autosomal Dominant Disease

- Incomplete penetrance
- Variable expressivity
- De novo mutations occur

Mutations in Types 4 and 13 Keratin Genes

- Keratin 4 and 13 are specific type I and type II keratin pairs that form spinous layer
  - Insertions, deletions, and substitutions of keratin 4 and 13 have been reported

CLINICAL ISSUES

Epidemiology

- Incidence
  - Unknown; autosomal dominant with variable expressivity
- Age
  - Onset in early childhood
    - Seldom declares during adolescence

Site

- Nonkeratinized squamous mucosa
- Buccal mucosa most common intraoral site
  - Other intraoral sites include lip, tongue, palate, and floor of mouth
- Extraoral mucosal sites have been reported but are not common
  - Larynx, esophagus, nasal, and anogenital mucosa

Presentation

- Asymptomatic

Natural History

- Periods of exacerbations
- Disease progression lessens after puberty

Treatment

- No standard treatment exists
  - Vitamin A and tretinoin creams may be used
  - Variable success with antibiotics
    - Antibiotics may exert anti-inflammatory effect
    - Penicillin, ampicillin, and tetracycline

Prognosis

- Disease progression usually stops after puberty
- No reports of malignant transformation

MICROSCOPIC PATHOLOGY

Histologic Features

- Marked parakeratosis and acanthosis
- Vacuolation or clearing of spinous cell layer
- Basement membrane intact
- Inflammation in connective tissue usually not present

ANCILLARY TESTS

Cytology

- Exfoliative studies with Papanicolaou staining
  - Pathognomonic perinuclear condensation of keratin tonofilaments

WHITE SPONGE NEVUS

Key Facts

Terminology

- Rare autosomal dominant genodermatosis exhibiting marked leukokeratosis

Clinical Issues

- Disease progression usually stops after puberty
- No reports of malignant transformation

Microscopic Pathology

- Marked parakeratosis and acanthosis
- Vacuolation or clearing of spinous cell layer

Ancillary Tests

- Pathognomonic perinuclear condensation of keratin tonofilaments on Pap stain

Top Differential Diagnoses

- Hereditary benign intraepithelial dyskeratosis
- Leukoedema
- Oral hairy leukoplakia

  - This feature is often better appreciated on cytology than on histologic sections

Electron Microscopy

- Perinuclear eosinophilic condensation represents masses of keratin tonofilaments
- Present only in superficial spinous layer

DIFFERENTIAL DIAGNOSIS

Hereditary Benign Intraepithelial Dyskeratosis

- Dyskeratotic cells seen in upper spinous layer
  - Dyskeratotic cell appears surrounded by adjacent epithelial cell (cell-within-cell)
- Conjunctival lesions presenting as gelatinous plaques

Leukoedema

- Common oral finding of buccal mucosa
  - Considered normal and represents edema
- Hyperparakeratosis
- Marked intracellular edema with large vacuolated cells
- No perinuclear eosinophilic condensation

Oral Hairy Leukoplakia

- Balloon cells in upper spinous layer
- Positive for Epstein-Barr virus (EBV)

DIAGNOSTIC CHECKLIST

Clinically Relevant Pathologic Features

- Age distribution
  - Usually noted incidentally in childhood
- Gross appearance
  - Diffuse thickened plaques with corrugated or folded surface

Pathologic Interpretation Pearls

- Superficial epithelium demonstrates perinuclear condensation
- No dysplasia noted
- Papanicolaou staining of exfoliative cytology pathognomonic

SELECTED REFERENCES

1. López Jornet P: White sponge nevus: presentation of a new family. Pediatr Dermatol. 25(1):116-7, 2008
2. Martelli H Jr et al: White sponge nevus: report of a three-generation family. Oral Surg Oral Med Oral Pathol Oral Radiol Endod. 103(1):43-7, 2007
3. Smith F: The molecular genetics of keratin disorders. Am J Clin Dermatol. 4(5):347-64, 2003
4. Richard G et al: Keratin 13 point mutation underlies the hereditary mucosal epithelial disorder white sponge nevus. Nat Genet. 11(4):453-5, 1995
5. Rugg EL et al: A mutation in the mucosal keratin K4 is associated with oral white sponge nevus. Nat Genet. 11(4):450-2, 1995

IMAGE GALLERY

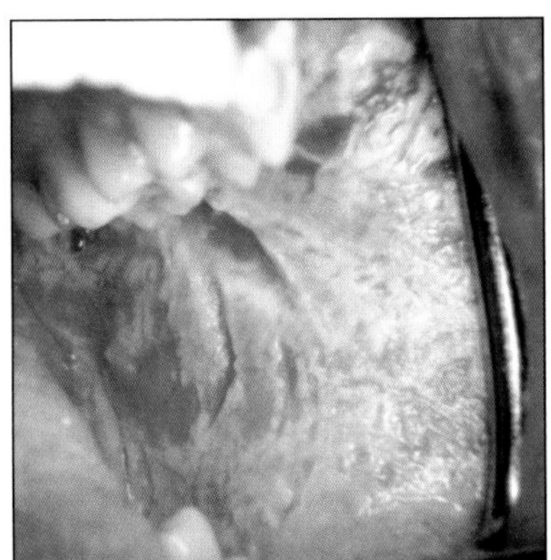

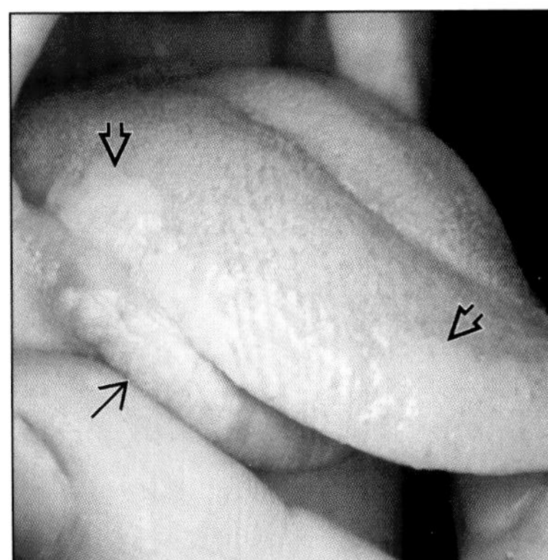

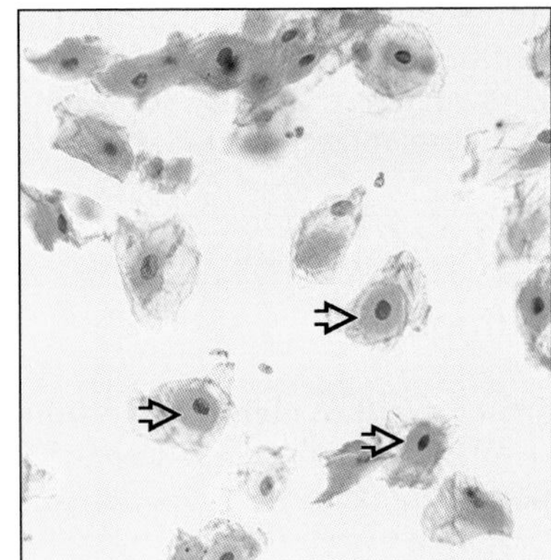

(Left) *Clinical photo shows a typical appearance of white sponge nevus of the buccal mucosa presenting as thick, white, folded plaques.* ***(Center)*** *Although not as common as the buccal mucosa, white sponge nevus can affect other oral sites, including the lip ➔ and tongue ➪ as shown here.* ***(Right)*** *Characteristic perinuclear eosinophilic condensation of the keratin tonofilaments ➪ are highlighted in a Papanicolaou-stained exfoliative cytology. (Courtesy B.W. Neville, DDS.)*

HAIRY LEUKOPLAKIA

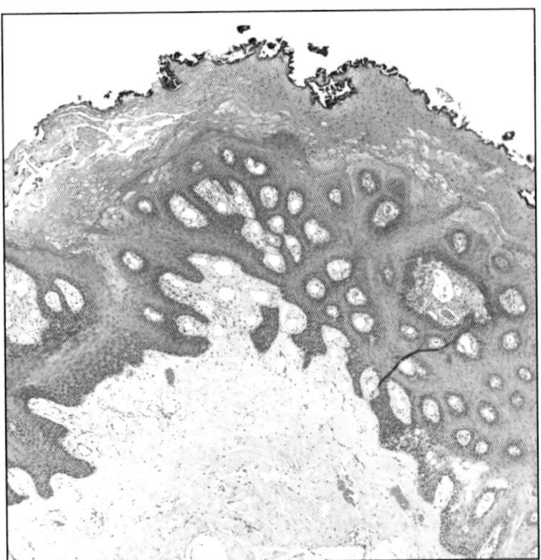

Oral hairy leukoplakia is characterized by an acanthotic, markedly parakeratotic corrugated epithelium. Note the relative lack of inflammation. Colonies of bacteria are noted on the epithelial surface.

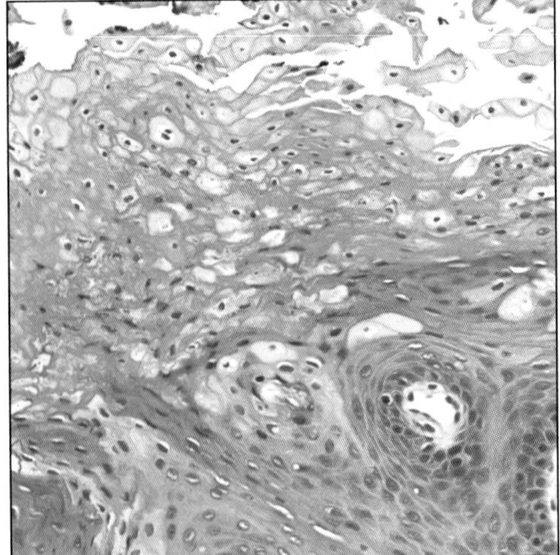

High-power photomicrograph shows "balloon" cells in the spinous layer of oral hairy leukoplakia. These features are indicative of a cytopathic viral effect.

TERMINOLOGY

Abbreviations

- Oral hairy leukoplakia (OHL)

Definitions

- EBV-associated epithelial hyperplasia usually on lateral tongue in immunocompromised patients

ETIOLOGY/PATHOGENESIS

Etiology

- OHL associated with HIV infection &/or immunosuppression
- Disease correlates with viral load and CD4 counts
- HIV(+) men who smoke > 1 pack per day have higher rates of OHL

Pathogenesis

- Epstein-Barr virus (EBV), herpes virus linked to OHL; usually latent infections
- Cytotoxic T-cells, which maintain EBV latent state decreased in HIV infection
  - Increased circulating EBV-infected B-cells
- Langerhans cells are decreased or absent in OHL
  - Antigen functions as immune cell present in epithelium
  - Decreased number may allow for persistent EBV infection and replication

CLINICAL ISSUES

Epidemiology

- Incidence
  - Since advent of highly active antiretroviral therapy (HAART), incidence has decreased to < 10% of HIV population
  - Cases have been reported in both solid organ and bone marrow transplant patients
    - Exact incidence unknown
- Age
  - All ages affected
- Gender
  - Most common in HIV(+) males

Site

- Lateral border of tongue most commonly affected

Presentation

- Epithelial hyperplasia with corrugated appearance
- Lesions are adherent and cannot be scraped off
- Appearance frequently changes, resolving then reappearing
  - Can be extensive, bilateral, and involve dorsal tongue
- Asymptomatic, unless superimposed *Candida* infection present
- Rarely other intraoral sites involved

Treatment

- No treatment is needed
- Antifungal therapy for superimposed candidiasis

Prognosis

- Although not an AIDS defining disease, it is marker of HIV disease progression
- AIDS patients with OHL have shorter lifespan than those who do not
- Some cases of OHL spontaneously resolve

MICROSCOPIC PATHOLOGY

Histologic Features

- Marked acanthosis and parakeratosis
- Epithelial hyperplasia with elongation of rete ridges
- Balloon cell in spinous layer
  - Viral cytopathic effect
    - Intracellular ballooning degeneration
    - Nuclear clearing with chromatin margination

HAIRY LEUKOPLAKIA

Key Facts

Terminology
- EBV-associated epithelial hyperplasia usually on lateral tongue in immunocompromised patients

Etiology/Pathogenesis
- OHL associated with HIV infection &/or immunosuppression

Microscopic Pathology
- Marked acanthosis and parakeratosis
- Balloon cell in spinous layer
- Coinfection with candidiasis
- EBER shows punctate nuclear staining of balloon cells in spinous layer

Top Differential Diagnoses
- Frictional keratosis
- Hyperplastic candidiasis
- Leukoplakia
- Lichen planus

- Candidal organisms can be seen in superficial keratin
- Very little if any inflammation
- No dysplasia should be seen

ANCILLARY TESTS

Histochemistry
- PAS-light green
  - Highlights candidal organisms

In Situ Hybridization
- Epstein-Barr virus encoded RNA (EBER) shows punctate nuclear staining of spinous layer balloon cells

DIFFERENTIAL DIAGNOSIS

Frictional Keratosis
- Lateral border of tongue is frequent site for inadvertent masticatory trauma
- No balloon cells seen in spinous layer

Hyperplastic Candidiasis
- Oral candidiasis can become hyperplastic and share similar clinical features
- PAS stains show numerous candidal organisms in superficial keratin

Leukoplakia
- Common location for oral leukoplakia
- No EBV etiology
- Various degrees of dysplasia may be seen

Lichen Planus
- Can appear hyperplastic clinically
- Basal cell liquefaction and dense band of lymphocytes and plasma cells adjacent to basal cells
- Dyskeratotic epithelial cell seen at epithelial-connective interface

DIAGNOSTIC CHECKLIST

Clinically Relevant Pathologic Features
- EBV-associated lesion generally present on lateral tongue in HIV(+) males

Pathologic Interpretation Pearls
- Layer of "balloon" cells in spinous layer positive for EBV by EBER staining
- May see coinfection with candidiasis

SELECTED REFERENCES

1. Mendoza N et al: Mucocutaneous manifestations of Epstein-Barr virus infection. Am J Clin Dermatol. 9(5):295-305, 2008
2. Coogan MM et al: Oral lesions in infection with human immunodeficiency virus. Bull World Health Organ. 83(9):700-6, 2005
3. Walling DM et al: Effect of Epstein-Barr virus replication on Langerhans cells in pathogenesis of oral hairy leukoplakia. J Infect Dis. 189(9):1656-63, 2004

IMAGE GALLERY

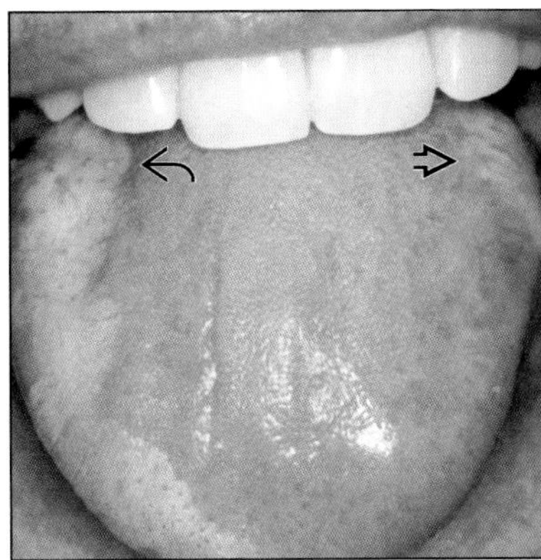

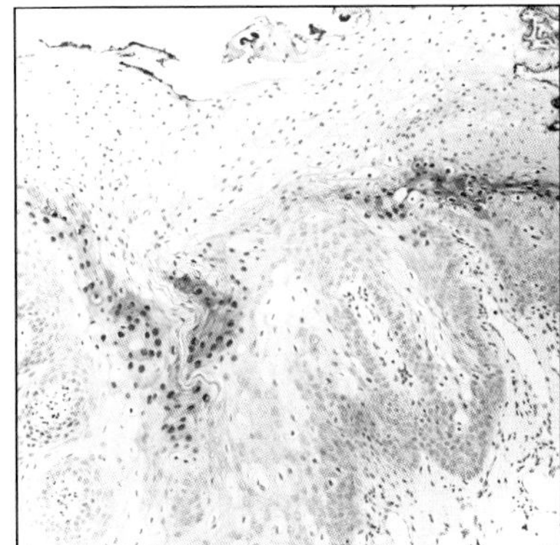

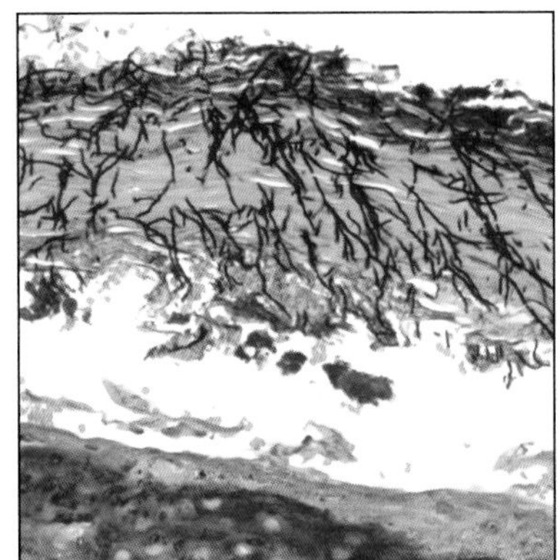

(Left) *Oral hairy leukoplakia is shown in an HIV(+) male. Note that the lesion is bilateral and diffuse ⇨. In some areas it becomes thickened ⇗.* ***(Center)*** *In situ hybridization for Epstein-Barr virus encoded RNA (EBER) shows strong punctate nuclear positivity in the area where the "balloon" cells were identified.* ***(Right)*** *PAS staining highlights the numerous candidal hyphae and spores in the superficial keratin. This co-infection is a common finding in OHL.*

ORAL INFECTIONS

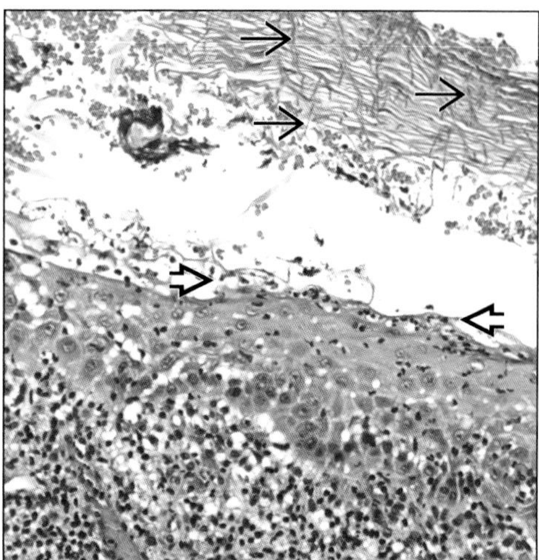

Hyperplastic candidiasis exhibits marked keratoses with neutrophilic microabscesses ⇨ in the superficial keratin. The detached keratin contains numerous fungal organisms →.

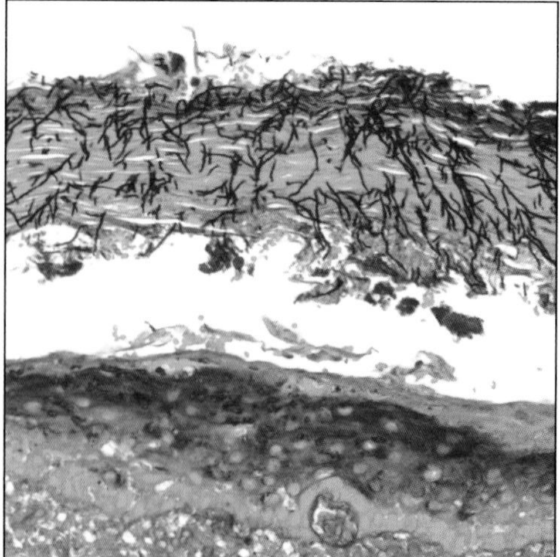

Periodic acid-Schiff stain of hyperplastic candidiasis highlights the numerous fungal hyphae and spores in the superficial keratin layer.

TERMINOLOGY

Abbreviations

- Herpes simplex virus type 1 (HSV1)
- Hand, foot, and mouth disease (HFMD)

Definitions

- Candidiasis: Most common oral fungal infection with diverse clinical presentation
  - Majority of cases associated with *C. albicans*
- Herpes simplex virus 1: DNA virus spread by direct contact or infected saliva
  - Most commonly seen in oral, ocular, or facial region, including pharynx, lips, intraoral area, and skin
- Actinomycosis: Normal saprophytic gram-positive anaerobic bacteria that can colonize bone and skin
- Herpangina: Common viral infection of young children associated with blisters of soft palate or tonsillar pillars
- Hand, foot, and mouth disease: Common viral illness of infants and children, which causes fever and blister eruptions of mouth &/or skin

ETIOLOGY/PATHOGENESIS

Candidiasis

- Overgrowth of fungal organisms that may be component of normal oral flora in up to 50% of population
  - Besides *C. albicans*, *C. tropicalis*, and *C. krusei* can also cause disease
- Caused by broad spectrum antibiotics, topical or systemic prednisone, anemia, xerostomia, impaired immune system, dentures

HSV1

- Acute herpetic gingivostomatitis (primary herpes)
  - Caused by human herpes simplex virus type I (a.k.a. HHV-1)
  - Transmission through direct contact of active perioral lesions or infected saliva
  - Incubation period 3-9 days
- Recurrent HSV1
  - Latent virus residing in sensory nerves becomes reactivated
    - Trigeminal ganglion is most common site of latency for head and neck HSV1
  - Reactivation of virus can be triggered by ultraviolet light, physical or mental stress, trauma, dental therapy

Actinomycosis

- Majority of cases caused by *A. israeli*
  - Other species include *A. viscous*, *A. naeslundii*
- Organisms generally enter soft tissue in area of trauma
- Associated with bisphosphonate-associated osteonecrosis of the jaws

Herpangina

- Caused by virus belonging to *Enterovirus* group (poliovirus, coxsackievirus, echovirus)
  - Coxsackie A16 virus is most common cause, but other coxsackie viruses can cause disease
    - Usually associated with coxsackievirus A1 to A6, A8, A10, or A22
- Transmission is direct contact, often oral-fecal route
- Epidemics every few years have been reported in many countries

HFMD

- Caused by virus belonging to *Enterovirus* group
- Transmission by direct contact from person to person
  - Virus found in secretions, including saliva, nose and throat secretions, blister fluid, and stools

ORAL INFECTIONS

Key Facts

Terminology

- Candidiasis: Most common oral fungal infection with diverse clinical presentation
- HSV1: Caused by human herpes virus, herpes simplex virus type I (a.k.a. HHV-1)
  - Transmission through direct contact of active perioral lesions or infected saliva
  - Recurrent HSV1: Latent virus resides in trigeminal ganglion and becomes reactivated
- Actinomycosis: Normal saprophytic gram-positive anaerobic bacteria that can colonize bone and skin
  - > 55% of cases involve cervicofacial region
- Herpangina: Common viral infection of young children associated with blisters of soft palate &/or tonsillar pillars
- Hand, foot, and mouth disease: Common viral illness of infants and children, which causes fever and blister eruptions of mouth &/or skin

Microscopic Pathology

- **Candidiasis:** Organisms can be seen in parakeratin layer highlighted by PAS staining
  - Neutrophilic microabscesses can be seen in keratin layer
- **HSV1:** Infected epithelial cells show acantholysis (Tzanck cells)
  - HSV1 in situ hybridization will demonstrate nuclear staining in virally infected cells
- **Actinomycosis:** Colonies of basophilic club-shaped bacteria arranged in radiating rosette pattern surrounded by neutrophils

CLINICAL ISSUES

Presentation

- **Candidiasis**: Numerous clinical presentations; patient may have more than 1 at the same time
- Pseudomembranous candidiasis (thrush) presents with white curd-like plaques that can be removed with scraping
- Erythematous candidiasis appears as reddened often atrophic mucosa with associated burning
  - **Median rhomboid glossitis** presents as central area of erythema on dorsal tongue with atrophic papillae
  - **Denture stomatitis** presents as erythema under full or partial denture
  - **Angular cheilitis** presents as erythematous fissured areas at corners of mouth
- Hyperplastic candidiasis composed of white plaques that cannot be wiped off
  - Can be difficult to separate from oral leukoplakia secondarily superimposed with *Candida*
- Mucocutaneous candidiasis
  - Seen in association with immunologic disorders involving endocrine system
- **HSV1**
  - Primary HSV1
    - < 15% of patients exhibit clinical manifestations of initial HSV1 infection
    - Abrupt onset of symptoms, including fever, nausea, chills, lymphadenopathy, and stomatitis
    - Gingiva becomes erythematous, painful, and enlarged
    - Numerous irregular coalescing ulcers throughout oral cavity
    - Generally, lesions are present intra-/periorally, pharynx, facial skin, and skin above waist
    - Halitosis
  - Recurrent HSV1
    - Most common site is vermillion border or surrounding skin of lip (herpes labialis, "fever blister")
    - Often experience prodrome of tingling, itching, and pain of affected site anywhere from 6-36 hours
    - Clusters of fluid-filled vesicles develop and rupture within 2 days, then form a crust
    - Intraoral recurrences are seen on keratinized mucosa, including hard palate and attached gingiva
- **Actinomycosis**
  - > 55% of actinomycosis involve cervicofacial region
  - May be a rapidly progressing acute infection or chronic
  - Suppurative abscesses may contain yellow flecks (**sulfur granules**), which are colonies of bacteria
  - Direct extension into soft tissue may result in sinus tract
  - Fibrosis of indurated soft tissue
  - Actinomycotic osteomyelitis of the jaws has been reported
- **Herpangina**
  - Disease begins with acute onset of fever and sore throat
    - Other symptoms include poor appetite, dysphagia, myalgia, diarrhea, vomiting, and headache
  - Small, 2-4 mm, red macules that form vesicles, numbering 2-6, occur in oropharynx
  - Constitutional symptoms resolve in days
  - Mouth ulcers resolve usually in 7-10 days
- **HFMD**
  - Disease usually presents with malaise, fever, and poor appetite
  - About 48 hours after fever onset, blisters develop in mouth (tongue, gums, and buccal mucosa)
  - Nonpruritic cutaneous rash may develop on palms and soles and sometimes buttocks and genitalia

Laboratory Tests

- **Candidiasis**
  - Culture can definitively identify organism
    - Specificity and sensitivity generally only needed in treatment-resistant cases

ORAL INFECTIONS

- **HSV1**
  - Virologic testing can be done but not as accurate as newer tests
  - Polymerase chain reaction (PCR) is used but more often reserved for spinal fluid
  - Serologic tests may be negative if testing right after initial exposure
    - To prevent false-negatives, testing should be done 12-16 weeks after exposure
    - Enzyme-linked immunosorbent assay (ELISA) highly accurate in typing HSV
- **Actinomycosis**
  - Isolation via culture is difficult because of other bacterial contaminants or prior antibiotic treatment
- **Herpangina**
  - Throat or stool samples can be sent for viral culture
  - PCR has been used to rapidly identify specific *Enterovirus*
- **HFMD**
  - Throat, cutaneous, or stool samples can be sent for laboratory testing to identify specific *Enterovirus*
    - Rarely done since test takes 2-4 weeks, and HFMD is self-limiting
    - PCR has been used to more rapidly identify specific *Enterovirus*

Treatment

- **Candidiasis**
  - Topical &/or systemic antifungal therapy
- **HSV1**
  - Systemic antivirals for primary HSV1
  - Topical &/or systemic antivirals for recurrent HSV1
- **Actinomycosis**
  - Incision and drainage of abscesses
  - Long-term intravenous antibiotic (penicillin, amoxicillin) for chronic cases or osteomyelitis
- **Herpangina**
  - Supportive therapy for constitutional symptoms
- **HFMD**
  - Supportive therapy for constitutional symptoms

MICROSCOPIC PATHOLOGY

Histologic Features

- **Candidiasis**
  - Organisms can be seen in parakeratin layer highlighted by PAS staining
    - Branching hyphae, 2 μm in diameter with ovoid spores
  - Neutrophilic microabscesses can be seen in keratin layer
  - Inflammatory cell exocytosis
- **HSV1**
  - Infected epithelial cells show acantholysis (Tzanck cells)
  - Ballooning degeneration of nuclei with chromatin condensation along periphery
  - Infected cells can fuse to form multinucleated cells
  - HSV1 in situ hybridization will demonstrate nuclear staining in virally infected cells
- **Actinomycosis**
  - Colonies of basophilic club-shaped bacteria arranged in radiating rosette pattern surrounded by neutrophils
  - Granulation tissue and nonvital bone
- **Herpangina and HFMD**
  - Self-limited disease and biopsy rarely done

DIFFERENTIAL DIAGNOSIS

Candidiasis

- Geographic tongue: Can see neutrophilic microabscesses in epithelium
- Oral dysplasia can be secondarily infected
  - Sometimes difficult to distinguish reactive atypia to fungal organisms and true dysplasia
  - Rebiopsy may be indicated after appropriate treatment
- Radiation mucositis: Bizarre epithelial and stromal cells
- *Candida* can be associated with intense inflammatory infiltrate mimicking lichen planus

HSV1

- Erythema multiforme (EM)
  - Need clinical correlation
  - Target lesions on skin in EM but not in HSV1
- Necrotizing ulcerative gingivitis
  - Lesions confined to gingiva
- Herpes zoster
  - Microscopically identical to HSV1
  - In situ hybridization will be able to distinguish between herpes virus subtypes

SELECTED REFERENCES

1. Allen MR et al: The pathogenesis of bisphosphonate-related osteonecrosis of the jaw: so many hypotheses, so few data. J Oral Maxillofac Surg. 67(5 Suppl):61-70, 2009
2. Lafleur MD et al: Patients with Long-term Oral Carriage Harbor High-persister Mutants of C. albicans. Antimicrob Agents Chemother. Epub ahead of print, 2009
3. Samaranayake LP et al: Oral mucosal fungal infections. Periodontol 2000. 49:39-59, 2009
4. Cernik C et al: The treatment of herpes simplex infections: an evidence-based review. Arch Intern Med. 168(11):1137-44, 2008
5. Nasser M et al: Acyclovir for treating primary herpetic gingivostomatitis. Cochrane Database Syst Rev. (4):CD006700, 2008
6. Fatahzadeh M et al: Human herpes simplex virus infections: epidemiology, pathogenesis, symptomatology, diagnosis, and management. J Am Acad Dermatol. 57(5):737-63; quiz 764-6, 2007
7. Sharkawy AA: Cervicofacial actinomycosis and mandibular osteomyelitis. Infect Dis Clin North Am. 21(2):543-56, viii, 2007
8. McCullough MJ et al: Oral viral infections and the therapeutic use of antiviral agents in dentistry. Aust Dent J. 50(4 Suppl 2):S31-5, 2005
9. Frydenberg A et al: Hand, foot and mouth disease. Aust Fam Physician. 32(8):594-5, 2003

Candida Species Infections

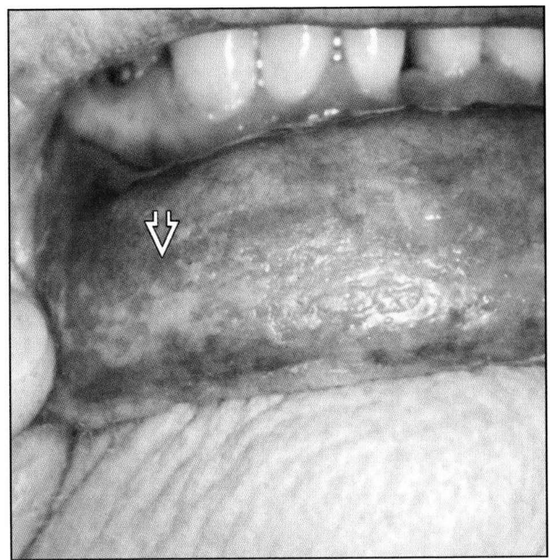

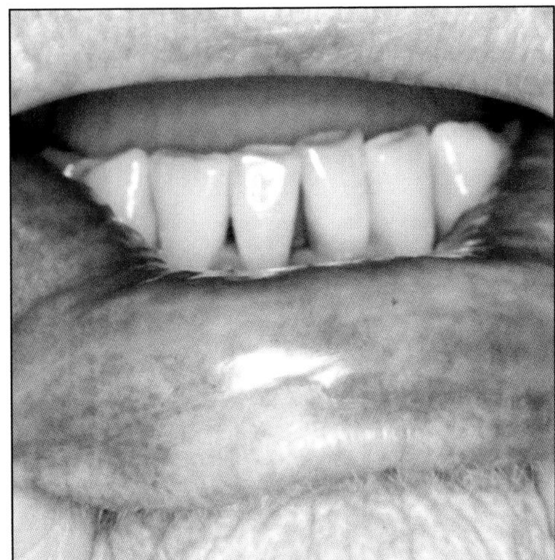

(Left) *Hyperplastic candidiasis ⇨ on the lower lip. Unlike pseudomembranous candidiasis, the white area does not scrape off and clinically resembles leukoplakia.* ***(Right)*** *After a 2 week treatment with clotrimazole troches, there is complete resolution of the white lesions. However, if any part of the lesion persisted, then biopsy would be indicated to rule out candidiasis superimposed on an area of leukoplakia.*

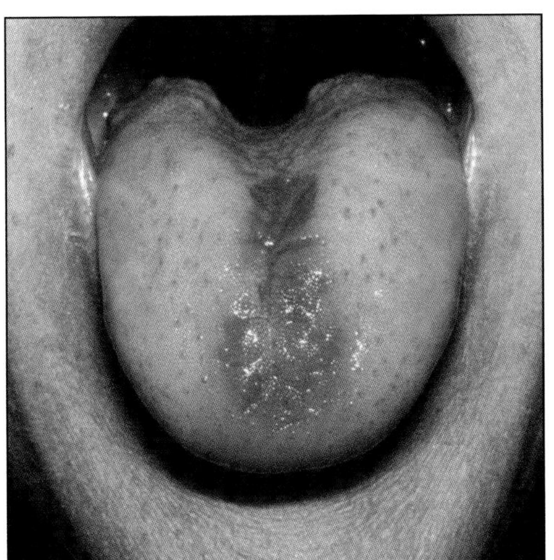

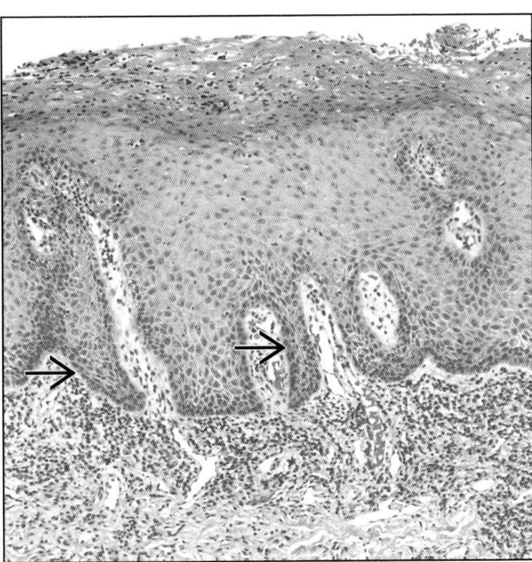

(Left) *Median rhomboid glossitis, a form of erythematous candidiasis, which affects the midline dorsal tongue, shows loss of the filiform papillae. This may be asymptomatic, or patients may experience generalized burning.* ***(Right)*** *Pathology of median rhomboid glossitis shows marked thickening of the parakeratin, inflammatory exocytosis, and elongated epithelial rete → along with subjacent chronic inflammation. PAS staining would demonstrate pseudo-hyphae and spores.*

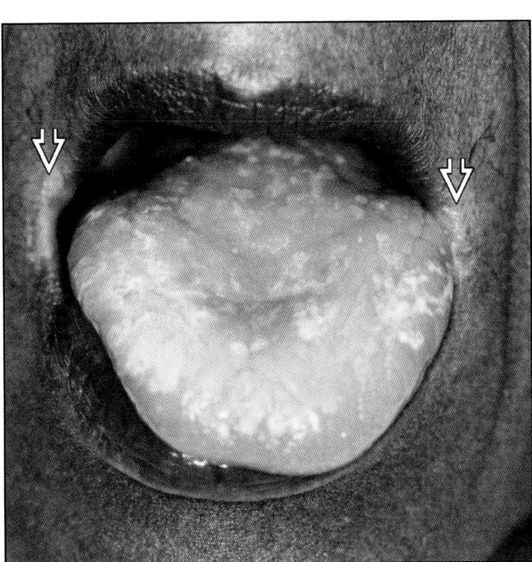

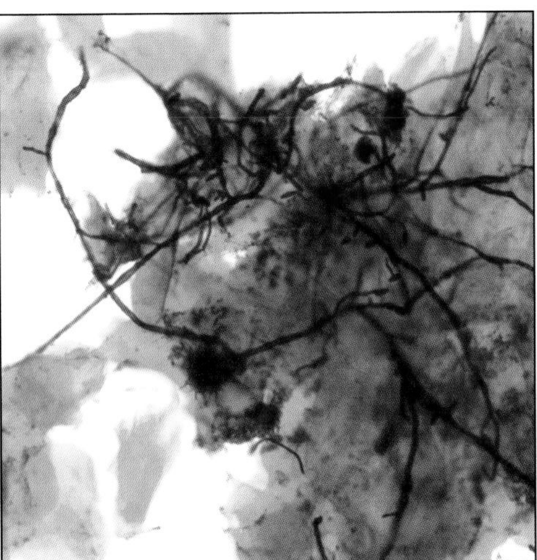

(Left) *Pseudomembranous candidiasis presenting as multiple white plaques on the dorsal tongue in an iron anemic patient. These plaques easily wipe off unlike hyperplastic candidiasis. The patient also has angular cheilitis ⇨ characterized by erythema and fissuring at the corners of the mouth.* ***(Right)*** *Exfoliative cytology with PAS stain demonstrates hyphae and pseudo-hyphae and budding spores typical of Candida albicans. Both squamous cells and inflammatory cells are seen.*

Herpes Simplex Virus Infections

(Left) *Primary HSV1 (acute herpetic gingivostomatitis) in a young person with numerous ulcers is noted on the lower lip and enlarged, erythematous painful gingiva ⇒. Depending on the severity of the outbreak, lesions last from 7-14 days.* ***(Right)*** *Multiple recurrent HSV1 herpes labialis are shown with characteristic vesicles on the lip vermilion ⇒. The extensive ulcerations present are due to mechanical rupture of the vesicles spreading the virus to other areas of the lip.*

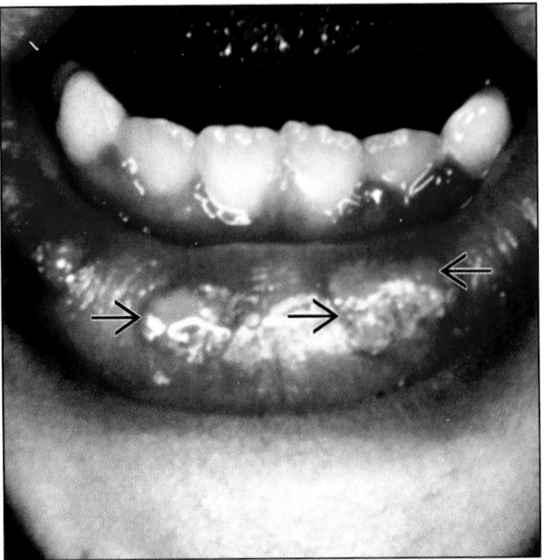

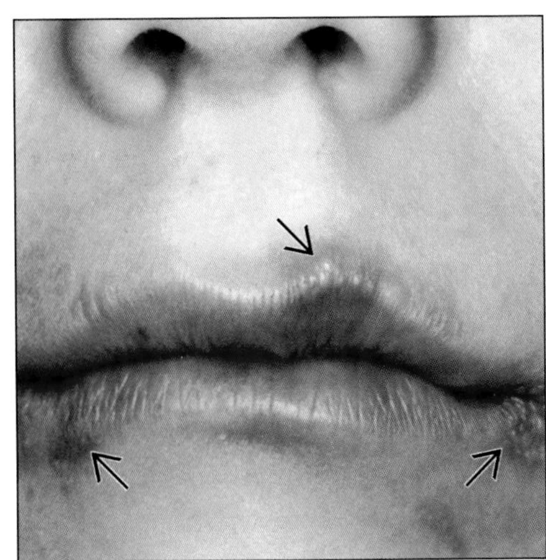

(Left) *Biopsy of HSV1 lesion shows in the superficial epithelium the ruptured vesicle with altered epithelial cells ⇨ and secondary inflammation. There is ulceration and exudate at the surface.* ***(Right)*** *High-power image of HSV1 from a ruptured vesicle shows virally altered acantholytic epithelial cells (Tzanck cells). Ballooning degeneration (nuclear enlargement) and chromatin condensation around the periphery of the nucleus is noted as well as multinucleation ⇒.*

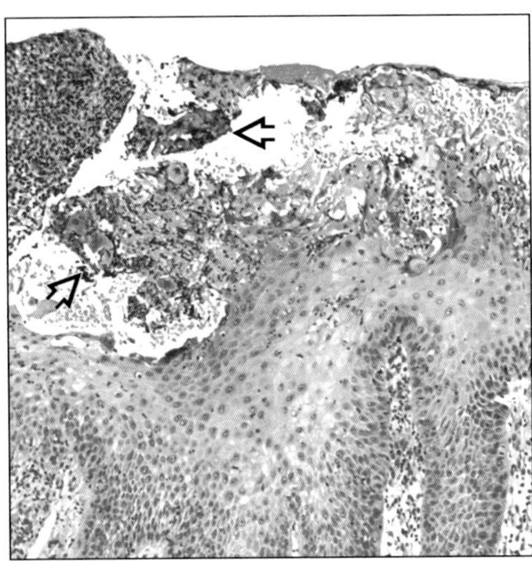

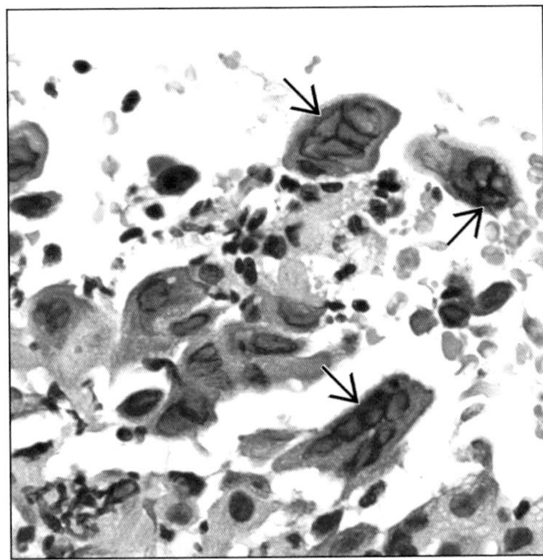

(Left) *In situ hybridization for HSV1 shows strong nuclear staining ⇒ in the virally altered acantholytic and multinucleated cells.* ***(Right)*** *Recurrent HSV1 can occur intraorally. It is generally seen on the keratinized tissue attached to bone, such as the hard palate and attached gingiva ⇒. Complete healing is usually in 7-10 days. In the immunosuppressed patient, lesions can occur anywhere in the oral cavity and may be chronic.*

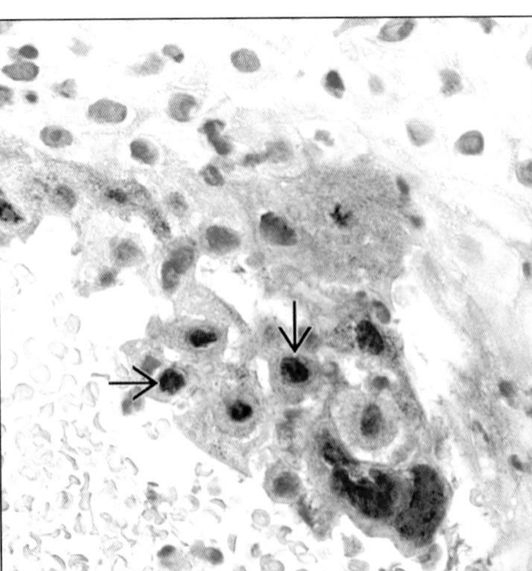

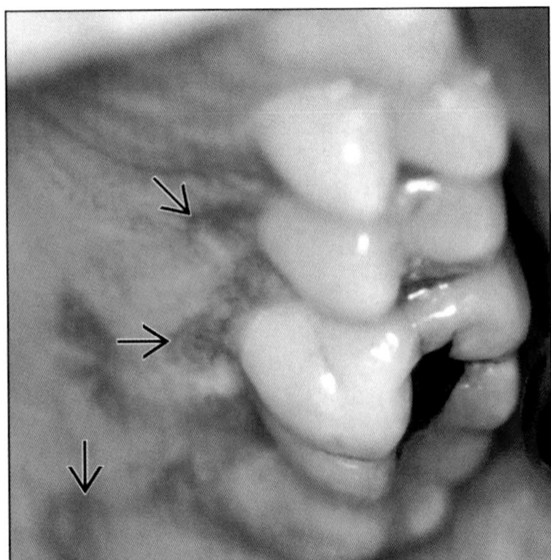

Actinomycosis and Hand, Foot, and Mouth Disease

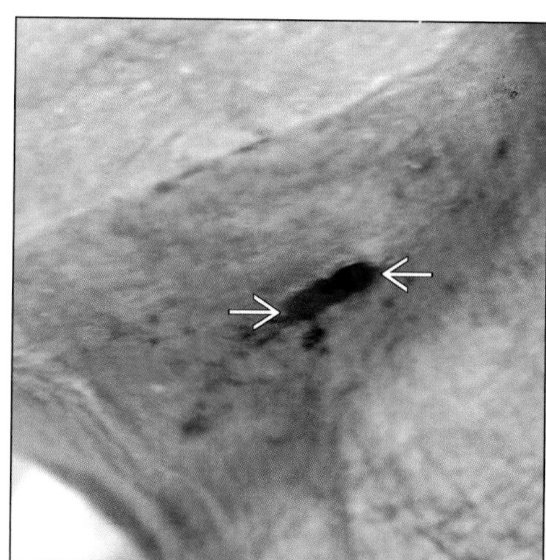

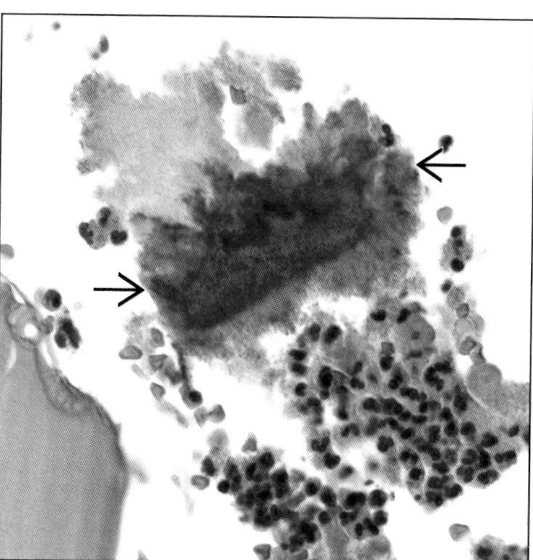

(Left) *Chronic draining fistula of the submandibular area* ➔ *is shown; culture was positive for actinomycosis. Yellowish flecks, which represent actinomycotic colonies (sulfur granules) may be noted in the suppurative area.* ***(Right)*** *Actinomycosis shows the characteristic club-shaped filamentous organisms arranged in a radiating rosette pattern* ➔*. Adjacent nonvital bone and neutrophils are noted. This was associated with osteonecrosis of the mandible.*

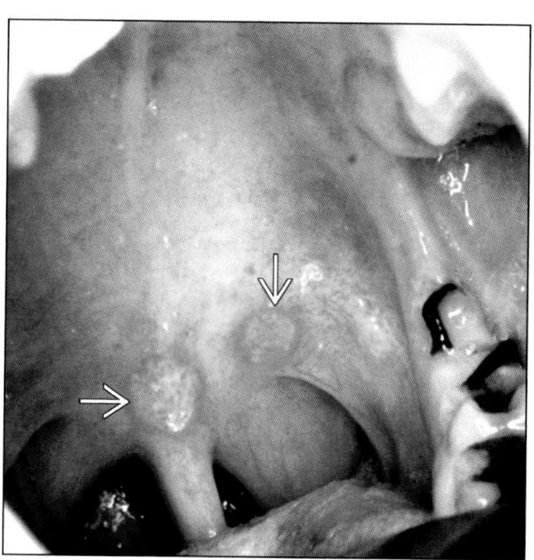

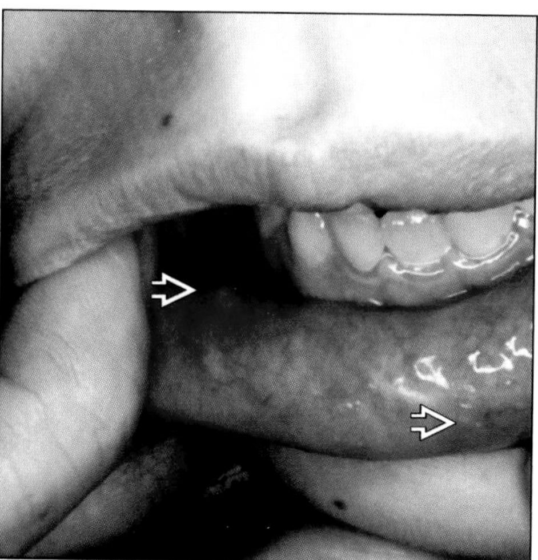

(Left) *Herpangina is seen as large aphthous-like ulcerations of the soft palate* ➔*. These areas start as small vesicles that rapidly ulcerate and last 7-10 days.* ***(Right)*** *Hand, foot, and mouth disease presents as multiple aphthous-like ulcerations on the labial mucosa* ➔*. The lesions resemble herpangina, but usually are more numerous and occur more frequently on the buccal mucosa, tongue, and labial mucosa. Oral lesions usually precede cutaneous lesions and generally resolve in 1 week.*

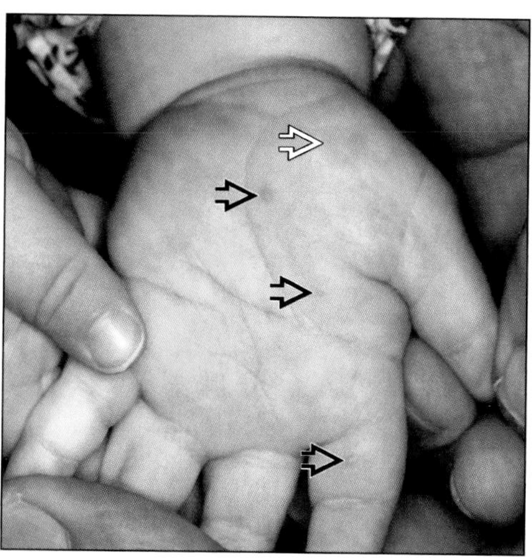

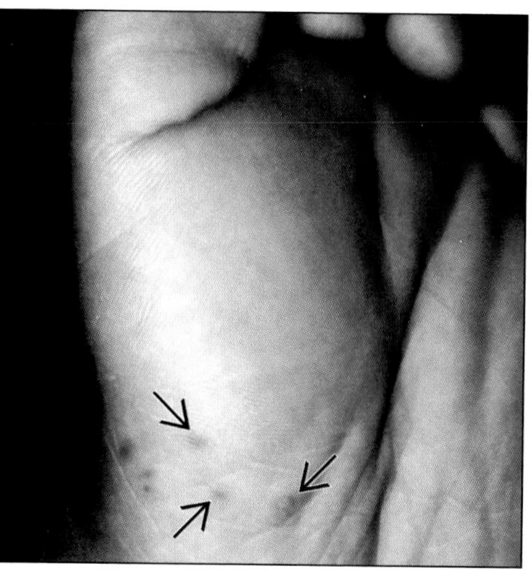

(Left) *Hand, foot, and mouth disease is shown with characteristic vesicles on the palm* ➔*. The lesions start as erythematous macules* ➔ *and then develop central vesicles, which heal without crusting. The ulcers are preceded by flu-like symptoms, including fever, sore throat, and myalgia.* ***(Right)*** *Hand, foot, and mouth disease is shown with numerous erythematous macules on the sole of the foot* ➔*. Rarely, other cutaneous sites may be involved, including buttocks, legs, and external genitalia.*

FOCAL EPITHELIAL HYPERPLASIA (HECK DISEASE)

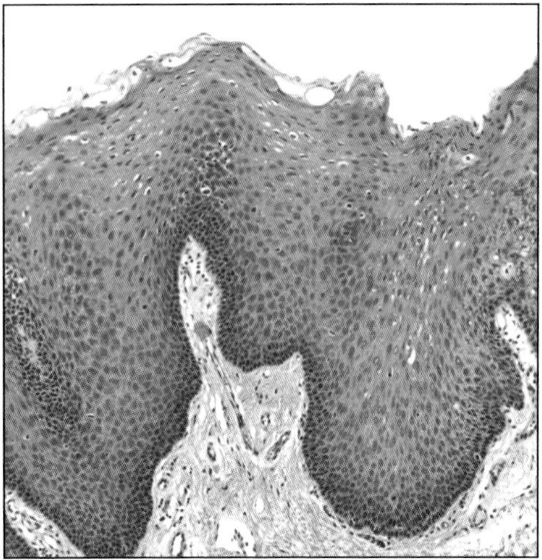

Focal epithelial hyperplasia with prominent acanthosis, elongated rete ridges, and a slightly papillary surface is shown. The papillary features are not always noted.

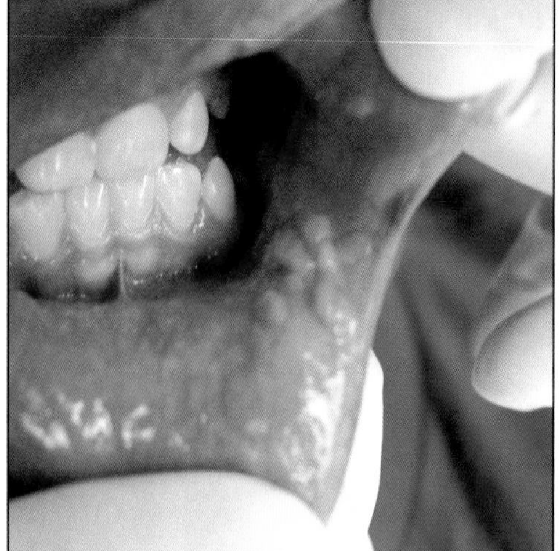

This focal epithelial hyperplasia presented as multiple mucosal colored papules and nodules of the lower lip. The lesions can appear papillary. (Courtesy D. Cox, MD.)

TERMINOLOGY

Synonyms

- Heck disease
- Multifocal epithelial hyperplasia

Definitions

- Benign, virus-induced epithelial proliferation of oral mucosa

ETIOLOGY/PATHOGENESIS

Infectious Agents

- Human papillomavirus (HPV) types 13 and 32
  - Often multiple family members infected
    - Uncertain as to whether this represents genetic vulnerability or viral transmission

Socioeconomic Factors

- Disease more common in communities with crowded living conditions and poor diet

Immunosuppression

- Focal epithelial hyperplasia (FEH) occurs in HIV-positive patients

Genetics

- HLA-DR4 (DRB1*0404) allele may play role in susceptibility
  - Frequent allele in Native American populations

CLINICAL ISSUES

Epidemiology

- Incidence
  - Exact incidence unknown
- Age
  - Majority of reported cases are in children (2-13 years of age)
- Gender
  - Suggestion of female predilection
- Ethnicity
  - 1st described in Native Americans and Inuit
    - Known to exist in North, South, and Central American Indians
    - Caucasians and blacks infrequently affected

Presentation

- Multiple 0.3-1.0 cm mucosal colored soft papules
  - Asymptomatic
  - Occur mostly on labial and buccal mucosa and tongue
  - Less likely noted on gingiva, palate, and oropharynx
- Papules can coalesce to form clusters with cobblestone appearance
- Usually surface is smooth, but can show papillary change
- Rarely affects other sites

Treatment

- Lesions often regress spontaneously
  - Can occur in months to years
  - Perhaps explains why few adults have disease
- Cryotherapy or carbon dioxide laser ablation have been used
  - Usually when lesions interfere with function or are traumatized, or for aesthetic purposes
  - Lesions may recur after treatment
- Medical therapy shows promise
  - Imiquimod 5% cream

Prognosis

- Exceedingly unlikely malignant potential

MICROSCOPIC PATHOLOGY

Histologic Features

- Prominent acanthosis
  - Thickened epithelium extends upward

FOCAL EPITHELIAL HYPERPLASIA (HECK DISEASE)

Key Facts

Terminology
- Benign, virus-induced epithelial proliferation of oral mucosa associated with HPV types 13 and 32

Clinical Issues
- Majority of reported cases are in children (2-13 years of age)
- Multiple 0.3-1.0 cm mucosal colored soft papules
- Occur mostly on labial and buccal mucosa and tongue
- Lesions often regress spontaneously
- No malignant potential has been reported

Microscopic Pathology
- Prominent acanthosis
- Elongated broad rete ridges
- Mitosoid cells
- Dyskeratosis &/or atypia should not be seen
- HPV13 or 32 detected in 75-100% of reported cases by DNA in situ hybridization

---

  - Rete noted at same depth as adjacent normal rete
- Elongated broad rete ridges
- May see papillary surface
- Koilocytic change in superficial keratinocytes can be noted
- **Mitosoid** cells
  - Represents ballooning and nuclear degeneration
  - Can be seen throughout epithelium
- Dyskeratosis &/or atypia should not be seen

In Situ Hybridization
- HPV13 or 32 detected in 75-100% of reported cases by DNA in situ hybridization

DIFFERENTIAL DIAGNOSIS

Clinical DDx
- Oral verruca vulgaris
  - Occurs mainly on keratinized mucosa
    - Vermilion of lip, hard palate, gingiva
  - White with papillary appearance
- Condyloma acuminatum
- Mucosal neuromas of MEN2

Microscopic DDx
- Papilloma
  - Pedunculated finger-like papillary projections with fibrovascular cores
  - Koilocytes can be seen in prickle layer
  - Associated with HPV6 &/or 11
- Condyloma acuminatum
  - Keratotic papillary surface
  - Numerous koilocytes in prickle layer
  - Associated with HPV6 &/or 11
- Oral verruca vulgaris
  - Multiple papillary projections with prominent granular layer (hypergranulosis)
  - Cupping effect of rete toward center of lesion seen
  - Associated inflammation often seen
  - Eosinophilic viral inclusions can be seen in granular layer
  - Associated with HPV types 2, 4, 6, 40, and 57

DIAGNOSTIC CHECKLIST

Pathologic Interpretation Pearls
- Since FEH extends upward, elongated rete are at same depth as adjacent normal rete ridges
- **Mitosoid** cells should not be interpreted as atypia

SELECTED REFERENCES

1. Bennett LK et al: Heck's disease: diagnosis and susceptibility. Pediatr Dermatol. 26(1):87-9, 2009
2. Durso BC et al: Extensive focal epithelial hyperplasia: case report. J Can Dent Assoc. 71(10):769-71, 2005
3. Bassioukas K et al: Oral focal epithelial hyperplasia. Eur J Dermatol. 10(5):395-7, 2000
4. Cohen PR et al: Focal epithelial hyperplasia: Heck disease. Pediatr Dermatol. 10(3):245-51, 1993

IMAGE GALLERY

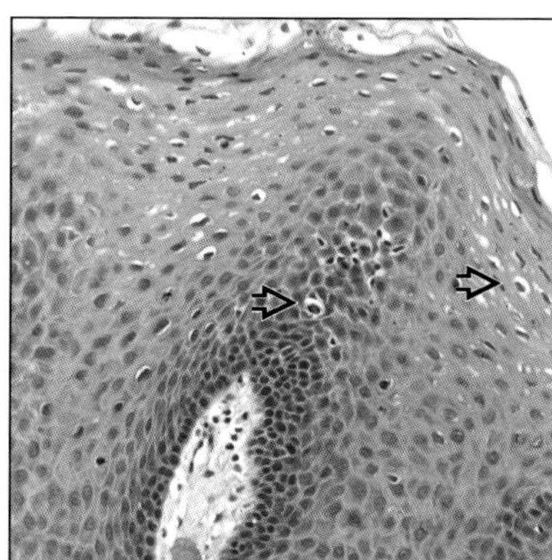

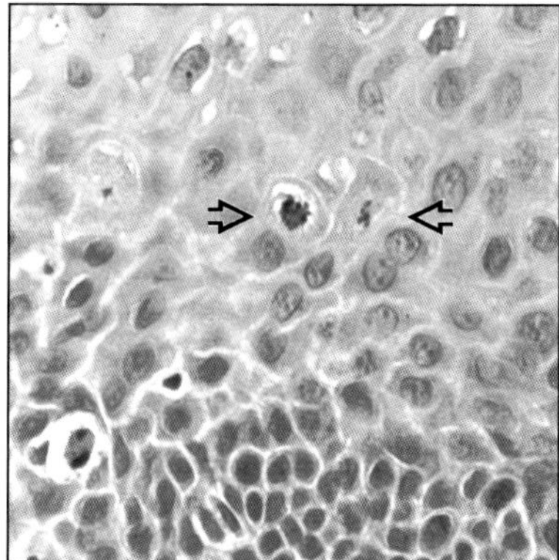

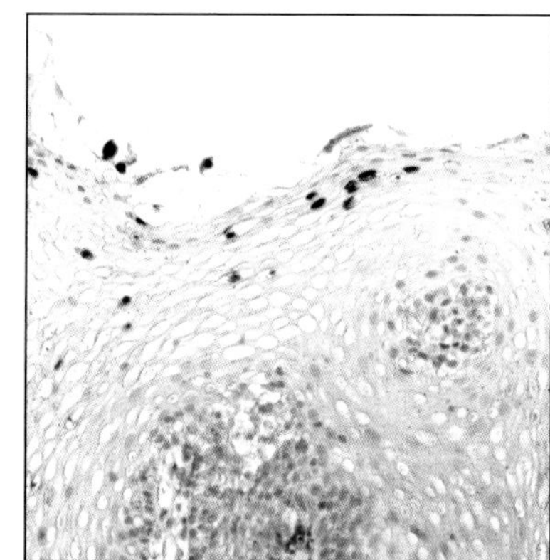

(Left) *High-power photomicrograph of focal epithelial hyperplasia with koilocytic change noted in some superficial keratinocytes ⇨, similar to other HPV-infected epithelium.* ***(Center)*** *Mitosoid cells ⇨ that represent an altered nucleus in an otherwise normal stratified squamous epithelium are seen.* ***(Right)*** *DNA in situ hybridization for HPV13 demonstrates numerous HPV-positive nuclei in the prickle layer of the epithelium.*

APHTHOUS STOMATITIS

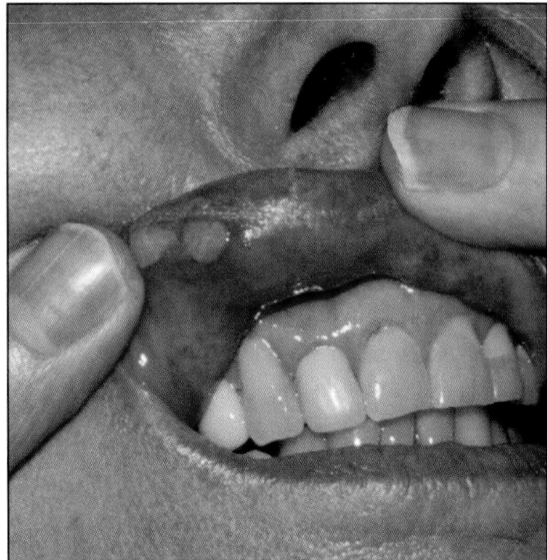

Clinical photograph shows minor recurrent aphthous ulcers. The 2 discrete ulcers, each under 1 cm, are noted in the upper labial mucosa. The ulcers may coalesce to form a larger ulcer.

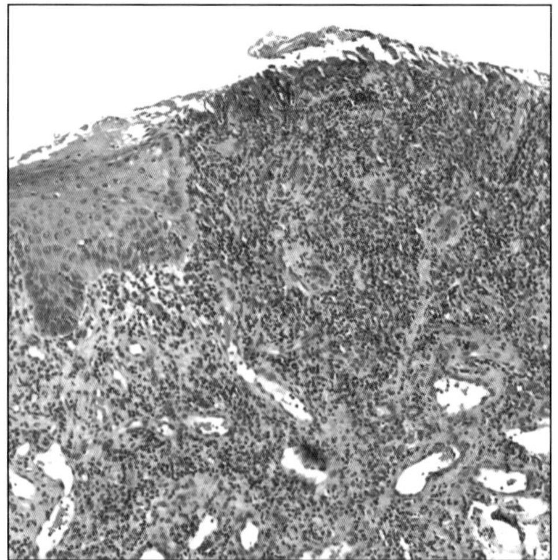

Hematoxylin & eosin shows an aphthous ulcer. Histology is that of a nonspecific ulcer with a fibrino-purulent membrane. A mixed inflammatory cell infiltrate is see beneath the ulcer bed.

TERMINOLOGY

Abbreviations

- Recurrent aphthous stomatitis (RAS)

Synonyms

- Recurrent aphthous ulcerations, canker sores

Definitions

- Noninfectious, common T-cell-mediated nonkeratinized mucosal ulceration

ETIOLOGY/PATHOGENESIS

Multifactorial

- Allergens thought to play role in triggering RAS
  - Cinnamon, cereal products, chocolate, nuts, and certain fruits and vegetables have been cited
- Mechanical trauma, such as orthodontia
- Stress and anxiety
- Nutritional deficiencies, including vitamin B12
- RAS demonstrates familial tendency
  - If both parents have RAS, 90% likelihood that offspring will develop RAS
- No known association with infectious agents, such as herpes, *Streptococcus,* and *Helicobacter pylori*

Immunology

- Precise initiating event unknown
- Peripheral blood in patients with RAS show decreased ratio of CD4 to CD8 cells and increased tumor necrosis factor-α
- Localized mucosal destruction due to local T-cell-mediated response
  - TNF-α generated by T-cells, macrophages, and mast cells result in tissue destruction

CLINICAL ISSUES

Epidemiology

- Incidence
  - Widely reported range (average: 35%)
- Age
  - RAS starts in childhood and adolescence and persists into adulthood
- Gender
  - Equal gender distribution

Presentation

- Minor RAS
  - Most common type; affects 80% of RAS patients
  - Lesions arise almost exclusively on nonkeratinized mucosa
  - Buccal mucosa and lip are most common locations
  - Often RAS present as multiple ulcers
  - May be preceded by prodrome of burning or stinging
  - Painful ulcer ≤ 1 cm, covered by yellow fibrinopurulent membrane surrounded by erythematous border
  - Heals without scarring in 7-14 days
  - Recurrences can be anywhere from every few weeks to every few years
    - Some patients who experienced very few aphthous ulcers in past may develop more frequent outbreaks for no known cause
- Major RAS
  - > 1 cm ulcers that can last for several weeks
  - Soft palate and tonsillar pillar are most common locations
  - May scar due to length of healing time
- Herpetiform RAS
  - Small ulcers ranging from 1-3 mm occurring in clusters
  - As many as 100 ulcers can present at single time
  - Variant most likely to have frequent recurrences

APHTHOUS STOMATITIS

Key Facts

Etiology/Pathogenesis

- Allergens thought to play role in triggering RAS
  - Cinnamon, cereal products, chocolate, nuts, and certain fruits and vegetables have been cited

Clinical Issues

- Widely reported incidence (average: 35%)
- Lesions arise almost exclusively on nonkeratinized mucosa
- Minor RAS: Most common type; affects 80% of RAS patients
- Major RAS: > 1 cm ulcers that can last for several weeks
- Herpetiform RAS present as clusters of small ulcers ranging from 1-3 mm
- Typically treated with topical and systemic corticosteroids

Microscopic Pathology

- No unique microscopic features
- Early lesions show ulceration with fibrinopurulent membrane cover

Top Differential Diagnoses

- Behçet disease (BD)
  - Microscopic features similar to RAS
- Reiter disease (reactive arthritis)
  - Oral lesions seen in < 20% of cases
  - Biopsy of circinate area of tongue similar in appearance to geographic tongue or psoriasis
- Crohn disease (regional ileitis; regional enteritis)
  - May see noncaseating granulomatous inflammation

  - Usually occur on nonkeratinized mucosa, but can appear anywhere
  - Name refers to herpes-like appearance only, as no herpes virus is identified
  - Heals without scarring in 7-14 days

Treatment

- Surgical approaches
  - Laser ablation
    - Shortens duration
- Drugs
  - Corticosteroids
    - Systemic therapy useful when numerous ulcers are present, especially in oropharynx
    - Intralesional steroid injections helpful in treating major RAS
    - Low potency topical steroids may decrease healing time
  - Dapsone
  - Colchicine
  - Pentoxifylline
  - Tetracycline
  - Thalidomide
    - Generally confined to HIV-associated major aphthous-like ulcers
- Chemical cautery
  - Usefulness antidotal

Prognosis

- Recurrences can occur sporadically for many years

MICROSCOPIC PATHOLOGY

Histologic Features

- No unique microscopic features
- Early lesions show ulceration with fibrinopurulent membrane cover
- Mixed inflammatory cell infiltrate beneath ulcer bed composed of lymphocytes, histiocytes, and neutrophils
- Increased vascularity

DIFFERENTIAL DIAGNOSIS

Behçet Disease (BD)

- Clinical features
  - Multisystem disorder involving ocular, mucocutaneous, cardiovascular, renal, and central nervous system
  - Not common disease in US, but more frequent in Mediterranean countries (1 in 10,000)
  - Male > > > > Female (16-24:1)
  - Disease usually presents in 3rd decade
  - Exact etiology unknown, but considered to be immunodysregulation disease
    - Proposed triggers include bacterial, viral, as well as environmental allergens
    - HLA-B51 frequently associated
    - TNF-α levels elevated
  - Oral and genital ulcers and posterior uveitis are common symptoms
  - Oral ulcerations often presenting symptom
  - Oral ulcers similar to RAS in both appearance, number, location, and duration
  - Genital ulcers similar in appearance to oral lesions and occur in 75% of patients
  - Cutaneous lesions include pustules, vesicles, folliculitis, acneiform eruptions, and pyoderma
    - Skin exhibits positive pathergy test, unique to BD
- Microscopic features
  - Similar to RAS, therefore diagnosis is based on clinical findings
  - Can observe leukocytoclastic vasculitis of small vessels
- Treatment of oral BD
  - Similar to RAS
  - Tetracycline mouthrinse is effective
- Prognosis
  - Clinical course variable, making predictions of long-term prognosis difficult
  - Disease more severe in men

Reiter Disease (Reactive Arthritis)

- Systemic disorder of unknown etiology

APHTHOUS STOMATITIS

- Most frequently seen in young men
- Male > > > Female (9:1)
- Usually triggered by urogenital or enteric infections
  - Bacteria include *Shigella*, *Salmonella*, *Streptococcus*, *Mycoplasma*, *Chlamydia*, and *Yersinia*
- Associated with HLA-B27
- Common in context of HIV infection

- Clinical features
  - Oral manifestations
    - Oral lesions seen in < 20% of cases
    - Oral and oropharyngeal erythema and ulceration
    - Circinate lesions of tongue similar in appearance to geographic tongue
  - Circinate balanitis, conjunctivitis, iritis, arthritis, keratotic plaques, and pustules on soles and palms
- Microscopic features
  - Biopsy of oral ulcer nonspecific and similar to RAS
  - Biopsy of circinate area of tongue similar in appearance to geographic tongue or psoriasis
    - Psoriasiform hyperkeratosis with elongated rete ridges
    - Neutrophilic microabscesses noted in superficial epithelium
- Treatment
  - Nonsteroidal anti-inflammatory drugs
    - Useful in managing arthritic component
  - Immunosuppressive agents
    - Corticosteroids, azathioprine, methotrexate
    - Use is limited in HIV-positive patients
- Prognosis
  - 2/3 of patients have self-limited course
  - Can have chronic recurrent ocular inflammation

Crohn Disease (Regional Ileitis; Regional Enteritis)

- Idiopathic inflammatory disorder of gastrointestinal tract
  - Primarily affects proximal colon and distal portion of small bowel
  - Most likely immune-mediated disease
    - Genetic, microbial, environmental, dietary, and vascular factors have been implicated
  - Incidence in US is 7/100,000 cases
    - Incidence increasing particularly in northern latitudes
  - More common in whites than blacks or Asians
    - 2-4x higher incidence in Jewish population
  - Female > Male (1.2:1)
  - Age of onset is bimodal: 15-30 years, 60-80 years
    - Most cases diagnosed by age 30
- Clinical features
  - Oral lesions
    - May be initial presentation of disease
    - Wide range of oral lesions have been reported
    - Aphthous-like ulcerations
    - Diffuse or nodular swelling of oral and perioral tissues termed orofacial granulomatosis
    - Patchy erythema of gingiva
- Microscopic features
  - Noncaseating granulomatous inflammation in superficial mucosa can be seen in oral biopsies
    - Feature can be variable
    - Special stain for organisms are negative
  - Nonspecific ulceration similar to RAS
- Treatment
  - Oral lesions may clear with treatment for gastrointestinal disease
  - Persistent oral ulcerations can be managed with topical corticosteroids
- Prognosis
  - Chronic disease with recurrent relapses
  - Mortality rate increases with disease duration
    - GI tract cancer is leading disease-related cause of death

Traumatic Ulcerative Granuloma

- Histologically, inflammation extends much deeper into striated muscle
- Sheets of histiocytes and lymphocytes with scattered eosinophils are seen

Herpes Simplex Virus (HSV), Type 1

- Most HSV ulcers occur on lip vermilion
- Intraoral HSV usually presents on keratinized mucosa (hard palate, attached gingiva)
- Acantholytic epithelial cells are seen in ulcer (Tzanck cells)
  - Ballooning degeneration of infected cell with margination of chromatin
  - Infected cells can fuse to form multinucleated cells
- HSV1 in situ hybridization will be positive in infected cells
- Older HSV1-associated lesions are indistinguishable from RAS

DIAGNOSTIC CHECKLIST

Clinically Relevant Pathologic Features

- Painful oral ulcers ranging in size from 1 mm to > 1 cm
- Ulcers usually last 7-14 days
- Noninfectious etiology

Pathologic Interpretation Pearls

- Microscopic findings are of nonspecific ulcer
- Clinical correlation required to make diagnosis

SELECTED REFERENCES

1. Keogan MT: Clinical Immunology Review Series: an approach to the patient with recurrent orogenital ulceration, including Behçet's syndrome. Clin Exp Immunol. 156(1):1-11, 2009
2. Oh SH et al: Comparison of the clinical features of recurrent aphthous stomatitis and Behçet's disease. Clin Exp Dermatol. 34(6):e208-12, 2009
3. Scully C et al: Oral mucosal disease: recurrent aphthous stomatitis. Br J Oral Maxillofac Surg. 46(3):198-206, 2008
4. Wu IB et al: Reiter's syndrome: the classic triad and more. J Am Acad Dermatol. 59(1):113-21, 2008
5. Harty S et al: A prospective study of the oral manifestations of Crohn's disease. Clin Gastroenterol Hepatol. 3(9):886-91, 2005

Clinical and Microscopic Features

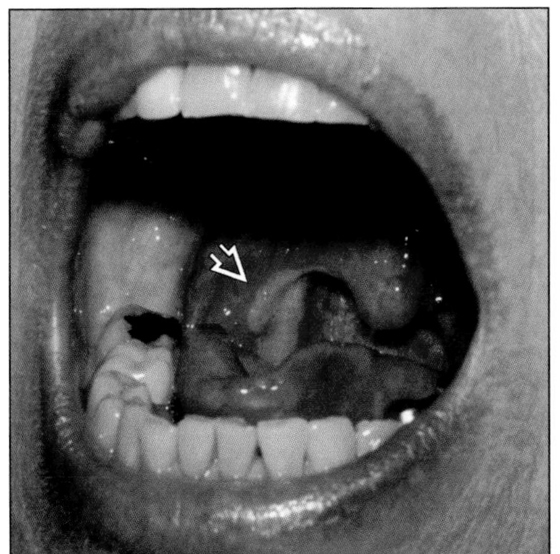

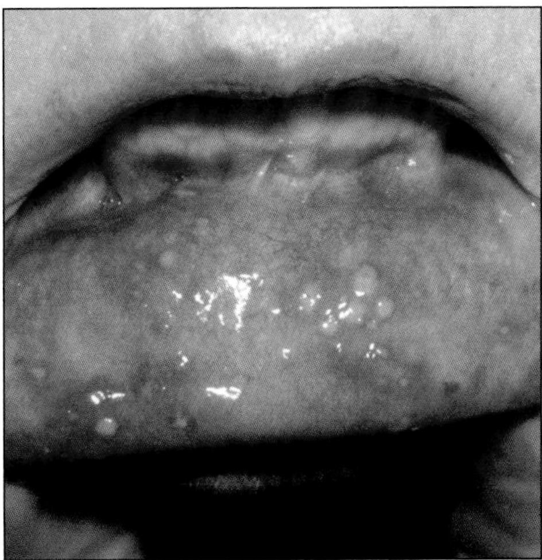

(Left) *Clinical photograph shows a major aphthous ulcer presenting on the tonsillar pillar ➡. These ulcers are quite painful and may produce reactive lymphadenopathy. Because of the ulcer size, resolution may take several weeks.* ***(Right)*** *Clinical photograph shows herpetiform aphthous ulcers. Despite the name, these ulcers do not have an infectious etiology. Clusters of numerous 1-3 mm ulcers are seen throughout the lower lip. Patients may experience as many as 100 ulcers at a time.*

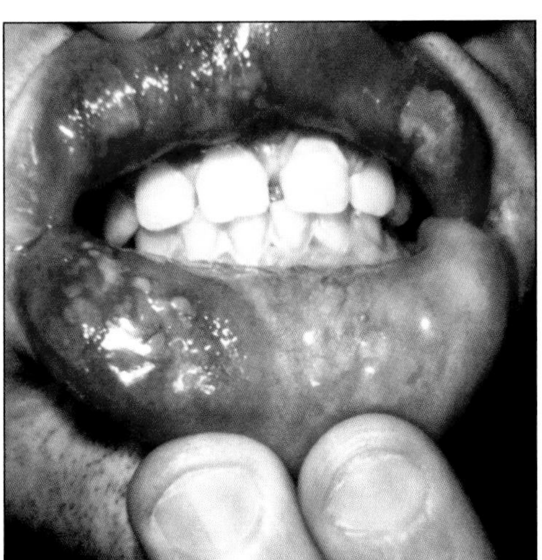

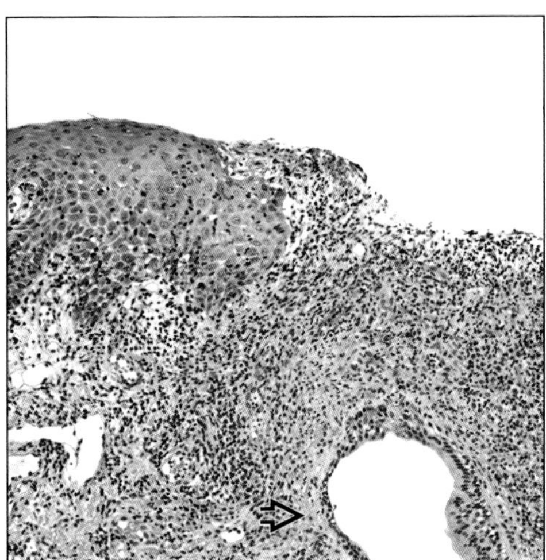

(Left) *Clinical photograph shows Behçet disease. Numerous ulcers 0.5 cm to > 1 cm are noted on both upper and lower lips. The ulcers of Behçet disease are indistinguishable from aphthous ulcers; therefore the diagnosis is based on clinical and not pathologic findings.* ***(Right)*** *Biopsy of a lip ulcer from a patient with Behçet disease shows salivary gland ductal hyperplasia ➡ adjacent to the inflammation. The microscopic findings are not unique and are similar to aphthous ulcers.*

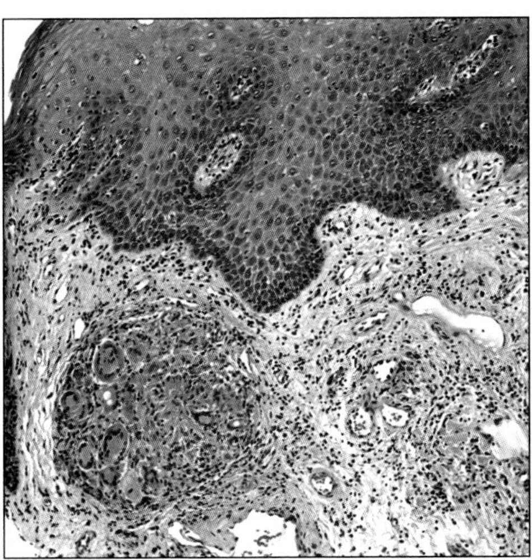

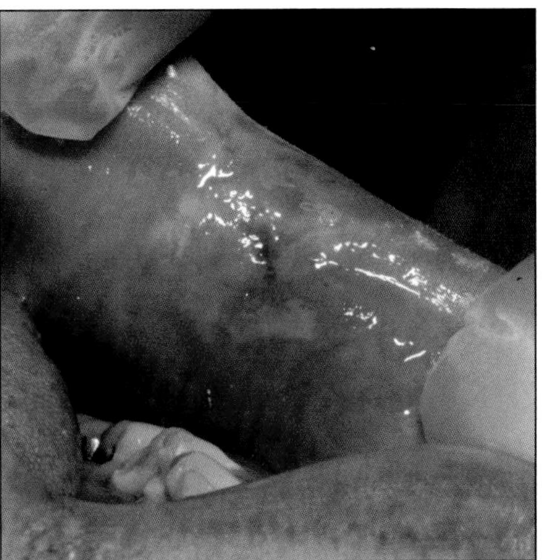

(Left) *Oral biopsy from a patient with Crohn disease shows nonnecrotizing granulomatous inflammation in the superficial lamina propria. Often granulomas are not seen in oral biopsy specimens.* ***(Right)*** *This clinical photograph is of a patient with reactive arthritis (Reiter disease) presenting with large aphthous-like ulcerations, acute onset of arthritis, and keratotic plaques of the soles. Microscopic examination revealed a nonspecific ulcer similar to aphthous ulcers.*

PEMPHIGUS VULGARIS

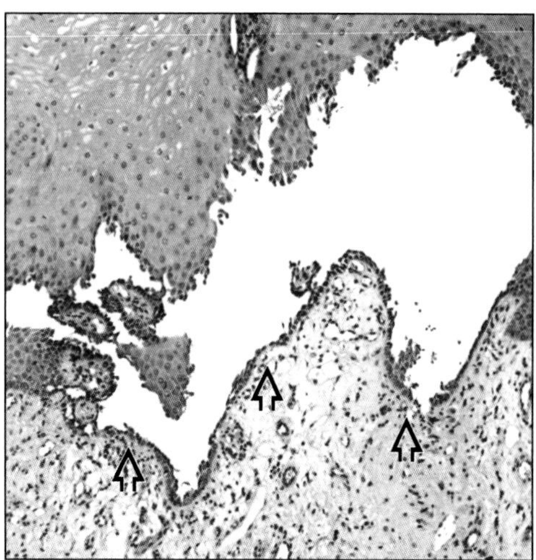

Low-power view of pemphigus vulgaris illustrates the typical intraepithelial clefting just above the basal layer ⊳. A mild to moderate chronic inflammatory cell infiltrate may be present.

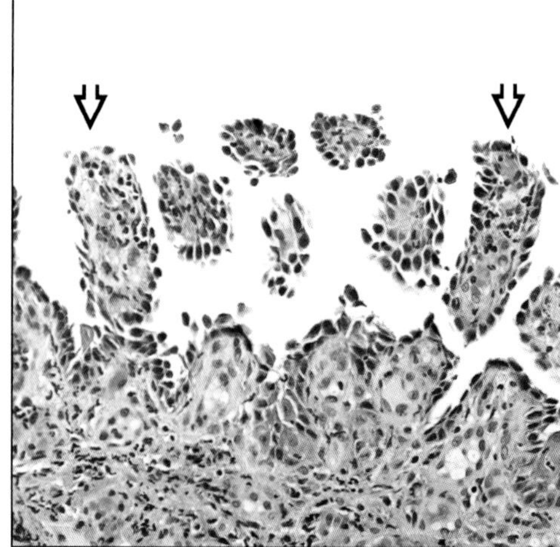

High-power view of pemphigus vulgaris shows irregular papillary projections of the submucosa with a single layer of cuboidal-shaped basal cells resembling a "row of tombstones" ⊳.

TERMINOLOGY

Abbreviations

- Pemphigus vulgaris (PV)

Definitions

- Autoimmune mucocutaneous disease characterized by intraepithelial blistering

ETIOLOGY/PATHOGENESIS

Etiology

- Circulating autoantibodies to desmoglein 1 and 3 adhesion molecules of squamous epithelium
  - Inhibits cell-cell adhesion resulting in acantholysis and blister formation

CLINICAL ISSUES

Epidemiology

- Incidence
  - Ranges up to 3.2/100,000 population
- Age
  - Most common in 4th-6th decade
    - Can be seen in all ages
- Gender
  - Equal sex distribution
- Ethnicity
  - Incidence higher in Ashkenazi Jews
  - Increased incidence in patients of Mediterranean descent

Site

- Mucous membranes: Oral, nasal, esophagus, larynx, nasopharynx, conjunctivae, genitalia, & anal mucosa
- Cutaneous sites mostly on intertriginous areas, trunk, head, and neck

Presentation

- Mucosal PV may be only manifestation of disease or precede cutaneous PV by average of 5 months
- Oral mucosal PV originates in 50-70% of patients
- Bullae &/or blisters which easily rupture, resulting in irregularly shaped, painful ulcers and erosions
- > 90% of patients will have oral involvement during disease course
- Oropharyngeal involvement can present as dysphagia
- Laryngeal involvement can present with hoarseness
- Cutaneous PV characterized by fluid-filled, flaccid blisters that rupture & leave painful ulcers
- Positive Nikolsky sign and Asboe-Hansen sign
  - Lateral pressure on a bullae causes extension into uninvolved mucosa

Natural History

- With treatment, complete remission has been reported, ranging from 2-10 years

Treatment

- Drugs
  - Local &/or systemic therapy depending on disease severity
  - Systemic &/or topical corticosteroids
  - Adjuvant immunosuppressants used for steroid sparing effect
    - Methotrexate, cyclophosphamide, cyclosporine, rituximab
  - Plasmapheresis
  - High-dose IV IgG
  - Anti-inflammatory drugs
    - Minocycline, dapsone, tetracycline

Prognosis

- Mortality reported in up to 6% of patients
  - Systemic infections most common cause of death
  - Mainly from complications due to long-term immunosuppressant therapy

PEMPHIGUS VULGARIS

Key Facts

Terminology
- Autoimmune mucocutaneous disease characterized by intraepithelial blistering

Clinical Issues
- Most common in 4th-6th decade
- Mucosal PV may be only manifestation of disease or precede cutaneous PV by average of 5 months
- Bullae &/or blisters which easily rupture, resulting in irregularly shaped, painful ulcers and erosions

Microscopic Pathology
- Suprabasal bullae formation with intraepithelial clefting

Ancillary Tests
- Exfoliative cytology specimens of blister will demonstrate acantholytic cells (Tzanck cells)
- Direct immunofluorescence of perilesional tissue will show homogeneous staining of IgG in intercellular spaces

MICROSCOPIC PATHOLOGY

Histologic Features
- Suprabasal bullae formation with intraepithelial clefting
- Round, swollen, hyperchromatic acantholytic (Tzanck) cells in cleft spaces
- Irregular papillary projections of the submucosa lined by single row of basal cells with cuboidal shape
- Little or no inflammation during early bullous phase

ANCILLARY TESTS

Cytology
- Exfoliative cytology specimens of blister will demonstrate acantholytic cells (Tzanck cells)

Immunofluorescence
- Direct immunofluorescence (DIF) of perilesional tissue will show homogeneous staining of IgG in intercellular spaces
  - May also see complement component C3 or IgA
- Indirect immunofluorescence (IIF) using serum from PV patients with monkey esophagus substrate
  - 80-90% of patients demonstrate circulating IgG antibodies against desmoglein 1 &/or 3
  - Antibody titers correlate with disease activity

DIFFERENTIAL DIAGNOSIS

Mucous Membrane Pemphigoid (MMP)
- Blistering disease characterized by sub-basal separation of epithelium
- DIF shows linear band of IgG(A) at basement membrane zone

Paraneoplastic Pemphigus
- Histology can be similar to PV, MMP, or EM
- Can be distinguished from PV by DIF and IIF

Erosive Lichen Planus
- Can be distinguished from PV by DIF and IIF

Erythema Multiforme (EM)
- Can be distinguished from PV by DIF

DIAGNOSTIC CHECKLIST

Pathologic Interpretation Pearls
- Acantholysis with suprabasal separation
- Immunofluorescence required for definitive diagnosis

SELECTED REFERENCES

1. Mignogna MD et al: Oropharyngeal pemphigus vulgaris and clinical remission: a long-term, longitudinal study. Am J Clin Dermatol. 11(2):137-45, 2010
2. Patrício P et al: Autoimmune bullous dermatoses: a review. Ann N Y Acad Sci. 1173:203-10, 2009

IMAGE GALLERY

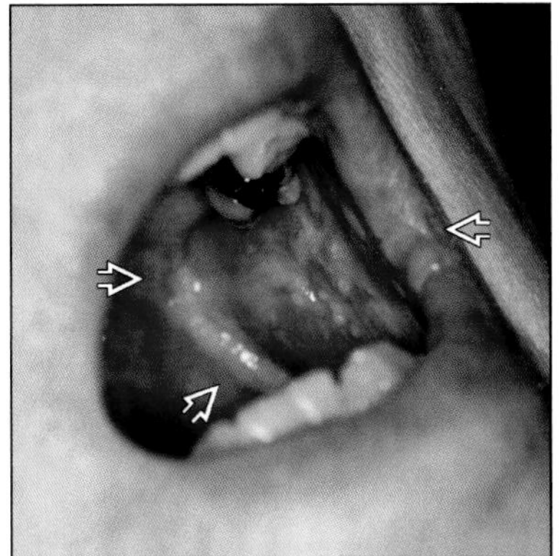

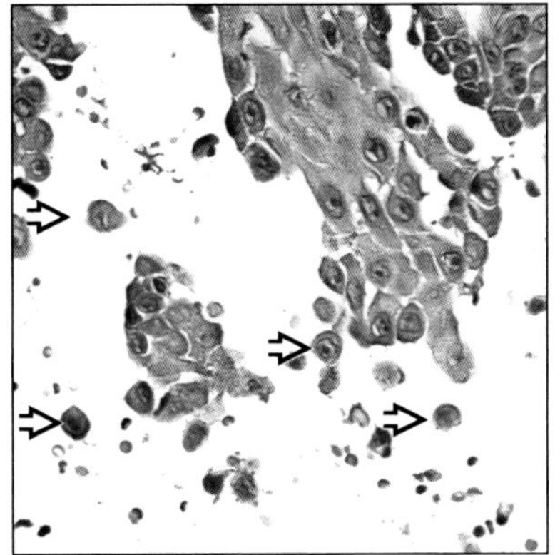

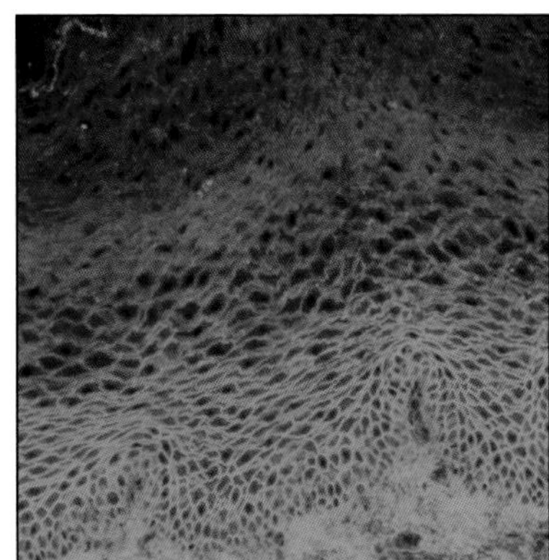

(Left) Clinical photo shows pemphigus vulgaris involving the buccal mucosa extending onto the vermillion border ➡. The white areas represent collapsed bullae and the red areas are mucosal erosions. *(Center)* Round, swollen, acantholytic cells (Tzanck cells) ➡ are often seen within the intraepithelial clefts in pemphigus vulgaris. *(Right)* Direct immunofluorescence of perilesional skin in pemphigus vulgaris shows a characteristic "fishnet" pattern of IgG deposits in the intercellular desmosomal areas at all levels of the epidermis.

MUCOUS MEMBRANE PEMPHIGOID (CICATRICIAL PEMPHIGOID)

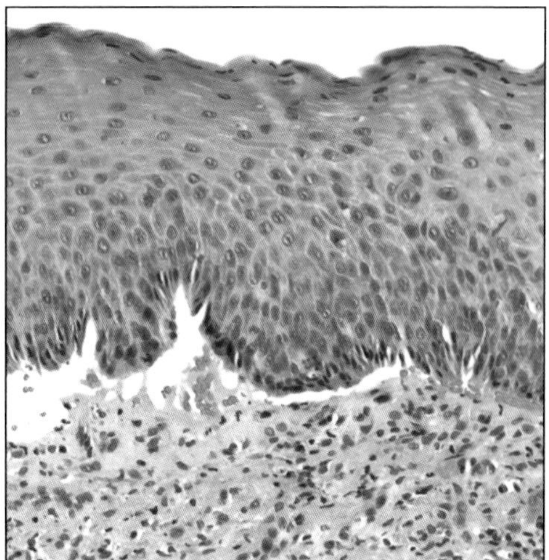

Mucous membrane pemphigoid with characteristic subepithelial clefting and intact basal cells is shown. A sparse inflammatory cell infiltrate is seen in the superficial lamina propria.

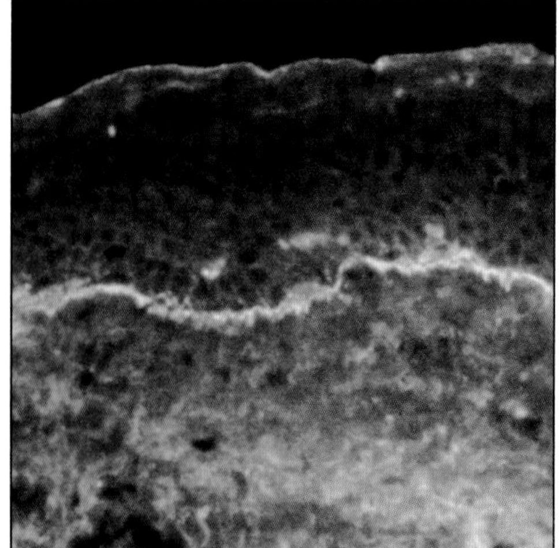

Direct immunofluorescence shows a perilesional mucosa from a patient with mucous membrane pemphigoid. A continuous linear deposit of IgG at the basement membrane zone is observed.

TERMINOLOGY

Abbreviations

- Mucous membrane pemphigoid (MMP)

Synonyms

- Cicatricial pemphigoid

Definitions

- Chronic, blistering mucocutaneous autoimmune disease

ETIOLOGY/PATHOGENESIS

Unknown

- Some studies show antibodies specific for hemidesmosomal antibodies BPAG1 or BPAG2
- Some patients have antibodies to β4 integrin subunit, laminin 5 and 6, and other antigens with unknown identity
- In USA, MMP associated with HLA-DQB1*0301

CLINICAL ISSUES

Epidemiology

- Incidence
  - Unknown, but 2x as common as pemphigus vulgaris
- Age
  - Generally presents in 6th or 7th decade
- Gender
  - Female > Male (2:1)

Presentation

- Oral lesions
  - Vesicles or blisters on mucosa, which erupt, leaving a raw area
  - Positive Nikolsky sign (induced trauma can elicit blister on clinically normal mucosa)
  - Gingival involvement seen in 64% of cases presenting as desquamative gingivitis
  - Also seen on buccal mucosa, palate, alveolus, tongue, and lower lip
- Ocular lesions
  - Occurs in up to 37% of patients with oral MMP
  - Chronic conjunctival irritation
    - Foreign body or burning sensation
  - Conjunctival ulcers develop with subsequent scarring
    - Adhesions (symblepharons) develop that fuse scleral and palpebral conjunctiva
    - With disease progression entropion formation causing eyelashes to rub against cornea
    - Blindness can occur if left untreated
- Upper aerodigestive tract
  - Esophageal involvement can result in esophageal stenosis from repeated untreated ulcers
  - Laryngeal involvement uncommon but can affect vocal cords leading to dysphonia and hoarseness
  - Nasal and nasopharyngeal involvement can cause epistaxis and mucosal scarring
- Other sites
  - Anus, rectum, and vagina can be affected
  - Cutaneous involvement reported in 10-43%

Treatment

- Surgical approaches
  - In ocular lesions, surgery to ablate ingrown eyelashes and release entropions
  - Esophageal strictures may require dilatation
  - Laryngeal stenosis may require tracheostomy
  - MMP should not be active during surgical intervention to prevent further disease exacerbation
- Medical approaches
  - Corticosteroids, both topical and systemic
  - Steroid-sparing therapy: Dapsone, cyclophosphamide, azathioprine, and cyclosporine
  - Intravenous Ig therapy
  - Anti-inflammatory drugs: Tetracycline

MUCOUS MEMBRANE PEMPHIGOID (CICATRICIAL PEMPHIGOID)

Key Facts

Terminology
- Chronic, blistering mucocutaneous autoimmune disease

Clinical Issues
- Generally presents in 6th or 7th decade
- Female > Male (2:1)
- Gingival involvement seen in 64% of cases
- Ocular lesions occurs in up to 37% of patients with oral MMP
- Chronic life-long disease with periods of remission

Microscopic Pathology
- Perilesional mucosa shows subepithelial clefting
- DIF shows continuous linear band IgG or C3 at basement membrane zone

Top Differential Diagnoses
- Erosive lichen planus
- Pemphigus vulgaris

Prognosis
- Chronic life-long disease with periods of remission

MICROSCOPIC PATHOLOGY

Histologic Features
- Perilesional mucosa shows subepithelial clefting
- Sparse inflammatory cell infiltrate, usually lymphocytes and plasma cells

Immunopathology
- Direct immunofluorescence (DIF)
  - Continuous linear band at basement membrane zone of fixed IgG or complement (C3)
  - Can also see IgM and IgA
- Indirect immunofluorescence
  - Salt-split skin can detect circulating antibodies to basement membrane zone
  - Not all patients have circulating antibodies
  - Antibody titer does not correlate with disease activity

DIFFERENTIAL DIAGNOSIS

Erosive Lichen Planus
- May share clinical and histologic features, but DIF will distinguish the 2 entities

Pemphigus Vulgaris
- Clinically similar but suprabasal separation seen

DIAGNOSTIC CHECKLIST

Clinically Relevant Pathologic Features
- Gingival involvement almost universal
- Ocular involvement results in scarring

Pathologic Interpretation Pearls
- Subepithelial clefting with sparse inflammatory cell infiltrate in superficial lamina propria
- DIF shows continuous linear band of IgG and C3 at basement membrane zone

SELECTED REFERENCES

1. Carrozzo M: A reappraisal of diagnostic criteria for mucous membrane pemphigoid. J Oral Pathol Med. 38(1):160, 2009
2. Olasz EB et al: Bullous pemphigoid and related subepidermal autoimmune blistering diseases. Curr Dir Autoimmun. 10:141-66, 2008
3. Scully C et al: Oral mucosal diseases: mucous membrane pemphigoid. Br J Oral Maxillofac Surg. 46(5):358-66, 2008
4. Bruch-Gerharz D et al: Mucous membrane pemphigoid: clinical aspects, immunopathological features and therapy. Eur J Dermatol. 17(3):191-200, 2007
5. Hertl M et al: T cell control in autoimmune bullous skin disorders. J Clin Invest. 116(5):1159-66, 2006
6. Rashid KA et al: Antigen specificity in subsets of mucous membrane pemphigoid. J Invest Dermatol. 126(12):2631-6, 2006
7. Sollecito TP et al: Mucous membrane pemphigoid. Dent Clin North Am. 49(1):91-106, viii, 2005

IMAGE GALLERY

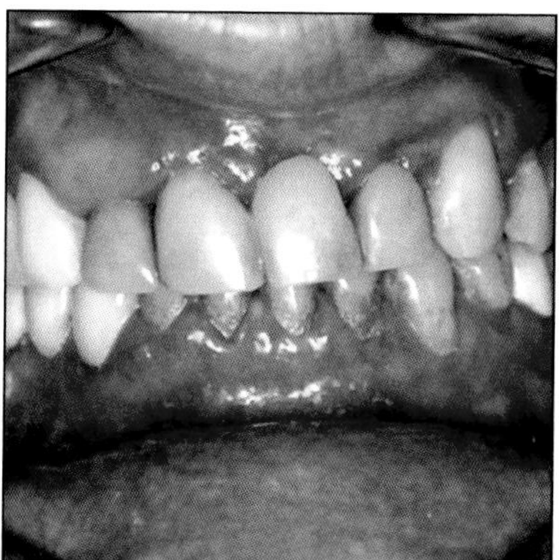

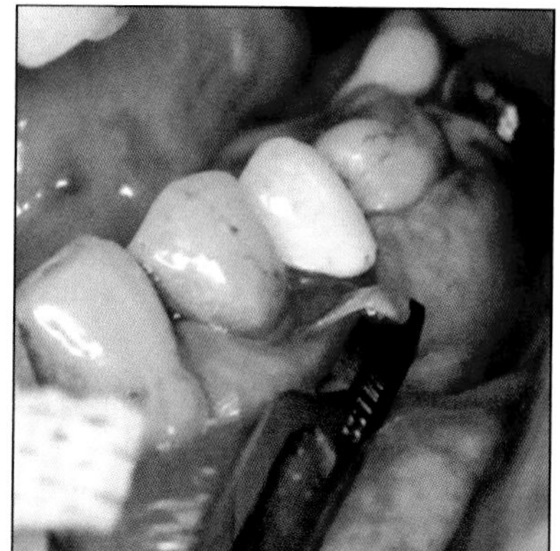

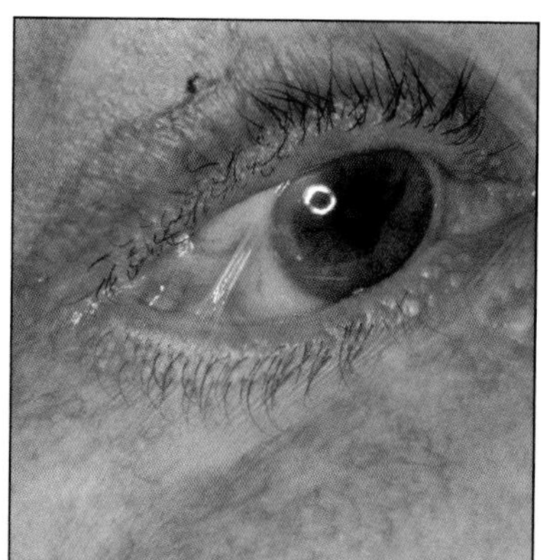

(Left) *Mucous membrane pemphigoid presents as desquamative gingivitis. This is one of the most common presentations for MMP.* ***(Center)*** *The mucosa in mucous membrane pemphigoid is very friable and can slough easily. Blister formation can be induced in clinically normal mucosa (positive Nikolsky sign).* ***(Right)*** *Symblepharon formation is seen between the bulbar and palpebral conjunctivae from a mucous membrane pemphigoid patient with ocular involvement.*

LICHEN PLANUS

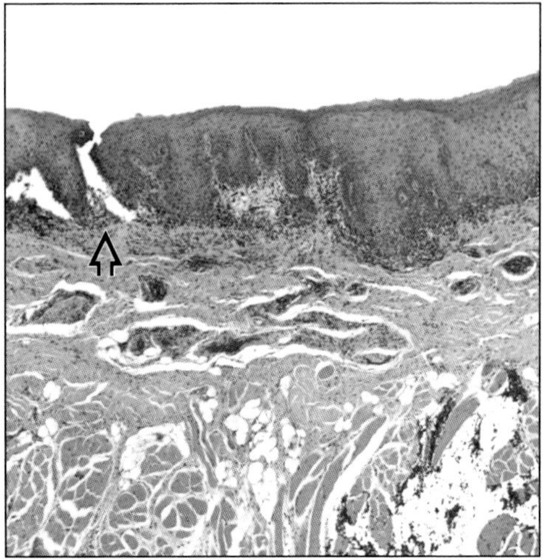

Lichen planus of oral mucosa shows acanthosis and "saw-tooth" rete ridges. At the edge of the specimen is a sub-basal separation, often seen in erosive lichen planus ⮚.

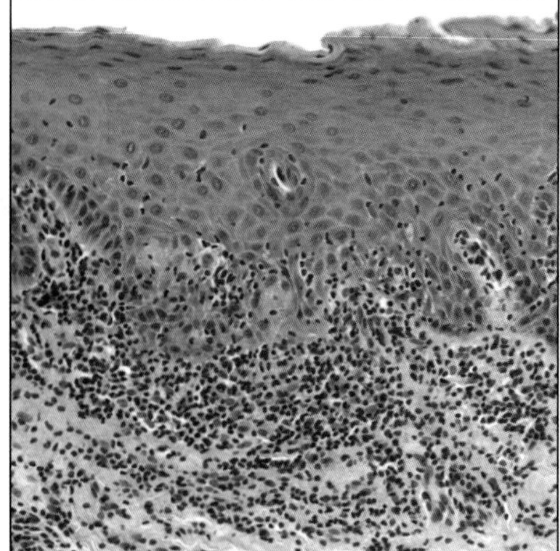

Band-like lymphocytic infiltrate is seen adjacent to the basement membrane with basal cell degeneration.

TERMINOLOGY

Abbreviations

- Lichen planus (LP)

Definitions

- Chronic, self-limited, inflammatory disorder that involves mucous membranes, skin, nails, and hair

ETIOLOGY/PATHOGENESIS

Etiology

- Precise cause unknown

Pathogenesis

- Thought to be T-cell immune-mediated response
  - Activated CD8(+) T-cells trigger basal cell apoptosis
  - Exact mechanism unknown and may involve mast cell chemotaxis or matrix metalloproteinases disrupting basement membrane
- No HLA association found
  - Genetic factors do not seem to be involved
- Drug reactions
  - Many drugs have been reported to be associated with onset of LP
    - Lesions do not always resolve when offending drug discontinued
- Hepatitis C
  - Association is controversial

CLINICAL ISSUES

Epidemiology

- Incidence
  - Between 1-2% of general population
- Age
  - Peaks in middle-aged adults
- Gender
  - Female > Male (3:2)

Presentation

- Reticular LP
  - Usually asymptomatic
  - Lesions involve multiple sites
  - Fine white lace-like striae (Wickham striae) on buccal mucosa, gingiva, and lip
  - White papules that can coalesce to form plaques
  - White plaques on dorsal tongue
  - Up to 44% of patients with oral LP will develop cutaneous LP
  - Scalp and nail involvement rare in patients with only oral LP
- Erosive LP
  - Complaints of pain while eating, particularly spicy foods
  - Atrophic erythematous mucosa with ulcerations
  - Periphery of lesion will show features of reticular LP
  - Can be confined to gingiva
    - LP confined to gingiva and genitals is recognized; more common in females
- Bullous LP
  - Unusual variant where bullae are formed during epithelial separation
  - Positive Nikolsky sign can be elicited

Treatment

- Adjuvant therapy
  - Reticular LP
    - No treatment is needed
  - Erosive LP
    - Topical or systemic corticosteroids
    - Topical antifungal drugs for secondary oral candidiasis
    - Tacrolimus has been used for steroid resistant LP

Prognosis

- Chronic disease
  - Symptoms wax and wane over patient lifetime
- Malignant transformation

Key Facts

Terminology
- Chronic, self-limited, inflammatory disorder that involves mucous membranes, skin, nails, and hair

Clinical Issues
- Between 1-2%
- Peaks in middle-aged adults
- Reticular LP usually asymptomatic
- Erosive LP exhibits atrophic erythematous mucosa with ulcerations

Microscopic Pathology
- Varying degrees of ortho or parakeratosis
- Rete ridges can demonstrate "saw-tooth" pattern
- Basal cell layer exhibits liquefaction (hydropic degeneration)
- Band-like, predominately T lymphocytes adjacent to basement membrane
- Ulceration or sub-basal separation seen in erosive LP
- Direct immunofluorescence of perilesional tissue
  - Not specific or diagnostic

Top Differential Diagnoses
- Mucous membrane pemphigoid
- Lichenoid reaction to dental amalgam
- Lichenoid reaction to drugs and topical agents

Diagnostic Checklist
- Oral LP should be multifocal and no significant dysplasia should be seen
- Sub-basal separation of epithelium from connective tissue

  - Controversial as some cases are not confirmed as LP histologically
  - Documented cases occur in atrophic or chronic ulcerative areas
  - Long-term clinical follow-up recommended for erosive LP

MICROSCOPIC PATHOLOGY

Histologic Features
- Varying degrees of orthokeratosis or parakeratosis
- Both atrophy and acanthosis can be seen
- Rete ridges can demonstrate "saw-tooth" pattern
- Basal cell layer exhibits liquefaction (hydropic degeneration)
- Degenerating keratinocytes (Civatte, hyaline, or colloid bodies) are noted at epithelial-connective tissue interface
- Band-like, predominately T lymphocytes adjacent to basement membrane
  - Plasma cells can also be present
- Ulceration or sub-basal separation seen in erosive LP
- No significant atypia should be seen
  - Superimposed candidiasis may cause reactive atypia

Immunopathology
- Direct immunofluorescence of perilesional tissue
  - Not specific or diagnostic
  - May show linear or granular deposits of fibrin or fibrinogen
  - Deposits of C3, IgM, IgG, and IgA occasionally seen
  - Colloid bodies

DIFFERENTIAL DIAGNOSIS

Mucous Membrane Pemphigoid
- Immunopathology useful in delineating disease from LP
  - Direct immunofluorescence shows continuous linear band at basement membrane zone of fixed IgG and C3
    - Occasionally IgA or IgM seen
  - Indirect immunofluorescence noted in sera, but studies show wide expression (5-90%)

Lichenoid Reaction to Dental Amalgam
- Noted only where there is direct contact of mucosa with dental amalgam
- Often lymphocytic infiltrate forms tertiary lymphoid follicles

Lichenoid Reaction to Drugs
- No specific differences
- May see more diffuse pattern of inflammation, including perivascular inflammation

Linear IgA Disease
- Direct immunofluorescence shows continuous linear band at basement membrane zone of IgA

Lupus Erythematosus
- Superficial and deep perivascular inflammatory infiltrate
- Immunopathology not specific

Cinnamon-induced Stomatitis
- Acanthosis with neutrophilic exocytosis
- Mixed inflammatory cell infiltrate in superficial lamina propria
- Marked interface change

Chronic Graft-vs.-Host Disease
- Epithelium exhibits basal cell liquefaction with numerous dyskeratotic keratinocytes
- Patchy moderate lymphocytic infiltrate in submucosa
- Diagnosis based on clinical history
  - Lesions present on average 6 months post transplantation

Oral Dysplasia
- Often see intense chronic inflammatory cell infiltrate mimicking LP
- Dyskeratotic epithelial cells can be noted
- Frank dysplasia seen that cannot be attributed to infection or ulceration

Causative Agents in Oral Lichenoid Reactions

Oral Lichenoid Drug Reactions	Oral Lichenoid Contact Reactions
Antihypertensives	**Dental materials**
Propranolol	Mercury
Hydrochlorothiazide	Nickel
Spironolactone	Palladium
Antimalarials	Silver
Chloroquine	Gold
Quinidine	Pallidum
Quinolone	Bismuth
Antibiotics	Glass Ionomer
Tetracycline	Composite
Ketoconazole	Porcelain
Nonsteroidal anti-inflammatory drugs	**Flavoring agents**
Naproxen	Cinnamon (cinnamic aldehyde)
Ibuprofen	Mint (mentha piperita)
Diclofenac	Tartar-control toothpaste
Miscellaneous	Eugenol
Gold	Balsam of Peru
Palladium	**Dental adhesives**
Penicillamine	Acrylate compounds
Allopurinol	Eugenol

Pemphigus Vulgaris

- Autoimmune-mediated disease that shares similar clinical findings
- Suprabasilar separation rather than sub-basal separation of epithelium
- Direct immunofluorescence shows IgG deposits in intercellular desmosomal areas
- Indirect immunofluorescence of patient sera shows circulating IgG antibodies in 80-90% of patients

DIAGNOSTIC CHECKLIST

Clinically Relevant Pathologic Features

- Oral LP should be multifocal
  - Solitary lesions may represent lichenoid keratoses

Pathologic Interpretation Pearls

- No significant dysplasia should be seen
  - Lichenoid lesions with dysplasia should not be diagnosed as LP with dysplasia
    - Multiple lichenoid lesions exhibiting varying degrees of dysplasia most likely represent proliferative verrucous leukoplakia

SELECTED REFERENCES

1. Buffon RB et al: Vulvovaginal-gingival lichen planus--a rare or underreported syndrome? Int J Dermatol. 48(3):322-4, 2009
2. Bidarra M et al: Oral lichen planus: a condition with more persistence and extra-oral involvement than suspected? J Oral Pathol Med. 37(10):582-6, 2008
3. Cooper SM et al: Vulvovaginal lichen planus treatment: a survey of current practices. Arch Dermatol. 144(11):1520-1, 2008
4. Leao JC et al: Desquamative gingivitis: retrospective analysis of disease associations of a large cohort. Oral Dis. 14(6):556-60, 2008
5. Lo Russo L et al: Diagnostic pathways and clinical significance of desquamative gingivitis. J Periodontol. 79(1):4-24, 2008
6. McCartan BE et al: The reported prevalence of oral lichen planus: a review and critique. J Oral Pathol Med. 37(8):447-53, 2008
7. Scully C et al: Oral mucosal disease: Lichen planus. Br J Oral Maxillofac Surg. 46(1):15-21, 2008
8. Thongprasom K et al: Steriods in the treatment of lichen planus: a review. J Oral Sci. 50(4):377-85, 2008
9. Al-Hashimi I et al: Oral lichen planus and oral lichenoid lesions: diagnostic and therapeutic considerations. Oral Surg Oral Med Oral Pathol Oral Radiol Endod. 103 Suppl:S25, 2007
10. Kulthanan K et al: Direct immunofluorescence study in patients with lichen planus. Int J Dermatol. 46(12):1237-41, 2007
11. Acay RR et al: Evaluation of proliferative potential in oral lichen planus and oral lichenoid lesions using immunohistochemical expression of p53 and Ki67. Oral Oncol. 42(5):475-80, 2006
12. van der Meij EH et al: The possible premalignant character of oral lichen planus and oral lichenoid lesions: a prospective study. Oral Surg Oral Med Oral Pathol Oral Radiol Endod. 96(2):164-71, 2003
13. Eisen D: The clinical features, malignant potential, and systemic associations of oral lichen planus: a study of 723 patients. J Am Acad Dermatol. 46(2):207-14, 2002
14. Fayyazi A et al: T lymphocytes and altered keratinocytes express interferon-gamma and interleukin 6 in lichen planus. Arch Dermatol Res. 291(9):485-90, 1999
15. Kirby AC et al: LFA-3 (CD58) mediates T-lymphocyte adhesion in chronic inflammatory infiltrates. Scand J Immunol. 50(5):469-74, 1999

LICHEN PLANUS

Clinical and Microscopic Features

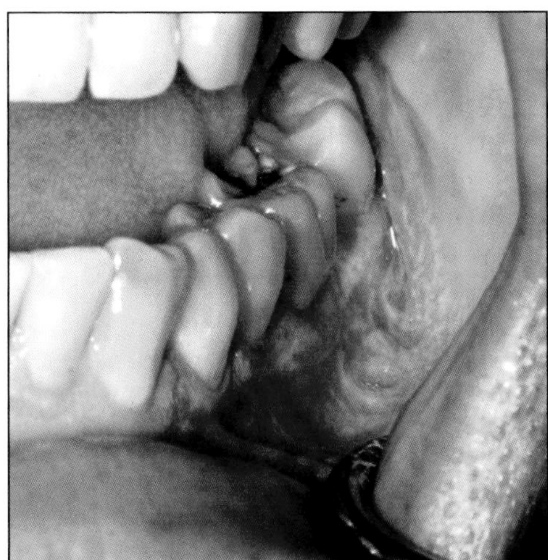

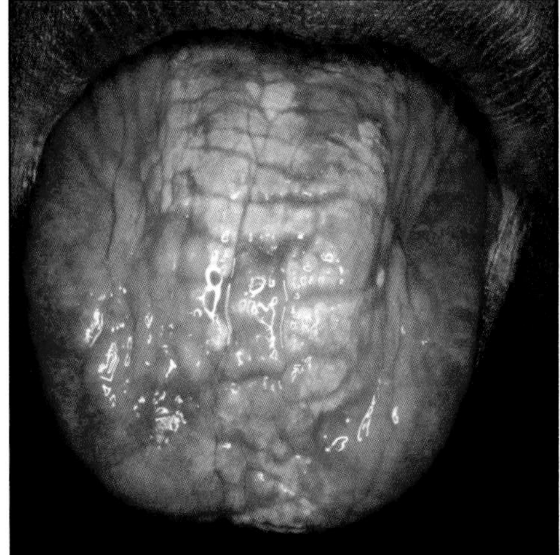

(Left) *Lichen planus of the buccal mucosa extends into the vestibule to involve the gingiva. Along the periphery of the lesion lace-like reticulations are noted. In the center area, focal erythema is noted.* ***(Right)*** *Lichen planus involves the dorsal tongue. In the central area, the lesion has white plaques, typical for this location. However, approaching the lateral borders of the tongue, areas of erythema are observed.*

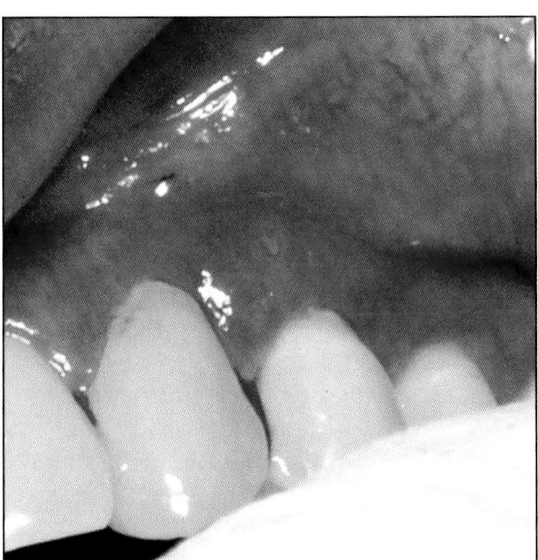

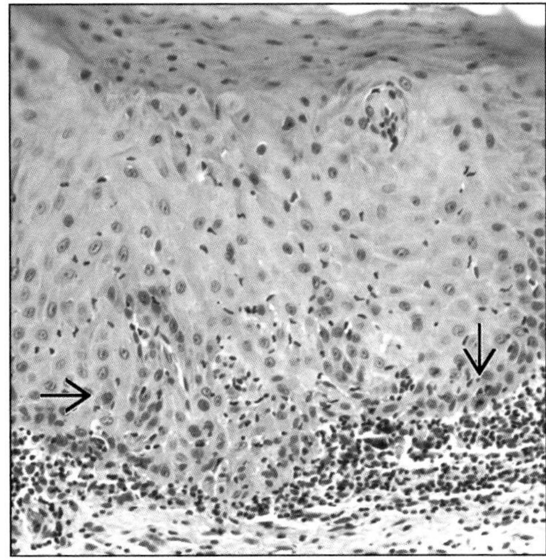

(Left) *Erosive lichen planus presents as desquamative gingivitis. When this is the only clinical finding, it is difficult to distinguish from mucous membrane pemphigoid or pemphigus vulgaris, and biopsy confirmation is required for diagnosis.* ***(Right)*** *High-power photomicrograph shows hydropic degeneration of the basal cells. Civatte or colloid bodies ⇒ are scattered at the epithelium-connective tissue interface. Inflammatory cell exocytosis is noted.*

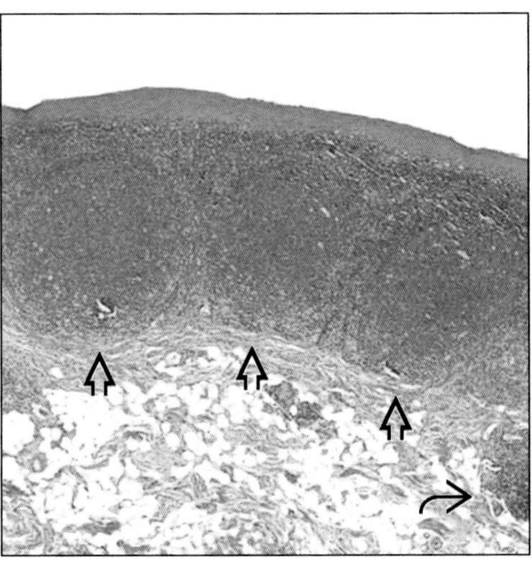

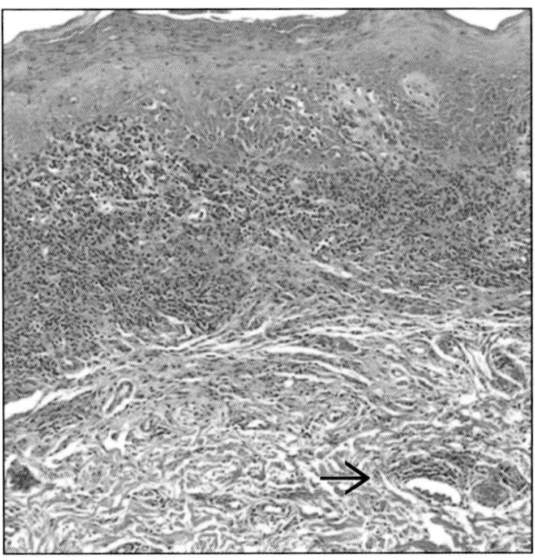

(Left) *The epithelium is atrophic and a dense lymphocytic infiltrate is seen in the lamina propria in this case of lichenoid reaction to dental amalgam. Numerous tertiary lymphoid follicles are present ⇨ as well as perivascular inflammation ↗.* ***(Right)*** *Marked acanthosis and inflammatory cell exocytosis is present in this case of cinnamon stomatitis. The inflammatory infiltrate in the submucosa is more mixed than in LP. Perivascular inflammation is frequently seen ⇒.*

ERYTHEMA MULTIFORME

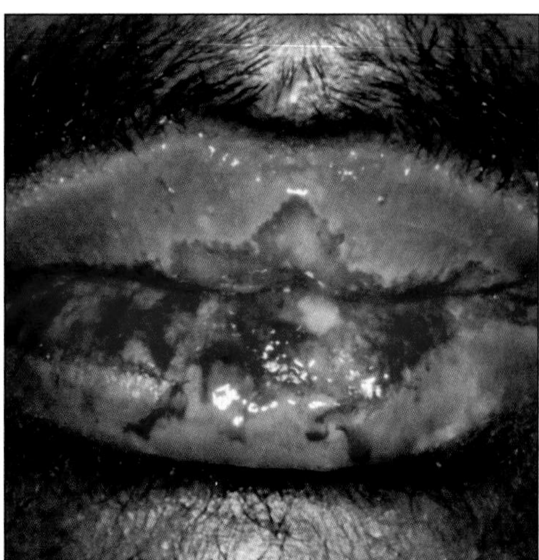

Erythema multiforme involving the lips shows large areas of ulceration and hemorrhage that eventually form characteristic crusts. The lips are the most common site of oral involvement.

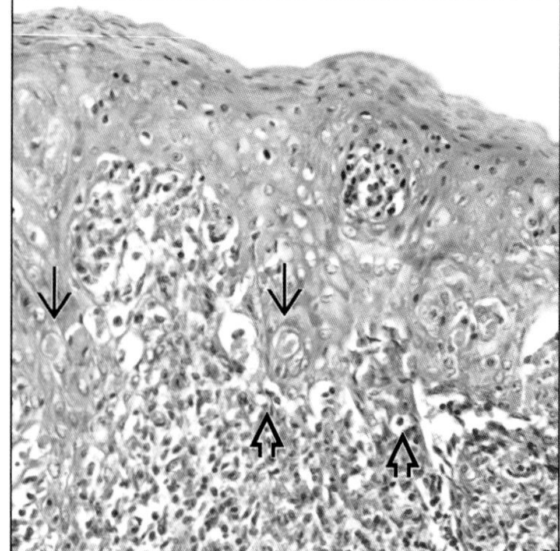

Vacuolar interface change at the stroma-epidermal junction ➡ along with hydropic changes of basal cells with dyskeratosis ➡ are typical of early erythema multiforme. Inflammation may be variable.

TERMINOLOGY

Abbreviations

- Erythema multiforme (EM)

Definitions

- Acute, immune-mediated, self-limiting mucocutaneous inflammatory disease

ETIOLOGY/PATHOGENESIS

Immune Reaction

- Most cases associated with T-cell mediated immune reaction to precipitating agent
  - Herpes simplex virus, *Mycoplasma pneumoniae*, and select drugs associated with triggering EM

CLINICAL ISSUES

Epidemiology

- Incidence
  - Unknown
- Age
  - Peak: 20-40 years
  - 20% of cases reported in children
- Gender
  - Male > Female in most reported series

Site

- EM minor: Primarily associated with target lesions of skin with involvement of no more than 1 mucous membrane (usually oral)
- EM major: Involvement of multiple mucous membranes, target lesions, and, infrequently, skin bulla

Presentation

- EM minor
  - Target or bull's-eye lesions of skin are hallmark of erythema multiforme
    - Begin as dusky-red flat macules or papules with regular round shape < 3 cm
    - Extremities most common site
  - Mucous membrane involvement, when present, is confined to 1 site
  - Oral involvement
    - Lip > buccal mucosa > labial mucosa > tongue > soft palate
    - Begins as erythematous patches that undergo necrosis and ulceration
    - Lip shows characteristic hemorrhagic crusting
- EM major
  - Skin lesions similar to EM minor, but may be raised or have bullae formation
  - Multiple mucous membranes involved
    - Oral, ocular, genital, laryngeal, esophageal

Natural History

- Self-limiting disease ranging from 2-6 weeks
- Subset of patients experience recurrent EM (20%)

Treatment

- Options, risks, complications
  - Offending agent or drug, if known, should be treated &/or stopped
  - Symptomatic treatment with analgesics
- Drugs
  - Herpes-associated EM can be treated with antiviral medication
    - Often used prophylactically in herpes-associated recurrent erythema multiforme
  - Cyclosporine, levamisole, dapsone, and cyclophosphamide used in severe outbreaks
  - Systemic corticosteroid commonly used
    - Lack of evidence substantiating efficacy, making use controversial

Prognosis

- Self-limiting disease

ERYTHEMA MULTIFORME

Key Facts

Terminology
- Acute, immune-mediated, self-limiting mucocutaneous inflammatory disease

Clinical Issues
- EM minor: Skin target lesions with only **1** mucous membrane site affected
- EM major: Skin target lesions with **multiple** mucous membranes affected

Microscopic Pathology
- Early: Upper lamina propria edema and blisters
- Mixed inflammatory cell infiltrate
- Hydropic degeneration of basal cells
- Individually necrotic keratinocytes within epithelium

Top Differential Diagnoses
- Primary herpes stomatitis, pemphigus vulgaris, mucous membrane pemphigoid, Behçet disease

MICROSCOPIC PATHOLOGY

Histologic Features
- Early lesions present with edema in upper lamina propria resulting in blister formation
  - May form both intra- and subepithelial blisters
- Mixed inflammatory cell infiltrate of lymphocytes, neutrophils, and occasionally, eosinophils
  - Perivascular location and in superficial lamina propria
- Inflammatory cell exocytosis with spongiosis and intracellular edema of epithelium
- Hydropic degeneration of basal cells
- Individually necrotic keratinocytes scattered throughout epithelium

ANCILLARY TESTS

Immunofluorescence
- IgM and C3 are found along basement membrane zone and in walls of blood vessels

DIFFERENTIAL DIAGNOSIS

Primary Herpes Stomatitis
- In absence of cutaneous lesions, diagnosis may be difficult
  - Gingiva often involved in primary herpes but not in erythema multiforme

Pemphigus Vulgaris
- Chronic mucocutaneous disease of older patients
- Suprabasilar separation with characteristic acantholytic cells
- Direct immunofluorescence diagnostic

Mucous Membrane Pemphigoid
- Chronic disease of older patients
- Subepithelial separation without neutrophils
- Direct immunofluorescence of IgG(A) along basement membrane

Behçet Disease
- No cutaneous lesions

DIAGNOSTIC CHECKLIST

Pathologic Interpretation Pearls
- Pathology relatively nonspecific and requires clinical correlation

SELECTED REFERENCES

1. Wetter DA et al: Recurrent erythema multiforme: clinical characteristics, etiologic associations, and treatment in a series of 48 patients at Mayo Clinic, 2000 to 2007. J Am Acad Dermatol. 62(1):45-53, 2010
2. Scully C et al: Oral mucosal diseases: erythema multiforme. Br J Oral Maxillofac Surg. 46(2):90-5, 2008
3. Ayangco L et al: Oral manifestations of erythema multiforme. Dermatol Clin. 21(1):195-205, 2003

IMAGE GALLERY

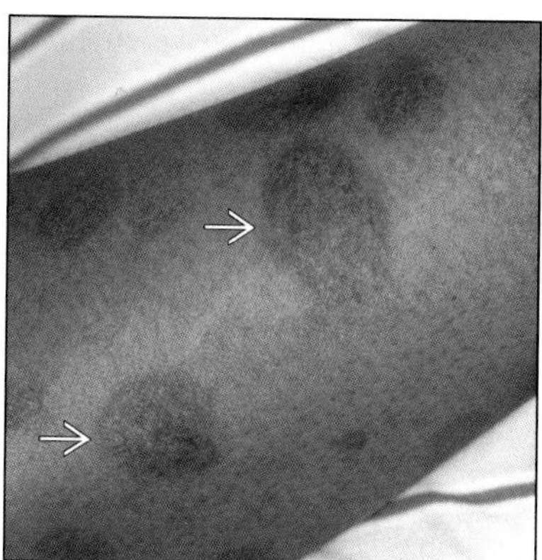
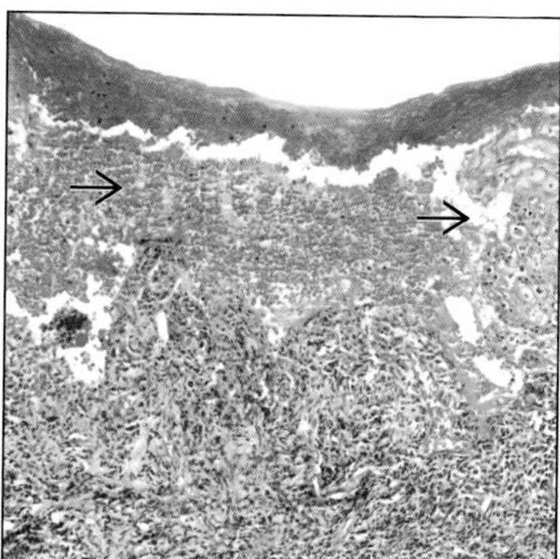
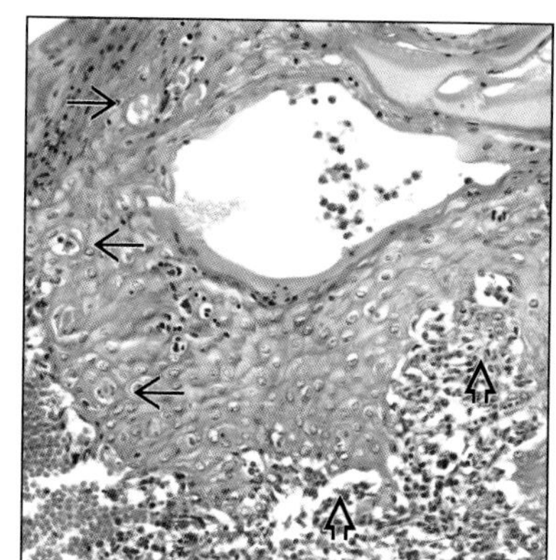

(Left) *Typical target or bull's-eye skin lesions ➡ are the hallmark of erythema multiforme. The extremities are the most common sites and usually have symmetrical involvement.* ***(Center)*** *This older lesion of erythema multiforme displays partial to full thickness necrosis ➡ along with a moderate inflammatory cell infiltrate.* ***(Right)*** *High-power view of erythema multiforme shows basal cell hydropic degeneration ⇨. Numerous scattered necrotic keratinocytes are present ➡.*

LUPUS ERYTHEMATOSUS

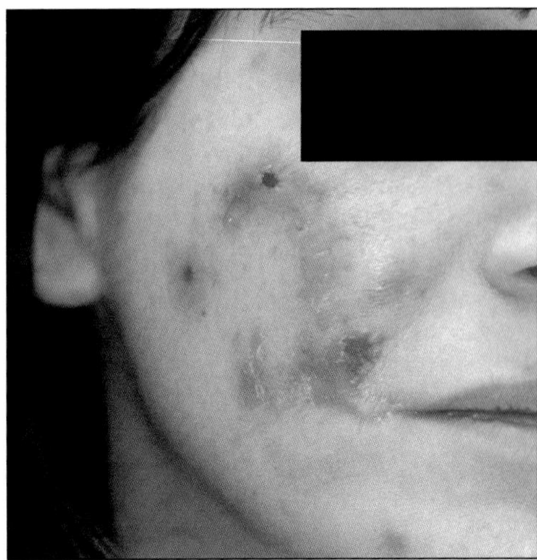

Chronic cutaneous (discoid) lupus occurring on the face is seen. The lesions often spread centrifugally with dilation of the follicle with a keratinous plug. Atrophy and scarring in older lesions is visible.

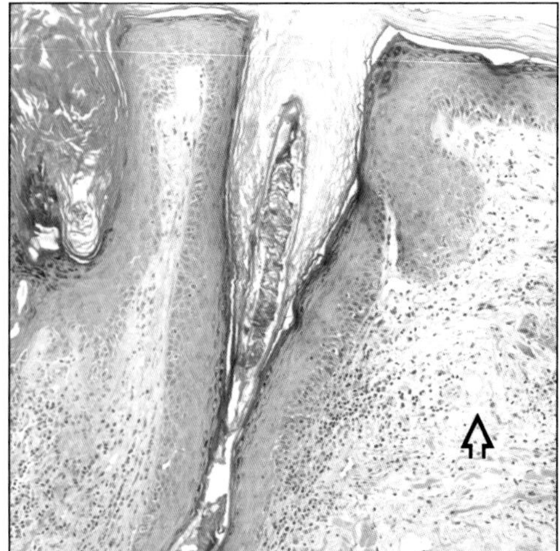

A biopsy of lupus erythematosus of the face with atrophic epidermis and keratotic plugging of the hair follicle shows a periappendiceal chronic inflammatory cell infiltrate in the dermis. Note increased dermal edema ⇨.

TERMINOLOGY

Abbreviations

- Lupus erythematosus (LE)
- Systemic lupus erythematosus (SLE)

Definitions

- Autoimmune disease affecting connective tissues and multiple organs divided into 3 major categories
  - Systemic LE (SLE) involves multiple organs with variety of cutaneous and oral manifestations
  - Chronic cutaneous LE (CCLE) or chronic discoid lupus consists primarily of cutaneous and oral manifestations
  - Subacute cutaneous LE (SCLE) has clinical features of both SLE and CCLE

ETIOLOGY/PATHOGENESIS

Etiology

- Unknown; however, circulating autoantibodies directed against nuclear material (ANA) are hallmark of SLE
- Drug-induced lupus reported
- Ultraviolet light may precipitate or aggravate LE

CLINICAL ISSUES

Epidemiology

- Incidence
  - Prevalence ranges from 15-50 cases per 100,000 population
- Age
  - Range: 15-40 years
  - Mean: 30 years
- Gender
  - Female > > > Male (5-10:1)
- Ethnicity
  - Black > > White (1:250 vs. 1:1,000)

Presentation

- SLE
  - Fatigue, myalgia, and joint pain
    - Common findings affecting up to 95% of patients
  - Mucocutaneous lesions in up to 85% of patients
    - Butterfly rash (malar region and nose bridge) in 40-50% of affected patients
  - Hematologic symptoms present in up to 85% of patients
  - Kidney affected in 30-50% of patients
    - Lupus nephritis and uremia are serious complications
  - Cardiopulmonary symptoms
    - Pericarditis most common complication
  - Neurological symptoms, including seizures and psychosis
  - Raynaud phenomenon
- CCLE
  - Cutaneous lesions are scaly, erythematous patches that heal with scarring and hypo- or hyperpigmentation
    - Mostly affect the face, particularly bridge of nose and malar area
    - Lesions tend to spread centrifugally
    - Follicular plugging and pigmentary changes are noted
  - About 50% of lesions present on hair-bearing areas of scalp or beard
  - Localized variant usually confined to head and neck region
    - Often this is only manifestation of LE
  - Oral lesions clinically resemble erosive lichen planus
    - Rarely present without cutaneous lesions
  - Patients with generalized CCLE involving areas below the neck have higher risk of developing SLE
- SCLE
  - Cutaneous lesions predominately on trunk and arms (80%)

LUPUS ERYTHEMATOSUS

Key Facts

Terminology
- Autoimmune disease affecting connective tissues and multiple organs divided into 3 major categories
  - Systemic LE involves multiple organs with variety of cutaneous and oral manifestations
  - Chronic cutaneous LE or discoid lupus consists primarily of cutaneous and oral manifestations
  - Subacute cutaneous LE overlaps SLE and CCLE

Clinical Issues
- 15-50 cases per 100,000 population
- Female > > > Male (5-10:1)
- Black > > White (1:250 vs. 1:1,000)

Microscopic Pathology
- Histology can vary depending on age of lesion
- Dermal edema with reticular mucin accumulation
- Hyperkeratosis with follicular plugging
- Superficial and deep perivascular and periadnexal infiltrate
- Incontinent melanin pigment in dermis
- Lymphocyte-rich interface dermatitis

Ancillary Tests
- Direct immunofluorescence of lesional tissue in SLE and CCLE show granular or shaggy deposits of IgG, IgM, or C3 at basement membrane zone

Diagnostic Checklist
- Diagnosis based on correlation of clinical findings with serological and pathologic findings
- Microscopic features overlap with many other diseases and are not specific

  - Mild systemic disease, usually arthralgia
  - Renal disease uncommon
  - Lesions on face and scalp occur in 20% of patients
  - Lesions usually heal without scarring
    - Hyper- or hypopigmentations may be seen

Laboratory Tests
- SLE
  - Positive ANA, anti-DNA, or anti-Sm antibodies
  - Proteinuria > 0.5g/24 hour or 3+, nephritic syndrome, cellular casts
  - Hemolytic anemia with reticulocytosis
  - Antiphospholipid antibodies
- CCLE
  - 25-80% of patients have positive ANA depending on sensitivity of test used
- SCLE
  - Most patients have positive ANA

Treatment
- Avoid excessive sunlight exposure since UV light may precipitate disease
- Systemic corticosteroids in combination with immunosuppressive drugs for more severe disease
- Topical steroids effective for both cutaneous and oral lesions
- NSAIDs and antimalarials are effective for mild disease

Prognosis
- Prognosis of SLE depends on disease severity and which organs are involved
  - Renal failure most common cause of death
  - Chronic immunosuppression increases mortality due to infection and risk of malignancy

MICROSCOPIC PATHOLOGY

Histologic Features
- SLE
  - Pauci-inflammatory cell interface dermatitis
  - Dermal edema with reticular mucin accumulation
  - Normal basement membrane zone
- CCLE
  - Hyperkeratosis with follicular plugging
  - Basement membrane thickening with PAS(+) material
  - Subepithelial edema
  - Lymphocyte rich interface dermatitis
  - Superficial and deep perivascular and periadnexal infiltrate
  - Dermal fibrosis
  - Incontinent melanin pigment in dermis
  - Histology can vary depending on age of lesion
- SCLE
  - Suprabasilar exocytosis of inflammatory cells
  - Mild to moderate inflammation in superficial dermis

ANCILLARY TESTS

Immunofluorescence
- Direct immunofluorescence (DIF) of lesional tissue in SLE and CCLE shows granular or shaggy deposits of IgG, IgM, or C3 at basement membrane zone
- Lupus band test (DIF) of normal uninvolved tissue is usually positive in SLE but not in CCLE
  - Not specific to SLE and can be seen in Sjögren syndrome, rheumatoid arthritis, and systemic sclerosis

DIFFERENTIAL DIAGNOSIS

Oral Lichen Planus
- Can see similar pathology to LE and requires clinical and laboratory correlation
- Subepithelial edema lacking
- No PAS(+) material in basement membrane zone
- DIF useful in differentiating these lesions

Drug Reaction
- Usually do not see dermal mucinosis, which is highlighted by Alcian blue-PAS staining
- Eosinophils, which are uncommon in LE, are usually seen

LUPUS ERYTHEMATOSUS

American College of Rheumatology Classification of Systemic Lupus Erythematosus (1997 Revised Criteria)

Site of Involvement	Findings
Mucocutaneous lesions	Malar rash
	Discoid rash
	Photosensitivity
	Oral or nasopharyngeal ulcers
Nonerosive arthritis	Involving 2 or more joints with swelling and tenderness
Cardiopulmonary disease	Pleuritis or pleural effusion
	OR
	Pericarditis
Renal disease	Proteinuria > 0.5 grams/day OR > 3+ if quantitation not performed
	OR
	Cellular casts
Neurologic disorders	Seizures in absence of offending drugs or metabolic disturbance
	OR
	Psychosis in absence of offending drugs or metabolic disturbance
Hematologic disorders	Hemolytic anemia
	OR
	Leukopenia < 4,000/mm³ on ≥ 2 occasions
	OR
	Lymphopenia < 1,500/mm on ≥ 2 occasions
	OR
	Thrombocytopenia < 100,000/mm³ in absence of offending drugs
Immunologic disorders	Anti-DNA antibody in abnormal titer
	OR
	Anti-Sm antibody to Sm nuclear antigen
	OR
	Positive antiphospholipid antibodies on
	Abnormal IgG or IgM anticardiolipin antibodies
	Positive lupus anticoagulant test
	OR
	False-positive test confirmed by *Treponema pallidum* immobilization or antibody
	Absorption test for at least 6 months
Positive antinuclear antibody	Abnormal titer of ANA by immunofluorescence or equivalent assay

The diagnosis of SLE is considered when 4 or more of the listed criteria are fulfilled.

DIAGNOSTIC CHECKLIST

Clinically Relevant Pathologic Features

- Diagnosis based on correlation of clinical findings with serological and pathologic findings

Pathologic Interpretation Pearls

- Microscopic features overlap with many other diseases and are not specific

SELECTED REFERENCES

1. Knott HM et al: Innovative management of lupus erythematosus. Dermatol Clin. 28(3):489-99, 2010
2. Pincus LB et al: Marked papillary dermal edema--an unreliable discriminator between polymorphous light eruption and lupus erythematosus or dermatomyositis. J Cutan Pathol. 37(4):416-25, 2010
3. Muñoz-Corcuera M et al: Oral ulcers: clinical aspects. A tool for dermatologists. Part II. Chronic ulcers. Clin Exp Dermatol. 34(4):456-61, 2009
4. Walling HW et al: Cutaneous lupus erythematosus: issues in diagnosis and treatment. Am J Clin Dermatol. 10(6):365-81, 2009
5. Nico MM et al: Oral lesions in lupus erythematosus: correlation with cutaneous lesions. Eur J Dermatol. 18(4):376-81, 2008
6. Brennan MT et al: Oral manifestations of patients with lupus erythematosus. Dent Clin North Am. 49(1):127-41, ix, 2005
7. Tebbe B: Clinical course and prognosis of cutaneous lupus erythematosus. Clin Dermatol. 22(2):121-4, 2004
8. Position paper: oral features of mucocutaneous disorders. J Periodontol. 74(10):1545-56, 2003
9. Crowson AN et al: The cutaneous pathology of lupus erythematosus: a review. J Cutan Pathol. 28(1):1-23, 2001

Clinical, Microscopic, and Immunofluorescence Features

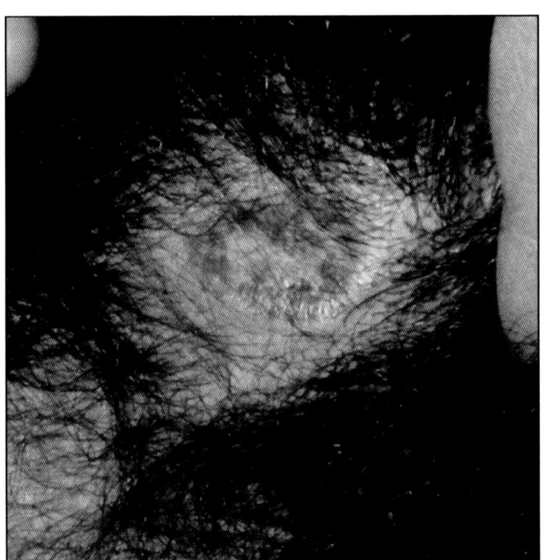

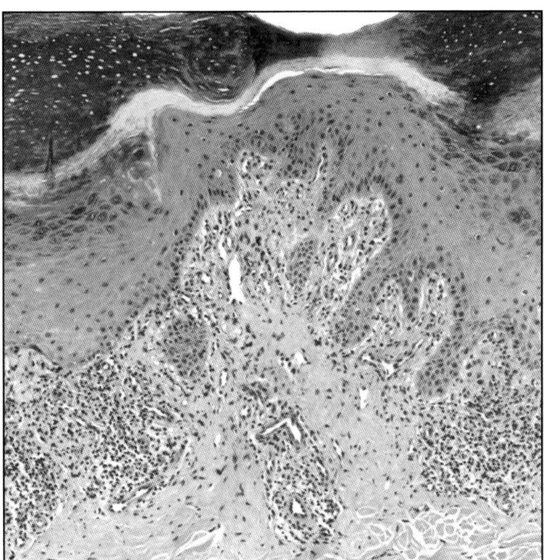

(Left) *Cicatricial scarring alopecia in a patient with chronic cutaneous discoid lupus with both hyper- and hypopigmentation shows fibrotic scarring and a depressed central atrophic area.* ***(Right)*** *Low-power image of hypertrophic chronic cutaneous (discoid) lupus erythematosus is shown. A patchy inflammatory cell infiltrate is seen with a superficial and deep perivascular pattern composed of lymphocytes and plasma cells. The band-like lymphocytic infiltrate of lichen planus is not seen.*

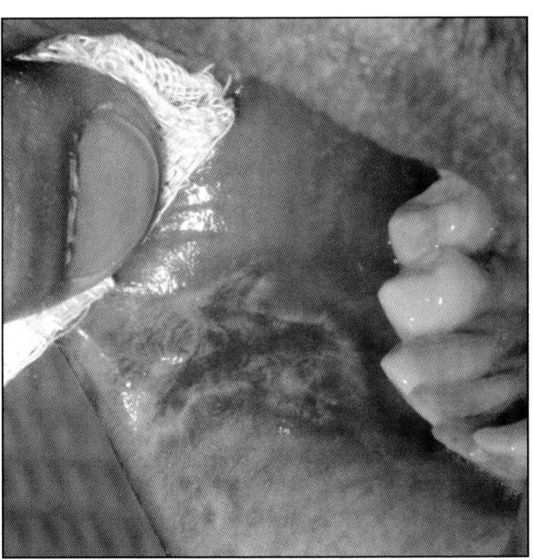

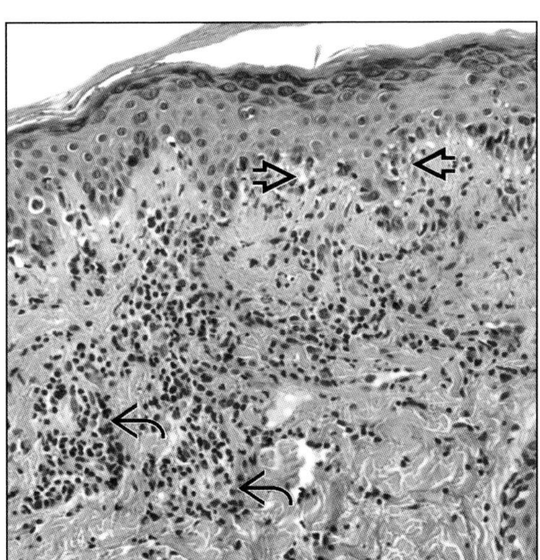

(Left) *Intraoral systemic lupus erythematosus (SLE) presents as a central erosive area surrounded by radiating keratotic striae mimicking lichen planus. SLE can also have a nonspecific presentation.* ***(Right)*** *Biopsy specimen of an oral lesion in a patient with systemic lupus erythematosus demonstrates vacuolar degeneration of the basal cells ⇨ as well as melanin pigment in basal cells. There is deeper lamina propria perivascular inflammation ↷.*

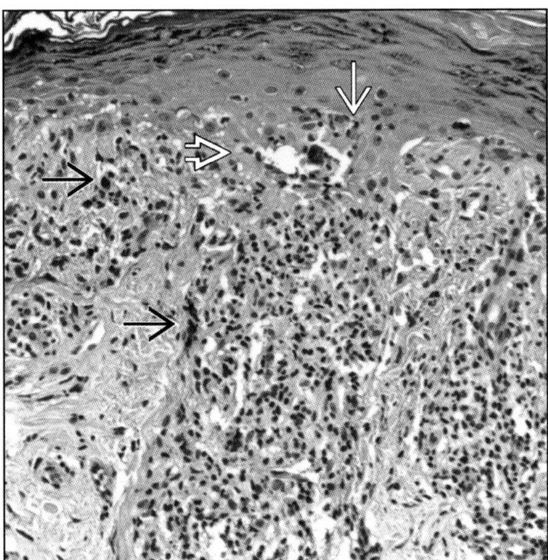

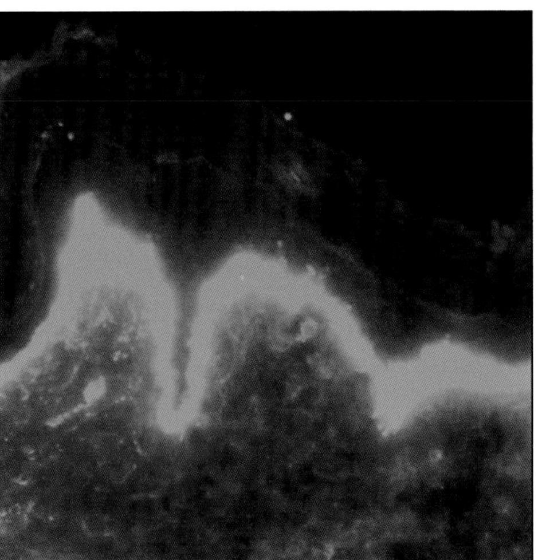

(Left) *High-power photomicrograph of lupus erythematosus shows prominent interface dermatitis with vacuolar change ➡ and a superficial and deep perivascular infiltrate. Degenerating keratinocytes ➡ and suprabasilar exocytosis are present. Older lesions often show pigment incontinence in the dermis →.* ***(Right)*** *Direct immunofluorescence of lesional tissue in lupus erythematosus shows a shaggy deposition of IgM at the basement membrane zone.*

TRAUMATIC ULCER

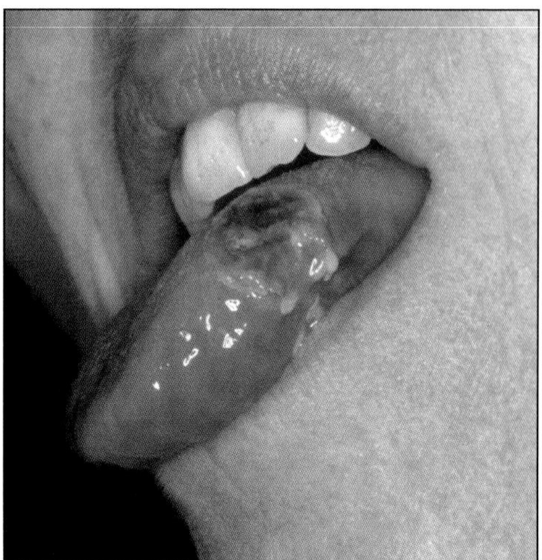

Clinical photograph shows a traumatic ulcer of the lateral tongue. The patient bit the tongue while anesthetized for dental treatment.

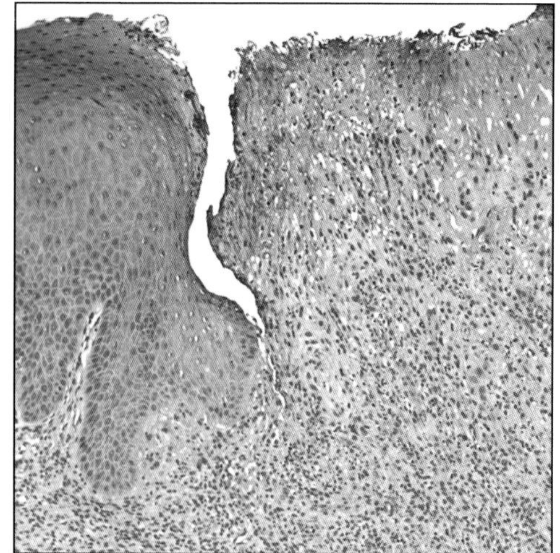

Higher power photomicrograph shows the thickened fibrino-purulent covering and granulation tissue composed of a mixed inflammatory cell infiltrate.

TERMINOLOGY

Synonyms

- Traumatic ulcer with stromal eosinophilia
- Eosinophilic granuloma of tongue
- Traumatic granuloma
- Atypical histiocytic granuloma
- Riga-Fede disease

Definitions

- Chronic traumatic ulceration of oral mucosa with unique histopathologic features

ETIOLOGY/PATHOGENESIS

Mechanical Damage

- Accidental trauma from biting
- Fractured or malposed teeth
- Sharp foodstuffs

Self-inflicted Wound

- Parafunctional habits
  - Nocturnal clenching
  - Tongue and lip biting
- Riga-Fede disease
  - Ulceration of ventral tongue caused by tongue thrusting
  - Occurs in infants with natal or neonatal teeth
- Electrical and thermal injury
  - Electrical cords
  - Hot foods and beverages
- Factitial injury
  - Lesch-Nyhan syndrome
  - Tourette syndrome
  - Obsessive compulsive disorder

CLINICAL ISSUES

Epidemiology

- Incidence
  - True incidence unknown as is under reported
  - Less common than recurrent aphthous stomatitis
- Age
  - Newborns and infants
    - Riga-Fede disease
  - Children
    - Thermal and electrical burns
    - Parafunctional habits
  - Adults
    - Fractured &/or malposed teeth
    - Parafunctional habits
- Gender
  - Male > Female

Site

- Can occur anywhere in oral cavity
- Lateral borders of tongue most common

Presentation

- Painful ulcer from 1 mm to > 1 cm
- Ulcer covered by fibrinopurulent membrane
- Usually see zone of hyperkeratosis surrounding ulcer
- Induration mimicking squamous cell carcinoma

Treatment

- Surgical approaches
  - Ulcers that do not resolve may need total excision
  - Biopsy of ulcer can initiate complete resolution
- Adjuvant therapy
  - Intralesional steroid injections

Prognosis

- Recurrence is common
- Source of trauma must be removed if possible

TRAUMATIC ULCER

Key Facts

Terminology
- Chronic traumatic ulceration of oral mucosa with unique histopathologic features

Etiology/Pathogenesis
- Accidental trauma from biting or fractured teeth
- Riga-Fede disease

Clinical Issues
- Can occur anywhere in oral cavity

Microscopic Pathology
- Ulcer bed composed of granulation tissue with mixed chronic inflammatory cell infiltrate lymphocytes, histiocytes, neutrophils, and occasionally plasma cells
- Inflammation including scattered eosinophils extends into underlying muscle

Top Differential Diagnoses
- Recurrent aphthous stomatitis

MICROSCOPIC PATHOLOGY

Histologic Features
- Ulcer covered by thickened fibrinopurulent membrane
- Pseudoepitheliomatous hyperplasia of adjacent epithelium can be seen
- Ulcer bed composed of granulation tissue with mixed chronic inflammatory cell infiltrate lymphocytes, histiocytes, neutrophils, and occasionally plasma cells
- Inflammation including scattered eosinophils extends into underlying muscle
- In subset of traumatic ulcers, atypical histiocytic cells are noted
  - Cells are pleomorphic and mitotic figures can be seen
  - Cells are CD30(+) and monoclonal rearrangement has been reported
  - Lymphocytes and eosinophils are admixed with atypical cells
  - Significance of these findings is uncertain
- Necrosis is a feature of traumatic ulcerations caused by thermal or electrical injury

DIFFERENTIAL DIAGNOSIS

Recurrent Aphthous Stomatitis
- Ulcer superficial and does not extend to muscle

Cutaneous CD30(+) T-cell Lymphoma
- Considered only in subset of cases with atypical histiocytes

SELECTED REFERENCES

1. Segura S et al: Eosinophilic ulcer of the oral mucosa: a distinct entity or a non-specific reactive pattern? Oral Dis. 14(4):287-95, 2008
2. Pilolli GP et al: Traumatic ulcerative granuloma with stromal eosinophilia of the oral mucosa: histological and immunohistochemical analysis of three cases. Minerva Stomatol. 56(1-2):73-9, 2007
3. Baroni A et al: Lingual traumatic ulceration (Riga-Fede disease). Int J Dermatol. 45(9):1096-7, 2006
4. Hirshberg A et al: Traumatic ulcerative granuloma with stromal eosinophilia: a reactive lesion of the oral mucosa. Am J Clin Pathol. 126(4):522-9, 2006
5. Segura S et al: Eosinophilic ulcer of the oral mucosa: another histological simulator of CD30+ lymphoproliferative disorders. Br J Dermatol. 155(2):460-3, 2006
6. Alobeid B et al: Eosinophil-rich CD30+ lymphoproliferative disorder of the oral mucosa. A form of "traumatic eosinophilic granuloma". Am J Clin Pathol. 121(1):43-50, 2004
7. Ficarra G et al: Traumatic eosinophilic granuloma of the oral mucosa: a CD30+(Ki-1) lymphoproliferative disorder? Oral Oncol. 33(5):375-9, 1997
8. el-Mofty SK et al: Eosinophilic ulcer of the oral mucosa. Report of 38 new cases with immunohistochemical observations. Oral Surg Oral Med Oral Pathol. 75(6):716-22, 1993

IMAGE GALLERY

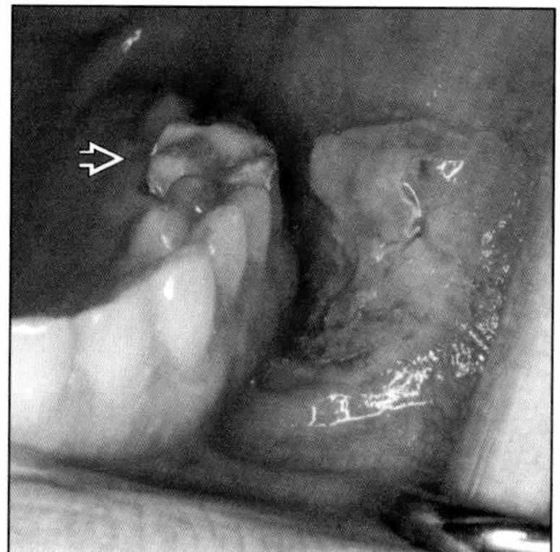

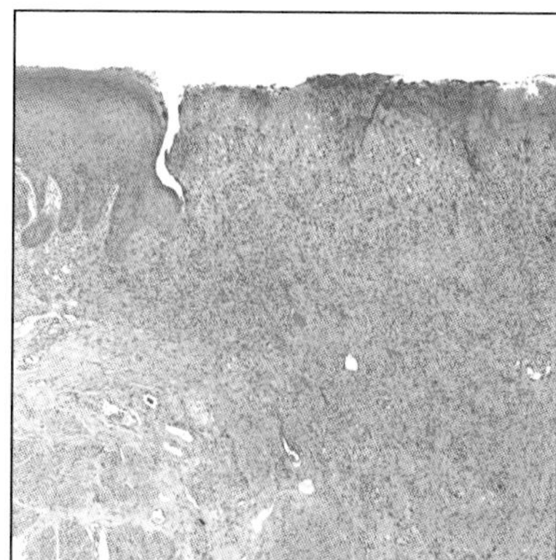

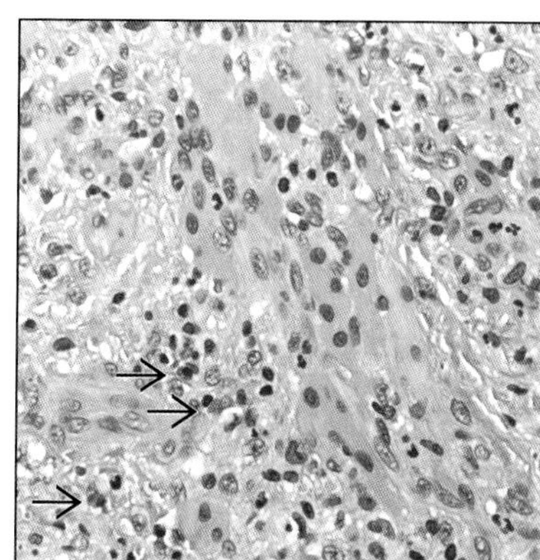

*(**Left**) Clinical photograph of a traumatic ulcer after dental treatment shows the tooth, which received treatment ➨. (**Center**) Hematoxylin and eosin shows traumatic ulcer of the lateral tongue. On low power, the inflammatory cell infiltrate is notable for the deep extension into the muscle. (**Right**) High-power photomicrograph demonstrates the mixed inflammatory cell infiltrate ➔. Numerous eosinophils are noted scattered throughout the striated muscle.*

FRICTIONAL HYPERKERATOSIS

Key Facts

Etiology/Pathogenesis

- Cheek, tongue, or lip biting
  - Morsicatio buccarum, morsicatio linguarum
- Toothbrush abrasion: Mostly seen on gingiva
- Ill-fitting dentures or malposed teeth

Clinical Issues

- **Presentation**
  - Most common presentation is **linea alba:** Single white line on buccal mucosa approximating occlusal (bite) plane
  - Thickened white areas of cheeks, tongue, or lips
  - Often affects > 1 site
  - Surface can have irregular or shredded appearance
  - Occasionally may see erythema or petechiae
- **Prognosis**
  - Reactive lesion with no malignant potential

Microscopic Pathology

- Acanthotic stratified squamous epithelium with marked para/orthokeratosis
- Orthokeratosis in gingiva and alveolar mucosa and biopsies of linea alba
- Keratin surface may be smooth
- Shaggy keratin associated with biting habit
- Bacterial colonies often seen on surface
- No atypia should be seen
- Variable amounts of chronic inflammation in superficial lamina propria

Top Differential Diagnoses

- **Oral hairy leukoplakia**
  - HIV-associated disease positive for EBER
- **Smokeless tobacco keratosis**
  - Vestibule is most frequent location
- **Cinnamon stomatitis**
  - Increased number of inflammatory cells, including eosinophils with exocytosis
- **Oral leukoplakia**
  - Clinical term for lesions that cannot be attributed to other diseases
  - Can see dysplasia

*(**Left**) Frictional hyperkeratosis of right lateral tongue is seen in a patient with chronic tongue biting habit. (**Right**) Note frictional hyperkeratosis of the buccal mucosa from cheek biting, usually seen along occlusal plane. This is termed linea alba when only a single, well-defined area of keratosis is seen along the occlusal plane. At times, lower labial mucosa is also involved & can be contiguous with buccal mucosa. Other common sites of frictional keratosis include attached gingiva from toothbrush abrasion & edentulous alveolus.*

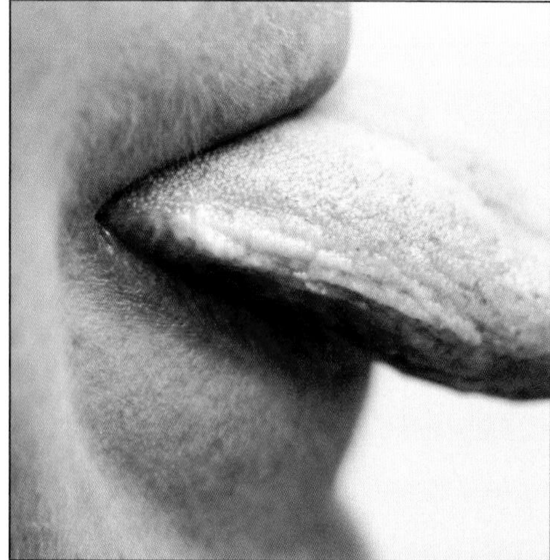

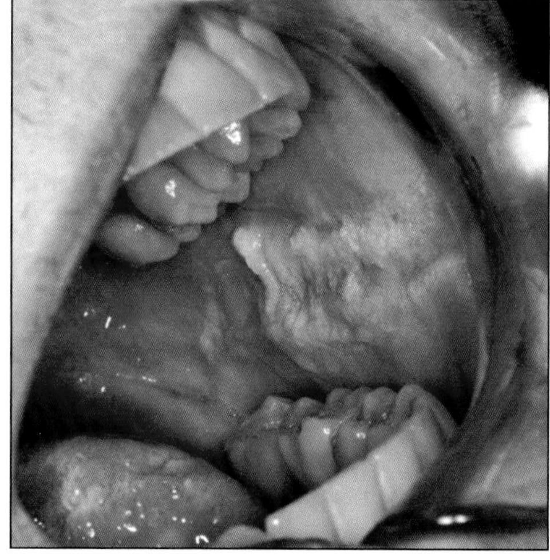

*(**Left**) Low-power microscopic image of oral frictional hyperkeratosis from the lateral border of the tongue composed of acanthotic stratified squamous epithelium exhibits marked parakeratosis. No atypia should be seen. (**Right**) High-power view of oral frictional keratosis shows a prominent granular cell layer. The superficial keratin has a shredded appearance along with a large number of bacteria colonies embedded within the surface keratin. Inflammation may or may not be present in examined specimens.*

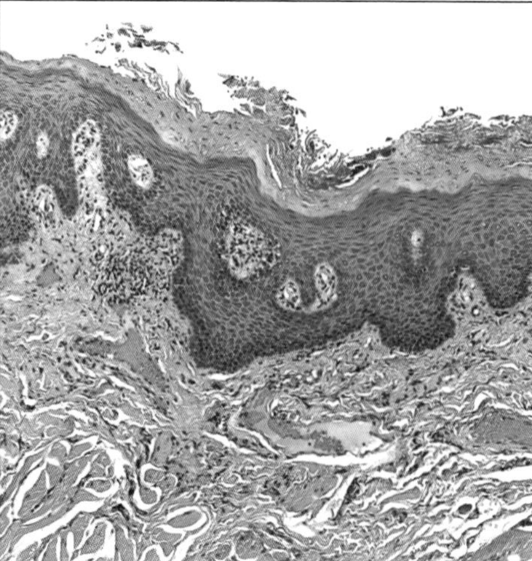

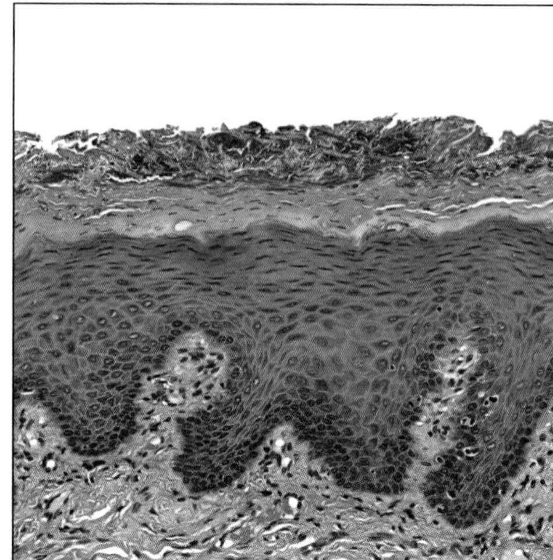

PSEUDOEPITHELIOMATOUS HYPERPLASIA

Key Facts

Terminology

- Reactive epithelial hyperplasia with extension of rete into deep lamina propria mimicking invasive squamous cell carcinoma
- **Abbreviations**
  - Pseudoepitheliomatous hyperplasia (PEH)
- **Synonyms**
  - Pseudocarcinomatous hyperplasia

Etiology/Pathogenesis

- **Lesions associated with PEH**
  - Granular cell tumor (GCT)
  - Hyperplastic candidiasis
  - Inflammatory papillary hyperplasia
  - Median rhomboid glossitis
  - Mucosal ulcers
  - Necrotizing sialometaplasia

Microscopic Pathology

- Marked epithelial hyperplasia
- Rete can extend deeply into lamina propria
  - Anastomoses of tongue-like projections
- Keratin pearl formation can occur
- No or very little cytologic atypia
- Mitotic figures may be present
  - Never atypical
- Neutrophilic microabscesses in keratin may be seen in candidiasis-associated PEH
- Infectious and ulcerative PEH will have inflammation

Top Differential Diagnoses

- **Well-differentiated squamous cell carcinoma**
  - Cytologic atypia is generally present
  - Nuclear pleomorphism and mitoses
- **GCT** often occurs on dorsal tongue, a rare site for oral cancer
- **Candidiasis**: Cellular atypia in PEH should be reevaluated clinically after antifungal treatment
- **Necrotizing sialometaplasia**
  - Superficial biopsies may only demonstrate metaplastic ducts of minor salivary glands
  - No cytologic atypia

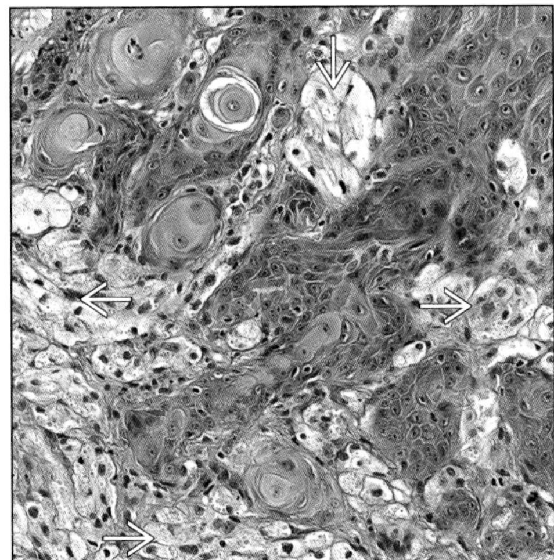

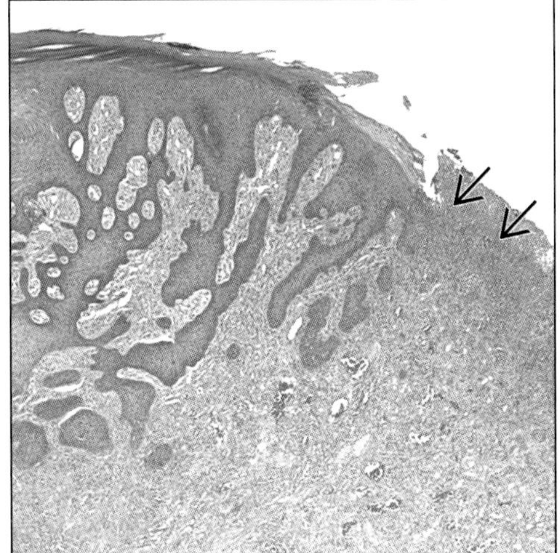

(Left) *GCT ➡ with florid pseudoepitheliomatous hyperplasia. Despite marked individual cell keratinization, no mitoses or cytologic atypia is present. Tongue-like projections show anastomoses mimicking carcinoma.* ***(Right)*** *Oral mucosal ulcer ➡ with adjacent pseudoepitheliomatous hyperplasia. This microscopic feature can be seen in a variety of ulcers, including aphthous ulcers, traumatic ulcers, herpetic ulcers, and nonhealing extraction sockets.*

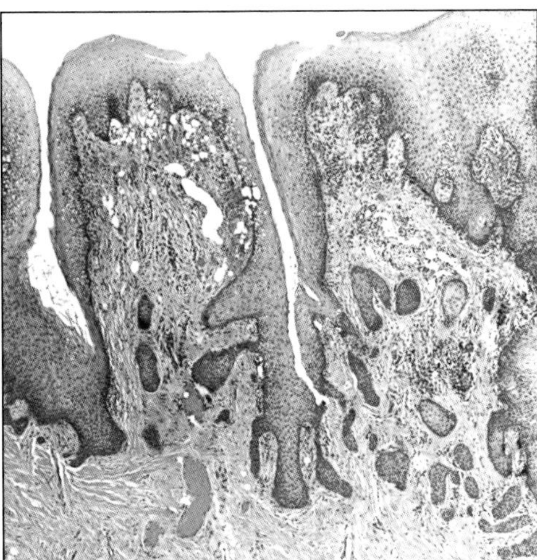

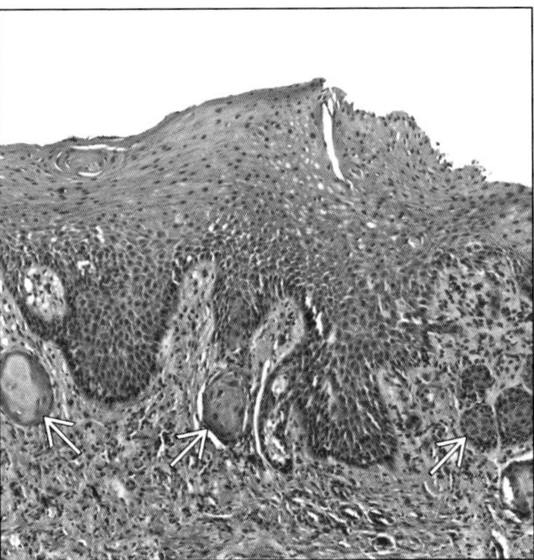

(Left) *Biopsy of the hard palate in a patient with ill-fitting dentures shows inflammatory hyperplasia exhibiting PEH. Periodic acid-Schiff staining will demonstrate spores and hyphae in the superficial keratin.* ***(Right)*** *Superficial biopsy of a non-healing ulcer on the hard palate shows necrotizing sialometaplasia. The metaplastic ducts ➡ can be mistaken for a superficial squamous cell carcinoma. This entity usually occurs on the hard palate, an unusual location for oral cancer.*

NECROTIZING SIALOMETAPLASIA

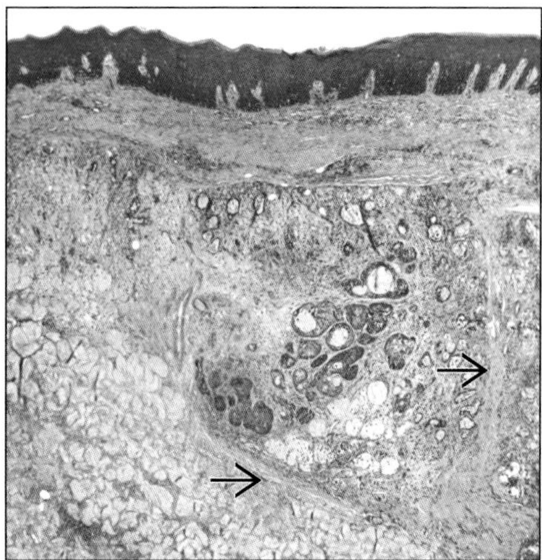

H&E shows necrotizing sialometaplasia associated with residual fibrous bands ⇒, which preserve the lobular architecture. Acinar coagulative necrosis and squamous epithelial nests are seen.

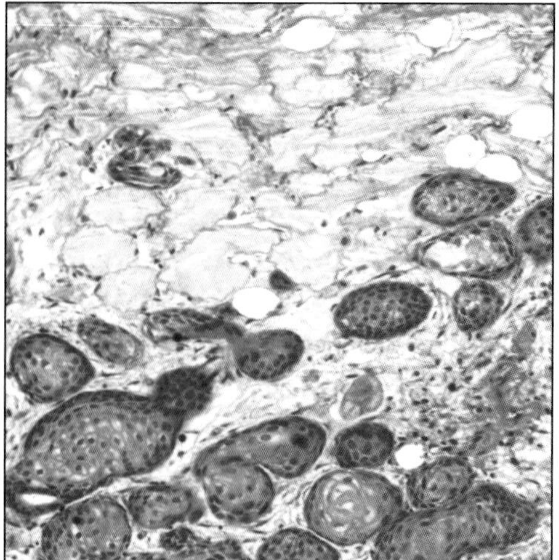

Outlines of necrotic salivary acini are present (center) along with ovoid nests of squamous epithelium. The generalized "lobular" architecture is preserved.

TERMINOLOGY

Abbreviations

- Necrotizing sialometaplasia (NSM)

Synonyms

- Adenometaplasia

Definitions

- Reactive, self-healing inflammatory condition of salivary glands leading to coagulative necrosis of salivary acini and squamous metaplasia of ductal structures

ETIOLOGY/PATHOGENESIS

Reactive/Inflammatory Condition

- Etiology is speculative
- Likely due to vascular compromise leading to ischemic necrosis
  - Commonly associated with trauma due to dental treatment, surgery, or other iatrogenic events
    - Ill-fitting dentures, upper respiratory tract infections, and adjacent neoplasms or cysts have also been implicated
  - Often, patient cannot recall inciting event

CLINICAL ISSUES

Epidemiology

- Age
  - Mean: 5th decade
  - Wide age range: 1st to 9th decades
- Gender
  - Male > Female

Site

- Majority of lesions affect minor salivary glands of oral cavity
  - Hard & soft palate most commonly affected (~ 75%)
    - Typically unilateral
    - Occasional bilateral or midline presentation
  - Lower lip, tongue, retromolar pad, and buccal mucosa occasionally affected
  - Upper aerodigestive tract sites may uncommonly be affected
    - Sinonasal tract and larynx
- < 10% of lesions involve major salivary glands

Presentation

- Initially presents as swelling of affected area
  - Swelling eventually replaced by crater-like ulcer
    - Rarely affects underlying palatal bone
  - May be associated with numbness or pain

Treatment

- No treatment required after diagnosis as lesions are self healing
  - Slowly heals in 3-12 weeks (average: 5-6 weeks)
  - Surgical debridement and sterile saline rinses may assist in healing

MACROSCOPIC FEATURES

General Features

- Crater-like ulcer

Size

- Usually 1-5 cm

MICROSCOPIC PATHOLOGY

Histologic Features

- Acinar coagulative necrosis and squamous metaplasia of salivary gland ducts
- Despite necrosis, **lobular architecture** of gland is maintained

NECROTIZING SIALOMETAPLASIA

Key Facts

Terminology

- Reactive inflammatory condition of salivary glands leading to coagulative necrosis of salivary acini and squamous metaplasia of ductal structures

Clinical Issues

- Majority of lesions affect minor salivary glands, especially of hard palate or junction of hard and soft palates

Microscopic Pathology

- Histologic picture is of acinar coagulative necrosis and squamous metaplasia of salivary gland ducts
- Variably dense subacute inflammatory infiltrate will be present in surrounding tissues &/or encompassing mucin pools
- Pseudoepitheliomatous hyperplasia of overlying squamous mucosal epithelium may be evident
  - May simulate malignancy

  - General outlines of necrotic salivary acini are present
- Squamous metaplasia of ductal structures presents as smooth, rounded nests of squamous epithelium
  - Residual ductal lumina and possible mucocytes may be present
    - May display mild ductal ectasia and small cyst-like formation
  - Dysplastic changes, such as pleomorphism, nuclear hyperchromasia, and abnormal mitotic figures, are rare to absent
- Variably dense, subacute inflammatory infiltrate may be present in surrounding tissues &/or encompassing mucin pools
- Pseudoepitheliomatous hyperplasia (PEH) of overlying squamous mucosal epithelium may be evident
  - PEH sometimes appears to merge with ductal squamous metaplasia, suggesting malignancy

DIFFERENTIAL DIAGNOSIS

Squamous Cell Carcinoma (SCC)

- PEH and nests of squamous epithelium in connective tissues may mimic SCC
  - Especially important when poorly oriented or inadequate biopsy
- Features favoring NSM vs. SCC
  - Maintained lobular salivary gland architecture
  - Presence of acinar coagulative necrosis
  - Round to ovoid nests of metaplastic squamous cells with smooth borders, lacking cytologic atypia
    - May show residual ductal lumina

Mucoepidermoid Carcinoma (MEC)

- Mucin pools and squamous epithelium may suggest MEC
- Features of NSM that may help distinguish from MEC
  - Maintained lobular salivary gland architecture
  - No invasion and minimal cyst formation
  - No intermediate or clear cell proliferations
  - Formation of true squamous islands
    - MEC tends to show epidermoid cells rather than true squamous cells

SELECTED REFERENCES

1. Carlson DL: Necrotizing sialometaplasia: a practical approach to the diagnosis. Arch Pathol Lab Med. 133(5):692-8, 2009
2. Komínek P et al: Necrotizing sialometaplasia: a potential diagnostic pitfall. Ear Nose Throat J. 85(9):604-5, 2006
3. Penner CR et al: Necrotizing sialometaplasia. Ear Nose Throat J. 82(7):493-4, 2003
4. Sandmeier D et al: Necrotizing sialometaplasia: a potential diagnostic pitfall. Histopathology. 40(2):200-1, 2002
5. Brannon RB et al: Necrotizing sialometaplasia. A clinicopathologic study of sixty-nine cases and review of the literature. Oral Surg Oral Med Oral Pathol. 72(3):317-25, 1991
6. Abrams AM et al: Necrotizing sialometaplasia. A disease simulating malignancy. Cancer. 32(1):130-5, 1973

IMAGE GALLERY

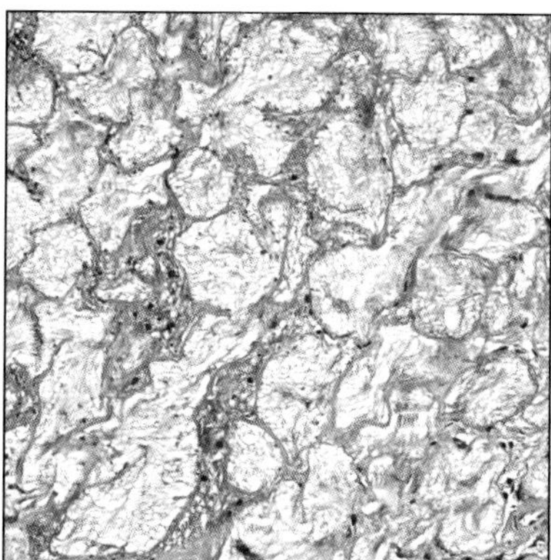

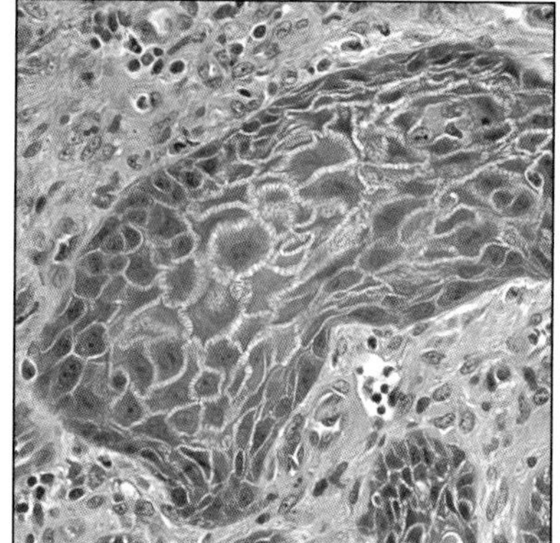

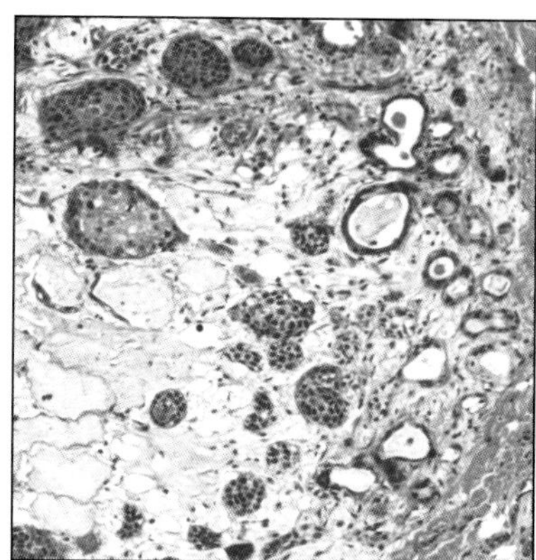

(Left) *Necrotizing sialometaplasia shows multiple necrotic mucinous acini. Note the loss of nuclei and cell borders, yet maintenance of the overall acinar architectural pattern.* ***(Center)*** *High-power view shows a metaplastic salivary duct. Note the squamous-type epithelium to include a well-defined basal cell layer and larger spinous layer cells.* ***(Right)*** *Cystic dilation of salivary ductal structures may be present, along with solid epithelial nests. Residual glands are noted.*

LYMPHANGIOMATOUS POLYP

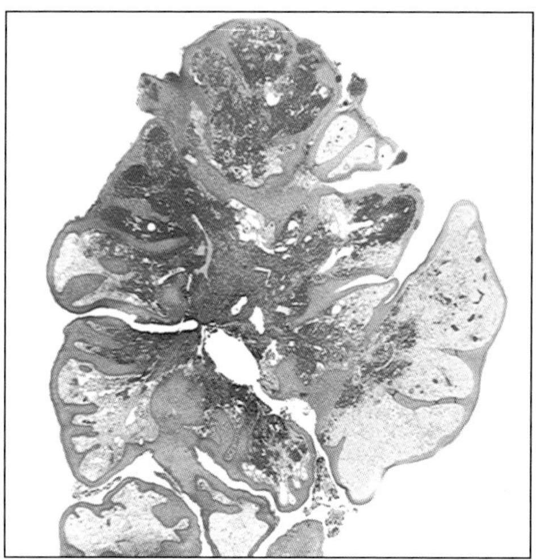

A low-power view demonstrates a polypoid structure with intact surface squamous epithelium. There are numerous vessels in the stroma, many associated with lymphocytes.

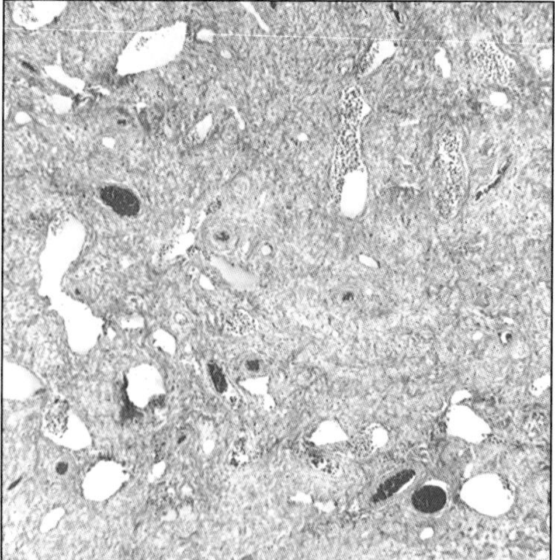

The stroma of a lymphangiomatous polyp can be quite fibrotic or sclerotic. Dilated vessels and lymphocytes are easily noted, although the density varies for each of these components.

TERMINOLOGY

Abbreviations

- Lymphangiomatous polyp (LAP)

Synonyms

- Lymphangiectatic fibrous polyp
- Fibrovascular polyp
- Polypoid lymphangioma
- Papillary lymphoid polyp
- Lymphoid papillary hyperplasia
- Angioma
- Angiofibroma
- Fibroangioma
- Fibrolipoma

Definitions

- Lymphangioma arising from palatine tonsil

ETIOLOGY/PATHOGENESIS

Developmental Anomaly

- Stroma is more abundant than vessels
- Probably hamartoma rather than neoplasm
  - Haphazard proliferation of elements normally present in tonsil

CLINICAL ISSUES

Epidemiology

- Incidence
  - Rare (about 2% of all tonsillar tumors)
  - > 90% of lymphangiomas develop in skin and subcutaneous tissues of head and neck
- Age
  - Mean: 25 years
  - Range: 3-50 years
- Gender
  - Equal gender distribution

Site

- Palatine tonsil

Presentation

- Dysphagia
- Sore throat
- Sensation of mass in throat (globus)
- Obstructive symptoms (size dependent)
- Lesions are frequently present for years

Treatment

- Surgical approaches
  - Simple excision

Prognosis

- Mass may cause "ball-valve" effect if not removed

MACROSCOPIC FEATURES

General Features

- Unilateral polyp

Size

- Mean: 1.6 cm
- Range: Up to 8 cm

MICROSCOPIC PATHOLOGY

Histologic Features

- Polypoid or papillary projections
- Prominent, dilated vascular channels
  - Usually not as prominent as typical lymphangioma
- Intact surface with hyperplasia
  - Lymphocytic epitheliotropism focally
- Vascular proteinaceous fluid with lymphocytes
- Variable stroma
  - Stroma consists of fibrous connective tissue and lymphoid elements
  - Fat and muscle may be present

LYMPHANGIOMATOUS POLYP

Key Facts

Terminology
- Lymphangioma arising from palatine tonsil

Clinical Issues
- Mean: 25 years; range: 3-50 years
- Obstructive symptoms (size dependent)

Macroscopic Features
- Unilateral, polyp

Microscopic Pathology
- Polypoid or papillary projections
- Prominent, dilated vascular channels
- Variable stroma
- Fibrous connective tissue and lymphoid elements

Ancillary Tests
- Endothelium positive with: CD31, CD34, FVIIIRAg, VEGF-1, podoplanin (D2-40)

  - Tends to be paucicellular fibrous background stroma

ANCILLARY TESTS

Immunohistochemistry
- Endothelium positive with: CD31, CD34, FVIIIRAg, VEGF-1, podoplanin (D2-40)
- Polytypic lymphoid cells, although T-cells (CD3) predominate

DIFFERENTIAL DIAGNOSIS

Juvenile Angiofibroma
- Males exclusively; nasopharynx, destructive large lesion, epistaxis, cellular stroma, variable vascular channels

Papillary Lymphoid Polyp
- Exclusively in children; papillary, prominent lymphoid follicles (development arc with LAP)

Hemangioma
- Dilated vessels with blood, no background stroma, lacks lymphocytes, tends to lack fibrosis

Fibroma
- No vascular component with heavily collagenized stroma

Squamous Papilloma
- Multiple exophytic projections covered with layers of squamous epithelium, koilocytic atypia, no lymphoid stroma, no vascular proliferation

SELECTED REFERENCES

1. Kardon DE et al: Tonsillar lymphangiomatous polyps: a clinicopathologic series of 26 cases. Mod Pathol. 13(10):1128-33, 2000
2. Sah SP et al: Lymphangiectatic fibrolipomatous polyp of the palatine tonsil. Indian J Pathol Microbiol. 43(4):449-51, 2000
3. Borges A et al: Giant fibrovascular polyp of the oropharynx. AJNR Am J Neuroradiol. 20(10):1979-82, 1999
4. Roth M: Lymphangiomatous polyp of the palatine tonsil. Otolaryngol Head Neck Surg. 115(1):172-3, 1996
5. Lupovitch A et al: Benign hamartomatous polyp of the palatine tonsil. J Laryngol Otol. 107(11):1073-5, 1993
6. Giusan AO: [2 cases of fibrous polyps of palatine tonsils] Vestn Otorinolaringol. (2):42, 1992
7. Shara KA et al: Hamartomatous tonsillar polyp. J Laryngol Otol. 105(12):1089-90, 1991
8. Heffner DK: Pathology of the tonsils and adenoids. Otolaryngol Clin North Am. 20(2):279-86, 1987
9. Al Samarrae SM et al: Polypoid lymphangioma of the tonsil: report of two cases and review of the literature. J Laryngol Otol. 99(8):819-23, 1985
10. Hiraide F et al: Lymphangiectatic fibrous polyp of the palatine tonsil. A report of three cases. J Laryngol Otol. 99(4):403-9, 1985
11. Pyun KS et al: Papillary lymphoid polyp of the palatine tonsil. Ear Nose Throat J. 64(5):243-5, 1985

IMAGE GALLERY

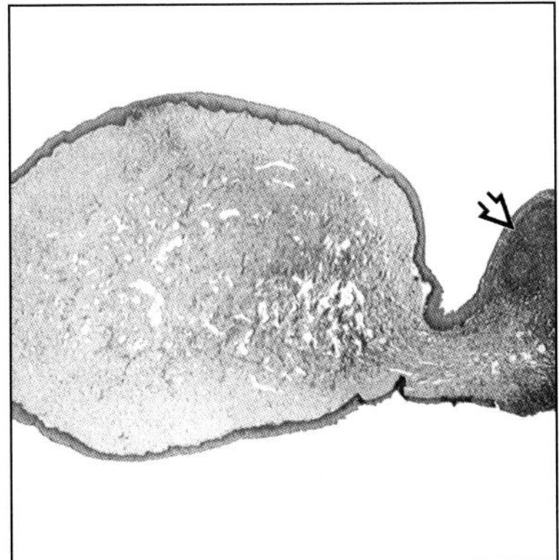
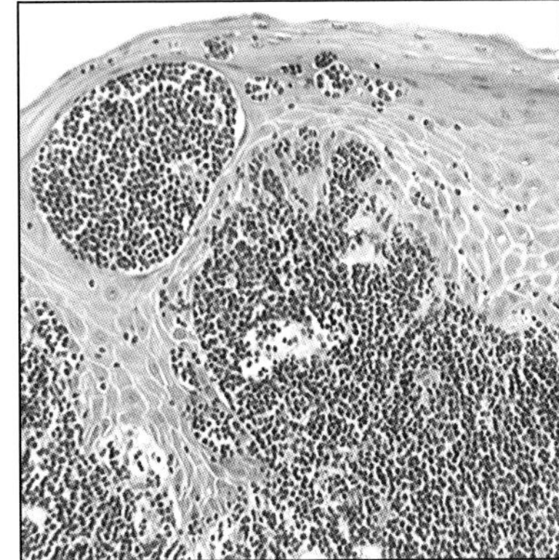
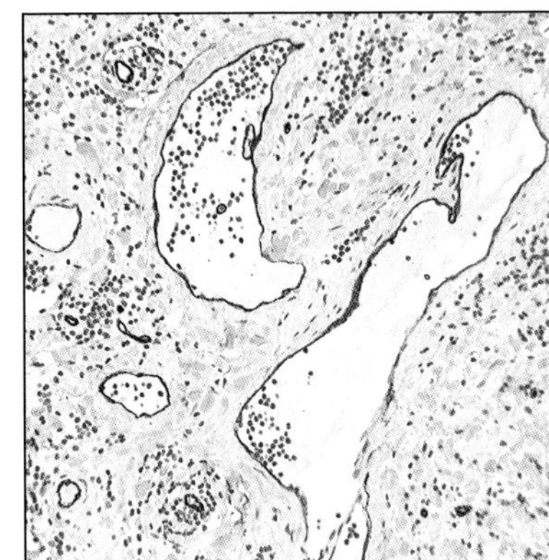

(Left) *A polypoid structure is noted protruding from the tonsil ⇒, a common finding in lymphangiomatous polyp. There is ample fibrosis associated with dilated vessels.* ***(Center)*** *The lymphocytes may display epidermotropism, aggregating in the epithelium in groups and clusters. The lymphocytes lack cytologic atypia.* ***(Right)*** *The rich vascular investment comprising the lesion can be highlighted with vascular markers, including CD34.*

AMALGAM TATTOO

Key Facts

Terminology

- Localized area of blue, gray, or black pigmentation caused by amalgam embedded into oral tissues, usually during dental procedures

Etiology/Pathogenesis

- Commonly used dental amalgam, which contains silver, tin, mercury, and other materials, can be embedded into tissue during dental procedures

Clinical Issues

- **Presentation**
  - Blue-gray to black pigment most common on gingiva and buccal mucosa
  - Asymptomatic flat macule ranging from a few mm to > 1 cm
- **Treatment**
  - Biopsy indicated if clinical diagnosis is uncertain
  - Can be removed for cosmesis

Image Findings

- Generally not visible radiographically

Microscopic Pathology

- Fine black granules scattered within superficial connective tissue
- Pigment can be seen in collagen, histocytes, fibroblasts, elastic fibers, and around blood vessel walls
- Usually no inflammation associated with pigment
- Foreign body multinucleated giant cell reaction reported in up to 38% of cases

Top Differential Diagnoses

- **Pigmented intraoral lesions**
  - Intraoral melanocytic nevus
  - Oral melanotic macule
  - Oral melanoma
- **Varicosities**
- **Unintentional mucosal tattoos**
  - Accidental placement of foreign material, such as pencil graphite

__(Left)__ Clinical photo shows diffuse blue-gray pigmentation typical for an amalgam tattoo. This tattoo could have been related to the missing teeth as well as to the premolar tooth with the amalgam restoration. (Courtesy X. Zornosa, DMD.) __(Right)__ H&E shows amalgam tattoo of the buccal vestibule with scattered large fragments of black material distributed in the lamina propria. The overlying epithelium is normal. Inflammation is noted, although many amalgam tattoos show little or no inflammation.

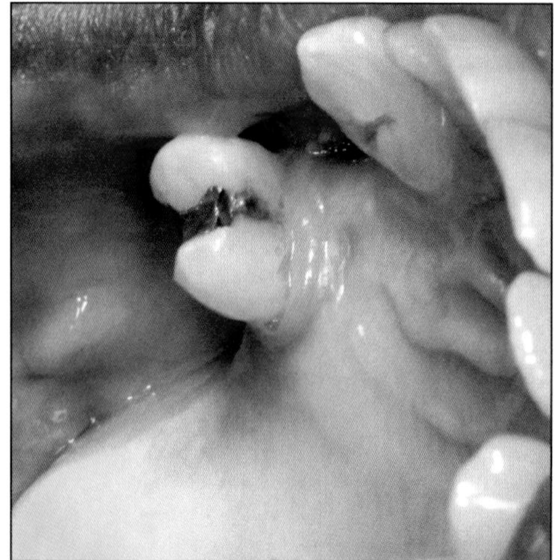

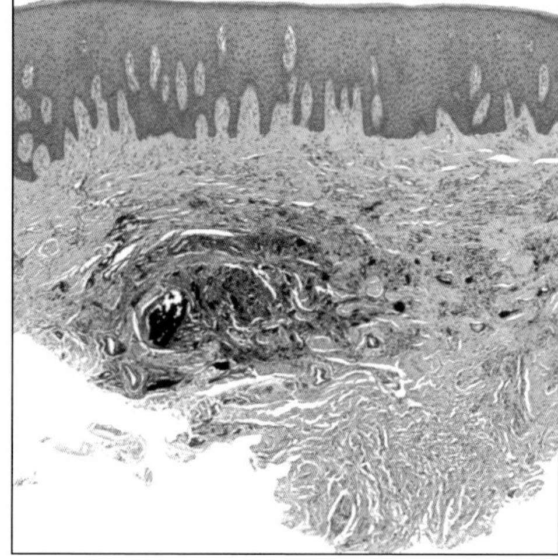

__(Left)__ High-power photomicrograph of an amalgam tattoo illustrates the perivascular location of the amalgam ⇨. The silver salts found in dental amalgam stain the reticulin fibers surrounding nerves and vessels. __(Right)__ H&E shows amalgam tattoo eliciting a foreign body giant cell reaction. Amalgam pigment is seen within the scattered giant cells with associated plasma cells and lymphocytes. Radiographs can at times confirm the metallic nature of the tattoo.

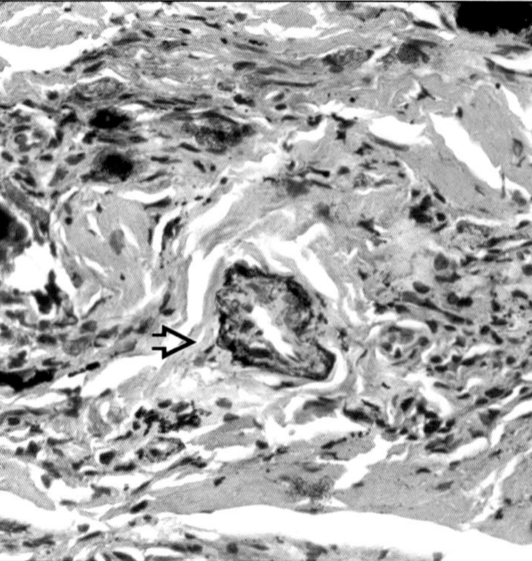

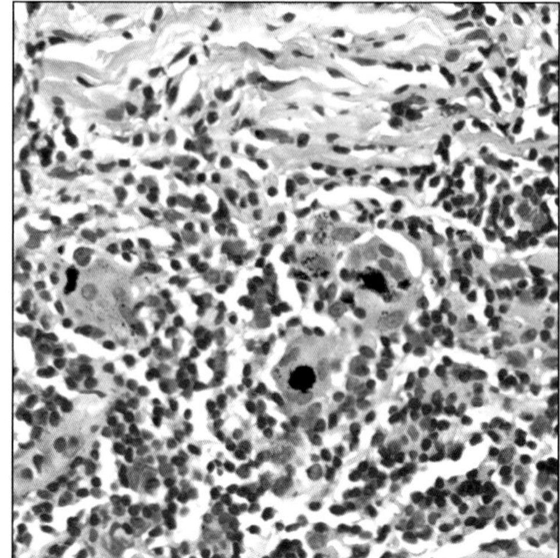

FORDYCE GRANULES

Key Facts

Terminology
- **Definition**
  - Benign, ectopic sebaceous glands
- **Synonyms**
  - Ectopic sebaceous glands, Fordyce condition or spots

Etiology/Pathogenesis
- Considered normal variant
  - Thought to arise from ectoderm inclusions during fusion of mandible and maxilla

Clinical Issues
- More commonly noted in adults than in children
- Equal gender distribution
- About 60% of children < 10 years of age have Fordyce granules
- Most common on lateral margins of upper and lower lip and buccal mucosa
- Less frequent on gingiva, retromolar area, and soft palate
- **Presentation**
  - Incidental, asymptomatic
  - Multiple uniform-sized 1-3 mm yellow papules &/ or plaques
  - Widely spaced or clustered to form plaques
- Normal variant and usually not treated
- Unassociated with other diseases

Microscopic Pathology
- Normal sebaceous glands lacking hair follicles
- Sebaceous hyperplasia can occur, particularly with advanced age
- May consist of only 1 lobule but usually multiple acinar lobules in superficial lamina propria
- Central duct extending to surface epithelium can be seen
- Each lobule is composed of peripheral layer of basophilic cuboidal cells
- Centrally located polygonal cells have abundant lipid-filled cytoplasm
- Glands can become obstructed forming pseudocysts
  - Cyst filled with mucin, sebum, &/or keratin

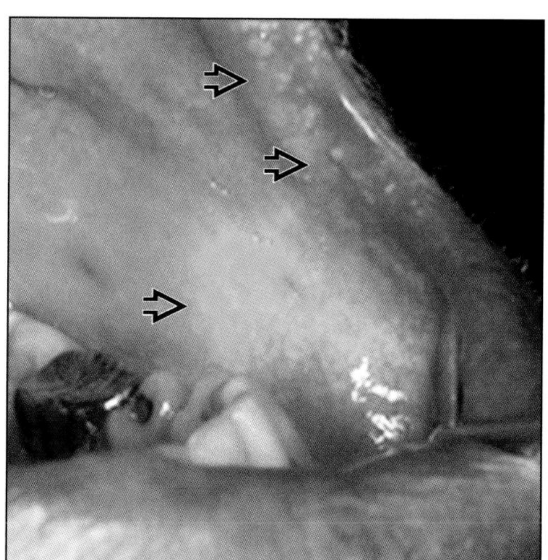

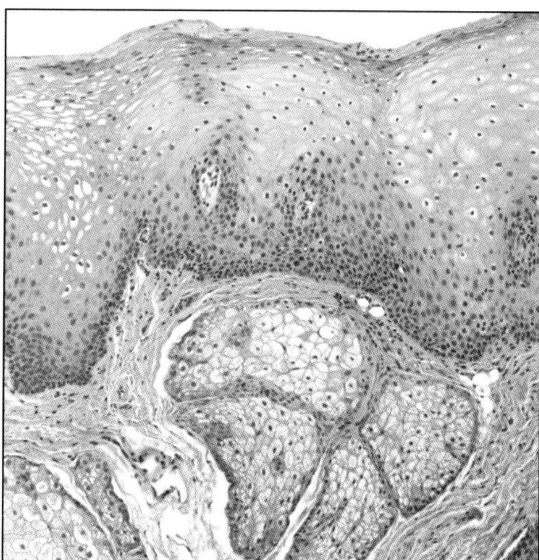

*(**Left**) Fordyce granules present as asymptomatic, yellow papules on labial & buccal mucosa ➲. This type of presentation is independent of age, although this photo is from an adult. (**Right**) Typical microscopic appearance of Fordyce granules from buccal mucosa. Sebaceous glands are composed of acinar lobules beneath normal-appearing epithelium. Usually < 15 lobules are seen per gland, and > 15 lobules per gland is considered to be sebaceous hyperplasia.*

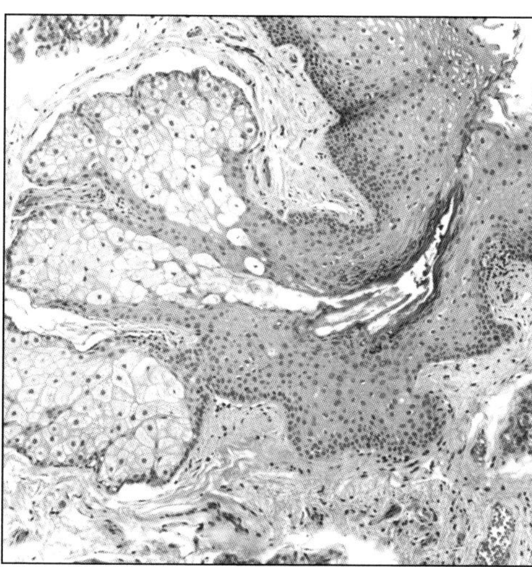

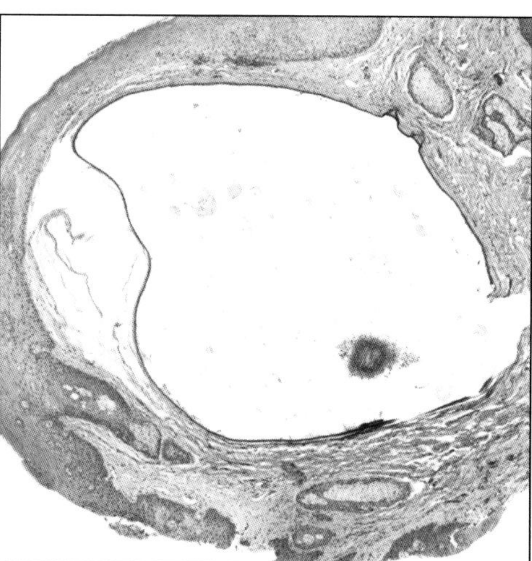

*(**Left**) High-power photomicrograph of Fordyce granules illustrates the central duct of the sebaceous lobule connecting the gland to the surface epithelium. (**Right**) Photomicrograph of a biopsy from the lip of Fordyce granules shows a pseudocyst; such a cyst generally develops in the excretory duct of the sebaceous gland. The cyst lumen generally contains keratin, sebum, &/or mucin. This is probably comparable to milia of the skin.*

GEOGRAPHIC TONGUE

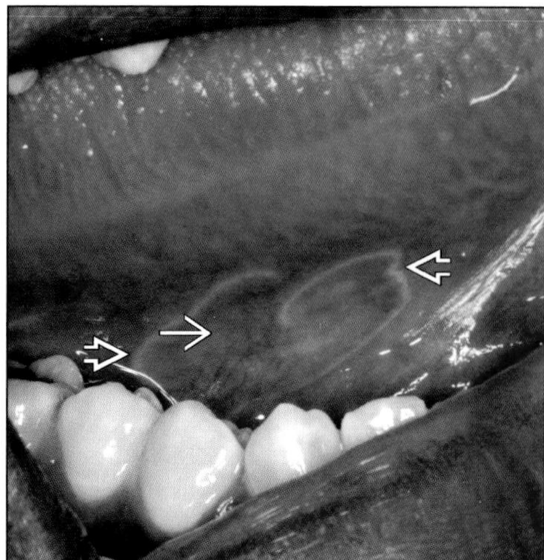

Clinical photograph of geographic tongue shows well-demarcated erythematous areas ➡ surrounded by a yellow-white border ➡. The ventral tongue location is a little unusual. (Courtesy K.M. Goodin, DDS.)

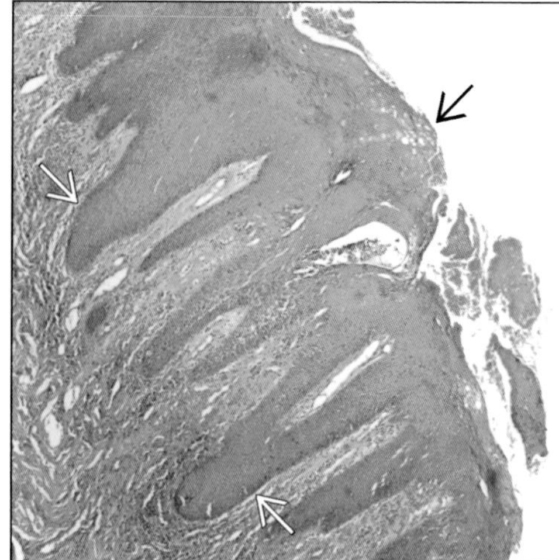

Hematoxylin and eosin shows the characteristic low-power presentation of geographic tongue with distinctive elongated rete ridges ➡ and parakeratosis ➡.

TERMINOLOGY

Synonyms

- Erythema migrans
- Benign migratory glossitis
- Psoriasiform mucositis

Definitions

- Benign inflammatory condition, primarily of the tongue with unknown etiology

ETIOLOGY/PATHOGENESIS

Unknown

- High association with fissured tongue
- Associated with atopy
  - Asthma
  - Rhinitis
- Smoking appears protective
- Possible familial predisposition
  - *HLA-Cw6* association
- May be associated with hormone use

CLINICAL ISSUES

Epidemiology

- Incidence
  - 1-2.5% of population
- Age
  - Wide age range
  - Most common in 2nd to 3rd decade
- Gender
  - Female > Male (1.5:1)

Site

- Primarily the tongue
  - Tip
  - Lateral borders
  - Dorsal
  - Rarely ventral
- Rarely other oral mucosal sites
  - Buccal
  - Labial
  - Soft palate

Presentation

- Usually asymptomatic
- Occasional reports of burning sensation with food
  - Sour
  - Spicy
  - Hot

Natural History

- Multiple, well-defined areas of erythema surrounded by raised, white-yellow borders that appear rapidly
- Healing occurs within days or weeks
- Lesion develops in another area
- Lesions appear to move or "migrate" around surface of tongue

Treatment

- No treatment in nearly all cases
  - Reassure patient
  - Explain condition
- Treatment rarely indicated
  - Severe burning sensation
    - Topical steroids
    - Avoiding trigger foods

Prognosis

- Excellent

MACROSCOPIC FEATURES

General Features

- Areas of erythema
  - Represents atrophy of filiform papillae
- Raised white-yellow borders

GEOGRAPHIC TONGUE

Key Facts

Terminology

- Benign inflammatory condition, primarily of the tongue with unknown etiology

Clinical Issues

- 1-2.5% of population
- Primarily the tongue
- Usually asymptomatic
- Multiple, well-defined areas of erythema surrounded by raised white-yellow borders that appear rapidly
- Lesions appear to move or "migrate" around surface of tongue

Microscopic Pathology

- Epithelium
  - Hyperparakeratosis
  - Acanthosis
  - Spongiosis
  - Elongated rete ridges
  - Munro abscesses

MICROSCOPIC PATHOLOGY

Histologic Features

- Epithelium
  - Hyperparakeratosis
  - Spongiosis
  - Acanthosis
  - Elongated rete ridges
  - Munro abscesses (collections of neutrophils)
- Lamina propria
  - Lymphocytic infiltration
  - Neutrophilic infiltration
- Reminiscent of psoriasis

DIFFERENTIAL DIAGNOSIS

Candidiasis

- Fungal elements are present

Lichen Planus

- Band-like lymphocytic infiltrate
- Destruction of basal cell layer
- Degenerating keratinocytes

Lichenoid Mucositis

- Associations
  - Dental amalgam
  - Medications
  - Foods
  - Oral hygiene products
- Nonspecific
- Band-like chronic inflammatory infiltrate

Psoriasis

- Exceedingly rare, considered by some not to affect oral cavity
- Correlation with skin disease

Contact Stomatitis

- Associated with cinnamon flavoring
  - Symptoms disappear with removal of causal agent
- Nonspecific
- Perivascular inflammation

SELECTED REFERENCES

1. Miloğlu O et al: The prevalence and risk factors associated with benign migratory glossitis lesions in 7619 Turkish dental outpatients. Oral Surg Oral Med Oral Pathol Oral Radiol Endod. 107(2):e29-33, 2009
2. Shulman JD et al: Prevalence and risk factors associated with geographic tongue among US adults. Oral Dis. 12(4):381-6, 2006
3. Jainkittivong A et al: Geographic tongue: clinical characteristics of 188 cases. J Contemp Dent Pract. 6(1):123-35, 2005
4. Pass B et al: Geographic tongue: literature review and case reports. Dent Today. 24(8):54, 56-7; quiz 57, 2005
5. Assimakopoulos D et al: Benign migratory glossitis or geographic tongue: an enigmatic oral lesion. Am J Med. 113(9):751-5, 2002

IMAGE GALLERY

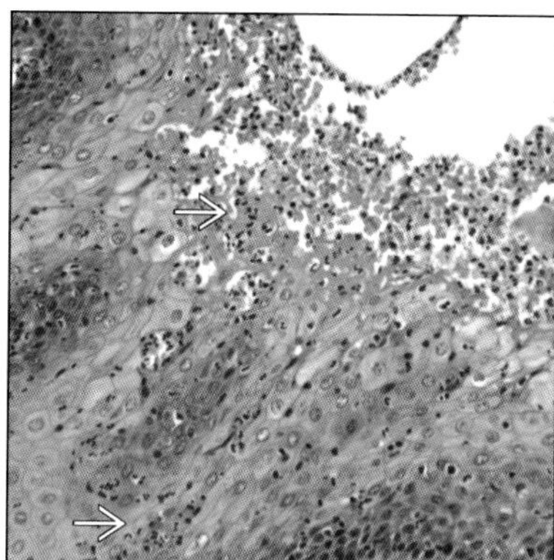

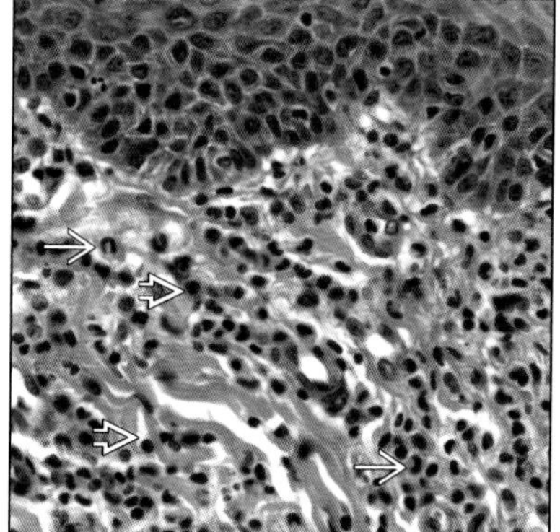

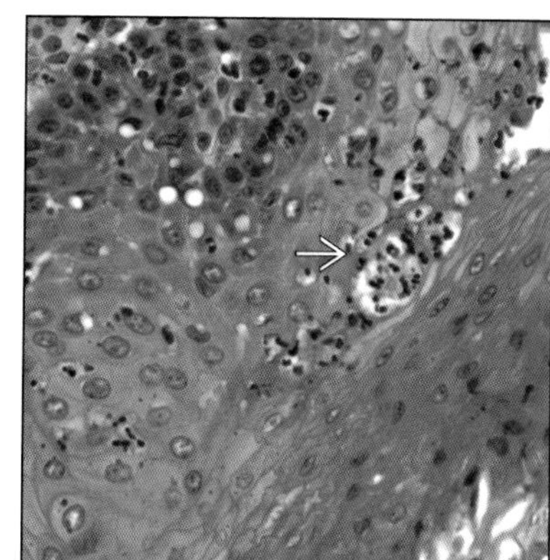

(Left) *High-power view shows a neutrophilic infiltration ➡. This infiltrate is responsible for the destruction of the epithelium, resulting in red lesions clinically.* *(Center)* *Hematoxylin and eosin shows the inflammatory infiltrate of the lamina propria, consisting primarily of lymphocytes ➡ and neutrophils ➡.* *(Right)* *High-power view shows the characteristic collections of neutrophils ➡, called Munro abscesses, within the epithelium.*

JUXTAORAL ORGAN OF CHIEVITZ

Key Facts

Terminology

- Normal structure located in buccotemporalis fascia bilaterally along medial surface of ascending ramus
  - Composed of nest of epithelial cells associated with small nerve branches of buccal nerve with supporting parenchyma

Etiology/Pathogenesis

- Normal anatomical structure
- First described by Danish histologist, J.H. Chievitz in 1885
- Persists throughout life
- No known function

Clinical Issues

- Rare reports of hyperplasia of juxtaoral organ of Chievitz have been reported
- No carcinoma has been reported arising from juxtaoral organ of Chievitz

Microscopic Pathology

- Not grossly apparent
- Size ranges from 0.7-1.7 cm in length and 0.1-0.2 cm in width
- Circumscribed nests of benign-appearing squamous cells within fibrous stroma
  - Cells are uniform and bland in appearance
  - No mitotic figures are seen
  - Desmoplasia is not present
  - No or little pleomorphism seen
  - Basement membrane noted around individual epithelial islands highlighted by PAS stain
- Keratinization is not seen
- Basaloid cells with nuclear palisading may be present
- Duct-like lumina may be present
  - Mucin negative
- Calcifications within epithelium have been noted
- Stroma rich in nerves
  - Epithelial islands often intimately associated with nerves
  - Both intra- and perineural epithelium may be present
- No inflammation
- Melanin deposits in surrounding stroma have been reported

Top Differential Diagnoses

- Invasive neurotropic squamous cell carcinoma
  - Lack of basement membrane
  - Pleomorphism
  - Keratinization or keratin pearls in keratinizing squamous cell cancer
  - Inflammatory cell response
  - Desmoplasia may be seen
  - Mitotic figures more common
- Mucoepidermoid carcinoma
  - Cystic, with mucocytes and epidermoid cells
  - Mucin-positive cells
- Adenoid cystic carcinoma
  - Strong perineural proclivity
  - Tends to have small, hyperchromatic nuclei with carrot- or peg-shaped cells
- Odontogenic carcinoma
  - Hyperchromatic palisaded basal cells mimic odontogenic epithelium
  - Intraosseous tumor

Diagnostic Checklist

- **Clinically relevant pathologic features**
  - Communication with surgeon crucial to avoid misdiagnosing structures as invasive carcinoma
- **Pathologic interpretation pearls**
  - Juxtaoral organ of Chievitz can exhibit both intra- and perineural invasion
  - SCC generally infiltrates nerve along perineural space with intraneural involvement rare
  - Keratinization not present

*(**Left**) Juxtaoral organ of Chievitz composed of nests of epithelial cells within a fibrofatty stroma. These nests are intimately associated with small nerves → (branches of the buccal nerve). (**Right**) High-power view of the juxtaoral organ of Chievitz highlighting the hyperchromatic basal cells, some exhibiting nuclear palisading →. A small nerve twig is also seen ▷.*

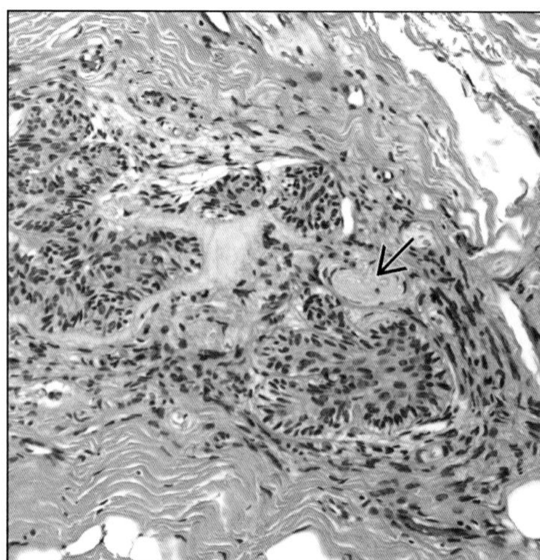

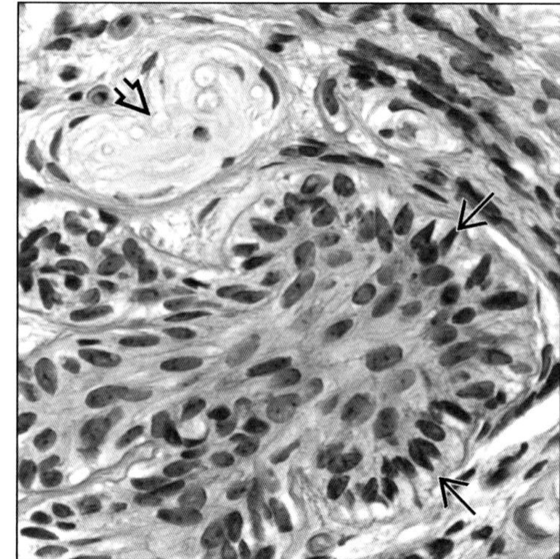

HETEROTOPIC SALIVARY GLANDS

Key Facts

Terminology

- Histologically normal salivary gland tissue located in unusual or abnormal anatomic location
- Synonyms
  - Salivary heterotopia, salivary gland choristoma, ectopic salivary glands

Clinical Issues

- Found incidentally
- Majority of heterotopic salivary glands located within structures of head and neck
  - Middle ear, external ear
  - Neck, thymus
  - Mandible (intraosseous)
  - Parathyroid gland
  - Cervical and periparotid lymph node
- Non-H&N sites may include
  - Mediastinum, stomach, prostate gland, rectum, or vulva
- May be discovered due to signs and symptoms associated with inflammation or neoplasia
- Heterotopic salivary gland tissue in neck may present as draining sinus
  - Most common on right side
  - Frequently associated with lower anterior sternocleidomastoid muscle
- No treatment required if incidental finding

Microscopic Pathology

- Histologic presentation akin to normal minor salivary gland tissue
  - Salivary lobules separated by fibrous septa
- Glandular cell types
  - Pure mucous
  - Pure serous
  - Combination of glandular acini (mucoserous)
- Associated pathologic conditions will be in keeping with specific diagnosis
  - May include cyst formation, oncocytic metaplasia/hyperplasia, benign or malignant neoplasms

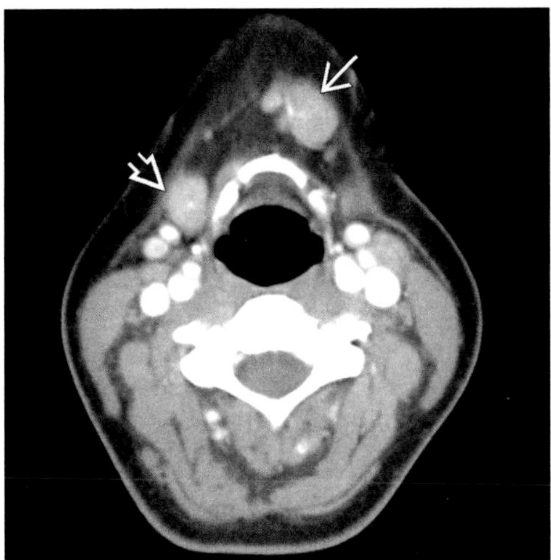

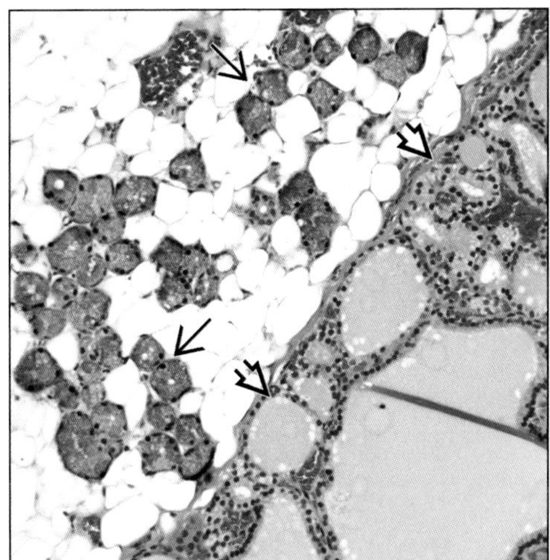

(Left) *Axial CECT shows accessory salivary gland tissue ➡ just to the left of midline within the soft tissue. The density and enhancement is similar to the normal submandibular gland ➡.* ***(Right)*** *The salivary gland parenchyma is normal in architecture and arrangement ➡, but it is identified immediately adjacent to the thyroid gland ➡. This is considered ectopic or heterotopic tissue.*

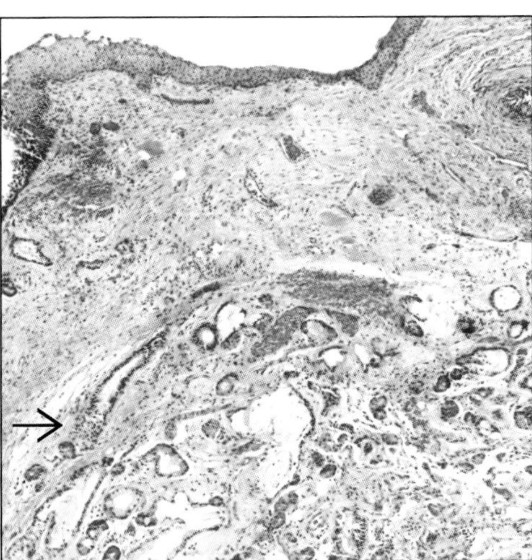

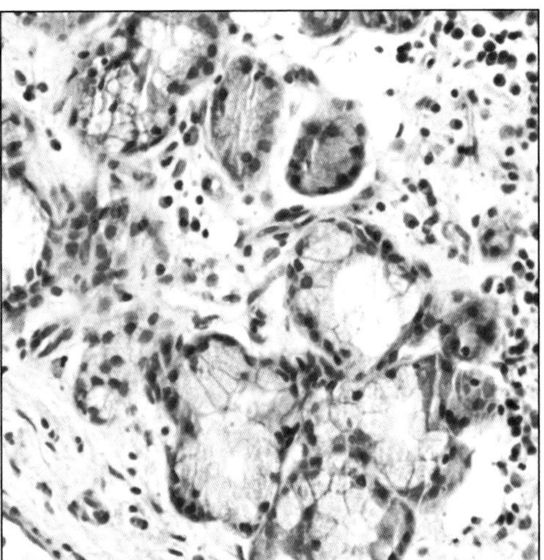

(Left) *H&E shows heterotopic minor salivary glands ➡ displaying ductal ectasia and sialadenitis. Seromucous glands are typical in the cartilaginous/nasopharynx portion of the eustachian tube but are not typical near the middle ear (pictured).* ***(Right)*** *High-power view shows primarily mucous acini and mild chronic sialadenitis.*

MUCOCELE AND RANULA

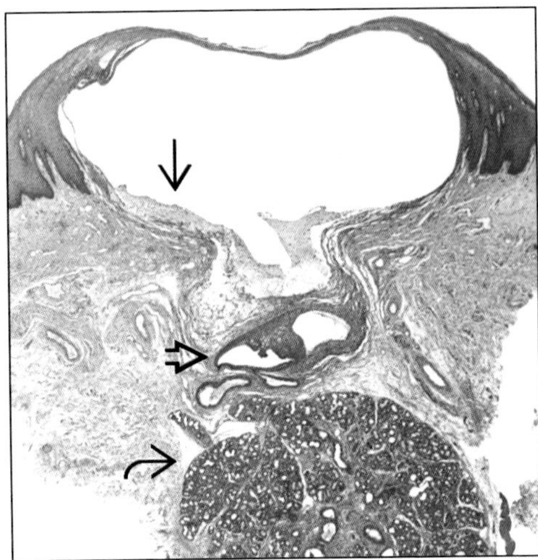

Lower lip mucocele is seen with extravasated mucin ➔ in superficial lamina propria and epithelial atrophy. Adjacent metaplastic ducts ➲ and glands with chronic sialadenitis ↗ are seen in deeper lamina propria.

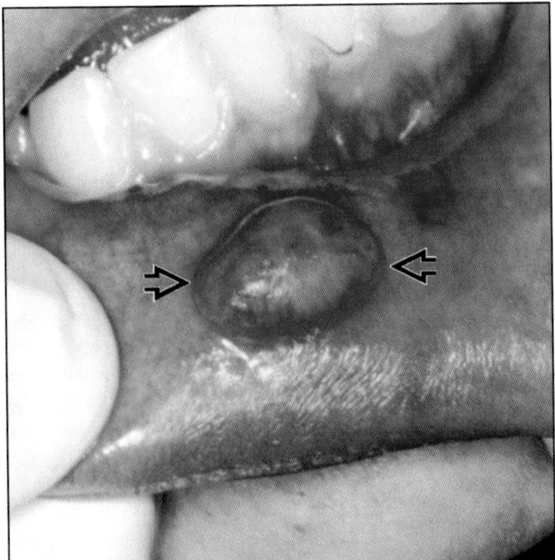

Clinical photo shows a blue, dome-shaped swelling on the lower lip ➲, which is the most common location for a mucocele. Mucoceles are generally fluctuant, although older lesions may be firmer on palpation.

TERMINOLOGY

Synonyms

- Mucus escape reaction
- Mucus retention phenomenon

Definitions

- Common lesion resulting from spillage of mucin into surrounding tissue from a ruptured salivary gland duct

ETIOLOGY/PATHOGENESIS

Pathogenesis

- Most likely localized trauma to salivary gland ducts

CLINICAL ISSUES

Epidemiology

- Incidence
  - Common
- Age
  - More frequent in children and young adults
    - Peak incidence in 2nd decade

Site

- Mucocele
  - Lower lip accounts for 70-81% of reported cases
  - Floor of mouth, ventral tongue, and palate are less frequently seen
- Plunging ranula
  - Floor of mouth
- Superficial mucocele
  - Soft palate and retromolar area

Presentation

- **Mucocele**
  - Most common on lower lip
  - Frequently presents as dome-shaped swelling with blue coloration due to extravasated mucin
- **Superficial mucocele**
  - Single or multiple blisters
- **Ranula**
  - Swelling in floor of mouth with bluish coloration
  - Large lesions can elevate tongue
  - Plunging ranulas result from mucin spillage dissecting the mylohyoid muscle producing neck swelling

Natural History

- Most mucoceles and ranulas need to be excised
  - Superficial mucoceles generally resolve in a few days, but often recur

Treatment

- Surgical approaches
  - **Mucoceles**
    - Chronic unresolving lesions require surgical excision
    - Adjacent glands need to be removed to minimize recurrences
  - **Ranula**
    - Marsupialization used for superficial lesions
    - Sublingual gland excision needed for larger lesions

Prognosis

- No sequelae

MACROSCOPIC FEATURES

Size

- **Mucocele**
  - Size ranges from a few millimeters to > 1 cm
- **Superficial mucocele**
  - Usually 1-3 mm

MUCOCELE AND RANULA

Key Facts

Terminology

- Common lesion resulting from spillage of mucin into surrounding tissue from ruptured salivary gland duct

Clinical Issues

- More frequent in children and young adults
- Lower lip accounts for 70-81% of reported cases
- Mucocele: Chronic lesions require surgical excision
- Ranula: Marsupialization for superficial lesions

Microscopic Pathology

- Normal overlying epithelium usually seen
- Mucin spillage surrounded by granulation tissue wall
- Adjacent glands exhibit chronic &/or sclerosing sialadenitis
- Instead of mucin spillage, ectatic ducts may contain mucin plugs termed mucous retention phenomenon or salivary ductal ectasia

MICROSCOPIC PATHOLOGY

Histologic Features

- Normal overlying epithelium usually seen
  - Surface ulceration may be present, particularly when mucocele has been secondarily traumatized
  - Extravasated mucin in superficial epithelium can be seen in superficial mucoceles
- Mucin spillage surrounded by granulation tissue wall
  - Inflammatory cells including foamy histiocytes are seen
  - Acute inflammation is not common feature
- Adjacent glands exhibit chronic &/or sclerosing sialadenitis
- Adjacent ducts may show epithelial or oncocytic metaplasia
- Instead of mucin spillage, ectatic ducts may contain mucin plugs termed mucous retention phenomenon or salivary ductal ectasia
  - Dilated ducts may produce papillary foldings into duct lumen
    - When oncocytic metaplasia is present, these features are similar to a Warthin tumor without lymphoid component

DIFFERENTIAL DIAGNOSIS

Mucous Duct Cyst

- Developmental, epithelial-lined cyst of uniform thickness
- Can occur in both major and minor salivary glands
- Clinically similar to mucoceles
- Lined by squamous, cuboidal, or columnar epithelium
- Little to no inflammation is seen in cyst wall

Low-Grade Mucoepidermoid Carcinoma

- Clinically can mimic mucocele
- Cyst lining not of uniform thickness
- Mucous cells can be readily identified in cyst lining
- Careful examination of surrounding cyst usually shows more typical areas of mucoepidermoid carcinoma
- Can be difficult on fine needle aspiration if only mucinous material is withdrawn

SELECTED REFERENCES

1. Harrison JD: Modern management and pathophysiology of ranula: literature review. Head Neck. 32(10):1310-20, 2010
2. Morton RP et al: Plunging ranula: congenital or acquired? Otolaryngol Head Neck Surg. 142(1):104-7, 2010
3. Granholm C et al: Oral mucoceles; extravasation cysts and retention cysts. A study of 298 cases. Swed Dent J. 33(3):125-30, 2009
4. Patel MR et al: Oral and plunging ranulas: What is the most effective treatment? Laryngoscope. 119(8):1501-9, 2009
5. Nico MM et al: Mucocele in pediatric patients: analysis of 36 children. Pediatr Dermatol. 25(3):308-11, 2008
6. Inoue A et al: Superficial mucoceles of the soft palate. Dermatology. 210(4):360-2, 2005

IMAGE GALLERY

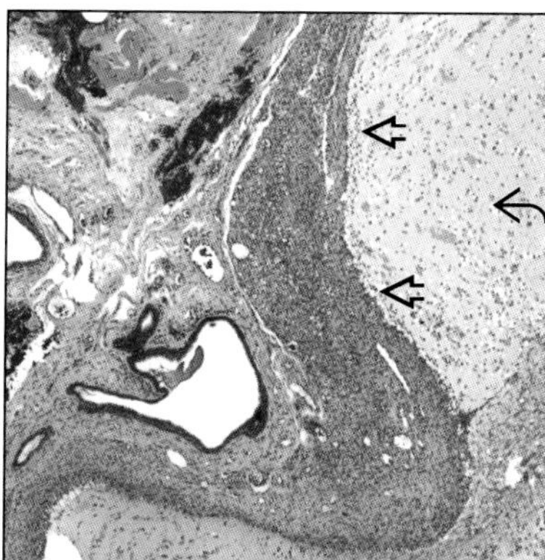

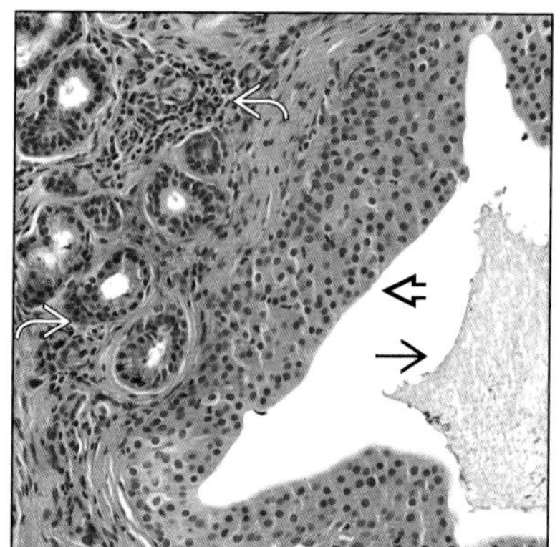

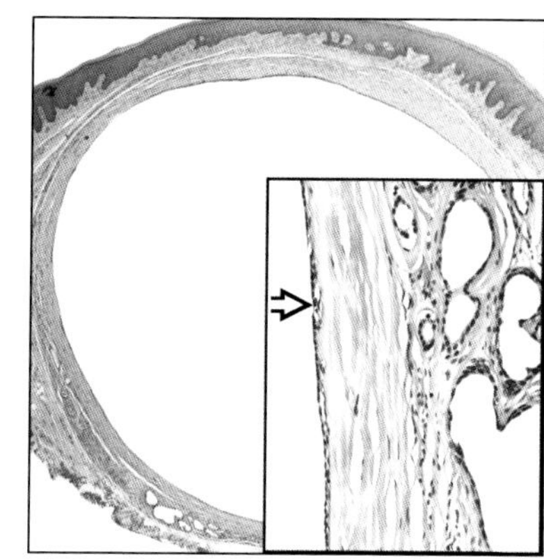

(Left) *H&E shows a typical histology of a ranula from the floor of the mouth with inspissated mucin ➔ eliciting a prominent granulation tissue wall response ➔.* ***(Center)*** *H&E shows mucocele presenting as a mucous retention phenomenon (cyst). Oncocytic metaplasia of the duct ➔ with mucin secretions in the lumen ➔ and adjacent sialadenitis ➔ is typical.* ***(Right)*** *H&E shows a mucus duct cyst composed of a uniform lining of flattened cuboidal epithelium ➔ surrounded by connective tissue devoid of inflammation.*

SQUAMOUS PAPILLOMA (INCLUDING VERRUCA AND CONDYLOMA)

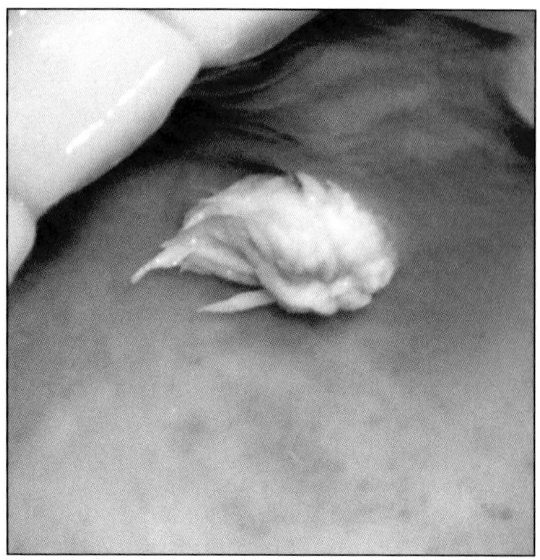

SP of the hard palate presents as a pedunculated lesion with numerous spike-like keratotic projections imparting a warty appearance. Depending on the degree of keratinization, SP can be white, red, or mucosal color.

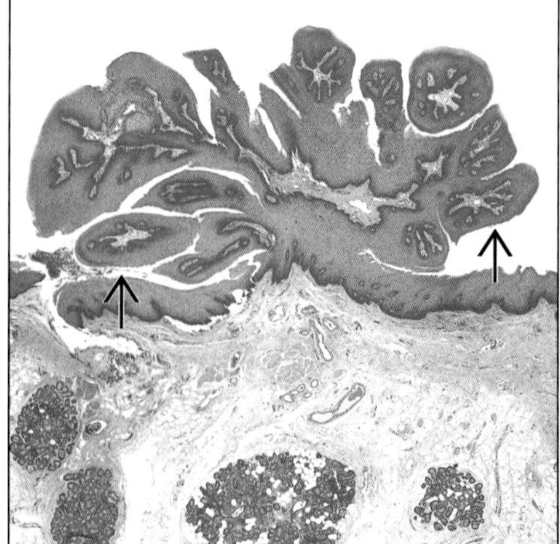

Low-power photomicrograph of squamous papilloma shows a pedunculated lesion with complex branching papillary structures supported by fibrovascular connective tissue cores ➔.

TERMINOLOGY

Abbreviations

- Squamous papilloma (SP)
- Verrucae vulgaris (VV)
- Condyloma acuminatum (CA)

Synonyms

- **VV**: Common wart, oral wart
- **CA**: Venereal wart

Definitions

- **SP**: Benign proliferation of squamous epithelium in exophytic pattern with branching fibrovascular tissue cores exhibiting papillary pattern causally related to human papillomavirus (HPV) infection
- **VV**: Benign, HPV-induced proliferation of squamous epithelium, usually on skin, but also in oral cavity
- **CA**: HPV-related proliferation of squamous epithelium of genitalia, perianal region, oral cavity, larynx

ETIOLOGY/PATHOGENESIS

Infectious Agents

- **SP**: HPV subtypes 6 and 11 have been detected in about 50% of cases
  - Virulence and infectivity rate thought to be low
  - Rarely HPV 16 detected
- **VV**: HPV subtypes 2, 4, 6, 40, or 57 detected in up to 100% of cases
  - Contagious and can spread to various body parts by autoinoculation
- **CA**: Considered a sexually transmitted disease
  - Lesions develop at site of contact or trauma
  - Usually HPV subtypes 2, 6, 11, 53, 54
    - Rarely high-risk HPV subtypes 16, 18, and 31 may be present (usually anogenital)
  - Oral CA may also arise from autoinoculation or maternal transmission

Pathogenesis

- HPV enters into epithelium at sites of trauma or wounds and infects actively dividing basal cells
- Viral altered epithelial cells in spinous layer (koilocytes)

CLINICAL ISSUES

Epidemiology

- Incidence
  - **SP**: Considered most frequent benign epithelial tumor of oral cavity
  - **VV**: Uncommon in oral cavity
  - **CA**: Uncommon in oral cavity
- Age
  - **SP**: Peak: 30-50 years but can affect all age groups
  - **VV**: More frequently seen in children or young adults
  - **CA**: Generally diagnosed in young adults and teenagers
    - Vertical transmission from mother to infant have been reported
    - CA in young children may represent sexual abuse
- Gender
  - **SP and VV**: Equal gender distribution

Site

- **SP**: May occur anywhere but most common sites include soft palate, uvula, hard palate, lingual frenum, and tongue
- **VV**: Oral lesions mostly occur on vermilion border, tongue, and labial mucosa
- **CA**: Oral lesions most frequently seen in soft palate, lingual frenum, and labial mucosa

Presentation

- **SP**
  - Usually presents as asymptomatic exophytic, pedunculated lesions

SQUAMOUS PAPILLOMA (INCLUDING VERRUCA AND CONDYLOMA)

Key Facts

Terminology
- Benign squamous epithelial proliferation in exophytic-papillary pattern with branching fibrovascular tissue cores causally related to HPV infection

Clinical Issues
- Asymptomatic exophytic lesion that can occur anywhere, although most common in soft palate, uvula, hard palate, lingual frenum, tongue
- **SP**: Most common oral benign epithelial tumor
- **SP**: Peak: 30-50 years
- **VV**: Peak: Children or young adults
- **CA**: Peak: Young adults and teenagers
- Conservative excision, laser ablation, or cryotherapy

Microscopic Pathology
- **SP**: Finger-like projections of squamous epithelium overlying fibrovascular stroma, basal/parabasal hyperchromasia, upper spinous layer koilocytes
- **VV**: Multiple papillary projections with hypergranulosis, marked hyperkeratosis, elongated rete, which tend to converge toward the center
- **CA**: Composed of acanthotic stratified squamous epithelium with papillary projections more blunted and broader than in squamous papilloma

Ancillary Tests
- HPV detection: In situ hybridization and PCR

Top Differential Diagnoses
- Proliferative verrucous leukoplakia, verrucous carcinoma, papillary squamous cell carcinoma

---

  - Color: White, red, or mucosal-colored depending on amount of surface keratinization
  - Generally ≤ 5 mm although can be larger
  - Spike-like or finger-like projections
  - Papillary projection can be blunted, imparting "cauliflower" appearance
- VV
  - Asymptomatic
  - Can be sessile or pedunculated
  - Oral: Generally white
    - Cutaneous: May be yellow, pink, or white
  - Generally ≤ 5 mm
  - Symmetrical round to ovoid papule or nodule with rough pebbly surface with central area of hyperkeratosis
  - Some lesions may have papillary projections
  - Well demarcated with abrupt margins
- CA
  - Generally sessile and mucosal-colored asymptomatic lesion
  - Multiple lesions often coalesce, forming larger mass
  - Generally 1-1.5 cm, although can be larger
  - Papillary projections are more blunted

Natural History
- Squamous papilloma and verruca vulgaris may spontaneously regress

Treatment
- Surgical approaches
  - Conservative surgical excision
  - Laser ablation
    - Possibility of aerosolized spread of HPV with this technique, especially in CA
  - Cryotherapy: Forms subepithelial blister leading to sloughing of lesion
- Drugs
  - Typical cutaneous treatments (intralesional bleomycin and 5-fluorouracil) **not** used for oral VV
  - Intralesional and topical cidofovir used for CA

Prognosis
- **Squamous papilloma and verruca vulgaris**
  - Recurrences have been reported
  - Some lesions will spontaneously resolve
- **Condyloma acuminatum**
  - No malignant transformation reported in oral CA, unlike anogenital area

MACROSCOPIC FEATURES

General Features
- Depends on type of lesion
- Sessile, exophytic to pedunculated mass
- Rough pebbly surface to multiple finger-like papillary projections, sometimes blunted

MICROSCOPIC PATHOLOGY

Histologic Features
- **Squamous papilloma**
  - Finger-like projections
  - Thin fibrovascular cores lined by squamous epithelium
  - Basal and parabasal hyperchromasia
    - Increased mitotic activity may be observed and not an indicator for dysplasia or malignancy
  - **Koilocytes** can be seen in prickle (spinous) layer
    - Hyperchromatic nucleus with wrinkled appearance
    - Perinuclear clearing
    - Well-defined, prominent intercellular borders
- **Verruca vulgaris**
  - Broad flat base
  - Multiple papillary projections with prominent granular layer (hypergranulosis) and marked hyperkeratosis
    - Coarse keratohyaline granules
  - Lack of branching of fibrovascular cores
  - Elongated rete ridges, which tend to converge toward the center
  - Koilocytes noted in superficial spinous layer
- **Condyloma acuminatum**

SQUAMOUS PAPILLOMA (INCLUDING VERRUCA AND CONDYLOMA)

- Acanthotic stratified squamous epithelium with papillary fronds
  - Projections more blunted and broader than in squamous papilloma
  - Appearance of keratin-filled crypts between projections into spinous layer
- Rete ridges often bulbous
- Variable number of koilocytes in prickle layer
  - Not as common in oral CA compared to anogenital lesions
- Surface keratinization less than in VV and most oral SP
- Underlying excretory ducts of minor salivary glands may be involved
  - Need to distinguish from salivary ductal papillomas

ANCILLARY TESTS

In Situ Hybridization

- Reliable method in paraffin-embedded tissue using type-specific probes
  - Not generally useful for diagnosis, treatment planning, or prognosis

PCR

- Most sensitive method for HPV detection and subtyping
  - Generally used only in research settings

DIFFERENTIAL DIAGNOSIS

Proliferative Verrucous Leukoplakia

- Lesions are multifocal and widespread
- Histologically variable
  - Early lesions may exhibit abundant keratosis with verrucous or papillary surface
  - Marked acanthosis
  - Dysplasia not a feature in early lesions
- Unrelenting progressive process that generally leads to conventional type squamous cell carcinoma

Verrucous Carcinoma

- Larger lesion
- Broad pushing border of infiltration at epithelial-stromal interface
- Marked parakeratosis with parakeratotic crypting and church-spire keratosis
- Normal epithelial maturation
- Occasional normal mitotic figure can be present in basal &/or parabasal layer
- No koilocytes

Papillary Squamous Cell Carcinoma

- Papillary projections lined by atypical to overtly malignant epithelium
- Hypercellular tumor
- Abnormal epithelial maturation
- Cellular pleomorphism
- Increased mitoses, including atypical mitotic figures
- Stromal invasion may or may not be seen

Focal Epithelial Hyperplasia (Heck Disease)

- Disease presents as multiple lesions generally in children and young adults
- Abrupt epithelial acanthosis
- Usually does not have papillary surface
- Elongated, broad rete ridges
- Scattered **mitosoid** cells
  - Altered nucleus resembling a mitotic figure

HIV-associated HPV Papillomas

- Usually multiple lesions
  - Present as mucosal-colored papules, cauliflower-like growths, or keratotic papillary projections
- Bizarre cellular atypia present in superficial spinous layer
  - Large pleomorphic nuclei and scattered giant cells
- Basal and parabasal layers generally unaffected
- Scattered koilocytes
  - HPV 7 and 32 have been isolated
- Malignant transformation has not been reported

DIAGNOSTIC CHECKLIST

Clinically Relevant Pathologic Features

- Nuclear features
  - Presence of koilocytes supports a viral etiology

SELECTED REFERENCES

1. Syrjänen S: Current concepts on human papillomavirus infections in children. APMIS. 118(6-7):494-509, 2010
2. Carneiro TE et al: Oral squamous papilloma: clinical, histologic and immunohistochemical analyses. J Oral Sci. 51(3):367-72, 2009
3. Trottier H et al: Epidemiology of mucosal human papillomavirus infection and associated diseases. Public Health Genomics. 12(5-6):291-307, 2009
4. Wang YP et al: Oral verrucous hyperplasia: histologic classification, prognosis, and clinical implications. J Oral Pathol Med. 38(8):651-6, 2009
5. Owotade FJ et al: Prevalence of oral disease among adults with primary HIV infection. Oral Dis. 14(6):497-9, 2008
6. Smith EM et al: Prevalence of human papillomavirus in the oral cavity/oropharynx in a large population of children and adolescents. Pediatr Infect Dis J. 26(9):836-40, 2007
7. Rinaggio J et al: Oral bowenoid papulosis in an HIV-positive male. Oral Surg Oral Med Oral Pathol Oral Radiol Endod. 101(3):328-32, 2006
8. Henley JD et al: Condyloma acuminatum and condyloma-like lesions of the oral cavity: a study of 11 cases with an intraductal component. Histopathology. 44(3):216-21, 2004
9. Anderson KM et al: The histologic differentiation of oral condyloma acuminatum from its mimics. Oral Surg Oral Med Oral Pathol Oral Radiol Endod. 96(4):420-8, 2003
10. Kui LL et al: Condyloma acuminatum and human papilloma virus infection in the oral mucosa of children. Pediatr Dent. 25(2):149-53, 2003
11. Syrjänen S: Human papillomavirus infections and oral tumors. Med Microbiol Immunol. 192(3):123-8, 2003
12. Flaitz CM: Condyloma acuminatum of the floor of the mouth. Am J Dent. 14(2):115-6, 2001
13. Garlick JA et al: Detection of human papillomavirus (HPV) DNA in focal epithelial hyperplasia. J Oral Pathol Med. 18(3):172-7, 1989

Microscopic and Clinical Features

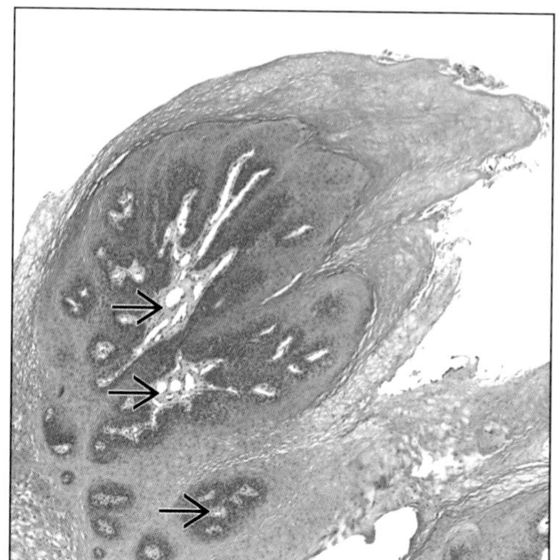

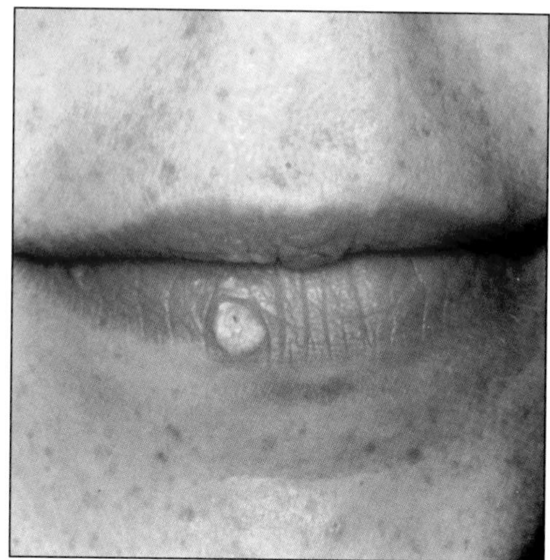

*(**Left**) High-power photomicrograph of squamous papilloma highlights the papillary frond supported by fibrovascular cores ➙. The surface keratin may be abundant as seen here, imparting a white appearance clinically. (**Right**) Verruca vulgaris of the lower lip in a child is shown. The vermilion border is a common location for verruca, which exhibits a rough, papillary surface. Verruca can also have papillary projections similar to squamous papillomas.*

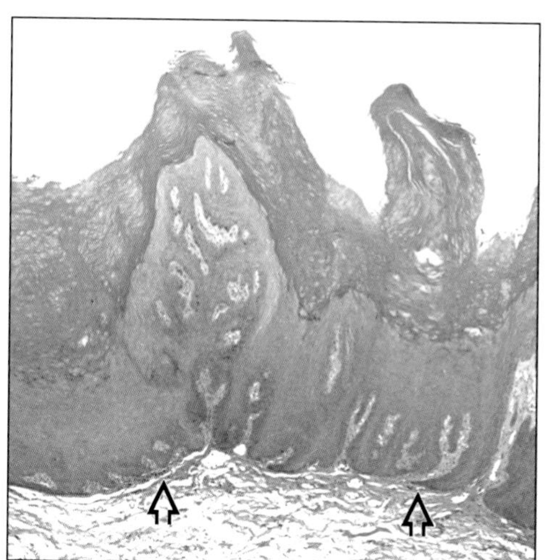

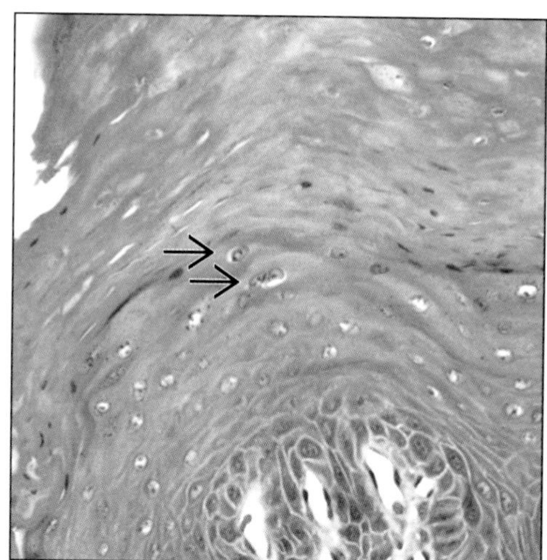

*(**Left**) Verruca vulgaris exhibits numerous papillary projections surfaced by a markedly keratotic squamous epithelium. Unlike squamous papillomas, which are pedunculated, verruca vulgaris has a broad flat base with elongated rete ridges that converge toward the center of the lesion ⇨. (**Right**) High-power view of a verruca vulgaris shows koilocytes ➙ in the superficial spinous layer characterized by dark condensed nuclei with cytoplasmic clearing.*

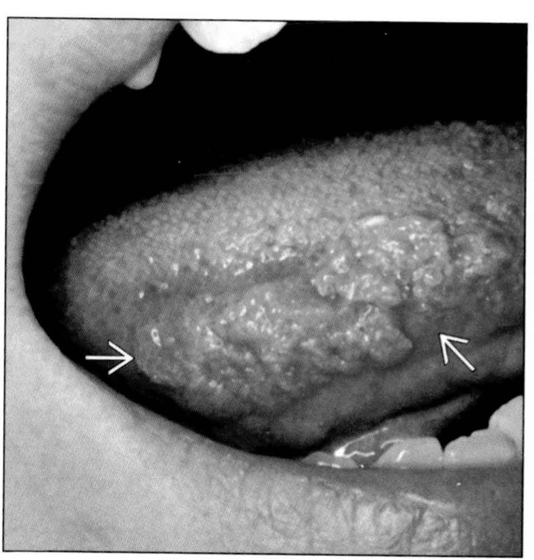

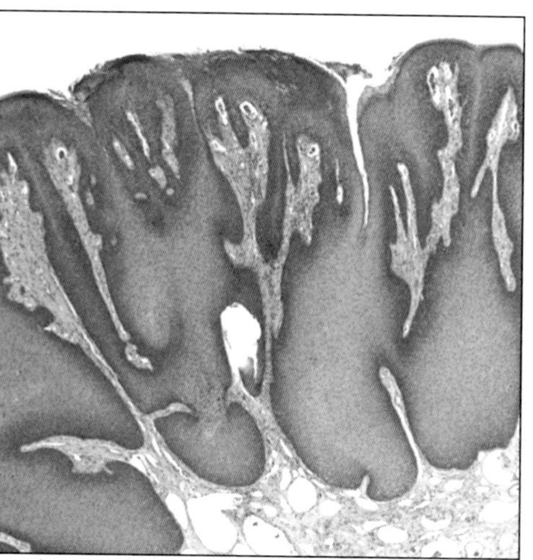

*(**Left**) Oral condyloma acuminatum of the lateral tongue presents as a pink, broad-based, sessile lesion with blunted surface projections ➡. The lesions are usually well demarcated from the surrounding normal tissue and may be multiple. (**Right**) Typical appearance of condyloma exhibits broader and more blunted papillary projections than squamous papillomas. The epithelium is markedly acanthotic. Koilocytes may be seen in the spinous layer but are more sparse than in genital condyloma.*

GRANULAR CELL TUMOR

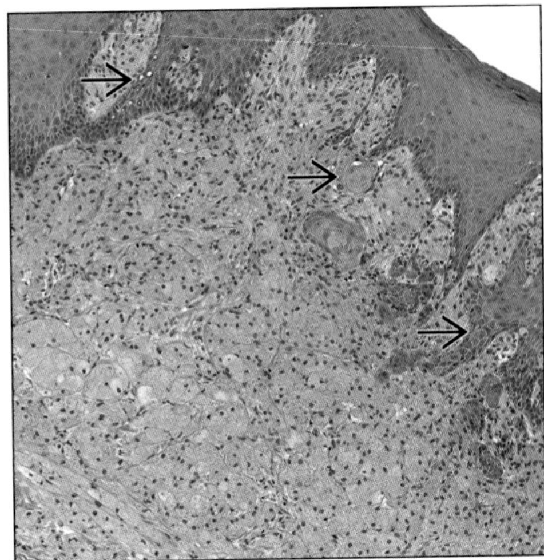

Prominent pseudoepitheliomatous hyperplasia ➔ is noted overlying the granular cell tumor. The tumor is unencapsulated, creating a sheet-like distribution of neoplastic granular cells.

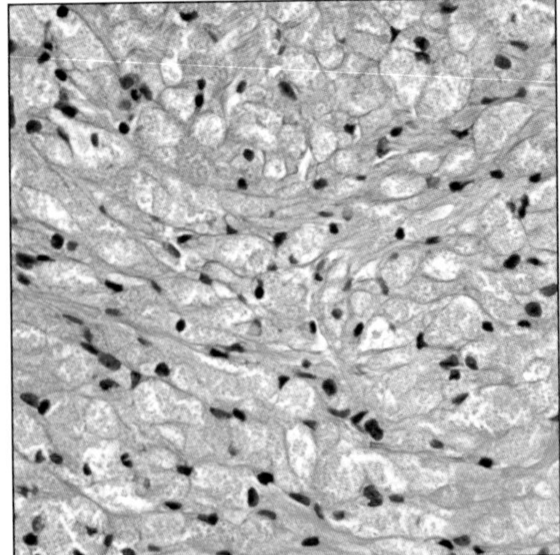

The granular cells are polygonal, showing a slightly spindled appearance. The cytoplasm contains numerous eosinophilic granules. The nuclei are small, round to oval, and hyperchromatic.

TERMINOLOGY

Abbreviations

- Granular cell tumor (GCT)

Synonyms

- Granular cell myoblastoma
- Abrikossoff tumor

Definitions

- Benign tumor composed of poorly demarcated accumulation of plump granular cells
  - Distinct from congenital epulis of newborn (gingival granular cell tumor of infancy)

ETIOLOGY/PATHOGENESIS

Schwann Cell Derivation

- Thought to arise from Schwann cells
  - Positive with neural-associated antibodies
  - Granules represent senescent change with accumulation of autophagocytic lysosomes

CLINICAL ISSUES

Epidemiology

- Incidence
  - Rare
    - < 1% of all head and neck tumors
- Age
  - All ages
    - Peak between 40 and 60 years
- Gender
  - Female > Male (2:1)
- Ethnicity
  - Blacks affected more often than whites

Site

- Over 50% of GCTs involve head and neck
  - Up to 70% of these develop in oral cavity (tongue, oral mucosa, hard palate)
- Tongue is most common single site (> 50% of all head and neck cases)
  - Dorsum > > lateral margin
- May develop in lips, buccal mucosa, floor of mouth, or palate
- Up to 20% of patients will have multifocal disease
  - Other oral sites or extraoral locations

Presentation

- Most present as painless mass
  - Usually have symptoms for < 12 months
- Rarely, may present with Eagle syndrome
  - Elicitation of pain on swallowing, turning head, or extending tongue
    - Syndrome is thought to be caused by irritation of glossopharyngeal nerve

Endoscopic Findings

- Overlying epithelium may be slightly pale
- Occasionally, there are concurrent candidal infections

Treatment

- Surgical approaches
  - Complete excision with narrow margins yields best outcome
  - Laser excision can be performed

Prognosis

- Excellent long-term prognosis
- Recurrence/relapse/persistence is uncommon (~ 10%)
- Malignant GCTs very rare in oral cavity

MACROSCOPIC FEATURES

General Features

- Smooth surfaced, submucosal swelling or nodule
  - Poorly demarcated lesion
- Cut surface has firm texture

GRANULAR CELL TUMOR

Key Facts

Terminology

- Benign tumor composed of poorly demarcated accumulation of plump granular cells
- Thought to arise from Schwann cells

Clinical Issues

- Female > Male (2:1)
- Blacks affected more often than whites
- Up to 70% of head and neck lesions develop in oral cavity (tongue most common)
- Up to 20% of patients will have multifocal disease
- Recurrence/relapse/persistence is uncommon (~ 10%)

Macroscopic Features

- Cut surface is firm, pale yellow or cream

Microscopic Pathology

- Unencapsulated plump polygonal to elongated granular cells blending with adjacent soft tissues, especially skeletal muscle
- Indistinct cell membranes surround abundant, granular, eosinophilic cytoplasm
- Overlying pseudoepitheliomatous hyperplasia is common

Ancillary Tests

- Granules are PAS positive, diastase resistant
- Strongly and uniformly positive for S100 protein

Top Differential Diagnoses

- Squamous cell carcinoma, rhabdomyoma, schwannoma, congenital epulis of newborn

---

- Pale yellow or cream
- Concurrent candidal infection may create a discrete, white plaque

Size

- Mean: 1-2 cm

MICROSCOPIC PATHOLOGY

Histologic Features

- Nonencapsulated
  - Blending with adjacent soft tissues, especially skeletal muscle is common
  - May extend up to epithelium, specifically papillae
  - Satellite nodules can develop
- Plump, polygonal to elongated eosinophilic cells
- Indistinct cell membranes, creating a syncytium
- Abundant, granular eosinophilic cytoplasm
  - Represent lysosomes
- Contain central small, dark to vesicular nuclei
- Overlying pseudoepitheliomatous hyperplasia (PEH)
  - Usually limited to epithelium immediately overlying tumor
  - Seen in about 30% of cases
- Rarely, marked stromal desmoplasia may be seen

ANCILLARY TESTS

Frozen Sections

- Pseudoepitheliomatous hyperplasia can mask tumor
- Granular, eosinophilic cytoplasm is usually easy to detect

Histochemistry

- Granules are periodic acid-Schiff (PAS) positive, diastase resistant

Immunohistochemistry

- Strongly and uniformly positive for S100 protein (nuclear and cytoplasmic)

Electron Microscopy

- Myelin-like figures, axon-like structures, angulate bodies, and basal lamina

DIFFERENTIAL DIAGNOSIS

Squamous Cell Carcinoma

- Pseudoepitheliomatous hyperplasia can mimic squamous cell carcinoma
  - PEH is only associated with GCT; it is not the tumor itself
- Small, superficial surface biopsy specimens can be difficult
- Must be properly oriented
- Squamous cell carcinoma usually shows p53 and E-cadherin immunoreactivity, a finding not seen in PEH
  - Immunohistochemistry does not replace properly oriented standard H&E material

Rhabdomyoma

- Uncommon in oral cavity
- Shows sheet-like distribution of polygonal cells with homogeneous, eosinophilic cytoplasm
- Cytoplasmic clearing with "spiderweb" cells is characteristic
- PTAH highlights cross striations in cytoplasm
- Does not have associated PEH

Schwannoma

- Often encapsulated, with well-defined border
- Has Antoni A and Antoni B areas, with Verocay bodies
- Much more spindled cellular arrangement
- Not associated with PEH
- Shows strong S100 protein staining, capsular EMA staining while lacking CD68

Congenital Epulis of Newborn

- Can be histologically indistinguishable from GCT
- Develops in newborns to infants only
- Lacks S100 protein immunoreactivity but is positive with vimentin and NSE

GRANULAR CELL TUMOR

Immunohistochemistry

Antibody	Reactivity	Staining Pattern	Comment
S100	Positive	Nuclear & cytoplasmic	Nearly all tumor cells
CD68	Positive	Cytoplasmic	Schwann cells of GCT and histiocytes (normal Schwann cells are negative)
Vimentin	Positive	Cytoplasmic	Strong and diffuse in all tumor cells
NSE	Positive	Cytoplasmic	Weak to strong in most tumor cells
CD57	Positive	Cytoplasmic	Weak reaction but in nearly all tumor cells
PGP9.5	Positive	Cytoplasmic	Most tumor cells
Inhibin-α	Positive	Cytoplasmic	Variably positive in most tumor cells
Calretinin	Positive	Nuclear & cytoplasmic	Variable in most tumor cells
NGFR	Positive	Cell membrane	Same as p75/NGFR
Collagen IV	Positive	Stromal matrix	Basement membrane positive, surrounding tumor cells
Ki-67	Positive	Nuclear	< 2% of nuclei in general
GFAP	Negative		
CK-PAN	Negative		
α-1-antitrypsin	Negative		
Desmin	Negative		

Leiomyoma
- Uncommon tumors of oral cavity
- Short to long, sweeping and interlacing fascicles
- Granular cells are uncommon in leiomyoma
- Tumor cells are positive with muscle markers, including actin-sm, actin-HHF-35, and desmin, while nonreactive for S100 protein

Nonneural Granular Cell Tumor
- Identical histologically but lacking S100 protein
- This is not a tumor seen in newborns, but in adults
- May occasionally show greater cytologic atypia than GCT

Lichen Planus Reaction
- Significant granular cells can be seen in association with oral lichen planus
  - Also called oral ceroid granuloma
- Characteristic interface inflammatory infiltrate with Civatte bodies
- Direct immunofluorescence characteristic for lichen planus
- Cells are positive with S100 protein
  - Thought to be reactive phenomenon triggered by inflammatory infiltrate
- Simultaneous presence of GCT and oral lichen planus may be possible

SELECTED REFERENCES

1. Fitzhugh VA et al: Fine-needle aspiration biopsy of granular cell tumor of the tongue: a technique for the aspiration of oral lesions. Diagn Cytopathol. 37(11):839-42, 2009
2. Vered M et al: Granular cell tumor of the oral cavity: updated immunohistochemical profile. J Oral Pathol Med. 38(1):150-9, 2009
3. Lerman M et al: Nonneural granular cell tumor of the oral cavity: a case report and review of the literature. Oral Surg Oral Med Oral Pathol Oral Radiol Endod. 103(3):382-4, 2007
4. Angiero F et al: Granular cells tumour in the oral cavity: report of eleven cases treated with laser surgery. Minerva Stomatol. 55(7-8):423-30, 2006
5. Eguia A et al: Granular cell tumor: report of 8 intraoral cases. Med Oral Patol Oral Cir Bucal. 11(5):E425-8, 2006
6. Zarovnaya E et al: Distinguishing pseudoepitheliomatous hyperplasia from squamous cell carcinoma in mucosal biopsy specimens from the head and neck. Arch Pathol Lab Med. 129(8):1032-6, 2005
7. Brannon RB et al: Oral granular cell tumors: an analysis of 10 new pediatric and adolescent cases and a review of the literature. J Clin Pediatr Dent. 29(1):69-74, 2004
8. van der Meij EH et al: Granular cells in oral lichen planus. Oral Dis. 7(2):116-8, 2001
9. Junquera LM et al: Granular-cell tumours: an immunohistochemical study. Br J Oral Maxillofac Surg. 35(3):180-4, 1997
10. Williams HK et al: Oral granular cell tumours: a histological and immunocytochemical study. J Oral Pathol Med. 26(4):164-9, 1997
11. Zangari F et al: Granular cell myoblastoma. Review of the literature and report of a case. Minerva Stomatol. 45(5):231-7, 1996
12. Collins BM et al: Multiple granular cell tumors of the oral cavity: report of a case and review of the literature. J Oral Maxillofac Surg. 53(6):707-11, 1995
13. Garlick JA et al: A desmoplastic granular cell tumour of the oral cavity: report of a case. Br J Oral Maxillofac Surg. 30(2):119-21, 1992
14. Okada H et al: Granular cell tumor of the tongue: an electron microscopical and immunohistochemical study. J Nihon Univ Sch Dent. 32(1):35-43, 1990
15. Payne-James JJ et al: Granular cell tumour (myoblastoma): two cases and a review of the literature. Br J Clin Pract. 44(8):334-6, 1990
16. Mirchandani R et al: Granular cell lesions of the jaws and oral cavity: a clinicopathologic, immunohistochemical, and ultrastructural study. J Oral Maxillofac Surg. 47(12):1248-55, 1989
17. Stewart CM et al: Oral granular cell tumors: a clinicopathologic and immunocytochemical study. Oral Surg Oral Med Oral Pathol. 65(4):427-35, 1988

GRANULAR CELL TUMOR

Clinical, Gross, Microscopic, and Ancillary Features

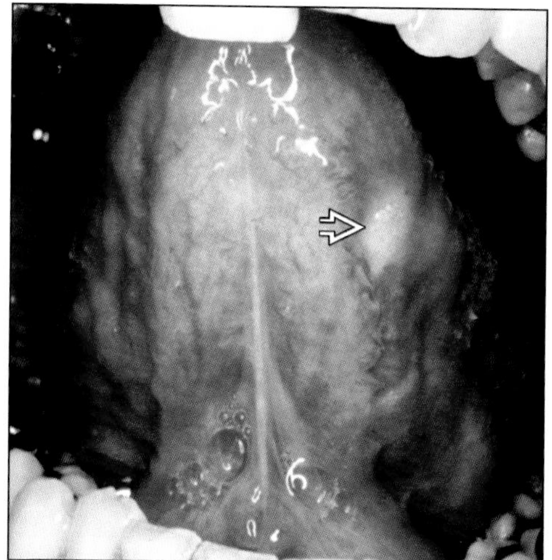

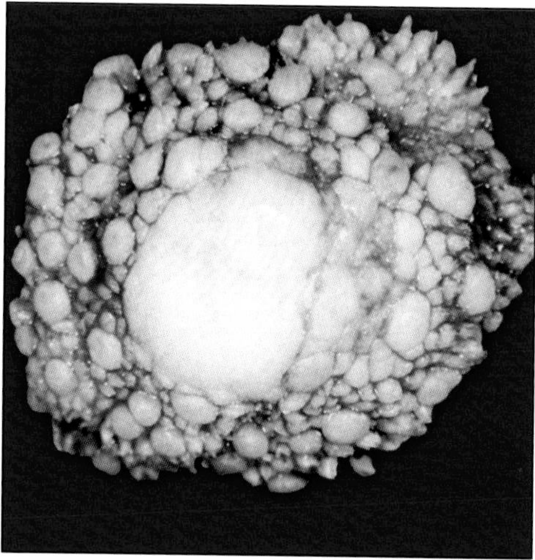

*(**Left**) Granular cell tumors present clinically as either a smooth-surfaced, submucosal swelling or nodule or as a pale to white, discrete, plaque-like lesion ➩. The overlying epithelium may be pale. A concurrent, secondary Candida infection may contribute to the pale, plaque-like appearance. (**Right**) This macroscopic photograph shows a smooth-surfaced, submucosal nodule, yielding a pale appearance. Note the remarkable number of papillary projections, part of concurrent PEH.*

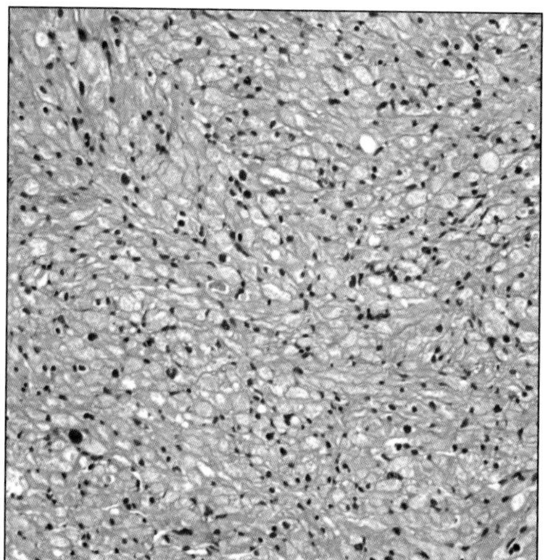

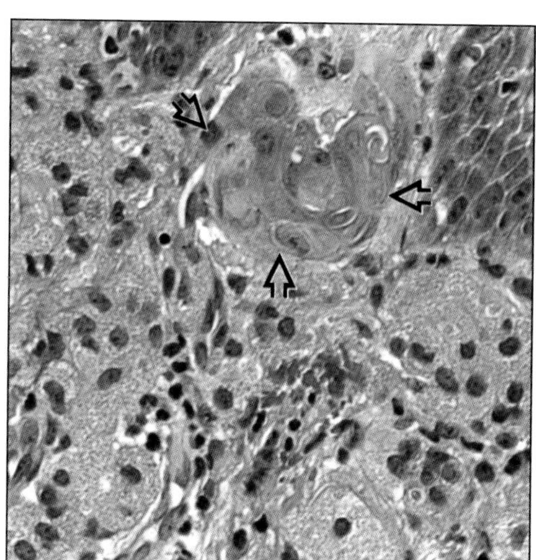

*(**Left**) There is a vaguely fascicular arrangement to these polygonal granular cells. Note abundant granular cytoplasm. The nuclei are small with hyperchromatic appearance from this intermediate power. (**Right**) Pseudoepitheliomatous hyperplasia can sometimes mimic squamous cell carcinoma ➩, as seen here. Note dyskeratosis and paradoxical maturation. Granular cells, in direct contact with areas of PEH, have granular cytoplasm with central, round nuclei.*

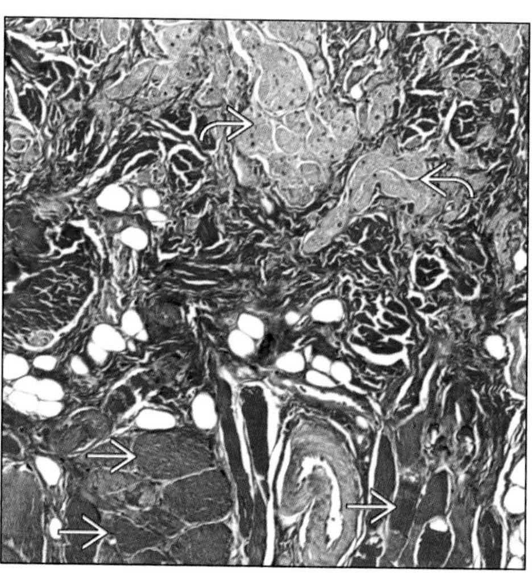

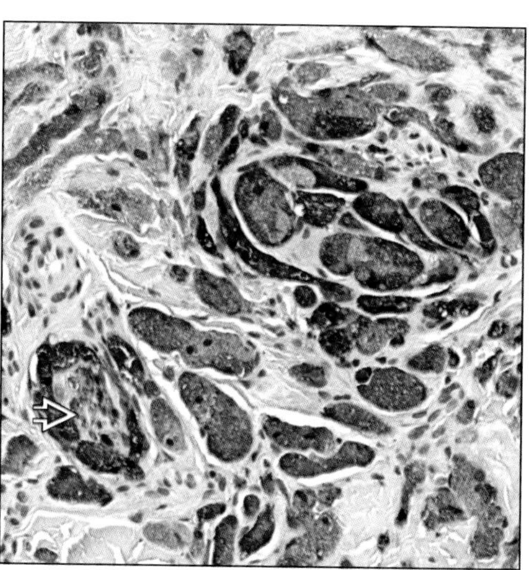

*(**Left**) A number of special stains may be of value in separating between soft tissue lesions of the oral cavity. A trichome stains the skeletal muscle brightly eosinophilic (red) ➔, while the fibrous connective tissue is blue. Note that the granular cells are lighter blue ➔. (**Right**) S100 protein strongly stains the cytoplasm and the nuclei of the granular cells. Note the entrapped peripheral nerve ➩. The tumor is derived from Schwann cells, so nerve association is common.*

CONGENITAL EPULIS OF THE NEWBORN

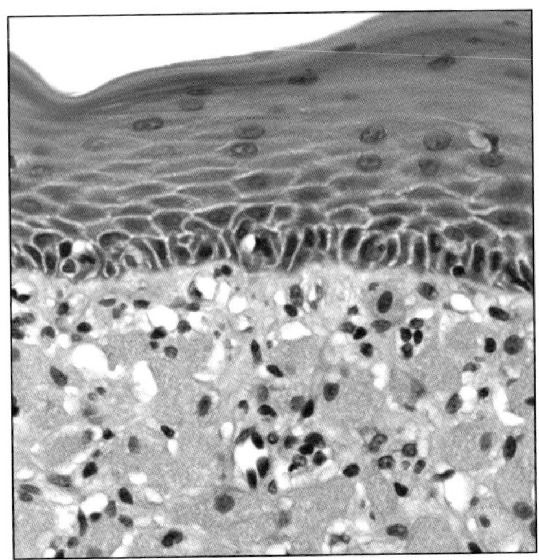

High-power photomicrograph of a congenital epulis shows a uniform epithelium with atrophy of the rete ridges. Cells with abundant granular cytoplasm and a basophilic nuclei are seen in the lamina propria.

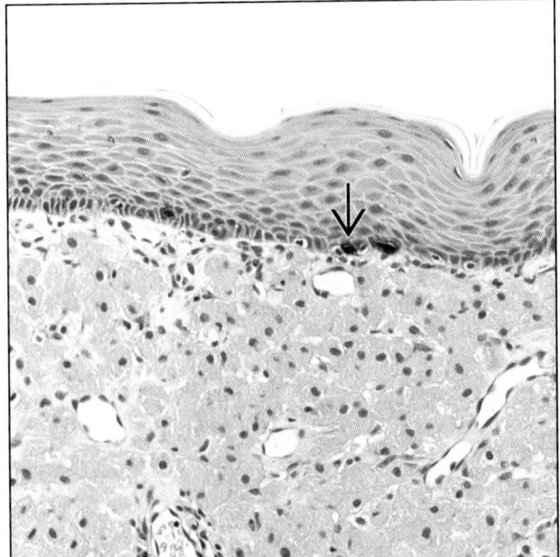

Unlike the granular cell tumor, the granular cells in congenital epulis are not immunoreactive for S100 protein. The overlying epithelium shows isolated melanocytes ⇨ positive with S100 protein.

TERMINOLOGY

Synonyms

- Neumann tumor
- Gingival granular cell tumor of infancy

Definitions

- Rare, benign congenital growth on alveolar mucosa in neonates

ETIOLOGY/PATHOGENESIS

Etiology

- Uncertain etiology, but possible nerve derivation

CLINICAL ISSUES

Epidemiology

- Incidence
  - Unknown
    - Estimated to be approximately 0.0006%
- Age
  - Neonates
- Gender
  - Female > > > > Male (8-10:1)

Site

- Gingival mucosa of maxilla or mandible
  - Maxilla > > mandible (3:1)
- Rare reports described on the tongue

Presentation

- Clinically presents at birth or within a few weeks
  - Some cases have been detected in utero by ultrasound
- Frequently occurs just lateral to midline in canine/lateral incisor region
- Smooth-surfaced
- Can cause respiratory obstruction
- Can cause feeding difficulties
- Generally presents as solitary mass
  - 10% of cases occur as multiple lesions

Natural History

- Lesions appear to regress after birth
- Rare: Complete regression without treatment

Treatment

- Surgical excision under local or general anesthesia

Prognosis

- Recurrences have not been reported even after incomplete excision
- No reports of malignant transformation

IMAGE FINDINGS

MR Findings

- Homogeneous mass without enhancement on T1WI
  - Generally excludes a vascular lesion
- Mass appears to arise from alveolus with no bone extension

MACROSCOPIC FEATURES

General Features

- Polypoid mass
- Color ranges from pink to red

Size

- Usually ≤ 2 cm
  - Reports of lesions up to 9 cm

MICROSCOPIC PATHOLOGY

Histologic Features

- Overlying epithelium is uniform in thickness, lacking rete ridges

CONGENITAL EPULIS OF THE NEWBORN

Key Facts

Terminology
- Rare, benign congenital growth on alveolar mucosa in neonates

Clinical Issues
- Female > > > > Male (8-10:1)
- Maxilla > > mandible (3:1)
- Clinically presents at birth to within a few weeks
- Lesions appear to regress after birth
- Surgical excision under anesthesia

Microscopic Pathology
- Stroma is composed of sheets of large polygonal cells
  - Abundant eosinophilic granular cytoplasm
  - Small round or oval basophilic nuclei
- Overlying epithelium is uniform in thickness

Diagnostic Checklist
- S100 protein(-) granular cells in soft tissue mass on alveolus of neonate are pathognomonic for congenital epulis

- Stroma is composed of sheets of large polygonal cells
  - Abundant eosinophilic granular cytoplasm
  - Small round or oval basophilic nuclei
- Small capillaries can be seen
- Older lesions may have fibrous septae with granular cells arranged in clusters

ANCILLARY TESTS

Immunohistochemistry
- Positive for vimentin and CD68
- Negative for S100 protein, cytokeratin, actin, desmin, estrogen and progesterone receptors

Electron Microscopy
- Granular cytoplasm shows heterogeneous electron-dense granules, lysosomes, and lipid droplets
- Cells have irregular cytoplasmic borders
- No evidence of schwannian or epithelial differentiation

DIFFERENTIAL DIAGNOSIS

Clinical DDx
- Melanotic neuroectodermal tumor of infancy
  - Midline lesion that shows melanin pigmentation
- Hemangiomas and vascular malformations
  - Usually red to blue-red in color
  - Ultrasonography findings can distinguish between the 2 entities
- Lymphatic malformations
  - Compressible mass, diagnosed by ultrasound

Granular Cell Tumor
- Has pseudoepitheliomatous hyperplasia
- Strong and diffuse S100 protein reactivity

DIAGNOSTIC CHECKLIST

Pathologic Interpretation Pearls
- Microscopic features of S100 protein(-) granular cells in soft tissue mass on alveolus of neonate are pathognomonic for congenital epulis

SELECTED REFERENCES

1. Bosanquet D et al: Congenital epulis: a case report and estimation of incidence. Int J Otolaryngol. 2009:508780, 2009
2. Eghbalian F et al: Congenital epulis in the newborn, review of the literature and a case report. J Pediatr Hematol Oncol. 31(3):198-9, 2009
3. Küpers AM et al: Congenital epulis of the jaw: a series of five cases and review of literature. Pediatr Surg Int. 25(2):207-10, 2009
4. Vered M et al: Congenital granular cell epulis presents an immunohistochemical profile that distinguishes it from the granular cell tumor of the adult. Virchows Arch. 454(3):303-10, 2009
5. Lazaris AC et al: Congenital epulis: an ultrastructural and immunohistochemical case study. Adv Clin Path. 4(4):159-63, 2000

IMAGE GALLERY

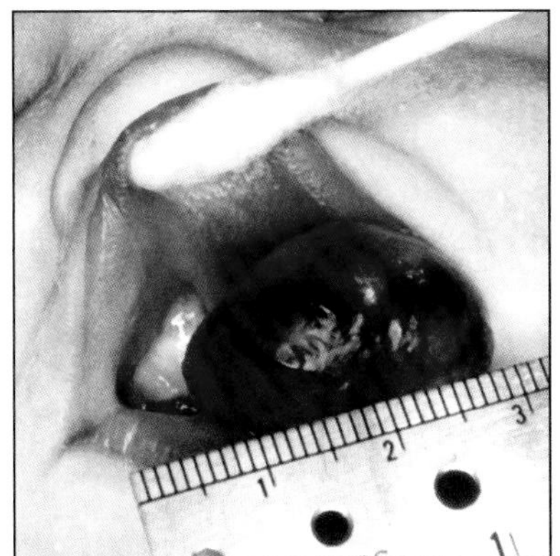

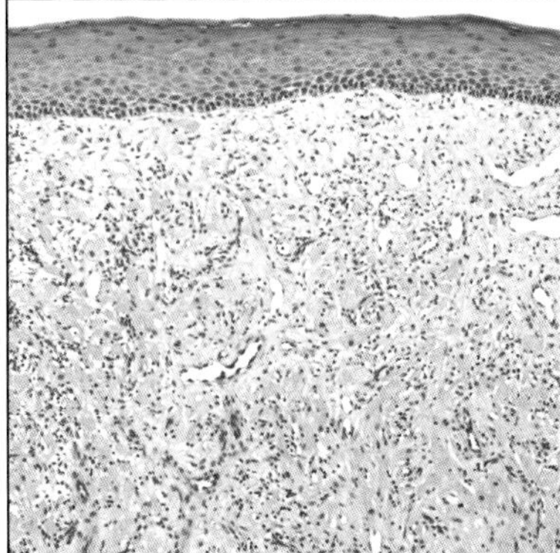
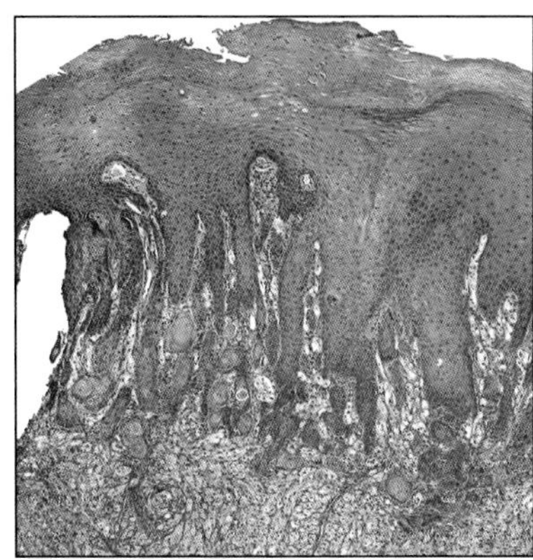

(Left) *Congenital epulis shows a red polypoid mass in the maxillary alveolus of a newborn. Most cases are ≤ 2 cm in size, and more than 90% develop in female patients.* ***(Center)*** *A low-power microscopic image of a congenital epulis shows that the epithelium of the congenital epulis is uniform and lacks rete ridges.* ***(Right)*** *More than 50% of granular cell tumors of the oral cavity exhibit pseudoepitheliomatous hyperplasia, a feature that is never seen in congenital epulis.*

PYOGENIC GRANULOMA

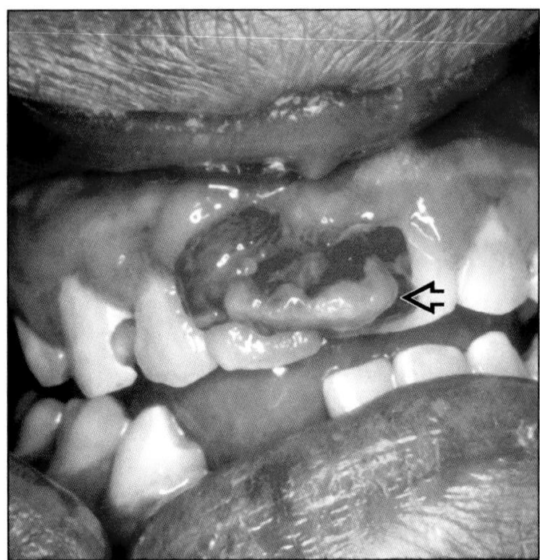

Pyogenic granuloma of the anterior maxillary gingiva in a pregnant patient presents as a red lobular mass with ulceration ➢, a common finding along with bleeding due to frequent trauma from eating or toothbrushing.

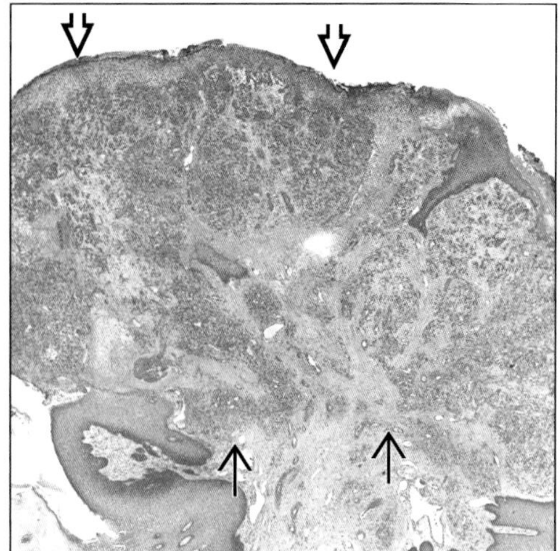

Low-power photomicrograph of an ulcerated ➢ pyogenic granuloma illustrates polypoid nature of the lesion as well as the zonal pattern of inflammation. The typical lobular pattern is more evident at the base →.

TERMINOLOGY

Abbreviations

- Pyogenic granuloma (PG)

Synonyms

- Lobular capillary hemangioma (LCH)
- Pregnancy tumor (epulis gravidarum)
- Epulis granulomatosus

Definitions

- Benign overgrowth of capillary loops with obviously vascular phenotype

ETIOLOGY/PATHOGENESIS

Etiology

- Poor oral hygiene
- Local irritants: Fractured tooth, poor restoration
- Localized trauma (biting)
- Hormones
  - Increased in pregnancy or oral contraceptive use

Pathogenesis

- Bicellular origin from endothelial and pericytic cells

CLINICAL ISSUES

Epidemiology

- Incidence
  - Common throughout the world
- Age
  - Wide range
  - Most common: Children and young adults
- Gender
  - Female > Male (2:1)
    - About 1% of pregnant women develop PG
    - Related to female hormonal influences on vessels
  - Pediatric age (up to 18 years): Male > Female

Site

- Gingiva
  - Most common (75%) site of oral cavity PG
  - Maxillary gingiva > mandibular gingiva
  - Anterior > posterior
  - Facial area > lingual or palatal gingiva
    - Some lesions however may extend from facial aspect to lingual or palatal tissue
  - Usual site in pregnant women
- Lips, tongue, and buccal mucosa are common sites
- Extraction socket (epulis granulomatosa)

Presentation

- Generally painless lobulated or polypoid mass
- Color varies with age of lesion
  - Earlier lesions tend to be highly vascular and will be purple to red
  - Older lesions become more fibrotic and appear pink
- Surface ulceration and bleeding
- Exuberant overgrowth of granulation tissue arising in recent extraction site
  - May be associated with sequestrum

Natural History

- PG in pregnancy can present in 1st trimester
  - Incidence increases throughout pregnancy
  - Often PG will spontaneously resolve after confinement

Treatment

- Surgical approaches
  - Conservative excision
    - Gingiva: Must extend to periosteum
- Remove inciting factor
  - Scaling of teeth and improve oral hygiene

Prognosis

- Excellent long-term clinical outcome
- Occasionally lesion recurs
  - PG removed during pregnancy often recurs
  - Recurrences more common in children

PYOGENIC GRANULOMA

Key Facts

Terminology
- Common, nonneoplastic polypoid growth of oral cavity

Etiology/Pathogenesis
- Poor oral hygiene
- Localized trauma (biting)

Clinical Issues
- Female predilection
- Gingiva most common location accounting for 75% of oral cavity PG
- About 1% of pregnant women develop PG (pregnancy tumor)

Microscopic Pathology
- Surface ulceration
- Small and large vessels often organized in lobular arrangement separated by fibrous septae
- Older lesions appear more collagenized

MACROSCOPIC FEATURES

General Features
- Polypoid (pedunculated), nodular or lobular mass often with surface ulceration
- May be connected by a stalk
- Soft and compressible

Size
- Range: 0.3-8 cm

MICROSCOPIC PATHOLOGY

Histologic Features
- Surface ulceration
  - Collarette of epithelium around ulcerated area
- Thickened fibrinopurulent membrane
- Below area of ulceration, mixed inflammation of neutrophils, lymphocytes, and plasma cells
  - Inflammation greater near surface and less at center
- Small and large vessels often organized in lobular arrangement separated by fibrous septae
  - When ulceration is present, this finding seen in deeper portion of lesion
  - Lumina can be absent, slit-like to prominent
  - Endothelial cells range from plump to flattened
  - Small capillaries and venules arranged around central vessel
- Vessels often are engorged with red blood cells
- Mitotic activity variable
  - Early: May have frequent but not atypical mitoses
- Older lesions appear more collagenized

DIFFERENTIAL DIAGNOSIS

Clinical Mimics
- Peripheral ossifying fibroma; peripheral giant cell granuloma
- All occur on gingiva and can become secondarily ulcerated
- Microscopically these 3 lesions are distinct

Kaposi Sarcoma
- Atypical mitoses and hyaline eosinophilic globules

Angiosarcoma
- Rare in oral cavity

SELECTED REFERENCES

1. Buchner A et al: Relative frequency of localized reactive hyperplastic lesions of the gingiva: a retrospective study of 1675 cases from Israel. J Oral Pathol Med. 39(8):631-8, 2010
2. Gordón-Núñez MA et al: Oral Pyogenic Granuloma: A Retrospective Analysis of 293 Cases in a Brazilian Population. J Oral Maxillofac Surg. Epub ahead of print, 2010
3. Saravana GH: Oral pyogenic granuloma: a review of 137 cases. Br J Oral Maxillofac Surg. 47(4):318-9, 2009
4. Zhang W et al: Reactive gingival lesions: a retrospective study of 2,439 cases. Quintessence Int. 38(2):103-10, 2007

IMAGE GALLERY

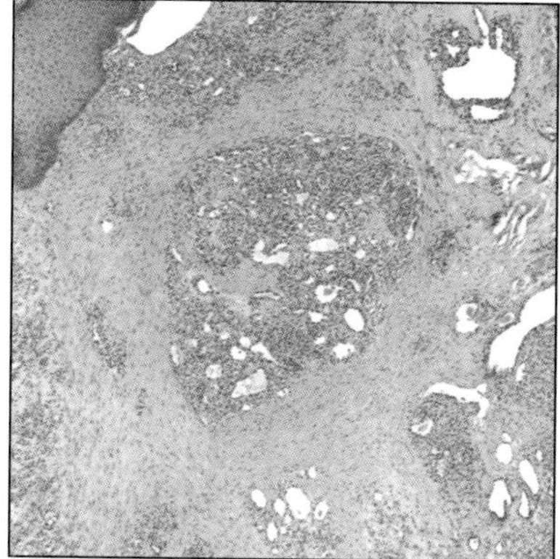

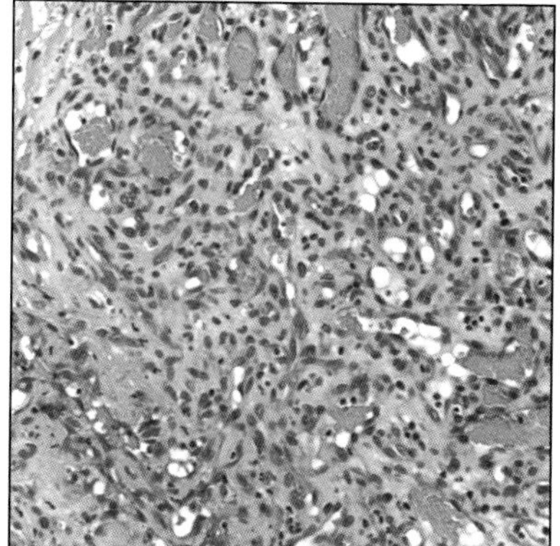

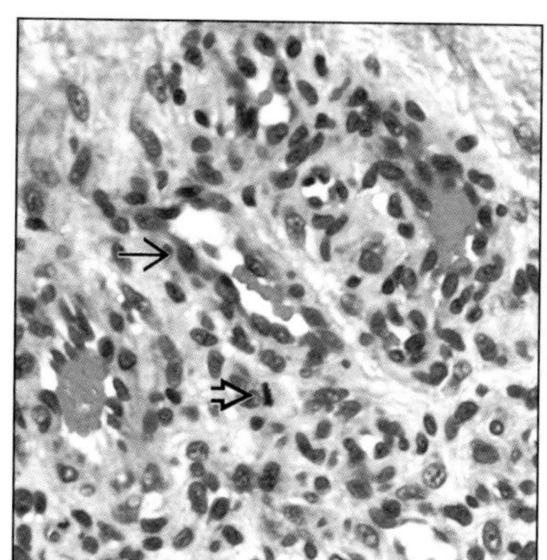

(Left) *A lobular proliferation of small and large endothelial-lined channels (surrounded by connective tissue) is noted. With age, the lesion becomes more fibrotic.* ***(Center)*** *Higher power view of pyogenic granuloma shows the numerous vessels engorged with red blood cells. Scattered inflammatory cells can be seen, especially in lesions that are ulcerated.* ***(Right)*** *Mitoses ⇨ can be seen in pyogenic granulomas, especially early lesions; however, atypical mitoses are not seen. Endothelial cells can be plump with an epithelioid appearance →.*

PERIPHERAL GIANT CELL GRANULOMA

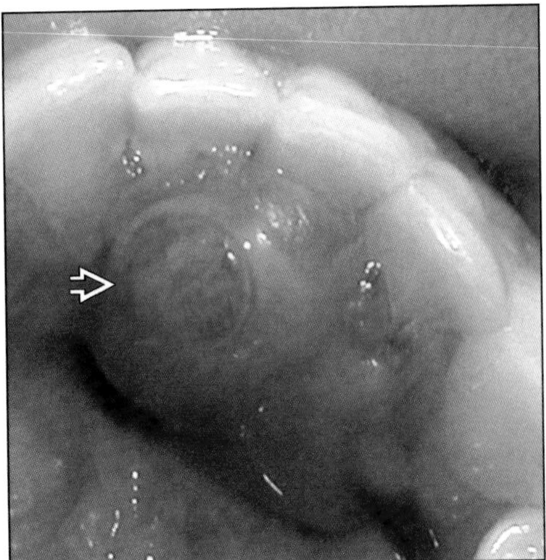

Clinical photograph shows a red nodular mass ➡ with surface ulceration.

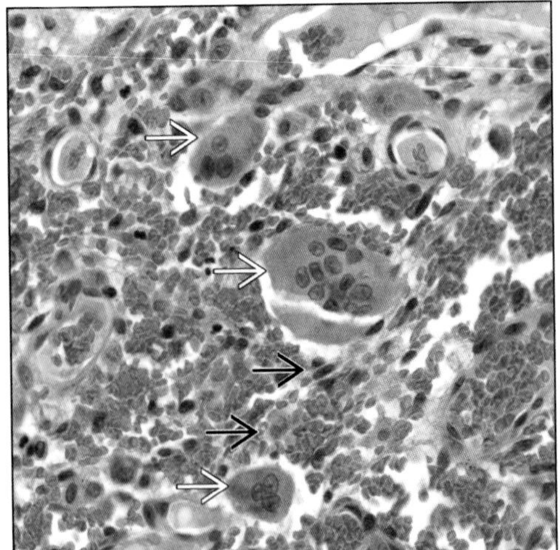

Hematoxylin & eosin shows several multinucleated giant cells ➡ with a background of oval to spindle-shaped stromal cells ⇨. Hemorrhage in the background is characteristic.

TERMINOLOGY

Abbreviations

- Peripheral giant cell granuloma (PGCG)

Synonyms

- Peripheral giant cell reparative granuloma
- Giant cell epulis

Definitions

- Reactive proliferation of multinucleated giant cells caused by trauma or irritation, exclusive to gingiva or alveolar ridge

ETIOLOGY/PATHOGENESIS

Etiology

- May arise from periodontal ligament or periosteum
- Giant cells show characteristics of osteoclasts

CLINICAL ISSUES

Epidemiology

- Incidence
  - Common
- Age
  - Wide range
  - Peak: 40-60 years
- Gender
  - Slight female predilection
    - Female > Male (1.5:1)

Site

- Exclusive to gingiva or alveolar ridge
  - Slight predilection for mandible > maxilla

Presentation

- Red to blue mass
- Sessile with smooth surface
- Pedunculated
- May be ulcerated

Treatment

- Surgical approaches
  - Excision down to periosteum
    - Follow patient for recurrences
- Dental hygiene
  - Scaling of adjacent teeth to remove local irritation

Prognosis

- Recurrences seen in approximately 10%

IMAGE FINDINGS

Radiographic Findings

- Rarely, "cupping" resorption of underlying bone (usually seen intraoperatively)
- Should not have intraosseous component

MACROSCOPIC FEATURES

General Features

- Nodular mass covered with mucosa
- Rubbery with soft consistency on cut surface

Size

- Usually < 2 cm

MICROSCOPIC PATHOLOGY

Histologic Features

- Nonencapsulated lesion
- Proliferation of multinucleated giant cells
  - Variable number of nuclei
  - Large vesicular nuclei or small nuclei
- Stroma
  - Plump to ovoid cells
  - Low mitotic index

PERIPHERAL GIANT CELL GRANULOMA

Key Facts

Terminology
- Reactive proliferation of multinucleated giant cells caused by trauma or irritation

Clinical Issues
- Common
- Exclusive to gingiva
- Often ulcerated
- Slight female predilection
- Wide age range with peak in 5th and 6th decade
- Treatment is excision down to underlying bone
- Recurrence rate is approximately 10%

Microscopic Pathology
- Proliferation of multinucleated giant cells

Top Differential Diagnoses
- Peripheral ossifying fibroma
- Pyogenic granuloma
- Fibroma

 - Hemorrhage (interstitial)
 - Hemosiderin pigment deposition
- Epithelium is frequently ulcerated
 - Fibropurulent membrane
 - Granulation tissue
- Acute and chronic inflammation
- Occasionally dystrophic mineralization or osteoid

DIFFERENTIAL DIAGNOSIS

Peripheral Ossifying Fibroma
- More cellular stroma, with predominantly spindled appearance
- May contain giant cells
- Mineralization (calcium or bone)

Pyogenic Granuloma
- Usually lobular arrangement of vessels around central vessel
- Vascular proliferation with rich inflammatory investment

Fibroma
- Haphazard arrangement of collagen bundles with scant fibroblasts

Parulis of Gingiva
- Distal opening of sinus tract from infected tooth
- Granulation tissue with acute inflammation

Central Giant Cell Lesion
- Central giant cell granuloma
 - Intraosseous, may perforate bone
- Brown tumor of hyperparathyroidism
 - Intraosseous, may perforate bone
 - Parathyroid hormone levels high
- Giant cell tumor
 - Occurs in epiphyses of long tubular bones
- Cherubism
 - Autosomal dominant bony lesion in children
 - Usually affects mandibles bilaterally

SELECTED REFERENCES

1. Salum FG et al: Pyogenic granuloma, peripheral giant cell granuloma and peripheral ossifying fibroma: retrospective analysis of 138 cases. Minerva Stomatol. 57(5):227-32, 2008
2. Mighell AJ et al: Peripheral giant cell granuloma: a clinical study of 77 cases from 62 patients, and literature review. Oral Dis. 1(1):12-9, 1995
3. Whitaker SB et al: Intraoral giant cell lesions: the peripheral and central forms of these entities. Pract Periodontics Aesthet Dent. 7(6):41-7; quiz 48, 1995
4. Shields JA: Peripheral giant-cell granuloma: a review. J Ir Dent Assoc. 40(2):39-41, 1994
5. Katsikeris N et al: Peripheral giant cell granuloma. Clinicopathologic study of 224 new cases and review of 956 reported cases. Int J Oral Maxillofac Surg. 17(2):94-9, 1988

IMAGE GALLERY

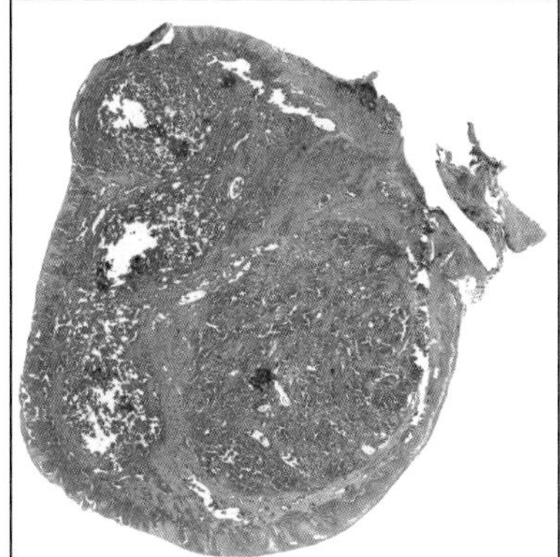

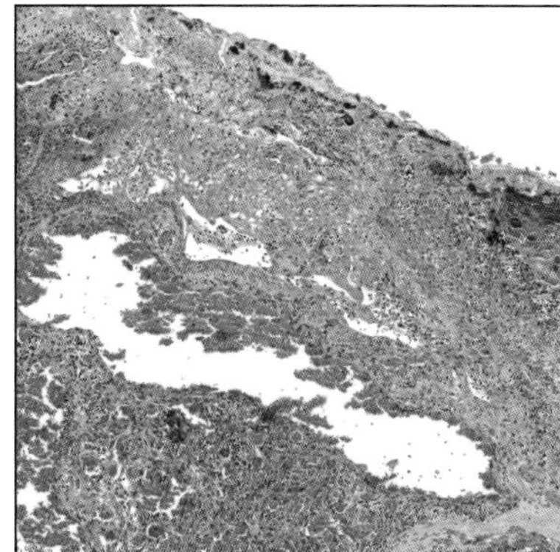

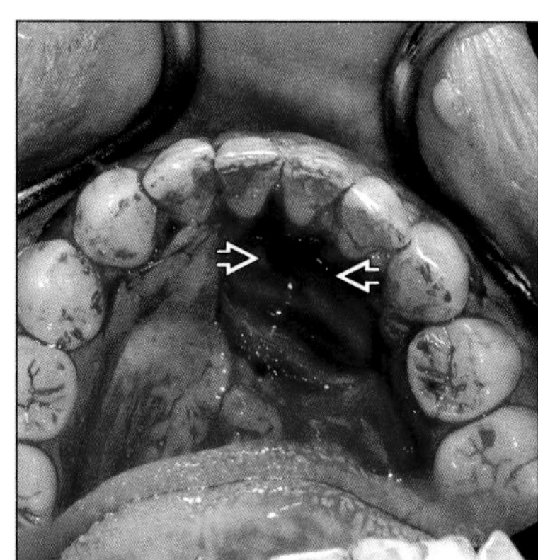

*(**Left**) Hematoxylin & eosin shows a low-power view of an exophytic soft tissue mass. Hemorrhage is easily seen. (**Center**) Hematoxylin & eosin shows an ulcer overlying a vascular stroma with a dense acute and chronic inflammatory infiltrate. (**Right**) Intraoperative photograph shows the lesion after removal of the peripheral giant cell granuloma. Note the slight erosion of bone that was underlying the lesion ⇨. (Courtesy J.T. Castle, DDS.)*

FIBROMA

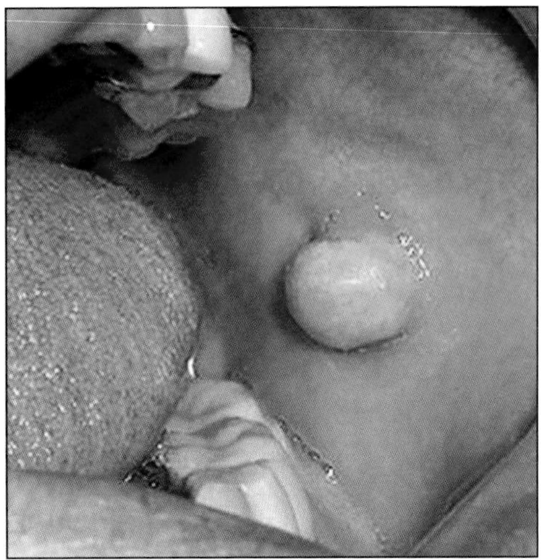

Clinical photograph shows a smooth-surfaced nodule on the buccal mucosa. Fibromas like these are often the result of occlusal trauma.

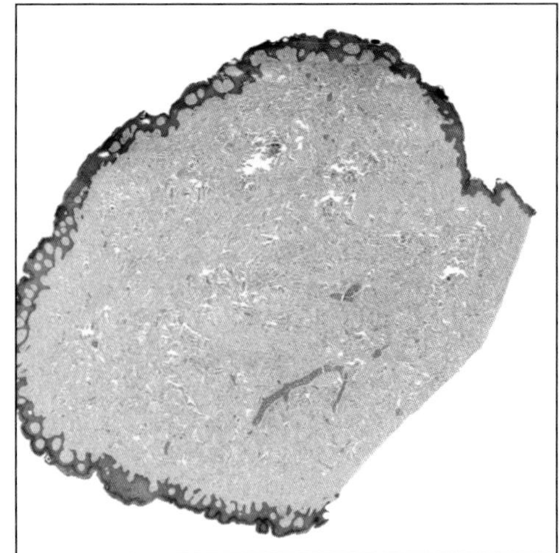

Hematoxylin & eosin shows a low-power view of an exophytic nodular mass composed of dense collagen.

TERMINOLOGY

Synonyms

- Irritation fibroma
- Traumatic fibroma
- Focal or localized hyperplasia

Definitions

- Proliferation of fibrous connective tissue in response to local irritation

ETIOLOGY/PATHOGENESIS

Etiology

- Reactive fibrous proliferation due to trauma or irritation
  - Trauma
    - Lip or cheek biting
    - Accidental injury
    - Factitious habits
  - Local irritation
    - Accumulation of plaque and calculus
    - Dental restorations with poor contours or margins
    - Orthodontic appliances
    - Dentures

CLINICAL ISSUES

Epidemiology

- Incidence
  - Most common oral cavity "tumor"
- Age
  - 4th to 6th decades
- Gender
  - Male > Female (2:1)

Site

- Free mucosal sites
  - Buccal, lip, tongue
- Fixed mucosal sites
  - Gingiva

Presentation

- Papillary or polypoid mass
  - Pain associated with secondary traumatic ulceration

Treatment

- Surgical approaches
  - Simple excision

Prognosis

- Recurrence is rare

MACROSCOPIC FEATURES

General Features

- Nodular mass surfaced by mucosa
- May be ulcerated

Size

- Usually > 1.5 cm

MICROSCOPIC PATHOLOGY

Histologic Features

- Collagen bundles arranged in haphazard fashion
- Unencapsulated
- Covered by stratified squamous epithelium
  - Epithelium may demonstrate atrophy
  - Secondary trauma may result in hyperkeratosis or ulcer

DIFFERENTIAL DIAGNOSIS

Peripheral Ossifying Fibroma

- Exclusive to gingiva
- More cellular stroma
- Mineralization or calcified spicules within stroma

FIBROMA

Key Facts

Terminology
- Focal proliferation of fibrous connective tissue in response to local irritation
- Synonyms: Irritation fibroma, traumatic fibroma, focal or localized fibrous hyperplasia

Clinical Issues
- Painful or painless mass
- Mucosa or gingiva
- Simple surgical excision

Microscopic Pathology
- Collagen bundles arranged in haphazard fashion
- Surfaced by stratified squamous epithelium
- 2° trauma may result in hyperkeratosis or ulcer

Top Differential Diagnoses
- Peripheral ossifying fibroma
- Granular cell tumor
- Peripheral giant cell granuloma
- Pyogenic granuloma

Granular Cell Tumor
- Granular eosinophilic cells are set in dense stroma but S100 protein positive

Peripheral Giant Cell Granuloma
- Exclusive to gingiva
- Proliferation of multinucleated giant cells
- Stroma contains plump to ovoid cells with erythrocytes

Pyogenic Granuloma
- Vascular proliferation, usually lobular
- Surface ulceration with rich inflammatory infiltrate

Mucocele (Retention vs. Extravasation)
- Mucin extravasated into stroma
- Adjacent inflamed minor salivary glands

Parulis of Gingiva
- Distal opening of sinus tract from infected tooth
- Granulation tissue with acute inflammation

Mesenchymal Tumors
- Lipoma
  - Lobular arrangement of fat cells
- Hemangioma
  - Vascular proliferation
- Neurofibroma
  - Interlacing bundles of spindle-shaped cells
  - Wavy nuclei
- Traumatic neuroma
  - Haphazard proliferation of mature nerve bundles

Giant Cell Fibroma
- Grossly appears papillary
- Numerous large, stellate fibroblasts

SELECTED REFERENCES

1. Stoopler ET et al: Clinicopathologic challenge: a solitary submucosal mass of the oral cavity. Int J Dermatol. 47(4):329-31, 2008
2. Torres-Domingo S et al: Benign tumors of the oral mucosa: a study of 300 patients. Med Oral Patol Oral Cir Bucal. 13(3):E161-6, 2008
3. Esmeili T et al: Common benign oral soft tissue masses. Dent Clin North Am. 49(1):223-40, x, 2005
4. Ono Y et al: Clinical study of benign lesions in the oral cavity. Acta Otolaryngol Suppl. (547):79-84, 2002
5. Satorres Nieto M et al: Prevalence of biopsied oral lesions in a service of oral surgery. Med Oral. 6(4):296-305, 2001
6. McGinnis JP Jr: Review of the clinical and histopathologic features of four exophytic gingival lesions--the pyogenic granuloma, irritation fibroma, peripheral giant cell granuloma, and peripheral ossifying fibroma. J Okla Dent Assoc. 77(3):25-30, 1987
7. Bouquot JE et al: Oral exophytic lesions in 23,616 white Americans over 35 years of age. Oral Surg Oral Med Oral Pathol. 62(3):284-91, 1986
8. Kornbrot A et al: Benign soft tissue tumors of the oral cavity. Int J Dermatol. 22(4):207-14, 1983
9. Buchner A et al: Localized hyperplastic lesions of the gingiva: a clinicopathological study of 302 lesions. J Periodontol. 48(2):101-4, 1977

IMAGE GALLERY

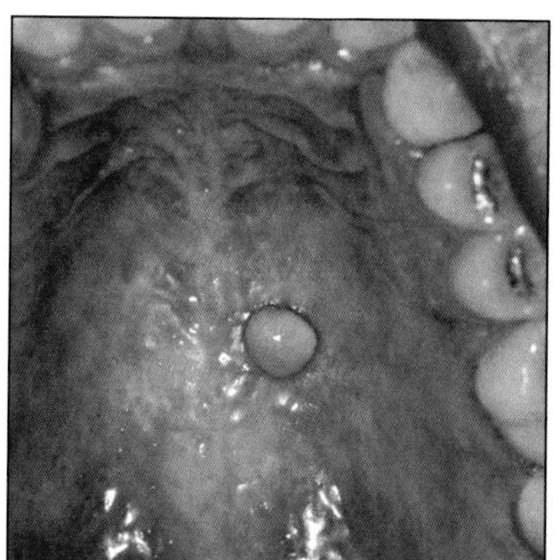

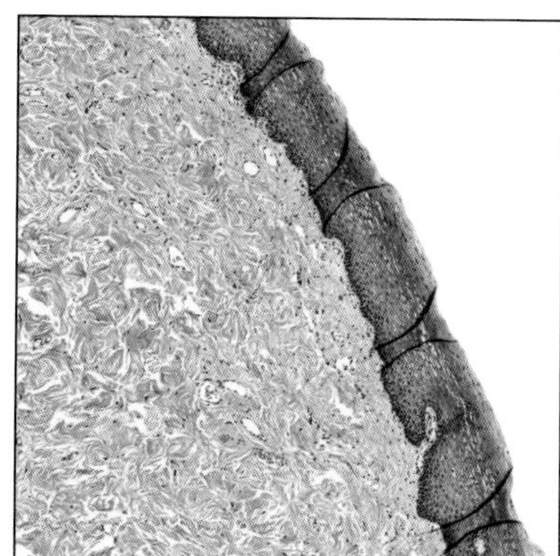

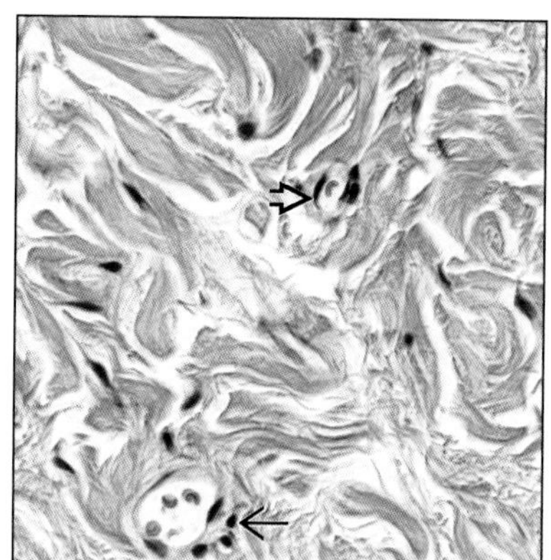

*(**Left**) Clinical photograph shows a smooth-surfaced pink nodule of the hard palate. (**Center**) Hematoxylin & eosin shows dense collagen beneath an epithelial surface that demonstrates atrophy of the rete ridges. (**Right**) Hematoxylin & eosin shows a high-power view of collagen bundles arranged in a haphazard fashion. Scattered inflammatory cells may be seen, usually lymphocytes ⇒ or plasma cells. Small blood vessels are seen throughout the specimen ⇒.*

PERIPHERAL OSSIFYING FIBROMA

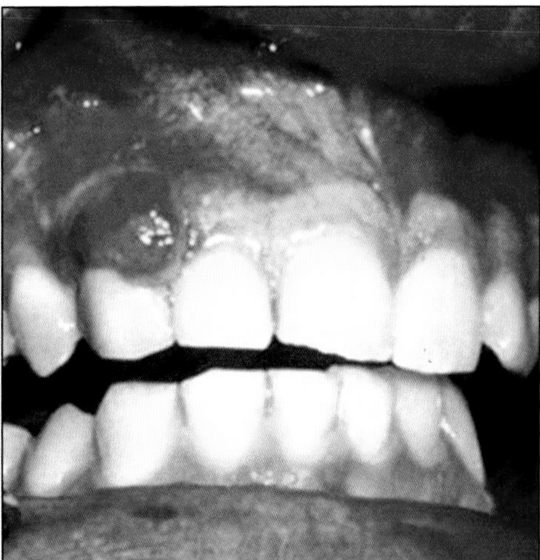

Clinical photograph shows a red-pink focally ulcerated mass of the maxillary gingiva.

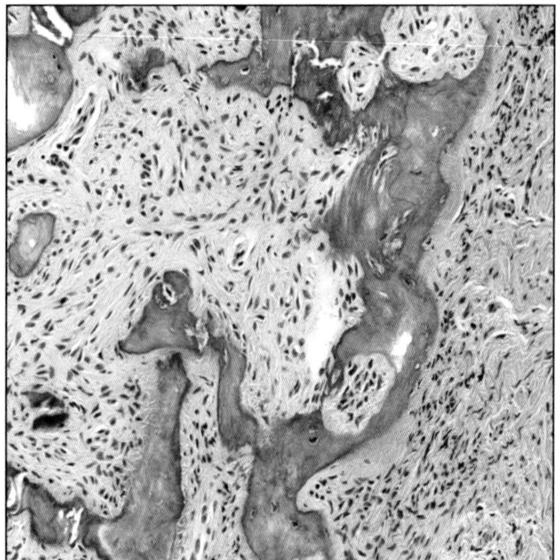

Hematoxylin & eosin shows a cellular fibroblastic proliferation associated with bone.

TERMINOLOGY

Abbreviations

- Peripheral ossifying fibroma (POF)

Synonyms

- Peripheral fibroma with calcification
- Peripheral odontogenic fibroma
  - Now considered a distinct entity

Definitions

- Reactive proliferation of fibrous tissue with mineralization exclusive to gingiva

ETIOLOGY/PATHOGENESIS

Etiology

- May be associated with chronic irritation
  - Poorly fitting dentures
  - Orthodontic appliances
  - Plaque and calculus

Origin

- Cells from periosteum
- Cells from periodontal ligament

CLINICAL ISSUES

Epidemiology

- Incidence
  - Common
- Age
  - Wide range, with peak in 2nd decade
- Gender
  - Female > Male (2:1)

Site

- Exclusive to gingiva, usually interdental papilla
  - More commonly affects maxilla
  - Incisor to canine region

Presentation

- Painful or painless mass
  - Pedunculated
  - Sessile
  - Red or pink
  - Often ulcerated

Treatment

- Surgical approaches
  - Surgical excision down to periosteum
- Dental hygiene
  - Complete scaling of adjacent teeth to remove local irritants

Prognosis

- Excellent
- Moderate rate of recurrence

MACROSCOPIC FEATURES

General Features

- Nodular mass
- Usually ulcerated
- Cut surfaces may reveal a gritty mineralized component

Size

- Variable, but usually < 2 cm

MICROSCOPIC PATHOLOGY

Histologic Features

- Cellular fibroblastic stroma
- Mineralized component
  - Bone, trabecular
  - Bone, woven
  - Dystrophic calcification
  - Cementum

PERIPHERAL OSSIFYING FIBROMA

Key Facts

Terminology
- Reactive proliferation of fibrous tissue with mineralization, exclusive to gingiva

Clinical Issues
- Exclusive to gingiva, usually interdental papilla
- Painful or painless mass
- Recurrences develop, but complete scaling of adjacent teeth to remove local irritants may help

Microscopic Pathology
- Cellular fibroblastic stroma
- Mineralized component, showing calcification, bone, or cementum

Top Differential Diagnoses
- Peripheral giant cell granuloma
- Pyogenic granuloma
- Irritation fibroma

  - Combination
  - Occasionally absent
- Surface may be ulcerated
  - Fibrinopurulent surface deposit
  - Granulation tissue

DIFFERENTIAL DIAGNOSIS

Peripheral Giant Cell Granuloma
- Proliferation of multinucleated giant cells
- Stroma containing plump to ovoid cells

Pyogenic Granuloma
- Vascular proliferation, usually lobular
- Reactive endothelial cells with inflammation

Irritation Fibroma
- Haphazard bundles of collagen
- Lack of calcification or bone

Parulis of Gingiva
- Distal opening of sinus tract from infected tooth
- Granulation tissue with acute inflammation

Giant Cell Fibroma
- Papillary appearance
- Numerous large, stellate fibroblasts

Epulis Fissuratum with Osseous and Chondromatous Metaplasia
- Caused by poorly fitting denture
- Multiple folds of hyperplastic tissue
- Variable chronic inflammatory infiltrate
- May show inflammatory papillary hyperplasia

SELECTED REFERENCES

1. García de Marcos JA et al: Peripheral ossifying fibroma: a clinical and immunohistochemical study of four cases. J Oral Sci. 52(1):95-9, 2010
2. Prasad S et al: Peripheral ossifying fibroma and pyogenic granuloma. Are they interrelated? N Y State Dent J. 74(2):50-2, 2008
3. Salum FG et al: Pyogenic granuloma, peripheral giant cell granuloma and peripheral ossifying fibroma: retrospective analysis of 138 cases. Minerva Stomatol. 57(5):227-32, 2008
4. Moon WJ et al: Peripheral ossifying fibroma in the oral cavity: CT and MR findings. Dentomaxillofac Radiol. 36(3):180-2, 2007
5. Zhang W et al: Reactive gingival lesions: a retrospective study of 2,439 cases. Quintessence Int. 38(2):103-10, 2007
6. Kumar SK et al: Multicentric peripheral ossifying fibroma. J Oral Sci. 48(4):239-43, 2006
7. Carrera Grañó I et al: Peripheral ossifying fibroma. Report of a case and review of the literature. Med Oral. 6(2):135-41, 2001
8. Cuisia ZE et al: Peripheral ossifying fibroma--a clinical evaluation of 134 pediatric cases. Pediatr Dent. 23(3):245-8, 2001
9. Buchner A et al: The histomorphologic spectrum of peripheral ossifying fibroma. Oral Surg Oral Med Oral Pathol. 63(4):452-61, 1987

IMAGE GALLERY

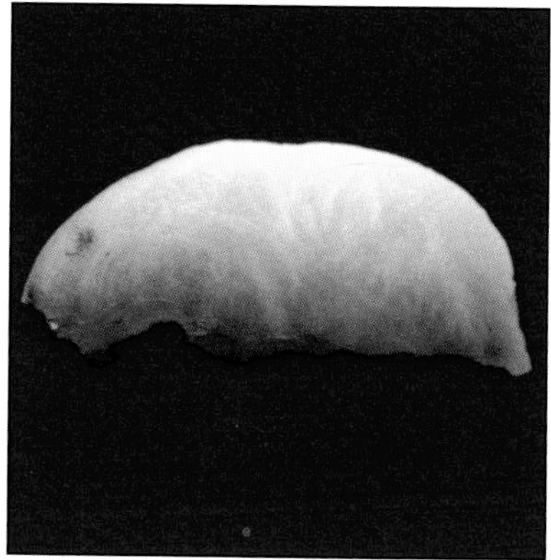

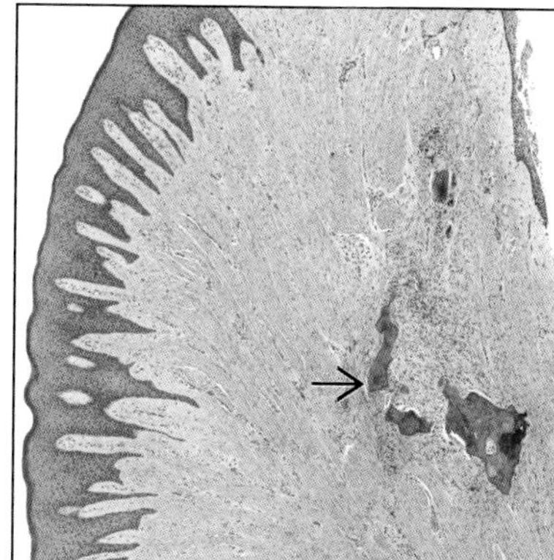

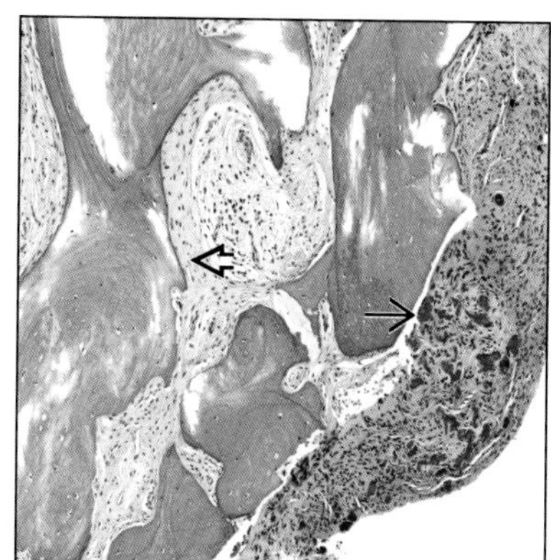

(Left) Gross photograph shows an intact squamous mucosa overlying a heavily fibrotic stroma with streaks of ossified material and fibrous connective tissue dissecting between the tissue. *(Center)* Hematoxylin & eosin shows a nonulcerated fibrous mass with central mineralization ➔. The lesion, in this case, is composed of only a small fraction of mineralized tissues. *(Right)* Hematoxylin & eosin shows well-formed bone ➪ with areas of dystrophic calcifications ➔ within the cellular fibrotic stroma.

MUCOSAL NEUROMA

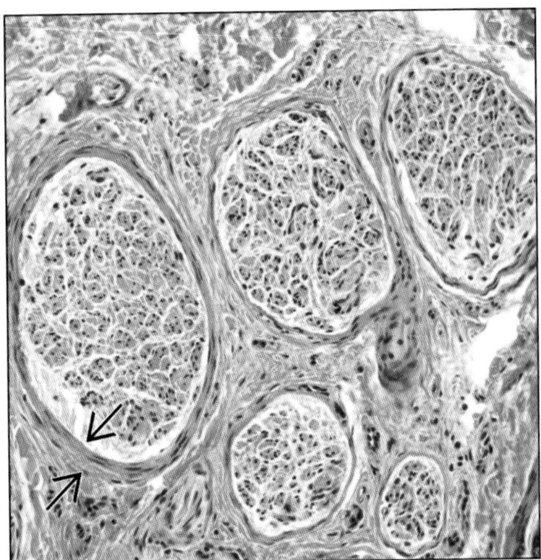

Hematoxylin and eosin shows a medium-power view of the hyperplastic nerve bundles characteristic of neuromas. The thickened perineurium ⇒ is readily seen at this power.

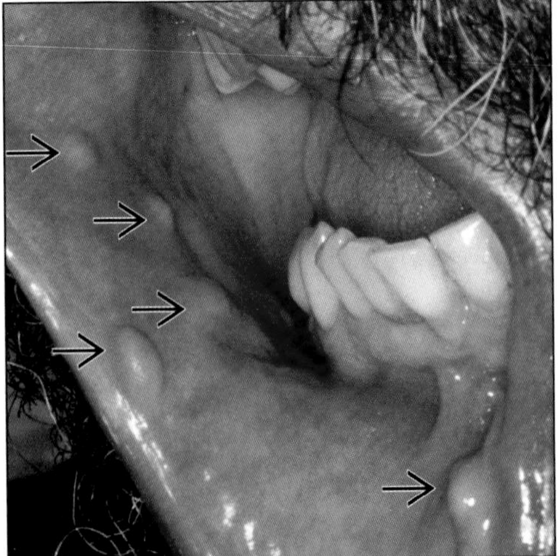

Clinical photo shows a patient with multiple endocrine neoplasia (MEN) type 2B. Numerous mucosal neuromas ⇒ are common in these patients, frequently the initial presentation of the disease.

TERMINOLOGY

Definitions

- Proliferation of nerves, often in plexiform pattern

ETIOLOGY/PATHOGENESIS

Syndrome Association

- Multiple endocrine neoplasia (specifically MEN2B)
  - Germline mutations of *RET* proto-oncogene on chromosome 10
  - Autosomal dominant
  - Spontaneous mutations in ~ 50%
- *PTEN* hamartoma tumor syndrome (PHTS)
  - Cowden syndrome
  - Bannayan-Riley-Ruvalcaba syndrome

CLINICAL ISSUES

Epidemiology

- Incidence
  - Most cases of multiple lesions are found in those with MEN2B
  - Rare solitary cases
- Age
  - First identified in childhood
- Gender
  - Equal gender distribution

Site

- Tongue
- Lips
  - Bilateral commissure is characteristic
- Less common
  - Gingiva, palate, buccal mucosa
- Extraoral sites
  - Conjunctiva and intestines

Presentation

- Soft, mucosa-colored papules

Laboratory Tests

- Serologic or genetic evaluation for MEN2B
  - Specifically, calcitonin levels to exclude medullary thyroid carcinoma

Natural History

- MEN2B
  - Mucosal neuromas
    - Often 1st sign of syndrome
  - Medullary thyroid carcinoma
    - Develops in 2nd or 3rd decade
    - Will occur in 90%
  - Pheochromocytoma (adrenal)
    - Risk increases with age
    - May be bilateral
  - Dysmorphic features
    - Marfanoid, thin face, thickened lips

Treatment

- No treatment indicated for mucosal neuromas
- Treatment for MEN2B
  - Prophylactic removal of thyroid gland
  - Close follow-up for development of pheochromocytomas

Prognosis

- Solitary lesions: Excellent
- MEN2B
  - Depends on early diagnosis
  - Specifically determined by associated malignancies

MACROSCOPIC FEATURES

General Features

- Mucosa-covered papule

MUCOSAL NEUROMA

Key Facts

Terminology
- Proliferation of nerves, often in plexiform pattern

Clinical Issues
- Rare solitary cases
- Tongue and lips most frequently
- Most cases of multiple lesions are found in patients with MEN2B
- Soft mucosa-colored papules

Microscopic Pathology
- Nonencapsulated
- Hyperplasia of nerve bundles
- Prominent thickening of perineurium

Top Differential Diagnoses
- Neurofibroma
- Traumatic neuroma
- Palisaded encapsulated neuroma
- Schwannoma (neurilemoma)

Size
- Small, usually 0.2-0.4 cm

MICROSCOPIC PATHOLOGY

Histologic Features
- Nonencapsulated, with haphazard distribution
- Hyperplasia of nerve bundles
- Prominent thickening of perineurium

ANCILLARY TESTS

Immunohistochemistry
- S100 protein positive

DIFFERENTIAL DIAGNOSIS

Neurofibroma
- May blend with surrounding tissue
- Spindle cells with variable collagen
- May be associated with neurofibromatosis

Traumatic Neuroma
- Lacks prominent perineurium
- History of trauma

Palisaded Encapsulated Neuroma
- Encapsulated, at least partially
- Spindle cells

Schwannoma (Neurilemoma)
- Characteristic Antoni A and B
- Verocay bodies
- Hyalinized vessels

DIAGNOSTIC CHECKLIST

Clinically Relevant Pathologic Features
- Multiple mucosal neuromas may indicate a syndromic association

SELECTED REFERENCES

1. Sallai A et al: Orolabial signs are important clues for diagnosis of the rare endocrine syndrome MEN 2B. Presentation of two unrelated cases. Eur J Pediatr. 167(4):441-6, 2008
2. Schaffer JV et al: Mucocutaneous neuromas: an underrecognized manifestation of PTEN hamartoma-tumor syndrome. Arch Dermatol. 142(5):625-32, 2006
3. Nishihara K et al: Solitary mucosal neuroma of the hard palate: a case report. Br J Oral Maxillofac Surg. 42(5):457-9, 2004
4. Toogood AA et al: No mutation at codon 918 of the RET gene in a family with multiple endocrine neoplasia type 2B. Clin Endocrinol (Oxf). 43(6):759-62, 1995
5. Cangiarella J et al: Mucosal neuromas and plexiform neurofibromas: an immunocytochemical study. Pediatr Pathol. 13(3):281-8, 1993

IMAGE GALLERY

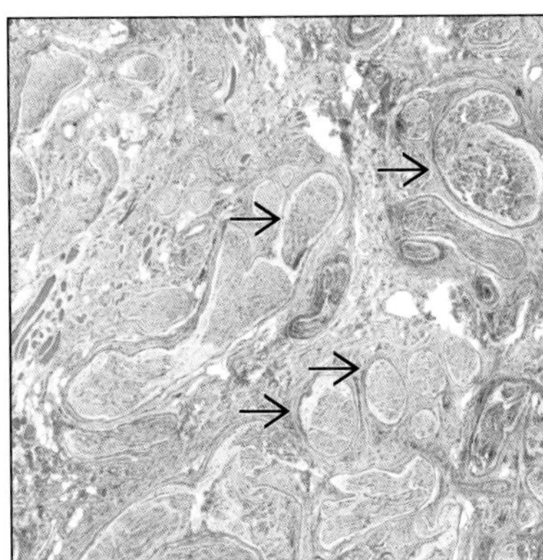

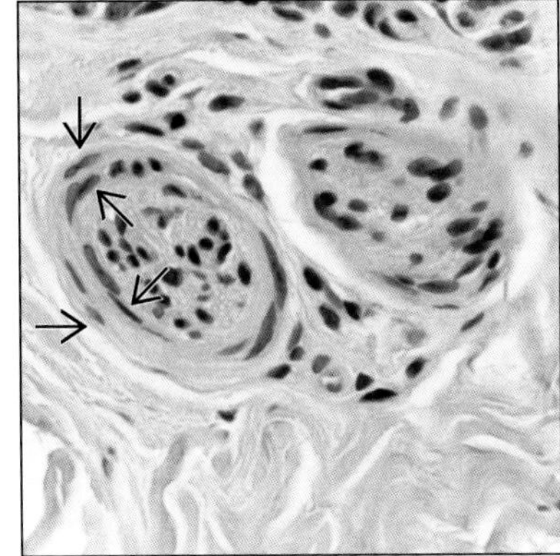

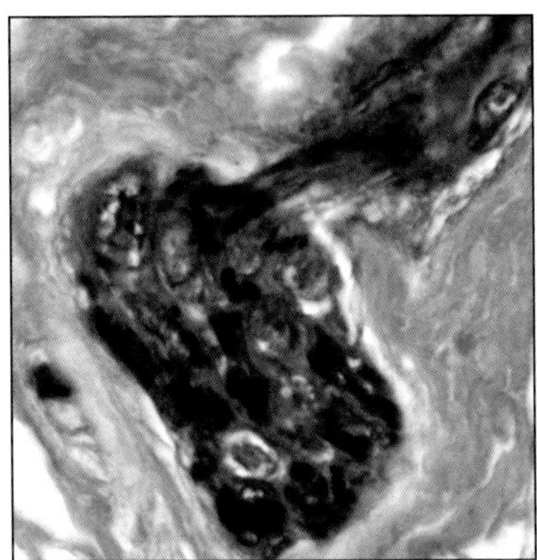

(Left) *Low-power view of a mucosal neuroma shows distinct nerve bundles ⇒ in a loose fibrovascular connective tissue background.* ***(Center)*** *High-power view shows the thickened perineurium ⇒ of a mucosal neuroma. A traumatic neuroma lacks this distinctive feature helping to distinguish the two entities, as they can be histologically similar.* ***(Right)*** *High-power view highlights the strong nuclear and cytoplasmic S100 protein reaction.*

ACQUIRED MELANOCYTIC NEVUS

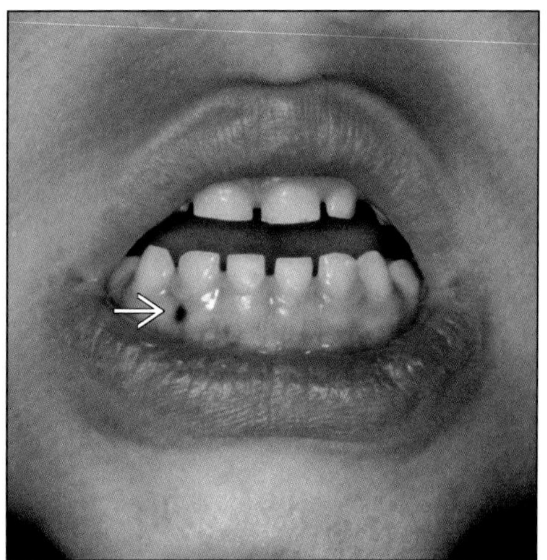

Junctional nevus in a 3-year-old child presents as an asymptomatic pigmented lesion of the attached gingiva ➔. This was noted by the mother within the 1st year of life.

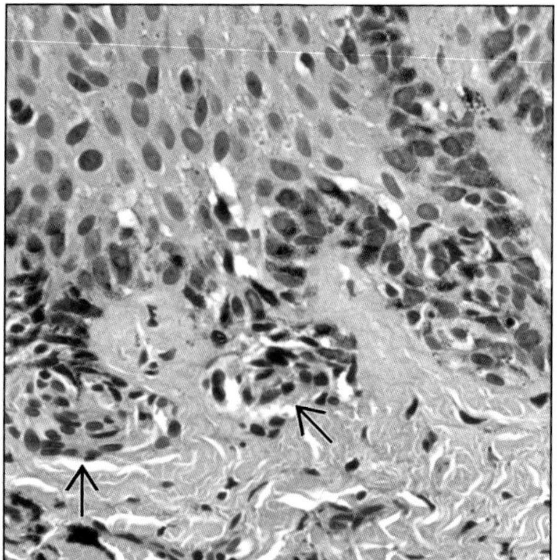

High-power photomicrograph of a junctional nevus shows abundant melanin pigment within the basal cells and nests of neval cells at the tip of the rete ridges ➔.

TERMINOLOGY

Synonyms
- Nevocellular nevus
- Mole

Definitions
- Localized proliferation of benign melanocytes that colonize the epithelium

ETIOLOGY/PATHOGENESIS

Pathogenesis
- Of neural crest origin, nevus cells migrate to select ectodermal structures during embryogenesis

CLINICAL ISSUES

Epidemiology
- Incidence
  - ~ 4.35 per 10,000,000 population/year
- Age
  - Wide range at diagnosis: 3-85 years
  - Average: 35 years
- Gender
  - Female > Male (1.5:1)
- Ethnicity
  - White patients have more nevi than blacks or Asians

Site
- Most common intraoral locations are
  - Palate, gingiva, buccal mucosa, lip
- Blue nevus: Most common on hard palate

Presentation
- Like cutaneous counterpart, oral melanocytic nevi have various stages, which correlate with specific microscopic findings
  - **Junctional nevus**
    - Brown to black macule
    - Well demarcated
    - Generally < 0.6 cm
  - **Compound nevus**
    - Painless tan to brown papule
    - Smooth epithelial surface
  - **Intramucosal (intradermal) nevus**
    - Most common intraoral melanocytic nevus
    - Can present as solitary sessile mass and be mistaken for fibroma
    - Up to 15% of intraoral nevi are amelanotic
    - Usually < 1 cm
    - May eventually involute
  - **Blue nevus**
    - 2nd most common intraoral melanocytic nevus
    - Blue coloration due to Tyndall effect
    - Dome-shaped or macule < 1 cm
    - Cellular variant of blue nevus less common, especially in oral cavity

Treatment
- Surgical approaches
  - Any oral pigmentation that cannot be reliably diagnosed based on clinical findings alone should be biopsied
    - There should be low threshold for biopsy, particularly if pigment is of recent onset
  - Small lesion size makes it amenable to excisional biopsy

Prognosis
- No reports of malignant transformation of intraoral melanocytic nevi or blue nevi
  - This is true, even in patients with multiple nevi

MACROSCOPIC FEATURES

Size
- Most are < 1 cm

ACQUIRED MELANOCYTIC NEVUS

Key Facts

Terminology

- Localized proliferation of benign melanocytes that colonize the epithelium

Clinical Issues

- Most common intraoral locations are palate, gingiva, buccal mucosa, and lip
- Blue nevus most commonly presents intraorally on hard palate
- Like cutaneous counterpart, oral melanocytic nevi have various stages, which correlate with specific microscopic findings
- Up to 15% of intraoral nevi are amelanotic
- Blue nevus 2nd most common intraoral melanocytic nevus
- Any oral pigmentation that cannot be reliably diagnosed based on clinical findings alone should be biopsied
- No reports of malignant transformation of intraoral melanocytic nevi or blue nevi

Microscopic Pathology

- Junctional nevus: Nests of melanocytic neval cells in basal cell layer
- Compound nevus: Nests of melanocytic neval cells in basal cell layer and in lamina propria
- Intramucosal nevus: Neval cells only present in lamina propria
- Blue nevus: Spindle-shaped melanocytes present deep in lamina propria parallel to epithelium
- Combined nevus with features of both blue nevus and melanocytic nevus have been reported

MICROSCOPIC PATHOLOGY

Histologic Features

- **Junctional nevus**
  - Nests or thèques of melanocytic neval cells in basal cell layer
  - Lack of dendritic processes
  - May see variation in nuclear size and shape, but no atypia present
  - Mitotic figures rare
- **Compound nevus**
  - Nests of melanocytic neval cells in basal cell layer
  - Groups of neval cells begin to "drop off" into superficial lamina propria
  - Pigment in both epithelium and submucosa variable
  - Rete may be elongated
  - Cellular atypia absent
- **Intramucosal (intradermal) nevus**
  - Thèques of nevocytes are no longer observed in epithelium
  - Nevocytes only present in lamina propria
  - Neval cells can be variably sized
  - More superficial neval cells can be larger, epithelioid in appearance forming nests (thèques)
    - Intracellular melanin frequently seen
  - Neval cells centrally located are smaller with less cytoplasm and usually lack pigment
    - Lymphocytic appearance
  - Deeper neval cells are often spindle-shaped similar to Schwann cells
- **Blue nevus**
  - Spindle-shaped melanocytes present deep in lamina propria
    - Cells arranged in parallel fashion to epithelium
    - Abundant melanin pigment
    - Branching dendritic extensions
  - Combined nevus with features of both blue nevus and melanocytic nevus are rare

DIFFERENTIAL DIAGNOSIS

Melanotic Macule/Focal Melanosis

- Melanin pigment in occasional basal cells
- Generally no significant increase in melanocytes
- Incontinent melanin &/or melanophages in superficial lamina propria

Physiologic Pigmentation

- Similar histology to melanotic macule

Melanoacanthoma

- Acanthotic epithelium with scattered dendritic melanocytes throughout
- No increase in melanocytes

Oral Melanoma

- Acral lentiginous and superficial spreading type
- Atypical melanocytes in basal layer invading superficial epithelium (Pagetoid spread)
- Invasion of melanocytes into lamina propria

SELECTED REFERENCES

1. Müller S: Melanin-associated pigmented lesions of the oral mucosa: presentation, differential diagnosis, and treatment. Dermatol Ther. 23(3):220-9, 2010
2. De Giorgi V et al: Prevalence and distribution of solitary oral pigmented lesions: a prospective study. J Eur Acad Dermatol Venereol. 23(11):1320-3, 2009
3. Meleti M et al: Pigmented lesions of the oral mucosa and perioral tissues: a flow-chart for the diagnosis and some recommendations for the management. Oral Surg Oral Med Oral Pathol Oral Radiol Endod. 105(5):606-16, 2008
4. Meleti M et al: Melanocytic nevi of the oral mucosa - no evidence of increased risk for oral malignant melanoma: an analysis of 119 cases. Oral Oncol. 43(10):976-81, 2007
5. Hatch CL: Pigmented lesions of the oral cavity. Dent Clin North Am. 49(1):185-201, ix-x, 2005
6. Kauzman A et al: Pigmented lesions of the oral cavity: review, differential diagnosis, and case presentations. J Can Dent Assoc. 70(10):682-3, 2004

ACQUIRED MELANOCYTIC NEVUS

Microscopic Features

(Left) Low-power image of a compound nevus of the lip shows uniform nests or thèques of neval cells in the epithelium. Neval nests are also noted in the superficial lamina propria. Zones of differentiation can be appreciated on this view with larger cells ➡ appearing closer to the epithelium; in the deeper area, the cells appear more spindled ➡. (Right) High-power image shows a compound nevus with neval cells "dropping off" from the epithelium into the lamina propria ➡.

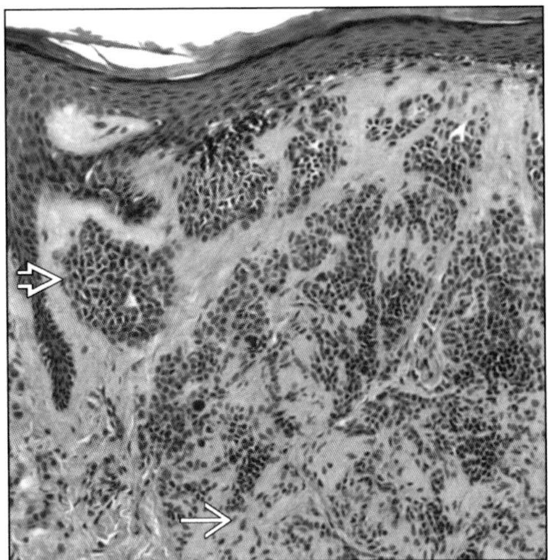

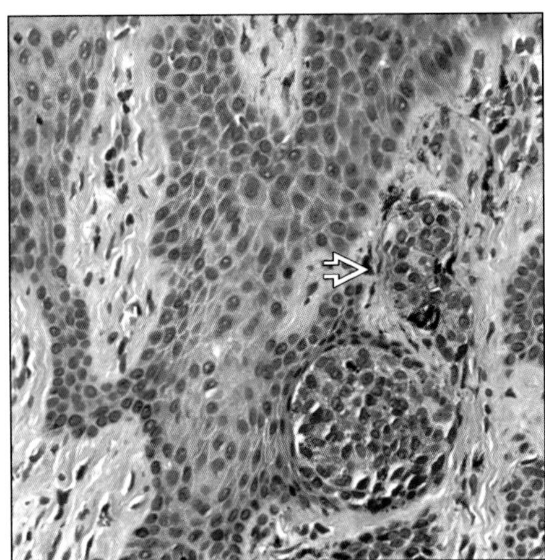

(Left) High-power photomicrograph of the superficial zone of a compound nevus shows epithelioid neval cells with abundant cytoplasm. The neval cells tend to form thèques ➡. (Right) Neval cells in the deepest portion of the lamina propria can appear spindled, similar to fibroblasts or Schwann cells. This is a feature of more mature nevi. The neval cells lack melanin and exhibit a neurotized appearance where the neval cells are palisaded and surrounded by wavy or mature collagen.

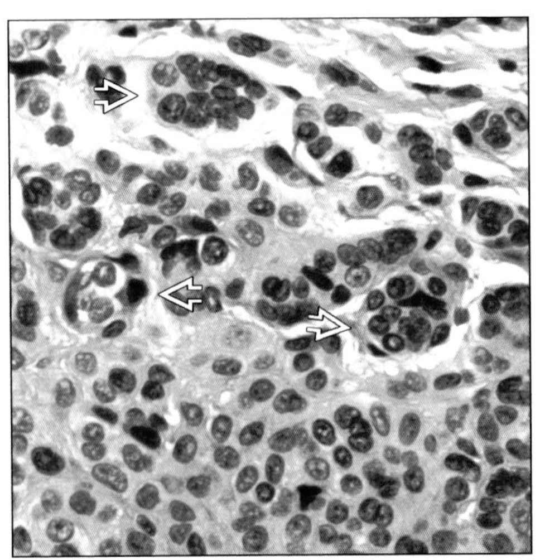

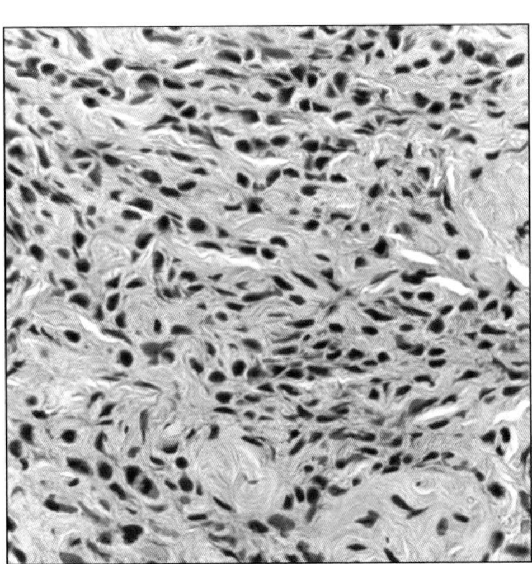

(Left) Pigmented intramucosal (intradermal) nevus of the buccal mucosa is seen. Abundant nests or thèques of pigmented neval cells are present in submucosa. Unlike compound nevus, no neval cells are found in epithelium. (Right) This intradermal nevus lacks melanin pigment as well as neval nests. The cells have less cytoplasm and appear more lymphocytic. This more mature type of nevus lacks cytologic atypia and can be confirmed by S100 protein immunohistochemistry.

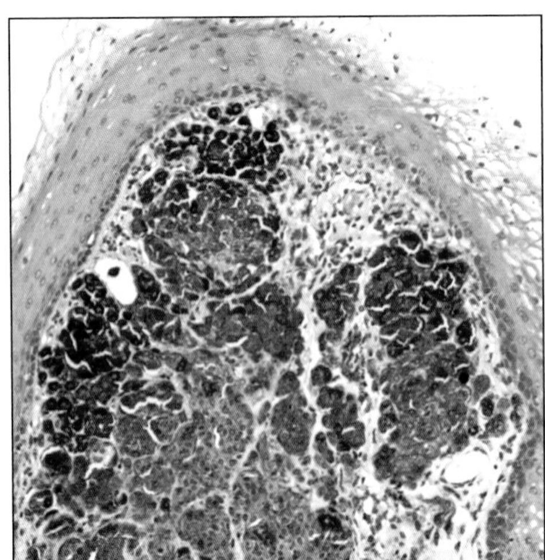

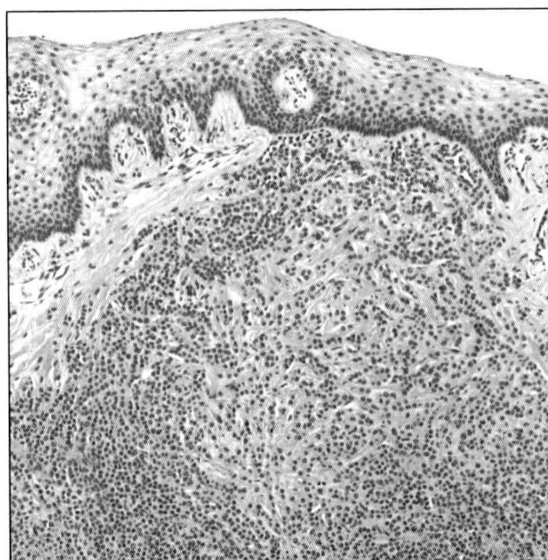

Microscopic Features and Differential Diagnosis

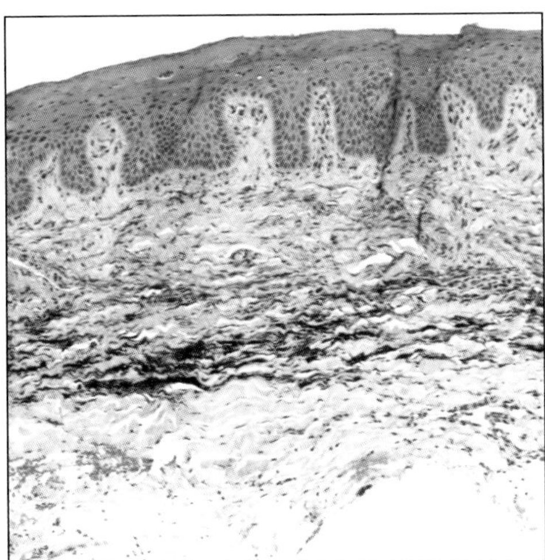

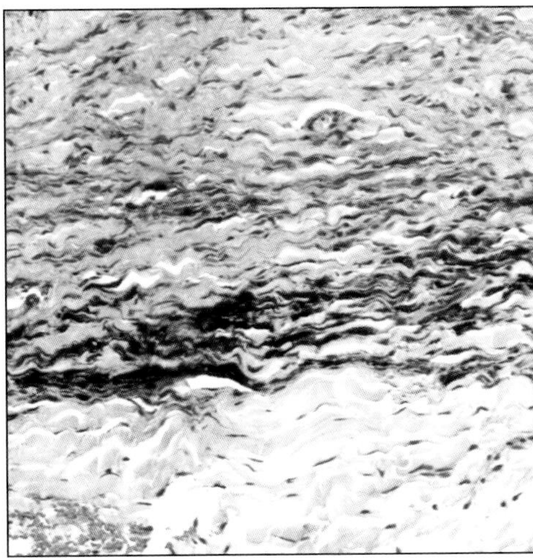

(Left) *Blue nevus of the hard palate shows melanin pigment in the deeper lamina propria parallel to the epithelial surface. The blue nevus is typically well delineated from the surrounding tissue.* ***(Right)*** *Deeply pigmented, elongated, spindle-shaped melanocytes in the lamina propria are characteristic of a blue nevus. The blue nevus can be associated with an overlying melanocytic nevus, termed a "combined nevus."*

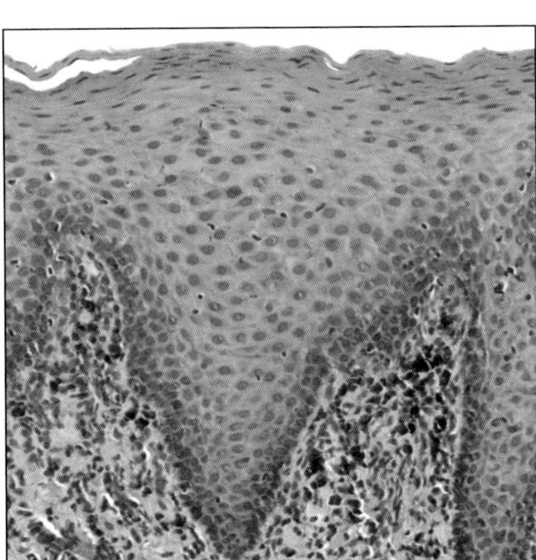

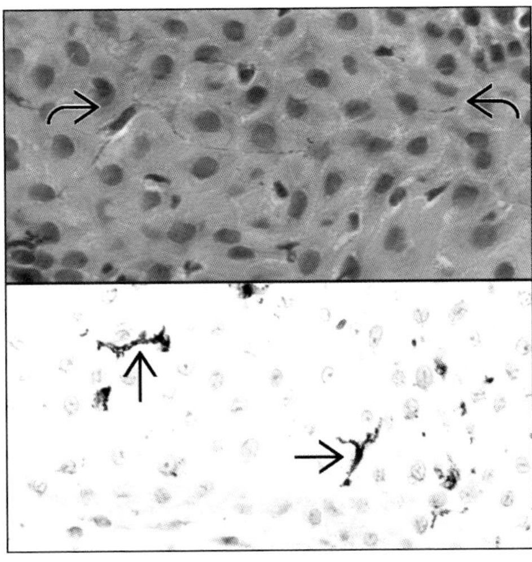

(Left) *Melanoacanthoma of the buccal mucosa demonstrates marked epithelial acanthosis and spongiosis and a chronic inflammatory cell infiltrate with melanin pigment in the superficial lamina propria.* ***(Right)*** *High-power image of melanoacanthoma shows dendritic melanocytes within the intercellular spaces of the acanthotic epithelium ↷. The melanocytes are highlighted by S100 protein immunohistochemistry (lower panel) →.*

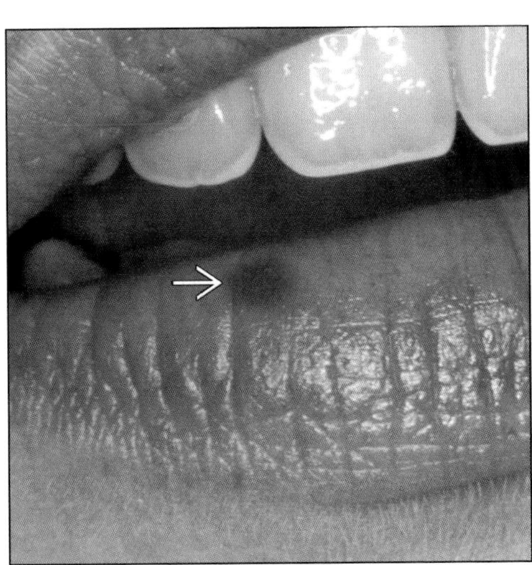

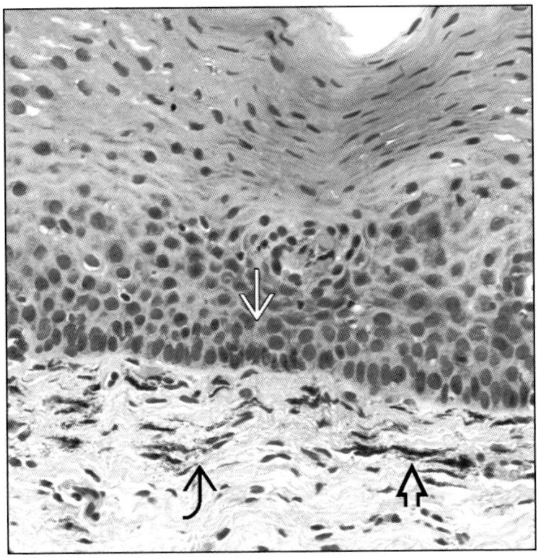

(Left) *Oral melanotic macule of the lower lip appears as a uniformly pigmented tan macule ➡. The lower lip is the most common location for melanotic macules, but they can occur anywhere in the oral cavity, including gingiva, palate, and cheek.* ***(Right)*** *The typical appearance of oral melanotic macules include melanin pigment noted in occasional basal cells ➡ and melanophages ⇨ and incontinent pigment in superficial submucosa ↷. Increased melanocytes may or may not be seen.*

TERATOMA

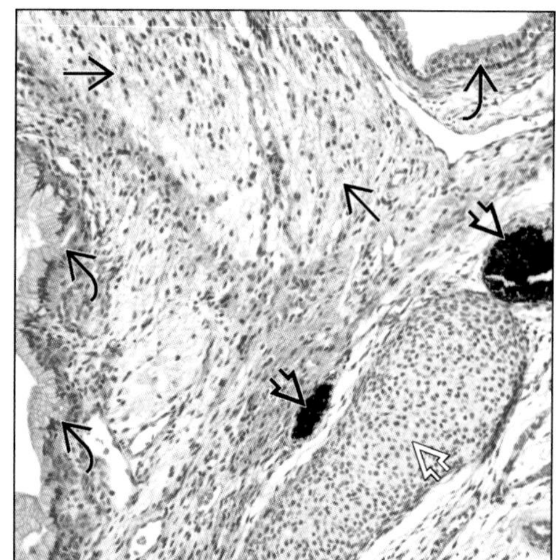

A haphazard arrangement is seen within this mature benign teratoma. There is glial tissue ⇨, retinal anlage epithelium ⇨, glandular elements ⇨, and immature cartilage ⇨.

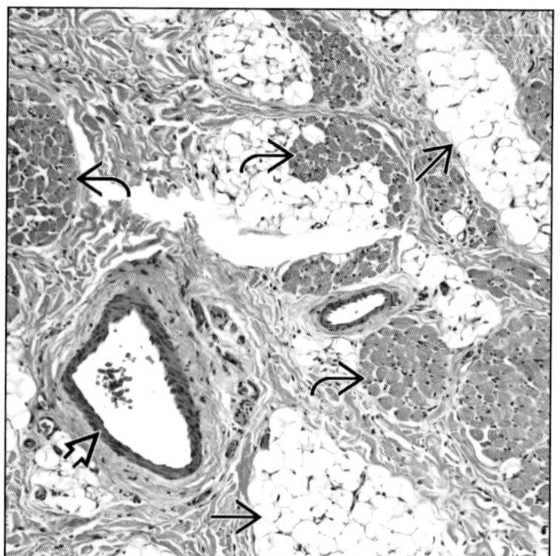

Virtually any tissue type can be seen in this section of a teratoma from a 2-day-old infant, showing mature skeletal muscle ⇨, adipose tissue ⇨, and a vessel ⇨.

TERMINOLOGY

Synonyms

- Epignathus: Teratoma that arises in oral cavity

Definitions

- Neoplasm of germ cell origin comprised of mature or immature tissues derived from all 3 germ cell layers: Ectoderm, endoderm, & mesoderm

ETIOLOGY/PATHOGENESIS

Pathogenesis

- Arise from pluripotent cells sequestered during embryogenesis
- Arise from misplaced embryonic germ cells (rests), which develop in the new location
- Incomplete division of twins (exceedingly rare)

CLINICAL ISSUES

Epidemiology

- Incidence
  - Rare
    - 1 in 4,000 live births have teratoma
    - 1-2% of these involve head and neck
- Age
  - Most are present at birth
    - May be identified during prenatal screening
- Gender
  - Female > Male

Site

- Oropharynx
  - Palate and tongue

Presentation

- At birth
  - Significant respiratory distress
  - Mass protruding from mouth
- Prenatal
  - Large mass detected by ultrasound
  - Polyhydramnios due to impaired fetal swallowing

Laboratory Tests

- Increased α-fetoprotein concentrations prenatally

Treatment

- Options, risks, complications
  - Respiratory distress
    - Tracheostomy or oral intubation
  - Unable to feed, requiring nasogastric tube
- Surgical approaches
  - Surgery must be instituted immediately in neonatal/antenatal cases to avoid morbidity or mortality
  - If mass is detected in utero, consider delivering fetus by ex utero intrapartum treatment (EXIT) procedure

Prognosis

- Even though by histology most are benign, bad outcome determined by
  - Large tumors
  - Intracranial involvement
- Concurrent germ cell tumors need to be excluded
  - Yolk sac tumor specifically is most significant
- Malignant transformation increases if tumors are not immediately resected
- Recurrences may be seen
  - Does not imply malignant transformation

IMAGE FINDINGS

Radiographic Findings

- Ultrasonographic images
  - Most common finding is multicystic mass with mixed echogenic signals

TERATOMA

Key Facts

Terminology

- Neoplasm of germ cell origin comprised of mature or immature tissues from all 3 germ cell layers

Clinical Issues

- Most tumors identified prenatally or at birth
  - Ultrasound: Multicystic mass; mixed echogenic signals
- Surgery must be instituted immediately, including EXIT procedure
- Worse outcome: Large tumor; intracranial extension

Microscopic Pathology

- Most are benign, with any tissue type identified
  - Ectoderm, mesoderm, endoderm derived
- Neural tissue is usually common
  - Primitive neural tissue may indicate malignancy

Top Differential Diagnoses

- Dermoid cyst, encephalocele

MACROSCOPIC FEATURES

General Features

- Heterogeneous tissues, firm to soft and cystic
  - Bone, cartilage, hair, teeth are frequently noted
- Gray-tan or yellow-white to translucent cut surface
- Multiloculated, cystic spaces
  - Spaces filled with white-tan creamy material, mucoid glairy material, or dark hemorrhagic fluid

Size

- Range: Up to 15 cm

MICROSCOPIC PATHOLOGY

Histologic Features

- Tissues from all 3 primordial layers: Ectoderm, mesoderm, & endoderm
- Wide array of any tissue type
- Variety of epithelial elements (squamous, respiratory, transitional, organs)
- Neural tissue is usually common
  - Brain, glial tissue, choroid plexus, pigmented retinal anlage
  - Primitive neural tissue may indicate malignancy
- Mesenchymal elements (cartilage, bone, muscle, fat)

DIFFERENTIAL DIAGNOSIS

Dermoid Cyst

- More common
- Histology limited to only skin elements
  - Cyst lined by epidermis with skin adnexal structures

Encephalocele

- Displaced neuroglial tissue
- Maintains connection to central nervous system

Glial Heterotopia

- Displaced neuroglial tissue
- No connection to central nervous system

Congential Rhabdomyosarcoma

- Malignant cells of muscular derivation
  - Positive: Desmin, myoglobin, myogenin, actins
- Lacks other tissue types

SELECTED REFERENCES

1. Benson RE et al: A large teratoma of the hard palate: a case report. Br J Oral Maxillofac Surg. 47(1):46-9, 2009
2. Freitas Rda S et al: Epignathus: two cases. Br J Oral Maxillofac Surg. 46(4):317-9, 2008
3. Hassan S et al: Massive lingual teratoma in a neonate. Singapore Med J. 48(8):e212-4, 2007
4. Celik M et al: Congenital teratoma of the tongue: a case report and review of the literature. J Pediatr Surg. 41(11):e25-8, 2006

IMAGE GALLERY

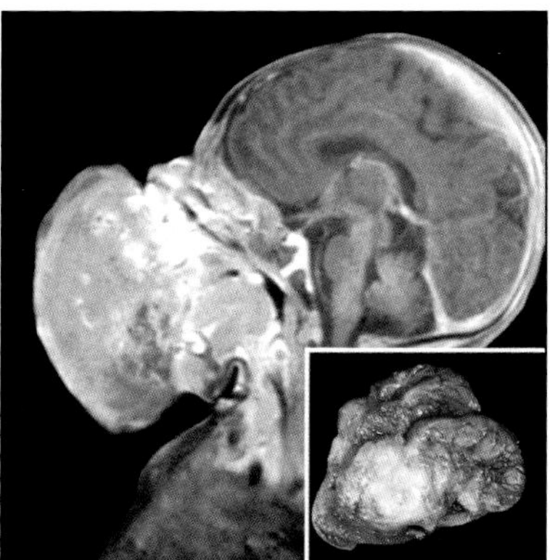

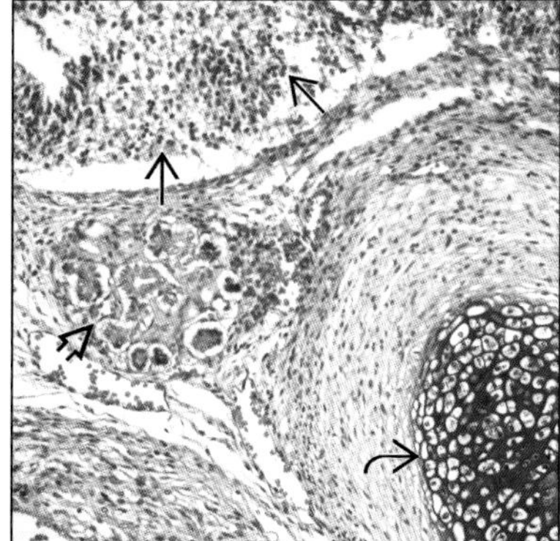

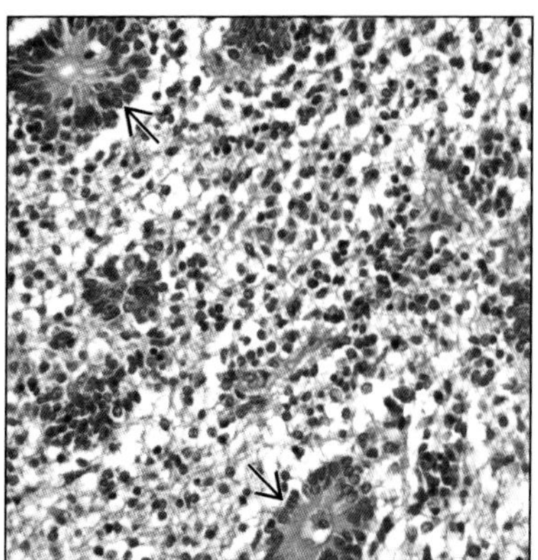

(Left) *Sagittal gadolinium-enhanced scan after delivery shows areas of enhancement within this large solid mass, which involved both the oro- and nasopharynx. The inset shows the resected mass with grumous material.* ***(Center)*** *Various neural ➔ and organ (pancreas) ⊳ elements are present in an immature mesenchyme. There is also mature cartilage ↗ in this teratoma.* ***(Right)*** *Sometimes primitive neural tissue is present, including rosette ➔ formation.*

ECTOMESENCHYMAL CHONDROMYXOID TUMOR

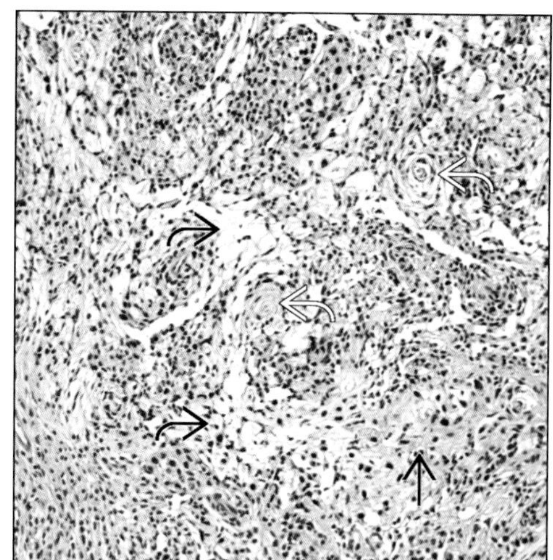

Cellular proliferation is arranged in net-like growth ➔ with associated myxoid and focally hyalinized stroma ➔. Swirling formation ➔ suggestive of neural differentiation is seen.

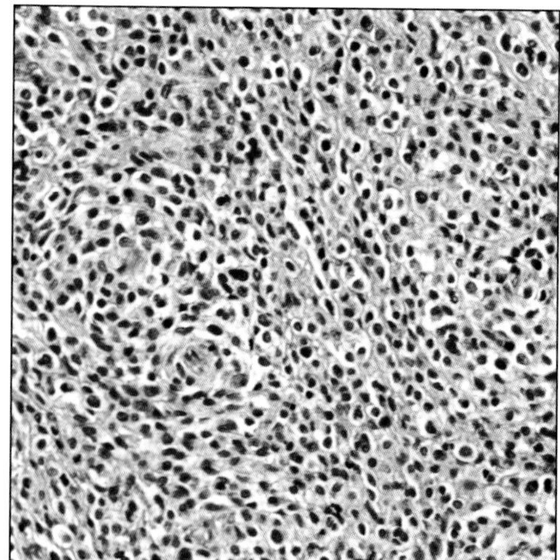

Cells are arranged in cords and strands composed of uniform-appearing small hyperchromatic nuclei and basophilic to eosinophilic to clear-appearing cytoplasm; hyalinized stroma is present.

TERMINOLOGY

Abbreviations

- Ectomesenchymal chondromyxoid tumor (ECT)

Definitions

- Benign intraoral tumor with presumed origin from undifferentiated (ecto)mesenchymal cell

ETIOLOGY/PATHOGENESIS

Controversial with Various Theories

- Derived by ectomesenchymal cells migrating from neural crest
  - Immunophenotype is supportive
- Minor salivary gland derivation
  - Lack of salivary gland tissue in these locations
- Myogenic origin
  - Immunophenotype is not supportive
- Equivalent to soft tissue myoepithelioma
  - Supported by morphologic and immunohistochemical similarities
  - Some authorities advocate using these designations interchangeably

CLINICAL ISSUES

Epidemiology

- Incidence
  - Rare
- Age
  - Occurs over wide range from 9-78 years old
    - Mean: 36.6 years
- Gender
  - Equal gender distribution

Site

- Anterior dorsal tongue is most common location
  - 1 reported case of base of tongue
  - 1 reported case of hard palate

Presentation

- Slow-growing mass
  - Submucosal with overlying intact surface without ulceration
- Painless

Treatment

- Surgical approaches
  - Excision is treatment of choice

Prognosis

- Excellent
  - Low recurrence rate likely due to inadequate excision

MACROSCOPIC FEATURES

General Features

- Submucosal circumscribed but not encapsulated nodular mass
  - May have entrapped muscle bundles at periphery
- Cut surface tan-yellow in color with gelatinous appearance

Size

- Ranges from 0.3-2.0 cm

MICROSCOPIC PATHOLOGY

Histologic Features

- Submucosal unencapsulated but well-delineated or circumscribed nodule(s) separated by fibrous stroma
- Proliferation of small round, oval, spindle, or stellate cells
  - Uniform-appearing small hyperchromatic nuclei and basophilic to eosinophilic to clear-appearing cytoplasm
  - Cells may be arranged in

ECTOMESENCHYMAL CHONDROMYXOID TUMOR

Key Facts

Terminology
- Benign intraoral tumor presumed origin from undifferentiated (ecto)mesenchymal cell

Clinical Issues
- Exclusively the tongue
  - Anterior dorsal most common location
- Slow-growing, painless mass
- Surgical excision is treatment of choice
- Excellent prognosis
  - Low recurrence rate likely due to inadequate excision

Microscopic Pathology
- Submucosal unencapsulated but well-delineated or circumscribed nodule(s) separated by fibrous stroma
- Proliferation of small round, oval, spindle or stellate cells
- Chondromyxoid to myxoid stroma, but hyalinized foci may be present
- Absence of glandular &/or myoepithelial components

Ancillary Tests
- Glial fibrillary acidic protein positive (100% of cases)
- Cytokeratin positive (92% of cases)
- S100 protein positive (60% of cases)
- Smooth muscle actin positive (54% of cases)
- Epithelial membrane antigen and desmin negative
- p63 and calponin negative

    - Cords
    - Strands
    - So-called net-like sheets
  - Nuclear pleomorphism, multinucleation, and mitotic figures typically not present
    - Cells with atypical pleomorphic hyperchromatic nuclei may be present
    - Absence of atypical mitoses and necrosis
- Chondromyxoid to myxoid stroma but hyalinized stroma may be present
  - Chondroid areas
    - Contain large cells
    - Usually a small component
- Swirling formations suggestive of neural differentiation may be present
- Absence of glandular &/or myoepithelial components
- May extend into and entrap soft tissue structures including
  - Skeletal muscle
  - Nerve branches

ANCILLARY TESTS

Histochemistry
- Alcian blue
  - Reactivity: Positive
  - Staining pattern
    - Stromal matrix
- Periodic acid-Schiff
  - Reactivity: Negative
- Mucicarmine
  - Reactivity: Positive
  - Staining pattern
    - Stromal matrix

Immunohistochemistry
- Glial fibrillary acidic protein (GFAP) positive in 100%
- Cytokeratin positive > 90%
- S100 protein positive > 60%
- Smooth muscle actin positive > 50%
- Epithelial membrane antigen and desmin negative
- p63 and calponin negative

Electron Microscopy
- Very few reports with ultrastructural findings
  - Presence of partial basal lamina
  - Absence of desmosomes or thin filaments

DIFFERENTIAL DIAGNOSIS

Myoepithelioma
- Rarely if ever localized to anterior tongue
  - Absence of adjacent salivary glands
- Usually show numerous patterns
- Characterized by presence of myoepithelial cells by light microscopy
  - Plasmacytoid &/or spindle-shaped
- More consistently positive for
  - p63
  - Calponin
  - Smooth muscle actin

Pleomorphic Adenoma
- Salivary gland tumors rarely localized to anterior dorsal tongue
- Presence of identifiable glandular differentiation by light microscopy
- Presence of immunohistochemical staining for myoepithelial cells
  - p63
  - Calponin

Myxoid Neurofibroma
- Wavy nuclei
- No chondroid areas
- Diffusely S100 protein immunoreactive

Nerve Sheath Myxoma (Classic Neurothekeoma)
- Typically located in dermis and subcutis
  - Rarely occur in association with mucous membranes
- Immunohistochemical staining limited to
  - S100 protein
  - PGP9.5

ECTOMESENCHYMAL CHONDROMYXOID TUMOR

Immunohistochemistry

Antibody	Reactivity	Staining Pattern	Comment
GFAP	Positive	Cytoplasmic	Diffuse and strong; 100% of cases
Vimentin	Positive	Cytoplasmic	Diffuse and strong; majority of cases
CK-PAN	Positive	Cytoplasmic	Variable staining (focal to diffuse) in > 90% of cases
S100	Positive	Nuclear & cytoplasmic	Focal moderate to strong in > 60% of cases
Desmin	Negative		Normal staining pattern is cytoplasmic
Calponin	Negative		Normal staining pattern is cytoplasmic
p63	Negative		Normal staining pattern is nuclear
EMA	Negative		Normal staining pattern is cytoplasmic
Actin-sm	Equivocal		Focal in 30-50% of cases

GFAP = glial fibrillary acidic protein; EMA = epithelial membrane antigen.

Ossifying Fibromyxoid Tumor of Soft Parts

- Typically located in subcutis although may occur in mucosal sites of head and neck
  - Sinonasal tract most common
  - No reported cases in anterior tongue
- Histologically associated with peripheral rim of lamellar bone
  - Up to 20% may be nonossifying
- Immunohistochemical staining includes
  - S100 protein
  - Leu-7
  - Neuron-specific enolase
  - Glial fibrillary acidic protein
  - May be desmin positive (20% of cases)
  - Typically negative for
    - Smooth muscle actin
    - Cytokeratin

Extraskeletal Myxoid Chondrosarcoma

- Location rare for chondrosarcomas of any type
- Histologically comprised of
  - Sheets of undifferentiated round, oval, or spindle-shaped cells
  - Abrupt transition to nodules of benign-appearing hyaline cartilage
  - Cartilage frequently contains central calcification and ossification
  - Hemangiopericytoma-like vascular pattern may be identified
- Undifferentiated cells immunoreactive for
  - Neuron specific enolase, Leu-7, CD99 (membranous)
  - Absence of cytokeratin, GFAP
- Cartilaginous component S100 protein positive

Chondroid Choristoma

- Predominately chondroid
- No atypia

Focal Oral Mucinosis

- Most common site is gingiva
- Myxomatous tissue with spindled and stellate fibroblasts

Mucous Retention Phenomenon (Mucocele)

- Presence of extravasated mucinous material with associated inflammatory cells
  - Numerous foamy macrophages
  - Mucicarmine strongly positive

SELECTED REFERENCES

1. Angiero F: Ectomesenchymal chondromyxoid tumour of the tongue. A review of histological and immunohistochemical features. Anticancer Res. 30(11):4685-9, 2010
2. Chopra R et al: Ectomesenchymal chondromyxoid tumor of the tongue masquerading as pleomorphic adenoma on fine needle aspiration cytology smears: a case report. Acta Cytol. 54(1):82-4, 2010
3. Seo SH et al: Reticulated myxoid tumor of the tongue: 2 cases supporting an expanded clinical and immunophenotypic spectrum of ectomesenchymal chondromyxoid tumor of the tongue. Am J Dermatopathol. 32(7):660-4, 2010
4. Pires FR et al: Clinical, histological and immunohistochemical features of ectomesenchymal chondromyxoid tumor. Oral Surg Oral Med Oral Pathol Oral Radiol Endod. 108(6):914-9, 2009
5. Portnof JE et al: Oral ectomesenchymal chondromyxoid tumor: case report and literature review. Oral Surg Oral Med Oral Pathol Oral Radiol Endod. 108(4):e20-4, 2009
6. Allen CM: The ectomesenchymal chondromyxoid tumor: a review. Oral Dis. 14(5):390-5, 2008
7. Goveas N et al: Ectomesenchymal chondromyxoid tumour of the tongue: Unlikely to originate from myoepithelial cells. Oral Oncol. 42(10):1026-8, 2006
8. Nigam S et al: Ectomesenchymal chondromyxoid tumor of the hard palate--a case report. J Oral Pathol Med. 35(2):126-8, 2006
9. Woo VL et al: Myoepithelioma of the tongue. Oral Surg Oral Med Oral Pathol Oral Radiol Endod. 99(5):581-9, 2005
10. Kaplan I et al: Ectomesenchymal chondromyxoid tumour of the anterior tongue. Int J Oral Maxillofac Surg. 33(4):404-7, 2004
11. de Visscher JG et al: Ectomesenchymal chondromyxoid tumor of the anterior tongue. Report of two cases. Oral Oncol. 39(1):83-6, 2003
12. Ide F et al: Ectomesenchymal chondromyxoid tumor of the anterior tongue with myxoglobulosislike change. Virchows Arch. 442(3):302-3, 2003
13. Kannan R et al: Ectomesenchymal chondromyxoid tumor of the anterior tongue: a report of three cases. Oral Surg Oral Med Oral Pathol Oral Radiol Endod. 82(4):417-22, 1996
14. Smith BC et al: Ectomesenchymal chondromyxoid tumor of the anterior tongue. Nineteen cases of a new clinicopathologic entity. Am J Surg Pathol. 19(5):519-30, 1995

ECTOMESENCHYMAL CHONDROMYXOID TUMOR

Clinical, Microscopic, and Immunohistochemical Features

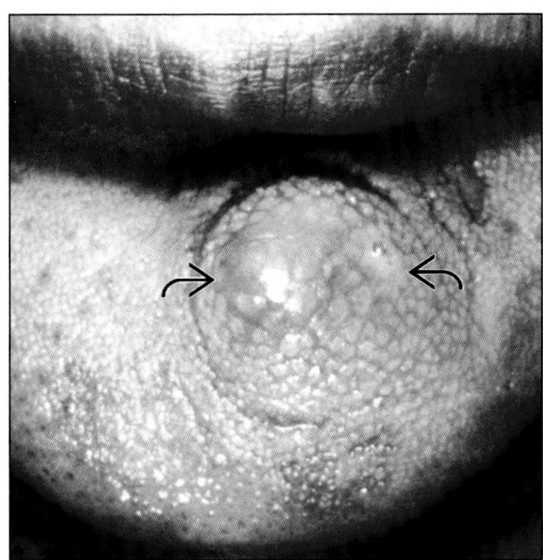

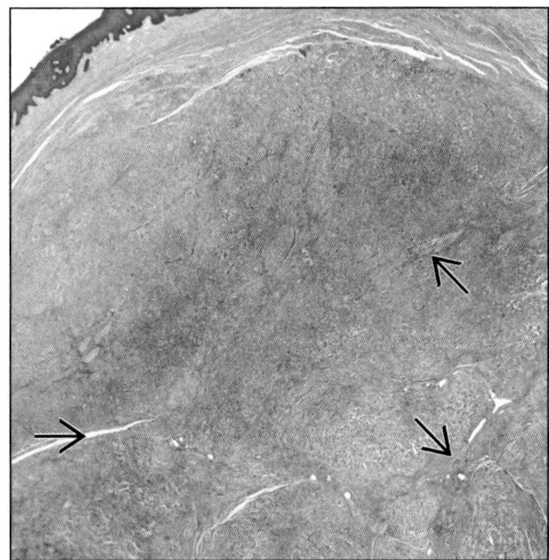

(Left) *The tumor appears as a submucosal nodule on anterior tongue ⮫ with intact overlying surface without ulceration.* ***(Right)*** *Submucosal circumscribed to well-delineated but unencapsulated hypercellular nodular proliferation with nodular foci is seen separated by fibrous stroma →. There is an absence of glandular &/or myoepithelial components.*

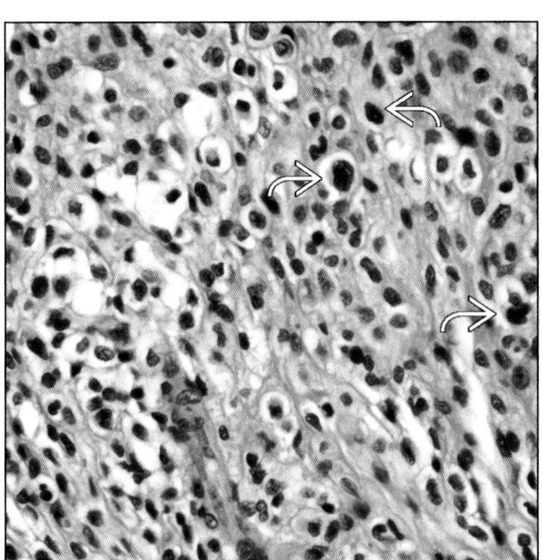

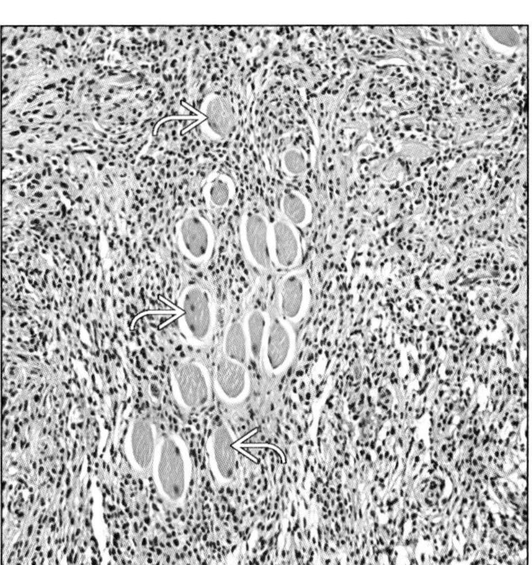

(Left) *The cells are round to oval, spindle or stellate-shaped with uniform, small, hyperchromatic nuclei arranged in cords. Occasional cells with nuclear pleomorphism may be seen ⮫.* ***(Right)*** *The neoplastic infiltrate envelops skeletal muscle ⮫ and may include nerve branches within neoplastic proliferation (not shown). The tumor typically lacks significant nuclear pleomorphism, increased mitotic activity, or necrosis.*

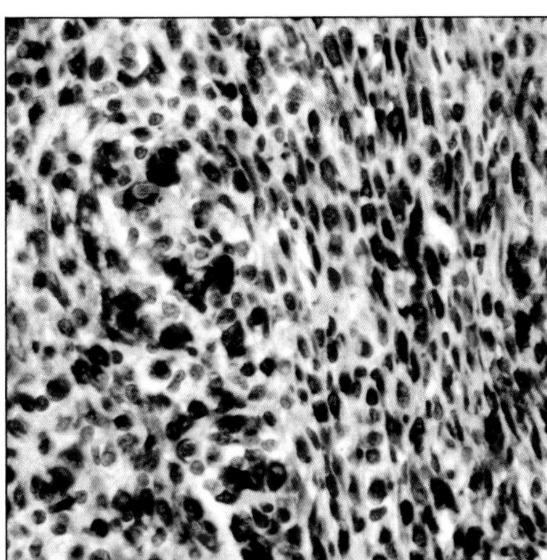

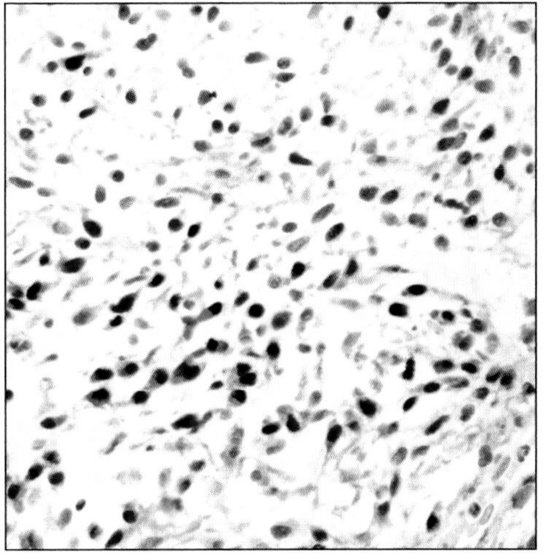

(Left) *The neoplastic cells are consistently immunoreactive for glial fibrillary acidic protein (GFAP), a finding identified in 100% of cases.* ***(Right)*** *In a majority of cases, the neoplastic cells are immunoreactive for S100 protein (nuclear and cytoplasmic). Additional immunomarkers that may be present include cytokeratin and smooth muscle actin (not shown). Lesional cells have not been reported to be immunoreactive for myoepithelial specific markers (e.g., p63, calponin).*

DYSPLASIA AND CARCINOMA IN SITU

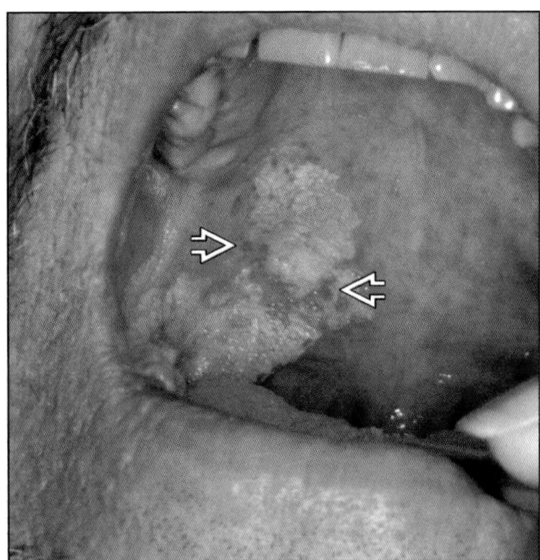

Erythroleukoplakia of the soft palate shows irregular areas of thickened homogeneous white plaques with speckled areas of erythema. Biopsy selection is important and should include the erythematous component.

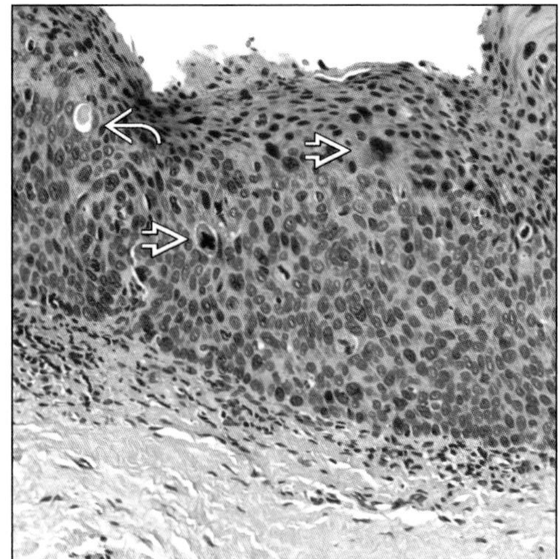

Carcinoma in situ of the soft palate exhibits full thickness cellular abnormalities, including marked pleomorphism, atypical mitotic figures, and dyskeratosis with an intact basement membrane.

TERMINOLOGY

Synonyms

- Dysplasia (mild, moderate, severe)
- Atypical epithelial hyperplasia
- Squamous intraepithelial lesion (SIL) or neoplasia (SIN)
- Leukoplakia
- Erythroplakia

Definitions

- **Dysplasia**
  - Morphologically altered epithelium with increased risk for malignant transformation than in its normal counterpart
- **Carcinoma in situ (CIS)**
  - Dysplasia involving full thickness of epithelium without evidence of invasion into lamina propria
  - Considered to be precancerous and will progress to invasive squamous cell carcinoma (SCC) if not treated
- **Oral leukoplakia**
  - Clinical term of exclusion and does not imply that microscopic tissue alteration is present
  - White patch that cannot be given another specific diagnostic name
  - Often divided into 2 subtypes
    - Homogeneous leukoplakia: Uniformly white
    - Nonhomogeneous or erythroleukoplakia: Has erythematous component
- **Oral erythroplakia (erythroplasia)**
  - Red patch or plaque that cannot be given another specific diagnostic name
- **Proliferative verrucous leukoplakia (PVL)**
  - Unique form of leukoplakia characterized by multiple flat keratoses that eventually develop verrucal or exophytic appearance
  - Almost 100% risk of malignant transformation

ETIOLOGY/PATHOGENESIS

Environmental Exposure

- Strong association with tobacco smoking
  - 70-90% of oral leukoplakias found in smokers
    - Heavy smokers have more numerous and larger lesions than light smokers
  - PVL does not have strong tobacco association
- Ultraviolet radiation
  - Leukoplakia of lower lip vermilion

Infectious Agents

- Candidal organisms
  - Often seen in association with dysplasia
    - Unknown whether organism is causative or secondarily infects dysplastic mucosa
- Human papillomavirus (HPV)
  - Not commonly seen in oral leukoplakia
  - Uncertain whether HPV infection is prognostic marker for malignant transformation

CLINICAL ISSUES

Epidemiology

- Incidence
  - Exact incidence of oral dysplasia unknown
    - Prevalence of oral leukoplakia in Western countries is around 2%
    - Dysplastic changes found in < 25% of leukoplakia biopsies
    - Erythroplakia significantly less common but > 90% of cases exhibit dysplasia, CIS, or invasive SCC
- Age
  - Usually > 40 years, increases rapidly with age
- Gender
  - Male > Female (2.3:1)
  - **PVL**: Female > Male (4:1)

DYSPLASIA AND CARCINOMA IN SITU

Key Facts

Terminology

- **Dysplasia**: Morphologically altered epithelium with increased risk for malignant transformation than in its normal counterpart
- **Carcinoma in situ**: Dysplasia involving full thickness of epithelium without evidence of invasion into lamina propria
  - Considered to be precancerous and will progress to invasive squamous cell carcinoma if not treated
- **Proliferative verrucous leukoplakia**: Unique form of leukoplakia characterized by multiple flat keratoses that eventually develop verrucal or exophytic appearance
  - Almost 100% risk of malignant transformation

Microscopic Pathology

- Both cellular abnormalities and maturation abnormalities are used in grading epithelial dysplasia
- **Hyperplasia**: Increased number of cells leading to acanthosis in basal/parabasal layer
- **Mild dysplasia**: Alteration limited to basal/parabasal layers
- **Moderate dysplasia**: Alterations from basal layer to midportion of spinous layer
  - If cytologic atypia is marked, then often lesion will be upgraded to severe dysplasia
- **Severe dysplasia**: Dysplasia involving 2/3 to almost complete thickness of epithelium
- **Carcinoma in situ**: Dysplastic epithelial cells extend from basal layer to mucosal surface

Site

- Can occur anywhere
  - Most common sites with highest risk of malignant transformation: Lateral and ventral tongue, floor of mouth, and lower lip
- Multifocal areas can occur, particularly in setting of PVL

Presentation

- White, red, or red and white patch

Natural History

- Risk of malignant transformation
  - Mild and moderate dysplasia: May be reversible
    - Reactive changes can be induced by candidiasis, ulcers, and mechanical irritation
  - Some reports of mild dysplasia progressing to SCC
  - Malignant transformation rates of leukoplakia (without dysplasia) range from 1-4%
  - Most erythroplasia will undergo malignant transformation if not excised

Treatment

- Options, risks, complications
  - Cessation of possible etiologies (tobacco smoking) may reverse clinical leukoplakia and mild to moderate dysplasia
- Surgical approaches
  - Excisional biopsy or laser ablation of abnormal area particularly in severe dysplasia or CIS

Prognosis

- No reliable marker to predict progression to SCC
- Recurrence rates after treatment: Up to 30%
  - No data on recurrence rate after erythroplakia excision
- Risk factors for malignant transformation of leukoplakia include
  - Long duration, erythroplasia, tongue or floor of mouth location, female, presence in nonsmokers

MACROSCOPIC FEATURES

General Features

- **Leukoplakia**
  - Thin white, gray or translucent plaque may be earliest presentation
  - Progresses to more thickened, white keratotic plaque that may have corrugated appearance
  - Nodular appearance with surface irregularities of verruciform appearance
  - Multiple white plaques, many with verruciform appearance are hallmark of PVL
    - Gingiva is frequent site of involvement in PVL
  - Can develop scattered areas of erythroplakia representing nonkeratinizing epithelium (speckled leukoplakia/erythroleukoplakia)
- **Erythroplakia**
  - Well-demarcated red plaque with soft, velvety texture

MICROSCOPIC PATHOLOGY

Histologic Features

- Cellular **and** maturation abnormalities are used in grading epithelial dysplasia
  - **Cellular abnormalities**
    - Nuclear pleomorphism
    - Nuclear hyperchromasia
    - Enlarged nucleoli (may be noted in reactive processes)
    - Increased nuclear to cytoplasmic ratio
    - Increased mitotic activity
    - Abnormal mitotic figures
    - Dyskeratosis
  - **Maturation abnormalities**
    - Drop-shaped rete ridges
    - Loss of polarity of basal cells
    - Loss of maturation with increased cellularity in spinous layer
    - Dysplastic process begins in basal/parabasal layer
- **Grading dysplasia**

DYSPLASIA AND CARCINOMA IN SITU

Classification Schemes for Oral Epithelial Dysplasia

WHO Classification	SIN	Ljubljana Classification: SIL*
Hyperplasia without dysplasia		Hyperplasia without dysplasia
Mild dysplasia	SIN1	Basal/parabasal hyperplasia
Moderate dysplasia	SIN2	Atypical hyperplasia**
Severe dysplasia	SIN3***	Atypical hyperplasia**
Carcinoma in situ	SIN3***	Carcinoma in situ

*SIN = squamous intraepithelial neoplasia; SIL = squamous intraepithelial lesion. *Developed for grading laryngeal dysplasia; **Considered to be high-grade dysplasia similar to moderate to severe dysplasia; ***Some authorities do not distinguish between severe dysplasia and carcinoma in situ.*

- **Hyperplasia**
  - Increased number of cells leading to acanthosis in basal/parabasal layer
  - Some leukoplakias exhibit epithelial atrophy
  - No cellular atypia
  - Normal maturation
  - May be either ortho- or parakeratinized or both
- **Mild dysplasia**
  - Alteration limited to basal/parabasal layers
  - Acanthosis
  - May have occasional lymphocytes
- **Moderate dysplasia**
  - Alterations from basal layer to midportion of spinous layer
  - Bulbous rete ridges
  - Moderate number of lymphocytes are often seen
  - If cytologic atypia is marked, then often lesion will be upgraded to severe dysplasia
- **Severe dysplasia**
  - Dysplasia involving 2/3 to almost complete thickness of epithelium
  - Epithelial atrophy
  - May have both keratinized and nonkeratinized areas
  - Dysplasia can be seen extending into underlying salivary gland ducts
  - Moderate to marked lymphocyte infiltrate in stroma subjacent to epithelium
  - Inflammatory cell exocytosis may be seen
  - Some experts feel severe dysplasia is synonymous with CIS

- **Carcinoma in situ**
  - Dysplastic epithelial cells extend from basal layer to mucosal surface
  - Basement membrane remains intact
  - Lesion is usually nonkeratinized
  - Keratin pearl formation unusual in CIS and may suggest invasive SCC in adjacent tissue
  - Dysplasia may extend into underlying salivary gland ducts
- **Proliferative verrucous leukoplakia**
  - Early lesions have unique pattern referred to as atypical epithelial (verrucous) hyperplasia
    - Marked keratosis with little to no dysplasia
    - Share some features with verrucous carcinoma (VC) although rete are usually not as bulbous
    - Often see superimposed candidiasis
  - Lesions generally progress to SCC or VC

DIFFERENTIAL DIAGNOSIS

Reactive Atypia

- Can be seen in epithelium adjacent to ulcers, including aphthous ulcers, herpetic lesion, and traumatic ulcers
- Neutrophilic infiltrate in superficial lamina propria may indicate presence of fungi, in particular *Candida* species
  - Special stains (periodic acid-Schiff) will highlight hyphae &/or spores on epithelial surface of superficial keratin

Microinvasive Carcinoma

- Biopsies of severe dysplasia or CIS should have multiple levels evaluated for definitive evidence of invasion into lamina propria
- Careful evaluation of epithelial/lamina propria interface needed
- If biopsy of severe dysplasia CIS represents a small sample of larger lesion, additional sampling or complete removal is recommended

Verrucous Carcinoma

- Verrucous leukoplakia share many histologic features with verrucous carcinoma and may be difficult to distinguish microscopically
- Verrucous carcinomas present as large, exophytic masses

SELECTED REFERENCES

1. Mehanna HM et al: Treatment and follow-up of oral dysplasia - a systematic review and meta-analysis. Head Neck. 31(12):1600-9, 2009
2. Smith J et al: Biomarkers in dysplasia of the oral cavity: a systematic review. Oral Oncol. 45(8):647-53, 2009
3. van der Waal I: Potentially malignant disorders of the oral and oropharyngeal mucosa; terminology, classification and present concepts of management. Oral Oncol. 45(4-5):317-23, 2009
4. Napier SS et al: Natural history of potentially malignant oral lesions and conditions: an overview of the literature. J Oral Pathol Med. 37(1):1-10, 2008
5. Warnakulasuriya S et al: Nomenclature and classification of potentially malignant disorders of the oral mucosa. J Oral Pathol Med. 36(10):575-80, 2007
6. Greer RO: Pathology of malignant and premalignant oral epithelial lesions. Otolaryngol Clin North Am. 39(2):249-75, v, 2006

Clinical and Microscopic Features

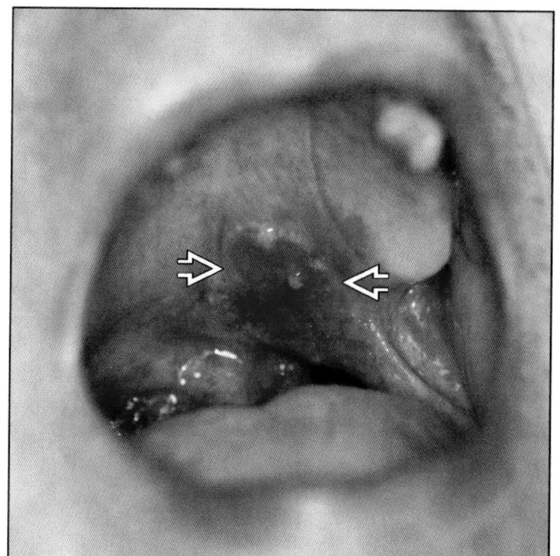

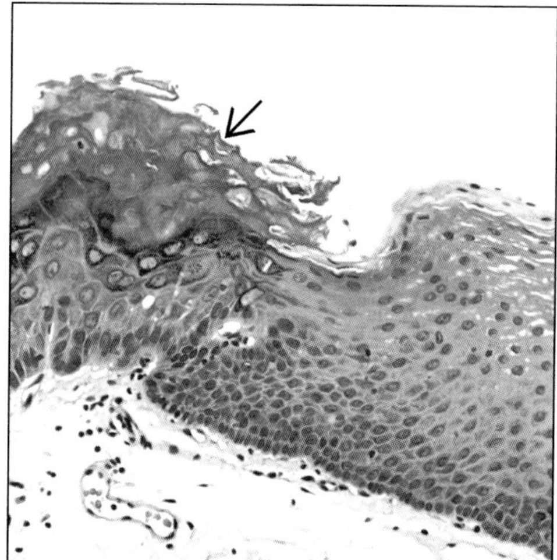

(Left) *Erythroplakia of the soft palate presents as a well-demarcated lesion with velvety surface* ➡. *Unlike oral leukoplakia in which most biopsies show no dysplasia, erythroplasia usually shows severe dysplasia, CIS, or SCC when biopsied.* ***(Right)*** *Biopsy of clinical leukoplakia shows areas of both parakeratosis and orthokeratosis* ➡ *without dysplasia. Although parakeratin is most frequently observed, the presence of orthokeratin does not have any prognostic implications.*

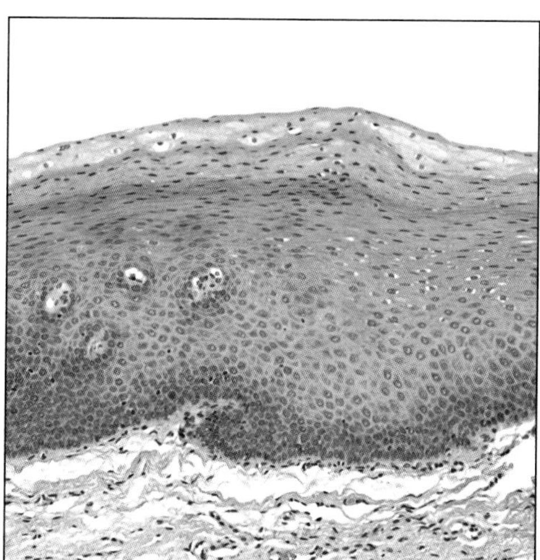

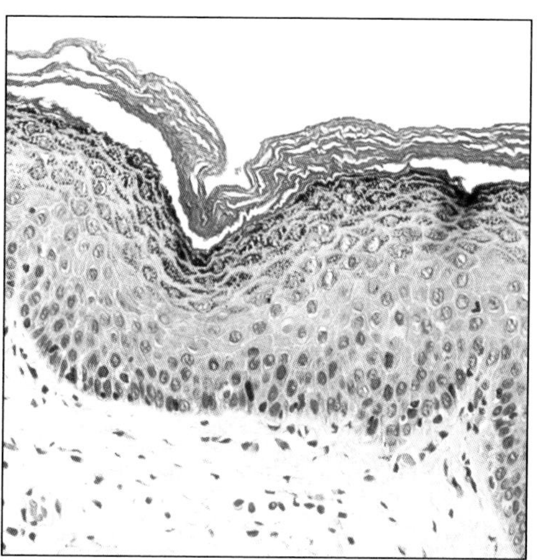

(Left) *Biopsy from a white lesion from the lateral tongue shows hyperparakeratosis and acanthosis without cytologic atypia. Simple hyperplasia such as this may be related to trauma and is readily reversible.* ***(Right)*** *Biopsy of the lateral tongue exhibits mild dysplasia with hyperchromatic nuclei present in the basal and parabasal layers but a normal maturation of epithelium. These lesions can revert to normal (similar to simple hyperplasia) or progress to a higher grade dysplasia.*

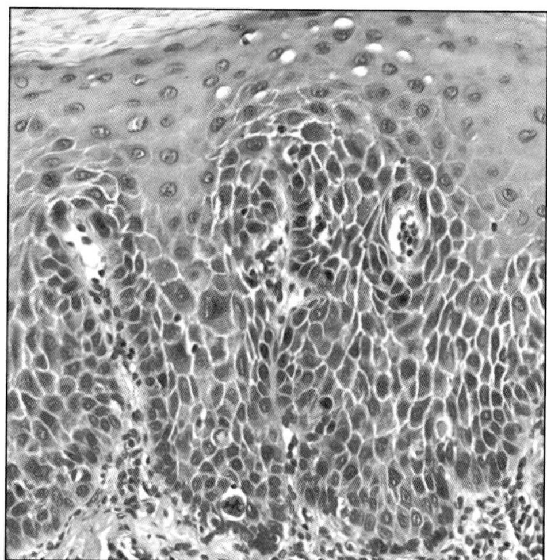

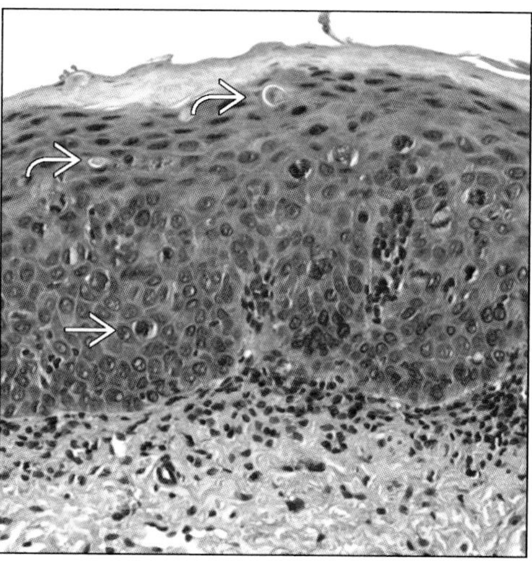

(Left) *Biopsy of moderate dysplasia shows elongated rete with marked acanthosis, nuclear pleomorphism, and mitoses extending to the middle 1/3 of the epithelium. Although potentially reversible, if possible, complete removal is warranted.* ***(Right)*** *Biopsy of the ventral tongue exhibits severe dysplasia with architectural disturbance involving most of the epithelium. Dyskeratosis* ➡*, nuclear pleomorphism, and numerous mitoses, including atypical forms* ➡*, are present.*

DYSPLASIA AND CARCINOMA IN SITU

Microscopic and Clinical Features

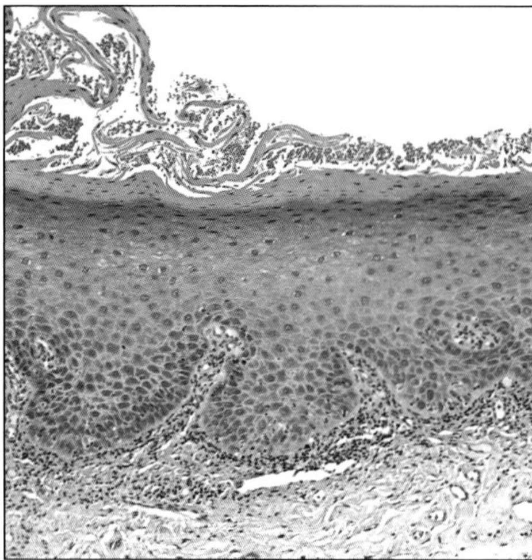

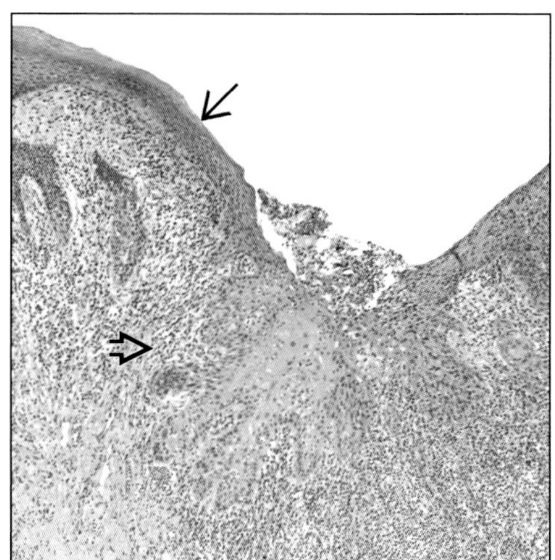

*(**Left**) Drop shape or budding of the rete ridges is a histomorphologic feature that can be seen even without any cytologic abnormalities. This feature, especially in combination with epithelial atrophy, and location on the tongue or floor of the mouth should upstage the grading. (**Right**) Invasive squamous cell carcinoma ⇨ arising adjacent to epithelium exhibits little to no dysplasia →. Although uncommon, malignant transformation can occur in nondysplastic oral leukoplakia.*

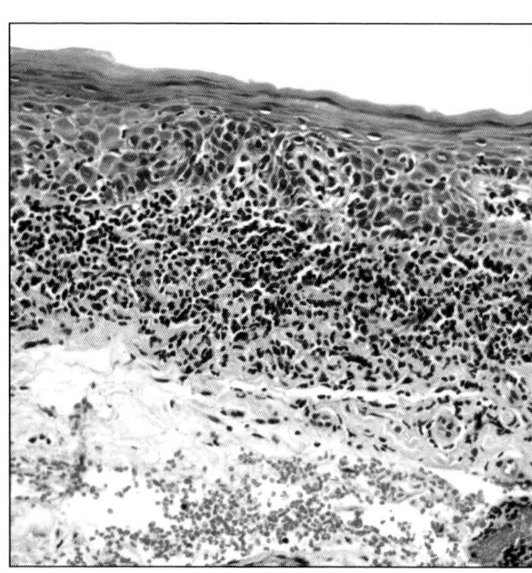

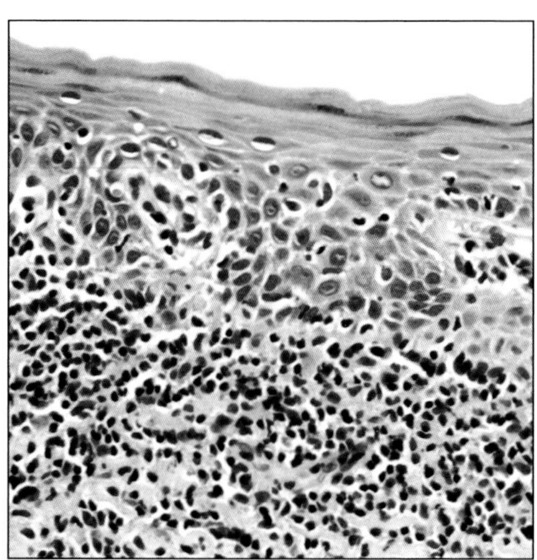

*(**Left**) Low-power photomicrograph of a white lesion on the ventral tongue exhibits epithelial atrophy with irregularly shaped rete. A prominent inflammatory cell infiltrate is subjacent to the basal cells imparting a "lichenoid" appearance. (**Right**) Higher power view shows features of moderate dysplasia, including hyperchromatic and pleomorphic nuclei extending to the midpoint of the epithelium. This should not be mistaken for lichen planus.*

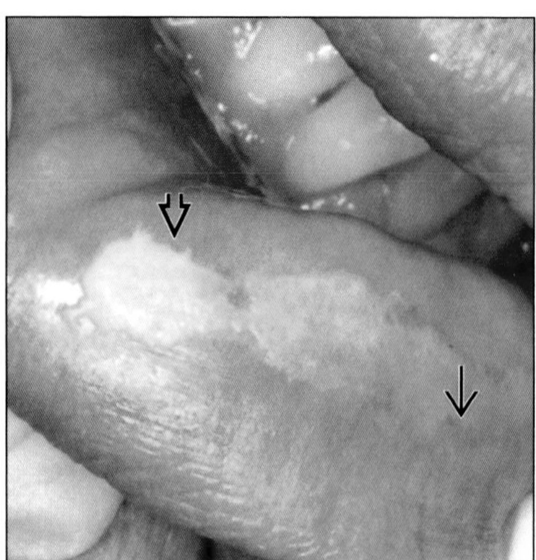

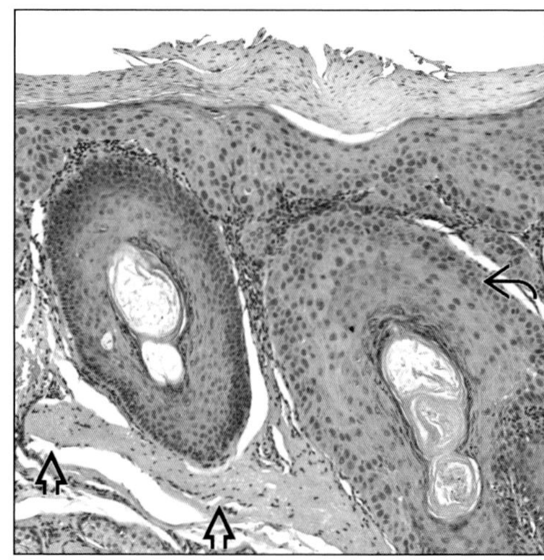

*(**Left**) Actinic cheilosis is a common precancerous condition associated with ultraviolet radiation. Blurring of the vermilion border and cutaneous portion → is seen along with thickened keratotic plaques ⇨. (**Right**) Biopsy of actinic cheilitis is characterized by atrophic epithelium with marked parakeratosis. The epithelium exhibits dysplastic changes that extend into the hair follicle ↪. Amorphous, basophilic alteration of the connective tissue (solar elastosis) is seen ⇨.*

DYSPLASIA AND CARCINOMA IN SITU

Clinical, Microscopic, and Histochemical Features

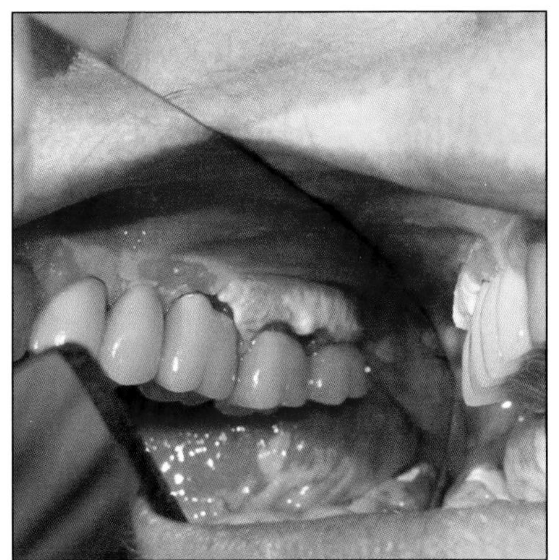

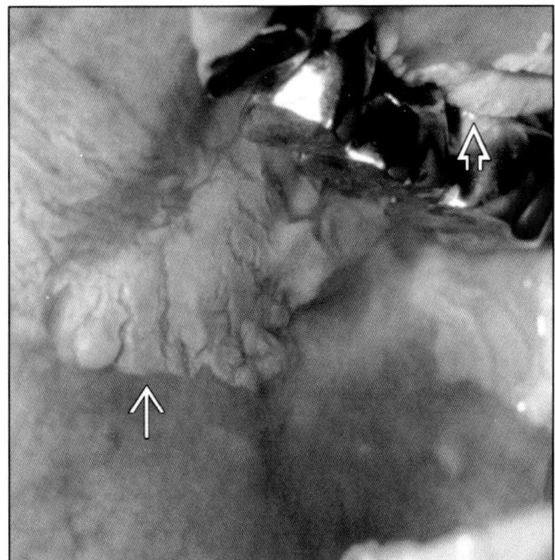

*(**Left**) Mirror photograph shows proliferative verrucous leukoplakia (PVL) in a 70-year-old woman with no history of smoking or alcohol abuse. PVL has a predilection for the gingiva, which is a common site for malignant transformation unlike more typical oral leukoplakia. Extensive, white, thickened and fissured areas are seen on the gingiva and tongue. (**Right**) Clinical photograph of PVL shows multiple keratotic plaques on the buccal mucosa → and the palatal gingiva ⇨.*

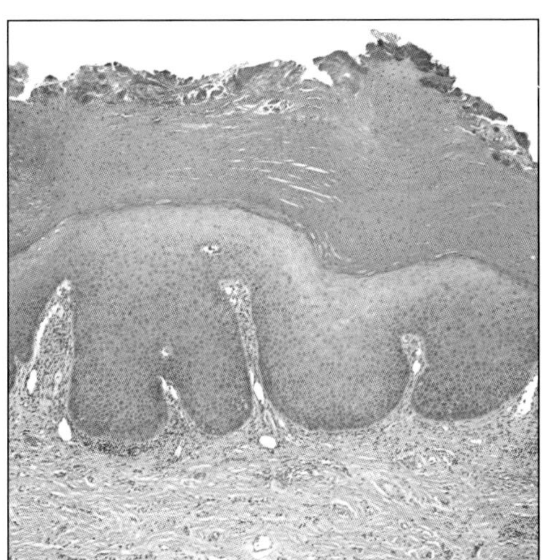

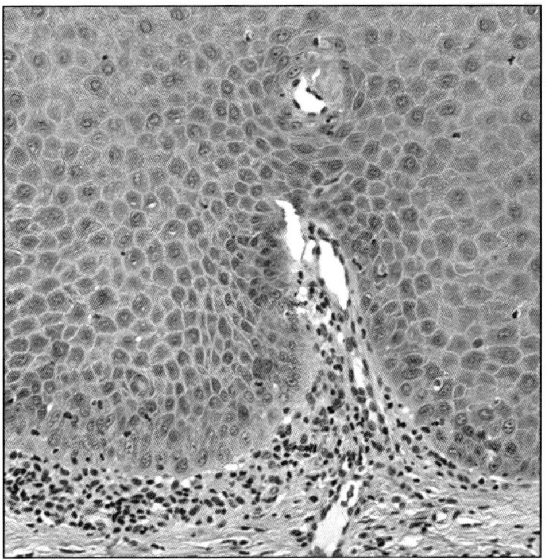

*(**Left**) Photomicrograph shows atypical epithelial (verrucous) hyperplasia in a patient with PVL. Marked parakeratosis corresponds to the clinical features of thickened and fissured mucosa. The rete are bulbous similar to verrucous carcinoma. (**Right**) High-power view demonstrates a lack of dysplastic features. Despite this finding, atypical epithelial hyperplasia is considered to be a potentially premalignant condition, and patients should be followed.*

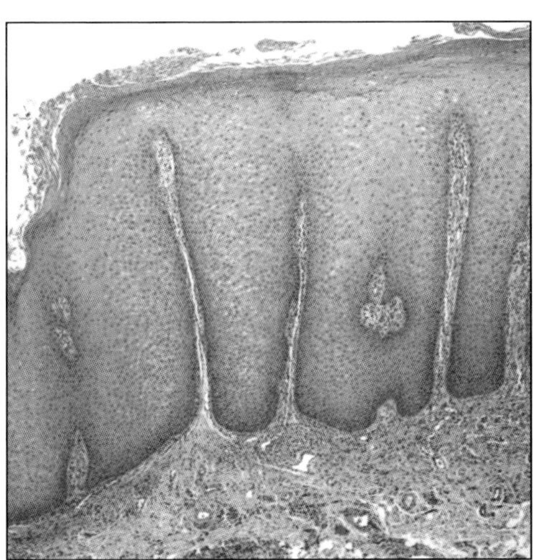

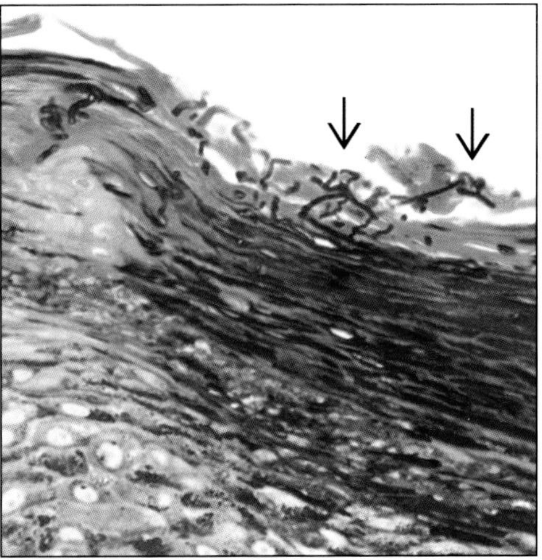

*(**Left**) Low-power image shows atypical epithelial hyperplasia in a patient with PVL. Surface keratinization in not abundant. Marked acanthosis is seen with elongated rete. No significant dysplastic findings are seen, but the overall architecture is worrisome for progression to cancer. (**Right**) Candidal overgrowth can be seen in leukoplakia as is shown here, highlighted by periodic acid-Schiff staining →. Candidiasis can frequently occur in lesions of PVL.*

SQUAMOUS CELL CARCINOMA

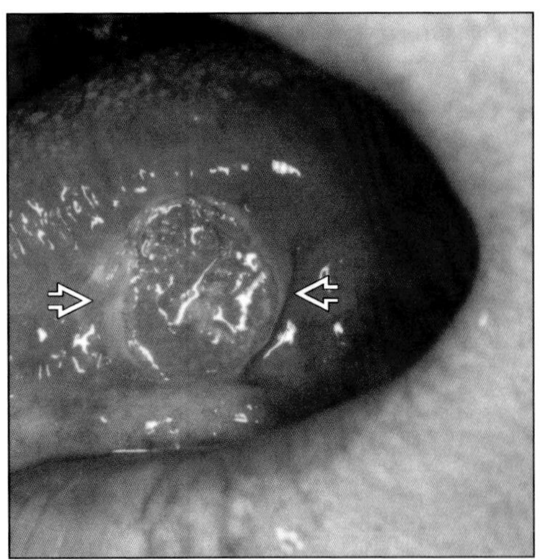

Squamous cell carcinoma arising on the posterior lateral border of the tongue presented as an exophytic mass with rolled borders ➡. On palpation, the lesion was firm and indurated.

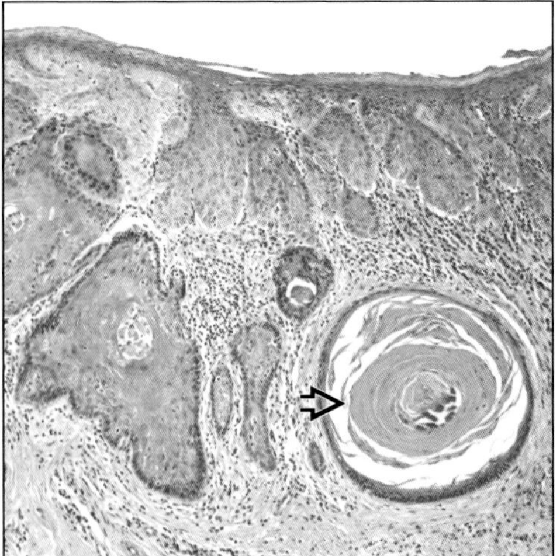

Well-differentiated squamous cell carcinoma shows islands of malignant epithelial cells arising from the overlying epithelium invading into the lamina propria with keratin pearl formation ➡.

TERMINOLOGY

Abbreviations

- Squamous cell carcinoma (SCC)
- Verrucous squamous cell carcinoma (VSCC)

Definitions

- Malignant neoplasm arising from squamous epithelium

ETIOLOGY/PATHOGENESIS

Environmental Exposure

- Tobacco use
- Betel quid (Paan): Combination of areca palm nuts, betel leaf, slaked lime, ± tobacco
  - Commonly used in south Asia
- Alcohol consumption
- Radiation exposure (ultraviolet and therapeutic)
- Nutritional deficiencies
  - Iron deficiency (Plummer-Vinson) associated with elevated risk of SCC

Infectious Agents

- Oncogenic virus: Human papillomavirus, high-risk type associated with development of tonsil and base of tongue cancer
  - Relationship to oral SCC is not as convincing

Immunosuppression

- HIV/AIDS patients have increased risk
- Organ transplant recipients

Precursor Lesions

- Can develop from area of leukoplakia or erythroplakia
  - Malignant transformation of severe dysplasia or carcinoma in situ

CLINICAL ISSUES

Epidemiology

- Incidence
  - About 35,000 new cases a year in USA (includes oropharynx)
  - > 400,000 new cases a year worldwide (includes pharynx)
    - Highest rates are in South Asia and account for 30% of all new cancer cases
- Age
  - Median: 62 years
  - Range: < 20-100 years
- Gender
  - Male > Female (2-3:1)
    - M:F ratio has decreased as more women smoke tobacco
- Ethnicity
  - Black > white (17/100,000 vs. 15.5/100,000) (USA men)
    - Survival differences also noted: 5-year survival in white vs. black men is 61% and 36%, respectively

Site

- Tongue (lateral and ventral) accounts for > 50% of cases
- Floor of mouth
- Lip (> 90% found on lower lip)
- Retromolar trigone
- Gingiva, buccal mucosa, palate less common in USA

Presentation

- Difficulty eating and swallowing
- Sore that does not heal
- Dentures that fit poorly
- Weight loss
- Earache
- Loose teeth

SQUAMOUS CELL CARCINOMA

Key Facts

Etiology/Pathogenesis

- Tobacco use, alcohol consumption, UV radiation, immunosuppression

Clinical Issues

- Accounts for > 90% of all oral cavity malignancies
- Most common in men in 6th and 7th decade
- Tongue (lateral and ventral) accounts for > 50% of cases
- Treatment includes surgery &/or radiation ± chemotherapy
- Disease-free survival and overall survival correlates with TNM staging
  - Resection margins, perineural and lymphovascular invasion
  - Lymph node metastases and extracapsular spread

Microscopic Pathology

- Majority of oral cavity SCC are conventional keratinizing type
- Histologic grade includes well, moderately, and poorly differentiated SCC
- Adjacent areas of dysplasia or CIS can be identified, but invasion can be seen without surface atypia
- Tumor spread influenced by anatomic location
- Variants of keratinizing SCC may be found
  - Verrucous carcinoma: > 75% found in oral cavity
  - Marked epithelial hyperplasia with broad elongated rete with pushing border

Top Differential Diagnoses

- Pseudoepitheliomatous hyperplasia, necrotizing sialometaplasia, radiation changes

Treatment

- Surgical approaches
  - Surgery remains mainstay of treatment of oral SCC ± lymph node dissection
  - Sentinal node biopsy
    - Experimental and used for staging a clinically N0 neck
- Adjuvant therapy
  - Induction and postoperative chemotherapy sometimes used
    - Cisplatin, 5-fluorouracil
    - Carboplatin and paclitaxel in combination
    - Few standardized control studies of oral cavity SCC
- Radiation
  - Postoperative radiotherapy dependent on tumor stage

Prognosis

- Disease-free survival and overall survival correlates with TNM staging
  - Stage 1-2: 5-year survival (82%)
  - Stage 3: 5-year survival (53%)
  - Metastatic disease at presentation: 5-year survival (28%)
- 2nd primary tumors
  - 10-35% increased risk of 2nd aerodigestive malignancy
  - May represent a new tumor or arise in same area (field effect)
- Resection margins
  - Positive surgical margins associated with decrease in overall survival
- Lymphovascular and perineural invasion
  - Associated with increased local recurrence and poorer overall survival
- Regional lymph node metastases
  - Associated with decrease in overall survival
  - Tumor thickness > 4-5 mm of lateral tongue cancer increases risk of nodal spread
    - Measurement taken from presumed original surface level to deepest tumor invasion
- Extracapsular spread in lymph node metastases
  - Associated with regional and distant metastases and poorer overall survival
- Advanced age associated with poorer prognosis

IMAGE FINDINGS

General Features

- Computed tomography (CT) &/or magnetic resonance imaging (MR) for preoperative tumor staging and treatment planning
- Chest CT or plain film to rule out lung metastases
- Positron emission tomography (PET) in evaluating distant metastases
  - Distant metastases uncommon in oral cavity cancer at presentation

MACROSCOPIC FEATURES

General Features

- Leukoplakia, erythroleukoplakia, or erythroplakia
  - Often cannot be distinguished clinically from hyperkeratoses or dysplasia
- **Exophytic** growth pattern
  - Tumor mass can be fungating, papillary, or verruciform
  - Surface often ulcerated
  - May be friable or firm
  - Typical growth pattern for verrucous carcinoma
- **Endophytic** growth pattern
  - Depressed, ulcerated lesion that is indurated
  - May see rolled border

MICROSCOPIC PATHOLOGY

Histologic Features

- Majority are conventional keratinizing SCC type
- Histologic grade includes well, moderately, and poorly differentiated SCC
- Adjacent areas of dysplasia or CIS can be identified

SQUAMOUS CELL CARCINOMA

- Invasion can be seen without any surface atypia
- **Patterns of invasion**
  - Superficial or microinvasive carcinoma
    - Basement membrane violated and tumor cells present in superficial lamina propria
    - Tumor depth only 1-2 mm as measured from adjacent intact basement membrane
  - Broad pushing front: Large tumor islands with well-defined margin
  - Jagged or irregular finger-like extensions into lamina propria
  - Small tumor islands, single filing pattern, individual cell infiltration, and widely dispersed pattern of infiltration
  - Pattern of infiltration is associated with prognosis
    - Irregular or jagged cords or small scattered tumor islands have worse prognosis
- Variable degrees of squamous differentiation
  - Dyskeratosis and squamous pearls
  - Pleomorphism
  - Mitoses, including atypical mitoses
- Perineural invasion should be documented
  - Correlates with recurrence and survival and impacts management
- Mitotic figures and necrosis increases with grade
- Inflammatory infiltrate
  - Lymphoid infiltrate at tumor/host interface common
    - Can appear "lichenoid"
  - Variable number of eosinophils
- Tumor spread influenced by anatomic location
  - Tongue SCC can spread beneath intact mucosa involving deeper intrinsic muscles
  - Gingival carcinoma can invade bone via periodontal ligament
  - Alveolar SCC in edentulous can invade bone directly through marrow spaces as bone resorbs intact cortex
  - Tumor can spread posteriorly in mandible along inferior alveolar nerve
  - Lip cancer spreads superficially in early stages
    - Advanced cases can invade mandible
  - Floor of mouth SCC spreads superficially in early stages but then extends into sublingual gland and mylohyoid muscle
  - Palatal tumors spread superficially

Lymphatic/Vascular Invasion

- Should be documented as it correlates with prognosis

Margins

- Margins (including bone) must be reported
- Shrinkage of up to 50% must be taken into consideration
  - This is particularly true of lateral tongue carcinoma where there is marked postsurgical retraction of muscle
- Bone beneath tumor needs to be sampled for invasion
  - Superficial erosion of mandible/maxilla does not constitute bone invasion and does not change stage

Lymph Nodes

- All lymph nodes removed should be evaluated
- Lymph nodes should be reported by level if identified surgically
- Presence of extracapsular spread (macroscopic/ microscopic) should be reported

Variants of Keratinizing SCC

- **Verrucous squamous cell carcinoma**
  - > 75% of all VSCC found in oral cavity
  - Marked epithelial hyperplasia with broad elongated rete with pushing border
  - Papillary surface with marked keratosis, keratin plugging, parakeratotic crypting
  - Normal epithelial maturation with little cytologic atypia
  - Mitoses rare and observed in basal/parabasal layer
  - Dense lymphoplasmacytic host response
  - Extensive sampling to rule out conventional-type SCC, which can occur in 20% of VSCC
- **Spindle cell "sarcomatoid" squamous cell carcinoma**
  - More common in larynx and pharynx
  - Often appears polypoid
  - Pleomorphic cells arranged in fascicles with numerous mitoses
  - May see CIS overlying tumor or areas of more conventional SCC
- **Basaloid squamous cell carcinoma**
  - More common in oropharynx, hypopharynx, and larynx
  - Superficial tumor shows typical squamous differentiation
  - Deeper tumor composed of sheets of basaloid cells with palisading of peripheral cells
  - Central (comedo) necrosis
  - High mitotic rate
- **Papillary squamous cell carcinoma**
  - Rarely found in oral cavity except as component of more conventional SCC
- **Lymphoepithelial carcinoma**
  - Rare in oral cavity
  - Morphologically similar to nasopharyngeal counterpart
- **Acantholytic squamous cell carcinoma (pseudoglandular or adenoid)**
  - Uncommon in oral cavity: Most cases reported on lower lip
  - Superficial area resembles conventional SCC
  - Deeper tumor has gland-like structures with scattered acantholytic cells
- **Carcinoma cuniculatum**
  - Primarily occurs on soles of feet but can present in oral cavity
  - Proliferation of epithelium with broad rete with keratin cores and crypts
  - Slow growing but deeply invasive; can burrow into bone or erode adjacent soft tissue structures
  - No cytologic atypia

ANCILLARY TESTS

Cytology

- Used in lymph node assessment

SQUAMOUS CELL CARCINOMA

Frozen Sections

- Useful to assess surgical soft tissue margins
- **Pitfalls**
  - Frozen section assessment of bone margins is problematic but imprints shown to be reliable indicator of margin status
  - Small specimen &/or poor orientation may result in over/under interpretation
  - Difficult to grade dysplasia by frozen section
    - Tissue distortion and artifactual changes make grading dysplasia challenging
    - Hyperplasia, pseudoepitheliomatous hyperplasia can be misinterpreted
    - Reactive epithelial changes adjacent to ulcer
    - Radiation changes: Knowledge of prior radiation is paramount
  - Juxtaoral organ of Chievitz
    - Normal structure located bilaterally at angle of mandible (retromolar trigone area)
    - Composed of nonkeratinizing, bland, uniform epithelial cells surrounded by basaloid cells associated with small nerves
    - Awareness of structure important to avoid misinterpretation of perineural invasion

Immunohistochemistry

- Epithelial cells positive for cytokeratin (CK) markers, including pancytokeratin and high molecular weight CK (cytoplasmic)
- High-grade tumors: Low molecular weight CK, CK8, CK18, CAM5.2, CK5/6 (cytoplasmic)
- CK7 and CK20 negative
- p53 (nuclear) is associated with a poor prognosis
- p53 (nuclear) overexpression, although in poorly differentiated SCC there may be little to no expression

Molecular Genetics

- Loss of heterozygosity commonly noted at 3p (*FHIT*), 9p (*CDKN2A*), 17p (*TP53*)
- Mutations in *TP53* (*P53*), a tumor suppressor gene located on short arm of 17 increases with tobacco smoking
  - Oral carcinomas in nonsmokers have fewer *P53* mutations
- Clonal proliferation of epithelial cells that harbor genetic mutations in one or more fields account for "field cancerization" that occurs in upper aerodigestive tract
  - Mutated *TP53* patches can be identified in mucosa adjacent to completely resected cancers, which may explain in part local tumor recurrences
- Overexpression of cyclooxygenase-2 (COX-2) may play a future role for targeted molecular therapy

DIFFERENTIAL DIAGNOSIS

Pseudoepitheliomatous Hyperplasia

- Benign reactive process lacking cellular atypia and nuclear pleomorphism

Necrotizing Sialometaplasia

- Requires adequate biopsy since overlying epithelium can exhibit pseudoepitheliomatous hyperplasia

Radiation Changes

- Can see marked pleomorphism of epithelial, endothelial, and stromal cells
- May require cytokeratin markers

DIAGNOSTIC CHECKLIST

Clinically Relevant Pathologic Features

- Clinical stage is most important predictor of prognosis
  - > 75% of oral SCC are diagnosed at advanced stage (III, IV), accounting for overall poor prognosis
  - Patients have increased risk of developing 2nd primary tumor of upper aerodigestive tract

Pathologic Interpretation Pearls

- Regardless of SCC variant, all are staged similarly

SELECTED REFERENCES

1. Al-Swiahb JN et al: Clinical, pathological and molecular determinants in squamous cell carcinoma of the oral cavity. Future Oncol. 6(5):837-50, 2010
2. Stucken E et al: Oral cavity risk factors: experts' opinions and literature support. J Otolaryngol Head Neck Surg. 39(1):76-89, 2010
3. Vered M et al: Oral tongue squamous cell carcinoma: recurrent disease is associated with histopathologic risk score and young age. J Cancer Res Clin Oncol. 136(7):1039-48, 2010
4. Stoeckli SJ et al: Sentinel node biopsy for early oral and oropharyngeal squamous cell carcinoma. Eur Arch Otorhinolaryngol. 266(6):787-93, 2009
5. Woolgar JA et al: Pitfalls and procedures in the histopathological diagnosis of oral and oropharyngeal squamous cell carcinoma and a review of the role of pathology in prognosis. Oral Oncol. 45(4-5):361-85, 2009
6. Müller S et al: Changing trends in oral squamous cell carcinoma with particular reference to young patients: 1971-2006. The Emory University experience. Head Neck Pathol. 2(2):60-6, 2008
7. Kowalski LP et al: Elective neck dissection in oral carcinoma: a critical review of the evidence. Acta Otorhinolaryngol Ital. 27(3):113-7, 2007
8. Woolgar JA: Histopathological prognosticators in oral and oropharyngeal squamous cell carcinoma. Oral Oncol. 42(3):229-39, 2006
9. Brandwein-Gensler M et al: Oral squamous cell carcinoma: histologic risk assessment, but not margin status, is strongly predictive of local disease-free and overall survival. Am J Surg Pathol. 29(2):167-78, 2005
10. Kademani D et al: Prognostic factors in intraoral squamous cell carcinoma: the influence of histologic grade. J Oral Maxillofac Surg. 63(11):1599-605, 2005
11. Ferlito A et al: The incidence of lymph node micrometastases in patients pathologically staged N0 in cancer of oral cavity and oropharynx. Oral Oncol. 38(1):3-5, 2002

SQUAMOUS CELL CARCINOMA

Imaging and Microscopic Features

(Left) *PET scan of a 35-year-old man with lateral tongue cancer presents at an advanced stage (stage IV) with numerous cervical lymph nodes. Lateral tongue SCC is the most common location in patients ≤ 40 years old, accounting for 80% of all oral cavity SCCs.* **(Right)** *This invasive squamous cell carcinoma appears to arise adjacent to epithelium with little cytologic atypia. This pattern of invasion with a broad pushing border at the advancing front is associated with a better prognosis.*

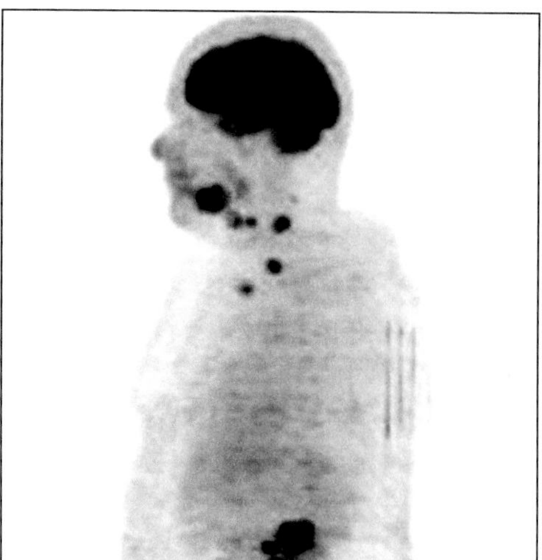

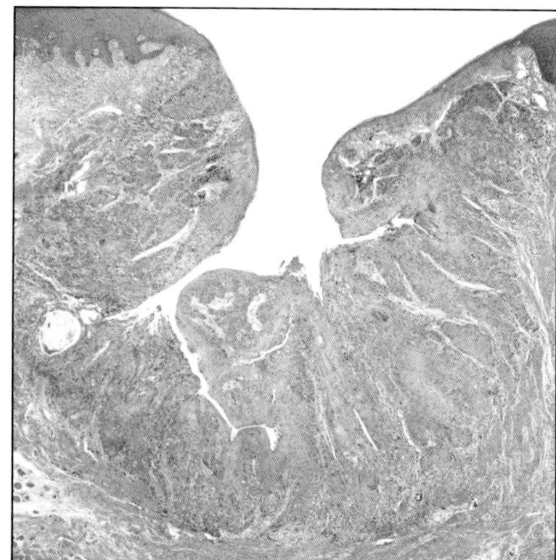

(Left) *Higher magnification shows violation of the basement membrane by scattered tongues of malignant epithelial cells ➙ associated with an inflammatory cell infiltrate. Individual dyskeratotic cells are scattered throughout ➙.* **(Right)** *SCC of the tongue with a prominent lymphocytic host response and keratin pearl formation is seen. The band-like lymphocytic infiltrate ➙ subjacent to surface basal cells can mimic lichen planus; in a superficial biopsy, close scrutiny is required to rule out dysplasia.*

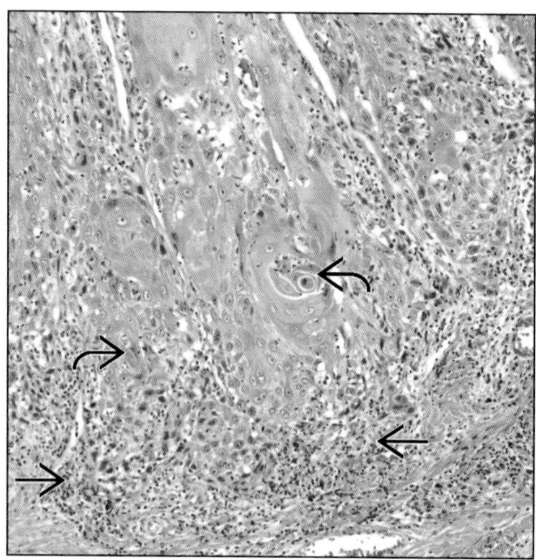

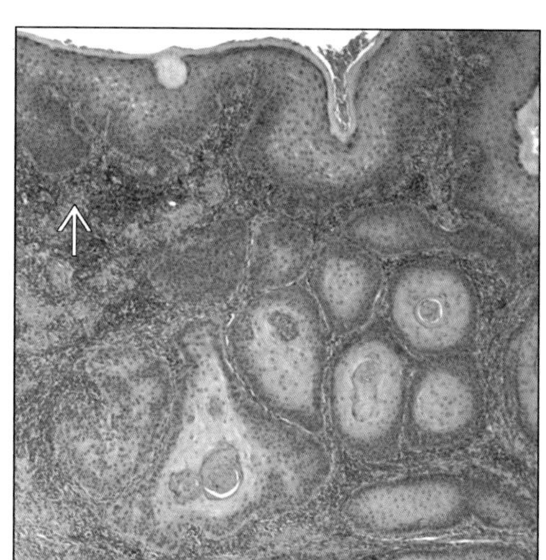

(Left) *Moderately differentiated SCC characterized by anastomosing strands of epithelial cells with little keratin pearl formation and cellular and nuclear pleomorphism is shown.* **(Right)** *Poorly differentiated SCC of the lower lip is seen with an acantholytic appearance in the deeper portion of tumor characterized by tumor nests with a glandular appearance lined by squamous epithelium ➙. The central spaces can contain acantholytic or dyskeratotic cells or cellular debris ➙.*

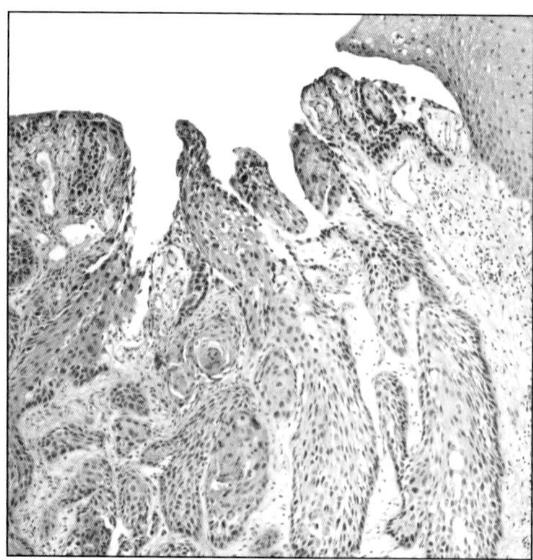

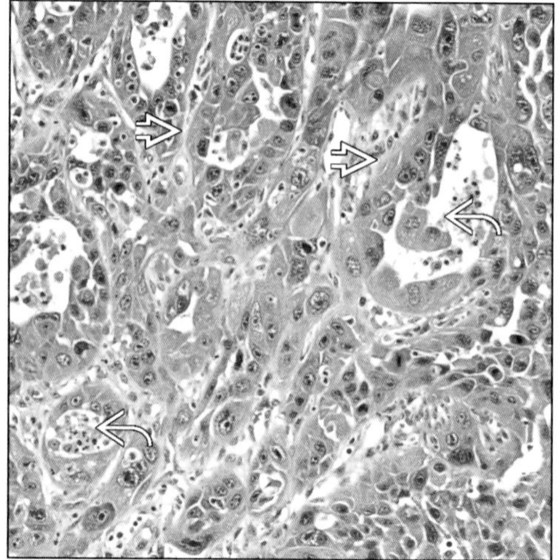

Microscopic and Clinical Features

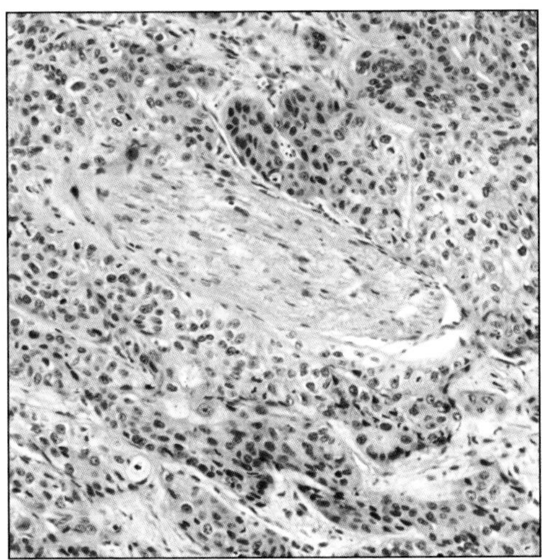

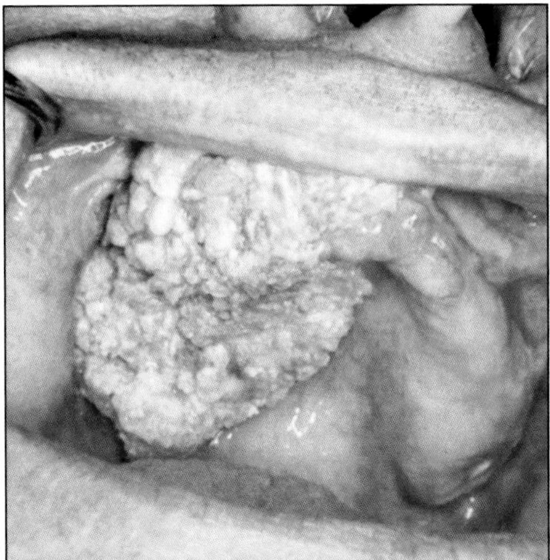

(Left) *Moderate differentiated SCC is seen surrounding a large caliber nerve. Perineural invasion is an adverse prognostic factor associated with recurrence and decreased survival.* ***(Right)*** *Verrucous squamous cell carcinoma of the maxilla is seen presenting as a well-demarcated carpet of epithelium with papillary projections with a lateral spread. The presence of surface ulceration in VC may indicate a conventional SCC component.*

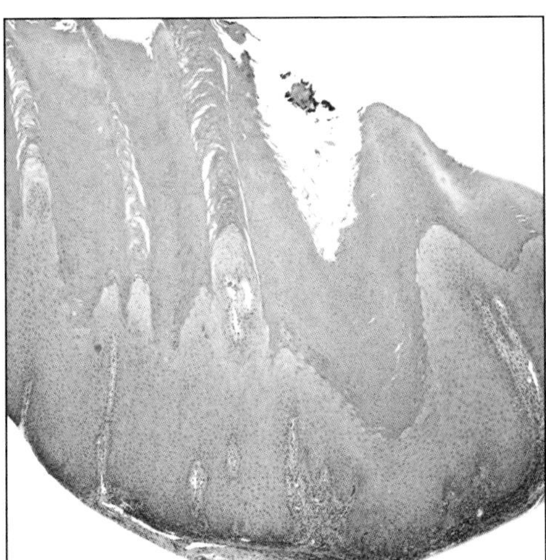

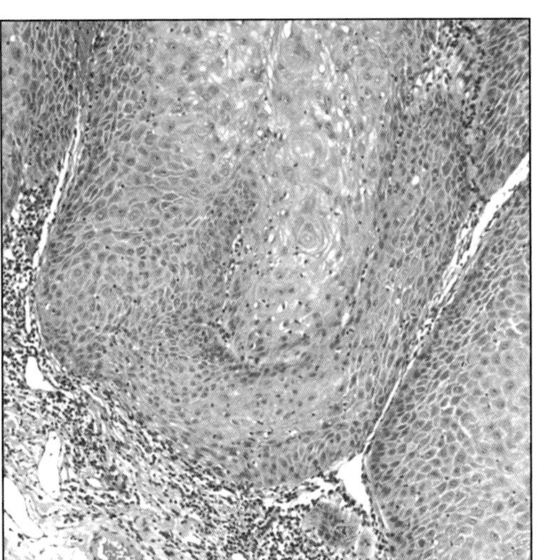

(Left) *Low-power image of VSCC illustrates a broad-based epithelial proliferation with marked parakeratosis with keratin plugging. The epithelium extends deeper into the submucosa than adjacent epithelium but without invasion. The bulbous rete ridges are associated with an intense inflammatory cell infiltrate at the tumor front.* ***(Right)*** *Higher power image of VSCC illustrates the broad, thickened epithelial rete, which lacks any cytologic atypia and exhibits a normal maturation.*

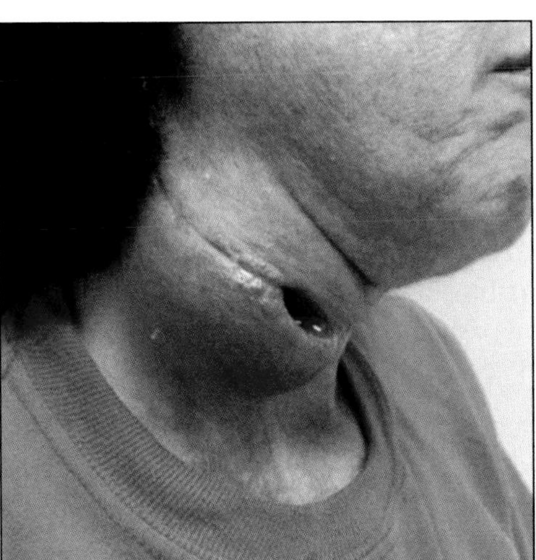

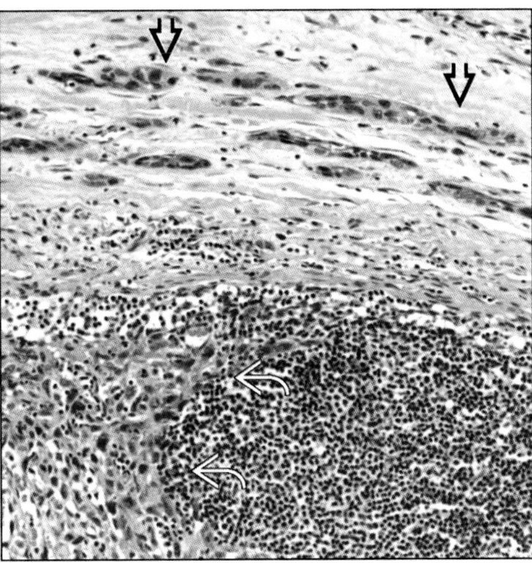

(Left) *A neck dissection from this patient shows extracapsular spread of SCC in a cervical lymph node. Despite postoperative radiation, persistent tumor growth is evident associated with a cutaneous fistula.* ***(Right)*** *Extracapsular spread in a cervical lymph node characterized by SCC is present within the lymph node ➡ and also outside the capsule ⇨. Extracapsular spread is an independent indicator of recurrent neck disease as well as overall patient survival.*

OROPHARYNGEAL CARCINOMA

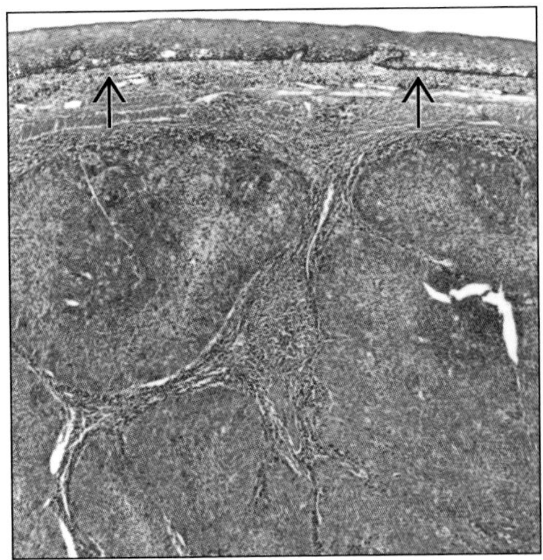

HPV-related nonkeratinizing SCC of the tonsil typically arises in the tonsillar crypts and the surface epithelium will often show no dysplastic changes ⇒. Note the marked basaloid appearance of the tumor.

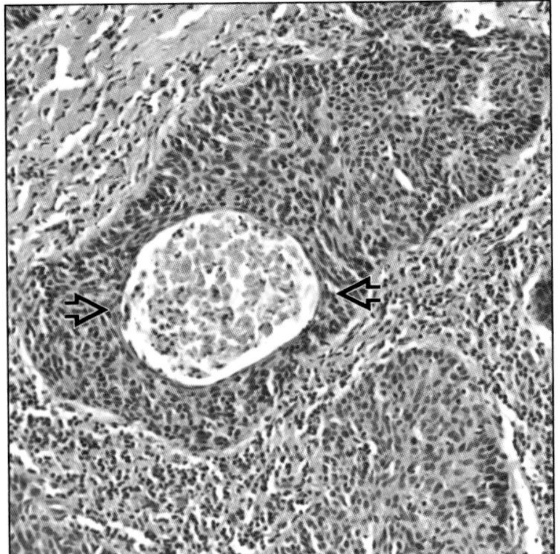

A common finding in nonkeratinizing SCC of the tonsil is comedo-type necrosis ⇒ as well as apoptosis and mitoses. These features should not be misinterpreted as basaloid squamous cell carcinoma.

TERMINOLOGY

Abbreviations

- Oropharyngeal squamous cell carcinoma (OPSCC)

Definitions

- Malignant epithelial neoplasm of oropharynx, including soft palate, tonsils, uvula, base of tongue, and oropharyngeal wall comprising Waldeyer ring

ETIOLOGY/PATHOGENESIS

Environmental Exposure

- Marijuana use greater in human papillomavirus (HPV)-positive OPSCC
- Tobacco smoking and alcohol use greater in HPV-negative OPSCC

Infectious Agents

- High-risk HPV associated with > 70% of cases OPSCC
  - HPV 16 predominant type, although other HPV high-risk types have been found

CLINICAL ISSUES

Epidemiology

- Incidence
  - OPSCC increased 1-2% annually in USA males in past 20 years, while rates of oral cavity carcinoma have decreased
- Gender
  - Male > Female (3:1)
- Ethnicity
  - HPV-positive OPSCC more common in whites

Site

- Anterior tonsillar pillar and fossa most common site followed by tongue base

Presentation

- Early lesions generally asymptomatic
- Tonsillar asymmetry
- Dysphagia
- Otalgia
- Trismus
- Enlarging cervical lymph node
  - Often presenting symptom
- > 70% of patients present with stage III or IV disease

Treatment

- Multiple approaches depending on clinical stage
  - Tonsillectomy for small T1 tumors confined to tonsil
  - Radiation therapy including intensity-modulated radiation therapy (IMRT)
  - Concurrent radiotherapy with multiagent chemotherapy
  - Targeted agents such as cetuximab
  - Salvage neck dissection when indicated

Prognosis

- HPV-positive OPSCC associated with improved survival outcomes
- Tumor size and presence of metastases influence prognosis

IMAGE FINDINGS

General Features

- PET/CT useful particularly when dealing with unknown primary

MACROSCOPIC FEATURES

General Features

- Exophytic or ulcerative
- May be clinical &/or radiographically undetected
- Cystic lymph node

OROPHARYNGEAL CARCINOMA

Key Facts

Terminology
- Malignant epithelial neoplasm of oropharynx, including soft palate, tonsils, uvula, base of tongue, and oropharyngeal wall comprising Waldeyer ring

Etiology/Pathogenesis
- High-risk HPV associated with > 70% of OPSCC cases

Clinical Issues
- OPSCC increased 1-2% annually in USA males in past 20 years
- Enlarged cervical lymph node often presenting symptom
- > 70% of patients present with stage III or IV disease
- HPV-positive OPSCC associated with improved survival outcomes

Microscopic Pathology
- **HPV-positive OPSCC**: Nonkeratinizing histology
  - Tumor often seen arising from epithelium of tonsillar crypts
  - Squamous maturation and focal areas of keratinization can be seen but should comprise < 10% of tumor
- **Lymphoepithelial-like OPSCC**: Similar to EBV-related nasopharyngeal carcinoma
  - p16(+) and EBV(-)
- **HPV-negative OPSCC**: Exhibits features of conventional-type SCC

Ancillary Tests
- p16 strongly positive in HPV-associated OPSCC
- HPV 16 correlates with p16 immunohistochemistry

- Base of tongue primary SCC can be deeply infiltrative with extension to oral tongue, vallecula, epiglottis, preepiglottic space, and tonsils

Sections to Be Submitted
- Entire tonsil should be submitted when trying to identify clinically occult primary &/or no mass noted grossly

MICROSCOPIC PATHOLOGY

Histologic Features
- **HPV-positive** OPSCC
  - **Nonkeratinizing** OPSCC
    - Tumor often seen arising from epithelium of tonsillar crypts rather than overlying epithelium
    - Basaloid oval to spindle-shaped cells with hyperchromatic nuclei and minimal cytoplasm forming trabeculae, sheets, or nests with sharply defined borders
    - Comedo-necrosis frequently present
    - Brisk mitotic rate and numerous scattered apoptotic cells
    - Permeated by lymphocytes
    - Squamous maturation and focal areas of keratinization can be seen but should comprise < 10% of tumor
  - **Hybrid-type** OPSCC
    - Has features of both nonkeratinizing OPSCC and keratinizing SCC
    - Amount of squamous maturation is > 10%
    - Not all cases show p16 immunoreactivity or HPV positivity by in situ hybridization
  - **Lymphoepithelial-like** OPSCC
    - Similar in histology to EBV-related nasopharyngeal carcinoma
    - Syncytial-appearing large tumor cells with indistinct cell borders and vesicular nuclei intermingled with lymphocytes and plasma cells
    - Tumor cells immunoreactive for cytokeratin
    - Positive for p16 by immunohistochemistry and negative for EBER by in situ hybridization
  - **Papillary** OPSCC
    - Uncommon morphologic variant of SCC that can occur in oropharynx
    - Finger-like projections of cytologically malignant epithelial cells with fibrovascular cores
    - Surface keratinization absent or limited
    - Definitive invasive SCC may be difficult to see, particularly on biopsy specimens
    - Up to 2/3 of cases reported to be p16 positive but < 50% positive for high-risk HPV
- **HPV-negative** OPSCC
  - **Keratinizing** SCC
    - Exhibits features of conventional-type SCC, including nests of epithelial cells with abundant eosinophilic cytoplasm and well-defined cell borders
    - Frank keratinization can be present
    - Basaloid morphology not seen
    - Tumors divided into well, moderately, and poorly differentiated

ANCILLARY TESTS

Cytology
- Fine needle aspiration of cervical lymph node may be initial biopsy
  - Nonkeratinizing OPSCC show cohesive groups of cells with distinct cell borders and hyperchromatic nuclei
    - Keratinization absent or minimal
    - Cellular debris and inflammatory cells
    - May be hypocellular because of cyst formation
    - Serous fluid in cystic lymph node metastasis
    - Distinct from metastatic lymph node with central necrosis

Immunohistochemistry
- p16 strongly positive in HPV-associated OPSCC
  - Both nuclear and cytoplasmic staining of tumor cells
  - Normal epithelium is negative or shows minimal patchy staining

- p16 considered reliable surrogate marker for high-risk HPV-associated OPSCC
- p16 useful on FNA cell block from occult neck mass to help localize tumor origin to oropharynx
- Strongly positive with cytokeratin(s)
  - Usually not required for diagnosis except in lymphoepithelial-like variant

In Situ Hybridization

- HPV 16 correlates with p16 immunohistochemistry
  - Positive test shows nuclear dots, which can range from strongly and diffusely positive to only a rare positive cell
  - May see single punctate nuclear dot or multiple nuclear dots in tumor cell
  - Not detected in normal tonsillar epithelium
  - May see hybridization signals in dysplastic epithelium
- Other HPV types have been detected, including HPV 6, 18, 33, 35, 45, and 52/58
- HPV ISH can be used on FNA cell block from metastatic lymph node

DIFFERENTIAL DIAGNOSIS

Basaloid Squamous Cell Carcinoma (BSCC)

- Highly aggressive tumor with propensity for oropharynx, hypopharynx, and larynx
- Growth pattern includes lobules and trabeculae that form "jigsaw" configuration
- Pleomorphic basaloid cells with numerous mitoses with peripheral nuclear palisading
- Hyaline or mucohyaline material can be seen intercellularly similar to duplicated basement membrane material seen in some salivary gland neoplasms
- Prominent comedo-type necrosis
- Squamous component is minor component and may be seen as dysplasia, CIS, or invasive SCC
- Frequent metastases to regional lymph nodes and lung
- HPV-negative
  - Detection of HPV in BSCC from oropharynx is associated with better prognosis; best to classify these tumors as nonkeratinizing SCC
- Immunoreactive for cytokeratins, variable expressivity for vimentin, neuron-specific enolase, S100 protein, and actins
- Poor prognosis

Nasopharyngeal Carcinoma (NPC)

- Share similar clinical presentation of enlarged cervical lymph node as initial manifestation of disease
  - Strong association with EBV
    - EBER in situ hybridization may be helpful in separating occult metastasis from either nasopharynx or oropharynx

DIAGNOSTIC CHECKLIST

Pathologic Interpretation Pearls

- When evaluating cystic neck mass in older individual, 1st diagnostic consideration should be cystic metastasis from oropharyngeal primary
  - Branchial cleft cysts are unusual in patients over 50 years of age
  - Branchial cleft cysts are p16 negative
- OPSCC should be evaluated for p16/HPV as it may direct treatment planning and prognosis

SELECTED REFERENCES

1. Allen CT et al: Human papillomavirus and oropharynx cancer: Biology, detection and clinical implications. Laryngoscope. 120(9):1756-72, 2010
2. Ang KK et al: Human papillomavirus and survival of patients with oropharyngeal cancer. N Engl J Med. 363(1):24-35, 2010
3. Evans M et al: The changing aetiology of head and neck cancer: the role of human papillomavirus. Clin Oncol (R Coll Radiol). 22(7):538-46, 2010
4. Singhi AD et al: Lymphoepithelial-like carcinoma of the oropharynx: a morphologic variant of HPV-related head and neck carcinoma. Am J Surg Pathol. 34(6):800-5, 2010
5. Stelow EB et al: Human papillomavirus-associated squamous cell carcinoma of the upper aerodigestive tract. Am J Surg Pathol. 34(7):e15-24, 2010
6. Chernock RD et al: HPV-related nonkeratinizing squamous cell carcinoma of the oropharynx: utility of microscopic features in predicting patient outcome. Head Neck Pathol. 3(3):186-94, 2009
7. Westra WH: The changing face of head and neck cancer in the 21st century: the impact of HPV on the epidemiology and pathology of oral cancer. Head Neck Pathol. 3(1):78-81, 2009
8. Begum S et al: Basaloid squamous cell carcinoma of the head and neck is a mixed variant that can be further resolved by HPV status. Am J Surg Pathol. 32(7):1044-50, 2008
9. Fakhry C et al: Improved survival of patients with human papillomavirus-positive head and neck squamous cell carcinoma in a prospective clinical trial. J Natl Cancer Inst. 100(4):261-9, 2008
10. Zhang MQ et al: Detection of human papillomavirus-related squamous cell carcinoma cytologically and by in situ hybridization in fine-needle aspiration biopsies of cervical metastasis: a tool for identifying the site of an occult head and neck primary. Cancer. 114(2):118-23, 2008
11. Begum S et al: Detection of human papillomavirus-16 in fine-needle aspirates to determine tumor origin in patients with metastatic squamous cell carcinoma of the head and neck. Clin Cancer Res. 13(4):1186-91, 2007
12. El-Mofty SK et al: Human papillomavirus (HPV)-related oropharyngeal nonkeratinizing squamous cell carcinoma: characterization of a distinct phenotype. Oral Surg Oral Med Oral Pathol Oral Radiol Endod. 101(3):339-45, 2006

Radiographic and Immunohistochemical Features

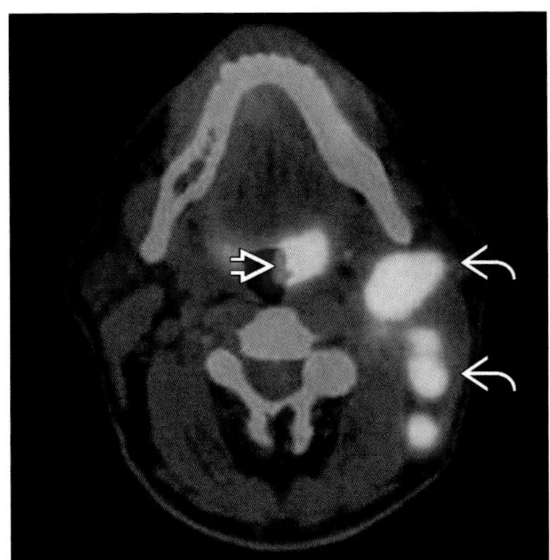

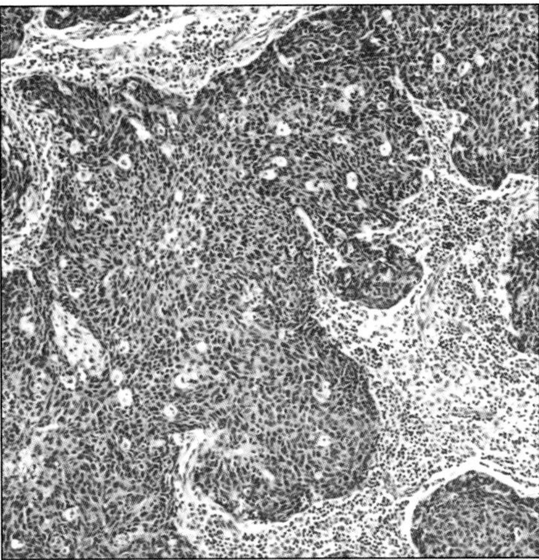

(Left) *Patients with tonsil SCC often present at an advanced stage as seen on this positron emission tomography (PET), which shows the primary in the tonsil ➡ along with numerous lymph node metastases ➦ in the cervical lymph node chain.* **(Right)** *Typical microscopic features of nonkeratinizing SCC of the tonsil are seen with sheets and nests of basaloid tumor cells with a sharply defined borders. No stromal reaction is seen to the tumor.*

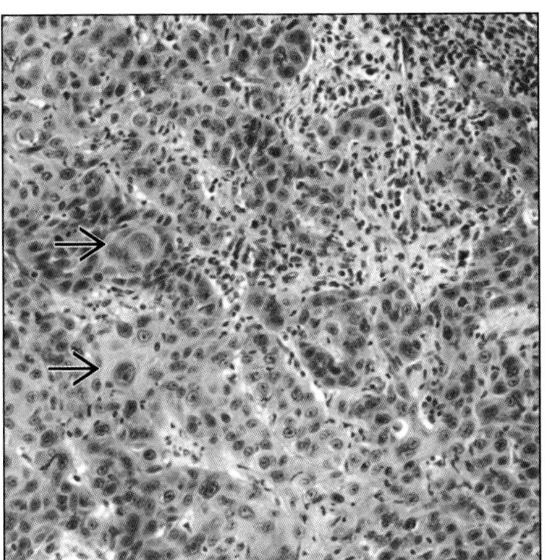

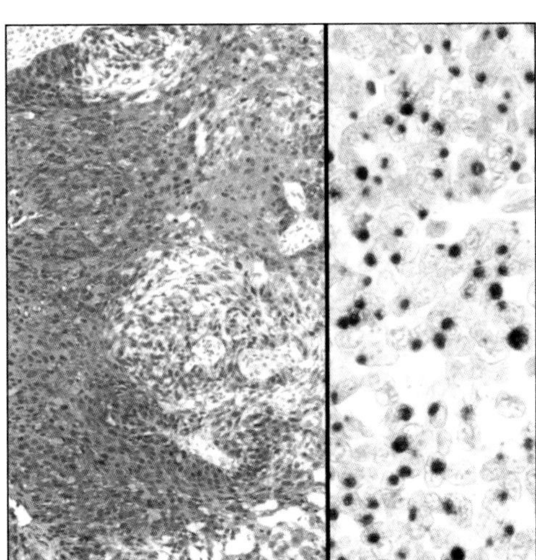

(Left) *Focal keratinization ➡ can be identified in some nonkeratinizing SCC of the tonsil but make up less than 10% of the tumor. Hybrid lesions can show basaloid morphology in the center with squamous differentiation toward the periphery.* **(Right)** *HPV-related nonkeratinizing SCC shows strong, diffuse nuclear and cytoplasmic immunoreactivity with p16 (left panel). In situ hybridization with HPV16/18 shows a strong signal characterized by nuclear dots (right panel).*

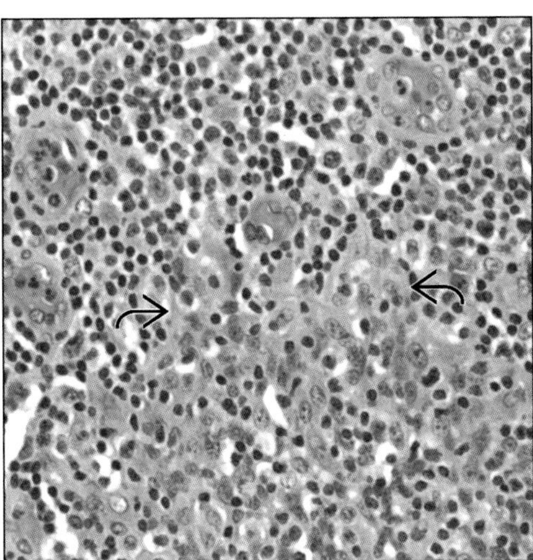

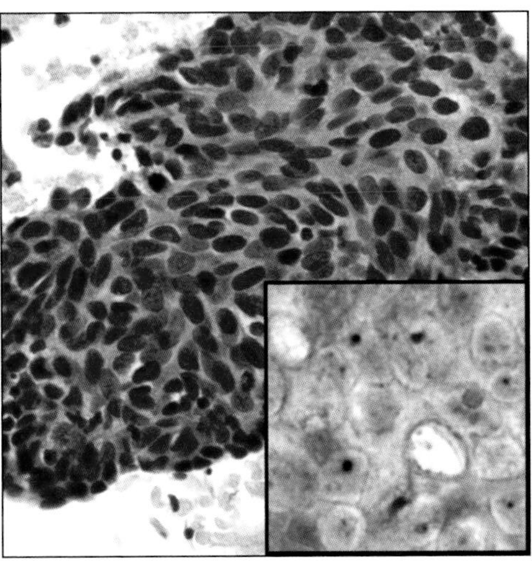

(Left) *A morphologic variant of HPV-related OPSCC is lymphoepithelial-like carcinoma, which is indistinguishable from nonkeratinizing nasopharyngeal carcinoma. The tumor cells have indistinct cell borders with a syncytial growth pattern ➦ and lymphoplasmacytic infiltrate.* **(Right)** *FNA of neck metastases is useful for diagnosis, as both p16 IHC and HPV ISH (inset) can be performed on the cell block, and if positive, can identify tumor origin in the oropharynx.*

MELANOMA

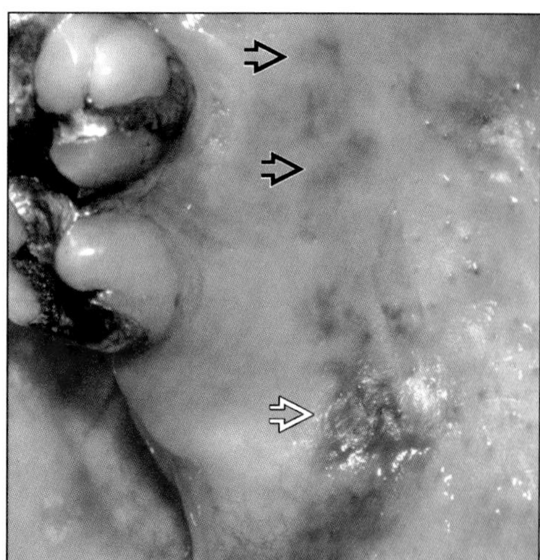

Primary melanoma of the hard palate presents as a diffuse, patchy area of heavy pigmentation with irregular borders ➡. Satellite lesions are noted away from the main area of pigmentation ⇨.

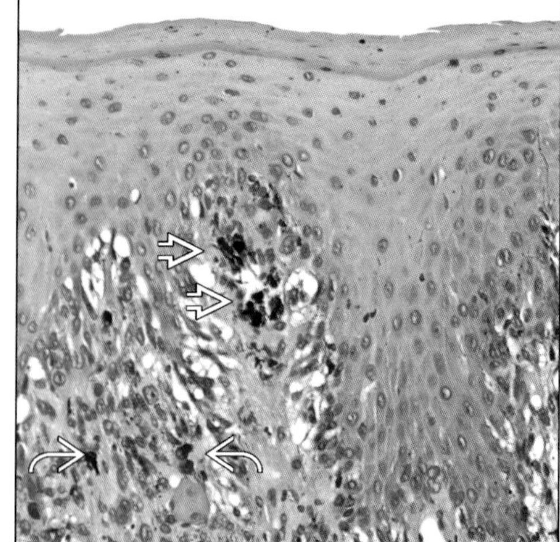

High-power histology shows acral lentiginous melanoma of the hard palate with numerous atypical melanocytes present in the basal epithelium ➡ with invasion into the superficial submucosa ➦.

TERMINOLOGY

Definitions

- Malignant neural crest-derived neoplasm with melanocytic differentiation
  - Atypical melanocytes at epithelial-connective tissue interface with upward migration or connective tissue invasion

ETIOLOGY/PATHOGENESIS

Etiology

- Unknown

CLINICAL ISSUES

Epidemiology

- Incidence
  - Extremely rare, accounting for < 1% of all melanomas
    - 0.02/100,000 population/year in USA
  - Represent about 50% of all head and neck mucosal melanomas
  - Represent < 0.5% of all oral malignancies
  - Unlike cutaneous melanoma, oral melanoma incidence has been stable
- Age
  - Mean in 6th-7th decades
  - Rare in pediatric age group
- Gender
  - Male > Female (2.5-3:1)
- Ethnicity
  - More common in Japan and western Africa

Site

- Hard palate and maxillary alveolus are most common sites of involvement (~ 80%)
- Remaining 20% include
  - Mandibular gingivae
  - Buccal mucosa
  - Floor of mouth and tongue

Presentation

- Most arise de novo, although 1/3 are preceded by pigmented lesion for a few months or years
  - "Melanosis" reported before development of melanoma
- Asymmetric, painless, pigmented lesion
  - Irregular borders or outlines
  - Black, purple, red, gray
    - 15% of oral melanomas are amelanotic
  - Macular, with nodular areas
- Many patients present at advanced stage with pain, ulceration, loose teeth
- Cervical lymph nodes metastases reported in up to 75% of cases at presentation
- Distant metastases seen in about 50% of patients at presentation

Treatment

- Surgical approaches
  - Radical surgical excision
    - Clear margins not always possible due to vital structures of this site
  - Many institutions recommend regional lymph node dissection, even in clinically negative neck
- Adjuvant therapy
  - No clear cut evidence that chemotherapy or immunotherapy for oral melanoma provides any survival benefits
    - Generally used for palliative purposes
  - Not recommended as a single modality treatment
- Radiation
  - May provide prolonged palliation but does not appear to provide any survival benefits

Prognosis

- Overall, poor prognosis
  - Median survival: 2 years

MELANOMA

Key Facts

Terminology
- Malignant neural crest-derived neoplasm with melanocytic differentiation

Clinical Issues
- Extremely rare accounting for < 1% of all melanomas
  - Represent < 0.5% of all oral malignancies
- Mean in 6th-7th decades
- Male > Female (2.5-3:1)
- Hard palate and maxillary alveolus are most common sites of involvement (~ 80%)
- Cervical lymph node metastases reported in more than 50% of cases at presentation
- Asymmetric, painless, pigmented lesion with irregular borders
- Radical surgical excision
- Overall, poor prognosis (median: 2 years)

Image Findings
- Oral cavity mass with high T1WI on MR

Microscopic Pathology
- Pagetoid spread or in situ component with single or multiple melanoma cells in superficial epithelium
- Epithelioid or spindle-shaped morphology to melanocytes containing fine melanin granules
- 1/3 of cases have bone/cartilage invasion

Ancillary Tests
- Generally diffuse and strong staining for S100 protein, HMB-45, and vimentin

Top Differential Diagnoses
- Metastatic melanoma, spindle cell squamous cell carcinoma, pleomorphic sarcoma

  - 5-year survival: 5-10%
- High rates of metastases to liver, brain, and lung
- Worse prognosis suggested by
  - Thickness of > 5 mm
  - Vascular invasion
  - Necrosis
  - Significant pleomorphism
  - Older age
  - High stage

IMAGE FINDINGS

MR Findings
- Best imaging study is multiplanar MR
- Oral cavity mass with high T1WI signal on MR
  - Melanotic melanomas show increased signal due to melanin, free radicals, metal ions, and hemorrhage, giving high or intermediate T1 signal

MACROSCOPIC FEATURES

General Features
- Brown to black pigmented lesion with irregular borders
- Flat macule extends laterally (radial growth phase); nodular lesion (vertical growth phase)
  - Some oral melanomas lack radial growth phase
- Satellite lesions of melanoma are common

Sections to Be Submitted
- Bone &/or cartilage for staging

Size
- Range: Up to 4 cm generally

MICROSCOPIC PATHOLOGY

Histologic Features
- Radial growth phase similar to acral lentiginous melanoma
  - Pagetoid spread (in situ): Single or multiple melanoma cells within epithelium
  - Atypical melanocytes in basal layer spreading laterally
  - Invasion of melanoma cells into lamina propria
  - Prominent dendritic processes may be seen
- Nodular growth phase
  - Epithelioid or spindle-shaped morphology to melanocytes containing fine melanin granules
    - 15% of oral melanomas have little to no melanin
  - 1/3 of cases have bone/cartilage invasion
  - Vascular and perineural invasion not readily noted
  - Mitoses tend to be infrequent but are increased in invasive tumors
  - Pleomorphic cells with atypical mitoses
  - Squamous surface ulceration or atrophy is common

ANCILLARY TESTS

Histochemistry
- Melanin can be highlighted with Masson-Fontana or Schmorl stains

Immunohistochemistry
- Generally diffuse and strong staining for S100 protein, HMB-45, and vimentin
  - Tyrosinase, Melan-A, and MITF are also positive
- Negative: Cytokeratin, myogenic markers, and epithelial membrane antigen

Molecular Genetics
- *NRAS* and *KIT* mutations have been identified in mucosal melanomas
  - May be useful for targeted therapies

DIFFERENTIAL DIAGNOSIS

Metastatic Melanoma
- Extremely rare with very few reported cases of metastases to oral cavity
- Most common: Tongue, buccal mucosa, lip

MELANOMA

Immunohistochemistry

Antibody	Reactivity	Staining Pattern	Comment
S100	Positive	Nuclear & cytoplasmic	Diffuse and strong
HMB-45	Positive	Cytoplasmic	Most tumor cells positive
Tyrosinase	Positive	Cytoplasmic	Variably reactive in most cases
melan-A103	Positive	Cytoplasmic	Variably reactive in most cases
MITF	Positive	Nuclear	Positive in most cases
Vimentin	Positive	Cytoplasmic	All tumor cells positive
CD117	Positive	Cytoplasmic	Isolated tumor cells positive
NSE	Positive	Cytoplasmic	Variably present in many cases
CK-PAN	Negative		
Desmin	Negative		
CD45RB	Negative		

AJCC TNM Staging Criteria for Oral Melanoma (2010)

TNM	Stage Categories	Definition
Primary tumor (T)	pT3	Mucosal disease only
	pT4a	Moderately advanced disease
		Tumor involving deep soft tissue, cartilage, bone, or overlying skin
	pT4b	Very advanced disease
		Tumor involving brain, dura, skull base, lower cranial nerves (IX, X, XI, XII), masticator space, carotid artery, prevertebral space, or mediastinal structures
Regional lymph nodes (N)	pNX	Regional lymph nodes cannot be assessed
	pN0	No regional lymph node metastases
	pN1	Regional lymph node metastasis present
Distant metastasis (M)		No distant metastasis (no pathologic M0; use clinical M to complete stage group)
	pM1	Distant metastasis

Adapted from 7th edition AJCC Staging Forms.

AJCC Pathologic Prognostic Groups for Oral Melanoma (2010)

Group	T	N	M
III	T3	N0	M0
IVA	T4a	N0	M0
	T3-T4a	N1	M0
IVB	T4b	Any N	M0
IVC	Any T	Any N	M1

Adapted from 7th edition AJCC Staging Forms.

- Clinical history required
- Special stains do not make a distinction

Spindle Cell Squamous Cell Carcinoma

- Should be considered when there is no pigmentation
- Junctional origin frequently present
- High-grade tumors, significant pleomorphism, increased mitoses
- Immunohistochemistry will separate these entities
  - Epithelial markers positive in up to 70% of cases
  - Lack melanoma markers

Pleomorphic Sarcoma

- High-grade spindled cell tumor
- Lacks surface origin or involvement
- By definition, lacks melanoma and epithelial markers

SELECTED REFERENCES

1. Moreno MA et al: Management of mucosal melanomas of the head and neck: did we make any progress? Curr Opin Otolaryngol Head Neck Surg. 18(2):101-6, 2010
2. Bachar G et al: Mucosal melanomas of the head and neck: experience of the Princess Margaret Hospital. Head Neck. 30(10):1325-31, 2008
3. Femiano F et al: Oral malignant melanoma: a review of the literature. J Oral Pathol Med. 37(7):383-8, 2008
4. Meleti M et al: Head and neck mucosal melanoma: experience with 42 patients, with emphasis on the role of postoperative radiotherapy. Head Neck. 30(12):1543-51, 2008
5. Wagner M et al: Mucosal melanoma of the head and neck. Am J Clin Oncol. 31(1):43-8, 2008

Microscopic and Immunohistochemical Features

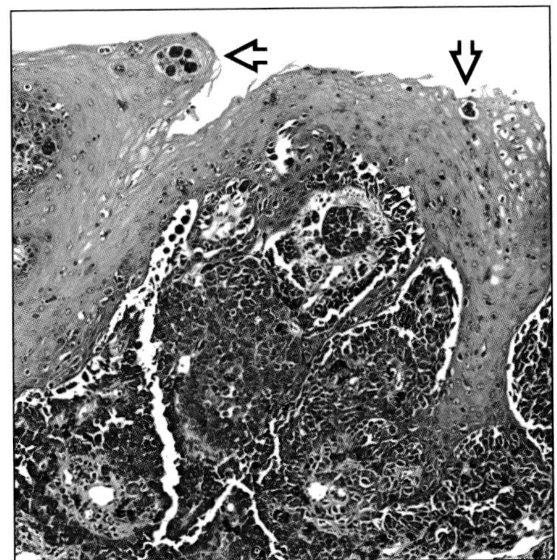

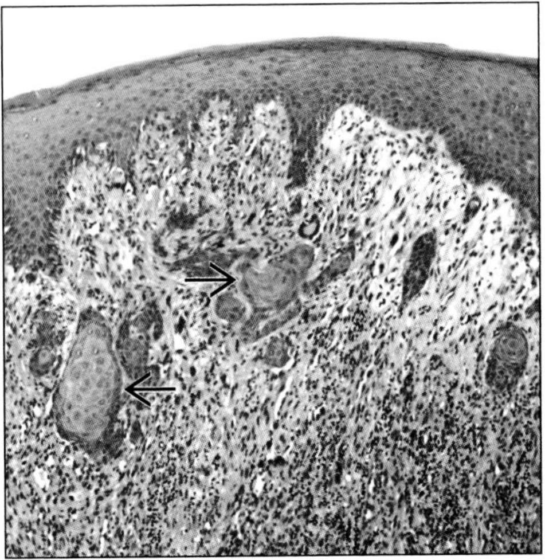

(Left) *Nodular melanoma of the hard palate with epithelioid malignant melanocytes is shown, some with melanin pigment present in the lamina propria. Individual melanocytes ⇨ are seen invading into the upper level of the epithelium.* ***(Right)*** *There is a concurrent pseudoepitheliomatous hyperplasia → present in association with the atypical melanocytic proliferation. An inflammatory infiltrate is also present. The melanoma may be obscured by this process or missed.*

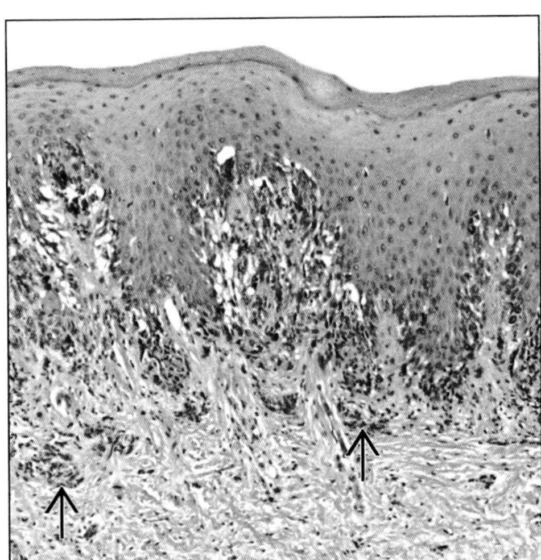

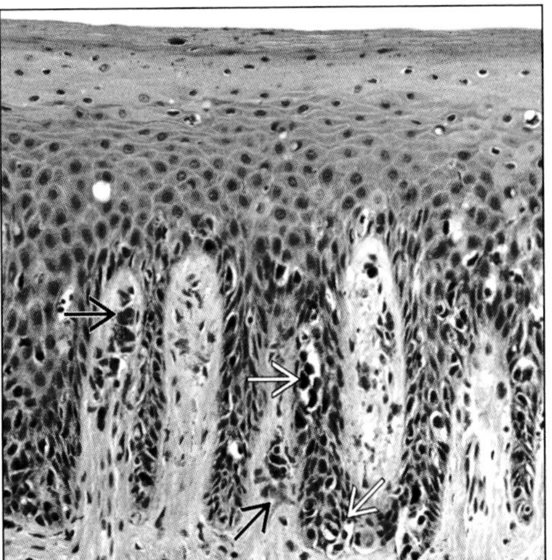

(Left) *The majority of the proliferation in this melanoma is noted at the epithelial to stromal junction. However, isolated nests of atypical melanocytes → are noted within the superficial region of the stroma. Inflammatory cells are inconspicuous.* ***(Right)*** *An in situ growth phase shows atypical and remarkably enlarged melanocytes at the epithelial to stromal junction. A number of melanophages → are present in the stroma with pigment. Nests of atypical melanocytes are obvious ➡.*

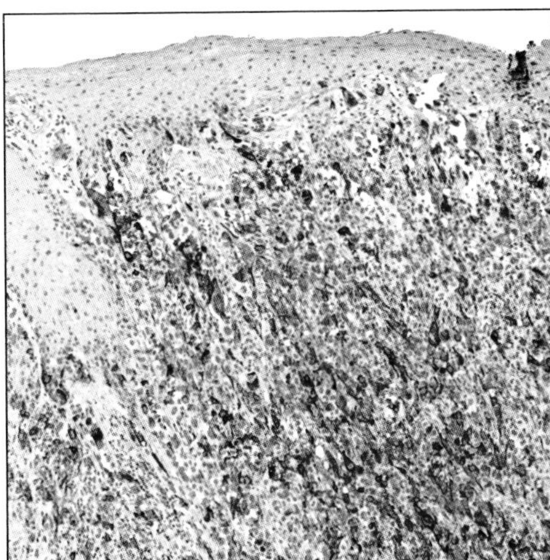

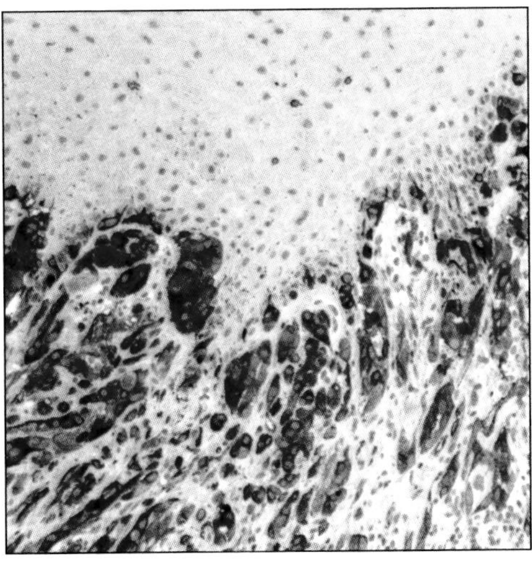

(Left) *S100 protein shows a very strong and diffuse nuclear and cytoplasmic reactivity in the neoplastic cells as they expand from the surface epithelium into the stroma. Depth of invasion is difficult to assess for oral melanoma.* ***(Right)*** *HMB-45 immunohistochemistry highlights the melanocytes present both in the basal layer as well as in the submucosa. This is one of the more specific markers for melanoma. It is important to know that staining can be patchy or focal.*

ANGIOSARCOMA

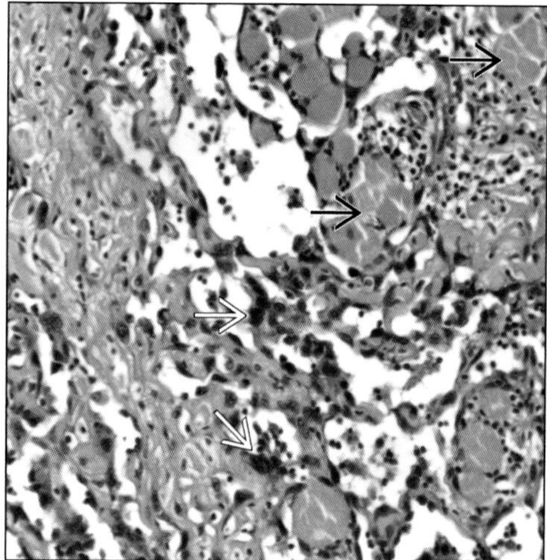

This moderately differentiated angiosarcoma is characterized by irregularly infiltrating vascular channels lined by atypical endothelial cells ➔. This tumor is invading surrounding muscle ⇨.

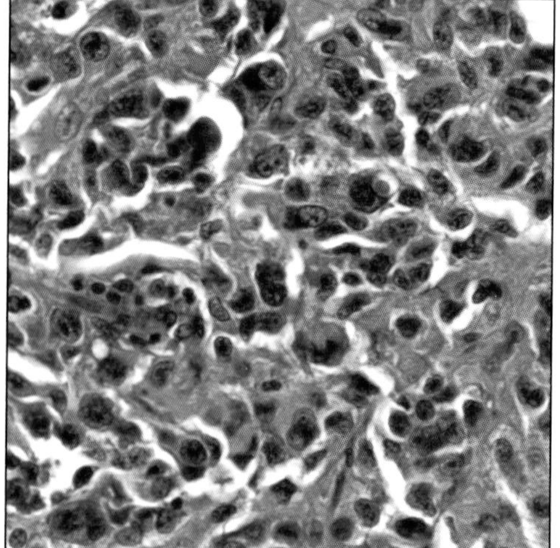

Poorly differentiated angiosarcoma shows atypical cells with little evidence of vascular channels. IHC staining (not shown) was needed to confirm the diagnosis.

TERMINOLOGY

Definitions

- Malignant neoplasm of vascular endothelium

ETIOLOGY/PATHOGENESIS

Associations

- Longstanding lymphedema
- Radiation treatment for other neoplasms
- Trauma/foreign body
- Immune system deficiency
- Preexisting benign vascular neoplasm

CLINICAL ISSUES

Epidemiology

- Incidence
  - Rare; oral tumors comprise ~ 1% of all angiosarcomas
    - Scalp skin is most common site (~ 50% of all angiosarcoma)
- Age
  - Wide range, with high incidence in elderly
- Gender
  - Male > Female (1.1:1)

Site

- Tongue > lip > gingiva > palate
  - Gingiva most common for secondary tumors

Presentation

- Bleeding is common presentation
- Painful mass, often with recent enlargement
  - Red to bluish-purple
- Ulceration is common

Treatment

- Options, risks, complications
  - Avoid biopsy due to bleeding risk
- Surgical approaches
  - Wide local excision
- Adjuvant therapy
  - Radiation and chemotherapy are considered ineffective

Prognosis

- Prognosis can be favorable
  - Lip and tongue primaries show relatively good prognosis
  - Seem to have better prognosis than other sites
- Metastasis and recurrence are common
  - Metastases to lung, liver, and bone

MACROSCOPIC FEATURES

General Features

- Invasive tumor with bloody cut surface
- Frequently multinodular

Size

- Range: Up to 7 cm (mean: 2.5 cm)

MICROSCOPIC PATHOLOGY

Histologic Features

- Wide spectrum of histologic patterns: Vasoformative, solid, papillary
- Anastomosing vascular channels
  - Lined by moderately atypical endothelial cells
  - Tumor cell spindling can be seen: Elongated nuclei with prominent nucleoli
- Papillary tufting often seen
- Intracytoplasmic vacuoles (neolumen) containing erythrocytes
- Epithelioid subtype
  - Large, polygonal eosinophilic cells, vesicular nuclei, prominent nucleoli, neolumen

ANGIOSARCOMA

Key Facts

Terminology
- Malignant neoplasm of vascular endothelium

Clinical Issues
- Oral tumors comprise ~ 1% of all angiosarcomas
- Wide age range, with high incidence in elderly
- Male > Female (1.1:1)
- Bleeding, painful mass
- Tongue > lip > gingiva > palate
- Wide local excision

Microscopic Pathology
- Wide spectrum of histologic patterns: Vasoformative, solid, papillary
- Anastomosing vascular channels
- Neolumen containing erythrocytes
- Large, polygonal eosinophilic cells, vesicular nuclei, prominent nucleoli

Ancillary Tests
- Positive with variety of vascular markers

Immunohistochemistry

Antibody	Reactivity	Staining Pattern	Comment
CD31	Positive	Cell membrane	More diffuse, more specific
CD34	Positive	Cell membrane	Focal
FVIIIRAg	Positive	Cytoplasmic	Diffuse, most tumor cells
Actin-sm	Positive	Cytoplasmic	Adjacent to vascular spaces
Ki-67	Positive	Nuclear	> 10% of cells
CK-PAN	Negative		± in soft tissue angiosarcomas

  - Epithelioid endothelial cells
- Mitotic rate varies based on tumor grade
- Prominent necrosis is often present
- Inflammatory infiltrate is usually absent or limited
- Tumor grade: Low, intermediate, high

ANCILLARY TESTS

Flow Cytometry
- Hypo- and hyperdiploid

Electron Microscopy
- Weibel-Palade bodies contain fine tubules and are intracytoplasmic storage granules of endothelial cells

DIFFERENTIAL DIAGNOSIS

Hemangiomas
- Lack pleomorphism and destructive growth

Spindle Cell Carcinoma
- Much more common than angiosarcoma
- **Negative**: Endothelial markers

Mucosal Malignant Melanoma
- Similar nuclear pleomorphism and large nucleoli
- **Positive**: Melanoma markers

Other Sarcomas
- **Negative**: Endothelial markers

SELECTED REFERENCES

1. Florescu M et al: Gingival angiosarcoma: histopathologic and immunohistochemical study. Rom J Morphol Embryol. 46(1):57-61, 2005
2. Fanburg-Smith JC et al: Oral and salivary gland angiosarcoma: a clinicopathologic study of 29 cases. Mod Pathol. 16(3):263-71, 2003

IMAGE GALLERY

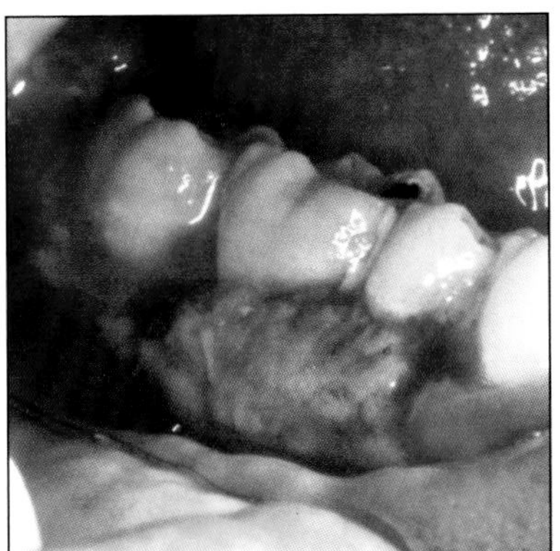

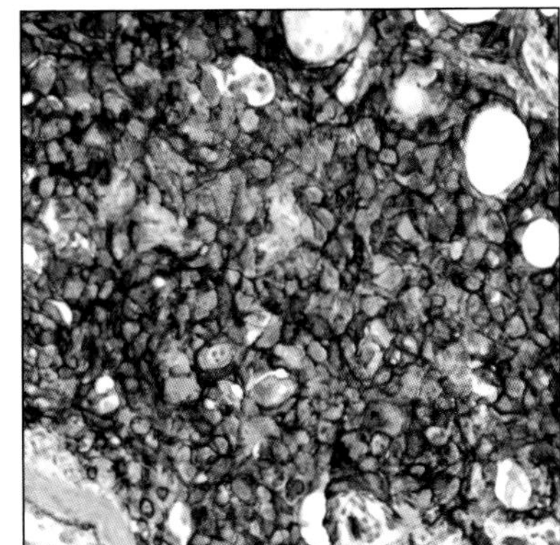

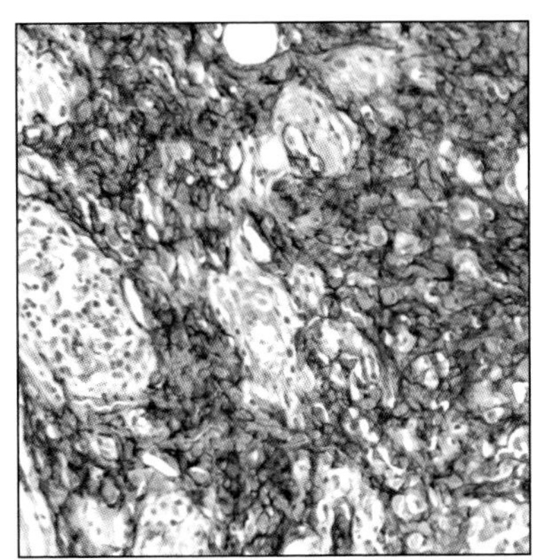

*(**Left**) This 15-year-old girl with gingival angiosarcoma presented with a bleeding mass, clinically thought to be a pyogenic granuloma. Subsequent biopsy was an angiosarcoma. The patient died of her disease 2 years later. (**Center**) An angiosarcoma with cytoplasmic reactivity to CD34 is shown. (**Right**) An angiosarcoma is seen with strong and diffuse cytoplasmic reactivity to CD31.*

KAPOSI SARCOMA

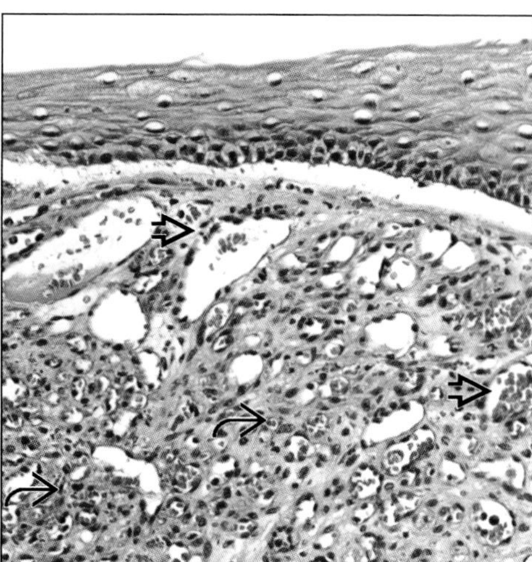

Kaposi sarcoma of the hard palate exhibits normal overlying mucosa and numerous vascular spaces of varying sizes in the submucosa. Erythrocytes are present within ⇨ and between the vessels ↪.

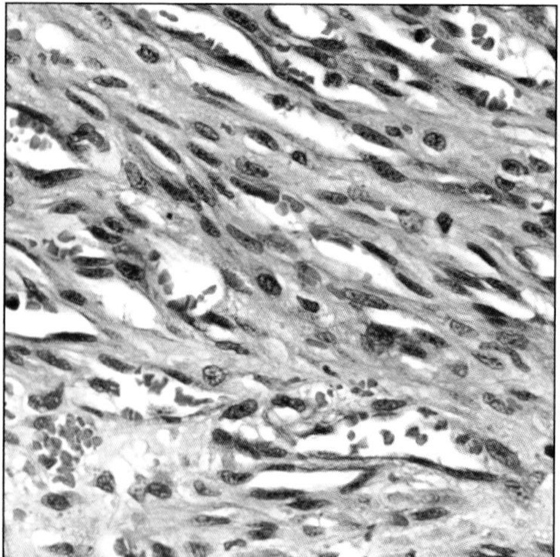

High-power photomicrograph shows a patch stage Kaposi sarcoma characterized by numerous slit-like spaces dissecting through the connective tissue. The vascular spaces often run parallel to the epithelium.

TERMINOLOGY

Abbreviations

- Kaposi sarcoma (KS)

Definitions

- Locally aggressive vascular neoplasm of intermediate type, which rarely metastasizes
  - Considered to be AIDS-defining illness

ETIOLOGY/PATHOGENESIS

Etiology

- Uniformly associated with human herpes virus 8 (HHV8)

CLINICAL ISSUES

Epidemiology

- Incidence
  - AIDS-associated KS seen in up to 20% of HIV-infected patients
- Age
  - AIDS-associated KS: 4th or 5th decade
- Gender
  - AIDS-associated KS: Primarily homo- and bisexual HIV-1 infected men in western countries

Site

- Oral cavity is common site for AIDS-associated KS
  - Hard palate most common location
    - Followed by gingiva and tongue

Presentation

- Multiple reddish to purple macules that eventually develop into plaques or nodules
- Bleeding, pain, and ulceration

Laboratory Tests

- HHV8 can be detected in peripheral blood

Treatment

- Surgical approaches
  - Surgery only done in cases where there is significant morbidity due to lesions
- Drugs
  - Single agent chemotherapy for aggressive forms of KS
    - Includes etoposide, bleomycin, paclitaxel
  - For small oral lesions
    - Intralesional injection with vinblastine
    - Cryotherapy may be used

Prognosis

- Dependent on immune status

MICROSCOPIC PATHOLOGY

Histologic Features

- Patch stage: Proliferation of small irregularly shaped vascular spaces, which often run parallel to epithelium
  - Extravasated erythrocytes and lymphocytes
  - Slit-like vascular spaces dissect collagen bundles
- Plaque stage: Further vascular proliferation along with spindle cell component
  - Intra- and extracellular hyaline globules
  - Denser inflammatory cell infiltrate
- Nodular stage: Unencapsulated infiltrating fascicles of spindled cells with atypia and mitoses

ANCILLARY TESTS

Histochemistry

- Hyaline globules are PAS-positive, diastase resistant

Immunohistochemistry

- HHV8 nuclear staining positive in all cases

KAPOSI SARCOMA

Key Facts

Terminology

- Locally aggressive vascular neoplasm of intermediate-type, which rarely metastasizes

Clinical Issues

- Oral cavity a common site for AIDS-associated KS
- Multiple reddish to purple macules that eventually develop into plaques or nodules
- HHV8 can be detected in peripheral blood

Microscopic Pathology

- Patch stage: Proliferation of small irregularly shaped vascular spaces, which often run parallel to epithelium
- Plaque stage: More vascular proliferation with spindle cell appearance; hyaline globules present
- Nodular stage: Infiltrating fascicles of spindled cells with atypia and mitoses

Clinical Forms of Kaposi Sarcoma

Type	Risk Group	Sites of Involvement	Clinical Course
Classic	> 70% elderly men of Slavic, Jewish, or Italian ancestry	Skin of lower extremities	Indolent
Endemic (African)	Children and middle-aged men	Skin of extremities; visceral involvement common; lymphadenopathic type common in children	Indolent in adults; aggressive in children
Iatrogenic or transplantation-associated	Solid organ transplant (0.5% of renal transplant patients); immunosuppressive therapy	Skin of extremities; may have visceral involvement	Variable; may resolve upon cessation of immunosuppressives
AIDS-related	HIV-infected patients; more commonly seen in male homo- and bisexuals at younger age group than classic KS	Skin of head and neck, extremities, genitals; mucosa of upper aerodigestive tract; lymph nodes	Aggressive

- Spindled cells usually positive for CD34 and CD31, but FVIIIRAg negative
- VEGFR-3, FLI-1 (nuclear transcription factor), and vimentin positive

DIFFERENTIAL DIAGNOSIS

Pyogenic Granuloma

- Lobular, endothelial growth, inflammation, no globules

Kaposiform Hemangioendothelioma

- Rare, usually occurs in 1st decade of life
- No association with HIV or HHV8 infection
- **Positive**: VEGFR-3, CD34, CD31; **negative**: FVIIIRAg

Spindle Cell Squamous Carcinoma

- Spindled cells; cytokeratin positive, HHV8 negative

Angiosarcoma

- Marked pleomorphism, mitoses, necrosis; no HHV8

SELECTED REFERENCES

1. Pantanowitz L et al: Immunohistochemistry in Kaposi's sarcoma. Clin Exp Dermatol. 35(1):68-72, 2010
2. Bagni R et al: Kaposi's sarcoma-associated herpesvirus transmission and primary infection. Curr Opin HIV AIDS. 4(1):22-6, 2009
3. Pantanowitz L et al: Pathology of Kaposi's sarcoma. J HIV Ther. 14(2):41-7, 2009
4. Laurent C et al: Human herpesvirus 8 infections in patients with immunodeficiencies. Hum Pathol. 39(7):983-93, 2008

IMAGE GALLERY

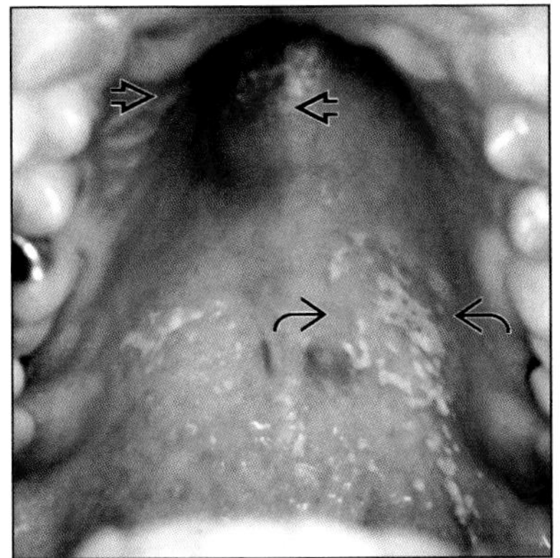

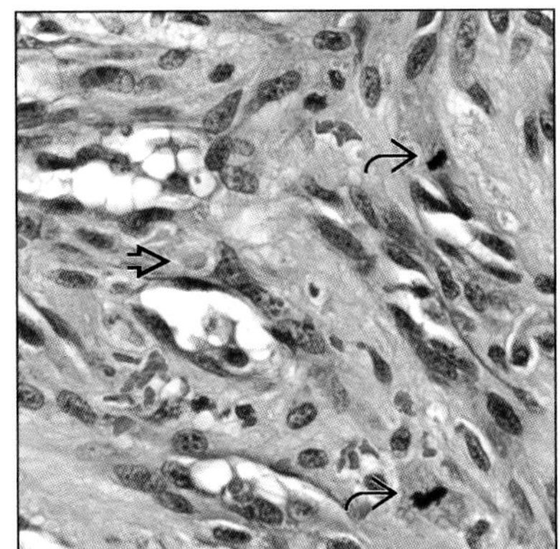

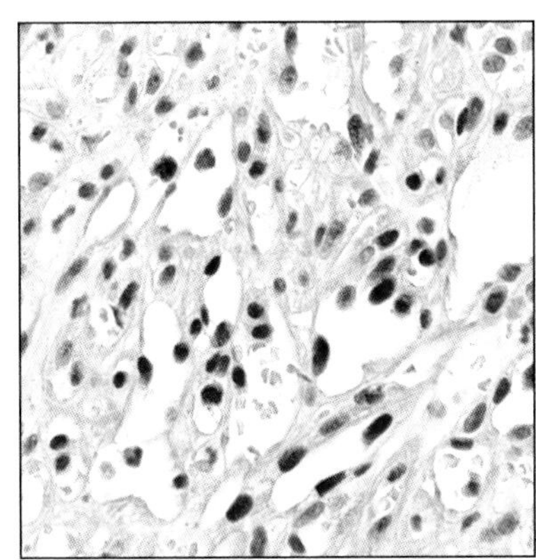

(Left) *HIV-associated Kaposi sarcoma presents as a brown/purple macule of the anterior hard palate ⇒. Concomitant oral pseudomembranous candidiasis is also noted ↗.* ***(Center)*** *High-power photomicrograph of Kaposi sarcoma shows spindled endothelial cells forming slit-like spaces. Hyaline globules ⇒ and mitotic figures ↗ are evident. These histologic findings are noted in both plaque and nodular stages.* ***(Right)*** *Tumor cells show strong diffuse nuclear immunoreactivity for human herpes virus type 8 (HHV8) latent nuclear antigen-1.*

METASTATIC/SECONDARY TUMORS

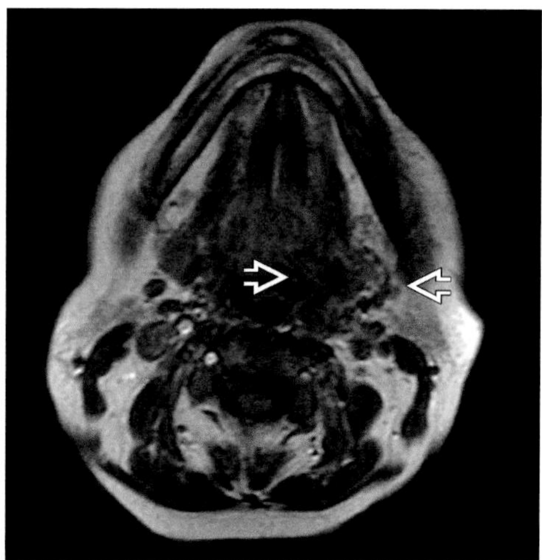

An 85-year-old woman presented with a 3-month history of jaw pain. A large destructive mass ➡ is noted on this T1WI MR in the retromolar trigone at the proximal ramus, with bone involvement.

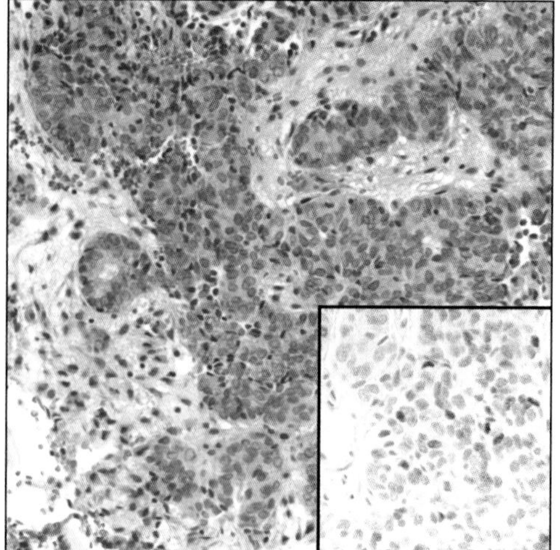

The patient had a history of endometrial adenocarcinoma, and a biopsy of a retromolar mass showed a metastatic tumor consistent with that diagnosis. The tumor was positive for ER (inset) and PR receptors.

TERMINOLOGY

Definitions

- Tumors secondarily involving oral mucosa and jaws that originate from, but are not in continuity with, primary malignancies of other anatomic sites
  - Lymphomas and leukemias are excluded by definition

ETIOLOGY/PATHOGENESIS

Pathogenesis

- Metastases involve various complex signaling pathways, including epithelial to mesenchymal transition, angiogenesis, growth factors, and inhibition of apoptosis

CLINICAL ISSUES

Epidemiology

- Incidence
  - Rare
    - Approximately 1% of oral malignancies
- Age
  - 5th to 7th decade
- Gender
  - Soft tissue: Male > Female (2:1)
  - Bone: Equal gender distribution

Site

- **Soft tissue**
  - Attached gingiva most common location accounting for > 50% of cases
  - Tongue 2nd most common site accounting for about 25% of cases
- **Bone**
  - Gnathic bone more frequently involved than soft tissue (2:1)
  - Mandible > > maxilla (4:1)
    - Molar area most common location
    - Rarely both jaws may be affected

Presentation

- Soft tissue location
  - Gingival metastases can resemble a reactive process, such as pyogenic granuloma
  - Hemorrhage
  - Submucosal mass
  - Occasionally surface ulceration
- Gnathic bone location
  - Rapid pain and swelling
  - Loose teeth
  - Nonhealing extraction site
    - Presumed that metastases was present prior to extraction and may have been underlying etiology
  - Paresthesia
  - Numb-chin syndrome: Loss of sensation to lower lip and chin due to involvement of inferior alveolar nerve
    - Not specific to metastases and may also be seen in inflammatory processes or primary jaw lesions

Natural History

- About 20-25% of metastases to oral cavity represent initial presentation of malignant disease
- Oral cavity may also be 1st sign of malignant disease

Treatment

- Surgical approaches
  - Surgery generally reserved for palliation
  - If oral metastases are isolated, local resection is sometimes advocated
- Adjuvant therapy
  - Treatment usually palliative and to improve quality of life
- Radiation
  - Used to control widespread disease and as palliative measure

METASTATIC/SECONDARY TUMORS

Key Facts

Terminology

- Tumors secondarily involving oral mucosa and jaws that originate from, but are not in continuity with, primary malignancies of other anatomic sites

Clinical Issues

- Approximately 1% of oral malignancies
- Attached gingiva most common soft tissue location accounting for > 50% of cases
- Gnathic bone more frequently involved than soft tissue (2:1)
- Mandible > > maxilla (4:1)

Microscopic Pathology

- Most common metastatic tumors to oral cavity in males are lung, kidney, and prostate
- Most common metastatic tumors to oral cavity in females are breast, genital organs, and kidney

Prognosis

- Poor; average survival time of 7 months

MICROSCOPIC PATHOLOGY

Histologic Features

- Metastatic tumor should be histologically similar to primary site of origin
- Metastases to soft tissue
  - Male: Lung (33%), renal (14%), colorectal (5%)
  - Female: Breast (25%), genital organs (15%), renal (12%), lung (9%)
- Metastases to gnathic bones
  - Male: Lung (22%), prostate (11%), renal (9%), adrenal (8%)
  - Female: Breast (41%), adrenal (8%), genital organs (8%), renal (7%)
- Other primary sites include skin, liver, prostate, thyroid, stomach, esophagus, bladder
- Adenocarcinoma most frequent tumor type
- Metastatic sarcomas to oral cavity are rare

ANCILLARY TESTS

Immunohistochemistry

- Markers specific to suspected primary tumor site are indicated, particularly when oral cavity is initial presentation of malignancy

DIFFERENTIAL DIAGNOSIS

Primary Tumor

- Poorly differentiated tumors of both soft tissue and bones may need to be distinguished from metastases
- Both soft tissue and intraosseous high-grade salivary gland carcinomas can share histologic features of metastatic tumors
  - Breast adenocarcinoma vs. salivary gland adenocarcinoma NOS
- Clear cell renal cell carcinoma shares features with intraosseous clear cell carcinoma
- Immunohistochemistry, clinical history, and radiographic imaging helpful
  - When exuberant tissue growth appears in post-extraction site, metastases should be considered
- When metastases represents initial presentation, PET scans may be indicated

SELECTED REFERENCES

1. Divya KS et al: Numb chin syndrome: a case series and discussion. Br Dent J. 208(4):157-60, 2010
2. Hirshberg A et al: Metastatic tumours to the oral cavity - pathogenesis and analysis of 673 cases. Oral Oncol. 44(8):743-52, 2008
3. van der Waal RI et al: Oral metastases: report of 24 cases. Br J Oral Maxillofac Surg. 41(1):3-6, 2003
4. Hirshberg A et al: Metastatic tumors to the jawbones: analysis of 390 cases. J Oral Pathol Med. 23(8):337-41, 1994

IMAGE GALLERY

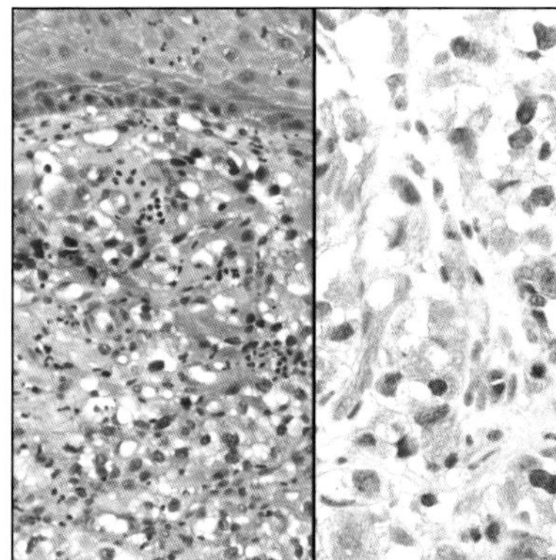

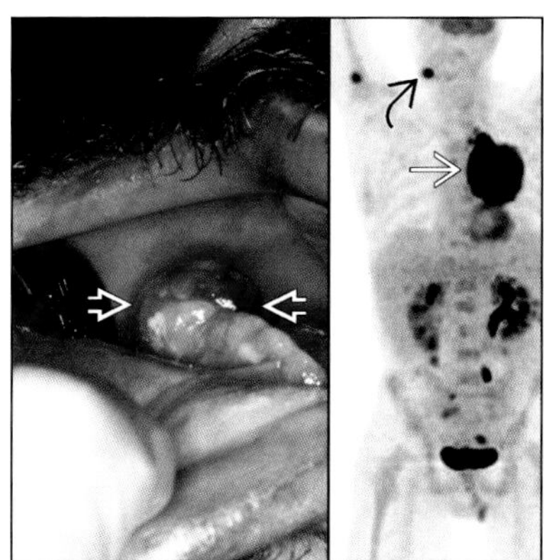

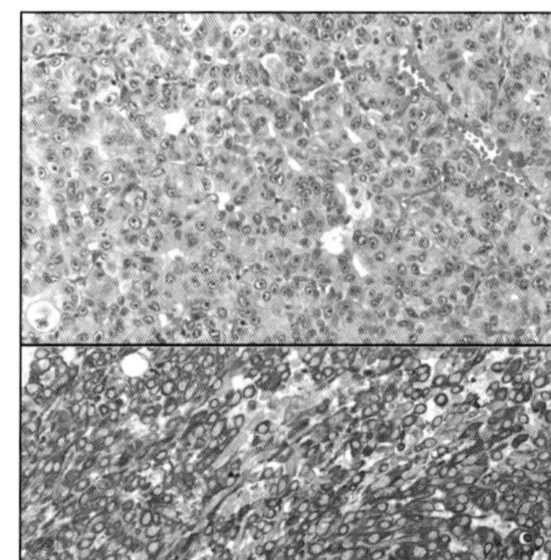

(Left) *Metastatic clear cell renal cell carcinoma to the mandibular attached gingiva is confirmed by immunostaining, including pax-2 (right).* ***(Center)*** *A 55-year-old man with a soft tissue mass ⇨ growing out of a recent extraction socket is the initial presentation of lung cancer. PET imaging showed a 10 cm lung mass ➡ and bone metastases to the humerus and mandible ↗.* ***(Right)*** *This adenocarcinoma is consistent with metastatic lung adenocarcinoma, confirmed by immunohistochemistry, including CK7 (lower).*

PROTOCOL FOR THE EXAMINATION OF LIP AND ORAL CAVITY SPECIMENS

Lip and Oral Cavity

Incisional Biopsy, Excisional Biopsy, Resection

Specimen (select all that apply)

___ Vermillion border of upper lip
___ Vermillion border of lower lip
___ Mucosa of upper lip
___ Mucosa of lower lip
___ Commissure of lip
___ Lateral border of tongue
___ Ventral surface of tongue, not otherwise specified (NOS)
___ Dorsal surface of tongue, NOS
___ Anterior 2/3 of tongue, NOS
___ Upper gingiva (gum)
___ Lower gingiva (gum)
___ Anterior floor of mouth
___ Floor of mouth, NOS
___ Hard palate
___ Buccal mucosa (inner cheek)
___ Vestibule of mouth
    ___ Upper
    ___ Lower
___ Alveolar process
    ___ Upper
    ___ Lower
___ Mandible
___ Maxilla
___ Other (specify): ___________________________
___ Not specified

Received

___ Fresh
___ In formalin
___ Other (specify): ___________________________

Procedure (select all that apply)

___ Incisional biopsy
___ Excisional biopsy
___ Resection
    ___ Glossectomy (specify): ___________________________
    ___ Mandibulectomy (specify): ___________________________
    ___ Maxillectomy (specify): ___________________________
    ___ Palatectomy
___ Neck (lymph node) dissection (specify): ___________________________
___ Other (specify): ___________________________
___ Not specified

**Specimen Integrity*

*___Intact
*___Fragmented

Specimen Size

Greatest dimensions: _________ x _________ x _________ cm
*Additional dimensions (if more than 1 part): _________ x _________ x _________ cm

Specimen Laterality

___ Right
___ Left

___ Bilateral
___ Midline
___ Not specified

Tumor Site (select all that apply)

___ Vermillion border of upper lip
___ Vermillion border of lower lip
___ Mucosa of upper lip
___ Mucosa of lower lip
___ Commissure of lip
___ Lateral border of tongue
___ Ventral surface of tongue, NOS
___ Dorsal surface of tongue, NOS
___ Anterior 2/3 of tongue, NOS
___ Upper gingiva (gum)
___ Lower gingiva (gum)
___ Anterior floor of mouth
___ Floor of mouth, NOS
___ Hard palate
___ Buccal mucosa (inner cheek)
___ Vestibule of mouth
  ___ Upper
  ___ Lower
___ Alveolar process
  ___ Upper
  ___ Lower
___ Mandible
___ Maxilla
___ Other (specify): ___________________________
___ Not specified

Tumor Focality

___ Single focus
___ Multifocal (specify): ___________________________

Tumor Size

Greatest dimension: _________ cm
*Additional dimensions: _________ x _________ cm

**Tumor Thickness (pT1 and pT2 tumors)*

*Tumor thickness: _________ mm
*Intact surface mucosa: _________ or ulcerated surface: _________

**Tumor Description (select all that apply)*

*Gross subtype
  *___ Polypoid
  *___ Exophytic
  *___ Endophytic
  *___ Ulcerated
  *___ Sessile
  *___ Other (specify): ___________________________

**Macroscopic Extent of Tumor*

*Specify: ___________________________

Histologic Type (select all that apply)

___ Squamous cell carcinoma, conventional
___ Variants of squamous cell carcinoma
  ___ Acantholytic squamous cell carcinoma

PROTOCOL FOR THE EXAMINATION OF LIP AND ORAL CAVITY SPECIMENS

- ____ Adenosquamous carcinoma
- ____ Basaloid squamous cell carcinoma
- ____ Carcinoma cuniculatum
- ____ Papillary squamous cell carcinoma
- ____ Spindle cell squamous carcinoma
- ____ Verrucous carcinoma

____ Lymphoepithelial carcinoma (non-nasopharyngeal)

____ Carcinomas of minor salivary glands

- ____ Acinic cell carcinoma
- ____ Adenoid cystic carcinoma
- ____ Adenocarcinoma, not otherwise specified (NOS)
  - ____ Low grade
  - ____ Intermediate grade
  - ____ High grade
- ____ Basal cell adenocarcinoma
- ____ Carcinoma ex-pleomorphic adenoma (malignant mixed tumor)
  - Grade
    - ____ Low grade
    - ____ High grade
  - Invasion
    - ____ Intracapsular (noninvasive)
    - ____ Minimally invasive
    - ____ Invasive
- ____ Carcinoma, type cannot be determined
- ____ Carcinosarcoma
- ____ Clear cell adenocarcinoma
- ____ Cystadenocarcinoma
- ____ Epithelial-myoepithelial carcinoma
- ____ Mucoepidermoid carcinoma
  - ____ Low grade
  - ____ Intermediate grade
  - ____ High grade
- ____ Mucinous adenocarcinoma (colloid carcinoma)
- ____ Myoepithelial carcinoma (malignant myoepithelioma)
- ____ Oncocytic carcinoma
- ____ Polymorphous low-grade adenocarcinoma
- ____ Salivary duct carcinoma
- ____ Other (specify): ____________________________

____ Adenocarcinoma, non-salivary gland type

- ____ Adenocarcinoma, not otherwise specified (NOS)
  - ____ Low grade
  - ____ Intermediate grade
  - ____ High grade
- ____ Other (specify): ____________________________

____ Neuroendocrine carcinoma

- ____ Typical carcinoid tumor (well-differentiated neuroendocrine carcinoma)
- ____ Atypical carcinoid tumor (moderately differentiated neuroendocrine carcinoma)
- ____ Small cell carcinoma (poorly differentiated neuroendocrine carcinoma)
- ____ Combined (or composite) small cell carcinoma, neuroendocrine type

____ Other (specify): ____________________________

____ Carcinoma, type cannot be determined

____ Mucosal malignant melanoma

Histologic Grade

____ Not applicable

___ GX: Cannot be assessed
___ G1: Well differentiated
___ G2: Moderately differentiated
___ G3: Poorly differentiated
___ Other (specify): ___________________________

*Microscopic Tumor Extension

*Specify: ___________________________

Margins (select all that apply)

___ Cannot be assessed
___ Margins uninvolved by invasive carcinoma
Distance from closest margin: _________ mm or _________ cm
Specify margin(s), per orientation, if possible: ___________________________
___ Margins involved by invasive carcinoma
Specify margin(s), per orientation, if possible: ___________________________
___ Margins uninvolved by carcinoma in situ (includes moderate and severe dysplasia†)
Distance from closest margin: _________ mm or _________ cm
Specify margin(s), per orientation, if possible: ___________________________
___ Margins involved by carcinoma in situ (includes moderate and severe dysplasia†)
Distance from closest margin: _________ mm or _________ cm
Specify margin(s), per orientation, if possible: ___________________________
___ Not applicable

*Treatment Effect (applicable to carcinomas treated with neoadjuvant therapy)

*___ Not identified
*___ Present (specify): ___________________________
*___ Indeterminate

Pathologic Staging (pTNM)

TNM descriptors (required only if applicable) (select all that apply)
___ m (multiple primary tumors)
___ r (recurrent)
___ y (post-treatment)

For all carcinomas (excluding mucosal malignant melanoma)

Primary tumor (pT)
___ pTX: Cannot be assessed
___ pT0: No evidence of primary tumor
___ pTis: Carcinoma in situ
___ pT1: Tumor ≤ 2 cm in greatest dimension
___ pT2: Tumor > 2 cm but ≤ 4 cm in greatest dimension
___ pT3: Tumor > 4 cm in greatest dimension
___ pT4a: Moderately advanced local disease

Lip: Tumor invades through cortical bone, inferior alveolar nerve, floor of mouth, or skin of face, i.e., chin or nose

Oral cavity: Tumor invades adjacent structures only (e.g., through cortical bone [mandible, maxilla], into deep [extrinsic] muscle of tongue [genioglossus, hyoglossus, palatoglossus, and styloglossus], maxillary sinus, skin of face)

___ pT4b: Very advanced local disease

Tumor invades masticator space, pterygoid plates, or skull base &/or encases internal carotid artery

Note: Superficial erosion alone of bone/tooth socket by gingival primary is not sufficient to classify a tumor as T4

Regional lymph nodes (pN)#
___ pNX: Cannot be assessed
___ pN0: No regional lymph node metastasis
___ pN1: Metastasis in single ipsilateral lymph node, ≤ 3 cm in greatest dimension
___ pN2a: Metastasis in single ipsilateral lymph node, > 3 cm but ≤ 6 cm in greatest dimension
___ pN2b: Metastasis in multiple ipsilateral lymph nodes, none > 6 cm in greatest dimension
___ pN2c: Metastasis in bilateral or contralateral lymph nodes, none > 6 cm in greatest dimension
___ pN3: Metastasis in lymph node > 6 cm in greatest dimension

PROTOCOL FOR THE EXAMINATION OF LIP AND ORAL CAVITY SPECIMENS

Specify: Number examined: ________

Number involved: ________

*Size (greatest dimension) of largest positive lymph node: ________

Distant metastasis (pM)

___ Not applicable

___ pM1: Distant metastasis

*Specify site(s), if known: ______________________

*Source of pathologic metastatic specimen (specify): ______________________

For mucosal malignant melanoma

Primary tumor (pT)

___ pT3: Mucosal disease

___ pT4a: Moderately advanced disease

Tumor involving deep soft tissue, cartilage, bone, or overlying skin

___ pT4b: Very advanced disease

Tumor involving brain, dura, skull base, lower cranial nerves (IX, X, XI, XII), masticator space, carotid artery, prevertebral space, or mediastinal structures

Regional lymph nodes (pN)

___ pNX: Regional lymph nodes cannot be assessed

___ pN0: No regional lymph node metastases

___ pN1: Regional lymph node metastases present

Distant metastases (pM)

___ Not applicable

___ pM1: Distant metastasis present

*Specify site(s), if known: ______________________

*Source of pathologic metastatic specimen (specify): ______________________

*Additional Pathologic Findings (select all that apply)

*___ None identified

*___ Keratinizing dysplasia

*___ Mild

*___ Moderate

*___ Severe (carcinoma in situ)

*___ Nonkeratinizing dysplasia

*___ Mild

*___ Moderate

*___ Severe (carcinoma in situ)

*___ Inflammation (specify type): ______________________

*___ Epithelial hyperplasia

*___ Colonization

*___ Fungal

*___ Bacterial

*___ Other (specify): ______________________

*Ancillary Studies

Specify type(s): ______________________

*Specify result(s): ______________________

*Clinical History (select all that apply)

*___ Neoadjuvant therapy

*___ Yes (specify type): ______________________

*___ No

*___ Indeterminate

*___ Other (specify): ______________________

**Data elements with asterisks are not required. However, these elements may be clinically important but are not yet validated or regularly used in patient management. †Applicable only to squamous cell carcinoma and histologic variants. #Superior mediastinal lymph nodes are considered regional lymph nodes (level VII). Midline nodes are considered ipsilateral nodes. Adapted with permission from College of American Pathologists, "Protocol for the Examination of Specimens from Patients with Carcinoma of the Lip and Oral Cavity." Web posting date October 2009, www.cap.org.*

Anatomic Stage/Prognostic Groups

Group	T	N	M
0	Tis	N0	M0
I	T1	N0	M0
II	T2	N0	M0
III	T3	N0	M0
	T1, T2, T3	N1	M0
	T1	N2	M0
	T2	N2	M0
	T3	N2	M0
IVA	T4a	N0	M0
	T4a	N1	M0
	T4a	N2	M0
	T4b	Any N	M0
IVB	Any T	N3	M0
IVC	Any T	Any N	M1

Adapted from 7th edition AJCC Staging Forms.

General Notes

Note	Description
m suffix	Indicates the presence of multiple primary tumors in a single site and is recorded in parentheses: pT(m)NM
y prefix	Indicates cases in which classification is performed during or following initial multimodality therapy. The cTNM or pTNM category is identified by a "y" prefix. The ycTNM or ypTNM categorizes the extent of tumor actually present at the time of that examination. The "y" categorization is not an estimate of tumor prior to multimodality therapy
r prefix	Indicates a recurrent tumor when staged after a disease-free interval, and is identified by the "r" prefix: rTNM
a prefix	Designates the stage determined at autopsy: aTNM
Surgical margins	Data field recorded by registrars describing the surgical margins of the resected primary site specimen as determined only by the pathology report
Neoadjuvant treatment	Radiation therapy or systemic therapy (consisting of chemotherapy, hormone therapy, or immunotherapy) administered prior to a definitive surgical procedure. If the surgical procedure is not performed, the administered therapy no longer meets the definition of neoadjuvant therapy

Adapted from 7th edition AJCC Staging Forms.

PROTOCOL FOR THE EXAMINATION OF LIP AND ORAL CAVITY SPECIMENS

Anatomic and Tumor Staging Graphics

*(**Left**) The anatomic divisions of the oral cavity (oropharynx) and lip are important parameters in separating tumors into specific prognostic categories. Dividing the tongue into halves, with anterior 2/3 and posterior 1/3 by the circumvallate papillae helps to predict metastatic patterns. (**Right**) This graphic shows a 2.8 cm dorsal anterior 2/3 of tongue tumor that also involves the lateral border. The tumor ends at the circumvallate papillae. This tumor would be a pT2.*

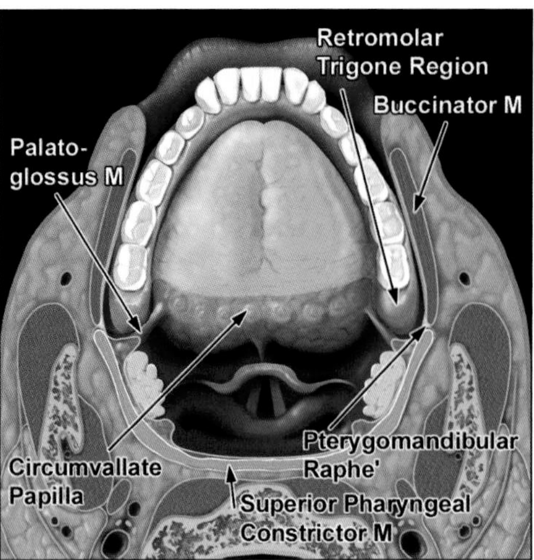

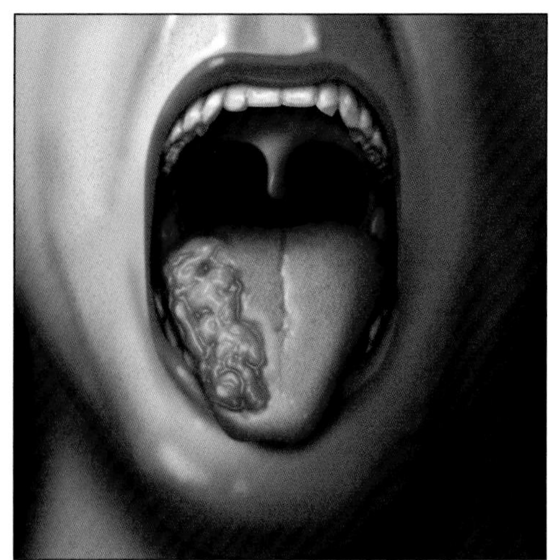

*(**Left**) Floor of the mouth cancers are known to behave in a more biologically aggressive fashion. Knowledge of the anatomy and muscles of the region help to correctly classify tumors (axial view). These parameters can be matched to radiographic findings. (**Right**) This midline mucosa of the lower lip tumor is identified expanding into the soft tissue and bone of the mandible, and expanding into the skin of the face. This tumor would be placed in the pT4a category.*

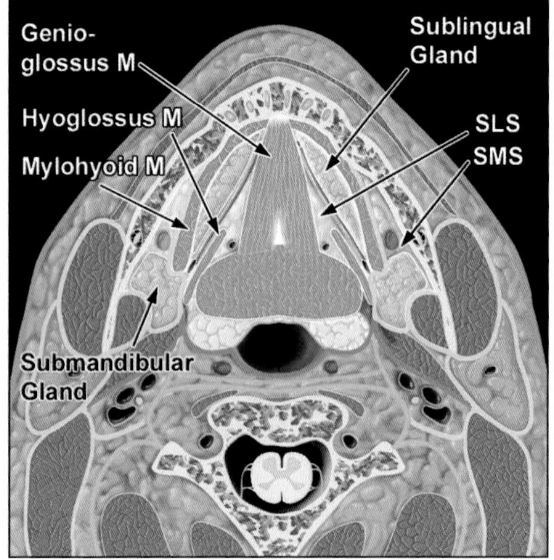

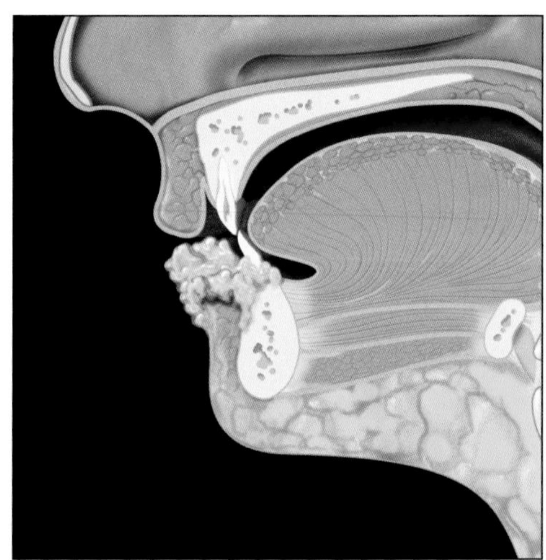

*(**Left**) A coronal view through the mid oral cavity helps to correlate the specific anatomic landmarks that can be seen on radiographic images as well as in the gross specimen. The nerves and vessels are important parameters in the staging of oral cavity tumors. (**Right**) Coronal view shows a lateral, dorsal squamous cell carcinoma that has grown into the deep muscles of the tongue and into the cortical bone of the mandible. This tumor would be classified as a pT4a tongue cancer.*

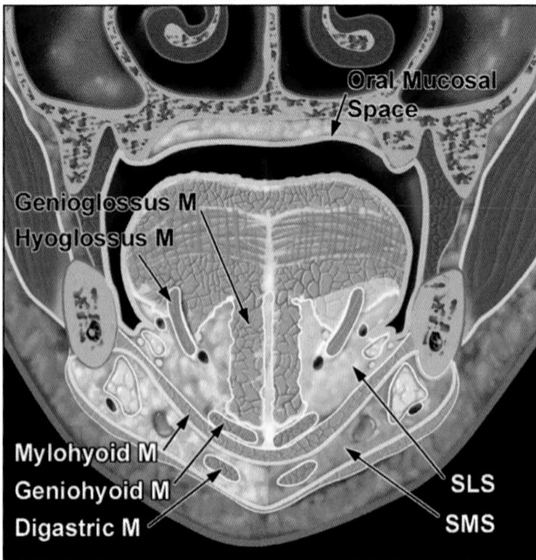

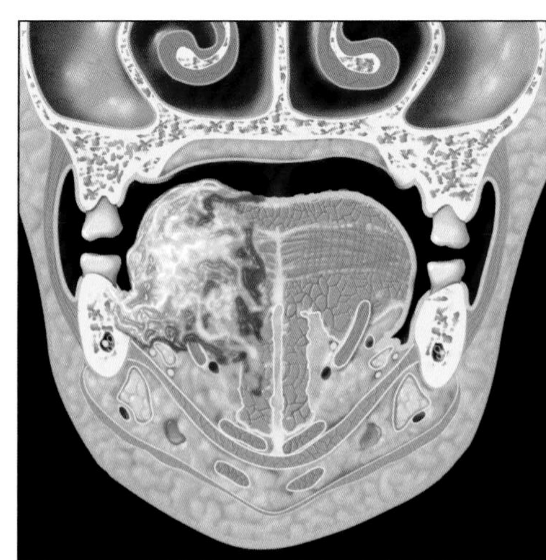

Anatomic and Tumor Staging Graphics

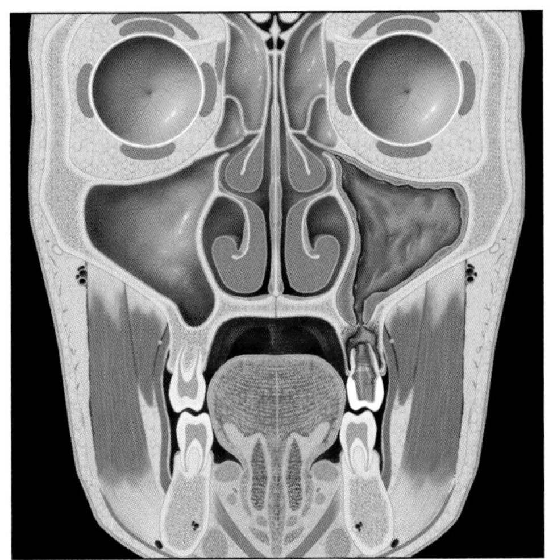

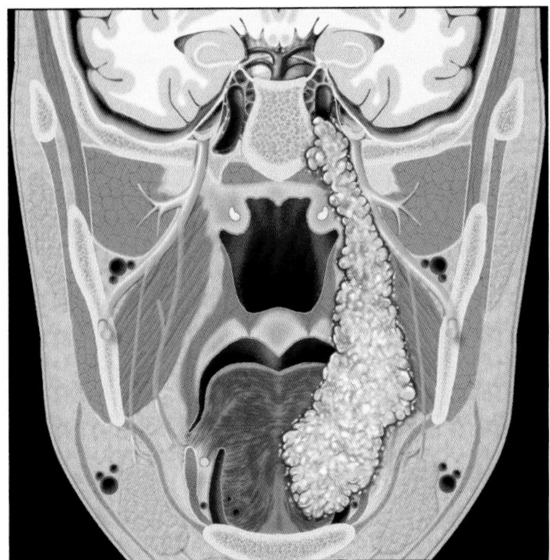

(Left) *Coronal graphic of the mid face demonstrates the relationship between the oral cavity, muscles of mastication, tooth structures, and the sinonasal complex. Tumors involving the palate and gnathic bones can easily cross into the adjacent structures.* ***(Right)*** *This is a very advanced tumor that started in the buccal mucosa, expanding into the tongue, floor of mouth, maxillary sinus, masticator space, and into the region of the sphenoid sinus (skull base). This is a pT4b tumor.*

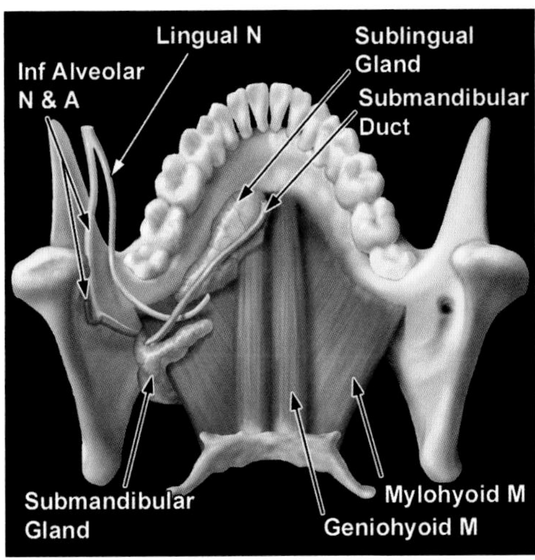

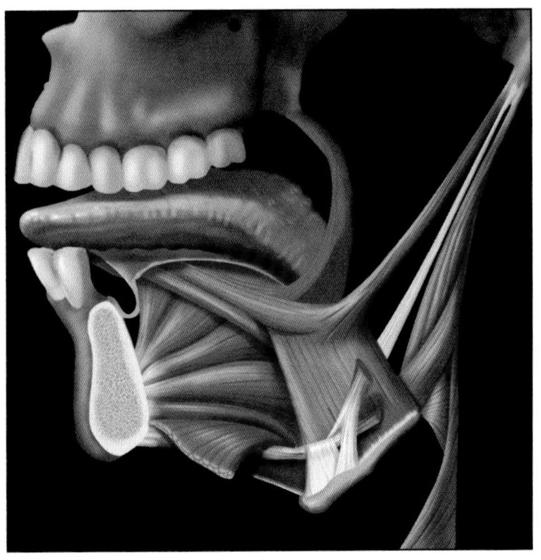

(Left) *Tumors of the minor salivary glands or of the submandibular/sublingual glands have a very intimate relationship with the muscles of the oral cavity, the bony structures of the jaw, and with nerves and vessels. Careful dissections are required to isolate these structures during examination.* ***(Right)*** *While the tongue is the major muscle of the oral cavity, many other muscles are associated with mastication and speech, highlighted in this graphic.*

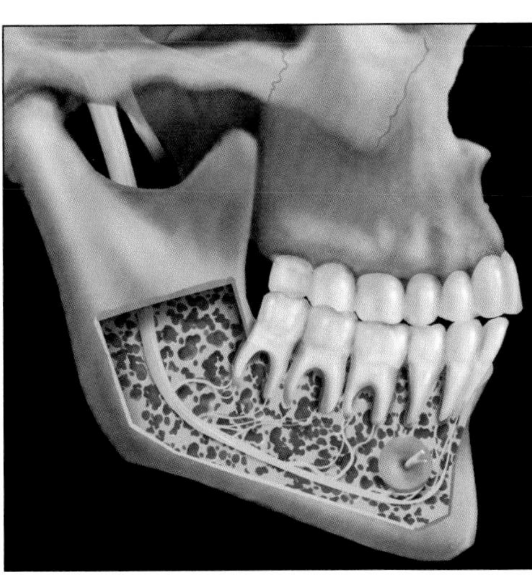

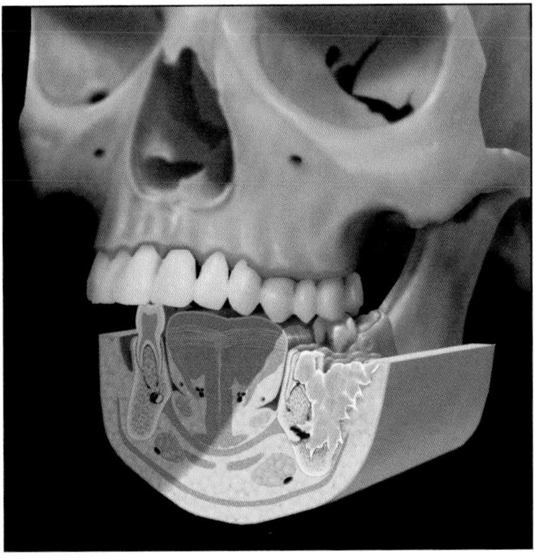

(Left) *The bones of the jaws are frequently involved by oral cavity tumors, or may be the source of a primary lesion (ameloblastoma, etc.). The relationship with the nerves (yellow) and teeth is quite important for classification and staging of these tumors.* ***(Right)*** *This cut-away shows a tumor that has expanded through the bone and muscles of the oral cavity, although it does not expand into the skin. This tumor is considered a pT4a lesion.*

Salivary Glands

POLYCYSTIC DISEASE OF THE PAROTID

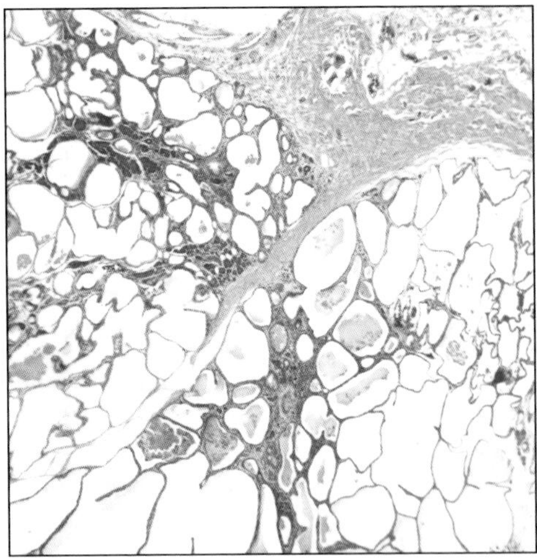

Low-power view shows polycystic disease of the parotid. The normal parenchyma of the parotid gland is replaced by variably sized cystic structures. Note the preservation of the lobular architecture.

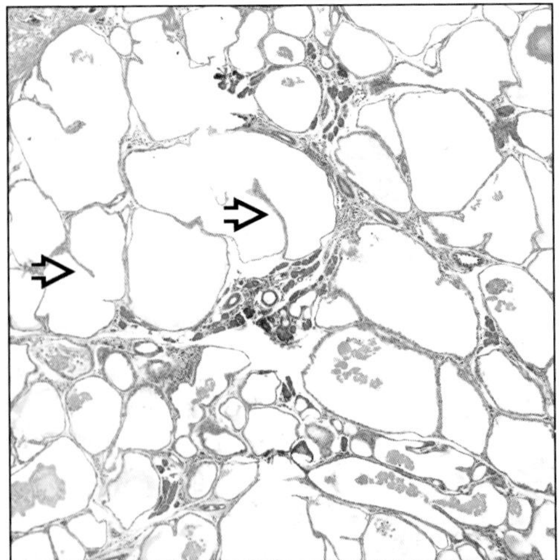

Low-power image shows multiple, variably sized cystic spaces within the parotid gland. Note the individual septations extending into the cystic lumina ⇨.

TERMINOLOGY

Synonyms

- Dysgenetic polycystic parotid gland disease

Definitions

- Marked dilation and cystic change within intercalated ducts of parotid gland
  - Striated and excretory ducts unaffected

ETIOLOGY/PATHOGENESIS

Inherited or Familial

- Might be sex linked
  - Vast majority in females

CLINICAL ISSUES

Epidemiology

- Incidence
  - Rare developmental anomaly
  - Not associated with polycystic disease of other organ systems
- Age
  - Typically becomes evident in childhood
    - However, overt clinical appearance may be delayed into adulthood
- Gender
  - Female > > > Male

Presentation

- Recurrent, fluctuating bilateral parotid gland swelling
- May be present for years prior to diagnosis
- Swelling not related to eating
- Typically not painful

Treatment

- Biopsy or excision only for diagnosis or cosmesis

Prognosis

- No malignant transformation
- No association with other cystic degenerative diseases

IMAGE FINDINGS

Radiographic Findings

- Bilateral, uniform, generalized post-contrast enhancement, reflecting multiple parenchymal cysts
- Main parotid duct is uninvolved

MACROSCOPIC FEATURES

General Features

- Exaggerated lobularity of glandular subcapsular surface
- Cut section may display mottled yellow nodules of spongy consistency

MICROSCOPIC PATHOLOGY

Histologic Features

- Salivary gland lobules are enlarged by multifocal to diffuse cystic dilation of intercalated ducts
  - Lobular architecture is maintained
    - Possible thickening of fibrous septa
    - Honeycomb or latticework-like architectural pattern within lobules
  - Lobules may be affected to different degree
    - Residual serous acinar structures may be present
- Cysts are irregularly sized and may be discreet or interconnected
  - Epithelial lining of variable morphology
    - Flattened and attenuated
    - Cuboidal
    - Apocrine-like
    - Polygonal with microvesicular cytoplasmic vacuolation

POLYCYSTIC DISEASE OF THE PAROTID

Key Facts

Terminology
- Marked dilation and cystic change within intercalated ducts of parotid gland

Clinical Issues
- Female > > > Male
- Recurrent, fluctuating bilateral parotid gland swelling

Microscopic Pathology
- Salivary gland lobules are enlarged by multifocal to diffuse cystic dilation of intercalated ducts
- Lobular architecture is maintained
- Cysts are irregularly sized and may be discreet or interconnected
- Epithelial lining of variable morphology
- Lumens may also contain proteinaceous, eosinophilic material, with variable inspissation

- Vesicular, vacuolated epithelial cells may be sloughed into cystic lumens
- Short, finger-like epithelial septations may extend into lumen
- Cysts may display direct communication with normal-appearing serous acini or striated ducts
    - In keeping with dilation of intercalated ducts
- Lumens may also contain proteinaceous, eosinophilic material, with variable inspissation
  - Secretions display variable morphology
    - Amorphous
    - Sialolith-like with concentric laminations
    - Crystaline and star-like with radiating projections
  - Luminal material may be reactive with Congo-Red and show apple-green birefringence under polarized light
    - Consistent with amyloid
- Minimal to absent inflammatory changes

ANCILLARY TESTS

Cytology
- Low cellularity with minimal proteinaceous background
- Scattered epithelial cell clusters, individual epithelial cells, red blood cells, and histiocytes
  - Polygonal epithelial cells with moderate cytoplasm
    - Nuclei round with small to inconspicuous nucleoli
    - Cytoplasm homogeneous to vacuolated
- Lack of lymphoid cell component

DIFFERENTIAL DIAGNOSIS

Cystic Salivary Gland Neoplasms
- Mucoepidermoid carcinoma or cystadenocarcinoma
- Not bilateral, multilobular, or with maintained lobular architecture

Sialodochiectasis or Chronic Sialectasis
- Duct dilatation or pooling of contrast in weakened ducts

SELECTED REFERENCES

1. Layfield LJ et al: Histologic and fine-needle aspiration cytologic features of polycystic disease of the parotid glands: case report and review of the literature. Diagn Cytopathol. 26(5):324-8, 2002
2. Brown E et al: Polycystic disease of the parotid glands. AJNR Am J Neuroradiol. 16(5):1128-31, 1995
3. Smyth AG et al: Polycystic disease of the parotid glands: two familial cases. Br J Oral Maxillofac Surg. 31(1):38-40, 1993
4. Batsakis JG et al: Polycystic (dysgenetic) disease of the parotid glands. Arch Otolaryngol Head Neck Surg. 114(10):1146-8, 1988
5. Dobson CM et al: Polycystic disease of the parotid glands: case report of a rare entity and review of the literature. Histopathology. 11(9):953-61, 1987
6. Seifert G et al: Bilateral dysgenetic polycystic parotid glands. Morphological analysis and differential diagnosis of a rare disease of the salivary glands. Virchows Arch A Pathol Anat Histol. 390(3):273-88, 1981

IMAGE GALLERY

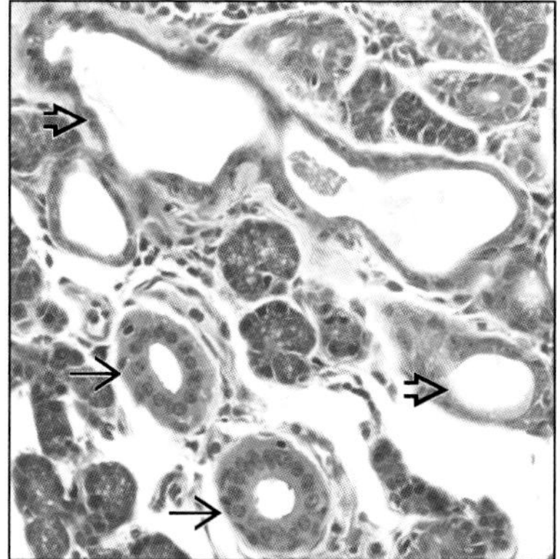

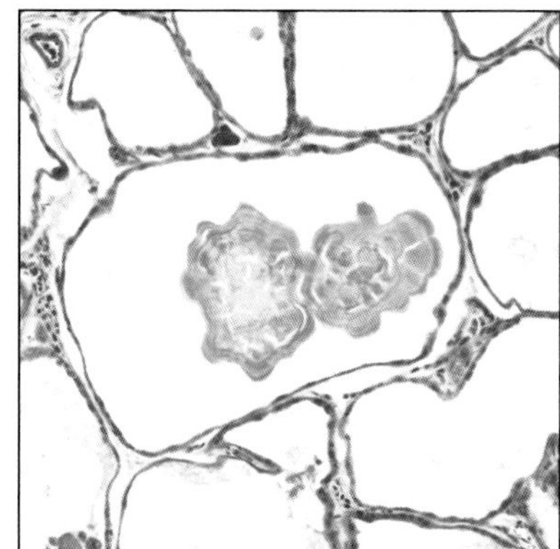

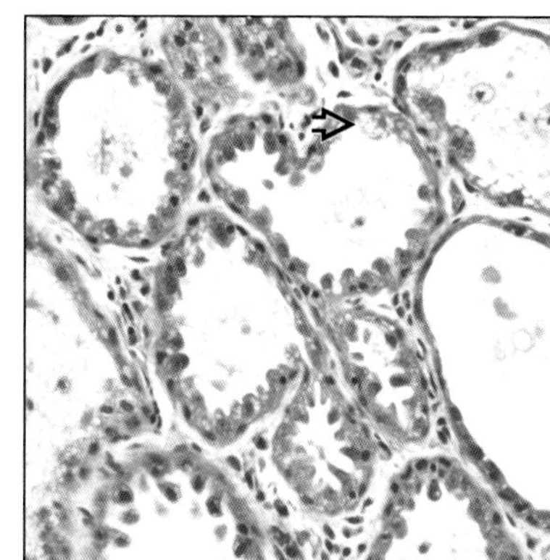

*(**Left**) Medium-power image demonstrates residual serous acini, 2 striated ducts ➔, and dilated intercalated ducts ⮚. Note that the striated ducts are not involved in the cystic process. (**Center**) The cystic structures are predominantly lined by flattened cuboidal epithelial cells. A small sialolith resides within the lumen of 1 cyst. (**Right**) Apocrine-like cytomorphology may be evident within the cystic epithelial lining. Microvesicular cytoplasmic vacuolation ⮚ is common in PDP.*

HIV SALIVARY GLAND DISEASE

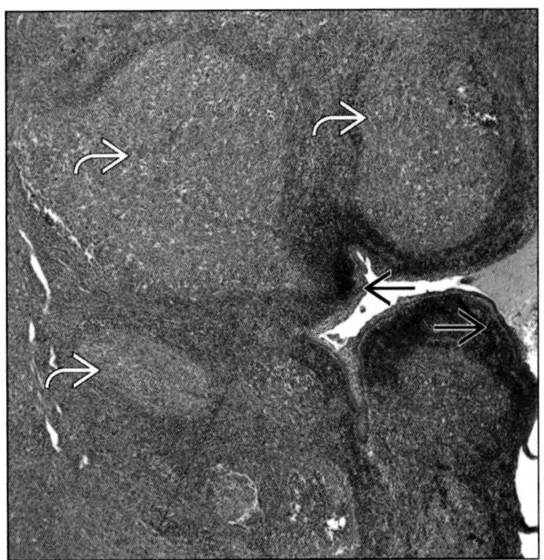

Parotid gland enlargement is characterized by the presence of intraparotid cystic epithelial proliferation ➩ with enlarged and irregularly shaped lymphoid follicles in the cyst wall ➦.

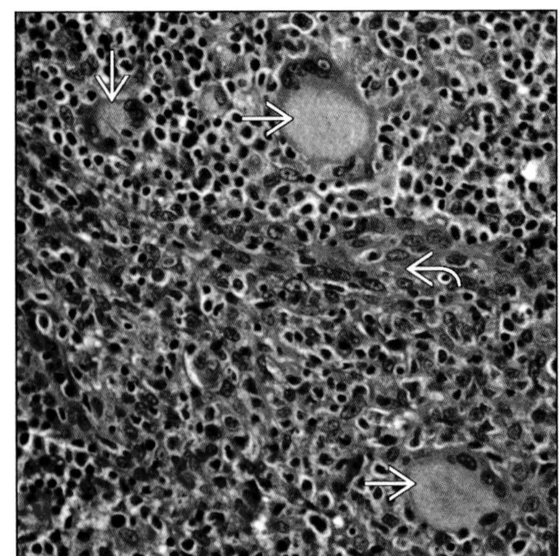

Multinucleated giant cells ➡, usually localized adjacent to epithelium ➦, in combination with the hyperplastic lymphoid follicles are features suggesting a diagnosis of HIV-SGD.

TERMINOLOGY

Abbreviations

- Human immunodeficiency virus salivary gland disease (HIV-SGD)

Synonyms

- AIDS-related parotid cyst (ARPC)

Definitions

- HIV-SGD includes HIV infected individuals with xerostomia, enlargement of one or more major salivary glands, or both

ETIOLOGY/PATHOGENESIS

Infectious Agents

- Caused by HIV infection

CLINICAL ISSUES

Epidemiology

- Incidence
  - Exact incidence of salivary gland enlargement in HIV-infected individuals not known but represents approximately 5% of adult patients
- Age
  - Primarily adult men aged 20-60 years
    - May occur in babies born of HIV-infected mothers
- Gender
  - Male > > > Female (9:1)
  - Equal gender distribution for babies born of HIV-infected mothers

Site

- Salivary gland involvement almost always parotid gland (98%)
  - Much less often submandibular gland (2%)
- Bilateral involvement in approximately 60% of cases

Presentation

- Symptoms include painless swelling of one or more salivary glands, xerostomia, dry eyes, arthralgias
- Salivary gland involvement typically occurs in early stages of HIV disease prior to development of AIDS
- Sjögren syndrome-like illness also identified in AIDS patients
  - Represents additional evidence of severely damaged immune system in HIV/AIDS patients
- Diffuse infiltrative lymphocytosis syndrome (DILS) and HIV-associated CD8(+) lymphocytosis syndrome
  - Primarily characterized by parotid gland enlargement, sicca symptoms, and pulmonary involvement in HIV infection
  - DILS associated with CD8 lymphocytosis and presence of HLA-DR5
  - Appears to be genetically determined host immune response to HIV
  - In DILS certain HIV-infected individuals develop oligoclonal expansion of CD8(+) lymphocytes characterized by persistent circulating CD8(+) lymphocytosis
  - Cells infiltrate multiple organs, but salivary glands and lung constitute major sites of involvement
  - Infiltrative process resembles Sjögren-like syndrome owing to visceral lymphocytic infiltration
  - Pulmonary process associated with DILS may mimic pneumonic process caused by *Pneumocystis carinii*
  - Other manifestations of DILS may include
    - Severe form of peripheral neuropathy
    - Lymphocytic infiltration of liver evident as hepatitis
    - Myositis
    - Lymphocytic interstitial nephritis
  - DILS may progress to development of parotid cysts

Laboratory Tests

- Serology evaluation will confirm HIV positivity
- Serologic markers present in Sjögren syndrome

HIV SALIVARY GLAND DISEASE

Key Facts

Terminology
- HIV-SGD includes HIV infected individuals with xerostomia, enlargement of one or more major salivary glands, or both

Etiology/Pathogenesis
- Caused by HIV infection

Clinical Issues
- Primarily adult men aged 20-60 years
- Salivary gland involvement almost always parotid gland (98%)
- Salivary gland involvement typically occurs in early stages of HIV disease prior to development of AIDS

Microscopic Pathology
- Early phases include florid follicular hyperplasia, attenuated to absent mantle lymphocytes, disruption of germinal centers (follicle lysis)
- Multinucleated giant cells (MGCs) localized to inter-/intrafollicular and periepithelial areas commonly seen
- Multiple squamous epithelial-lined cysts and epimyoepithelial islands present

Ancillary Tests
- HIV p24 core antigen immunoreactivity found in germinal centers (follicular dendritic cells), scattered lymphoid cells, and multinucleated giant cells

---

  - e.g., anti-salivary duct autoantibodies, anti-nuclear antibodies (ANA), anti-RO (SS-A), anti-LA (SS-B) commonly absent in HIV-SGD

Treatment
- Options, risks, complications
  - Treatment options for HIV-SGD vary, including surgical resection (parotidectomy, conservative excision, curettage), radiation, and symptomatic relief
- Drugs
  - Highly active antiretroviral treatment (HAART) shown to reduce size of parotid swellings and even result in regression of HIV-SGD
  - Prevalence of DILS significantly decreased in post-HAART era suggesting DILS is an antigen (viral)-driven response and primary treatment for it is anti-HIV therapy

Prognosis
- Parotid gland involvement does not appear to play any role in course of disease or progression to AIDS
- Successful outcome using HAART is reflected by diminution in viral load and immune restoration
- HIV-SGD is benign but hematologic malignancies may occur in association with HIV-SGD or develop subsequently
  - Polymorphic B-cell lymphoproliferative disorders also occur in association with HIV infection
  - Biologic significance and malignant status of polymorphic B-cell lymphoproliferative disorders remain unclear
  - Comparable morphologically and molecularly to polymorphic B-cell lymphoproliferative disorders arising after solid organ transplantation

IMAGE FINDINGS

Radiographic Findings
- CT scan and MR show unilateral or bilateral multicentric cysts of varying sizes

MICROSCOPIC PATHOLOGY

Histologic Features
- Lymphoid-related changes
  - Similar to changes seen in lymph nodes with early to chronic phases including
    - Florid follicular hyperplasia with attenuated to absent mantle lymphocytes
    - Disruption of germinal centers (follicle lysis)
    - Presence of multinucleated giant cells (MGCs) localized to inter- and intrafollicular areas, adjacent to or within epithelial component
  - Monomorphic round cells with clear cytoplasm (monocytoid B-cells) can be found in clusters
  - Interfollicular mixed (benign) inflammatory cell infiltrate with mature lymphocytes, histiocytes, neutrophils, and plasma cells present
- Cystic epithelial changes
  - Multiple squamous epithelial-lined cysts and epimyoepithelial islands present
  - Squamous epithelial-lined cysts and epimyoepithelial islands typically permeated by mature lymphocytes
    - Typically monocytoid B-cells in epimyoepithelial islands
- Origin of these cysts appears to be from salivary gland (parotid) epithelial structures arising in intra- or peri-parotid lymph nodes accounting for lymphoid component

ANCILLARY TESTS

Cytology
- Combination of features
  - Heterogeneous lymphoid population
  - Scattered single &/or clustered foamy macrophages
  - Numerous multinucleated giant cells
  - Superficial &/or anucleated squamous cells

HIV SALIVARY GLAND DISEASE

Immunohistochemistry

- Lymphoid component includes reactivity for B-cell lineage and T-cell lineage markers
- Epithelial markers (e.g., cytokeratins, EMA, others) delineate squamous epithelial-lined cysts and epimyoepithelial islands
- HIV p24 core antigen immunoreactivity found in germinal centers (follicular dendritic cells), scattered lymphoid cells, and multinucleated giant cells
  - Multinucleated giant cells also S100 protein and p55 (actin bundling protein) positive

Molecular Genetics

- Monoclonal *TCR* gene found in DILS and HIV-associated CD8(+) lymphocytosis syndrome
  - Despite presence of monoclonal *TCR* gene
    - CD8(+) expansions are reactive cell populations believed to represent immune response to viral infection rather than malignant disorder
    - CD8(+) expansions capable of mediating noncytotoxic inhibition of HIV replication

DIFFERENTIAL DIAGNOSIS

Infectious Disease

- No specific infectious agent
- Combination of cystic epithelial proliferation, multinucleated giant cells, and lymphoid component not typically seen in infectious diseases other than HIV-SGD

Lymphoepithelial Cyst

- Cystic epithelial proliferation similar to HIV-SGD but lacks alterations of lymphoid follicles/germinal centers and absence of multinucleated giant cells
- Absent p24 immunoreactivity

Benign Lymphoepithelial Lesion

- Shares some features with HIV-SGD but lacks alterations of lymphoid follicles/germinal centers and absence of multinucleated giant cells
- Absent p24 immunoreactivity

Sjögren Syndrome

- Serologic markers present in Sjögren syndrome commonly absent in HIV-SGD
- DILS in HIV may share similarities to classic Sjögren syndrome manifested by distinctive clinical, serologic, immunologic, and immunogenetic characteristics
- Findings to distinguish DILS from classic Sjögren syndrome include
  - Greater degree of salivary gland enlargement and extraglandular disease (pulmonary, renal, gastrointestinal, breast muscle)
  - Low frequency of autoantibodies
  - Differing HLA associations

Cystic Salivary Gland Neoplasms

- Differentiation from salivary gland neoplasms (benign and malignant) straightforward, as cellular components diagnostic for a given cystic salivary gland neoplasm are absent in HIV-SGD

Malignant Lymphoma (ML)

- In contrast to HIV-SGD, MLs show presence of monomorphic cell population, cytologically malignant cells, and clonal cell population by ancillary testing (immunohistochemical &/or molecular diagnostics)

SELECTED REFERENCES

1. Gupta N et al: Multinucleated giant cells in HIV-associated benign lymphoepithelial cyst-like lesions of the parotid gland on FNAC. Diagn Cytopathol. 37(3):203-4, 2009
2. Shanti RM et al: HIV-associated salivary gland disease. Oral Maxillofac Surg Clin North Am. 21(3):339-43, 2009
3. Franco-Paredes C et al: Diagnosis of diffuse CD8+ lymphocytosis syndrome in HIV-infected patients. AIDS Read. 12(9):408-13, 2002
4. Chhieng DC et al: Utility of fine-needle aspiration in the diagnosis of salivary gland lesions in patients infected with human immunodeficiency virus. Diagn Cytopathol. 21(4):260-4, 1999
5. Vicandi B et al: HIV-1 (p24)-positive multinucleated giant cells in HIV-associated lymphoepithelial lesion of the parotid gland. A report of two cases. Acta Cytol. 43(2):247-51, 1999
6. Kordossis T et al: Prevalence of Sjögren's-like syndrome in a cohort of HIV-1-positive patients: descriptive pathology and immunopathology. Br J Rheumatol. 37(6):691-5, 1998
7. Mandel L et al: Parotid gland swelling in HIV diffuse infiltrative CD8 lymphocytosis syndrome. Oral Surg Oral Med Oral Pathol Oral Radiol Endod. 85(5):565-8, 1998
8. Williams FM et al: Prevalence of the diffuse infiltrative lymphocytosis syndrome among human immunodeficiency virus type 1-positive outpatients. Arthritis Rheum. 41(5):863-8, 1998
9. Kazi S et al: The diffuse infiltrative lymphocytosis syndrome. Clinical and immunogenetic features in 35 patients. AIDS. 10(4):385-91, 1996
10. Itescu S et al: Tissue infiltration in a CD8 lymphocytosis syndrome associated with human immunodeficiency virus-1 infection has the phenotypic appearance of an antigenically driven response. J Clin Invest. 91(5):2216-25, 1993
11. Itescu S et al: Diffuse infiltrative lymphocytosis syndrome: a disorder occurring in human immunodeficiency virus-1 infection that may present as a sicca syndrome. Rheum Dis Clin North Am. 18(3):683-97, 1992
12. Schiødt M et al: Natural history of HIV-associated salivary gland disease. Oral Surg Oral Med Oral Pathol. 74(3):326-31, 1992
13. Schiødt M: HIV-associated salivary gland disease: a review. Oral Surg Oral Med Oral Pathol. 73(2):164-7, 1992
14. Strigle SM et al: A review of the fine-needle aspiration cytology findings in human immunodeficiency virus infection. Diagn Cytopathol. 8(1):41-52, 1992
15. Itescu S et al: A diffuse infiltrative CD8 lymphocytosis syndrome in human immunodeficiency virus (HIV) infection: a host immune response associated with HLA-DR5. Ann Intern Med. 112(1):3-10, 1990
16. Bruner JM et al: Immunocytochemical identification of HIV (p24) antigen in parotid lymphoid lesions. J Laryngol Otol. 103(11):1063-6, 1989

Imaging, Microscopic Features and Ancillary Techniques

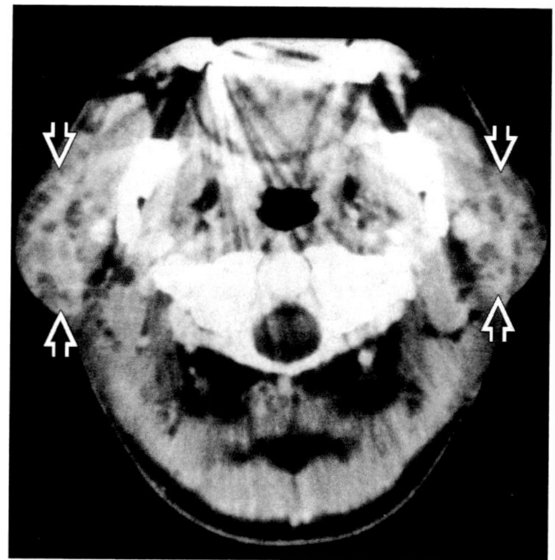

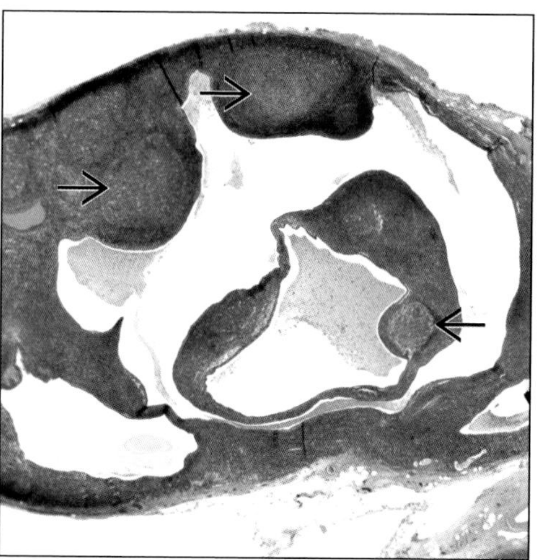

(Left) *Radiographic (CT scan) imaging in a young adult male shows the presence of bilateral multicentric variable-sized cysts* ⇨*. These image findings in this clinical setting raise concern for a possible diagnosis of HIV SGD.* ***(Right)*** *Intraparotid multicystic lesion in which the cysts prove to be lined by benign epithelium and enlarged, irregularly shaped lymphoid follicles* → *are present within the wall of the cyst.*

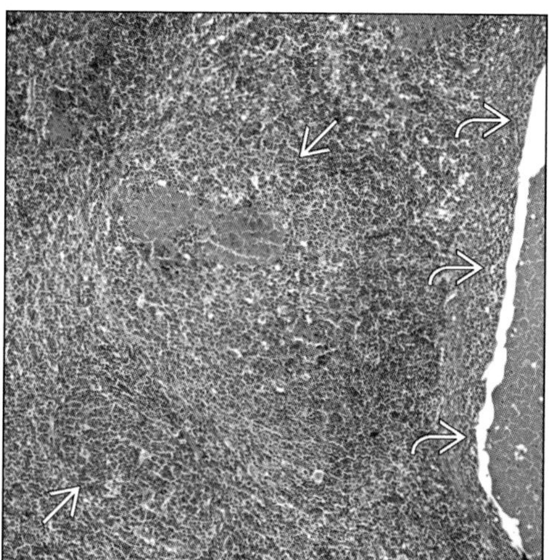

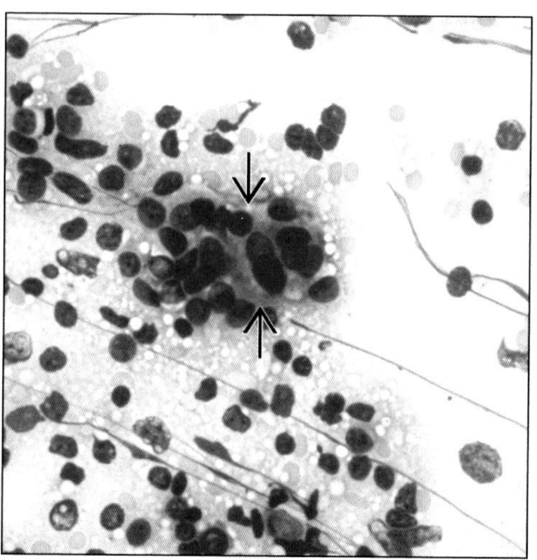

(Left) *In the wall of the cyst, there are irregularly shaped lymphoid follicles* ➔ *with attenuated to absent mantle lymphocytes and follicle lysis. The cyst is lined by epithelium* ➔*, which is obscured secondary to lymphoid cell infiltration.* ***(Right)*** *Fine needle aspirate biopsy of patient with HIV-SGD shows a heterogeneous population of lymphoid cells and a multinucleated giant cell* →*. In the appropriate clinical setting, these cytologic findings would be consistent with HIV infection.*

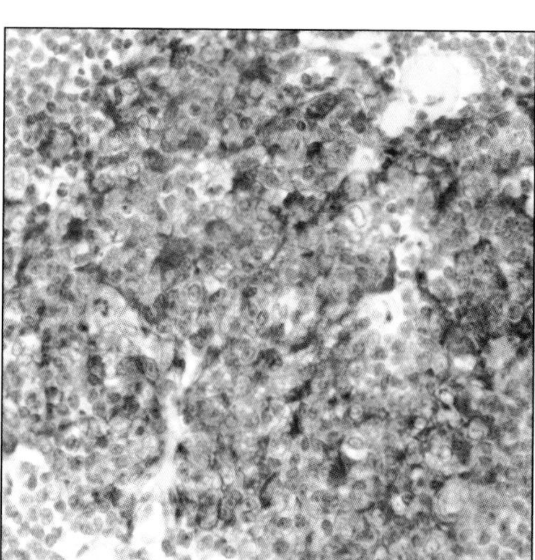

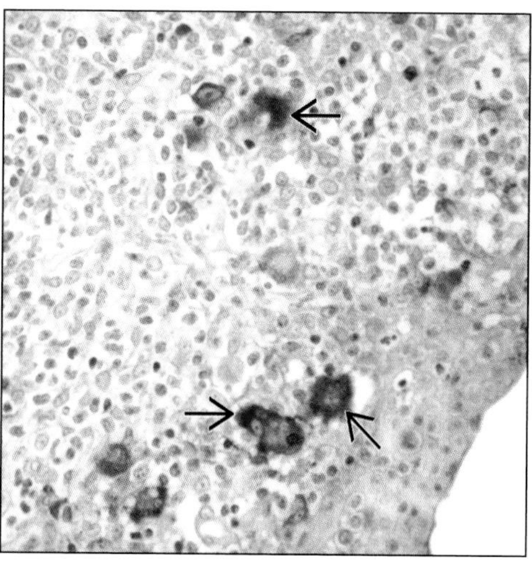

(Left) *Immunoreactivity with HIV p24 core antigen is identified in the germinal centers (follicular dendritic cells), a primary location where the virus replicates.* ***(Right)*** *The multinucleated giant cells are immunoreactive with HIV p24 core antigen* →*. In conjunction with the clinical history, presence of cystic lesions of one or more salivary glands, light microscopic features, and HIV p24 immunoreactivity, the diagnosis of HIV-SGD is established.*

CHRONIC SCLEROSING SIALADENITIS

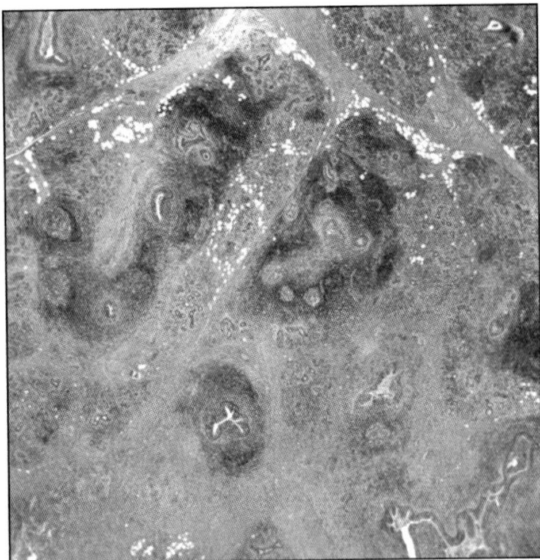

Submandibular chronic sclerosing sialadenitis is characterized by retention of the lobular architecture, dense inflammatory infiltrate, acinar atrophy, and interlobular fibrosis.

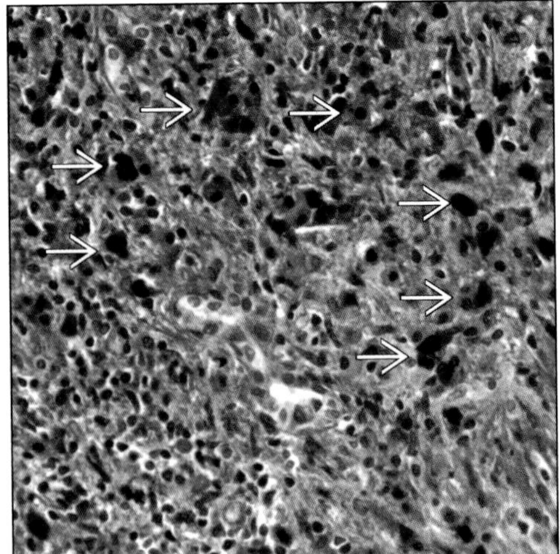

It is now recognized that submandibular chronic sclerosing sialadenitis may be an IgG4-related disease, confirmed by the presence of abundant IgG4 immunoreactive plasma cells ➡.

TERMINOLOGY

Abbreviations

- Chronic sclerosing sialadenitis (CSS)

Synonyms

- Küttner tumor
- IgG4-associated sialadenitis
- Punctate parotitis

Definitions

- Chronic fibroinflammatory salivary gland disease with characteristic morphology that may represent IgG4-associated disease

ETIOLOGY/PATHOGENESIS

Immune-Mediated

- Increasing evidence that CSS, if IgG4 related, may be component of IgG4-related systemic disease
  - IgG4-related diseases include
    - Autoimmune pancreatitis
    - Involvement of extrapancreatic organs including kidney, lung, retroperitoneum, liver, gallbladder, lymph nodes, breast, salivary glands, lacrimal gland, aorta
  - Morphologic features in CSS suggesting immune-mediated process include
    - Presence of prominent lymphoplasmacytic infiltrate and lymphoid follicles
    - Presence of unusual cytotoxic T-cell populations

Obstructive Sialadenitis

- Prior to IgG4 association, sialolithiasis felt to be commonly associated with CSS of submandibular gland
  - May be true in percentage of non-IgG4-related cases

CLINICAL ISSUES

Epidemiology

- Incidence
  - Unknown, but under recognized
- Age
  - Most often occurs in 4th to 7th decades
- Gender
  - Affects males slightly more often than females

Site

- Primarily affects submandibular gland
  - Rarely, multiple salivary glands (major and minor) may be affected in single patient

Presentation

- Pain and swelling of affected gland common
  - Often associated with ingestion of food
- Patients may present with asymptomatic swelling of affected gland
- May be localized to salivary gland involvement
- May be associated with sclerosing lesions in extrasalivary gland tissues (systemic IgG4-related disease)

Laboratory Tests

- Serum IgG4, IgG, IgG4/IgG ratio (normally 3-6%) typically elevated
- Antibodies present in Sjögren syndrome including anti-SS-A, anti-SS-B not found in CSS
- Absence of antineutrophilic antibodies (cytoplasmic and perinuclear)
- Eosinophilia, hypergammaglobulinemia, and antinuclear antibodies (ANA) may be present in systemic but not localized disease

Treatment

- Options, risks, complications
  - IgG4-related sialadenitis steroid sensitive
- Surgical approaches

CHRONIC SCLEROSING SIALADENITIS

Key Facts

Terminology
- Chronic fibroinflammatory salivary gland disease with characteristic morphology that may represent IgG4-associated disease

Etiology/Pathogenesis
- Increasing evidence that CSS, if IgG4 related, may be component of IgG4-related systemic disease
- Prior to IgG4 association, sialolithiasis felt to be commonly associated with CSS of submandibular gland
  - May be true in percentage of non-IgG4-related cases

Clinical Issues
- Primarily affects submandibular gland
- IgG4-related sialadenitis steroid sensitive

Microscopic Pathology
- Preservation of lobular architecture
- Dense lymphoplasmacytic infiltrate within lobules
- Large irregular lymphoid follicles with expanded geographic germinal centers
- Sheets of mature plasma cells
- Acinar atrophy
- Lobules separated by fibrosis composed of fibroblasts and chronic inflammatory cells
- Phlebitis (obliterative or nonobliterative) may or may not be identified

Ancillary Tests
- Abundant IgG4(+) plasma cells present
- IgG4(+) plasma cells present in inflamed lobules, interlobular septae, occasionally in germinal centers

---

  - CSS associated with sialolithiasis
    - Removal of stone by surgery, endoscopy or lithotripsy
    - In approximately 20% of cases, symptoms persist, necessitating surgical resection of involved gland

Prognosis
- IgG4-related
  - Excellent response to steroid
- Sialolithiasis-related
  - Removal of stone results in reduction in swelling and pain
- Rarely, extranodal marginal zone B-cell lymphoma (MALT) of salivary gland and salivary duct carcinoma may arise in background of CSS

IMAGE FINDINGS

Radiographic Findings
- Sonographic findings usually show diffuse involvement of submandibular gland
  - Less often, focal involvement may occur
- Diffuse involvement of gland may simulate sonographic appearance of "cirrhotic" liver
  - Less often, diffuse heterogeneous involvement with duct dilatation and calculi may be identified
- Focal lesions appear as hypoechoic, heterogeneous "masses," with radial branching vascular pattern

MICROSCOPIC PATHOLOGY

Histologic Features
- Well-defined to circumscribed lesion involving variable proportion of gland or entire gland
- Characteristic features include
  - Preservation of lobular architecture
  - Dense lymphoplasmacytic infiltrate within lobules
  - Large irregular lymphoid follicles with expanded geographic germinal centers
  - Sheets of mature plasma cells
  - Acinar atrophy
  - Lobules separated by fibrosis composed of fibroblasts and chronic inflammatory cells
- Phlebitis (obliterative or nonobliterative) may or may not be identified
- Thickening of interlobular septa by sclerotic tissue
- Metaplastic changes of ducts may be present including squamous &/or mucous metaplasia
  - Mucous metaplasia may include ciliated cells and goblet cells
- Noncaseating granulomas may be seen
  - Likely result of mucus extravasation from ducts in cases associated with sialolithiasis

ANCILLARY TESTS

Cytology
- In combination with clinical findings, cytologic findings can strongly suggest diagnosis
  - Paucicellular to moderately cellular aspirate characterized by scattered tubular/ductal structures
  - Paucity or absence of acini
  - Tubular/ductal structures often enveloped by collagen bundles or lymphoplasmacytic infiltrate
  - Isolated fragments of fibrous stroma may be identified
  - Background rich in lymphoid and plasma cells

Immunohistochemistry
- Abundant cytotoxic T-cells, especially in association with ducts and acini
- B-cells mostly restricted to lymphoid follicles
- IgG4-related sialadenitis
  - Abundant IgG4 immunoreactive plasma cells present
  - Proportion of IgG4/IgG-positive plasma cells > 45%
  - IgG4-positive plasma cells present in inflamed lobules, interlobular septae, occasionally in germinal centers

Cytogenetics
- Immunoglobulin heavy chain includes polyclonal rearrangement in majority of case

- Suggests CSS may be result of immune process possibly triggered by intraductal agents

DIFFERENTIAL DIAGNOSIS

Chronic Sialadenitis, Not Otherwise Specified

- Shares overlapping histologic features with CSS but lacks uniform presence of increased IgG4 plasma cells
- May be associated with sialolithiasis

Sialolithiasis

- Caused by calcareous concretions within salivary gland ducts &/or parenchyma as result of mineralization of debris accumulated within duct lumina
- Calculi particularly common in submandibular gland (Wharton duct) accounting for 80-90% of cases
  - Parotid gland (Stensen duct) involvement in 10-20% of cases
- Radiographic analysis represents most reliable means to detect presence of calculi
- Microscopic features include
  - Calculi seen in parenchyma or ducts
  - With time, parenchymal changes include fibrosis, parenchymal atrophy with loss of acini, chronic inflammation, ductal dilatation, scarring
- Shares overlapping histologic features with CSS but lacks uniform presence of increased IgG4 plasma cells

Sarcoidosis of Salivary Glands

- Most often involves parotid gland as isolated process or as part of syndrome termed uveoparotid fever (Heerfordt disease) characterized by
  - Parotitis, xerostomia, uveitis and facial nerve palsy
- Presence of noncaseating granulomatous inflammation: Finding not seen in CSS

Sjögren Syndrome

- Typically, disease of parotid gland that rarely (if ever) presents as isolated submandibular gland disease as occurs in CSS
- Does not show features associated with CSS including interlobular fibrosis, dense lymphoplasmacytic cell infiltrate with sheets of plasma cells, and lymphoid hyperplasia

Lymphoepithelial Sialadenitis (LESA)

- Does not show features associated with CSS including interlobular fibrosis, dense lymphoplasmacytic cell infiltrate with sheets of plasma cells, and lymphoid hyperplasia

Sialadenosis

- Nonneoplastic, noninflammatory enlargement of salivary glands (parotid in particular) almost always associated with underlying systemic disorder or secretory dysfunction
- In contrast to CSS, histomorphologic features include acinar cell enlargement with absent inflammatory cell infiltrate

SELECTED REFERENCES

1. Geyer JT et al: Chronic sclerosing sialadenitis (Küttner tumor) is an IgG4-associated disease. Am J Surg Pathol. 34(2):202-10, 2010
2. Dhobale S et al: IgG4 related sclerosing disease with multiple organ involvements and response to corticosteroid treatment. J Clin Rheumatol. 15(7):354-7, 2009
3. Gill J et al: Salivary duct carcinoma arising in IgG4-related autoimmune disease of the parotid gland. Hum Pathol. 40(6):881-6, 2009
4. Kamisawa T et al: Lacrimal gland function in autoimmune pancreatitis. Intern Med. 48(12):939-43, 2009
5. Tabata T et al: Serum IgG4 concentrations and IgG4-related sclerosing disease. Clin Chim Acta. 408(1-2):25-8, 2009
6. Van Moerkercke W et al: A case of IgG4-related sclerosing disease with retroperitoneal fibrosis, autoimmune pancreatitis and bilateral focal nephritis. Pancreas. 38(7):825-32, 2009
7. Cheuk W et al: Lymphadenopathy of IgG4-related sclerosing disease. Am J Surg Pathol. 32(5):671-81, 2008
8. Chow TL et al: Kuttner's tumour (chronic sclerosing sialadenitis) of the submandibular gland: a clinical perspective. Hong Kong Med J. 14(1):46-9, 2008
9. Kamisawa T et al: IgG4-related sclerosing disease. World J Gastroenterol. 14(25):3948-55, 2008
10. Cheuk W et al: Advances in salivary gland pathology. Histopathology. 51(1):1-20, 2007
11. Kamisawa T et al: IgG4-related sclerosing disease incorporating sclerosing pancreatitis, cholangitis, sialadenitis and retroperitoneal fibrosis with lymphadenopathy. Pancreatology. 6(1-2):132-7, 2006
12. Yamamoto M et al: A new conceptualization for Mikulicz's disease as an IgG4-related plasmacytic disease. Mod Rheumatol. 16(6):335-40, 2006
13. Kitagawa S et al: Abundant IgG4-positive plasma cell infiltration characterizes chronic sclerosing sialadenitis (Küttner's tumor). Am J Surg Pathol. 29(6):783-91, 2005
14. Ahuja AT et al: Kuttner tumour (chronic sclerosing sialadenitis) of the submandibular gland: sonographic appearances. Ultrasound Med Biol. 29(7):913-9, 2003
15. Kamisawa T et al: A new clinicopathological entity of IgG4-related autoimmune disease. J Gastroenterol. 38(10):982-4, 2003
16. Cheuk W et al: Kuttner tumor of the submandibular gland: fine-needle aspiration cytologic findings of seven cases. Am J Clin Pathol. 117(1):103-8, 2002
17. Tiemann M et al: Chronic sclerosing sialadenitis of the submandibular gland is mainly due to a T lymphocyte immune reaction. Mod Pathol. 15(8):845-52, 2002
18. Ochoa ER et al: Marginal zone B-cell lymphoma of the salivary gland arising in chronic sclerosing sialadenitis (Küttner tumor). Am J Surg Pathol. 25(12):1546-50, 2001
19. Chan JK: Kuttner tumor (chronic sclerosing sialadenitis) of the submandibular gland: an underrecognized entity. Adv Anat Pathol. 5(4):239-51, 1998
20. Isacsson G et al: Salivary calculi as an aetiological factor in chronic sialadenitis of the submandibular gland. Clin Otolaryngol Allied Sci. 7(4):231-6, 1982

Imaging and Microscopic Features

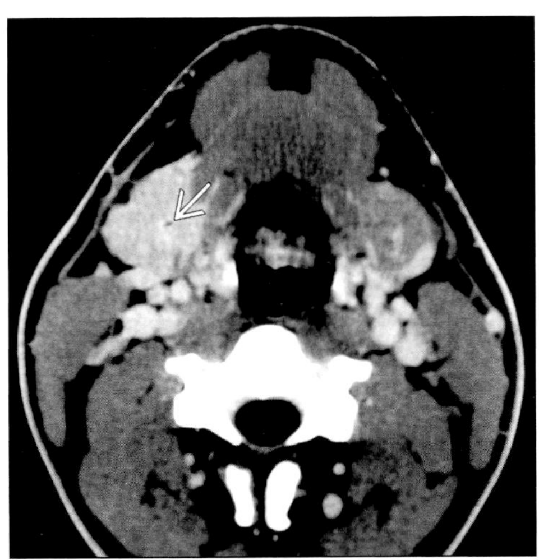

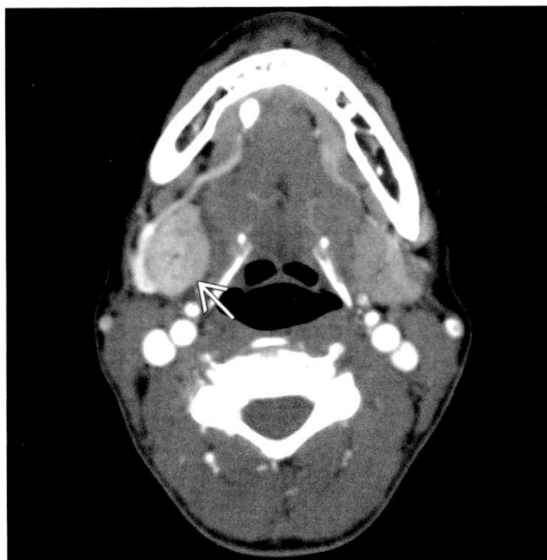

(Left) *Chronic sclerosing sialadenitis may result 2° to sialolithiasis. Asymmetric enhancement of right enlarged submandibular gland is seen. Note slight dilatation of submandibular duct hilum ➔.* ***(Right)*** *Axial CECT shows an enhancing, enlarged right submandibular gland ➔ secondary to a stone in the distal duct at the level of the ductal papilla. Histologically, evidence of stone formation was present with secondary chronic sclerosing sialadenitis (not shown).*

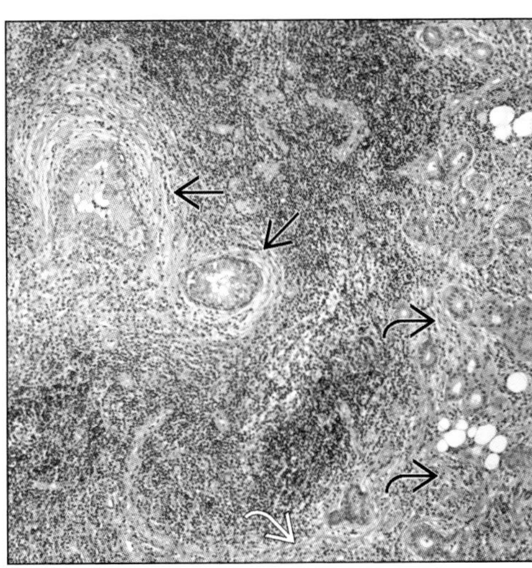

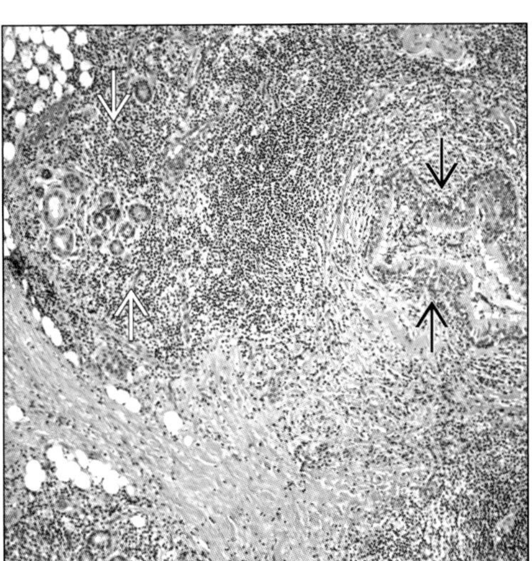

(Left) *The fibrosis in chronic sclerosing sialadenitis is present around ducts ➔ as well as around lobules ➔. Additional findings include dense inflammatory infiltrate and acinar atrophy ➔.* ***(Right)*** *The dense inflammatory infiltrate is present around ducts ➔ and within the lobules ➔, the latter characterized by acinar atrophy. The inflammatory component also involves perilobular fibrotic bands. These are the features of chronic sclerosing sialadenitis.*

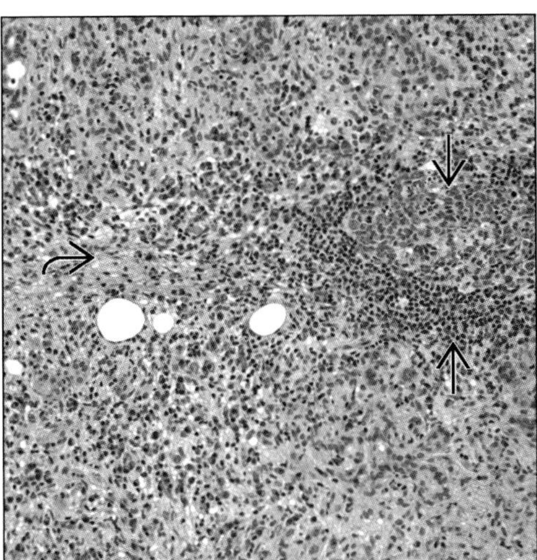

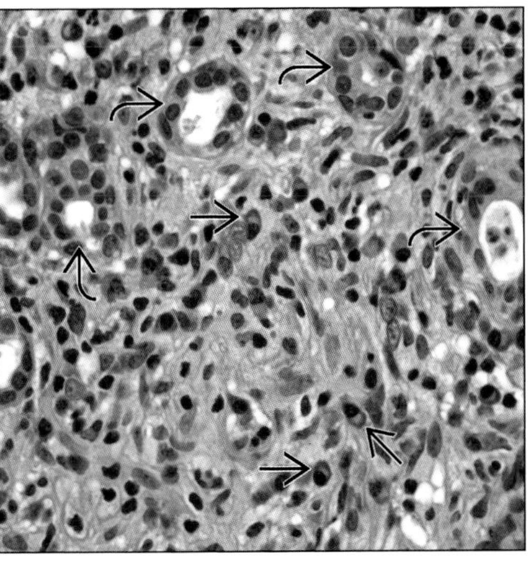

(Left) *The submandibular gland shows a dense inflammatory cell infiltrate throughout the parenchyma, including into perilobular fibrosis ➔ as well as germinal centers ➔.* ***(Right)*** *The nature of the inflammatory cell infiltrate can be seen, including mature lymphocytes and mature plasma cells, the latter characterized by the presence of perinuclear "hof" ➔ representing the Golgi apparatus. Residual acini are present ➔, but there is marked glandular atrophy.*

BENIGN LYMPHOEPITHELIAL CYST

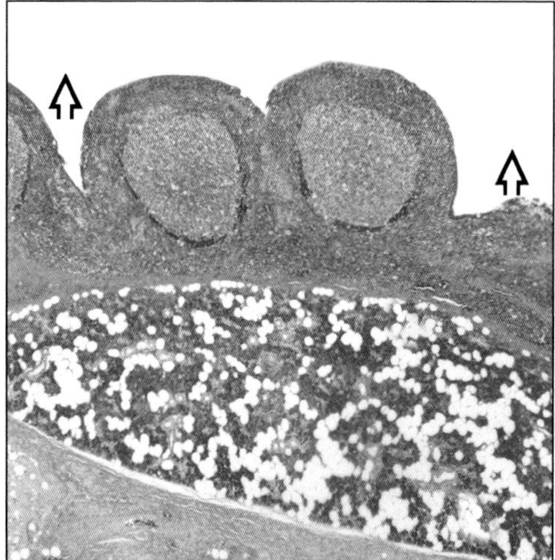

This benign lymphoepithelial cyst of the parotid gland has a corrugated architectural pattern due to the germinal center formations. The lumen of the cyst ⇨ shows an empty space.

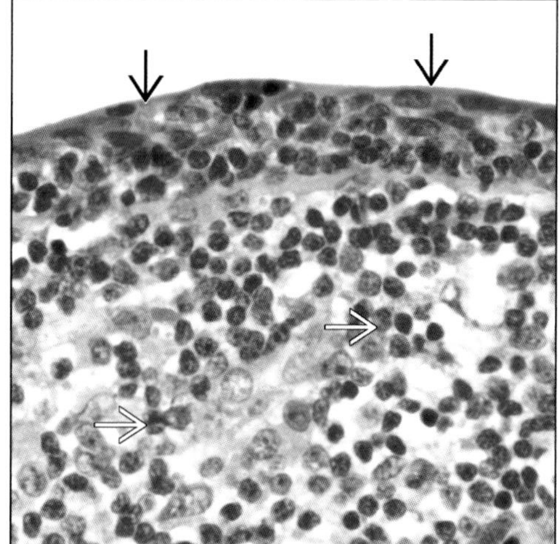

This high-power view demonstrates a flattened, squamous epithelial lining ⇨, which shows an intimate association with the lymphoid population ➡, a common finding in BLEC.

TERMINOLOGY

Abbreviations

- Benign lymphoepithelial cyst (BLEC)

Definitions

- Benign, cystic epithelial lesion intimately associated with lymphocytic proliferation within cyst wall

ETIOLOGY/PATHOGENESIS

Developmental Anomaly

- Theories attempt to explain dual population of cystic salivary epithelium and distinct lymphoid component
  - Possibly derived from embryologic branchial cleft remnants, representing intraparotid branchial cleft cysts
  - Entrapped salivary epithelium within intraparotid/periparotid lymph node
  - Salivary duct cyst that recruits lymphoid component
    - Akin to tumor-associated lymphoid proliferation (TALP) seen with salivary gland malignancies (e.g., acinic cell carcinoma, mucoepidermoid carcinoma)

Infectious

- If bilateral, there is a strong human immunodeficiency virus type-1 (HIV-1) association

CLINICAL ISSUES

Epidemiology

- Incidence
  - Rare
    - Develops in 3-6% of early HIV-infected patients
- Age
  - Occurs over a very wide range
  - Average: 5th to 6th decades
- Gender
  - Historically, more common in males
  - Recent studies show BLECs to occur with slightly greater frequency in females

Site

- Nearly all BLECs are found within parotid gland
  - Although histologically similar, intraoral lymphoepithelial cysts are considered of tonsillar origin (not considered further here)
- Typically unilateral
  - If bilateral, HIV association should be considered

Presentation

- Usually asymptomatic
- Usually has compressible, unilateral swelling
- Occasional patients complain of tenderness, pain, or facial nerve palsy

Treatment

- Surgical excision treatment of choice

Prognosis

- BLECs are not known to recur

MACROSCOPIC FEATURES

Size

- Mean: 3 cm

MICROSCOPIC PATHOLOGY

Histologic Features

- Unilocular and unicystic lesion that is typically well demarcated within parotid gland
- Cysts are ordinarily lined by stratified squamous epithelium
  - Cuboidal, columnar, or pseudostratified epithelium may line cyst
  - Goblet cells, oncocytes, or sebaceous cells may be seen

BENIGN LYMPHOEPITHELIAL CYST

Key Facts

Terminology
- Benign cystic epithelial lesion intimately associated with lymphocytic proliferation within cyst wall

Clinical Issues
- Practically all salivary lymphoepithelial cysts are found within parotid gland
- Surgical excision treatment of choice

Microscopic Pathology
- Unilocular and unicystic lesion that is typically well demarcated within parotid gland
- Ordinarily lined by stratified squamous epithelium, although cuboidal, columnar, or pseudostratified epithelial types may occasionally be seen
- Lymphoid component, to include germinal center formation, is dense and found within wall of cyst

- Dense lymphoid component within cyst wall
  - Germinal center formation is regularly identified

DIFFERENTIAL DIAGNOSIS

HIV-associated Salivary Gland Disease
- HIV-associated cystic lesions are typically multiple, possibly bilateral, and also contain lymphoepithelial islands
- Germinal centers are larger and more irregular
  - Interfollicular tissue contains numerous plasma cells, neutrophils, histiocytes, and large, irregular mononuclear or multinuclear cells

Cystic Squamous Cell Carcinoma (SCC)
- Lymph node architecture, with cyst lined by "ribbon" of atypical epithelium, including mitotic figures and keratinaceous debris

Papillary Cystadenoma Lymphomatosum
- a.k.a. Warthin tumor
- Cystic epithelial proliferation with papillary infolding and intimate lymphoid component
- Papillae are lined with bilayered, oncocytic epithelium

Mucoepidermoid Carcinoma
- Often has cystic component and possible TALP
- BLECs lack solid epidermoid nests, intermediate cells, or infiltrative architectural pattern of MEC

SELECTED REFERENCES

1. Kojima M et al: HIV-unrelated benign lymphoepithelial cyst of the parotid glands containing lymphoepithelial lesion--like structures: a report of 3 cases. Int J Surg Pathol. 17(6):421-5, 2009
2. Wu L et al: Lymphoepithelial cyst of the parotid gland: its possible histopathogenesis based on clinicopathologic analysis of 64 cases. Hum Pathol. 40(5):683-92, 2009
3. Varnholt H et al: Salivary gland lymphoepithelial cysts. Ear Nose Throat J. 86(5):265, 2007
4. Layfield LJ et al: Cystic lesions of the salivary glands: cytologic features in fine-needle aspiration biopsies. Diagn Cytopathol. 27(4):197-204, 2002
5. Som PM et al: Nodal inclusion cysts of the parotid gland and parapharyngeal space: a discussion of lymphoepithelial, AIDS-related parotid, and branchial cysts, cystic Warthin's tumors, and cysts in Sjögren's syndrome. Laryngoscope. 105(10):1122-8, 1995
6. Auclair PL: Tumor-associated lymphoid proliferation in the parotid gland. A potential diagnostic pitfall. Oral Surg Oral Med Oral Pathol. 77(1):19-26, 1994
7. Cleary KR et al: Lymphoepithelial cysts of the parotid region: a "new face" on an old lesion. Ann Otol Rhinol Laryngol. 99(2 Pt 1):162-4, 1990
8. Elliott JN et al: Lymphoepithelial cysts of the salivary glands. Histologic and cytologic features. Am J Clin Pathol. 93(1):39-43, 1990
9. Fujibayashi T et al: Lymphoepithelial (so-called branchial) cyst within the parotid gland. Report of a case and review of the literature. Int J Oral Surg. 10(4):283-92, 1981
10. Stewart S et al: Lymphoepithelial (branchial) cyst of the parotid gland. J Oral Surg. 32(2):100-6, 1974
11. Weitzner S: Lymphoepithelial (branchial) cyst of parotid gland. Oral Surg Oral Med Oral Pathol. 35(1):85-8, 1973

IMAGE GALLERY

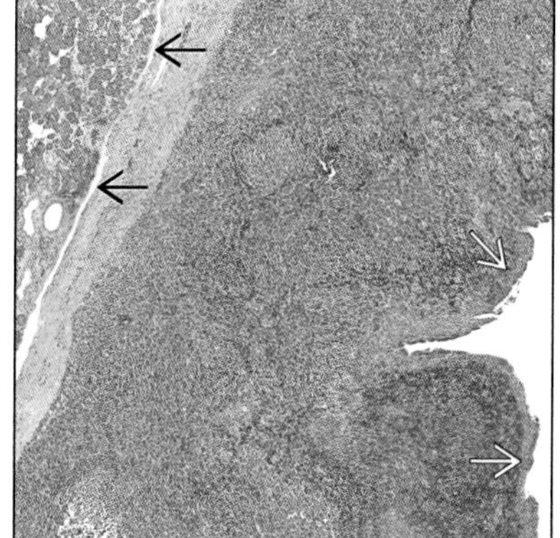
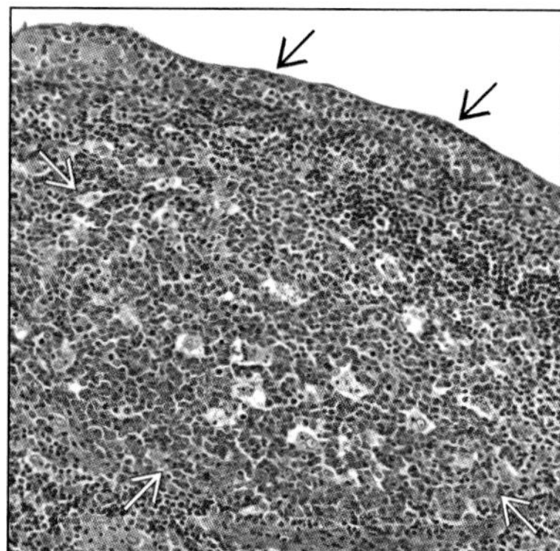
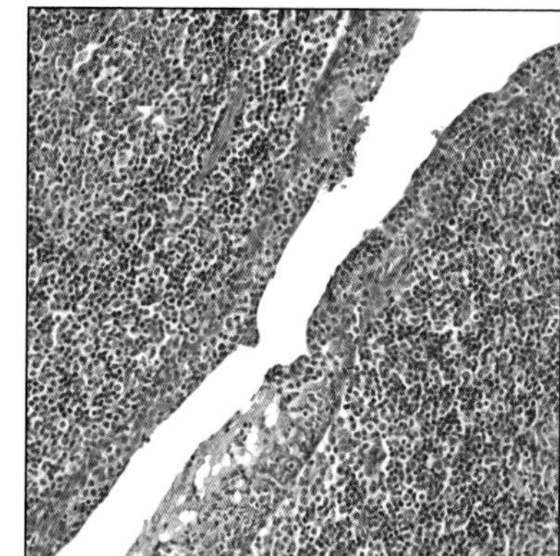

(Left) There is a well-demarcated junction between the lymphoid population and the fibrous connective tissue separating the cyst from the normal salivary gland ⇒. The epithelium lines the cyst ➡. *(Center)* Medium-power view shows a lymphocytic germinal center ➡ underlying the squamous epithelial cystic lining ⇒. *(Right)* Medium-power view shows squamous epithelial cystic lining of an LEC. Portions of the epithelium demonstrate an irregular parakeratinized surface.

BENIGN LYMPHOEPITHELIAL LESION

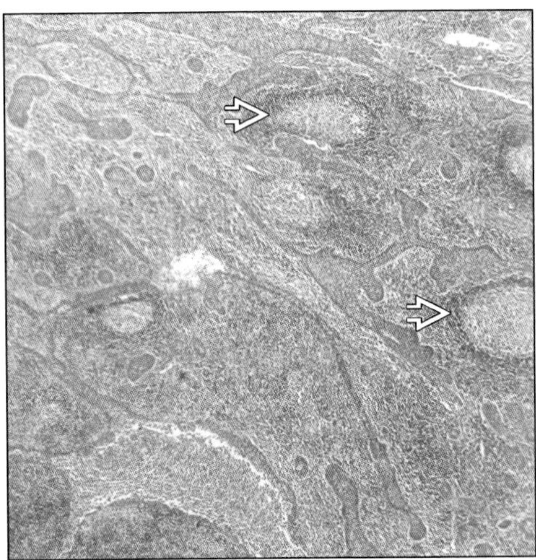

This image of a parotid gland shows variable effacement of the salivary gland lobules by a chronic inflammatory infiltrate. There are germinal centers ➡ associated with lymphoepithelial complexes.

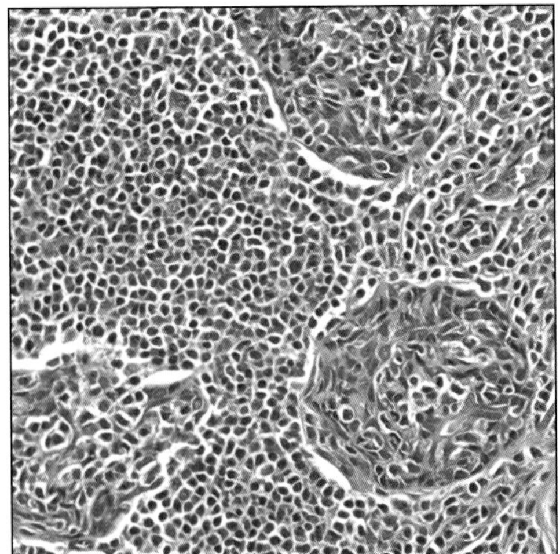

Lymphoepithelial complexes within BLEL are shown. The nests are variable in size and surrounded by a dense lymphoid cell population. Lymphocytic clonality was not evident in this case, confirming a benign lesion.

TERMINOLOGY

Abbreviations

- Benign lymphoepithelial lesion (BLEL)

Synonyms

- Lymphoepithelial sialadenitis (LESA)
- Myoepithelial sialadenitis (MESA)

Definitions

- Reactive, focal to diffuse lymphoid infiltrate of salivary glands leading to parenchymal atrophy and degeneration of glandular elements into irregular epithelial complexes

ETIOLOGY/PATHOGENESIS

Association

- Strong association with Sjögren syndrome (SS)
  - Majority of patients with SS also have BLEL of parotid glands
  - Typically bilateral

CLINICAL ISSUES

Epidemiology

- Incidence
  - Uncommon
  - Most cases associated with SS
  - BLEL occasionally seen independent of SS
    - Usually unilateral
    - May be secondary to obstruction
- Age
  - Mean: 5th-6th decade
- Gender
  - Female > Male (3:1)

Site

- Vast majority affect parotid gland
- Commonly bilateral

Presentation

- Recurrent, firm, diffuse enlargement or swelling of affected gland
- With or without pain

Treatment

- Excision of affected gland may be required

Prognosis

- Excellent in most cases
- Potential evolution to extranodal marginal zone B-cell lymphoma (EMZBCL)

MACROSCOPIC FEATURES

General Features

- Salivary gland capsule is intact
- Multinodular diffuse enlargement to discrete micronodules

MICROSCOPIC PATHOLOGY

Histologic Features

- Effacement of salivary parenchyma by dense infiltrate of lymphocytes and plasma cells
  - Lobular architecture preserved
    - Distinct separation of lobules by fibrous septa
  - Lobular effacement variable
    - May be completely effaced in advanced disease
  - Eosinophils and neutrophils usually absent
- Atrophy of glandular and ductal epithelium
- Formation of "lymphoepithelial complexes"
  - Also termed "epimyoepithelial islands"
  - Complexes of irregular size and morphology
  - Epithelial component composed of small, irregular cells with scant cytoplasm
    - Polygonal or spindled

BENIGN LYMPHOEPITHELIAL LESION

Key Facts

Terminology
- Reactive, focal to diffuse polyclonal lymphoid infiltrate of salivary glands leading to parenchymal atrophy and degeneration of glandular elements into irregular epithelial complexes

Clinical Issues
- Strong association with Sjögren syndrome (SS)
- Mean: 5th to 6th decade
- Female > Male (3:1)
- Vast majority affect parotid gland
- Recurrent, firm, diffuse enlargement of affected gland

Microscopic Pathology
- Effacement of salivary parenchyma by dense infiltrate of lymphocytes and plasma cells
- Lobular architecture preserved
- Formation of "lymphoepithelial complexes"
- Mixture of polyclonal T and B lymphocytes

        - Cell borders may be indistinct
    - Variable permeation by B lymphocytes
        - Intracomplex lymphocytes may be small and inconspicuous, to relatively large with clear surrounding halo
- Deposits of extracellular, eosinophilic hyaline material
    - Often located within lymphoepithelial complex
- Germinal center formation rare to significant

ANCILLARY TESTS

Cytology
- Cellular smears with mixed inflammatory infiltrate and histiocytes
- Myoepithelial and ductal epithelial cells interspersed with lymphoid infiltrate
- Calcific bodies may be aspirated

Immunohistochemistry
- Mixture of T and B lymphocytes
- Clonality studies (κ and λ) show polyclonal population

Flow Cytometry
- Fresh tissue (at initial biopsy) for flow cytometry

DIFFERENTIAL DIAGNOSIS

Sjögren Syndrome (SS)
- BLEL is highly suggestive but not pathognomic of SS
- Ocular and oral signs and symptoms, combined with SS-A/SS-B autoantibodies

Extranodal Marginal Zone B-cell Lymphoma
- Loss of lobular architecture with destroyed fibrous septae
- Extension beyond gland capsule into adjacent tissues
- Sheets of medium-sized atypical B-cells
    - Invasion of epithelial complexes by clonal monocytoid B-cells
- Sheets of plasma cells

Tumor-associated Lymphoid Proliferation
- Secondary lymphoid infiltration associated with salivary malignant neoplasm
- Present at advancing edge or within tumor

Benign Lymphoepithelial Cyst
- Squamous-lined cystic space within lymphoid stroma

SELECTED REFERENCES

1. Ellis GL: Lymphoid lesions of salivary glands: malignant and benign. Med Oral Patol Oral Cir Bucal. 12(7):E479-85, 2007
2. Quintana PG et al: Salivary gland lymphoid infiltrates associated with lymphoepithelial lesions: a clinicopathologic, immunophenotypic, and genotypic study. Hum Pathol. 28(7):850-61, 1997
3. DiGiuseppe JA et al: Lymphoid infiltrates of the salivary glands: pathology, biology and clinical significance. Curr Opin Oncol. 8(3):232-7, 1996

IMAGE GALLERY

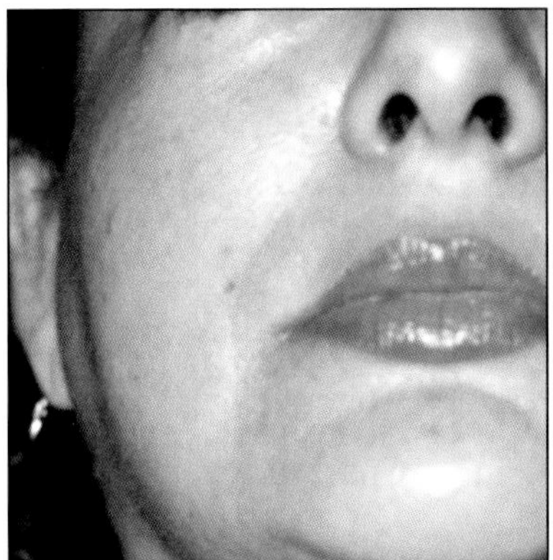

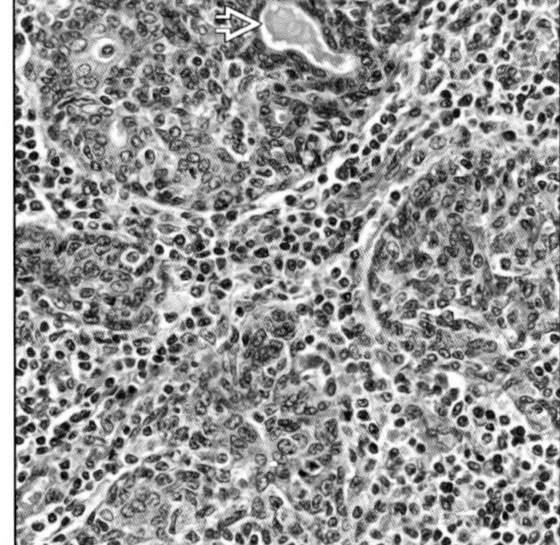

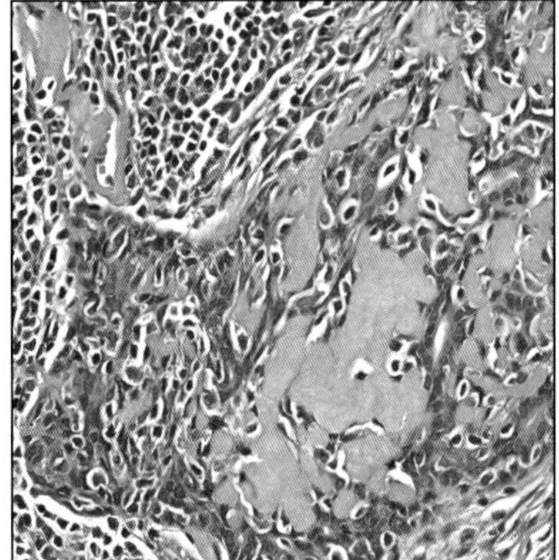

(Left) *This clinical photograph shows a patient with bilateral enlargement of parotid glands (right side shown). (Courtesy E. Childers, DDS.)* ***(Center)*** *Epithelial complexes composed of small, irregular cells with scant cytoplasm display variable infiltration by small lymphocytes. A small collection of hyaline material ⇨ is evident.* ***(Right)*** *Abundant eosinophilic hyaline material is present in this lymphoepithelial complex, as are numerous scattered lymphoid cells with surrounding clear halos.*

SJOGREN SYNDROME

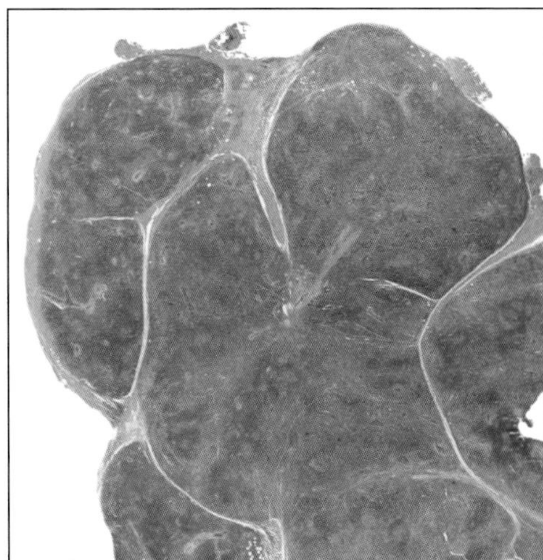

The parotid gland is diffusely infiltrated by chronic inflammatory cells. The normal architectural morphology is intact, with fibrous septae separating the glandular lobules. Glandular effacement is not present.

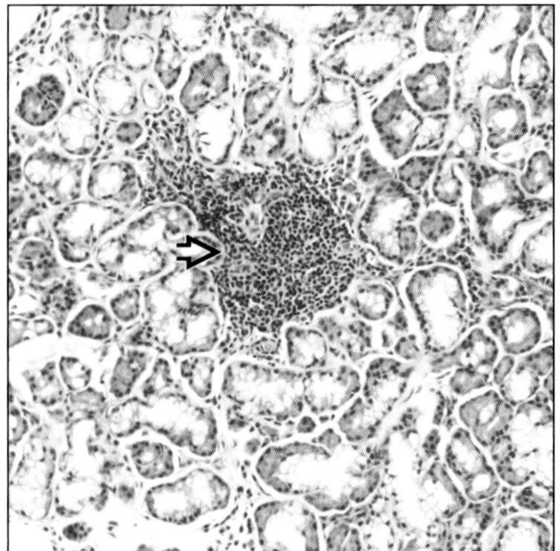

Labial minor salivary gland biopsy shows a lymphoid aggregate ➪ within the salivary acini. One or more foci within 4 mm² of salivary gland tissue is supportive of a diagnosis of Sjögren syndrome.

TERMINOLOGY

Abbreviations

- Sjögren syndrome (SS)

Synonyms

- Mikulicz disease, Sicca syndrome

Definitions

- **Primary SS**: Chronic, systemic autoimmune disease primarily affecting parotid and lacrimal excretory glands, leading to xerostomia and xerophthalmia, respectively
- **Secondary SS**: Above in association with another autoimmune, connective tissue disorder
  - Typically rheumatoid arthritis or systemic lupus erythematosus

ETIOLOGY/PATHOGENESIS

Primary Sjögren Syndrome

- Etiology unknown, yet likely multifactorial and complex
  - Endocrine: Systemic and local androgen deficiencies
  - Genetics
    - 1° SS associated with *HLA-B8* and *HLA-Dw3*
    - 2° SS associated with *HLA-DRw4*
  - Viral infection: EBV, Coxsackievirus, and HTLV-1
  - Autonomic nervous system
    - Blockage of receptor sites by antimuscarinic antibodies (anti-M3R)
  - Upregulation of INFα and β-cell activating factor

CLINICAL ISSUES

Epidemiology

- Incidence
  - 0.5-3% of population
    - May be undiagnosed in nearly half of affected patients
- Age
  - Mean: 5th-7th decades
    - Peaks at menarche and menopause
- Gender
  - Female > > > Male (9:1)
    - Males may be more common in juvenile presentation
- Ethnicity
  - No racial predilection

Site

- Lacrimal and parotid glands most severely affected
  - Commonly bilateral
- Submandibular, sublingual, and minor salivary glands affected to lesser degree
- Upper respiratory tract
  - Sinonasal mucosa, eustachian tube, and larynx
- Multiple other organ systems possibly affected

Presentation

- Xerostomia (dry mouth)
  - Typically noted after saliva production falls below 50% of normal
  - Taste alterations
  - Difficulties in speech and mastication
  - Possible burning sensation
  - Less frequently associated with
    - Dental caries
    - Dry, cracked lips, angular cheilitis
    - Fissured or depapillated tongue
    - Chronic candidiasis
    - Oral ulcerations
- Xerophthalmia (dry eyes, keratoconjunctivitis sicca)
  - Pain and foreign body sensation
  - Photosensitivity, ocular fatigue
  - Redness, loss of visual acuity, filamentary keratitis
- Parotid gland

SJOGREN SYNDROME

Key Facts

Terminology
- Reactive, focal to diffuse lymphoid infiltrate of salivary glands leading to parenchymal atrophy and degeneration of glandular elements into irregular epithelial complexes
- **Primary SS**: Chronic, systemic autoimmune disease primarily affecting parotid and lacrimal glands
- **Secondary SS**: Above in association with another autoimmune disorder

Clinical Issues
- Mean age: 5th-7th decades
- Female > > > Male (9:1)
- Lacrimal and parotid glands most severely affected, commonly bilateral
- Recurrent, firm, diffuse parotid enlargement lasting weeks to months, with occasional remission
  - Typically painless, bilateral swellings of lateral orbital margin
- Diagnosis based upon results of multiple tests
  - Positive anti-SS-A (RO) &/or anti-SS-B (LA)
  - Rheumatoid factor positive in up to 95%
- Treatment mostly supportive
  - 44x increased risk of developing lymphoma

Image Findings
- MR sialography is best diagnostic study

Microscopic Pathology
- Minor salivary glands with lymphocytic and plasma cell infiltrate
  - Lymphoid aggregate = ≥ 50 lymphocytes
- Lymphocytic infiltration, acinar atrophy, and formation of epimyoepithelial islands

---

  - Recurrent, firm, diffuse parotid enlargement lasting weeks to months, with occasional remission
    - Enlargement correlated with increased disease severity
    - Persistent swelling may indicate transformation into low-grade lymphoma
  - Possible discomfort/pain, which may increase with eating
  - Potential retrograde infections with suppuration from Stensen duct
- Lacrimal gland
  - Typically painless, bilateral swellings of lateral orbital margin
  - Associated with chronic dacryoadenitis
  - Associated with infection (especially viral), sarcoidosis, Graves disease, and orbital inflammatory syndrome
- Other presentations based upon affected system
- Many patients have other connective tissue, autoimmune, or rheumatologic disorders
  - Diabetes, sarcoidosis, malnutrition, infection, alcoholism, bulimia
  - Medications can be related to disorder development

Laboratory Tests
- Diagnosis based upon results of multiple tests
  - Ocular
    - Schirmer test: Decreased tear secretion
    - Rose bengal and lissamine green: Dyes used to examine eye surface for dry spots
  - Salivary flow tests (sialometry)
  - Serology
    - Positive anti-SS-A (RO) &/or anti-SS-B (LA)
    - Also autoantibodies for muscarinic receptor M3, IFI16, KLHL12, or KLHL7
    - Rheumatoid factor positive in up to 95%
    - Anti-nuclear antibody (ANA) positive in up to 80%
    - Erythrocyte sedimentation rate (ESR) usually elevated
    - Immunoglobulins: Usually elevated in SS patients

Treatment
- Treatment mostly supportive
- Xerostomia: Adequate hydration and stimulation of salivary flow
  - Topical stimulation: Sugar-free gum, candies, or lozenges
  - Systemic stimulation: Pilocarpine, cevimeline, bromhexine, tibolone
- Xerophthalmia
  - Topical: Artificial tears, including eye drops or ointments
  - Systemic: Androgens (methyl-testosterone) or cyclosporine
- Oral hygiene instruction, topical fluoride, and chlorhexidine rinses
- Antifungal therapy for chronic candidiasis

Prognosis
- Slowly progressive, evolving over decades
  - May wax and wane over time
- Most serious complication is lymphoma development
  - 44x increased risk of developing lymphoma
    - Approximately 4-10% of SS patients
  - Typically low grade
    - Extranodal marginal zone B-cell lymphoma (EMZBCL) of mucosa-associated lymphoid tissue (MALT) is most common
    - Represents approximately 85% of lymphomas in SS patients
    - Good prognosis unless transformation into diffuse large B-cell lymphoma
- Juvenile cases may resolve spontaneously at puberty

IMAGE FINDINGS

Radiographic Findings
- Sialography
  - Dilation of ducts (sialodochiectasis) and punctate collections of contrast medium
  - "Fruit-laden branchless tree"
- Scintigraphy

SJOGREN SYNDROME

- Noninvasive nuclear medicine technique measuring salivary gland function
  - Uptake and secretion of (Tc-99m) pertechnetate
  - Low values in keeping with loss of salivary gland function

MR Findings

- MR sialography is best diagnostic study
  - Punctate, globular, cavitary, or destructive parotid distal duct changes show high T2 signal
- STIR MR sequence makes findings more conspicuous
- T1WI: Discrete collections of low signal intensity
- T2WI: Diffuse, bilateral high T2 1-2 mm up to > 2 mm foci

CT Findings

- Bilateral enlarged parotids with multiple cystic and solid intraparotid lesions with or without punctate calcifications
  - Lacrimal glands frequently involved
- "Miliary pattern" of small cysts diffusely throughout both parotids seen in intermediate stage
- Cysts and solid masses (lymphoid aggregates) in late stage

MACROSCOPIC FEATURES

General Features

- Overall gland enlargement
- Intact salivary gland capsule
- Multinodular to diffuse with or without micronodules

Size

- Variable gland size, although overall enlargement

MICROSCOPIC PATHOLOGY

Histologic Features

- Major salivary glands with lymphocytic infiltration, acinar atrophy, and formation of epimyoepithelial islands
  - i.e., benign lymphoepithelial lesion
- Lacrimal gland with lymphocytic and plasma cell infiltrate
- Labial minor salivary gland biopsy
  - Minor salivary glands with focal lymphocytic infiltration
    - Infiltrate adjacent to normal appearing acini
    - Parenchymal acinar atrophy, fibrosis, duct ectasia (chronic sclerosing sialadenitis), or acute inflammation not in keeping with SS
  - Lymphoid aggregate = ≥ 50 lymphocytes
    - Periductal lymphoid aggregates (sialodochitis) not counted in test
  - Minimum of 4 mm² of minor salivary gland parenchyma required (5-10 minor salivary glands)
  - Focus score = number of lymphoid aggregates per 4 mm² of salivary gland tissue
    - Focus score of ≥ 1 supportive of SS
    - Correlation increases with greater focus score

ANCILLARY TESTS

Cytology

- Cellular smears with mixed inflammatory infiltrate and histiocytes
- Myoepithelial and ductal epithelial cells interspersed with lymphoid infiltrate

Immunohistochemistry

- Mixed population of B and T lymphocytes
  - CD4(+) T-cell lymphocytes
- Clonal studies (κ and λ) show polyclonal population

Flow Cytometry

- Fresh tissue (at initial biopsy) for flow cytometry
  - Polyclonal population helps exclude possibility of lymphoma

Cytogenetics

- Gene rearrangement studies to exclude lymphoma

DIFFERENTIAL DIAGNOSIS

Benign Lymphoepithelial Lesion

- BLEL is highly suggestive of SS, especially if bilateral
- Ocular and oral signs and symptoms, when combined with SS-A/SS-B autoantibodies, support SS rather than BLEL

Benign Lymphoepithelial Cyst

- Benign, cystic epithelial lesion intimately associated with lymphocytic proliferation within cyst wall
- Unilocular and unicystic lesion that is typically well demarcated within parotid gland
- Cysts are ordinarily lined by stratified squamous epithelium
  - Cuboidal, columnar, or pseudostratified epithelium may line cyst
- Dense lymphoid component within cyst wall
  - Germinal center formation is regularly identified

Chronic Sialadenitis

- Mixed chronic inflammatory infiltrate containing plasma cells, lymphocytes, and neutrophils
- Prominent periductal and acinar fibrosis
- Parenchymal acinar atrophy
- Duct ectasia (chronic sclerosing sialadenitis) or acute inflammation not in keeping with SS
- Lobular architecture is maintained
- Lack of lymphoepithelial lesions

Sarcoidosis

- Tight, well-formed, epithelioid histiocyte aggregates
  - Palisade of histiocytes at periphery
- Giant cells may be present
- Noncaseating for most cases
- Lymphocytes and plasma cells usually present

Warthin Tumor

- Defined tumor with capsule &/or circumscription
- Papillary, oncocytic epithelium arranged with cyst
- Lymphoid aggregates around periphery, often with germinal center formation

SJOGREN SYNDROME

Revised American-European Classification Criteria* for Sjögren Syndrome

Symptom or Test	Result or Interpretation
I. Ocular symptoms (1 of 3)	Foreign body sensation within eye
	Daily, persistent dry eyes for greater than 3 months
	Artificial tear uses greater than 3x per day
II. Oral symptoms (1 of 3)	Daily, persistent dry mouth for greater than 3 months
	Recurrent or persistent enlargement of salivary glands
	Requiring liquids to promote swallowing
III. Ocular tests (1 of 2)	Unanesthetized Schirmer test (< 5 mm in 5 minutes)
	Vital dye (1% rose Bengal) staining (≥ 4 according to van Bijsterveld scoring system)
IV. Positive lip biopsy	Focus score of 1 or greater (> 1 lymphocytic aggregate [50+] per 4 mm^2 of salivary gland tissue)
V. Oral tests (1 of 3)	Sialometry: Unstimulated salivary flow < 0.1 mL per minute
	Abnormal parotid gland sialography
	Abnormal salivary scintigraphy
VI. Serology	Positive anti-SS-A (RO) &/or anti-SS-B (LA)
Primary Sjögren syndrome	Requires 4 of the 6 criteria, to include either positive lip biopsy or positive serology, or
	Requires 3 of the 6 objective criteria (III, IV, V, VI)
Secondary Sjögren syndrome	Presence of autoimmune connective tissue disease (e.g., rheumatoid arthritis, systemic lupus erythematosus), and
	Presence of criteria I or II , plus any 2 objective criteria (III, IV, V)

**Adapted from Vitali C et al: Classification criteria for Sjögren's syndrome. Ann Rheum Dis. 61(6):554-8, 2002.*

Extraglandular Manifestations of Sjögren Syndrome

Organ and System	Disease Entity
Thyroid	Autoimmune thyroiditis
Liver	Primary biliary cirrhosis
Lung	Interstitial fibrosis
Kidney	Glomerulonephritis and interstitial nephritis
Skin	Dryness, vasculitis, and peripheral neuropathies
Neurologic	Peripheral neuropathy, carpal tunnel syndrome
Joints	Pain and arthritis
Gastrointestinal	Dysphagia, reflux, pernicious anemia

Extranodal Marginal Zone B-cell Lymphoma

- Loss of lobular architecture with destroyed fibrous septae
- Extension beyond gland capsule into adjacent tissues
- Sheets of medium-sized atypical B-cells
  - Invasion of epithelial complexes by clonal monocytoid B-cells
- Sheets of plasma cells

Tumor-associated Lymphoid Proliferation

- Secondary lymphoid infiltration associated with a number of salivary epithelial malignant neoplasms
- Present at advancing edge or within tumor

Metastatic Carcinoma

- Destructive growth of cytologic atypical cells without myoepithelial islands

STAGING

Based on MR Sialography

- I: Punctate contrast/high signal ≤ 1 mm
- II: Globular contrast/high signal 1-2 mm
- III: Cavitary contrast/high signal > 2 mm
- IV: Complete destruction of parotid parenchyma

SELECTED REFERENCES

1. Margaix-Muñoz M et al: Sjögren's syndrome of the oral cavity. Review and update. Med Oral Patol Oral Cir Bucal. 14(7):E325-30, 2009
2. Nikolov NP et al: Pathogenesis of Sjögren's syndrome. Curr Opin Rheumatol. 21(5):465-70, 2009
3. Gutta R et al: Sjögren syndrome: a review for the maxillofacial surgeon. Oral Maxillofac Surg Clin North Am. 20(4):567-75, 2008
4. Vitali C et al: Classification criteria for Sjögren's syndrome: a revised version of the European criteria proposed by the American-European Consensus Group. Ann Rheum Dis. 61(6):554-8, 2002
5. Quintana PG et al: Salivary gland lymphoid infiltrates associated with lymphoepithelial lesions: a clinicopathologic, immunophenotypic, and genotypic study. Hum Pathol. 28(7):850-61, 1997
6. Andrade RE et al: Distribution and immunophenotype of the inflammatory cell population in the benign lymphoepithelial lesion (Mikulicz's disease). Hum Pathol. 19(8):932-41, 1988

SJOGREN SYNDROME

Diagrammatic, Clinical, and Imaging Features

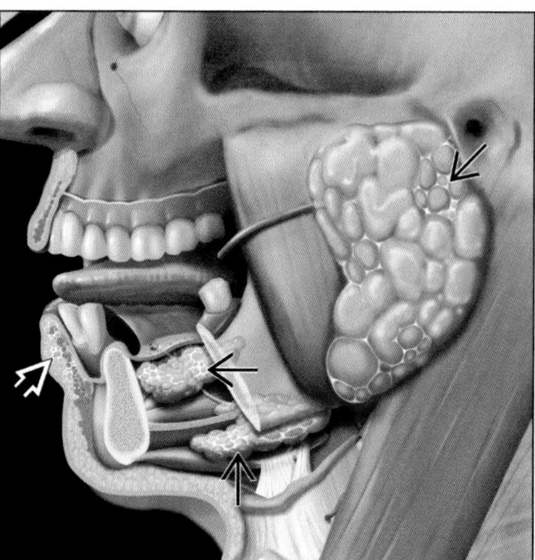

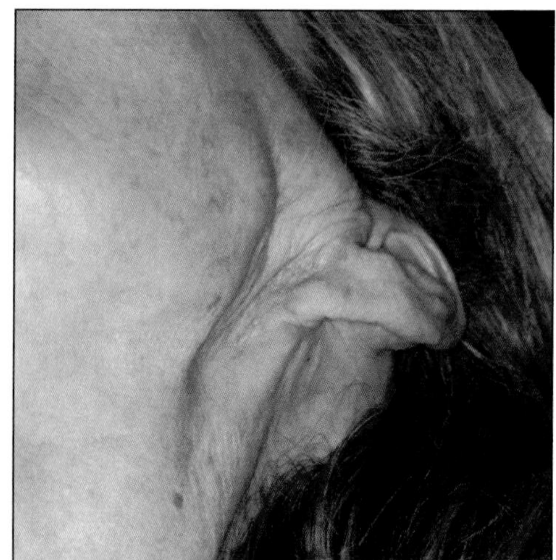

(Left) *This graphic demonstrates inflammatory-related enlargement of the major salivary glands ➔ and minor glands of the lip ➔.* *There is still preservation of the lobular architecture.* ***(Right)*** *Sjögren syndrome with parotid gland enlargement shows that the process is typically bilateral and may show intermittent resolution. Depending on the duration of symptoms, persistent enlargement may indicate malignant transformation. (Courtesy G. Illei, DDS.)*

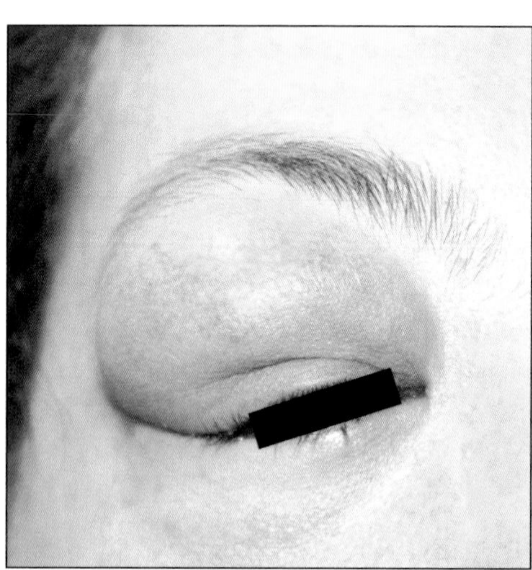

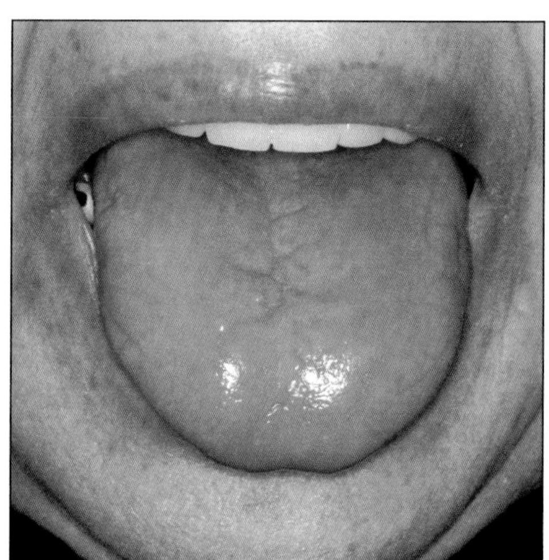

(Left) *Clinical swelling of the lacrimal gland, palpebral lobe is shown in a patient with Sjögren syndrome. Serologic and radiographic evaluation will help to confirm the diagnosis. (Courtesy G. Illei, DDS.)* ***(Right)*** *Loss of filiform papillae on the dorsum of the tongue, secondary to xerostomia, is shown in a patient with Sjögren syndrome. This may be accompanied by burning sensation or alteration in taste. (Courtesy G. Illei, DDS.)*

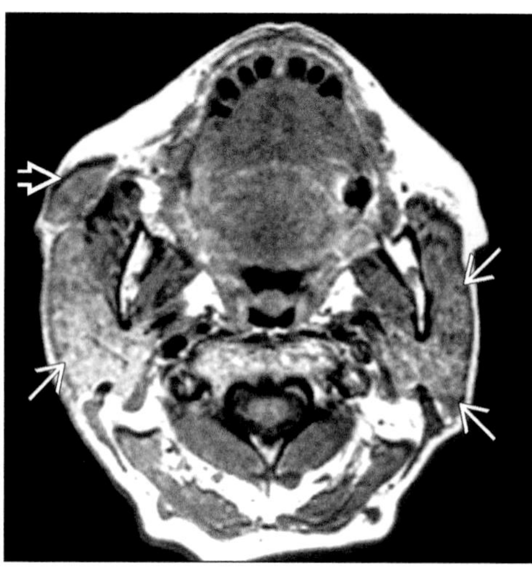

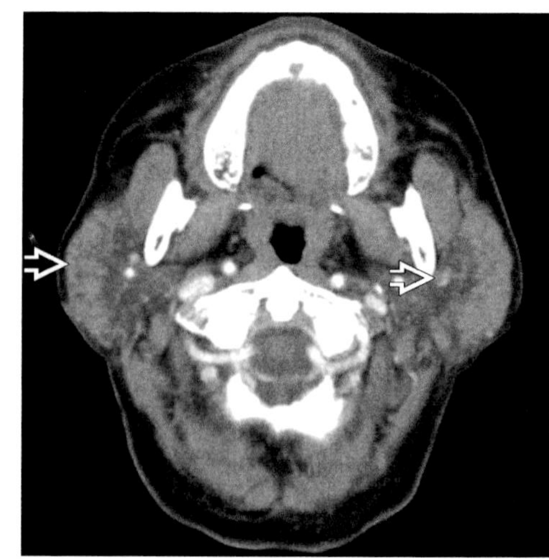

(Left) *Axial T1WI MR shows bilateral parotid gland enlargement ➔ with a diffusely heterogeneous appearance of 1-2 mm foci of altered signal intensity. The accessory lobes on the superficial aspect of the masseter muscles are also involved ➔. MR with sialography is the study of choice for Sjögren syndrome.* ***(Right)*** *Computed tomography examination shows bilateral enlargement of the parotid glands ➔. There is a vague "miliary pattern" of small cysts diffusely throughout the parotids.*

SJOGREN SYNDROME

Imaging and Microscopic Features

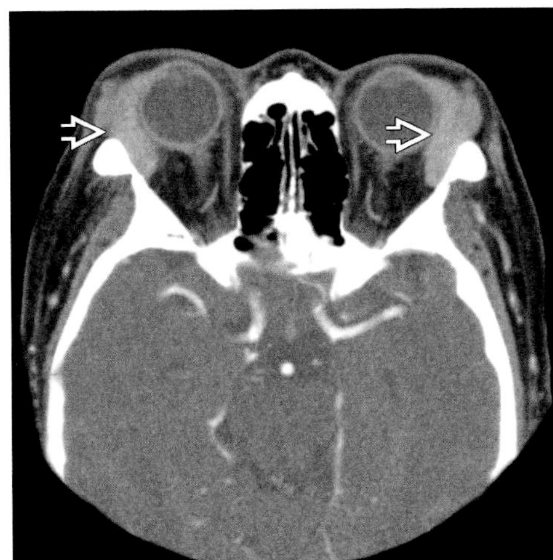

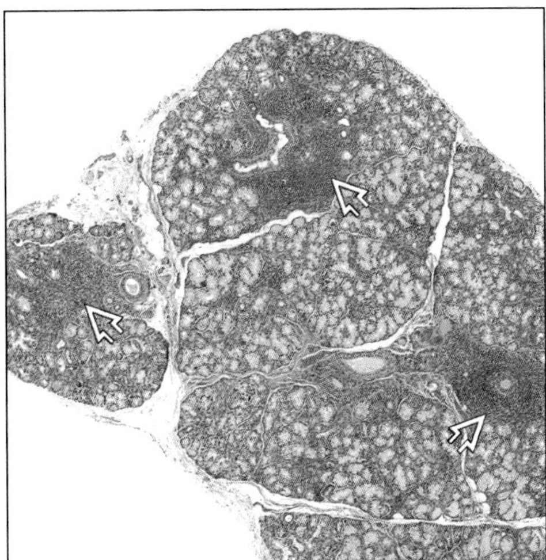

(Left) *Computed tomography examination shows bilateral enlargement of the lacrimal glands ⇨. The differential consideration for this type of change is broad but is diagnostic in the correct serologic and biopsy setting.* ***(Right)*** *A biopsy taken from the lip includes many lobules of salivary gland tissue (4 mm² is required), with a number of foci of > 50 lymphocytes/plasma cells ⇨. Periductal foci do not count toward focus score.*

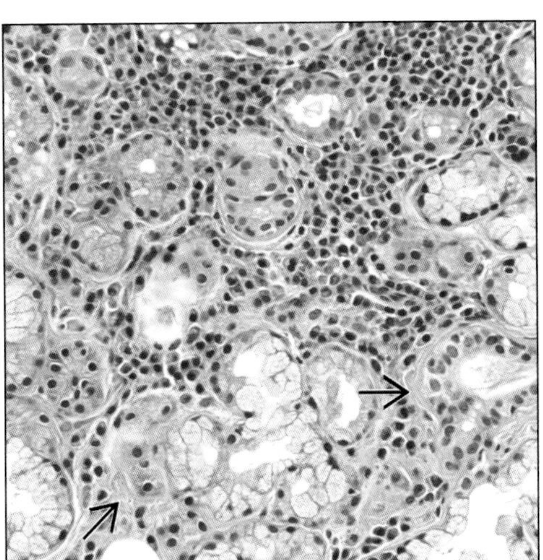

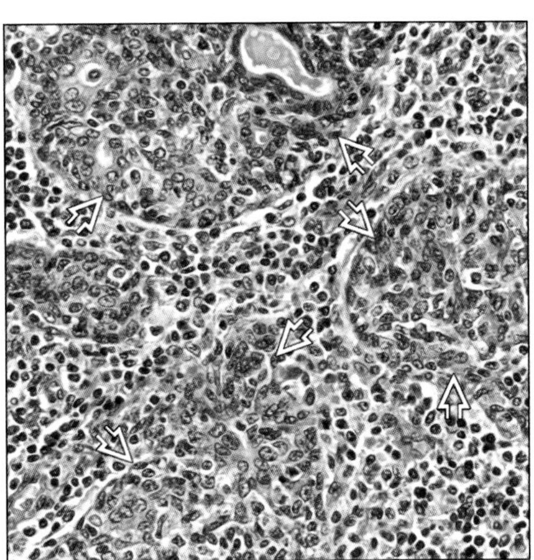

(Left) *An increased number of lymphocytes and plasma cells are seen juxtaposed to the normal, nonatrophic salivary gland parenchyma. There are thin wisps of fibrosis → but no ectasia or neutrophils.* ***(Right)*** *In some cases, there are well-developed lymphoepithelial lesions (epimyoepithelial complexes ⇨), in which there is a mixture of lymphoid elements with the epithelial-myoepithelial islands. BLEL are seen in most patients with well-developed Sjögren syndrome.*

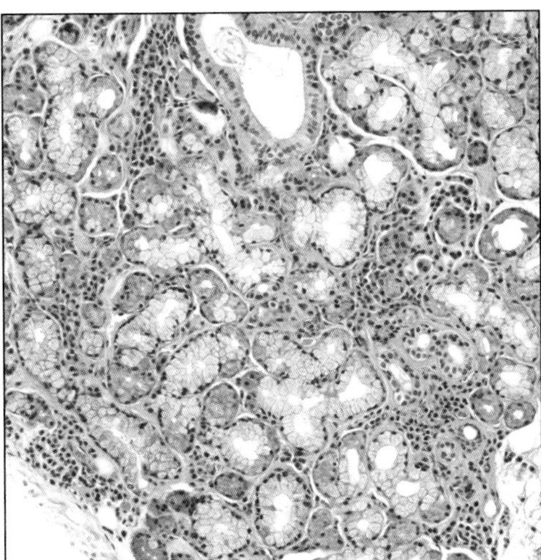

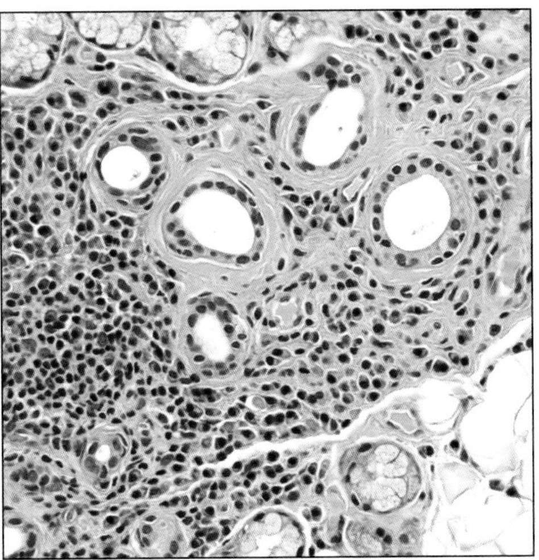

(Left) *Within this salivary gland lobule, there are significantly more than 50 lymphocytes and plasma cells. While there is focal fibrosis, there is no dilatation or acinar atrophy. Acute inflammatory cells are not present. The patient had positive SS-A antibodies.* ***(Right)*** *In this case of chronic sclerosing sialadenitis, a differential for SS, there is strong periductal and periacinar fibrosis, with duct dilatation with a rich inflammatory infiltrate of lymphocytes and plasma cells.*

ONCOCYTOSIS (ONCOCYTIC HYPERPLASIA)

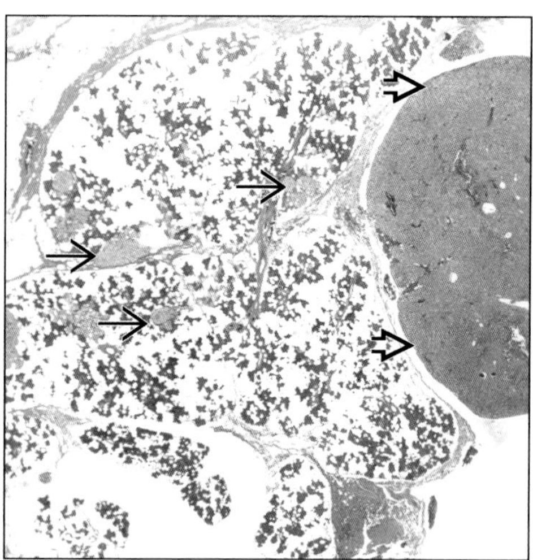

Multiple small foci ➔ of oncocytic hyperplasia are highlighted in this parotid gland. A larger hyperplastic nodule is present in the right portion of the field ⇨.

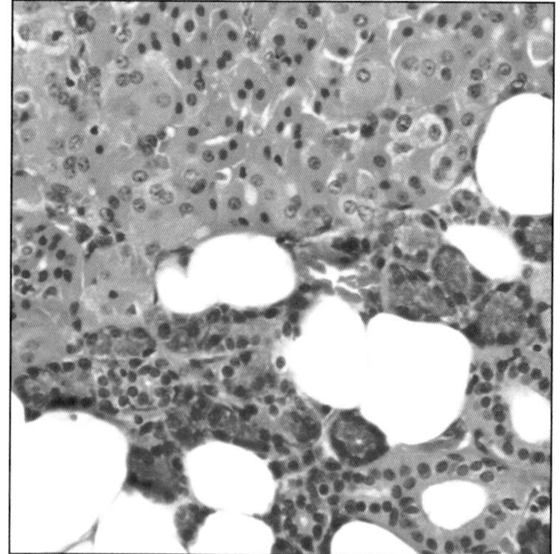

Note the intimate interface between the metaplastic oncocytic cells (top half) and the normal parotid gland parenchyma (bottom half). There is a lack of capsule.

TERMINOLOGY

Synonyms

- Oncocytic hyperplasia

Definitions

- **Oncocytes** are altered epithelial cells whose cytoplasm contains vast numbers of abnormal mitochondria
  - Cell is large and polygonal, with well-defined borders, and has granular appearing acidophilic cytoplasm
- **Oncocytic metaplasia** is non-mass-forming alteration/transformation of glandular epithelial cells into oncocytes
- **Oncocytosis** (a.k.a. **oncocytic hyperplasia**) is a nonneoplastic proliferation of oncocytes, which may be localized, multifocal, or diffuse (**diffuse oncocytosis**)
  - May produce unencapsulated nodules (**nodular oncocytic hyperplasia**) in lobular distribution

ETIOLOGY/PATHOGENESIS

Aging

- Oncocytic change associated with normal aging

CLINICAL ISSUES

Epidemiology

- Incidence
  - Occurrence increases with age
    - Focal oncocytic metaplasia almost universal after 70 years
- Age
  - Normally seen after 50 years

Site

- May be noted in any salivary gland
  - Parotid gland is affected more frequently

Presentation

- Oncocytic metaplasia and oncocytosis are generally asymptomatic
  - Tenderness of affected gland is possible
- Nodular oncocytic hyperplasia may present as clinically evident mass

Treatment

- Surgical approaches
  - No treatment necessary for oncocytic metaplasia
  - Oncocytic hyperplasia is benign process
    - No further treatment is required after diagnosis

Prognosis

- Due to possible multifocal nature of oncocytosis, clinical "recurrence" may be noted

MACROSCOPIC FEATURES

General Features

- Oncocytic metaplasia may be difficult to identify macroscopically
- Specimens with diffuse or nodular oncocytic hyperplasia may show grossly evident small nodules

MICROSCOPIC PATHOLOGY

Histologic Features

- Oncocytes are large, polygonal cells with abundant finely granular acidophilic/eosinophilic cytoplasm
  - Oncocytic change may involve salivary acini, intercalated ducts, or striated ducts
  - Nuclei are round to oval, centrally placed, and may contain one or more prominent nucleoli
    - Nuclei may be shrunken and pyknotic
    - Binucleated cells may be seen
  - Cytoplasmic glycogen accumulation may peripheralize intracytoplasmic mitochondria
    - Results in clear cytoplasm (**clear cell oncocytosis**)

ONCOCYTOSIS (ONCOCYTIC HYPERPLASIA)

Key Facts

Terminology

- Oncocyte: Altered epithelial cell whose cytoplasm contains vast numbers of abnormal mitochondria

Microscopic Pathology

- Oncocytes are large and polygonal with granular cytoplasm
- Oncocytic metaplasia shows intimate, direct apposition of oncocytic cells with normal salivary gland parenchyma
- Oncocytic hyperplasia may range from small collections to larger, unencapsulated nodules

Ancillary Tests

- Phosphotungstic acid hematoxylin (PTAH), Novelli, Luxol fast blue, and Cresylecht violet V all highlight cytoplasmic mitochondria

- Oncocytic metaplasia shows intimate, direct apposition of oncocytic cells with normal salivary gland parenchyma and stroma
- Oncocytic hyperplasia may range from small collections of cells to larger, unencapsulated nodules
  - May be singular or multifocal
  - Diffuse oncocytic hyperplasia (diffuse oncocytosis) involves nearly all of salivary gland parenchyma with no nodule or tumor formation

ANCILLARY TESTS

Histochemistry

- Phosphotungstic acid hematoxylin (PTAH) stains cytoplasmic mitochondria dark blue-black
- Novelli stains cytoplasmic mitochondria blue-purple
- Luxol fast blue shows metachromatically positive mitochondria in cytoplasm
- Cresylecht violet V reaction shows metachromatically positive cytoplasmic granules

DIFFERENTIAL DIAGNOSIS

Oncocytoma

- Differences between oncocytoma and clinically evident nodular oncocytic hyperplasia are vague
- Features favoring oncocytoma include partial or full encapsulation, and lack of included ductal structures

Other Salivary Gland Neoplasms

- Oncocytic change may be seen in many salivary gland neoplasms
  - Including Warthin tumor, pleomorphic adenoma, and mucoepidermoid carcinoma
  - Oncocytic metaplasia/hyperplasia lacks papillary cystic architecture and dense lymphoid infiltrate
  - Presence of other cell types (myoepithelial, mucocytes, epidermoid cells) favors other neoplasms

SELECTED REFERENCES

1. Capone RB et al: Oncocytic neoplasms of the parotid gland: a 16-year institutional review. Otolaryngol Head Neck Surg. 126(6):657-62, 2002
2. Loreti A et al: Diffuse hyperplastic oncocytosis of the parotid gland. Br J Plast Surg. 55(2):151-2, 2002
3. Dardick I et al: Differentiation and the cytomorphology of salivary gland tumors with specific reference to oncocytic metaplasia. Oral Surg Oral Med Oral Pathol Oral Radiol Endod. 88(6):691-701, 1999
4. Chang A et al: Oncocytes, oncocytosis, and oncocytic tumors. Pathol Annu. 27 Pt 1:263-304, 1992
5. Brandwein MS et al: Oncocytic tumors of major salivary glands. A study of 68 cases with follow-up of 44 patients. Am J Surg Pathol. 15(6):514-28, 1991
6. Palmer TJ et al: Oncocytic adenomas and oncocytic hyperplasia of salivary glands: a clinicopathological study of 26 cases. Histopathology. 16(5):487-93, 1990

IMAGE GALLERY

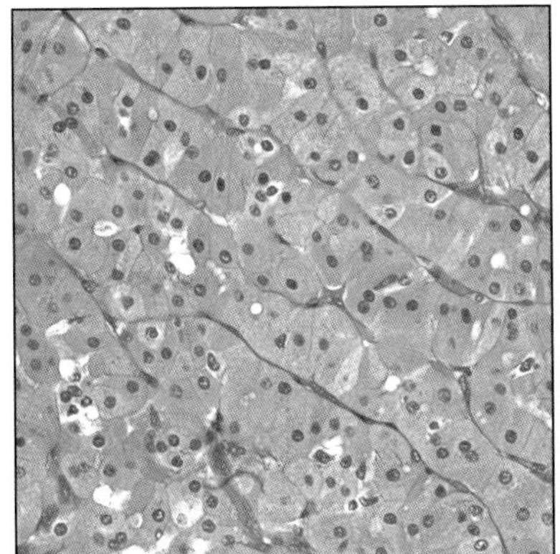
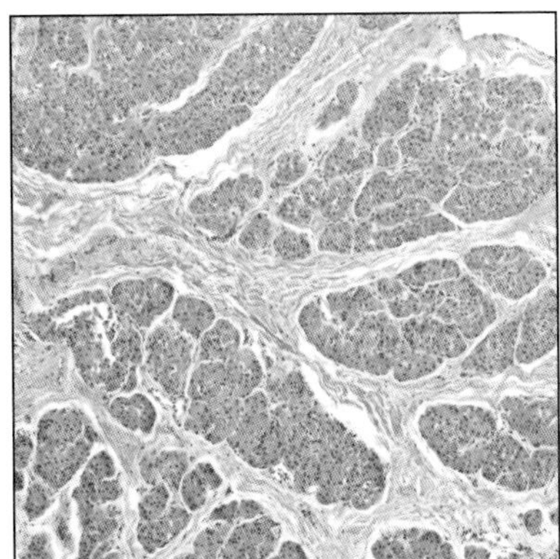
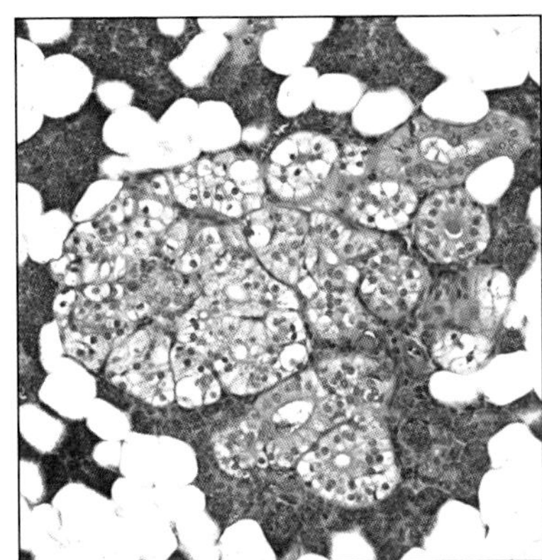

(Left) *Oncocytes are characterized by abundant granular eosinophilic cytoplasm, round to oval nuclei, and polygonal morphology.* ***(Center)*** *Diffuse oncocytic hyperplasia (diffuse oncocytosis) is characterized by complete replacement of the salivary gland acini by oncocytes. Note the preservation of the lobular architecture.* ***(Right)*** *Clear cell oncocytosis is characterized by cytoplasmic glycogen accumulation and peripheralization of the intracytoplasmic mitochondria.*

SCLEROSING POLYCYSTIC ADENOSIS

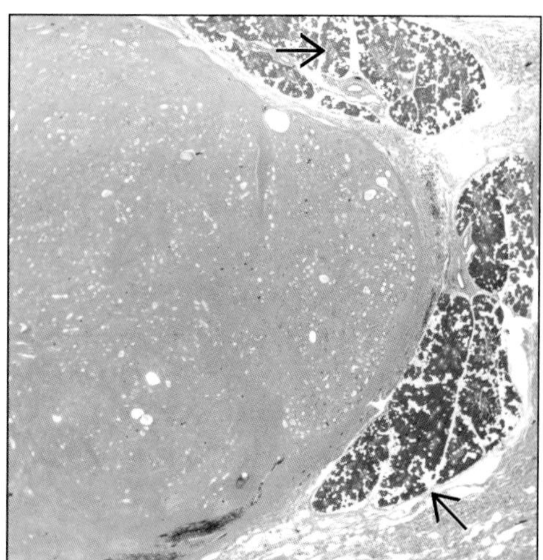

Low-power view shows a well-circumscribed, lobular epithelial proliferation with intervening fibrous bands. The surrounding salivary gland parenchyma ⇒ is unremarkable.

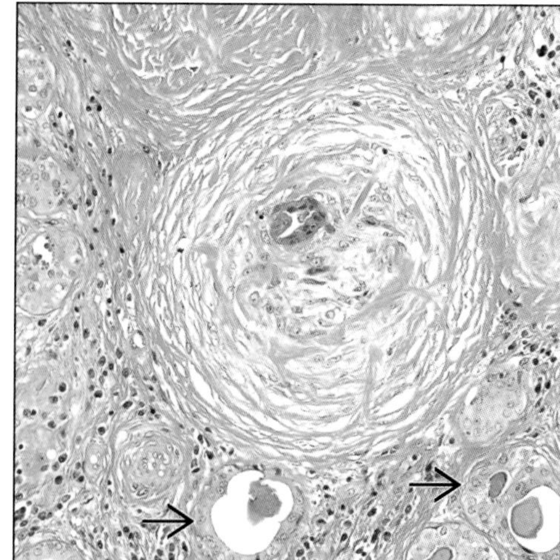

Medium-power view shows a fibrotic nodule within sclerosing polycystic adenosis. Hyperplastic ductal epithelium in solid nests and ducts are also present ⇒.

TERMINOLOGY

Abbreviations

- Sclerosing polycystic adenosis (SPA)

Synonyms

- Smith tumor

Definitions

- Pseudoneoplastic inflammatory lesion of salivary glands that histologically resembles breast fibrocystic disease

CLINICAL ISSUES

Epidemiology

- Incidence
  - Rare lesion of salivary glands
- Age
  - Children to elderly
  - Mean presentation in 4th to 5th decades
- Gender
  - Females slightly more often than males

Site

- Majority in parotid gland
  - Occasionally located in submandibular or minor salivary glands

Presentation

- Slow-growing, usually asymptomatic mass

Treatment

- Surgical approaches
  - Complete, conservative local surgical excision
  - Conservation of facial nerve in parotid lesions

Prognosis

- Recurrence possible in approximately 1/3 of cases
  - Usually related to incomplete excision or possible multifocal disease
- No reports of metastatic spread or related mortality

MACROSCOPIC FEATURES

General Features

- Circumscribed, pale, rubbery mass
- May appear multinodular

Size

- Range: 1-12 cm

MICROSCOPIC PATHOLOGY

Histologic Features

- Circumscribed but unencapsulated
  - Often surrounded by normal salivary gland tissue
- Prominent fibrous sclerosis with focal formation of hyalinized sclerotic nodules
- Hyperplastic epithelial proliferation of ductal, tubular, and acinar cells in lobular pattern
  - May form solid or cribriform nests
    - Cystic dilation may be evident
    - Eosinophilic, spherical, laminated hyaline globules ("collagenous spherulosis") may be noted within epithelial nests
- Glandular epithelial cells vary in appearance
  - May include flattened cuboidal, columnar, apocrine-like, mucinous, squamous, and foamy cells
  - Acinar-like cells with prominent eosinophilic, periodic acid-Schiff (PAS) positive cytoplasmic granules
    - Histologically reminiscent of Paneth cells of intestine
  - Foamy epithelial cytoplasm likely due to degenerative changes
    - May resemble sebaceous cells
- Nests of xanthomatous macrophages may be present associated with areas of epithelial degeneration

Key Facts

Terminology

- Pseudoneoplastic inflammatory salivary gland lesion resembling breast fibrocystic disease

Microscopic Pathology

- Acinar-like cells with prominent eosinophilic cytoplasmic granules
  - Similar to Paneth cells of intestine
- Circumscribed but unencapsulated
- Lobulated
- Hyperplastic epithelial proliferation of ductal, tubular, and acinar cells in lobular pattern
- Circumscribed but unencapsulated
- Surrounded by normal salivary gland tissue
- Prominent fibrous sclerosis with focal formation of hyalinized sclerotic nodules

Top Differential Diagnoses

- Pleomorphic adenoma and chronic sclerosing sialadenitis

- Epithelial atypia or dysplasia (up to carcinoma in situ) has been noted
  - No reports of invasive malignant disease

ANCILLARY TESTS

Immunohistochemistry

- Epithelial cells reactive with pan-cytokeratin
- Myoepithelial cells reactive with S100 protein, smooth muscle actin, and calponin
- Luminal epithelial cells reactive for estrogen receptors (20%) and progesterone receptors (80%)

DIFFERENTIAL DIAGNOSIS

Pleomorphic Adenoma (PA)

- Definitive lobular growth pattern of sclerosing polycystic adenosis is not normally seen in pleomorphic adenoma (PA)
- Acinar Paneth-like epithelial cells of SPA are not seen in PA
- SPA lacks prominent myoepithelial component of PA
- SPA lacks myxochondroid background and scattered, noncohesive myoepithelial cells

Chronic Sclerosing Sialadenitis

- Although fibrosis occurs in both conditions, chronic sclerosing sialadenitis lacks nodular fibrotic pattern of SPA
- Acinar Paneth-like epithelial cells are not seen in chronic sclerosing sialadenitis

SELECTED REFERENCES

1. Gupta R et al: Sclerosing polycystic adenosis of parotid gland: a cytological diagnostic dilemma. Cytopathology. 20(2):130-2, 2009
2. Cheuk W et al: Advances in salivary gland pathology. Histopathology. 51(1):1-20, 2007
3. Noonan VL et al: Sclerosing polycystic adenosis of minor salivary glands: report of three cases and review of the literature. Oral Surg Oral Med Oral Pathol Oral Radiol Endod. 104(4):516-20, 2007
4. Gnepp DR: Sclerosing polycystic adenosis of the salivary gland: a lesion that may be associated with dysplasia and carcinoma in situ. Adv Anat Pathol. 10(4):218-22, 2003
5. Skálová A et al: Sclerosing polycystic adenosis of parotid gland with dysplasia and ductal carcinoma in situ. Report of three cases with immunohistochemical and ultrastructural examination. Virchows Arch. 440(1):29-35, 2002
6. Smith BC et al: Sclerosing polycystic adenosis of major salivary glands. A clinicopathologic analysis of nine cases. Am J Surg Pathol. 20(2):161-70, 1996

IMAGE GALLERY

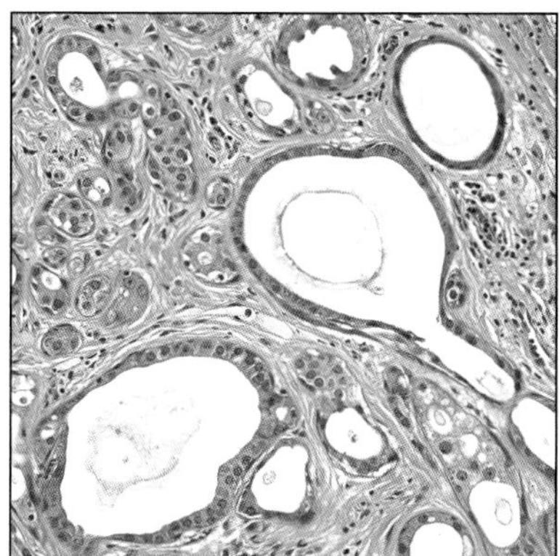

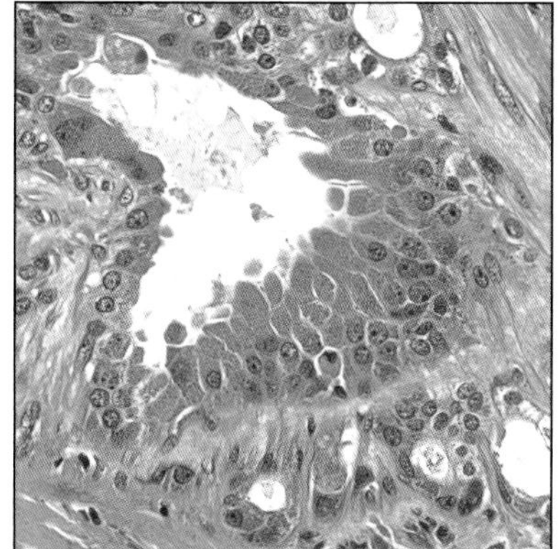

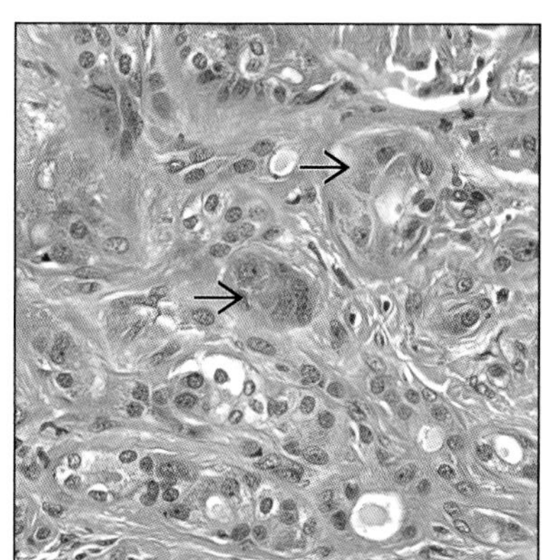

(Left) *Medium-power view displays an epithelial proliferation in small nests, ducts, and dilated cystic structures, surrounded by dense fibrous connective tissue.* ***(Center)*** *High-power view shows a ductal structure composed of glandular epithelial cells with bright eosinophilic cytoplasmic granules.* ***(Right)*** *High-power view shows numerous small duct-like structures. Focal ductal epithelial cells contain eosinophilic granules →. Note the fibrosis between the epithelial cells.*

SIALOLITHIASIS

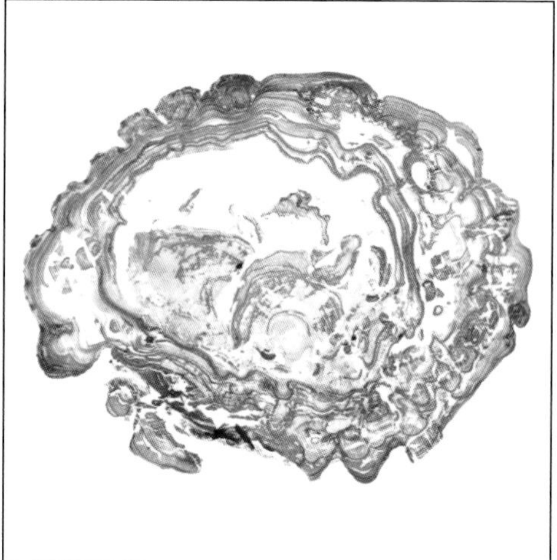

In this low-power view of a sialolith, stones develop due to multiple laminar calcifications around a central nidus of debris.

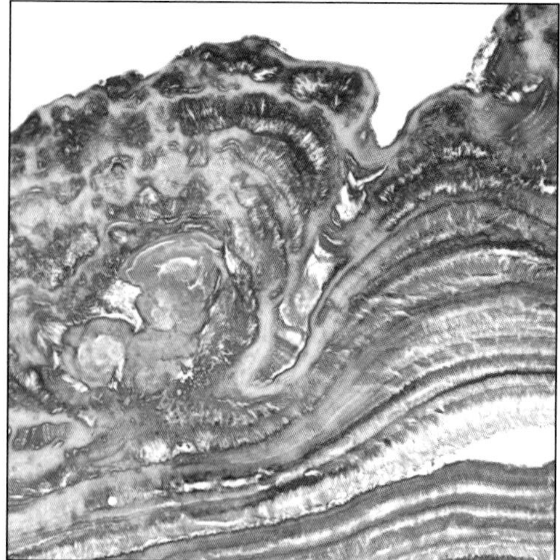

In this high-power view of a sialolith, note the laminar architectural pattern of the calcifications. The concentric layering suggests a certain length of time for stone formation.

TERMINOLOGY

Synonyms

- Salivary duct stone
- Salivary calculus

Definitions

- Detached calcified mass within salivary ductal structures or parenchyma resulting from mineralization of entrapped debris
  - Debris may include central focus of bacteria, inspissated mucus, or foreign material

CLINICAL ISSUES

Epidemiology

- Incidence
  - Uncommon
- Age
  - Middle-aged adults are most commonly affected
    - Average age: ~ 50 years old
    - Uncommon in children
- Gender
  - Slight male predilection

Site

- Salivary stones are most common in ductal structure of submandibular gland (Wharton duct)
  - Location in Wharton duct likely due to higher content of mucinous saliva
  - Stone formation within Stensen duct of parotid gland is uncommon
  - Rare formation in sublingual or minor salivary glands

Presentation

- Symptoms depend upon degree and duration of obstruction and size of stone
  - Initial presentation may include recurrent episodes of pain and swelling
    - Symptoms usually associated with eating
  - Longstanding obstruction may lead to chronic sialadenitis with possible bacterial infection
- Calculi may be physically detectable if of sufficient size and close to ductal orifice

Treatment

- Small stones may be removed by manual manipulation
  - May be aided by moist heat, sialogogues, &/or increased fluid intake
- Larger stones may require surgical excision
- Other treatments include
  - Extracorporeal shockwave lithotripsy
  - Laser lithotripsy via endoscopy
  - Wire basket extraction via interventional radiology
- Affected gland may need to be excised if significant inflammatory changes have occurred

Prognosis

- Degree of morbidity depends upon size of stone and duration of blockage
- No mortality

IMAGE FINDINGS

General Features

- If sufficiently calcified, radiographic studies may demonstrate radiopaque mass
  - Identified in soft tissue of salivary gland or floor of mouth
- In panoramic radiography, radiopaque calcification may be superimposed over mandibular body
  - May mimic intraosseous lesion, such as osteoma

MACROSCOPIC FEATURES

General Features

- Affected salivary gland may be enlarged and firm

Key Facts

Terminology
- Detached calcified mass within salivary ductal structures or parenchyma
- Formed by accumulation of calcium salts around central focus of bacteria, inspissated mucous, or foreign material

Clinical Issues
- Most commonly located in ductal structure of submandibular gland
- Symptoms may include recurrent episodes of pain and swelling, usually associated with eating

Microscopic Pathology
- Salivary stones are round to ovoid with concentric calcified layers
- Surrounding duct (if present) may display squamous, mucous, or oncocytic metaplastic change
- Glandular parenchyma may show fibrosis, acinar atrophy, and mucositis

- Sialoliths are hard, round to ovoid, white to yellow-tan masses

Size
- Varies
- Submandibular gland calculi tend to be larger than those from other salivary gland sites

MICROSCOPIC PATHOLOGY

Histologic Features
- Salivary stones may be located in ductal lumina or within salivary gland parenchyma
- Salivary stones are round to ovoid with concentric calcified layers
  - Central area of debris may be evident
- Surrounding duct (if present) may display squamous, mucous, or oncocytic metaplastic change
- Glandular parenchyma may show fibrosis, acinar atrophy, and mucositis

DIFFERENTIAL DIAGNOSIS

Chronic Sclerosing Sialadenitis (CSS)
- May be part and parcel with sialolithiasis
  - However, both CSS and sialolithiasis can be stand alone diagnoses

Intraosseous Radiopacity
- Radiographic superimposition over mandibular body or ramus may erroneously suggest intrabony pathology
- Multiple radiographic angles should elucidate true soft tissue location of radiopacity

SELECTED REFERENCES

1. Harrison JD: Causes, natural history, and incidence of salivary stones and obstructions. Otolaryngol Clin North Am. 42(6):927-47, Table of Contents, 2009
2. Iro H et al: Outcome of minimally invasive management of salivary calculi in 4,691 patients. Laryngoscope. 119(2):263-8, 2009
3. Su YX et al: Sialoliths or phleboliths? Laryngoscope. 119(7):1344-7, 2009
4. Walvekar RR et al: Combined approach technique for the management of large salivary stones. Laryngoscope. 119(6):1125-9, 2009
5. Walvekar RR et al: Endoscopic sialolith removal: orientation and shape as predictors of success. Am J Otolaryngol. 30(3):153-6, 2009
6. Angiero F et al: Sialolithiasis of the submandibular salivary gland treated with the 810- to 830-nm diode laser. Photomed Laser Surg. 26(6):517-21, 2008
7. Alves de Matos AP et al: On the structural diversity of sialoliths. Microsc Microanal. 13(5):390-6, 2007
8. Damm DD: Oral diagnosis. Panoramic radiopacities. Sialolithiasis. Gen Dent. 55(6):592, 595, 2007
9. Shah D et al: Salivary sialoliths. Br Dent J. 203(6):295, 2007

IMAGE GALLERY

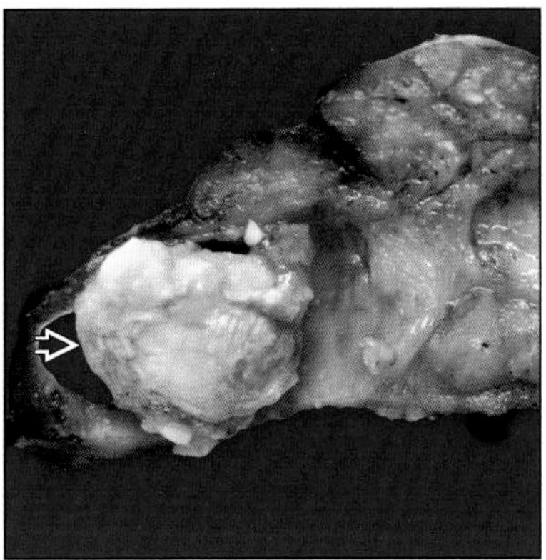
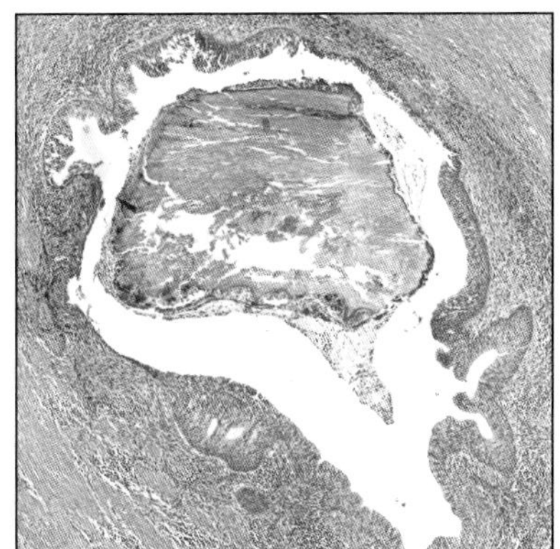
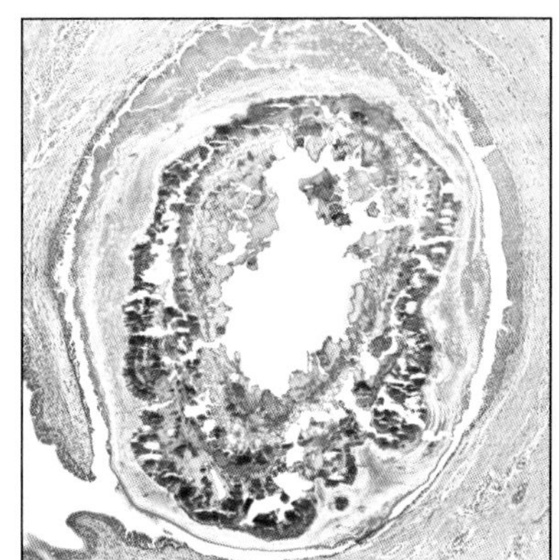

(Left) Gross photograph shows a sialolith within a dilated duct from the parotid gland. The calculus is yellow, with some crumbling and breakdown seen ⊳. (Center) A small sialolith is present within Wharton duct. A prominent chronic inflammatory cell infiltrate surrounds the dilated duct. (Right) Medium-power view shows a sialolith within an ectatic salivary duct lumen. The laminar accretion pattern is easily seen in this example.

PLEOMORPHIC ADENOMA

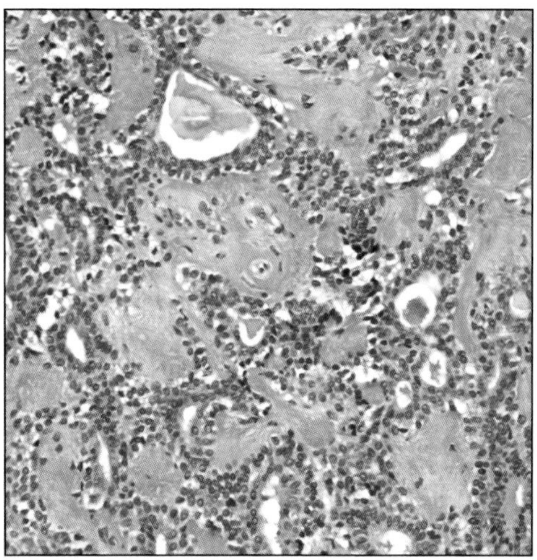

This tumor shows characteristic areas of tubular and ductal structures with a background of hyaline stroma. Pleomorphic adenomas show amazing microscopic diversity.

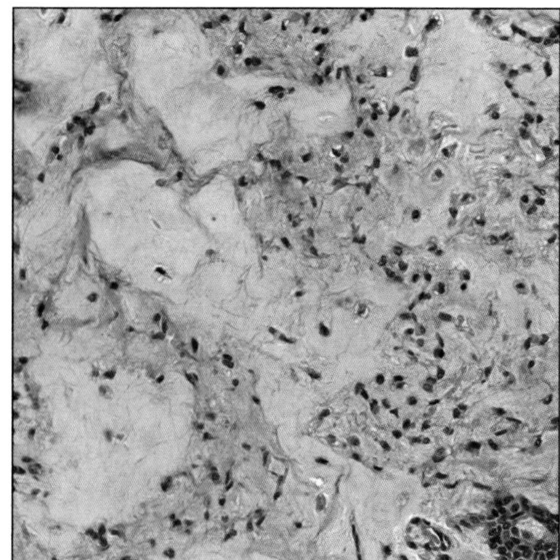

Hematoxylin & eosin shows a tumor with predominant myxoid stroma with focal epithelial structures. The ratio of epithelium and stroma can vary widely among tumors.

TERMINOLOGY

Abbreviations

- Pleomorphic adenoma (PA)

Synonyms

- Benign mixed tumor (BMT)
- Mixed tumor
- Chondroid syringoma
  - Only used if skin/dermis based primary

Definitions

- Benign epithelial tumor that shows both epithelial and modified myoepithelial elements mixed with mesenchymal myxoid, mucoid, or chondroid appearing material
  - Significant architectural diversity rather than cytologic pleomorphism

CLINICAL ISSUES

Epidemiology

- Incidence
  - Most common neoplasm of salivary gland origin
    - 45-76% of all salivary gland neoplasms
    - Comprises about 75% of all major salivary gland neoplasms
    - Comprises about 40% of all minor salivary gland neoplasms
  - Approximately 3/100,000 population
- Age
  - Wide age range
    - Peak in 4th-6th decade
    - Most common benign salivary gland tumor in children
- Gender
  - Female > Male (slightly) in adults
  - Male > Female in children (< 18 years)

Site

- Parotid gland most common site (approximately 80%)
  - Most commonly superficial lobe
    - Inferior (lower pole) or "tail" of parotid gland
  - Deep lobe less frequently
    - Large lesions may compromise airway
- Minor salivary glands 2nd most common site
  - Palate
    - Most common minor salivary gland site
    - Involves junction of hard and soft palate
    - Unilateral, fixed mass (no soft tissue to allow mobility)
  - Buccal mucosa
  - Upper lip
  - Rarely affects lower lip and tongue
- Uncommon in submandibular and sublingual glands
- Can affect larynx, nasal cavity, ear, orbit, upper aerodigestive tract, gastrointestinal tract
- Rarely, may develop within ectopic salivary gland tissue

Presentation

- Usually, painless, slow-growing mass
- Single, smooth, mobile, firm nodule
  - Rarely, a 2nd tumor is found
    - Metachronous vs. synchronous
    - May be identified concurrently with Warthin tumor
- Mucosal ulceration is uncommon
- Paresthesia due to nerve compression is rare finding
- If pain is present, tumor is more likely to be infarcted

Natural History

- Slow growing
- Asymptomatic
- May reach enormous size if neglected
- Uncommon malignant transformation
  - Up to 7% of cases

PLEOMORPHIC ADENOMA

Key Facts

Terminology
- Synonym: Benign mixed tumor
- Benign epithelial tumor that shows epithelial, myoepithelial, and mesenchymal differentiation

Clinical Issues
- Most common neoplasm of salivary gland origin
- Parotid gland most common site
- Slow growing
- Minor salivary glands 2nd most frequent site affected

Macroscopic Features
- Recurrent tumors are generally multinodular
- Irregular mass
- Parotid gland
  - Variably thick capsule
  - Rarely unencapsulated
- Minor glands
  - Poorly developed to absent capsule

Microscopic Pathology
- Innumerable cytologic and architectural patterns
- Epithelial tissue
- Mesenchymal-like tissue

Top Differential Diagnoses
- Myoepithelioma
- Basal cell adenoma
- Adenoid cystic carcinoma
- Polymorphous low-grade adenocarcinoma
- Carcinoma ex-pleomorphic adenoma

Diagnostic Checklist
- No two look alike

Treatment
- Options, risks, complications
  - Surgical complications
    - Frey syndrome (gustatory sweating)
    - Decreased muscle control of face (if facial nerve is sacrificed)
    - Capsule disruption may result in "seeding" of tumor (increases likelihood of recurrence)
    - Enucleation only results in high recurrence rate (up to 50%)
- Surgical approaches
  - Parotid gland
    - Superficial parotidectomy
    - Extracapsular dissection (include rim of uninvolved tissue)
    - Facial nerve preservation when possible
  - Minor glands
    - Conservative, complete surgical excision
  - Submandibular gland
    - Complete excision

Prognosis
- Excellent long-term prognosis, although limited by recurrence and malignant transformation
  - Overall recurrence rate: Up to 2.5%, most developing within 10 years
- Parotid gland tumors have recurrence rate as high as 8%
  - Recurrences tend to be multinodular or multifocal
- Submandibular and minor salivary gland tumors rarely recur
- Malignant transformation in up to 7% of cases, with the following risk factors
  - Long history of untreated tumor
  - Multiple recurrences
  - Age of patient (usually > 40 years)
  - Male gender
  - Tumors > 2 cm in greatest dimension
  - Deep lobe tumors
  - More common in parotid gland

IMAGE FINDINGS

General Features
- Imaging provides information about exact anatomic site, extent of disease, and possible invasion or nodal metastases
- Ultrasound or CT are complimentary and allow for image-guided fine needle aspiration
  - Excellent resolution and tissue characterization without radiation hazard, especially for superficial lobe lesions
- MR or CT is mandatory to evaluate tumor extent and exclude local invasion
  - Unilateral mass, which shows post-contrast enhancement, has high T2 signal, and does not invade surrounding tissue planes, is most likely PA
  - MR spectroscopy may separate Warthin from PA, although not yet well accepted
- Ultrasonography is especially valuable in children, since most tumors are benign and many are cystic or vascular (color Doppler for latter)
  - High-resolution sonography has nearly 100% sensitivity in detecting intraparotid tumors
  - Precisely outlines tumor borders
  - Can detect multiple or bilateral lesions
- Sialography delineates ductal system but is limited in tumor assessment

MACROSCOPIC FEATURES

General Features
- Irregular mass
- Fibrous capsule
  - Parotid gland
    - Variably thick incomplete capsule but rarely unencapsulated
  - Minor glands
    - Poorly developed to absent
- Cut surface homogeneous, white to white-tan
- Recurrent tumors are generally multinodular
- Hemorrhage

PLEOMORPHIC ADENOMA

  - Secondary to FNA or previous surgical procedures
- Infarction
  - Secondary to FNA or previous surgical procedures

Size

- Majority between 2-5 cm
- Rarely, may be enormous

MICROSCOPIC PATHOLOGY

Histologic Features

- Innumerable architectural patterns
  - Solid
  - Tubular or trabecular
  - Cystic
- Epithelial tissue shows variable morphology
  - Spindle
  - Clear
  - Squamous
  - Basaloid
  - Plasmacytoid
- Mesenchymal-like tissue
  - Myxoid stroma
  - Myxochondroid
  - Hyaline stroma
  - Rarely lipomatous
  - Bone
- Duct structures
  - Lined by cuboidal epithelium
  - Lined by columnar epithelium
- Rarely, crystals are present
  - Collagenous crystalloids: Eosinophilic needle shapes arranged radially
  - Tyrosine-rich crystalloids: Eosinophilic bunted shapes arranged tubularly
  - Crystalloids resembling oxalate crystals
- Occasionally squamous metaplasia is identified
- Rarely necrosis
- Rarely sebaceous cells

ANCILLARY TESTS

Cytology

- Findings are variable
- Cellular smears with epithelial and mesenchymal cells and background
- Clusters or cohesive groups of epithelial cells
  - Branching trabeculae of cells that drop off into stroma
  - Plasmacytoid or spindle cells
    - Bipolar myoepithelial cells with eccentric round nuclei
    - Spindled cells tend to embed within stroma
  - Round, ovoid to fusiform nuclei
  - Delicate nuclear chromatin distribution
  - Squamous and sebaceous cells may be seen
  - Atypia can be seen but tends to be single cell
- Fibrillar myxochondroid stroma
  - Feathered edge that blends and surrounds epithelial/myoepithelial cells
  - Cells may line up along edge of matrix, mimicking adenoid cystic carcinoma
  - Pale green with alcohol fixed Papanicolaou stains
  - Deep purple to magenta with air dried Romanowsky stains (Diff-Quik, Giemsa)
    - Striking metachromasia with Giemsa
  - Appears different from mucus, necrotic material, or inflammatory debris
- High cellularity with limited stroma should be diagnosed as "salivary gland neoplasm" to avoid misdiagnosis

Immunohistochemistry

- Immunohistochemistry is sensitive but not specific
- Panel of cytokeratin, p63, GFAP, S100 protein, and SMA is recommended, as all will be variably positive

Cytogenetics

- 4 major cytogenetic abnormalities, with rearrangements involving
  - 8q12 (39%)
    - t(3;8)(p21;q12) and t(5;8)(p13;q12) are most frequently identified translocations
    - Target gene is pleomorphic adenoma gene 1 (*PLAG1*), a zinc finger transcription factor
    - Consistently rearranged and activated, resulting in overexpression in about 50% of cases
  - 12q13-15 (8%)
    - t(9;12)(p24;q14-15) or ins(9;12)(p24;q12q15) most frequently identified translocation
    - Target gene is high mobility group protein gene, *HMGA2* (or *HMGIC*), which is overexpressed
    - *HMGA2* encodes architectural transcription factor that promotes activation of gene expression
  - Sporadic clonal rearrangements of other genes (23%)
  - Normal karyotype (30%)
    - More often are stroma rich than tumors with 8q12 abnormalities
- Currently identified 5 *PLAG1*- and *HMGA2*-containing fusion genes are tumor specific
- Infrequent overexpression of p53 oncoprotein (about 15% of cases), perhaps an early event in malignant transformation

Electron Microscopy

- Structurally modified myoepithelial cells show basal lamina, small microvilli, and well-developed desmosomes
- Cell arrangement and ultrastructure mimics normal salivary gland ducts
- Mesenchymal cells give modified myoepithelial cell appearance with tonofilaments, microfilaments, linear densities of plasma membrane, pinocytotic vesicles, and residua of basement membrane
- Elastic fibers are usually close to neoplastic myoepithelial-like cells

DIFFERENTIAL DIAGNOSIS

Myoepithelioma

- Essentially a cellular mixed tumor with no glandular differentiation and no myxochondroid matrix
- Perhaps part of pleomorphic adenoma spectrum

Immunohistochemistry

Antibody	Reactivity	Staining Pattern	Comment
CK-PAN	Positive	Cytoplasmic	Both ductal epithelial cells and spindle cells
S100	Positive	Nuclear & cytoplasmic	Myoepithelial cells
GFAP	Positive	Cytoplasmic	Myoepithelial cells and myxoid areas
Actin-sm	Positive	Cytoplasmic	Periductal and spindle cells; negative in plasmacytoid cells
Calponin	Positive	Cytoplasmic	Plasmacytoid cells
CK7	Positive	Cytoplasmic	Plasmacytoid cells
Vimentin	Positive	Cytoplasmic	Both epithelial and myoepithelial cells
p63	Positive	Nuclear	
SMHC	Positive	Cytoplasmic	Myoepithelial cells
CD10	Positive	Cytoplasmic	Myoepithelial cells
CD117	Negative		
CK20	Negative		

- Less common

Basal Cell Adenoma
- Uniform proliferation of basaloid cells
- Absence of myxochondroid stroma
- Prominent basal lamina encircle nests of cells

Adenoid Cystic Carcinoma
- Cells are predominately uniform in size with oval to angulated shape
- Variable patterns but most have areas of amorphous eosinophilic hyalinized stroma
- Infiltrative margins
- Perineurial invasion

Polymorphous Low-Grade Adenocarcinoma
- Uniform oval cells
- Numerous growth patterns
- Unencapsulated
- Perineural invasion
- Almost exclusive to minor salivary glands

Carcinoma Ex-Pleomorphic Adenoma
- Infiltrative margins, perineural and vascular invasion
- Marked pleomorphism, mitotic figures, necrosis
- Adenocarcinoma, NOS, but salivary duct carcinoma common also

Mixed Tumor of Skin (Chondroid Syringoma)
- Essentially same histology but arising from skin

SELECTED REFERENCES

1. Ito FA et al: Histopathological findings of pleomorphic adenomas of the salivary glands. Med Oral Patol Oral Cir Bucal. 14(2):E57-61, 2009
2. Shah SS et al: Glial fibrillary acidic protein and CD57 immunolocalization in cell block preparations is a useful adjunct in the diagnosis of pleomorphic adenoma. Arch Pathol Lab Med. 131(9):1373-7, 2007
3. da Cruz Perez DE et al: Salivary gland tumors in children and adolescents: a clinicopathologic and immunohistochemical study of fifty-three cases. Int J Pediatr Otorhinolaryngol. 68(7):895-902, 2004
4. Stennert E et al: Recurrent pleomorphic adenoma of the parotid gland: a prospective histopathological and immunohistochemical study. Laryngoscope. 114(1):158-63, 2004
5. Alves FA et al: Pleomorphic adenoma of the submandibular gland: clinicopathological and immunohistochemical features of 60 cases in Brazil. Arch Otolaryngol Head Neck Surg. 128(12):1400-3, 2002
6. Hill AG: Major salivary gland tumours in a rural Kenyan hospital. East Afr Med J. 79(1):8-10, 2002
7. Verma K et al: Role of fine needle aspiration cytology in diagnosis of pleomorphic adenomas. Cytopathology. 13(2):121-7, 2002
8. Pinkston JA et al: Incidence rates of salivary gland tumors: results from a population-based study. Otolaryngol Head Neck Surg. 120(6):834-40, 1999
9. Yamamoto Y et al: DNA analysis at p53 locus in carcinomas arising from pleomorphic adenomas of salivary glands: comparison of molecular study and p53 immunostaining. Pathol Int. 48(4):265-72, 1998
10. Kilpatrick SE et al: Mixed tumors and myoepitheliomas of soft tissue: a clinicopathologic study of 19 cases with a unifying concept. Am J Surg Pathol. 21(1):13-22, 1997
11. Auclair PL et al: Atypical features in salivary gland mixed tumors: their relationship to malignant transformation. Mod Pathol. 9(6):652-7, 1996
12. Renehan A et al: An analysis of the treatment of 114 patients with recurrent pleomorphic adenomas of the parotid gland. Am J Surg. 172(6):710-4, 1996
13. Takai Y et al: Diagnostic criteria for neoplastic myoepithelial cells in pleomorphic adenomas and myoepitheliomas. Immunocytochemical detection of muscle-specific actin, cytokeratin 14, vimentin, and glial fibrillary acidic protein. Oral Surg Oral Med Oral Pathol Oral Radiol Endod. 79(3):330-41, 1995
14. Allen CM et al: Necrosis in benign salivary gland neoplasms. Not necessarily a sign of malignant transformation. Oral Surg Oral Med Oral Pathol. 78(4):455-61, 1994
15. Humphrey PA et al: Crystalloids in salivary gland pleomorphic adenomas. Arch Pathol Lab Med. 113(4):390-3, 1989
16. Campbell WG Jr et al: Characterization of two types of crystalloids in pleomorphic adenomas of minor salivary glands. A light-microscopic, electron-microscopic, and histochemical study. Am J Pathol. 118(2):194-202, 1985
17. Eveson JW et al: Salivary gland tumours. A review of 2410 cases with particular reference to histological types, site, age and sex distribution. J Pathol. 146(1):51-8, 1985

PLEOMORPHIC ADENOMA

Imaging, Clinical, and Gross Features

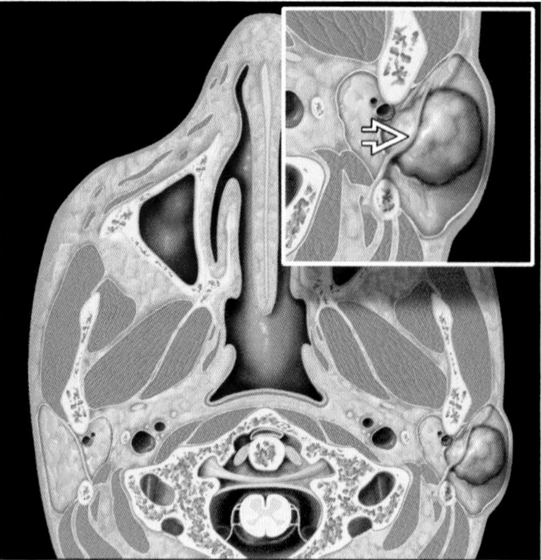

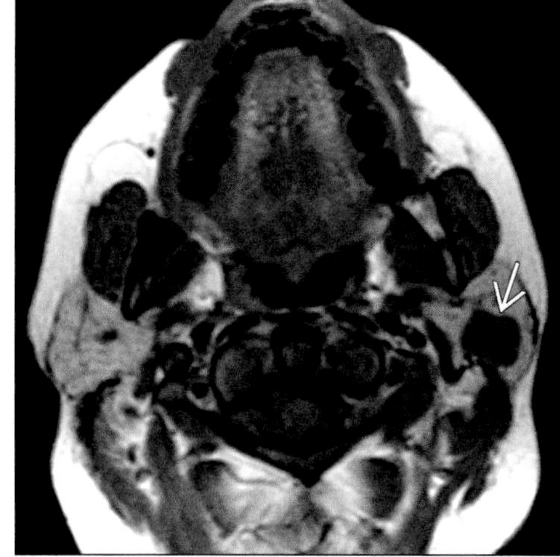

(Left) *Axial graphic shows the close relationship of the facial nerve ➡ to the parotid gland. Surgical excision requires the identification and preservation of the facial nerve; damage of the nerve can result in decreased muscle control of the face and Frey syndrome.* ***(Right)*** *T1 nonenhanced MR reveals a well-circumscribed hypointense tumor ➡ within the superficial lobe of the parotid gland. This tumor enhances with contrast and is commonly hyperintense on T2 MR sequences.*

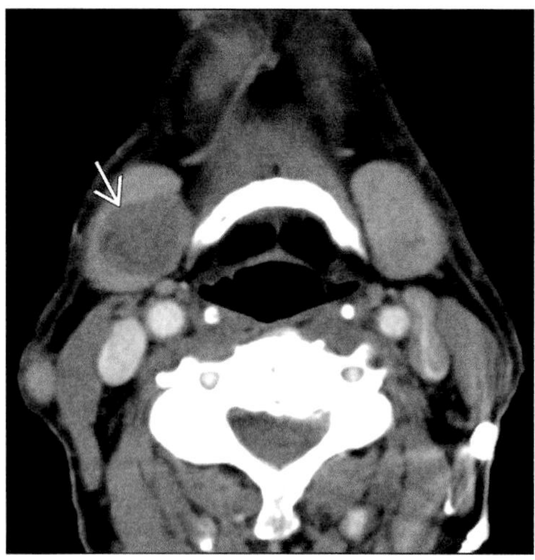

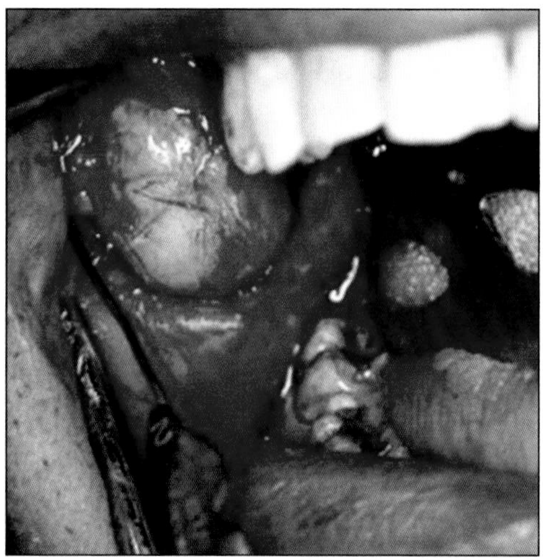

(Left) *CT with contrast shows a pleomorphic adenoma within the right submandibular gland ➡. The gland enhances more than the tumor, making identification on CT simple. About 50% of tumors of the submandibular gland are pleomorphic adenomas.* ***(Right)*** *Intraoperative photograph shows the removal of a pleomorphic adenoma of minor salivary gland origin via an intraoral approach. This patient had been aware of this tumor for over 3 years prior to consenting to surgery.*

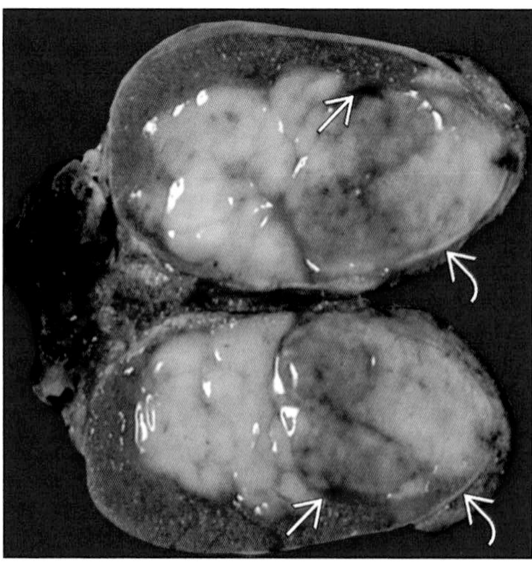

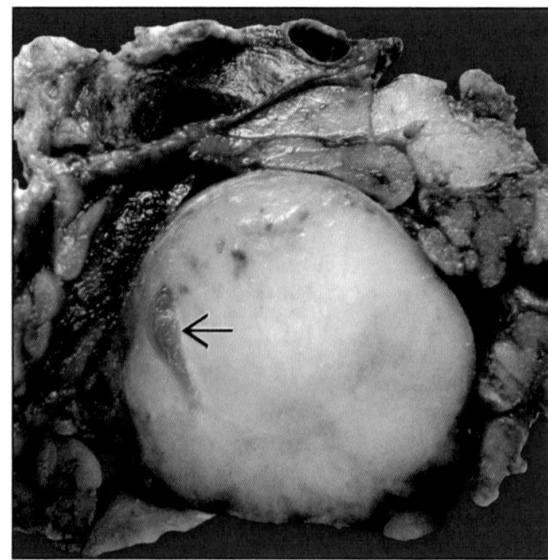

(Left) *Gross photograph shows a well-circumscribed, oval pleomorphic adenoma. Bisection shows a tan-pink to white surface and a thin fibrous capsule ➡. Focal hemorrhage may be seen secondary to a fine needle aspiration ➡.* ***(Right)*** *Gross photograph shows a formalin fixed pleomorphic adenoma with well-defined borders surrounded by normal gland and soft tissue. Note the focus of translucent tissue ➡, representing an area of myxochondroid tissue.*

Microscopic Features

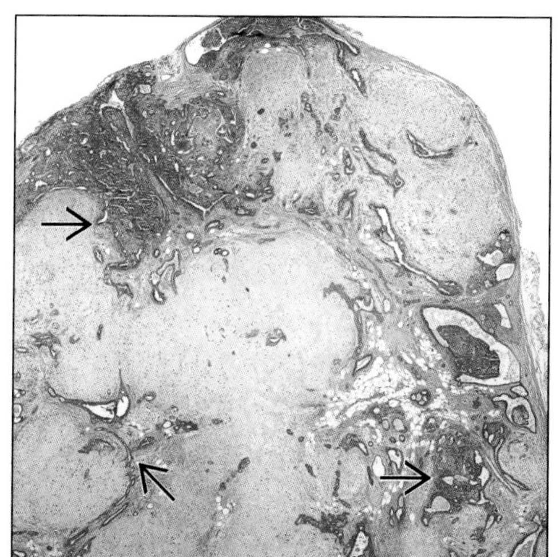

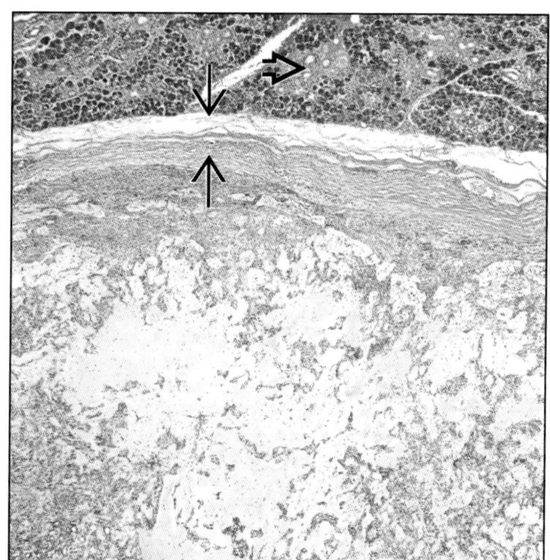

(Left) Hematoxylin & eosin shows a characteristic pleomorphic adenoma with varying patterns within a single section. Areas with ductal structures ➔ are closely associated with a myxomatous stroma. *(Right)* Pleomorphic adenoma of a major gland shows a distinctive fibrous capsule ➔ separating it from the associated salivary gland ➔. Tumors of minor salivary glands may have an incomplete to absent capsule; this is especially common in palatal tumors.

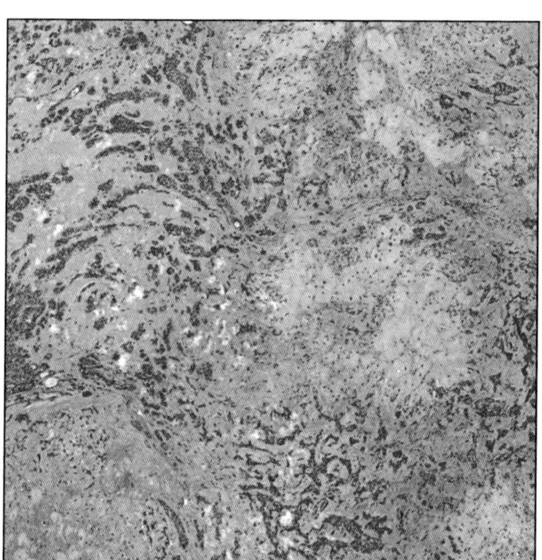

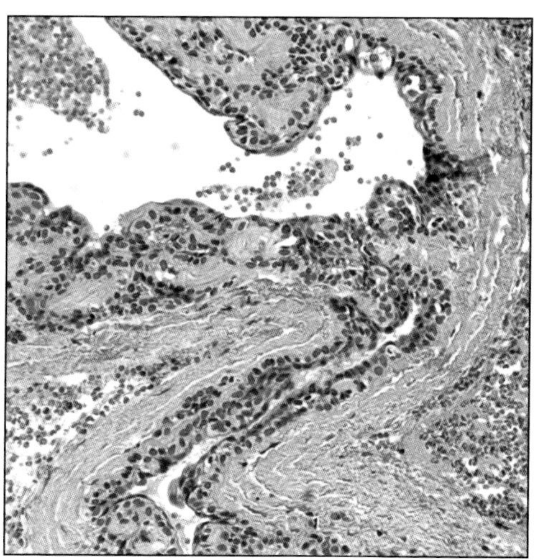

(Left) Hematoxylin & eosin shows myxoid background with islands and anastomosing strands of epithelial cells. This case was accurately diagnosed, prior to excision, based on the aspirate obtained from a fine needle biopsy. *(Right)* Pleomorphic adenoma shows a central cyst. Small cystic spaces may contain keratin. Numerous cystic areas are a feature of mucoepidermoid carcinoma, and this malignant tumor should be ruled out.

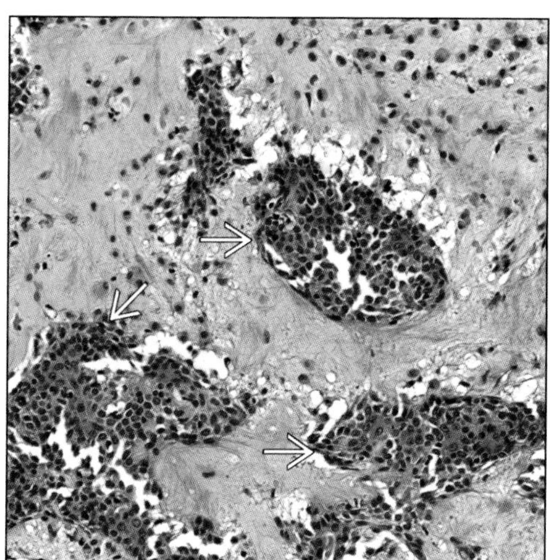

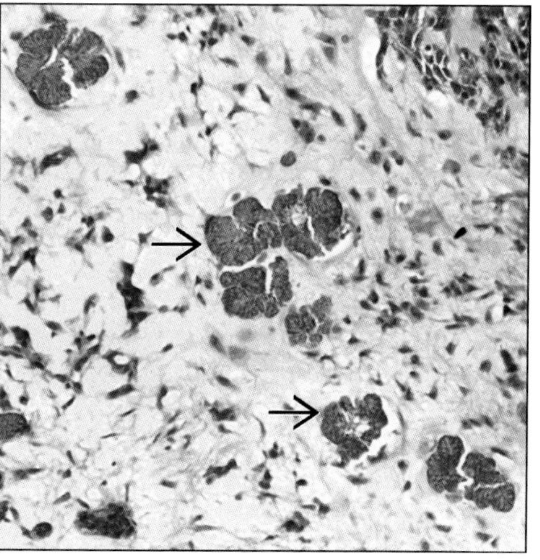

(Left) PA shows focal solid areas composed of oval plasmacytoid cells ➔. A myoepithelioma must be considered in the differential diagnosis when ductal structures are lacking. Ducts were numerous in other areas of this tumor. Also, the myxochondroid stroma seen is not a feature of monomorphic adenomas. *(Right)* Hematoxylin & eosin shows tyrosine-rich crystals ➔ scattered in a myxoid stroma. Of all salivary gland tumors, PAs are the most common tumors to have crystalloids.

PLEOMORPHIC ADENOMA

Microscopic and Cytologic Features

*(**Left**) Hematoxylin & eosin shows a high-power view of a duct lined by round to cuboidal luminal cells adjacent to a focus of myxoid stroma. (**Right**) A high-power view of a pleomorphic adenoma shows a cartilaginous-like focus. While chondroid areas are not uncommon, tumors rarely have areas that resemble mature cartilage. Bone is occasionally seen.*

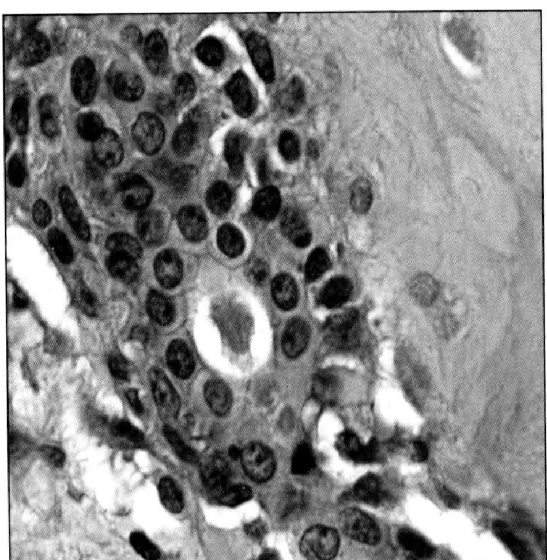

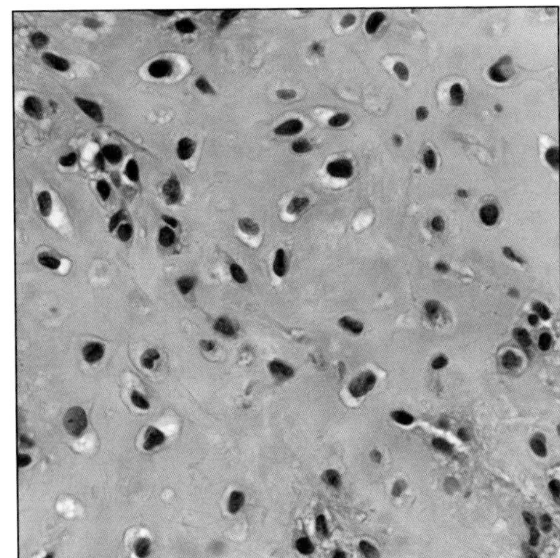

*(**Left**) Hematoxylin & eosin shows the blending of the epithelial cells with the mucinous-myxoid matrix material. (**Right**) Prominent zone of hypocellular hyalinized fibroconnective tissue in a PA. The presence of hypocellular hyalinized stroma is an atypical feature associated with increased risk of malignant transformation to carcinoma ex-pleomorphic adenoma as compared to PAs without this feature. Additional sections to exclude malignancy are recommended when this feature is present.*

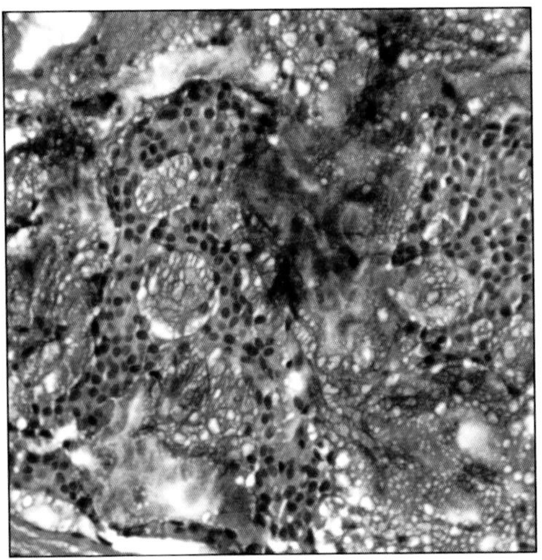

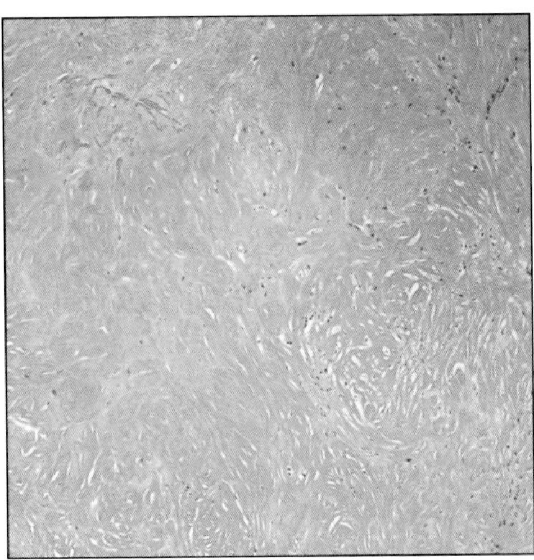

*(**Left**) Diff-Quik shows a fibrillar background stroma and a streaming of epithelial nuclei within the material. There are small collections of epithelial cells intermingled with the background myxoid-matrix material. (**Right**) Diff-Quik shows a bright magenta appearance to the fibrillar myxochondroid matrix material. Note how the epithelial-myoepithelial cells blend with the matrix, although a single focus ⇨ shows a peripheral palisade of nuclei.*

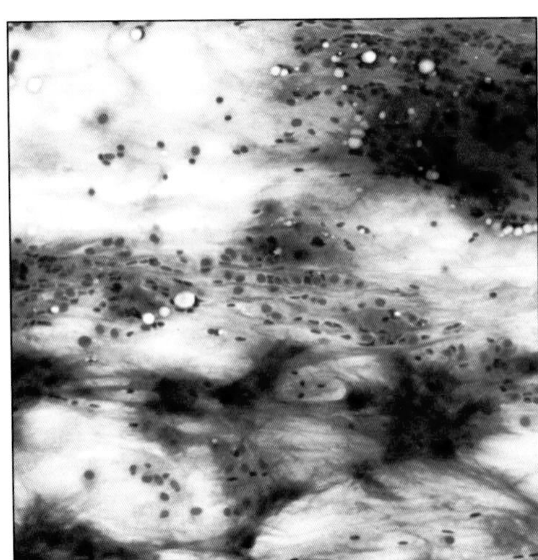

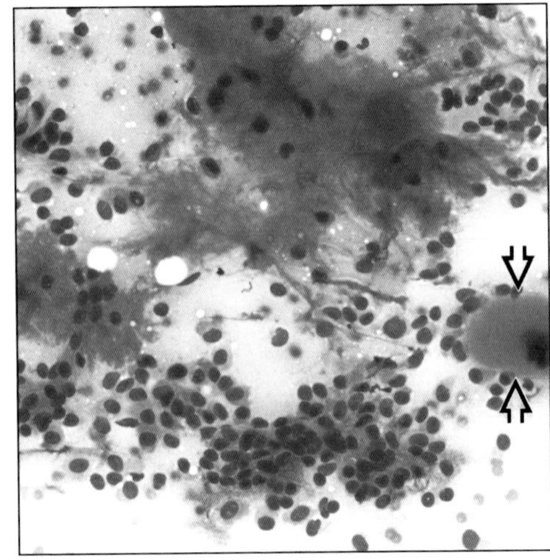

Cytologic and Immunohistochemical Features

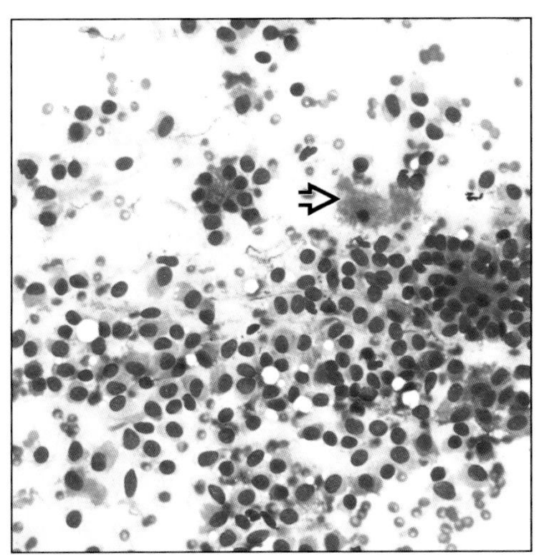

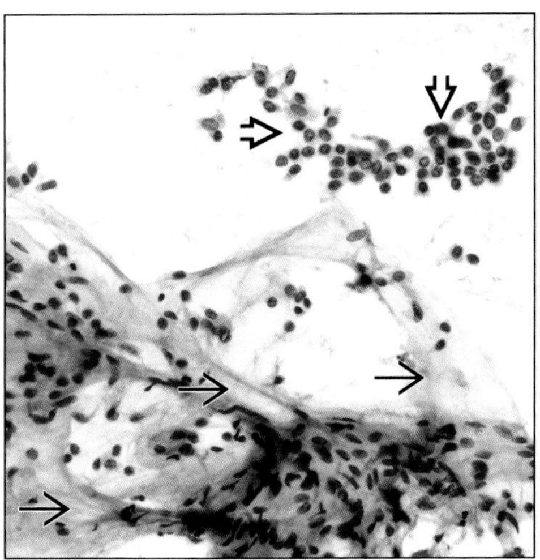

*(**Left**) Diff-Quik shows a much more cellular neoplastic proliferation with only a few foci of matrix material ⇨ in this cellular pleomorphic adenoma. The cells have a plasmacytoid appearance, with eccentric nuclei that are round and regular. (**Right**) Papanicolaou stain shows the epithelial groups ⇨ as well as the background stroma →, although the stroma is much less easy to definitively identify in comparison to the Diff-Quik preparations.*

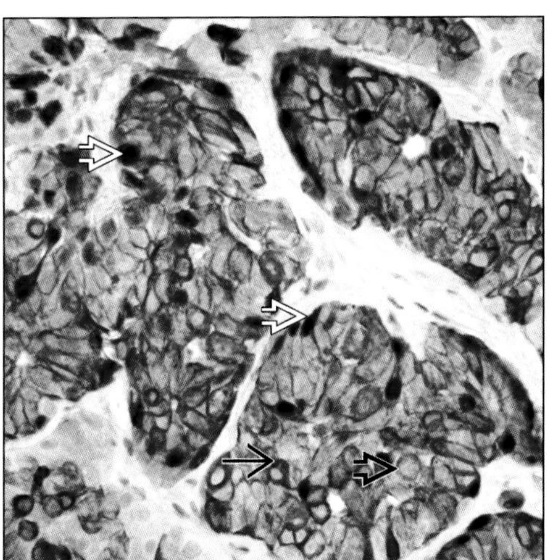

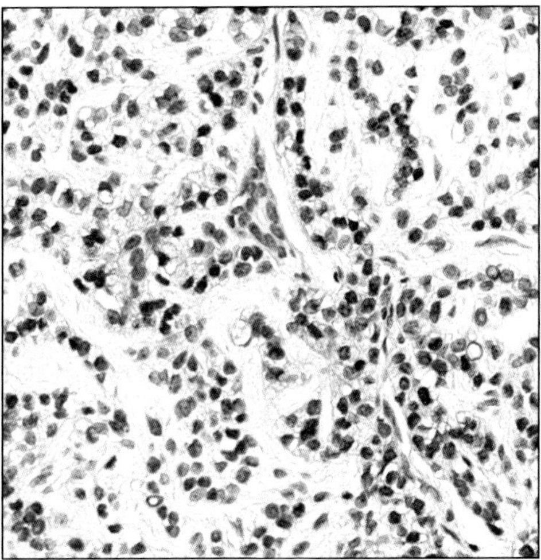

*(**Left**) Triple immunohistochemistry cocktail highlights the membrane of the epithelial cells (EMA) ⇨, while the cytoplasm of the neoplastic cells is stained light brown (CK5/6) →, and the nuclei of the basal-myoepithelial cells are highlighted with p63 ➡. (**Right**) S100 protein shows nuclear and cytoplasmic reactivity for myoepithelial cells but has variable reactivity for other cells.*

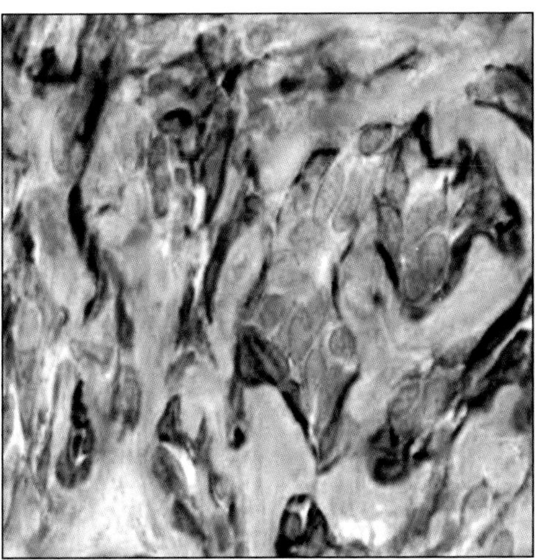

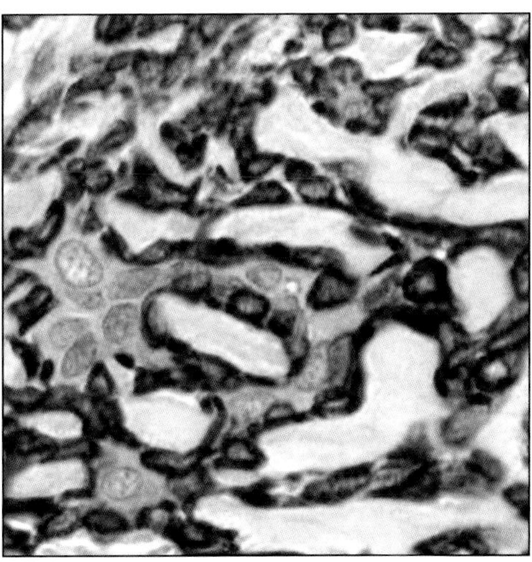

*(**Left**) Smooth muscle actin (SMA) shows reactivity in spindle and polygonal myoepithelial cells. (**Right**) Glial fibrillary acidic protein (GFAP) shows dense reactivity for myoepithelial cells in the myxoid areas of the tumor.*

MYOEPITHELIOMA

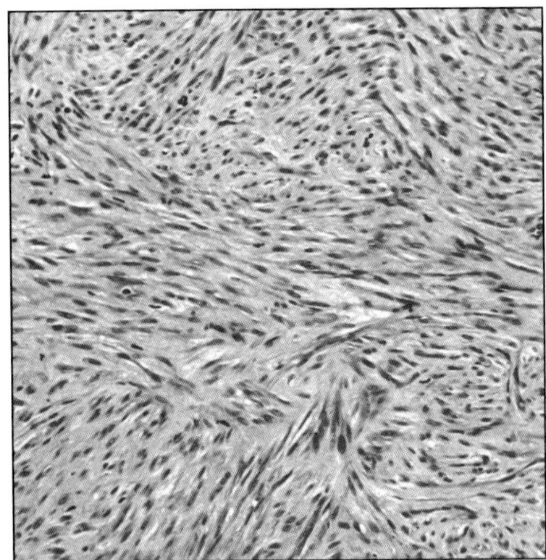

Myoepithelioma shows a predominant spindle cell morphology. Tumors of this type are more commonly noted in the major salivary glands. This could be easily confused with leiomyoma or schwannoma.

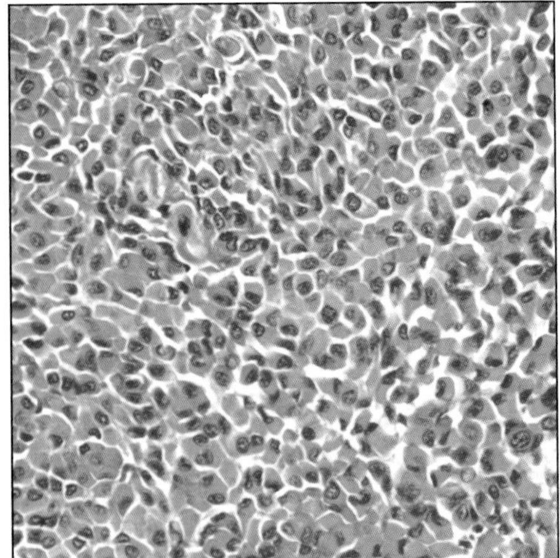

Plasmacytoid predominant variant of myoepithelioma is located in the hard palate, a common place for this histologic type. The nuclei are eccentric, surrounded by eosinophilic cytoplasm.

TERMINOLOGY

Synonyms

- Myoepithelial adenoma
- Benign myoepithelial tumor

Definitions

- Benign salivary gland neoplasm composed entirely of myoepithelial differentiated cells
  - No ductal cells allowed

CLINICAL ISSUES

Epidemiology

- Incidence
  - ~ 2% of all salivary gland neoplasms
    - ~ 6% of minor salivary gland neoplasms
- Age
  - Wide range affected
  - Average: 5th decade (44 years)
    - Peak in 3rd to 4th decade
- Gender
  - Equal gender distribution

Site

- About 1/2 occur in parotid gland
- Palate (hard or soft) affected next most frequently

Presentation

- Typically asymptomatic
- Slowly growing swelling of affected region
- Painless mass

Treatment

- Surgical approaches
  - Surgical excision with tumor-free margins
    - Superficial parotidectomy, wide local excision, or submandibulectomy

Prognosis

- Less likely to recur than pleomorphic adenoma
- Clinical recurrence associated with positive surgical margins
- Benign myoepitheliomas can undergo malignant transformation
  - Especially in longstanding tumors or in tumors with multiple recurrences

MACROSCOPIC FEATURES

General Features

- Well demarcated yet variably encapsulated
- Soft gray, white, or yellow-tan mass
- May have rubbery to solid consistency

Size

- Usually < 3 cm

MICROSCOPIC PATHOLOGY

Histologic Features

- Well circumscribed but variably encapsulated
- Broad range of appearances due to multiple architectural patterns
  - Solid, myxoid, reticular, nested, cord-like
- Typically composed of spindled or plasmacytoid cells
  - May have dominant cell type or mixed morphology
  - Plasmacytoid cells with hyperchromatic, round to oval nuclei and abundant, eccentric eosinophilic cytoplasm
    - Characteristic but not pathognomonic
    - Seen in myoepithelioma and pleomorphic adenoma of palate
  - Although not common, clear, polygonal (epithelioid), or stellate cells may be seen
- Background with variable collagenization
  - May contain abundant acellular mucoid stroma

Key Facts

Terminology

- Benign salivary gland neoplasm composed entirely of myoepithelial differentiated cells

Microscopic Pathology

- Typically composed of spindled or plasmacytoid cells
- Background with variable collagenization
- Chondroid or myxochondroid areas are absent

Ancillary Tests

- Reactive with CK-pan, CK7, CK14, p63, GFAP, S100 protein, actins, and calponin

Top Differential Diagnoses

- Pleomorphic adenoma (PA)
  - If ductal structures present, use cellular PA
- Myoepithelial carcinoma
- Plasmacytoma

- Lacks chondroid or myxochondroid matrix
- Lacks infiltration, perineural invasion, profound pleomorphism, necrosis, increased mitotic figures

ANCILLARY TESTS

Immunohistochemistry

- Reactive with CK-pan, CK7, CK14, p63, GFAP, and S100 protein
- Variable reactivity with actin-sm, actin-HHF-35, SMHC, and calponin
  - Actins reactive in spindled cells but typically nonreactive in plasmacytoid cells
- Mutations of *p53* have been observed

Electron Microscopy

- Shows epithelial and myoepithelial differentiation

DIFFERENTIAL DIAGNOSIS

Pleomorphic Adenoma (PA)

- If ductal structures are present, diagnose as cellular (myoepithelial-predominant) pleomorphic adenoma
- Myxochondroid matrix is typically seen in PA

Myoepithelial Carcinoma

- Myoepithelioma lacks necrosis, atypical mitotic figures, or invasion into surrounding parenchyma
  - Biopsy site changes due to fine needle aspiration may mimic malignant degeneration

Spindled Soft Tissue Neoplasm

- Neural, smooth muscle, or other spindled soft tissue neoplasms may be considered
- Cytokeratin supports epithelial differentiation

Plasmacytoma

- Perinuclear cytoplasmic clearing ("hof") in plasma cells
- Lacks myoepithelial immunohistochemistry

SELECTED REFERENCES

1. Bakshi J et al: Plasmacytoid myoepithelioma of palate: three rare cases and literature review. J Laryngol Otol. 121(9):e13, 2007
2. Cuadra Zelaya F et al: Plasmacytoid myoepithelioma of the palate. Report of one case and review of the literature. Med Oral Patol Oral Cir Bucal. 12(8):E552-5, 2007
3. Furuse C et al: Myoepithelial cell markers in salivary gland neoplasms. Int J Surg Pathol. 13(1):57-65, 2005
4. Sugiura R et al: Myoepithelioma arising from the buccal gland: histopathological and immunohistochemical studies. J Oral Sci. 42(1):39-42, 2000
5. Dardick I: Myoepithelioma: definitions and diagnostic criteria. Ultrastruct Pathol. 19(5):335-45, 1995
6. Takai Y et al: Diagnostic criteria for neoplastic myoepithelial cells in pleomorphic adenomas and myoepitheliomas. Immunocytochemical detection of muscle-specific actin, cytokeratin 14, vimentin, and glial fibrillary acidic protein. Oral Surg Oral Med Oral Pathol Oral Radiol Endod. 79(3):330-41, 1995
7. Sciubba JJ et al: Myoepithelioma of salivary glands: report of 23 cases. Cancer. 49(3):562-72, 1982

IMAGE GALLERY

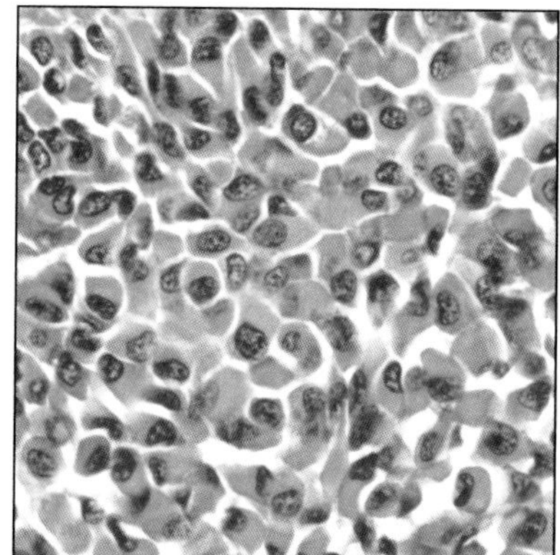

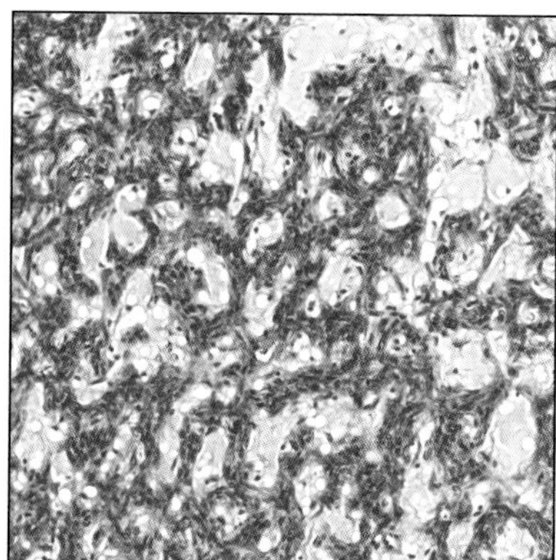

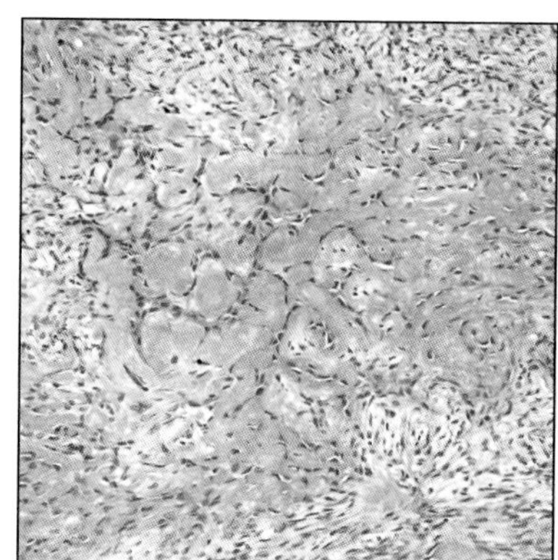

(Left) *The nuclei in the plasmacytoid cells are eccentric, surrounded by amorphous eosinophilic cytoplasm. The cytoplasm lacks a "hof" zone of clearing. There is no pleomorphism or necrosis.* ***(Center)*** *Myoepithelioma displaying a somewhat reticular architectural pattern is composed of spindled-to-basaloid cells. There is a myxoid background.* ***(Right)*** *A myoepithelioma composed predominantly of spindle cells is shown. Hyalinization and nuclear palisading are suggestive of a neural neoplasm.*

BASAL CELL ADENOMA

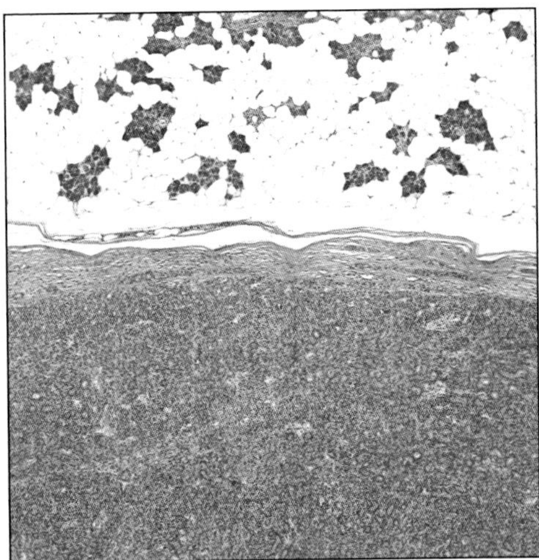

Basal cell adenoma, solid type is an encapsulated proliferation of small basaloid cells in large sheets and nests. Lack of invasion into the surrounding salivary parenchyma defines benignancy.

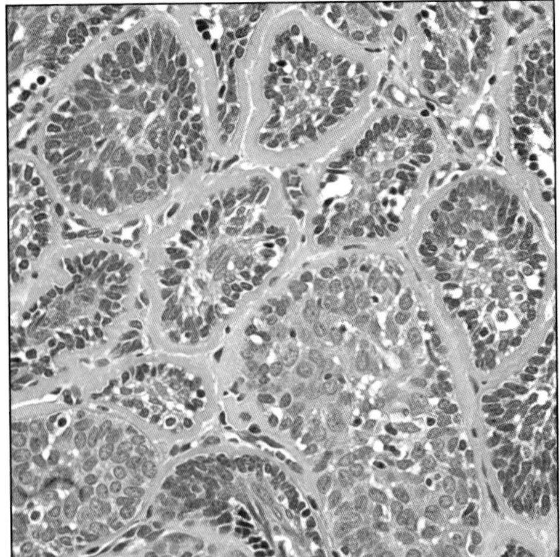

Basal cell adenoma, membranous type is characterized by variably sized islands of basaloid cells in a jigsaw puzzle-like pattern surrounded by eosinophilic hyaline material that is PAS(+) (not shown).

TERMINOLOGY

Abbreviations

- Basal cell adenoma (BCA)

Synonyms

- Membranous subtype: Dermal analogue tumor

Definitions

- Benign salivary epithelial neoplasm composed of basaloid cells lacking chondromyxoid stroma

CLINICAL ISSUES

Epidemiology

- Incidence
  - Represents ~ 2-3% of all salivary gland neoplasia
- Age
  - Wide range
  - Peak: 6th to 7th decades
- Gender
  - Female > Male (2:1)
  - Membranous type: Slight male predominance

Site

- Approximately 75% occur in parotid gland
- Remainder evenly distributed between submandibular gland and minor salivary glands
  - Minor salivary glands regions include lip, palate, and buccal mucosa

Presentation

- Typically asymptomatic, unilateral, solitary mobile swelling of affected gland
- Membranous variant relatively unique
  - May display multicentric or multifocal growth
  - Potentially associated with concomitant skin adnexal neoplasms
    - Dermal cylindroma (most common), trichoepithelioma, eccrine spiradenoma

Treatment

- Complete surgical excision
  - Solid, trabecular and tubular variants: Conservative excision with rim of normal tissue
  - Membranous variant: Parotidectomy (superficial to total) due to possible multifocality

Prognosis

- Recurrence unusual, except for membranous subtype
  - Membranous subtype recurs in up to 25%
    - Evaluate for potential skin adnexal neoplasms
- Malignant transformation possible
  - Highest in membranous type (up to 28%)
  - Otherwise, risk approximately 4%

MACROSCOPIC FEATURES

General Features

- Well-circumscribed encapsulated nodule
- Membranous type may be multinodular or multifocal
- Cut surface is solid and homogeneous to cystic

Size

- Range: 1-3 cm

MICROSCOPIC PATHOLOGY

Histologic Features

- All subtypes composed of basaloid cells
  - May display 2 cell morphologies
    - Small cells with scant eosinophilic cytoplasm and round-to-oval deeply basophilic nuclei
    - Slightly larger cells with more abundant cytoplasm and pale staining nuclei
  - Smaller cells may palisade at periphery of nests or trabeculae and surround larger, central cells
    - Especially in solid and membranous patterns
- Squamous eddies and small ductal structures possible
- Multiple architectural subtypes

BASAL CELL ADENOMA

Key Facts

Terminology

- Benign salivary epithelial neoplasm of small basaloid cells without myxochondroid matrix

Clinical Issues

- Membranous variant may be associated with concomitant skin adnexal neoplasms

Microscopic Pathology

- 2 possible subtypes of basaloid cells
  - Smaller cells at periphery of tumor nests
  - Larger cells in interior of tumor nests
- Solid, trabecular, tubular, and membranous morphologic patterns
  - Membranous pattern may show multinodular growth

Top Differential Diagnoses

- Basal cell adenocarcinoma, canalicular adenoma, adenoid cystic carcinoma

---

- **Solid pattern**
  - Basaloid epithelial sheets or nests of variable size
- **Trabecular pattern**
  - Plexiform bands of basaloid cells
- **Tubular pattern**
  - Numerous small ductal lumens connected by bands of basaloid cells
  - Often seen in concert with trabecular pattern, hence "**tubulotrabecular**" moniker
- **Membranous pattern**
  - Variably sized islands of basaloid cells surrounded by eosinophilic hyaline material
  - Peripheral palisading may be conspicuous
  - Nests form **jigsaw puzzle-like** pattern
  - Nests may contain drop-like hyaline material
  - Most common type to display multifocal growth
- All patterns demonstrate stroma of variable amount and collagenous density
- Tumors of major salivary glands may be circumscribed and encapsulated
  - Multinodular growth may simulate invasion

ANCILLARY TESTS

Immunohistochemistry

- Keratin variably reactive in all epithelial cells
  - Strongest in inner, larger basaloid cells
- Actin-sm, p63, and calponin reactivity in peripheral, smaller basaloid cells
- S100 protein may be variably reactive in both epithelial cell types

DIFFERENTIAL DIAGNOSIS

Basal Cell Adenocarcinoma

- Parenchymal invasion, necrosis, numerous mitotic figures
- Must differentiate invasion from multinodular/ multifocal growth

Canalicular Adenoma

- Usually upper lip; composed of "beaded" chains of short columnar cells

Adenoid Cystic Carcinoma

- Clear cells with angular pyknotic nuclei
- Parenchymal &/or perineural invasion
- Cribriform pattern rare in BCA

SELECTED REFERENCES

1. Machado de Sousa SO et al: Immunohistochemical aspects of basal cell adenoma and canalicular adenoma of salivary glands. Oral Oncol. 37(4):365-8, 2001
2. Yu GY et al: Histogenesis and development of membranous basal cell adenoma. Oral Surg Oral Med Oral Pathol Oral Radiol Endod. 86(4):446-51, 1998
3. Nagao T et al: Carcinoma in basal cell adenoma of the parotid gland. Pathol Res Pract. 193(3):171-8, 1997
4. Batsakis JG et al: Basaloid monomorphic adenomas. Ann Otol Rhinol Laryngol. 100(8):687-90, 1991

IMAGE GALLERY

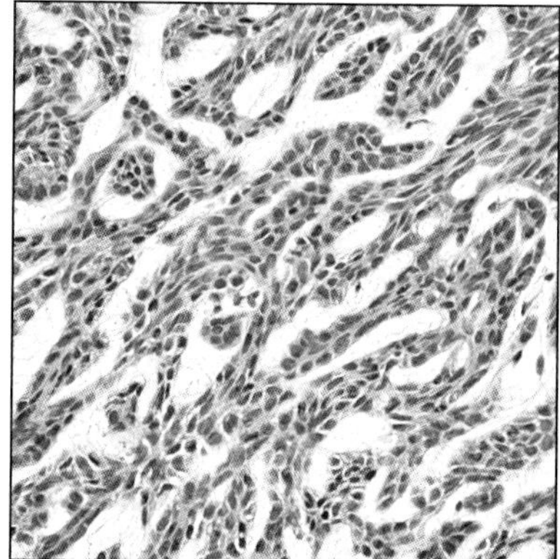

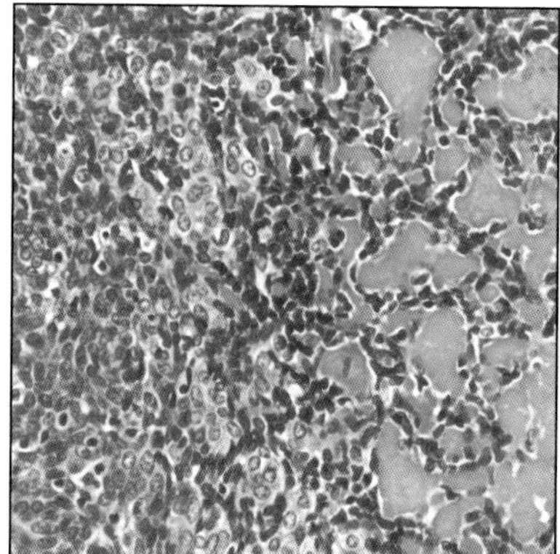

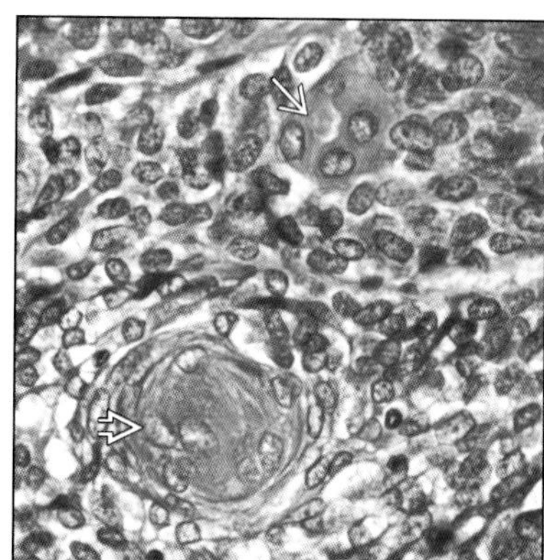

*(**Left**) Basal cell adenoma, trabecular pattern is composed of strands and cords of basaloid cells within loose stroma. Peripheral palisading may be uncommon in this pattern. (**Center**) Drop-like eosinophilic hyaline material may be variably present in basal cell adenoma and be surrounded by small basaloid epithelial cells. (**Right**) Basal cell adenoma, solid type include foci of squamous eddies ➡ and small ducts ➡ surrounded by basaloid cells.*

WARTHIN TUMOR (PAPILLARY CYSTADENOMA LYMPHOMATOSUM)

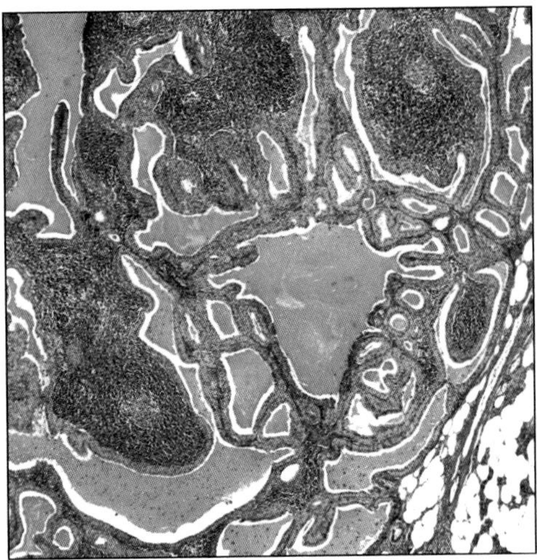

Classic histology of Warthin tumor includes cyst formation, papillary architecture, oncocytic epithelium, and an inflammatory cell infiltrate in the walls of the cysts.

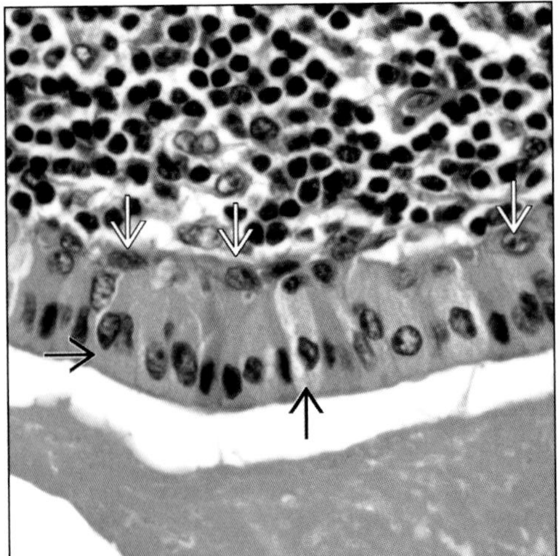

Granular eosinophilic (oncocytic) cells are composed of luminal columnar cells with hyperchromatic nuclei aligned toward the luminal aspect ⇨ and basal cuboidal cells with vesicular nuclei ➡.

TERMINOLOGY

Abbreviations

- Warthin tumor (WT)

Synonyms

- Adenolymphoma, cystadenolymphoma, papillary cystadenoma lymphomatosum

Definitions

- Benign salivary gland tumor characterized by
  - Cystic and papillary growth
  - Presence of bilayered epithelial proliferation
  - Presence of associated mature lymphocytic cell stroma

ETIOLOGY/PATHOGENESIS

Environmental Exposure

- Strong link between WT and cigarette smoking

Infectious Agents

- Role of Epstein-Barr virus (EBV) and human herpes virus 8 (HHV8) in development of Warthin tumor suggested but not substantiated

Pathogenesis

- Felt to develop from neoplastic transformation of entrapped salivary duct epithelium within intra- and periparotid lymph nodes
  - Ontogenically, parotid gland last of the salivary glands to be encapsulated resulting in
    - Incorporation or entrapment of lymphoid tissue within parotid or incorporation/entrapment of parotid parenchyma within periparotid lymph nodes
    - Presence of subcapsular sinus(es) confirms lymph node as such structures not a feature of non-lymph-node tissues
    - Presence of B- and T-cell markers in lymphoid component of WT

CLINICAL ISSUES

Epidemiology

- Incidence
  - 2nd most common benign salivary gland tumor (following pleomorphic adenoma)
    - Accounts for approximately 5-6% of all salivary gland tumors
    - Represents up to 12% of benign parotid gland tumors
- Age
  - Occurs over wide range, but most common in 5th-7th decades of life
    - Uncommon in first 3 decades of life
- Gender
  - Male > Female, but
    - Evidence shows marked decline in incidence in men with increased prevalence in women
    - Demographic changes linked to smoking habits (declining use by men, increasing use by women)

Site

- Almost exclusively involves parotid gland, particularly in superficial lobe along inferior pole adjacent to angle of mandible
  - Rare cases reported in submandibular gland, palate, lip, tonsil, larynx, and maxillary sinus
- Bilateral tumors seen in up to 10% of cases and multifocal tumors in up to 12% of cases
  - Bilateral or multifocal tumors may occur synchronously or metachronously

Presentation

- Most common symptom is painless mass
  - Rarely, pain is associated complaint

WARTHIN TUMOR (PAPILLARY CYSTADENOMA LYMPHOMATOSUM)

Key Facts

Terminology

- Benign salivary gland tumor characterized by
  - Cystic and papillary growth
  - Presence of bilayered epithelial proliferation
  - Presence of associated mature lymphocytic cell stroma

Etiology/Pathogenesis

- Strong link between Warthin tumor and cigarette smoking

Clinical Issues

- 2nd most common benign salivary gland tumor (following pleomorphic adenoma)
- Almost exclusively involves parotid gland, particularly in superficial lobe along inferior pole adjacent to angle of mandible
- Complete surgical excision is treatment of choice
- Locally recurrent tumor may occur related to inadequate excision or to multicentrically occurring neoplasms

Microscopic Pathology

- Epithelial component lining the papillary projections composed of double layer of granular eosinophilic cells (referred to as oncocytic epithelia)
- Lymphoid component predominantly composed of mature lymphocytes containing lymphoid follicles with germinal centers
- May undergo degenerative alterations, spontaneously or following manipulation (e.g., post-fine needle aspiration biopsy), including
  - Infarction/necrosis, squamous metaplasia, and cytologic atypia

Natural History

- May occur synchronously or metachronously with other salivary gland tumors including
  - Pleomorphic adenoma (most common), monomorphic adenomas, oncocytoma, basal cell adenoma
  - Acinic cell adenocarcinoma, ductal adenocarcinoma, and adenoid cystic carcinoma

Treatment

- Surgical approaches
  - Complete surgical excision is treatment of choice
    - Should include adequate margin of uninvolved tissue
    - Facial nerve should be preserved

Prognosis

- Locally recurrent tumor may occur related to inadequate excision or to multicentrically occurring neoplasms
- Transformation to malignant WT exceedingly rare (incidence of < 0.1%) and may include
  - Epithelial component (carcinoma ex Warthin tumor)
    - Squamous cell carcinoma (most common), oncocytic carcinoma, adenocarcinoma not otherwise specified, undifferentiated carcinoma, mucoepidermoid carcinoma
    - May metastasize to regional lymph nodes; distant metastasis rare
  - Lymphoid component
    - Malignant lymphoma, usually non-Hodgkin type

IMAGE FINDINGS

Radiographic Findings

- Radionucleotide imaging
  - Increased uptake of Tc-99m, which does not wash out following sialogue administration
  - Plays important role in diagnosis and is related to presence of oncocytes and their increased mitochondrial content

CT Findings

- Well-defined area of increased density in posteroinferior segment of superficial lobe of parotid

MACROSCOPIC FEATURES

General Features

- Encapsulated, soft and fluctuant, round to oval mass with smooth or lobulated surface
- On cut section, appears tan-brown with multiple cystic spaces within which papillary projections may be seen
  - Mucoid or brown exudate may be expressed from cysts
- Solid areas can be identified and are noted for white nodular appearance representative of lymphoid follicles

Size

- 1-8 cm in diameter

MICROSCOPIC PATHOLOGY

Histologic Features

- Papillary and cystic lesion composed of epithelial and lymphoid components
- Epithelial component lining the papillary projections composed of double layer of granular eosinophilic cells (referred to as oncocytic epithelia)
  - Inner or luminal cells: Nonciliated, tall columnar cells with nuclei aligned toward luminal aspect
  - Outer or basal cells: Round, cuboidal, or polygonal cells with vesicular nuclei
  - Prominent oncocytic appearance of cells is due to presence of increased mitochondrial content
- Lymphoid component predominantly composed of mature lymphocytes containing lymphoid follicles with germinal centers

- Epithelial component is sharply demarcated from lymphoid component
  - Other inflammatory cells may be seen, including plasma cells, histiocytes, mast cells, and occasional multinucleated (Langhans-type) giant cells
- Lumens of cysts may contain thick secretions, cholesterol crystals, cellular debris, or corpora amylacea-like laminated bodies
- Squamous metaplasia and focal necrosis may be seen in association with secondary inflammation
- Due to presence of oncocytic cells, WT is subject to degenerative alterations
  - Occurs spontaneously or following manipulation (e.g., post-fine needle aspiration biopsy) including
    - Infarction and necrosis
    - Cytologic atypia
    - Squamous metaplasia
    - Granulation tissue, inflammation, fibrosis, hemorrhage
    - Pseudoinfiltrative growth pattern
- Metaplastic or infarcted variant of WT
  - Accounts for < 10% of all WT
  - Most likely develops following prior manipulation (e.g., fine needle aspiration biopsy)
  - Extensive necrosis with ghost-like papillary structures remaining
  - Squamous metaplasia (nonkeratinizing)
  - Cytologic atypia may be prominent, as well as increased mitotic figures but absence of atypical mitoses
  - Extensive fibrosis with dense collagen and reactive myofibroblasts may be seen along periphery
  - Mixed acute and chronic inflammation
  - Lipogranulomas, cholesterol granulomas may be present
  - Residual noninfarcted foci of Warthin tumor may be present

ANCILLARY TESTS

Cytology

- Aspiration may yield thick, tannish-brownish fluid; fluid may suggest presence of mucus
- Combination of oncocytic-appearing epithelial cells and mature lymphocytes
- Oncocytic epithelial cells appear in cohesive clusters as well as individual cells and may take on a honeycomb arrangement characterized by
  - Abundant granular and eosinophilic cytoplasm
  - Uniform round nuclei with identifiable nucleoli
  - Distinct cell borders
  - Absence of lymphocytes in epithelial clusters
- Squamous (metaplastic) cells may be identified
- Background of aspirate may appear "dirty" with cellular debris and associated lymphoid cells

Histochemistry

- Phosphotungstic acid-hematoxylin (PTAH) stains demonstrate mitochondria as blue-black granules in cytoplasm of both epithelial cell layers

Immunohistochemistry

- All epithelial cells are (pan)cytokeratin positive
  - Luminal (or inner) epithelial cells are CK7, CK8 and CK18, and EMA positive
- S100 protein, p63, calponin, GFAP, and actin negative
- Lymphoid cells reactive for B-cell (CD20) and T-cell (CD3) markers, as well as CD56, CD4 (helper cells) and CD8 (suppressor cells)

Cytogenetics

- t(11;19) translocation and *CRTC1/MAML2* fusion transcript identified in WT
  - Many mucoepidermoid carcinomas have t(11;19) translocation and *CRTC1/MAML2* fusion transcript
  - Similar translocation and fusion transcript in WT and mucoepidermoid carcinoma suggest evidence for common genetic association

DIFFERENTIAL DIAGNOSIS

Cystadenoma

- Lack characteristic features associated with WT including
  - Bilayered epithelial layer and prominent dense lymphoid stroma with germinal centers

Salivary Gland Tumors with Oncocytic Cells

- Oncocytes may be seen in a wide variety of tumors/ lesions (e.g., oncocytoma, mucoepidermoid carcinoma, acinic cell carcinoma, others)
  - Absence of characteristic bilayered epithelial layer and prominent dense lymphoid stroma of WT

SELECTED REFERENCES

1. Bell D et al: CRTC1/MAML2 fusion transcript in Warthin's tumor and mucoepidermoid carcinoma: evidence for a common genetic association. Genes Chromosomes Cancer. 47(4):309-14, 2008
2. Dalpa E et al: High prevalence of Human Herpes Virus 8 (HHV-8) in patients with Warthin's tumors of the salivary gland. J Clin Virol. 42(2):182-5, 2008
3. Fehr A et al: A closer look at Warthin tumors and the t(11;19). Cancer Genet Cytogenet. 180(2):135-9, 2008
4. Sadetzki S et al: Smoking and risk of parotid gland tumors: a nationwide case-control study. Cancer. 2008 May 1;112(9):1974-82. Erratum in: Cancer. 113(3):662-3, 2008
5. Maiorano E et al: Warthin's tumour: a study of 78 cases with emphasis on bilaterality, multifocality and association with other malignancies. Oral Oncol. 38(1):35-40, 2002
6. Di Palma S et al: Metaplastic (infarcted) Warthin's tumour of the parotid gland: a possible consequence of fine needle aspiration biopsy. Histopathology. 35(5):432-8, 1999
7. Ballo MS et al: Sources of diagnostic error in the fine-needle aspiration diagnosis of Warthin's tumor and clues to a correct diagnosis. Diagn Cytopathol. 17(3):230-4, 1997
8. Klijanienko J et al: Fine-needle sampling of salivary gland lesions. II. Cytology and histology correlation of 71 cases of Warthin's tumor (adenolymphoma). Diagn Cytopathol. 16(3):221-5, 1997
9. Eveson JW et al: Infarcted ('infected') adenolymphomas. A clinicopathological study of 20 cases. Clin Otolaryngol Allied Sci. 14(3):205-10, 1989

Imaging, Cytologic, Gross, and Varied Histology

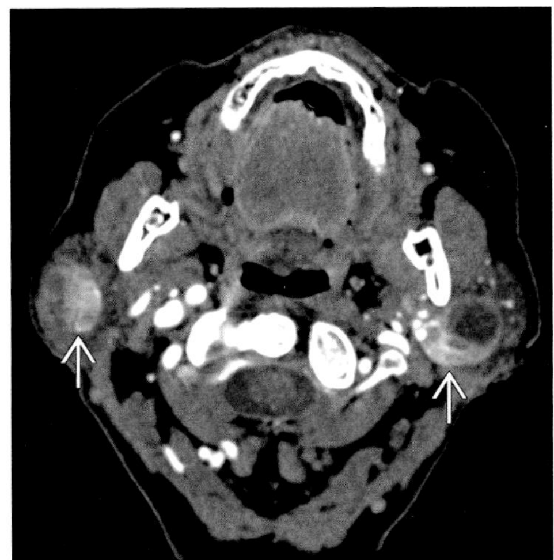

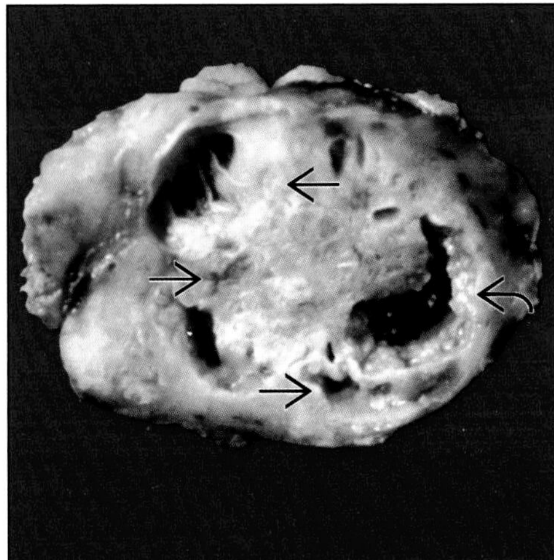

(Left) *Axial CECT through the parotid glands shows bilateral heterogeneous masses* ➔ *of varying size. The lesions show classic marked heterogeneity and heterogeneous contrast enhancement.* ***(Right)*** *Resected WT of the parotid gland shows cystic, solid, and focal papillary* ➔ *growth. The central area has the flesh-colored appearance of lymphoid tissue. There are foci of necrosis* ➔ *that occurred secondary to a prior fine needle aspiration.*

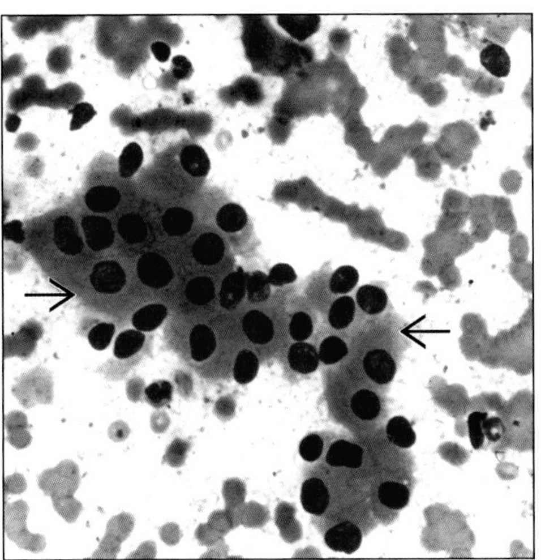

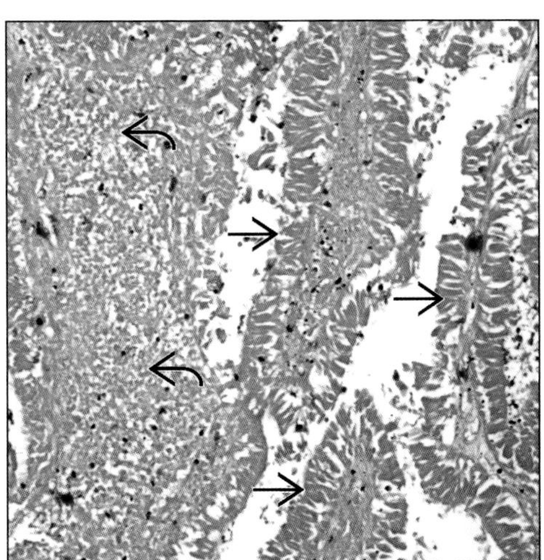

(Left) *Primary diagnostic evaluation of salivary gland lesions includes fine needle aspiration. The presence of clusters of oncocytic-appearing epithelial cells* ➔ *with scattered mature lymphocytes in the background supports a diagnosis of WT (Diff-Quik).* ***(Right)*** *Metaplastic or infarcted variant of Warthin tumor shows extensive necrosis with residual ghost-like papillary structures including oncocytic epithelium* ➔ *and lymphoid cell component* ➔*.*

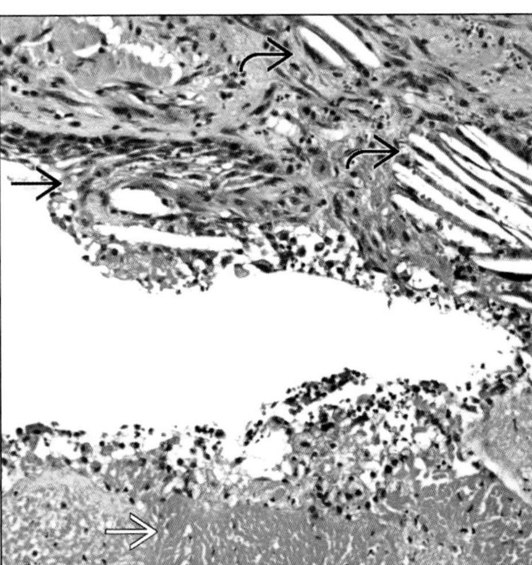

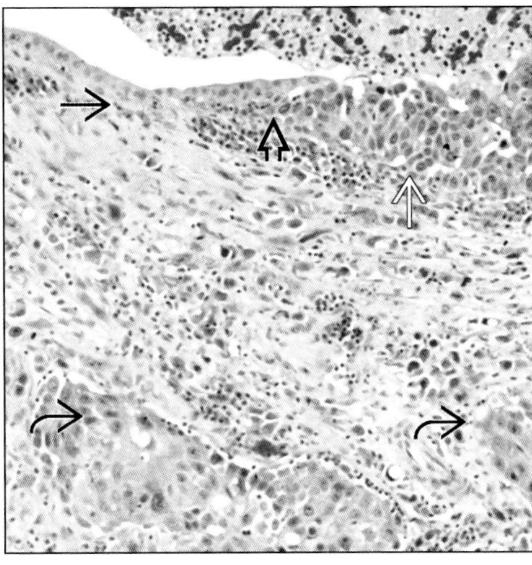

(Left) *Infarcted Warthin tumor shows squamous metaplasia* ➔ *and cholesterol granulomas* ➔*. Necrosis is present* ➔*. In such examples, cytologic atypia may be prominent and mitotic figures may be seen, but atypical mitoses and invasive growth are not present, excluding a possible diagnosis of carcinoma.* ***(Right)*** *Malignant transformation of WT shows transition* ➔ *from benign epithelium of WT* ➔ *to carcinoma* ➔ *and invasive undifferentiated carcinoma* ➔*.*

ONCOCYTOMA

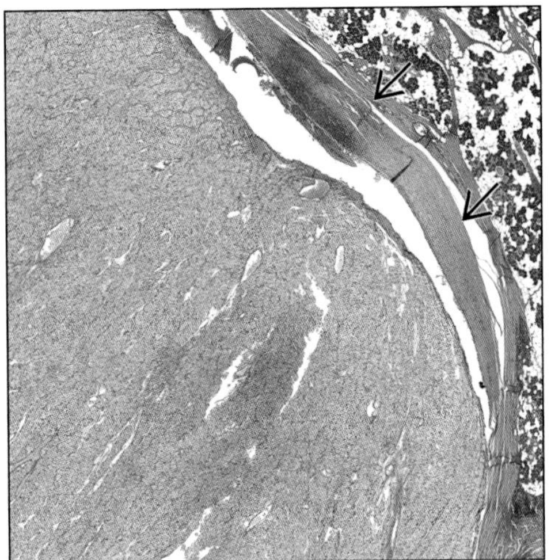

There is an encapsulated tumor, separated from the surrounding parotid parenchyma by a thick and well-formed fibrous connective tissue capsule ⇒. The tumor is composed of only oncocytes.

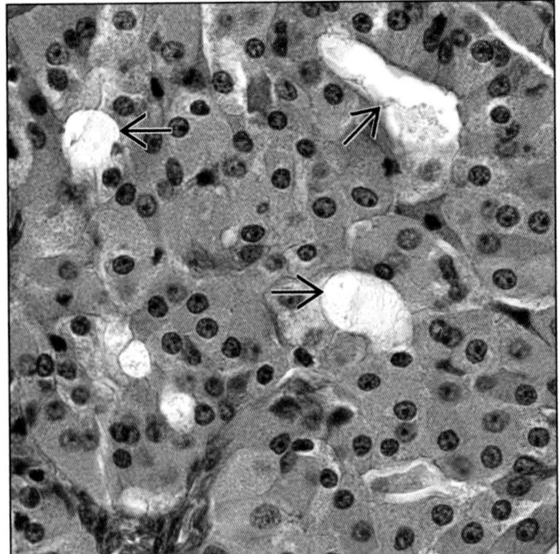

At high power, the oncocytoma shows a glandular architecture, with the lumen easily identified ⇒. The cells are polygonal, containing abundant eosinophilic, granular cytoplasm. The nuclei are round.

TERMINOLOGY

Synonyms

- Oncocytic adenoma
- Oxyphilic adenoma

Definitions

- Benign salivary gland neoplasm composed exclusively of large polygonal epithelial cells containing abundant, abnormal mitochondria (oncocytes)
  - By definition, no features of other types of salivary gland neoplasms

ETIOLOGY/PATHOGENESIS

Environmental Exposure

- Ionizing radiation (about 20% of patients)
  - Therapeutic or occupational, usually 5 or more years earlier
  - Patients with radiation exposure present on average 20 years younger than patients without radiation exposure

Pathogenesis

- Striated ducts
  - Normally contain many mitochondria
- Aging
  - Oncocytic metaplasia increases with advancing age (especially in parotid)
  - May be internal derangement or reaction to extracellular environment

CLINICAL ISSUES

Epidemiology

- Incidence
  - Approximately 1.5% of all salivary gland neoplasms
    - Up to 3% of parotid gland neoplasms
- Age
  - Mean: 6th-8th decades
    - About 20 years younger for radiation-exposed patients
    - Younger (mean: 58 years) for submandibular tumors
  - Not a tumor that develops in children
- Gender
  - Slight female predominance
    - Significant female bias for clear cell type oncocytoma
- Ethnicity
  - Predominantly affects whites

Site

- Parotid > > > submandibular gland
- Minor salivary glands: Lower lip, palate, pharynx, buccal mucosa

Presentation

- Asymptomatic, slow-growing swelling or mass
- ~ 7% of patients have bilateral tumors
- Pain or discomfort rarely reported
- Symptoms usually present for long duration (2 years)

Treatment

- Options, risks, complications
  - May have multifocal or bilateral disease
- Surgical approaches
  - Complete surgical excision is curative (parotidectomy)
- Radiation
  - Not employed, as oncocytes are radioresistant

Prognosis

- Minimal recurrence with adequate excision
  - Local recurrence may be multiple and bilateral
  - Recurrence may develop after a long delay (13 years)
- If tumors are bilateral, there is increased risk of recurrence
- Questionable malignant transformation

ONCOCYTOMA

Key Facts

Terminology
- Benign salivary gland neoplasm composed exclusively of large polygonal epithelial cells containing abundant, abnormal mitochondria (oncocytes)

Clinical Issues
- Mean: 6th-8th decades
- Parotid > > > submandibular gland
- Asymptomatic, slow-growing swelling or mass
  - ~ 7% of patients have bilateral tumors

Macroscopic Features
- Usually solitary, soft, well circumscribed

Microscopic Pathology
- Single nodule, distinct from surrounding parenchyma
- Variable architecture: Solid, acinar, trabecular
- Composed entirely of oncocytes or oxyphilic cells
  - Large, polygonal cells (2x size of acinar cells)
  - Abundant, eosinophilic, finely granular cytoplasm
  - Distinctive and prominent cell borders
- Intracytoplasmic glycogen may accumulate, giving a clear appearance
- Lymphocytes are focally minimal to absent

Ancillary Tests
- Mitochondrial stains are positive: PTAH, Novelli
- EM shows cytoplasm filled by mitochondria
  - ~ 60% of volume

Top Differential Diagnoses
- Nodular oncocytic hyperplasia, oncocytic metaplasia
- Warthin tumor, mucoepidermoid carcinoma, clear cell tumors

IMAGE FINDINGS

Radiographic Findings
- Tc-99m increased uptake and prolonged retention, retained after sialogogue administration
  - Related to increased mitochondrial content

CT Findings
- Usually shows well-defined area of increased density

MACROSCOPIC FEATURES

General Features
- Usually solitary
  - Different from nodular oncocytic hyperplasia: Multiple small nodules
- Soft, well circumscribed to partially encapsulated
- Tan to light brown nodule
- Rarely cystic

Size
- Range: 0.5-7 cm
- Mean: 3.5 cm

MICROSCOPIC PATHOLOGY

Histologic Features
- Well circumscribed with variably thick capsule
- Should be single nodule, distinct from surrounding parenchyma
  - Rare oncocytes can be seen in surrounding parenchyma but not in nodules
- No evidence of invasion
- Variable architecture
  - Solid, acinar or ducts (small lumen), trabecular (serpentine cords), papillary, cystic, follicular
- Composed entirely of oncocytes or oxyphilic cells
  - Large polygonal cells (2x size of acinar cells)
  - Lacking pleomorphism
  - Abundant, eosinophilic, finely granular cytoplasm
    - Due to high numbers of mitochondria
  - Uniform, central nuclei with coarse chromatin
  - Prominent nucleoli may be seen
  - 2 cell types can be seen, depending on eosinophilia
    - **Light cells**: Abundant oncocytic cytoplasm surrounding oval vesicular nucleus
    - **Dark cells**: Brightly eosinophilic cytoplasm with pyknotic nucleus
  - Distinctive and prominent cell borders
- Intracytoplasmic glycogen may accumulate, giving a clear appearance
- Delicate, fibrovascular stroma
  - Stromal hyalinization, vascularity, or degeneration is possible
- Lymphocytes are focally minimal to absent
- Mitoses are uncommon

Clear Cell Variant
- If clear cells predominate: **Clear cell oncocytoma**
  - Clearing is a fixation artifact &/or intracytoplasmic glycogen deposition

ANCILLARY TESTS

Cytology
- Usually cellular aspirates
- Show polygonal epithelial cells in papillary fragments, sheets, acinar-like structures, or singly
- Large cells with abundant granular cytoplasm
- Prominent nucleoli may be noted
- There are **no** background lymphocytes

Histochemistry
- Mitochondrial stains are positive
  - Phosphotungstic acid-hematoxylin (48 hour incubation; deep blue granules)
  - Novelli
  - Cresylecht violet V
  - Klüver-Barrera Luxol fast blue
- PAS ± diastase highlights glycogen in clear cells

Immunohistochemistry
- Positive

- Keratins: CK5/6, CK8/18, CK19
  - EMA
  - Anti-mitochondrial antibody
  - p63 (basal cells)
- Negative
  - S100 protein
  - Actins (SMA, MSA)
  - Calponin, p63
  - GFAP

Cytogenetics

- Rarely, mitochondrial DNA mutations may be detected

Electron Microscopy

- Cytoplasm is filled by mitochondria (~ 60% of volume)
  - Irregularly shaped mitochondria frequently show abnormal, elongated cristae with partial lamellar substructure
- Irregular nuclei with inclusions and glycogen granules

DIFFERENTIAL DIAGNOSIS

Nodular Oncocytic Hyperplasia

- Separation of hyperplasia from neoplasia is arbitrary in many cases
  - Distinction is clinically irrelevant
- Generally not a clinical mass
  - Generalized gland involvement (bilateral) can be seen
- Lacks well-developed capsule
- Multiple, topographically distinctive, variably sized nodules
- Rarely, diffuse process affecting entire gland (oncocytosis)
- Involves all cell types, including striated ducts, acinar cells
  - Intermingling of oncocytes with normal acinar elements

Oncocytic Metaplasia

- Normal salivary gland elements and tumors can have areas of oncocytic metaplasia
- Pleomorphic adenoma, basal cell adenoma, cystadenoma, mucoepidermoid carcinoma, and polymorphous low-grade adenocarcinoma are tumors that most frequently have oncocytic metaplasia
  - Myoepithelial features, chondromyxoid stroma, and other features help to separate

Papillary Cystadenoma Lymphomatosum

- a.k.a. Warthin tumor
- Characteristic papillary-cystic architecture
  - Bilayered epithelium
- Oncocytes make up epithelial component of tumor
- Lymphoid stroma (even on FNA material) is hardly ever seen in oncocytoma

Mucoepidermoid Carcinoma (MEC)

- Mucocytes are very rare in oncocytoma but required for MEC as are epidermoid and intermediate cells
- Epidermoid pattern with cystic changes are usually present
- Organoid architecture not usually present in MEC

Clear Cell Tumors

- Specifically for differential considerations for clear cell variant
- Clear cell mucoepidermoid carcinoma (MEC), epithelial-myoepithelial carcinoma (EMC), clear cell acinic cell adenocarcinoma, metastatic renal cell carcinoma (RCC)
  - All are malignant with infiltrative growth
  - None of these tumors tends to be completely composed of clear cells
  - Specific characteristics of each tumor help with separation
    - Epidermoid cells, mucocytes, and intermediate cells for MEC
    - Biphasic appearance of EMC
    - Basophilic cytoplasmic granules for acinic cell adenocarcinoma, lacking glycogen and PTAH reactions
    - Nuclear irregularities, prominent vascularity and extravasated erythrocytes, CD10(+), RCC(+), pax-2, and clinical history for RCC
- Clear cell myoepithelioma has myoepithelial markers by immunohistochemistry

SELECTED REFERENCES

1. Wakely PE Jr: Oncocytic and oncocyte-like lesions of the head and neck. Ann Diagn Pathol. 12(3):222-30, 2008
2. Hughes JH et al: Pitfalls in salivary gland fine-needle aspiration cytology: lessons from the College of American Pathologists Interlaboratory Comparison Program in Nongynecologic Cytology. Arch Pathol Lab Med. 129(1):26-31, 2005
3. Verma K et al: Salivary gland tumors with a prominent oncocytic component. Cytologic findings and differential diagnosis of oncocytomas and Warthin's tumor on fine needle aspirates. Acta Cytol. 47(2):221-6, 2003
4. Capone RB et al: Oncocytic neoplasms of the parotid gland: a 16-year institutional review. Otolaryngol Head Neck Surg. 126(6):657-62, 2002
5. Dardick I et al: Differentiation and the cytomorphology of salivary gland tumors with specific reference to oncocytic metaplasia. Oral Surg Oral Med Oral Pathol Oral Radiol Endod. 88(6):691-701, 1999
6. Paulino AF et al: Oncocytic and oncocytoid tumors of the salivary glands. Semin Diagn Pathol. 16(2):98-104, 1999
7. Ellis GL: Clear cell neoplasms in salivary glands: clearly a diagnostic challenge. Ann Diagn Pathol. 2(1):61-78, 1998
8. Thompson LD et al: Oncocytomas of the submandibular gland. A series of 22 cases and a review of the literature. Cancer. 78(11):2281-7, 1996
9. Damm DD et al: Benign solid oncocytoma of intraoral minor salivary glands. Oral Surg Oral Med Oral Pathol. 67(1):84-6, 1989

ONCOCYTOMA

Radiographic, Gross, and Microscopic Features

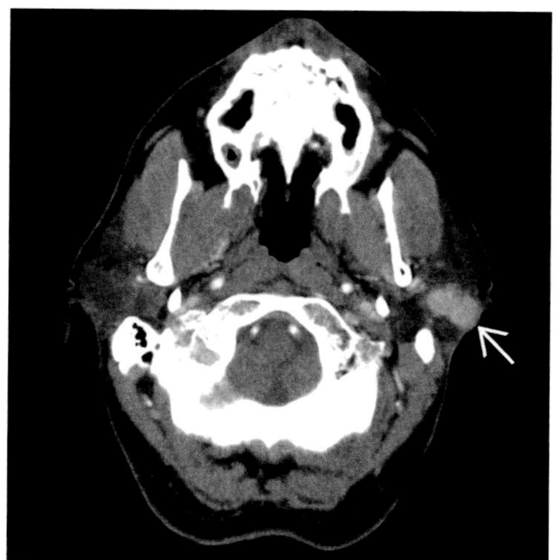

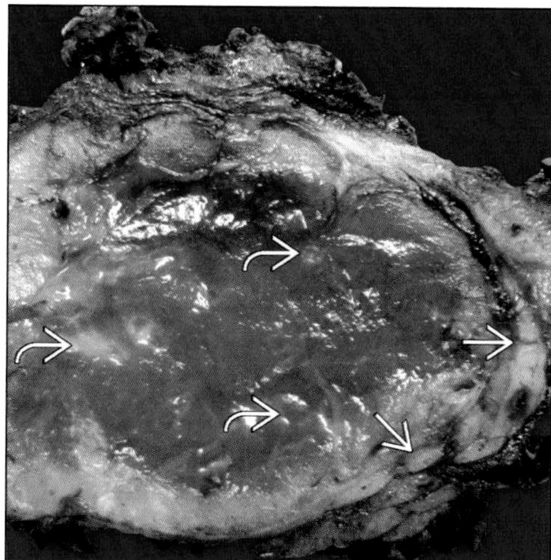

(Left) There is a bright signal intensity in the mass identified within the left parotid gland ➡. There are some differences in signal intensity and quality based on tumor type, but most of these findings are subtle. **(Right)** The parotid gland parenchyma ➡ at the periphery is compressed by the neoplasm. The cut surface is tan to reddish-brown, focally showing areas of degeneration or cystic change ➡. The mahogany color is quite characteristic of oncocytoma.

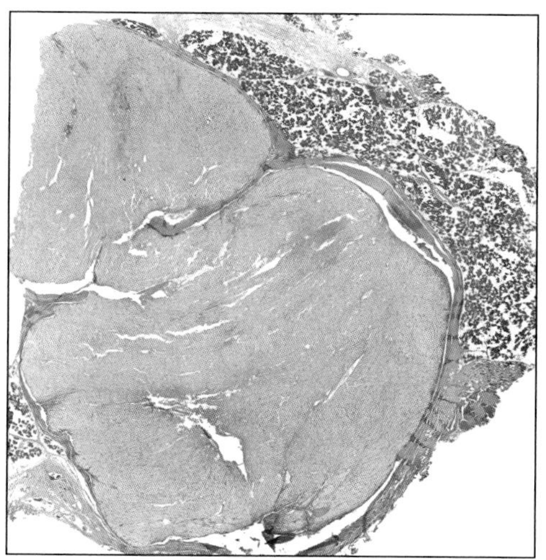

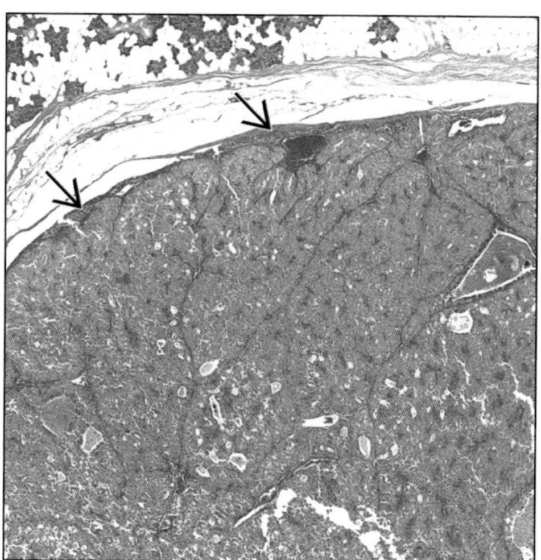

(Left) There is a single well-circumscribed and encapsulated tumor in the parotid salivary gland. The tumor shows a brightly eosinophilic appearance even at low power. No oncocytic nodules are identified in the salivary gland parenchyma. **(Right)** This well-circumscribed oncocytoma is distinctly separate from the salivary gland parenchyma. There is a very thin band of lymphocytes at the edge ➡, an uncommon finding. There is a solid to glandular architecture.

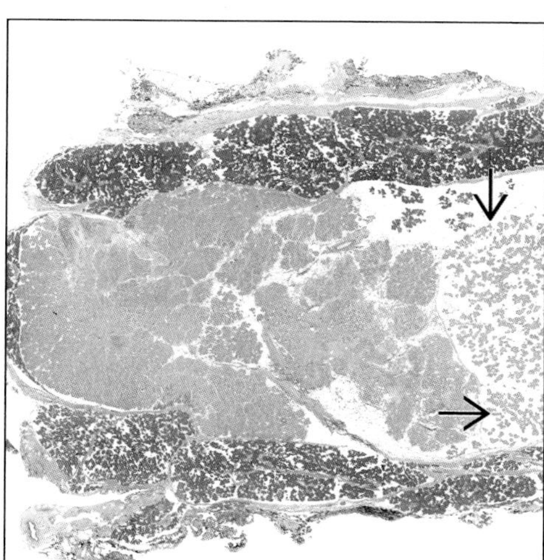

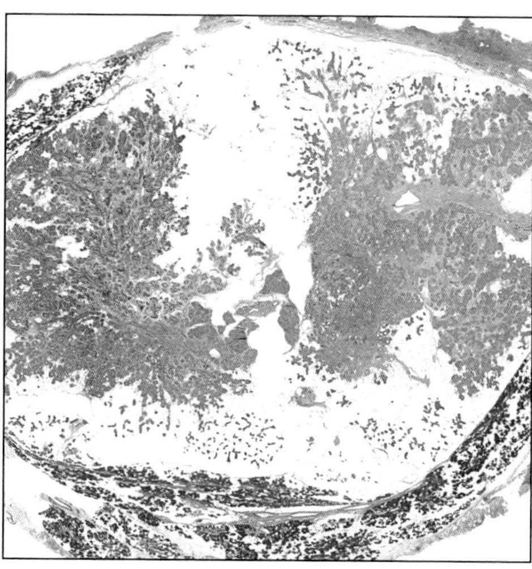

(Left) The oncocytoma is composed of a dominant nodule within the parotid gland. However, areas of fatty change are noted within the tumor, creating a less cellular appearance ➡. The tumor cells are oncocytes. **(Right)** This tumor is a single nodule composed of oncocytes and fat. However, a core needle biopsy through this lesion may suggest a diagnosis of diffuse oncocytosis or nodular oncocytic hyperplasia. The tumor is circumscribed but is not well encapsulated.

ONCOCYTOMA

Microscopic Features

(Left) *The neoplastic cells are large polygonal cells with brightly eosinophilic granular cytoplasm. The nuclei are round and regular with coarse to vesicular nuclear chromatin distribution. A delicate fibrovascular stroma separates the cells.* ***(Right)*** *A glandular or acinar appearance can be seen in this tumor composed exclusively of oncocytes. There is a lack of cytologic atypia, and the nuclei are round and regular.*

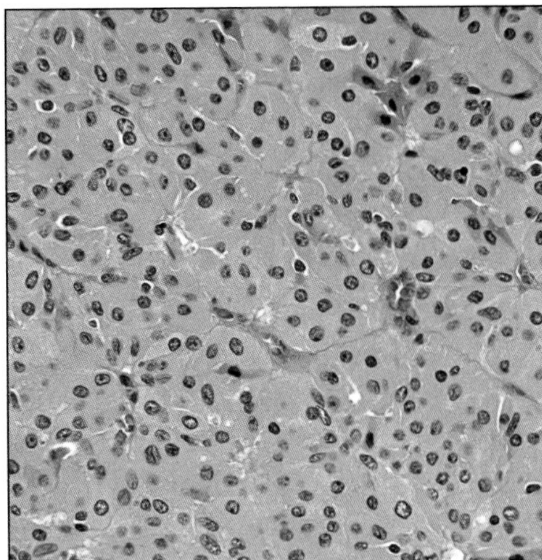

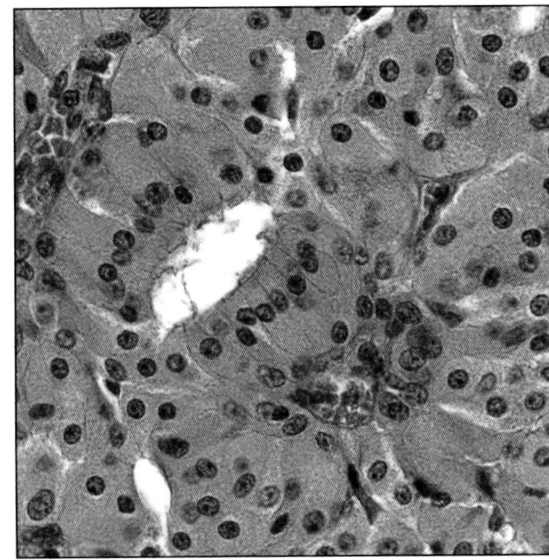

(Left) *In a number of cases the fibrous connective tissue stroma can be more loose and prominent, creating small nodules or gland-like spaces in an oncocytoma. There is still a monotony to the cells and a lack of pleomorphism.* ***(Right)*** *A paraganglioma-like pattern can sometimes be seen in oncocytoma. Note very well-formed fibrous connective tissue stroma separating this tumor in small nests or zellballen-like nests. The cytoplasm is granular and eosinophilic.*

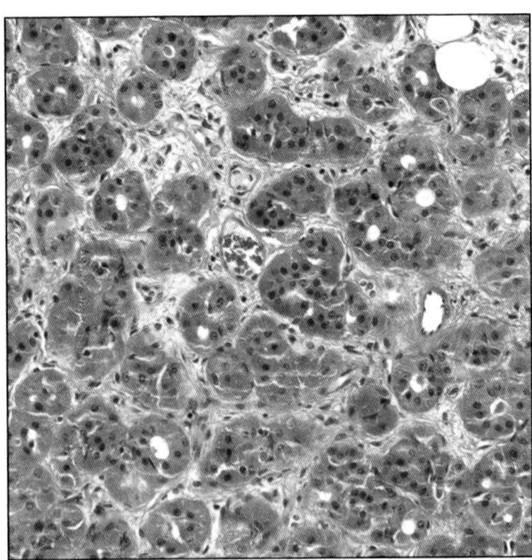

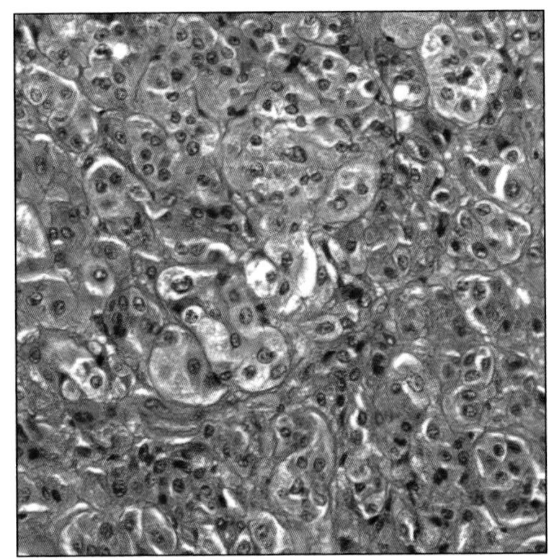

(Left) *A slight clearing of the cytoplasm can be seen in this oncocytoma. Note the very prominent cell borders. The very well-developed fibrovascular stroma separates the tumor cells into a trabecular architecture.* ***(Right)*** *Oncocytoma may undergo cystic change. There is a flocculent-serous material within the cysts, lined by oncocytes. The cysts vary in size and shape. There is a generalized lack of lymphocytes, a helpful feature in differentiating oncocytoma from Warthin tumor.*

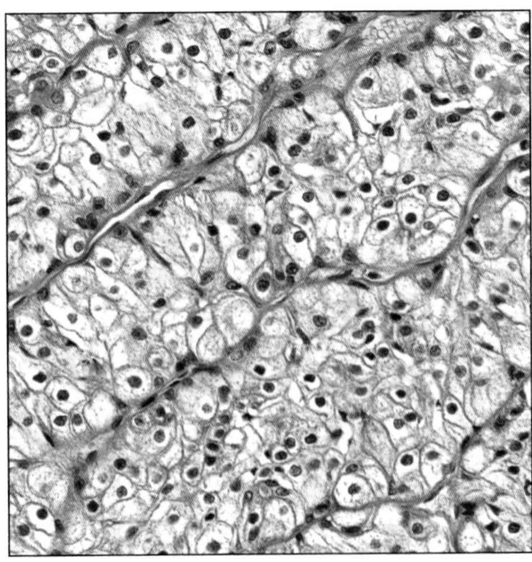

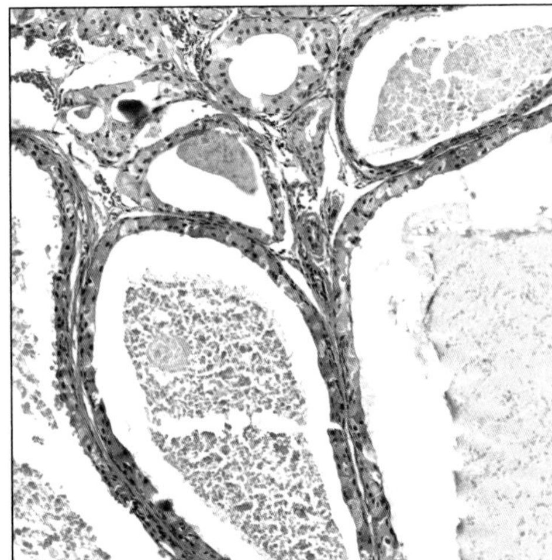

Ancillary Techniques

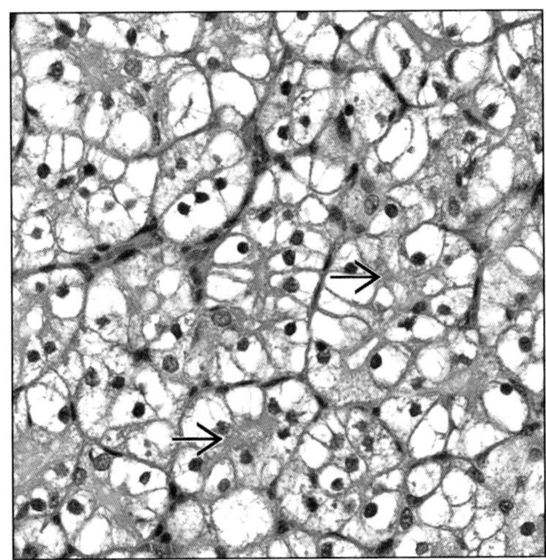

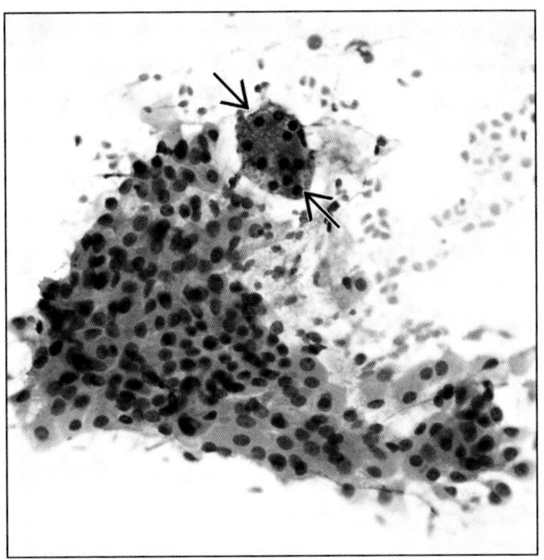

(Left) *The clear cell oncocytoma has cleared cytoplasm, creating very prominent and well-formed cell borders. Note a few areas still show oncocytic features ➔. This is a mimic of metastatic renal cell carcinoma.* ***(Right)*** *This smear demonstrates a sheet of oncocytic cells. There is slight overlapping, with small, round, hyperchromatic nuclei identified. There is an acinus ➔ as a point of comparison to the oncocytic cells. Lymphocytes are absent from the background.*

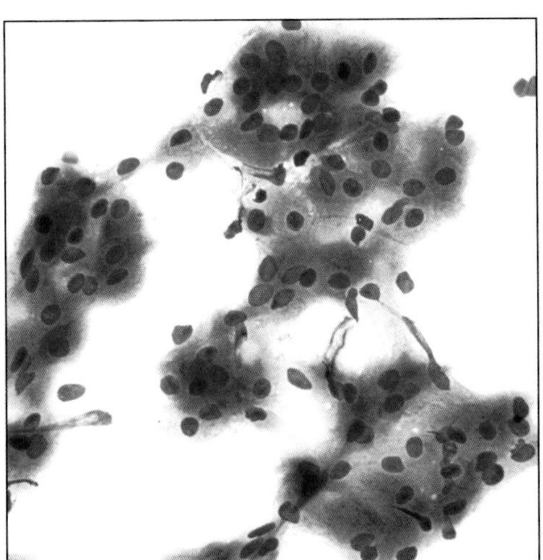

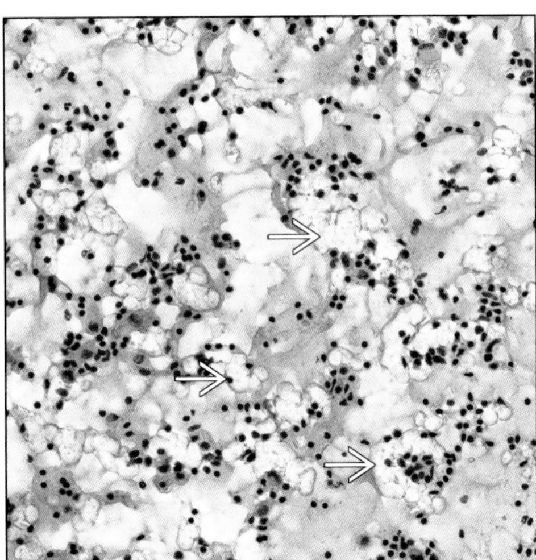

(Left) *This Diff-Quik stained smear shows the purple appearance of oncocytes. There is abundant cytoplasm surrounding the round and regular nuclei. Note the lack of pleomorphism and lymphocytes.* ***(Right)*** *This clear cell oncocytoma FNA smear shows a very cellular aspirate. The clear cytoplasm creates a clearing in the background serum ➔. The nuclei are small and round. The background lacks erythrocytes and lymphocytes, helping eliminate other tumors from the differential diagnosis.*

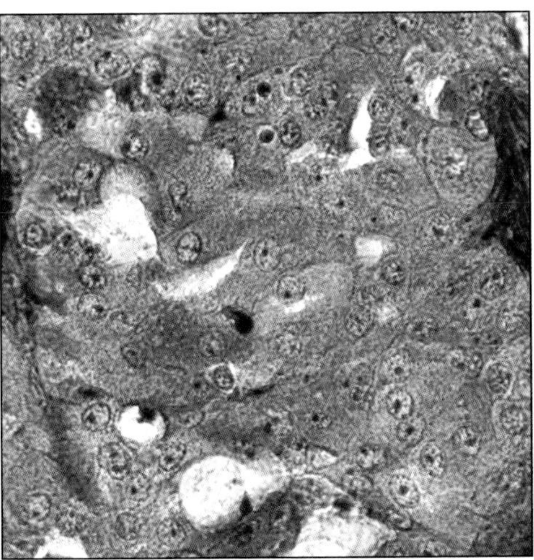

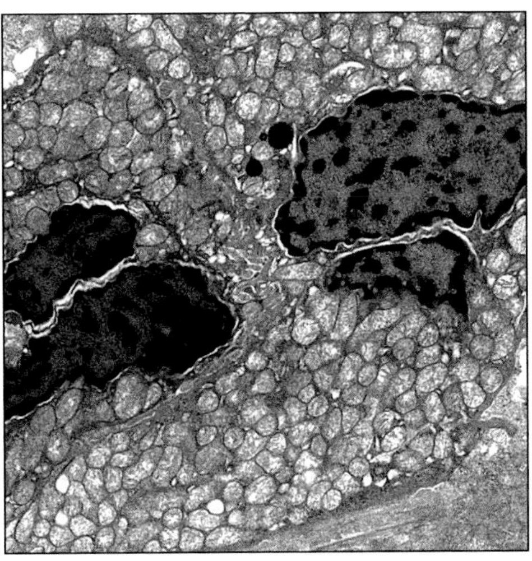

(Left) *The PTAH stain accentuates the abnormal mitochondria by staining them as dark blue granules. This stain can be difficult to perform.* ***(Right)*** *The cytoplasm of this oncocyte is filled with round to oval to irregular-shaped mitochondria, pushing against themselves and the nucleus. The mitochondria show abnormal, elongated cristae with a partial lamellar substructure. This electron microscopic appearance is characteristic for an oncocytoma. (Courtesy S. Bhuta, MD.)*

CANALICULAR ADENOMA

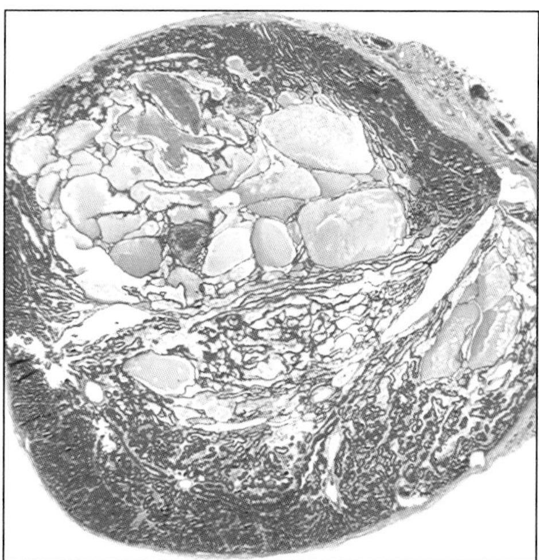

Hematoxylin & eosin shows a well-defined mass surrounded by a capsule with cystic spaces filled with proteinaceous fluid.

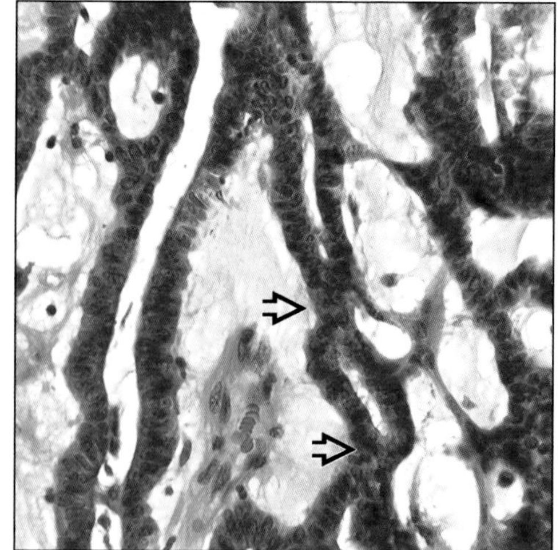

Hematoxylin & eosin shows canalicular architecture with "beading" ⇨, characteristic of canalicular adenoma.

TERMINOLOGY

Synonyms

- Monomorphic adenoma

Definitions

- Benign epithelial salivary gland neoplasm arranged in interconnecting cords of columnar cells

CLINICAL ISSUES

Epidemiology

- Incidence
  - Uncommon
    - About 2% of all salivary gland tumors; 4% of all benign tumors
    - About 20% of all lip salivary gland tumors
- Age
  - Wide range: 3rd to 9th decades
  - Mean: 65 years
- Gender
  - Female > Male (2:1)

Site

- Vast majority in **upper** lip
  - Buccal mucosa and palate rarely affected

Presentation

- Slowly enlarging mass
- Mobile, compressible, frequently slightly blue, submucosal nodules
- Multifocality common
  - Most common benign multifocal tumor

Treatment

- Surgical approaches
  - Conservative local excision, including multifocal tumors

Prognosis

- Excellent
  - Recurrences may represent incompletely excised multifocal tumors

MACROSCOPIC FEATURES

General Features

- Well circumscribed
- Light yellow/tan/brown nodules
- Cut surface frequently has cysts with gelatinous material

Sections to Be Submitted

- Include multifocal tumors, if present
- Borders with surrounding mucosa/stroma included

Size

- Range: 0.5-4 cm, but most are < 1 cm

MICROSCOPIC PATHOLOGY

Histologic Features

- Encapsulated
- Canalicular pattern with cords and ribbons showing connection points between opposing columnar cells within spaces
  - Beading: Columnar cells abutting one another within tubules
- Tubules interconnect in lattice-like architecture
- Cuboidal to columnar cells
- Basaloid cells with round to oval nuclei
- Scant, slightly eosinophilic cytoplasm
- No mitotic figures
- Loose, fibrillar stroma; rich in hyaluronic acid and chondroitin sulphate
- Calcifications may be seen (microliths)

CANALICULAR ADENOMA

Key Facts

Terminology
- Benign epithelial salivary gland neoplasm arranged in interconnecting cords of columnar cells

Clinical Issues
- Vast majority in upper lip
- Multifocality common (most common benign multifocal tumor)
- Recurrences may represent incompletely excised multifocal tumors

Microscopic Pathology
- Canalicular pattern with connection points (beading) between opposing columnar cells within tubular spaces
- Loose, fibrillar stroma; rich in hyaluronic acid and chondroitin sulphate

Top Differential Diagnoses
- Basal cell adenoma
- Adenoid cystic carcinoma

Margins
- May be "involved" due to multifocality

ANCILLARY TESTS

Immunohistochemistry
- Various keratins are immunoreactive
  - Includes AE1/AE3 and CK7
- Positive: S100 protein and CD117
- Negative: Smooth muscle actin, calponin, smooth muscle myosin heavy chain, p63, GFAP

DIFFERENTIAL DIAGNOSIS

Basal Cell Adenoma
- Multiple patterns
- No beading
- Almost exclusively basaloid cells
- Columnar cells not identified
- Has characteristic collagenized stroma

Adenoid Cystic Carcinoma
- Linear arrangement of columnar cells is absent
- Cell borders are indistinct
- Nuclei are
  - Peg-shaped
  - Angular
  - Irregular
- Borders are infiltrative
- Perineural invasion common
- Background stroma or reduplicated basal lamina lacks capillaries

DIAGNOSTIC CHECKLIST

Pathologic Interpretation Pearls
- Beading of columnar cells is characteristic

SELECTED REFERENCES

1. Machado de Sousa SO et al: Immunohistochemical aspects of basal cell adenoma and canalicular adenoma of salivary glands. Oral Oncol. 37(4):365-8, 2001
2. Zarbo RJ et al: Salivary gland basal cell and canalicular adenomas: immunohistochemical demonstration of myoepithelial cell participation and morphogenetic considerations. Arch Pathol Lab Med. 124(3):401-5, 2000
3. Ferreiro JA: Immunohistochemical analysis of salivary gland canalicular adenoma. Oral Surg Oral Med Oral Pathol. 78(6):761-5, 1994
4. Waldron CA et al: Tumors of the intraoral minor salivary glands: a demographic and histologic study of 426 cases. Oral Surg Oral Med Oral Pathol. 66(3):323-33, 1988
5. Daley TD et al: Canalicular adenoma: not a basal cell adenoma. Oral Surg Oral Med Oral Pathol. 57(2):181-8, 1984
6. Gardner DG et al: The use of the terms monomorphic adenoma, basal cell adenoma, and canalicular adenoma as applied to salivary gland tumors. Oral Surg Oral Med Oral Pathol. 56(6):608-15, 1983
7. Nelson JF et al: Monomorphic adenoma (canalicular type). Report of 29 cases. Cancer. 31(6):1511-3, 1973

IMAGE GALLERY

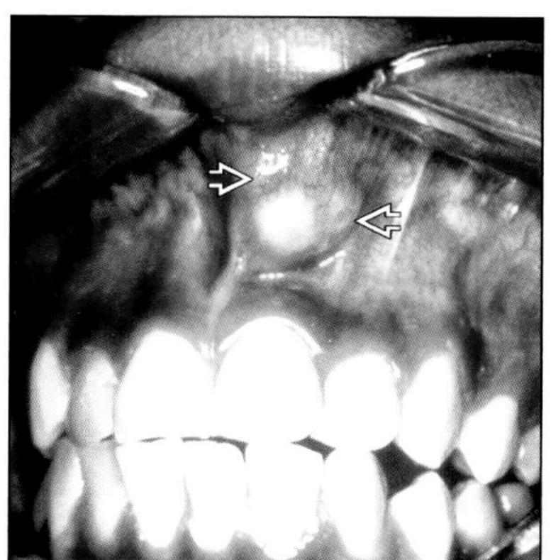

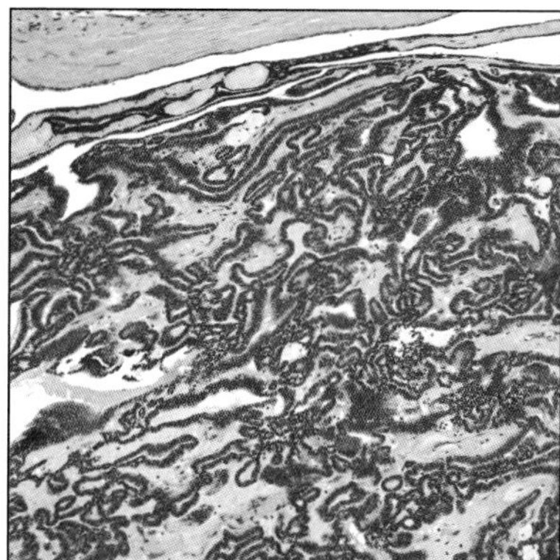

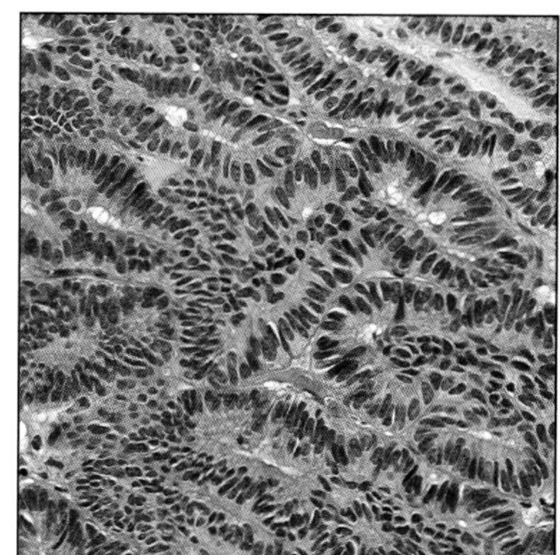

(Left) *Clinical photograph shows a well-defined nodule within the gingiva-lip junction* ⇒. ***(Center)*** *Hematoxylin & eosin shows multiple channels (canaliculi) with a nonspecific vascular stroma. The cells have a columnar, basaloid phenotype.* ***(Right)*** *Hematoxylin & eosin shows basaloid columnar cells arranged in loose canals with focal stroma.*

LYMPHADENOMA AND SEBACEOUS LYMPHADENOMA

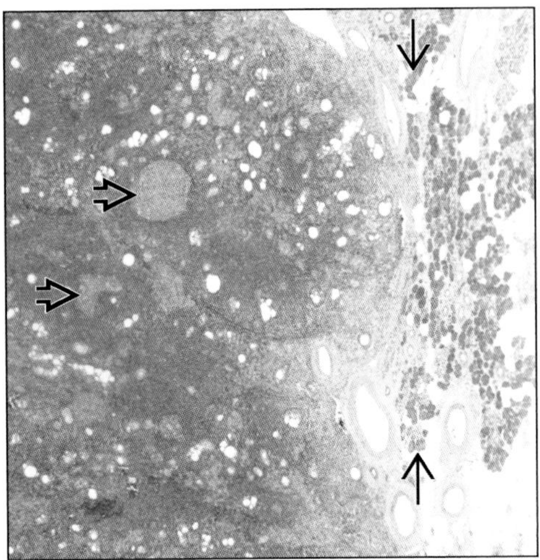

Sebaceous lymphadenoma demonstrates a pushing border into the parotid parenchyma ➔. Small cysts are present within a dense lymphoid stroma, which contains germinal centers ➩.

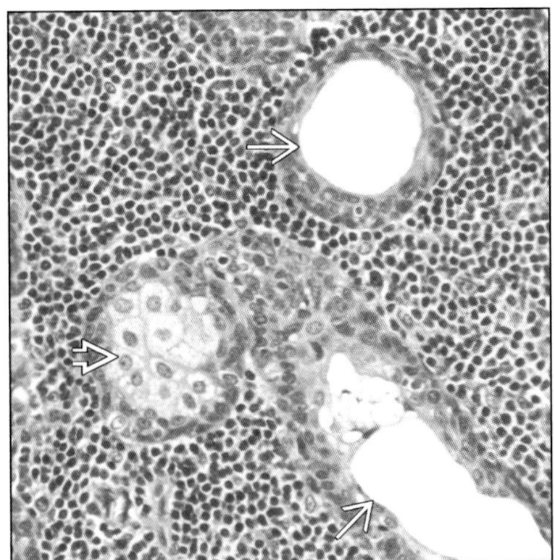

Sebaceous lymphadenoma demonstrates small nests of sebaceous cells ➩, variably sized cysts ➔, and a dense lymphoid stroma. Sebaceous cells may also be seen within cyst walls.

TERMINOLOGY

Abbreviations

- Sebaceous lymphadenoma (SLA)
- Lymphadenoma (LA)

Definitions

- **Sebaceous lymphadenoma**
  - Rare salivary gland neoplasm composed of epithelial nests and cysts with focal sebaceous differentiation distributed within dense hyperplastic lymphoid tissue
- **Lymphadenoma**
  - Histologically similar to sebaceous lymphadenoma but devoid of sebaceous elements

CLINICAL ISSUES

Epidemiology

- Incidence
  - Very rare
    - < 0.2% of all parotid gland neoplasms
- Age
  - Average: 6th to 8th decades
- Gender
  - Equal gender distribution

Site

- > 90% in parotid gland or surrounding tissues
- Rare reports in minor salivary glands

Presentation

- Asymptomatic mass in parotid gland
  - Duration of symptoms: Ranges from 1 month to 15 years

Treatment

- Conservative surgical excision

Prognosis

- No recurrences reported following adequate resection

MACROSCOPIC FEATURES

General Features

- Round to oval soft mass
- Solid and homogeneous to cystic
- Yellow to cream color

Size

- Range: 1-6 cm

MICROSCOPIC PATHOLOGY

Histologic Features

- Well circumscribed
  - Typically encapsulated
  - Pushing, yet noninfiltrative border
- Epithelial element
  - Evenly dispersed solid epithelial nests and cysts
  - Cysts of variable size
    - Squamoid, columnar, or cuboidal lining
    - May contain secreted material
  - SLA: Sebaceous cells in solid nests or within cyst walls
  - LA: Lack of sebaceous component
  - Bland cytology
- Lymphoid component
  - Uniformly dense
  - Germinal centers may be focal to numerous
  - **No** infiltration/invasion of epithelial component
- Foreign body reaction may be present due to cyst rupture

LYMPHADENOMA AND SEBACEOUS LYMPHADENOMA

Key Facts

Terminology

- Sebaceous lymphadenoma
  - Epithelial nests and cysts with focal sebaceous differentiation distributed within dense hyperplastic lymphoid tissue
- Lymphadenoma histologically similar yet devoid of sebaceous elements

Clinical Issues

- Conservative surgical excision
- No recurrences reported following parotidectomy
- Majority in parotid gland or surrounding tissues

Microscopic Pathology

- Well circumscribed, partial to fully encapsulated
- Bland cytology

Top Differential Diagnoses

- Warthin tumor, tumor-associated lymphoid proliferation (TALP), metastatic carcinoma

ANCILLARY TESTS

Immunohistochemistry

- Pancytokeratin reactivity in epithelial component
- p63 reactive in basal layer of sebaceous nests
- Lymphoid markers (CD3, CD20, Bcl-2, etc.) confirm reactive, hyperplastic lymphoid population

DIFFERENTIAL DIAGNOSIS

Warthin Tumor

- Papillary-cystic architectural pattern
- Cysts lined by bilayered oncocytic epithelium
- Sebaceous elements rare to nonexistent in Warthin tumor

Tumor-associated Lymphoid Proliferation (TALP)

- Reactive lymphoid infiltrate commonly seen associated with mucoepidermoid carcinoma and acinic cell adenocarcinoma
- TALP infiltrate poorly circumscribed and with variable density
- SLA and LA show well-defined borders and even lymphoid dispersion

Metastatic Carcinoma

- Sebaceous adenoma and lymphadenoma may mimic metastatic disease to lymph nodes
- Bland cytology, even epithelial distribution, and relative morphologic consistency of nests and cysts favor SLA and LA

SELECTED REFERENCES

1. Gallego L et al: Non-sebaceous lymphadenoma of the parotid gland: immunohistochemical study and DNA ploidy analysis. Oral Surg Oral Med Oral Pathol Oral Radiol Endod. 107(4):555-8, 2009
2. Dardick I et al: Lymphadenoma of parotid gland: Two additional cases and a literature review. Oral Surg Oral Med Oral Pathol Oral Radiol Endod. 105(4):491-4, 2008
3. Hayashi D et al: Sebaceous lymphadenoma of the parotid gland: report of two cases and review of the literature. Acta Otorhinolaryngol Ital. 27(3):144-6, 2007
4. Maffini F et al: Sebaceous lymphadenoma of salivary gland: a case report and a review of the literature. Acta Otorhinolaryngol Ital. 27(3):147-50, 2007
5. Yang S et al: Non-sebaceous lymphadenoma of the salivary gland: case report with immunohistochemical investigation. Virchows Arch. 450(5):595-9, 2007
6. Maruyama S et al: Sebaceous lymphadenoma of the lip: report of a case of minor salivary gland origin. J Oral Pathol Med. 31(4):242-3, 2002
7. Auclair PL: Tumor-associated lymphoid proliferation in the parotid gland. A potential diagnostic pitfall. Oral Surg Oral Med Oral Pathol. 77(1):19-26, 1994
8. Batsakis JG et al: Sebaceous lesions of salivary glands and oral cavity. Ann Otol Rhinol Laryngol. 99(5 Pt 1):416-8, 1990
9. Gnepp DR et al: Sebaceous neoplasms of salivary gland origin. Report of 21 cases. Cancer. 53(10):2155-70, 1984

IMAGE GALLERY

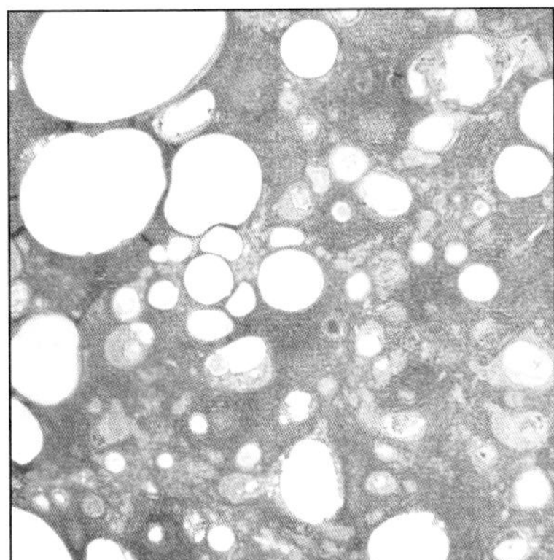

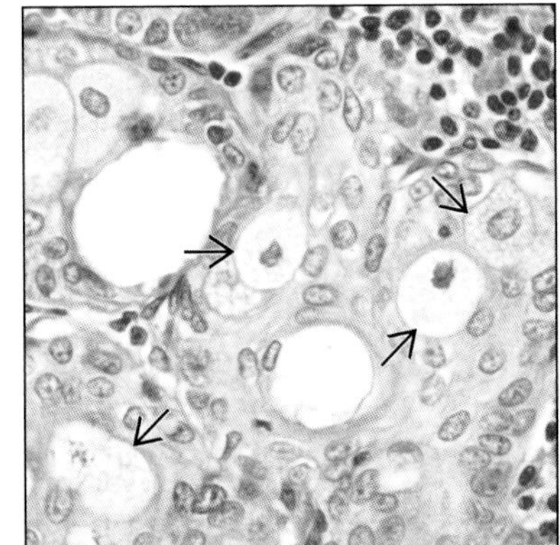

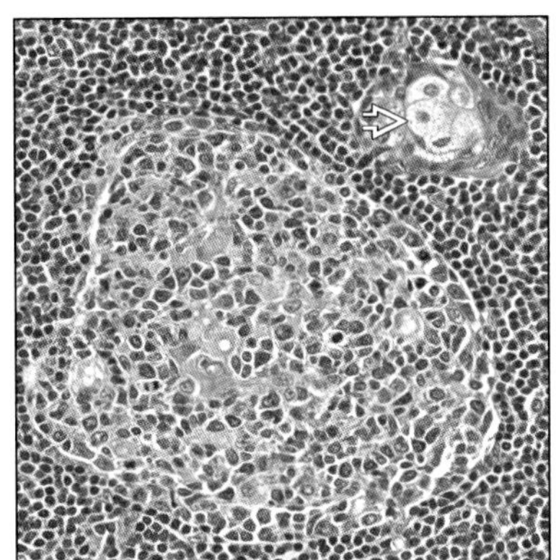

*(**Left**) Sebaceous lymphadenoma with numerous variably sized cysts and solid nests supported by a dense lymphoid population. The epithelial population is evenly distributed within the neoplasm. (**Center**) Well-differentiated sebaceous cells may be found in nests or in cyst walls ⇒. Two small cystic spaces are evident. (**Right**) Variably sized reactive lymphoid germinal centers may be present in both entities and can be few to numerous. Note the sebaceous cells ⇒.*

SEBACEOUS ADENOMA

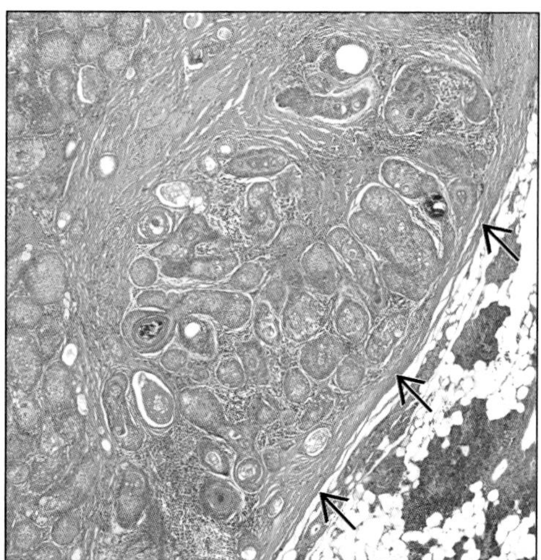

Low-power view shows sebaceous adenoma. This predominantly solid example is well circumscribed and encapsulated ⇨. Mainly cystic lesions may display an irregular interface with the surrounding parenchyma.

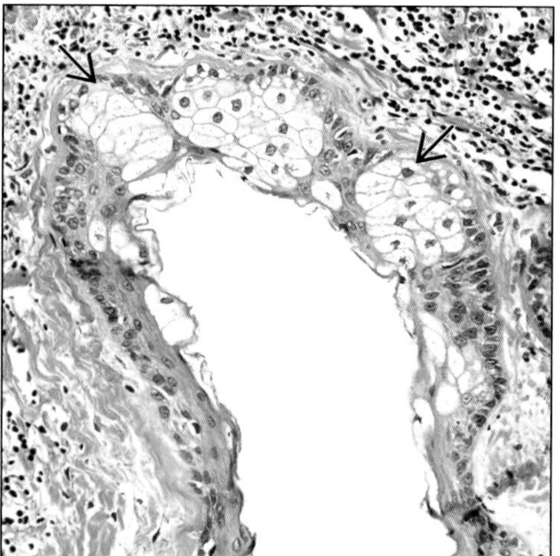

Sebaceous adenoma, cystic variant, is shown. Variably sized nests of sebaceous cells ⇨ are located within the wall of a cystic space lined by stratified squamous epithelium.

TERMINOLOGY

Abbreviations

- Sebaceous adenoma (SA)

Definitions

- Rare, benign salivary gland neoplasm composed of proliferating epithelial cells with focal sebaceous differentiation

CLINICAL ISSUES

Epidemiology

- Incidence
  - < 1% of all salivary gland neoplasia
- Age
  - Wide age range
    - Mainly adults, average in 6th to 7th decade
- Gender
  - Male > Female

Site

- Most often in parotid gland
  - Rare reports in submandibular gland
  - Intraoral tumors may be salivary gland origin or associated with Fordyce granules

Presentation

- Asymptomatic
- Firm, slowly growing mass

Treatment

- Conservative, yet total surgical excision

Prognosis

- No reports of recurrence or malignant degeneration
- Possible association with Muir-Torre syndrome
  - Genodermatosis characterized by sebaceous neoplasms of skin and visceral malignancies (gastrointestinal or genitourinary carcinomas)
    - *MLH1* and *MSH2* (on chromosomes 3 and 2, respectively) are abnormal
    - Unknown if salivary gland-based sebaceous neoplasms are part of this syndrome
    - May be difficult to differentiate adnexal-based lesions from salivary gland in buccal mucosa

MACROSCOPIC FEATURES

General Features

- Firm, well-circumscribed, pinkish gray to white mass
- Solid or cystic

Size

- Typically 1-3 cm

MICROSCOPIC PATHOLOGY

Histologic Features

- Epithelial proliferation forming variably sized solid nests or cysts
- Well circumscribed with inconsistent encapsulation
  - Cystic areas may show haphazard boundary with surrounding parenchyma
- Peripheral epithelial cells are immature and surround variably developed sebaceous cells
  - Quantity of well-differentiated sebaceous cells varies from minimal to abundant
- Squamous differentiation also observed
  - Especially identified lining cystic spaces
- Occasional oncocytes or mucocytes
  - Will be highlighted with PTAH or mucicarmine, respectively
  - Sebaceous cells will be nonreactive with these histochemical stains
- Foreign body reaction may be noted surrounding extravasated cystic material

SEBACEOUS ADENOMA

Key Facts

Terminology

- Rare, benign salivary gland neoplasm composed of proliferating epithelial cells with focal sebaceous differentiation

Clinical Issues

- Most often in parotid gland
- Conservative yet total surgical excision
- No reports of recurrence or malignant degeneration

Microscopic Pathology

- Epithelial proliferation forming variably sized solid nests or cysts
- Well circumscribed with inconsistent encapsulation
- Peripheral epithelial cells are immature and surround variably mature sebaceous cells
- Quantity of well-differentiated sebaceous cells varies from minimal to abundant
- Squamous differentiation also observed

ANCILLARY TESTS

Immunohistochemistry

- Reactive with pancytokeratin and epithelial membrane antigen
- Nonreactive with actin-sm and S100 protein

DIFFERENTIAL DIAGNOSIS

Mucoepidermoid Carcinoma

- Focal mucocytes and squamous differentiation may suggest mucoepidermoid carcinoma (MEC)
- Sebaceous adenoma is usually circumscribed and noninfiltrative
- Nests with well-differentiated sebaceous cells are rare to nonexistent in MEC
- Although epidermoid cytomorphology is present, MEC lacks true squamous differentiation
- Clear cells and intermediate cells of MEC not seen in sebaceous adenoma

Sebaceous Adenocarcinoma

- Due to partial encapsulation, infiltration into surrounding parenchyma may be simulated, suggesting malignancy
- Sebaceous adenoma lacks significant mitotic activity
  - Aberrant, atypical mitoses are not found
- Other features of malignancy (necrosis, perineural invasion, or significant pleomorphism) not seen in sebaceous adenoma

Sebaceous Hyperplasia

- Lobules in sebaceous hyperplasia are few in number and surround excretory duct
- Sebaceous adenoma lacks presence of excretory duct and epithelial nests may number in hundreds

SELECTED REFERENCES

1. Apple SK et al: Sebaceous adenoma of the parotid gland: a case report with fine needle aspiration findings and histologic correlation. Acta Cytol. 53(4):419-22, 2009
2. Welch KC et al: Sebaceous adenoma of the parotid gland in a 2-year-old male. Otolaryngol Head Neck Surg. 136(4):672-3, 2007
3. de Vicente Rodríguez JC et al: Sebaceous adenoma of the parotid gland. Med Oral Patol Oral Cir Bucal. 11(5):E446-8, 2006
4. Izutsu T et al: Sebaceous adenoma in the retromolar region: report of a case with a review of the English literature. Int J Oral Maxillofac Surg. 32(4):423-6, 2003
5. Iezzi G et al: Sebaceous adenoma of the cheek. Oral Oncol. 38(1):111-3, 2002
6. Liu CY et al: Sebaceous adenoma in the submandibular gland. Otolaryngol Head Neck Surg. 126(2):199-200, 2002
7. Batsakis JG et al: Sebaceous lesions of salivary glands and oral cavity. Ann Otol Rhinol Laryngol. 99(5 Pt 1):416-8, 1990
8. Gnepp DR et al: Sebaceous neoplasms of salivary gland origin. Report of 21 cases. Cancer. 53(10):2155-70, 1984

IMAGE GALLERY

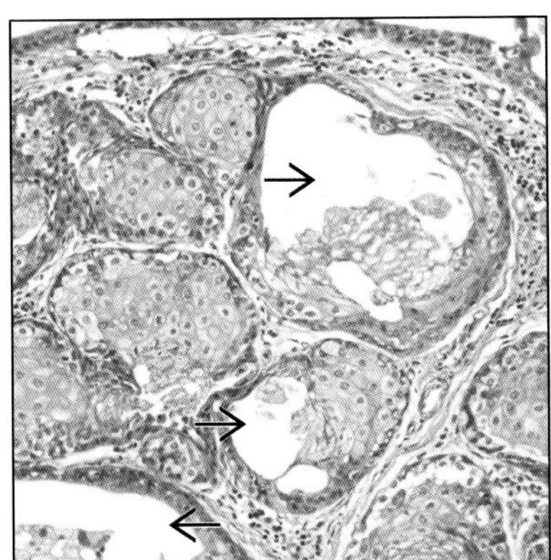

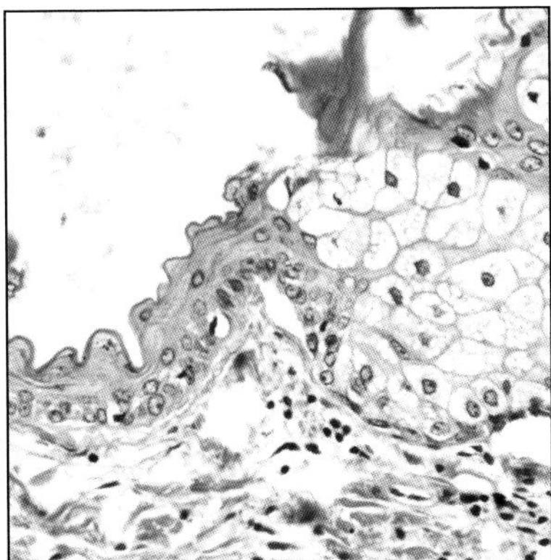

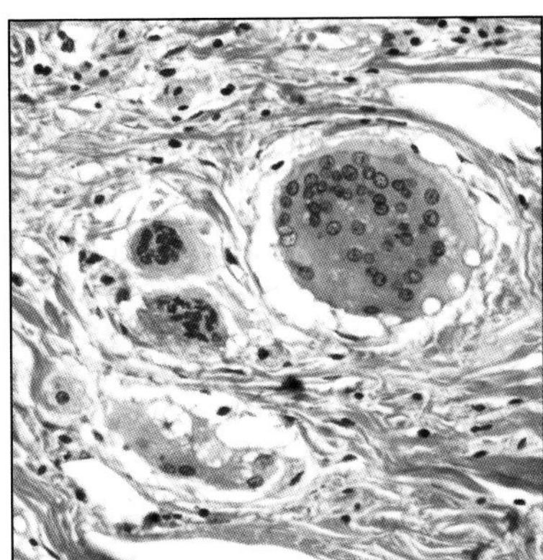

(Left) *In this sebaceous adenoma, solid nests of sebaceous cells may undergo cystic degeneration* ⇒*. Small primitive basaloid cells surround the periphery of the solid nests and cysts.* ***(Center)*** *Sebaceous cells are shown within a squamous epithelial cyst wall. Note the corrugated squamous lining.* ***(Right)*** *A foreign body giant cell reaction may be noted in response to extravasated cystic contents. A fine needle aspiration had been previously performed on this sebaceous adenoma.*

DUCTAL PAPILLOMAS

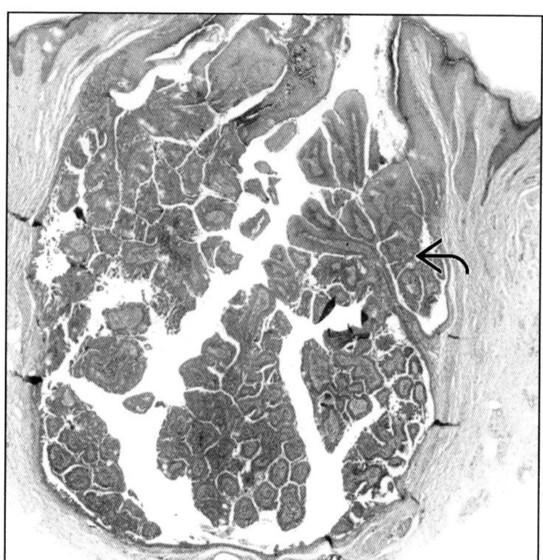

SP characterized by endophytic cavity of papillary (ductal) epithelium merging with surface squamous epithelium is shown; abrupt transition from squamous epithelium to mucosal proliferation is present.

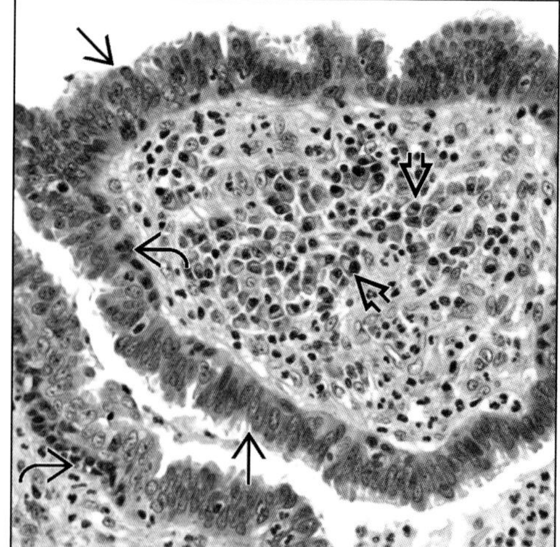

SP ductal epithelium includes an outer layer of columnar cells and an inner layer of cuboidal (basal) cells; the stroma includes an admixture of mature plasma cells and lymphocytes.

TERMINOLOGY

Abbreviations

- Sialadenoma papilliferum (SP)
- Inverted ductal papilloma (IDP)
- Intraductal papilloma (IP)

Synonyms

- Epidermoid papillary adenoma (for IDP)
  - IDP shares histologic features with sinonasal (schneiderian) inverted papilloma but does not share in biologic behavior of sinonasal (schneiderian) inverted papilloma
- Called SP due to similarity to cutaneous syringocystadenoma papilliferum

Definitions

- Ductal papillomas: Group of uncommon benign epithelial salivary gland neoplasms with unique histologic features that includes SP, IP, IDP
  - SP: Benign salivary gland tumor characterized by exophytic (papillary) and endophytic epithelial proliferation of mucosa or salivary duct origin
  - IP: Benign salivary gland neoplasm characterized by unicystic duct dilatation of luminal papillary proliferation arising from segment of interlobular or excretory duct
  - IDP: Benign salivary gland neoplasm characterized by
    - Luminal papillary projection arising at junction of salivary gland duct and oral mucosal surface epithelium with characteristic inverted (endophytic) growth

CLINICAL ISSUES

Epidemiology

- Incidence
  - SP, IP: Uncommon
  - IDP: Rare
- Age
  - SP, IDP: Occurs primarily in adults over wide range but most frequent in 6th-7th decades
  - IP: Primarily affects adults in 4th-7th decades
- Gender
  - SP: Male > Female
  - IDP, IP: Equal gender distribution

Site

- SP: Most common site of occurrence is palate (> 80%), particularly junction of hard and soft palates
  - Other minor salivary glands sites involved may include buccal mucosa, retromolar region, tonsillar pillar, lip, and nasopharynx (adenoids)
  - Major gland involvement rare; when involved, parotid gland most commonly affected
- IP: Intraoral minor salivary glands are most frequently involved
  - Buccal mucosa and lips most commonly affected
  - Other less common sites include floor of mouth, soft palate, and tongue
  - Involvement of major glands rare
- IDP: Most common sites of occurrence include lower lip and buccal (vestibular) mucosa
  - Other sites of involvement include upper lip, floor of mouth, and soft palate

Presentation

- SP: Asymptomatic (painless) lesion generally discovered incidentally
  - Clinical appearance often mistaken for papilloma
  - Duration of symptoms may be from months to years
- IP: Painless mass
- IDP: Generally asymptomatic; may present as slow-growing painless, nodular submucosal swelling

Treatment

- Surgical approaches
  - SP, IP, IDP: Conservative but complete surgical excision treatment of choice

DUCTAL PAPILLOMAS

Key Facts

Terminology

- Ductal papillomas represent group of uncommon benign epithelial salivary gland neoplasms with unique histologic features including
  - Sialadenoma papilliferum (SP)
  - Intraductal papilloma (IP)
  - Inverted ductal papilloma (IDP)

Clinical Issues

- SP: Palate most common site (> 80%), particularly junction of hard and soft palates
- IDP: Lower lip and buccal (vestibular) mucosa most common sites of occurrence
- IP: Buccal mucosa and lips most commonly affected
- Conservative but complete surgical excision treatment of choice and is curative for all ductal papillomas

Microscopic Pathology

- SP
  - Exophytic and endophytic proliferation of squamous and ductal epithelium
- IP
  - Unicystic cavity lined by cuboidal to columnar epithelial cells giving rise to papillary fronds filling cavity
- IDP
  - Unencapsulated but well-demarcated, endophytic basaloid and squamous/epidermoid cell growth

Top Differential Diagnoses

- Mucoepidermoid carcinoma, papillary cystadenoma, verrucous carcinoma

Prognosis

- SP, IP, IDP: Cured following complete excision
  - Recurrence rare
  - Malignant transformation of SP rarely occurs but not known to occur in IP, IDP

MACROSCOPIC FEATURES

General Features

- SP: Well-circumscribed, papillary or verrucoid, round to oval, tan-pink-appearing lesion
  - Base of lesion is broad or pedunculated
- IP: Well-circumscribed, mucosa-covered (nonulcerated) nodule
  - Cut section reveals unicystic lesion containing friable tissue
- IDP: Submucosal firm nodule
  - Small surface pore may be seen, which is contiguous with lumen of tumor

Size

- SP: Measures from few mm to as large as 7 cm
- IP: Measures from 0.5-2 cm in greatest dimension
- IDP: Measures up to 1.5 cm in greatest dimension

MICROSCOPIC PATHOLOGY

Histologic Features

- SP: Exophytic and endophytic proliferation of surface and ductal epithelium
  - Papillary to verrucoid growth composed of stratified squamous epithelium with fibrovascular connective tissue core
    - Acanthosis and parakeratosis of squamous epithelium seen
  - Endophytic proliferation of ductal epithelium present lying immediately subjacent to and merging with surface squamous epithelium
    - Abrupt transition from stratified squamous epithelium covering mucosal papillary proliferation to columnar epithelium lining ducts
    - Ductal epithelium unencapsulated forming dilated and tortuous structures
    - Deeper portions ductal structures have papillary luminal projections and microcysts
    - Absence of encapsulation and presence of poor circumscription at base of lesion may simulate presence of invasive growth
  - Ductal epithelium composed of 2 cell layers
    - Outer or luminal layer composed of tall columnar cells with eosinophilic granular cytoplasm
    - Inner or basal cell composed of cuboidal cells with eosinophilic granular cytoplasm
  - Interspersed mucous cells and oncocytic cells may be seen
  - Chronic inflammatory cell infiltrate predominantly plasma cells admixed with mature lymphocytes present in lamina propria of squamous component and in stroma of glandular component
- IP: Unicystic cavity lined by 1 or 2 layers of epithelial cells giving rise to numerous papillary fronds with thin fibrovascular core filling cavity
  - Epithelial cells comprised of 1 or 2 layers of cuboidal or columnar epithelium with eosinophilic cytoplasm
    - Papillations are covered by similar epithelium
    - Cytologic atypia is absent with no significant increase in mitotic activity
    - Mucocytes in form of goblet cells seen admixed within ductal epithelium
  - Continuity of papillary projections to cyst wall present, but depending on sections papillae may not be seen in continuity to cyst wall and appear to float within lumen
  - Epithelial component confined to cyst cavity without extension into adjacent stromal tissue
- IDP: Unencapsulated but well-demarcated, endophytic epithelial growth
  - Composed of thick, bulbous proliferations contiguous with but not protruding from surface epithelium
  - Communication with surface by narrow opening may be seen

DUCTAL PAPILLOMAS

Ductal Papillomas

	SP	IP	IDP
Gender	M > F	M = F	M = F
Age	Most frequent 6th-7th decades	Most frequent 4th-7th decades	Most frequent 6th decade
Site	Palate (> 80%), particularly junction of hard and soft palates	Buccal mucosa, lips	Lower lip, buccal (vestibular) mucosa
Presentation	Painless lesion discovered incidentally	Painless (submucosal) mass	Painless, nodular submucosal swelling
Histology	Exophytic squamous epithelial proliferation merging with endophytic ductal epithelial proliferation forming dilated and tortuous papillary structures	Unicystic cavity lined by cuboidal to columnar epithelial cells giving rise to papillary fronds filling cavity	Unencapsulated, well-demarcated, endophytic basaloid and squamous/epidermoid epithelial growth composed of thick, bulbous proliferations contiguous with but not protruding from surface epithelium
Treatment	Complete surgical excision	Complete surgical excision	Complete surgical excision
Prognosis	Rarely recurs; malignant transformation rarely occurs	Rarely recurs; malignant transformation does not occur	Rarely recurs; malignant transformation does not occur

SP = sialadenoma papilliferum; IP = intraductal papilloma; IDP = inverted ductal papilloma.

- Downward (endophytic) growth appears to fill luminal cavity
  - Endophytic growth is "pushing" into submucosa rather than demonstrating invasion or infiltration
- Consists of basaloid and squamous/epidermoid cells with interspersed mucous cells and microcytes
- Cytologic atypia is absent with no significant increase in mitotic activity
- Luminal surface epithelium composed of cuboidal or columnar cells with papillary appearance

ANCILLARY TESTS

Histochemistry

- Mucous cells: Intracytoplasmic mucicarmine and diastase-resistant, PAS(+) material

Immunohistochemistry

- SP ductal luminal cells reactive for cytokeratins (AE1/AE3, CK7, CK19, CAM5.2), CEA, EMA, S100 protein
- SP basal cells reactive for CK7, CK14, S100 protein, vimentin
- Langerhans cells in SP S100 protein and CD1a positive

DIFFERENTIAL DIAGNOSIS

Mucoepidermoid Carcinoma (MEC)

- Characteristic cell types, including epidermoid cells, mucocytes, and intermediate cells, often with proliferative (thickened appearance) in MEC but absent in SP, IP, IDP
- Presence of invasive tumor in MEC not a feature of SP, IP, or IDP
  - Diagnosis of MEC can be made in the absence of invasive tumor only if requisite cell types (epidermoid cells, mucocytes and intermediate cells) identified

Papillary Cystadenoma (PC)

- Possible differential diagnosis with IP; differentiating features include
  - IP: Almost invariably unicystic lesion; PC: Most multicystic
  - IP: Occurs in associated with dilated salivary gland duct; PC: No association with salivary gland duct
  - Intraluminal papillations of IP more complex and numerous than papillae of PC

Verrucous Carcinoma (VC)

- Possible differential diagnosis with SP, differentiating features include
  - Presence of tiered keratosis in VC absent in SP
  - Absence of ductal component in VC present in SP

SELECTED REFERENCES

1. Kubota N et al: Inverted ductal papilloma of minor salivary gland: case report with immunohistochemical study and literature review. Pathol Int. 56(8):457-61, 2006
2. Cabov T et al: Oral inverted ductal papilloma. Br J Oral Maxillofac Surg. 42(1):75-7, 2004
3. Gomes AP et al: Sialadenoma papilliferum: immunohistochemical study. Int J Oral Maxillofac Surg. 33(6):621-4, 2004
4. Brannon RB et al: Ductal papillomas of salivary gland origin: A report of 19 cases and a review of the literature. Oral Surg Oral Med Oral Pathol Oral Radiol Endod. 92(1):68-77, 2001
5. Ubaidat MA et al: Sialadenoma papilliferum of the hard palate: report of 2 cases and immunohistochemical evaluation. Arch Pathol Lab Med. 125(12):1595-7, 2001
6. Mirza S et al: Intraductal papilloma of the submandibular gland. J Laryngol Otol. 114(6):481-3, 2000
7. Nagao T et al: Intraductal papillary tumors of the major salivary glands: case reports of benign and malignant variants. Arch Pathol Lab Med. 124(2):291-5, 2000
8. Maiorano E et al: Sialadenoma papilliferum: an immunohistochemical study of five cases. J Oral Pathol Med. 25(6):336-42, 1996
9. de Sousa SO et al: Inverted ductal papilloma of minor salivary gland origin: morphological aspects and cytokeratin expression. Eur Arch Otorhinolaryngol. 252(6):370-3, 1995
10. Koutlas IG et al: Immunohistochemical evaluation and in situ hybridization in a case of oral inverted ductal papilloma. J Oral Maxillofac Surg. 52(5):503-6, 1994
11. Waldron CA et al: Tumors of the intraoral minor salivary glands: a demographic and histologic study of 426 cases. Oral Surg Oral Med Oral Pathol. 66(3):323-33, 1988

DUCTAL PAPILLOMAS

Microscopic Features

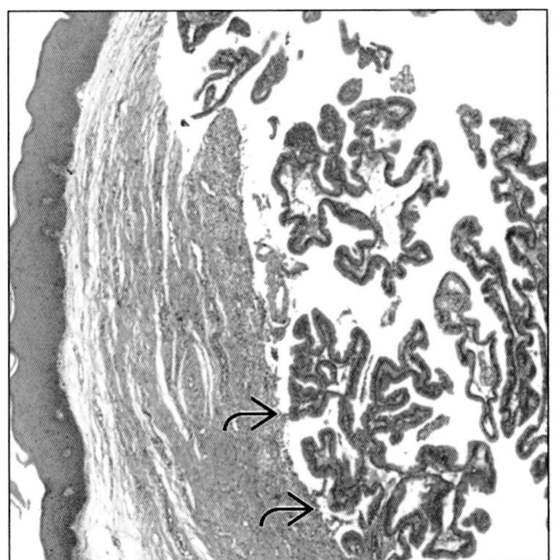
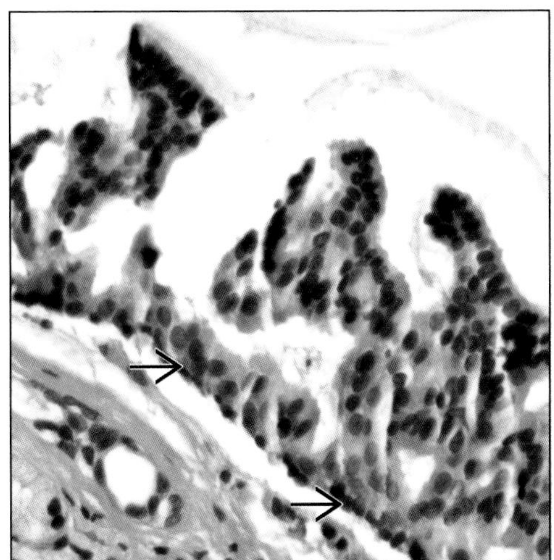

(Left) *Intraductal papilloma is characterized here by a submucosal unicystic epithelial-lined cavity giving rise ↷ to a papillary epithelial proliferation with fibrovascular cores filling the cystic cavity.* ***(Right)*** *At higher magnification, the cyst is lined by 1 or 2 layers of epithelial cells → that give rise to a proliferation comprised of cuboidal to columnar epithelium with eosinophilic cytoplasm within the cyst cavity.*

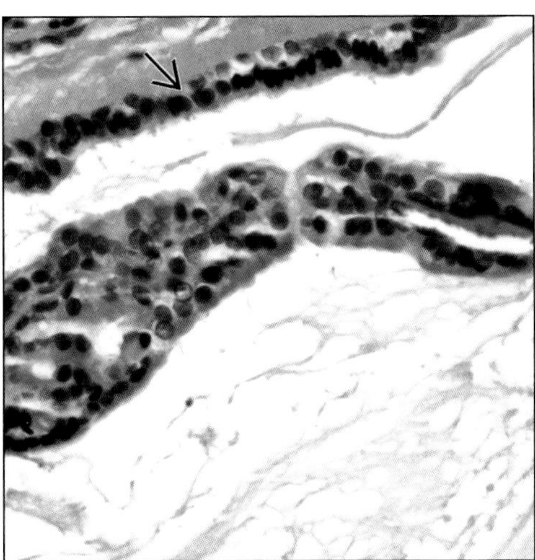
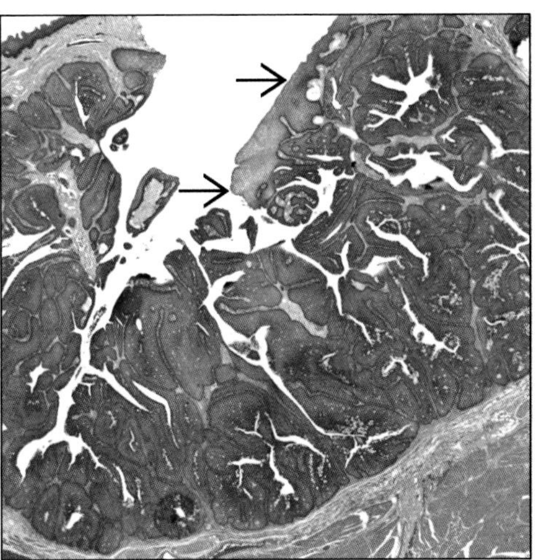

(Left) *Another area of the intraductal papilloma shows the cyst lining cells → and intracystic papillary structure comprised of cuboidal to columnar epithelium with eosinophilic cytoplasm.* ***(Right)*** *Inverted ductal papilloma appears as an unencapsulated but well-demarcated, endophytic epithelial growth composed of thick, bulbous proliferation contiguous with → but not protruding from the surface epithelium. The downward (endophytic) growth appears to fill a luminal cavity.*

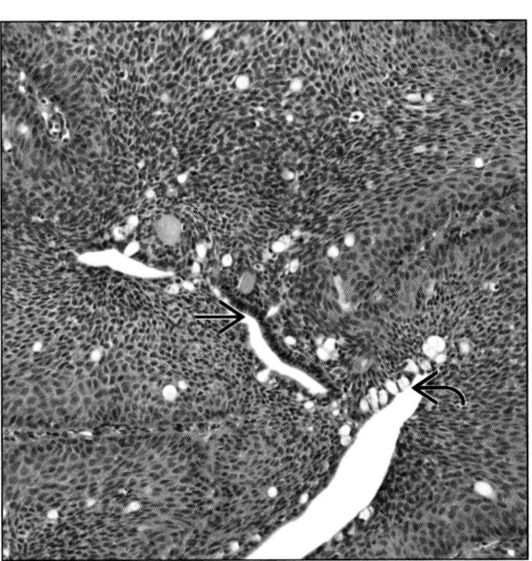
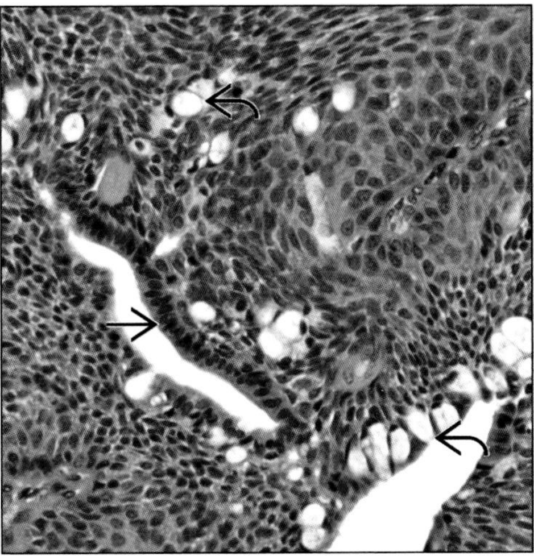

(Left) *Inverted ductal papilloma consists of a predominantly basaloid and squamous/epidermoid cell proliferation with interspersed mucous cells ↷ and luminal surface epithelium with cuboidal or columnar cells →.* ***(Right)*** *At higher magnification, the predominant basaloid and squamous/epidermoid cell component is evident lacking cytologic atypia and increased mitotic activity. Mucocytes ↷ and luminal surface cuboidal or columnar cells are evident →.*

CYSTADENOMA

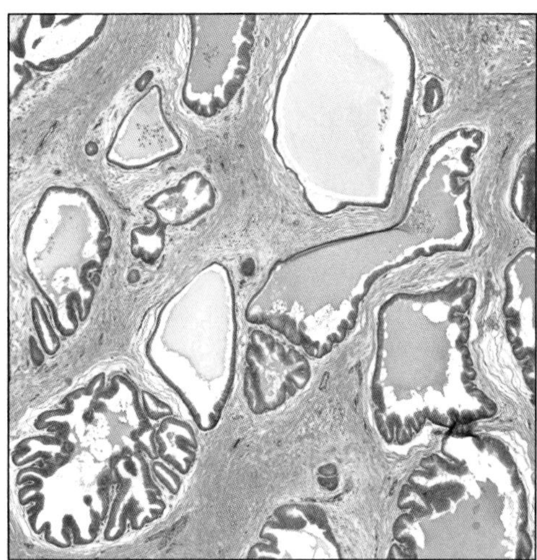

Cystadenoma demonstrates multiple, variably sized cystic spaces supported by fibrous connective tissue. Papillary infoldings and an eosinophilic fluid are evident within many cystic spaces.

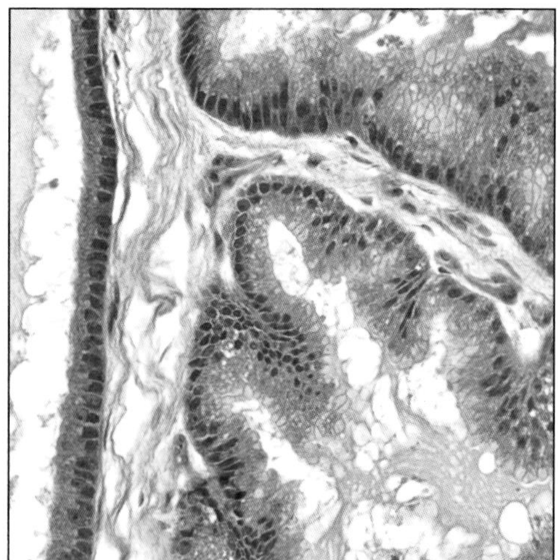

The epithelial lining of cystadenoma typically varies from cuboidal to columnar epithelial cells. This example demonstrates short to tall columnar epithelial cells with a mucinous cytomorphology.

TERMINOLOGY

Synonyms

- Cystic duct adenoma

Definitions

- Benign unicystic or multicystic epithelial neoplasm devoid of extraluminal solid growth

CLINICAL ISSUES

Epidemiology

- Incidence
  - Approximately 4% of all benign epithelial salivary gland neoplasms
  - Roughly 10% of all minor salivary gland adenomas
- Age
  - Wide range
  - Average: 6th to 7th decades
- Gender
  - Female > Male (2-3:1)

Site

- Location and relative frequency vary depending upon study
- Parotid gland affected in about 50% of cases
- Minor salivary glands next most common
  - Lips > buccal mucosa > palate
- Occasional submandibular gland involvement

Presentation

- Slowly growing painless mass
- Mucosal lesions may simulate mucoceles

Treatment

- Conservative surgical excision

Prognosis

- Recurrence uncommon after complete removal
- Rare malignant transformation

MACROSCOPIC FEATURES

General Features

- Single to multiple cystic spaces of variable size
- Possible intraluminal proliferation

MICROSCOPIC PATHOLOGY

Histologic Features

- Well circumscribed but variable encapsulation
  - Possible irregular interface with surrounding parenchyma
  - Cysts separated by fibrous connective tissue
  - Focal to spotty inflammatory element may be present in connective tissues
- Cystic spaces of variable number and size
  - Epithelial lining typically composed of cuboidal to columnar cells
    - Occasional mucinous or oncocytic epithelial lining, which may be focal or diffuse
    - Squamoid lining rare and typically focal
  - Intraluminal papillary proliferation may be evident
    - Especially common in unicystic lesions
  - **Papillary oncocytic cystadenoma**
    - Cystadenoma with significant intraluminal papillary projections surfaced by a single or bilayered oncocytic epithelial lining
    - Epithelial component may resemble Warthin tumor
  - Cysts may contain eosinophilic fluid &/or scattered detached cells
- Cytology bland with rare mitotic figures
- Extraluminal solid growth is not typical
  - Presence should raise suspicion for malignancy, especially if abnormal cytology evident

CYSTADENOMA

Key Facts

Terminology
- Benign unicystic or multicystic epithelial neoplasm devoid of extraluminal solid growth

Clinical Issues
- Primary location in parotid gland and minor salivary glands of lips, buccal mucosa, and palate
- Conservative surgical excision
- Recurrence uncommon after complete removal

Microscopic Pathology
- Well circumscribed but variable encapsulation
- Cystic spaces of variable number and size
- Epithelial lining typically composed of cuboidal to columnar cells
- Intraluminal papillary proliferation may be evident

Top Differential Diagnoses
- Mucoepidermoid carcinoma, salivary duct cyst, cystadenocarcinoma, Warthin tumor

DIFFERENTIAL DIAGNOSIS

Mucoepidermoid Carcinoma
- May contain significant cystic component and papillary growth
- Features favoring mucoepidermoid carcinoma include
  - Extraluminal solid growth of epidermoid, intermediate, &/or clear cells
  - Infiltrative border

Salivary Duct Cyst
- Composed of markedly dilated salivary gland duct
  - Majority in parotid gland
  - Typically unicystic
  - Flattened epithelial lining surrounded by dense fibrous connective tissue
- Unicystic cystadenoma favored if intraluminal epithelial proliferation present

Cystadenocarcinoma
- Cystadenoma and low-grade cystadenocarcinoma may be cytologically and architecturally similar
- Malignancy in cystadenocarcinoma mainly defined by frank invasion of salivary parenchyma

Warthin Tumor (Papillary Cystadenoma Lymphomatosum)
- Multiple cystic spaces lined by bilayered oncocytic epithelium
  - Similar to papillary oncocytic cystadenoma
- Prominent dense lymphoid stroma is absent in cystadenoma

SELECTED REFERENCES

1. Zhang S et al: Papillary oncocytic cystadenoma of the parotid glands: a report of 2 cases with varied cytologic features. Acta Cytol. 53(4):445-8, 2009
2. Lim CS et al: Papillary cystadenoma of a minor salivary gland: report of a case involving cytological analysis and review of the literature. Oral Surg Oral Med Oral Pathol Oral Radiol Endod. 105(1):e28-33, 2008
3. Buchner A et al: Relative frequency of intra-oral minor salivary gland tumors: a study of 380 cases from northern California and comparison to reports from other parts of the world. J Oral Pathol Med. 36(4):207-14, 2007
4. Toida M et al: Intraoral minor salivary gland tumors: a clinicopathological study of 82 cases. Int J Oral Maxillofac Surg. 34(5):528-32, 2005
5. Michal M et al: Micropapillary carcinoma of the parotid gland arising in mucinous cystadenoma. Virchows Arch. 437(4):465-8, 2000
6. Simionescu C et al: Histopathologic and immunohistochemical study in one case of cystadenoma of parotid gland becoming malignant. Rom J Morphol Embryol. 45:159-64, 1999
7. Alexis JB et al: Papillary cystadenoma of a minor salivary gland. J Oral Maxillofac Surg. 53(1):70-2; discussion 73, 1995
8. Waldron CA et al: Tumors of the intraoral minor salivary glands: a demographic and histologic study of 426 cases. Oral Surg Oral Med Oral Pathol. 66(3):323-33, 1988

IMAGE GALLERY

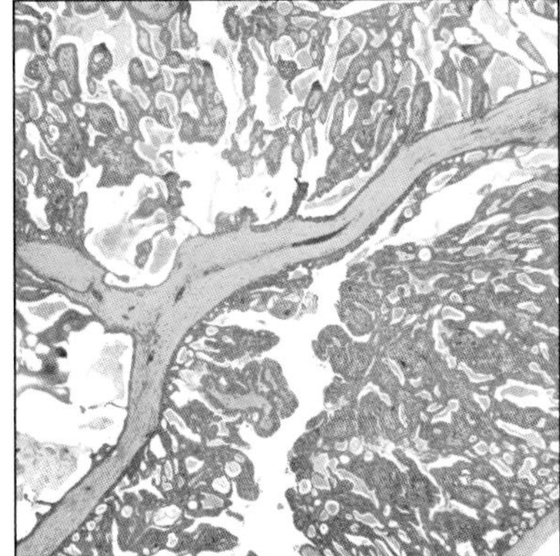
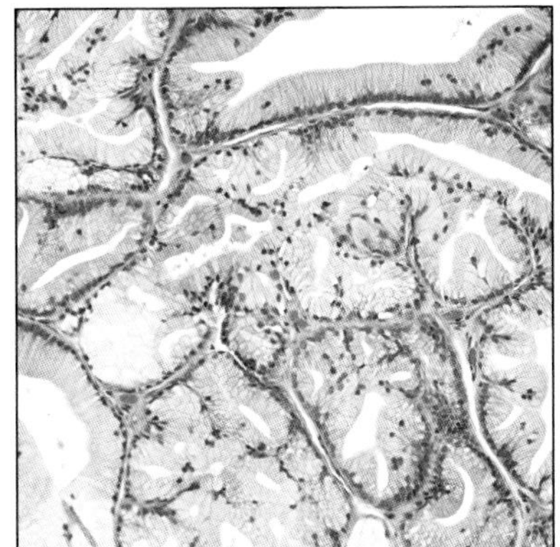
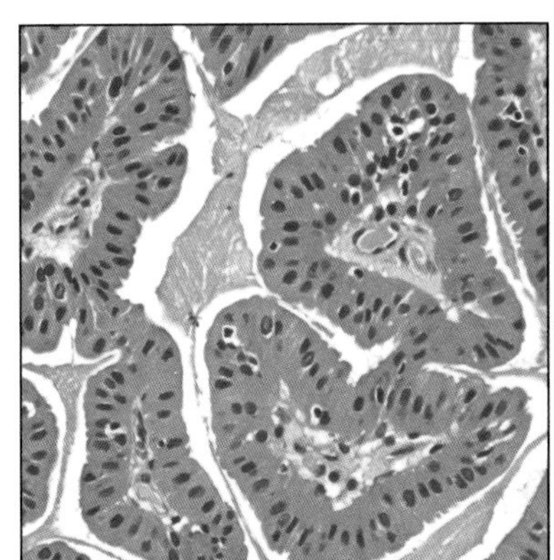

*(**Left**) Relatively large cystic spaces containing a papillary intraluminal epithelial proliferation. The cysts are separated by fibrous connective tissue. (**Center**) A cystadenoma composed of tall columnar mucocytes is shown. This rare form has been termed "mucinous cystadenoma" or "cystadenoma, mucous cell type." (**Right**) A papillary oncocytic cystadenoma demonstrates intraluminal papillary projections composed of bilayered oncocytic epithelium, similar to Warthin tumor.*

HEMANGIOMA

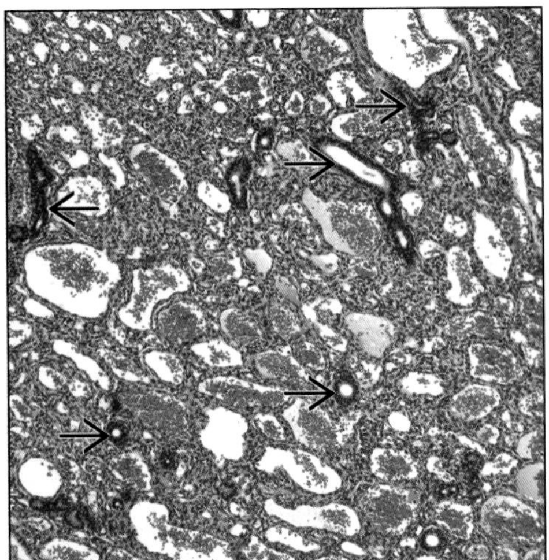

A juvenile capillary hemangioma shows salivary gland ducts ⇒ associated with innumerable endothelial-lined vascular spaces. The duct architecture is intact, but the glandular tissue is replaced.

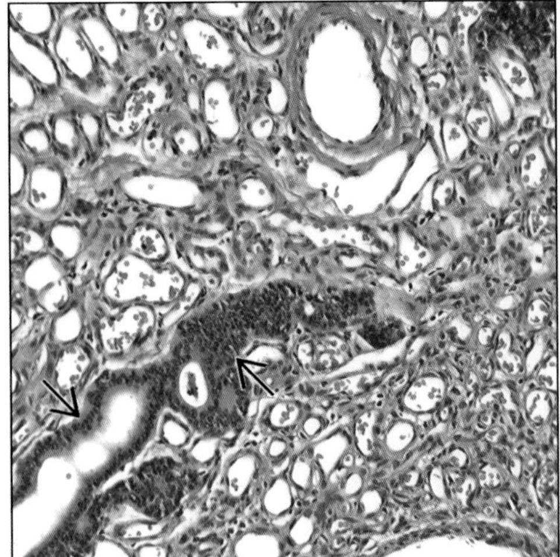

An excretory duct of the parotid gland ⇒ is almost completely surrounded by a vascular proliferation. There are extravasated erythrocytes in the lumen. There is no atypia or anastomosing spaces.

TERMINOLOGY

Synonyms

- Benign infantile hemangioendothelioma (discouraged)
- Infantile hemangioma
- Cellular hemangioma
- Immature capillary hemangioma
- Juvenile hemangioma

Definitions

- Tumor composed of proliferation of endothelial cells forming variably mature blood vessels
  - All histologic variants of hemangioma occur in salivary glands, but capillary (juvenile) hemangioma is most common

CLINICAL ISSUES

Epidemiology

- Incidence
  - Rare
    - Account for < 0.5% of salivary tumors
    - Mesenchymal tumors account for about 3.5% of salivary gland tumors
    - < 1% of all hemangiomas develop in salivary gland
    - Schwannomas and lipomas are most common followed by hemangiomas
- Age
  - Majority (up to 90%) diagnosed in 1st 2 decades
    - Highest in perinatal or neonatal period
  - > 90% of parotid gland tumors in infants < 1 year old are hemangioma
  - Cavernous hemangioma: Usually seen in adolescents or adults
- Gender
  - Female > > Male (2-4:1)
    - **Capillary (juvenile)** hemangioma shows this ratio
    - **Cavernous** hemangioma tends to be seen more frequently in older males

Site

- Parotid gland is most common location (~ 90%)
  - Very rare in submandibular, sublingual, or minor salivary glands
- Slight predilection for left side
- Up to 25% are bilateral

Presentation

- Usually asymptomatic soft tissue parotid swelling
- Arc of development is seen
  - Small swelling few weeks after birth
    - 1/2 of patients have "cutaneous" lesion at birth
    - Gives bluish discoloration of overlying skin
    - Accentuated when infant cries (baby becomes hypoxemic, so "blue" appearance is highlighted)
  - Mass detected by 6 months
    - Often shows rapid enlargement
    - During proliferative phase, 50-60% show skin surface ulceration
    - Overlying skin is usually not directly affected, but hemangioma "pushes" up
    - Facial asymmetry and deformity may be present
  - Sometime after 1st year, slow regression (involution) begins
    - May take years to completely involute (into teens): Very slow involutional phase
- Frequently, hemangiomas become large and involve adjacent structures
  - Ear, hypopharynx, parapharyngeal space, base of skull, subglottis, lip, eye, nose
- Pain and tenderness are not typical
- Consumptive coagulopathy (Kasabach-Merritt syndrome) **not** associated with salivary gland hemangiomas
- Complications may arise and include cutaneous ulceration, bleeding, airway compression, congestive heart failure

HEMANGIOMA

Key Facts

Terminology
- Tumor composed of proliferation of endothelial cells forming variably mature blood vessels
  - Capillary (juvenile) hemangioma is most common

Clinical Issues
- 90% diagnosed in 1st 2 decades (neonatal period)
- Female > > Male (2-4:1)
- Parotid gland is most common location (~ 90%)
  - Up to 25% are bilateral
- Gives bluish discoloration of overlying skin, especially when baby cries
- May show rapid enlargement during proliferative phase, involving adjacent structures
- Can be managed by observation, pharmacologic therapy, &/or surgery
- Majority spontaneously involute before 7 years (75-95%), many earlier
- Pharmacological therapy yields excellent response

Microscopic Pathology
- Diffuse gland enlargement, with lobular expansion
- Gland replaced by closely packed endothelial cells and small immature capillaries, leaving ducts intact
- Variably sized and shaped vessels
- Mitoses often increased but never atypical

Ancillary Tests
- Endothelial cells positive: CD31, CD34, FVIIIRAg
- Residual ducts are keratin positive

Top Differential Diagnoses
- Angiosarcoma, Kaposi sarcoma

- Rarely, may have "turkey wattle" sign: Enlargement of facial mass on dependency of head
  - Considered pathognomonic of vascular malformation or hemangioma
- Exceedingly rare malignant transformation

Treatment
- Options, risks, complications
  - Can be managed by observation, pharmacologic therapy, &/or surgery
  - Delay any definitive treatment in hope of spontaneous resolution
  - Biologically benign but occasionally associated with extensive and life-threatening growth
    - Uncommonly, tracheostomy may be required
    - Congestive heart failure due to shunting
  - Complications may include failure to thrive, scarring, facial nerve injury (during surgery), hematoma, blood loss, facial deformity, and death
  - Pressure (compression) therapy or embolization if tumor is large
  - Do not lend themselves to fine needle aspiration or biopsy due to bleeding complications
- Surgical approaches
  - Early cosmetic resection can cure disfiguring tumors
    - Cavernous hemangiomas in adults should be excised (do not spontaneously involute)
  - Reconstructive procedure may be necessary after involution or pharmacologic therapy
    - Removal of redundant skin &/or soft tissue or auricular reconstruction
- Drugs
  - Pharmacological therapy (corticosteroids and interferon) yields a response in up to 98% of cases
    - May take several years to completely involute/resolve/regress
    - No major complications with pharmacologic management
  - Corticosteroids result in regression or stabilization in about 80%
  - Interferon-α 2a or 2b gives additional regression in corticosteroid-resistant cases (95% of cases)
- Other
  - Laser (thermocautery) and radiotherapy only employed in rare, life-threatening cases
  - Alcohol injection no longer used

Prognosis
- Pediatric tumors initially grow rapidly, but vast majority involute
  - Majority spontaneously involute before 7 years (75-95%), many earlier
- Very rare malignant transformation to angiosarcoma
- Reconstruction frequently required after involution

IMAGE FINDINGS

Radiographic Findings
- Ultrasonography favored as initial imaging study because lesions are cystic
  - Vascular lesions can be demonstrated with color Doppler imaging
- Tc-99m labeled red blood cell (RBC) scintigraphy can be used

MR Findings
- T1-weighted images: Masses are isointense to muscle
- T2-weighted images: Masses are hyperintense with numerous small vessels
- Strong enhancement with gadolinium
- Extent of lesion easily documented, helping to guide management

MACROSCOPIC FEATURES

General Features
- Diffuse gland enlargement, with expansion of lobules
  - Discrete or distinct tumor mass is not seen
- Hemorrhagic
- Red to brown

Size
- Frequently large (up to 10 cm)

HEMANGIOMA

MICROSCOPIC PATHOLOGY

Histologic Features

- Expand salivary gland lobules and replace parenchyma
- Separated into hemangioma (> 90%) and lymphangioma (< 10%) (not considered here)
- Hemangiomas divided into juvenile (infantile) capillary hemangioma, cavernous hemangioma, and arteriovenous malformation (latter not further considered)

Juvenile (Infantile) Capillary Hemangioma

- Lobular architecture of gland is intact, separated by septa, but lobules are enlarged
- Salivary acini diffusely replaced by endothelial cells and small immature capillaries
  - Salivary gland ducts stand out, surrounded by proliferation
  - Peripheral nerves are not involved
- Closely packed sheets of endothelial cells and pericytes
- Vascular differentiation may be limited to small, inconspicuous lumina
  - During arc of development, lumina become dominant feature
- Variably sized and shaped vessels
  - Small capillary channels lined by plump, round to ovoid endothelial cells
    - Indistinct cell borders
    - Oval nuclei, occasional groove, and small nucleoli
  - Larger, thin-walled vessels often accentuated at tumor periphery
- Mitoses often increased but never atypical
- Diffuse interstitial fibrosis and infarction seen in regression
  - Thrombi and phleboliths may be present

Cavernous Hemangioma

- Large, expanding, cystic cavities, filled with blood
- Expanded and compressed parotid parenchyma at periphery
  - Lacks retained salivary gland ducts
- Lined by plump to flattened endothelial cells

ANCILLARY TESTS

Cytology

- Usually **not** performed since there is high index of clinical accuracy and desire to avoid bleeding
- Bloody aspirates with groups and clusters of spindle-shaped cells and bland endothelial cells
  - Cells have limited cytoplasm and oval nuclei
- Isolated ductal structures may be noted

Histochemistry

- Reticulin highlights small fibers encircling vessels

Immunohistochemistry

- Endothelial cells positive: CD31, CD34, and FVIIIRAg
- Glucose transporter 1 protein (GLUT1) positive in juvenile hemangiomas

DIFFERENTIAL DIAGNOSIS

Angiosarcoma

- Exceedingly rare in age group affected by hemangioma
- Freely anastomosing vascular channels, pleomorphic cells, increased mitoses, atypical mitoses, necrosis, invasion and destructive growth (glandular architecture destroyed)

Kaposi Sarcoma

- Seen in acquired immune deficiency syndrome (AIDS), males predominantly, and older age at presentation
- Involves submandibular or parotid gland, showing spindle cell vascular proliferation arranged in fasciculated bundles, variable nuclear pleomorphism, mitotic figures, extravasated erythrocytes, and hyaline globules
- Human herpes virus 8 (HHV8) will be positive

Phleboliths and Angiolithiasis

- May mimic sialoliths, although exceedingly uncommon in young patients
- Angiolithiasis are structures showing laminations of alternating low and high mineral content (apatite) associated with blood and fibroblasts
  - Thought to develop in regressed hemangioma

SELECTED REFERENCES

1. Sinno H et al: Management of infantile parotid gland hemangiomas: a 40-year experience. Plast Reconstr Surg. 125(1):265-73, 2010
2. Greene AK et al: Management of parotid hemangioma in 100 children. Plast Reconstr Surg. 113(1):53-60, 2004
3. Wong KT et al: Vascular lesions of parotid gland in adult patients: diagnosis with high-resolution ultrasound and MRI. Br J Radiol. 77(919):600-6, 2004
4. Fanburg-Smith JC et al: Oral and salivary gland angiosarcoma: a clinicopathologic study of 29 cases. Mod Pathol. 16(3):263-71, 2003
5. Childers EL et al: Hemangioma of the salivary gland: a study of ten cases of a rarely biopsied/excised lesion. Ann Diagn Pathol. 6(6):339-44, 2002
6. Thompson LD: Hemangioma of the parotid. Ear Nose Throat J. 81(11):769, 2002
7. Khurana KK et al: The role of fine-needle aspiration biopsy in the diagnosis and management of juvenile hemangioma of the parotid gland and cheek. Arch Pathol Lab Med. 125(10):1340-3, 2001
8. Castle JT et al: Kaposi sarcoma of major salivary gland origin: A clinicopathologic series of six cases. Cancer. 88(1):15-23, 2000
9. North PE et al: GLUT1: a newly discovered immunohistochemical marker for juvenile hemangiomas. Hum Pathol. 31(1):11-22, 2000
10. Lack EE et al: Histopathologic review of salivary gland tumors in childhood. Arch Otolaryngol Head Neck Surg. 114(8):898-906, 1988
11. Batsakis JG: Vascular tumors of the salivary glands. Ann Otol Rhinol Laryngol. 95(6 Pt 1):649-50, 1986
12. Seifert G et al: [Mesenchymal (non-epithelial) salivary gland tumors. Analysis of 167 tumor cases of the salivary gland register.] Laryngol Rhinol Otol (Stuttg). 65(9):485-91, 1986
13. Schuller DE et al: Salivary gland neoplasms in children. Otolaryngol Clin North Am. 10(2):399-412, 1977

HEMANGIOMA

Microscopic Features

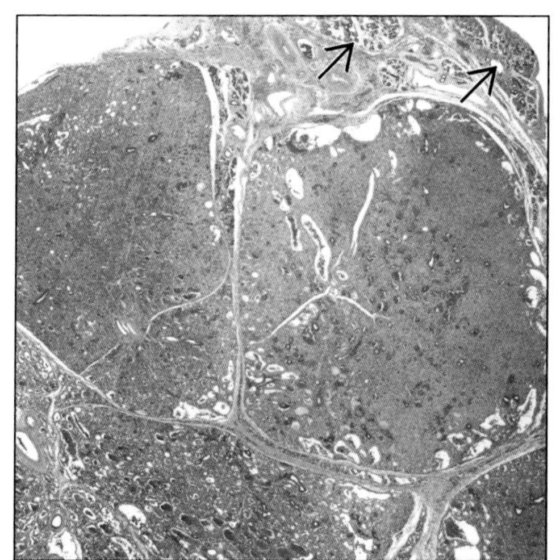

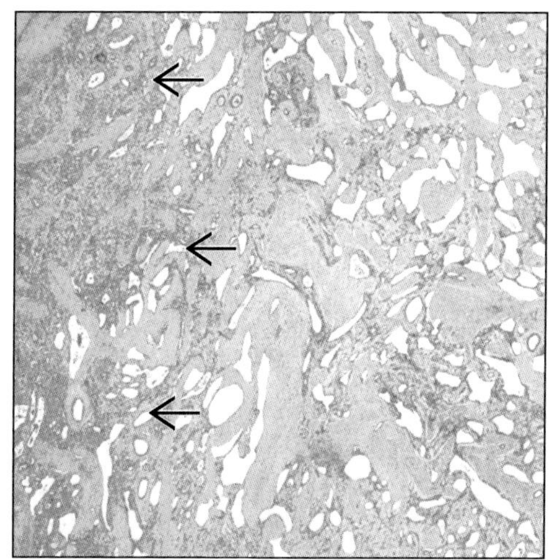

*(**Left**) On low power, residual salivary gland parenchyma is present →. Note the maintained lobular architecture, with fibrous septa creating the separation. There are many vascular channels identified (filled with blood) even at low power. (**Right**) Residual salivary gland is noted →, although the vascular channels in this hemangioma are accompanied by more fibrosis. This is a tumor that has started to involute. Dilated vascular spaces are easily identified.*

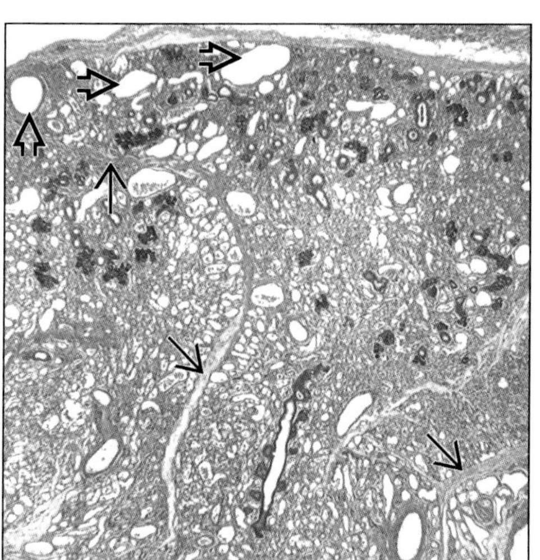

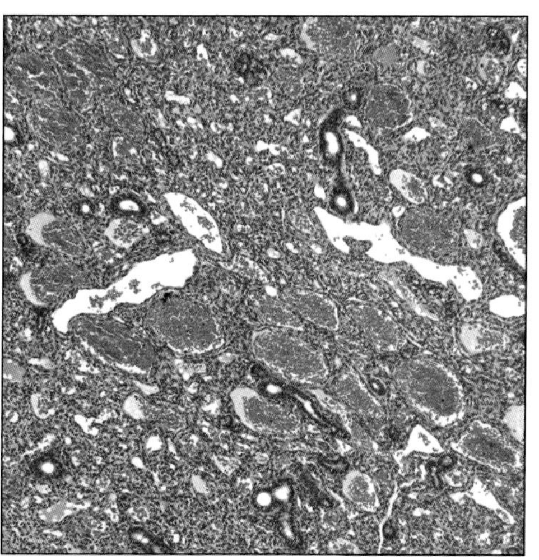

*(**Left**) On low power, the dark blue residual salivary gland ducts stand out against the background of the vascular proliferation. Fibrous septa → are easily identified. The vascular spaces are variably sized, with larger vessels noted at the periphery ⇨. (**Right**) An intermediate magnification shows large vessels filled with erythrocytes. Some of the vessels are empty. Note the more "solid" proliferation of vessels in the background. The ducts (dark blue) are not destroyed.*

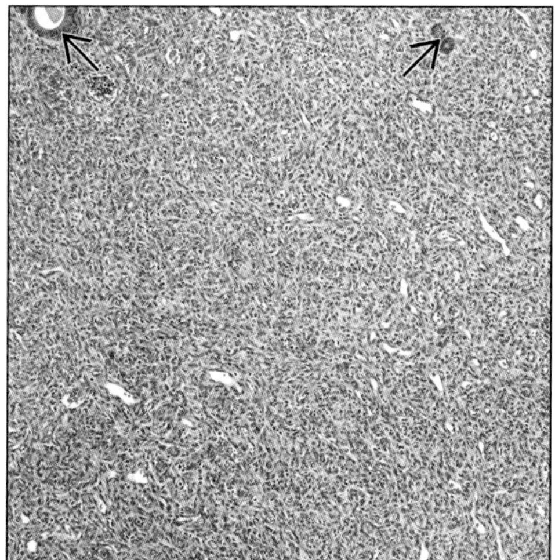

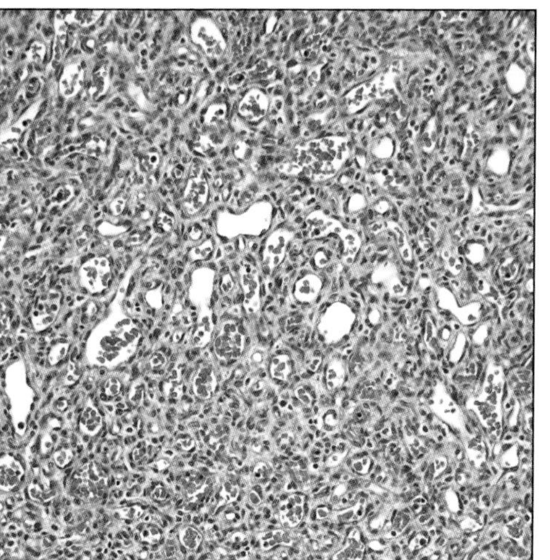

*(**Left**) A highly cellular proliferation replaces the salivary gland acini in this case. Isolated ducts are noted →. Small slit-like spaces hint at the vascular nature of the lesion. However, the majority of this lesion is comprised of immature vascular channels and endothelial cells. (**Right**) Numerous capillary-sized vessels are lined by unremarkable endothelial cells. Erythrocytes are noted within the lumen of many of the vessels. There is no atypia.*

MUCOEPIDERMOID CARCINOMA

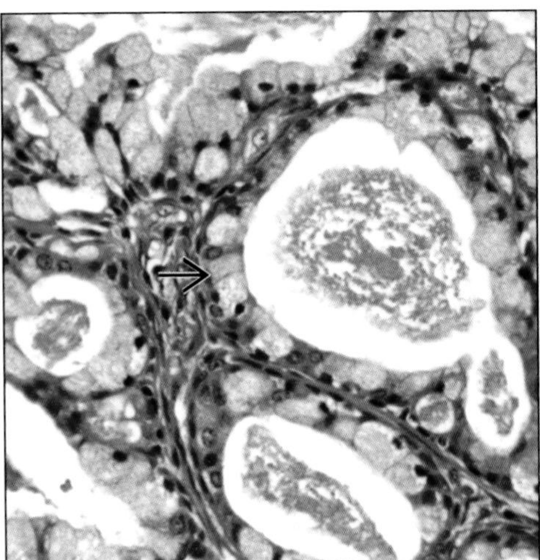

Hematoxylin & eosin shows small cystic spaces lined by mucous cells ⇨. These cells are large, ovoid, and have abundant foamy cytoplasm. The nuclei are frequently "squashed" toward the periphery.

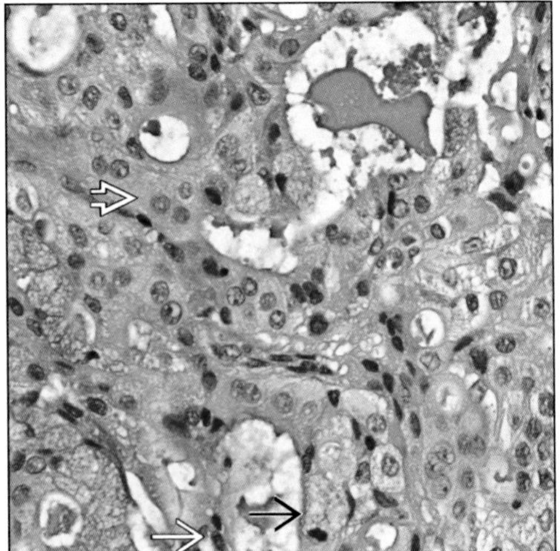

There are epithelial cells ➡, intermediate cells ➡, and mucocytes ⇨. This is the required triad of cell types for the diagnosis of mucoepidermoid carcinoma, although cell types are variably present.

TERMINOLOGY

Abbreviations

- Mucoepidermoid carcinoma (MEC)

Definitions

- Malignant epithelial tumor with variable components of mucous, epidermoid, and intermediate cells

ETIOLOGY/PATHOGENESIS

Environmental Exposure

- Ionizing radiation
  - Latent period between irradiation to malignancy varies
    - Long-term follow-up is required

Pathogenesis of Primary Intraosseous Tumors

- Malignant transformation of epithelial lining of odontogenic cysts
  - Favored mechanism
- Malignant transformation of ectopic salivary gland tissue

CLINICAL ISSUES

Epidemiology

- Incidence
  - Salivary gland carcinomas are rare, comprising ~ 0.3% of all cancers
  - Most common malignant salivary gland tumor
    - Represents ~ 16% of all salivary gland tumors
  - Most common salivary gland tumor to arise in gnathic bones
- Age
  - Wide range
  - Most common malignant salivary gland tumor in children
- Gender
  - Female > Male

Site

- Major glands
  - Parotid gland is most common location
- Minor glands
  - Palate or buccal mucosa
- Central (primary intraosseous)
  - Originates within jaws
    - Predilection for mandible

Presentation

- Painless, slow-growing mass
- Parotid gland
  - Usually asymptomatic solitary mass
  - Symptomatic
    - Pain, facial numbness and paralysis
    - Drainage from ipsilateral ear
    - Dysphagia, trismus
    - Rapid increase in size
- Minor glands
  - May be misdiagnosed clinically as reactive or inflammatory lesion
  - Swelling, fluctuant, red-blue mass
  - Secondary ulceration occasionally
  - Bleeding or drainage
  - Dysphagia, paresthesia
- Primary intraosseous
  - Radiolucent lesion on dental radiograph
  - Swelling, pain, facial asymmetry, trismus
- Rarely associated with other benign salivary gland tumors
  - Can be metachronous or synchronous
  - Pleomorphic adenoma, Warthin tumor, oncocytoma

Treatment

- Surgical approaches
  - Major glands

MUCOEPIDERMOID CARCINOMA

Key Facts

Terminology
- Malignant epithelial tumor with variable components of mucous, epidermoid, and intermediate cells

Clinical Issues
- Most common malignant salivary gland tumor
- Major glands most commonly affected, followed by minor salivary glands
- Low-grade tumors rarely metastasize
- Positive surgical margins are predictive of recurrence or residual tumor

Macroscopic Features
- Circumscribed, partially encapsulated, or poorly defined periphery

Microscopic Pathology
- Variably sized cystic spaces
- Contains intermediate cells, epidermoid cells, and mucocytes
  - Mucocytes are arranged in nests or scattered
- Clear cells may be predominant
- Tumor-associated lymphoid proliferation (TALP)
- Tumor grading very helpful in predicting outcome and management

Ancillary Tests
- Mucicarmine positive mucocytes

Top Differential Diagnoses
- Sialometaplasia
- Mucus extravasation reaction
- Squamous cell carcinoma
- Clear cell adenocarcinoma and epithelial-myoepithelial carcinoma

---

    - Conservative excision for stage I and II parotid gland tumors
    - Preservation of facial nerve, if possible
    - Complete resection of submandibular gland
    - Neck dissection for metastatic disease, large tumors, or high-grade tumors
  - Minor glands
    - Excision with wide margin
    - Lesion infiltrating or closely abutting bone may require resection of bone
    - Neck dissection for metastatic disease, large tumors, or high-grade tumors
  - Primary intraosseous
    - Enucleation or curettage
    - Segmental resection
    - Neck dissection based on clinical findings
- Adjuvant therapy
  - Radiotherapy
    - Used when inoperable; positive margins
    - High-stage disease
  - Chemotherapy
    - May be useful for high-grade tumors

Prognosis
- Low-grade tumors
  - Rarely metastasize
  - Only 2.5% result in death
- High-grade tumors
  - 55-80% metastasize or result in death
- Positive surgical margins are predictive of recurrence
- Metastases
  - Predictive of poor prognosis
    - Lung, bone, brain
- Sites of aggressive tumors regardless of grade
  - Submandibular gland has prognosis similar to high-grade lesion
  - Tongue and floor of mouth
- Primary intraosseous rarely metastasize

IMAGE FINDINGS

General Features
- MR, CT, and radiographs used for major glands
- Minor gland tumors may show erosion of adjacent bone
- Primary intraosseous tumors are generally well-circumscribed radiolucencies

MACROSCOPIC FEATURES

General Features
- Circumscribed, partially encapsulated, or poorly defined periphery
- Cut surface
  - Pink, tan, or yellow
  - Cystic, sometimes with blood

Size
- Highly variable
  - < 1 cm to large disfiguring masses

MICROSCOPIC PATHOLOGY

Histologic Features
- Cystic spaces
  - Often filled with mucin
  - Occasionally papillary projections are present
- Epidermoid cells
  - Nests or scattered
  - Polygonal cells
- Intermediate cells
  - Large polygonal epidermoid cells
  - Small basal cells
  - Often found in nests or sheets
- Mucous cells
  - Intracytoplasmic mucin
  - Large or ovoid
  - Vacuolated or clear cytoplasm
  - In groups or individually scattered
- Clear cells

MUCOEPIDERMOID CARCINOMA

- Usually < 10% of cells but can be dominant finding
- Contain glycogen or mucin
- Spilled mucus
  - Incites inflammatory response
  - May be misinterpreted as mucous escape reaction
- Tumor-associated lymphoid proliferation (TALP)
  - Lymphoid cells with occasional germinal centers
  - May be confused with metastatic disease to a lymph node
- Necrosis, anaplasia, and mitoses variably present
- Perineural and vascular invasion can be seen
- Grading used for prognosis and management
- Sarcomatoid transformation may rarely be seen
- Sclerosing mucoepidermoid carcinoma
  - Fibrous stroma is plentiful and can be hyalinized
  - Inflammatory cells (eosinophils included) may be seen

ANCILLARY TESTS

Cytology

- Clusters of bland intermediate or epithelial cells
- Mucocytes within clusters
- Variable amounts of mucin in background
- May be hypocellular or acellular if cystic areas are sampled
- Papanicolaou stain: Epithelial cells with dense, green-blue cytoplasm
- Diff-Quik: Mucocytes with intracellular, red-granular mucin droplet
  - Epithelial cells with light pink-purple cytoplasm

Frozen Sections

- Usually quite distinctive
- High-grade lesions may be misdiagnosed as squamous cell carcinoma

Immunohistochemistry

- p63
  - Strong, basal cell nuclear reaction
  - May highlight intermediate as well as epidermoid cells
  - Highly reactive lesions may indicate poor prognosis
- CK5/6
  - Highlights epidermoid-type cells but is often negative in transitional cells
- Ki-67
  - High expression seen with increased proliferation, usually indicative of high-grade tumor
  - Overexpression may serve as indicator of poor prognosis
- HER2
  - Tends to be strongly reactive in high-grade tumors
  - Overexpression may serve as indication for poor prognosis
  - Reactivity may guide future therapy with Herceptin

Cytogenetics

- t(11;19)(q21-22;p13)
  - This translocation fuses mucoepidermoid carcinoma translocated 1 (*MECT1*) (exon 1 of gene at 19p13) with Mastermind-like gene family (*MAML2*) (exons 2-5 of gene at 11q21)
  - Identified in low- to intermediate-grade tumors only
- Variable losses of 2q, 5p, 12p, and 16p
- Aneuploid tumors
  - Higher recurrence rate and decreased survival
  - Increased cervical lymph node involvement

DIFFERENTIAL DIAGNOSIS

Sialometaplasia

- Usually in lobular pattern, lacking cystic growth, no intermediate cells
- Mucocytes are residual to salivary gland

Mucus Extravasation Reaction

- Lacks intermediate cells and epithelial cells
- Mucus found primarily in macrophages

Squamous Cell Carcinoma

- Usually has keratinization and well-developed intercellular bridges
- Lacks intermediate cells

Clear Cell Malignancies

- Clear cell adenocarcinoma
  - Lacks intermediate cells or mucocyte differentiation
- Epithelial-myoepithelial carcinoma
  - Lacks intermediate cells, mucocyte differentiation
  - Shows distinct and characteristic biphasic glandular proliferation

Cystadenoma

- Not infiltrative
- Lacks sheets of epithelial proliferations and intermediate cells
- Focal rare mucocytes

Cystadenocarcinoma

- Lacks intermediate cells
- Focal rare mucocytes

DDx of Primary Intraosseous Tumors

- Glandular odontogenic tumor
- Reactive cyst with mucous metaplasia
- Clear cell odontogenic carcinoma

SELECTED REFERENCES

1. Cheuk W et al: Advances in salivary gland pathology. Histopathology. 51(1):1-20, 2007
2. do Prado RF et al: Calcifications in a clear cell mucoepidermoid carcinoma: a case report with histological and immunohistochemical findings. Oral Surg Oral Med Oral Pathol Oral Radiol Endod. 104(5):e40-4, 2007
3. Triantafillidou K et al: Mucoepidermoid carcinoma of minor salivary glands: a clinical study of 16 cases and review of the literature. Oral Dis. 12(4):364-70, 2006
4. Haddad R et al: Herceptin in patients with advanced or metastatic salivary gland carcinomas. A phase II study. Oral Oncol. 39(7):724-7, 2003
5. Nguyen LH et al: HER2/neu and Ki-67 as prognostic indicators in mucoepidermoid carcinoma of salivary glands. J Otolaryngol. 32(5):328-31, 2003

MUCOEPIDERMOID CARCINOMA

Immunohistochemistry

Antibody	Reactivity	Staining Pattern	Comment
CK-PAN	Positive	Cytoplasmic	Most cells, although only focally for mucocytes
CK5/6	Positive	Cytoplasmic	More common in epidermoid than transitional cells
CK7	Positive	Cytoplasmic	More intense staining for intermediate/transitional cells
p63	Positive	Nuclear	Basal cell reaction; strong staining suggests worse prognosis
CK14	Positive	Cytoplasmic	
CK19	Positive	Cytoplasmic	
CK17	Positive	Cytoplasmic	
EpCAM/BER-EP4/ CD326	Positive	Cell membrane & cytoplasm	
HER2	Positive	Cell membrane	Greater degree of positivity, suggests higher grade tumor
Ki-67	Positive	Nuclear	The higher the proliferation index, the higher the grade of tumor and the worse the prognosis
CK20	Negative	Cytoplasmic	
S100	Negative	Nuclear & cytoplasmic	
GFAP	Negative	Cytoplasmic	
Actin-HHF-35	Equivocal	Cytoplasmic	5% positivity

Tumor Grading

Parameter	Point Value
Intracystic component less than 20%	2
Neural invasion present	2
Necrosis present	3
Four or more mitoses per 10 high power fields	3
Anaplasia	4
Grade	**Total Point Score**
Low grade	0-4
Intermediate grade	5-6
High grade	7 or more

Adapted from Auclair PL et al: Mucoepidermoid carcinoma of intraoral salivary glands: evaluation and application of grading criteria in 143 cases. Cancer. 69(8):1217-24, 1998.

Histochemical Studies

Histochemical Stain	Reactivity	Staining Pattern	Comment
Mucicarmine	Positive	Cytoplasmic	Identifies mucocytes
Periodic acid-Schiff (PAS)	Positive	Cytoplasmic	Identifies glycogen
Alcian blue	Positive	Cytoplasmic	Identifies mucocytes
Periodic acid-Schiff with diastase	Negative		

6. Curry JL et al: Synchronous benign and malignant salivary gland tumors in ipsilateral glands: a report of two cases and a review of literature. Head Neck. 24(3):301-6, 2002
7. Foschini MP et al: Low-grade mucoepidermoid carcinoma of salivary glands: characteristic immunohistochemical profile and evidence of striated duct differentiation. Virchows Arch. 440(5):536-42, 2002
8. Guzzo M et al: Mucoepidermoid carcinoma of the salivary glands: clinicopathologic review of 108 patients treated at the National Cancer Institute of Milan. Ann Surg Oncol. 9(7):688-95, 2002
9. Brandwein MS et al: Mucoepidermoid carcinoma: a clinicopathologic study of 80 patients with special reference to histological grading. Am J Surg Pathol. 25(7):835-45, 2001
10. Ellis GL: Clear cell neoplasms in salivary glands: clearly a diagnostic challenge. Ann Diagn Pathol. 2(1):61-78, 1998
11. Goode RK et al: Mucoepidermoid carcinoma of the major salivary glands: clinical and histopathologic analysis of 234 cases with evaluation of grading criteria. Cancer. 82(7):1217-24, 1998
12. Loyola AM et al: Study of minor salivary gland mucoepidermoid carcinoma differentiation based on immunohistochemical expression of cytokeratins, vimentin and muscle-specific actin. Oral Oncol. 34(2):112-8, 1998
13. Auclair PL: Tumor-associated lymphoid proliferation in the parotid gland. A potential diagnostic pitfall. Oral Surg Oral Med Oral Pathol. 77(1):19-26, 1994
14. Auclair PL et al: Mucoepidermoid carcinoma of intraoral salivary glands. Evaluation and application of grading criteria in 143 cases. Cancer. 69(8):2021-30, 1992

MUCOEPIDERMOID CARCINOMA

Radiographic, Clinical, and Gross Features

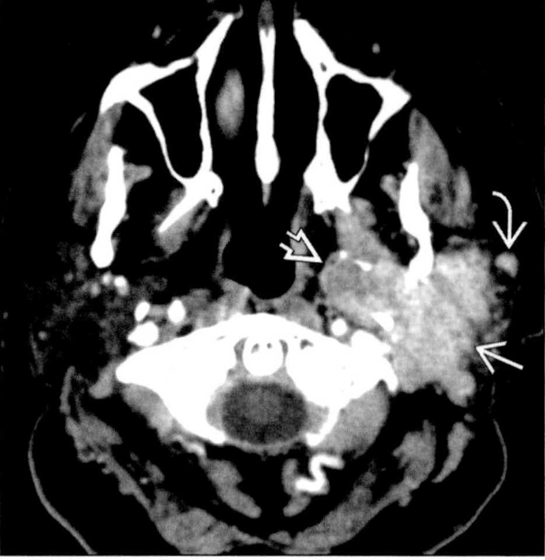

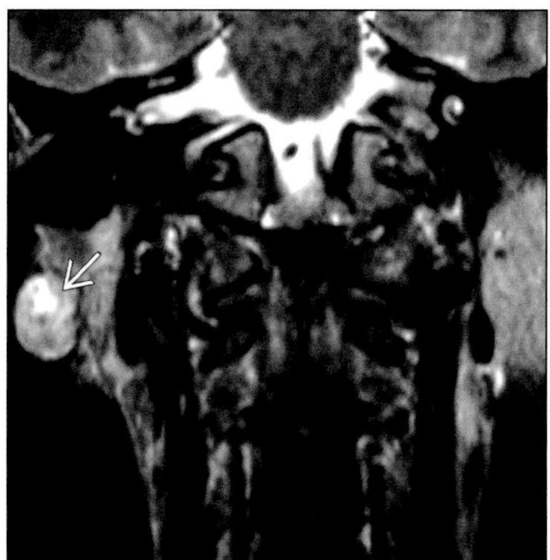

(Left) *Axial contrast-enhanced computed tomography shows an invasive high-grade mucoepidermoid carcinoma involving the superficial lobe ➔ and deep lobe ➔. There is significant destruction of the parotid parenchyma by the tumor. Notice the single intraparotid lymph node ➔.* ***(Right)*** *Corresponding coronal T2-weighted magnetic resonance image shows a well-defined, high signal tumor with cystic necrosis ➔. This could be easily mistaken for another tumor type.*

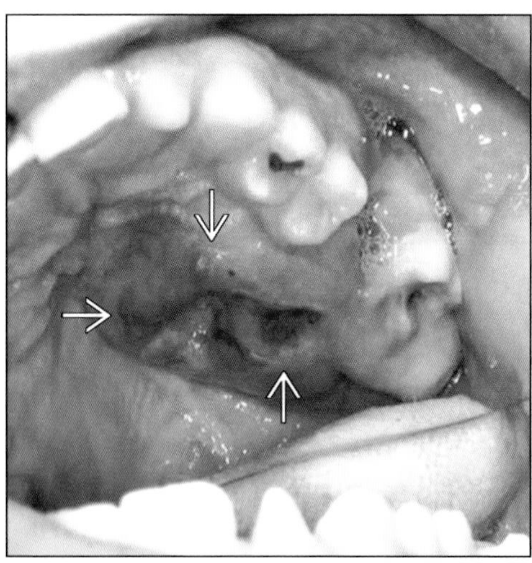

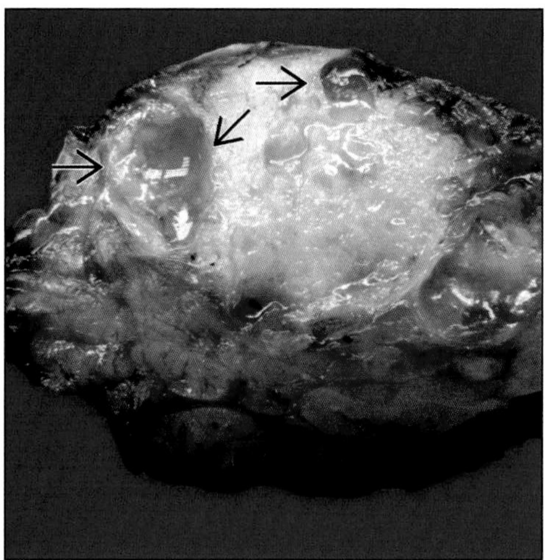

(Left) *Clinical photograph shows an ulcerated red mass of the posterior lateral hard palate ➔. Microscopic review confirmed a low-grade mucoepidermoid carcinoma arising from a minor salivary gland. Palate primaries usually do not have a capsule.* ***(Right)*** *Gross photograph shows a tumor with a tan-yellow cut surface. Mucoid material can be seen in the cystic spaces ➔. The remaining parenchyma is compressed toward the periphery.*

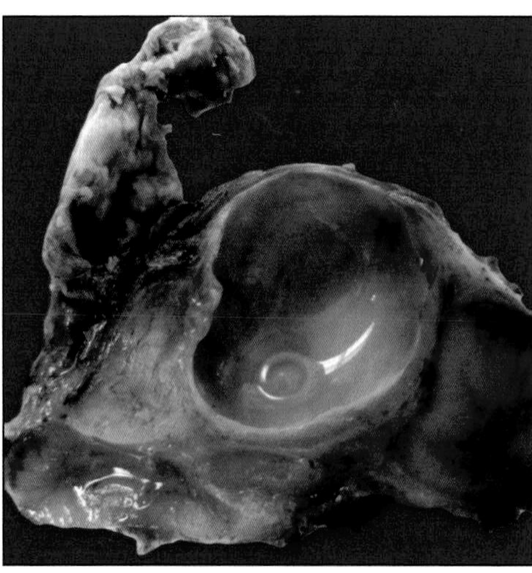

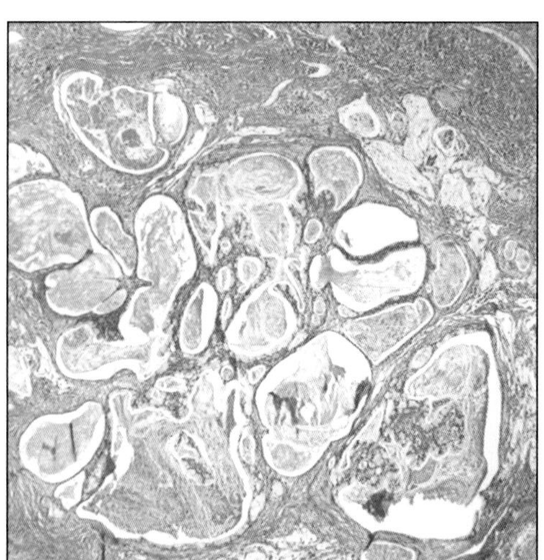

(Left) *Gross photograph shows a predominately unicystic mucoepidermoid carcinoma. The lumen was filled with thick, tenacious, mucoid material. This type of lesion can easily mimic a mucocele, clinically and macroscopically.* ***(Right)*** *Hematoxylin & eosin shows a neoplasm comprised of numerous, variably sized cystic spaces lined by epithelium. Based on the greater than 20% cystic component, this pattern suggests a low-grade tumor (assuming a total score of 4 or less.)*

Microscopic Features

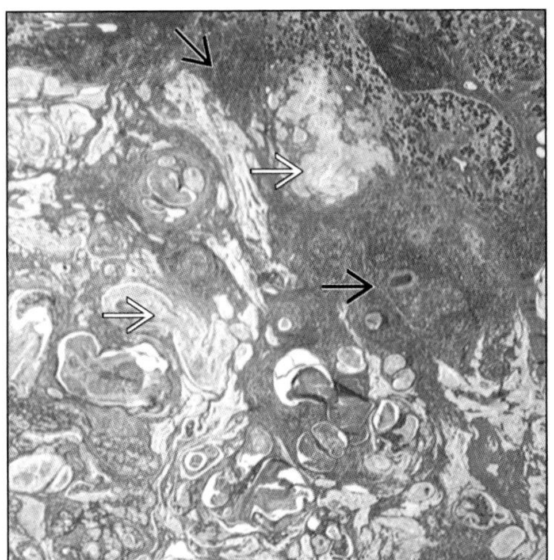

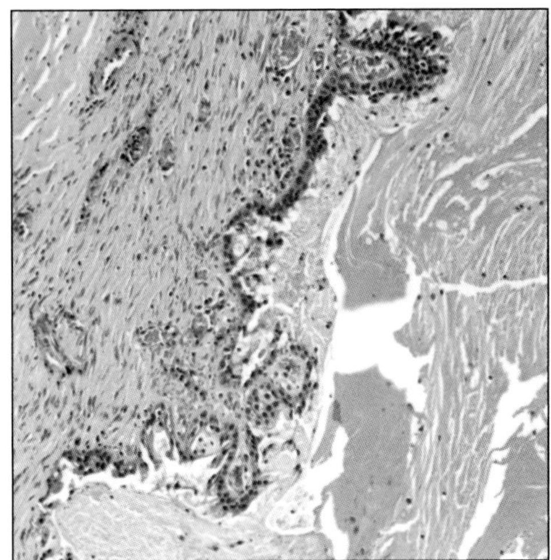

(Left) *Hematoxylin & eosin shows a cystic tumor with areas of spilled mucus ➡. It is not uncommon to have cysts of the tumor rupture, yielding free mucus, which incites an inflammatory response ⇨. In small biopsies, these features may be misdiagnosed as a mucous escape reaction (mucocele).* ***(Right)*** *Shown here is a unicystic tumor in the parotid. Clinically it was thought to be a branchial cleft cyst.*

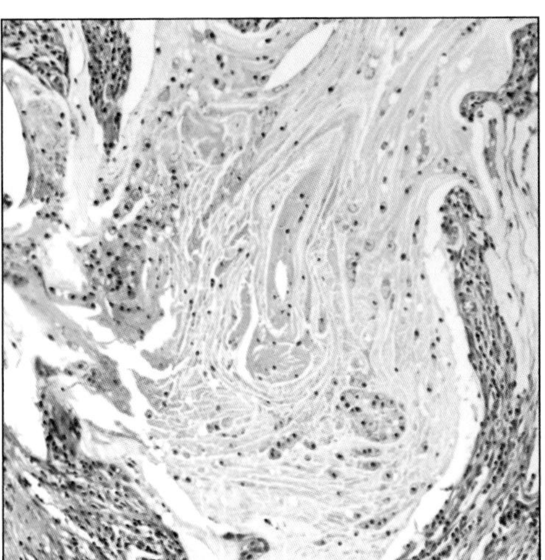

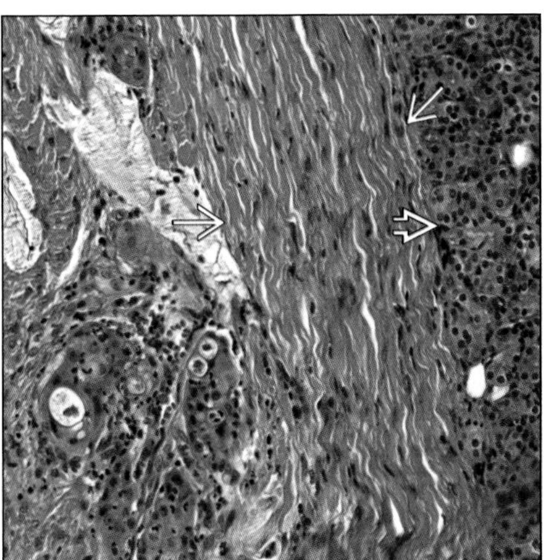

(Left) *Hematoxylin & eosin shows a pool of free mucus that has caused an inflammatory response. The mucinous material may contain inflammatory debris and histiocytes. These should not be mistaken for true "mucocytes," which should be sought in the lining epithelium.* ***(Right)*** *Hematoxylin & eosin shows an area of partial encapsulation ➡ separating the parotid gland ➡ from the tumor. Note the small cyst-gland spaces and extravasated mucus material within the tumor.*

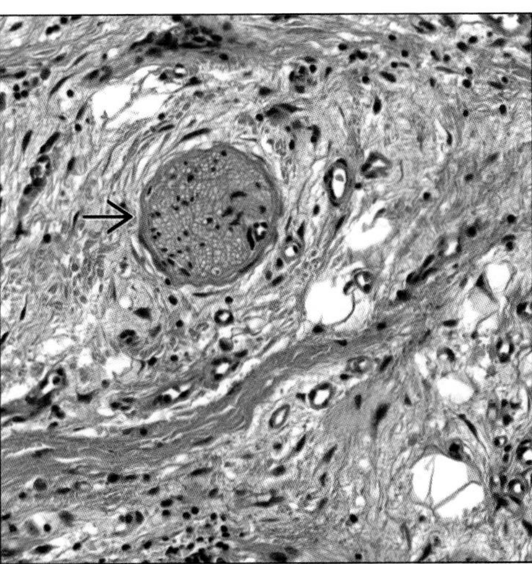

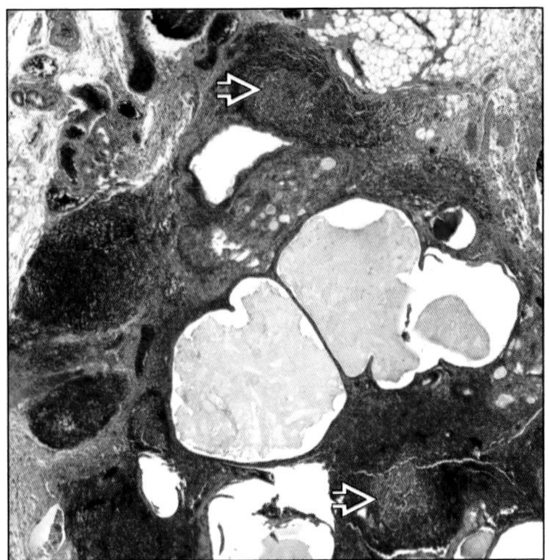

(Left) *The neoplastic cells invade beyond the contours of the tumor into the adjacent soft tissue. Sometimes, mucinous material will be present around nerves ⇨. Isolated epithelial cells are frequently suspended in the mucus pools.* ***(Right)*** *This mucoepidermoid tumor has tumor-associated lymphoid proliferation (TALP). Well-formed germinal centers are easily identified ➡, but no capsule is seen, indicating this in not metastatic disease to a lymph node.*

MUCOEPIDERMOID CARCINOMA

Microscopic Features

*(**Left**) The epidermoid and intermediate cell component of a mucoepidermoid carcinoma may undergo clear cell change. Sometimes, as in this case, it can be the dominant finding. The differential diagnosis expands when this is the case. (**Right**) Hematoxylin & eosin shows a tumor with a focus of clear cells. There are prominent intercellular borders, with small hyperchromatic nuclei. Clear cells contain glycogen and occasionally mucin. A PAS or mucicarmine stain may be helpful.*

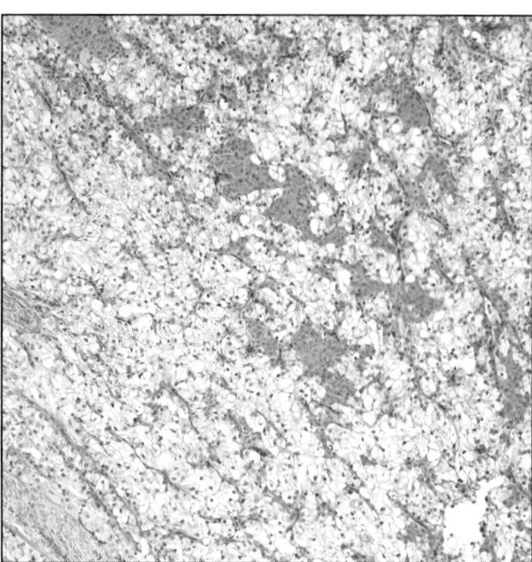

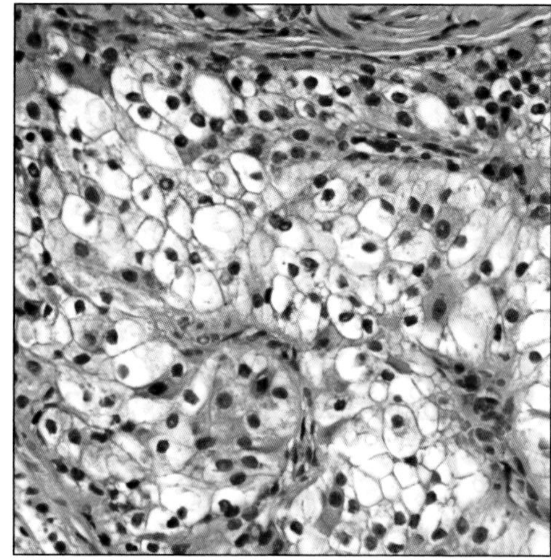

*(**Left**) The components of mucoepidermoid carcinoma are frequently intermingled and blended. The mucocytes ⇒ are sometimes quite prominent but identified as single cells within the epidermoid/transitional cell component. There are no well-formed cystic spaces in this field. Inflammatory cells are frequently present. (**Right**) Hematoxylin & eosin shows cellular anaplasia and focal acute inflammation. Mucocytes can be seen ➡. These features are suggestive of a high-grade tumor.*

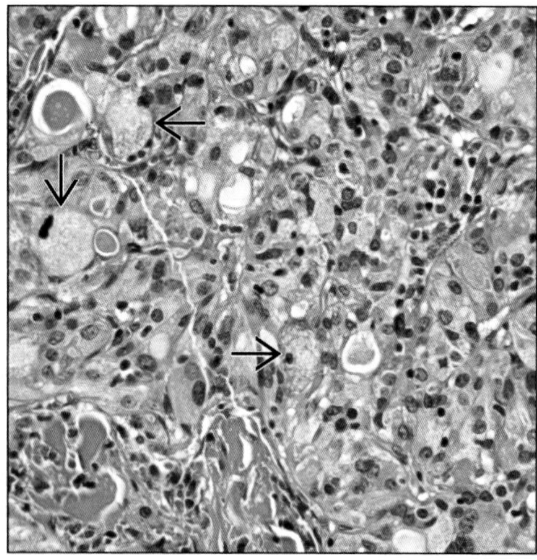

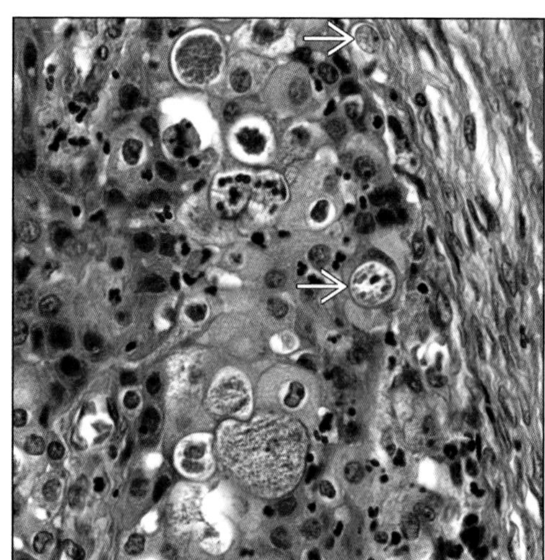

*(**Left**) Hematoxylin & eosin shows a high-power view of an atypical mitotic figure ⇒ within a pleomorphic high-grade tumor. There is a transitional epithelial proliferation immediately adjacent to this atypical mitotic figure. (**Right**) Hematoxylin & eosin shows a collection of mucous cells with foamy cytoplasm. The foamy cytoplasm can also be seen in histiocytes. It is for this reason that mucicarmine or other mucin stains need to be performed to confirm the diagnosis.*

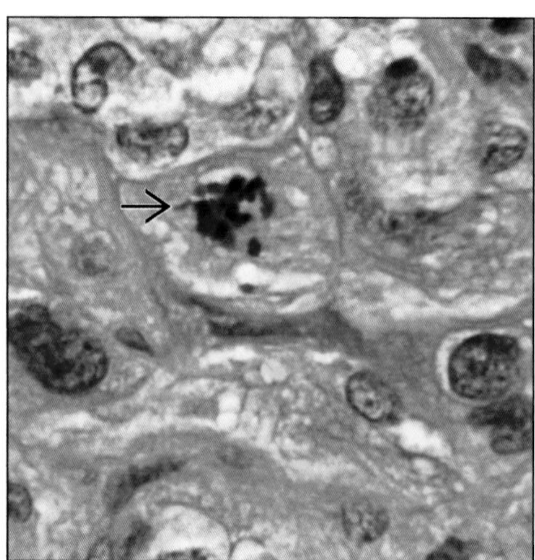

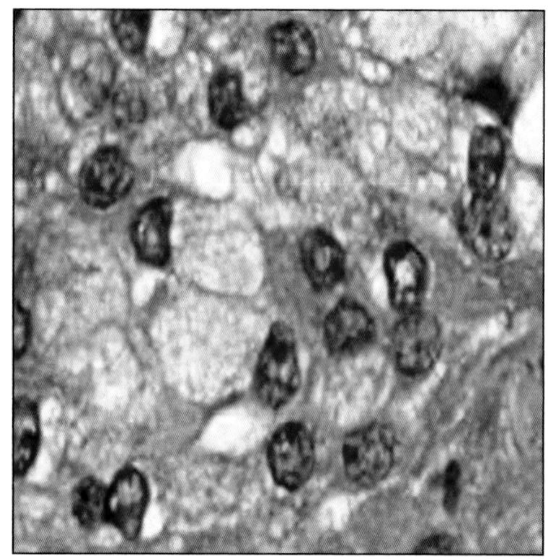

Ancillary Techniques

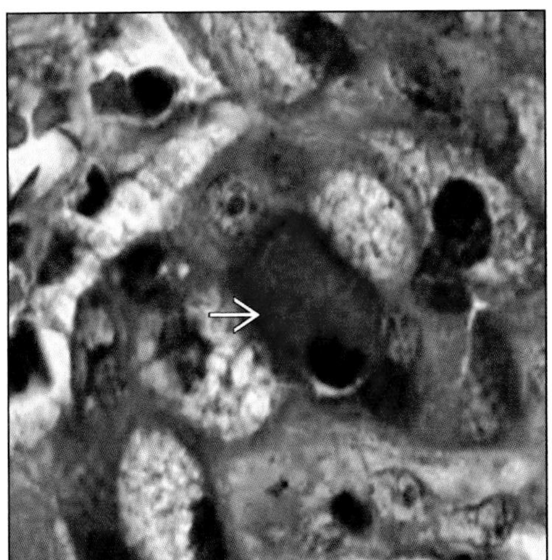
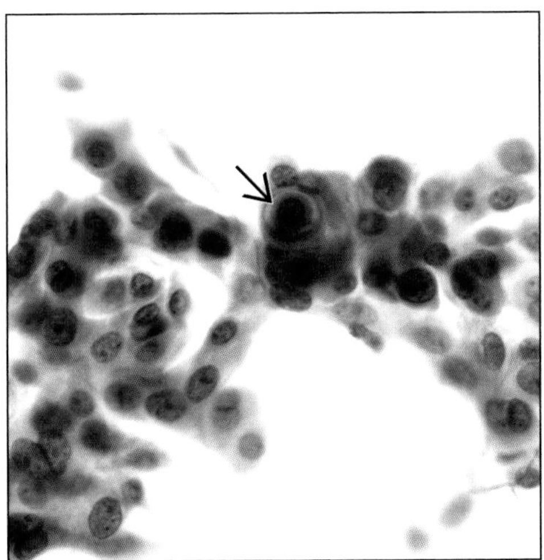

(Left) *Mucicarmine stain helps confirm intracytoplasmic mucin ➔. It can be difficult to identify these cells with H&E staining. The surrounding cells also have a "vacuolated" appearance but do not contain mucin, highlighting the need to perform histochemical stains.* **(Right)** *The cytology smear demonstrates sheets and clusters of epidermoid-transitional cells with opaque cytoplasm. There is a suggestion of a vacuole within the cytoplasm ➔ of one of the neoplastic cells.*

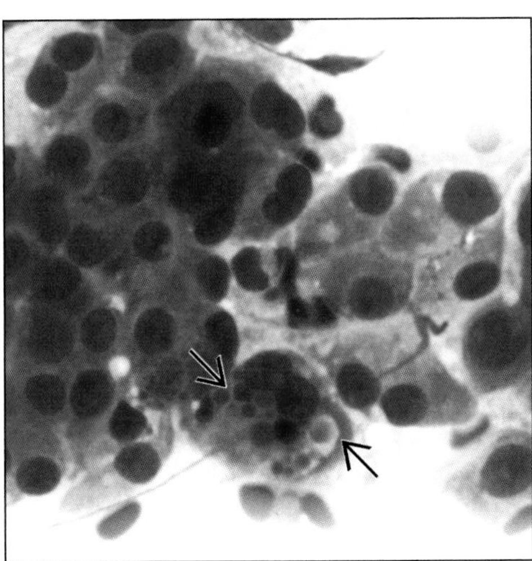
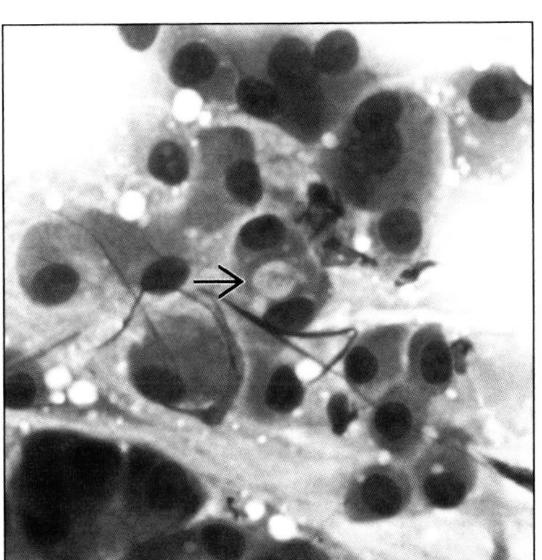

(Left) *There is a sheet-like distribution to these neoplastic epithelioid cells, making up the epidermoid component of this tumor. Note the mucin-filled cytoplasm ➔ highlighting a mucocyte in this smear. Mucin is usually a deep magenta. Often, it is present in the background.* **(Right)** *There is a well-formed mucocyte ➔ in the center of the field, surrounded by epidermoid or transitional cells. Note the "bluish" appearance to the cytoplasm, similar to squamous cells.*

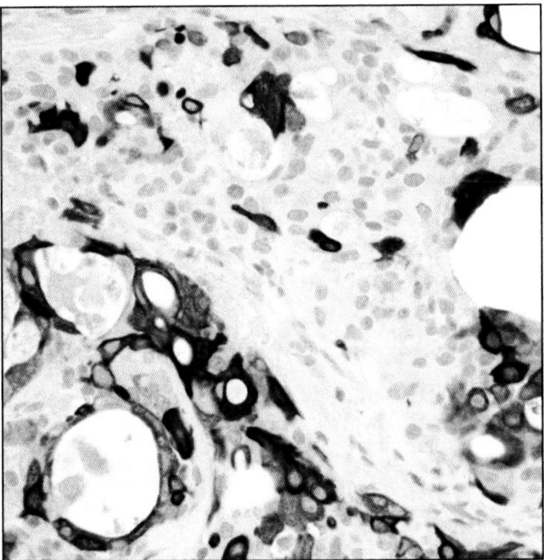
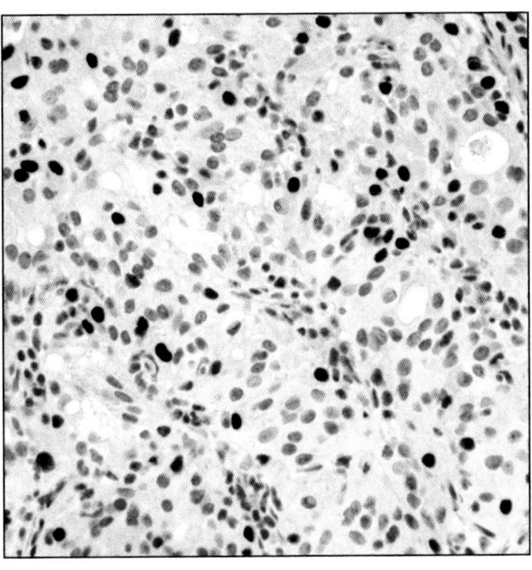

(Left) *CK5/6 highlights the epithelial cells associated with the duct-like structures. There is a variable intensity to the staining.* **(Right)** *Immunohistochemistry studies are usually not required and often unhelpful in confirming the diagnosis of a mucoepidermoid carcinoma. However, p63 will highlight the nuclei of intermediate cells. There is not usually reactivity with mucocytes or epidermoid cells.*

ADENOID CYSTIC CARCINOMA

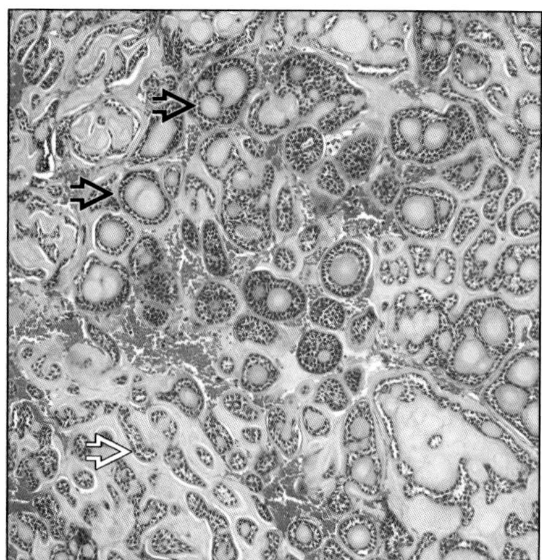

Hematoxylin & eosin shows an adenoid cystic carcinoma with areas of cribriform ⇨ and tubular patterns ➡. These tumors may have multiple patterns, although a single pattern usually predominates.

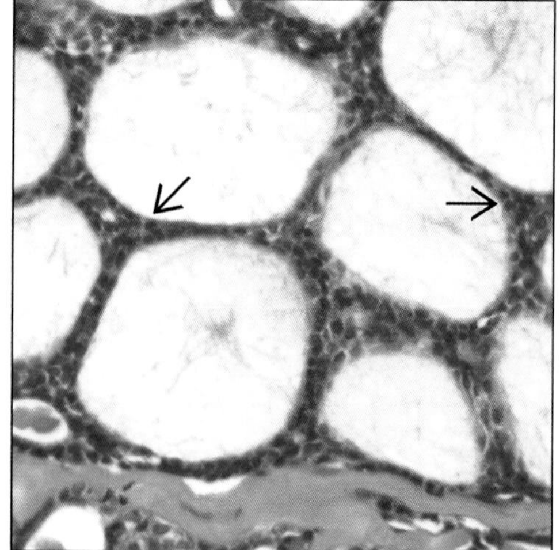

Hematoxylin and eosin shows a tumor with a cribriform pattern. This pattern is the most common and is often said to look like "Swiss cheese" or a "telephone dial." Note the dark angulated cells →.

TERMINOLOGY

Abbreviations

- Adenoid cystic carcinoma (ACC or ACCa)

Synonyms

- Cylindroma
  - Outdated terminology
  - May be confused with benign dermal tumor with same name
- Adenocystic carcinoma
  - Outdated terminology
  - May be confused with carcinoma of eccrine origin

Definitions

- Malignant epithelial tumor with myoepithelial and ductal differentiation

CLINICAL ISSUES

Epidemiology

- Incidence
  - 4th most common malignant salivary gland tumor
- Age
  - Adults, peak in 6th decade
  - Rare in children
- Gender
  - Female > Male (3:2)

Site

- Found with essentially equal frequency in major and minor salivary glands
- Major
  - Parotid gland most frequently affected
  - Sublingual gland
- Minor
  - Palate most frequently affected
  - Tongue
  - Lip
- Other
  - Sinonasal
  - Nasopharynx
  - Larynx/trachea
  - Lacrimal gland
  - Other sites in body
    - Breast and lung

Presentation

- Mass
- Tenderness or pain
- Swelling
- Facial paralysis
- Intraoral lesions may be ulcerated

Treatment

- Options, risks, complications
  - Extensive resections may result in significant cosmetic issues
- Surgical approaches
  - Radical excision
  - Reconstruction when indicated
- Adjuvant therapy
  - Chemotherapy is occasionally used for large tumors or late stage tumors
    - No definitive protocols
- Radiation
  - Conflicting reports on effectiveness

Prognosis

- Clinical stage predicts outcome and survival
- High incidence of recurrence
- Characterized by late onset metastases
  - 5-year survival rate is good
  - 20-year survival rate is poor
- Patients with solid pattern tumors have worse prognosis
- Poor prognostic factors
  - Large tumors, greater than 4 cm
  - Regional lymph node metastasis
  - Distant metastasis
    - Lungs and bone

ADENOID CYSTIC CARCINOMA

Key Facts

Terminology
- Malignant epithelial tumor with myoepithelial and ductal differentiation

Clinical Issues
- 4th most common malignant salivary gland tumor
- Found with nearly equal frequency in major and minor salivary glands
- Adults primarily, with peak in 6th decade
- Presentation
  - Mass
  - Tenderness or pain
  - Facial paralysis
- Tumors commonly recur and may develop late onset metastases
- Treated with radical excision

Microscopic Pathology
- Present with variety of patterns
  - Cribriform, tubular, solid, or combination
- Cells are usually small, with limited eosinophilic to clear cytoplasm
- Nuclei are oval to sharply angulated (peg-shaped), with coarse chromatin and small nucleoli
- Mitotic figures are rare

Ancillary Tests
- Multiple nerve sections may be submitted for frozen section: Tumor may "skip"

Top Differential Diagnoses
- Polymorphous low-grade adenocarcinoma, pleomorphic adenoma, basal cell adenoma/ adenocarcinoma, epithelial-myoepithelial carcinoma

- High reactivity to Ki-67 is indicator of poor prognosis
- Perineural invasion associated with variable outcome data
  - May be one reason why tumors recur
- Surgical margin status does not affect survival
- Anatomic site affects outcome
  - Palatal lesions have best outcome
  - Parotid gland tumors have better prognosis than submandibular gland tumors

IMAGE FINDINGS

Radiographic Findings
- Bone destruction may be present

MACROSCOPIC FEATURES

General Features
- Poorly circumscribed
- Unencapsulated
  - Rarely encapsulated
- White-gray cut surface
- Firm

Size
- Quite variable, although can be large

MICROSCOPIC PATHOLOGY

Histologic Features
- Infiltrative
  - Perineural invasion commonly seen
  - Infiltrative edges into fat, skeletal muscle, soft tissue
- Combinations of patterns usually present, although one predominates
- **Cribriform** pattern
  - Like "Swiss cheese" or "telephone dial"
  - Epithelial nests contain pseudocysts
    - Pseudocysts are not true glandular lumens but are part of tumor stroma
  - Pseudocysts contain one or both of
    - Amorphous glycosaminoglycans
    - Hyalinized basal lamina
- **Tubular** pattern
  - Lumens are more conspicuous
  - True lumens surrounded by ductal cells with myoepithelial cells forming 2nd layer
  - Small nests separated by eosinophilic hyalinized stroma
- **Solid** pattern
  - Minimum of 30% solid growth required
  - Greater degree of nuclear pleomorphism than in other types
  - Associated with increased mitotic activity
  - Necrosis may be present
- **Cytologic** features
  - Small to medium cells with eosinophilic to clear cytoplasm
  - Nuclei are oval to sharply angulated with coarse, basophilic chromatin
    - Occasional small nucleoli
  - Mitotic figures are rare
    - Except for the solid pattern

ANCILLARY TESTS

Cytology
- May be difficult to distinguish from other salivary gland tumors
- Cohesive cellular clusters surrounding "balls" of mucopolysaccharide material
- Peg- or carrot-shaped nuclei
- High nuclear to cytoplasmic ratio
- Coarse nuclear chromatin
- Characteristic round, scattered fragments of mucopolysaccharide material surrounded by cells
  - Diff-Quik: Purple-pink to magenta bubblegum-like
  - Papanicolaou: Light green, orange, or clear
  - Cells are at periphery, not embedded within stroma

Frozen Sections
- Multiple peripheral nerve sections are often submitted

- Tumor may "skip" along nerve

Histochemistry

- Alcian blue: Highlights basement membrane material of pseudolumina
- Periodic acid-Schiff (PAS): Highlights basement membrane material of pseudolumina

Immunohistochemistry

- May have limited practical use
  - Tumors in differential diagnosis often react similarly
- MCM2: Expressed in G1/G2/S and labels cells enabled to proliferate
  - Minichromosome maintenance proteins
  - Family of 6 proteins that form complex to allow DNA replication
  - Enables cell to divide; expressed throughout cell cycle
  - Overexpressed in many tumors, but MCM2 has highest expression in ACC (> 10%) and is low to absent in PLGA and PA (< 10%)

Cytogenetics

- No particular gene profile identified
- 30% have evidence of translocations involving chromosome 9p13-23 and 6q
- About 50% have loss of chromosome 12q12
- LOH at 6q23-25: Associated with poorer prognosis
- Alteration of p53: Associated with tumor recurrence and progression to solid type

Electron Microscopy

- Shows luminal and abluminal differentiation, with epithelial and myoepithelial features

DIFFERENTIAL DIAGNOSIS

Polymorphous Low-Grade Adenocarcinoma

- Most difficult to distinguish from ACC
- Only identified in minor salivary glands
- Low-power pattern shows
  - Single cell invasion, often in columns
  - Targetoid, swirling, or "eye of storm" patterns around nerves
- Bland uniform oval to round cells
  - Lacks pleomorphism
  - Lacks mitotic figures
  - Nuclear chromatin is vesicular to delicate
- Immunohistochemistry does not help to separate
  - Proliferation markers, including MCM2, may help with separation from ACC

Pleomorphic Adenoma (PA)

- Lacks infiltration, especially perineural invasion
- Myxochondroid matrix material is different, with blending of epithelial cells into matrix
- Plasmacytoid and spindled cells common
- Ducts are present
- Squamous and oncocytic metaplasia more common

Basal Cell Adenocarcinoma

- Shows well-developed peripheral palisading
- Invasive growth defines this tumor
- Lacks pleomorphism
- Rare mitotic figures
- Lacks glycosaminoglycan material, although does have basal lamina

Basal Cell Adenoma

- Lacks infiltrative growth
- Shows well-developed peripheral palisading
- Lacks pleomorphism
- Lacks mitoses

Epithelial-Myoepithelial Carcinoma

- Periductal cells are large, nonangulated, and clear
- Lacks pleomorphism
- Lacks mitoses

Carcinoma Ex-Pleomorphic Adenoma

- Features of pleomorphic adenoma are present (or there is clinical history)
- ACC may be malignant component of carcinoma ex-pleomorphic adenoma

Basaloid Squamous Cell Carcinoma

- May be associated with overlying epithelial dysplasia
- Usually found in base of tongue or hypopharynx
- Distinctive comedonecrosis
- Squamous differentiation is required, a feature not seen in ACC

Cylindroma

- Skin tumor, common in head and neck
- Epithelial islands arranged in "jigsaw" pattern surrounded by thickened basement membrane
- Cytologically bland

Sialoblastoma

- Develops almost exclusively in children
- Basaloid cells with vesicular nuclei
- Peripheral palisading of nuclei is common

Neuroendocrine Carcinoma

- Difficult to diagnose with small biopsies
- Rare in salivary gland
- No cribriform pattern
- Immunoreactivity for neuroendocrine markers

DIAGNOSTIC CHECKLIST

Pathologic Interpretation Pearls

- Stage is more meaningful than grade for predicting long-term prognosis

SELECTED REFERENCES

1. Dardick I et al: Sialoblastoma in adults: distinction from adenoid cystic carcinoma. Oral Surg Oral Med Oral Pathol Oral Radiol Endod. 109(1):109-16, 2010
2. Oplatek A et al: Patterns of recurrence and survival of head and neck adenoid cystic carcinoma after definitive resection. Laryngoscope. 120(1):65-70, 2010
3. Barrett AW et al: Perineural invasion in adenoid cystic carcinoma of the salivary glands: a valid prognostic indicator? Oral Oncol. 45(11):936-40, 2009

ADENOID CYSTIC CARCINOMA

Immunohistochemistry

Antibody	Reactivity	Staining Pattern	Comment
CK-PAN	Positive	Cytoplasmic	All tumor cells, although can be differentially expressed
CD117	Positive	Cell membrane & cytoplasm	Solid type more reactive than tubular type
Actin-sm	Positive	Cytoplasmic	Abluminal cells
Calponin	Positive	Cytoplasmic	Abluminal cells
p63	Positive	Nuclear	Abluminal cells
CK7	Positive	Cytoplasmic	All tumor cells
SMHC	Positive	Cytoplasmic	Abluminal cells
S100	Positive	Nuclear & cytoplasmic	Abluminal cells
MCM2	Positive	Nuclear	Usually > 10% of nuclei react
TTF-1	Negative		
CD56	Negative		
GFAP	Equivocal	Cytoplasmic	Limited reactivity in only isolated cells

Grading of Adenoid Cystic Carcinoma

Parameter	Grade 1	Grade 2	Grade 3
Percentage of tumors in each grade	45%	35%	20%
Circumscription	Good	Deceptive or irregular	Never
Necrosis	Absent	May be present	Easily identified
Bone invasion	Absent	May be present	Often present
Perineural invasion (nerves beyond the gland raise the grade)	Present	Easily identified	Significant, including large nerves
Dominant pattern	Tubular	Cribriform	Solid
Pleomorphism	Limited	Present	Profound variability
Mitoses	Rare	Few	Many
Recurrences	50%	80%	100%
15-year survival	39%	26%	5%

Survival Rates Based on Stage

Stage	10-Year Survival Rate
I	75%
II	43%
III & IV	15%

Adapted from Spiro RH et al: Stage means more than grade in adenoid cystic carcinoma. Am J Surg. 164(6):623-8, 1992.

4. Friedrich RE et al: Adenoid cystic carcinoma of salivary and lacrimal gland origin: localization, classification, clinical pathological correlation, treatment results and long-term follow-up control in 84 patients. Anticancer Res. 23(2A):931-40, 2003
5. Penner CR et al: C-kit expression distinguishes salivary gland adenoid cystic carcinoma from polymorphous low-grade adenocarcinoma. Mod Pathol. 15(7):687-91, 2002
6. Araújo VC et al: The cribriform features of adenoid cystic carcinoma and polymorphous low-grade adenocarcinoma: cytokeratin and integrin expression. Ann Diagn Pathol. 5(6):330-4, 2001
7. Jeng YM et al: Expression of the c-kit protein is associated with certain subtypes of salivary gland carcinoma. Cancer Lett. 154(1):107-11, 2000
8. Norberg-Spaak L et al: Adenoid cystic carcinoma: use of cell proliferation, BCL-2 expression, histologic grade, and clinical stage as predictors of clinical outcome. Head Neck. 22(5):489-97, 2000
9. Jones AS et al: Tumours of the minor salivary glands. Clin Otolaryngol Allied Sci. 23(1):27-33, 1998
10. Jones AS et al: Adenoid cystic carcinoma of the head and neck. Clin Otolaryngol Allied Sci. 22(5):434-43, 1997
11. Kapadia SB et al: Fine needle aspiration of pleomorphic adenoma and adenoid cystic carcinoma of salivary gland origin. Acta Cytol. 41(2):487-92, 1997
12. Spiro RH: Distant metastasis in adenoid cystic carcinoma of salivary origin. Am J Surg. 174(5):495-8, 1997
13. Jin Y et al: Characteristic karyotypic features in lacrimal and salivary gland carcinomas. Br J Cancer. 70(1):42-7, 1994
14. Spiro RH et al: Stage means more than grade in adenoid cystic carcinoma. Am J Surg. 164(6):623-8, 1992
15. Hamper K et al: Prognostic factors for adenoid cystic carcinoma of the head and neck: a retrospective evaluation of 96 cases. J Oral Pathol Med. 19(3):101-7, 1990
16. Waldron CA et al: Tumors of the intraoral minor salivary glands: a demographic and histologic study of 426 cases. Oral Surg Oral Med Oral Pathol. 66(3):323-33, 1988

ADENOID CYSTIC CARCINOMA

Imaging and Macroscopic Features

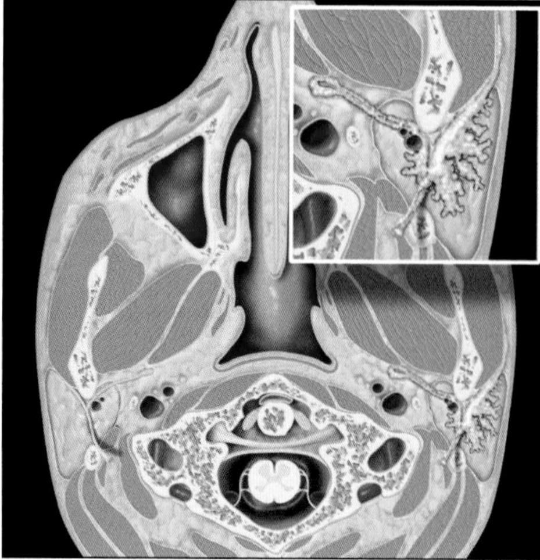

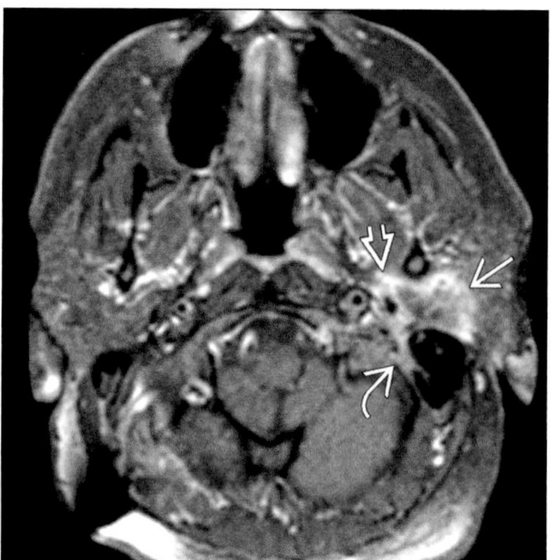

*(**Left**) This graphic demonstrates the proclivity of adenoid cystic carcinoma for perineural invasion. This feature is not exclusive to this particular tumor, however. The tumor often "skips" along the nerve, making frozen section margins very challenging and perhaps unreliable. (**Right**) Axial T1 enhanced fat-saturated MR image demonstrates an invasive deep and superficial lobe parotid adenoid cystic carcinoma involving the stylomastoid foramen.*

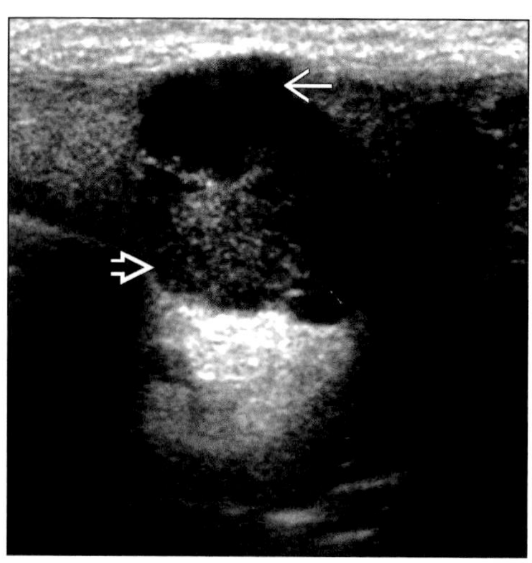

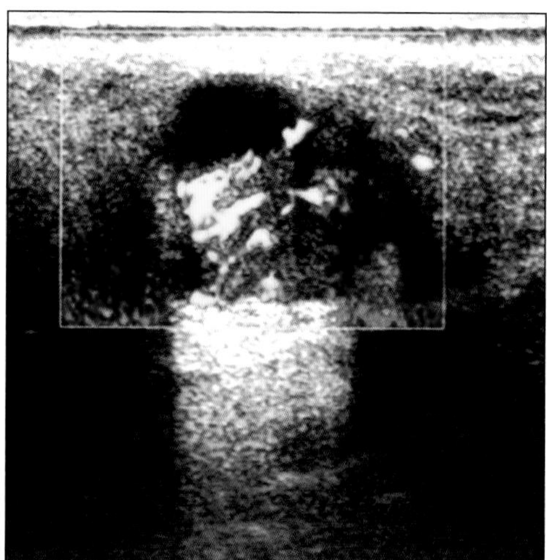

*(**Left**) Longitudinal grayscale US shows an adenoid cystic carcinoma as a hypoechoic, heterogeneous tumor with cystic necrosis. The tumor just bulges out of the glandular contour. Still, this tumor is fairly well defined & simulates a pleomorphic adenoma radiographically. (**Right**) Power Doppler US in the same patient shows prominent vessels in the solid portion of the tumor. This increased flow is not unique to ACC, but it does raise the possibility of a malignancy.*

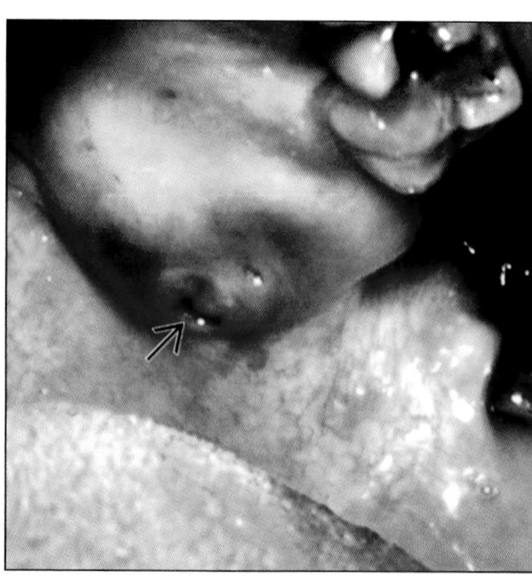

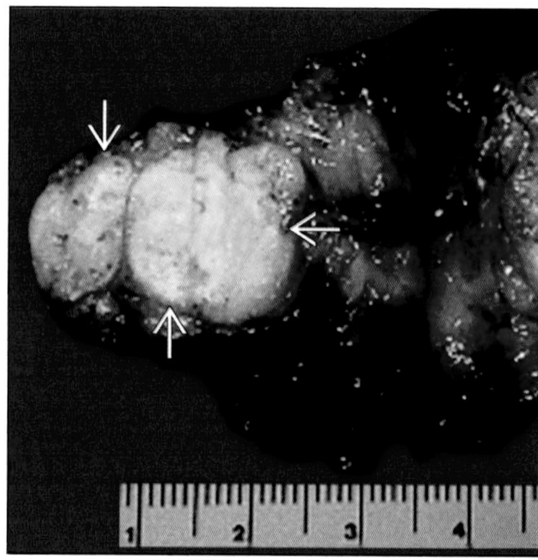

*(**Left**) Clinical photograph shows a large adenoid cystic carcinoma of the palate. The surface is ulcerated due to trauma during eating. This lesion was repeatedly treated as an infection before a biopsy revealed a solid variant of adenoid cystic carcinoma. (**Right**) Gross photograph shows a multinodular focally circumscribed tumor of the parotid gland. The gross appearance of circumscription or encapsulation is not representative of the histologic findings of invasion.*

Microscopic Features

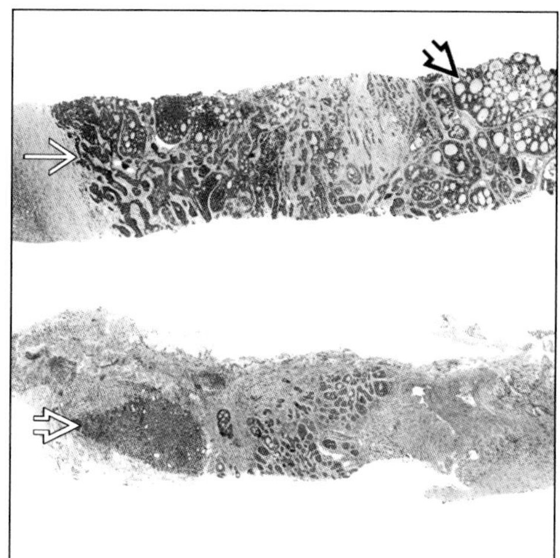

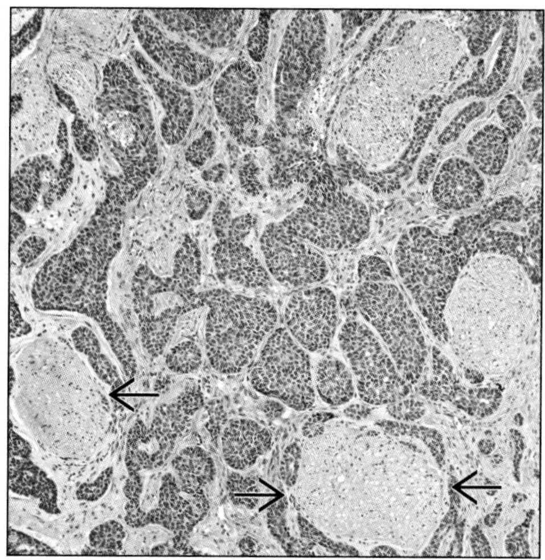

(Left) Needle biopsy of an adenoid cystic carcinoma shows areas of solid ➡, cribriform ➡, and tubular patterns ➡. Core biopsies can be difficult to confidently diagnose as ACC, but "malignant salivary gland neoplasm" may help in guiding therapy. **(Right)** Hematoxylin & eosin shows tumor cells encircling small nerve twigs ➡. This is a characteristic feature of adenoid cystic carcinoma, although it may be found in other tumors, and may result in nerve paralysis.

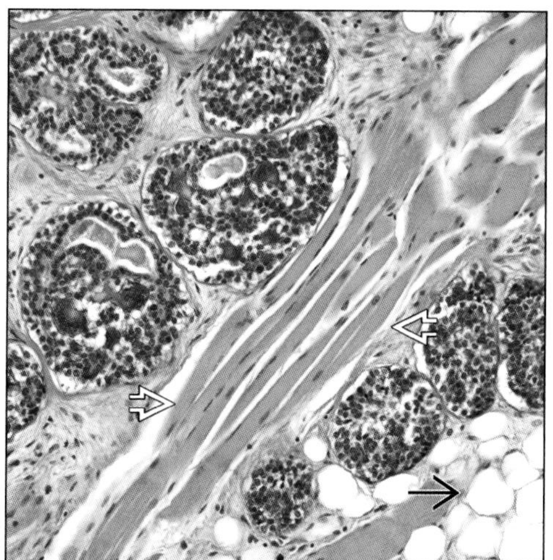

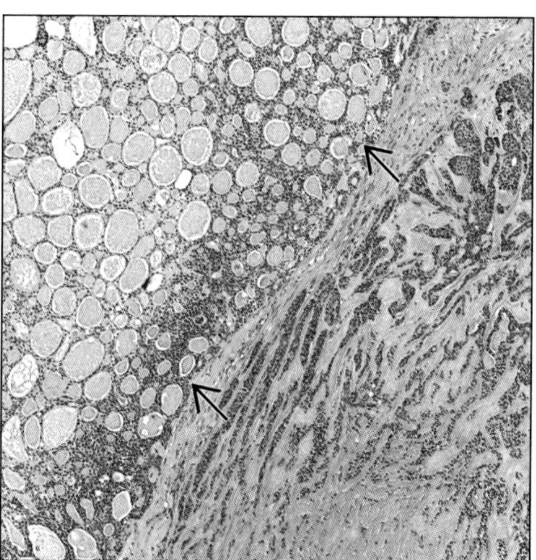

(Left) Hematoxylin & eosin shows tumor islands invading into surrounding muscle ➡ and fat ➡. Extensive surgeries may result in increased morbidity and mortality. Additionally, patients may refuse treatment due to devastating cosmetic defects. **(Right)** The classic cribriform pattern of adenoid cystic carcinoma ➡ is identified immediately adjacent to areas of single cell infiltration. This pattern can also be seen in PLGA. Nuclear features help make a correct diagnosis.

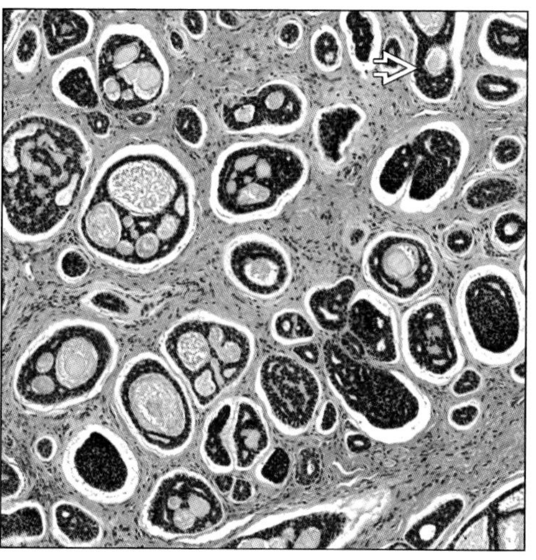

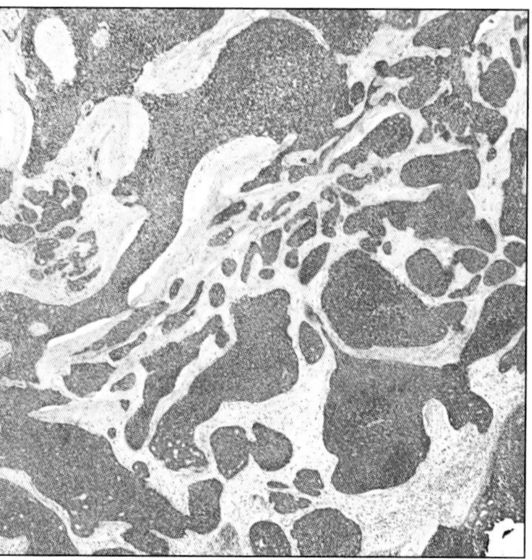

(Left) This tumor highlights a cribriform pattern. Despite the appearance, the cyst-like spaces are actually connected to the surrounding stroma. The tumor cells are often described as creating "C" shapes ➡ that partially encircle the stroma. **(Right)** Large tumor nests are seen in the solid pattern of ACC. The solid pattern tends to be more mitotically active and has a poorer prognosis than other types of adenoid cystic carcinoma.

ADENOID CYSTIC CARCINOMA

Microscopic Features

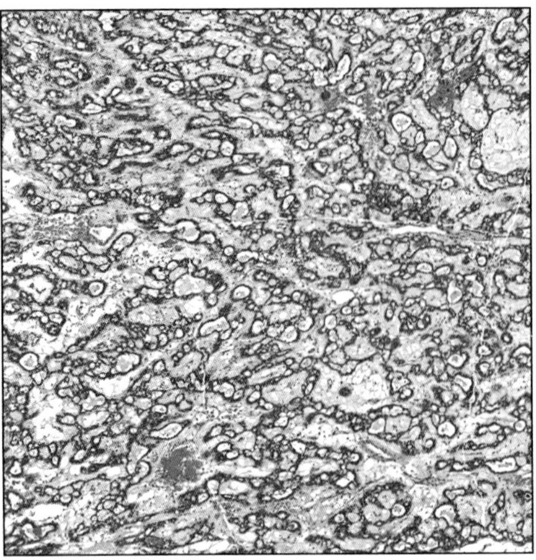

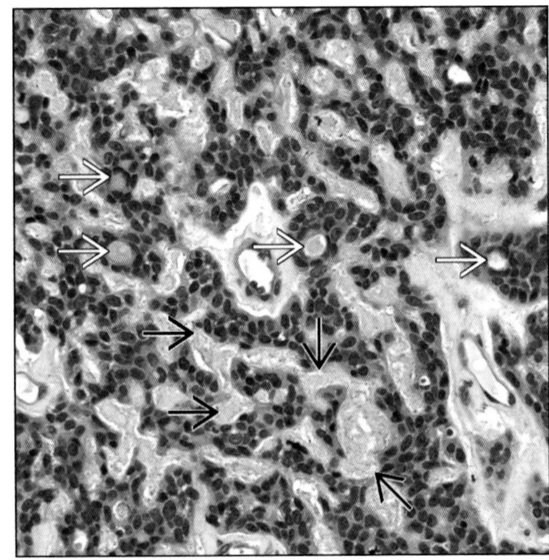

(Left) *A low-power view of an adenoid cystic carcinoma shows myriad spaces with cystic material separated by a loose to collagenized fibrous connective tissue stroma. The cells are basophilic at this magnification.* ***(Right)*** *The cyst-like spaces are in fact in continuity ⇒ with each other, a feature helpful in the diagnosis of ACC. The spaces are filled with stroma made of amorphous glycosaminoglycans, hyalinized basal lamina, or a combination of both. Note the tubules ➡.*

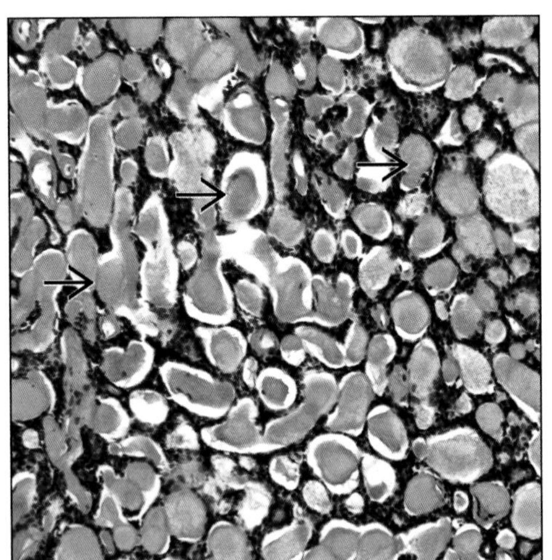

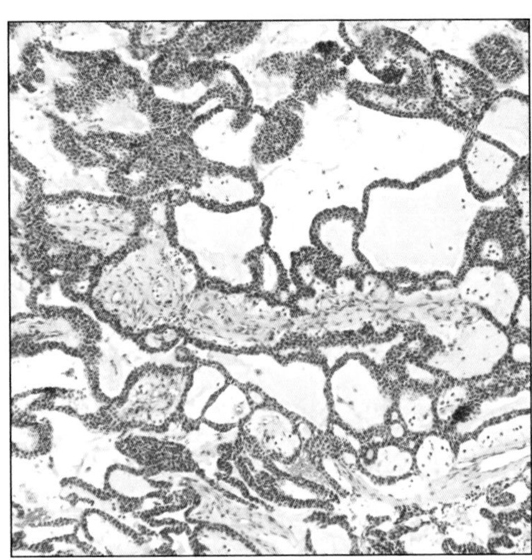

(Left) *The tumor cells are set within a dense, brightly eosinophilic, hyalinized stroma ⇒. The stroma is composed of basal lamina. This same stroma can be seen in cytology specimens and may be helpful in making a definitive diagnosis for ACC.* ***(Right)*** *ACC can demonstrate a number of different patterns. The cystic pattern in this tumor simulates a canalicular adenoma or perhaps a cystadenoma. However, high power would help to make the separation among these tumor types.*

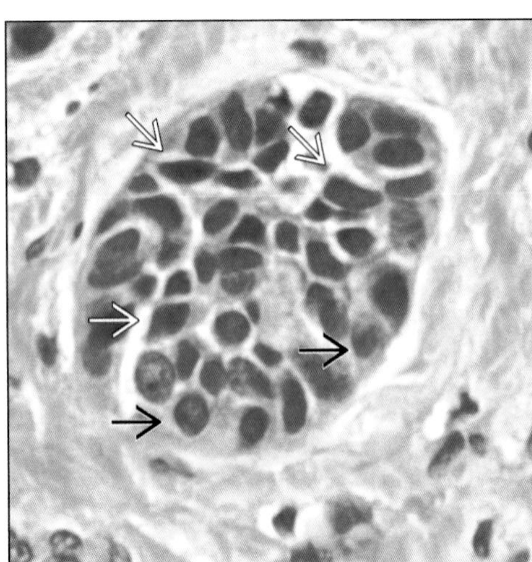

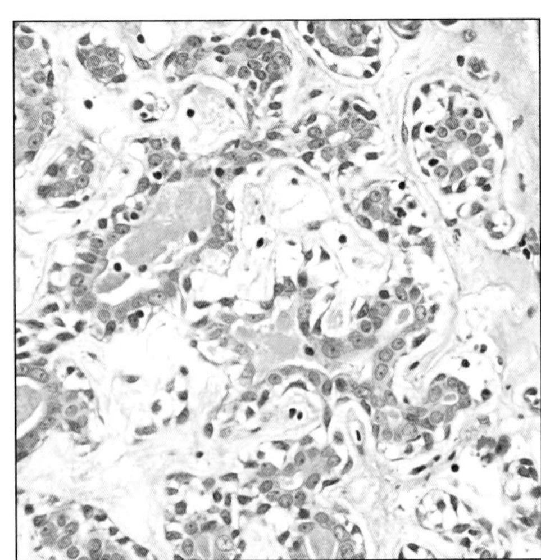

(Left) *Hematoxylin & eosin shows an island of tumor cells with angular cells with clear cytoplasm ➡ and more ovoid cells with less characteristic eosinophilic cytoplasm ⇒. The angular cells are helpful in differentiating this tumor from a polymorphous low-grade adenocarcinoma, which classically has bland, ovoid vesicular nuclei.* ***(Right)*** *Clear cell change is noted within a myoepithelial focus in this ACC. This focus was found among others that showed histologically characteristic features of ACC.*

Ancillary Techniques

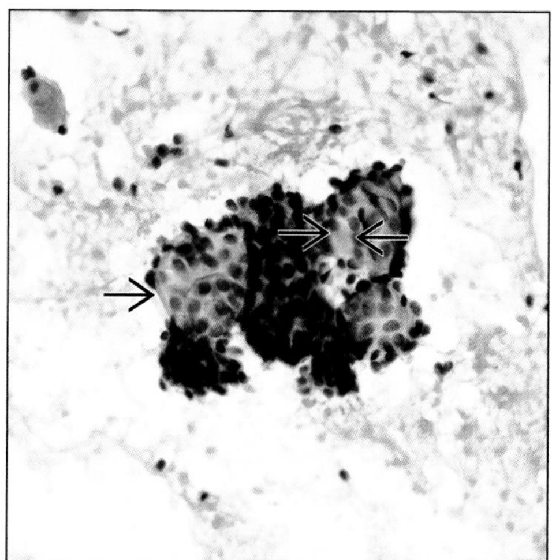

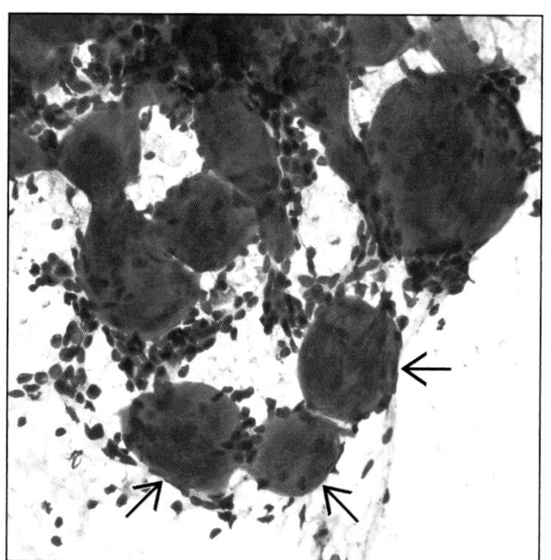

(Left) *This Papanicolaou stain shows an aggregate of small round to oval cells with hyaline material that is clear to pale green ⇨. Note the cells are surrounding the material.* ***(Right)*** *Diff-Quik (air-dried) shows a cluster of cells with round nuclei and purple hyaline spheres ⇨. These purple areas are sometimes referred to as bubblegum-like and are helpful when considering ACC. The cells surround the hyaline material rather than merging with it, as would be seen in pleomorphic adenoma.*

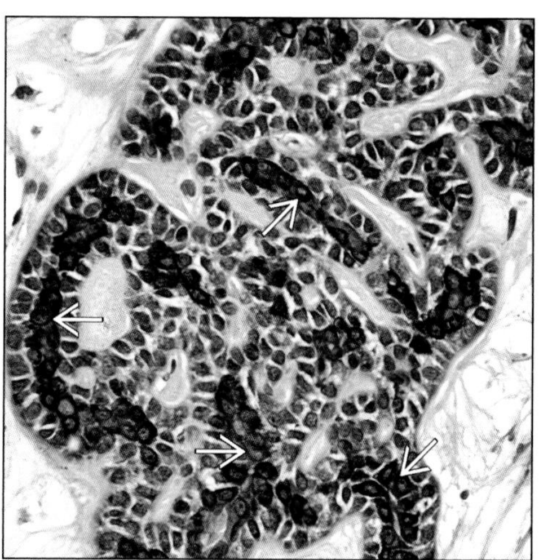

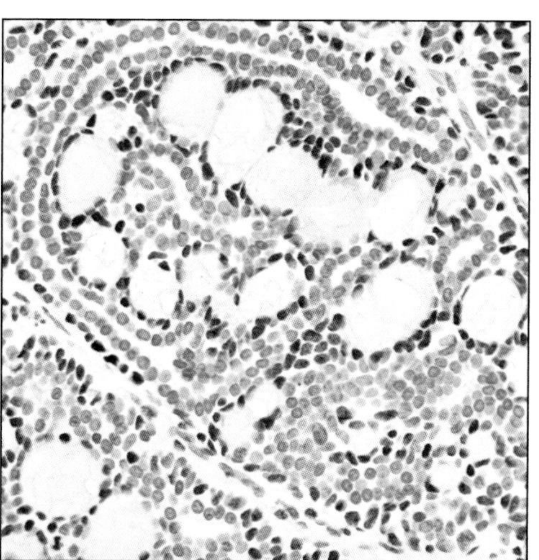

(Left) *CK-PAN is reactive in this adenoid cystic carcinoma. Staining intensity may vary among different tumors and even within a single neoplasm. Staining is cytoplasmic; in this particular tumor, staining is rather intense but greater in the luminal cells ➡.* ***(Right)*** *p63 shows strong nuclear reactivity in abluminal cells of ACC. The 2nd population of cells lacks reactivity, a feature that highlights the epithelial-myoepithelial phenotype of the tumor.*

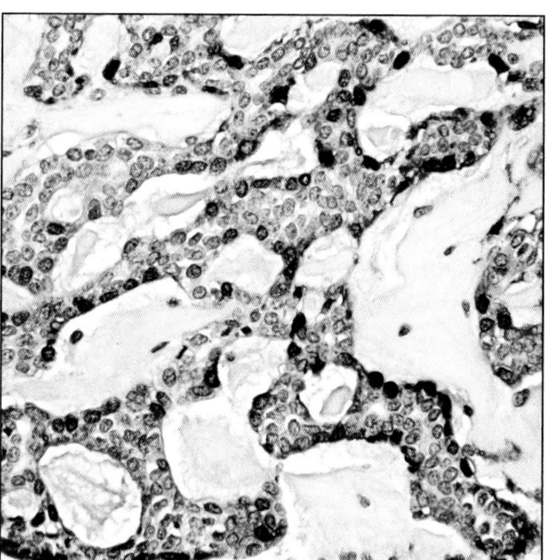

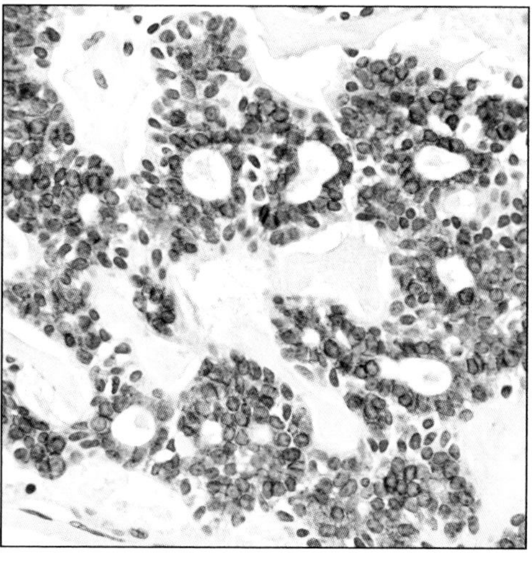

(Left) *S100 protein shows primarily nuclear reactivity in this adenoid cystic carcinoma. S100 protein has variable nuclear and cytoplasmic reactivity and may show remarkable intensity among different tumors and even in the same tumor.* ***(Right)*** *CD117 (C-KIT) is consistently reactive in the cell membrane and cytoplasm of adenoid cystic carcinoma, with the solid variant being more reactive than the tubular variant. Note the differential immunoreactivity, with luminal cells highlighted.*

ACINIC CELL CARCINOMA

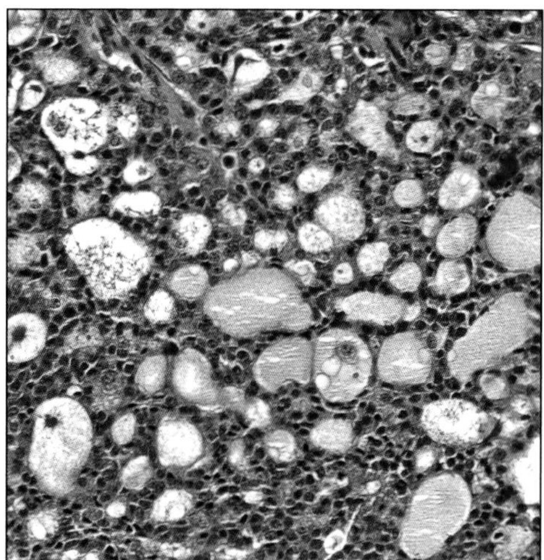

Acinic cell carcinoma shows multiple small cysts, creating a microcystic pattern. This lattice-like or sieve-like appearance is quite characteristic. There are secretions within the lumen.

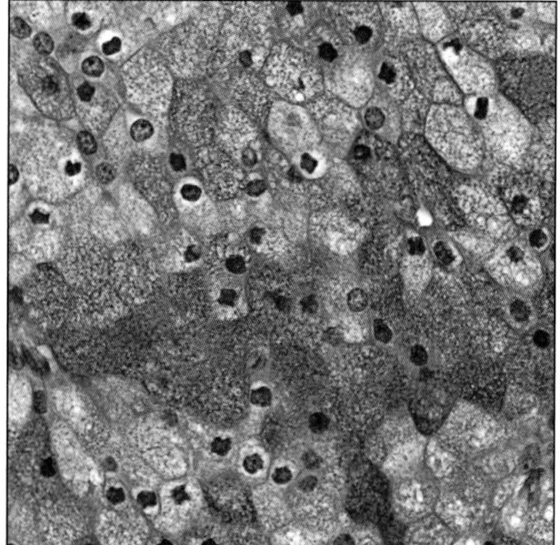

Serous acinar cells (most characteristic for AcCC) are large, polygonal with abundant light to dark basophilic, granular cytoplasm. Dense, blue to purple, fine to coarse zymogen granules are seen.

TERMINOLOGY

Abbreviations

- Acinic cell carcinoma (AcCC)

Synonyms

- Acinic cell adenocarcinoma
- Acinous cell carcinoma
- Acinic cell tumor
  - Discouraged, as malignancy is well established

Definitions

- Malignant epithelial salivary gland neoplasm demonstrating serous acinar cell differentiation with cytoplasmic zymogen secretory granules
  - Is **not** exclusively, nor even necessarily predominantly, serous type cells
  - Salivary ductal cells are also part of this neoplasm

ETIOLOGY/PATHOGENESIS

Environmental Exposure

- Radiation exposure possible factor

Pathogenesis

- Serous acinar cell with zymogen secretory granules
- Arise from intercalated duct cells with differentiation toward serous acinar cells

CLINICAL ISSUES

Epidemiology

- Incidence
  - Accounts for about 6% of salivary gland tumors
  - Represents approximately 10-12% of all malignant salivary gland tumors
  - 2nd to mucoepidermoid carcinoma in frequency
- Age
  - Wide range
    - Even distribution from 2nd to 7th decades
    - Mean: Mid 40s
  - 2nd most common malignant salivary gland tumor in children (2nd decade)
- Gender
  - Female > Male (3:2)

Site

- Parotid gland most common (80%)
  - Parotid is largest salivary gland, comprised nearly exclusively of serous type acini
- Minor salivary glands 2nd most common site
  - Intraoral, buccal mucosa, upper lip, and palate specifically (6-15%)
- Submandibular (4%) and sublingual (1%)
  - Despite high serous type acini in sublingual gland
- Rare: Lacrimal gland, larynx, pharynx, nasal cavity
- Most common bilateral salivary gland malignancy
  - Dwarfed by bilateral Warthin tumors and pleomorphic adenomas

Presentation

- History of slowly enlarging solitary parotid/facial mass, which may be mobile or fixed
  - Duration varies from weeks to several decades
- Pain (vague, intermittent) or tenderness is present in up to half of patients
- Facial nerve paralysis present in 5-10% of cases
  - Facial muscle weakness and tingling
- Uncommonly multinodular
- Uncommonly fixed to skin or muscle

Treatment

- Surgical approaches
  - Complete surgical excision treatment of choice
    - Incomplete excision portends poor prognosis
- Radiation
  - Not presently used in primary management
  - Improved survival for incompletely excised tumors or advanced stage disease
    - Valuable for occult metastases

ACINIC CELL CARCINOMA

Key Facts

Terminology
- Malignant neoplasm of serous acinar cell differentiation

Clinical Issues
- ~ 10% of all malignant salivary gland tumors
- Parotid gland most commonly affected (80%)
- Generally good prognosis (5-year survival: 80-90%)
- Recurrences (locally) in about 35% of cases

Microscopic Pathology
- Circumscribed, solitary, oval to round masses
- **Patterns (in order of frequency)**
  - Solid/lobular, papillary-cystic, microcystic
  - Follicular is rare
- Multiple cell types
  - **Serous acinar**: Large, polygonal cells
  - Abundant lightly basophilic, granular cytoplasm
  - **Intercalated duct type**: Smaller, eosinophilic to amphophilic cells
  - **Vacuolated**: Clear, cytoplasmic vacuoles
  - **Nonspecific glandular**: Round to polygonal, often syncytial, and smaller than acinar cells
  - **Clear cells**: Nonstaining cytoplasm and prominent cell borders
- Associated with lymphoid infiltrate, sometimes prominent

Ancillary Tests
- PAS(+), diastase-resistant zymogen granules

Top Differential Diagnoses
- Normal salivary gland, papillary cystadenocarcinoma, mucoepidermoid carcinoma, clear cell tumors

Prognosis
- Generally, good prognosis
  - 5-year survival: 80-90% (disease specific)
  - 10-year survival: 65%
- Clinical stage more reliable than histologic grading in determining outcome
- Recurrences (locally) in about 35% of cases
  - Most develop within 5 years of diagnosis
- Behavior does not correlate with grade or growth pattern
- Poor prognosis (including tumor recurrence) associated with
  - Regional lymph node and distant metastases
    - Cervical lymph node metastases initially
    - Lung and bone most common distant sites (about 15% of cases)
  - Multiple recurrences
  - Incomplete resection
  - Submandibular gland location or deep lobe of parotid involvement
    - Minor salivary gland location has better prognosis than major glands
  - Age > 30 years
  - Short symptom duration
  - Large size
  - Multinodularity
  - Histology: Cellular pleomorphism, necrosis, perineural invasion, stromal hyalinization, no lymphoid infiltrate, dedifferentiation
  - Increased mitoses (> 10% Ki-67 labeling)

MACROSCOPIC FEATURES

General Features
- Circumscribed, solitary oval to round masses
  - Occasionally ill defined with irregular peripheries
  - Not usually encapsulated
  - Bilateral and multifocal tumors are rare
- Multinodularity is uncommon
- Cut surface is lobular and tan to red
- Rubbery to firm
- Solid to cystic (hemorrhagic)

Size
- Range: 0.5-13 cm
- Mean: 1-3 cm

MICROSCOPIC PATHOLOGY

Histologic Features
- Tumor extension into normal tissue is common, although "apparent" encapsulation is present
- Although one pattern and cell type often dominate, combination and spectrum is common
- **Patterns (in order of frequency)**
  - Sheets, nodules, or aggregates in **solid/lobular** pattern (most readily recognized pattern)
    - **Blue dot tumor**: Basophilic, granular cytoplasm and round, basophilic nuclei
  - Small spaces in **microcystic** pattern
    - Yields lattice-like or sieve-like appearance
    - May represent coalescence of ruptured and degenerated vacuolated cells
  - Large cyst cavities with papillary projections of epithelial cells comprise **papillary-cystic** pattern
    - Due to complexity and sectioning, papillae appear to be "floating" within cystic spaces
    - Delicate fibrovascular cores are noted
    - Often vascular and hemorrhagic, with hemosiderin identified in cytoplasm of luminal cells
    - Luminal epithelial cells can have "hobnail" or "tombstone row" appearance
    - Usually intercalated duct-type and vacuolated cells
  - Multiple, epithelial-lined cystic spaces filled with eosinophilic proteinaceous material found in **follicular** pattern
    - Only prominent in ~ 5% of tumors
    - Usually intercalated duct-type cells
    - Psammoma bodies can be seen
    - Eosinophilic, homogeneous, proteinaceous fluid mimics thyroid colloid (hence "follicular")
- **Many cell types (in order of frequency)**

ACINIC CELL CARCINOMA

- **Serous acinar** cells are large, polygonal cells with abundant lightly basophilic, granular cytoplasm
  - Most common cell type
  - Strong resemblance to normal serous acini cells
  - Round, uniform, slightly eccentric nuclei, hyperchromatic to vesicular
  - Dense, gray to blue to purple, fine to coarse zymogen granules
  - Granules are often accentuated at lumen
  - Cytoplasm may be finely reticular or foamy
- **Intercalated duct type** cells surround luminal spaces and tend to be smaller, eosinophilic to amphophilic cells
  - Cuboidal with centrally located nuclei
- **Vacuolated** cells have clear, cytoplasmic vacuoles
  - Majority cellular component in ~ 10% of tumors
  - Vacuoles fill most of cytoplasm, are variable in size, and tend to be smaller the greater the number present within cytoplasm
  - Vacuoles are negative with PAS and mucicarmine
  - Remaining cytoplasm is eosinophilic to amphophilic
- **Nonspecific glandular** cells are round to polygonal, often syncytial, and smaller than acinar cells
  - Majority cellular component in ~ 15% of tumors
  - Amphophilic to eosinophilic cytoplasm with round nuclei
  - Granules are lacking
  - Nuclei are more variable
- **Clear cells** have nonstaining cytoplasm with prominent cell borders
  - Present in ~ 6%; majority cellular component in < 1%
  - No glycogen identified (therefore, clearing is probably processing artifact)
  - Usually show small collections and are seldom dominant finding
- Lymphoid infiltrate, sometimes prominent with germinal center formation, can be seen
  - Part of "tumor-associated lymphoid proliferation" (TALP) concept
  - Sometimes it simulates a lymph node but should not be misinterpreted as metastasis
- Stromal fibrosis or desmoplasia is uncommon
- High-grade transformation (dedifferentiation) into high-grade carcinoma (including small cell carcinoma) is rare and heralds poor prognosis

Variants

- Specific pattern is dominant or only finding
  - **Solid, microcystic, papillary-cystic, follicular**
- Specific cell type is dominant or only finding
  - **Intercalated ductal, vacuolated cell, nonspecific glandular, and clear cell types**

ANCILLARY TESTS

Cytology

- High false-negative rate (interpreted as normal)
- Cellular smears with clean background
- Cohesive, small, tight clusters resembling normal acini
  - Fibrovascular core may be noted
- Ducts and adipocytes are absent
- Large, uniform cells with small, round and regular nuclei with coarse chromatin (lymphocyte-like nuclei)
  - Serous acinar cells with central nuclei
- Ample, granular to vacuolated cytoplasm, lacking coarse granules
  - Stripped cytoplasm creates naked nuclei
- Lymphocytes may be prominent component of stroma

Histochemistry

- PAS(+), diastase-resistant zymogen granules
  - Reaction can be patchy and limited
  - No glycogen identified
- Negative or only focally positive granules with mucicarmine

Immunohistochemistry

- Immunoprofile is nonspecific and unpredictable, so seldom of diagnostic value

Flow Cytometry

- DNA ploidy does not predict outcome

Cytogenetics

- No consistent or specific structural chromosomal alterations
- Deletions of chromosome 6q, loss of Y and trisomy 21 have been reported
- LOH most frequently at chromosomes 4p, 5q, 6p, and 17p regions
  - Chromosomes 4p15-16, 6p25-qter, and 17p11 show highest incidence of alterations

Electron Microscopy

- Both acinar type and ductal type cells identified
- Secretory zymogen granules in cytoplasm
  - Round, variably electron dense secretory granules
  - Rough endoplasmic reticulum usually present
- Basal lamina separates epithelium from stroma
- Clear cells are due to dilatations of rough endoplasmic reticulum, lipid inclusions, autophagic vacuoles, or intracytoplasmic pseudolumina
- Ductal cells lack secretory granules and have apical junctional complexes and microvilli

DIFFERENTIAL DIAGNOSIS

Normal Salivary Gland

- Lobular, with striated and interlobular ducts, acini, and adipocytes
- Stromal fibrosis is often detected
- Very well-differentiated tumors may be difficult to diagnose on core needle biopsy specimens

Papillary Cystadenocarcinoma

- Arranged in papillary and microcystic pattern, similar to AcCC
- Lacks zymogen granules (acinar cells), vacuolated cells, and intercalated ductal differentiation
- Lacks mucocytes (mucicarmine[+])

Mucoepidermoid Carcinoma

- Specifically, microcystic pattern can cause confusion with AcCC (although rare)

ACINIC CELL CARCINOMA

Immunohistochemistry

Antibody	Reactivity	Staining Pattern	Comment
CK-PAN	Positive	Cytoplasmic	All tumor cells
α-1-antitrypsin	Positive	Cytoplasmic	Most tumor cells
α-1-antichymotrypsin	Positive	Cytoplasmic	Most tumor cells
CEA-M	Positive	Cytoplasmic	Many tumor cells
Amylase	Positive	Cytoplasmic	Weak and patchy, although positive in most tumors
LF	Positive	Cytoplasmic	Lactoferrin; positive in most tumors
S100	Positive	Nuclear & cytoplasmic	Seen in about 10% of tumors
α-amylase	Negative		Enzyme (+) in normal serous acinar cells but not in neoplastic cells
p63	Negative		
Calponin	Negative		
Actin-sm	Negative		

- Mucicarmine(+) material must be within cell cytoplasm, not just in cystic spaces
- No serous acinar cells identified

Metastatic Thyroid Carcinoma

- Follicular pattern of AcCC mimics thyroid carcinoma
- Colloid and both thyroglobulin and TTF-1 reactivity confirm metastatic disease

Clear Cell Tumors

- Clear cell variant of AcCC is rare, and clear cells are usually limited and focal
- Differential diagnoses include
  - Epithelial-myoepithelial carcinoma: Usually biphasic, lacking serous acinar cell differentiation
  - Clear cell adenocarcinoma: Associated with heavy fibrosis and strong glycogen content
  - Clear cell oncocytoma: Oncocytes are present somewhere in tumor, with (+) mitochondrial stains
  - Metastatic renal cell carcinoma: Shows a pseudoalveolar pattern, prominent intercellular borders, significant glycogen, and usually pleomorphism

Polymorphous Low-Grade Adenocarcinoma

- Minor salivary gland location; multiple patterns of growth; single file infiltration; perineural proclivity; bland cells with vesicular nuclei; no serous acinar differentiation

SELECTED REFERENCES

1. Al-Zaher N et al: Acinic cell carcinoma of the salivary glands: a literature review. Hematol Oncol Stem Cell Ther. 2(1):259-64, 2009
2. Daneshbod Y et al: Diagnostic difficulties in the interpretation of fine needle aspirate samples in salivary lesions: diagnostic pitfalls revisited. Acta Cytol. 53(1):53-70, 2009
3. Skálová A et al: Acinic cell carcinoma with high-grade transformation: a report of 9 cases with immunohistochemical study and analysis of TP53 and HER-2/neu genes. Am J Surg Pathol. 33(8):1137-45, 2009
4. Rau AR et al: Infarction of acinic cell carcinoma in a patient infected with HIV: a complication of fine-needle aspiration cytology obscuring definitive diagnosis. Diagn Cytopathol. 29(4):222-4, 2003
5. Ali SZ: Acinic-cell carcinoma, papillary-cystic variant: a diagnostic dilemma in salivary gland aspiration. Diagn Cytopathol. 27(4):244-50, 2002
6. Hoffman HT et al: National Cancer Data Base report on cancer of the head and neck: acinic cell carcinoma. Head Neck. 21(4):297-309, 1999
7. Ellis GL: Clear cell neoplasms in salivary glands: clearly a diagnostic challenge. Ann Diagn Pathol. 2(1):61-78, 1998
8. Slater LJ: Acinic cell carcinoma and PAS-positive granules. Oral Surg Oral Med Oral Pathol Oral Radiol Endod. 86(5):507-8, 1998
9. Crivelini MM et al: Immunohistochemical study of acinic cell carcinoma of minor salivary gland. Oral Oncol. 33(3):204-8, 1997
10. Michal M et al: Well-differentiated acinic cell carcinoma of salivary glands associated with lymphoid stroma. Hum Pathol. 28(5):595-600, 1997
11. Napier SS et al: Acinic cell carcinoma in Northern Ireland: a 10-year review. Br J Oral Maxillofac Surg. 33(3):145-8, 1995
12. Skalova A et al: Cell proliferation correlates with prognosis in acinic cell carcinomas of salivary gland origin. Immunohistochemical study of 30 cases using the MIB 1 antibody in formalin-fixed paraffin sections. J Pathol. 173(1):13-21, 1994
13. Oliveira P et al: Acinic cell carcinoma of the salivary glands. A long term follow-up study of 15 cases. Eur J Surg Oncol. 18(1):7-15, 1992
14. Colmenero C et al: Acinic cell carcinoma of the salivary glands. A review of 20 new cases. J Craniomaxillofac Surg. 19(6):260-6, 1991
15. Hiratsuka H et al: Acinic cell carcinoma of minor salivary gland origin. Oral Surg Oral Med Oral Pathol. 63(6):704-8, 1987
16. Chaudhry AP et al: Histogenesis of acinic cell carcinoma of the major and minor salivary glands. An ultrastructural study. J Pathol. 148(4):307-20, 1986
17. Ferlito A: Acinic cell carcinoma of minor salivary glands. Histopathology. 4(3):331-43, 1980
18. Chen SY et al: Acinic cell adenocarcinoma of minor salivary glands. Cancer. 42(2):678-85, 1978
19. Batsakis JG et al: Acinous cell carcinoma: a histogenetic hypothesis. J Oral Surg. 35(11):904-6, 1977
20. Seifert G et al: Classification of the pathohistology of diseases of the salivary glands - review of 2,600 cases in the Salivary Gland Register. Beitr Pathol. 159(1):1-32, 1976

ACINIC CELL CARCINOMA

Microscopic and Invasive Features

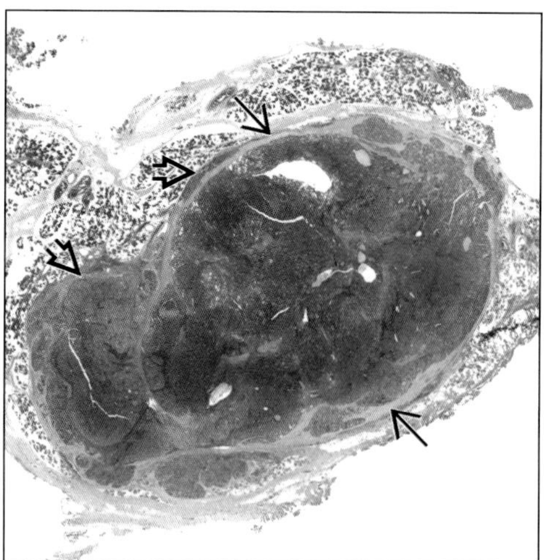

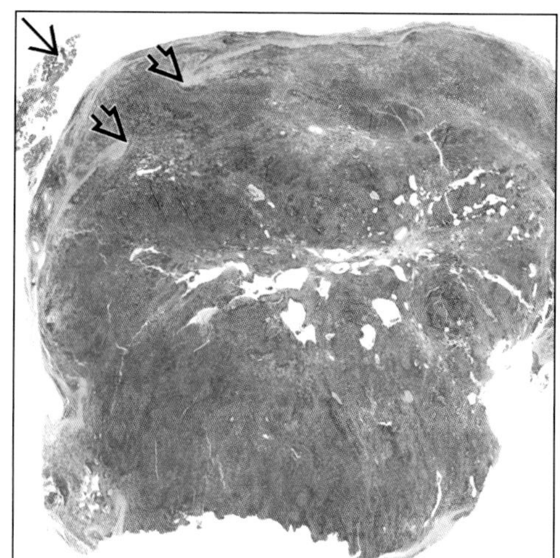

(Left) *The tumors are usually circumscribed with an irregular periphery. This multinodular tumor has a suggestion of an incomplete fibrous connective tissue capsule ⇒ surrounding it. Invasion into the parenchyma is suggested ⇨.* ***(Right)*** *Tumor-associated lymphoid proliferation (TALP) can be a conspicuous finding, as shown in this tumor. Salivary gland tissue is noted ⇒, but the pattern simulates a lymph node. Note the invasion through the "capsule" ⇨.*

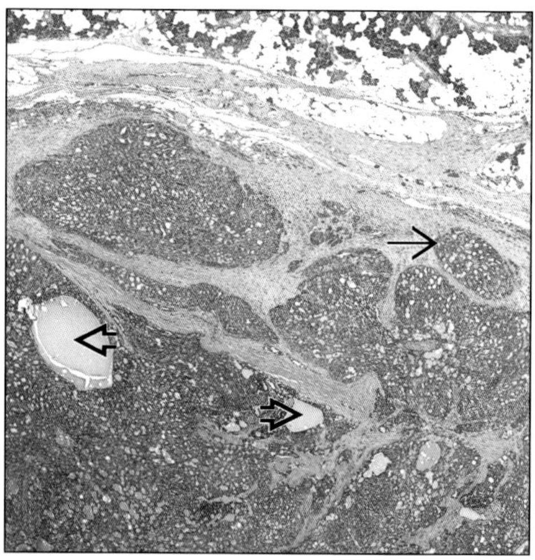

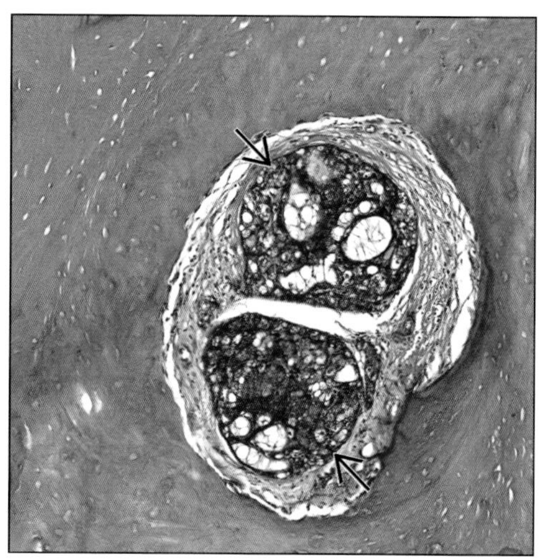

(Left) *The periphery of the tumor is irregular, with a solid-lobular to nodular pattern. Areas suggesting vascular invasion ⇒ are noted, but the separation from a nodule or tumor is sometimes challenging. Note the cysts within the tumor ⇨.* ***(Right)*** *While infrequent, minor salivary gland tumors may infiltrate into the adjacent bone ⇒, as shown in this micrograph. The tumor islands are noted with a fragment of bone taken from the mandible in a floor of the mouth primary tumor.*

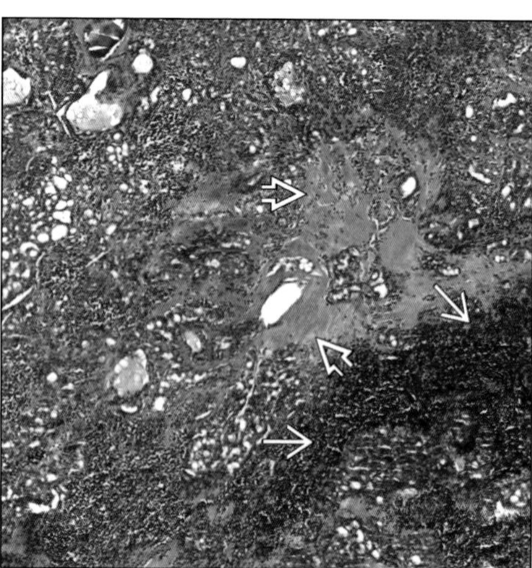

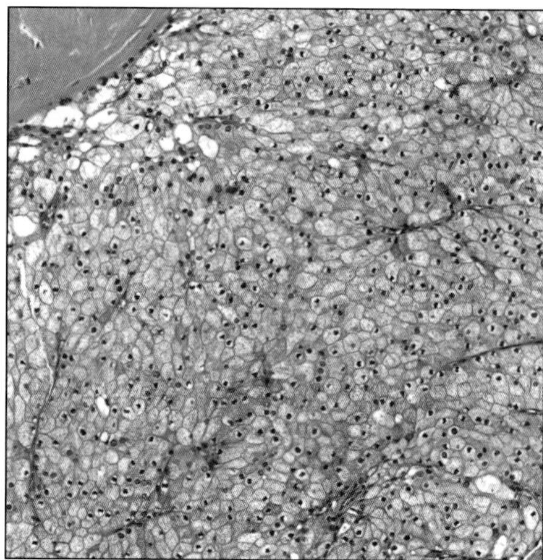

(Left) *There are many times when there is a spectrum of patterns and cell types within a single tumor. In this case areas of solid, microcystic, and follicular architecture are seen, along with a prominent lymphoid infiltrate ➡. Intratumoral fibrosis is easily identified ➡.* ***(Right)*** *The solid sheet of basophilic cells with granular, basophilic cytoplasm surrounding round basophilic nuclei result in the colloquial "blue dot tumor" designation for this tumor.*

Patterns of Growth

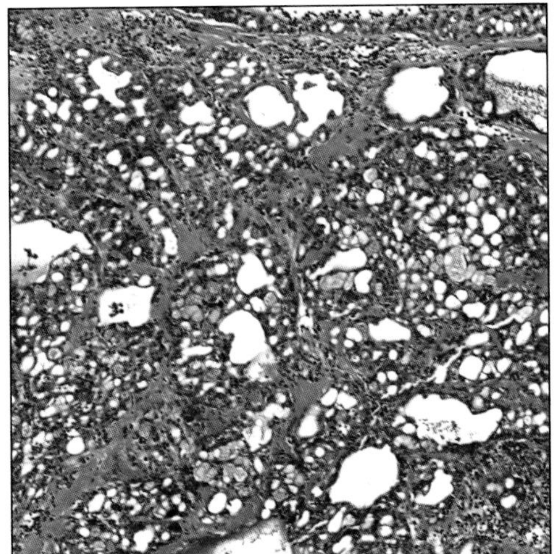

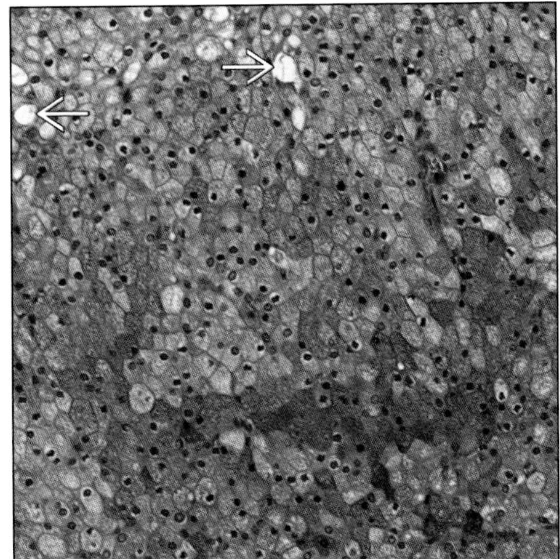

***(Left)** There are a variety of different cystic spaces in this tumor, although the pattern of a microcystic appearance predominates. Fibrovascular septae are noted separating the tumor cells. Some of the cells are made up of the "vacuolated" cell type, further accentuating the "cystic" appearance. **(Right)** There are frequently slight variations in cytoplasmic appearance, where some cells have darker cytoplasm than others. There are a few foamy ➔ or finely reticular cells in this tumor.*

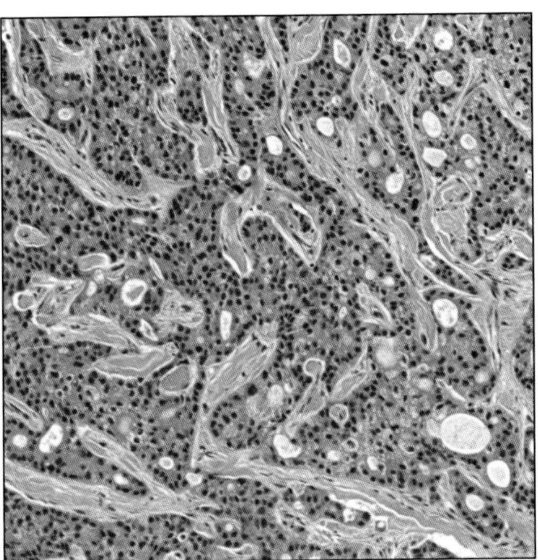

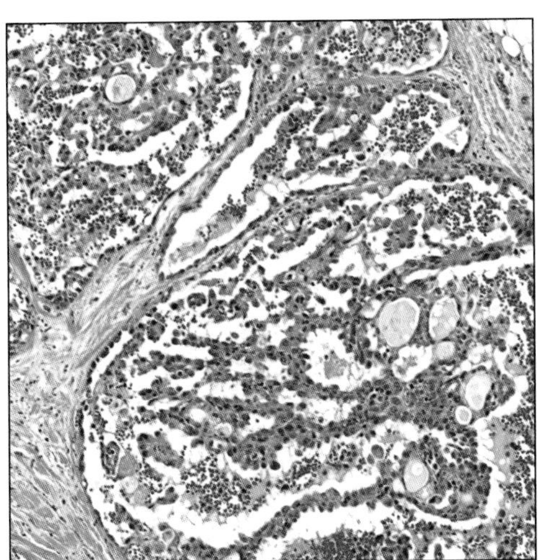

***(Left)** This tumor is arranged in a predominantly lobular and glandular pattern, with intratumoral fibrosis. The intercalated duct type cells are dominant in this tumor, with short cuboidal cells exhibiting central nuclei. **(Right)** The papillary-cystic pattern of growth yields a complex arrangement of papillae within a cystic space. The papillae show a "hobnail" or "tombstone row" appearance of the luminal cells. Extravasated erythrocytes are seen throughout.*

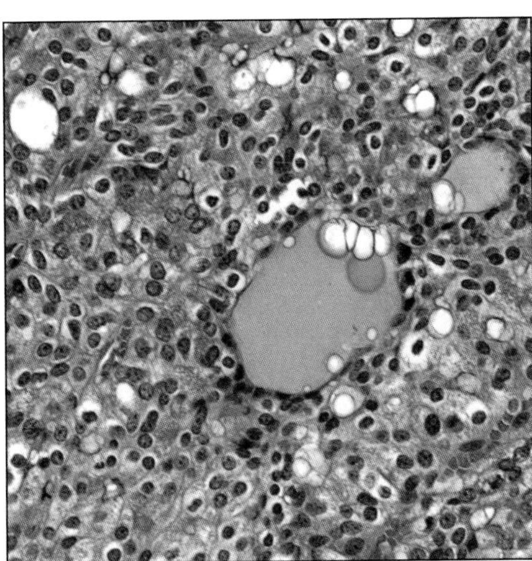

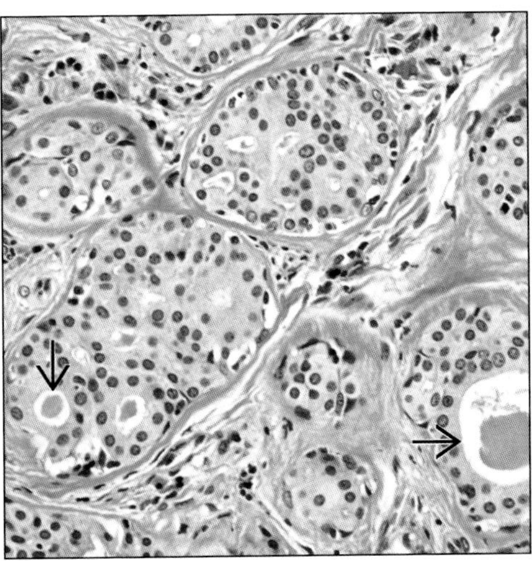

***(Left)** This field shows serous acinar cells as well as a few intercalated duct-type cells. Vacuolated cells are not identified in this case. **(Right)** This tumor shows a follicular-type pattern. There are small glandular-like cells arranged around the periphery of a gland, with concretions present in the center ➔. The histologic similarity to a thyroid follicular tumor can be seen.*

ACINIC CELL CARCINOMA

Uncommon Histologic Features

(Left) Abundant granular, basophilic cytoplasm is present in these serous acinar cells. The nuclei are hyperchromatic, round, and have a slightly eccentric placement within the cell. *(Right)* The lymphoid infiltrate in this acinic cell carcinoma shows a well-formed germinal center ➡ surrounded by smaller lymphoid cells. The tumor is present at the periphery of this lymphoid follicle. This pattern does not mimic a lymph node architecture.

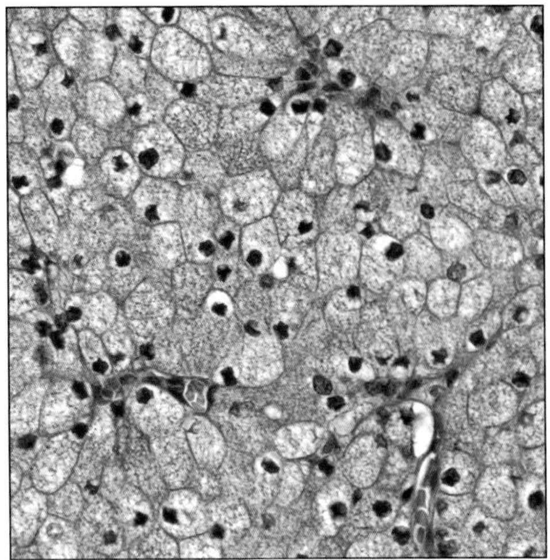

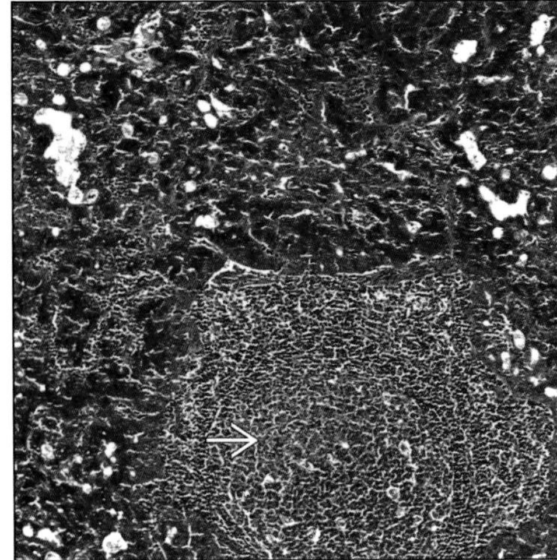

(Left) The blending of the acinar cells ➡ with the background lymphoid elements is very subtle in this tumor. At low power the epithelial elements may be inconspicuous, simulating the presence of a lymph node. There are secretions ⇨, which may help with the diagnosis of AcCC. *(Right)* The acinar cells ➡ are surrounding a reactive metaplastic squamous proliferation. This is an uncommon reactive finding after fine needle aspiration. The degree of cytologic atypia can be remarkable.

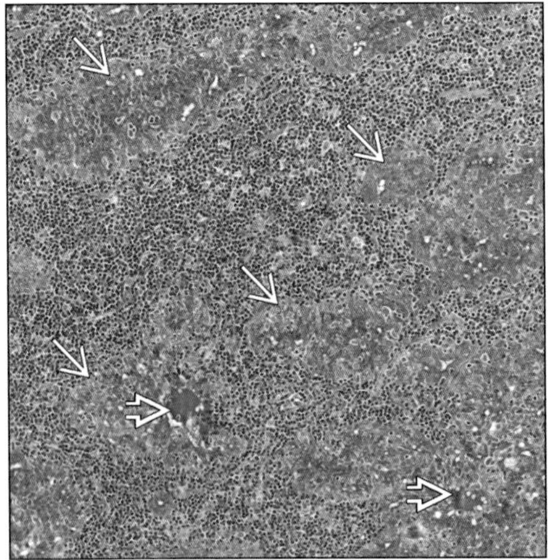

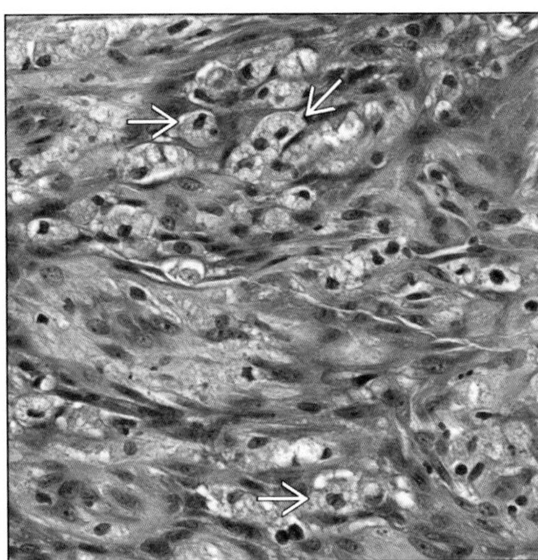

(Left) High-grade transformation (dedifferentiation) can be seen in AcCC. In this case, the acinar cell component ➡ is juxtaposed to the sheet-like appearance of a poorly differentiated carcinoma. Subtle gland-like or duct-like profiles are noted ⇨. *(Right)* Higher grade tumors are frequently associated with areas of necrosis ➡ and degeneration. There are still multiple areas within the tumor that show the characteristic acinar cell appearance ⇨.

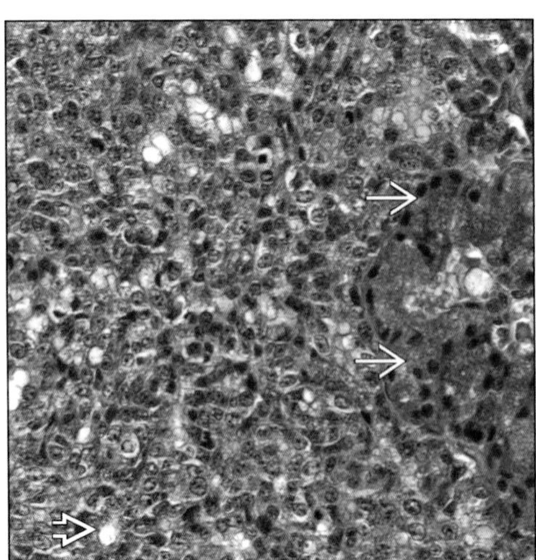

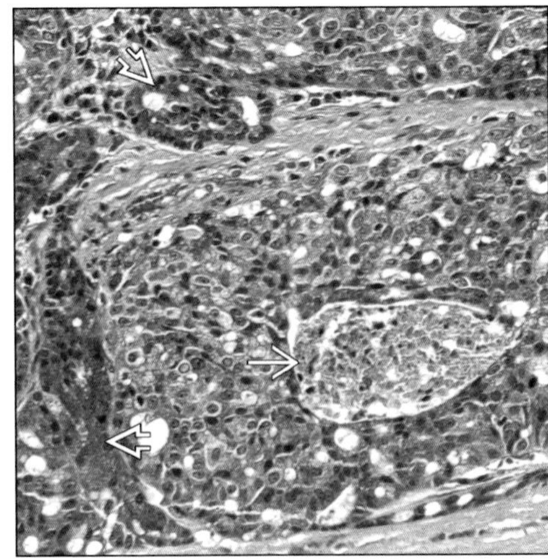

Microscopic Features and Ancillary Techniques

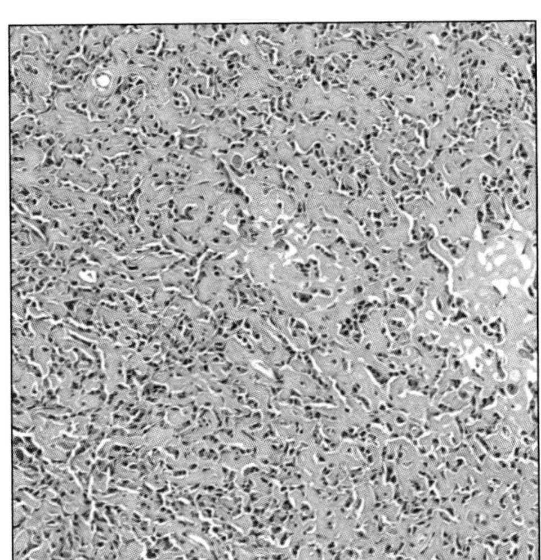

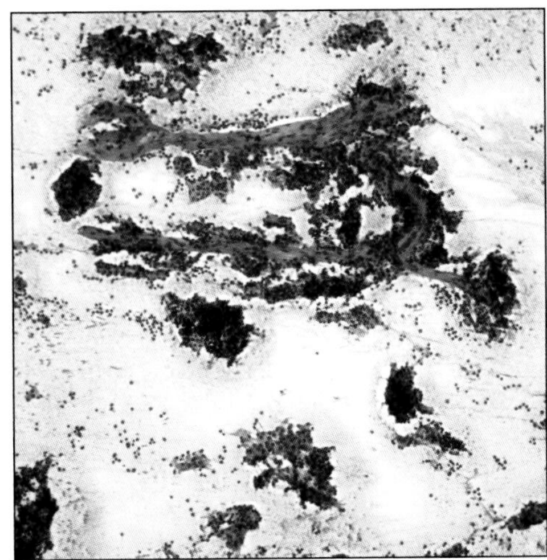

(Left) *This tumor is associated with a very dense stromal fibrosis. The fibrosis has compressed the neoplastic cells into cords and nests. At this magnification, a specific tumor type cannot be confirmed. However, the characteristic cellular components were present in other fields.* ***(Right)*** *There is a cellular smear, showing cohesive, small, tight clusters associated with a fibrovascular core. The background shows some naked nuclei and proteinaceous fluid.*

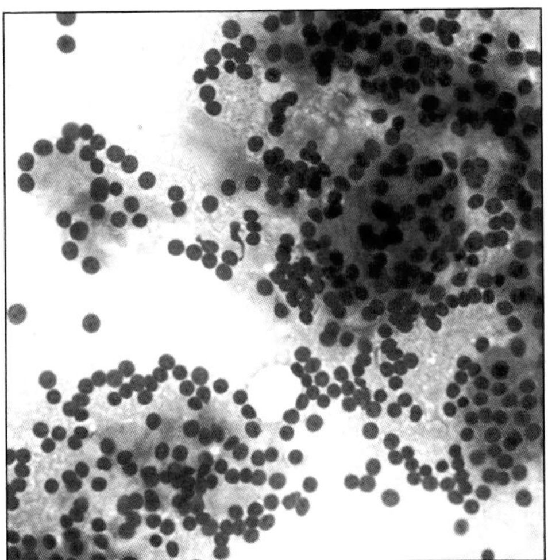

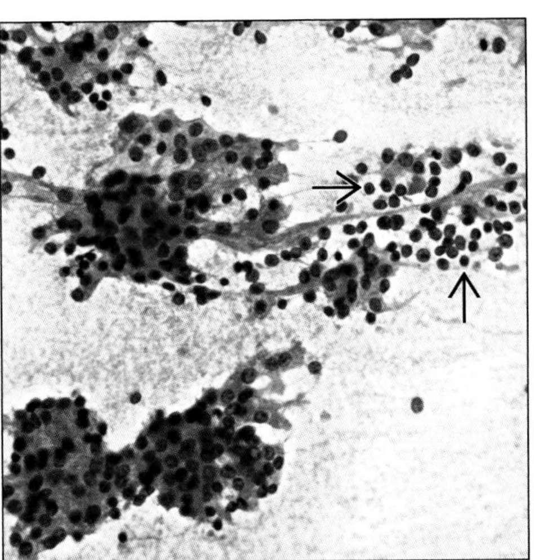

(Left) *This Diff-Quik preparation shows cohesive, small, tight clusters of cells resembling normal acini. The nuclei are round and regular with coarse nuclear chromatin distribution. The cytoplasm is delicately vacuolated.* ***(Right)*** *The tight acinar cells are associated with stripped cells, showing naked nuclei ➔. There is limited to no cytologic atypia. The nuclei are about the size of lymphocytes, but there are no lymphoglandular bodies in the background.*

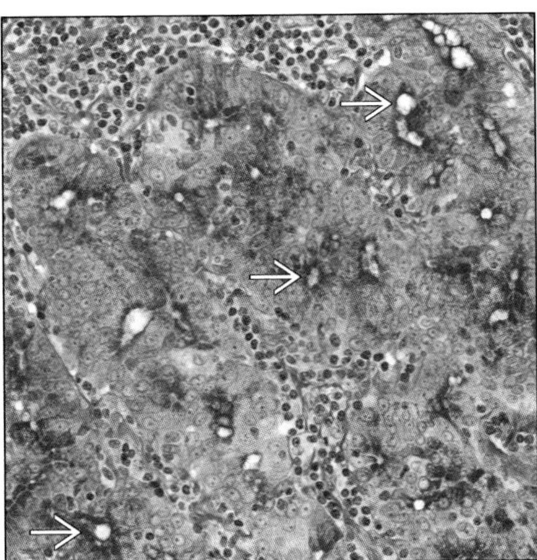

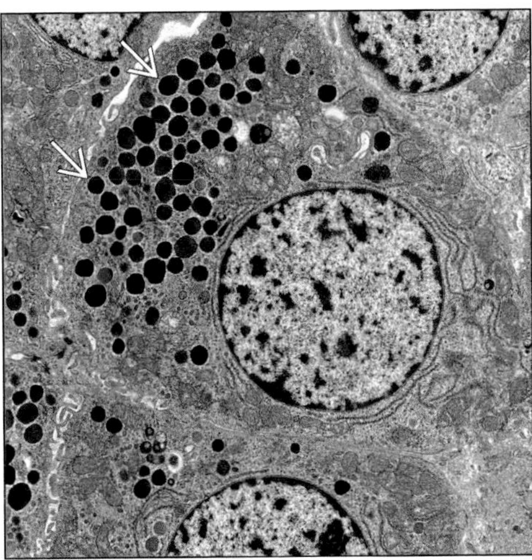

(Left) *PAS(+), diastase-resistant zymogen granules are accentuated at the lumen ➔ in this AcCC. This pattern of distribution is quite common.* ***(Right)*** *An electron micrograph demonstrates the characteristic zymogen granules in the cytoplasm of a serous acinar cell. They are electron-dense, showing slight variability in shape and size ➔. There are other cytoplasmic organelles, including mitochondria and endoplasmic reticulum. (Courtesy S. Bhuta, MD.)*

POLYMORPHOUS LOW-GRADE ADENOCARCINOMA

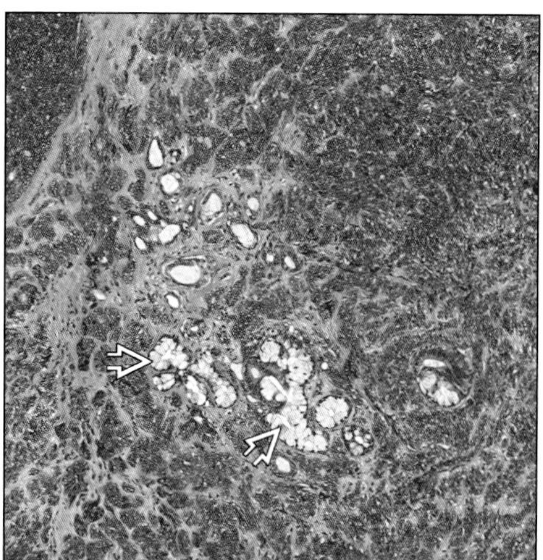

The tumor is unencapsulated, showing encasement or "entombment" of the residual minor salivary gland tissue ➡. The tumor surrounds but does not destroy the salivary gland tissue.

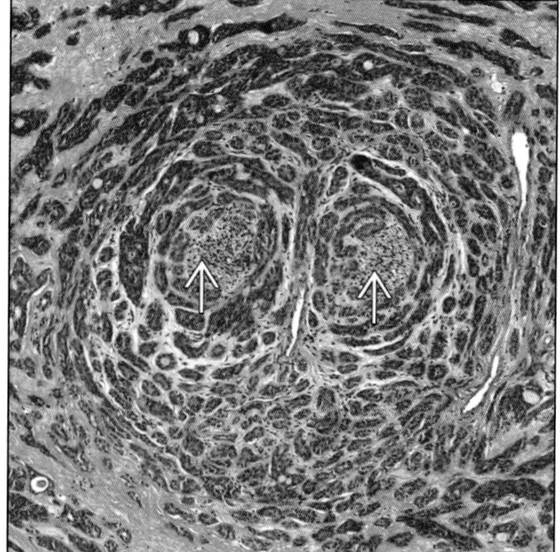

An intermediate power demonstrates 2 nerves ➡ creating a nidus with concentrically arranged tumor cells in thin strands. This targetoid appearance around a peripheral nerve is quite characteristic.

TERMINOLOGY

Abbreviations

- Polymorphous low-grade adenocarcinoma (PLGA)

Synonyms

- Terminal duct carcinoma
- Lobular carcinoma

Definitions

- Malignant epithelial tumor characterized by infiltrative growth of cytologically uniform cells arranged in architecturally diverse patterns

ETIOLOGY/PATHOGENESIS

Pathogenesis

- Intercalated/terminal duct derivation is presumptive

CLINICAL ISSUES

Epidemiology

- Incidence
  - Uncommon: ~ 2% of all salivary gland tumors
  - 2nd most common intraoral minor salivary gland malignant tumor (~ 25%)
- Age
  - Wide range: 16-95 years
  - Mean: 60 years
    - Vast majority are between 50 and 70 years
  - Exceedingly rare in children
- Gender
  - Female > Male (2:1)
- Ethnicity
  - Predilection for black patients

Site

- Almost **always** in minor glands
- Order of frequency
  - Palate (60%), especially at mucosal junction of hard and soft palates
  - Buccal (cheek) mucosa (~ 15%)
  - Lip (particularly upper) (~ 10%)
  - Retromolar areas
  - Floor of mouth, tongue (posterior 3rd specifically), oropharynx, tonsil
  - Other sites: Lacrimal gland, sinonasal tract, nasopharynx, and upper/lower respiratory tracts
- Multifocal synchronous primaries are rare

Presentation

- Usually forms slow-growing, firm, nontender mass
  - "Dentures not fitting"
- Discovered incidentally during routine dental examination
- Ulceration, bleeding, or telangiectasia and pain are uncommon
- Bone erosion or infiltration is uncommon
- Tumors may be mobile or fixed
- Neck mass rarely seen in patients with floor of mouth tumors
- Duration of symptoms varies from a few days up to 40 years
  - Mean: 2 years

Treatment

- Options, risks, complications
  - Long-term clinical follow-up is warranted due to indolent nature and prolonged latent period
- Surgical approaches
  - Complete, but conservative surgical excision is treatment of choice
  - Wide excision due to frequent perineural invasion
  - Neck dissection for proven regional metastases
- Radiation
  - Uncommonly, postoperative radiation used for recalcitrant recurrences
    - Palliative rather than curative

POLYMORPHOUS LOW-GRADE ADENOCARCINOMA

Key Facts

Terminology
- Malignant epithelial tumor characterized by infiltrative growth of cytologically uniform cells arranged in architecturally diverse patterns

Clinical Issues
- 2nd most common intraoral minor salivary gland malignant tumor (~ 25%)
- Female > Male (2:1)
- Almost **always** in minor glands (palate: 60%)
- Usually forms slow-growing, firm, nontender mass
- Complete, but conservative surgical excision is treatment of choice
- Overall excellent long-term prognosis

Microscopic Pathology
- Unencapsulated, although well circumscribed
- Infiltrative growth
  - Incarcerated minor salivary glands
  - Significant perineural invasion
- Striking variety of growth patterns
  - "Eye of the storm" or "whorled" appearance
  - Concentric layering of cells around central nidus, creating **targetoid** tableau
- Uniformly bland round to polygonal or fusiform tumor cells
- Slate gray-blue stroma usually only focal

Ancillary Tests
- Expression of epithelial and myoepithelial markers

Top Differential Diagnoses
- Pleomorphic adenoma, adenoid cystic carcinoma, papillary cystadenocarcinoma

Prognosis
- Overall excellent long-term prognosis
  - ~ 95% 10-year survival
  - Patients may die **with** tumor, but generally not **from** tumor
- Local recurrences in 9-15% of cases
  - Hard palate tumors especially
  - Recurrences may develop many years after primary (mean: 5-7 years)
  - Women are more likely to develop recurrences than men
- Spread to regional lymph nodes in 9-15% of cases
  - Increased risk of metastases with positive surgical margins
- Distant metastases are rare
  - Lung is most commonly affected site

IMAGE FINDINGS

Radiographic Findings
- Radiographs performed for mucosal tumors overlying bone to determine extent of surgery

MACROSCOPIC FEATURES

General Features
- Uniformly firm to solid, ovoid masses
- Characteristically unencapsulated, although well circumscribed
- Tumor approximates overlying surface epithelium, which is seldom ulcerated
- Cut surface is homogeneous, pale-yellow to tan

Size
- Range: 0.4-6 cm
- Mean: 2 cm
- Lip tumors tend to be smaller
  - More easily detected clinically rather than difference in biology
- Size does not influence prognosis

MICROSCOPIC PATHOLOGY

Histologic Features
- Infiltrative growth, architectural diversity, and cytologic uniformity, set in characteristic matrix
- **Infiltrative** growth
  - Unencapsulated, but usually well circumscribed
  - Uninvolved, usually intact surface epithelium
  - Encased, entombed, incarcerated, or completely surrounded minor salivary glands, with wrapping around, but not destruction by neoplastic cells
  - Invades into soft tissues, especially fat; less frequently skeletal muscle
  - Significant perineural invasion
  - Bone invasion is seen, especially with palate tumors
- **Patterns** of growth
  - Striking variety of growth patterns
  - Low power gives "eye of the storm," "streaming" or "whorled" appearance
  - Characteristic concentric layering of cells around central nidus, creating targetoid tableau
    - Nidus formed by small nerve twigs
  - Periphery often shows linear, single-file cell infiltration
  - Arranged in lobules, thèques, glandular profiles, tubules, trabeculae, and cribriform nests
    - Interconnecting cords parallel to more solid, convex nests of tumor
    - Small tubules lined by single layer of cuboidal cells
  - Papillae, if identified, are focal and not dominant pattern
- **Cellular** features
  - Uniformly bland (isomorphic) round to polygonal or fusiform tumor cells
  - Small to medium, with indistinct cellular borders
  - Ample pale to eosinophilic cytoplasm
  - Round to oval nuclei with open, vesicular nuclear chromatin
  - Inconspicuous to small nucleoli
- **Matrix** material

POLYMORPHOUS LOW-GRADE ADENOCARCINOMA

Immunohistochemistry

Antibody	Reactivity	Staining Pattern	Comment
CK-PAN	Positive	Cytoplasmic	All tumor cells positive in all cases
Vimentin	Positive	Cytoplasmic	Nearly all tumor cells
p63	Positive	Nuclear	Strong and diffuse, localized to peripheral tumor cells adjacent to connective tissue stroma
S100	Positive	Nuclear & cytoplasmic	Nearly 100% of all tumor cells in all cases
CEA-M	Positive	Cytoplasmic	Approximately 55% of tumor cells positive
EMA	Positive	Cytoplasmic	Most tumor cells reactive
CD117	Positive	Cytoplasmic	Nearly all tumors are variably immunoreactive
Actin-sm	Positive	Cytoplasmic	Approximately 10-15% of tumor cells positive
Actin-HHF-35	Positive	Cytoplasmic	Variable
GFAP	Positive	Cytoplasmic	Approximately 10-15% of tumor cells show faint, focal, or weak reactivity in luminal cells
Bcl-2	Positive	Nuclear	All tumor cells positive
Ki-67	Positive	Nuclear	Low proliferation index (< 6%)
p53	Positive	Nuclear	Only in rare isolated cells
MCM2	Positive	Nuclear	Usually < 9%
Galectin-3	Positive	Cytoplasmic	Variably positive in many cases

  - Slate gray-blue stroma usually only focal
  - Hyalinized, slightly eosinophilic stroma separates cells
- Inconspicuous mitoses
- Tyrosine-like crystals are uncommonly identified (< 5%)
- Rare metaplastic changes: Squamous, sebaceous, mucous, clear, oncocytic

ANCILLARY TESTS

Cytology
- Limited experience, as minor salivary gland tumors are infrequently sampled

Immunohistochemistry
- Variable expression of epithelial and myoepithelial markers

Cytogenetics
- Chromosome 12 abnormalities are most common: p or q arms (12q22 and 12p12.3)

DIFFERENTIAL DIAGNOSIS

Pleomorphic Adenoma (PA)
- Very difficult with small biopsies
- Minor salivary gland PAs are **not** encapsulated but are nodular or bosselated
- Lack perineural invasion
- Plasmacytoid cells are common but lacking in PLGA
- Myxochondroid matrix usually present (except in cellular tumors)
  - Both have hyaline or mucohyaline stroma
- Strong and diffuse GFAP seen in epithelial cells and in mesenchymal cells
  - PLGA shows faint, focal, or weak reactivity in epithelial luminal cells only

Adenoid Cystic Carcinoma (ACC)
- Multiple growth patterns mimic PLGA, although cribriform pattern much more common in ACC
  - Fascicular pattern is not seen in ACC
- Nuclei are peg-shaped, carrot-shaped, or angular, with hyperchromasia
- Pseudocystic spaces with glycosaminoglycans
  - Slate blue-gray background matrix is not seen
- Proliferation index usually higher than PLGA

Papillary Cystadenocarcinoma
- Papillary pattern is dominant
- Tumor is cystic, while this is not true of PLGA
- More frequent pleomorphism and mitoses

SELECTED REFERENCES

1. Thompson LD. Polymorphous low grade adenocarcinoma. Pathol Case Rev. 9(6):259-63, 2004
2. Evans HL et al: Polymorphous low-grade adenocarcinoma: a study of 40 cases with long-term follow up and an evaluation of the importance of papillary areas. Am J Surg Pathol. 24(10):1319-28, 2000
3. Castle JT et al: Polymorphous low grade adenocarcinoma: a clinicopathologic study of 164 cases. Cancer. 86(2):207-19, 1999
4. Gnepp DR et al: Polymorphous low-grade adenocarcinoma: glial fibrillary acidic protein staining in the differential diagnosis with cellular mixed tumors. Oral Surg Oral Med Oral Pathol Oral Radiol Endod. 83(6):691-5, 1997
5. Kelsch RD et al: Polymorphous low-grade adenocarcinoma: flow cytometric, p53, and PCNA analysis. Oral Surg Oral Med Oral Pathol Oral Radiol Endod. 84(4):391-9, 1997
6. Simpson RH et al: Polymorphous low-grade adenocarcinoma of the salivary glands: a clinicopathological comparison with adenoid cystic carcinoma. Histopathology. 19(2):121-9, 1991
7. Gnepp DR et al: Polymorphous low-grade adenocarcinoma of minor salivary gland. An immunohistochemical and clinicopathologic study. Am J Surg Pathol. 12(6):461-8, 1988

POLYMORPHOUS LOW-GRADE ADENOCARCINOMA

Clinical and Microscopic Features

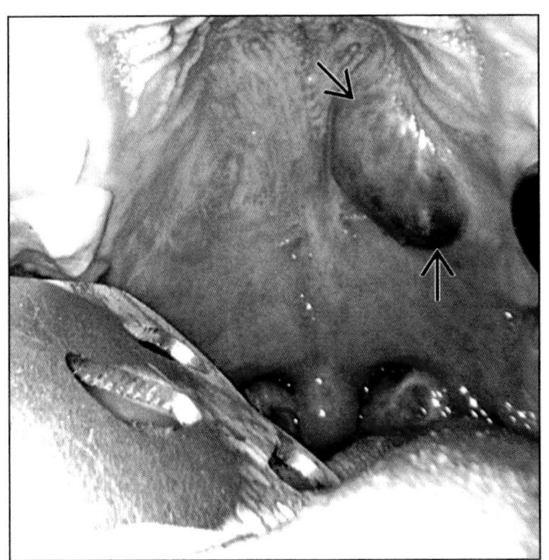

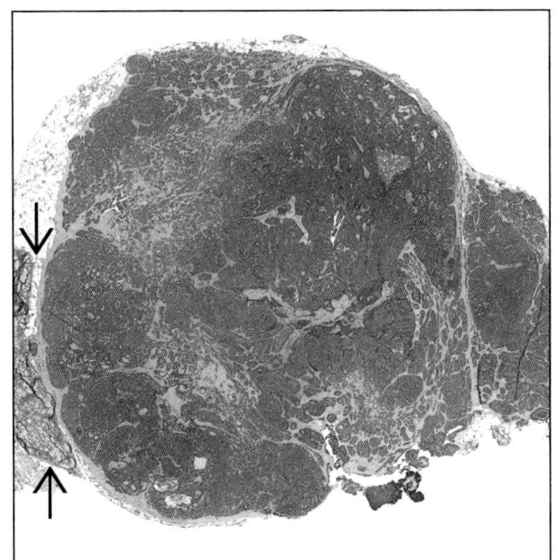

(Left) *Clinical photograph demonstrates a palate mass →. There is no ulceration, although mottling of the surface is present. These changes are nonspecific and by themselves do not confirm malignancy. (Courtesy G.G. Calzada, MD.)* ***(Right)*** *This unencapsulated tumor shows a small residuum of salivary gland tissue → at the periphery. Note the tumor at many of the margins of this wide excision. A multinodular appearance is seen.*

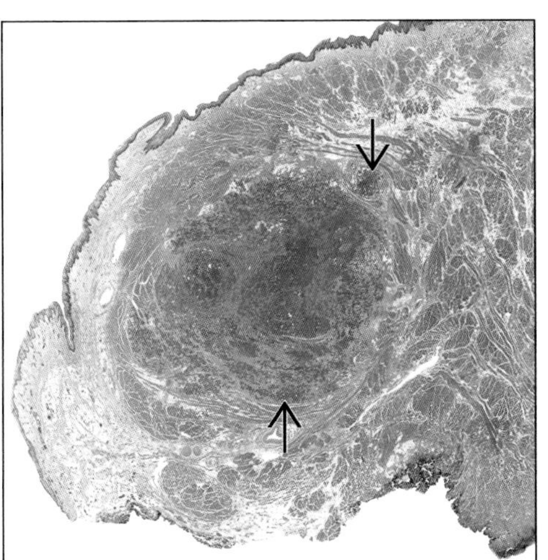

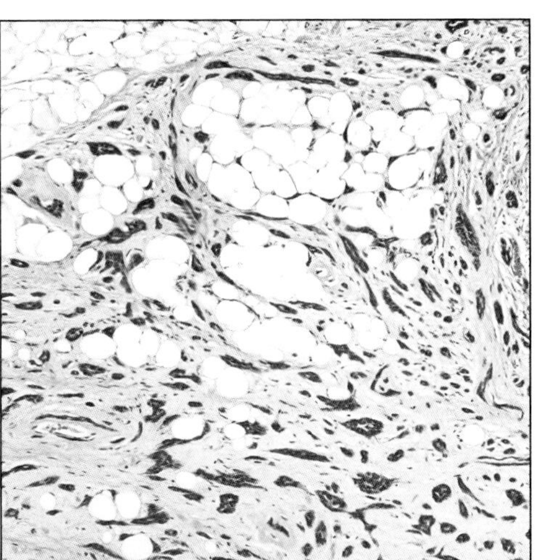

(Left) *There is a tumor nodule within this tongue resection. Note the lack of capsule, although the tumor is quite well defined. Areas of extension are present →.* ***(Right)*** *Single cells and small "strands" of neoplastic cells are extending into the adjacent adipose connective tissue. There is a background of bluish-gray matrix. The cells are small and bland, even at this low magnification.*

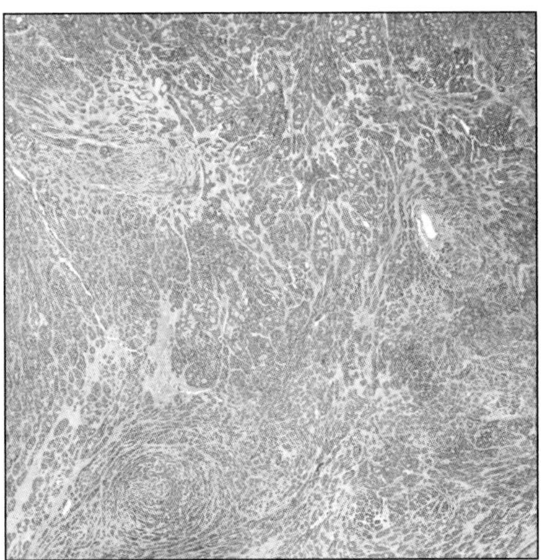

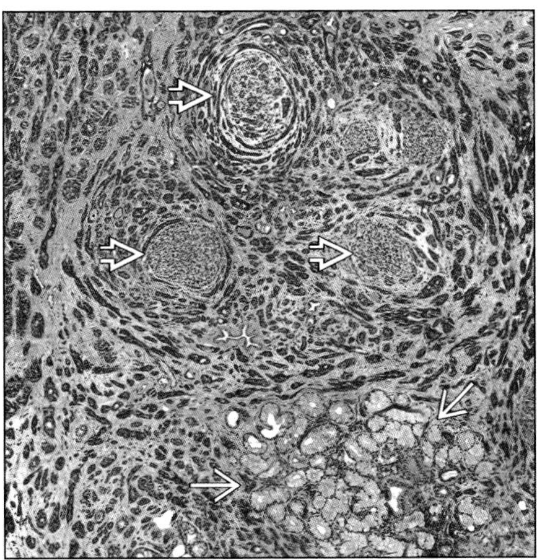

(Left) *The low-power appearance of these tumors is that of multiple different patterns, hence the name "polymorphous." A "swirling" or "eye of the storm" pattern is quite characteristic for this neoplasm.* ***(Right)*** *This tumor shows 2 of the low-power histologic features so characteristic for PLGA: Encasement of the minor salivary gland tissue → and the concentric arrangement around nerves, creating a targetoid pattern ⇒.*

POLYMORPHOUS LOW-GRADE ADENOCARCINOMA

Microscopic Features

(Left) A minor salivary gland and duct are present in the center of this field ⇨, entirely surrounded, although not destroyed by the neoplasm. There is densely collagenized stroma as well as areas of bluish myxoid stroma. *(Right)* There is a central tumor nidus with concentrically arranged tumor cells in thin strands. Although a nerve is suggested, it cannot be confirmed at this power.

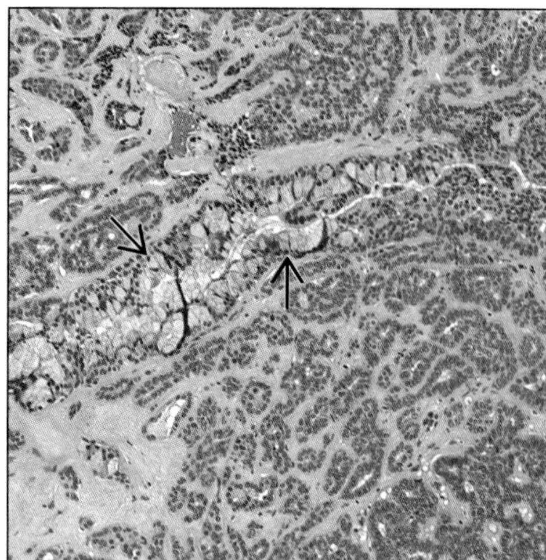

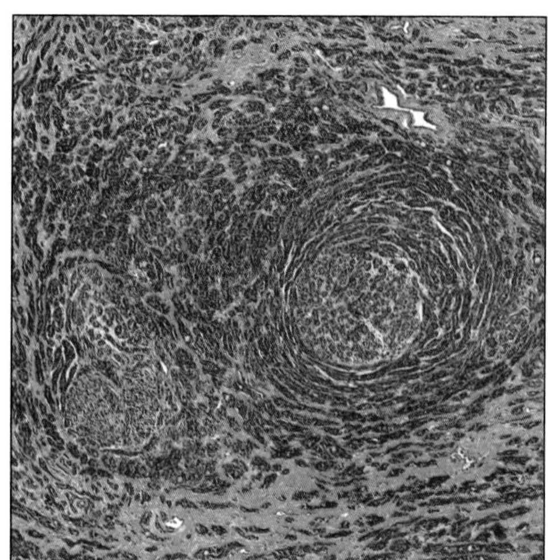

(Left) This high-power photomicrograph shows tumor cells infiltrating a peripheral nerve, creating a targetoid appearance. Note the appearance of small "glands" or "tubules" ➡ within the nerve. *(Right)* These neoplastic cells are cytologically bland and quite monotonous. There is a sheet-like to solid arrangement in this field. The nerve ➡ is surrounded by the tumor cells, although not infiltrated by them.

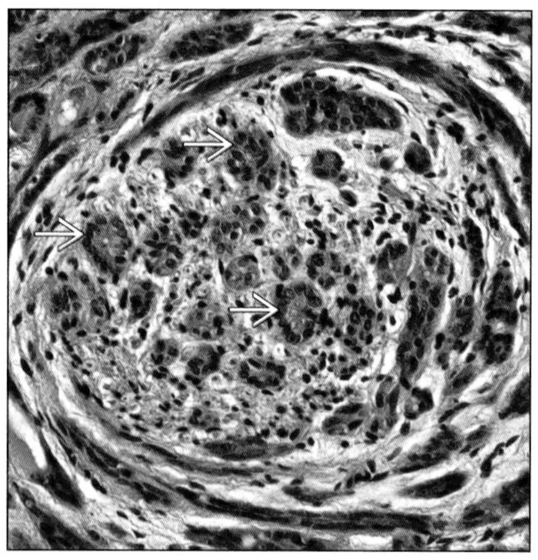

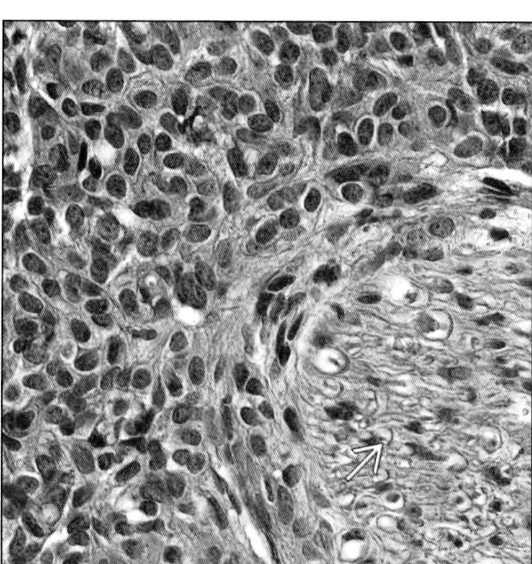

(Left) The tumor cells are frequently arranged in a single file ("Indian-filing") pattern, reminiscent of infiltrating lobular breast carcinoma (hence the previous name). Heavy fibrosis separates the tumor cells. *(Right)* A cribriform pattern of growth ➡ along with a tubular/trabecular pattern is frequently observed in PLGA. The patterns are often juxtaposed to one another, as in this case, although blending is also common.

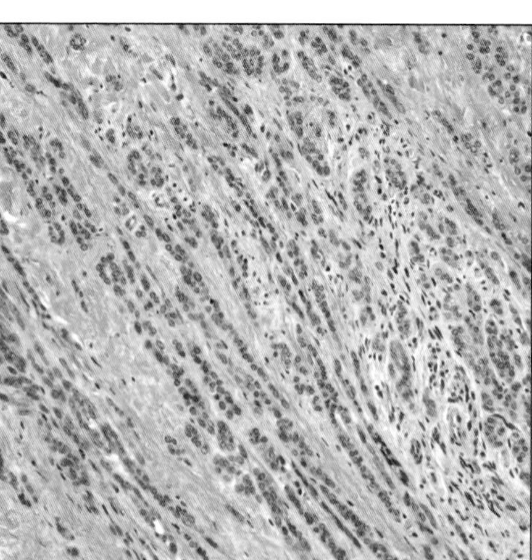

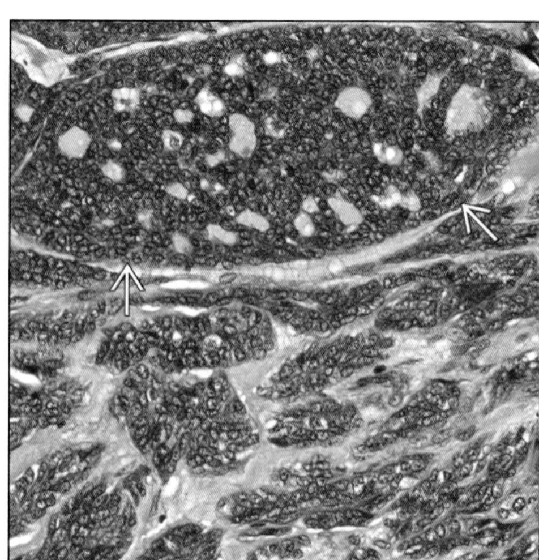

Microscopic and Immunohistochemical Features

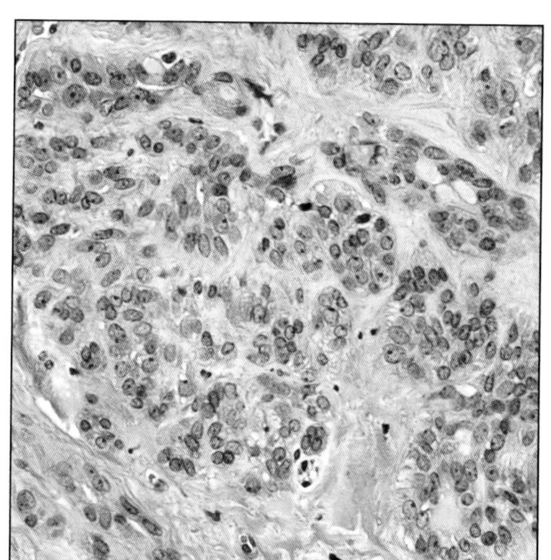

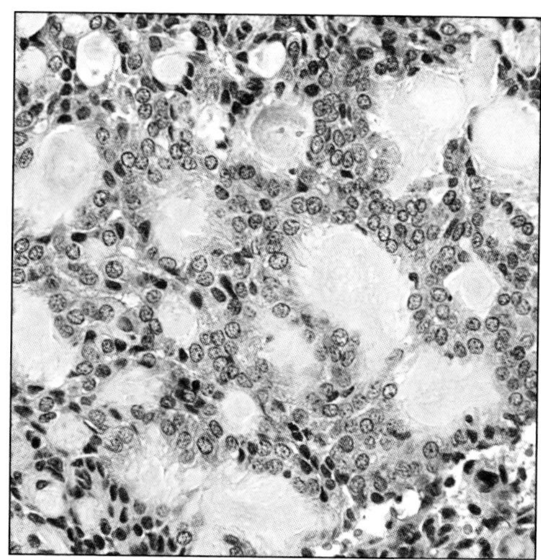

*(**Left**) The neoplastic cells are cytologically bland, arranged in vague nested or glandular patterns. There is open, delicate vesicular nuclear chromatin. Nucleoli are small and inconspicuous. (**Right**) A cribriform architectural arrangement of the tumor cells around reduplicated basement membrane material mimics the appearance of adenoid cystic carcinoma, although the cytologic features are different. The chromatin is delicate and even rather than heavy and coarse.*

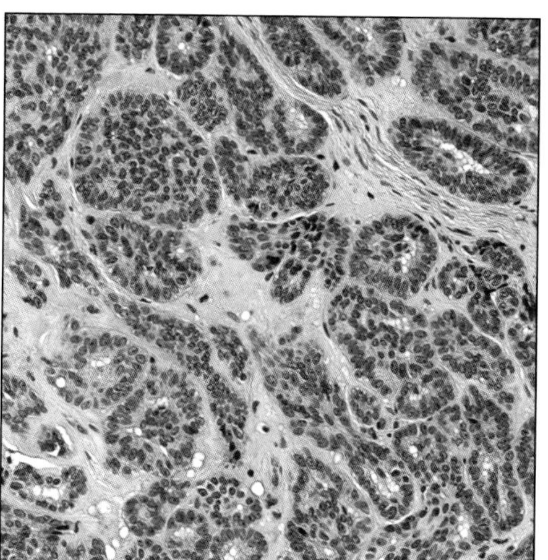

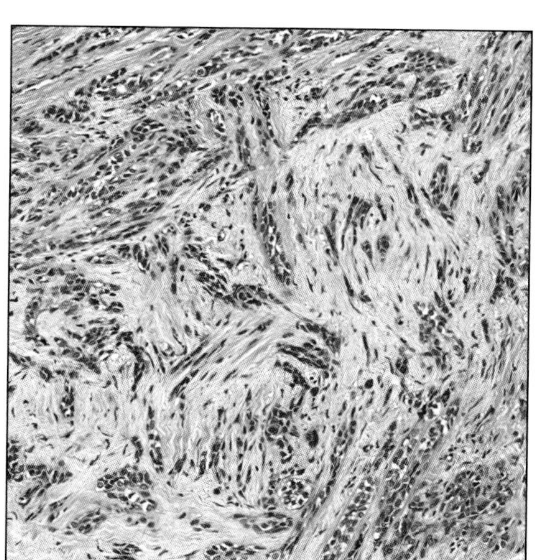

*(**Left**) A slate gray-blue myxoid change in the background stroma is an almost constant feature in polymorphous low-grade adenocarcinoma. The neoplastic cells are arranged in glands and tubules. (**Right**) The tumor cells are spindled to stranded in this neoplasm. The characteristic slate gray-blue myxoid change in the background is different from pleomorphic adenoma. Note the abruptness between the cells and the stroma, rather than blending, as is seen in pleomorphic adenoma.*

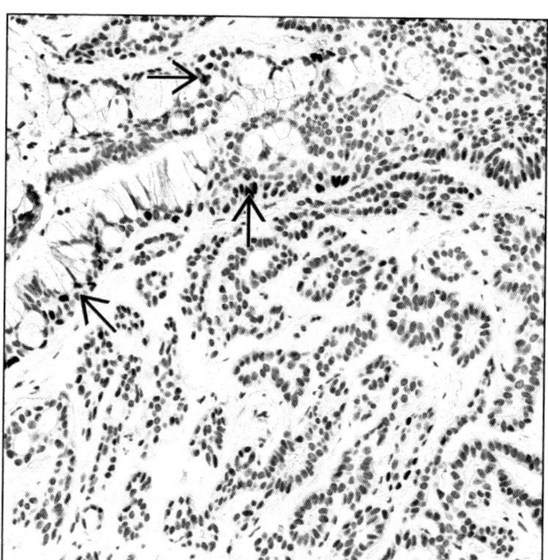

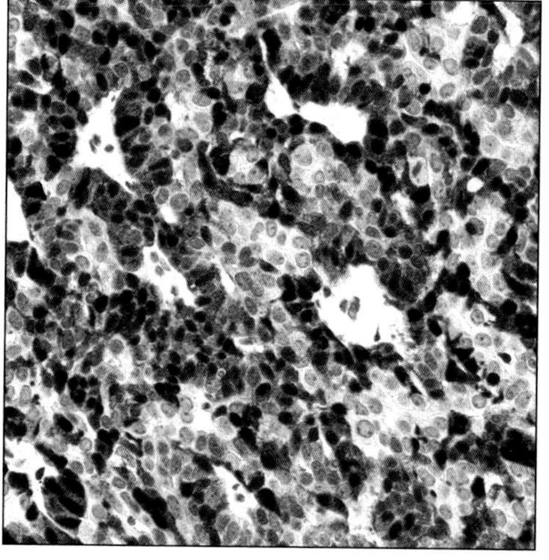

*(**Left**) The neoplastic cells are interpreted to be epithelial and myoepithelial, which is why they will show strong and diffuse immunoreactivity with p63, S100 protein, keratin, and CEA. In this case, the native duct shows residual p63 immunoreactive basal/myoepithelial cells ⇒. (**Right**) Nearly all of the tumor cells are immunoreactive with S100 protein, showing nuclear and cytoplasmic reactivity. However, the "glandular" profiles are not stained in this example.*

CARCINOMA EX-PLEOMORPHIC ADENOMA

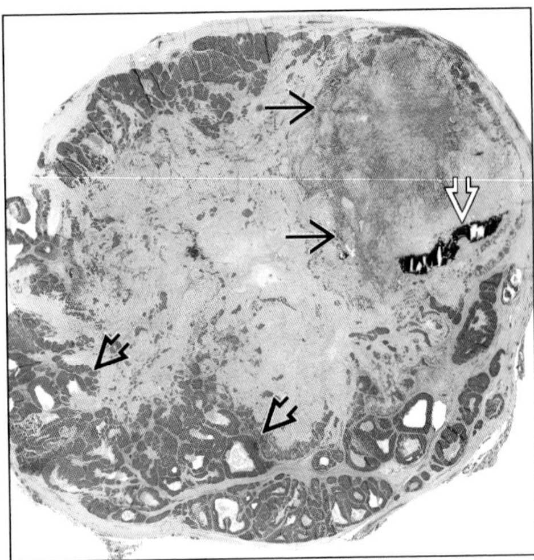

There is a well-circumscribed tumor, with areas of residual pleomorphic adenoma ➔ and calcifications ➔. However, even at low power, the areas of carcinoma ➔ are more cellular, with a glandular architecture.

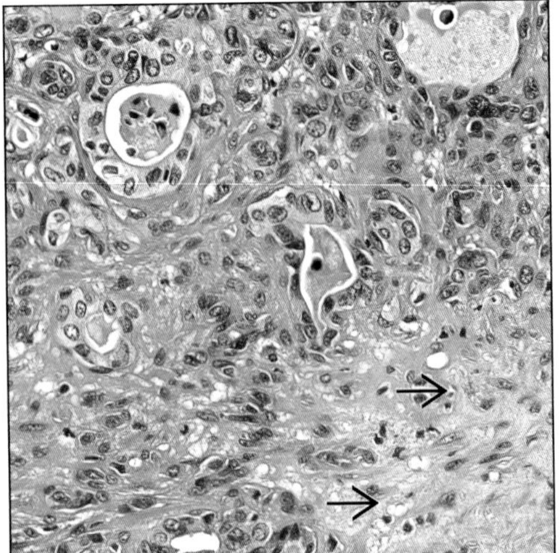

There is a remarkable degree of cytologic pleomorphism with a sclerotic background stroma. Areas suggestive of residual pleomorphic adenoma ➔ are seen, although limited by this high-power view.

TERMINOLOGY

Abbreviations

- Carcinoma ex-pleomorphic adenoma (Ca ex-PA)

Synonyms

- Carcinoma ex benign mixed tumor
- Malignant mixed tumor

Definitions

- Presence of carcinoma arising from pleomorphic adenoma (PA)
  - Requires concurrent pleomorphic adenoma histologically or history of pleomorphic adenoma at same site
  - Carcinoma can be any epithelial neoplasm

ETIOLOGY/PATHOGENESIS

Pathogenesis

- There is malignant transformation of epithelial component
- Areas of transition help to substantiate a continuum

CLINICAL ISSUES

Epidemiology

- Incidence
  - Accounts for about 4% of all salivary tumors
    - 12% of all salivary malignancies
    - 7% of all pleomorphic adenomas
- Age
  - Usually in 6th and 7th decades
    - About 10-12 years older than age at presentation of pleomorphic adenoma
    - Exceptional in children
- Gender
  - Probably equal gender distribution

Site

- Major salivary glands most often (80%)
  - Parotid (80%) > submandibular (18%) > > sublingual gland (< 2%)
  - May be due to large tumor size and increased recurrence rate for major gland location
- Minor glands (20%)
  - Palate > > nasopharynx > nasal cavity > > larynx

Presentation

- Long clinical history of pleomorphic adenoma
  - The greater the length of time with tumor, the higher the risk of malignant transformation
    - 5 years: 1.6%; 15 years: 9.6%
    - Symptoms/mass present for up to 44 years
  - Need to have well-documented previous tumor in same anatomic site if there is no histologic evidence of benign PA
    - Some tumors are slow growing and asymptomatic, so long history of mass by itself is insufficient
- May have had multiple surgeries
  - About 20% have had previous surgery
- Usually, recent rapid enlargement
- Nerve palsies are common (40%)
- Majority are painless
- Rare: Skin ulceration, soft tissue attachment, bone invasion

Treatment

- Surgical approaches
  - Complete surgical eradication
  - Lymph node dissection often required (~ 20%)
    - Some recommend neck dissection for all major gland tumors
    - Lymph node dissection may not be necessary for low-grade carcinomas or those with limited invasion
- Radiation
  - Majority receive postoperative radiation therapy

CARCINOMA EX-PLEOMORPHIC ADENOMA

Key Facts

Terminology

- Presence of carcinoma arising from pleomorphic adenoma

Clinical Issues

- Usually 6th to 7th decades, about 10 years older than PA
- Parotid > > minor salivary glands
- Long clinical history of painless mass with recent rapid enlargement and nerve palsy
- Complete surgical resection
- Local recurrence is common (up to 50%)
- Local or distant metastases are common (up to 70%)
- Poor overall survival
- Prognostically significant factors include grade, stage, proportion of carcinoma, extent of invasion

Microscopic Pathology

- Carcinoma may be specific tumor type
- Carcinoma shows significant pleomorphism, increased mitoses, necrosis, destructive growth
- Relative proportions of carcinoma and adenoma vary widely
- Separated into low and high grade
- PA is very frequently extensively hyalinized (fibrotic, scarred)

Reporting Considerations

- Must report extent of invasion
  - Noninvasive (encapsulated) carcinoma without evidence of capsular invasion
  - Minimally invasive (≤ 1.5 mm)
  - Invasive (> 1.5 mm)

    - Especially used for widely invasive &/or high-grade tumors
    - May be useful in controlling local disease

Prognosis

- Local recurrence can be seen (range of 25-50%)
  - Majority are seen within 5 years of diagnosis
  - Many patients experience more than 1 recurrence
  - Recurrence rates tend to be lower for minor salivary gland primaries
  - Higher percentage of patients die with disease if they have local recurrence
- Local or distant metastases are common (range of 50-70%)
  - Local lymph node metastases: Up to 25%
    - May be higher if there was previous surgery
  - Distant sites: Lung, bone (spine), liver, brain, skin
    - Most common in patients with local recurrence
- Poor overall survival
  - Majority die of disease (60%)
  - 5-year survival (30%)
- Prognostically significant factors (order of importance)
  - **Grade**
    - Low grade: Tend not to die of tumor
    - High grade: Majority die from tumor
  - **Stage**
  - **Proportion of tumor that is carcinoma**
  - **Extent of invasion**
    - Noninvasive (encapsulated): Excellent long-term outcome (identical to conventional PA)
    - Minimally invasive tumors (≤ 1.5 mm): Good outcome (75-85% at 5 years)
    - Widely invasive (> 1.5 mm): Poor outcome (25-65% at 5 years)
  - **Large tumor size**
  - **Histologic subtype**
    - Polymorphous low-grade adenocarcinoma: 96% 5-year survival
    - Salivary duct carcinoma: 62% 5-year survival
    - Myoepithelial carcinoma: 50% 5-year survival
    - Undifferentiated carcinoma: 30% 5-year survival
  - **High proliferation index**
  - **Margin status**
    - Positive margins predict higher recurrence rate and higher death rate from tumor

IMAGE FINDINGS

Radiographic Findings

- Location, extent, and lymph node status can be established
- Areas of benign PA may be identified
  - Areas of calcification more common in PA
- Ill-defined margin or loss of sharp margin is often a clue to malignancy
- Low T2 MR signal in solid mass is worrisome for malignancy
- Perineural spread along CN VII in temporal bone
  - Facial nerve plane separating superficial and deep lobes of parotid may be lost

MACROSCOPIC FEATURES

General Features

- Circumscribed and encapsulated tumors may be seen
- Most tumors are poorly circumscribed with invasion easily identified
  - Area of circumscription may represent residual PA
  - Area of scarring may also represent residual PA
- Necrosis and hemorrhage may be present
- Benign areas: Translucent gray-blue
- Carcinoma areas: Firm, white, tan or gray

Sections to Be Submitted

- Must submit areas of transition between possible benign and malignant zones
- Must submit from periphery to be able to measure extent of invasion

Size

- Range: Up to 25 cm
- Mean: About 5 cm
- Average size is about 2x that of PA

CARCINOMA EX-PLEOMORPHIC ADENOMA

MICROSCOPIC PATHOLOGY

Histologic Features

- Carcinomatous component may be part of specific tumor type
  - Adenocarcinoma, NOS, salivary duct carcinoma, adenoid cystic carcinoma, mucoepidermoid carcinoma, myoepithelial carcinoma, polymorphous low-grade adenocarcinoma, epithelial-myoepithelial carcinoma
    - Epithelial and myoepithelial components together
    - Epithelial component only
  - Carcinoma shows
    - Significant pleomorphism (enlarged pleomorphic cells with hyperchromatic nuclei, prominent nucleoli)
    - Increased mitotic figures
    - Areas of necrosis
    - Destructive growth
- Relative proportions of carcinoma and adenoma vary widely
  - Malignant and benign juxtaposed
  - Malignant and benign blended
  - Sclerotic nodule in malignant tumor suggests residual PA
  - Multifocal, distinct and separate malignant nodules
  - Carcinoma ranges from focal to diffuse
    - In majority of cases, carcinoma represents > 50% of tumor volume
  - Malignant cells replace inner duct layer, leaving peripheral myoepithelial layer intact
  - Extensive sampling may be required to document PA
    - Carcinoma frequently overgrows and replaces benign areas
    - In rare cases, clinical history of a tumor at the same site may be only PA documentation
- Separated into low and high grade
  - Based on degree of pleomorphism, necrosis, increased mitoses
- Concurrent PA is very frequently extensively hyalinized (fibrotic, scarred)
- Separation based on invasion
  - Noninvasive (encapsulated) carcinoma without evidence of capsular invasion
  - Minimally invasive: Distance from capsule to distant extent of tumor is ≤ 1.5 mm
  - Invasive: Distance from capsule to distant extent of tumor is > 1.5 mm
- Destructive soft tissue (fat, skeletal muscle) invasion is common
- Widely invasive tumors tend to be myoepithelial carcinomas
- Perineural and vascular invasion are routinely seen
- "Poorly differentiated" high-grade adenocarcinoma that is difficult to classify raises the possibility of Ca ex-PA

Lymphatic/Vascular Invasion

- Must be certain it is "atypical" epithelium in vascular spaces

Carcinosarcoma

- A **true** malignant mixed tumor
- Pleomorphic adenoma with carcinoma and sarcoma concurrently present
- Much more aggressive than Ca ex-PA
- Most common elements are chondrosarcoma and carcinoma
  - Osteosarcoma, fibrosarcoma, and rhabdomyosarcoma can be seen

Benign Metastasizing Pleomorphic Adenoma

- Benign pleomorphic adenoma in distant site
  - Lung, liver, kidney, and lymph nodes
- Believed to be iatrogenic in patient with history of multiple recurrences and multiple surgeries for PA
- Benign epithelial elements within vessels adjacent to pleomorphic adenoma
- Histologically benign without any cytologic atypia in distant foci
- Most follow similar outcome as PA, but adverse behavior may occur

ANCILLARY TESTS

Cytology

- Marked variation in type and grade of carcinoma, coupled with unknown benign and malignant proportions, make FNA interpretation difficult
- Adequate sampling is critical
  - Must be extensively sampled to exclude malignant transformation
    - Large lesions, recurrent lesions, or tumors of long duration
  - Grade of malignant tumor may help with separation
    - Highly malignant epithelial cells (salivary duct carcinoma) are relatively straight forward (especially with cell block material)
    - Low-grade carcinoma (mucoepidermoid, adenocarcinoma, NOS) may be more difficult to separate
- Cellular smears, with epithelial predominant population
- May show 2 distinct patterns
  - Unequivocal groups and single malignant cells admixed with benign epithelial and stromal components of PA
    - Groups, sheets, papillary structures, cribriform pattern
    - Large cells, pleomorphic nuclei, prominent nucleoli, increased mitotic figures, necrosis
  - Variably pleomorphic cells, without clear-cut malignant criteria, with mixture of epithelial and stromal components of PA

Immunohistochemistry

- Carcinomas separated into
  - Epithelial only (majority): AE1/AE3, EMA, CK7, CK8, CK19 positive
  - Epithelial and myoepithelial (~ 25%)
    - AE1/AE3, EMA, CK7, CK8, CK19: Ductal
    - α-SMA, CK14, vimentin: Myoepithelial
- S100 protein, GFAP: Helps confirm PA component

CARCINOMA EX-PLEOMORPHIC ADENOMA

- Increased frequency **in carcinoma areas** with
  - Ki-67 (MIB-1)
  - Epidermal growth factor receptor (EGFR)
  - Strong overexpression and amplification of HER-2/neu
  - Minichromosome maintenance protein-2 (MCM2) (higher labeling index [20%] than PA [7%])
- Laminin, collagen IV, tenascin, and fibronectin are variably expressed based on type and degree of invasion present
- Neural cell adhesion molecule (NCAM) is absent or weak in carcinoma component

Flow Cytometry
- Aneuploid population may be identified in high-grade Ca ex-PA
- Ploidy results do not appear to be predictive of tumor behavior

Cytogenetics
- Multiple structural, numeric, and chromosome deletions reported
  - 6q, 8q, 12q
    - Alterations at 12q13-15 (amplification of *HMGIC* and *MDM2* genes)
- LOH identified at chromosome 8q, 12q, and 17p
  - Specifically: 8q11.23-q12, 12q23-qter, 17p13, 17p11
  - Frequently show alterations in all 3 chromosomal arms
  - 17p alterations may correlate with disease stage and proliferation rate

DIFFERENTIAL DIAGNOSIS

Pleomorphic Adenoma (PA)
- Completely encapsulated, although bosselated and nodular periphery
- Recurrent tumors are frequently multinodular and multifocal
- Frank anaplasia is absent
- Chondroid material usually identified
- In tumors with extensive sclerosis/hyalinization, additional sampling is recommended to exclude carcinoma
- PAs with high mitotic index are more likely to transform to carcinoma
- Degeneration in PA may have hemorrhage, necrosis, inflammation, and squamous metaplasia
- PA must be identified in Ca ex-PA in order to qualify for designation

Metastatic Carcinoma
- Tends to be multifocal
- Shows distinct morphology within background of pleomorphic adenoma
- Lymph-vascular emboli are easily identified
- Clinical history is frequently known

Salivary Duct Carcinoma (SDC)
- High-grade malignancy
- May be malignant component of Ca ex-PA
  - Prognosis for primary and transformed SDC is uniformly bad

REPORTING CONSIDERATIONS

Key Elements to Report
- Histologic subtype
- Degree of differentiation (tumor grade)
- Must report extent of invasion
  - In situ, intracapsular, noninvasive, pre-invasive carcinoma; severely dysplastic PA
  - Minimally invasive (≤ 1.5 mm)
  - Invasive (> 1.5 mm)

STAGING

AJCC
- T: Based on tumor size (< 2 cm, 2-4 cm, > 4 cm) and extraparenchymal extension
- N: Based on lymph node size (< 3 cm, 3-6 cm, > 6 cm), number of lymph nodes, and whether ipsilateral/bilateral
- M: Distant metastases present

SELECTED REFERENCES

1. Katabi N et al: Prognostic factors of recurrence in salivary carcinoma ex pleomorphic adenoma, with emphasis on the carcinoma histologic subtype: a clinicopathologic study of 43 cases. Hum Pathol. 41(7):927-34, 2010
2. Altemani A et al: Carcinoma ex pleomorphic adenoma (CXPA): immunoprofile of the cells involved in carcinomatous progression. Histopathology. 46(6):635-41, 2005
3. Di Palma S et al: Non-invasive (intracapsular) carcinoma ex pleomorphic adenoma: recognition of focal carcinoma by HER-2/neu and MIB1 immunohistochemistry. Histopathology. 46(2):144-52, 2005
4. Wahlberg P et al: Carcinoma of the parotid and submandibular glands--a study of survival in 2465 patients. Oral Oncol. 38(7):706-13, 2002
5. Olsen KD et al: Carcinoma ex pleomorphic adenoma: a clinicopathologic review. Head Neck. 23(9):705-12, 2001
6. Auclair PL et al: Atypical features in salivary gland mixed tumors: their relationship to malignant transformation. Mod Pathol. 9(6):652-7, 1996
7. Brandwein M et al: Noninvasive and minimally invasive carcinoma ex mixed tumor: a clinicopathologic and ploidy study of 12 patients with major salivary tumors of low (or no?) malignant potential. Oral Surg Oral Med Oral Pathol Oral Radiol Endod. 81(6):655-64, 1996
8. Wenig BM et al: Metastasizing mixed tumor of salivary glands. A clinicopathologic and flow cytometric analysis. Am J Surg Pathol. 16(9):845-58, 1992
9. Garner SL et al: Salivary gland carcinosarcoma: true malignant mixed tumor. Ann Otol Rhinol Laryngol. 98(8 Pt 1):611-4, 1989
10. Hellquist H et al: Malignant mixed tumour. A salivary gland tumour showing both carcinomatous and sarcomatous features. Virchows Arch A Pathol Anat Histopathol. 409(1):93-103, 1986
11. Eneroth CM et al: Malignancy in pleomorphic adenoma. A clinical and microspectrophotometric study. Acta Otolaryngol. 77(6):426-32, 1974

CARCINOMA EX-PLEOMORPHIC ADENOMA

Radiographic, Clinical, Gross, and Microscopic Features

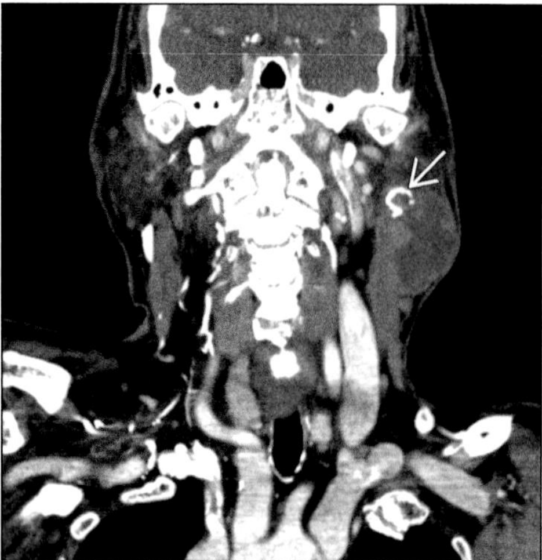

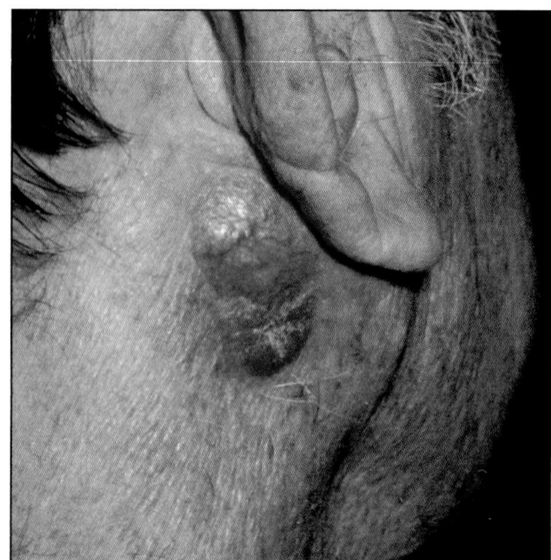

*(**Left**) A mass in the superficial lobe of the parotid gland shows focal osseous metaplasia ➔. Areas of calcification are common in pleomorphic adenoma (PA). However, there is cystic change and destructive growth, a feature of carcinoma ex-pleomorphic adenoma (salivary duct carcinoma). (**Right**) This retroauricular tumor shows remarkable skin erythema. Ulceration has not yet developed but is likely to develop if left unmanaged. The patient had a history of pleomorphic adenoma.*

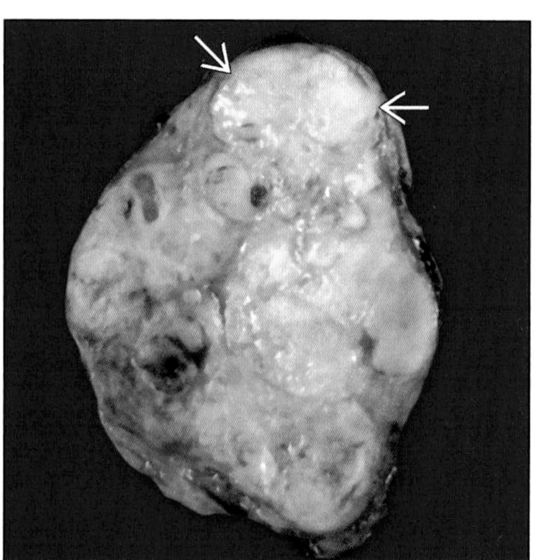

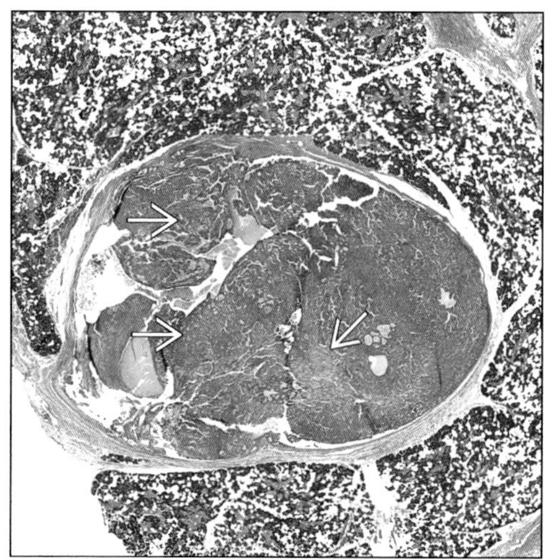

*(**Left**) The neoplasm shows a very fleshy appearance with areas of yellow degeneration, focal cystic change, and hemorrhage. Areas of pale-shiny residual pleomorphic adenoma are noted ➔. It is not uncommon to be able to detect areas of residual pleomorphic adenoma during gross examination. (**Right**) This is an example of encapsulated Ca ex-PA. The PA is quite cellular, showing isolated ➔, multifocal areas of carcinoma, which were confirmed at high power.*

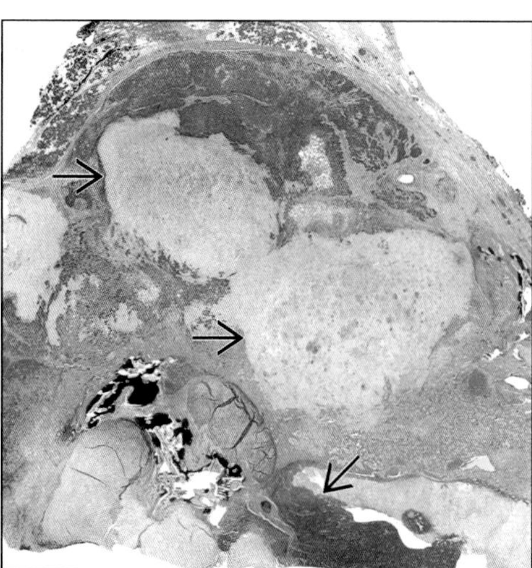

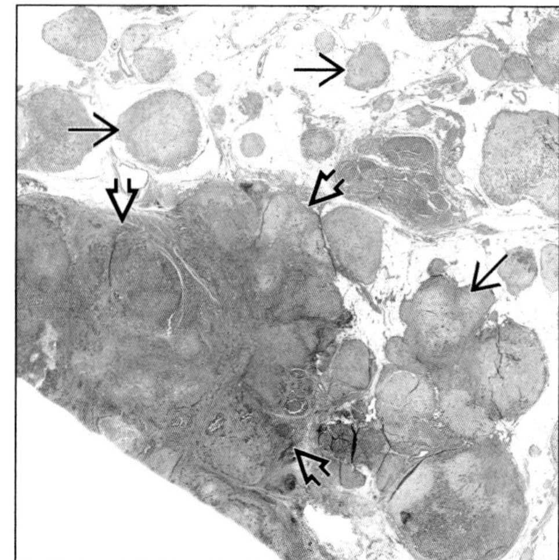

*(**Left**) The degree of cellularity and variability in this case is worrisome for carcinoma. Note the differences in cartilaginous matrix ➔. (**Right**) Multiple distinct nodules of PA are noted in the fat ➔, a characteristic feature of recurrent PA. However, there is a cellular destructive nodule that shows carcinomatous transformation ⇨. Multiple recurrences are common in tumors that undergo malignant transformation.*

CARCINOMA EX-PLEOMORPHIC ADENOMA

Microscopic Features

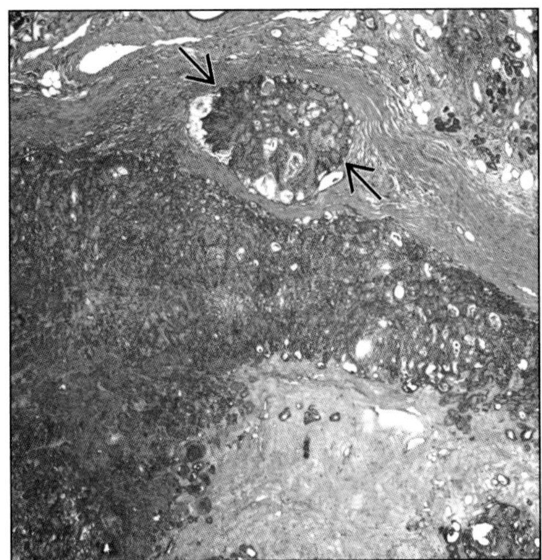

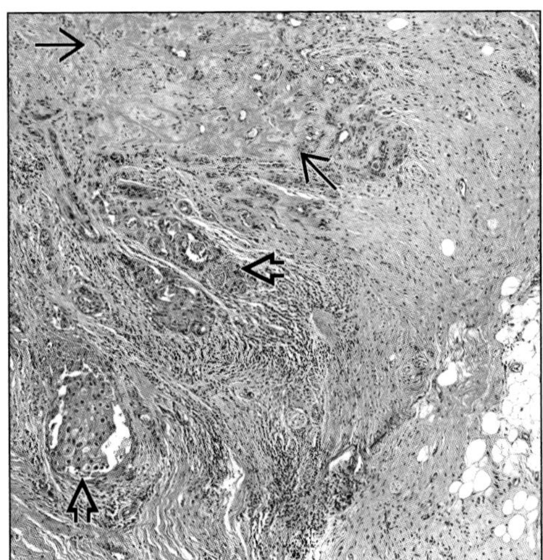

(Left) *This carcinoma has invaded into and through the capsule → but does not extend > 1.5 mm. This would be considered a minimally invasive tumor.* **(Right)** *There is benign PA → juxtaposed with areas of carcinoma ⇨ in this Ca ex-PA. There is extension of the tumor in the adjacent fatty tissue. The extent of invasion, specifically whether > or ≤ 1.5 mm, is an important prognostic indicator, as is tumor grade. The tumor in this lesion is high grade.*

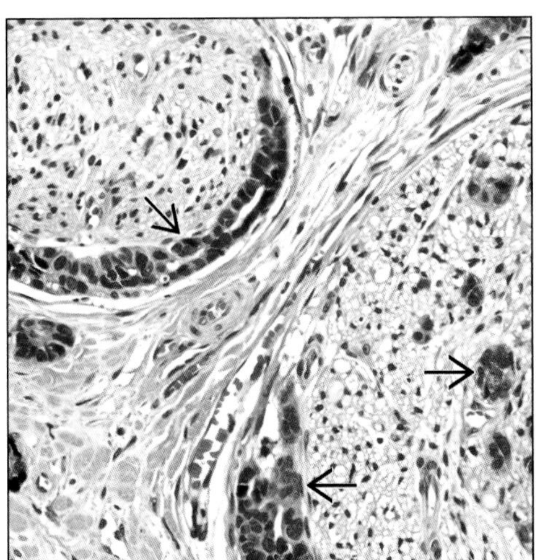

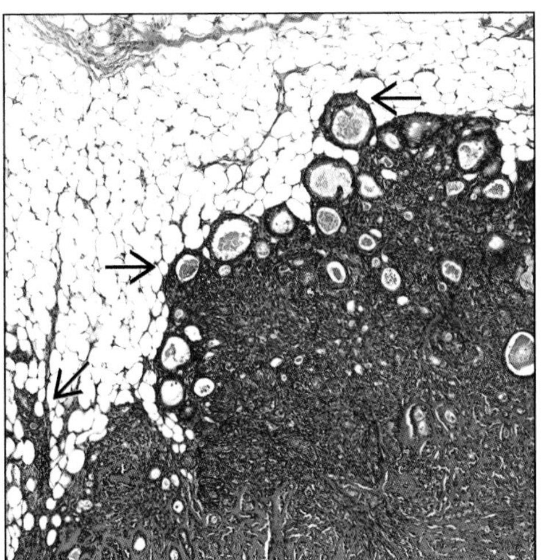

(Left) *The neoplastic glandular elements are intimately associated with the nerve, with both perineural and intraneural invasion →. Perineural and intravascular invasion are frequent findings in Ca ex-PA, although not necessarily tumor specific.* **(Right)** *Carcinoma, showing glandular differentiation, is invading out into the adjacent adipose tissue →. There is a background of benign pleomorphic adenoma associated with hyalinization.*

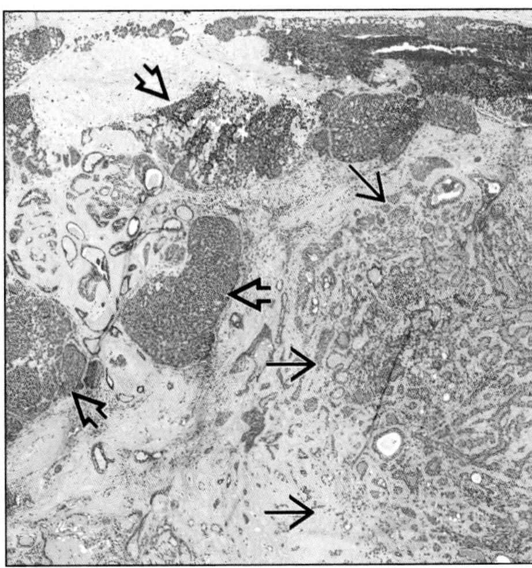

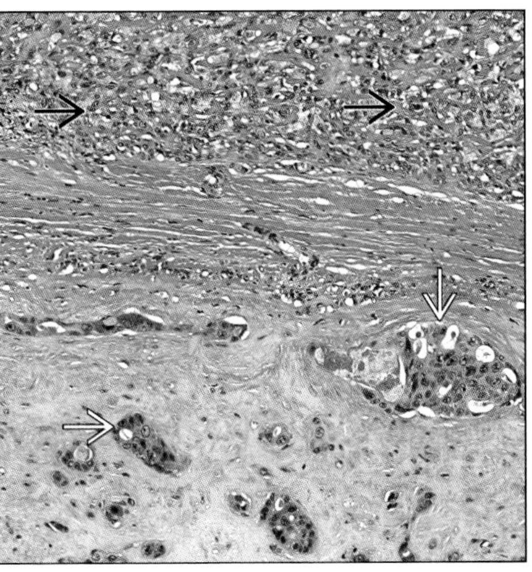

(Left) *It is important to document areas of both benign and malignant tumor within the same lesion. The benign PA → in this tumor has a different cellularity and degree of cytologic atypia in comparison to the areas of carcinoma ⇨.* **(Right)** *The PA area is cellular, although showing remarkable sclerosis or fibrosis →. This fibrosis blends imperceptibly with the areas of frankly pleomorphic carcinoma ➡. Atypia and necrosis are common in carcinoma.*

CARCINOMA EX-PLEOMORPHIC ADENOMA

Microscopic Features

*(**Left**) The carcinomatous elements of a Ca ex-PA can be a variety of different tumor types, both within and between tumors. In this case, the carcinoma appears to be an adenoid cystic pattern ➔, blending with areas of PA. (**Right**) The malignancy in this case was an adenocarcinoma, NOS. It is easy to see the malignant epithelial component ➔ juxtaposed to the areas of benign PA. Adenocarcinoma, NOS, is the most common malignant tumor type, followed by salivary duct carcinoma.*

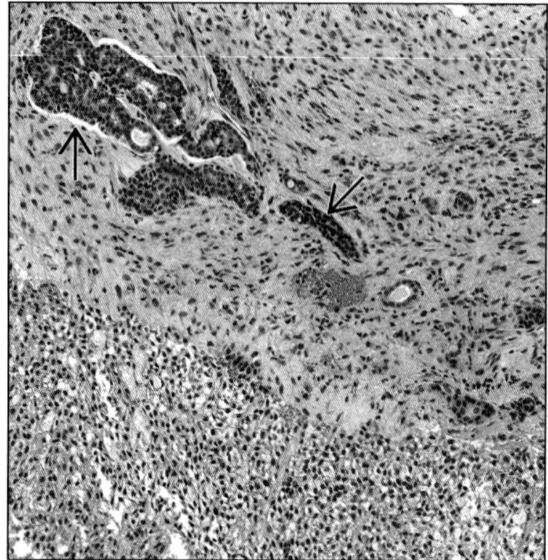

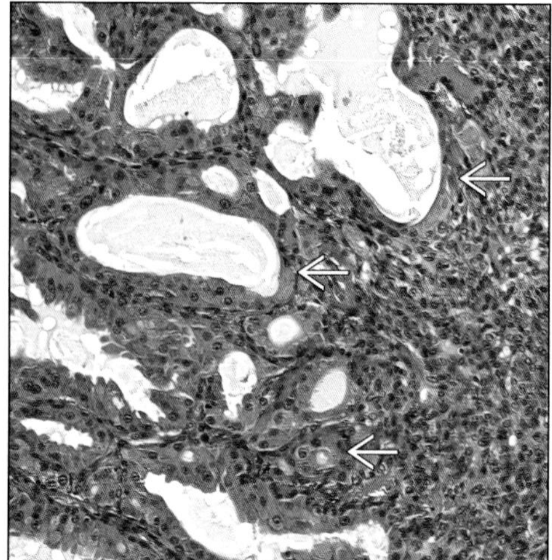

*(**Left**) A variety of different patterns of growth are common for PA, but the degree of cytologic atypia in the carcinomatous areas is beyond the spectrum of a benign neoplasm. This carcinoma has a degree of hyperchromasia that is beyond the benign tumor. Fat invasion is noted. (**Right**) There is a high-grade adenocarcinoma in this field, changes most consistent with a salivary duct carcinoma type. Note the areas of comedonecrosis ➔ as well as increased fibrosis.*

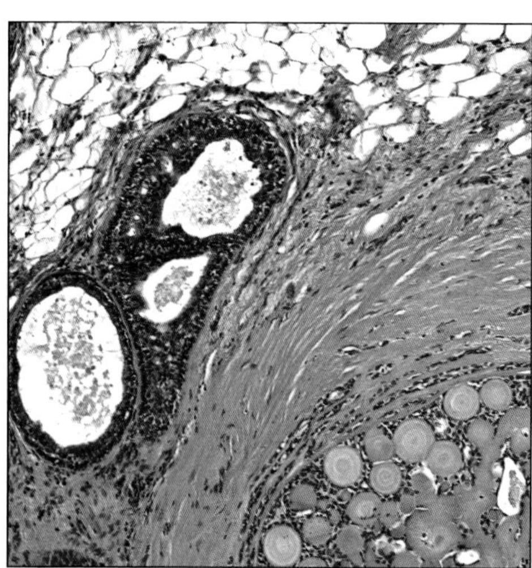

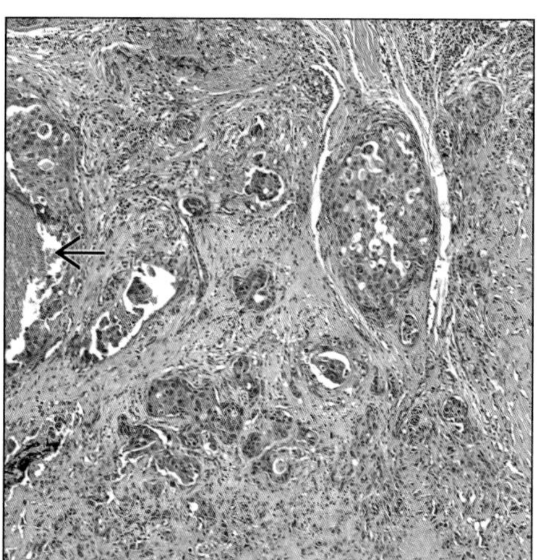

*(**Left**) In many tumors, the malignant transformation begins with the luminal duct-like areas, filling in along the myoepithelial-lined spaces. This feature can be highlighted with immunohistochemistry. (**Right**) This degree of stromal hyalinization or scarring in a PA must alert the pathologist to the possibility of a malignant transformation. Whenever this type of fibrosis is found, additional or deeper sections are recommended to exclude concurrent carcinoma.*

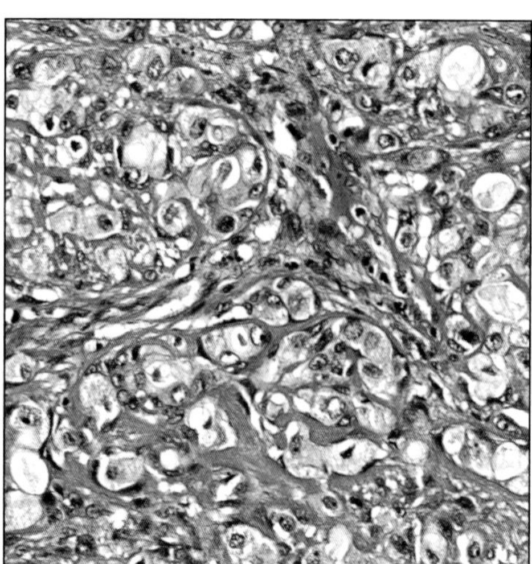

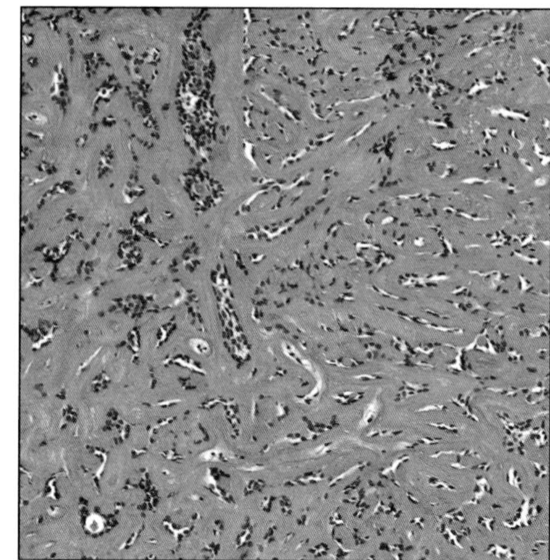

Microscopic, Variant, and Immunohistochemical Features

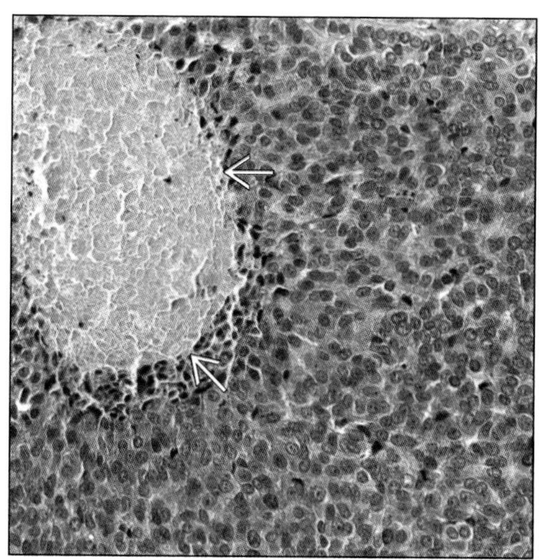

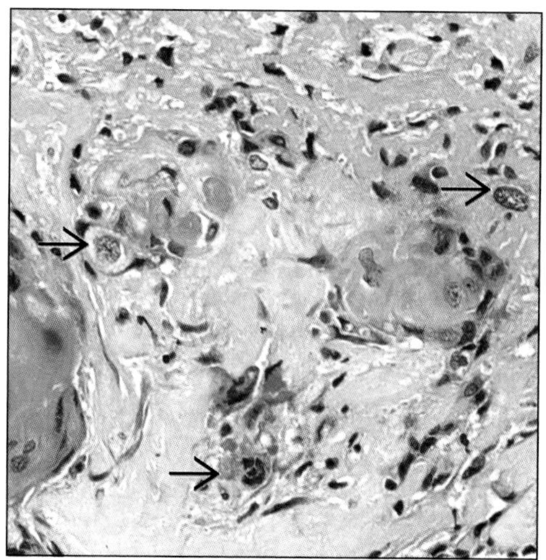

(Left) An area of comedonecrosis ➔ is found in this Ca ex-PA focus. There is a very high cellularity, associated with increased mitoses. There is a very high nuclear to cytoplasmic ratio and cellular atypia. ***(Right)*** *Within a densely hyalinized background, islands of metaplastic squamous epithelium are noted. There are many isolated, highly atypical epithelial cells ➔. These features are quite characteristic of a Ca ex-PA.*

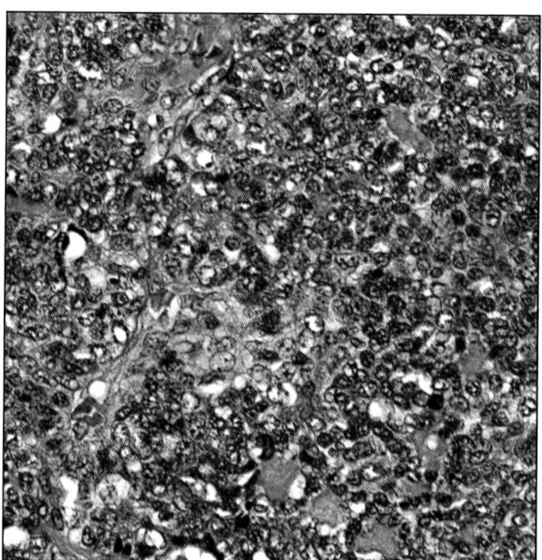

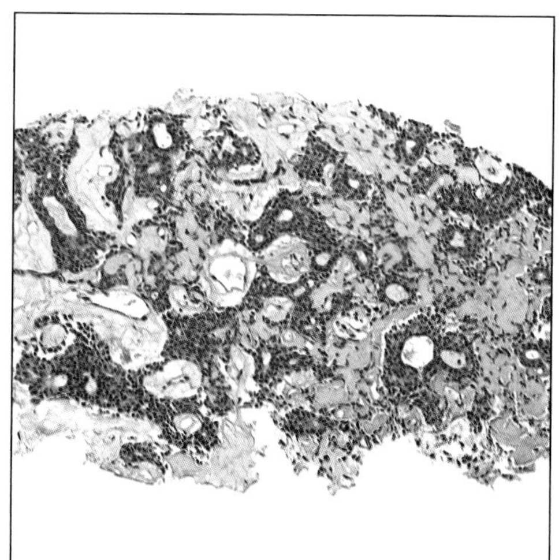

(Left) *Undifferentiated or poorly differentiated carcinomas can be seen within Ca ex-PA. There is a very high nuclear to cytoplasmic ratio. There is no residual PA in this field.* ***(Right)*** *A core needle biopsy of the kidney shows a "benign" pleomorphic adenoma. There is an unremarkable epithelial proliferation set in a myxochondroid matrix. The patient had multiple previous surgeries for parotid gland PA, and this is an example of "benign metastasizing PA."*

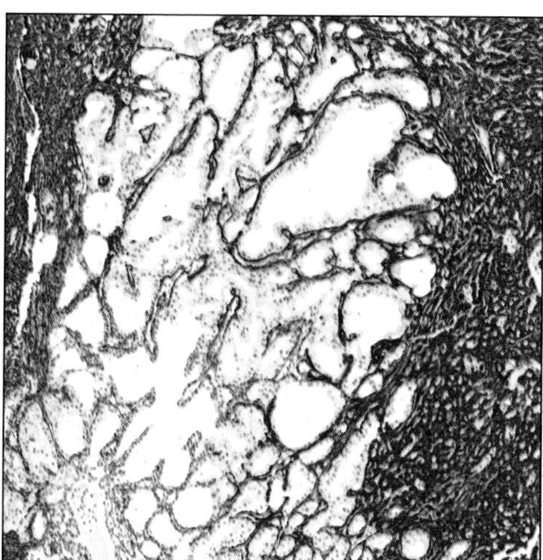

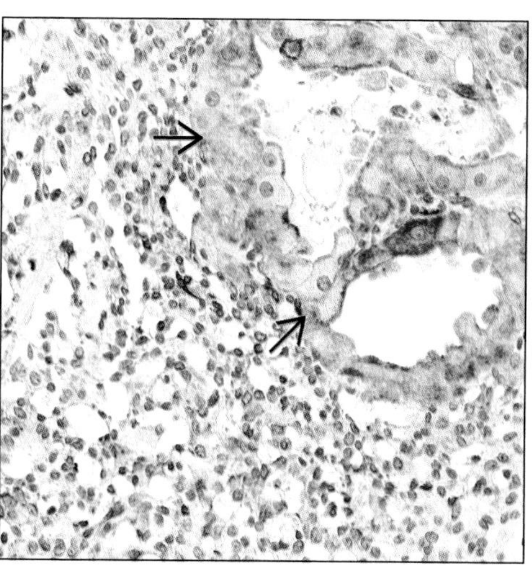

(Left) *CK14 is a basal/myoepithelial marker, shown highlighting much of the background PA, but lacking reaction within the cells showing carcinomatous transformation.* ***(Right)*** *PA usually shows well-developed S100 protein immunoreactivity in the myoepithelial component. However, the cytoplasmic-only uptake by the carcinoma ➔ area is distinct and different from the surrounding nuclear and cytoplasmic immunoreactivity in areas of PA.*

SALIVARY DUCT CARCINOMA

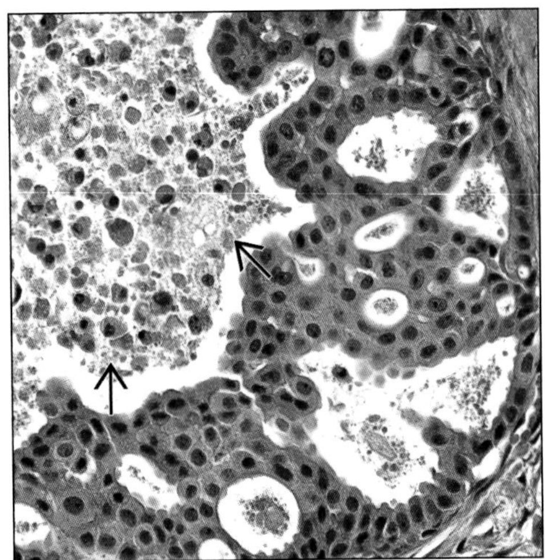

A large duct is filled with a neoplastic proliferation that is arranged in the classic "Roman bridge" architecture. The center of the duct contains an area of comedonecrosis ⇒.

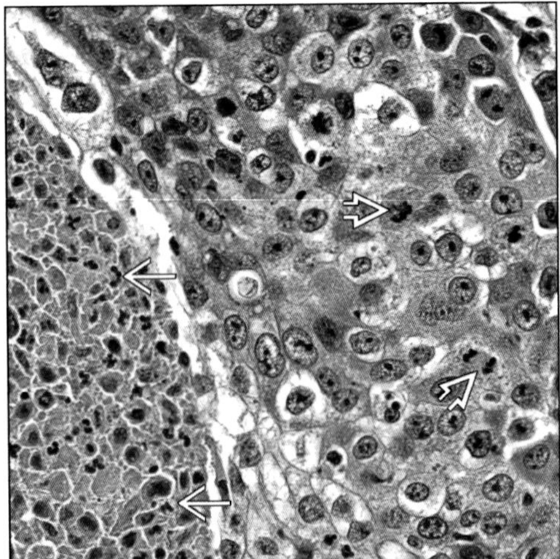

An area of comedonecrosis ➡ fills the center of this tumor nest. The cells show remarkable pleomorphism, prominent nucleoli, and mitotic figures ➡.

TERMINOLOGY

Abbreviations

- Salivary duct carcinoma (SDC)

Synonyms

- Cribriform salivary carcinoma of excretory ducts
- High-grade salivary duct carcinoma
- Cribriform carcinoma

Definitions

- High-grade adenocarcinoma resembling high-grade breast ductal carcinoma thought to be derived from intralobular and interlobular excretory ducts
  - Important to recognize as specific category/entity with clinical implications
- Low-grade cribriform cystadenocarcinoma is a unique entity, perhaps not a low-grade variant of salivary duct carcinoma

ETIOLOGY/PATHOGENESIS

Possible Chronic Stimulation

- SDC arising in longstanding chronic obstructive sialadenitis has been reported
- SDC is common tumor in carcinoma ex-pleomorphic adenoma

CLINICAL ISSUES

Epidemiology

- Incidence
  - Uncommon salivary gland malignancy
    - De novo &/or part of carcinoma ex-pleomorphic adenoma
  - Up to 9% of malignant salivary gland neoplasms
- Age
  - Older at initial presentation (usually > 50 years)
  - Peak: 7th decade
- Gender
  - Male > Female (2-4:1)

Site

- Parotid gland is most commonly involved (about 70-95% of cases)
- Submandibular, minor salivary gland (palate specifically), and rarely sublingual gland
- Maxillary sinus and larynx very uncommon

Presentation

- Swelling of parotid gland is most frequent sign
  - Recent rapid growth is common finding
- Majority of patients experience facial nerve paresthesia, pain, paresis, palsy, or paralysis
- Surface ulceration can be seen
- Cervical lymphadenopathy is present in about 1/3 of patients at initial presentation
  - Subsequently, most patients will develop lymph node metastases
- Since SDC develops within pleomorphic adenoma, symptom durations can be deceiving

Treatment

- Options, risks, complications
  - Aggressive multimodality therapy required
  - Surgery and radiation combined
    - Chemotherapy and trastuzumab (Herceptin) are experimental
- Surgical approaches
  - Wide excision to include lymph node dissection
- Drugs
  - Trastuzumab (Herceptin) may be used as adjuvant therapy in patients with FISH (or CISH) positive HER-2/neu tumors
- Radiation
  - Adjuvant radiotherapy combined with surgery

Prognosis

- Poor prognosis overall (< 35% 5-year survival)

SALIVARY DUCT CARCINOMA

Key Facts

Terminology

- High-grade adenocarcinoma resembling high-grade breast ductal carcinoma

Clinical Issues

- Peak: 7th decade
- Male > Female (2-4:1)
- Parotid gland is most commonly involved
- Recent rapid growth, facial nerve involvement
- Most patients present with stage III or IV disease
- Aggressive multimodality therapy required
- Poor prognosis overall (< 35% 5-year survival)

Microscopic Pathology

- Perineural and lymph-vascular invasion are common
- Comedonecrosis is conspicuous
- Rounded, solid or cystic nodules of tumor cells
- Arranged in solid, papillary, and cribriform patterns
  - "Roman bridge" architecture is classic
- Polygonal cells show moderate to marked pleomorphism with ample eosinophilic, granular cytoplasm
- Numerous mitoses, including atypical forms
- **Variants**: Sarcomatoid, micropapillary, mucin-rich, osteoclast-type giant cell

Ancillary Tests

- Immunoreactive for epithelial markers, androgen receptor, HER-2/neu

Top Differential Diagnoses

- Metastatic breast carcinoma, cystadenocarcinoma, polymorphous low-grade adenocarcinoma, oncocytic carcinoma, mucoepidermoid carcinoma

  - One of the most aggressive salivary gland malignancies
  - Local invasion, frequent lymph-vascular metastases
- Local recurrences in up to 50%
- High rates of lymph node and distant metastases (60-70%)
  - Early distant metastases is the rule
  - Lymph node metastases correlate with worse prognosis
    - Presence of nodal metastases predicts distant metastases
  - Distant sites include lung, bone, liver, spleen, skin, adrenal glands, kidney, and brain
- Most patients present with stage III or IV disease
- Poor prognostic indicators
  - Size > 3 cm; positive surgical margin status
  - Lymph-vascular &/or perineural invasion; lymph node &/or distant metastases; micropapillary pattern
  - Positive HER-2/neu overexpression, lack of ERP-β expression
- **No** correlation with outcome: p53 protein, DNA aneuploidy, increased proliferative activity

IMAGE FINDINGS

Radiographic Findings

- Ill-defined margins, frequently showing necrosis
- Useful to identify metastatic disease

MR Findings

- Low to moderate high signal intensity in comparison to contralateral parotid gland on T2-weighted images
- Early enhancement with low washout ratio suggests malignant salivary gland tumor (but nonspecific)

MACROSCOPIC FEATURES

General Features

- Unencapsulated and poorly circumscribed
  - Infiltration of adjacent parenchyma can be seen
- Multinodularity is common
- Cut surface is firm, solid, grayish white to yellowish white
- Cysts and foci of necrosis are frequently seen
- Fibrosis is often prominent
- Macroscopic features of concurrent/preexisting pleomorphic adenoma may be seen

Size

- Average: 3.5 cm
- Range: 1-10 cm

MICROSCOPIC PATHOLOGY

Histologic Features

- Variably sized, rounded, solid or cystic nodules of tumor cells that resemble intraductal or infiltrating ductal carcinoma of the breast
- Small nodules (2x the diameter of interlobular salivary gland ducts) are filled with neoplastic cells
- Larger cystic nodules with irregular shape
- Comedonecrosis is conspicuous (central-intraductal type or filling cystic spaces)
- Perineural invasion (60%) and vascular invasion (31%) are frequent
- Marked, dense, desmoplastic (hyalinized) fibrosis is conspicuous
- Lymphoplasmacytic inflammatory cell infiltrate is frequently present
- Cells are arranged in cribriform, band-like solid, and papillary patterns
  - "Roman bridge" architecture is classic
- Small tumor nests infiltrate between larger nodules
  - Nonneoplastic glandular parenchyma is absent between nodules
- Epithelial cells have moderate to marked pleomorphism, are cuboidal to polygonal, with ample eosinophilic, granular, oncocytic cytoplasm
  - Although often monotonous in any single tumor
- Nuclei are round, centrally located, with large, prominent nucleoli and hyperchromatic chromatin
- Mitotic figures are usually easily identified, including atypical forms

SALIVARY DUCT CARCINOMA

- Psammoma bodies and areas of squamous differentiation are uncommon
- Often, SDC is malignant component of carcinoma ex-pleomorphic adenoma

Lymphatic/Vascular Invasion

- Frequently extensive

Margins

- Often positive, as tumors are infiltrative and unencapsulated

Lymph Nodes

- Positive in 60-70% of cases, many at presentation

Variants

- All variants still have histopathologic features of typical salivary duct carcinoma
- **Sarcomatoid**
  - Biphasic neoplasm composed of both SDC and sarcomatoid (spindle cell) elements
  - Dyscohesive, pleomorphic population, predominantly spindled
  - Concurrent heterologous elements (bone, cartilage) can be seen
  - Pleomorphic adenoma is concurrently detected
  - Sarcomatous areas positive: EMA; CK4 (focal in ~ 50%); p53 (diffuse in ~ 30%)
- **Micropapillary**
  - Invasive micropapillary architecture
    - Morula-like small epithelial cell clusters without fibrovascular cores surrounded by clear space
  - Eosinophilic cytoplasm, with apocrine-type apical globules of cytoplasm
  - Immunoreactivity: CK7, EMA (distinctive "inside-out" pattern), HER-2/neu, p53, Ki-67 (high index)
  - More aggressive biologic behavior (high lymph node metastases) than other variants of SDC with shorter mean survival than conventional SDC
- **Mucin-rich**
  - SDC with malignant cell nests floating in pools of extracellular epithelial mucin
- **Osteoclast-type giant cell**
  - Osteoclast-like giant cells resembling giant cell tumor of bone
  - Mononuclear cells are immunoreactive for epithelial markers and androgen receptors
- **Low-grade SDC**
  - Controversial entity (cribriform cystadenocarcinoma)
    - May be part of papillary cystadenocarcinoma
  - Shows cribriform and "Roman bridge" architecture
  - Low nuclear grade and lacks necrosis
  - Much better prognosis than conventional SDC

ANCILLARY TESTS

Cytology

- Cellular smears with abundant background debris and necrotic material
- Epithelial tumor cells arranged in cohesive clusters
- Cribriform pattern in sheets or 3-dimensional papillary clusters
- Isolated, individual atypical epithelial cells scattered at periphery of clusters
- Round, polygonal to spindled tumor cells with abundant, finely granular to vacuolated cytoplasm
- Medium to large, pleomorphic, and hyperchromatic nuclei
- Nucleoli prominent
- Mitotic figures can be seen
- Androgen receptor can be performed on smears to confirm diagnosis

Histochemistry

- Nonreactive with mucicarmine and Alcian blue

Immunohistochemistry

- Immunoreactive for epithelial markers, androgen receptor, HER-2/neu
  - Breast epithelial markers are positive in many

Flow Cytometry

- High frequency of DNA aneuploidy

Cytogenetics

- Frequent LOH involving 9p21, 6q, 16q, 17p, and 17q regions
  - Locus on 9q21 contains *CDKN2A/p16* tumor suppressor gene, with inactivation associated with progression

Electron Microscopy

- Basal lamina, desmosomes, tight junctions, and luminal cells with microvilli
- Basally located myoepithelial cells occasionally present

DIFFERENTIAL DIAGNOSIS

Metastatic Breast Carcinoma

- Very rare and would have clinical/radiographic history of breast primary
- Circumscribed tumor nodules, "Roman bridge" cribriform architecture, ductal structures, comedonecrosis, and pleomorphism seen in both
  - Sialodochodysplasia would exclude metastatic disease
- Positive with ER and PR, but negative with AR (usually)

Cystadenocarcinoma

- Different from **cribriform cystadenocarcinoma**
- Predominantly papillary, cystic tumor, with low-grade cytologic features
- Absent comedonecrosis
- Lacks infiltration

Polymorphous Low-Grade Adenocarcinoma

- Minor salivary gland location
- May have focal cribriform pattern but usually many patterns
- Cytologically bland, no necrosis, inconspicuous mitoses

Oncocytic Carcinoma

- Abundant, granular eosinophilic cytoplasm can be seen in both

Immunohistochemistry

Antibody	Reactivity	Staining Pattern	Comment
CK-PAN	Positive	Cytoplasmic	Most tumor cells
CK7	Positive	Cytoplasmic	Most tumor cells
EMA	Positive	Cell membrane & cytoplasm	
CEA-M	Positive	Cytoplasmic	
Androgen receptor	Positive	Nuclear	Strong reaction in up to 90% of tumors; more common in men than in women (80% vs. 30%)
HER2	Positive	Cell membrane	Strong, diffuse, linear membrane reactivity in > 30% of tumor cells; present in up to 50% of tumors
EGFR	Positive	Cell membrane	Up to 50% of tumors have positive reaction
p53	Positive	Nuclear	Strong in most tumor cells, but range of 20-80% of tumors
GCDFP-15	Positive	Cytoplasmic	Strong, but focally immunoreactive
Cyclin-D1	Positive	Nuclear	Strongly overexpressed in most tumor cells
ERP-β	Positive	Nuclear	Variable, up to 70% of tumors
PRP	Positive	Nuclear	< 5% of tumors
PSA	Positive	Cytoplasmic	< 5% of tumors
PAP	Positive	Cytoplasmic	< 5% of tumors
TGF-α	Positive	Cytoplasmic	About 2/3 of tumors will show positive reaction
p63	Positive	Nuclear	Highlights myoepithelial/basal cells in most tumors
CK14	Positive	Cytoplasmic	Only in myoepithelial cells surrounding "ducts" or large spaces (but interpret with caution)
Calponin	Positive	Cytoplasmic	Only in myoepithelial cells surrounding "ducts" or large spaces (but interpret with caution)
Actin-sm	Positive	Cytoplasmic	Only of myoepithelial cells surrounding "ducts" or large spaces (but interpret with caution)
PPAR-γ	Positive	Cytoplasmic	Approximately 70% of cases will be positive
S100	Negative		
Bcl-2	Negative		

- Lacks cystic, papillary, and cribriform patterns
- Oncocytes tend to be large
- Comedonecrosis usually absent
- Plentiful mitochondria (PTAH or EM)

Adenoid Cystic Carcinoma

- Cribriform pattern is common but not "Roman bridge" pattern
- Comedonecrosis is usually absent
- Shows ductal and myoepithelial type cells
  - Small, angular nuclei with hyperchromasia
- Background of pseudolumina with glycosaminoglycans &/or hyalinized basal lamina
- Prominent myoepithelial immunohistochemistry

Mucoepidermoid Carcinoma, High Grade

- Lacks prominent papillary or cribriform patterns
- Presence of mucocytes (goblet cells), epidermoid cells, and transitional areas

SELECTED REFERENCES

1. Kashiwagi N et al: Salivary duct carcinoma of the parotid gland: clinical and MR features in six patients. Br J Radiol. 82(982):800-4, 2009
2. Johnson CJ et al: Her-2/neu expression in salivary duct carcinoma: an immunohistochemical and chromogenic in situ hybridization study. Appl Immunohistochem Mol Morphol. 16(1):54-8, 2008
3. Simpson RH et al: Salivary duct carcinoma in situ of the parotid gland. Histopathology. 53(4):416-25, 2008
4. Nabili V et al: Salivary duct carcinoma: a clinical and histologic review with implications for trastuzumab therapy. Head Neck. 29(10):907-12, 2007
5. Jaehne M et al: Clinical and immunohistologic typing of salivary duct carcinoma: a report of 50 cases. Cancer. 103(12):2526-33, 2005
6. Brandwein-Gensler M et al: Low-grade salivary duct carcinoma: description of 16 cases. Am J Surg Pathol. 28(8):1040-4, 2004
7. Nagao T et al: Invasive micropapillary salivary duct carcinoma: a distinct histologic variant with biologic significance. Am J Surg Pathol. 28(3):319-26, 2004
8. Nagao T et al: Sarcomatoid variant of salivary duct carcinoma: clinicopathologic and immunohistochemical study of eight cases with review of the literature. Am J Clin Pathol. 122(2):222-31, 2004
9. Etges A et al: Salivary duct carcinoma: immunohistochemical profile of an aggressive salivary gland tumour. J Clin Pathol. 56(12):914-8, 2003
10. van Heerden WF et al: Intraoral salivary duct carcinoma: a report of 5 cases. J Oral Maxillofac Surg. 61(1):126-31, 2003
11. Hoang MP et al: Molecular and biomarker analyses of salivary duct carcinomas: comparison with mammary duct carcinoma. Int J Oncol. 19(4):865-71, 2001

SALIVARY DUCT CARCINOMA

Radiographic and Microscopic Features

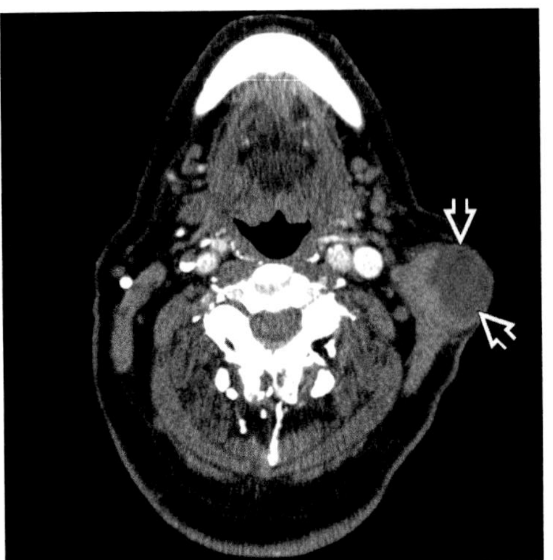

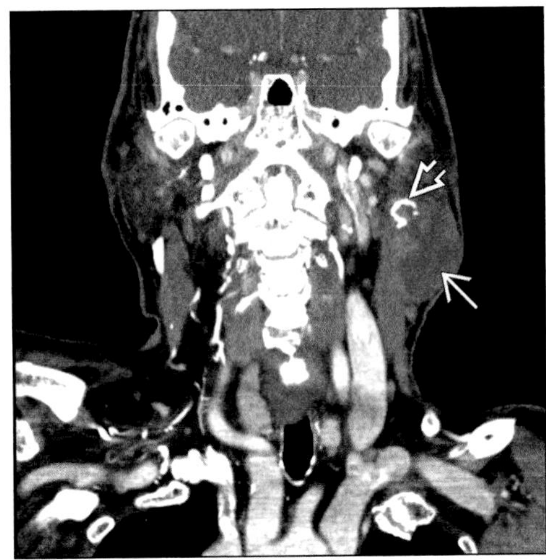

(Left) Computed tomography image shows a left parotid gland mass. There is cystic degeneration ➡ within the central portion of the mass. This is characteristic of a high-grade neoplasm, although it is not specific as to type. *(Right)* Computed tomography image shows a left parotid gland mass. There is cystic degeneration within the central portion of the mass ➡. Note the calcification ➡, which suggests a previous pleomorphic adenoma.

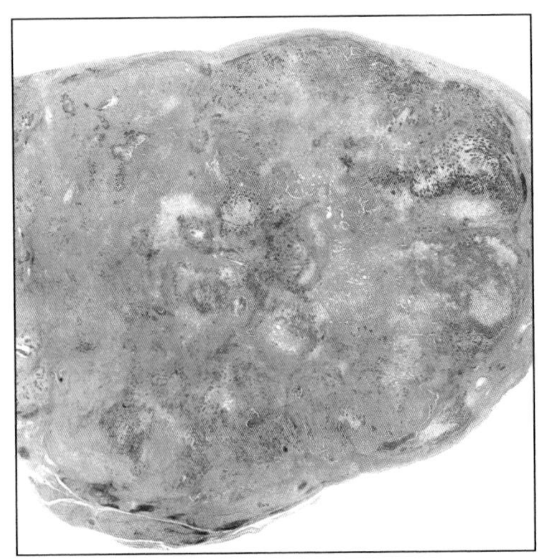

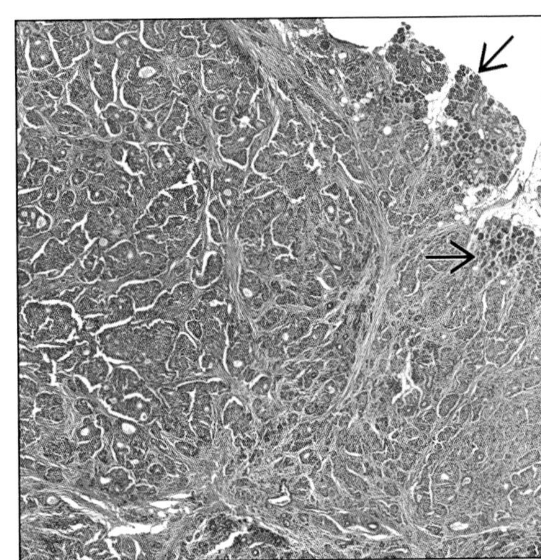

(Left) The tumors are usually large, nearly completely replacing the entire gland. There are frequently areas of necrosis and fibrosis, as shown in this low-power view. A vague nodularity to the tumor is noted. *(Right)* There is a micropapillary pattern to this SDC that demonstrates infiltration into the adjacent parotid gland parenchyma →. The tumors tend to lack well-formed capsules and are widely invasive.

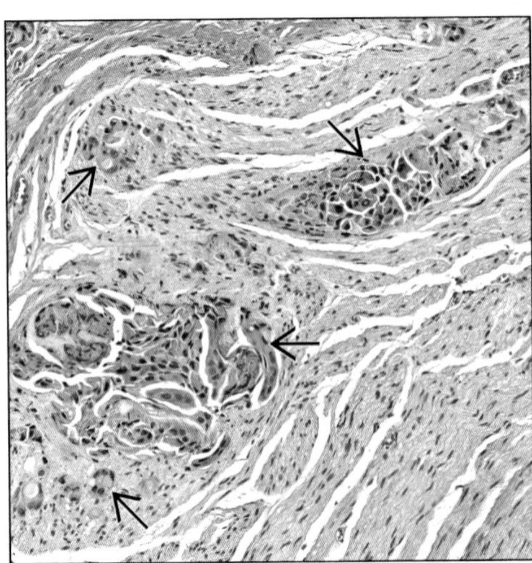

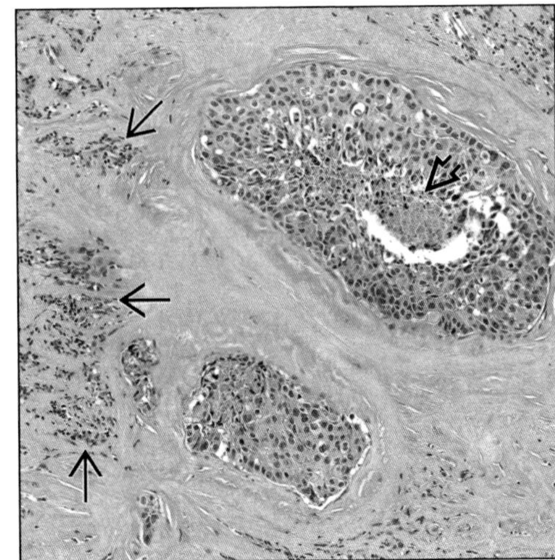

(Left) Perineural and intraneural invasion are conspicuous findings in SDC. Here, a large nerve contains neoplastic cells → within the substance of the nerve bundles. *(Right)* Islands and nests of tumor cells give the appearance of ducts. There is significant desmoplastic fibrosis separating the tumor islands. However, there are also many areas of more individual cell infiltration →, a finding commonly seen in SDC. Note the comedonecrosis ➡, also a frequent finding.

Microscopic Features

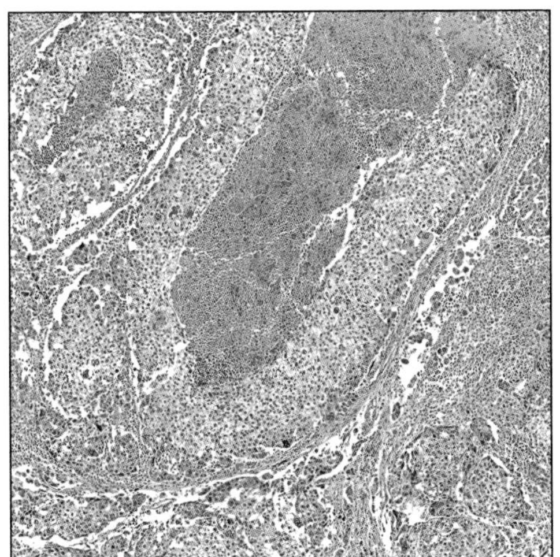

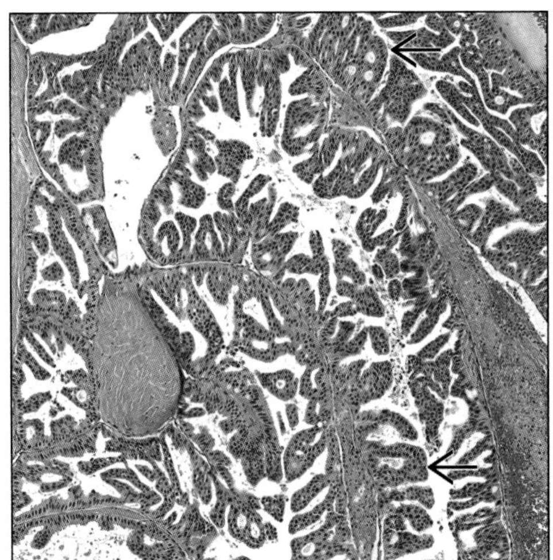

(Left) *Sheets of neoplastic cells show multiple areas of large comedonecrosis, which are composed of central-intraductal type necrosis filling the cystic area. This particular pattern is not readily seen in other salivary gland malignancies.* ***(Right)*** *The neoplasm is typically arranged in cribriform, band-like solid regions and papillary patterns. This field demonstrates a large number of papillae, although areas of "Roman bridge" formation are also noted ➙.*

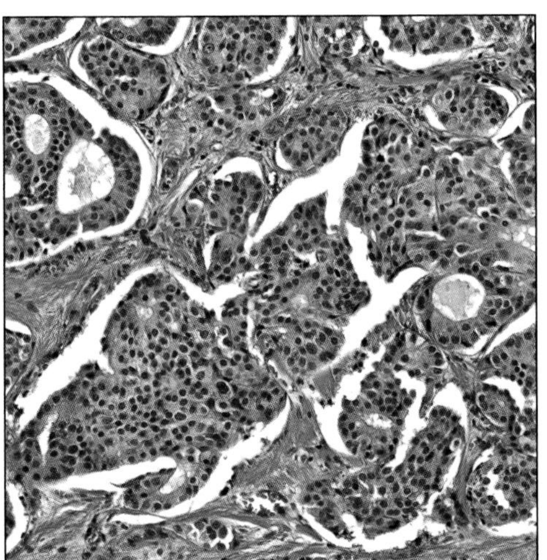

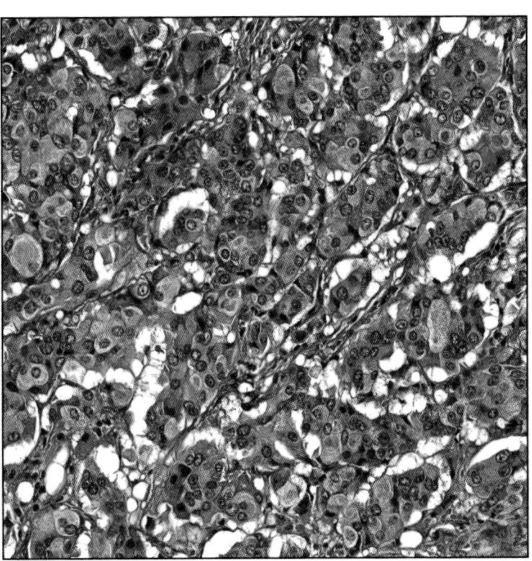

(Left) *Small nodules of tumor cells create a ductal appearance. Note the separation by heavy fibrous connective tissue stroma. There is cellular monotony in this area, even though all the cells are atypical.* ***(Right)*** *Multiple small packets of neoplastic cells are noted in this area. This is not the micropapillary pattern but instead an example of the retraction artifacts that are commonly seen in SDC.*

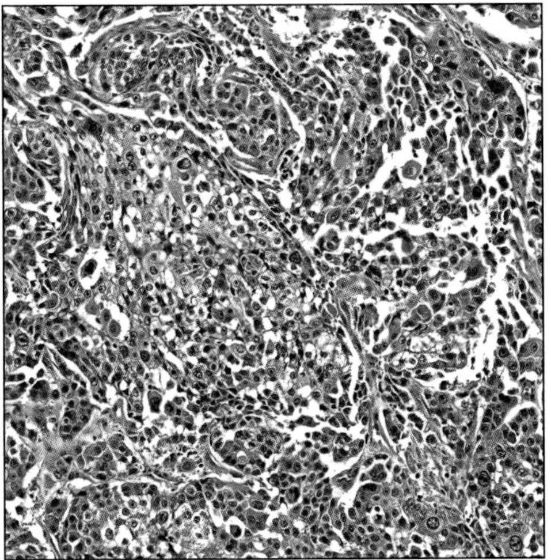

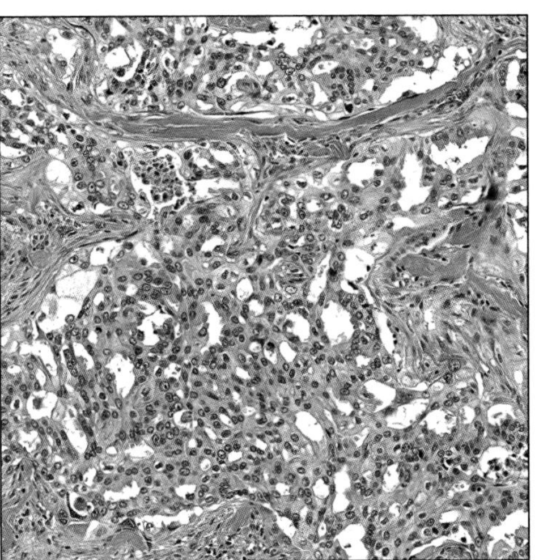

(Left) *The large cystic area is filled with a solid to pseudopapillary proliferation of highly atypical cells. This appearance is that of a high-grade malignancy.* ***(Right)*** *The cells are arranged in a cribriform pattern, with fibrovascular stroma separating the tumor nodules. The cystic spaces are easily identified and give an appearance similar to a ductal carcinoma in situ of the breast. The degree of cytologic atypia is beyond what would be seen in papillary cystadenocarcinoma.*

SALIVARY DUCT CARCINOMA

Microscopic Features

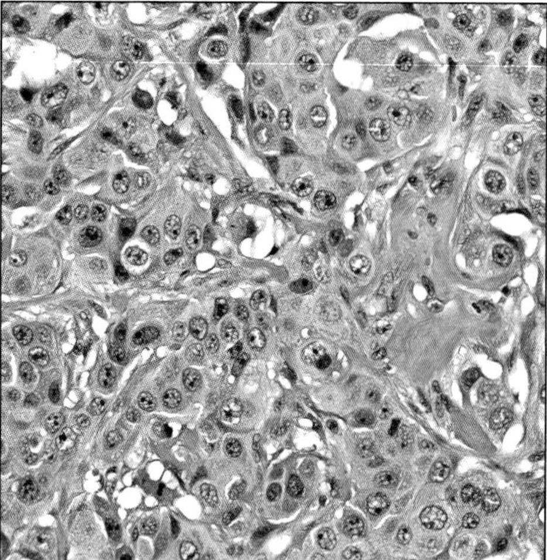

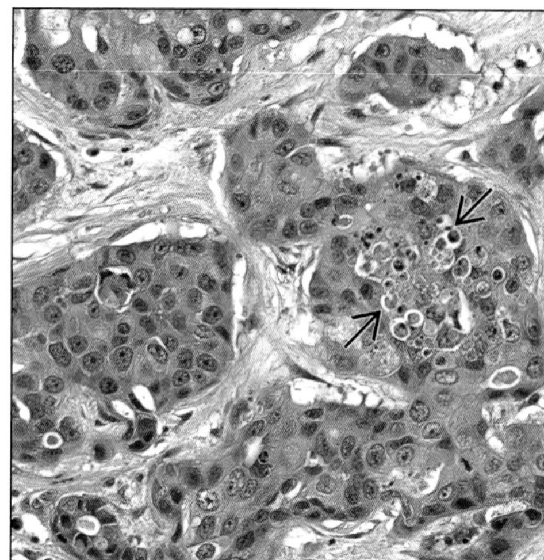

(Left) *The epithelial cells have moderate to marked pleomorphism, showing polygonal cells with ample eosinophilic, granular cytoplasm. Nucleoli are easily identified in most of the tumor cells.* ***(Right)*** *The neoplastic cells are arranged in small nests with the polygonal cells showing moderate pleomorphism. The cytoplasm is granular to opacified. Note the area of early degeneration or comedonecrosis* ➙.

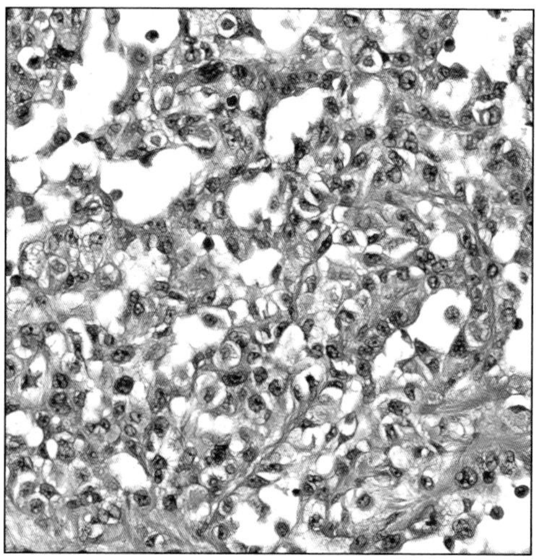

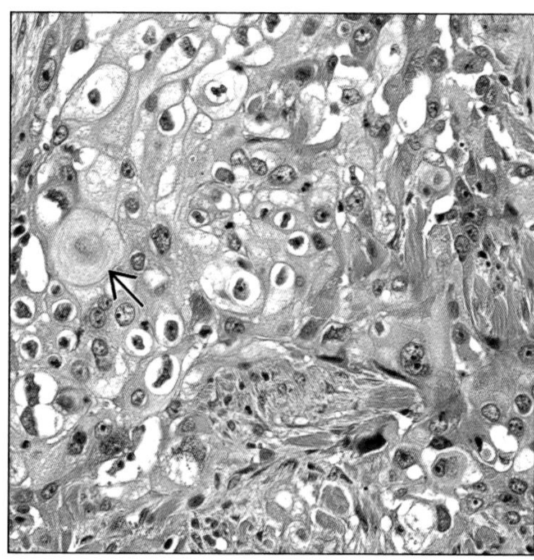

(Left) *There is a clearing to the cytoplasm in this particular area of an SDC, although it is infrequently observed. The tumor is arranged in a cribriform to glandular pattern.* ***(Right)*** *This tumor focus shows an infiltrating pattern of cells with a squamous appearance. There is even a suggestion of keratinization* ➙ *in one of the cells. Note significant pleomorphism in this area.*

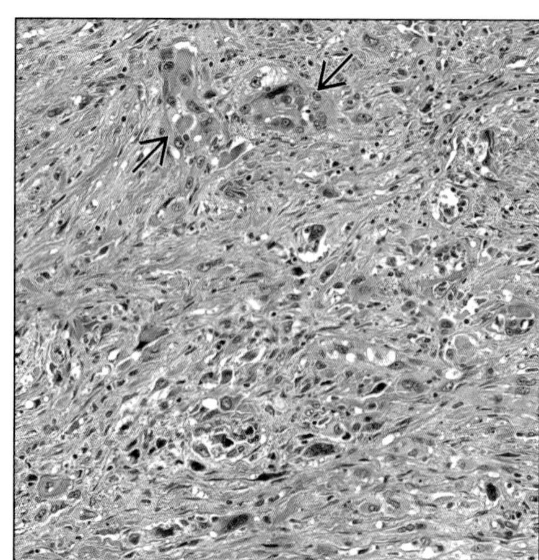

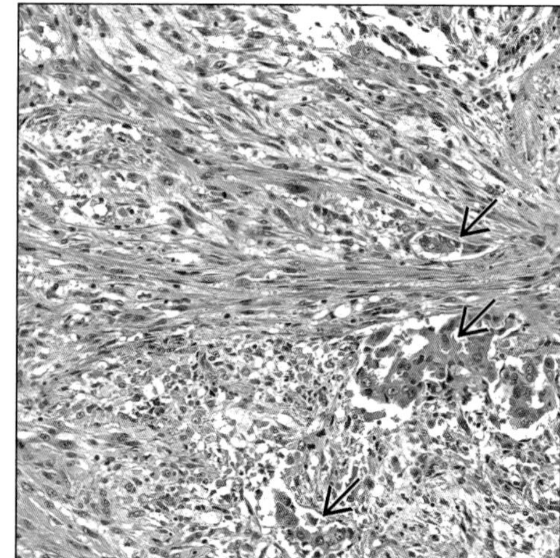

(Left) *The neoplastic cells show a biphasic appearance with dyscohesive pleomorphic epithelioid cells* ➙ *immediately juxtaposed and blending with sarcomatoid (spindle cell) elements that predominate in this tumor. There is profound pleomorphism.* ***(Right)*** *Biphasic neoplasms, such as this one, are composed of epithelial and spindle cell elements in a sarcomatoid SDC. The epithelial cells* ➙ *are dyscohesive, mixed with the fascicles of spindled cells. There is a background myxoid degeneration.*

Ancillary Techniques

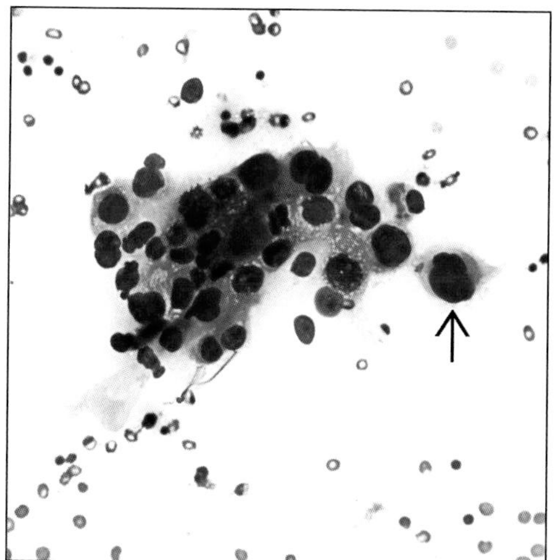
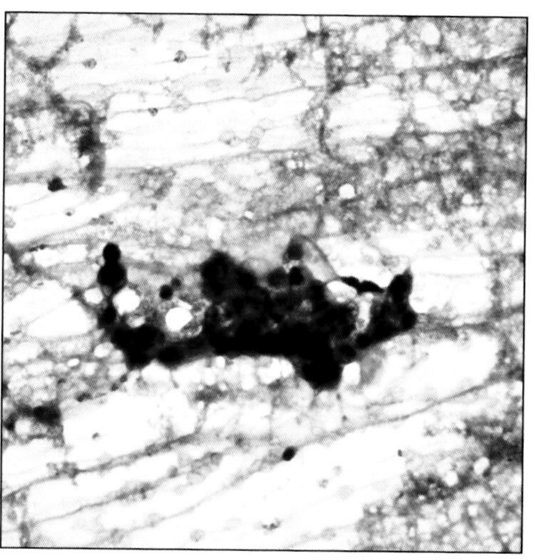

(Left) *This smear shows a cohesive cluster of epithelial tumor cells with an isolated atypical epithelial cell ⊡ at the periphery of the cluster. The tumor cells are polygonal with finely vacuolated cytoplasm.* ***(Right)*** *This cribriform epithelial cluster is identified in a background of debris and necrotic material. It is common to see this background in a high-grade neoplasm. High-power examination shows pleomorphism and prominent nucleoli.*

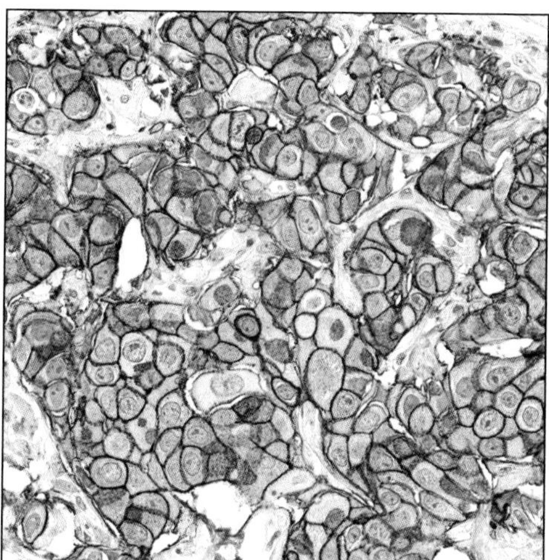
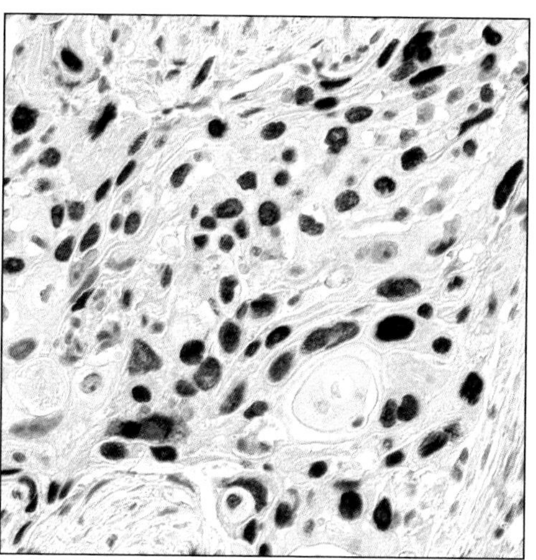

(Left) *Similar to breast carcinoma, SDC with HER-2/neu staining shows a strong, diffuse membrane reactivity circumferentially highlighting the neoplastic cells in > 30% of the tumor cells. There may be a few cases where only isolated cells show this pattern.* ***(Right)*** *Although p63 is usually in the basal or myoepithelial cell compartment, the very strong and diffuse immunoreactivity in this field highlights many pleomorphic cells in this SDC.*

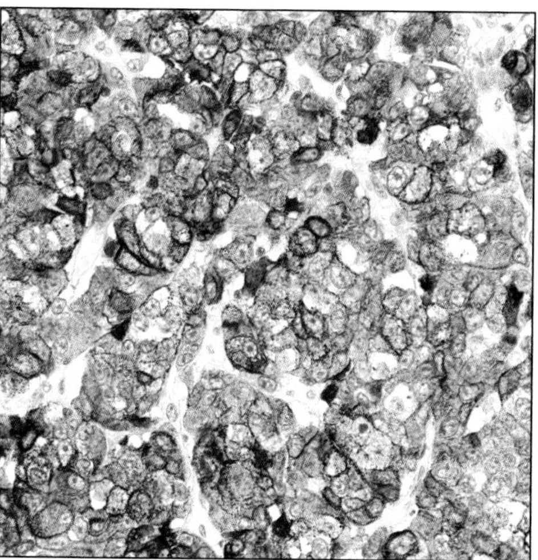
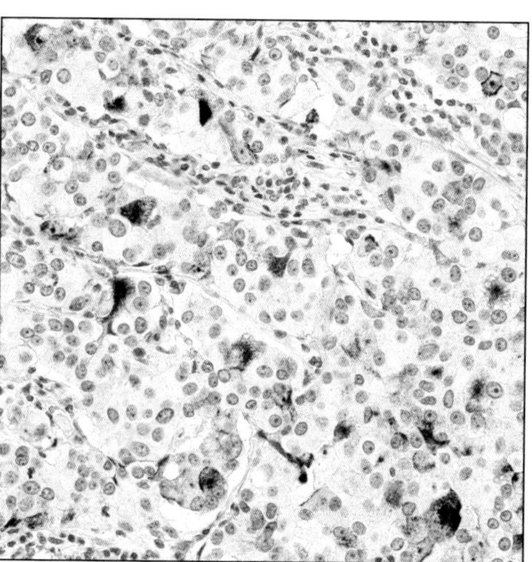

(Left) *EMA usually shows a very strong cell membrane reactivity, but there is also a frequent cytoplasmic blush or granular reactivity. This epithelial marker is quite characteristic for SDC.* ***(Right)*** *BRST-2 (GCDFP-15) often highlights only isolated neoplastic cells in SDC. It is quite common that only rare cells will be positive in the neoplastic proliferation, a feature that can help confirm the diagnosis.*

EPITHELIAL-MYOEPITHELIAL CARCINOMA

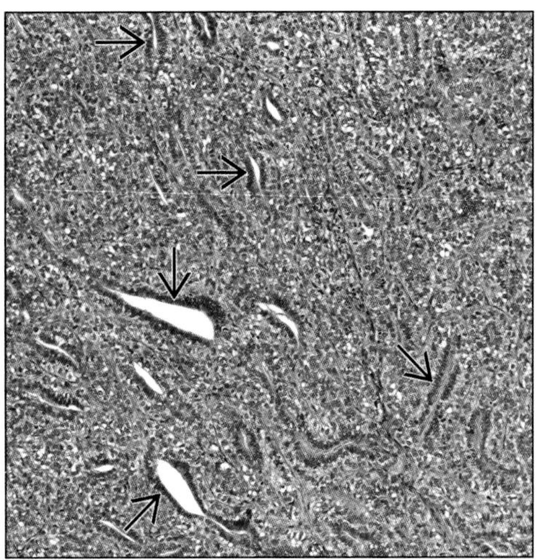

EMC shows classic biphasic (bilayered) tubular histology. More hyperchromatic, inner ductal cells are noted ➔ surrounded by myoepithelial clear cells.

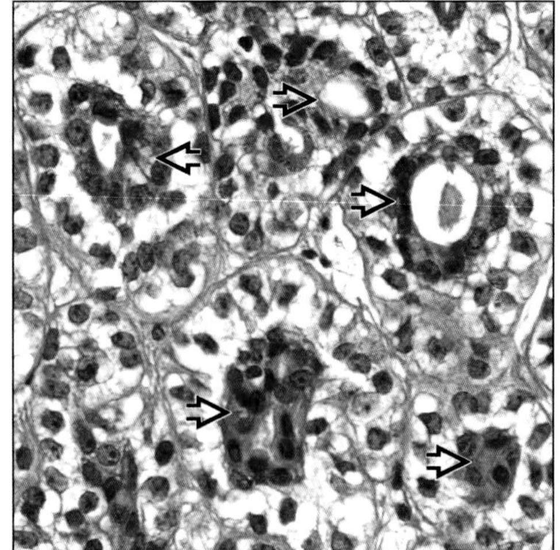

The inner layer is formed by a single row of cuboidal epithelial cells ➲ around a lumen. The outer layer is formed by large polygonal myoepithelial cells with clear cytoplasm and indistinct borders.

TERMINOLOGY

Abbreviations

- Epithelial-myoepithelial carcinoma (EMC)

Synonyms

- Adenomyoepithelioma
- Glycogen-rich adenocarcinoma
- Clear cell carcinoma
- Tubular solid adenoma
- Monomorphic clear cell tumor

Definitions

- Malignant neoplasm demonstrating variable proportions of biphasic pattern of inner luminal epithelial duct-like cells and outer abluminal layer of myoepithelial-like cells

ETIOLOGY/PATHOGENESIS

Cell of Origin

- Presumed to be of intercalated duct origin (biphasic)

CLINICAL ISSUES

Epidemiology

- Incidence
  - About 1% of all salivary gland tumors
  - About 2% of all salivary gland malignancies
- Age
  - Range: Teens to 90s; peak: 6th to 7th decades
  - Rare in children
- Gender
  - Female > Male (2:1)

Site

- Major salivary glands most commonly
  - Parotid gland: About 70%
  - Submandibular gland: About 12%
- Minor salivary glands also affected (about 18%)
  - Upper and lower respiratory tracts, palate

Presentation

- Slow-growing, painless mass
- Tumors are frequently present for years
- Minor salivary gland lesions present as submucosal nodule
  - May be ulcerated and less well defined than their major gland counterparts
- Rarely, tumors with high-grade transformation may present with rapid growth and pain, along with facial nerve palsy
- Synchronous bilateral tumors are very rare

Treatment

- Surgical approaches
  - Complete excision
    - Parotidectomy or wide excision
- Radiation
  - Only used with suboptimal resection

Prognosis

- Usually good overall prognosis (low-grade tumor)
  - 90% 5-year survival
  - 75% 10-year survival
- Recurrences in up to 50%
  - Recurrences usually develop within 5 years
  - Univariate predictors of recurrence
    - Margin status, angiolymphatic invasion, tumor necrosis, myoepithelial anaplasia
- Distant metastases in up to 20%
  - Cervical lymph nodes, lung, liver, and kidney
- Death from disease in about 10% of cases
- Poorer prognosis associated with
  - Minor salivary gland tumors
  - Rapid tumor growth
  - Large tumor size
  - Solid growth, nuclear atypia
  - High proliferation index, aneuploidy
  - High-grade transformation

EPITHELIAL-MYOEPITHELIAL CARCINOMA

Key Facts

Terminology
- Malignant neoplasm demonstrating biphasic pattern of inner duct-like and outer layer of myoepithelial-like cells

Clinical Issues
- About 1% of all salivary gland tumors
- Female > Male (2:1)
- Major salivary glands most commonly
- Good overall prognosis
  - Recurrences in up to 50%

Macroscopic Features
- Nodular or multinodular mass, with irregular borders

Microscopic Pathology
- Classic features of biphasic (bilayered) tubular histology, which predominates
- **Inner layer** formed by single row of cuboidal to columnar epithelial cells
- **Outer layer** formed by myoepithelial cells arranged in multiple layers of large polygonal cells with indistinct borders
  - Cytoplasm is clear, surrounding vesicular nucleus
- Basement membrane-like hyalinized material may separate duct-like structures

Ancillary Tests
- Epithelial and myoepithelial markers highlight dual population

Top Differential Diagnoses
- Pleomorphic adenoma, myoepithelioma
- Myoepithelial carcinoma, clear cell acinic cell carcinoma, clear cell adenocarcinoma

MACROSCOPIC FEATURES

General Features
- Well-defined but unencapsulated mass
- Nodular or multinodular mass, with irregular borders
- Minor salivary gland tumors are poorly defined
- Tumors are firm, gray-tan-white
- Cystic areas may be seen on cut surface

Sections to Be Submitted
- Tumor junction with salivary gland parenchyma

Size
- Range: 2-12 cm; mean: 2.5 cm

MICROSCOPIC PATHOLOGY

Histologic Features
- Lobules of tumor
- Surface ulceration (minor salivary gland tumors) in about 40% of cases
- Classic features of biphasic (bilayered) tubular histology, which predominates
  - **Inner layer** formed by single row of cuboidal to columnar epithelial cells
    - Dense to finely granular cytoplasm surrounding round to oval nucleus
    - Duct cells are intercalated duct-like
  - **Outer layer** formed by myoepithelial cells
    - Large polygonal cells with indistinct borders arranged in multiple layers
    - Clear cytoplasm around eccentric, vesicular nucleus
    - Rich in glycogen (diastase-sensitive PAS[+])
- Clear cells may dominate, with only isolated duct-lining cells (without canalization)
  - Luminal cells comprise up to about 1/3 of cell population
- Proteinaceous material may be seen in lumen
  - PAS positive but not mucicarmine positive
- Mixture of tubular, glandular, and solid patterns
  - Organoid or thèque-like pattern can be seen
  - Solid, spindled cell population may be present
- Papillary and cystic areas comprise small proportion of some tumors (20%)
- Pleomorphism is mild for vast majority
- Basement membrane-like hyalinized material may separate duct-like structures
- Perineural and vascular invasion are common
  - Bone invasion is uncommon
- Mitotic figures are sparse (1-2/10 HPFs)
- **Rare** findings
  - Squamous &/or sebaceous differentiation
  - Spindle cell pattern
  - Ancient change
  - Oncocytic luminal cells
  - Verocay-like change
  - High-grade transformation (dedifferentiation) (~ 2%)
    - Sheets and nests of markedly atypical cells showing necrosis, increased mitoses
    - Areas of typical EMC still identified
  - May represent component in carcinoma ex-pleomorphic adenoma (~ 1%)

ANCILLARY TESTS

Cytology
- One of the tumors with high false-negative rate
- Biphasic smears with ductal cells and larger clear cells
- Larger cells are fragile, creating naked nuclei
- Hyalinized basal lamina can create globules

Histochemistry
- PAS highlights basement membrane material and glycogen (with diastase) in myoepithelial cells

Immunohistochemistry
- Epithelial and myoepithelial dualism highlighted by appropriate selected immunohistochemistry

Flow Cytometry
- Aneuploidy associated with worse prognosis

EPITHELIAL-MYOEPITHELIAL CARCINOMA

Immunohistochemistry

Antibody	Reactivity	Staining Pattern	Comment
CK-PAN	Positive	Cytoplasmic	Ductal cells specifically
EMA	Positive	Cytoplasmic	Ductal cell specifically
CK5/6	Positive	Cytoplasmic	Variably present, ductal and myoepithelial cells
p63	Positive	Nuclear	Myoepithelial cells only
Actin-sm	Positive	Cytoplasmic	Myoepithelial cells only
Calponin	Positive	Cytoplasmic	Myoepithelial cells only
CK14	Positive	Cytoplasmic	Myoepithelial cells only
SMHC	Positive	Cytoplasmic	Myoepithelial cells only
S100	Positive	Nuclear & cytoplasmic	Myoepithelial cells predominantly
Vimentin	Positive	Cytoplasmic	Preferentially myoepithelial cells
CD117	Positive	Cytoplasmic	Variably present, highlighting myoepithelial cells specifically
p53	Positive	Nuclear	Only in tumors with dedifferentiation
GFAP	Equivocal	Cytoplasmic	Myoepithelial cells occasionally

Electron Microscopy

- Ductal cells have microvilli on luminal surface, attached with junctional complexes and desmosomes
- Electron lucent myoepithelial cells surround ductal cells, contain abundant glycogen and have cytokeratin filaments, subplasmalemmal plaques, and multilayered basal lamina

DIFFERENTIAL DIAGNOSIS

Pleomorphic Adenoma

- Multinodular and bosselated growth with biphasic epithelial/myoepithelial populations
- Myxochondroid matrix material merged or blended with epithelial population
  - EMC cells sharply separated from matrix material
- Bilayered tubule formation is **not** prominent, nor is clear cell population

Adenoid Cystic Carcinoma (ACC)

- Cribriform pattern (most common in ACC) is not seen in EMC
- Cells are small, with peg-shaped or carrot-shaped very hyperchromatic nuclei

Myoepithelioma/Myoepithelial Carcinoma

- Spindled cell neoplasm **without** ductal or tubule formation (by definition)

Mucoepidermoid Carcinoma

- Problems with clear cell variant, specifically
- Cyst formation, mucocytes, and transitional pattern seen somewhere in tumor
  - Lacks biphasic pattern

Clear Cell Acinic Cell Carcinoma

- Lacks biphasic appearance
- Clear cell areas tend to be small and nondominant
- Basophilic, granular cytoplasm predominates in most
- High glycogen content is not seen
- No myoepithelial phenotype immunohistochemically

Clear Cell Adenocarcinoma

- Predilection for minor salivary gland (intraoral) sites
- Monotonous cell population, lacking myoepithelial differentiation
- Small islands and single cell infiltration associated with prominent fibrous connective tissue stroma

Oncocytoma, Clear Cell Type

- Large polygonal cells without biphasic appearance
- Clear cell changes may predominate, but oncocytic, granular cytoplasm is still found

SELECTED REFERENCES

1. Kusafuka K et al: Dedifferentiated epithelial-myoepithelial carcinoma of the parotid gland: a rare case report of immunohistochemical analysis and review of the literature. Oral Surg Oral Med Oral Pathol Oral Radiol Endod. 106(1):85-91, 2008
2. Seethala RR et al: Epithelial-myoepithelial carcinoma: a review of the clinicopathologic spectrum and immunophenotypic characteristics in 61 tumors of the salivary glands and upper aerodigestive tract. Am J Surg Pathol. 2007 Jan;31(1):44-57. Erratum in: Am J Surg Pathol. 32(12):1923, 2008
3. Wang B et al: Primary salivary clear cell tumors--a diagnostic approach: a clinicopathologic and immunohistochemical study of 20 patients with clear cell carcinoma, clear cell myoepithelial carcinoma, and epithelial-myoepithelial carcinoma. Arch Pathol Lab Med. 126(6):676-85, 2002
4. Tralongo V et al: Epithelial-myoepithelial carcinoma of the salivary glands: a review of literature. Anticancer Res. 18(1B):603-8, 1998
5. Maiorano E et al: Clear cell tumors of the salivary glands, jaws, and oral mucosa. Semin Diagn Pathol. 14(3):203-12, 1997
6. Brocheriou C et al: [Epithelial-myoepithelial carcinoma of the salivary glands. Study of 15 cases and review of the literature.] Ann Pathol. 11(5-6):316-25, 1991
7. Dardick I et al: Myoepithelial cells in salivary gland tumors--revisited. Head Neck Surg. 7(5):395-408, 1985
8. Corio RL et al: Epithelial-myoepithelial carcinoma of intercalated duct origin. A clinicopathologic and ultrastructural assessment of sixteen cases. Oral Surg Oral Med Oral Pathol. 53(3):280-7, 1982

Microscopic Features

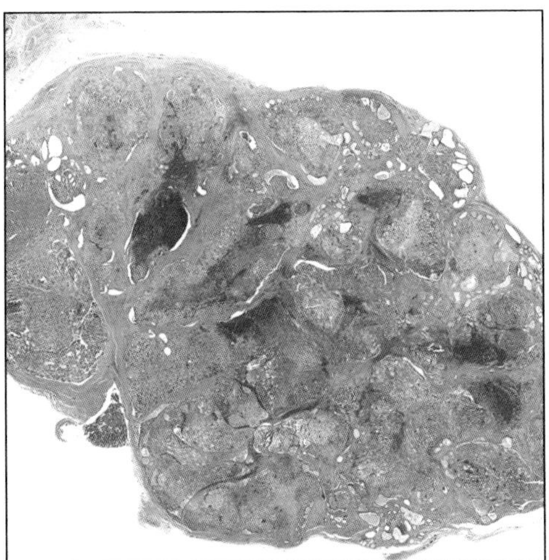

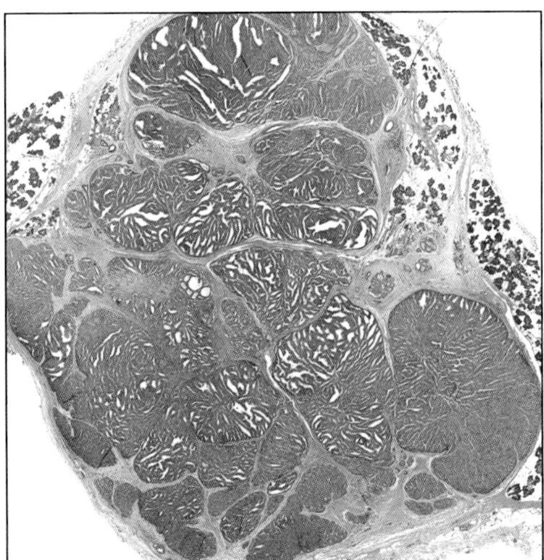

(Left) *On low power, there is a well-defined but unencapsulated tumor showing a multinodular appearance with irregular borders.* ***(Right)*** *There is an irregular periphery as the tumor confronts the salivary gland parenchyma. A capsule is not appreciated. The multinodular tumor shows fibrous septae as well as a few areas of cystic change. Invasion is a helpful feature in defining this tumor, although it may be difficult to detect on low power.*

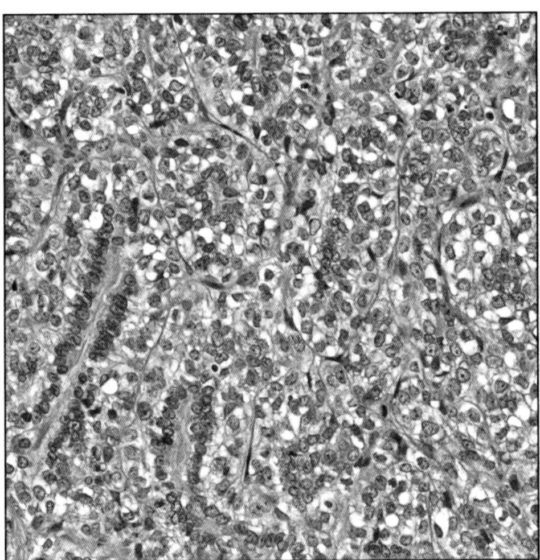

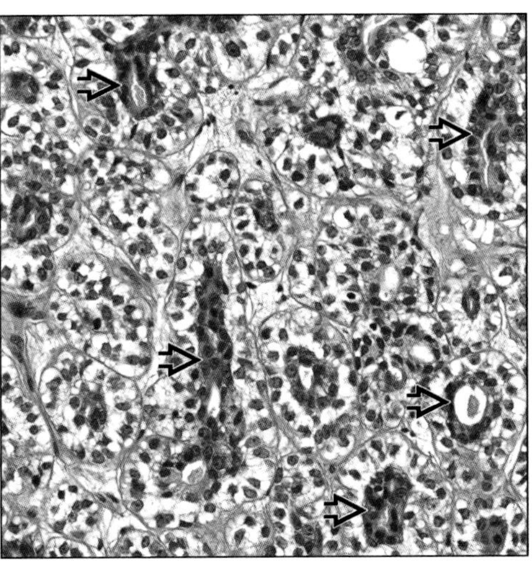

(Left) *The tumor will frequently display a cellular, solid pattern. However, the characteristic bilayered tubule formation is easily detected. The outer myoepithelial cells have cleared cytoplasm.* ***(Right)*** *Delicate wisps of stroma surround the tumor nests. They have the characteristic central duct-like structures (cuboidal cells) ⇨, which are surrounded by the syncytial arrangement of myoepithelial cells with clear cytoplasm.*

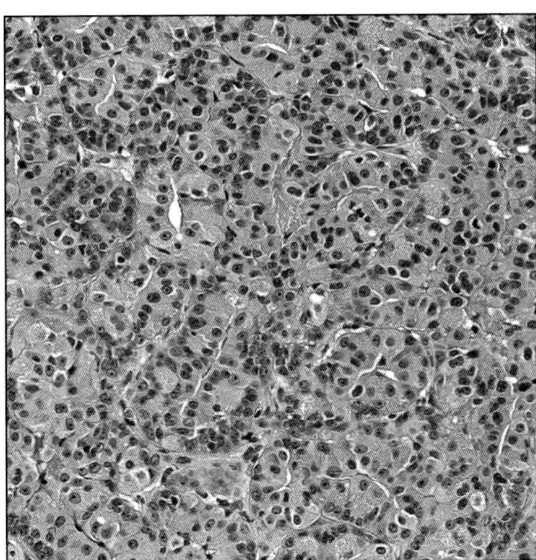

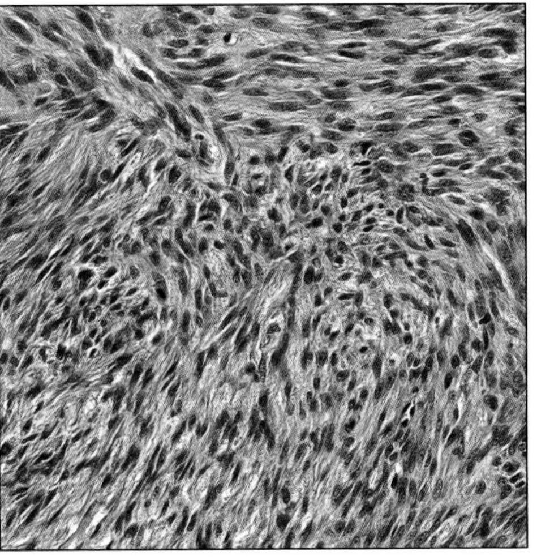

(Left) *There is a more sheet-like or solid pattern to this tumor. However, darker cells are noted adjacent to the areas of more eosinophilic appearance. This tumor had areas of more classic biphasic appearance elsewhere.* ***(Right)*** *Spindled myoepithelial cells are a common finding, although in general this is not a dominant pattern of growth. A vaguely fascicular architecture is suggested here. If this was the only pattern in the tumor, it would be a myoepithelioma/ myoepithelial carcinoma.*

EPITHELIAL-MYOEPITHELIAL CARCINOMA

Variant Microscopic Features

*(**Left**) The characteristic biphasic appearance is present in the left side, but a cystic appearance is also noted ⇨. This is not a common pattern in EMC. (**Right**) The ductal, luminal cells may have an oncocytic appearance in a few tumors. The biphasic appearance is still appreciated in this tumor, with the darker nuclei of the myoepithelial cells present at the periphery of the tubules. Immunohistochemistry would help to highlight this separation.*

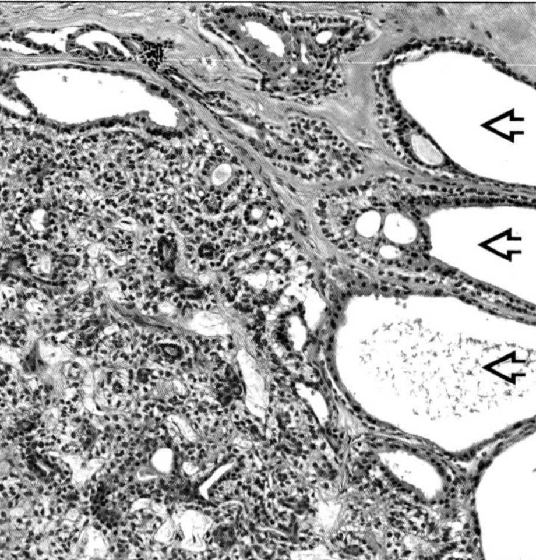

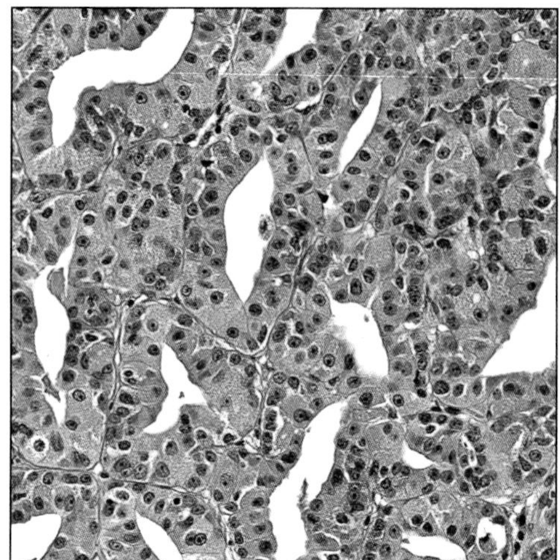

*(**Left**) Although the clear cell change in the myoepithelial cells should predominate, there are tumors that lack this feature. Secretions in the lumen of these ducts do not stain with mucicarmine. There is a moderate degree of nuclear pleomorphism. (**Right**) In a solid area like this, only isolated "tubules" are present ➡. The luminal cells have an oncocytic or granular cytoplasm. The myoepithelial cells appear more "basaloid" in this field.*

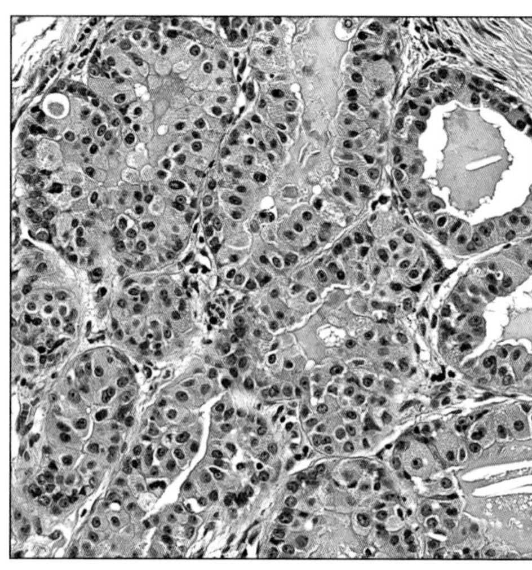

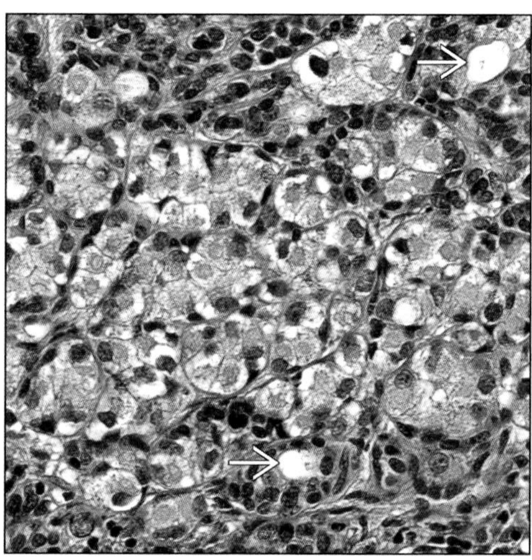

*(**Left**) The histologic resemblance of this single high-power field to a basal cell adenoma is quite remarkable. Basement membrane-like hyalinized material is seen separating the duct-like structures. However, the biphasic appearance can still be seen ➡ if carefully evaluated. (**Right**) Tumor cell necrosis ⇨ is not a frequent feature in this tumor, although there can be foci in a few tumors. Note the characteristic biphasic tubule formation elsewhere →.*

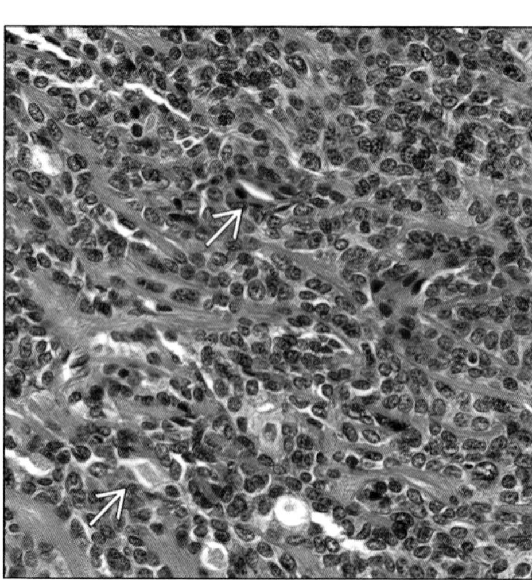

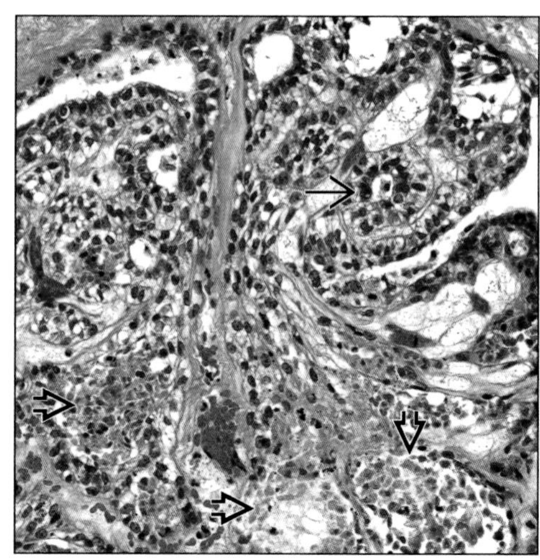

Immunohistochemical Features

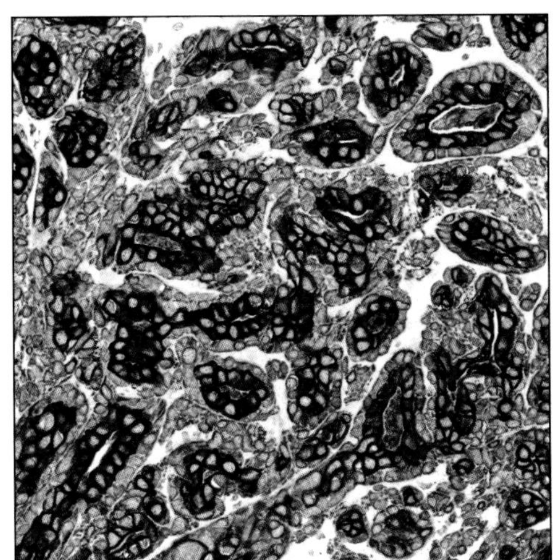

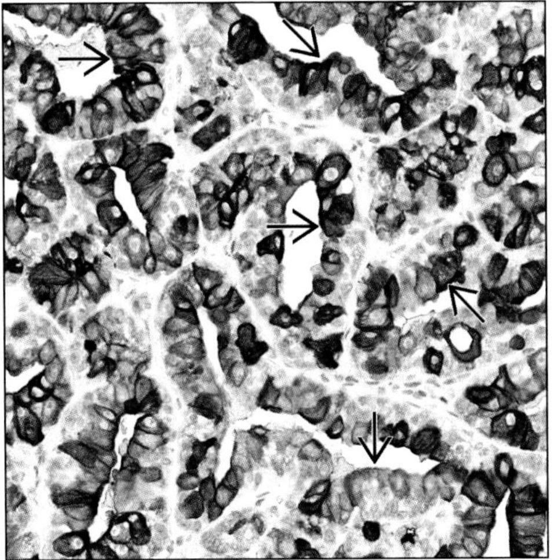

(Left) *Both the epithelial and myoepithelial cells are highlighted with a pan-keratin. However, there is an accentuation with a darker reactivity of the ductal-luminal cells than the myoepithelial cells.* ***(Right)*** *In many tumors, the keratin (in this case, CK7) highlights only the ductal-tubule inner luminal cells ⇒. This type of staining helps to reinforce the histologic duality of this neoplasm.*

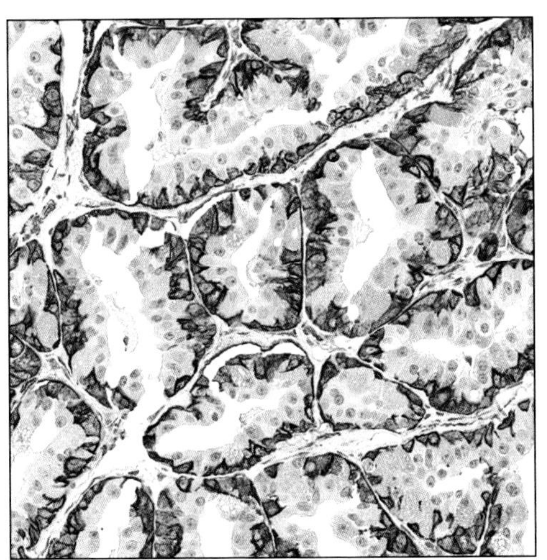

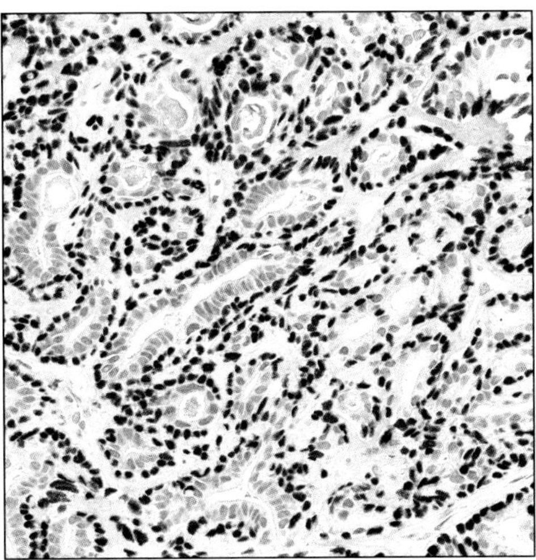

(Left) *The myoepithelial cells react with a variety of immunohistochemistry studies, although the smooth muscle actin often gives the most characteristic and strong reactivity. Calponin, muscle specific actin, and CK14 give a similar result.* ***(Right)*** *p63 strongly and diffusely highlights the nuclei of neoplastic myoepithelial cells in this EMC. Note that the inner luminal/ductal cells are not stained with this marker. Of course, p63 is immunoreactive in many salivary gland neoplasms.*

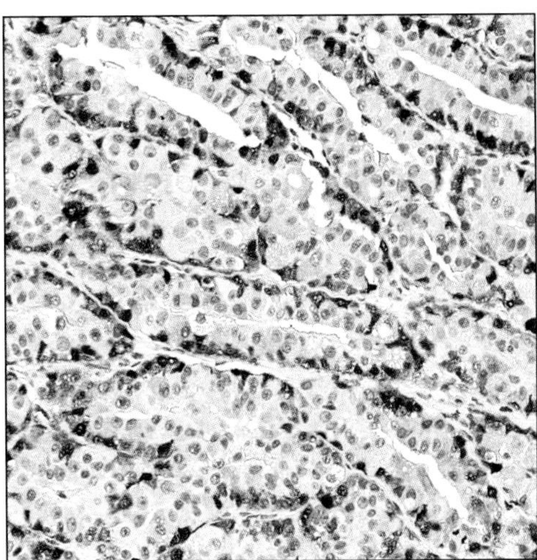

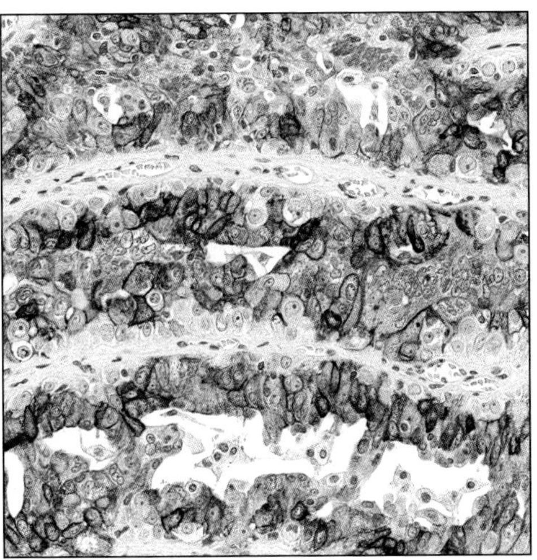

(Left) *S100 protein highlights both the cytoplasm and nuclei of the myoepithelial cells predominantly. However, a few ductal cells may be positive with this marker also. It is not a unique nor specific marker.* ***(Right)*** *CD117 is a marker that has been applied to many salivary gland neoplasms. Unfortunately, the specificity and sensitivity for any one tumor type is absent. As can be seen here, there is myoepithelial as well as ductal cell immunoreactivity.*

ADENOCARCINOMA, NOT OTHERWISE SPECIFIED

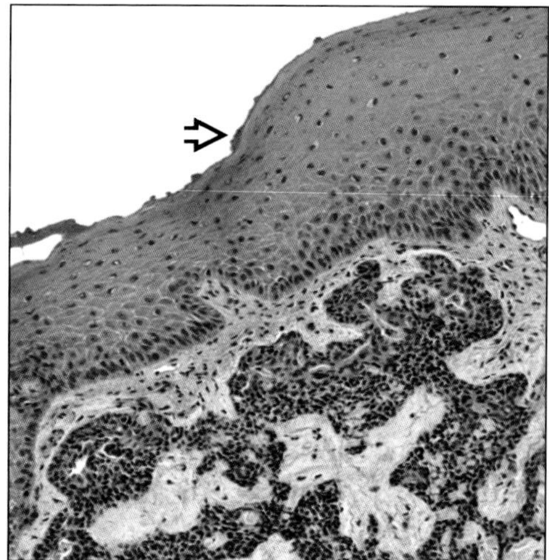

Hematoxylin & eosin shows a gland-forming tumor with overlying mucosa ⇨. This tumor is of minor salivary gland origin and would be a grade 2 tumor.

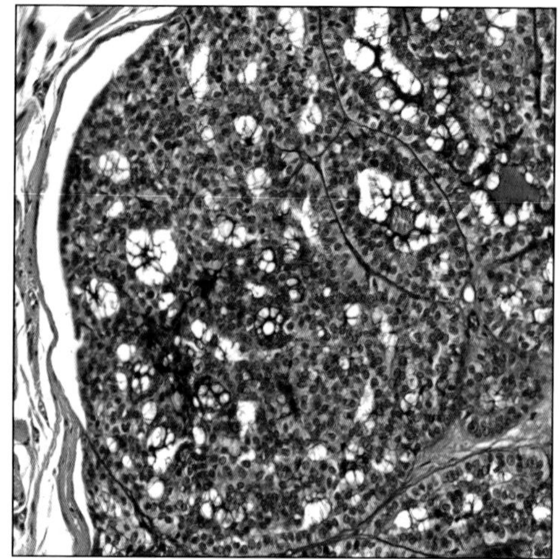

Hematoxylin & eosin shows organoid islands of tumor cells with complex glandular growth and little to no intervening stroma. This tumor would be a grade 1 tumor.

TERMINOLOGY

Abbreviations

- Adenocarcinoma, not otherwise specified (NOS)

Definitions

- Malignant salivary gland neoplasm with ductal differentiation that lacks distinctive histologic features of other salivary gland carcinomas

CLINICAL ISSUES

Epidemiology

- Incidence
  - Depending on reporting, may represent 3rd most common malignant salivary gland tumor
  - Inconsistent reporting and selection criteria limits results
- Age
  - Wide age range
  - Peak in 6th to 7th decades
- Gender
  - Females slightly more common than males

Site

- Majority in major glands (parotid specifically)
- Minor glands accounts for about 40% of cases
  - Hard palate, buccal mucosa, lips

Presentation

- Solitary, asymptomatic mass
- Pain (20% of patients)
  - More often in submandibular gland tumors
- Facial weakness (20% of patients)
- Minor salivary gland tumors may show ulceration
- Palate tumors may destroy bone (up to 25%)
- Wide range for duration of symptoms (up to 10 years)

Treatment

- Surgical approaches
  - Complete excision is primary treatment
  - Approach dependent on tumor location
- Adjuvant therapy
  - Postoperative radiotherapy may be indicated for intermediate to high-grade tumors

Prognosis

- Difficult to predict, due to limited studies
- Clinical stage, site of involvement, and tumor grade all influence prognosis
- **Site**
  - Intraoral tumors have better prognosis
  - Major gland tumors show decreased survival
- **Tumor grade**
  - Low-grade tumors
    - Longer time periods without disease
    - Fewer distant metastases
    - No change in overall survival, however
  - High-grade tumors
    - Recurrences develop more commonly
    - More likely to have distant metastases

MACROSCOPIC FEATURES

General Features

- Focally or partially circumscribed
- Irregular and ill-defined invasive edges
- Cut surface
  - Yellow-white
  - Necrosis and hemorrhage contrasts with tumor

MICROSCOPIC PATHOLOGY

Histologic Features

- Variety of patterns of growth
  - Nests, islands, cords, tubules, solid sheets
  - Ducts: Much more common in low- to intermediate-grade tumors
    - Cysts may sometimes be present

Key Facts

Terminology

- Salivary gland carcinoma with ductal differentiation that lacks distinctive features of other salivary gland cancers

Clinical Issues

- 3rd most common malignant salivary gland tumor
- Favors parotid gland
- Usually asymptomatic

Macroscopic Features

- Irregular invasive margins

Microscopic Pathology

- May have very small areas characteristic of specific salivary gland tumor
- Grade reflects cytologic atypia

Top Differential Diagnoses

- Diagnosis of exclusion

    - Presence of ducts helps in separation from other tumor types
- Neoplastic epithelium
    - Cuboidal to oval to columnar cells
    - Distinct cell borders
    - Occasional clear cells
    - Occasional oncocytes
- Cells display variable pleomorphism, mitotic figures, and nucleoli
- Stroma can be collagenized or myxoid
- Eosinophilic, extracellular matrix, or extracellular mucin may be present
- Tumors are usually invasive
    - Perivascular or intravascular, perineural invasion
- May have necrosis and hemorrhage
- May have very small areas characteristic of specific salivary gland tumor

DIFFERENTIAL DIAGNOSIS

Other Salivary Gland Tumors

- Adenocarcinoma, NOS is diagnosis of exclusion

Metastatic Disease

- History of other malignancy
- Immunohistochemistry helps to confirm specific sites of origin

GRADING

Reflected by Cytologic Atypia

- Separated into 3 grades based on increased pleomorphism, less ductal differentiation, and increased mitoses
    - **Grade 1**: Well-formed ductal/tubular structures; mild pleomorphism; small nucleoli; few mitoses
    - **Grade 2**: Less ductal/tubular structures; moderate pleomorphism; increased mitoses
    - **Grade 3**: Limited ductal/tubular structures (sufficient to diagnose adenocarcinoma); moderate to severe pleomorphism; hyperchromasia; increased mitoses, including atypical forms; necrosis and hemorrhage

SELECTED REFERENCES

1. Buchner A et al: Relative frequency of intra-oral minor salivary gland tumors: a study of 380 cases from northern California and comparison to reports from other parts of the world. J Oral Pathol Med. 36(4):207-14, 2007
2. Li J et al: Salivary adenocarcinoma, not otherwise specified: a collection of orphans. Arch Pathol Lab Med. 128(12):1385-94, 2004
3. Ihrler S et al: Differential diagnosis of salivary acinic cell carcinoma and adenocarcinoma (NOS). A comparison of (immuno-)histochemical markers. Pathol Res Pract. 198(12):777-83, 2002
4. Neely MM et al: Tumors of minor salivary glands and the analysis of 106 cases. J Okla Dent Assoc. 86(4):50-2, 1996

IMAGE GALLERY

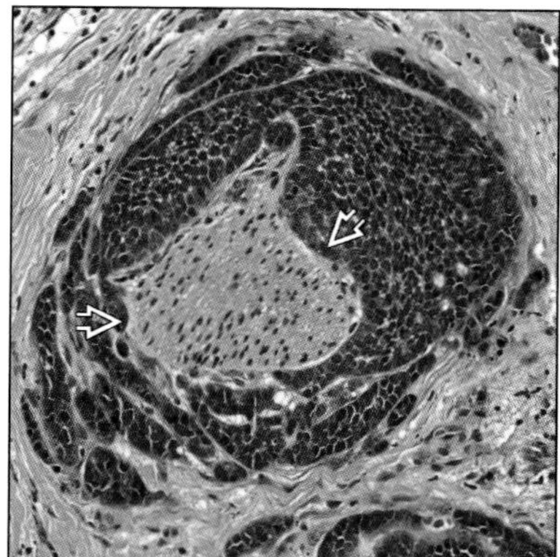

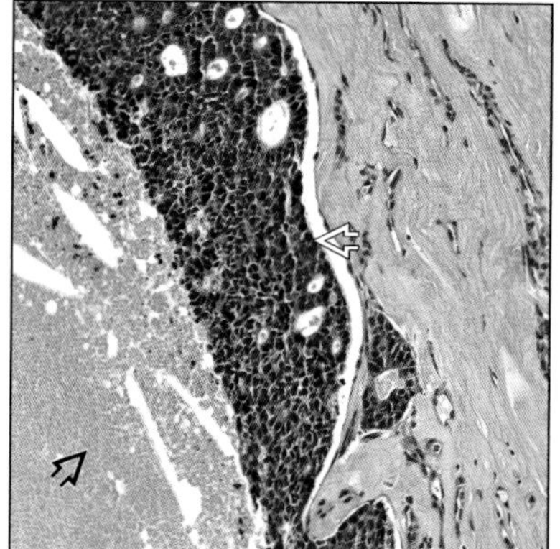

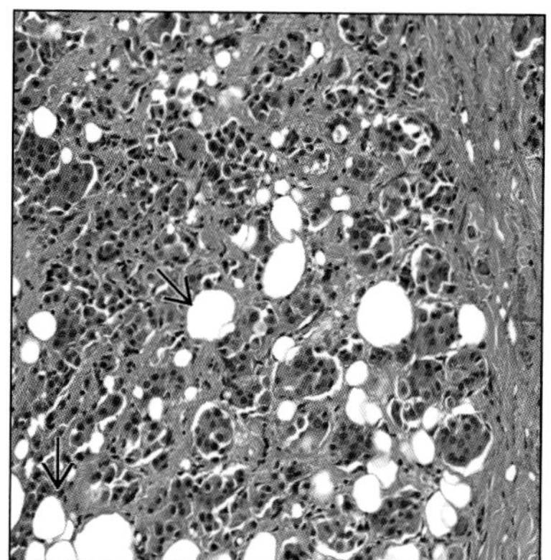

*(**Left**) Hematoxylin & eosin shows a focus of perineural invasion ➡. This is often a feature of a high-grade tumor. (**Center**) Hematoxylin & eosin shows hyperchromatic tumor cells ➡ abutting an area of necrosis ⇨. (**Right**) Hematoxylin & eosin shows a tumor with closely apposed organoid islands. This tumor is invading the fat → adjacent to the involved salivary gland.*

CLEAR CELL CARCINOMA (HYALINIZING/SCLEROSING)

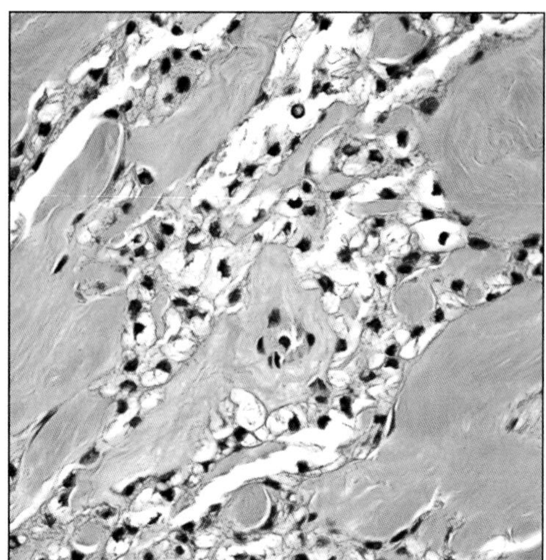

A high magnification of clear cell carcinoma displays cords and trabeculae of epithelial cells with variably clear cytoplasm, set within a densely collagenized, acellular stroma.

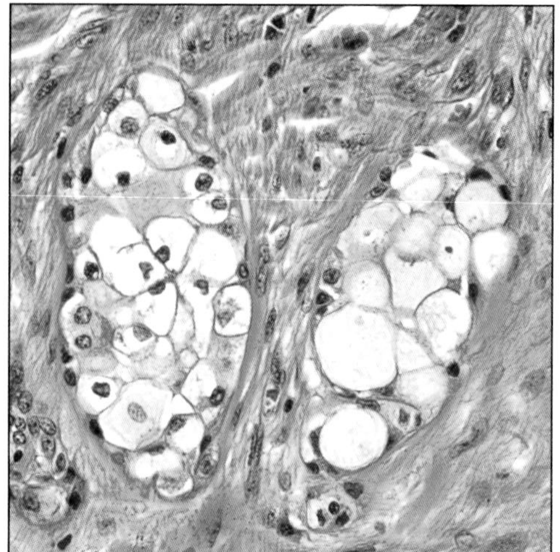

The epithelial cells are round to polygonal with well-defined cytoplasmic borders. Intracytoplasmic glycogen accumulation accounts for cell expansion and clear presentation.

TERMINOLOGY

Abbreviations

- Clear cell carcinoma (CCC)

Synonyms

- Clear cell adenocarcinoma
- Hyalinizing clear cell carcinoma

Definitions

- Epithelial malignant salivary gland neoplasm characterized by proliferation of clear cells set within loose to densely hyalinized stroma
    - By definition, absence of features characteristic for other salivary gland neoplasms that have clear cells

ETIOLOGY/PATHOGENESIS

Cell of Origin

- Glandular (ductal) or squamous derivation
- Absence of myoepithelial component

CLINICAL ISSUES

Epidemiology

- Incidence
    - Rare (< 1% of all salivary gland tumors)
- Age
    - Mean: 6th decade; range: 24-78 years
- Gender
    - Female > Male (1.2:1)

Site

- Minor salivary glands predominate (~ 80%)
    - Tongue, palate, floor of mouth, buccal mucosa, lip, and tonsillar area (in descending order)
- Minority in major glands
    - Parotid > > submandibular gland

Presentation

- Swelling or mass lesion
    - Dome-shaped or sessile
    - Possible mucosal surface ulceration
- May erode or extend into underlying bone
- Occasional association with pain
- Duration of symptoms: 1 month to 15 years
    - Typically show slow growth
- ~ 25% have regional nodal metastasis at presentation
    - Minority may have distant metastases to lung or bone

Treatment

- Surgical approaches
    - Wide surgical excision with clear margins
    - Selective neck dissection should be considered due to propensity for local nodal spread
- Adjuvant therapy
    - Pending adequacy of excision and presence of mets

Prognosis

- Excellent survival
    - Approximately 11% recurrence rate
- Nearly no patients die from disease
- Long-term follow-up due to possibility of recurrence and regional nodal metastasis

IMAGE FINDINGS

Radiographic Findings

- Submucosal mass at hard-soft palate junction
- MR is best imaging modality; less affected by dental amalgam

MACROSCOPIC FEATURES

General Features

- Poorly circumscribed, infiltrating into adjacent tissues
- Cut surface is grayish-white

CLEAR CELL CARCINOMA (HYALINIZING/SCLEROSING)

Key Facts

Terminology
- Epithelial malignant salivary gland neoplasm characterized by proliferation of clear cells set within loose to densely hyalinized stroma

Clinical Issues
- Minor salivary glands predominate (~ 80%)
- ~ 25% have regional nodal metastasis at presentation

Microscopic Pathology
- Infiltrative mass composed of sheets, cords, nests, or trabeculae of monotonous epithelial cells with variably clear cytoplasm
- Stroma loose and myxoid to dense and hyalinized

Ancillary Tests
- **Positive**: AE1/AE3, 34βE12, CAM5.2, CK7, EMA
- **Negative**: S100 protein, α-SMA, MSA, myosin, calponin, GFAP, CK20

Size
- Mean: 2 cm (most < 3 cm)

MICROSCOPIC PATHOLOGY

Histologic Features
- Infiltrative mass composed of sheets, cords, nests, or trabeculae of monotonous epithelial cells with variably clear cytoplasm
  - Majority of cells round to polygonal with eccentric nuclei
    - Well-defined cell borders
  - Minority of cells are relatively small with eosinophilic cytoplasm
    - May be admixed or at periphery of clear cell nests
    - May also form small groups or islands
  - Glandular duct formation typically absent
  - Rare mitotic activity
  - Perineural invasion in about 1/3 of cases
  - Rare, focal squamous differentiation
- Stroma
  - Loose and myxoid to dense and hyalinized
  - Dense hyalinization most common

ANCILLARY TESTS

Histochemistry
- Clear cells reactive with PAS and diastase sensitive
  - Indicating intracytoplasmic glycogen accumulation
- Mucicarmine negative

Immunohistochemistry
- **Positive**: AE1/AE3, 34βE12, CAM5.2, CK7, EMA (75%)
- **Negative**: S100 protein, α-SMA, muscle specific actin, myosin, calponin, GFAP, CK20

DIFFERENTIAL DIAGNOSIS

Salivary Gland Neoplasms With Clear Cells
- **Malignant**: Mucoepidermoid carcinoma, epithelial-myoepithelial carcinoma, acinic cell carcinoma, myoepithelial carcinoma
- **Benign**: Oncocytoma, myoepithelioma, pleomorphic adenoma

Metastatic Renal Cell Carcinoma (RCC)
- Prominent sinusoidal vessels, hemorrhage; and IHC coexpression of keratin and vimentin, with CD10, pax-2, and anti-RCC reactivity, favoring a renal primary

SELECTED REFERENCES

1. Dardick I et al: Clear cell carcinoma: review of its histomorphogenesis and classification as a squamous cell lesion. Oral Surg Oral Med Oral Pathol Oral Radiol Endod. 108(3):399-405, 2009
2. Solar AA et al: Hyalinizing clear cell carcinoma: case series and comprehensive review of the literature. Cancer. 115(1):75-83, 2009

IMAGE GALLERY

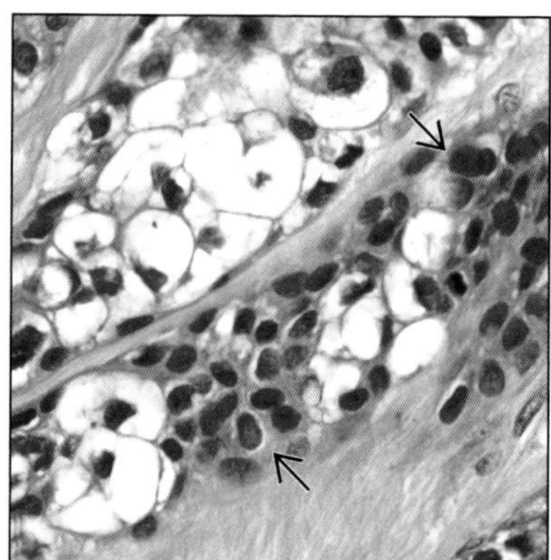

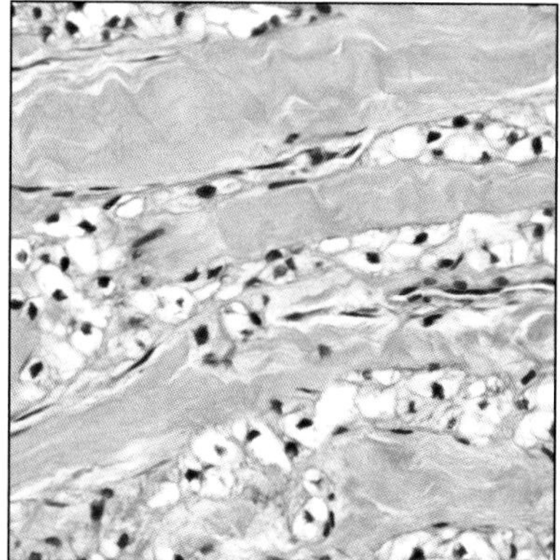

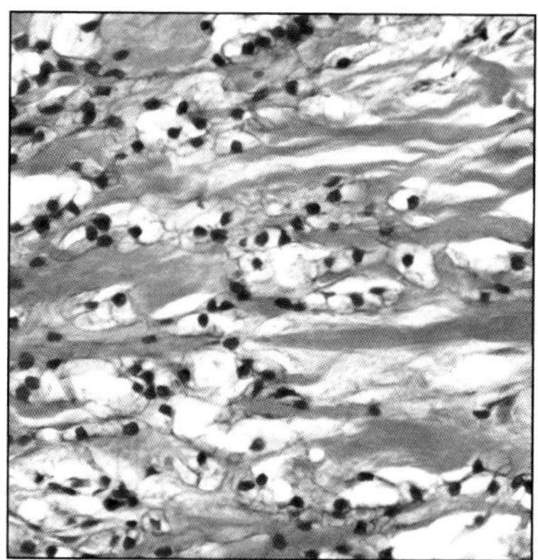

(Left) *At high power, 2 cell types are evident: Smaller polygonal epithelial cells ⇒ are seen admixed with relatively large clear cells.* ***(Center)*** *Cords and nests of clear cells are present within a hyalinized stroma. Epithelial cells display eccentric, hyperchromatic nuclei and well-defined cell borders.* ***(Right)*** *The collagenous stroma in this example varies from loose and feathery to dense and band-like. The epithelial portion is in small nests, cords, and individual cells.*

CYSTADENOCARCINOMA (PAPILLARY)

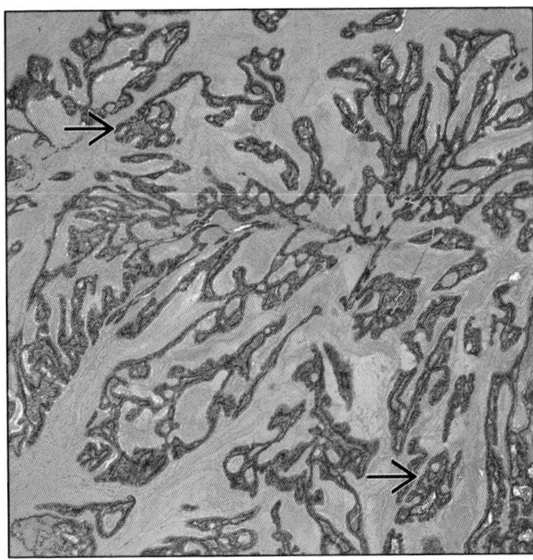

Low-power magnification shows a number of variably complex papillary structures in a mucinous to serous fluid. The papillary structures are thin and delicate to focally cribriform ⇒.

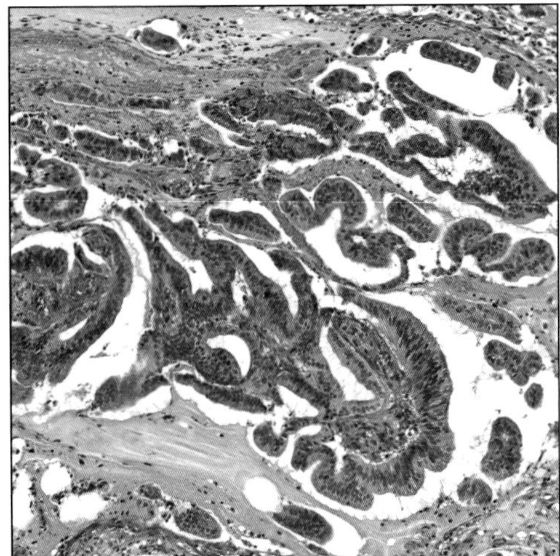

Neoplastic proliferation shows a number of duct-like structures and papillae suspended in a mucinous background. The cells lining the papillary structures are columnar, with multiple layers of cells.

TERMINOLOGY

Synonyms

- Low-grade papillary adenocarcinoma

Definitions

- Malignant epithelial salivary gland neoplasm characterized by predominantly cystic growth with intraluminal papillae
  - Malignant counterpart of cystadenoma
  - Lacks specific histopathologic features of other salivary carcinomas with cystic growth
  - A few cases are not papillary

CLINICAL ISSUES

Epidemiology

- Incidence
  - Rare (< 1%)
- Age
  - Wide range at presentation (20-86 years)
    - Mean: 6th decade
    - ~ 75% of patients are > 50 years old
- Gender
  - Equal gender distribution

Site

- Parotid is most commonly affected (~ 70%)
- Minor salivary glands (~ 25%)
  - Order of frequency: Buccal mucosa, lips, palate, floor of mouth, tongue, retromolar region

Presentation

- Slowly growing, painless swelling or mass
- Tumors may be compressible
- Palate tumors may erode bone and extend into nasal cavity/paranasal sinuses
- Symptoms present for long duration (mean: 4 years)

Treatment

- Surgical approaches
  - Complete surgical excision
    - Wide excision for minor salivary glands

Prognosis

- Excellent overall prognosis (indolent, low grade)
  - Approaching 100% 5-year survival
- Recurrences are uncommon (~ 10%)
  - Develop up to 10 years after primary
- Lymph node metastases are uncommon (~ 10%)

MACROSCOPIC FEATURES

General Features

- Partially circumscribed but unencapsulated
- Multicystic, often filled with fluid or mucin

Size

- Range: 0.5-6 cm

MICROSCOPIC PATHOLOGY

Histologic Features

- Well circumscribed but not usually encapsulated
- Invasion into surrounding parenchyma or soft tissue, nerves, &/or vessels is often limited
  - Invading islands may be solid
  - Cysts may appear quite a distance from main tumor mass
- Prominent cystic appearance
  - Haphazard cysts, sometimes filled with mucin
  - Cysts may be back to back or show limited fibrous connective tissue stroma
  - Duct-like structures may be part of "cystic" appearance
  - Relatively few, large cysts may be seen
  - Dystrophic calcification may be present
- Papillary growth is almost always present

CYSTADENOCARCINOMA (PAPILLARY)

Key Facts

Terminology
- Malignant epithelial salivary gland neoplasm characterized by predominantly cystic growth with intraluminal papillae

Clinical Issues
- Slowly growing, painless swelling or compressible mass
- Usually a tumor of older age (6th decade)
- Parotid is most commonly affected (~ 70%)
- Complete surgical excision
- Excellent overall prognosis (indolent, low grade)

Microscopic Pathology
- Partially circumscribed and encapsulated
- Prominent cystic appearance
  - Haphazard cysts, sometimes filled with mucin
  - Cysts may be back to back or show limited fibrous connective tissue stroma
- Papillary growth is almost always present
  - Papillae vary from single simple projections with delicate fibrovascular cores to complex, arborizing structures filling the lumen
- Cysts and papillae lined by small and large cuboidal to columnar cells
- Cells are cytologically bland
- Mitotic figures are uncommon
- Tumor-associated lymphoid proliferation (TALP) is frequently present

Top Differential Diagnoses
- Cystadenoma, acinic cell carcinoma (papillary-cystic variant), mucoepidermoid carcinoma, salivary duct carcinoma, polymorphous low-grade adenocarcinoma

  - Papillae vary from single simple projections with delicate fibrovascular cores to complex, arborizing structures filling the lumen
- Cysts and papillae lined by small and large cuboidal to columnar cells
  - Can be mucinous, clear, or oncocytic (rare)
  - Columnar cells usually line papillae
  - Multiple cell layers can be seen, including "cribriform" pattern
  - Rarely, epidermoid cells can be seen focally
- Cells are cytologically bland
  - Nucleoli may be present
  - Cytoplasm may be vacuolated or "soap-bubble" in appearance
- Mitotic figures are usually infrequent
- Ruptured cysts elicit granulation tissue or foreign body giant cell reaction
- Tumor-associated lymphoid proliferation (TALP) is frequently present
- Necrosis is uncommon
- Pure mucinous cystadenocarcinoma is rare, similar to gastrointestinal primaries

ANCILLARY TESTS

Cytology
- Background of fluid, inflammatory cells; occasionally mucinous
- Variable cellularity with small number of cohesive tumor cell clusters and micropapillae
- Tumor cells are small to medium, possibly showing overlapping
  - Bland appearance of cells with vacuolated cytoplasm
  - Round nuclei are frequently eccentric

Immunohistochemistry
- Keratin, CK7, CEA-M, EMA positive

DIFFERENTIAL DIAGNOSIS

Cystadenoma
- Frequently unencapsulated, lacking invasion
- Multicystic appearance does not equate with invasion

Acinic Cell Carcinoma, Papillary-Cystic Type
- Microcystic growth with papillae lined by vacuolated small cells
- Solid areas with larger cells showing acinar cells with basophilic, granular cytoplasm

Mucoepidermoid Carcinoma
- Cystic appearance is characteristic (low-grade tumors)
- 3 cell types lining the cysts: Mucocyte, intermediate, epidermoid
- Solid areas tend to predominate
- Epidermoid features rare in cystadenocarcinoma

Salivary Duct Carcinoma (SDC)
- Cystic appearance can be prominent
- Large, pleomorphic cells with abundant cytoplasm
- Mitoses and necrosis easily identified
- Low-grade SDC: "Cribriform" pattern

Polymorphous Low-Grade Adenocarcinoma
- Focal cysts with papillae can be seen but are not dominant pattern
- Single cell infiltration, targetoid growth, "eye of whirlwind" appearance, and perineural invasion

SELECTED REFERENCES

1. Kawahara A et al: Cytological features of cystadenocarcinoma in cyst fluid of the parotid gland: Diagnostic pitfalls and literature review. Diagn Cytopathol. 38(5):377-81, 2010
2. Koc M et al: MRI findings of papillary cystadenocarcinoma of the submandibular gland. Diagn Interv Radiol. 16(1):20-3, 2010
3. Foss RD et al: Salivary gland cystadenocarcinomas. A clinicopathologic study of 57 cases. Am J Surg Pathol. 20(12):1440-7, 1996

CYSTADENOCARCINOMA (PAPILLARY)

Microscopic Features

*(**Left**) Although there is an artifactual space, the cystic spaces can be seen filled with papillary tumor projections ➔. This is a case from the tongue and floor of mouth. The surface mucosa is uninvolved. (**Right**) There is a circumscribed tumor with a large cyst filled by complex, arborizing papillary structures. Invasion is not appreciated in this field. Note the mucinous material in the cystic spaces.*

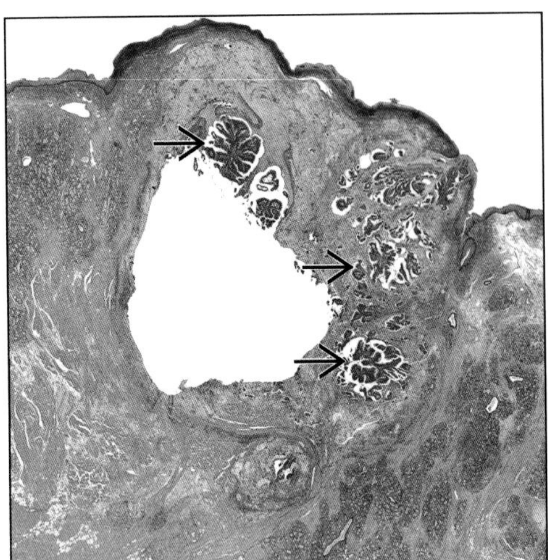

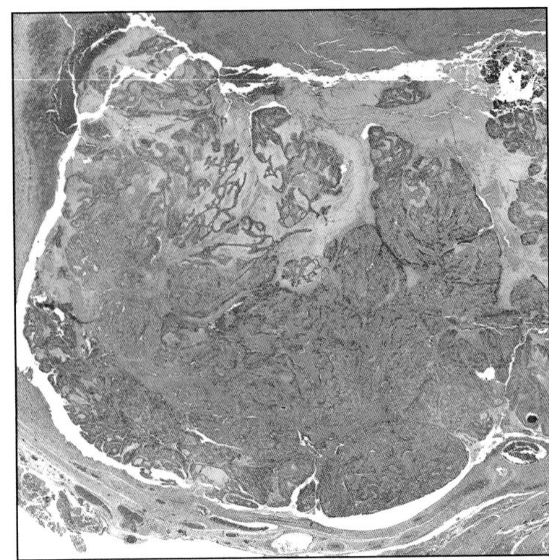

*(**Left**) Fibrous connective tissue may be seen at the periphery ➲, but a well-formed capsule is usually absent. The epithelial proliferation is arranged in complex and arborizing to pencil-like papillary projections. (**Right**) There is an "infiltration" of the epithelial groups ➔ into the surrounding parenchyma and soft tissue. Cystic spaces are present, but this lesion shows a slightly more "solid" appearance. The papillae are lined by columnar cells.*

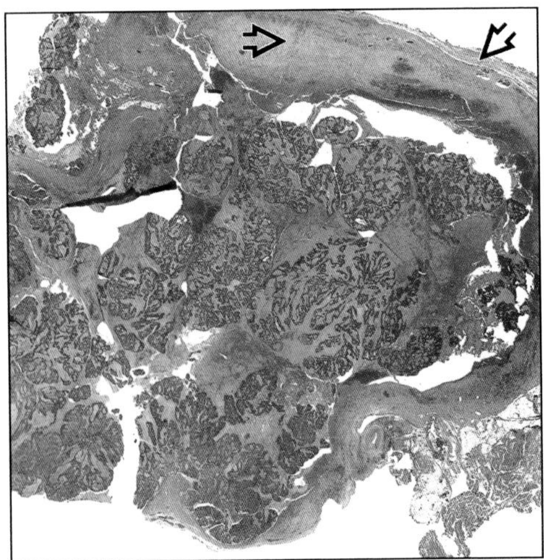

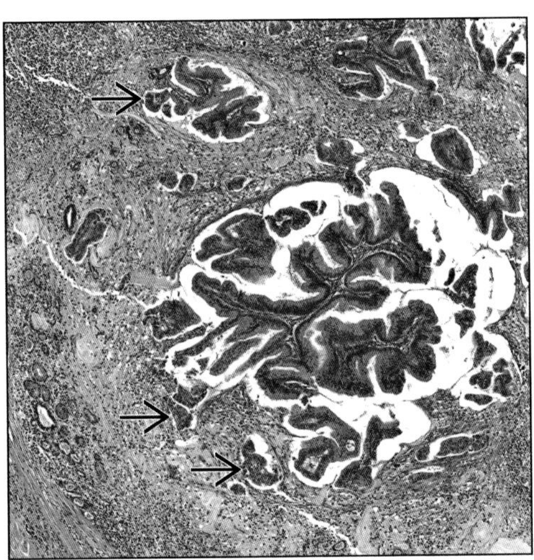

*(**Left**) This tumor shows a significantly complex papillary architecture. Free floating papillae attest to the complexity of the structures. The cells lining the spaces are cuboidal to low columnar. The differential with acinic cell carcinoma is obvious with a case at this magnification. (**Right**) There is a more stout or thick appearance to the papillae in this case. However, the columnar cells lining the papillae show cuboidal cells with limited to absent cytologic atypia.*

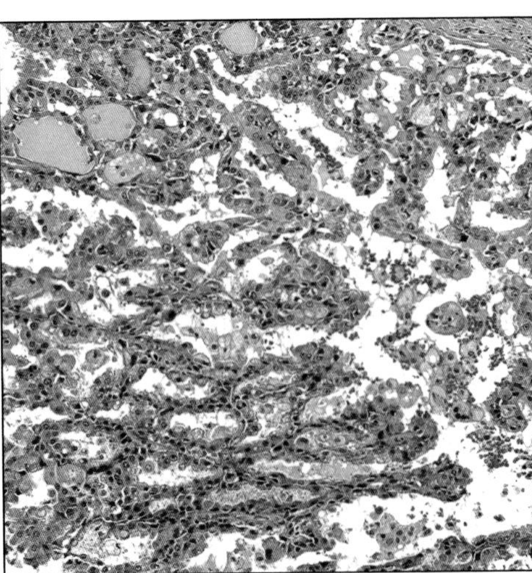

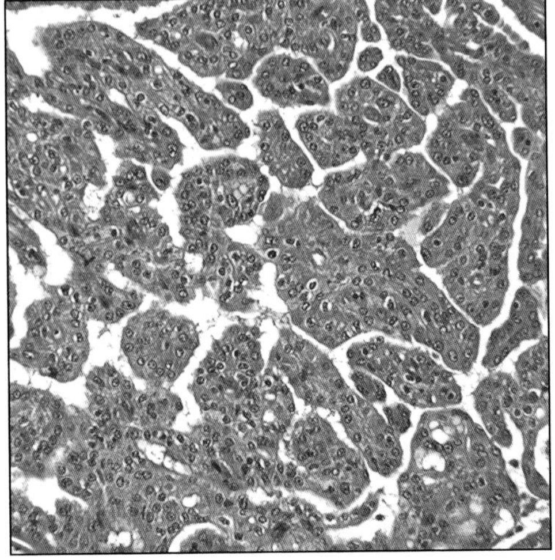

Microscopic Features and Ancillary Techniques

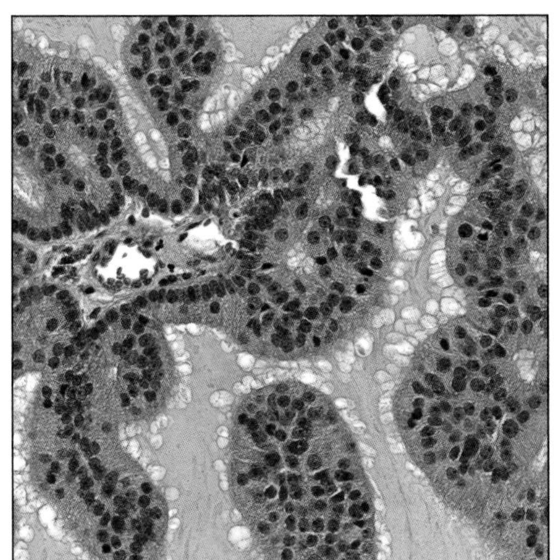

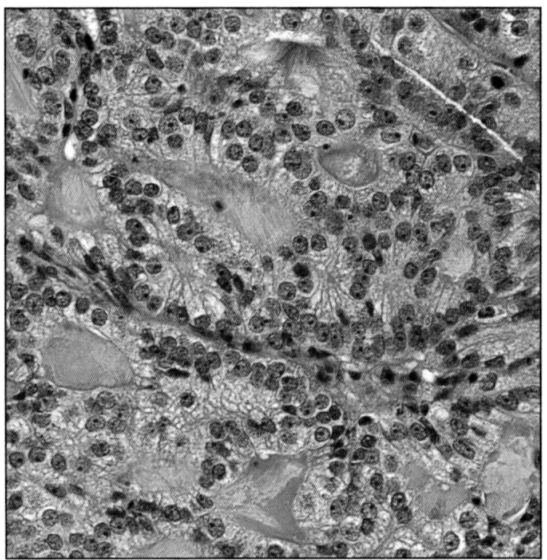

***(Left)** High-power magnification shows the cuboidal to columnar appearance of the epithelial cells. There are basally located round and regular nuclei with slightly eosinophilic cytoplasm. **(Right)** These cytologically bland cells show the "glandular" appearance or duct-like appearance that can be seen in cystadenocarcinoma. The cytoplasm is slightly vacuolated to "soap-bubble" in appearance. Nucleoli are small and inconspicuous. Mitoses are absent.*

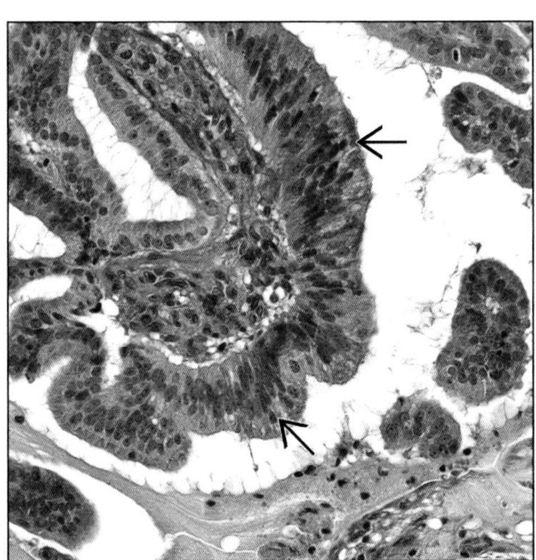

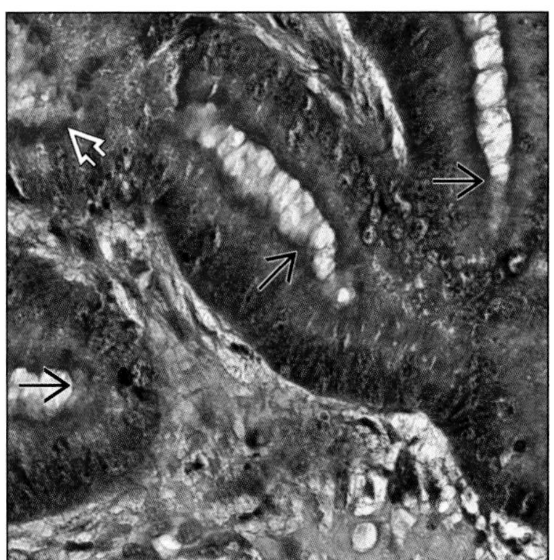

***(Left)** A stratified nuclear appearance → is quite prominent in this papillary structure. However, the nuclei are quite bland. There is a vague mucinous quality to the cystic material. **(Right)** A mucicarmine stain highlights a luminal mucinous material →, which is also noted within the apical cytoplasm of a few of the cells ➡. The mucinous material can be highlighted with mucicarmine or with PAS, although it is uncommon to have a strong reaction like this case demonstrates.*

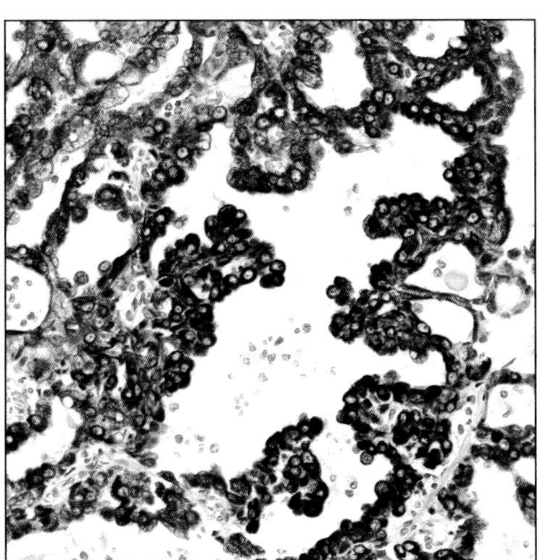

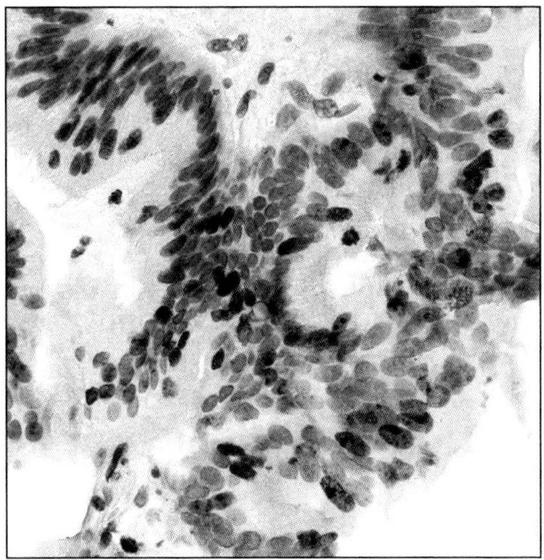

***(Left)** Immunohistochemistry studies are seldom of value in making this diagnosis. However, CK7 (shown), keratin, EMA, and CEA are all positive to a variable degree in these tumors. The results do not really help make a separation between benign and malignant tumors. **(Right)** The mitotic index is usually limited to absent. However, a Ki-67 labeling index can sometimes highlight foci with increased proliferation. In this case, there were isolated foci in the tumor that showed increased reactivity.*

MYOEPITHELIAL CARCINOMA

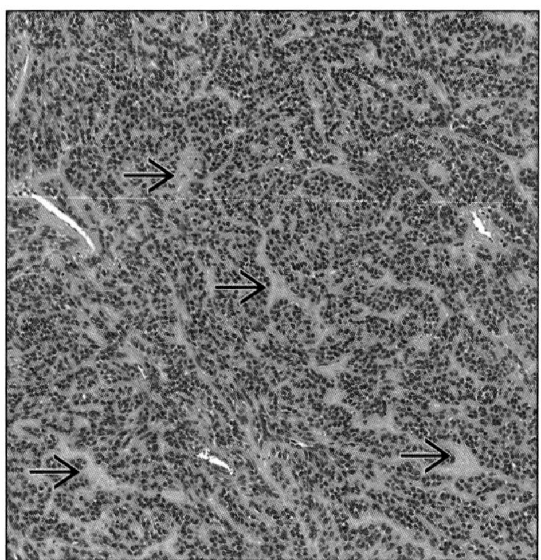

There are a number of patterns of growth in this myoepithelial carcinoma. There is a prominent eosinophilic basal lamina ➔ surrounding many of the tumor nests/islands.

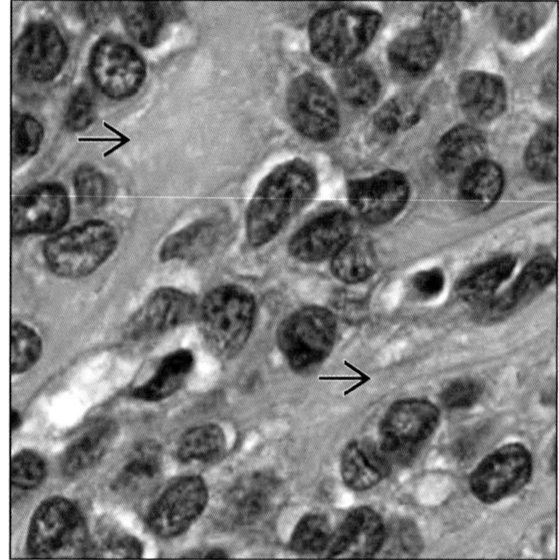

High-power image shows epithelioid cells with a high nuclear to cytoplasmic ratio and slightly cleared cytoplasm. A background of eosinophilic basal lamina material ➔ is also present.

TERMINOLOGY

Synonyms

- Malignant myoepithelioma

Definitions

- Malignant tumor of exclusively myoepithelial differentiation
- Malignant counterpart to myoepithelioma

ETIOLOGY/PATHOGENESIS

Pathogenesis

- About 1/2 of myoepithelial carcinomas develop within preexisting pleomorphic adenoma or from myoepithelioma

CLINICAL ISSUES

Epidemiology

- Incidence
  - Uncommon
    - < 2% of malignant salivary gland neoplasms
  - Likely to be under reported
    - Included in World Health Organization classification in 1991
- Age
  - Wide age range
    - Mean: 6th decade
  - Rare in children
- Gender
  - Equal gender distribution

Site

- Most occur in parotid gland (~ 75%)
- Submandibular gland and minor salivary glands less commonly affected

Presentation

- Usually present with rapidly expanding, painless mass
- Tumors tend to be locally destructive
- Occasionally will be painful or tender
- Dysphagia uncommon
- Weight loss can be seen

Natural History

- Some patients report rapid increase in a previous benign tumor (like pleomorphic adenoma)
- Multiple recurrences of pleomorphic adenoma or myoepithelioma are risk factor

Treatment

- Surgical approaches
  - Complete resection
    - Major glands: Parotidectomy or submandibulectomy
    - Minor glands: Wide local excision
- Adjuvant therapy
  - Chemotherapy and radiation yield mixed, debatable results

Prognosis

- Tumors may be locally aggressive
- Regarded as intermediate- to high-grade tumor
  - Approximately 1/3 of patients die of disease
    - Marked cellular pleomorphism and high proliferation index suggest worse clinical outcome
- Recurrences are common (approximately 1/3), frequently multiple times
- Regional and distant metastases are uncommon at presentation but may occur late in course of disease
- Cervical metastases before distant metastases
  - Lung and other sites
- No difference in outcome between "de novo" vs. those arising from pleomorphic adenoma or myoepithelioma

MYOEPITHELIAL CARCINOMA

Key Facts

Terminology

- Malignant tumor of exclusively myoepithelial differentiation
- Malignant counterpart to myoepithelioma

Clinical Issues

- Uncommon; most occur in parotid gland
- Complete resection
- Multiple recurrences of pleomorphic adenoma or myoepithelioma is risk factor
- Wide age range

Macroscopic Features

- Most unencapsulated
- Nodular

Microscopic Pathology

- Variable patterns of growth
- Invasive growth
- Myoepithelial cells: Plasmacytoid, epithelioid, or spindled showing pleomorphism
- Mucoid or myxoid stroma
- May be carcinoma of carcinoma ex-pleomorphic adenoma
- No ducts identified

Ancillary Tests

- Combinations of IHCs most useful
- May not be of much practical use
  - CK5/6(+)
  - S100 protein(+)
  - GFAP(+)
  - Vimentin(+)

IMAGE FINDINGS

Radiographic Findings

- Bone destruction is most often seen in minor salivary gland disease

MACROSCOPIC FEATURES

General Features

- Most tumors are unencapsulated, usually well defined
- Nodular or bosselated surface
- Gray-white, firm, "glassy" cut surface
- Cystic degeneration and necrosis are uncommon

Size

- Range: 2-10 cm

MICROSCOPIC PATHOLOGY

Histologic Features

- Invasive growth
  - Most helpful feature in separation from benign tumor
  - Adjacent bone may be involved
  - Perineural and vascular invasion frequent
- Patterns
  - Nodular to diffuse
  - Tumor cells arranged in nests, sheets, or cords
  - Usually highly cellular, but hypocellular lesions can be seen
- Ducts are not present (by definition)
- Myoepithelial cells
  - Range from plasmacytoid to epithelioid to spindled, in various combinations
  - Marked pleomorphism can be seen but is usually limited
  - Cytoplasm can be clear
- Stroma
  - Mucoid or myxoid
    - Due to accumulation of proteoglycans
  - Basal lamina can be present
  - Cartilaginous tissue is rare
- Mitotic figures are usually easy to find, including atypical forms
- Necrosis is uncommon
  - May be associated with biopsy or FNA
- May be the malignant component within a carcinoma ex-pleomorphic adenoma
  - PA may include ducts
- Rare squamous differentiation

ANCILLARY TESTS

Cytology

- Features are diverse and may lack characteristics of malignancy
- Cells are arranged in small clusters
- Cells appear epithelioid, plasmacytoid, spindled, or clear
  - Frequently mixture of cell types

Immunohistochemistry

- Nonneoplastic myoepithelial cells will react with many of same antigens
- Generally of limited practical use
  - Exception is separation from sarcoma
- Combinations or limited panels are most useful
  - Positive with CK5/6, S100 protein, GFAP, and vimentin

Cytogenetics

- Up to 1/2 may have aberrations
  - Chromosome 8 alterations are most frequently identified

Electron Microscopy

- May demonstrate
  - Actin filaments, pinocytotic vesicles, desmosomes, and basal lamina
    - Longitudinally oriented 6-8 nm cytoplasmic microfilaments with focal dense bodies
- Infrequently utilized for diagnostic purposes

MYOEPITHELIAL CARCINOMA

Immunohistochemistry

Antibody	Reactivity	Staining Pattern	Comment
Vimentin	Positive	Cytoplasmic	Strong and diffuse
S100	Positive	Nuclear & cytoplasmic	Usually strong and diffuse in all neoplastic cells
Calponin	Positive	Cytoplasmic	Not as frequently positive as S100 protein
CK-PAN	Positive	Cytoplasmic	Usually majority of cells are positive
SMHC	Positive	Cytoplasmic	Variable intensity
Actin-sm	Positive	Cytoplasmic	
CK5/6	Positive	Cytoplasmic	
GFAP	Positive	Cytoplasmic	Usually highlights only isolated cells
CK14	Equivocal	Cytoplasmic	Variable expression
CK7	Equivocal	Cytoplasmic	Variable expression

DIFFERENTIAL DIAGNOSIS

Myoepithelioma

- Lacks infiltrative growth
- Lacks cytologic atypia

Sarcomas

- Synovial sarcoma
  - Biphasic type has glandular structures
  - Distinctive chromosomal translocation t(X;18)
  - GFAP negative
- Leiomyosarcoma
  - Cellular tumor comprised of interlacing fascicles
  - Perinuclear cytoplasmic clearing adjacent to cigar-shaped nuclei
  - Negative with S100 protein, GFAP, and CD117

Epithelial-Myoepithelial Carcinoma

- Numerous ducts
  - Lumen lined by eosinophilic, cuboidal duct cells
  - Duct cells surrounded by large polygonal clear myoepithelial cells
- Usually shows biphasic nature with immunohistochemistry

Plasmacytoma

- Plasmacytoid cells with clock-face nuclear chromatin distribution
- Perinuclear "Hoff" or clearing is characteristic
- Positive with CD138, CD79-α, showing κ or λ restriction
- Negative with S100 protein, GFAP, actins (smooth muscle, muscle specific), and smooth muscle myosin heavy chain (SMHC)

DIAGNOSTIC CHECKLIST

Clinically Relevant Pathologic Features

- Myoepithelial carcinoma is distinctive from myoepithelioma
  - Invasive growth with atypical cytologic features

Pathologic Interpretation Pearls

- Diagnosis requires interpretation of tumor morphology and immunohistochemistry

SELECTED REFERENCES

1. Yang S et al: Myoepithelial carcinoma of intraoral minor salivary glands: a clinicopathological study of 7 cases and review of the literature. Oral Surg Oral Med Oral Pathol Oral Radiol Endod. 110(1):85-93, 2010
2. Losito NS et al: Clear-cell myoepithelial carcinoma of the salivary glands: a clinicopathologic, immunohistochemical, and ultrastructural study of two cases involving the submandibular gland with review of the literature. Pathol Res Pract. 204(5):335-44, 2008
3. Losito NS et al: Clear-cell myoepithelial carcinoma of the salivary glands: a clinicopathologic, immunohistochemical, and ultrastructural study of two cases involving the submandibular gland with review of the literature. Pathol Res Pract. 204(5):335-44, 2008
4. Said S et al: Myoepithelial carcinoma ex pleomorphic adenoma of salivary glands: a problematic diagnosis. Oral Surg Oral Med Oral Pathol Oral Radiol Endod. 99(2):196-201, 2005
5. Ogawa I et al: Dedifferentiated malignant myoepithelioma of the parotid gland. Pathol Int. 53(10):704-9, 2003
6. Yu G et al: Myoepithelial carcinoma of the salivary glands: behavior and management. Chin Med J (Engl). 116(2):163-5, 2003
7. Chhieng DC et al: Cytology of myoepithelial carcinoma of the salivary gland. Cancer. 96(1):32-6, 2002
8. Savera AT et al: Myoepithelial carcinoma of the salivary glands: a clinicopathologic study of 25 patients. Am J Surg Pathol. 24(6):761-74, 2000
9. Di Palma S et al: Myoepithelial carcinoma with predominance of plasmacytoid cells arising in a pleomorphic adenoma of the parotid gland. Histopathology. 33(5):485, 1998
10. Nagao T et al: Salivary gland malignant myoepithelioma: a clinicopathologic and immunohistochemical study of ten cases. Cancer. 83(7):1292-9, 1998
11. Alós L et al: Myoepithelial tumors of salivary glands: a clinicopathologic, immunohistochemical, ultrastructural, and flow-cytometric study. Semin Diagn Pathol. 13(2):138-47, 1996
12. Bombí JA et al: Myoepithelial carcinoma arising in a benign myoepithelioma: immunohistochemical, ultrastructural, and flow-cytometrical study. Ultrastruct Pathol. 20(2):145-54, 1996
13. Wang J et al: Quantitative multivariate analysis of myoepithelioma and myoepithelial carcinoma. Int J Oral Maxillofac Surg. 24(2):153-7, 1995
14. Dardick I et al: Myoepithelial cells in salivary gland tumors--revisited. Head Neck Surg. 7(5):395-408, 1985

MYOEPITHELIAL CARCINOMA

Microscopic Features

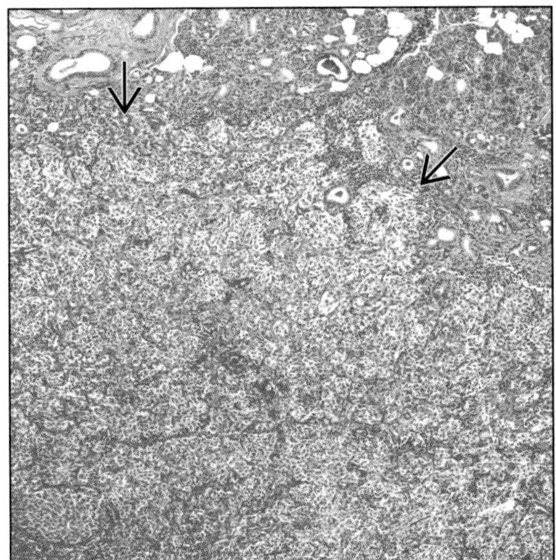

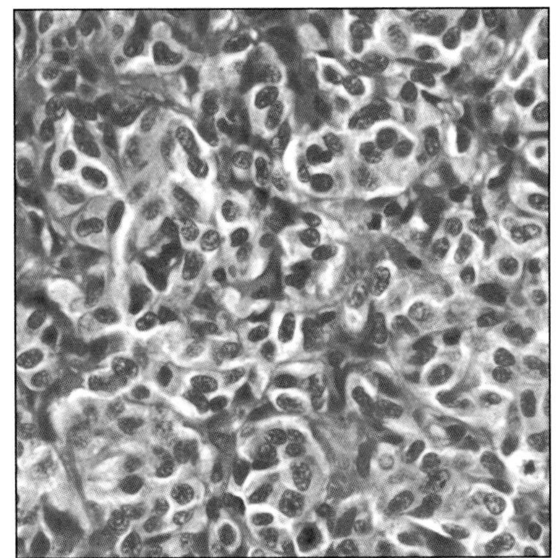

(Left) *Hematoxylin & eosin shows a low-power view of a predominately clear cell tumor. The tumor lacks a well-defined capsule but is seen invading into the native salivary gland →. Other clear cell salivary gland tumors should be considered in the differential diagnosis.* ***(Right)*** *A high-power view shows a clear cell tumor. There is a delicate, even nuclear chromatin distribution. In other areas of this tumor, epithelioid and plasmacytoid cell types were seen.*

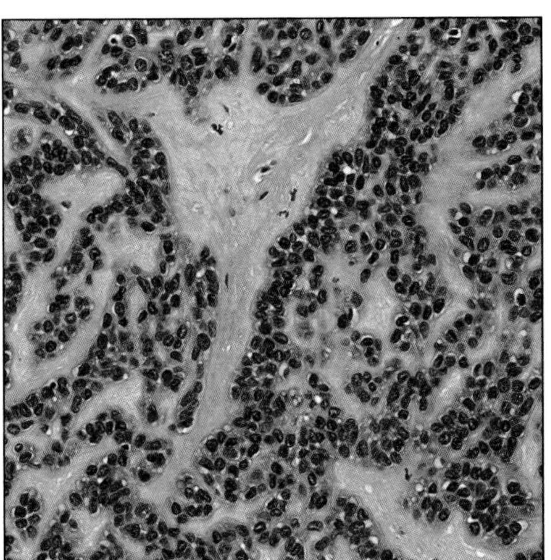

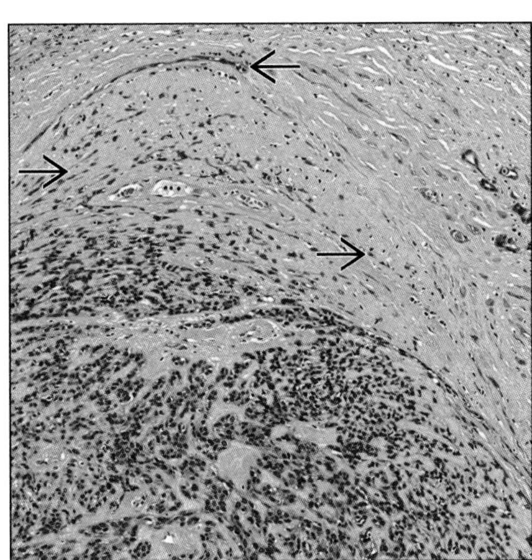

(Left) *Hematoxylin & eosin shows a trabecular arrangement to uniform neoplastic basaloid cells in a background of eosinophilic hyalinized stroma.* ***(Right)*** *There is infiltration by the neoplastic cells into the adjacent parenchyma and fibrous connective tissue →. The cells are slightly compressed, giving a single file infiltrative pattern. Note the lack of glandular profiles and the basal lamina material.*

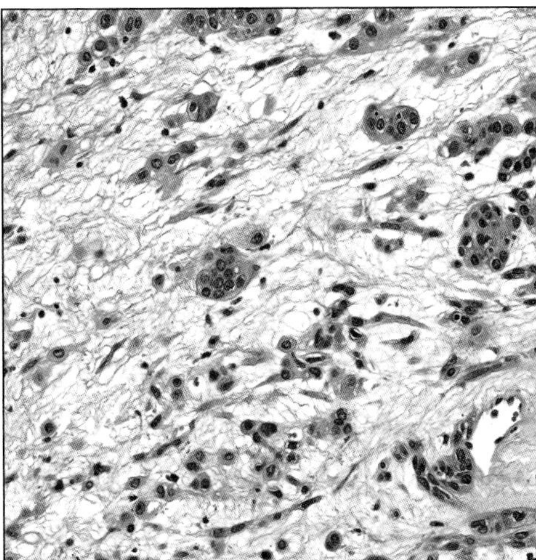

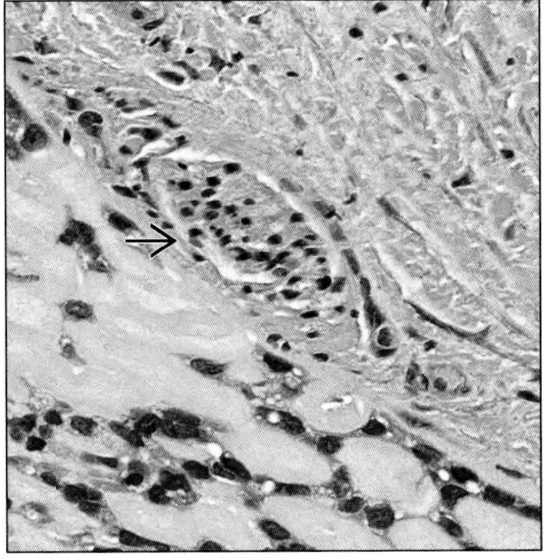

(Left) *This tumor shows a myxoid stroma instead of a hyalinized appearance. The cells have a haphazard distribution. The cells are epithelioid, although focally a suggestion of plasmacytoid features is noted.* ***(Right)*** *The myoepithelial nature of the tumor is difficult to appreciate on this high-power field. However, there is a very prominent eosinophilic basal lamina surrounding and separating the tumor cells. Note the nerve twig → immediately adjacent to the epithelial proliferation.*

SMALL CELL UNDIFFERENTIATED CARCINOMA

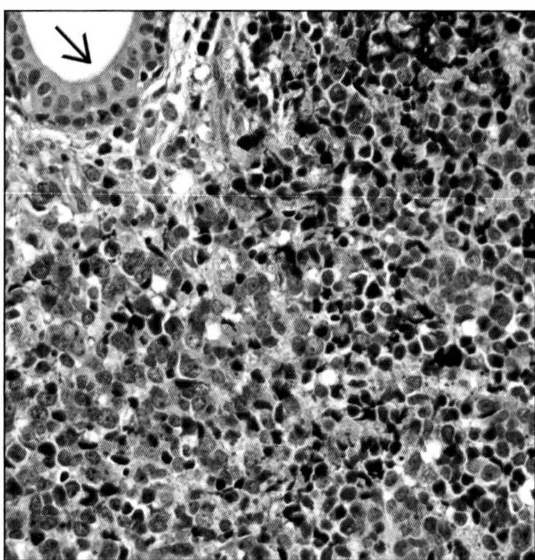

There is a "small blue round cell" neoplastic infiltrate adjacent to a salivary gland duct ⇒. Apoptosis and crushed nuclei are seen throughout this neoplasm. The chromatin is smudged and even.

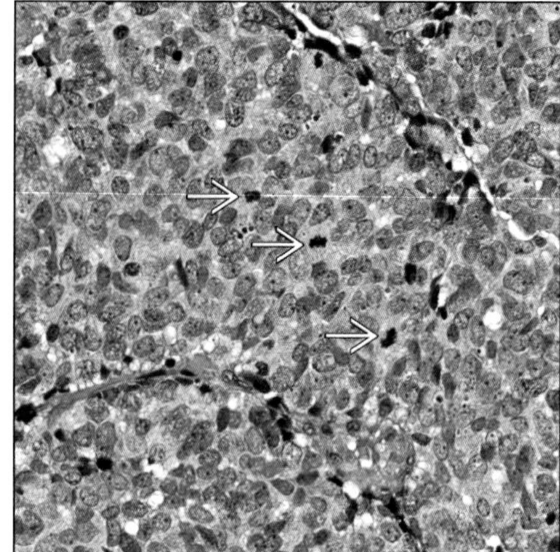

There is a vague trabecular arrangement, with a syncytium of cells that have a very high nuclear to cytoplasmic ratio. The nuclear chromatin is even, without nucleoli. Mitotic figures are noted ⇒.

TERMINOLOGY

Abbreviations

- Small cell undifferentiated carcinoma (SCUC)

Synonyms

- Neuroendocrine carcinoma

Definitions

- Malignant epithelial neoplasm characterized by small, undifferentiated cells with scant cytoplasm, fine nuclear chromatin, and inconspicuous nucleoli
  - Demonstrates neuroendocrine differentiation
  - Lacks histomorphologic features of either glandular or epidermoid differentiation

ETIOLOGY/PATHOGENESIS

Histogenesis

- Proposed hypothetical multipotential ductal stem cell gives rise to tumor

CLINICAL ISSUES

Epidemiology

- Incidence
  - Rare: ~ 1% of all salivary gland neoplasms and < 3% of salivary gland malignancies
- Age
  - Wide range: 5-90 years
  - Mean: 6th-8th decades
- Gender
  - Male > Female (2:1)

Site

- Vast majority affect parotid gland (~ 80%)
  - Submandibular gland > > intraoral minor salivary glands (buccal mucosa, tongue, tonsillar area)

Presentation

- Painless, rapidly growing, firm mass
  - Symptoms present for short duration (< 3 months)
- Fixed to adjacent tissues, including skin
- Facial nerve palsy can be seen
- Cervical lymphadenopathy is common
- Syndrome of inappropriate antidiuretic hormone production (Schwartz-Bartter syndrome) is unusual as paraneoplastic syndrome

Treatment

- Options, risks, complications
  - Combination aggressive management yields best outcome
- Surgical approaches
  - Wide surgical excision, with ipsilateral neck dissection (in clinically positive cases)
- Drugs
  - Chemotherapy employed for regional recurrences or distant metastases
- Radiation
  - Postoperative radiation (up to 600 cG)

Prognosis

- Highly aggressive tumor with poor overall long-term prognosis
  - Slightly better outcome than pulmonary counterparts
- Approximately 70% mortality (5-year survival 10-45%)
- Local recurrence develops in ~ 50% of patients
- Metastatic disease seen in > 50% of patients
  - Most common sites include liver, brain, and mediastinum (hematogenous spread)
  - Cervical lymph node metastases less common (lymphatic spread)
- Poor prognostic factors: Large tumor size (> 3 cm), negative CK20 immunoreactivity, limited number of neuroendocrine markers positive
  - Tumor size is most important prognostic factor

SMALL CELL UNDIFFERENTIATED CARCINOMA

Key Facts

Terminology
- Malignant epithelial neoplasm characterized by small, undifferentiated cells with scant cytoplasm, fine nuclear chromatin, and inconspicuous nucleoli
  - Demonstrates neuroendocrine differentiation

Clinical Issues
- Male > Female (2:1)
- Vast majority affect parotid gland (~ 80%)
- Painless, rapidly growing, firm mass
  - Cervical lymphadenopathy is common
- Combination aggressive management yields best outcome
- Highly aggressive tumor with poor overall long-term prognosis

Microscopic Pathology
- Extensive infiltration
- Arranged in solid sheets, nests, and irregular cords
  - Well-formed, small areas of crushed nuclei give a dark "blue" appearance
- Poorly differentiated tumor cells slightly larger than lymphocytes
- Uniform cells with dense nuclear chromatin and small, inconspicuous nucleoli
- Necrosis and mitoses are frequent

Ancillary Tests
- CK20 perinuclear dot-like reaction

Top Differential Diagnoses
- Skin Merkel cell carcinoma, metastatic small cell carcinoma, lymphoma, melanoma

  - Larger tumors are associated with perineural invasion, extrasalivary gland extension, and recurrence

MACROSCOPIC FEATURES

General Features
- Poorly circumscribed, lobulated, infiltrating adjacent structures
- Firm, solid to fleshy
- Gray-white to yellow-tan, with necrosis and hemorrhage

Size
- Range: 2-10 cm, usually > 3 cm

MICROSCOPIC PATHOLOGY

Histologic Features
- Extensive infiltration
  - Adjacent parenchyma
  - Muscle, fat, dermis, bone
  - Perineural invasion and vascular invasion are frequently identified
- Arranged in solid sheets, nests, and irregular cords
  - Cellular dyscohesion may create pseudoglandular or ductal appearance
  - Rosette formation or peripheral palisading is occasionally identified
- Well-formed, small areas of crushed nuclei give dark "blue" appearance
- Abundant, dense fibrosis may separate tumor into islands or nests
  - Fibrosis may be vascularized or hyalinized
- Poorly differentiated tumor cells slightly larger than lymphocytes
  - Uniform cells with dense nuclear chromatin and small, inconspicuous nucleoli
  - Nuclear molding can be seen
  - Scant cytoplasm, although occasionally more cytoplasm can be seen
- Coagulative &/or comedonecrosis is seen
- Lymphoid infiltrate is limited and patchy
- Mitoses are frequent
- Rare spindled tumor cells may be present
- Isolated areas with squamous differentiation have been reported

Variant
- Large cell type
  - Same criteria as used for large cell neuroendocrine carcinoma (LCNEC) of lung
  - Significant necrosis and high mitotic rate
  - Prominent perineural and vascular invasion
  - Large, polygonal pleomorphic cells arranged in organoid, solid, trabecular, rosette-like, and dyscohesive patterns
    - Moderate nuclear to cytoplasmic ratio, ample cytoplasm, coarse chromatin, conspicuous nucleoli
    - Cytoplasm is clear to eosinophilic
  - Lack CK20 immunoreactivity

ANCILLARY TESTS

Cytology
- Cellular smears with dispersed to loose clusters of small to intermediate-sized cells
- Mild to moderate pleomorphism, scant cytoplasm, and nuclear molding
  - Smudged nuclei may be present
- Rosettes or pseudorosettes may be noted
- Multinucleated tumor cells or macrophages are uncommon

Immunohistochemistry
- CK20 perinuclear dot-like reaction is most sensitive and specific reaction
  - Present in skin Merkel cell carcinoma also
  - Not seen in other salivary gland tumors nor in pulmonary small cell carcinoma

SMALL CELL UNDIFFERENTIATED CARCINOMA

Immunohistochemistry

Antibody	Reactivity	Staining Pattern	Comment
CK-PAN	Positive	Dot positivity	Perinuclear globular or dot-like positive
CK20	Positive	Dot positivity	Perinuclear globular or dot-like positive (Merkel type)
Chromogranin-A	Positive	Cytoplasmic	Granular reactivity
Synaptophysin	Positive	Cytoplasmic	Granular reactivity
CD56	Positive	Cell membrane & cytoplasm	Most tumor cells
NSE	Positive	Cytoplasmic	Most tumor cells, but nonspecific
CD57	Positive	Cytoplasmic	Most tumor cells
CK7	Positive	Cytoplasmic	Some cases positive
EMA	Positive	Cell membrane	Most tumor cells
NFP	Positive	Cytoplasmic	Only rare and isolated tumor cells positive
Ki-67	Positive	Nuclear	> 50% tumor cells positive
S100	Negative		
HMB-45	Negative		
TTF-1	Equivocal	Nuclear	Up to 20% of cells may be positive in some cases

- Panel of neuroendocrine markers recommended: Chromogranin, synaptophysin, CD56, CD57, NSE, NFP (prognostic significance)

Cytogenetics

- Only isolated cases studied, with markedly reduced expressions of p21Waf1 and p27Kip1
- Loss of heterozygosity at chromosome 9p21 has been reported for large cell type

Electron Microscopy

- About 20-30% of cases show membrane-bound cytoplasmic neuroendocrine granules

DIFFERENTIAL DIAGNOSIS

Merkel Cell Carcinoma (Skin)

- Direct extension from skin primary or metastasis to parotid/lymph nodes
  - Skin of scalp, neck, and face may metastasize to parotid lesion
- Paranuclear keratin immunoreactivity, especially CK20; NFP globular(+); TTF-1(-)

Metastases

- Metastatic small cell carcinoma from lung to salivary gland is uncommon
- Histologically identical
- Immunohistochemistry may help: TTF-1(+), CK20(-) favors lung primary
  - Keratin is usually paranuclear dot-like in small cell carcinoma

Lymphoma

- Tend to be sheet-like, infiltrating between glands and ducts
- Lack pseudoglandular spaces, ductal-type structures, rosettes
- Variable necrosis and mitotic figures
- Smaller cells than seen in SCUC, but with irregular contours, lacking molding
- Strongly positive for lymphoma immunohistochemistry (i.e., CD45RB, CD20, CD3, CD30, CD43, CD56, ALK, TIA-1)

Melanoma

- Skin melanomas frequently metastasize to intraparotid lymph nodes
- Tumor cells tend to be larger, lack molding, have prominent nucleoli and intranuclear cytoplasmic inclusions
- Melanin pigment may help with separation
- Positive for melanoma markers (S100 protein, Melan-A, HMB-45, tyrosinase)

SELECTED REFERENCES

1. Jorcano S et al: Primary neuroendocrine small cell undifferentiated carcinoma of the parotid gland. Clin Transl Oncol. 10(5):303-6, 2008
2. Nagao T et al: Small cell carcinoma of the major salivary glands: clinicopathologic study with emphasis on cytokeratin 20 immunoreactivity and clinical outcome. Am J Surg Pathol. 28(6):762-70, 2004
3. Pontius AT et al: Metastatic neuroendocrine tumors of the parotid gland. Am J Otolaryngol. 25(2):129-33, 2004
4. Klijanienko J et al: Fine-needle sampling of primary neuroendocrine carcinomas of salivary glands: cytohistological correlations and clinical analysis. Diagn Cytopathol. 24(3):163-6, 2001
5. Nagao T et al: Primary large-cell neuroendocrine carcinoma of the parotid gland: immunohistochemical and molecular analysis of two cases. Mod Pathol. 13(5):554-61, 2000
6. Ordóñez NG: Value of thyroid transcription factor-1 immunostaining in distinguishing small cell lung carcinomas from other small cell carcinomas. Am J Surg Pathol. 24(9):1217-23, 2000
7. Toyosawa S et al: Small cell undifferentiated carcinoma of the submandibular gland: immunohistochemical evidence of myoepithelial, basal and luminal cell features. Pathol Int. 49(10):887-92, 1999
8. Chan JK et al: Cytokeratin 20 immunoreactivity distinguishes Merkel cell (primary cutaneous neuroendocrine) carcinomas and salivary gland small cell carcinomas from small cell carcinomas of various sites. Am J Surg Pathol. 21(2):226-34, 1997

Microscopic Features and Ancillary Techniques

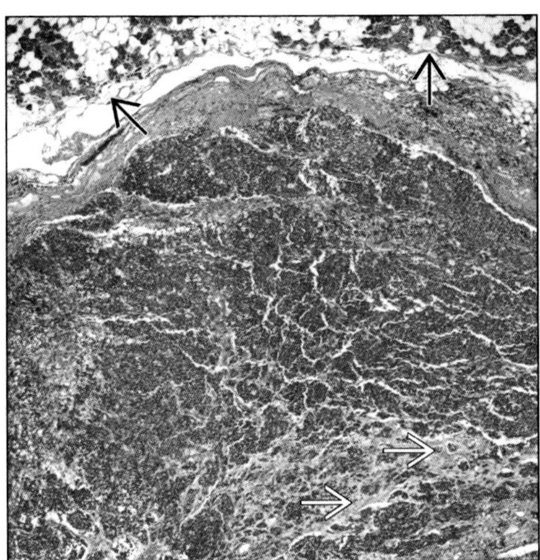

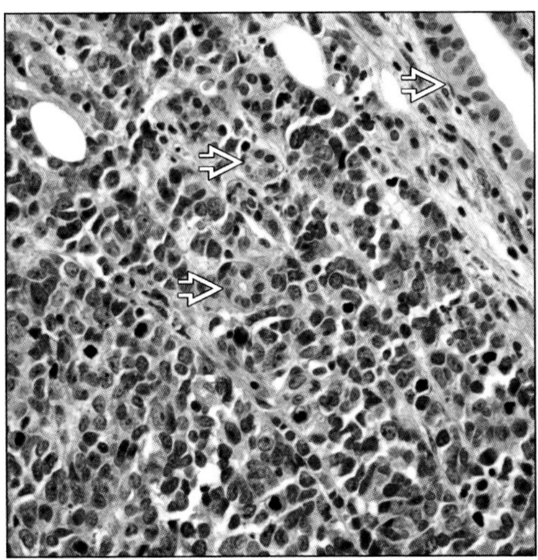

(Left) *The parotid parenchyma ➞ is noted at the periphery. The neoplasm has a vague lobular architecture, with areas of smudged cells, characteristic of SCUC. Areas of degeneration are noted ➞.* ***(Right)*** *The small cells have cytologic isomorphism, with apoptotic cells seen. The cells invade between the salivary gland ducts and acini ➞. This is a characteristic pattern for this tumor type. There is some nuclear molding, with dense nuclear chromatin distribution.*

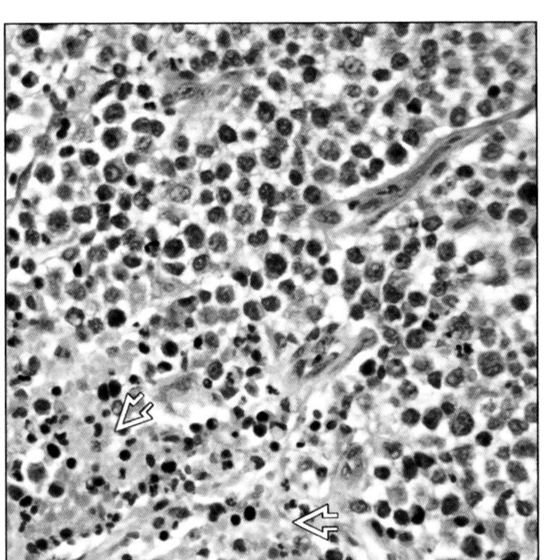

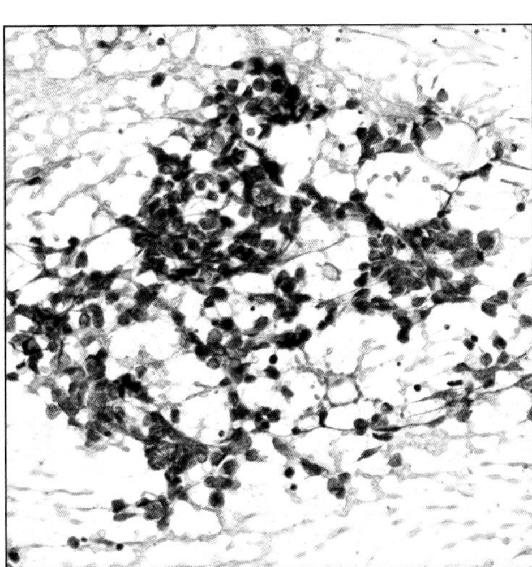

(Left) *An area of comedonecrosis ➞ is noted in this sheet of small neoplastic cells. These cells have scant slightly cleared to eosinophilic cytoplasm. The chromatin is dense, but even.* ***(Right)*** *There is a cellular smear with dispersed to loose clusters of small to intermediate-sized cells. Mild pleomorphism is noted in cells that have scant cytoplasm and nuclear molding. Lymphoglandular bodies are absent. These findings on FNA can be seen in pulmonary small cell carcinoma also.*

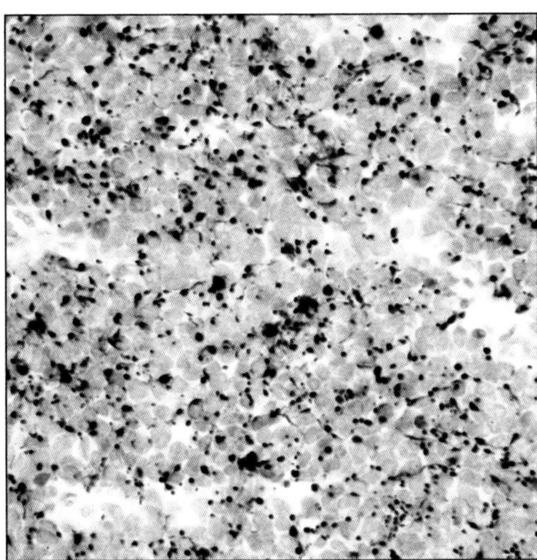

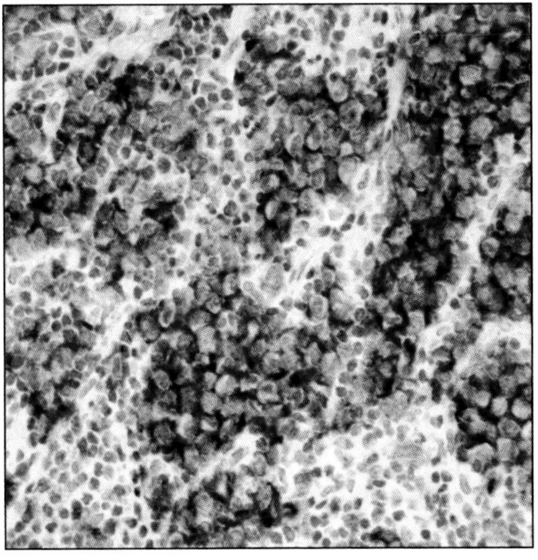

(Left) *The CK20 immunohistochemistry yields a characteristic perinuclear dot-like reaction in the cytoplasm of nearly all of the cells. This is one of the most sensitive and specific reactions, as it is seen neither in other salivary gland tumors nor in pulmonary small cell carcinoma. It can be seen in Merkel cell carcinoma, however.* ***(Right)*** *A panel of neuroendocrine markers is recommended, as the more neuroendocrine markers that are positive (CD56 in this image), the better the prognosis.*

LYMPHOEPITHELIAL CARCINOMA

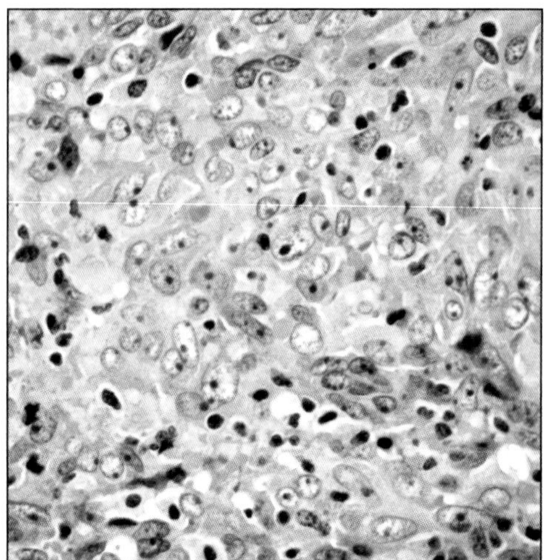

The neoplastic cells are characterized by enlarged nuclei with vesicular chromatin, prominent nucleoli, and indistinct borders, the latter creating a syncytial pattern of growth.

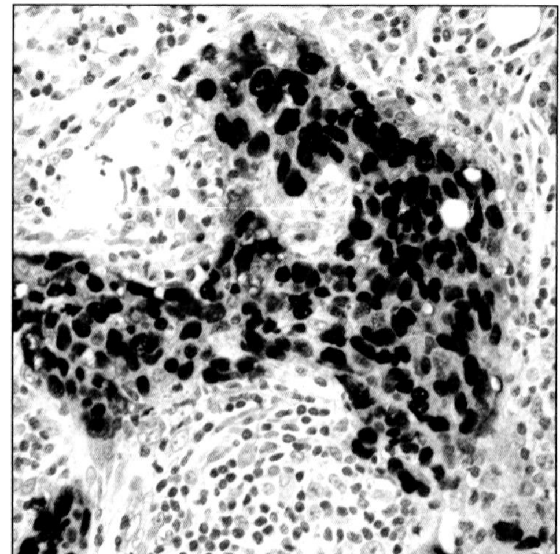

In situ hybridization for Epstein-Barr encoded RNA (EBER) shows the neoplastic cells to be diffusely positive (nuclear staining) supporting the diagnosis of lymphoepithelial carcinoma.

TERMINOLOGY

Abbreviations

- Lymphoepithelial carcinoma (LEC)

Synonyms

- Undifferentiated carcinoma
- Lymphoepithelioma-like carcinoma
- Lymphoepithelial-like carcinoma
- Undifferentiated carcinoma with lymphoid stroma
- Malignant lymphoepithelial lesion
- Carcinoma ex lymphoepithelial lesion

Definitions

- Undifferentiated carcinoma with associated prominent nonneoplastic lymphoplasmacytic cell infiltrate

ETIOLOGY/PATHOGENESIS

Infectious Agents

- Etiology linked to Epstein-Barr virus (EBV)
  - Near 100% association in patients in endemic areas
  - In nonendemic areas, EBV usually absent but rarely may be identified
  - Presence of EBV in clonal episomal form suggests role in tumor development

Familial

- Inherited trichoepitheliomas reported in setting of LEC suggesting hereditary predisposition

CLINICAL ISSUES

Epidemiology

- Incidence
  - Rare salivary gland tumor accounting for < 1% of all salivary gland tumors
    - Highest incidence worldwide in Eskimo/Inuit population
- Age
  - Occurs over wide age range with most patients in 5th decade of life
- Gender
  - In Eskimos/Inuits, more common in females
- Ethnicity
  - Predilection for Arctic region natives (Eskimos/Inuits from Alaska, Canada, Greenland), southeastern Chinese, and Japanese

Site

- Parotid gland most common site of occurrence (80%) followed by submandibular gland
  - Rare occurrence in minor salivary glands throughout upper aerodigestive tract

Presentation

- Mass swelling with or without associated pain &/or facial nerve paralysis
  - Fixation to skin &/or underlying structures seen in advanced tumors
  - High frequency (10-40%) of concurrent cervical lymphadenopathy

Laboratory Tests

- Elevated anti-EBV viral capsid antigen IgA, anti-EBV nuclear antigen IgG in patients from endemic regions

Natural History

- Most develop de novo but may arise in association with lymphoepithelial sialadenitis
  - No known association with other autoimmune disorders
    - e.g., Sjögren disease

Treatment

- Options, risks, complications
  - Combined (multimodality) therapy treatment of choice
    - Surgical resection
    - Neck dissection

LYMPHOEPITHELIAL CARCINOMA

Key Facts

Terminology
- Undifferentiated carcinoma with associated prominent nonneoplastic lymphoplasmacytic cell infiltrate

Etiology/Pathogenesis
- Etiology linked to Epstein-Barr virus (EBV)
- Near 100% association in patients in endemic areas; in nonendemic areas, EBV usually absent

Clinical Issues
- Predilection for Arctic region natives (Eskimos/Inuits from Alaska, Canada, Greenland), southeastern Chinese, and Japanese
- Parotid gland most common site of occurrence (80%)
- Combined (multimodality) therapy treatment of choice (surgical resection, neck dissection, radiation therapy)
- 5-year survival rate: 75-85%

Microscopic Pathology
- Infiltrative tumor characterized by polygonal to spindle-shaped cells with large round to oval, basophilic to vesicular-appearing nuclei separated or overrun by nonneoplastic lymphoid stroma

Ancillary Tests
- Cytokeratins, epithelial membrane antigen (EMA), p63 positive
- EBER nearly always positive (endemic cases)

    - Radiation therapy
- Surgical approaches
  - Total parotidectomy
  - Regional neck dissection indicated given high frequency of nodal metastasis

Prognosis
- 5-year survival rate reported to be 75-85%
- Prognosis linked to clinical stage
- In Eskimos/Inuits, reported more aggressive clinical course and higher clinical stage disease at presentation

MACROSCOPIC FEATURES

General Features
- Circumscribed but unencapsulated, lobulated, firm, tan-white mass

Size
- 1-10 cm in greatest dimension

MICROSCOPIC PATHOLOGY

Histologic Features
- Infiltrative tumor characterized by
  - Lobules
  - Sheets
  - Nests
  - Islands
  - Trabeculae
  - Cords of neoplastic cells separated or overrun by lymphoid stroma
- Neoplastic cells include
  - Polygonal to spindle-shaped with large round to oval, basophilic to vesicular-appearing nuclei
  - One or more prominent nucleoli
  - Abundant amphophilic to lightly eosinophilic cytoplasm
  - Cells have indistinct cell borders and syncytial growth usually evident
- Moderate to marked nuclear pleomorphism present
- Increased mitotic activity and necrosis
- Nonneoplastic lymphoplasmacytic cell infiltrate with or without germinal centers present
  - Present in between and around tumor nests or may overrun and obscure epithelial component
  - Abundant histiocytes may be seen creating "starry sky" appearance
  - Noncaseating granulomatous inflammation may be identified
- Amyloid stroma may also be present
- Invasion into
  - Nonneoplastic salivary gland parenchyma
  - Surrounding connective tissues
  - Nerves (neurotropism)
  - Vessels (angioinvasion)

ANCILLARY TESTS

Cytology
- Cohesive aggregates or individual neoplastic cells include
  - Medium to large cells with large vesicular-appearing nuclei
  - One or more prominent nucleoli
  - High nuclear to cytoplasmic ratio
- Associated mature lymphocytes and plasma cells are typically numerous

Immunohistochemistry
- Cytokeratins, epithelial membrane antigen (EMA), p63 positive
- In situ hybridization detects EBV-encoded RNA (EBER)
- p16 negative
- Lymphoid cells reactive for B-cell (CD20) and T-cell (CD3) markers

Molecular Genetics
- SLEC-LMP1 and B95-8-LMP1 nucleotide sequences and molecular clone of LMP1 directly isolated from SLEC may be a useful tool to identify high-pathogenic EBV strain(s)

  - Associated with salivary gland lymphoepithelial carcinoma

DIFFERENTIAL DIAGNOSIS

Metastatic Undifferentiated Carcinoma

- Waldeyer tonsillar ring origin
  - Nasopharynx
  - Base of tongue
  - Tonsil
- Overlapping histologic, immunohistochemical, ultrastructural, and molecular features
- Differentiation predicated on clinical evaluation to exclude metastasis from primary Waldeyer ring carcinoma

Malignant Lymphoma

- Hematolymphoid immunomarkers positive
- Epithelial immunomarkers negative

Malignant Melanoma

- Melanocytic immunomarkers positive
  - S100 protein
  - HMB-45
  - Melan-A
  - Tyrosinase
- Epithelial immunomarkers negative

Lymphoepithelial Sialadenitis (LESA)

- Characterized by
  - Presence of lymphoepithelial islands
  - Mixed inflammatory cells
  - Absence of malignant cells

SELECTED REFERENCES

1. Schneider M et al: Lymphoepithelial carcinoma of the parotid glands and its relationship with benign lymphoepithelial lesions. Arch Pathol Lab Med. 132(2):278-82, 2008
2. Ellis GL: Lymphoid lesions of salivary glands: malignant and benign. Med Oral Patol Oral Cir Bucal. 12(7):E479-85, 2007
3. Manganaris A et al: Lymphoepithelial carcinoma of the parotid gland: is an association with Epstein-Barr virus possible in non-endemic areas? Int J Oral Maxillofac Surg. 36(6):556-9, 2007
4. Larbcharoensub N et al: Epstein-Barr virus associated lymphoepithelial carcinoma of the parotid gland; a clinicopathological report of three cases. J Med Assoc Thai. 89(9):1536-41, 2006
5. Wang CP et al: Lymphoepithelial carcinoma versus large cell undifferentiated carcinoma of the major salivary glands. Cancer. 101(9):2020-7, 2004
6. Saku T et al: Epstein-Barr virus infected lymphoepithelial carcinomas of the salivary gland in the Russia-Asia area: a clinicopathologic study of 160 cases. Arkh Patol. 65(2):35-9, 2003
7. Jayaram G et al: Lymphoepithelial carcinoma of salivary gland - cytologic, histologic, immunocytochemical, and in situ hybridization features in a case. Diagn Cytopathol. 22(6):400-2, 2000
8. Jang SJ et al: Lymphoepithelial carcinoma of the submandibular gland--a case report. J Korean Med Sci. 12(3):252-5, 1997
9. Safneck JR et al: Fine needle aspiration biopsy findings in lymphoepithelial carcinoma of salivary gland. Acta Cytol. 41(4):1023-30, 1997
10. Worley NK et al: Lymphoepithelial carcinoma of the minor salivary gland. Arch Otolaryngol Head Neck Surg. 123(6):638-40, 1997
11. Abdulla AK et al: Lymphoepithelial carcinoma of salivary glands. Head Neck. 18(6):577-81, 1996
12. Nagao T et al: Epstein-Barr virus-associated undifferentiated carcinoma with lymphoid stroma of the salivary gland in Japanese patients. Comparison with benign lymphoepithelial lesion. Cancer. 78(4):695-703, 1996
13. Christiansen MS et al: Spindle cell malignant lymphoepithelial lesion of the parotid gland: clinical, light microscopic, ultrastructural, and in situ hybridization findings in one case. Mod Pathol. 8(7):711-5, 1995
14. Leung SY et al: Lymphoepithelial carcinoma of the salivary gland: in situ detection of Epstein-Barr virus. J Clin Pathol. 48(11):1022-7, 1995
15. Chan JK et al: Specific association of Epstein-Barr virus with lymphoepithelial carcinoma among tumors and tumorlike lesions of the salivary gland. Arch Pathol Lab Med. 118(10):994-7, 1994
16. Hamilton-Dutoit SJ et al: Undifferentiated carcinoma of the salivary gland in Greenlandic Eskimos: demonstration of Epstein-Barr virus DNA by in situ nucleic acid hybridization. Hum Pathol. 22(8):811-5, 1991
17. Cleary KR et al: Undifferentiated carcinoma with lymphoid stroma of the major salivary glands. Ann Otol Rhinol Laryngol. 99(3 Pt 1):236-8, 1990
18. Kott ET et al: Lymphoepithelial carcinoma (malignant lymphoepithelial lesion) of the salivary glands. Arch Otolaryngol. 110(1):50-3, 1984
19. Hanji D et al: Malignant lymphoepithelial lesions of the salivary glands with anaplastic carcinomatous change. Report of nine cases and review of literature. Cancer. 52(12):2245-52, 1983

Microscopic and Immunohistochemical Features

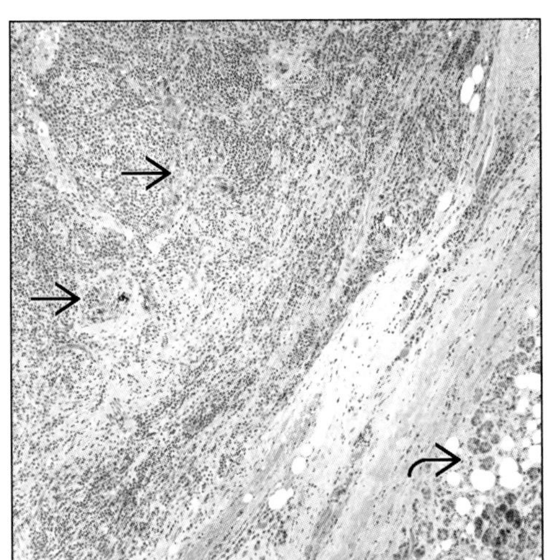

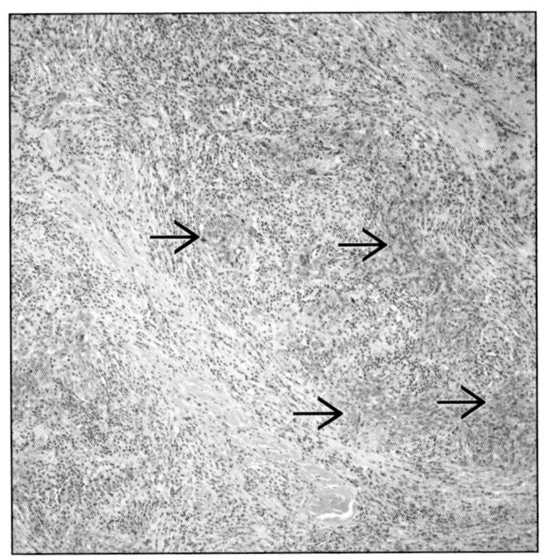

(Left) *Cellular proliferation is comprised of cohesive tumor nests ⇒ with associated dense lymphoid proliferation that is demarcated from residual parotid gland parenchyma ⇗.* ***(Right)*** *Cohesive nests of carcinoma ⇒ with associated fibrosis are readily identifiable even in the presence of a dense nonneoplastic lymphocytic cell proliferation. Not all cases of lymphoepithelial carcinoma will be associated with a desmoplastic reaction.*

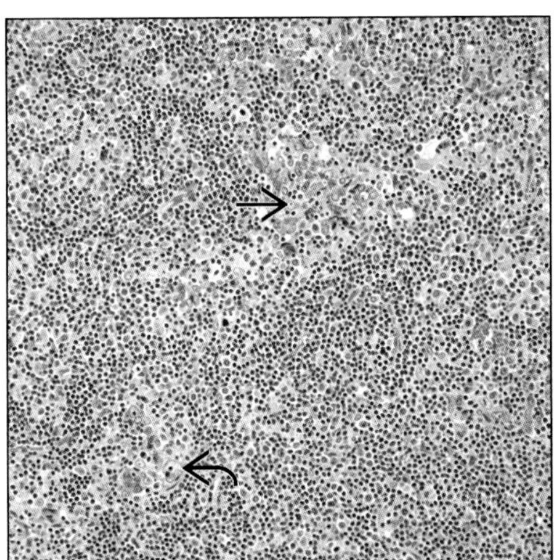

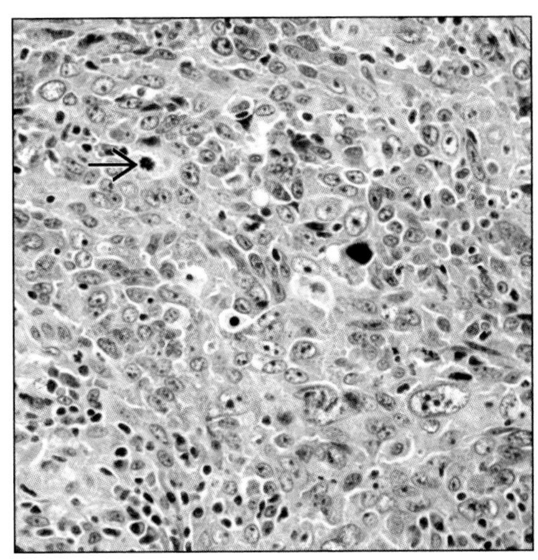

(Left) *The absence of desmoplasia coupled with the presence of a dense nonneoplastic lymphocytic cell infiltrate may overrun the invasive carcinoma, potentially resulting in diagnostic difficulties. The invasive carcinoma may appear in nests ⇒ or as individual cells ⇗.* ***(Right)*** *Irrespective of the setting, the neoplastic cells have enlarged vesicular nuclei with prominent nucleoli and indistinct borders. Nuclear pleomorphism and increased mitotic figures ⇒ may be present.*

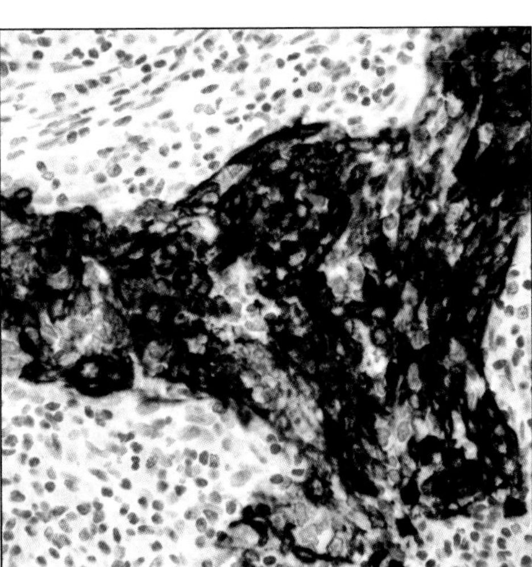

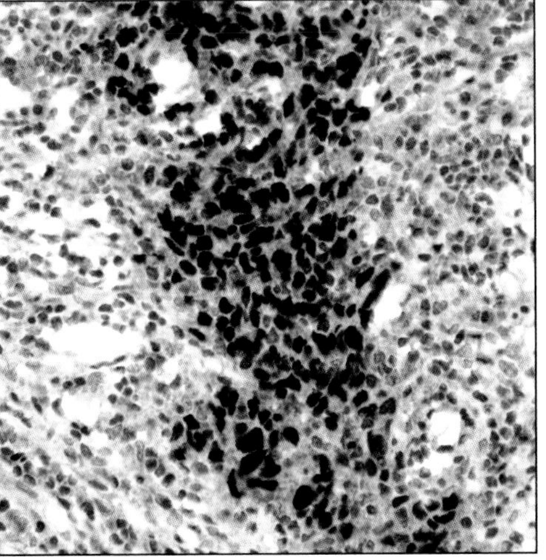

(Left) *IHC staining is essential in differentiating a salivary gland epithelial malignancy from malignant lymphoma. To this end, neoplastic cells of lymphoepithelial carcinoma are immunoreactive for a variety of epithelial markers, including diffuse and intense reactivity for pan-cytokeratin.* ***(Right)*** *In addition to cytokeratins, neoplastic cells are p63 immunoreactive (nuclear and cytoplasmic) representing a marker of squamous epithelial cell origin.*

BASAL CELL ADENOCARCINOMA

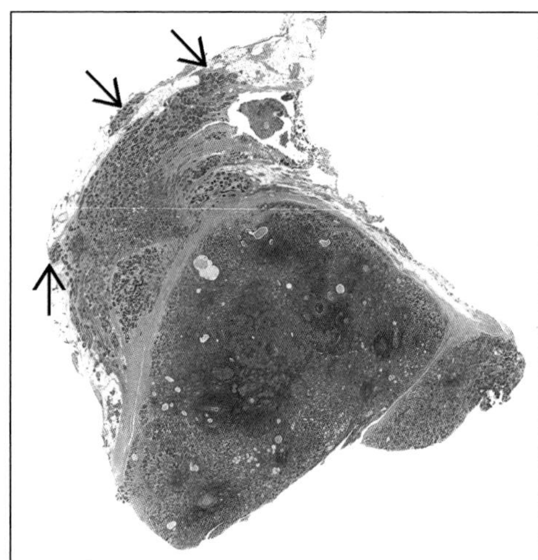

The tumor is well circumscribed, showing an irregular fibrous capsule. The tumor invades into the adjacent fat ⇒, a finding helpful in confirming the diagnosis of a basal cell adenocarcinoma.

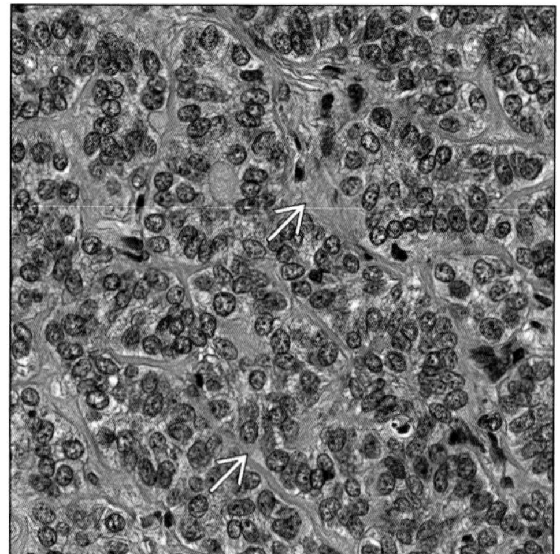

The neoplastic nests are separated by eosinophilic basement membrane-like material ⇒. The cells are small, uniform, dark, basaloid cells, showing scant cytoplasm and indistinct cell borders.

TERMINOLOGY

Synonyms

- Malignant basal cell adenoma
- Basal cell carcinoma
- Malignant basal cell tumor
- Basaloid salivary carcinoma
- Carcinoma ex monomorphic adenoma

Definitions

- Malignant basaloid salivary gland tumor identical to basal cell adenoma, except showing invasion and capacity for metastasis
  - Conceptionally malignant counterpart of basal cell adenoma
  - Initially included in WHO classification in 1991, but 1st used by Ellis and Gnepp in 1988

ETIOLOGY/PATHOGENESIS

Inherited

- Autosomal dominant inherited Brooke-Spiegler syndrome
  - Multiple benign skin tumors (spiradenoma or cylindroma) with rare malignant transformation into possible basal cell adenocarcinoma, among other tumor types

Precursor

- In a few cases, basal cell adenocarcinoma develops from basal cell adenoma
- Most arise de novo

Histogenesis

- Arises from pluripotential cells
- Arises from ductal and myoepithelial cells

CLINICAL ISSUES

Epidemiology

- Incidence
  - Rare, approximately 1-2% of all salivary gland tumors
- Age
  - Wide range, although usually in adults
    - Mean: 7th-8th decades
  - Rare, if at all, in children (probably represents sialoblastoma)
- Gender
  - Female > Male (1.2:1)

Site

- Parotid gland most commonly affected (85-90%)
  - Usually superficial lobe
- Submandibular gland (~ 10%)
- Minor salivary glands (oral cavity usually), rare

Presentation

- Painless swelling, enlargement or mass
- Pain or tenderness is uncommon
- Symptoms may be present for long duration (years)
- Brooke-Spiegler syndrome
  - Multiple skin adnexal tumors concurrent with basal cell adenocarcinoma (BCAC)

Treatment

- Surgical approaches
  - Complete local excision with free margins
    - May be more difficult to achieve in minor salivary gland locations
    - **No** enucleation or curettage
  - Neck dissection only in clinically positive cases
- Radiation
  - May be used for minor salivary gland tumors

BASAL CELL ADENOCARCINOMA

Key Facts

Terminology
- Malignant basaloid salivary gland tumor identical to basal cell adenoma, except showing invasion and capacity for metastasis

Clinical Issues
- Mean age: 7th-8th decades
- Parotid gland most commonly affected (85-90%)
- Painless swelling, enlargement, or mass
- Considered low-grade malignant tumor, with good long-term prognosis
- May be locally destructive with recurrence

Microscopic Pathology
- Unencapsulated, circumscribed to infiltrative
- Invasion into parenchyma, fat, skeletal muscle, vessels, nerves
- Necrosis can be seen (~ 45%)
- Mitotic figures increased
- Multiple patterns of growth: Solid, membranous, tubulo-trabecular
- Nests separated by eosinophilic basement membrane-like material
- **Small**, **dark**, basaloid cells predominate
- **Large**, **polygonal** cells
- Peripheral nuclear palisading at junction with stroma

Ancillary Tests
- Immunohistochemistry identifies dual differentiation: Ductal epithelial and myoepithelial

Top Differential Diagnoses
- Basal cell adenoma, adenoid cystic carcinoma, pleomorphic adenoma

Prognosis
- Considered low-grade malignant tumor, with good long-term prognosis
- May be locally destructive with recurrence
  - Up to 50% have recurrences
  - Highest in tumors of minor salivary glands
  - Recurrences up to 10 years after primary (indolent)
- Uncommon metastases
  - Most are to cervical lymph nodes (up to 15%)
  - Lung very uncommon
- Death from disease is rare (< 4%)
- Worse prognosis
  - Minor salivary gland, advanced stage, residual tumor at surgery, tumor recurrence

MACROSCOPIC FEATURES

General Features
- Cut surface is homogeneous to focally cystic, gray-white to tan-brown
- Unencapsulated, circumscribed to infiltrative

Sections to Be Submitted
- Must include periphery to document invasion (parenchyma, soft tissue, nerve, vessels)

Size
- Variable, usually < 5 cm

MICROSCOPIC PATHOLOGY

Histologic Features
- Identical to basal cell adenoma, except for invasion
- Circumscribed, but tend to lack capsule
- Invasion required for diagnosis
  - Adjacent parenchyma, fat, skeletal muscle, dermis
  - Vascular invasion (~ 75% of cases)
  - Perineural invasion (~ 40% of cases)
- Necrosis can be seen (~ 45%)
  - Comedonecrosis, coagulative necrosis, apoptosis
- Multiple patterns of growth
  - Solid (most common)
  - Membranous (very thick collagenized matrix)
  - Tubulo-trabecular
- Nests separated by eosinophilic basement membrane-like material
  - Collagenous septations
  - Thick, densely hyalinized basal lamina
  - Hyaline droplets within tumor nests
- Cluster or lobule formed by 2 cell populations
  - **Small**, **dark**, basaloid cells predominate
    - Uniform population
    - Scant cytoplasm
    - Indistinct cell borders
    - Round to oval basophilic nuclei
  - **Large**, **polygonal** cells
    - Ample eosinophilic to amphophilic cytoplasm
- Peripheral nuclear palisading at junction with stroma less conspicuous than in adenoma
- Luminal differentiation seen (usually in tubulo-trabecular pattern)
  - Cuboidal, ductal cells surrounding lumen
- Nuclear pleomorphism is uncommon
- Mitotic figures
  - May be difficult to find
  - Range from 1-10/10 HPFs
- Squamous differentiation is infrequently observed
- Lymphocytic and plasma cell infiltrate frequently present
- Hybrid tumors (BCAC with another tumor) are exceedingly rare
  - 2 histologically distinctive tumors in same area
    - BCAC and adenoid cystic carcinoma
    - BCAC and epithelial-myoepithelial carcinoma
  - Proportion must be ≥ 10%

ANCILLARY TESTS

Cytology
- Separation from basal cell adenoma is nearly impossible

BASAL CELL ADENOCARCINOMA

- Smears are cellular, with irregular cohesive sheets, trabeculae and tubules, 3-dimensional clusters, and individual cells
  - Peripheral palisading may be noted
- Homogeneous population of small, basaloid cells with high nuclear to cytoplasmic ratio
  - Nuclei are dense, round to ovoid
  - Pleomorphism and nucleoli help to confirm malignant diagnosis
  - Naked nuclei are frequently present
- Globules or spheres of amorphous eosinophilic matrix material surrounded by tumor cells may be present
- Necrosis, if present, helps with diagnosis
- Mitoses are sometimes present

Immunohistochemistry

- Identifies dual differentiation: Ductal epithelial and myoepithelial
- Variable reactivity both within and between tumors
- Increased Ki-67 labeling index (> 5%) suggests carcinoma

Flow Cytometry

- Nearly all tumors are diploid

Cytogenetics

- No unique or specific chromosomal abnormalities reported

Electron Microscopy

- Ultrastructural features identical for basal cell adenoma and BCAC
- Demonstrate basal, myoepithelial, and ductal differentiation
  - Basal cells (nonluminal) have tonofilaments, desmosome
  - Ductal cells have luminal microvilli, tight junctions
  - Myoepithelial cells have cytoplasmic myofilaments, plasmalemmal extensions, and desmosomes
- Excess basal lamina, marginally and intercellularly seen around nonluminal cells

DIFFERENTIAL DIAGNOSIS

Basal Cell Adenoma

- Circumscribed, without soft tissue infiltration, vascular &/or perineural invasion
- Multifocal or membranous type can simulate "invasion"
- Lacking in cellular atypia
- Limited to absent mitoses (< 3/10 HPF)
- Immunohistochemistry generally not helpful

Adenoid Cystic Carcinoma (ACC)

- ACC has much worse prognosis
- Very difficult to separate by core needle biopsy or FNA, because both have uniform basaloid cells
- Solid variant of adenoid cystic specifically
  - Areas of characteristic ACC usually present somewhere in tumor
- Cribriform pattern and pseudocysts filled with basophilic glycosaminoglycans
- Palisading is not a prominent feature
- Lacks "large pale and small dark" cells common in BCAC
- High nuclear to cytoplasmic ratio; carrot-shaped, peg-shaped, or angular nuclei
- Coarse nuclear chromatin, high mitotic rate, necrosis

Pleomorphic Adenoma

- Multinodular and bosselated growth may simulate invasion
- Presence of myxochondroid matrix
  - Cellular variants may have limited stroma
- Plasmacytoid and spindled cells are frequent (absent in BCAC)
- Epithelial/myoepithelial cells blend into stroma
  - BCAC has abrupt border with matrix
- Tends to lack palisading, necrosis, and high mitotic index

Basaloid Squamous Cell Carcinoma

- High-grade neoplasm, not considered primary salivary gland tumor, but in minor salivary gland locations, distinction is more difficult
- Basaloid phenotype can be seen in both tumors
- Both have comedonecrosis and eosinophilic hyaline-type material
- Abrupt squamous differentiation: Keratinization, squamous cell carcinoma in situ, squamous cell carcinoma
  - Usually involves overlying surface mucosa also

Metastatic Basal Cell Carcinoma

- Skin tumors may metastasize to intraparotid lymph nodes
- Palisading, basaloid architecture, necrosis, and increased mitotic figures
- Lacks biphasic appearance, with myoepithelial cell differentiation

SELECTED REFERENCES

1. Klijanienko J et al: Comparative cytologic and histologic study of fifteen salivary basal-cell tumors: differential diagnostic considerations. Diagn Cytopathol. 21(1):30-4, 1999
2. Quddus MR et al: Basal cell adenocarcinoma of the salivary gland: an ultrastructural and immunohistochemical study. Oral Surg Oral Med Oral Pathol Oral Radiol Endod. 87(4):485-92, 1999
3. Nagao T et al: Basal cell adenocarcinoma of the salivary glands: comparison with basal cell adenoma through assessment of cell proliferation, apoptosis, and expression of p53 and bcl-2. Cancer. 82(3):439-47, 1998
4. Fonseca I et al: Basal cell adenocarcinoma of minor salivary and seromucous glands of the head and neck region. Semin Diagn Pathol. 13(2):128-37, 1996
5. Müller S et al: Basal cell adenocarcinoma of the salivary glands. Report of seven cases and review of the literature. Cancer. 78(12):2471-7, 1996
6. Williams SB et al: Immunohistochemical analysis of basal cell adenocarcinoma. Oral Surg Oral Med Oral Pathol. 75(1):64-9, 1993

BASAL CELL ADENOCARCINOMA

Immunohistochemistry

Antibody	Reactivity	Staining Pattern	Comment
CK-PAN	Positive	Cytoplasmic	All cells, but luminal and ductal cells stronger
AE1/AE3	Positive	Cytoplasmic	Highlights central and luminal cells preferentially
CK7	Positive	Cytoplasmic	Positive in many cases
EMA	Positive	Cell membrane & cytoplasm	Highlights luminal cells preferentially
CEA-M	Positive	Cytoplasmic	Highlights luminal cells preferentially
p63	Positive	Nuclear	Basal/myoepithelial cells
S100	Positive	Nuclear & cytoplasmic	Basal and myoepithelial cells; variable staining intensity
Calponin	Positive	Cytoplasmic	Basal/myoepithelial cells
Actin-sm	Positive	Cytoplasmic	Basal/myoepithelial cells
Actin-HHF-35	Positive	Cytoplasmic	Basal/myoepithelial cells
CK14	Positive	Cytoplasmic	Basal/myoepithelial cells
Vimentin	Positive	Cytoplasmic	Diffusely immunoreactive
CD117	Positive	Cytoplasmic	Random cells positive in about 30% of cases
EGFR	Positive	Cell membrane & cytoplasm	> 50% of cells to be called positive; only about 25% of tumors
p53	Positive	Nuclear	> 10% of tumor cells interpreted to be positive; about 30-50% of cases
Ki-67	Positive	Nuclear	> 5% suggest basal cell adenocarcinoma
Androgen receptor	Positive	Nuclear	Rare tumor cells and only limited cases
Bcl-2	Positive	Nuclear	> 50% of tumor cells in most cases
TAG72	Negative		B72.3
HER2	Negative		
HMFG	Equivocal		Milk fat globulin

BASAL CELL ADENOCARCINOMA

Microscopic Features

*(**Left**) Basal cell adenocarcinoma demonstrates an area of vascular invasion ⇨, along with an irregular periphery with extension and infiltration into the adjacent adipose connective tissue ⇨. (**Right**) This tumor shows an area of fibrosis but is also associated with multiple small nests of tumor that extend into the adjacent fat ⇨. Unremarkable salivary gland parenchyma is present ⇨.*

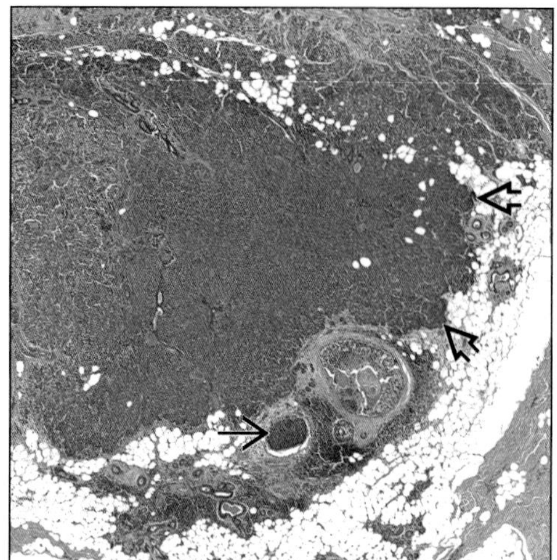

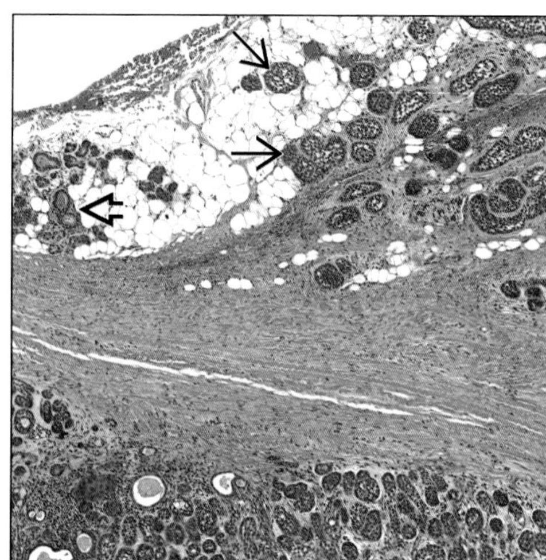

*(**Left**) Sometimes the foci of invasion are larger than small cell nests, as illustrated in this case. There is a large nest of tumor expanding beyond the contour of the tumor ⇨ and through an area of fibrosis. (**Right**) Basal cell adenocarcinoma are cellular tumors, showing a variety of different growth patterns. In this case, the solid to trabecular architecture is the dominant finding. A very delicate connective tissue stroma is noted in this case.*

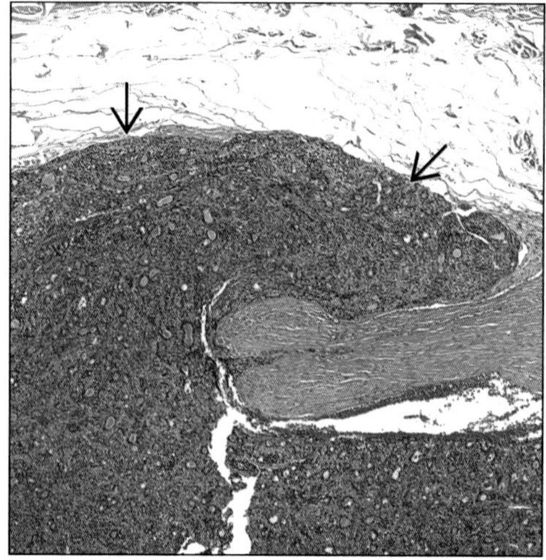

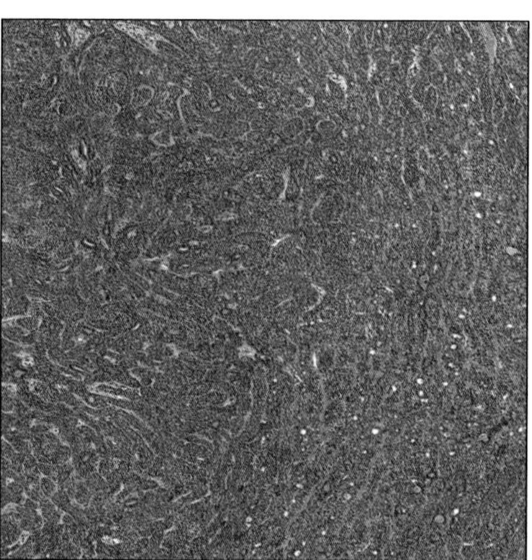

*(**Left**) The eosinophilic basal lamina separates these tumor nests into islands. The cells show a suggestion of palisading. Tubules with lumen are noted ➡ throughout this neoplasm. (**Right**) There are lobules of basaloid cells predominating in this tumor. There is a slightly basophilic substance within this neoplasm. This tumor has some architecture features that are similar to adenoid cystic carcinoma, one of the tumors in the differential diagnosis.*

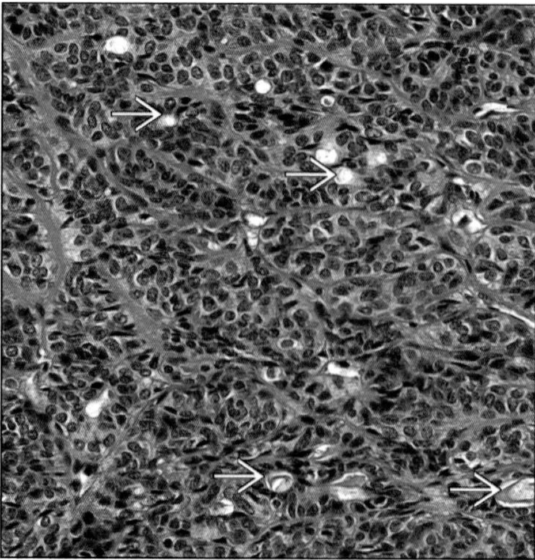

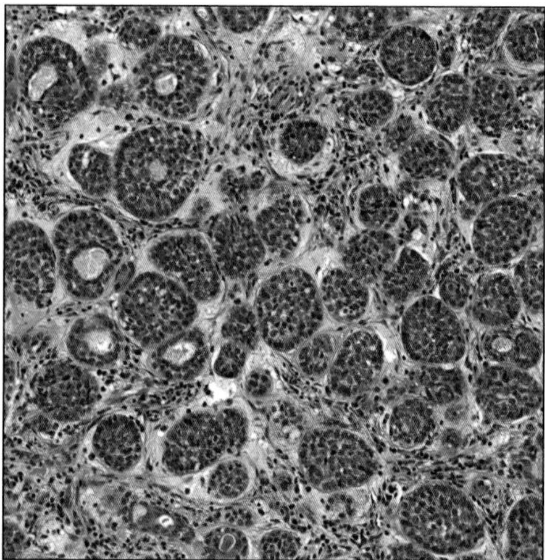

Immunohistochemical Features

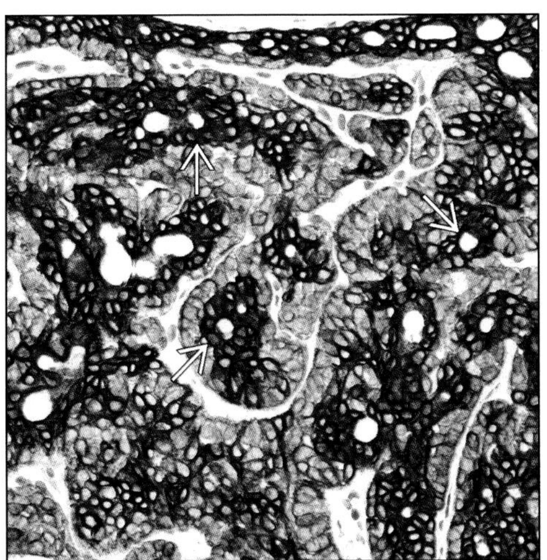

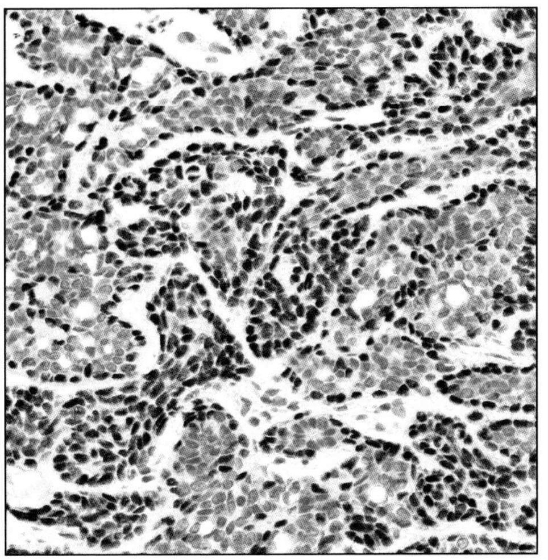

(Left) *The keratin immunohistochemistry study highlights the luminal or tubular cells ➡ within the islands of the tumor. Keratin does not separate between the various cellular components of BCAC.* ***(Right)*** *p63 highlights the basaloid or myoepithelial cells in BCAC, while the luminal or central cells are not highlighted. This finding is identical to what is seen in basal cell adenoma.*

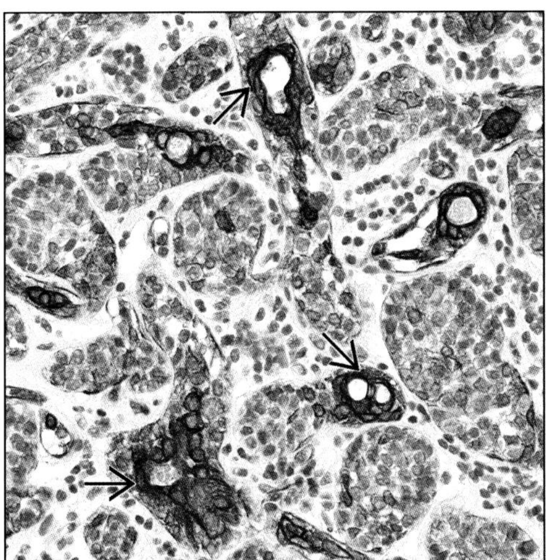

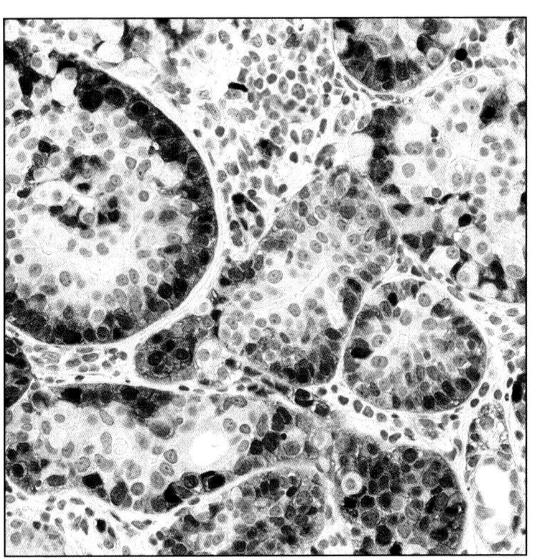

(Left) *A variety of different keratins can be seen in BCAC. In this case, the CK5/6 can be seen specifically highlighting areas of squamous differentiation ➡ in this tumor.* ***(Right)*** *S100 protein accentuated the myoepithelial cells in BCAC, and so will be noted at the periphery of the cell clusters. The central, luminal cells are not accentuated by this marker. Further, it could be used to highlight nerves around the tumor and document perineural invasion.*

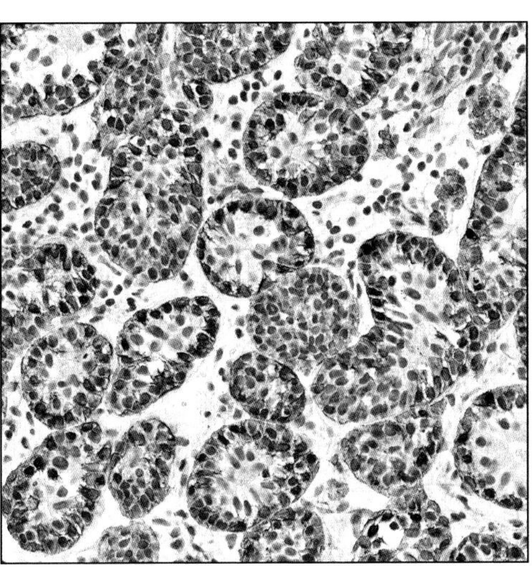

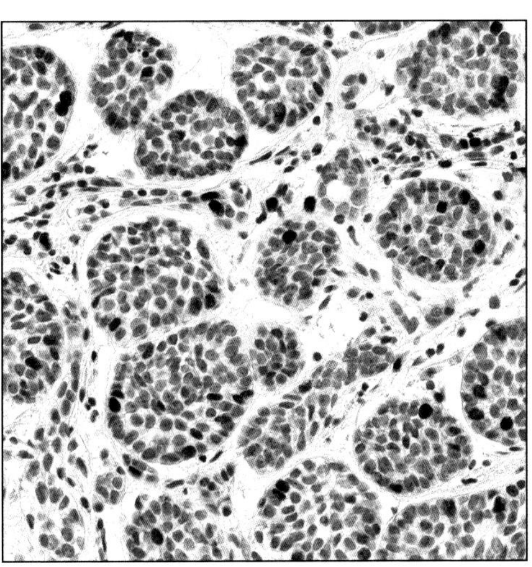

(Left) *A variety of different muscle markers can be used to highlight the myoepithelial differentiation of this tumor. Muscle specific actin, smooth muscle actin (shown), calponin, and CK903 can all highlight this population.* ***(Right)*** *Ki-67 can be used to accentuate the proliferating cells. The separation of benign from malignant, trying to use a cutoff of 5% or 10% of cells, is arbitrary. Most authors have used > 5% proliferation index to suggest malignancy.*

ONCOCYTIC CARCINOMA

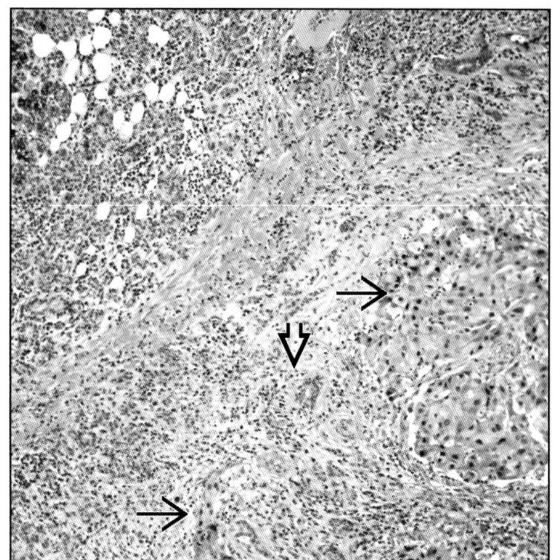

Oncocytic carcinoma is characterized by the presence of an unencapsulated neoplastic proliferation composed of solid cellular nests ⇒ with infiltration into parotid parenchyma ⇨.

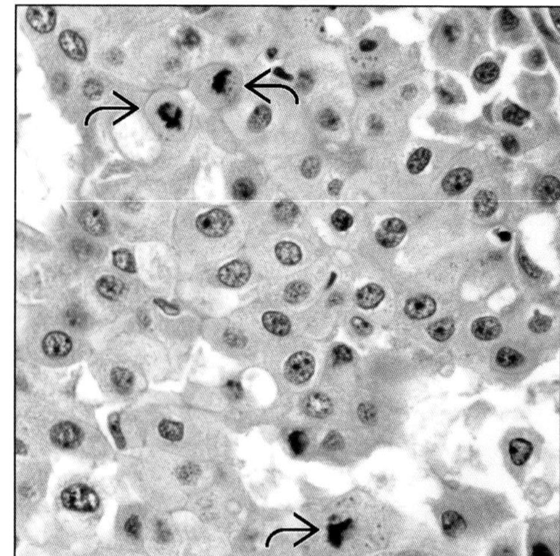

The neoplastic cells are characterized by prominent granular eosinophilic cytoplasm with centrally located round to oval nuclei, some with prominent nucleoli; mitotic figures are present ↗.

TERMINOLOGY

Synonyms

- Malignant oncocytoma
- Oncocytic adenocarcinoma

Definitions

- Malignant salivary gland epithelial tumor predominantly or exclusively composed of oncocytic cells with cytomorphologic features of malignancy (adenocarcinomatous features) and invasive growth

CLINICAL ISSUES

Epidemiology

- Incidence
  - Exceedingly rare tumor type representing < 1% of all salivary gland tumors
- Age
  - Most frequently occurs in 5th-8th decades of life
- Gender
  - Male > Female

Site

- Occurs predominantly but not exclusively in parotid gland (80%)
  - Other sites of occurrence may include submandibular gland
  - Much less often in minor salivary glands

Presentation

- Mass or swelling with or without associated pain &/or facial nerve paralysis
- May arise from a longstanding benign oncocytoma or occur de novo
  - In association with oncocytoma, presents with rapid enlargement of preexisting mass lesion
  - Rare example arising from Warthin tumor
- Cervical lymphadenopathy at presentation fairly common

Treatment

- Surgical approaches
  - Total parotidectomy
  - Nodal dissection is advocated given high incidence of regional (nodal) metastasis
- Radiation
  - Efficacy of radiotherapy not definitively proven

Prognosis

- Guarded
  - Tendency to recur
  - Tendency to metastasize including regional lymph nodes and distant metastases
  - Distant metastases occur to
    - Lungs
    - Kidney
    - Mediastinum
    - Liver
    - Bone
    - Thyroid gland
  - Distant metastasis is associated with poor prognosis, resulting in tumor-related death within 4 years

MACROSCOPIC FEATURES

General Features

- Unencapsulated, single or multinodular, firm mass with tan-gray appearance
- Foci of necrosis may be present

MICROSCOPIC PATHOLOGY

Histologic Features

- Partially encapsulated or unencapsulated lesion showing varied growth patterns
  - Sheets and nests of neoplastic cells infiltrating surrounding tissues with loss of normal lobular architecture

ONCOCYTIC CARCINOMA

Key Facts

Terminology

- Malignant salivary gland epithelial tumor predominantly or exclusively composed of oncocytic cells with cytomorphologic features of malignancy (adenocarcinomatous features) and invasive growth

Clinical Issues

- Occurs predominantly but not exclusively in parotid gland (80%)
- Mass or swelling with or without associated pain &/or facial nerve paralysis
- May arise from longstanding benign oncocytoma or occur de novo
  - In association with oncocytoma, presents with rapid enlargement of preexisting mass lesion
- Total parotidectomy
- Nodal dissection is advocated given high incidence of regional (nodal) metastasis

Microscopic Pathology

- Neoplastic cells are characterized by large, round to oval cells with abundant granular eosinophilic cytoplasm
- Invasion includes infiltration of nonneoplastic salivary gland parenchyma, surrounding connective tissues, neurotropism, &/or angioinvasion

Ancillary Tests

- Electron microscopy
  - Numerous mitochondria that vary in size and shape

- Neoplastic cells are characterized by large, round to oval cells with abundant granular eosinophilic cytoplasm
  - Nuclei enlarged, centrally located, round to oval with vesicular chromatin, often with prominent nucleoli
- Nuclear pleomorphism varies from case to case and even within same case
  - Foci with absent nuclear pleomorphism may be seen near to or admixed with cells showing moderate to marked nuclear pleomorphism
    - These features raise possibility of oncocytic carcinoma arising in association with oncocytoma
- Clear cell change may be focal or more widespread
- Increased mitotic activity and necrosis may be present
- Invasion includes infiltration of nonneoplastic salivary gland parenchyma, surrounding connective tissues, neurotropism, &/or angioinvasion

ANCILLARY TESTS

Cytology

- Aspirates show similar findings to those seen in oncocytoma
- Cytologic features indicative of malignancy include
  - Marked nuclear pleomorphism
  - Increased mitotic activity with atypical mitoses
  - Necrosis

Histochemistry

- Stains for mitochondria, including Novelli and phosphotungstinic acid hematoxylin (PTAH), show purplish and blue cytoplasmic granules, respectively
- Stains for epithelial mucin negative

Immunohistochemistry

- Cytokeratins including pancytokeratin (AE1/AE3), CK7, CK8, CK19 positive
- CEA, EMA positive
- S100 protein, p63, calponin, smooth muscle actin negative
- Increased proliferative activity as determined by Ki-67 (MIB-1) staining may be present

Electron Microscopy

- Numerous mitochondria that vary in size and shape
- Desmosomes, nearly continuous basal lamina, and lumina with microvilli are present

DIFFERENTIAL DIAGNOSIS

Oncocytoma

- Circumscribed to encapsulated lesion lacking
  - Significant nuclear pleomorphism
  - Increased mitotic activity
  - Invasive growth
- Oncocytic carcinoma with limited nuclear pleomorphism and mitotic activity occur but evidence of invasive growth is present

Oncocytosis

- Histologically, oncocytotic foci are
  - Unencapsulated
  - Appear in multiple (often 2 or more) separate nodules
  - Contain residual (nononcocytic) salivary gland parenchyma including
    - Ductular epithelium and serous acinar cells
  - Lack significant nuclear pleomorphism, mitotic activity, and invasive growth

Oncocytic Variants of Specific Malignant Salivary Gland Carcinomas

- Category of tumors that may include (among others)
  - Mucoepidermoid carcinoma
  - Acinic cell adenocarcinoma
  - Salivary duct carcinoma
- In order to render a diagnosis of clear cell variant of specific malignant salivary gland tumor
  - Residual evidence of specific tumor type (e.g., mucoepidermoid carcinoma, others) must be identified

ONCOCYTIC CARCINOMA

- Acceptable even if residual focus of specific tumor type is only focally identified
- Salivary duct carcinoma
  - Often immunoreactive for androgen receptor &/or Her-2/neu
    - Such immunoreactivity not present in oncocytic carcinoma

Clear Cell Variants of Specific Malignant Salivary Gland Carcinomas

- Category of tumors that may include
  - Mucoepidermoid carcinoma
  - Acinic cell adenocarcinoma
  - Myoepithelial carcinoma
- In order to render a diagnosis of clear cell variant of specific malignant salivary gland tumor
  - Residual evidence of specific tumor type (e.g., mucoepidermoid carcinoma, others) must be identified
  - Acceptable even if residual focus of specific tumor type is only focally identified

Metastatic Carcinoma

- Rare occurrence of metastatic carcinoma to salivary gland with oncocytic &/or clear cells
- Primarily includes renal cell carcinoma and less often thyroid carcinoma
- Metastatic renal cell carcinoma characterized by
  - Fibrovascular cores and centrally located red blood cells
  - Immunohistochemical reactivity for
    - CD10
    - pax-2
    - Renal cell carcinoma marker
- Metastatic thyroid carcinoma shows
  - Immunohistochemical reactivity for
    - Thyroglobulin
    - Thyroid transcription factor 1 (TTF-1)

SELECTED REFERENCES

1. Weinreb I et al: Oncocytic mucoepidermoid carcinoma: clinicopathologic description in a series of 12 cases. Am J Surg Pathol. 33(3):409-16, 2009
2. Di Palma S et al: Oncocytic change in pleomorphic adenoma: molecular evidence in support of an origin in neoplastic cells. J Clin Pathol. 60(5):492-9, 2007
3. Caloglu M et al: Oncocytic carcinoma of the parotid gland. Onkologie. 29(8-9):388-90, 2006
4. Giordano G et al: Oncocytic carcinoma of parotid gland: a case report with clinical, immunohistochemical and ultrastructural features. World J Surg Oncol. 4:54, 2006
5. Guclu E et al: A rare malignancy of the parotid gland: oncocytic carcinoma. Eur Arch Otorhinolaryngol. 262(7):567-9, 2005
6. Brannon RB et al: Oncocytic mucoepidermoid carcinoma of parotid gland origin. Oral Surg Oral Med Oral Pathol Oral Radiol Endod. 96(6):727-33, 2003
7. Cinar U et al: Oncocytic carcinoma of the parotid gland: report of a new case. Ear Nose Throat J. 82(9):699-701, 2003
8. Kimura M et al: Oncocytic carcinoma of the parotid gland. A case report. Acta Cytol. 47(6):1099-102, 2003
9. Capone RB et al: Oncocytic neoplasms of the parotid gland: a 16-year institutional review. Otolaryngol Head Neck Surg. 126(6):657-62, 2002
10. Stanley MW: Selected problems in fine needle aspiration of head and neck masses. Mod Pathol. 15(3):342-50, 2002
11. Alberty J et al: [Oncocytic neoplasms of the parotid gland. Differential diagnosis, clinical course and review of the literature.] HNO. 49(2):109-17, 2001
12. Jahan-Parwar B et al: Oncocytic mucoepidermoid carcinoma of the salivary glands. Am J Surg Pathol. 23(5):523-9, 1999
13. Paulino AF et al: Oncocytic and oncocytoid tumors of the salivary glands. Semin Diagn Pathol. 16(2):98-104, 1999
14. Nakada M et al: Oncocytic carcinoma of the submandibular gland: a case report and literature review. J Oral Pathol Med. 27(5):225-8, 1998
15. Shintaku M et al: Identification of oncocytic lesions of salivary glands by anti-mitochondrial immunohistochemistry. Histopathology. 31(5):408-11, 1997
16. Brandwein MS et al: Oncocytic tumors of major salivary glands. A study of 68 cases with follow-up of 44 patients. Am J Surg Pathol. 15(6):514-28, 1991
17. Bengoechea O et al: Oncocytic adenocarcinoma arising in Warthin's tumor. Pathol Res Pract. 185(6):907-11; discussion 911-4, 1989
18. Ellis GL: "Clear cell" oncocytoma of salivary gland. Hum Pathol. 19(7):862-7, 1988
19. Goode RK et al: Oncocytic adenocarcinoma of salivary glands. Oral Surg Oral Med Oral Pathol. 65(1):61-6, 1988
20. Austin MB et al: Oncocytoid adenocarcinoma of the parotid gland. Cytologic, histologic and ultrastructural findings. Acta Cytol. 31(3):351-6, 1987
21. Johns ME et al: Oncocytic neoplasms of salivary glands: an ultrastructural study. Laryngoscope. 87(6):862-71, 1977
22. Gray SR et al: Oncocytic neoplasms of salivary glands: a report of fifteen cases including two malignant oncocytomas. Cancer. 38(3):1306-17, 1976
23. Lee SC et al: Malignant oncocytoma of the parotid gland. A light and electron microscopic study. Cancer. 37(3):1606-14, 1976
24. Johns ME et al: Oncocytic and oncocytoid tumors of the salivary glands. Laryngoscope. 83(12):1940-52, 1973

ONCOCYTIC CARCINOMA

Microscopic and Histochemical Features

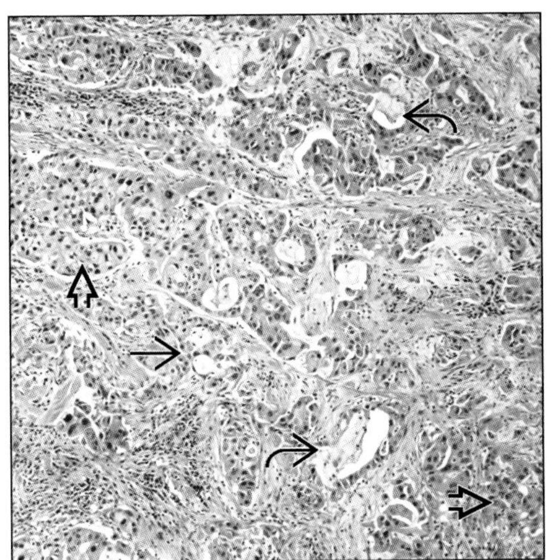

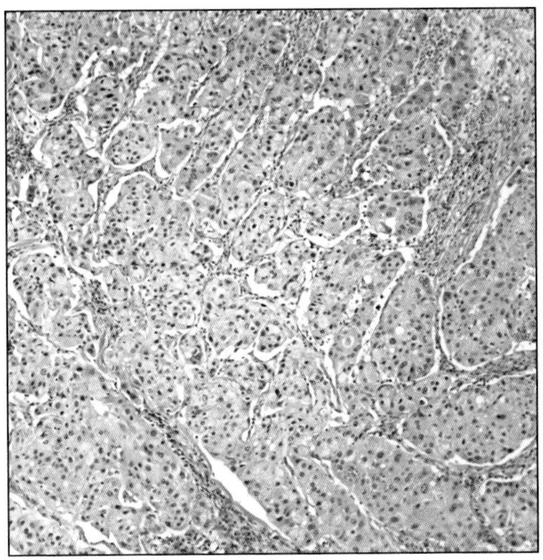

(Left) *The neoplasm is infiltrative with desmoplastic stroma and shows a variety of growth patterns, including glandular → and solid →. Complex growth with back-to-back glands → is focally present.* ***(Right)*** *Additional growth patterns may include trabecular and organoid. Irrespective of the pattern of growth, the neoplastic proliferation is entirely composed of oncocytic cells characterized by the presence of a prominent granular eosinophilic-appearing cytoplasm.*

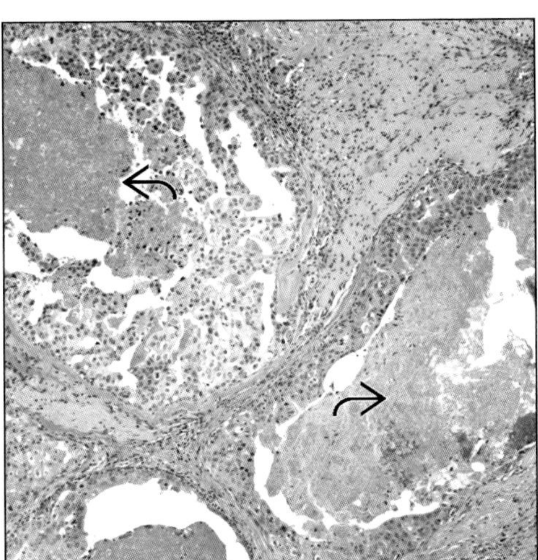

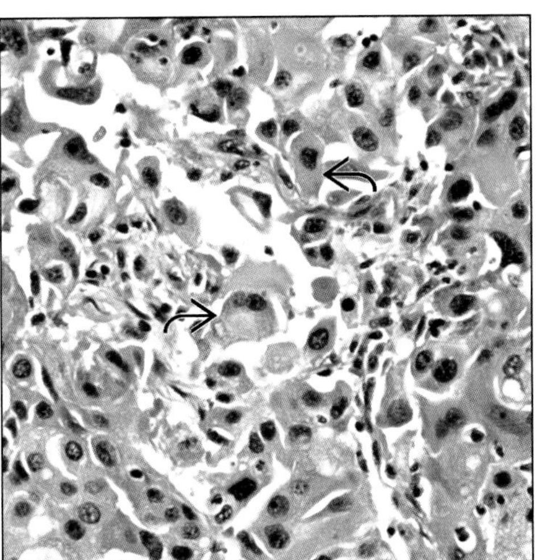

(Left) *Cystic growth and central (comedotype) necrosis → in oncocytic carcinoma may suggest a diagnosis of salivary duct carcinoma (SDC). In contrast to SDC, oncocytic carcinoma is entirely composed of oncocytes and lack immunostaining for androgen receptor and Her-2/neu.* ***(Right)*** *Oncocytic carcinoma is comprised of cells with prominent granular eosinophilic-appearing cytoplasm →. Nuclear pleomorphism and hyperchromasia are present.*

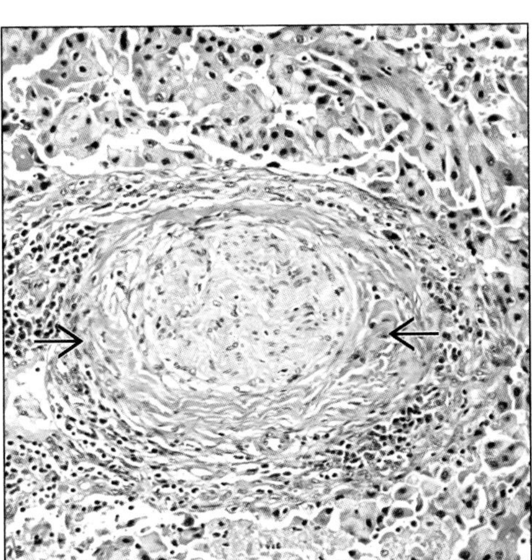

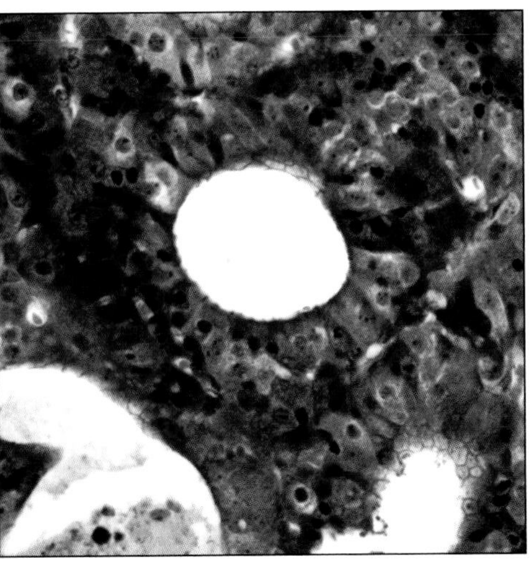

(Left) *In any case, the cellular features of oncocytic carcinomas may be similar to oncocytomas. Differentiation may thus be predicated on the presence of invasion growth that may include invasion into adjacent salivary gland parenchyma, lymph-vascular invasion, and invasion into soft tissues, including around nerves →.* ***(Right)*** *Phosphotungstic acid-hematoxylin (PTAH) stain demonstrates mitochondria as seen by intracytoplasmic (blue-black) granules in the oncocytic cells.*

SEBACEOUS CARCINOMA AND SEBACEOUS LYMPHADENOCARCINOMA

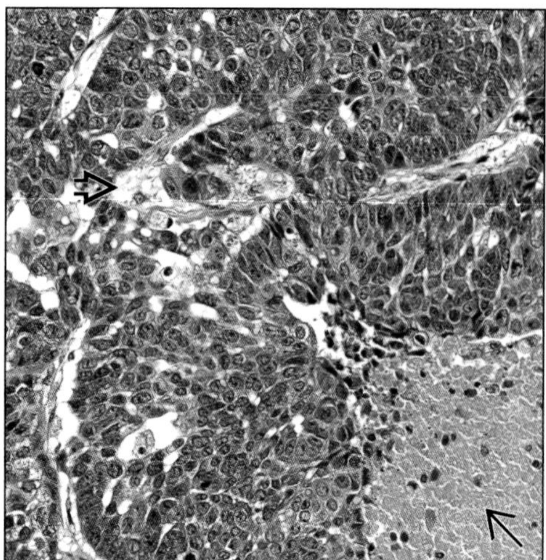

A solid to trabecular sheet of basaloid neoplastic cells with an area of comedonecrosis ⇒ comprise this sebaceous carcinoma. Sebocytes ⇒ are infrequent in this area.

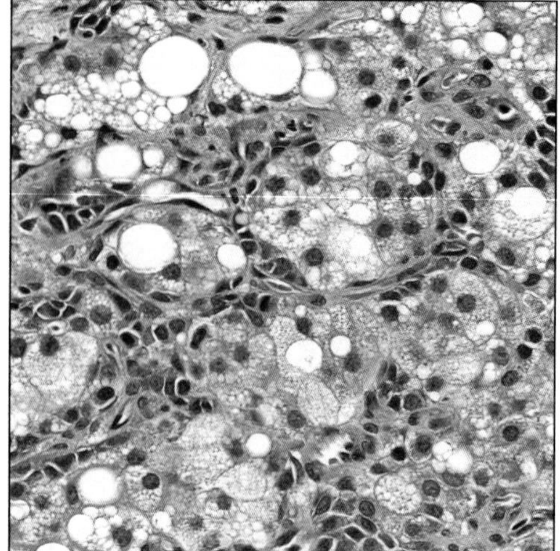

In this area of tumor, a basaloid periphery is noted surrounding large cells with multivesicular or multivacuolated cytoplasm. There is limited pleomorphism in this field.

TERMINOLOGY

Synonyms

- Sebaceous adenocarcinoma

Definitions

- Sebaceous carcinoma (SC): Malignant epithelial neoplasm with focal areas of sebaceous differentiation
- Sebaceous lymphadenocarcinoma: Carcinoma arising from sebaceous lymphadenoma

ETIOLOGY/PATHOGENESIS

Cell of Origin

- Pluripotential cell
  - Sebaceous and glandular differentiation in same cell suggests pluripotential cell origin
  - Sebaceous cells can be identified in many different salivary gland tumors

CLINICAL ISSUES

Epidemiology

- Incidence
  - Very rare
- Age
  - Wide range: Teens to 93 years
  - Bimodal peak: 3rd and 7th decades
- Gender
  - Equal gender distribution

Site

- Overwhelming majority in parotid gland (> 90%)
  - Rare in minor salivary glands (oral cavity)

Presentation

- Presentation is variable
  - Painless, slow-growing, asymptomatic swelling
  - Painful mass
  - Possible facial nerve paralysis
  - Occasional fixation to skin
- No relationship to Muir-Torre
  - No increased risk of developing visceral malignancy

Treatment

- Surgical approaches
  - Wide surgical excision is treatment of choice
  - Radical surgery, including elective neck dissection, should be considered for poor prognostic tumors
- Radiation
  - Postoperative radiotherapy recommended for high-stage and high-grade tumors

Prognosis

- Considered intermediate-grade malignancy with guarded prognosis
- Approximately 60-70% 5-year survival
  - Worse than 85% 5-year survival for skin primaries
- Recurrences develop in about 30%
- Metastases (regional lymph nodes and distant sites) are uncommon
- Poor prognostic indicators: Cytologic atypia, facial nerve involvement

MACROSCOPIC FEATURES

General Features

- Partially encapsulated, often well circumscribed
- Pushing or locally infiltrating margins
- Variably yellow, tan or gray-white

Size

- Range: 0.6-8.5 cm

MICROSCOPIC PATHOLOGY

Sebaceous Carcinoma

- Perineural invasion may be seen (~ 20%)

SEBACEOUS CARCINOMA AND SEBACEOUS LYMPHADENOCARCINOMA

Key Facts

Terminology
- Sebaceous carcinoma (SC): Malignant epithelial neoplasm with focal areas of sebaceous differentiation

Clinical Issues
- Bimodal peak: 3rd and 7th decades
- Overwhelming majority in parotid gland (> 90%)
- Painless, slow-growing, asymptomatic swelling or painful mass
- No relationship to Muir-Torre
- Approximately 60-70% 5-year survival

Microscopic Pathology
- Partially encapsulated, often well circumscribed
- Perineural invasion may be seen (~ 20%)
- Comedonecrosis may be seen
- Tumors form sheets, irregular islands, trabeculae, and large nests
- Ductal structures are common and may become cystic
- Sebocytes: Isolated, small clusters, large islands
  - Multivesicular and vacuolated clear cytoplasm
- Basaloid or squamous areas predominate
  - Basaloid areas predominate at nest periphery

Ancillary Tests
- Sebocytes: EMA (cytoplasmic vesicles highlighted), CD15, GCDFP-2

Top Differential Diagnoses
- Sebaceous adenoma
- Sebaceous lymphadenoma
- Direct extension from skin

- Vascular invasion is uncommon
- Tumors form sheets, irregular islands, trabeculae, and large nests
- Cords of tumor cells may extend into adjacent tissue
- Ductal structures are common and may become cystic
  - Lining cells are cuboidal to low columnar without significant atypia
- Degree of sebaceous differentiation is very variable
  - Sebocytes: Isolated, small clusters, large islands
  - Multivesicular and vacuolated clear cytoplasm
    - Not just clear cytoplasm
- Basaloid or squamous areas predominate
  - Cellular pleomorphism is variable
  - Most cells have large, hyperchromatic nuclei and clear to eosinophilic cytoplasm
  - Nucleoli are often conspicuous
  - Basaloid areas predominate at periphery of nests
  - Isolated mucocytes may be present
- Comedonecrosis (center of tumor islands) may be seen
- Lymphocytes may be present but not arranged in germinal centers

Sebaceous Lymphadenocarcinoma
- Arise in association with sebaceous lymphadenoma or lymphadenoma
- Carcinoma is demarcated, lacking lymphoid stroma, showing invasion, pleomorphism, increased mitoses

ANCILLARY TESTS

Histochemistry
- Sebocytes positive with fat stains (oil red O, Sudan)

Immunohistochemistry
- Sebocytes mainly: EMA (cytoplasmic vesicles), CD15, lactoferrin, GCDFP-2, androgen receptor

DIFFERENTIAL DIAGNOSIS

Sebaceous Adenoma
- Well-circumscribed tumor with variably sized solid nests or cysts
- Peripheral epithelial cells are immature and surround variably developed sebaceous cells
- Lack cytologic atypia, invasion, and increased mitoses

Sebaceous Lymphadenoma
- Evenly distributed solid epithelial nests and cysts
- Cysts lined by bland squamoid, columnar, or cuboidal lining
- Sebaceous cells in solid nests or within cyst walls
- Background of uniformly dense lymphoid cells, often arranged in germinal centers

Direct Extension from Skin Primary
- Skin SC may directly invade salivary gland
- Clinical &/or radiographic separation required

Sebaceous EMC
- Sebaceous differentiation intermingled with areas of epithelial-myoepithelial carcinoma (EMC)
  - May be diffuse or focal
- Characteristic bilayered tubular structures
- Limited cytologic atypia
- SC lacks myoepithelial markers (smooth muscle actin, calponin)

SELECTED REFERENCES

1. Ahn SH et al: Sebaceous lymphadenocarcinoma of parotid gland. Eur Arch Otorhinolaryngol. 263(10):940-2, 2006
2. Croitoru CM et al: Sebaceous lymphadenocarcinoma of salivary glands. Ann Diagn Pathol. 7(4):236-9, 2003
3. Gnepp DR et al: Sebaceous neoplasms of salivary gland origin. Report of 21 cases. Cancer. 53(10):2155-70, 1984
4. Gnepp DR: Sebaceous neoplasms of salivary gland origin: a review. Pathol Annu. 18 Pt 1:71-102, 1983

SEBACEOUS CARCINOMA AND SEBACEOUS LYMPHADENOCARCINOMA

Imaging and Microscopic Features

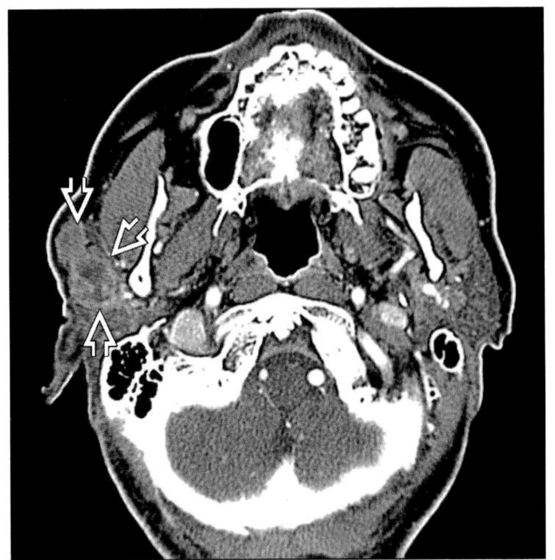

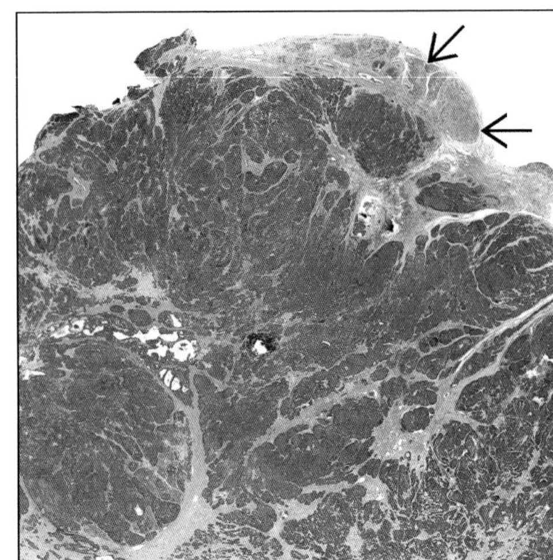

(Left) *The computed tomography image demonstrates a tumor within the right parotid gland ➡ showing an area of cystic degeneration. However, this is nonspecific and does not help define the tumor type.* ***(Right)*** *A small portion of salivary gland parenchyma is present ➡. The tumor is unencapsulated and noncircumscribed. There is a lobular to sheet-like pattern, with bands of fibrosis dissecting between the tumor nests.*

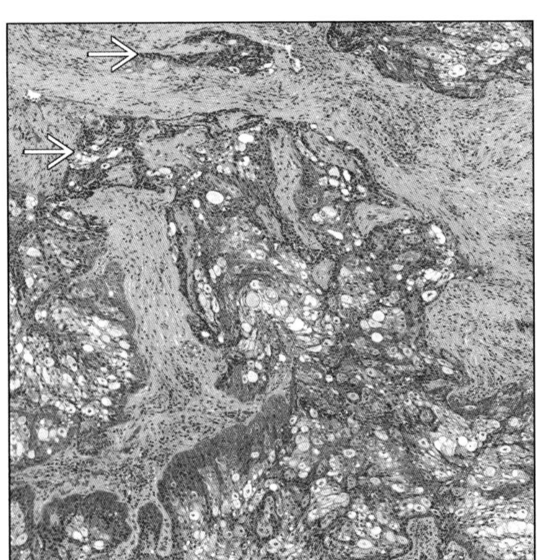

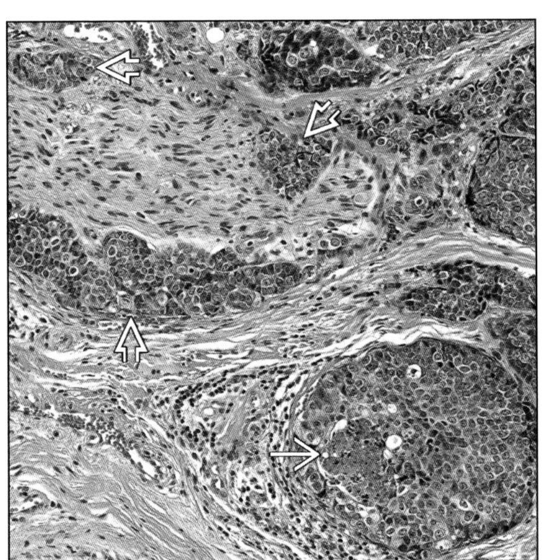

(Left) *Infiltration into the adjacent stroma is noted ➡, along with a very heavy fibrosis. Even at this low magnification, cleared microvesicular cytoplasm can be seen as part of the sebaceous differentiation.* ***(Right)*** *This case highlights a nerve showing multiple areas of perineural invasion ➡, a feature seen in about 20% of tumors. There is also an area of comedonecrosis ➡, identified at the center of a tumor nest. These are helpful in confirming a malignant diagnosis.*

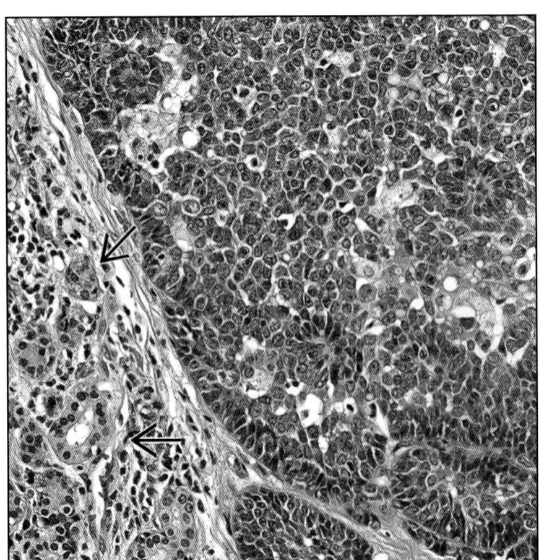

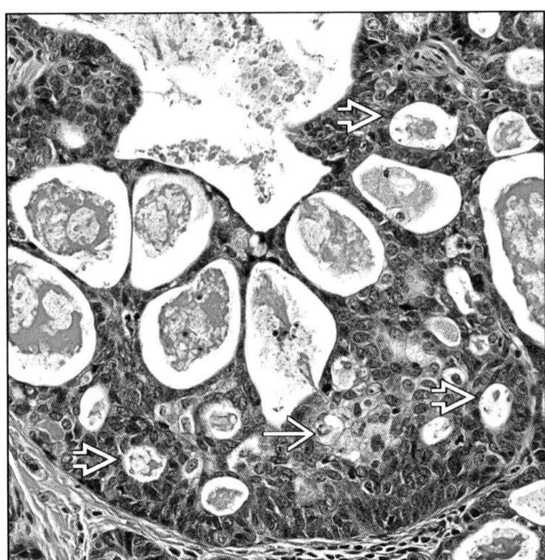

(Left) *A remnant of salivary gland tissue ➡ is seen adjacent to the basaloid neoplastic proliferation. There is a vague palisading at the periphery of the tumor islands. While histiocytes are seen, no well-developed sebocytes are in this field.* ***(Right)*** *Areas of cyst formation are common in sebaceous carcinoma. Secretions are noted within the lumina. A rare sebocyte ➡ is noted in this area of basaloid and ductal ➡ differentiation.*

Microscopic and Immunohistochemical Features

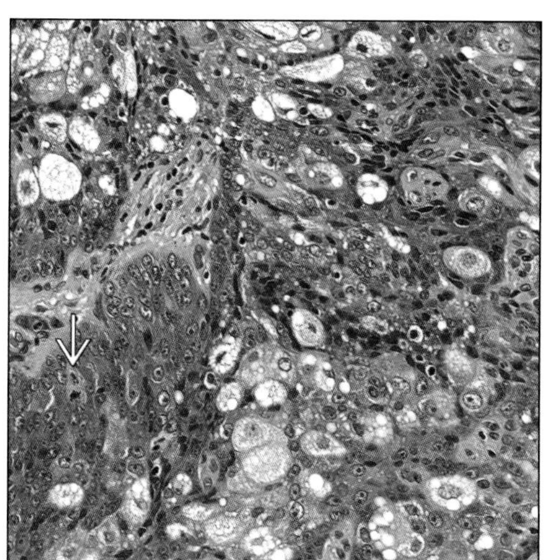

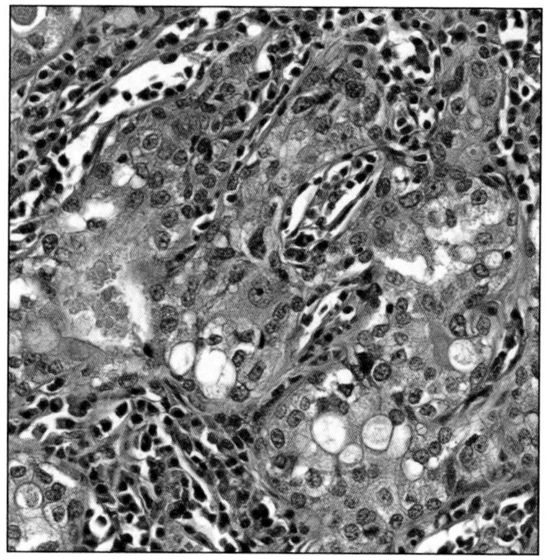

(Left) *There is well-developed pleomorphism in this area of tumor, showing predominantly a basaloid phenotype. Sebocytes in clusters and individually are noted throughout. A mitosis is seen ➡.* **(Right)** *This area shows a background of inflammatory elements intermingled with the neoplastic proliferation. This area shows a predominantly ductal and squamous appearance without well-developed sebaceous differentiation in this area.*

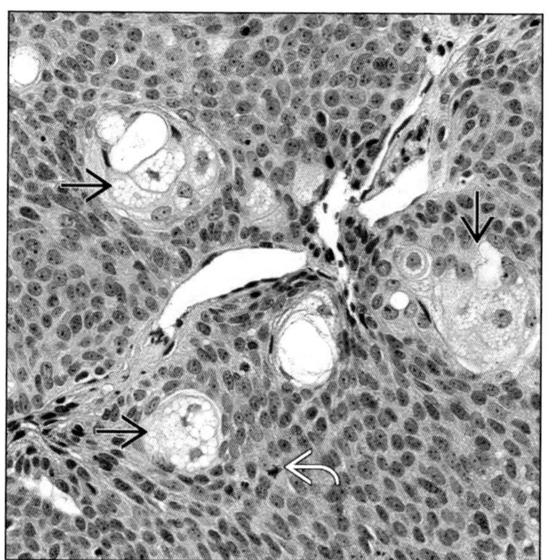

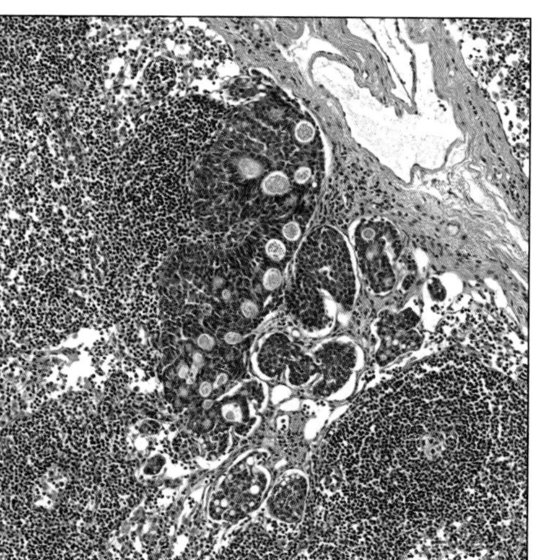

(Left) *There are small collections of sebocytes ➡ set in a tumor showing a predominantly squamoid appearance. The sheet of neoplastic cells has a "pavement" appearance, with isolated mitoses ➡.* **(Right)** *The periparotid lymph nodes should be carefully examined, as metastatic foci from sebaceous carcinoma may be identified, as shown here. This tumor shows a basaloid and cystic pattern similar to what was seen in parts of the primary tumor.*

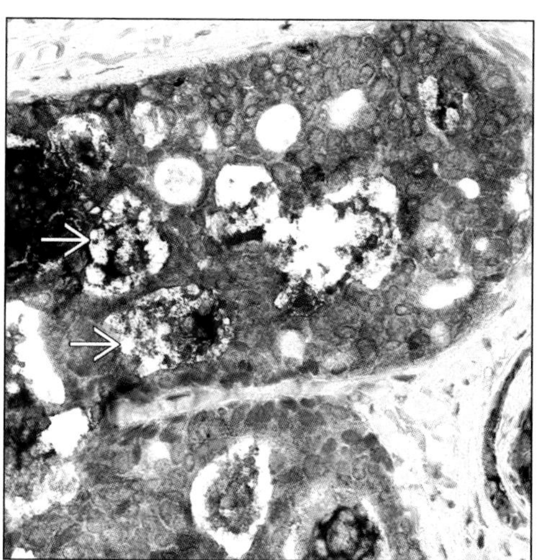

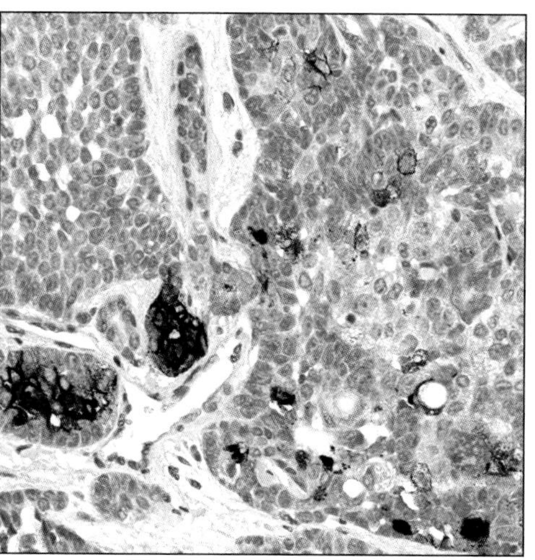

(Left) *EMA can be used to highlight areas of sebocytic differentiation, which show prominent deposition. In many cases there is an accentuation of the cytoplasmic vesiculation ➡, as noted here.* **(Right)** *BRST-2 (GCDFP-15) is also used to highlight the sebocytes, as shown in this area. The background basaloid or squamoid cells do not stain with this marker. Therefore, it is important to review the entire tumor to find these areas of isolated immunoreactivity.*

SIALOBLASTOMA

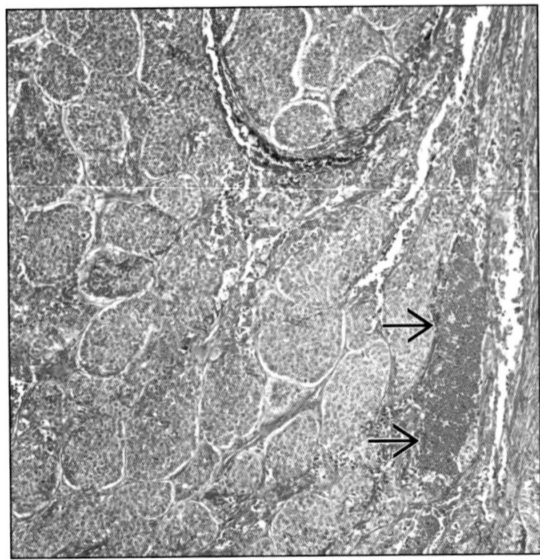

The tumor shows a lobular architecture with a slight cracking artifact around the lobules. An area of comedonecrosis ➔ is present with the tumor trabeculae.

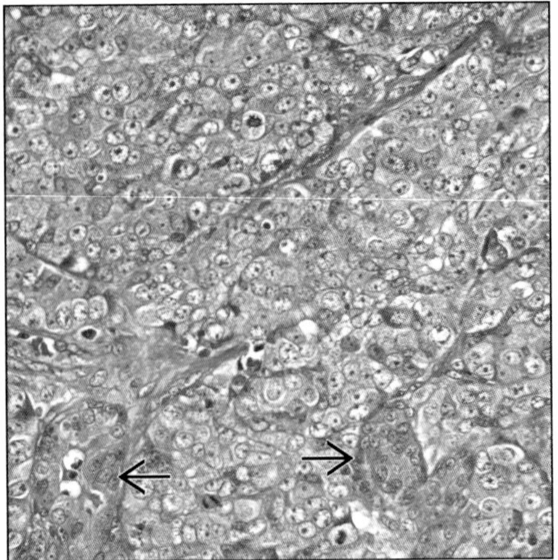

There is a syncytial arrangement of these basaloid cells, showing vesicular to delicate nuclear chromatin. Small duct-like cuboidal cells ➔ are noted within the tumor.

TERMINOLOGY

Synonyms

- Congenital basal cell adenoma
- Embryoma
- Congenital hybrid basal cell adenoma-adenoid cystic carcinoma
- Basaloid adenocarcinoma

Definitions

- Sialoblastoma is low-grade malignant epithelial and myoepithelial neoplasm recapitulating primitive salivary gland anlage

ETIOLOGY/PATHOGENESIS

Reserve Cell Origin

- May arise from retained blastema cells
  - Dysembryogenic changes in parenchyma adjacent to tumor
  - Focal proliferation of terminal ductal epithelial bulbs
  - Salivary anlage at arrested state of differentiation
- May arise from basal reserve cells

CLINICAL ISSUES

Epidemiology

- Incidence
  - Extremely rare congenital tumor
    - < 100 cases worldwide
- Age
  - Prenatal, perinatal, to neonatal period
    - Very rare after 2 years
- Gender
  - Male > Female (1.2:1)

Site

- Parotid > submandibular gland (3:1)

Presentation

- Mass in cheek or submandibular gland region
- If tumors are large, skin ulceration may be seen
- Rapid growth is common
- Infrequently associated with nevus sebaceous and hepatoblastoma
  - Also considered congenital lesions

Treatment

- Options, risks, complications
  - Chemotherapy has untoward long-term sequelae, especially in patients so young
- Surgical approaches
  - Complete surgical excision
- Adjuvant therapy
  - May be used, but complications hamper use in the very young
  - If primary tumor is unresectable, consider chemotherapy

Prognosis

- Biologic behavior is unpredictable and variable
  - Tumor may be benign, indolent, or aggressive
- In **most** patients, surgery is curative
- Recurrences develop in up to 30% of all patients
  - Usually manifests within 4 years of diagnosis
- Regional metastases may be seen in up to 10%
- Distant metastases uncommon
  - Tend to develop in lung most frequently
- Aggressive clinical course suggested by unfavorable histology
  - Perineural &/or vascular invasion, necrosis, significant pleomorphism

IMAGE FINDINGS

Radiographic Findings

- Prenatal sonography may identify tumor
- Expansile, large, lobulated masses

SIALOBLASTOMA

Key Facts

Terminology
- Sialoblastoma is low-grade malignant epithelial and myoepithelial neoplasm recapitulating primitive salivary gland anlage

Clinical Issues
- Age: Prenatal, perinatal, to neonatal period
- Site: Parotid > submandibular gland (3:1)
- Rapid growth is common
- Complete surgical excision, possible chemotherapy
- Biologic behavior is unpredictable and variable
- Aggressive clinical course suggested by
  - Perineural &/or vascular invasion, necrosis, significant pleomorphism

Microscopic Pathology
- Size range: 2-7 cm
- Patterns of growth include
  - Solid nests, cribriform, trabeculae, nodules
- Basaloid epithelial cells with scanty cytoplasm
  - Oval nuclei, single nucleoli, fine chromatin
- More mature cuboidal cells forming ductules
- Myoepithelial spindle-shaped cells are inconspicuous
- Mitoses are usually easy to find
- Necrosis (comedonecrosis) can be detected

Ancillary Tests
- Biphasic immunohistochemistry for ductal and basaloid cells

Top Differential Diagnoses
- Pleomorphic adenoma, basal cell adenoma
- Adenoid cystic carcinoma

- Hemorrhage and necrosis may be useful findings

MACROSCOPIC FEATURES

General Features
- Lobular, multinodular, partially circumscribed mass
- Gray, yellow, or white
- Focal necrosis and hemorrhage may be present

Sections to Be Submitted
- Preoperative core-needle biopsy helps to exclude other lesions that require different management

Size
- Range: 2-7 cm

MICROSCOPIC PATHOLOGY

Histologic Features
- Approximately recapitulates embryologic development of salivary glands at 3rd month
- 2 major patterns of growth, prognostically significant
  - **Favorable pattern**
    - Partial encapsulation
    - Bland basaloid tumor cells with intervening stroma
  - **Unfavorable pattern**
    - Broad pushing to infiltrative borders
    - Perineural or vascular invasion
    - Anaplastic basaloid tumor cells with scant stroma
- Patterns of growth include
  - Solid nests
  - Cribriform
  - Trabeculae or nodules with peripheral palisading
- Basaloid epithelial cells with scanty cytoplasm
- Round to oval nuclei
  - Usually single nucleolus with gossamer-fine chromatin pattern
  - Multiple nucleoli can be seen
- More mature cuboidal cells forming ductules are sometimes seen
  - Peripheral palisading can be present
- Nuclear pleomorphism can be focally recognized
- Stroma is usually loose, immature, and myxoid
- Myoepithelial spindle-shaped cells are inconspicuous
- Mitoses are usually easy to find
  - Seem to increase with recurrent disease
- Necrosis (comedonecrosis) can be detected

ANCILLARY TESTS

Cytology
- Variably arranged, cohesive, solid clusters of basaloid cells
  - Clusters are mixture of ductal cells and rounded, dense, hyaline globular material
    - Globules are magenta on Diff-Quik
- Background with single myoepithelial and epithelial cells

Histochemistry
- PAS-positive secretion in cystic spaces

Immunohistochemistry
- Tumors show biphasic expression
  - Ductal cells: Cytokeratin, CK7, CK19
  - Basaloid/myoepithelial cells: S100 protein, actin, calponin, p63
- p53 overexpressed in tumors with more aggressive biologic behavior
- Increasing Ki-67 labeling associated with unfavorable outcome

DIFFERENTIAL DIAGNOSIS

Pleomorphic Adenoma
- Exceedingly rare in neonatal age group
- Combination of epithelial and myoepithelial cells, with ductal cells
- Chondromyxoid matrix or stroma
- Squamous metaplasia
- Oncocytic change

SIALOBLASTOMA

Immunohistochemistry

Antibody	Reactivity	Staining Pattern	Comment
S100	Positive	Nuclear & cytoplasmic	Nearly all tumor cells but more intensely in spindle cells
Vimentin	Positive	Cytoplasmic	Nearly all tumor cells
CK-PAN	Positive	Cytoplasmic	Accentuates ductal cells but can be seen in all cells
CK7	Positive	Cell membrane	Luminal or duct-like cells
CK19	Positive	Cell membrane	Luminal or duct-like cells
p63	Positive	Nuclear	Variable degree but especially basaloid cells
Actin-sm	Positive	Cytoplasmic	Highlights myoepithelial/basaloid cells
Calponin	Positive	Cytoplasmic	Highlights myoepithelial/basaloid cells
p53	Positive	Nuclear	Increased expression associated with worse clinical outcome
α-fetoprotein	Positive	Cytoplasmic	Rarely detected but seen in tumors with unfavorable outcome
HER2	Positive	Cell membrane	Moderate staining in limited population of cells
Ki-67	Positive	Nuclear	< 2% index: Favorable outcome; 40-80% index: Unfavorable outcome

- No invasion

Basal Cell Adenoma

- Very rare in neonatal age group
- Monotonous population of basaloid cells
- Lack mitoses
- Lacks pleomorphism
- May have excess basal lamina material, a hyaline PAS-positive tissue

Adenoid Cystic Carcinoma

- Exceedingly rare in neonatal age group
- Invasive lesion, with strong perineural proclivity
- Cribriform and sieve-like pattern is common
- Peg/carrot-shaped cells, often arranged in palisade
- Reduplicated basement membrane material
- Mucopolysaccharide secretions

Teratoma

- Tumors show elements from all 3 germinative layers
  - Endoderm
  - Ectoderm
  - Mesoderm
- Immature tumors
  - Highly malignant
  - Cellular pleomorphism
  - Necrosis
  - Increased mitoses

SELECTED REFERENCES

1. Dardick I et al: Sialoblastoma in adults: distinction from adenoid cystic carcinoma. Oral Surg Oral Med Oral Pathol Oral Radiol Endod. 109(1):109-16, 2010
2. Patil DT et al: Sialoblastoma: utility of Ki-67 and p53 as a prognostic tool and review of literature. Pediatr Dev Pathol. 13(1):32-8, 2010
3. Mertens F et al: Clonal chromosome aberrations in a sialoblastoma. Cancer Genet Cytogenet. 189(1):68-9, 2009
4. Scott JX et al: Treatment of metastatic sialoblastoma with chemotherapy and surgery. Pediatr Blood Cancer. 50(1):134-7, 2008
5. Williams SB et al: Sialoblastoma: a clinicopathologic and immunohistochemical study of 7 cases. Ann Diagn Pathol. 10(6):320-6, 2006
6. Herrmann BW et al: Congenital salivary gland anlage tumor: a case series and review of the literature. Int J Pediatr Otorhinolaryngol. 69(2):149-56, 2005
7. Yekeler E et al: Sialoblastoma: MRI findings. Pediatr Radiol. 34(12):1005-7, 2004
8. Huang R et al: Imprint cytology of metastatic sialoblastoma. A case report. Acta Cytol. 47(6):1123-6, 2003
9. Mostafapour SP et al: Sialoblastoma of the submandibular gland: report of a case and review of the literature. Int J Pediatr Otorhinolaryngol. 53(2):157-61, 2000
10. Brandwein M et al: Sialoblastoma: clinicopathological/ immunohistochemical study. Am J Surg Pathol. 23(3):342-8, 1999
11. Seifert G et al: The congenital basal cell adenoma of salivary glands. Contribution to the differential diagnosis of congenital salivary gland tumours. Virchows Arch. 430(4):311-9, 1997
12. Som PM et al: Sialoblastoma (embryoma): MR findings of a rare pediatric salivary gland tumor. AJNR Am J Neuroradiol. 18(5):847-50, 1997
13. Dehner LP et al: Salivary gland anlage tumor ("congenital pleomorphic adenoma"). A clinicopathologic, immunohistochemical and ultrastructural study of nine cases. Am J Surg Pathol. 18(1):25-36, 1994
14. Batsakis JG et al: Embryoma (sialoblastoma) of salivary glands. Ann Otol Rhinol Laryngol. 101(11):958-60, 1992
15. Taylor GP: Congenital epithelial tumor of the parotid-sialoblastoma. Pediatr Pathol. 8(4):447-52, 1988

SIALOBLASTOMA

Clinical, Microscopic, and Immunohistochemical Features

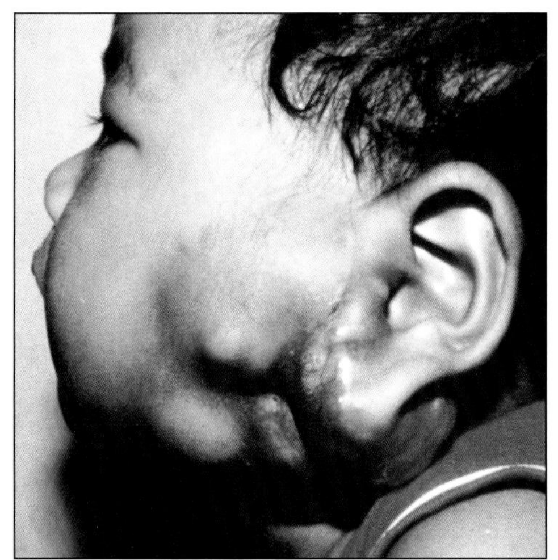

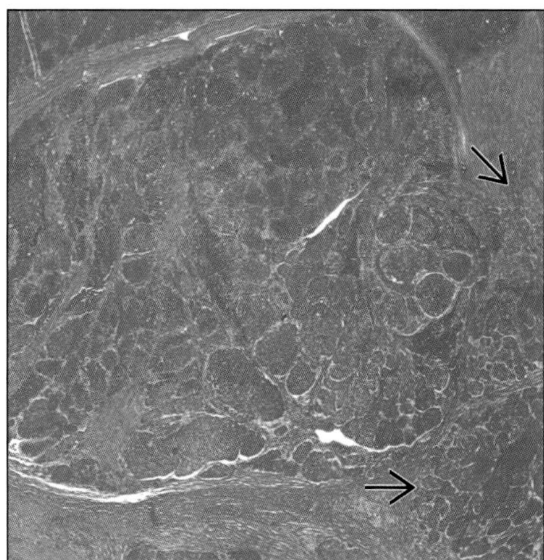

*(**Left**) This boy, less than 1 year old, was noted to have a rapidly enlarging mass in the region of the parotid gland. Note the surface ulceration and involvement of the preauricular, retroauricular, and superior cervical regions. This is a typical presentation of this uncommon neoplasm. (**Right**) There is a multinodular appearance to this tumor, showing heavy fibrous connective tissue. There is extension of the tumor into the fibrous connective tissue capsule ⇒. (Courtesy R. Foss, DDS.)*

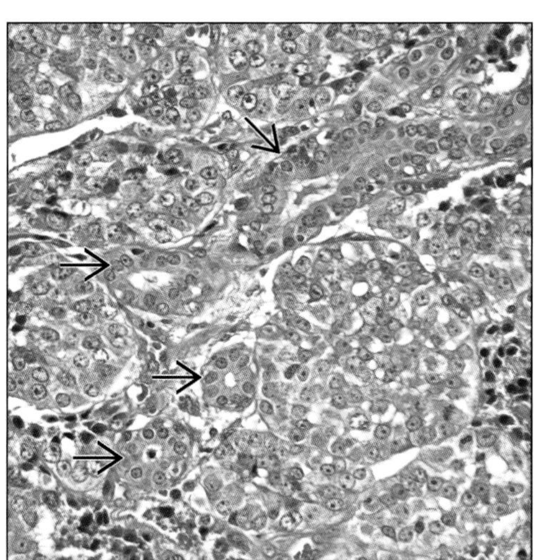

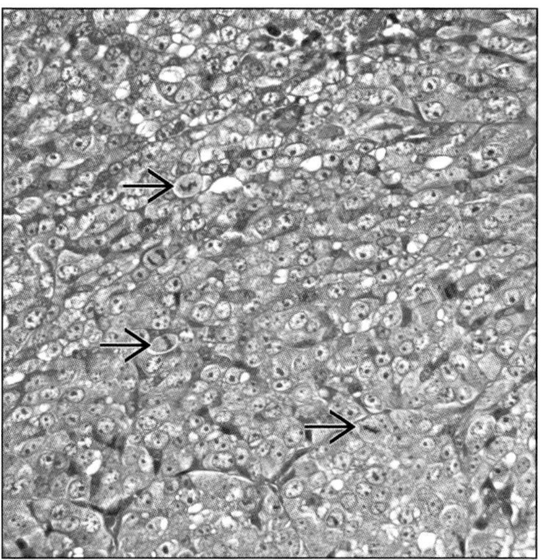

*(**Left**) This image highlights the biphasic appearance of the tumor. There are nests of basaloid cells juxtaposed with more mature cuboidal cells, which are forming ductules ⇒. A hint of palisading is noted. (**Right**) A sheet-like to focally nodular pattern is present in this tumor. Note the vesicular nuclear chromatin distribution and the single prominent nucleoli. Mitotic figures ⇒ are easily identified in this tumor.*

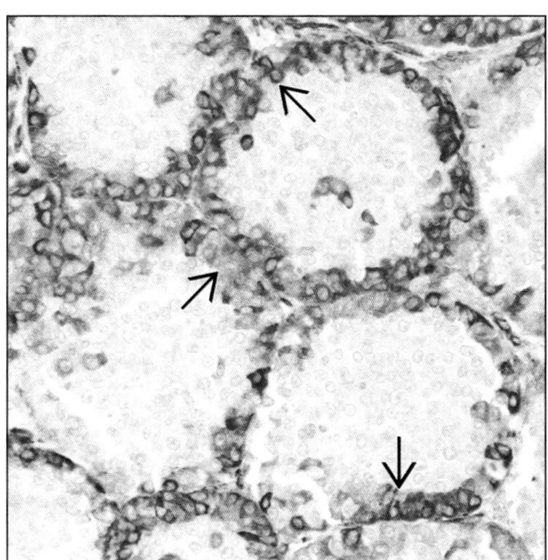

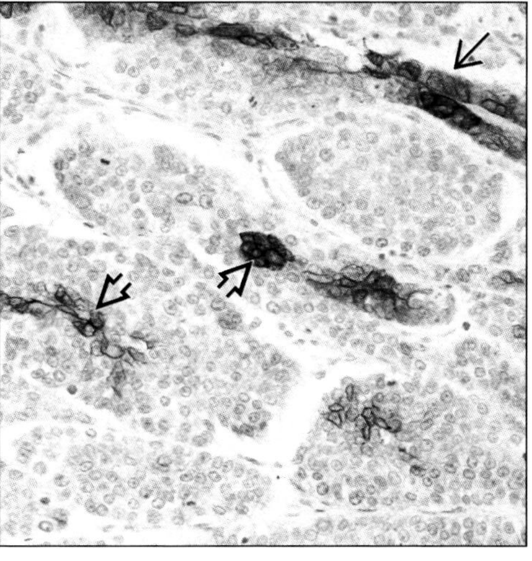

*(**Left**) Smooth muscle actin shows a very strong decoration of the peripheral cells ⇒ in each of the lobules of this sialoblastoma. Other markers (S100 protein, calponin, p63) may also be used to highlight the myoepithelial cells. (Courtesy R. Foss, DDS.) (**Right**) The ductal ⇒ and luminal ⇨ cells are highlighted with a pan-cytokeratin immunohistochemistry. Focal reactivity is noted in other cells, but the biphasic appearance is accentuated with this stain. (Courtesy R. Foss, DDS.)*

PROTOCOL FOR THE EXAMINATION OF SALIVARY GLAND SPECIMENS

Major Salivary Glands

Incisional Biopsy, Excisional Biopsy, Resection

Specimen

___ Parotid gland

  ___ Superficial lobe only

  ___ Deep lobe only

  ___ Total parotid gland

___ Submandibular gland

___ Sublingual gland

Received

___ Fresh

___ In formalin

___ Other (specify): ____________________________

Procedure (select all that apply)

___ Incisional biopsy

___ Excisional biopsy

___ Resection, parotid gland

  ___ Superficial parotidectomy

  ___ Total parotidectomy

___ Resection, submandibular gland

___ Resection, sublingual gland

___ Neck (lymph node) dissection (specify): ____________________________

___ Other (specify): ____________________________

___ Not specified

**Specimen Integrity*

*___ Intact

*___ Fragmented

Specimen Size

Greatest dimensions: _________ x _________ x _________ cm

*Additional dimensions (if more than 1 part): _________ x _________ x _________ cm

Specimen Laterality

___ Right

___ Left

___ Bilateral

___ Not specified

Tumor Site (select all that apply)

___ Parotid gland

  ___ Superficial lobe

  ___ Deep lobe

  ___ Entire parotid gland

___ Submandibular gland

___ Sublingual gland

___ Other (specify): ____________________________

___ Not specified

Tumor Focality

___ Single focus

___ Bilateral

___ Multifocal (specify): ____________________________

Tumor Size

Greatest dimension: _________ cm

*Additional dimensions: _________ x _________ cm

___ Cannot be determined

*Tumor Description (select all that apply)

*___ Encapsulated/circumscribed
*___ Invasive
*___ Solid
*___ Cystic
*___ Other (specify): ___________________________

*Macroscopic Extent of Tumor (extent of invasion)

*Specify: ___________________________

Histologic Type (select all that apply)

___ Acinic cell carcinoma
___ Adenoid cystic carcinoma
___ Adenocarcinoma, not otherwise specified (NOS)
  ___ Low grade
  ___ Intermediate grade
  ___ High grade
___ Basal cell adenocarcinoma
___ Carcinoma ex-pleomorphic adenoma (malignant mixed tumor)
  ___ Grade
    ___ Low grade
    ___ High grade
  ___ Invasion
    ___ Intracapsular (noninvasive)
    ___ Minimally invasive
    ___ Invasive
___ Carcinosarcoma (true malignant mixed tumor)
___ Clear cell adenocarcinoma
___ Cystadenocarcinoma
___ Epithelial-myoepithelial carcinoma
___ Large cell carcinoma
___ Low-grade cribriform cystadenocarcinoma
___ Lymphoepithelial carcinoma
___ Metastasizing pleomorphic adenoma
___ Mucoepidermoid carcinoma
  ___ Low grade
  ___ Intermediate grade
  ___ High grade
___ Mucinous adenocarcinoma (colloid carcinoma)
___ Myoepithelial carcinoma (malignant myoepithelioma)
___ Oncocytic carcinoma
___ Polymorphous low-grade adenocarcinoma
___ Salivary duct carcinoma
___ Sebaceous adenocarcinomas
  ___ Sebaceous adenocarcinoma
  ___ Sebaceous lymphadenocarcinoma
___ Sialoblastoma
___ Small cell (neuroendocrine) carcinoma
___ Squamous cell carcinoma, primary
___ Undifferentiated carcinoma, large cell type
___ Other (specify): ___________________________
___ Carcinoma, type cannot be determined

Histologic Grade

___ Not applicable

PROTOCOL FOR THE EXAMINATION OF SALIVARY GLAND SPECIMENS

___ GX: Cannot be assessed
___ G1: Well differentiated
___ G2: Moderately differentiated
___ G3: Poorly differentiated
___ Other (specify): ___________________________

Microscopic Tumor Extension

*Specify: ___________________________

Margins

___ Cannot be assessed
___ Margins uninvolved by carcinoma
Distance of tumor from closest margin: ________ mm or ________ cm
Specify margin, if possible: ___________________________
___ Margin(s) involved by carcinoma
Specify margin(s) if possible: ___________________________

Treatment Effect (applicable to carcinomas treated with neoadjuvant therapy)

*___Not identified
*___Present (specify): ___________________________
*___Indeterminate

Lymph-Vascular Invasion

___ Not identified
___ Present
___ Indeterminate

Perineural Invasion

___ Not identified
___ Present
___ Indeterminate

Lymph Nodes, Extranodal Extension

___ Not identified
___ Present
___ Indeterminate

Pathologic Staging (pTNM)

TNM Descriptors (required only if applicable) (select all that apply)
___ m (multiple primary tumors)
___ r (recurrent)
___ y (post-treatment)

Primary Tumor (pT)†
___ pTX: Cannot be assessed
___ pT0: No evidence of primary tumor
___ pT1: Tumor ≤ 2 cm in greatest dimension **without extraparenchymal extension**
___ pT2: Tumor > 2 cm but ≤ 4 cm in greatest dimension **without extraparenchymal extension**
___ pT3: Tumor > 4 cm &/or tumor **with extraparenchymal extension**
___ pT4a: Moderately advanced tumor
Tumor invades skin, mandible, ear canal, &/or facial nerve
___ pT4b: Very advanced local disease
Tumor invades skull base &/or pterygoid plates &/or encases carotid artery

Regional Lymph Nodes (pN)#
___ pNX: Cannot be assessed
___ pN0: No regional lymph node metastasis
___ pN1: Metastasis in single ipsilateral lymph node, ≤ 3 cm in greatest dimension
___ pN2: Metastasis in a single ipsilateral lymph node, > 3 cm but ≤ 6 cm in greatest dimension, or in multiple lymph nodes none > 6 cm in greate4st dimension, or in bilateral or contralateral lymoph nodes, none > 6 cm in greatest dimension
___ pN2a: Metastasis in single ipsilateral lymph node, > 3 cm but ≤ 6 cm in greatest dimension

____ pN2b: Metastasis in multiple ipsilateral lymph nodes, none > 6 cm in greatest dimension

____ pN2c: Metastasis in bilateral or contralateral lymph nodes, none > 6 cm in greatest dimension

____ pN3: Metastasis in lymph node, > 6 cm in greatest dimension

Specify: Number examined: ________

Number involved: ________

*Size (greatest dimension) of largest positive lymph node: ________

Distant Metastasis (pM)

____ Not applicable

____ pM1: Distant metastasis

*Specify site(s), if known: ____________________

*Additional Pathologic Findings (select all that apply)

*____ Sialadenitis

*____ Tumor associated lymphoid proliferation (TALP)

*____ Other (specify): ____________________

*Ancillary Studies

*Specify type(s): ____________________

*Specify result(s): ____________________

*Clinical History (select all that apply)

*____ Neoadjuvant therapy

*____ Yes (specify type): ____________________

*____ No

*____ Indeterminate

*____ Other (specify): ____________________

*Data elements with asterisks are not required. However, these elements may be clinically important but are not yet validated or regularly used in patient management. †There is no category of carcinoma in situ (pTis) relative to carcinomas of salivary glands (major, minor). #Superior mediastinal lymph nodes are considered regional lymph nodes (level VII). Midline nodes are considered ipsilateral nodes. Adapted with permission from College of American Pathologists, "Protocol for the Examination of Specimens from Patients with Carcinomas of the Salivary Glands." Web posting date October 2009, www.cap.org.

Anatomic Stage/Prognostic Groups

Group	T	N	M
I	T1	N0	M0
II	T2	N0	M0
III	T1, T2, T3	N1	M0
	T3	N0	M0
IVA	T1, T2, T3	N2	M0
	T4a	N0, N1, N2	M0
IVB	T4b	Any N	M0
	Any T	N3	M0
IVC	Any T	Any N	M1

Adapted from 7th edition AJCC Staging Forms.

General Notes

Note	Description
m suffix	Indicates the presence of multiple primary tumors in a single site and is recorded in parentheses: pT(m)NM
y prefix	Indicates cases in which classification is performed during or following initial multimodality therapy. The cTNM or pTNM category is identified by a "y" prefix. The ycTNM or ypTNM categorizes the extent of tumor actually present at the time of that examination. They "y" categorization is not an estimate of tumor prior to multimodality therapy
r prefix	Indicates a recurrent tumor when staged after a disease-free interval and is identified by the "r" prefix: rTNM
a prefix	Designates the stage determined at autopsy: aTNM

Adapted from 7th edition AJCC Staging Forms.

PROTOCOL FOR THE EXAMINATION OF SALIVARY GLAND SPECIMENS

Anatomic and Tumor Staging Graphics

*(**Left**) The major salivary glands are surrounded by a rich plexus of lymphatics and lymph nodes. Many lymph nodes are within the parotid gland, as illustrated here. (**Right**) Graphic shows a large tumor in the parotid salivary gland. This tumor shows extension into the ear canal and facial nerve, placing it in the pT4a category. The lymph nodes would also need to be evaluated to place the tumor in the correct TNM classification.*

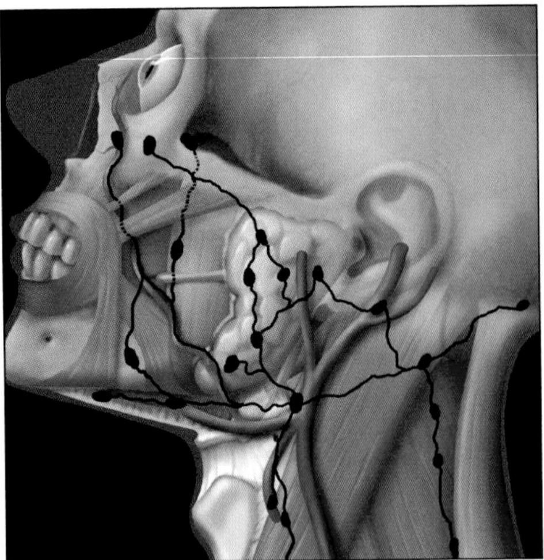

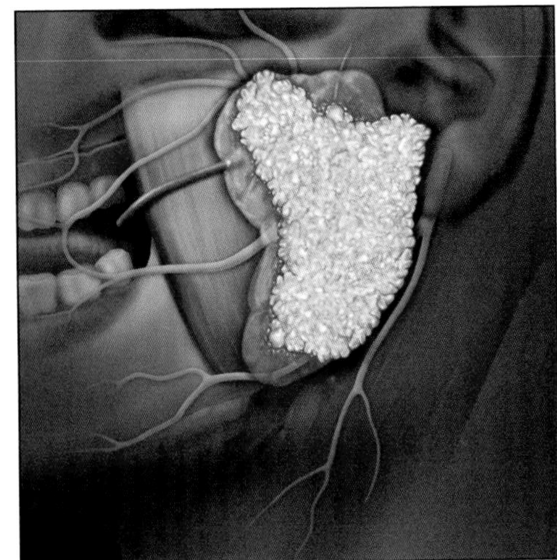

*(**Left**) The intimate relationship between the superficial and deep lobe of the parotid gland with the surrounding bone, nerves, and vessels is very important in the accurate staging of salivary gland neoplasms. (**Right**) There is a 1.8 cm tumor identified in the superficial lobe of the parotid gland. There is no extraparenchymal extension and no perineural invasion. This tumor would be placed in the pT1 category.*

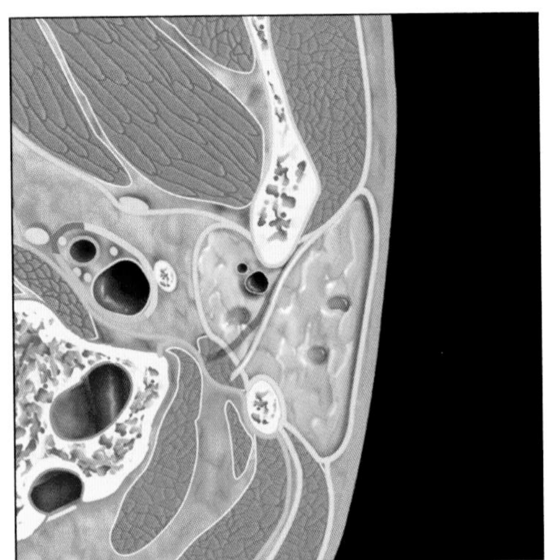

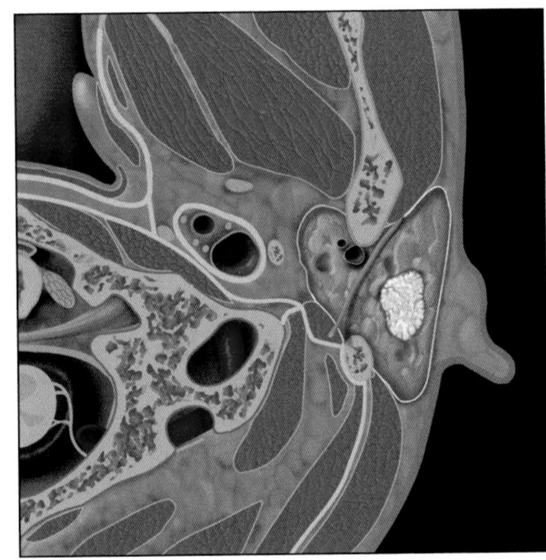

*(**Left**) Axial graphic highlights the multiple compartments of the neck at the level of the parotid space (PS). The carotid space (CS) and masticator space (MS) are quite close, highlighting the need for very careful clinical, radiographic, and gross evaluation of parotid tumors for accurate staging. (**Right**) This large tumor originated in the deep lobe of the parotid gland, but has expanded to fill into the space of the masticator muscle and carotid sheath, placing this tumor in the pT4b category.*

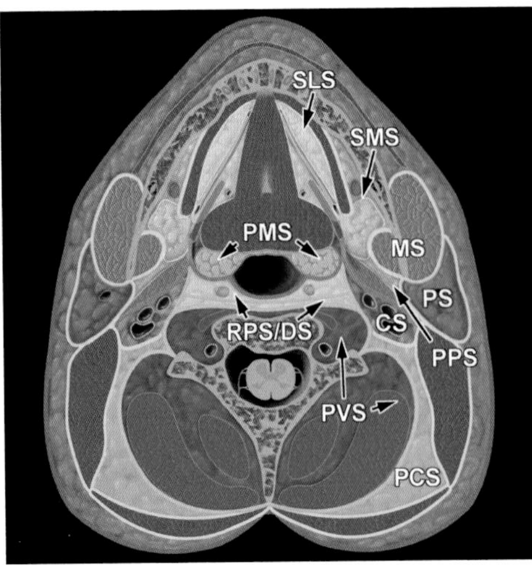

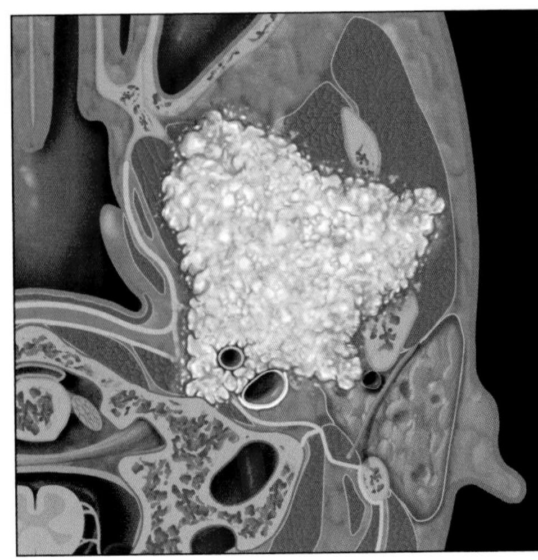

Anatomic and Tumor Staging Graphics

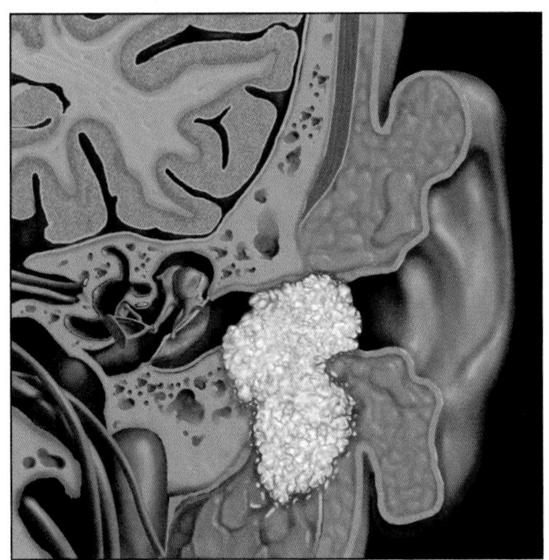

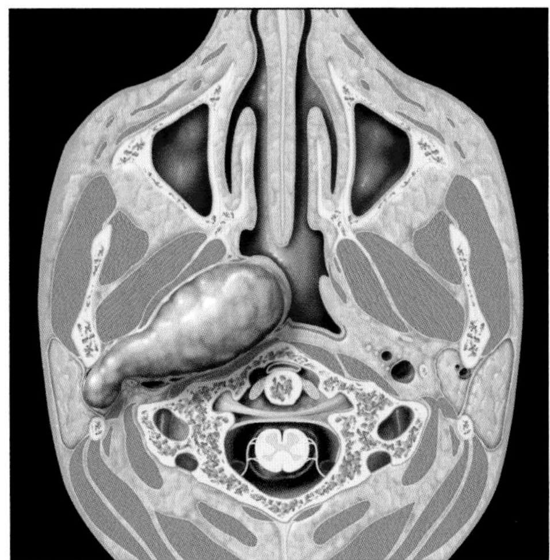

(Left) *In some patients, a parotid gland tumor may present as an external auditory canal mass, as illustrated here. The tumor may be benign (pleomorphic adenoma), but that is quite uncommon.* ***(Right)*** *Axial graphic demonstrates how a deep lobe of the parotid tumor has expanded into the oropharynx/nasopharynx, presenting as a submucosal mass. The carotid sheath is compressed, but it is not invaded by this pleomorphic adenoma.*

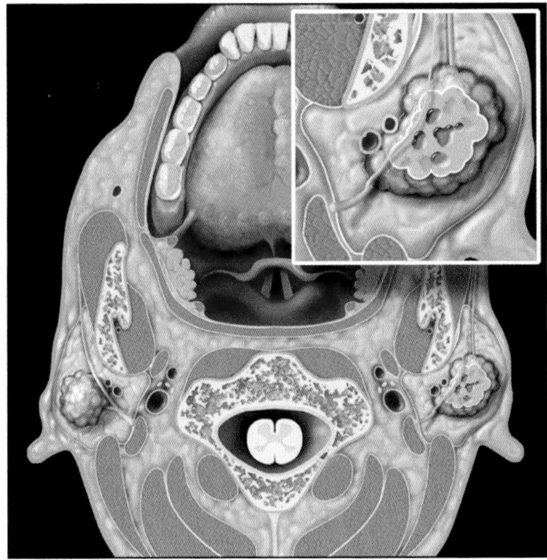

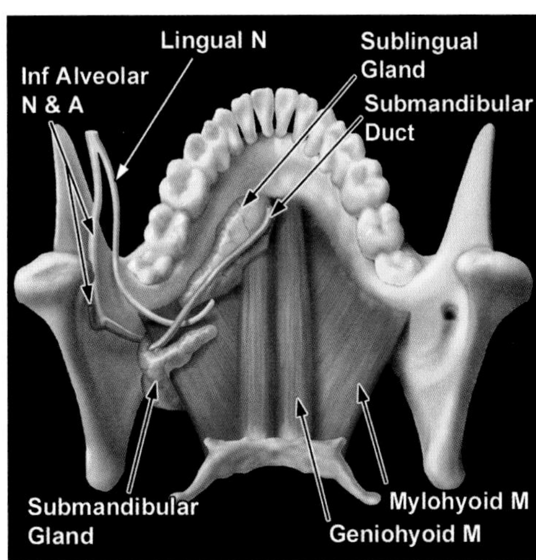

(Left) *Bilateral tumors are not infrequent in the salivary glands, although they are more commonly benign than malignant. It is important to realize that nerve compression or entrapment by the tumor is not the same as perineural invasion.* ***(Right)*** *An anatomic depiction of the submandibular and sublingual glands and their relationship to the surrounding muscles, bones, and nerves. Careful evaluation of these areas is required in staging tumors of these glands.*

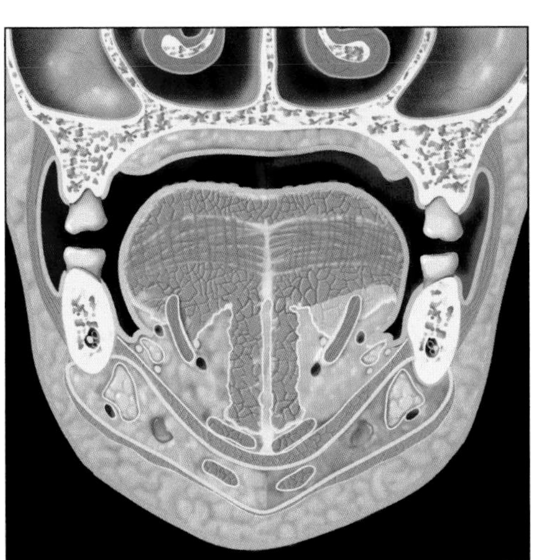

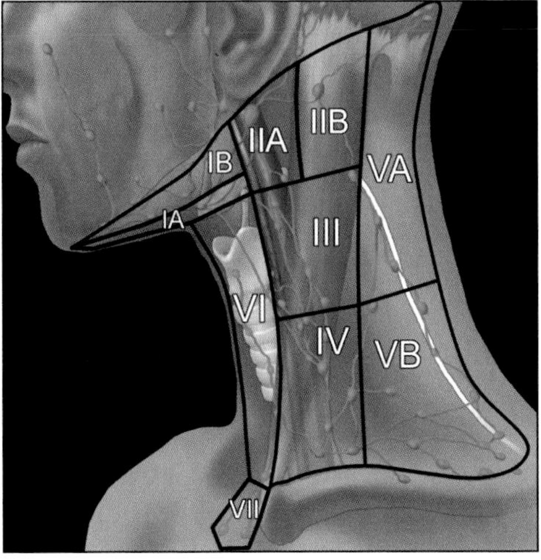

(Left) *This coronal view highlights the many anatomic relationships between tumors of minor salivary glands that may develop within the oral cavity, tongue, and soft tissues.* ***(Right)*** *Neck lymph node dissection is frequently employed for malignancies of the head and neck. The neck lymph nodes are separated into compartments (I-VII), each affected more frequently by specific tumor primary sites or tumor types. Each compartment is usually reported separately.*

Jaw

Congenital/Genetic/Hereditary

Infectious

Reactive

Cysts

Benign Neoplasm

Malignant Neoplasm

CHERUBISM

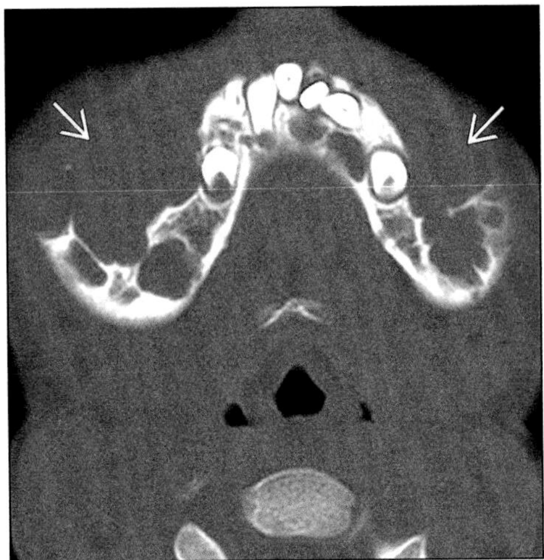

This CT shows bilateral, multilocular, radiolucent areas ➔ within the mandible. The cortex is perforated, resulting in associated teeth displacement.

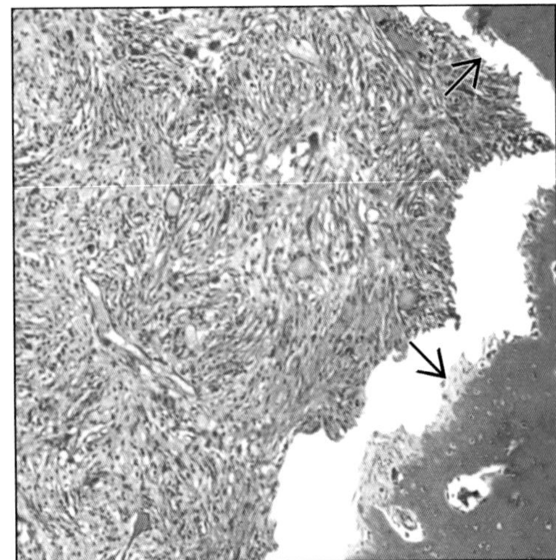

Cherubism often appears as a spindle cell lesion with resorption of the adjacent bone ➔ and subsequent re-formation of the bone, leading to "expansion" of the bone clinically and radiographically.

TERMINOLOGY

Definitions

- Inherited disease characterized by progressive, painless, symmetrical expansion of the jaws, resulting in cherubic facial appearance
  - Characterized by loss of bone, restricted to the jaws, and by replacement with fibrous tissue
  - Affected patients resemble **cherubs** (putti) in Renaissance paintings: Round face and upward gaze toward heaven

ETIOLOGY/PATHOGENESIS

Inherited

- Autosomal-dominant hereditary childhood disease with variable expression causing self-limiting fibro-osseous dysplasia affecting the jaws bilaterally
  - No relationship to fibrous dysplasia
- Sporadic cases are described

CLINICAL ISSUES

Epidemiology

- Incidence
  - Rare disorder
- Age
  - Nearly always identified before 5 years
    - Most often between 12- 24 months
    - No cases reported at birth
- Gender
  - Male > Female (2:1)
    - 100% penetrance in males
    - 50-70% penetrance in females

Site

- Jaws bilaterally
- Mandible affected most commonly
  - Particularly ascending rami, retromolar area, and molar area
  - Coronoid process can be involved
  - Condyles are always spared
- Posterior maxilla less frequently affected

Presentation

- Initially described by Jones in 1933 as **familial multilocular cystic disease of the jaws**
- Significant clinical variation
  - Symptoms and signs depend on severity of condition
    - No clinical or radiologic features
    - Grotesquely deforming mandibular and maxillary overgrowth
  - Respiratory distress and impaired vision and hearing
  - The younger the age at initial presentation, the faster it seems to grow
  - Cervical adenopathy is occasionally present
- Symmetrical, hard, and painless swelling of the jaws described as angel-like
  - Extragnathic bony involvement is rare (ribs, humerus, femur, tibia)
- Usually isolated disease in otherwise mentally and physically normal child
  - Often history of another afflicted family member
- With florid infraorbital maxillary involvement, inferior rim of sclera appears more prominent, giving classic "eye to heaven" appearance
- Malaligned teeth, impacted teeth, or delayed dentition may be seen due to the jaw disorder
- Rarely associated with Noonan syndrome, Ramon syndrome, and fragile X syndrome

Laboratory Tests

- Serum phosphorus and calcium usually normal
- Alkaline phosphatase may be high during active stages of the disease

CHERUBISM

Key Facts

Terminology
- Inherited disease characterized by progressive, painless, symmetrical expansion of the jaws, resulting in a cherubic facial appearance

Clinical Issues
- Autosomal-dominant hereditary childhood disease with variable expression
- Nearly always identified before 5 years of age
- Male > Female (2:1)
- Mandible affected most commonly
- Great variation in clinical expression
- Symmetrical, hard, and painless swelling of the jaws described as angel-like
- No specific uniform treatment
  - Generally, watchful waiting for spontaneous regression/involution in adulthood
  - Radiation absolutely **contraindicated**

Image Findings
- Bilateral, multilocular, radiolucent areas within gnathic bones

Microscopic Pathology
- Histologic appearance is **not** diagnostic without clinical and radiographic findings
- Highly vascular fibrous stroma (fibroblasts) arranged in whorled pattern
- Numerous osteoclastic-type multinucleated giant cells with prominent nucleoli
  - Giant cells arranged near hemorrhagic foci

Top Differential Diagnoses
- Fibrous dysplasia, infantile cortical hyperostosis, hyperparathyroidism, giant cell tumor

Natural History
- Bone is replaced by proliferating fibrous tissue that contains giant cells
- Maxilla responds before mandible
  - Reappearance of maxillary antra
- Affected children appear normal at birth
- Maximum enlargement usually develops within 2 years of onset
- Disease may undergo spontaneous involution during teen years
  - Maxillary lesions tend to regress earlier than mandible lesions
  - Disease may stabilize at end of puberty
- Facial appearance may return to normal by 4th or 5th decade

Treatment
- Options, risks, complications
  - No uniform treatment
  - Generally, watchful waiting for spontaneous regression/involution in adulthood
  - Considered a self-limited condition
    - Treatment depends on patients' functional and esthetic needs
- Surgical approaches
  - Early surgical intervention is contraindicated because it seems to predispose to recurrences
  - Surgery limited to patients with
    - Impaired speech, chewing or swallowing difficulties
    - Major deformities that may cause psychological problems
  - Cosmetic surgery in only a few cases
- Radiation
  - Absolutely **contraindicated** due to potential risk of osteoradionecrosis and fibrosarcoma development

Prognosis
- Excellent long-term prognosis
- Vast majority of cases show no residual disease after 30 years
  - Minor jaw enlargement may remain

IMAGE FINDINGS

Radiographic Findings
- Bilateral, multilocular, radiolucent areas within gnathic bones
- Extent of lesions varies from minor to massive involvement of both jaws
- Anatomic location
  - Usually appear at mandibular angle, then spread to ascending rami and body
  - Maxillary processes may also be involved
  - Other facial bones may be affected
- In adults, multilocular rarefactions become sclerotic with progressive calcification
- Roentgenograms occasionally provide only sign of disease
  - Diagnostic when bilateral
- Cortex may be perforated
- Teeth may be displaced, unerupted, and appear to be floating in cyst-like spaces
- Inferior alveolar canal (mandible) may be displaced, with lesions occupying alveolar process, angle, and ramus
- May advance toward incisors, obliterating sigmoid notch, but condyles are spared
- Maxilla: Alveolar widening may result in narrow V-shaped palate
  - May cause backward displacement of tongue
  - Palatal vault may be obliterated in severe cases
    - May cause dysarthria, dysphagia, dyspnea

MACROSCOPIC FEATURES

General Features
- Unencapsulated, periosteum not normally found
- Appears reddish, gray, yellowish, or bluish
- Consistency varies from hard, semi-hard to soft, jelly-like

Size
- Variable depending on clinical presentation

CHERUBISM

MICROSCOPIC PATHOLOGY

Histologic Features

- Histologic appearance is **not** diagnostic without clinical and radiographic findings
- Highly vascular fibrous stroma arranged in whorled pattern
  - Contains large numbers of fibroblasts
  - Mitoses may be present but are neither increased nor atypical
  - Blood vessels are well formed with enlarged endothelial cells
- Numerous osteoclastic-type multinucleated giant cells
  - Prominent nucleoli
  - Mainly arranged near hemorrhagic foci and degenerating hemosiderin
- Perivascular collagen cuffing around small capillaries primarily
- Mature lesions exhibit more dense fibrous tissue, with fewer multinucleated giant cells
- Bone remodeling can be seen at periphery
  - Bone represents remodeled trabeculae, not primary bone formation
  - Polarized light will highlight woven bone appearance
- In a few cases, immature odontogenic material may be found
  - Tooth germs may be entrapped by process
- In a few cases, giant cells may be abundant
  - May cause confusion with central giant cell granuloma or brown tumor of hyperparathyroidism

ANCILLARY TESTS

Cytogenetics

- Point mutations in *SH3BP2* gene

Molecular Genetics

- Germline mutations in *SH3BP2* gene encoding adapter protein
  - Chromosome 4p16.3
  - Mutations cause dysregulation of *Msx-1* gene, involved in regulating mesenchymal interaction in craniofacial morphogenesis
  - Mutations are not detected in all cases

DIFFERENTIAL DIAGNOSIS

Fibrous Dysplasia

- Not usually familial
- Appears between 10-30 years
- Seldom bilateral
- Bony abnormality with prominent, "alphabet letters" slender bone in background stroma

Infantile Cortical Hyperostosis

- Presents in 1st 6 months of life
- Not bilateral
- Radiographically does not produce cystic areas
- Thickening of mandibular lower border

Hyperparathyroidism

- Rare in patients younger than 30 years
- Generally is not bilateral or symmetrical
- Increased serum alkaline phosphatase, increased serum calcium, decreased phosphorus, and increased urine phosphorus

Giant Cell Tumor

- Unusual in the jaws
- Giant cell reparative granuloma is usually not bilateral, appears different radiographically, may be peripheral

Odontogenic Lesions

- Bilateral cysts are uncommon
- Rare in 1st 5 years of life
- Ameloblastoma: Large cystic lesion showing ameloblastic epithelium, stellate reticulum, and reverse polarity of nuclei
- Odontogenic fibroma: Unique radiographic findings, small odontogenic islands within heavy fibrosis, lacking giant cells

GRADING

Proposed Grading for Clinical Presentation

- Grade 1
  - Limited to both ascending rami of mandible
- Grade 2
  - Involvement of maxillary tuberosities and mandibular ascending rami (congenital absence of 3rd molars)
- Grade 3
  - Massive involvement of both jaws except coronoid processes and condyles

SELECTED REFERENCES

1. Carvalho VM et al: Novel mutations in the SH3BP2 gene associated with sporadic central giant cell lesions and cherubism. Oral Dis. 15(1):106-10, 2009
2. Mortellaro C et al: Diagnosis and treatment of familial cherubism characterized by early onset and rapid development. J Craniofac Surg. 20(1):116-20, 2009
3. Hatani T et al: Adaptor protein 3BP2 and cherubism. Curr Med Chem. 15(6):549-54, 2008
4. Jing X et al: Fine-needle aspiration cytological features of Cherubism. Diagn Cytopathol. 36(3):188-9, 2008
5. Carvalho Silva E et al: Cherubism: clinicoradiographic features, treatment, and long-term follow-up of 8 cases. J Oral Maxillofac Surg. 65(3):517-22, 2007
6. Peñarrocha M et al: Cherubism: a clinical, radiographic, and histopathologic comparison of 7 cases. J Oral Maxillofac Surg. 64(6):924-30, 2006
7. Beaman FD et al: Imaging characteristics of cherubism. AJR Am J Roentgenol. 182(4):1051-4, 2004
8. Kozakiewicz M et al: Cherubism--clinical picture and treatment. Oral Dis. 7(2):123-30, 2001
9. Von Wowern N: Cherubism: a 36-year long-term follow-up of 2 generations in different families and review of the literature. Oral Surg Oral Med Oral Pathol Oral Radiol Endod. 90(6):765-72, 2000
10. Yamaguchi T et al: Cherubism: clinicopathologic features. Skeletal Radiol. 28(6):350-3, 1999

Diagrammatic, Microscopic, and Molecular Features

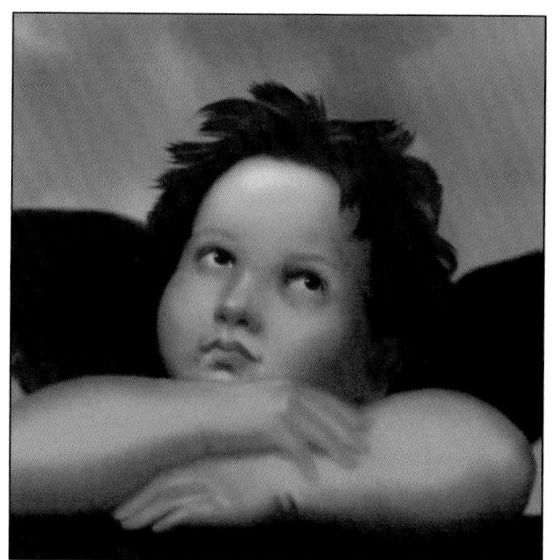

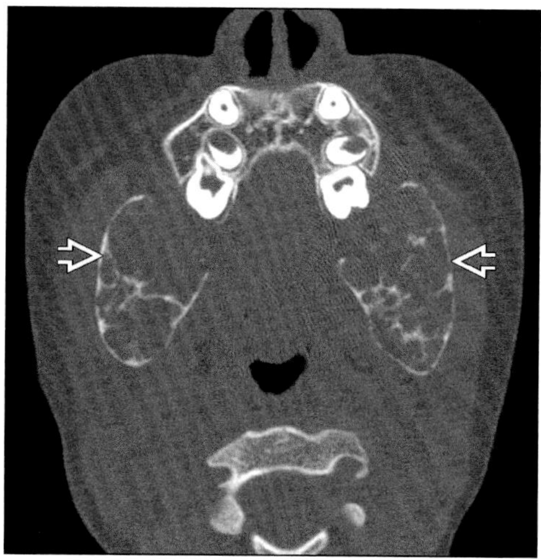

(Left) *This graphic shows a cherub from which the name for this syndrome was modeled. The eyes are slightly directed upward and there is an asymmetry of the cheeks due the underlying changes in the bone. Clinical images testify to this likeness.* ***(Right)*** *Axial bone CT shows a case of cherubism involving the mandible to a greater degree than the maxilla. The bones are expanded and replaced by multiple fibrous-filled cysts ➪. Note the symmetrical bone involvement.*

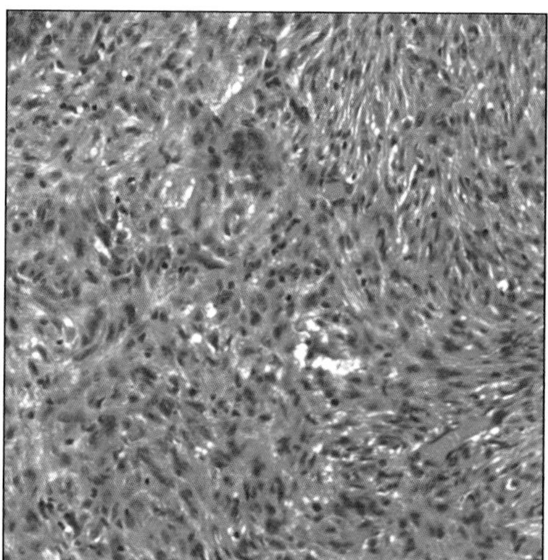

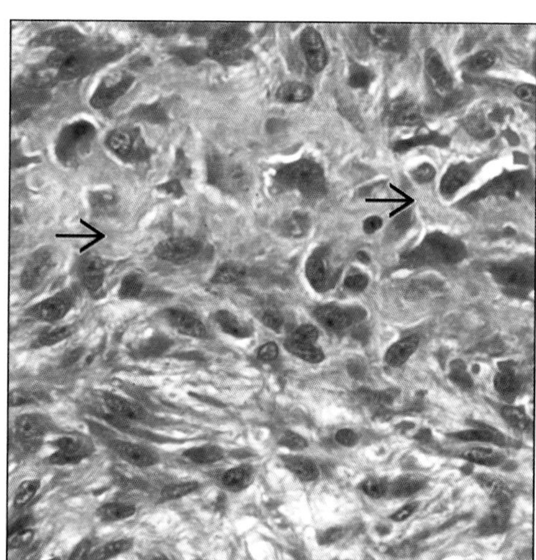

(Left) *The histology in cherubism often appears similar to that of giant cell reparative granuloma with bland spindle cells, often in a storiform pattern, with delicate vessels, scattered inflammation, and occasionally hemosiderin.* ***(Right)*** *High power shows a very delicate osseous matrix forming → directly out of the mononuclear cells. There is blending of the process into the more spindled fibroblasts. Extravasated erythrocytes are noted, often showing hemosiderin as well.*

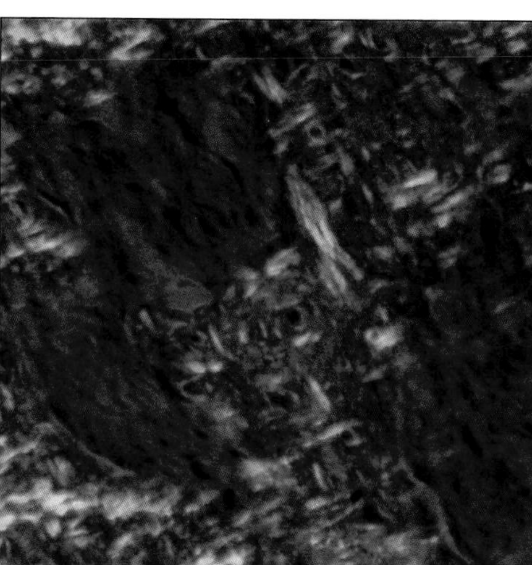

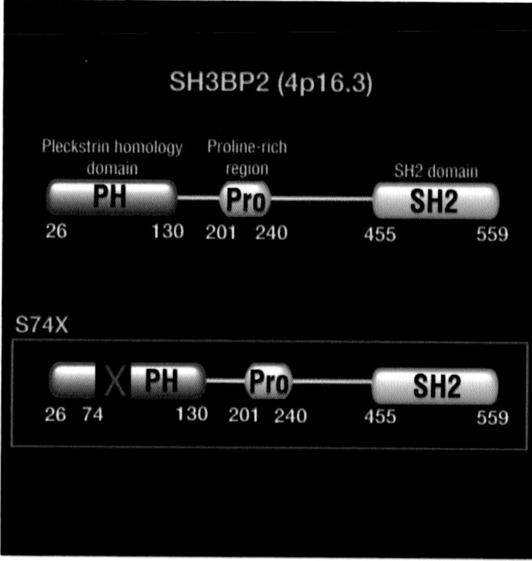

(Left) *Polarized light examination of lesional material demonstrates a woven pattern to the collagen bundles, characteristic of the osseous matrix in this condition.* ***(Right)*** *A schematic diagram of the genetic abnormality identified in this disease shows alterations in the c-Abl-binding protein SH3BP2 gene. Usually a point mutation in the pleckstrin homology domain region, this results in production of an overly active variant of the protein.*

OSTEOMYELITIS

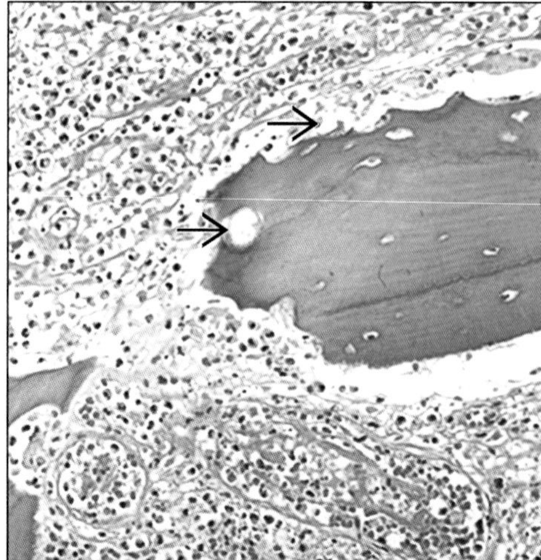

Infection of bone manifests itself as inflammation and necrosis of the marrow with secondary destruction of the adjacent bone ⇒. Acute inflammatory cells place this into the acute osteomyelitis category.

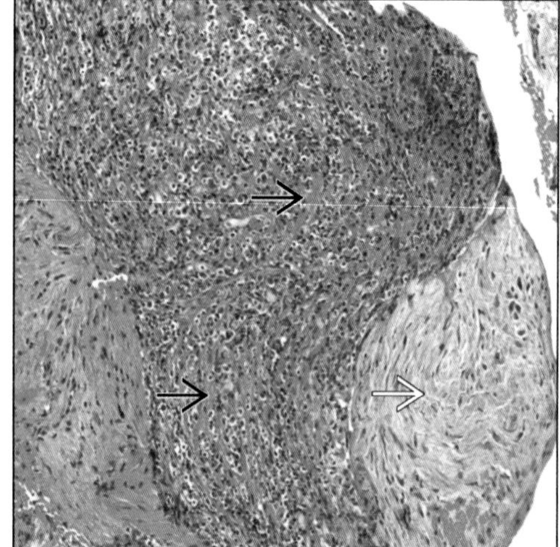

Inflammation, especially acute, is often associated with fibrin deposition ⇒ and associated delicate fibrosis ➡. Bone is not visible, as it may be completely resorbed.

TERMINOLOGY

Synonyms

- Osteitis

Definitions

- Osteomyelitis is inflammation or infection of bone and bone marrow
- Multiple classification schemes
  - **Composition of infiltrate**
    - **Acute**: Neutrophils
    - **Subacute**: Mix of neutrophils and chronic inflammatory cells (lymphocytes, monocytes, plasma cells)
    - **Chronic**: Chronic inflammatory cells and fibrosis
    - **Granulomatous**: Histiocytes, giant cells, and either acute or chronic inflammation
  - **Infectious agent**
    - Bacterial, fungal, viral, parasitic
  - **Method of acquisition**
    - Hematogenous (blood stream infection spread from distant site, such as lung, urinary bladder)
    - Direct extension from contiguous site (oral cavity into jaws; mucosa into paranasal sinuses)
    - Direct contamination (broken bone, direct injury)
  - **Site of involvement**
    - Gnathic (jaw)
    - Paranasal sinuses
    - Mastoid/temporal bone
    - Vertebrae

ETIOLOGY/PATHOGENESIS

Pathogenesis

- Originates as inflammation of vascularized connective tissue in bone marrow
  - Begins in organic bone matrix
  - Spreads along marrow cavity
  - Results in osteoclastic bone resorption
  - Bone necrosis
  - Reactive reformation by osteoblasts
- Chronicity is multifactorial
  - Avascular and ischemic nature of sequestrum produces area of lowered oxygen tension
  - Antibiotics cannot penetrate
  - Lowered oxygen tension effectively reduces bacteriocidal activities of neutrophils
  - Favors conversion of aerobic to anaerobic infection

Risk Factors

- **Injury**
  - Bone fracture or deep penetrating puncture wounds
  - Iatrogenic (during teeth cleaning, dental work, following surgery)
  - Intravenous drug use (nonsterile needles)
- **Circulation limitations**
  - Diabetes, peripheral arterial disease, sickle cell disease, atherosclerosis, hypertension
- **Iatrogenic causes**
  - Indwelling urinary catheters, central lines, respirators, dialysis machines

CLINICAL ISSUES

Epidemiology

- Incidence
  - In general, uncommon disease in head and neck
  - Increased frequency of osteomyelitis in
    - Chronic systemic diseases, diabetes mellitus, poor oral hygiene, tobacco use, alcoholism, immunosuppression, malnutrition, intravenous drug abuse, malignancy
    - Gram-negative aerobic bacteria and *Candida* species more common in intravenous drug users and immunosuppressed
- Age
  - In general, all ages can be affected
  - Jaw: Usually 6th to 7th decades

OSTEOMYELITIS

Key Facts

Terminology
- Osteomyelitis is infection of bone and bone marrow with multiple classification schemes

Etiology/Pathogenesis
- Injury, intravenous drug use (nonsterile needles), iatrogenic causes

Clinical Issues
- Fever, chills, irritability or lethargy, malaise, pain, headache, cranial neuropathy
  - Subacute/chronic symptoms are not characteristic
- Bone scan is most sensitive study for early disease
- Important to culture offending organism by percutaneous or open biopsy
- Surgery to remove dead bone with targeted intravenous antimicrobial therapy

Microscopic Pathology
- Marrow fibrosis or edema is hallmark
- Bone marrow fibrosis, bone death, and resorption
- Acute: Neutrophilic infiltrate with delicate marrow fibrosis or edema
- Subacute: Infiltrate of both neutrophils and chronic inflammatory cells
- Chronic: Chronic inflammatory infiltrate

Ancillary Tests
- Gram, acid-fast, fluorostain, GMS, and PAS-LG (among others) highlight organisms

Top Differential Diagnoses
- Inflammatory reaction, lymphoma, sarcoid, bisphosphonate therapy, radiation

- Gender
  - In general, equal gender distribution
  - Jaw osteomyelitis: Male > Female

Site
- Mandible
  - Most commonly affected maxillofacial area
  - Odontogenic infections and fractures are predisposing factors
  - Posterior body most commonly affected
  - Oral flora (usually commensal)
- Maxilla: More commonly affected in children
- Other bones: Paranasal sinuses, temporal, skull base, cervical spine

Presentation
- General findings
  - Fever, chills, irritability or lethargy, malaise, pain, headache, cranial neuropathy
  - Swelling, warmth, or redness over infected area
  - Must have high index of suspicion in patients with persistent neck pain &/or dysphagia
- Subacute or chronic type symptoms are not characteristic, making diagnosis difficult
- **Jaw**
  - Arise as complication of dental extractions and surgery, trauma, or fracture mismanagement
  - In infancy, maxilla is more commonly affected due to greater surface area and more extensive blood supply
- **Sinuses**
  - Sinusitis can lead to orbital cellulitis, subperiosteal abscess, orbital abscess, facial osteomyelitis, cavernous sinus/cortical vein thrombosis
- **Orbit**
  - More often in children, orbit is susceptible to contiguous spread from sinuses
- **Mastoiditis and skull base**
  - Starting with otitis externa ("malignant" or necrotizing), it evolves into cellulitis, chondritis, and via Haversian system, into osteomyelitis
  - Patients are usually immunocompromised: Diabetes, leukemia, AIDS, prior treatment with cytotoxic medication &/or corticosteroids
  - *Pseudomonas aeruginosa* is most frequent organism (rarely, mucormycosis, aspergillosis)
    - Must discriminate between these organisms as treatment is completely different, avoiding life-threatening outcome

Laboratory Tests
- Important to culture offending organism
  - Percutaneous or open biopsy
- Blood cultures are often negative

Treatment
- Options, risks, complications
  - Treatment is based on causative organism, but specifics are beyond scope of this book
    - Surgery to remove dead bone with targeted intravenous antimicrobial therapy
  - Complications
    - Osteonecrosis, septic arthritis, impaired growth, nerve paralysis (skull base), rare development of squamous cell carcinoma (overlying draining fistula)
- Surgical approaches
  - Surgical treatment involves
    - Debridement of necrotic bone and tissue
    - Drainage of pus/fluid
    - Obtaining appropriate culture
    - Removal of foreign objects (potential nidus for recurrent infection)
    - Achieving bone stability, including bone grafting
  - Can be difficult given head and neck anatomy
- Drugs
  - Drug regimens depend on organisms involved
  - Treatment usually involves 6-12 weeks of targeted antimicrobial therapy

Prognosis
- Most cases are self limited and cured
  - Early diagnosis and aggressive treatment important
- Treatment for < 4 weeks has 25% relapse rate

OSTEOMYELITIS

- Exacerbations require additional combination therapy
- Skull base osteomyelitis has poor prognosis: Requires high-dose intravenous antibiotic therapy

IMAGE FINDINGS

Radiographic Findings

- Conventional radiographs are diagnostic from 3rd week of disease forward
- Plain films very difficult to diagnose due to anatomy

MR Findings

- Standard of care for diagnosis, without radiation exposure
- Establishes extent of disease, shows bone marrow changes and soft tissue involvement

CT Findings

- Not as useful as MR or scintigraphy

Bone Scan

- Most sensitive study (gold standard for initial diagnosis)
  - Hyperperfused inflammatory stage 2-3 days after infection starts
  - Low specificity and limited spatial resolution
  - Does not separate between osteomyelitis and bone tumors with increased bone metabolism

MACROSCOPIC FEATURES

General Features

- Tend to be curettings

Size

- Range: 1-5 cm
  - Abscesses may be larger (soft tissues involved)

MICROSCOPIC PATHOLOGY

Histologic Features

- Marrow fibrosis or edema is hallmark
  - Bone death assessed by marrow fibrosis and inflammation
  - Lack of osteocytes can be due to overdecalcification
- **Acute**
  - Neutrophilic infiltrate with delicate marrow fibrosis or edema
  - Bone death and bone resorption
    - Osteoclastic resorption due to pressure of infiltrate
    - Micro-resorption due to released neutrophil neutral proteases
- **Subacute**
  - Infiltrate of both neutrophils and chronic inflammatory cells
  - Bone marrow fibrosis, bone death, and resorption
- **Chronic**
  - Chronic inflammatory infiltrate
  - Dense fibrosis
  - Bone death with foci of new bone formation
- **Granulomatous**
  - Monocytoid histiocytes with/without caseation (necrosis) and peripheral lymphoplasmacytic cuff

ANCILLARY TESTS

Histochemistry

- Gram, acid-fast, fluorostain, GMS, and PAS-LG (among others) highlight organisms
  - Axiomatic, fails to give antimicrobial sensitivities

Immunohistochemistry

- Antibodies to certain infectious agents are available

DIFFERENTIAL DIAGNOSIS

Inflammatory Reaction

- Inflammation part of fracture repair
- Present at tumor borders
- Lack of acute inflammation and dead bone

Lymphoma

- Atypical lymphoid infiltrate with bone remodeling and dense fibrosis
- Monoclonal immunohistochemistry reactions

Sarcoid

- Noncaseating, tight, well-formed granulomas
- Concurrent disease in lung, mediastinum, and other locations

Bisphosphonate Therapy

- Bone necrosis with death, followed by active remodeling
- More often a chronic process

Radiation Osteitis

- Bone necrosis and death with chronic inflammation
- History usually known

SELECTED REFERENCES

1. Sethi A et al: Tubercular and chronic pyogenic osteomyelitis of cranio-facial bones: a retrospective analysis. J Laryngol Otol. 122(8):799-804, 2008
2. Prasad KC et al: Osteomyelitis in the head and neck. Acta Otolaryngol. 127(2):194-205, 2007
3. Sharkawy AA: Cervicofacial actinomycosis and mandibular osteomyelitis. Infect Dis Clin North Am. 21(2):543-56, viii, 2007
4. Otto KJ et al: Invasive fungal rhinosinusitis: what is the appropriate follow-up? Am J Rhinol. 20(6):582-5, 2006
5. Dudkiewicz M et al: Acute mastoiditis and osteomyelitis of the temporal bone. Int J Pediatr Otorhinolaryngol. 69(10):1399-405, 2005
6. Marshall AH et al: Osteomyelitis of the frontal bone secondary to frontal sinusitis. J Laryngol Otol. 114(12):944-6, 2000
7. Perloff JR et al: Bone involvement in sinusitis: an apparent pathway for the spread of disease. Laryngoscope. 110(12):2095-9, 2000
8. Aitasalo K et al: A modified protocol for early treatment of osteomyelitis and osteoradionecrosis of the mandible. Head Neck. 20(5):411-7, 1998

Diagrammatic, Imaging, and Microscopic Features

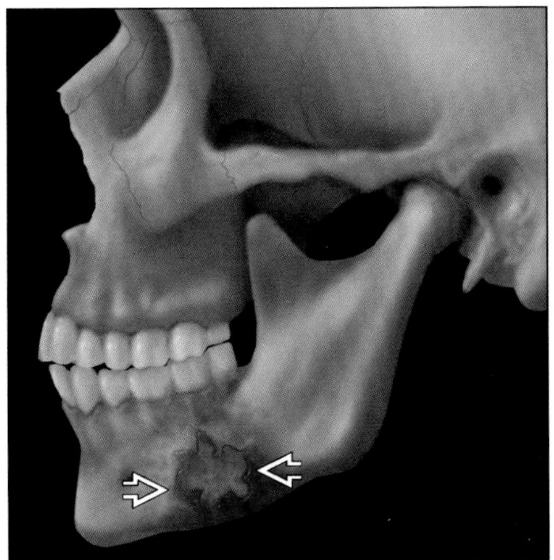

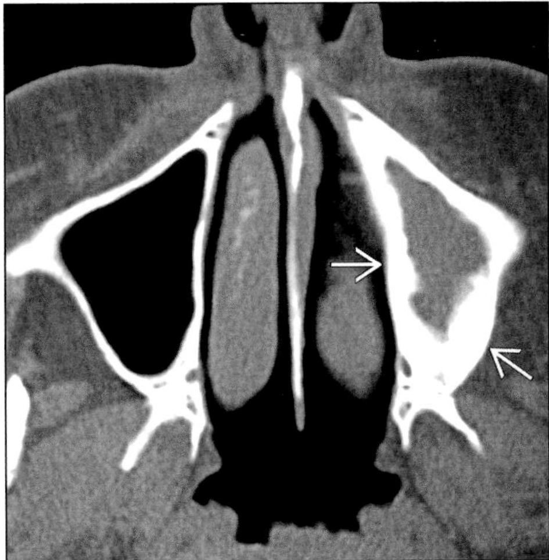

*(**Left**) This graphic shows osteomyelitis ⇨ resulting in destruction of the mandible and extension into the adjacent soft tissues. The destruction is largely a result of the release of neutral proteases, primarily collagenase, from the neutrophils. (**Right**) Axial bone CT shows opacification of the left maxillary sinus without expansion. Thickening of the sinus walls → is seen, consistent with chronic osteomyelitis. There is a background setting of chronic rhinosinusitis.*

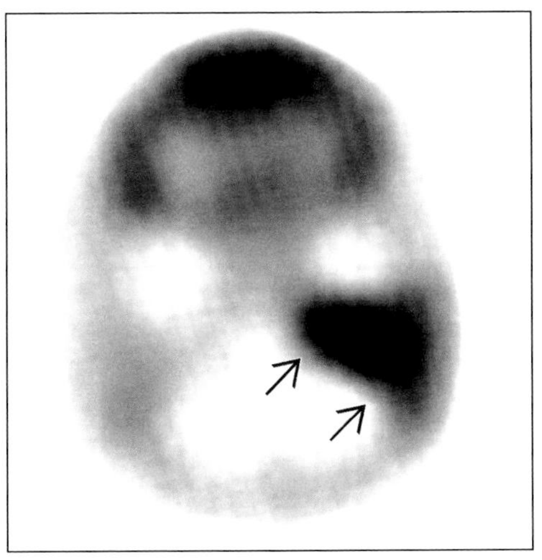

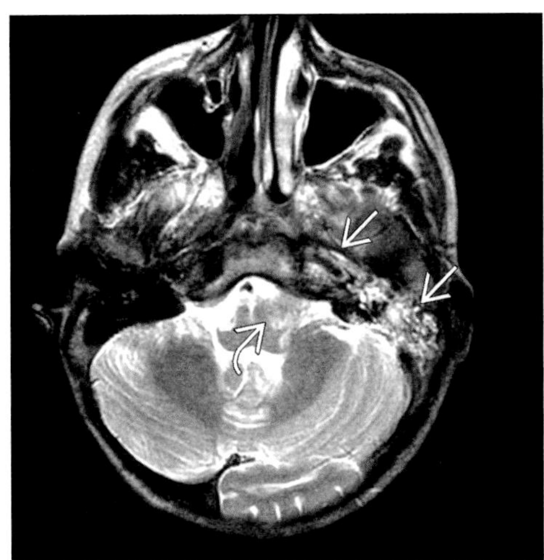

*(**Left**) Axial Tc-99m MDP SPECT of the skull shows increased uptake in the left temporal bone →, extending to the petrous apex. This appearance is nonspecific but helps in a patient being treated for "malignant" otitis externa. (**Right**) Axial T2WI MR shows diffuse opacification of the left mastoid and petrous air cells → as well as abnormal signal related to pus in the left CPA subarachnoid space ↷. These findings correspond to increased uptake in scintigraphic studies.*

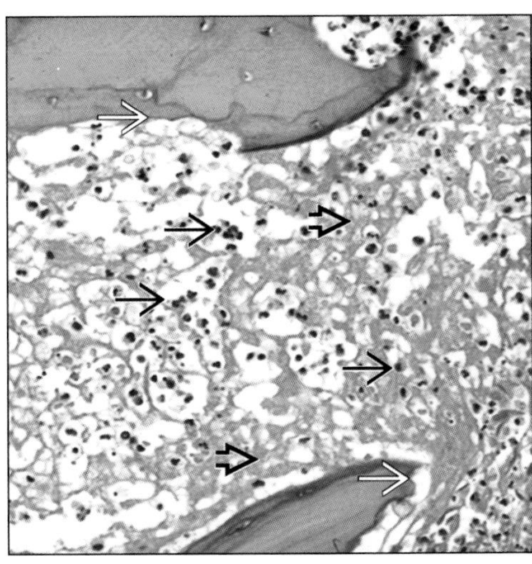

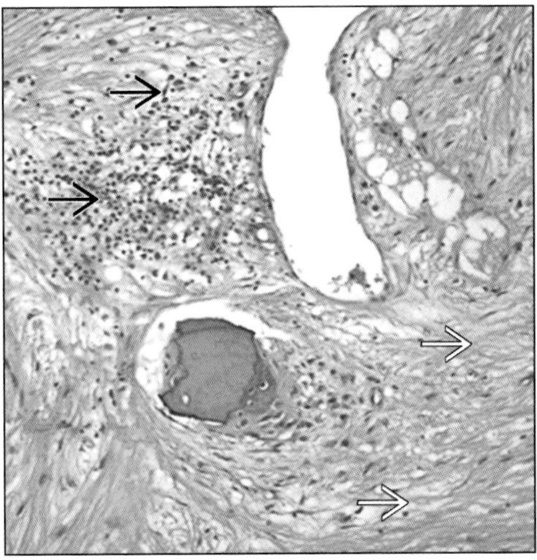

*(**Left**) Acute inflammation is composed of neutrophils → often with necrosis ⇨. Degranulation of the neutrophils releases neutral proteases resulting in bone destruction → in the areas of inflammation. This bone resorption is distinct from that seen as a result of osteoclastic resorption. (**Right**) Chronic osteomyelitis is noted by the presence of mononuclear inflammatory cells → (lymphocytes, plasma cells, macrophages) with a background of dense fibrosis →.*

TORI

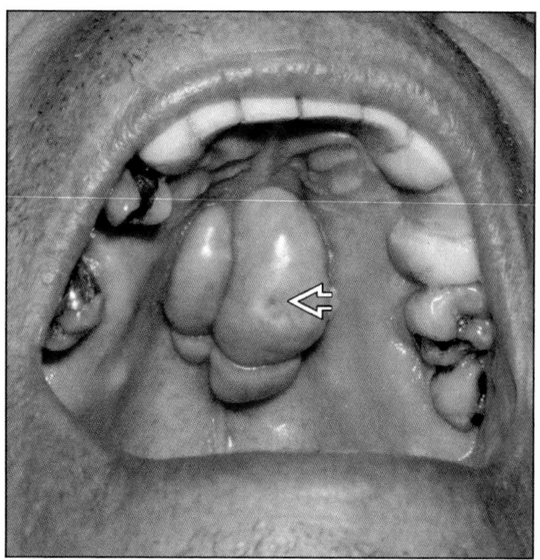

Torus palatinus presents as a large, lobulated palatal mass that is bony hard. Because of the large size of this torus, it is subject to trauma; the thin overlying mucosa can ulcerate ➡.

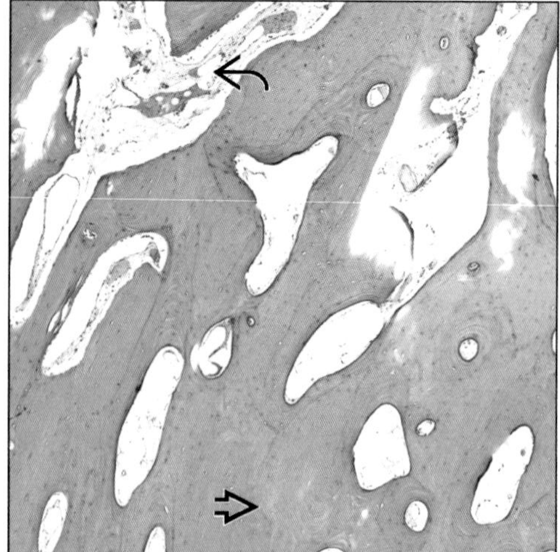

High-power photomicrograph of a decalcified torus is composed of dense cortical lamellar bone ➡. Fatty marrow is evident associated with trabecular bone, a feature not always present ➡.

TERMINOLOGY

Abbreviations

- Torus palatinus (TP)
- Torus mandibularis (TM)

Synonyms

- Exostoses

Definitions

- Localized benign hyperostotic bony growths, which arise from cortical plate
  - Torus palatinus: Bony growth arising from hard palate midline
  - Torus mandibularis: Bony growth arising from lingual mandible above mylohyoid bone

ETIOLOGY/PATHOGENESIS

Etiology

- Exact etiology unknown but includes both environmental and genetic factors

CLINICAL ISSUES

Epidemiology

- Incidence
  - TP: Exact incidence unknown, but common (25-40% prevalence in USA)
    - Much higher in certain ethnic groups (> 50%)
  - TM: Prevalence between 5-10%
    - Related to masticatory forces, such as bruxism
- Age
  - Usually early adult life
- Gender
  - TP: Female > Male (2:1)
  - TM: Slight Male > Female (1.1:1)
- Ethnicity
  - TP: Inuit and Asian populations reportedly have higher incidence

Site

- TP: Midline of hard palate
- TM: Lingual mandible generally in molar-premolar area

Presentation

- Bony mass in oral cavity

Natural History

- TP and TM: Usually 1st present in young adulthood
  - May increase in size over many decades
  - May also undergo resorption and decrease in size

Treatment

- Options, risks, complications
  - TP and TM: Lesions can usually be diagnosed clinically and are asymptomatic
    - May become ulcerated due to masticatory trauma
  - Bisphosphonate related osteonecrosis can involve tori similar to jaws
- Surgical approaches
  - Surgical removal necessary only when bony protuberance interferes with dental function
  - May experience regrowth after removal

Prognosis

- TP: High bone mineral density correlating with presence of large palatal tori in white women
- No reports of malignant transformation

IMAGE FINDINGS

Radiographic Findings

- TP: Generally not seen on routine dental films
  - Depending on size, can be seen on CT and MR scans
- TM: Large lesions can be visualized on periapical and occlusal films
  - Can be seen on both CT and MR scans

TORI

Key Facts

Terminology

- Torus palatinus (TP) refers to bony growth arising in midline of hard palate
- Torus mandibularis (TM) refers to bony growth arising in lingual mandible above mylohyoid bone

Clinical Issues

- Usually 1st noted in early adult life
- TP and TM: Lesions can usually be diagnosed clinically and are asymptomatic
- No reports of malignant transformation

Microscopic Pathology

- Dense, mature lamellar bone with minimal osteoblastic activity
- May have small fibrofatty marrow spaces
- Some cases may have dense cortical bone overlying trabecular (cancellous) bone

MACROSCOPIC FEATURES

General Features

- TP: Most are < 2 cm
  - Gross appearance variable
    - May have subtle symmetrically raised area with broad base
    - Large lobulated lesions arising from single base, which may be either symmetric or asymmetric
    - Multinodular tori, which arise from multiple bony protuberances that coalesce
- TM: May be unilateral or bilateral
  - Generally single protuberance, but multiple protuberances can be seen
  - Can become large and multilobulated

Size

- Range: 0.2 cm up to 4 cm

MICROSCOPIC PATHOLOGY

Histologic Features

- Dense mature lamellar bone
- Scattered osteocytes
- May have small fibrofatty marrow spaces
- Minimal osteoblastic activity
- Some cases may have dense cortical bone overlying trabecular (cancellous) bone

DIFFERENTIAL DIAGNOSIS

Buccal Exostosis

- Common bony growths along facial aspect of maxilla &/or mandible
- Diagnosis made on clinical presentation
- Histology identical to TP and TM

Osteoma

- Seen in craniofacial skeleton, including jaws
- Usually solitary and asymptomatic
  - Multiple osteomas are associated with Gardner syndrome
- May be exophytic (periosteal) or endophytic (endosteal)
- Well-circumscribed sclerotic bone on radiographs
- Histology identical to TP and TM, although perhaps with more osteoblastic activity

SELECTED REFERENCES

1. Jainkittivong A et al: Prevalence and clinical characteristics of oral tori in 1,520 Chulalongkorn University Dental School patients. Surg Radiol Anat. 29(2):125-31, 2007
2. Chohayeb AA et al: Occurrence of torus palatinus and mandibularis among women of different ethnic groups. Am J Dent. 14(5):278-80, 2001
3. Jainkittivong A et al: Buccal and palatal exostoses: prevalence and concurrence with tori. Oral Surg Oral Med Oral Pathol Oral Radiol Endod. 90(1):48-53, 2000

IMAGE GALLERY

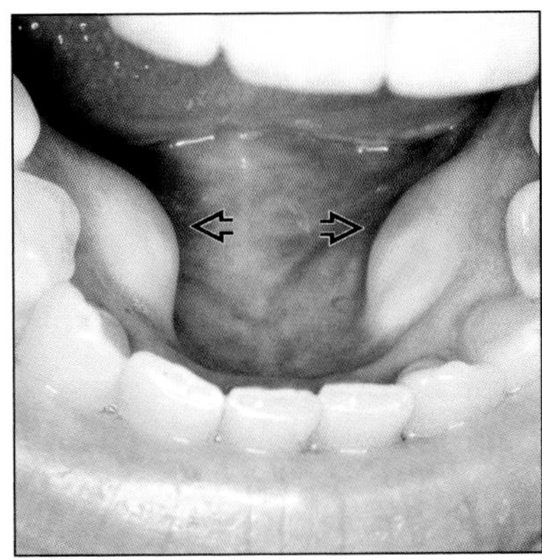
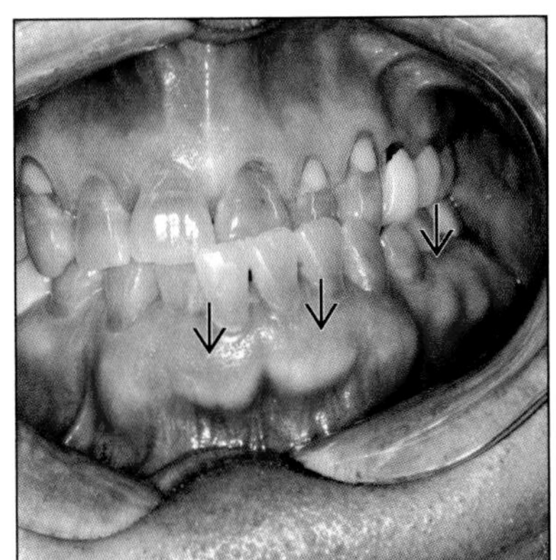
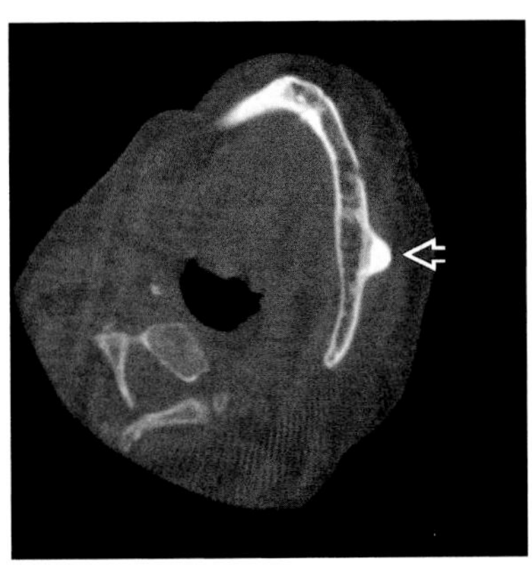

*(**Left**) Torus mandibularis or lingual tori are present as bilateral bony protuberances of the mandibular alveolar ridge ⇨. These lesions can become quite large and lobulated. (**Center**) Multiple buccal exostoses of the mandibular ridge → are seen. Generally these are asymptomatic unless secondarily ulcerated. (**Right**) CT scan shows an osteoma arising on the periosteal buccal surface of the mandible ➡. Unlike exostoses, which are multiple, osteomas are usually solitary. Histologically they are similar to exostoses.*

FIBROUS DYSPLASIA

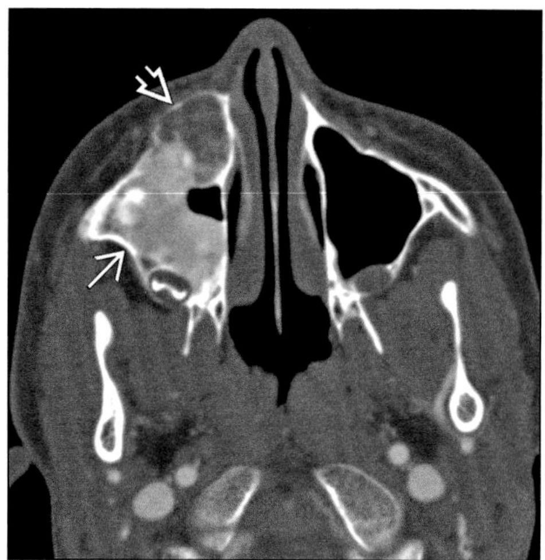

CT demonstrates expanded bone, with areas of characteristic "ground-glass" density ➡ with prominent cortex, interspersed with more cystic-appearing areas ➡ showing cortical attenuation.

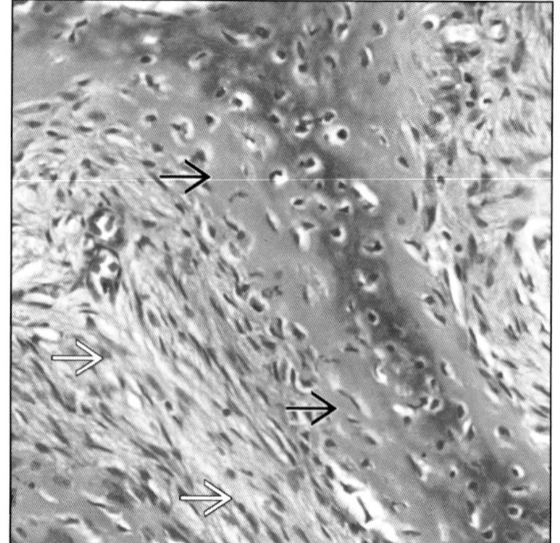

The osseous matrix ➡ arises directly out of the background bland, mononuclear, spindle cell stroma ➡. There is an absence of osteoblastic rimming. There is no cytologic atypia.

TERMINOLOGY

Abbreviations

- Fibrous dysplasia (FD)

Synonyms

- Osteitis fibrosa
- Osteodystrophia fibrosa
- Fibrous osteoma
- Ossifying fibroma
- Unilateral von Recklinghausen disease

Definitions

- Fibrous dysplasia is genetically based sporadic disease that occurs in 3 clinical subtypes
  - Monostotic (1 bone)
  - Polyostotic (multiple bones)
  - McCune-Albright syndrome
    - Initially identified as distinct entity by Donovan McCune and Fuller Albright
    - Multiple bones with FD, skin hyperpigmentation, and hyperfunctioning endocrinologic disturbances
- Term **fibrous dysplasia** introduced by Lichtenstein in 1938

ETIOLOGY/PATHOGENESIS

Genetic

- Activating missense mutations in *GNAS1* gene coding for α subunit of stimulatory G protein are a consistent finding
- Clonal chromosomal aberrations suggest lesion is neoplastic

CLINICAL ISSUES

Epidemiology

- Incidence
  - Uncommon disorder
    - Involvement of craniofacial bones is common
  - Incidence varies depending on monostotic vs. polyostotic cases
    - Monostotic form accounts for 80-85% of cases
    - Severe polyostotic cases, craniofacial involvement approaches 100%
- Age
  - Children and young adults
  - Occasionally seen in older patients
- Gender
  - Craniofacial disease shows equal gender distribution
    - Monostotic form: Equal gender distribution
    - Polyostotic form: Female > Male

Site

- Craniofacial bones are typically involved in ~ 10% of patients with monostotic form and in up to 100% with polyostotic form
- Skull base is skeletal site most commonly affected
- Maxilla and paranasal regions more frequently affected than mandible
  - May be extension across suture lines to involve adjacent bones
- Term "monostotic" not usually employed for maxilla or face

Presentation

- Painless swelling of jaws leading to facial asymmetry
- Maxilla swelling may lead to nasal obstruction and chronic sinusitis
- When skull base is affected, compression of cranial nerves may cause visual impairment or hearing loss
  - Craniofacial involvement can be asymptomatic and detected incidentally
  - Skull disease sometimes associated with pain
    - Neither extent nor location seem to account for pain
- About 3% of patients with polyostotic form have endocrinopathies

FIBROUS DYSPLASIA

Key Facts

Terminology
- Fibrous dysplasia is genetically based sporadic disease that occurs in 3 clinical subtypes

Clinical Issues
- Children and young adults
- Painless swellings of jaws leading to facial asymmetry, nasal obstruction, chronic sinusitis
- Monostotic form accounts for 80-85% of cases
- Skull base > maxilla > paranasal regions
- Skull base lesions may cause visual impairment or hearing loss (cranial nerves affected)
- ~ 3% of patients with polyostotic form have endocrinopathies (McCune-Albright syndrome)

Image Findings
- Abnormal opacification, with numerous small to diffusely distributed opacities ("cotton wool," "ground-glass"), merging with adjacent bone

Microscopic Pathology
- Moderately cellular fibrous tissue containing fine branching, curvilinear trabeculae of woven bone
- Nearly complete lack of osteoblast rimming
- Bony spicules merge with adjacent bone

Ancillary Tests
- Activating missense mutations in *GNAS1* gene

Top Differential Diagnoses
- Ossifying fibroma, osseous dysplasia, osteosarcoma, osteomyelitis

---

- McCune-Albright syndrome
  - Hyperfunctioning endocrinopathies, including precocious puberty, fluctuating thelarche, hyperthyroidism, growth hormone excess, rickets/osteomalacia
  - Café au lait spots
- When associated with intramuscular myxomas, called Mazabraud syndrome
- Accurate classification depends on clinical, radiological, and histomorphological features

Natural History
- Tendency to slow or stop disease progression after skeletal maturation
- Can cause severe deformity and asymmetry
  - Most significant: Blindness

Treatment
- Options, risks, complications
  - Treatment with bisphosphonates usually relieves pain
    - Tends not to affect natural history of disorder
- Surgical approaches
  - Generally employed to achieve cosmetic results or functional status
  - Fractures through area of FD in craniofacial bones are uncommon

Prognosis
- Considered a self-limiting disease
- Rarely, osteosarcoma may arise

IMAGE FINDINGS

Radiographic Findings
- Radiographic appearance is variable based on patient age
- Craniofacial disease differs from axial skeleton findings
- Craniofacial FD is poorly defined and more radiopaque
  - Axial FD frequently shows circumscribed radiolucency with thin sclerotic periphery
- Abnormal opacification, especially monostotic form
  - Numerous small to diffusely distributed opacities ("cotton wool")
  - Yields characteristic "ground-glass" or "orange skin" appearance
- Early lesions may be radiolucent
  - Become increasingly radiopaque
  - Gradual merging of radiologically abnormal bone with adjacent bone
- Subclassified into 3 different patterns
  - Pagetoid (56%)
  - Cystic (21%)
  - Sclerotic (23%)
    - Preferentially involves facial bones and skull base

CT Findings
- Poorly defined lesion merging with adjacent bone

MACROSCOPIC FEATURES

General Features
- Gritty, nondescript fragments of bone

MICROSCOPIC PATHOLOGY

Histologic Features
- Normal bone replaced by moderately cellular fibrous tissue
  - Spindled fibroblasts with moderate amount of collagen
- Stroma contains fine branching, curvilinear trabeculae of woven bone
  - Irregular shapes (alphabet soup, Chinese characters)
- Nearly complete lack of osteoblast rimming of bony trabeculae
- Bony spicules merge imperceptibly with adjacent cancellous bone or overlying cortex
- Jaw lesions may show lamellar bone
- Rarely, tiny calcified spherules may be present

- Using polarized light, woven bone has disorganized collagen bundles
- Possible reasons for difference between maxillofacial vs. long bone FD
  - Maxillofacial derivation from membranous bone, a network of broad trabeculae
  - Lamellar bone occurs occasionally in FD

ANCILLARY TESTS

Molecular Genetics

- Sporadic, congenital mutations in cAMP regulating protein, Gsa
  - Example of somatic mosaicism in which wide spectrum of disease is possible
- Activating missense mutations in *GNAS1* gene
  - *GNAS1* codes for α subunit of stimulatory G protein
- Gsa is central in cell signaling pathway that leads to generation of intracellular 2nd messenger, cAMP
- Activating mutations lead to ligand-independent cAMP/protein kinase A signaling
- Cyclic AMP is involved in signal transduction from multiple cell surface receptors including
  - Parathyroid hormone (PTH)
  - Follicle stimulating hormone (FSH)
  - Luteinizing hormone (LH)
  - Thyroid stimulating hormone (TSH)
- All of the mutations thus far identified are at 201 Arg position
  - In > 95%, arginine is replaced by either cysteine or histidine (R201C or R201H)
- These mutations result in inhibition of intrinsic GTPase activity of Gsa protein
  - This aspect leads to constitutive, ligand-independent generation of intracellular cAMP
- Detected using genomic DNA and allele specific polymerase chain reaction (PCR)
  - Usually exons 8 and 9 of *GNAS1* gene

DIFFERENTIAL DIAGNOSIS

Ossifying Fibroma

- Radiographic correlation is absolutely required
  - Clearly demarcated lesion
  - FD tends to be diffuse with blending into surrounding bone
- Will have bony spicules that have osteoblastic rimming
- Stromal cellularity is variable

Osseous Dysplasia

- Has many different types of mineralized material
- Stromal cellularity is quite variable
- Lacks woven bone trabeculae fusing to uninvolved bone

Osteosarcoma (Low Grade)

- Invades through cortical bone into soft tissues
- Osteoid in background, usually with osteoblastic rimming
- Lacks woven bone trabeculae fusing to uninvolved bone

Osteomyelitis, Sclerosing Type

- Coarse trabeculae of lamellar bone
- Edematous stroma containing lymphocytes
- Lacks woven bone trabeculae fusing to uninvolved bone

SELECTED REFERENCES

1. Kim YH et al: Role of surgical management in temporal bone fibrous dysplasia. Acta Otolaryngol. 129(12):1374-9, 2009
2. Mendonça Caridad JJ et al: Fibrous dysplasia of the mandible: Surgical treatment with platelet-rich plasma and a corticocancellous iliac crest graft-report of a case. Oral Surg Oral Med Oral Pathol Oral Radiol Endod. 105(4):e12-8, 2008
3. Menezes AH: Craniovertebral junction neoplasms in the pediatric population. Childs Nerv Syst. 24(10):1173-86, 2008
4. Mäkitie AA et al: Bisphosphonate treatment in craniofacial fibrous dysplasia--a case report and review of the literature. Clin Rheumatol. 27(6):809-12, 2008
5. Yu Hon Wan A et al: Fibrous dysplasia of the temporal bone presenting with facial nerve palsy and conductive hearing loss. Otol Neurotol. 29(7):1039-40, 2008
6. Conejero JA et al: Management of incidental fibrous dysplasia of the maxilla in a patient with facial fractures. J Craniofac Surg. 18(6):1463-4, 2007
7. Galvan O et al: Fibro-osseous lesion of the middle turbinate: ossifying fibroma or fibrous dysplasia? J Laryngol Otol. 121(12):1201-3, 2007
8. Panda NK et al: A clinicoradiologic analysis of symptomatic craniofacial fibro-osseous lesions. Otolaryngol Head Neck Surg. 136(6):928-33, 2007
9. Gerceker M et al: Fibrous dysplasia in the retropharyngeal area. Ear Nose Throat J. 85(7):446-7, 2006
10. Hempel JM et al: Fibrous dysplasia of the frontal bone. Ear Nose Throat J. 85(10):654, 656-7, 2006
11. Mendonça-Caridad JJ et al: Frontal sinus obliteration and craniofacial reconstruction with platelet rich plasma in a patient with fibrous dysplasia. Int J Oral Maxillofac Surg. 35(1):88-91, 2006
12. Berlucchi M et al: Endoscopic surgery for fibrous dysplasia of the sinonasal tract in pediatric patients. Int J Pediatr Otorhinolaryngol. 69(1):43-8, 2005
13. Chan EK: Ethmoid fibrous dysplasia with anterior skull base and intraorbital extension. Ear Nose Throat J. 84(10):627-8, 2005
14. Post G et al: Endoscopic resection of large sinonasal ossifying fibroma. Am J Otolaryngol. 26(1):54-6, 2005
15. Song JJ et al: Monostotic fibrous dysplasia of temporal bone: report of two cases and review of its characteristics. Acta Otolaryngol. 125(10):1126-9, 2005
16. Hullar TE et al: Paget's disease and fibrous dysplasia. Otolaryngol Clin North Am. 36(4):707-32, 2003
17. Nelson BL et al: Fibrous dysplasia of bone. Ear Nose Throat J. 82(4):259, 2003
18. Ozbek C et al: Fibrous dysplasia of the temporal bone. Ann Otol Rhinol Laryngol. 112(7):654-6, 2003
19. Wenig BM et al: Fibro-osseous, osseous, and cartilaginous lesions of the orbit and paraorbital region. Correlative clinicopathologic and radiographic features, including the diagnostic role of CT and MR imaging. Radiol Clin North Am. 36(6):1241-59, xii, 1998

Imaging, Microscopic, and Molecular Features

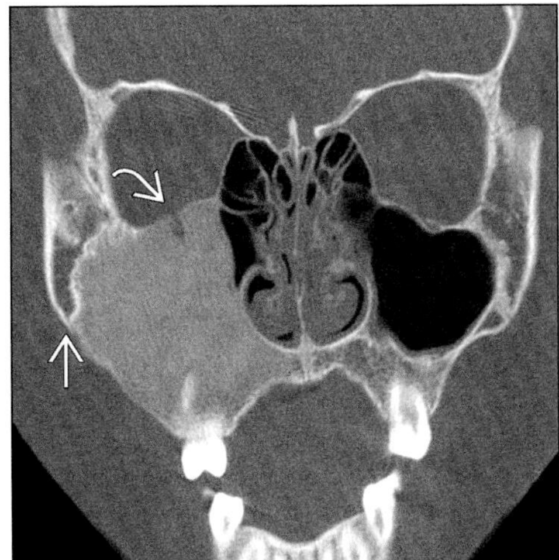

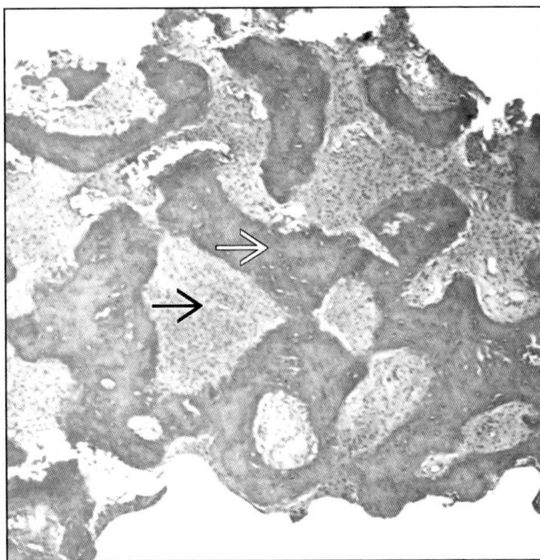

(Left) *The maxillary sinus is expanded by monostotic fibrous dysplasia (FD). There is extension to zygomaticomaxillary synchondrosis ➔ and infraorbital nerve engulfment ↷. The opacification is nonspecific on CT images, as opposed to the appearance on plain films.* ***(Right)*** *Low-power view demonstrates irregularly shaped islands and formations of woven bone ➔ with a bland, mononuclear, spindle cell background ⇨. Note the absence of osteoblastic rimming.*

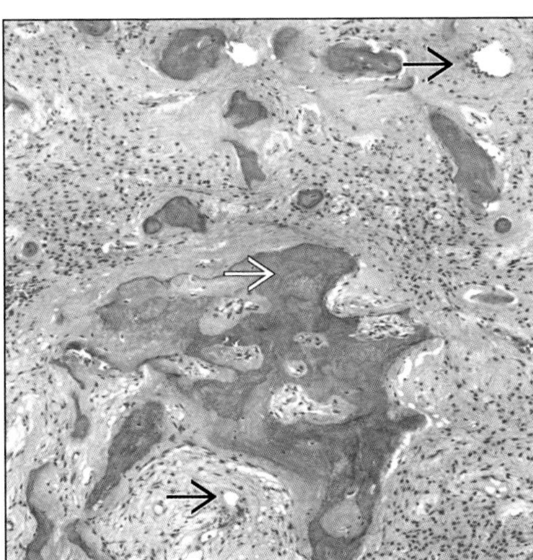

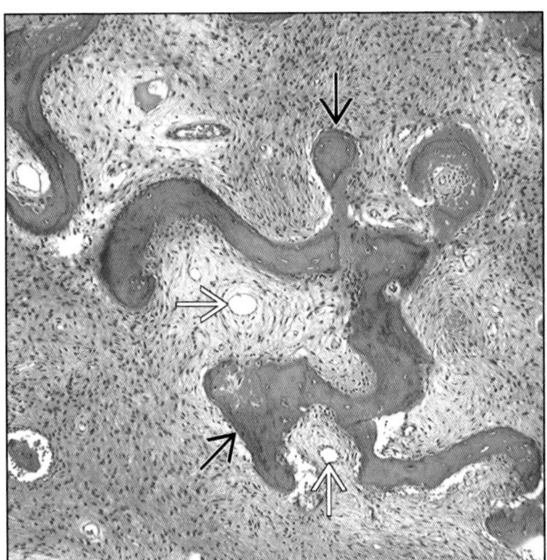

(Left) *An older fibrous dysplasia lesion demonstrates larger islands as discrete bone formations that are merging as a result of remodeling ➔. The background stroma contains numerous vessels of small to medium size ⇨. The stroma is variably cellular.* ***(Right)*** *A high power shows curvilinear "alphabet" pieces of woven bone ⇨ arising directly out of the spindle cell background with small, delicate vessels ➔. This blending without osteoblastic rimming is a helpful feature.*

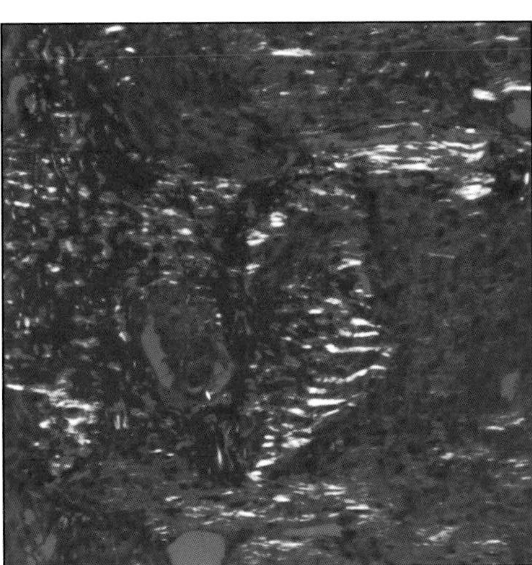

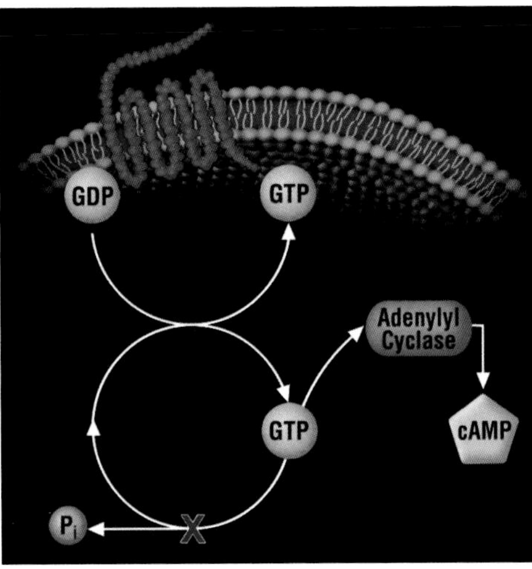

(Left) *Using polarized light shows the disorganized, yellow to orange collagen bundles characteristic of woven bone. There is no order or Haversian/ lamellar appearance.* ***(Right)*** *Mutations inactivate the intrinsic GTPase activity, preventing the inactivation of the Gs α subunit. Once activated, the mutated Gs α subunit is able to continuously stimulate adenylyl cyclase, increasing intracellular cAMP and causing continual stimulation of downstream cAMP signaling cascades.*

OSTEORADIONECROSIS

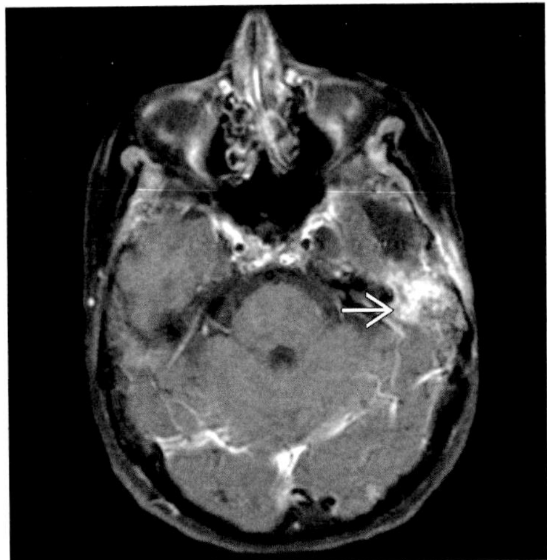

Axial T1WI post-contrast MR reveals a typical ill-defined mottled pattern, in which the debris enhances intensely throughout ➡. This is nonspecific, although characteristic.

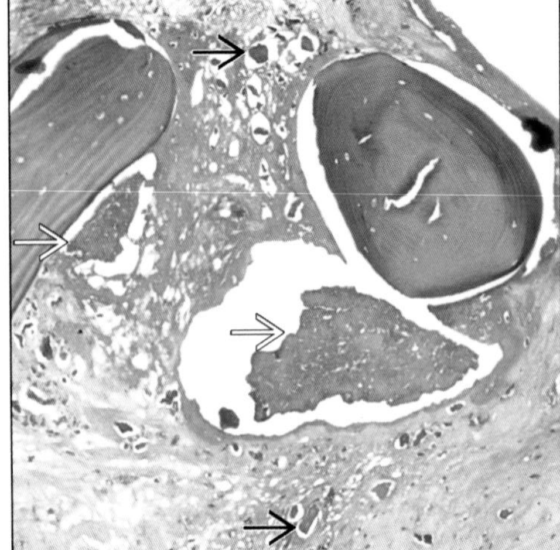

Lamellar trabecular bone is shown with complete marrow fibrosis & collections of bone fragments ⇨ & amorphous debris ➡. This combination of findings is quite supportive of the diagnosis of ORN.

TERMINOLOGY

Abbreviations

- Osteoradionecrosis (ORN)

Synonyms

- Radiation osteitis
- Radio-osteonecrosis
- Radiation osteomyelitis
- Osteonecrosis

Definitions

- Avascular bone necrosis due to irradiation

ETIOLOGY/PATHOGENESIS

Etiology

- Several theories
  - **Release of histamine**
    - Histamine damages surrounding tissues
  - **Radiation injury**
    - Radiation directly damages regenerating tissues
    - Key to progression is activation and dysregulation of fibroblastic activity, which leads to atrophic tissue within previously irradiated area
    - Indirect damage by radiation generated reactive oxygen species or free radicals
    - Reduction in bony matrix and its replacement with fibrous tissues
    - Combination of death of osteoblasts after irradiation, failure of osteoblasts to repopulate, and excessive proliferation of myofibroblasts
  - **Trauma**
    - Surgical manipulation impairs healing process
  - **Infection**
    - Interferes with normal regenerative response
  - **Hypoxia, hypovascularity, and hypocellularity**
    - Synergy of issues leads to death and subsequent fibrosis
    - Destruction of endothelial cells
    - Vascular thrombosis
    - Leads to necrosis of microvessels, local ischemia, and tissue loss
  - **Reactive oxygen species mediates release of cytokines**
    - Tumor necrosis factor
    - Platelet-derived growth factor
    - Fibroblast growth factor
    - Interleukins 1, 4, and 6
    - Transforming growth factor
    - Connective tissue growth factor
  - **Injured endothelial cells**
    - Produce chemotactic cytokines that trigger acute inflammatory response
    - Generates further release of reactive oxygen species from neutrophils and phagocytes
- All result in unregulated fibroblastic activation, and myofibroblast phenotype persists
  - Characterized by high rates of proliferation
  - Secretion of abnormal products of extracellular matrix
  - Reduced ability to degrade such components

CLINICAL ISSUES

Epidemiology

- Incidence
  - Develops in up to 30% of patients treated by radiation
    - Generally about 5% of patients
  - No significant decrease despite improvements in pre-radiotherapy oral and dental care
- Age
  - Generally older patients
    - Similar to age of head and neck cancers
- Gender
  - Male > Female in general
    - Depends on reason for radiation treatment

OSTEORADIONECROSIS

Key Facts

Terminology

- Avascular bone necrosis due to irradiation

Etiology/Pathogenesis

- Several theories to explain cause
  - Radiation injury, trauma, infection, hypoxia, release of cytokines, injury of endothelial cells

Clinical Issues

- No significant decrease in incidence
  - Develops in about 5% of patients treated by radiation
  - Tend to be rare with doses less than 60 Gy
  - More common when brachytherapy is used
- Patients present with pain, which can be severe and intractable
- Ulceration or necrosis of mucosa
- Exposure of necrotic bone for longer than 3 months
- Mandible is affected more often than maxilla
  - Body most often
- Several different approaches to management
  - Conservative management, invasive surgery, and hyperbaric oxygen therapy

Image Findings

- Ill-defined mottled radiolucent/radio-opaque

Microscopic Pathology

- Overlap with osteomyelitis, with histologic phase matching those of healing traumatic wounds
- Endothelial changes with inflammatory response
- Necrotic and devitalized bone
- Abnormal fibroblastic activity predominates with disorganization of extracellular matrix

Site

- Mandible more often than maxilla
  - Most often affects the body

Presentation

- One of the most severe and serious oral complications of head and neck radiation
  - Regaud published 1st report in 1922 on ORN of jaws after radiotherapy
- Most patients experience severe pain
  - Pain can be intractable
- Trismus
- Ulceration or necrosis of mucosa
- Exposure of necrotic bone for longer than 3 months
- Local infection, often with intraoral/extraoral fistulas
- Pathologic fractures may be seen
- Masticatory difficulties
- Other associated findings include
  - Dysesthesia
  - Halitosis
  - Dysgeusia
  - Food impaction in area of exposed sequestra
- Early lesions may be asymptomatic
  - In spite of seeing exposed devitalized bone through ulcerated mucosa or skin
- Factors that may contribute to development of ORN include
  - Size and site of primary tumor treated by radiation
  - Dose of radiation
  - Type of mandibular resection, injury, or dental extractions
  - Infection
  - Immune deficiencies
  - Malnutrition

Natural History

- Arc of development defined by sequence of events
  - Radiation
    - Less common after hyperfractionated radiotherapy at 72-80 Gy
  - Hypovascular + hypocellular + hypoxic tissue formation
  - Trauma-induced or spontaneous mucosa breakdown
  - Nonhealing wound
- Rare with less than 60 Gy of radiation exposure
  - More common when brachytherapy is used
- When chemotherapy is added to radiotherapy, incidence of ORN may be increased
- Documented incidence after dental extractions is about 5%
  - 3x higher in dentate than in edentulous patients
  - Mainly as a result of injury from extractions and infection from periodontal disease
- Interval between radiotherapy and onset of ORN can vary
  - Most occur between 4 months and 2 years
- Risk remains for life, albeit to a lesser degree
  - May present much earlier after local traumatic event

Treatment

- Options, risks, complications
  - ORN is irreversible and extremely difficult to treat
  - Several different approaches
    - Conservative management (only indicated in small necrotic bone areas)
    - Invasive surgery
    - Hyperbaric oxygen therapy (HBO)
- Surgical approaches
  - Severe, intractable pain is primary reason for surgery
  - Variable surgical approaches
    - Simple sequestrectomy to hemimandibulectomy
  - Sequestrectomies should be delayed until necrotic bone can be lifted free easily
    - Leaves delicate granulation tissue in the bed undamaged
  - Unless radical resection is planned, surgery should be designed to create as little trauma to bone as possible
  - Healing will often be problematic without measures to improve vascularity

Prognosis

- Progression can lead to pathologic fracture
- Outcome often based on reason for radiation

OSTEORADIONECROSIS

- Intraoral &/or extraoral fistula may also be seen
- Symptoms may never be completely eliminated

IMAGE FINDINGS

Radiographic Findings

- Panoramic radiographs demonstrate osteolysis
  - Show typical ill-defined mottled pattern
    - Radiolucent areas alternating with radiopaque areas

MR Findings

- Low signal intensity on T1WI
- Post-contrast T1WI show contrast enhancement
- Variable T2 signal intensity
  - High T2 signal intensity and contrast enhancement identified when there is infection

MACROSCOPIC FEATURES

General Features

- Irregular fragments of bone
- May be softened due to nonviability

Size

- Range up to several centimeters

MICROSCOPIC PATHOLOGY

Histologic Features

- Overlap with osteomyelitis
- Histopathological phases closely resemble healing of traumatic wounds
- 3 distinct phases are seen
  - **Initial prefibrotic** phase
    - Changes in endothelial cells predominate with associated inflammatory response
  - **Constitutive organized** phase
    - Abnormal fibroblastic activity predominates with disorganization of extracellular matrix
  - **Fibroatrophic** phase
    - Tissue remodeling occurs
- In general, a number of nonspecific features are present
  - Extravasated erythrocytes
  - Hypovascularity with vessel thrombosis
  - Endarteritis may be present
  - Hyalinization and fibrosis
  - Necrotic and devitalized bone
- Sclerotic bone with empty osteocyte lacunae
- With time, secondary infection may be seen
- Reactive, metaplastic squamous mucosa may line a fistula

DIFFERENTIAL DIAGNOSIS

Bisphosphonate Osteonecrosis

- Bisphosphonate used primarily to treat bone metastases of solid tumors and multiple myeloma
- Intravenous preparations seem to have higher incidence of osteonecrosis than oral preparations
- Develops in up to 12% of patients on therapy
- Mandible affected more frequently than maxilla (2:1)
- Often associated with preceding dental procedure (dental extraction)
- Clinical features include nonhealing ulcers, loose teeth, and infections
- Histological overlap: Necrotic bone, fibrinous exudate, and mixed inflammatory infiltrate, often accompanied by bacterial colonization
- **Differences**: Necrotic bone alternating with areas of vital bone; no decrease in number of capillaries

Recurrent Carcinoma

- If radiation was given for squamous cell carcinoma, atypia in squamous-lined fistula may be worrisome
- Squamous epithelium immediately associated with granulation tissue and necrotic bone favor fistula
- Careful review shows reactive changes rather than pleomorphism of carcinoma

Radiation Changes

- Cytologic atypia from radiation changes can also mimic malignancy
- Fibroblastic, endothelial, and squamous/epithelia all affected by radiation
- History will generally help to make the separation

SELECTED REFERENCES

1. Benlier E et al: Massive osteoradionecrosis of facial bones and soft tissues. J BUON. 14(3):523-7, 2009
2. Freiberger JJ et al: Multimodality surgical and hyperbaric management of mandibular osteoradionecrosis. Int J Radiat Oncol Biol Phys. 75(3):717-24, 2009
3. Kelishadi SS et al: Is simultaneous surgical management of advanced craniofacial osteoradionecrosis cost-effective? Plast Reconstr Surg. 123(3):1010-7, 2009
4. Le Stanc E et al: Mandibular lesion differential diagnoses in a patient with a previous history of locally advanced head and neck carcinoma. Clin Nucl Med. 34(7):435-8, 2009
5. McLeod NM et al: Management of patients at risk of osteoradionecrosis: results of survey of dentists and oral & maxillofacial surgery units in the United Kingdom, and suggestions for best practice. Br J Oral Maxillofac Surg. Epub ahead of print, 2009
6. Zevallos JP et al: Complications of radiotherapy in laryngopharyngeal cancer: effects of a prospective smoking cessation program. Cancer. 115(19):4636-44, 2009
7. Gevorgyan A et al: Bisphosphonate-induced necrosis of the jaws: a reconstructive nightmare. Curr Opin Otolaryngol Head Neck Surg. 16(4):325-30, 2008
8. Lyons A et al: Osteoradionecrosis of the jaws: current understanding of its pathophysiology and treatment. Br J Oral Maxillofac Surg. 46(8):653-60, 2008
9. Ferguson HW et al: Advances in head and neck radiotherapy to the mandible. Oral Maxillofac Surg Clin North Am. 19(4):553-63, vii, 2007
10. Otmani N: Oral and maxillofacial side effects of radiation therapy on children. J Can Dent Assoc. 73(3):257-61, 2007
11. Sandel HD 4th et al: Microsurgical reconstruction for radiation necrosis: an evolving disease. J Reconstr Microsurg. 23(4):225-30, 2007

Imaging and Microscopic Features

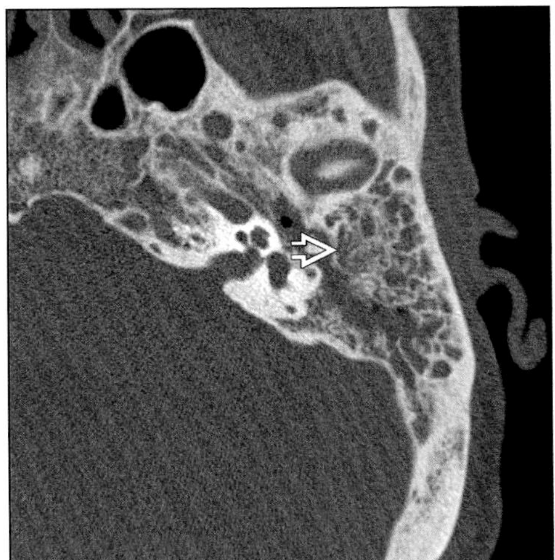

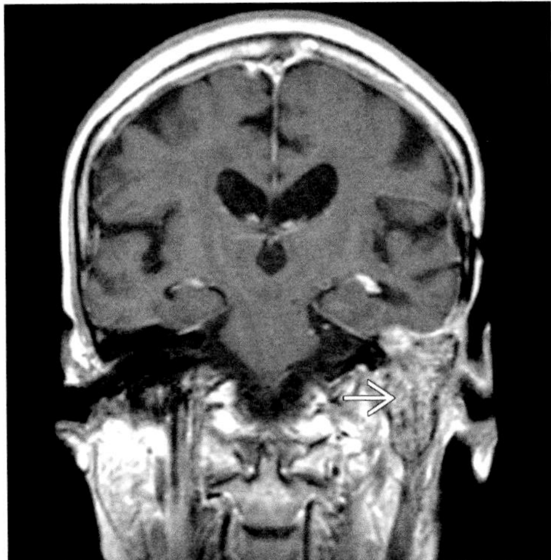

*(**Left**) Axial CT reveals debris throughout the middle ear cleft. Examination of mastoid septations reveals coalescent changes ⇨ with large defects in lateral cortex. This pattern suggests osteoradionecrosis. (**Right**) Axial MR T1WI post contrast reveals that the debris enhances intensely throughout →. Note the destruction of the bone and surrounding soft tissue.*

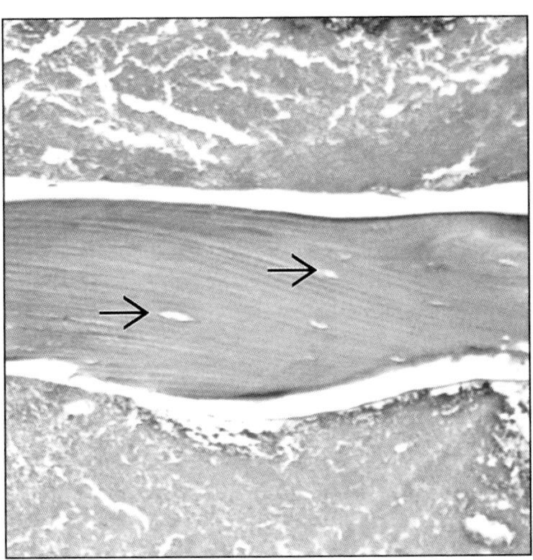

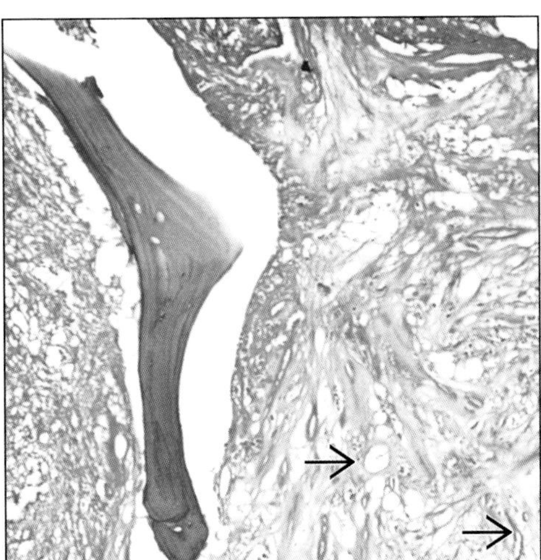

*(**Left**) Trabecular bone is seen with missing osteocytes and empty lacunae →. This is an indication of bone death. There is abundant necrotic debris surrounding this process. Many times these areas can become secondarily infected. (**Right**) The bone is necrotic, showing a lack of nuclei within the lacunar spaces. The marrow is heavily fibrotic with abundant vessels →. There are a number of inflammatory elements present, usually chronic if not secondarily infected.*

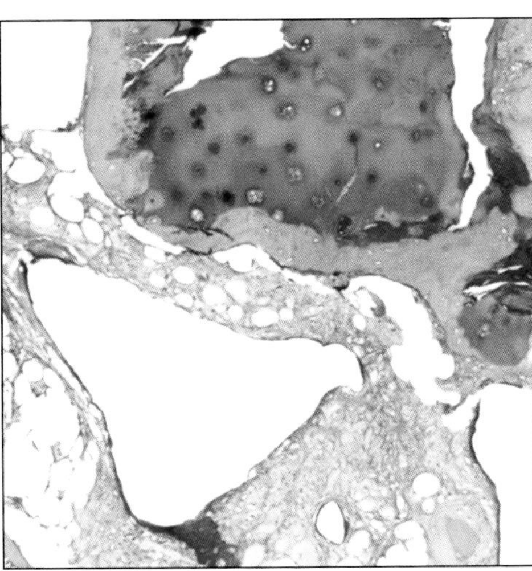

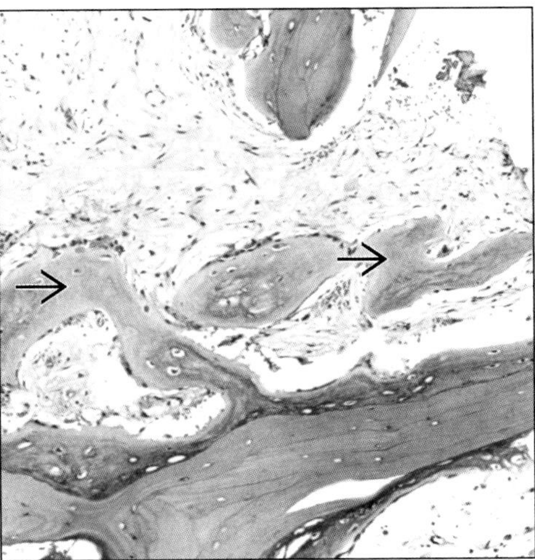

*(**Left**) Marrow necrosis can be fibromyxoid or edematous in nature in the early stages, making diagnosis challenging. However, when any marrow changes are noted in the correct clinical setting, the diagnosis can be reliably made. (**Right**) Later in the repair stages of radiation osteitis, new bone formation → can be noted around the nonviable trabeculae. Reversal lines may be quite prominent. There is often associated scattered chronic inflammation, helping to confirm the diagnosis.*

PAGET DISEASE OF BONE

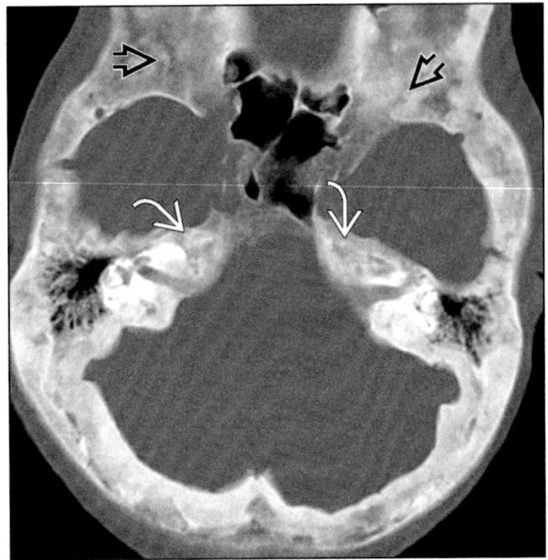

Axial image demonstrates to excellent advantage some patchy residual demineralization at the petrous apex ➔ and at the floor of the anterior cranial fossa ⊳.

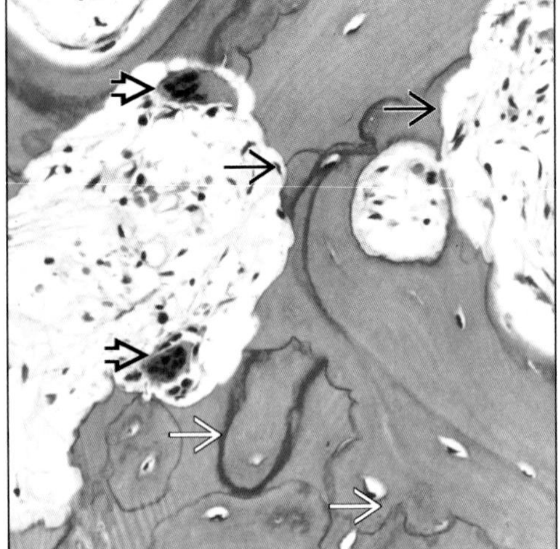

A section shows bone with irregular, scalloped edges → with multiple reversal lines ➔ and osteoclasts ⊳. This change can be seen in other disorders and thus requires radiographic correlation.

TERMINOLOGY

Synonyms

- Osteitis deformans

Definitions

- Paget disease of bone is localized skeletal disorder characterized by osteoclasts of increased number and size containing multiple nuclei
  - Excessive breakdown and formation of bone tissue
  - Named after Sir James Paget, who initially described the disease in 1877

ETIOLOGY/PATHOGENESIS

Infectious Agents

- Have been proposed based on electron microscopy data
- No conclusive proof for infectious agent

CLINICAL ISSUES

Epidemiology

- Incidence
  - Occurs in familial clusters and sporadically
  - 15-40% of patients have positive family history
  - Nongenetic factors are also involved in appearance of the disease
    - Variable penetrance in families
    - Highly localized nature of the disease
    - Epidemiologic data over the past 25 years
  - Estimated that 1 in 100-150 individuals over age of 45 has Paget
- Age
  - Usually seen in patients over the age of 40 years
- Gender
  - Equal gender distribution
- Ethnicity
  - Asian populations tend to be less commonly affected

Site

- Can affect any bones
  - Monostotic: 1 bone
  - Polyostotic: Multiple bones
- Most common sites are
  - Pelvis (70%)
  - Femur (55%)
  - Lumbar spine (50-55%)
  - Skull (40%)
  - Tibia (30%)
  - Feet, hands, and **facial** bones are rarely affected but are seen in some patients

Presentation

- Tends to be nonspecific
- Disease weakens bones
- Results in a number of symptoms
  - Bone pain is most common (often joint associated)
  - Headaches
  - Hearing loss
  - Drowsiness due to vascular steal syndrome
  - Deformities: Increased head size, change in curvature of spine
    - Changes in vision if orbits are affected
  - Fractures
  - Arthritis: Joint cartilage damage
  - Teeth spread: Muscles pull abnormally on bone, resulting in intraoral displacement of teeth, malocclusion, and chewing difficulties
  - Teeth may show hypercementosis (increased cementum deposition at tooth root)
- Cardiovascular disease is common
- Kidney stones are more common
- Central nervous system affected by pressure of bone on brain, spinal cord, and nerves

PAGET DISEASE OF BONE

Key Facts

Terminology

- Paget disease of bone is localized skeletal disorder characterized by osteoclasts of increased number and size containing multiple nuclei

Clinical Issues

- Occurs in familial clusters
- Usually seen in patients over the age of 40
- Can be monostotic or polyostotic
- Biochemical markers of bone turnover (alkaline phosphatase) are key in disease monitoring
- Oral bisphosphonates are mainstay of therapy

Image Findings

- Plain films: "Blade of grass" sign
- Typical "cotton wool" or "ground-glass" appearance
- Late stages: Predominantly sclerotic

Microscopic Pathology

- Affected bones will have enlarged pumice-like gross morphology
- Mid-stage: Osteoblastic and osteoclastic activity
  - Osteoclasts are larger in size and have large number of nuclei
- Numerous reversal lines are noted as a result of increased remodeling
- High degree of vascularity noted in intervening intertrabecular spaces
- Initially, osteoporosis predominates

Top Differential Diagnoses

- Renal osteodystrophy, hyperparathyroidism, ossifying hemangioma

Laboratory Tests

- Biochemical markers of bone turnover are key in monitoring disease progression and response to therapy
- Total serum alkaline phosphatase (ALP) may be useful in monitoring the disease
  - Elevated in over 85% of Paget patients
- Serum calcium, phosphorous, and aminotransferase are normal in Paget

Natural History

- Excessive osteoclastic activity in Paget disease causes accelerated bone resorption
- Tightly coupled to recruitment of osteoblasts in that area
- Result is rapid formation of disorganized bone tissue that is mechanically weaker than native bone
  - Fractures and deformity result
- High output cardiac failure in some patients
  - High vascularity in lesions can sequester large amounts of circulating blood in larger bones
- Low percentage of patients can develop secondary sarcoma
  - Osteosarcoma
  - Malignant fibrous histiocytoma
  - Fibrosarcoma
  - Giant cell tumor of bone
  - Secondary sarcomas are generally high grade

Treatment

- Options, risks, complications
  - Bisphosphonates are one of the mainstays
    - Osteonecrosis can be complication of this therapy
  - Risk of fracture remains high
    - Calcium and vitamin D supplementation to manage osteoporosis
    - Must be used with caution in bisphosphonate therapy and kidney stone patients
  - Risk of secondary sarcoma is 4-10%
- Surgical approaches
  - Joint replacement can be difficult due to underlying abnormal bone
  - Fracture repair is often difficult due to underlying nature of bone
  - Oncologic surgery needed with secondary sarcomas
- Drugs
  - Oral bisphosphonates are most widely prescribed agents for Paget disease
    - Use may be limited by complicated dosing requirements and poor gastrointestinal absorption
    - Drug therapy regimens can result in mandibular osteonecrosis in some cases
  - Calcitonin analogues are infrequently used

Prognosis

- Poor prognosis with secondary sarcoma
  - Malignant fibrous histiocytoma and osteosarcoma most common secondary sarcomas
- High output cardiac failure difficult to manage

IMAGE FINDINGS

Radiographic Findings

- Initial work-up should include skeletal survey and bone scan
- Initial presentation on plain films will show osteoporosis
- Affected bones will be enlarged and thickened
- Plain films will often show "blade of grass" sign as initial presentation
  - Caused by advancing waves of osteoclasts resorbing bone along long axis of bone
- As disease progresses, typical "cotton wool" or "ground-glass" appearance is noted
  - Appearance due to presence of osteoblasts synthesizing osseous matrix
- Late stages of the disease are predominantly sclerotic
- Dental radiographs show loss of lamina dura, hypercementosis, and calcified pulp chambers

Bone Scan

- Intense uptake of tracer at affected sites
  - Due to increased metabolic activity from osteoblastic activity

PAGET DISEASE OF BONE

- Useful in identifying polyostotic involvement

MACROSCOPIC FEATURES

General Features

- Affected bones will have enlarged pumice-like gross morphology
- Bone can be grossly friable

Sections to Be Submitted

- 1 per centimeter if sarcoma is involved

Size

- Variable depending on bone involved

MICROSCOPIC PATHOLOGY

Histologic Features

- Findings reflect stage of disease
  - Initial stages are reflective of osteoclastic activity
    - Numerous osteoclasts
    - Increased vascularity
    - Numerous resorptive surfaces
  - Mid stage shows a mix of patterns
    - Osteoclastic resorption
    - Increased vascularity
    - Numerous surfaces covered with active osteoblasts
  - End stage is primarily sclerotic
- Osteoclasts are larger in size and have large number of nuclei
- Numerous reversal lines are noted as a result of increased remodeling
- High degree of vascularity noted in intervening intertrabecular spaces
- Initially osteoporosis predominates
- Middle stage reveals both osteoblastic and osteoclastic activity
- As disease becomes less active, marrow appears fibrotic

ANCILLARY TESTS

Histochemistry

- Alkaline phosphatase staining in osteoblasts in these specimens

Cytogenetics

- Familial cases display autosomal dominant pattern of inheritance with variable penetrance
- Studies of families with Paget have identified several loci
  - 2q36
  - 5q31
  - 5q35
  - 10p13
  - 18q22, 13,14
  - *SQSTSM1* gene on chromosome 5

DIFFERENTIAL DIAGNOSIS

Renal Osteodystrophy

- High osteoclastic activity due to secondary hyperparathyroidism
- Low intervening vascularity
- Marked increase in osteoid seam production
- Paratrabecular fibrosis often noted
- High percentage of resorptive surfaces without reversal lines
- Mosaic morphology usually not noted

Hyperparathyroidism

- Increased number of osteoclasts
- Increased resorptive surfaces

Ossifying Hemangioma

- Variable amounts of delicate, well-formed vessels
- Small area involved rather than larger areas of Paget
- Bone forms in thin boundaries around vessels
- Mosaic pattern unusual

DIAGNOSTIC CHECKLIST

Pathologic Interpretation Pearls

- Reversal lines in bone present in a number of diseases
- Need to see constellation of clinical and pathological signs
- Radiology key to interpreting biopsy specimens
- Need to rule out forms of hyperparathyroidism before diagnosis
- Any presence of atypia should be followed up to rule out secondary sarcoma

SELECTED REFERENCES

1. Goytia RN et al: Bisphosphonates and osteonecrosis: potential treatment or serious complication? Orthop Clin North Am. 40(2):223-34, 2009
2. McNeill G et al: Re: Paget's disease of the bone: a review. Rheumatol Int. 29(10):1253-4, 2009
3. Singer FR: Paget disease: when to treat and when not to treat. Nat Rev Rheumatol. 5(9):483-9, 2009
4. Colina M et al: Paget's disease of bone: a review. Rheumatol Int. 28(11):1069-75, 2008
5. Cundy T et al: Paget disease of bone. Trends Endocrinol Metab. 19(7):246-53, 2008
6. Haugeberg G: Imaging of metabolic bone diseases. Best Pract Res Clin Rheumatol. 22(6):1127-39, 2008
7. Ralston SH et al: Pathogenesis and management of Paget's disease of bone. Lancet. 372(9633):155-63, 2008
8. Ralston SH: Pathogenesis of Paget's disease of bone. Bone. 43(5):819-25, 2008
9. Silverman SL: Paget disease of bone: therapeutic options. J Clin Rheumatol. 14(5):299-305, 2008
10. Monsell EM: The mechanism of hearing loss in Paget's disease of bone. Laryngoscope. 114(4):598-606, 2004
11. Hullar TE et al: Paget's disease and fibrous dysplasia. Otolaryngol Clin North Am. 36(4):707-32, 2003
12. Carter LC: Paget's disease: important features for the general practitioner. Compendium. 11(11):662, 664-5, 668-9, 1990

Diagrammatic, Radiographic, and Microscopic Features

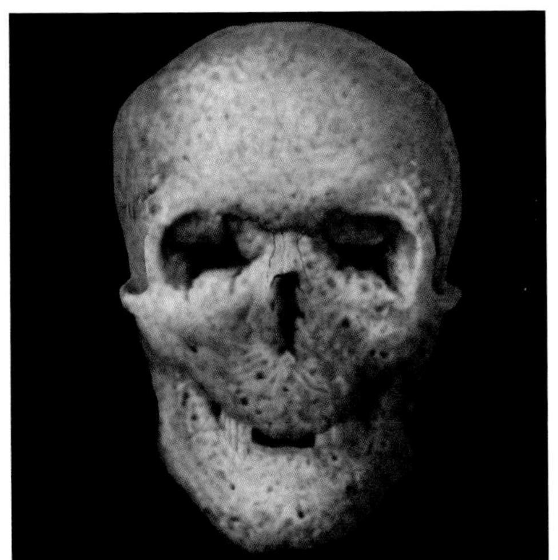

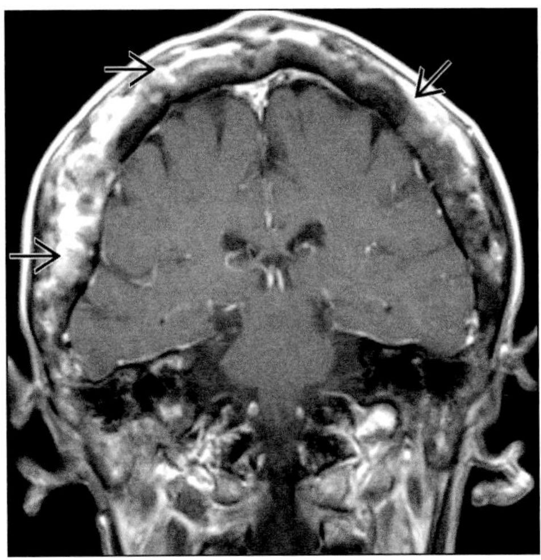

(Left) *This graphic represents a patient with Paget disease involving multiple bones of the head. The bones are misshapen and widened, with a gross appearance resembling the porosity of volcanic or pumice stone.* ***(Right)*** *Enhanced T1-weighted MR image reveals intense heterogeneous enhancement of the vascularized connective tissue ⇒ throughout the visualized calvarium. This is appreciated to best advantage on coronal post-contrast images.*

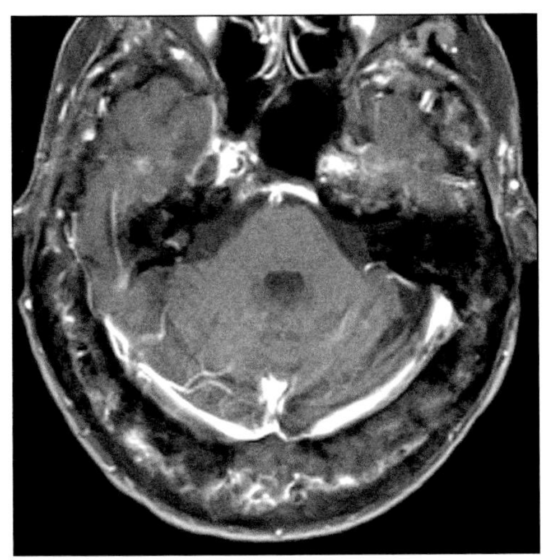

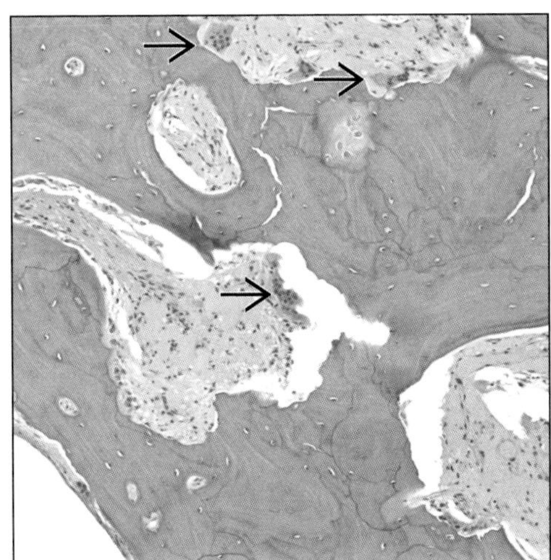

(Left) *Enhanced T1-weighted MR image reveals intense heterogeneous enhancement of the vascularized connective tissue throughout the visualized calvarium of skull base. This is a typical appearance of Paget disease of bone.* ***(Right)*** *The image demonstrates thickened trabecular struts of bone with prominent reversal lines. There are numerous osteoclasts ⇒, while osteoblasts are not as commonly present.*

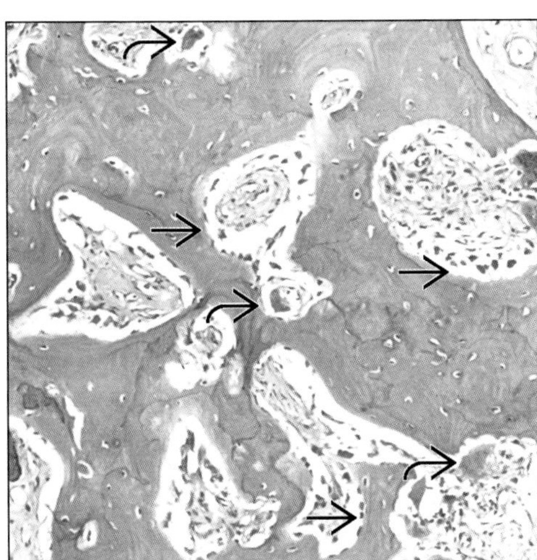

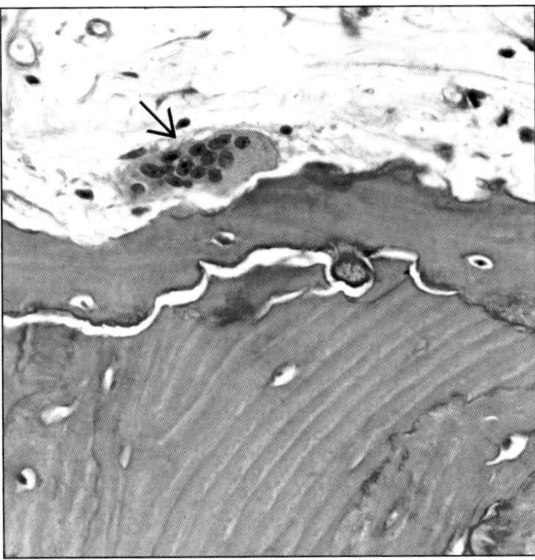

(Left) *This is a representation of the middle stage of Paget disease. The figure shows extensive woven bone, with numerous osteoclasts ↗ and active osteoblasts ⇒. Reversal lines are present but are not as prominent as some cases. These changes are nonspecific. Clinical and radiographic correlation are required.* ***(Right)*** *The osteoclasts ⇒ in Paget disease are larger than normal osteoclasts, as well as showing an increased number of nuclei.*

CENTRAL GIANT CELL LESION

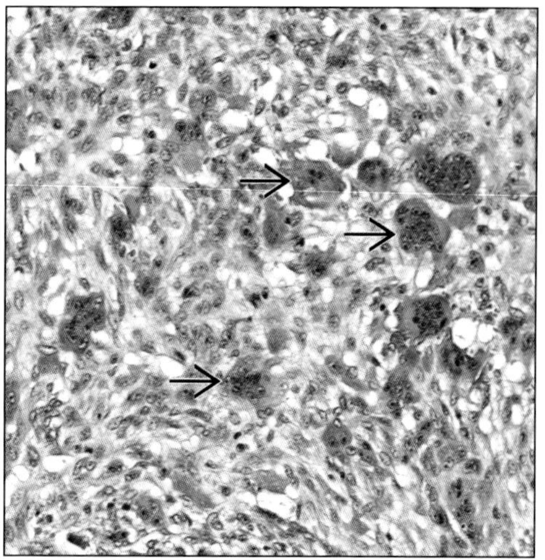

Hematoxylin & eosin shows numerous multinucleated giant cells associated with red blood cell extravasation. The nuclei of the multinucleated giant cells ➔ are similar to those of the stroma.

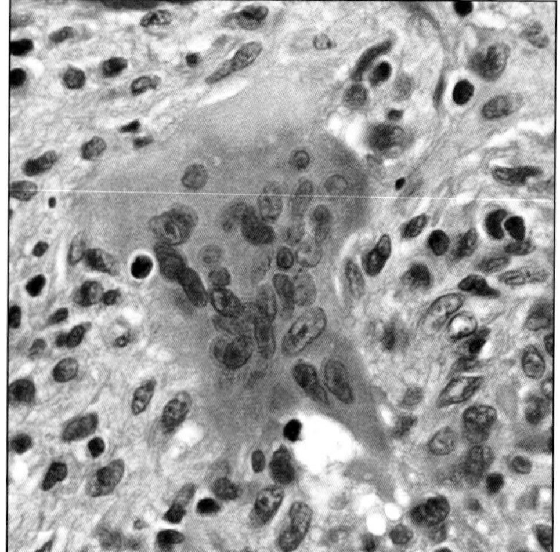

Hematoxylin & eosin shows the variability in size and shape of the giant cells within a giant cell lesion.

TERMINOLOGY

Synonyms

- Central giant cell granuloma
- Giant cell tumor
- Giant cell reparative granuloma

Definitions

- Potentially locally aggressive osteolytic lesion of gnathic bones

ETIOLOGY/PATHOGENESIS

Pathogenesis

- Controversial
  - Neoplastic
    - Aggressive vs. nonaggressive
  - Reactive (not favored)

CLINICAL ISSUES

Epidemiology

- Incidence
  - Uncommon
- Age
  - Wide range
    - Peak in mid to late teens
- Gender
  - Female > Male (2:1)

Site

- Mandible more commonly affected
  - More common in anterior region
  - Frequently crosses midline

Presentation

- Nonaggressive
  - Asymptomatic, detected on routine dental radiographs
  - Few symptoms
    - Slow-growing, painless expansion of bone
- Aggressive
  - Pain &/or paresthesia
  - Erosion of cortical plates, resorption of adjacent roots, and tooth displacement

Treatment

- Surgical approaches
  - Curettage
  - Rarely resection for large aggressive lesions
    - Reconstruction
- Drugs
  - Corticosteroid (such as triamcinolone)
    - Weekly injections into lesion
  - Calcitonin
    - Subcutaneous injection or nasal spray
  - Interferon-α injections

Prognosis

- Commonly recur

IMAGE FINDINGS

Radiographic Findings

- Expansile, radiolucent defect
  - Unilocular
  - Multilocular
- Well delineated
- May resorb nearby roots
- Occasionally crosses midline of jaw

MACROSCOPIC FEATURES

General Features

- Friable, brown, and hemorrhagic

CENTRAL GIANT CELL LESION

Key Facts

Terminology
- Potentially locally aggressive osteolytic lesion of gnathic bones

Clinical Issues
- Favors mandible
- Surgical curettage, rarely resection for large aggressive lesions
- Alternative treatments: Corticosteroid, calcitonin, and interferon-α
- Commonly recur

Image Findings
- Radiolucent defect

Microscopic Pathology
- Giant cells
  - Most likely related to osteoclasts
  - Few to upward of 20 nuclei
- Stroma

MICROSCOPIC PATHOLOGY

Histologic Features
- Giant cells
  - Most likely related to osteoclasts
  - Focal collections to diffuse distribution
  - Variable size and shape
  - Up to 20 nuclei per cell
- Stroma
  - Loosely arranged to fibrous
  - Cellular
  - Erythrocyte extravasation with hemosiderin
- Correlation of histology with aggressive nature
  - Debatable, with mixed results
  - Cellular stroma, uniformly distributed giant cells with increased mitotic figures (not atypical)

ANCILLARY TESTS

Molecular Genetics
- No mutations of *SH3BP2* gene (known to cause cherubism), making this a distinct entity

DIFFERENTIAL DIAGNOSIS

Brown Tumor of Hyperparathyroidism
- Signs and symptoms of parathyroid dysfunction
- Serum calcium and parathyroid hormone levels abnormal

Cherubism
- Distinctive clinically; familial; manifests in early childhood with bilateral jaw involvement

Aneurysmal Bone Cyst
- More cystic and more hemorrhagic

Giant Cell Tumor
- Believed to occur exclusively in long bones

SELECTED REFERENCES

1. de Lange J et al: Central giant cell granuloma of the jaw: a review of the literature with emphasis on therapy options. Oral Surg Oral Med Oral Pathol Oral Radiol Endod. 104(5):603-15, 2007
2. Motamedi MH et al: Peripheral and central giant cell granulomas of the jaws: a demographic study. Oral Surg Oral Med Oral Pathol Oral Radiol Endod. 103(6):e39-43, 2007
3. Comert E et al: Oral and intralesional steroid therapy in giant cell granuloma. Acta Otolaryngol. 126(6):664-6, 2006
4. de Lange J et al: Calcitonin therapy in central giant cell granuloma of the jaw: a randomized double-blind placebo-controlled study. Int J Oral Maxillofac Surg. 35(9):791-5, 2006
5. Farrier SL et al: A 10-year review of the occurrence and treatment of central giant cell granulomas, in a District General Hospital. J Oral Pathol Med. 35(6):332-7, 2006
6. De Lange J et al: Clinical and radiological features of central giant-cell lesions of the jaw. Oral Surg Oral Med Oral Pathol Oral Radiol Endod. 99(4):464-70, 2005

IMAGE GALLERY

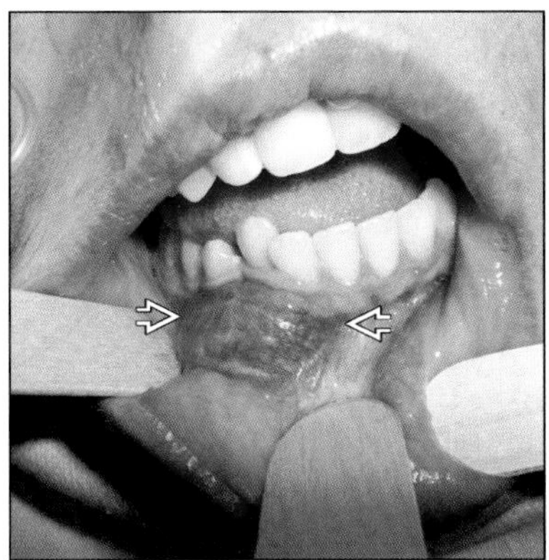

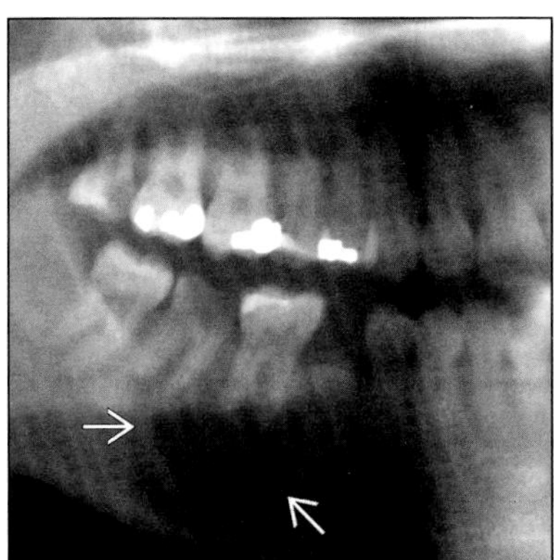

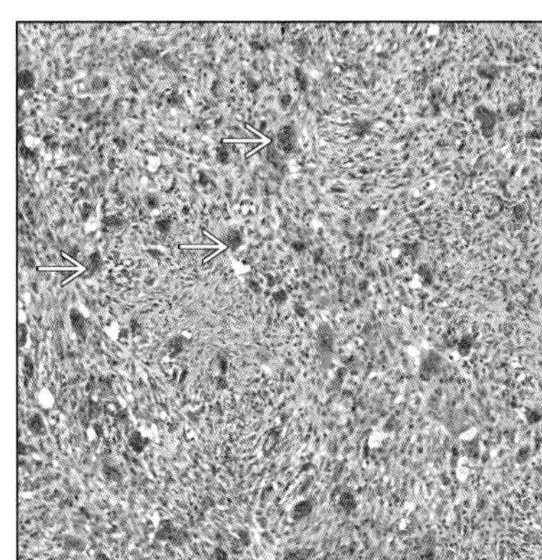

(Left) *Clinical photograph shows a mass in the gingiva ⇨, an extension from the mandible in this patient with a central giant cell lesion. (Courtesy B.W. Walline, MD.)* ***(Center)*** *Radiograph shows a unilocular radiolucent area associated with the apex of the 1st and 2nd molar →. This was considered preoperatively to be a periapical granuloma or periapical cyst.* ***(Right)*** *Hematoxylin & eosin shows evenly distributed giant cells ⇨ in a fibrovascular stroma. The stroma is cellular, without showing a significant amount of extravasated erythrocytes.*

SIMPLE BONE CYST

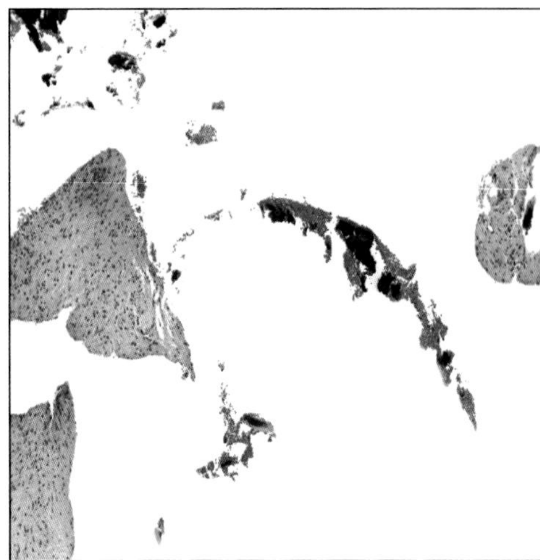

Hematoxylin & eosin shows scant fragments of fibrovascular connective tissue and bone. Lack of submitted tissue is characteristic of a simple bone cyst.

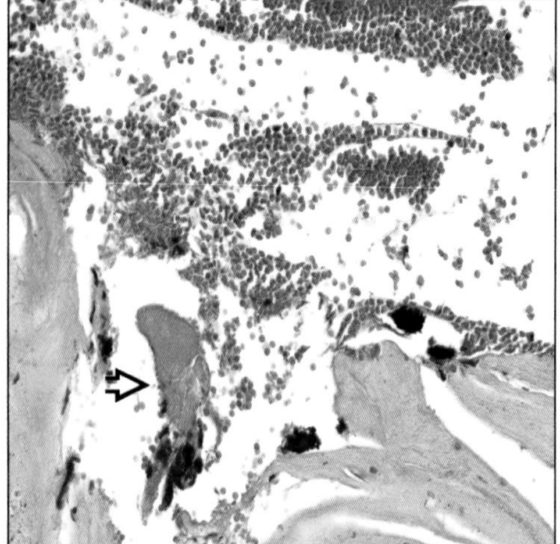

Hematoxylin & eosin shows scant fibrovascular connective tissue and numerous red blood cells. A small fragment of bone ⇨ is identified.

TERMINOLOGY

Synonyms

- Traumatic bone cyst
- Traumatic bone cavity
- Solitary bone cyst
- Hemorrhagic cyst

Definitions

- Benign empty or fluid-filled cavity within bone

ETIOLOGY/PATHOGENESIS

Pathogenesis

- Controversial, although unknown
- Trauma (reported infrequently)
  - Causes intraosseous hematoma
  - Hematoma fails to involute resulting in cyst/cavity
- Disturbance in bone growth
- Vascular anomalies
- Result of low-grade infection

CLINICAL ISSUES

Epidemiology

- Incidence
  - Common
- Age
  - Found primarily in 1st 2 decades of life
- Gender
  - Male > Female

Site

- Mandible
  - Premolar-molar region
- Lesions of maxilla are rare

Presentation

- Most are asymptomatic
  - Discovered with routine dental radiographs
- Pain
- Swelling
- Sensitivity of nearby teeth
  - Teeth test vital
- Rare: Paresthesia; pathologic fracture; expansile

Treatment

- Surgical approaches
  - Open cavity to confirm biopsy
  - Curettage of bony wall
  - Large lesion may require bone graft

Prognosis

- After surgery, defect generally resolves
- Recurrence may develop
  - Tends to be higher if there are multiple cysts
  - Usually develops within 3 years, if it is going to occur

IMAGE FINDINGS

Radiographic Findings

- Well-defined radiolucency
- Defect often shows "scalloping" between tooth roots
  - 50% of cases
- Rarely, multifocal
- Rarely, associated with benign fibro-osseous lesion
  - Cemento-osseous dysplasia

MACROSCOPIC FEATURES

General Features

- Clinically, empty or containing blood or straw-colored fluid
- Scant fragments of friable soft tissue
- Small bone fragments
- Larger bone fragments

SIMPLE BONE CYST

Key Facts

Terminology
- Benign empty or fluid-filled cavity in bone

Clinical Issues
- Common lesion, affecting males in 1st 2 decades
- Most are asymptomatic
- Mandible, specifically premolar-molar region

Image Findings
- Radiolucent
- Defect often shows "scalloping" between tooth roots

Microscopic Pathology
- Small fragments of fibrovascular connective tissue
- Small fragments of bone

Top Differential Diagnoses
- Developmental odontogenic cysts
  - Dentigerous cyst; lateral periodontal cyst
- Reactive odontogenic lesions (radicular cyst, periapical granuloma)

  - May represent bone removed to gain access to cavity, creating a "bone window"

Size
- Range: 1-10 cm

MICROSCOPIC PATHOLOGY

Histologic Features
- Small fragments of fibrovascular connective tissue
- Small fragments of bone
  - Reactive with cellular trabeculae
- Red blood cells
- Rare giant cells
- No epithelial lining
- Dystrophic calcifications

DIFFERENTIAL DIAGNOSIS

Developmental Odontogenic Cysts
- Dentigerous cyst
  - Associated with crown of unerupted tooth
  - Cyst lining
- Lateral periodontal cyst
  - Associated with lateral aspect of tooth root
  - Cyst lining

Reactive Odontogenic Lesions
- Radicular cyst
  - Cyst lining
  - Associated with root of nonvital tooth
- Periapical granuloma
  - Dense inflammatory infiltrate
  - Associated with root of nonvital tooth

DIAGNOSTIC CHECKLIST

Clinically Relevant Pathologic Features
- Radiolucent "scalloping" between tooth roots

SELECTED REFERENCES

1. Cortell-Ballester I et al: Traumatic bone cyst: a retrospective study of 21 cases. Med Oral Patol Oral Cir Bucal. 14(5):E239-43, 2009
2. Slootweg PJ: Lesions of the jaws. Histopathology. 54(4):401-18, 2009
3. Harnet JC et al: Solitary bone cyst of the jaws: a review of the etiopathogenic hypotheses. J Oral Maxillofac Surg. 66(11):2345-8, 2008
4. Suei Y et al: A comparative study of simple bone cysts of the jaw and extracranial bones. Dentomaxillofac Radiol. 36(3):125-9, 2007
5. Suei Y et al: Simple bone cyst of the jaws: evaluation of treatment outcome by review of 132 cases. J Oral Maxillofac Surg. 65(5):918-23, 2007
6. Shimoyama T et al: So-called simple bone cyst of the jaw: a family of pseudocysts of diverse nature and etiology. J Oral Sci. 41(2):93-8, 1999
7. Copete MA et al: Solitary bone cyst of the jaws: radiographic review of 44 cases. Oral Surg Oral Med Oral Pathol Oral Radiol Endod. 85(2):221-5, 1998

IMAGE GALLERY

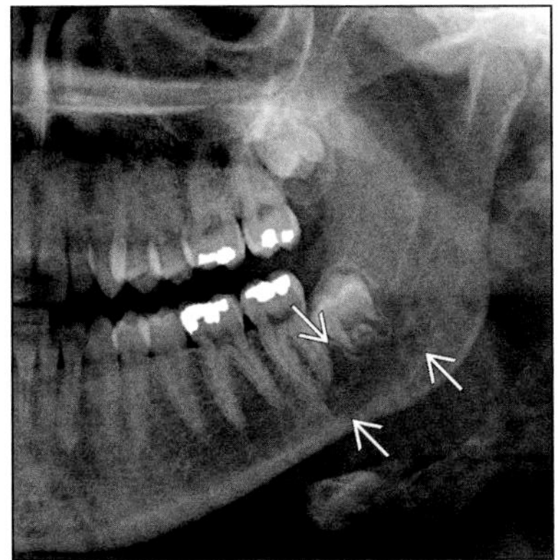

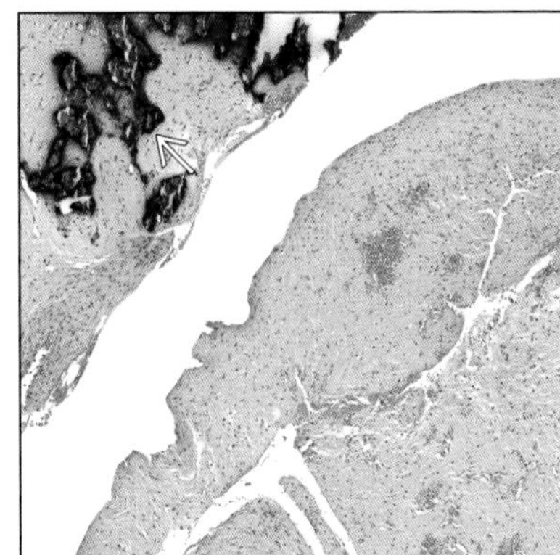

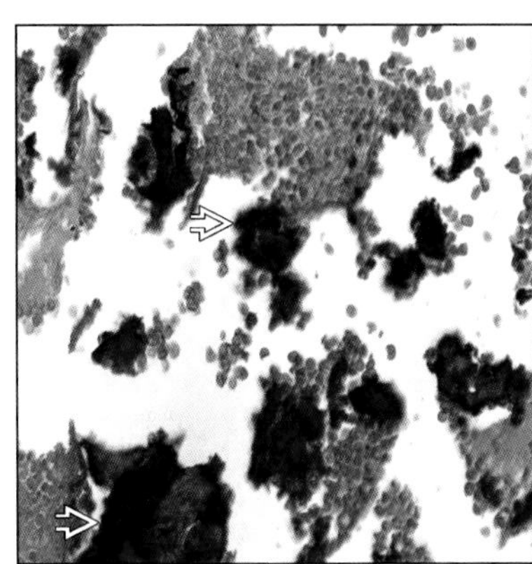

*(**Left**) Radiograph shows a simple bone cyst at the angle of the mandible. Note the cyst ➡ has a scalloped margin that projects between the roots of the 2nd molar and the impacted 3rd molar. (**Center**) Hematoxylin & eosin shows loose fibrovascular connective tissue that was curetted from the walls of the essentially empty bony cavity. An area of dystrophic calcification ➡ is present in the soft tissue. (**Right**) Hematoxylin & eosin shows scattered red blood cells and dystrophic calcifications ➡.*

DENTIGEROUS CYST

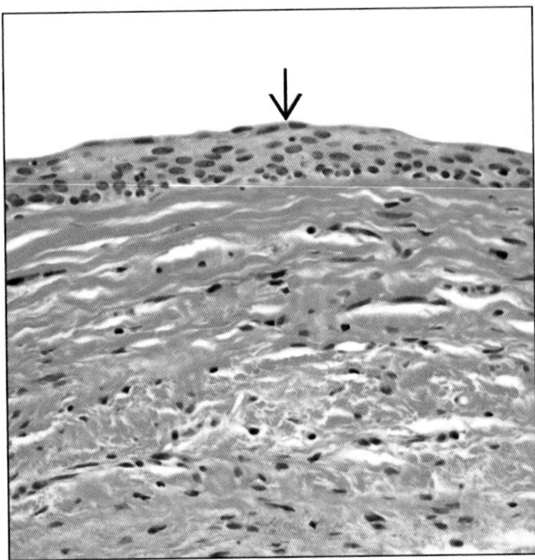

Hematoxylin & eosin shows a noninflamed dentigerous cyst with a thin keratinized epithelial lining ➔. There is no basal palisading, no refractile keratin layer, and separation artifact.

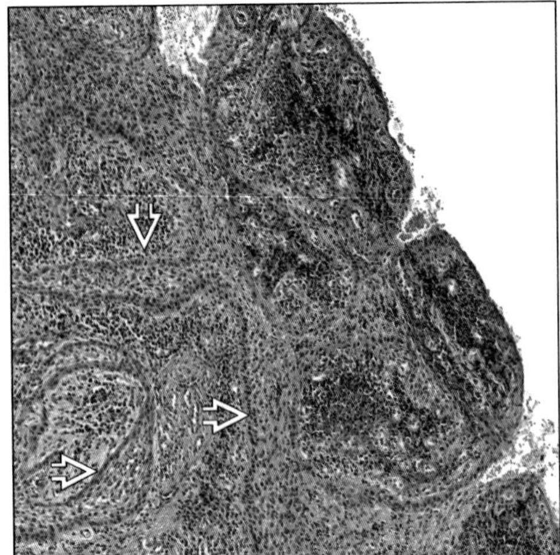

Hematoxylin & eosin shows an inflamed dentigerous cyst with hyperplastic rete ridges ➔ and a dense inflammatory infiltrate. This is a common finding with secondarily inflamed or infected cysts.

TERMINOLOGY

Abbreviations

- Dentigerous cyst (DC)

Synonyms

- Follicular cyst

Definitions

- Developmental cyst surrounding the crown of impacted tooth and attached to cemento-enamel junction

ETIOLOGY/PATHOGENESIS

Pathogenesis

- Develops by accumulation of fluid between reduced enamel epithelium and crown of a tooth

CLINICAL ISSUES

Epidemiology

- Incidence
  - Most common developmental cyst
    - 25% of all jaw cysts
- Age
  - Wide range
  - Peak incidence: 2nd to 3rd decade
- Gender
  - Slight male predilection

Site

- Most commonly associated with mandibular 3rd molars
- Maxillary canines
- Maxillary 3rd molars
- Mandibular 2nd premolars

Presentation

- Small cyst may be asymptomatic
  - Discovered on routine dental radiographs
- Expansion of bone
- Resorption of adjacent teeth
- Pain
- Infection
  - Usually associated with oral communication

Treatment

- Careful enucleation of cyst
- Extraction
  - Prosthodontic replacement if needed
- Preservation of tooth may be indicated
- Large cysts are occasionally treated with marsupialization

Prognosis

- Excellent
- Recurrence is rare
- Rare cases of malignant transformation

IMAGE FINDINGS

Radiographic Findings

- Usually unilocular radiolucency around the crown of affected tooth
- Well-defined sclerotic border
- Larger lesions may appear multilocular
- May displace involved tooth
  - Mandibular 3rd molars
    - Angle of mandible
    - Ascending ramus
  - Maxillary canines
    - Floor of nose
    - Floor of sinus
    - Rarely orbit
- Relationship to tooth
  - Central

DENTIGEROUS CYST

Key Facts

Terminology
- Developmental cyst surrounding crown of impacted tooth and attached to cemento-enamel junction

Clinical Issues
- Most common developmental cyst
- Most commonly associated with mandibular 3rd molars or maxillary canines
- Careful enucleation of cyst

Image Findings
- Usually unilocular radiolucency around crown of affected tooth, with well-defined sclerotic border

Microscopic Pathology
- Noninflamed: 2-3 layers of cuboidal cells, with occasional mucus or ciliated cells
- Inflamed: Proliferative epithelium with chronic inflammatory cells

---

    - Surrounds crown of tooth
  - Lateral
    - Cyst grows laterally along root and partially surrounds crown
  - Circumferential
    - Surrounds crown and much of root

MACROSCOPIC FEATURES

General Features
- Fibrous tan friable soft tissue
- Extracted tooth
  - Relationship to tooth is usually lost with extraction procedure

MICROSCOPIC PATHOLOGY

Histologic Features
- Noninflamed
  - Fibrous to fibromyxoid connective tissue
  - 2-3 layers of cuboidal to ovoid epithelium
  - Occasional mucous cells
  - Rare ciliated cells
  - Occasional dystrophic calcifications
  - Odontogenic epithelial rests
- Inflamed
  - Fibrous connective tissue
  - Proliferative epithelium
  - Hyperplastic rete ridges
  - Chronic inflammatory cells
  - Acute inflammatory cells, usually associated with oral communication
  - Cholesterol clefts
  - Rushton bodies
  - Rare mucous cells
  - Rare ciliated cells
  - Rare sebaceous cells

DIFFERENTIAL DIAGNOSIS

Enlarged Dental Follicle
- Usually < 3-4 mm radiographically
- No cystic epithelium

SELECTED REFERENCES

1. Grossmann SM et al: Demographic profile of odontogenic and selected nonodontogenic cysts in a Brazilian population. Oral Surg Oral Med Oral Pathol Oral Radiol Endod. 104(6):e35-41, 2007
2. Yeo JF et al: Clinicopathological study of dentigerous cysts in Singapore and Malaysia. Malays J Pathol. 29(1):41-7, 2007
3. Dunsche A et al: Dentigerous cyst versus unicystic ameloblastoma--differential diagnosis in routine histology. J Oral Pathol Med. 32(8):486-91, 2003
4. Farah CS et al: Pericoronal radiolucencies and the significance of early detection. Aust Dent J. 47(3):262-5, 2002
5. Mosqueda-Taylor A et al: Odontogenic cysts. Analysis of 856 cases. Med Oral. 7(2):89-96, 2002

IMAGE GALLERY

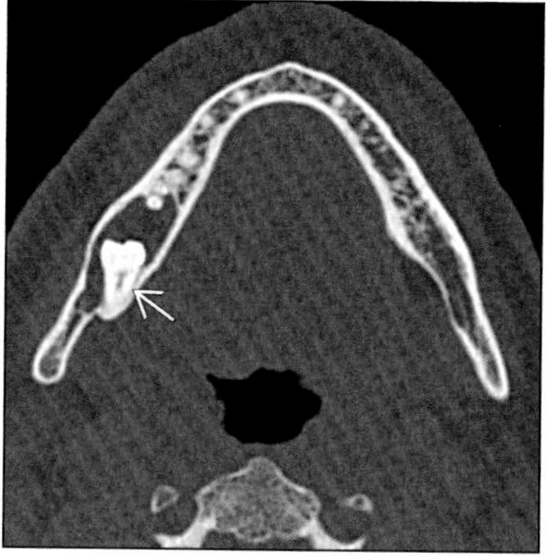

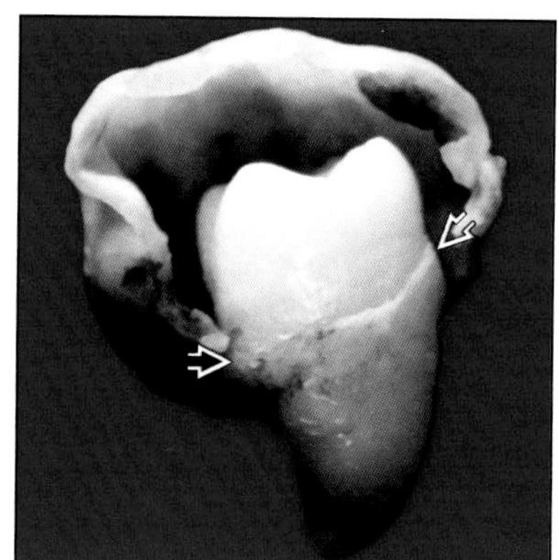

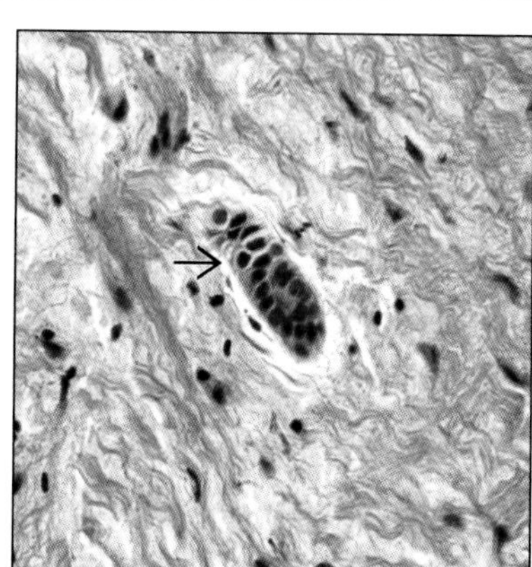

(Left) *Axial bone CT shows a classic dentigerous cyst arising from an unerupted 3rd mandibular molar ➔. Slight expansion of mandibular cortical walls is also typical.* ***(Center)*** *Gross photograph shows the crown of the tooth within the cyst. The cyst wall is attached to the tooth at the cemento-enamel junction ➔ and forms a collar. This feature is seldom preserved, unless the sample is carefully removed and dissected.* ***(Right)*** *Hematoxylin & eosin shows epithelial odontogenic rests in the connective tissue wall of a dentigerous cyst ➔.*

PERIAPICAL CYST/GRANULOMA

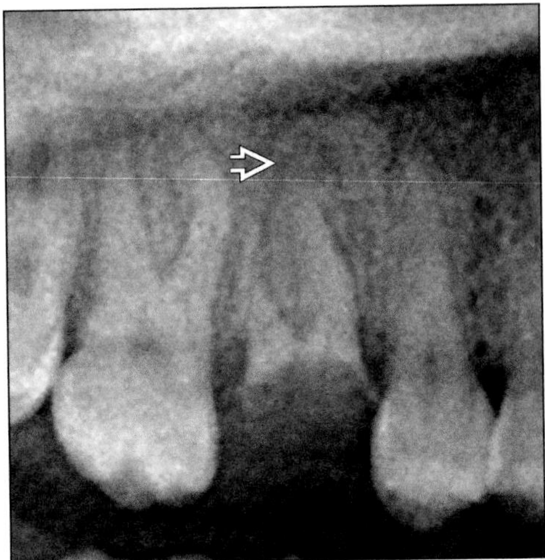

Radiograph shows a decayed tooth with a poorly defined radiolucency at the apex of the root ➔. This tooth tested nonvital and was subsequently extracted.

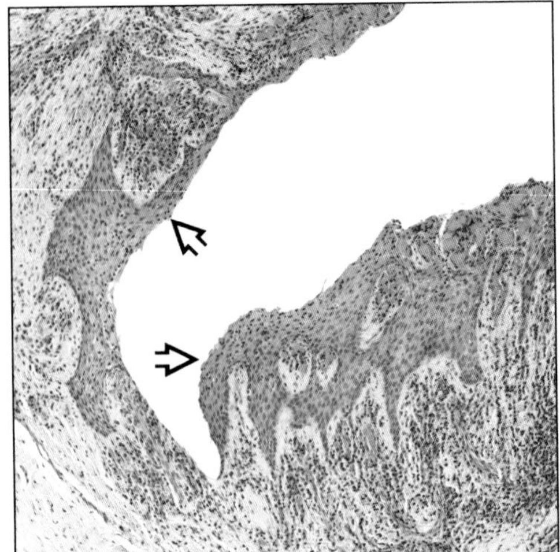

Hematoxylin & eosin shows the stratified squamous epithelial lining ➔ of a periapical cyst. A dense inflammatory infiltrate can be seen in the fibrous wall.

TERMINOLOGY

Synonyms

- Periapical cyst
  - Periradicular cyst
  - Apical periodontal cyst
- Periapical granuloma
  - Periradicular granuloma
  - Periradicular periodontitis

Definitions

- Inflamed tissue associated with apex or root surface of nonvital tooth

CLINICAL ISSUES

Epidemiology

- Incidence
  - Periapical cyst
    - Approximately 75% periapical lesions
    - Most common cyst of jaw
  - Periapical granuloma
    - Less common
- Age
  - Wide range
- Gender
  - Equal gender distribution

Site

- Always associated with root surface of tooth

Presentation

- Asymptomatic
  - May be detected during routine dental radiographs
- Symptomatic
  - Pain
  - Sensitivity to temperature changes
  - Mobility of affected teeth
  - Responds abnormally to clinical testing
    - Electric pulp test
    - Percussion

Natural History

- Caries causes cavitation of tooth
- Bacterial invasion of pulp tissue
- Toxins are generated
- Pulp tissue becomes devitalized

Treatment

- Endodontic treatment
  - Nonsurgical endodontic therapy (root canal)
  - Surgical endodontic therapy
    - For teeth that fail to respond to conventional endodontic treatment
    - Very large lesions
  - Restoration of associated tooth
  - Periodic follow-up
- Extraction of associated tooth or teeth
- Antibiotic treatment
  - For lesions with acute infections
  - Lesions with actinomycosis

Prognosis

- Good with appropriate treatment

IMAGE FINDINGS

Radiographic Findings

- Radiolucency
  - Variable size
  - Circumscribed to poorly circumscribed
  - Associated with apex or root surface
  - May cause root resorption
- Associated tooth conditions
  - Carious or fractured
  - Large restoration
  - Evidence of previous endodontic therapy
  - No significant pathology evident

PERIAPICAL CYST/GRANULOMA

Key Facts

Terminology
- Inflamed tissue associated with apex or root surface of nonvital tooth

Clinical Issues
- Periapical cyst is most common cyst of jaw
- Asymptomatic or symptomatic
- Endodontic treatment, extraction, or antibiotic therapy

Image Findings
- Radiolucency
- Associated with apex or root surface

Microscopic Pathology
- Periapical cyst
  - Stratified squamous epithelium
- Inflammation is variable
- Dystrophic calcifications

MACROSCOPIC FEATURES

General Features
- May be submitted as attached apical tissue on extracted tooth

MICROSCOPIC PATHOLOGY

Histologic Features
- Fibrous tissue
- Periapical cyst
  - Stratified squamous epithelial lining
- Inflammation is variable
  - Chronic and acute: Lymphocytes, plasma cells, multinucleated giant cells, histocytes, eosinophils, and neutrophils
- Dystrophic calcifications
- Cholesterol clefts
- Foreign material if previously endodontically treated

DIFFERENTIAL DIAGNOSIS

Scar
- Dense fibrous connective tissue with little inflammation

Keratinizing Odontogenic Tumor (Odontogenic Keratocyst)
- Usually lacks inflammation
- Epithelial surface
  - Lack of rete ridges
  - Parakeratotic with corrugated appearance
  - 6-8 cells thick with palisaded, hyperchromatic basal layer

Orthokeratinized Odontogenic Cyst
- Usually lacks inflammation
- Orthokeratinized epithelial surface

Lateral Periodontal Cyst
- Usually lacks inflammation
- Thin epithelial lining with focal thickenings

Nasopalatine Duct Cyst
- Limited to anterior palate
- Variety of epithelial types
- Associated with blood vessels, nerves, and occasionally minor salivary glands

SELECTED REFERENCES

1. Siqueira JF Jr et al: Bacteria in the apical root canal of teeth with primary apical periodontitis. Oral Surg Oral Med Oral Pathol Oral Radiol Endod. 107(5):721-6, 2009
2. Dammaschke T et al: Long-term survival of root-canal-treated teeth: a retrospective study over 10 years. J Endod. 29(10):638-43, 2003
3. Kirkevang LL et al: Frequency and distribution of endodontically treated teeth and apical periodontitis in an urban Danish population. Int Endod J. 34(3):198-205, 2001

IMAGE GALLERY

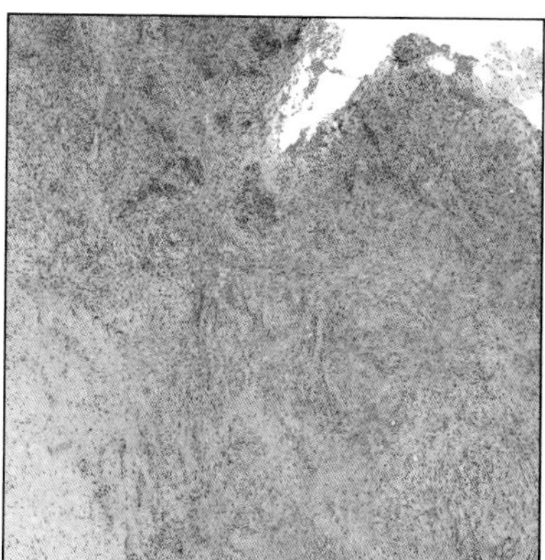

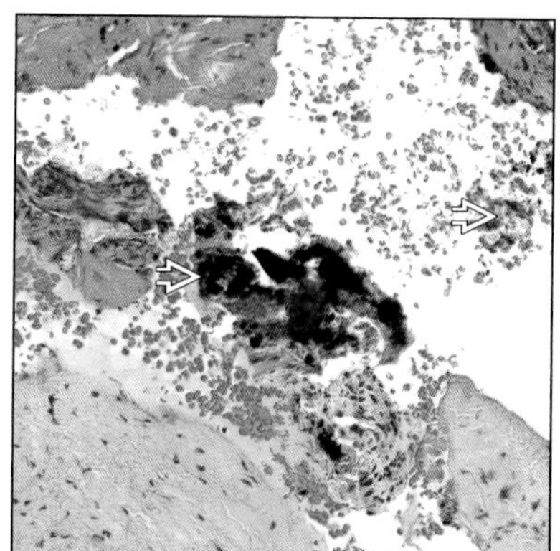

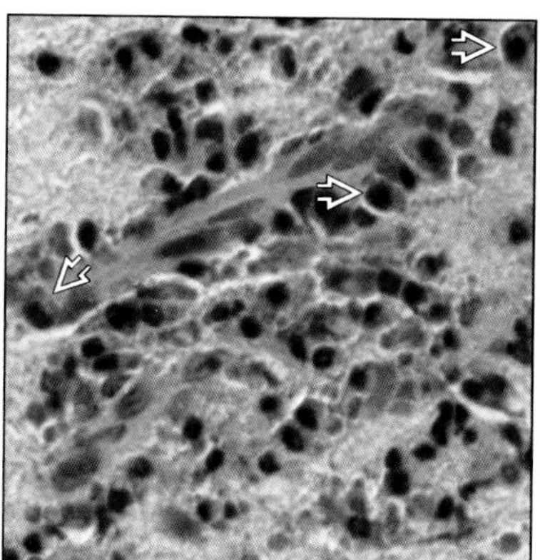

*(**Left**) A low-power view shows periapical granuloma with a mixed inflammatory infiltrate consisting of primarily lymphocytes, plasma cells, histocytes, and neutrophils. (**Center**) Hematoxylin & eosin shows a focus of foreign material ⇨ associated with a previous endodontic procedure. (**Right**) Hematoxylin & eosin shows the chronic inflammatory infiltrate that can be associated with either a periapical granuloma or cyst. This focus shows primarily plasma cells ⇨.*

AMELOBLASTOMA

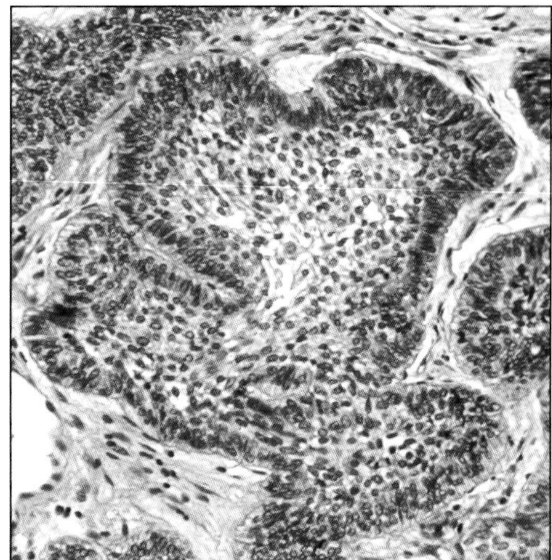

Hematoxylin & eosin shows the follicular variant of ameloblastoma. The follicular pattern is by far the most common and recognizable type of ameloblastoma. Basal palisading is noted.

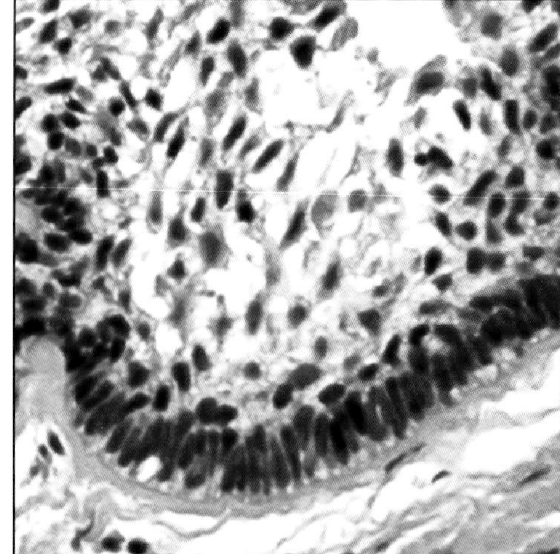

The classic characteristics of an ameloblastoma include islands of epithelium with central stellate reticulum surrounded by tall ameloblast-like cells. Note the reverse polarization of the nuclei.

TERMINOLOGY

Definitions

- Benign, slowly growing, locally aggressive neoplasm of odontogenic epithelium

ETIOLOGY/PATHOGENESIS

Origin

- Not definitively determined
  - Cell rests of enamel organ
  - Dental lamina
  - Epithelial lining of odontogenic cysts
  - Basal cells of oral mucosa

CLINICAL ISSUES

Epidemiology

- Incidence
  - Most common odontogenic tumor
    - Excluding odontomas
  - Incidence is equal to all other odontogenic tumors combined
  - Peripheral ameloblastoma is most common peripheral odontogenic tumor
- Age
  - Intraosseous
    - Wide range: 2nd to 6th decade
    - Average: 36 years
    - Rare before 10 years
  - Unicystic
    - Tend to develop at younger age
    - 75% found in 2nd to 3rd decade
  - Peripheral
    - Average: 51 years
- Gender
  - Equal gender distribution
- Ethnicity
  - Suggestion of ethnic variation requires further study

Site

- 80-85% occur in posterior mandible
- Peripheral variant found on gingiva
  - Usually anterior mandible
- Rare in sinonasal tract

Presentation

- Usually asymptomatic
  - Oftentimes incidental finding on routine dental radiographs
- Painless swelling
- Expansion of jaw
- Large lesions may present as disfiguring masses
- Pain is unusual

Treatment

- Surgical approaches
  - Conventional ameloblastomas generally require en bloc resection
    - Surgical margins extend at least 1 cm beyond radiographic evidence of tumor
    - Maxillary tumors may require more radical approach due to proximity to vital structures
    - Postsurgical reconstruction when needed
  - Unicystic lesions are treated with local enucleation
  - Peripheral lesions are easily treated with local excision
- Close clinical follow-up required for all ameloblastomas

Prognosis

- Conventional ameloblastoma
  - Recurrence rate as high as 35%
  - Persistent and infiltrating behavior
  - May kill patient by invading vital structures
    - Particularly tumors of posterior maxilla
- Unicystic ameloblastoma
  - Recurrence rates of 5-10%
- Peripheral ameloblastoma

AMELOBLASTOMA

Key Facts

Terminology
- Benign, locally aggressive neoplasm of odontogenic epithelium

Clinical Issues
- Most common odontogenic tumor (excluding odontomas)
- 80-85% occur in posterior mandible
- Peripheral variant found on gingiva
- Usually asymptomatic, oftentimes incidental finding on routine dental radiographs
- Large lesions may present as disfiguring masses
- Conventional ameloblastomas generally require en bloc resection
- Unicystic lesions are treated with local enucleation
- Peripheral lesions are easily treated with local excision
- Conventional ameloblastomas have recurrence rate as high as 35%

Image Findings
- Conventional types usually appear as multilocular radiolucencies

Microscopic Pathology
- Long anastomosing cords or sheets of odontogenic epithelium
- Stellate reticulum
- Subnuclear vacuolization
- Reverse polarity of nuclei (Vickers-Gorlin change)
- Many variants
  - Plexiform, follicular, basaloid, granular cell, acanthomatous, unicystic

  - Recurrence rates as high as 25%
  - Easily re-treated with local excision
- Histologic subtypes do not affect prognosis
- Rare transformation to ameloblastic carcinoma
  - Locally invasive with poor survival
- Rarely undergoes transformation to malignant ameloblastoma
  - Associated with poor survival
  - Metastases
    - 75% of patients have pulmonary metastases
    - Liver, skull, brain, and kidney less often

IMAGE FINDINGS

General Features
- Conventional types usually appear as multilocular radiolucencies
  - Multilocular
    - "Soap bubble" or "honeycomb" appearance
- Unilocular or unicystic
  - Unicystic tumors lack loculations
- Often associated with impacted tooth
- Peripheral lesions may show some underlying erosion of bone
  - Should not invade bone
- Desmoplastic variant usually appears as mixed radiopaque/radiolucent lesion
  - Oftentimes thought to be benign fibro-osseous lesion
- Cortical expansion is frequent finding
- Tumor may cause resorption of adjacent teeth

MACROSCOPIC FEATURES

General Features
- Solid to cystic
- Small lesions may appear circumscribed
- Larger lesions will infiltrate or expand surrounding bone
- Unicystic lesions, by definition, must be grossly unicystic

Sections to Be Submitted
- Bone margins

Size
- Broad range
  - Has potential for massive growth

MICROSCOPIC PATHOLOGY

Histologic Features
- Odontogenic epithelial islands
  - Centrally, stellate reticulum composed of loosely arranged angular cells
  - Surrounded by single layer of ameloblast-like cells
  - Nuclei are located away from basement membrane: Reverse polarity
    - Vickers-Gorlin change
  - Basal cytoplasmic vacuolization
- Stroma is variable
  - Loose
  - Dense
- Numerous patterns can be seen
  - Single pattern may predominate
  - Combination of patterns
- Invasive

Variants
- Plexiform
  - Long anastomosing cords or sheets of odontogenic epithelium
  - Peripheral palisading
  - Loose stroma
- Follicular
  - Islands of odontogenic epithelium
  - Peripheral palisading
  - Fibrous stroma
- Desmoplastic
  - Dense angular islands of odontogenic epithelium
  - Peripheral palisading found only focally
  - Dense collagen stroma
- Basaloid

- Nest of uniform basal cells
- No central stellate reticulum
- Granular cell
  - Central epithelial cells have granular eosinophilic cytoplasm
- Acanthomatous
  - Squamous metaplasia within odontogenic epithelial islands
  - Keratin formation
- Unicystic
  - Tumor confined to luminal wall of single cyst

ANCILLARY TESTS

Molecular Genetics

- *ING* family of tumor suppressor gene has high frequency loss of heterozygosity (LOH)
  - ING5 locus LOH correlated to solid tumor type
- Notch signaling molecules may be associated with specific tumor phenotypes
- Dysregulation of a number of genes involved in normal tooth development may play a role
  - FOS oncogene most overexpressed gene
  - Underexpressed genes include:
    - SHH, TRAF3, DCC, CDH12, TDGF1, TGFB1

DIFFERENTIAL DIAGNOSIS

Ameloblastic Fibroma

- Younger patients
- Mesenchymal stroma resembling dental papilla
  - Plump cells
  - Stellate-shaped cells
  - Loose matrix
- Epithelial component
  - Thin cords or strands
  - Small islands

Ameloblastic Fibro-odontoma

- Younger patients
- Mesenchymal stroma resembling dental papilla
  - Plump cells
  - Stellate-shaped cells
  - Loose matrix
- Epithelial component
  - Thin cords or strands of odontogenic epithelium
  - Small discrete islands of odontogenic epithelium
- Mineralized tissue
  - Enamel matrix
  - Dentin
  - Cementum

Adenomatoid Odontogenic Tumor

- Favors anterior maxilla
- Encapsulated
- Duct-like spaces
- Nodular swirling pattern
- Amorphous amyloid-like material
- Calcifications

Calcifying Odontogenic Cyst

- Presence of ghost cells
- Calcifications

Ameloblastic Carcinoma

- Destructive growth
- Cytologic features of malignancy, including pleomorphism and increased mitotic figures

Malignant Ameloblastoma

- Requires development of metastatic deposits
  - Usually in lung

Squamous Odontogenic Tumor

- Rarely cystic
- Peripheral cells in epithelial island do not show polarization

Squamous Cell Carcinoma

- Acanthomatous ameloblastoma may have similarities
- Cytologic features of malignancy

Odontoameloblastoma

- Essentially ameloblastoma with concurrent odontoma

Basal Cell Carcinoma

- Peripheral tumors may have similar histologic appearance
- Do not occur in gingiva

Dentigerous Cyst

- Always associated with unerupted tooth
- May have similarities to unicystic tumors
- Lacks reverse polarity and subnuclear vacuolization

SELECTED REFERENCES

1. Adeline VL et al: Clinicopathologic features of ameloblastoma in Kenya: a 10-year audit. J Craniofac Surg. 19(6):1589-93, 2008
2. Odukoya O et al: Clinicopathological study of 100 Nigerian cases of ameloblastoma. Niger Postgrad Med J. 15(1):1-5, 2008
3. Scheper MA et al: Expression and alterations of the PTEN / AKT / mTOR pathway in ameloblastomas. Oral Dis. 14(6):561-8, 2008
4. Heikinheimo K et al: Gene expression profiling of ameloblastoma and human tooth germ by means of a cDNA microarray. J Dent Res. 81(8):525-30, 2002
5. Ord RA et al: Ameloblastoma in children. J Oral Maxillofac Surg. 60(7):762-70; discussion, 770-1, 2002
6. Philipsen HP et al: Peripheral ameloblastoma: biological profile based on 160 cases from the literature. Oral Oncol. 37(1):17-27, 2001
7. Philipsen HP et al: Unicystic ameloblastoma. A review of 193 cases from the literature. Oral Oncol. 34(5):317-25, 1998
8. Reichart PA et al: Ameloblastoma: biological profile of 3677 cases. Eur J Cancer B Oral Oncol. 31B(2):86-99, 1995
9. Siar CH et al: Ameloblastoma in Malaysia--a 25-year review. Ann Acad Med Singapore. 22(6):856-60, 1993
10. Waldron CA et al: A histopathologic study of 116 ameloblastomas with special reference to the desmoplastic variant. Oral Surg Oral Med Oral Pathol. 63(4):441-51, 1987

Imaging, Gross, and Microscopic Features

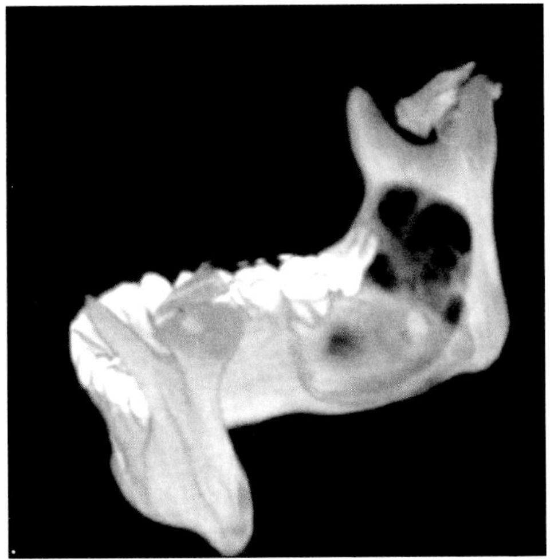

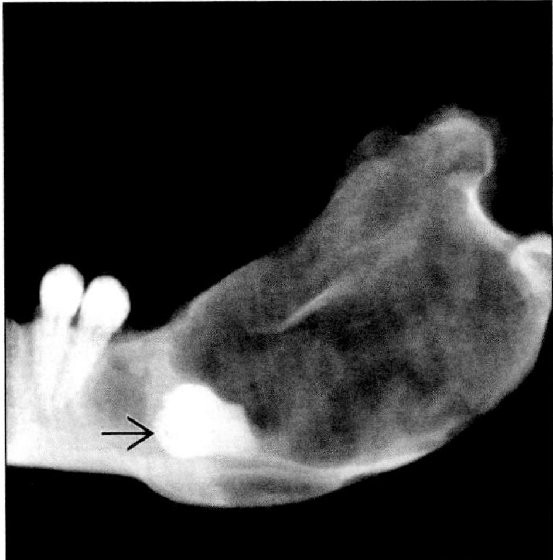

(Left) *This 3D reconstructed image highlights the multicystic nature of most ameloblastomas. The ramus and body of the mandible is nearly completely replaced and expanded by the tumor.* ***(Right)*** *This specimen radiograph highlights the radiolucent appearance of the tumor. Note the tooth ⇨ at the periphery of the tumor. The "soap bubble" appearance of the sample is easily identified.*

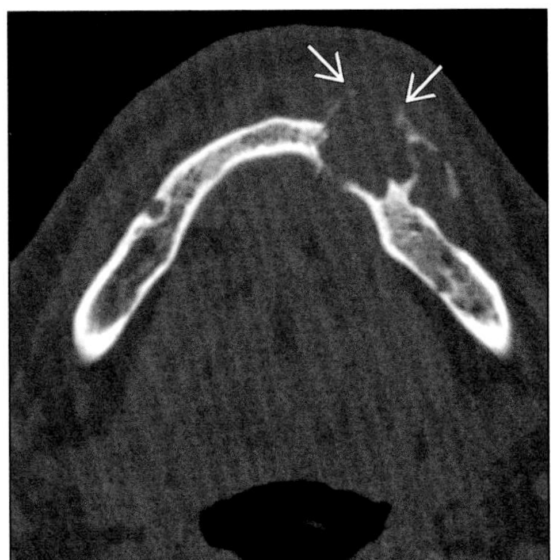

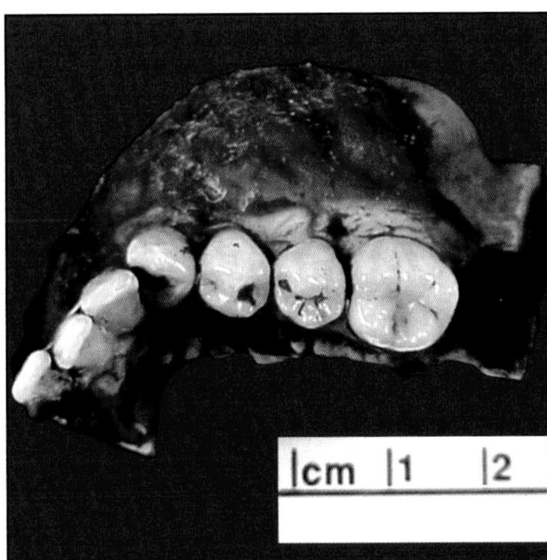

(Left) *This computed tomography scan shows an ameloblastoma that has perforated the bone and invaded soft tissue ➡. This is an uncommon finding, as usually the bone is remodeled or sclerotic at the periphery of the tumor.* ***(Right)*** *Gross photograph shows the extent of the resection required to completely remove the tumor, even though it is a benign lesion. Patients with this type of resection will require reconstruction and very close follow-up to identify recurrence.*

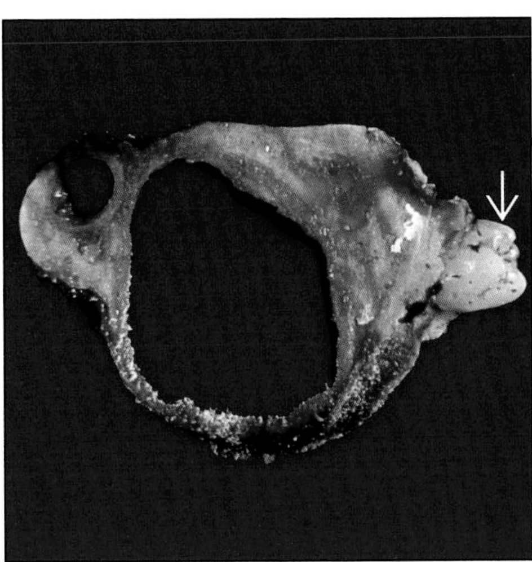

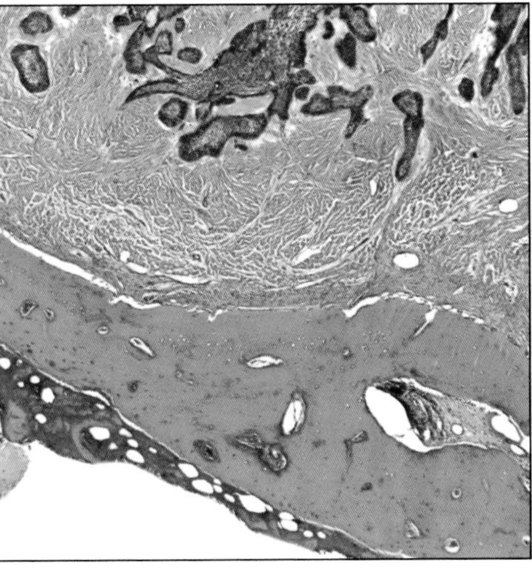

(Left) *Gross photograph shows a large, multi-cystic lesion of the mandible. It is not uncommon to have this type of empty cyst at macroscopic examination. Note the tooth included with the resection ➡. The diagnosis in this case was conventional follicular ameloblastoma.* ***(Right)*** *Hematoxylin & eosin shows tumor at a bone margin. Intraoperatively and radiologically, this margin was thought to be negative. The tumor often goes beyond any radiologic evidence of the disease.*

AMELOBLASTOMA

Microscopic and Radiographic Features

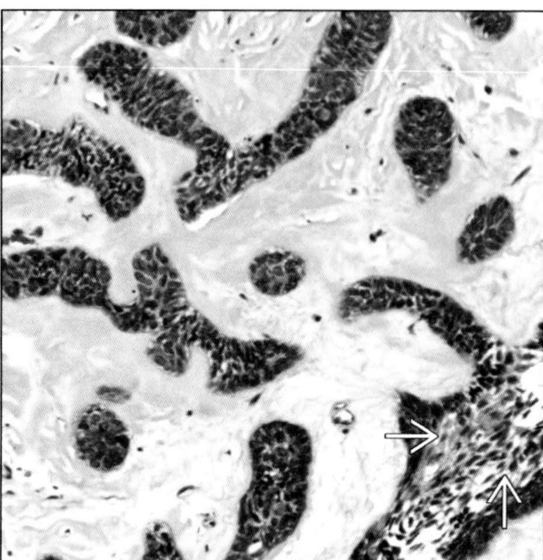

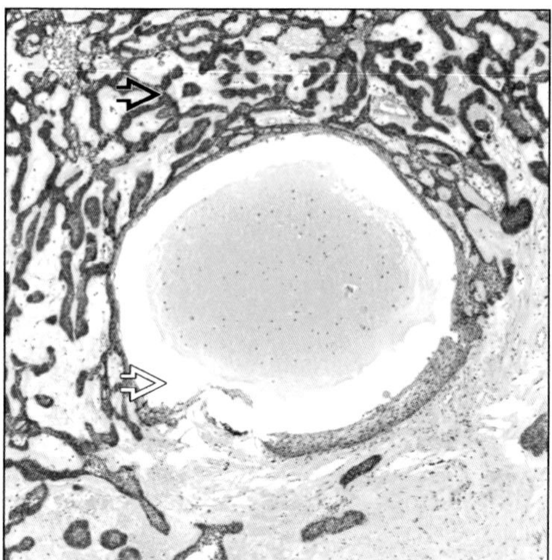

(Left) *Hematoxylin & eosin shows islands of odontogenic epithelium in a dense collagenous stroma. There is still well-developed stellate reticulum ➔ in this image, even though peripheral palisading of basaloid cells is not present.* ***(Right)*** *Hematoxylin & eosin shows cystic degeneration ➔ of a large tumor with a primarily plexiform pattern ➔. Cyst formation is relatively uncommon in this histologic pattern, and is instead more frequent in the follicular type.*

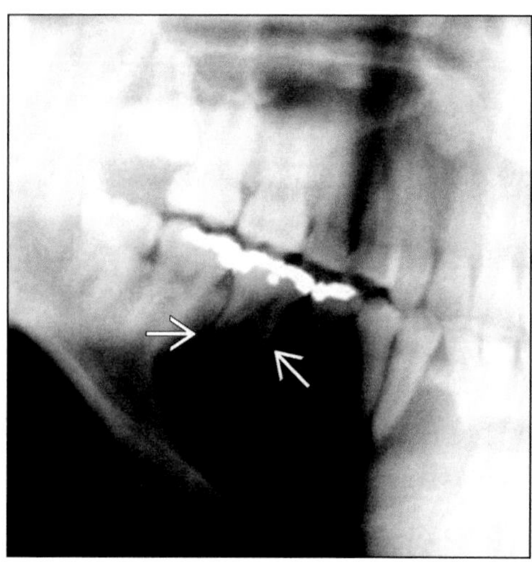

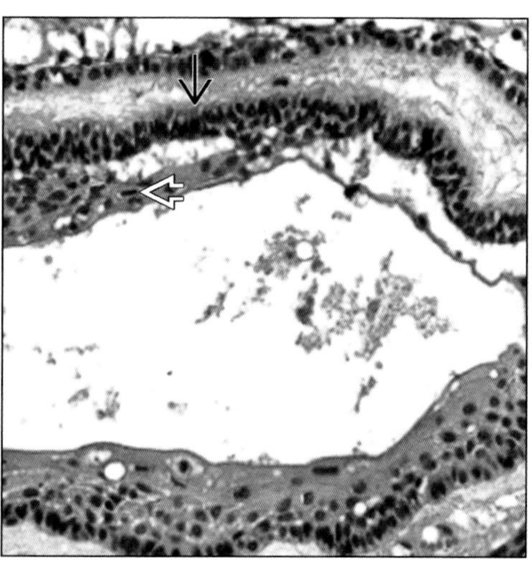

(Left) *Radiograph shows a unicystic ameloblastoma. There is a well-defined, unilocular cystic space within the bony interstices. Note the root resorption ➔, a finding frequently seen in ameloblastoma.* ***(Right)*** *Hematoxylin & eosin shows the distinct basal cell layer ➔ of a unicystic ameloblastoma. The stellate reticulum-like cells ➔ are on the surface of the cystic epithelium. On low power, this could be mistaken for an inflammatory or developmental odontogenic cyst.*

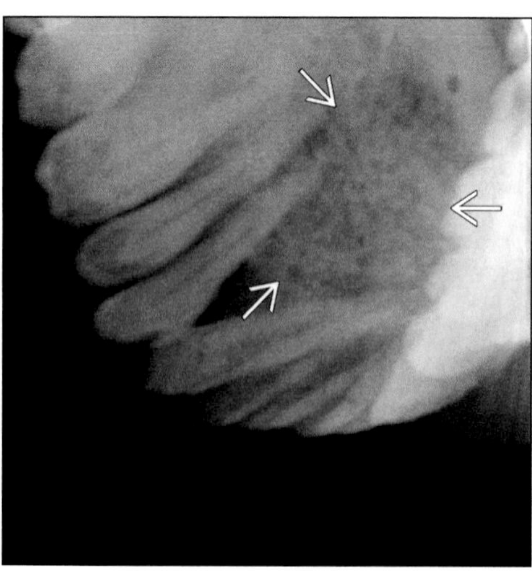

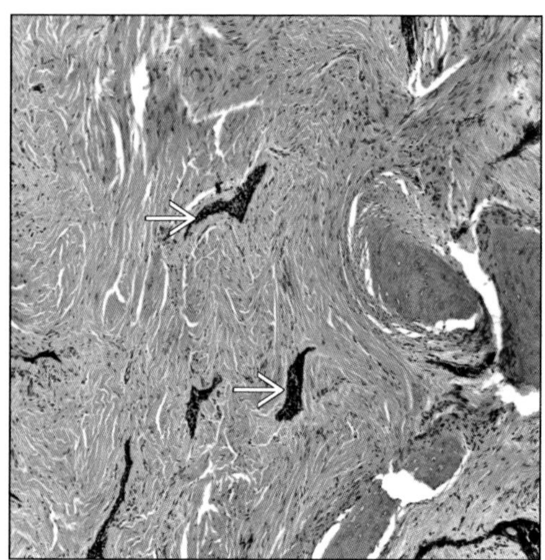

(Left) *Radiograph shows a desmoplastic ameloblastoma, characterized by a mixed radiolucent and radiopaque appearance ➔. Desmoplastic ameloblastomas have a predilection for the anterior maxilla, seen here splaying the tooth roots.* ***(Right)*** *Hematoxylin & eosin shows the desmoplastic variant of ameloblastoma. The islands of odontogenic epithelium ➔ appear squeezed by the dense collagenous stroma. The ameloblasts, reverse polarity, and stellate reticulum are difficult to see.*

Variant Microscopic Features

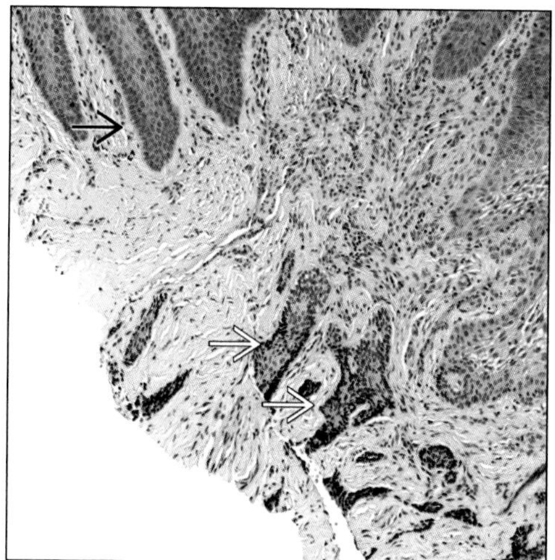

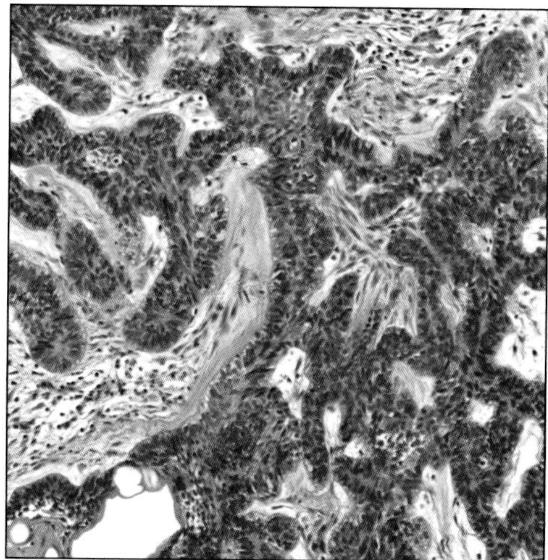

(Left) *Hematoxylin & eosin shows a peripheral ameloblastoma with distinct islands of odontogenic epithelium ➡ within the lamina propria. Note the overlying epithelium of the gingiva ⇨. The separation between invasive squamous cell carcinoma can be difficult.* ***(Right)*** *Hematoxylin & eosin shows the plexiform variant of ameloblastoma. This pattern is characterized by anastomosing cords and islands of odontogenic epithelium. Little stellate reticulum can be seen.*

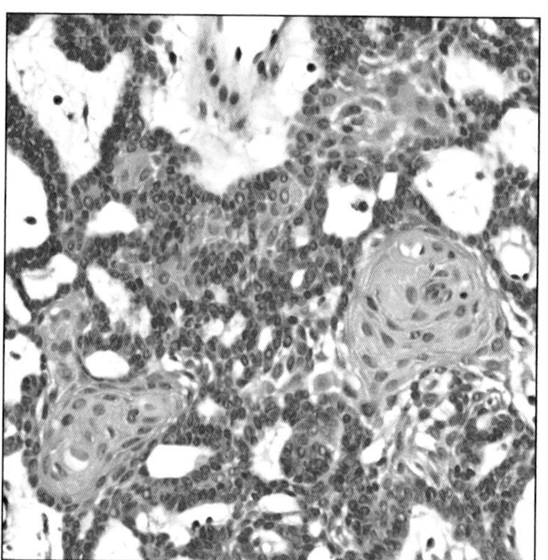

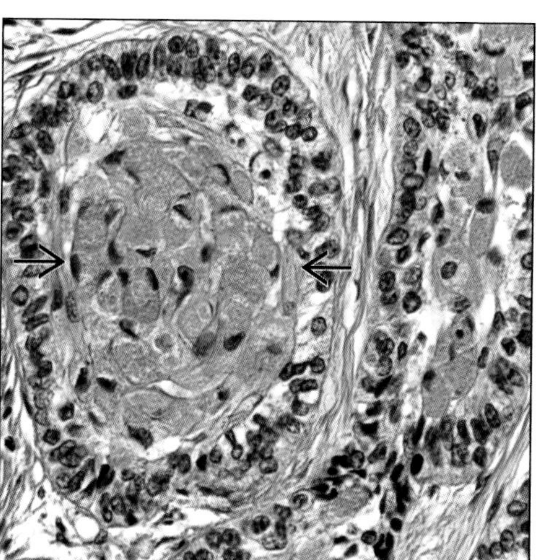

(Left) *Hematoxylin & eosin shows the acanthomatous variant of ameloblastoma. The islands show central areas of squamous differentiation, which need to predominate in order to apply this variant classification.* ***(Right)*** *Hematoxylin & eosin shows granular variant of ameloblastoma. Note the prominent granular cytoplasm of the cells within the islands ⇨. Similar to other variants, this finding needs to be the major pattern within the tumor.*

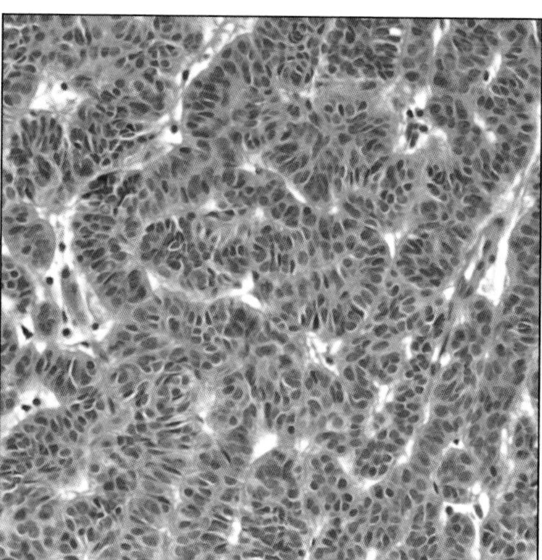

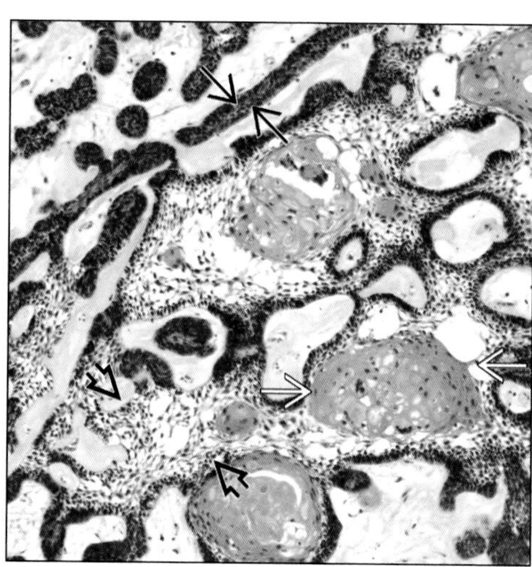

(Left) *Hematoxylin & eosin shows the basal cell variant of ameloblastoma. Note the more cuboidal, peripheral cells with nuclei that show hyperchromasia and lack of stellate reticulum. This is the least common variant of ameloblastoma, and is quite difficult to diagnose.* ***(Right)*** *Hematoxylin & eosin shows a tumor with areas of plexiform ⇨, acanthomatous ➡, and follicular patterns ⇨. It is not unusual, especially in large tumors, to have more than 1 histologic pattern.*

SQUAMOUS ODONTOGENIC TUMOR

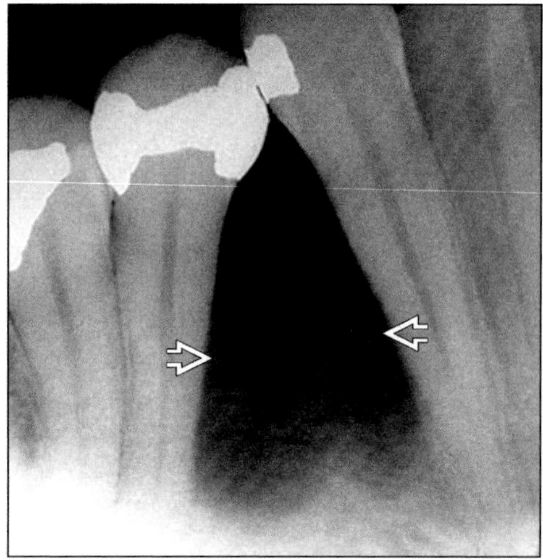

Radiograph reveals a triangular radiolucent defect ⇨ between the premolar and canine. This example was treated as periodontal disease but failed to respond so was subsequently biopsied.

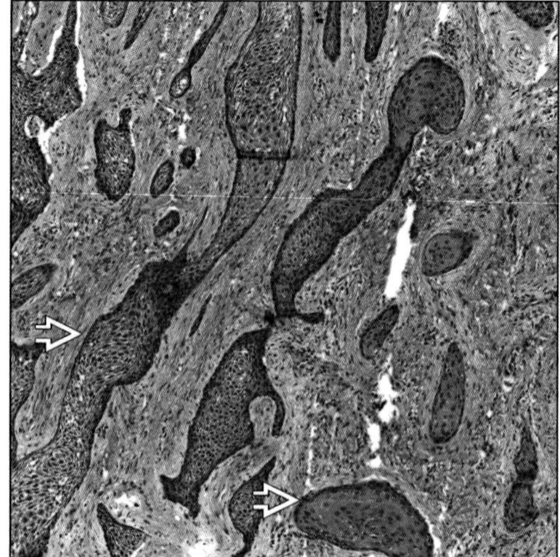

Hematoxylin & eosin shows islands of bland squamous epithelium ⇨ within a fibrous stroma. At low power the differential diagnosis may include squamous cell carcinoma.

TERMINOLOGY

Abbreviations

- Squamous odontogenic tumor (SOT)

Definitions

- Benign odontogenic neoplasm of squamous epithelium that may demonstrate locally aggressive behavior

ETIOLOGY/PATHOGENESIS

Pathogenesis

- Believed to arise from rest of Malassez in periodontal ligament
- Peripheral lesions may arise from surface epithelium

CLINICAL ISSUES

Epidemiology

- Incidence
  - Very rare
    - 1st described in 1975
- Age
  - Wide range
    - 2nd to 7th decades

Site

- Anterior maxilla
- Posterior mandible
- Rarely reported as peripheral lesion in gingiva

Presentation

- Localized loosening of teeth in absence of periodontal disease
  - Deep periodontal pocket
- Gingival swelling
- Pain
- Asymptomatic
  - Incidental finding on routine dental radiographs
- Rarely multifocal
- Associated teeth generally test vital

Treatment

- Surgical approaches
  - Conservative removal of lesion and any affected teeth
    - Aggressive curettage of affected bone
  - Scaling and root planing of adjacent teeth
  - Prosthetic restoration of extracted teeth
  - Peripheral lesions may be excised down to periosteum

Prognosis

- Rarely recur
- Maxillary lesions may require closer follow-up as they have been reported to be more aggressive
  - Anatomy of region
  - Porous bone making removal difficult
- Multifocal lesions have been reported as less aggressive
- Very rare cases of malignant transformation

IMAGE FINDINGS

Radiographic Findings

- Not specific but usually consist of triangular radiolucent defect lateral to tooth
  - May suggest loss of bone from periodontal disease
- Ill- and well-defined radiolucency
- Sclerotic margins
- Occasional cortical erosion
- May occasionally displace adjacent teeth

MACROSCOPIC FEATURES

General Features

- Gross specimen may consist of fragmented curettings
- Fragments of bone

SQUAMOUS ODONTOGENIC TUMOR

Key Facts

Terminology
- Benign odontogenic neoplasm of squamous epithelium that may demonstrate locally aggressive behavior

Clinical Issues
- Very rare
- Conservative removal of lesion and any affected teeth
- Rarely recur

Image Findings
- Not specific but usually consist of triangular radiolucent defect lateral to tooth

Microscopic Pathology
- Epithelial nest and islands
  - Bland
- Stroma
  - Fibrous connective tissue

- Extracted teeth

MICROSCOPIC PATHOLOGY

Histologic Features
- Epithelial nest and islands
  - Varying shapes
  - Bland
  - Single cell keratinization may be seen
  - Microcysts
  - Laminated calcifications
- Stroma
  - Fibrous connective tissue
  - Hyalinization may be seen around islands

DIFFERENTIAL DIAGNOSIS

Ameloblastoma
- More common
- More destructive
- Peripheral palisading nuclei
- Stellate reticulum

Squamous Cell Carcinoma
- Frequently, may have soft tissue component
- Cytologically atypical, including atypical mitotic figures

Metastatic Carcinoma
- History of primary disease
- Cytologically atypical

Odontogenic Epithelial Rests
- Small collections of odontogenic epithelium
- Usually found incidentally in other conditions
  - Dental follicular tissue
  - Dentigerous cysts
  - Other odontogenic cyst and tumors

Organ of Chievitz
- a.k.a. juxtaoral organ of Chievitz
- Most commonly found in retromolar pad area
- Collection of discrete nest of cells with distinct squamous appearance

SELECTED REFERENCES

1. Kim K et al: Squamous odontogenic tumor causing erosion of the lingual cortical plate in the mandible: a report of 2 cases. J Oral Maxillofac Surg. 65(6):1227-31, 2007
2. Haghighat K et al: Squamous odontogenic tumor: diagnosis and management. J Periodontol. 73(6):653-6, 2002
3. Regezi JA: Odontogenic cysts, odontogenic tumors, fibroosseous, and giant cell lesions of the jaws. Mod Pathol. 15(3):331-41, 2002
4. Melrose RJ: Benign epithelial odontogenic tumors. Semin Diagn Pathol. 16(4):271-87, 1999
5. Philipsen HP et al: Squamous odontogenic tumor (SOT): a benign neoplasm of the periodontium. A review of 36 reported cases. J Clin Periodontol. 23(10):922-6, 1996
6. Baden E et al: Squamous odontogenic tumor. Report of three cases including the first extraosseous case. Oral Surg Oral Med Oral Pathol. 75(6):733-8, 1993

IMAGE GALLERY

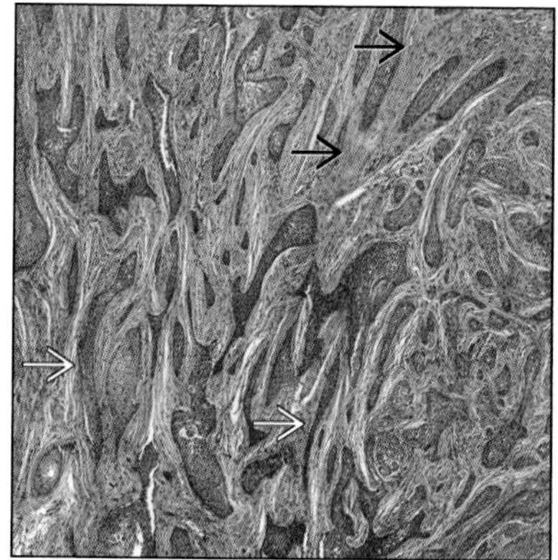

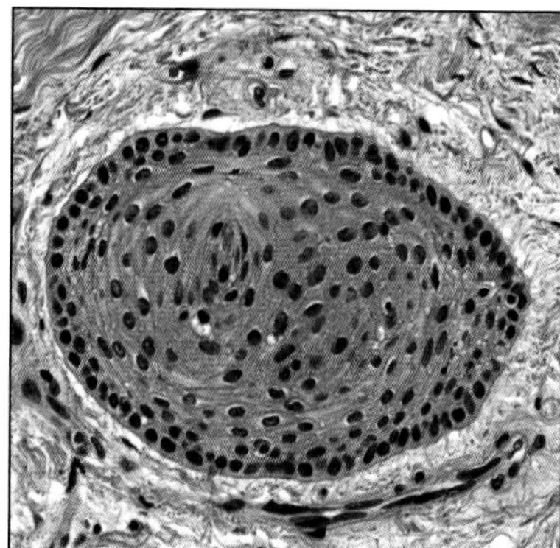

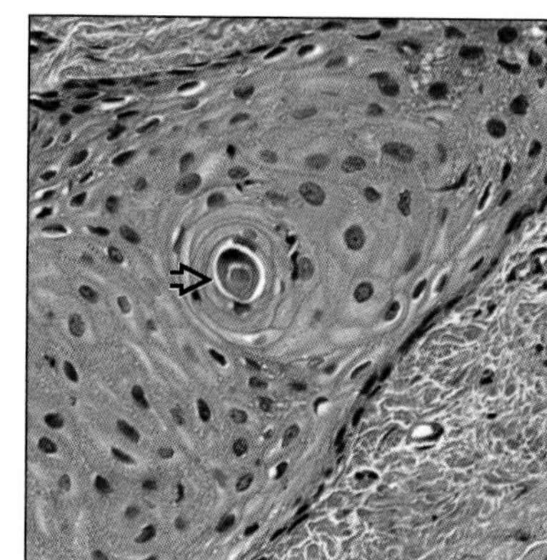

*(**Left**) This squamous odontogenic tumor is composed predominantly of cord-like nests of bland squamous epithelium ➡. Note the fibrous stroma ⇒. (**Center**) High-power view of a tumor island shows the lack of cytologic atypia that one would expect with a carcinoma. Additionally, the peripheral cells show no sign of reverse polarity, characteristic of an ameloblastoma. (**Right**) Hematoxylin & eosin shows an island with a small laminated calcified structure ⇒.*

CALCIFYING EPITHELIAL ODONTOGENIC TUMOR

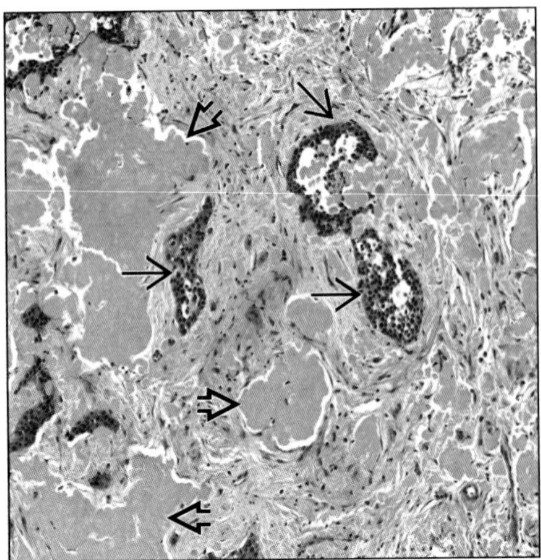

Low-power view shows islands of polyhedral epithelial cells ⇒ in a fibrous stroma. Areas of amorphous, eosinophilic, amyloid-like material ⇨ are readily identifiable in this tumor.

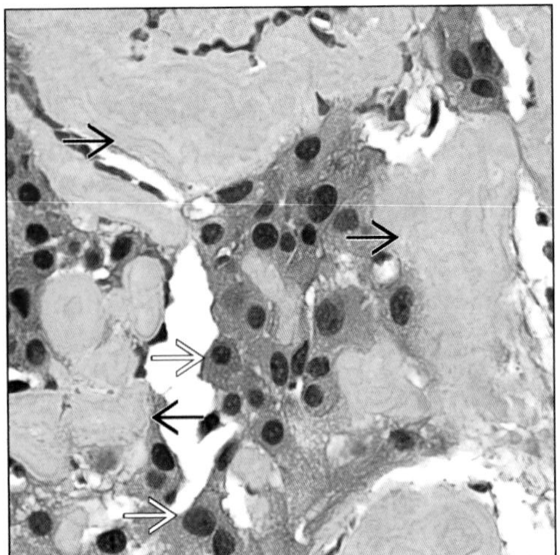

A collection of polyhedral tumor cells with distinctive eosinophilic cytoplasm ➡ shows areas of amorphous, eosinophilic, amyloid-like material ⇒ located throughout the tumor, which is quite characteristic.

TERMINOLOGY

Abbreviations

- Calcifying epithelial odontogenetic tumor (CEOT)

Synonyms

- Pindborg tumor

Definitions

- Epithelial odontogenic neoplasm with local invasion, characterized by amyloid-like material and calcifications

CLINICAL ISSUES

Epidemiology

- Incidence
  - Rare
  - < 1% of all odontogenic tumors
- Age
  - Wide range: 20-60 years most common
  - Average: 40 years
- Gender
  - Equal gender distribution

Site

- Vast majority are intraosseous
  - ~ 75% arise in mandible
    - Usually posterior: Molar or premolar area
  - Remainder arise in mandible
- Extraosseous: Peripheral variant
  - About 5% of cases, involving anterior gingiva

Presentation

- Asymptomatic, painless expansile mass
- Slowly growing swelling
- Firm, painless mass on gingiva

Treatment

- Surgical approaches
  - Local resection, including narrow rim of bone
  - Peripheral variant excised to periosteum

Prognosis

- Recurrence rate: 15%
  - Slightly higher in clear cell variant (22%)
- Long-term follow-up recommended
- Malignant transformation is rare

IMAGE FINDINGS

Radiographic Findings

- Considerable variation of mixed radiolucent-radiopaque lesions
- Unilocular or multilocular radiolucency
- Contains calcifications
  - Oftentimes aggregating around crown of unerupted teeth
- Associated with impacted tooth in > 50% of cases
  - Most common mandibular 3rd molar
- Peripheral variant may show cupping of underlying bone

MACROSCOPIC FEATURES

General Features

- Solid tumor (no cyst formation)
- Varying amounts of calcifications

Sections to Be Submitted

- Bone margins

MICROSCOPIC PATHOLOGY

Histologic Features

- Epithelial cells
  - Sheets, cords, or islands of cells
  - Polyhedral cells with abundant eosinophilic cytoplasm

CALCIFYING EPITHELIAL ODONTOGENIC TUMOR

Key Facts

Terminology
- Rare epithelial odontogenic neoplasm with amyloid-like material and calcifications

Clinical Issues
- Rare
- 75% found in mandible
- Peripheral variant excised to periosteum
- Local resection, including narrow rim of bone

Image Findings
- Unilocular radiolucency

Microscopic Pathology
- Sheets, cords, or islands of polyhedral epithelial cells
- Abundant eosinophilic cytoplasm with prominent cell borders and intercellular bridges
- Hyalinized, eosinophilic homogeneous stroma: Amyloid
- Liesegang rings: Basophilic concentric calcified layers

  - Intracellular bridges well developed
  - Prominent, well-defined cell borders
  - Pleomorphism usually present
    - Giant tumor nuclei occasionally seen
  - Mitotic figures rare
  - Clear cell variant uncommon
- Matrix
  - Hyalinized or fibrous connective tissue stroma
  - Eosinophilic and homogeneous
- Calcification
  - Liesegang rings: Basophilic concentric layers
  - Usually adjacent to tumor cells
  - Noncalcifying variant
- Rarely associated with adenomatoid odontogenic tumor

ANCILLARY TESTS

Histochemistry
- Matrix positive with Congo red and thioflavin T (amyloid)

DIFFERENTIAL DIAGNOSIS

Squamous Cell Carcinoma
- Lacks amyloid and calcifications
- Generally shows more cellular pleomorphism

Clear Cell Odontogenic Carcinoma
- Lacks amyloid and calcifications

Metastatic Tumors
- **Squamous cell carcinoma**
  - Primary site must be identified
  - Lacks amyloid and calcifications
  - Generally shows more cellular pleomorphism
- **Renal cell carcinoma** (clear cell variant)
  - Primary site must be identified
  - Vascular pattern with extravasated erythrocytes
  - Lacks amyloid and calcifications
  - Immunoreactivity for CD10, pax-2, renal cell carcinoma marker

SELECTED REFERENCES

1. Cicconetti A et al: Calcifying epithelial odontogenic (Pindborg) tumor. A clinical case. Minerva Stomatol. 53(6):379-87, 2004
2. Belmonte-Caro R et al: Calcifying epithelial odontogenic tumor (Pindborg tumor). Med Oral. 7(4):309-15, 2002
3. Kaplan I et al: Radiological and clinical features of calcifying epithelial odontogenic tumour. Dentomaxillofac Radiol. 30(1):22-8, 2001
4. Aviel-Ronen S et al: The amyloid deposit in calcifying epithelial odontogenic tumor is immunoreactive for cytokeratins. Arch Pathol Lab Med. 124(6):872-6, 2000
5. Cross JJ et al: Value of computed tomography and magnetic resonance imaging in the treatment of a calcifying epithelial odontogenic (Pindborg) tumour. Br J Oral Maxillofac Surg. 38(2):154-7, 2000
6. Philipsen HP et al: Calcifying epithelial odontogenic tumour: biological profile based on 181 cases from the literature. Oral Oncol. 36(1):17-26, 2000

IMAGE GALLERY

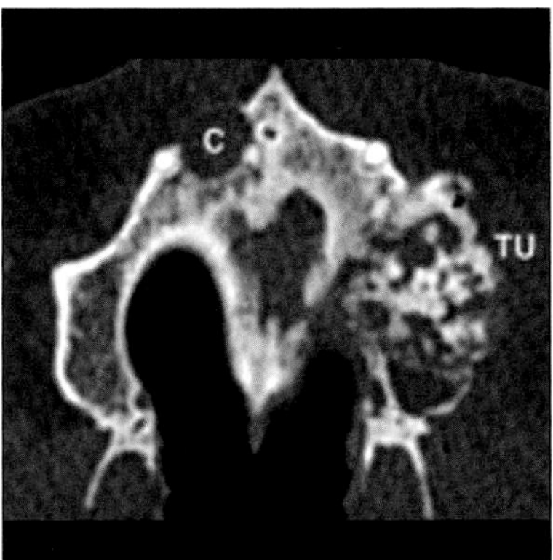

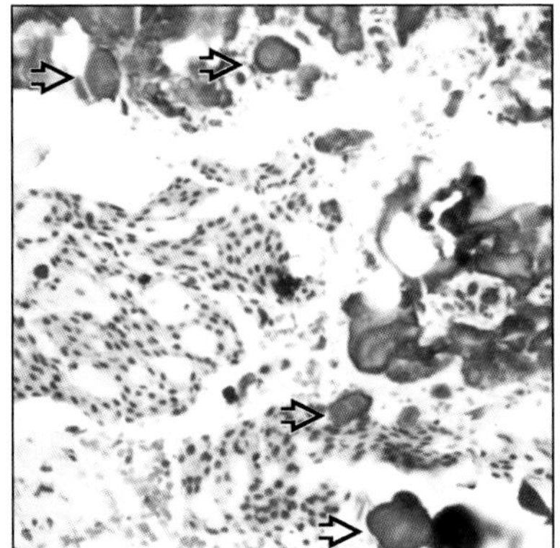

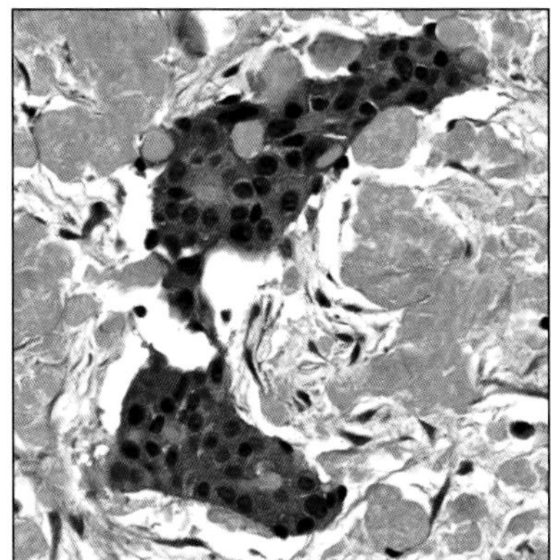

*(**Left**) CT of the left maxilla shows mixed radiolucency and radiopacities (TU). In addition, the right maxilla shows a radicular cyst (C), which is not related but just happens to be present. (**Center**) This tumor has dense calcifications with distinctive concentric laminations called Liesegang rings ⇨. (**Right**) Hematoxylin and eosin shows islands of epithelial cells with characteristic pleomorphism, a feature that may be misinterpreted as a feature of malignancy.*

ADENOMATOID ODONTOGENIC TUMOR

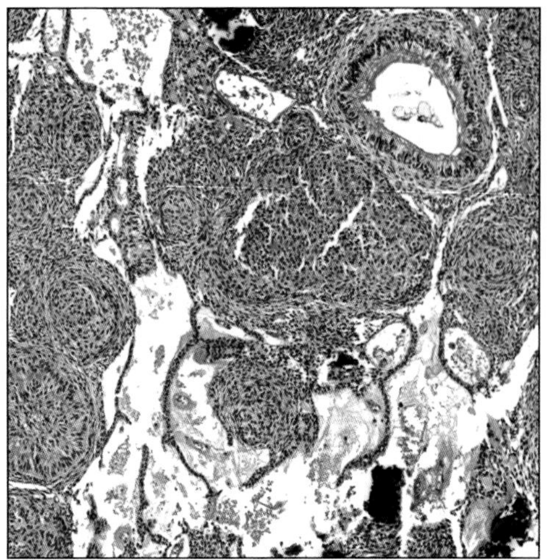

Hematoxylin & eosin shows whorling masses of cells with some gland-like structures admixed. Small foci of calcification are scattered throughout the tumor.

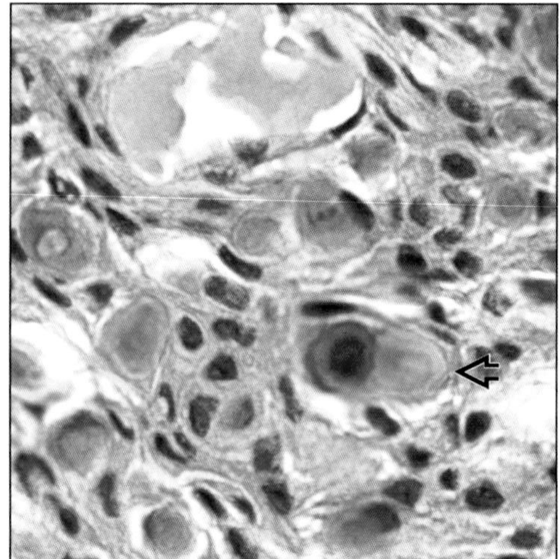

Hematoxylin & eosin shows an area of calcification with distinct laminations ⊳.

TERMINOLOGY

Abbreviations

- Adenomatoid odontogenic tumor (AOT)

Synonyms

- Formerly known as adenoameloblastoma
  - Confusion with ameloblastoma should be avoided

Definitions

- Benign tumor of odontogenic epithelium with distinct duct-like appearance embedded in mature connective tissue stroma

ETIOLOGY/PATHOGENESIS

Developmental Anomaly

- May derive from epithelium of enamel organ

CLINICAL ISSUES

Epidemiology

- Incidence
  - 3-7% of odontogenic tumors
- Age
  - Most common in 2nd decade
    - > 90% found before age 30
- Gender
  - Female > Male (2:1)

Site

- Most common in anterior maxilla
- Rare extraosseous variant
  - Gingiva
  - Favors maxilla

Presentation

- Usually asymptomatic
- Painless expansion of bone
- Associated with unerupted teeth
- May displace adjacent teeth
- Extraosseous variants
  - Small, sessile
  - May be ulcerated due to secondary trauma
- May occasionally be seen in association with calcifying epithelial odontogenic tumor

Treatment

- Surgical approaches
  - Enucleation from bone
- Orthodontics to correct malocclusion

Prognosis

- Recurrences are exceedingly rare to nonexistent

IMAGE FINDINGS

Radiographic Findings

- Well-defined radiolucency, usually unilocular
- Often associated with unerupted tooth
  - Usually maxillary canine
- May contain fine calcifications, "snow flakes"

MACROSCOPIC FEATURES

General Features

- Usually surrounded by thick, well-defined capsule
- Cut section may reveal
  - Cysts or solid pattern
  - Calcifications
  - Unerupted tooth

Size

- Usually < 3 cm

ADENOMATOID ODONTOGENIC TUMOR

Key Facts

Terminology
- Benign tumor of odontogenic epithelium with distinct duct-like appearance

Macroscopic Features
- Usually surrounded by thick well-defined capsule

Microscopic Pathology
- Duct-like nests or cords lined by cuboidal to columnar cells
- Reversed nuclear polarity away from central lumen-like space
- Duct-like spaces are pseudolumina containing eosinophilic secretions
- Contains amorphous amyloid-like material and mineralizations

Diagnostic Checklist
- 2/3 tumor

MICROSCOPIC PATHOLOGY

Histologic Features
- Nodules of odontogenic epithelium
  - Duct-like nests or cords lined by cuboidal to columnar cells
  - Reversed nuclear polarity away from central lumen-like space
  - Duct-like spaces are pseudolumina containing eosinophilic secretions
- Stroma
  - Spindle to polyhedral eosinophilic cells
  - Swirling to nodular pattern
  - Contains amorphous amyloid-like material (tumor droplets)
  - Mineralizations
  - Small vessels
- Melanin pigmentation of both odontogenic and stroma cells has been described

DIFFERENTIAL DIAGNOSIS

Ameloblastoma
- Lacks gland-like structures
- Usually larger and more invasive
- Lacks capsule

Salivary Gland Tumor
- Rare location, usually without calcifications
- Lacks reverse polarity and stroma is not prominent

DIAGNOSTIC CHECKLIST

Clinically Relevant Pathologic Features
- Tumor of 2/3
  - 2/3 women, in 2nd decade, in anterior maxilla, in association with impacted tooth

SELECTED REFERENCES

1. Philipsen HP et al: An updated clinical and epidemiological profile of the adenomatoid odontogenic tumour: a collaborative retrospective study. J Oral Pathol Med. 36(7):383-93, 2007
2. Philipsen HP et al: Adenomatoid odontogenic tumour: facts and figures. Oral Oncol. 35(2):125-31, 1999
3. Arotiba GT et al: The adenomatoid odontogenic tumor: an analysis of 57 cases in a black African population. J Oral Maxillofac Surg. 55(2):146-8; discussion 149-50, 1997
4. Buchner A et al: Pigmented lateral periodontal cyst and other pigmented odontogenic lesions. Oral Dis. 2(4):299-302, 1996
5. Chattopadhyay A: Adenomatoid odontogenic tumour. Review of literature and report of 30 cases from India. Indian J Dent Res. 5(3):89-95, 1994
6. Montes Ledesma C et al: Adenomatoid odontogenic tumour with features of calcifying epithelial odontogenic tumour. (The so-called combined epithelial odontogenic tumour.) Clinico-pathological report of 12 cases. Eur J Cancer B Oral Oncol. 29B(3):221-4, 1993
7. Philipsen HP et al: Adenomatoid odontogenic tumor: biologic profile based on 499 cases. J Oral Pathol Med. 20(4):149-58, 1991

IMAGE GALLERY

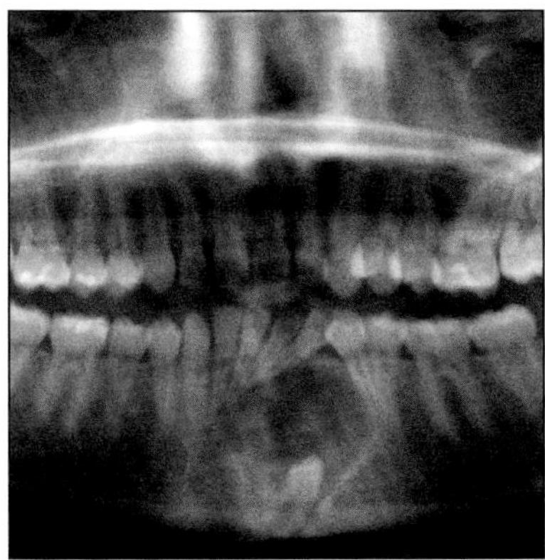

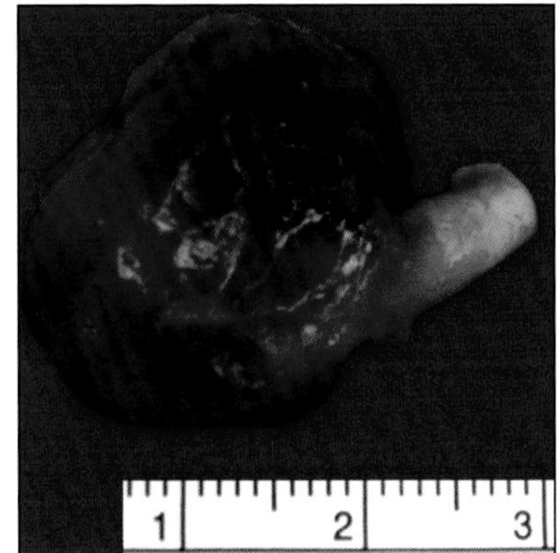

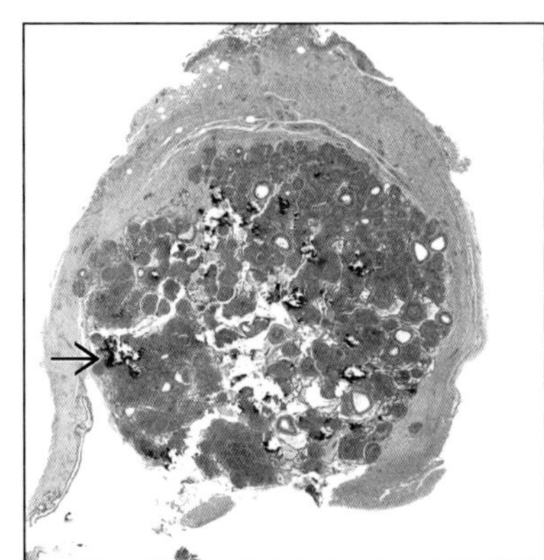

(Left) Radiograph shows a radiolucency associated with the crown of the unerupted mandibular canine. This lesion was thought to be a dentigerous cyst. (Center) Gross image shows a well-circumscribed solid mass enveloping the crown of the mandibular canine. The lesion "shells out" from the surrounding bone. (Right) Hematoxylin & eosin shows a low-power view demonstrating a thick capsule surrounding the tumor. Mineralization can be seen throughout the specimen ⇒.

KERATOCYSTIC ODONTOGENIC TUMOR (ODONTOGENIC KERATOCYST)

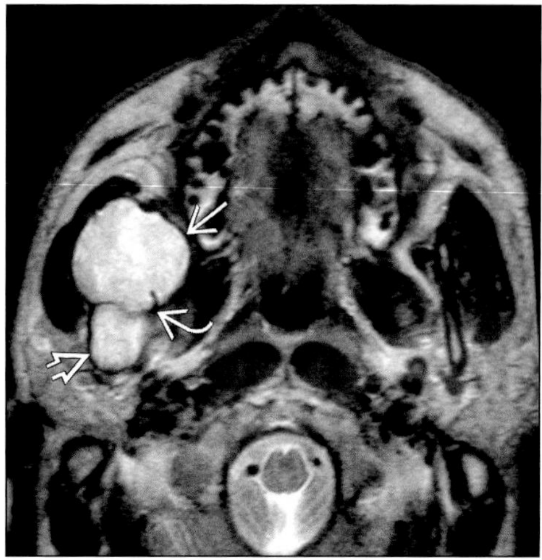

Axial T2 MR reveals a mandibular odontogenic keratocyst as a high signal, expansile mass within the coronoid process ➔ and ramus ⊳. Internal septation ↷ is noted.

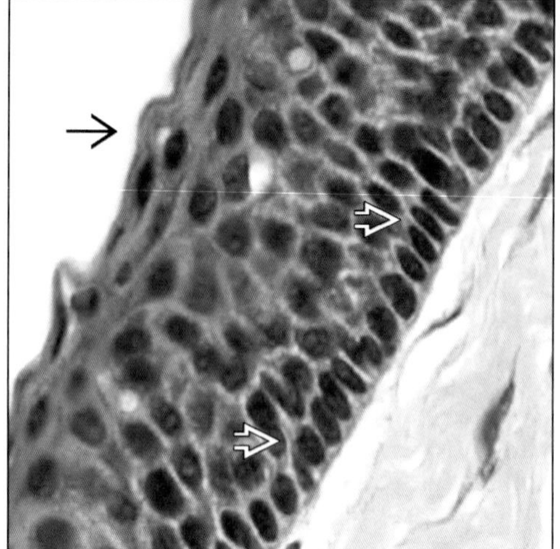

Cells of the basal layer of the epithelium show characteristic palisading and hyperchromaticity ⊳. The epithelium is 6-8 cells thick and demonstrates a wavy, parakeratinized surface →.

TERMINOLOGY

Synonyms

- Odontogenic keratocyst (OKC)
- Primordial cyst
- Odontogenic keratocystoma

Definitions

- Distinct developmental odontogenic cyst that may be locally aggressive

ETIOLOGY/PATHOGENESIS

Histogenesis

- May arise from cells of dental lamina
- May arise from extensions of basal cells from overlying oral epithelium

Inherited Condition

- Nevoid basal cell carcinoma syndrome (NBCCS; Gorlin syndrome)
  - Autosomal dominant trait
    - High penetrance, variable expression
  - Spontaneous mutations
  - 9q22, involving *PTCH* gene

CLINICAL ISSUES

Epidemiology

- Incidence
  - 4-12% of developmental cysts
- Age
  - Wide range, usually 10-40 years
  - Cysts found at earlier age in those with NBCCS
- Gender
  - Slight male predilection
- Ethnicity
  - Caucasians affected most commonly

Site

- Predilection for mandible (60-80%)
  - Posterior and ascending ramus
- Maxillary lesions tend to be smaller

Presentation

- Asymptomatic
- Pain, discomfort, and swelling
- Rarely, intraoral drainage and neurologic symptoms due to nerve compression
- Nevoid basal cell carcinoma syndrome (NBCCS)
  - Multiple keratocystic odontogenic tumors (KOT)
    - Consistent feature, seen in ~ 75% of patients
  - Basal cell carcinomas
    - Young age, located in areas not typically exposed to sun
  - Palmar and plantar pits
  - Skeletal anomalies
    - Bifid ribs, kyphoscoliosis, mild mandibular prognathism, and calcification of falx cerebri
  - Other tumors
    - Medulloblastoma and ovarian fibromas
  - Other characteristics
    - Hypertelorism, epidermal cysts of skin

Treatment

- Surgical approaches
  - Enucleation or curettage
  - Marsupialization
  - En bloc resection followed by reconstruction

Prognosis

- Multiple recurrences (about 30% of cases)
  - More common in NBCCS
- Malignant transformation is rare

IMAGE FINDINGS

Radiographic Findings

- Well-defined, unilocular radiolucency

KERATOCYSTIC ODONTOGENIC TUMOR (ODONTOGENIC KERATOCYST)

Key Facts

Terminology
- Odontogenic keratocyst (OKC)
- Distinct developmental odontogenic cyst that may be locally aggressive

Etiology/Pathogenesis
- Arise from cells of dental lamina
- Nevoid basal cell carcinoma syndrome (Gorlin syndrome) is associated with multiple odontogenic keratocysts

Clinical Issues
- Predilection for mandible
- Multiple recurrences
- Ovarian fibromas

Image Findings
- Well-defined, unilocular radiolucency
- Smooth, corticated borders

Macroscopic Features
- Thin, friable soft tissue
- Keratinaceous debris

Microscopic Pathology
- Epithelial lining
- 6-8 cells thick
- Lacks rete ridges
- Parakeratotic epithelial cells
- Wavy or corrugated surface
- Basal layer shows palisading and hyperchromicity
- Inflammation may alter characteristic histology

Top Differential Diagnoses
- Orthokeratinized odontogenic cyst
- Dentigerous cyst

- Smooth, corticated borders
- Larger lesions may be multilocular
- Minimal bone expansion
- Often associated with unerupted tooth
  - Teeth displaced rather than resorbed

MACROSCOPIC FEATURES

General Features
- Thin, friable soft tissue
- Keratinaceous debris in cyst lumen
- Bone fragments and unerupted tooth

MICROSCOPIC PATHOLOGY

Histologic Features
- Epithelial lining
  - 6-8 cells thick
  - Lacks rete ridges
    - Epithelium often detached from fibrous wall, creating cleft
  - Basal layer shows palisading and hyperchromicity
  - Parakeratotic epithelial cells
  - Wavy or corrugated surface keratinization (refractile)
  - Keratinaceous debris in lumen
  - Nevoid basal cell carcinoma syndrome
    - More satellite cysts, daughter cysts, budding, and proliferative odontogenic epithelial rests
- Fibrous connective tissue
  - May be detached from overlying epithelium
- When inflamed, epithelium is altered
  - Acute and chronic inflammatory cells
  - Characteristic histology altered, with rete noted
- Epithelial hyaline bodies (Rushton bodies) may be seen
  - Refractile, brightly eosinophilic curvilinear bodies in keratin
- Rarely, malignant transformation

ANCILLARY TESTS

Immunohistochemistry
- High *Ki-67* labeling confirms proliferation
- *TP53* overexpressed

Molecular Genetics
- *PTCH* gene (chromosome 9q22.3-q31) a tumor suppressor gene, with loss of function
  - Results in overexpression of *BCL-1* and *TP53*

DIFFERENTIAL DIAGNOSIS

Orthokeratinized Odontogenic Cyst
- Orthokeratotic epithelial lumen surface
- Prominent keratohyaline granules
- Basal layer lacks palisading

Dentigerous Cyst
- Always associated with unerupted tooth
- Thin, nonkeratinized epithelial lumen surface

Periapical Cyst
- Always associated with radicular surface of nonvital tooth
- Stratified squamous epithelial lumen surface
- Dense inflammation

DIAGNOSTIC CHECKLIST

Pathologic Interpretation Pearls
- Multiple odontogenic keratocysts indicate work-up for nevoid basal cell carcinoma syndrome

SELECTED REFERENCES

1. García de Marcos JA et al: Basal cell nevus syndrome: clinical and genetic diagnosis. Oral Maxillofac Surg. 13(4):225-30, 2009
2. González-Alva P et al: Keratocystic odontogenic tumor: a retrospective study of 183 cases. J Oral Sci. 50(2):205-12, 2008

KERATOCYSTIC ODONTOGENIC TUMOR (ODONTOGENIC KERATOCYST)

Clinical Presentation of Gorlin Syndrome

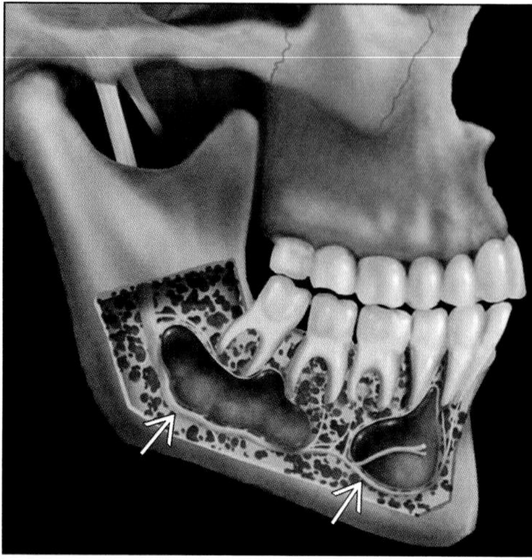

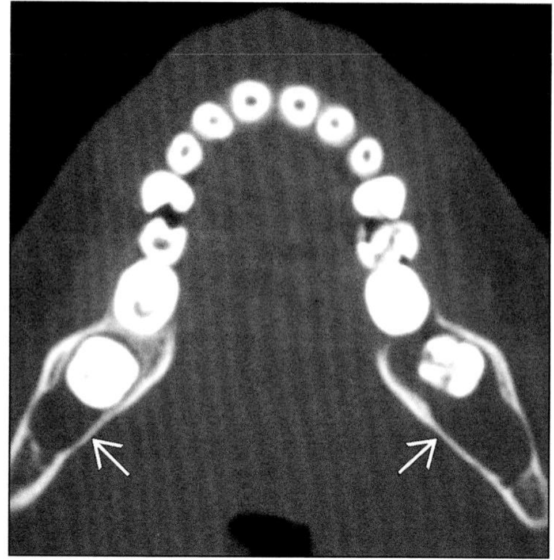

(Left) *Lateral graphic with outer mandibular cortex removed shows the classic appearance of multiple OKCs in NBCCS. Lesions splay teeth roots and displace ➔ the inferior alveolar nerve. Tooth resorption is not a common finding.* ***(Right)*** *Axial CT shows bilateral expansile OKCs ➔ containing unerupted molars in the area of the retromolar triangles. This is a patient with known NBCCS. Keratocystic odontogenic tumors are one of the most consistent findings in this syndrome.*

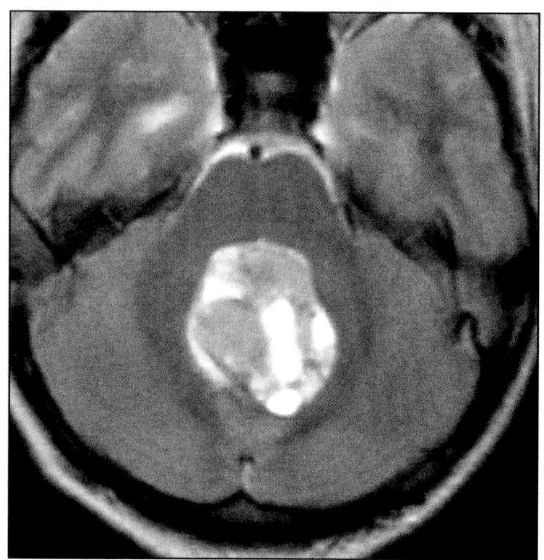

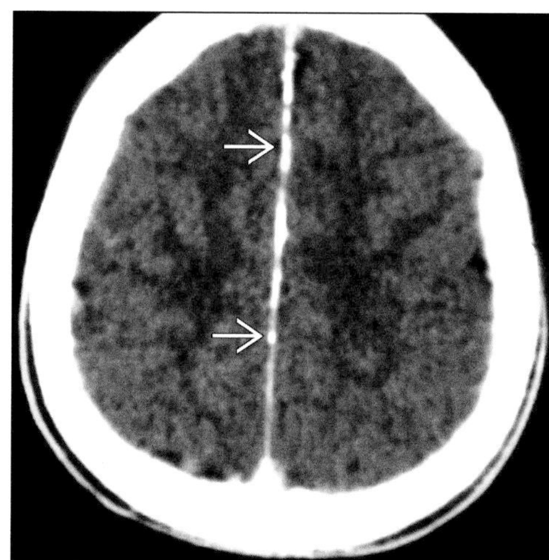

(Left) *Axial T2 MR image reveals a 4th ventricular medulloblastoma in a child with nevoid basal cell carcinoma syndrome. After identification of this tumor, the odontogenic cysts were identified.* ***(Right)*** *Axial NECT shows calcified falx cerebri ➔ in a child with nevoid basal cell carcinoma syndrome. Skeletal abnormalities are a common finding in those affected by the syndrome and include bifid ribs and kyphoscoliosis.*

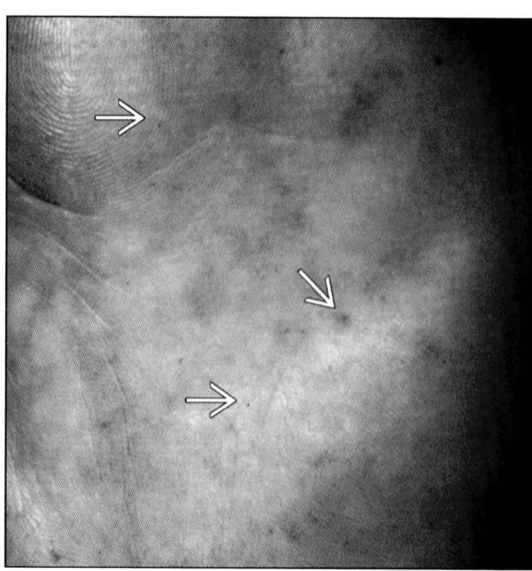

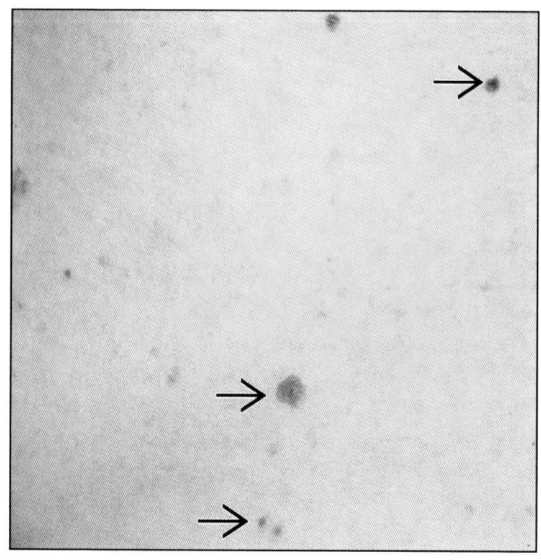

(Left) *Plantar and palmar pits ➔ are a common finding in nevoid basal cell carcinoma syndrome. These pits are a result of the alteration in the development of the basal epithelial cells.* ***(Right)*** *Clinical photo shows multiple basal cell carcinomas ➔ in a patient with nevoid basal cell carcinoma syndrome. These skin lesions are a major component of the syndrome and can number in the hundreds. Treatment of multiple basal cell carcinomas all over the body can lead to considerable cosmetic disfigurement.*

Microscopic Features

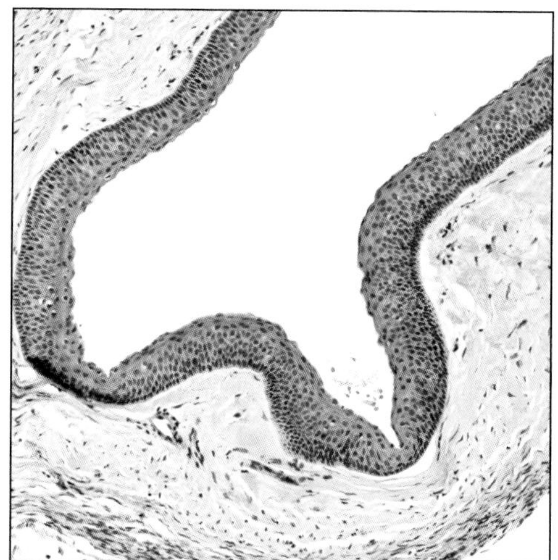

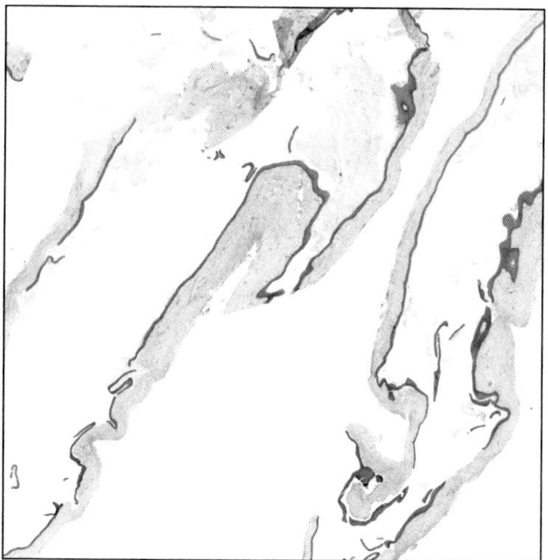

(Left) *This cyst is lined by a relatively thin epithelium, showing a flat interface with the fibrous connective tissue. A cleft is often present, an artifact of processing resulting from the lack of well-developed rete ridges. This lesion is readily identified, even on low to moderate magnification.* ***(Right)*** *Keratocystic odontogenic tumors generally have thin friable walls and a distinctive lumen.*

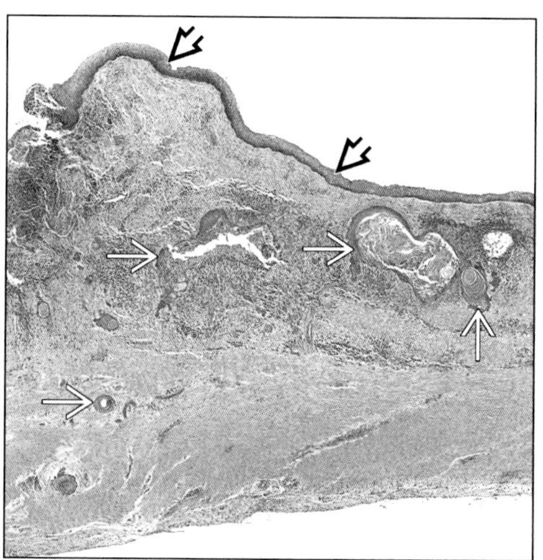

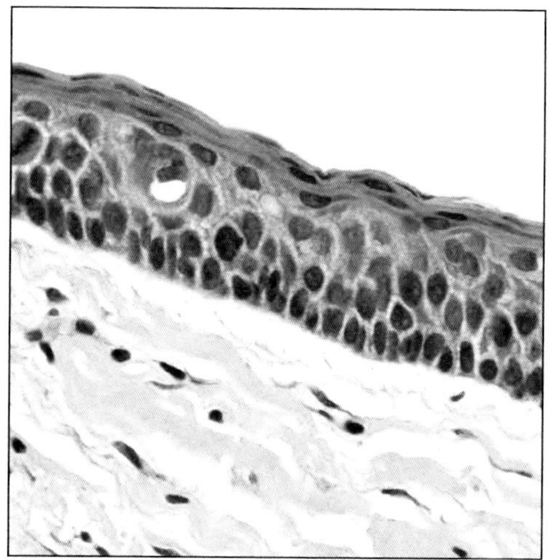

(Left) *Daughter or satellite cysts ➔, seen in this keratocytic odontogenic tumor ➢, are more frequently seen in patients with Gorlin syndrome, or nevoid basal cell carcinoma syndrome. This lesion is also notable for the dense inflammatory infiltrate within the fibrous stroma.* ***(Right)*** *A thin portion of epithelium has become detached from the underlying fibrovascular connective tissue, a common finding in this lesion because of the lack of rete ridges.*

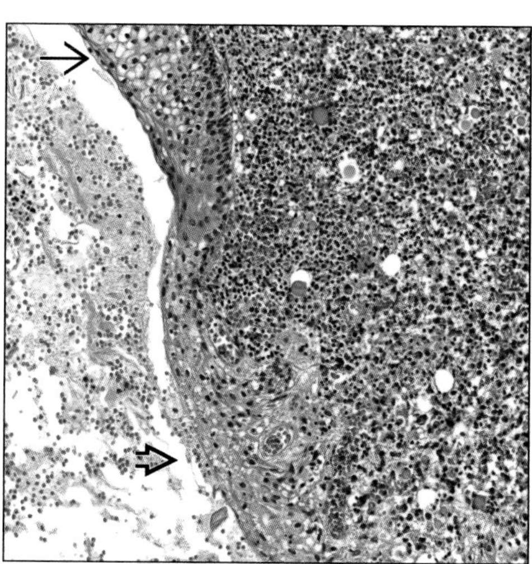

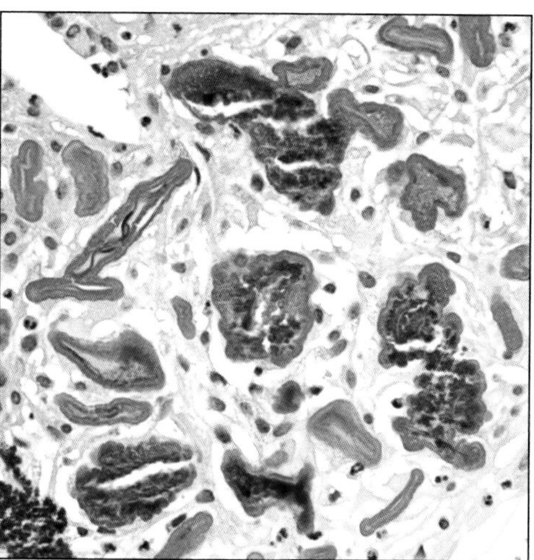

(Left) *Note the transition of the epithelium from the characteristic, well-organized, noninflamed area ➔ into an area of dense inflammation ➢.* ***(Right)*** *Rushton bodies are not pathognomonic of this tumor but are a useful finding. They represent a breakdown product (of keratin) combined with debris, calcified material, and products of blood. This refractile material is most commonly identified in areas of inflammation.*

AMELOBLASTIC FIBROMA/FIBRO-ODONTOMA

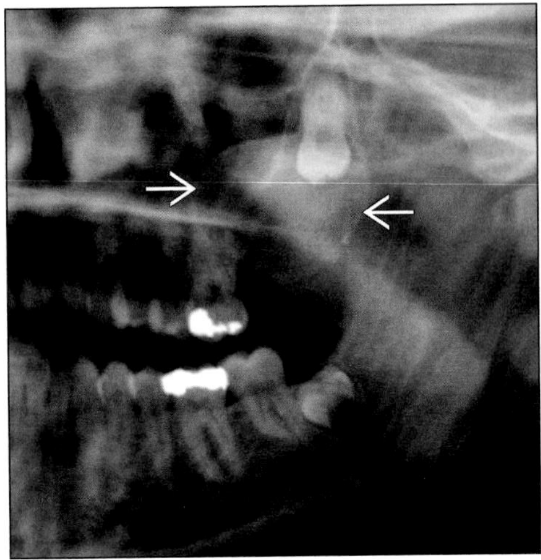

Radiograph shows a large radiolucent lesion ➡ associated with an impacted maxillary 3rd molar. Sclerosis is lacking. Developing dentition supports the young age of the patient.

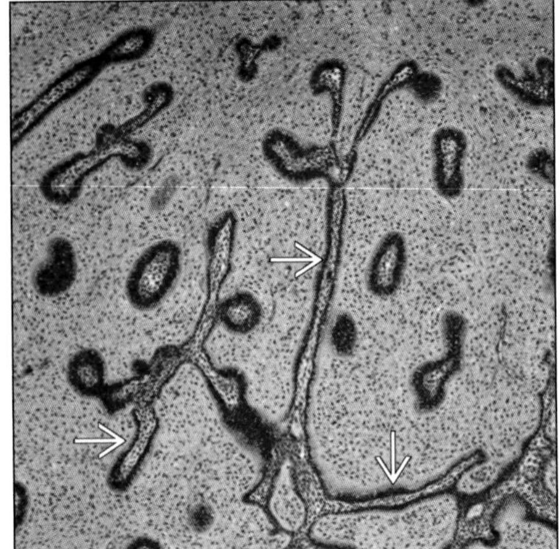

Hematoxylin and eosin shows long, narrow cords of odontogenic epithelium ➡. The stroma is a loose matrix that resembles the dental papilla of a developing tooth, showing low cellularity.

TERMINOLOGY

Abbreviations

- Ameloblastic fibroma (AF)
- Ameloblastic fibro-odontoma (AFO)

Definitions

- Ameloblastic fibroma
  - True neoplasm composed of a mixture of odontogenic epithelial and mesenchymal tissues
- Ameloblastic fibro-odontoma
  - Tumor composed of a mixture of odontogenic epithelial and mesenchymal tissues that also contains dentin and enamel

ETIOLOGY/PATHOGENESIS

Ameloblastic Fibroma

- True neoplasm

Ameloblastic Fibro-odontoma

- May represent a stage of developing odontoma
- Hamartoma
- Rare familial adenomatous polyposis (FAP) association

CLINICAL ISSUES

Epidemiology

- Incidence
  - Rare, even though initially described in 1891
- Age
  - Most common in 1st 2 decades of life
  - Rare in adults
- Gender
  - AF: Slight male predilection
  - AFO: Equal gender distribution

Site

- Posterior mandible is most common location
- Posterior maxilla
- Anterior jaw

Presentation

- Small lesions
  - Usually asymptomatic
  - Found on routine radiographs
- Larger lesions
  - Swelling
  - May prevent eruption of teeth

Treatment

- Surgical approaches
  - Radical vs. conservative management depends on age at presentation
    - Curettage vs. resection
  - Conservative resection for AF, especially in young people

Prognosis

- Ameloblastic fibroma
  - Longer, recurrence-free survival when managed by radical procedures compared to conservative methods
  - Recurrence is variable
    - Highest in cases managed conservatively (up to 90%) vs. radical resection (< 10%)
  - Uncommon malignant transformation (~ 10%) to ameloblastic fibrosarcoma
    - 45% of ameloblastic sarcomas develop in association with recurrent ameloblastic fibromas
  - Close follow-up is indicated
- Ameloblastic fibro-odontoma
  - Recurrences have not been documented

IMAGE FINDINGS

Radiographic Findings

- Radiolucent
  - Unilocular or multilocular

AMELOBLASTIC FIBROMA/FIBRO-ODONTOMA

Key Facts

Terminology
- AF: True mixed odontogenic neoplasm
- AFO: Mixed odontogenic lesion containing dentin and enamel

Clinical Issues
- 1st 2 decades of life

Image Findings
- Radiolucent
- AFO has variable amounts of calcified materials

Microscopic Pathology
- Composed of small islands, cords, or strands of odontogenic epithelium
- Stroma resembles the dental papilla of embryologic tooth development
- Mineralized tissue in AFO only
  - Enamel, dentin, calcified material
- High mesenchymal MIB-1 in recurrent/malignant AF

- Well-circumscribed to sclerotic margin
- Frequently associated with unerupted tooth
- Ameloblastic fibro-odontoma will have variable amounts of calcified materials
  - Flake-like or solid dense masses

MACROSCOPIC FEATURES

Ameloblastic Fibroma
- White to tan, translucent

Ameloblastic Fibro-odontoma
- White to tan, translucent
- Mineralized tooth structure

MICROSCOPIC PATHOLOGY

Histologic Features
- Epithelial component
  - Small islands, cords, or strands of odontogenic epithelium
    - Peripheral cells are columnar and ameloblast-like
    - Scant central areas of stellate reticulum-like tissue
- Stroma
  - Cellular, myxoid tissue resembling developing dental papilla
    - Cytologically bland round to angulated cells
  - Few to no mitotic figures
- Mineralized tissue: Ameloblastic fibro-odontoma only
  - Enamel, dentin, calcified material

ANCILLARY TESTS

Immunohistochemistry
- Increased MIB-1 in mesenchyme of recurrent and malignant AF

DIFFERENTIAL DIAGNOSIS

Ameloblastoma
- Variable patterns, with loose to collagenous stroma

Odontoma
- Small odontogenic epithelial rests within normal dental follicular tissue
- No epithelium strands or pale myxoid stroma

Ameloblastic Fibrosarcoma
- Hypercellular stroma with increased mitoses

SELECTED REFERENCES

1. Chen Y et al: Ameloblastic fibroma: a review of published studies with special reference to its nature and biological behavior. Oral Oncol. 43(10):960-9, 2007
2. Gyulai-Gaál S et al: Mixed odontogenic tumors in children and adolescents. J Craniofac Surg. 18(6):1338-42, 2007
3. Cohen DM et al: Ameloblastic fibroma, ameloblastic fibro-odontoma, and odontoma. Oral Maxillofac Surg Clin North Am. 16(3):375-84, 2004
4. Takeda Y: Ameloblastic fibroma and related lesions: current pathologic concept. Oral Oncol. 35(6):535-40, 1999

IMAGE GALLERY

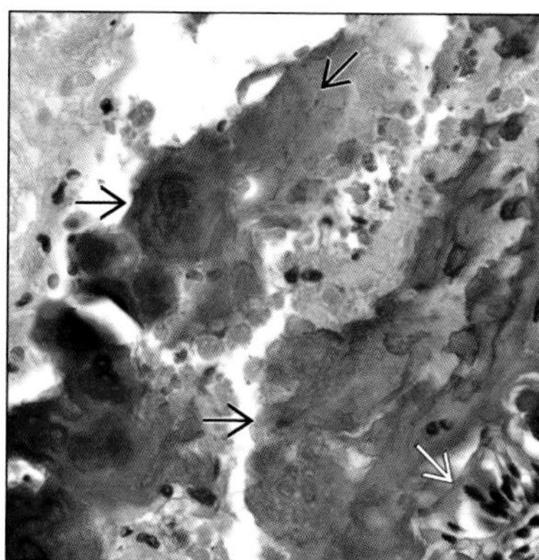

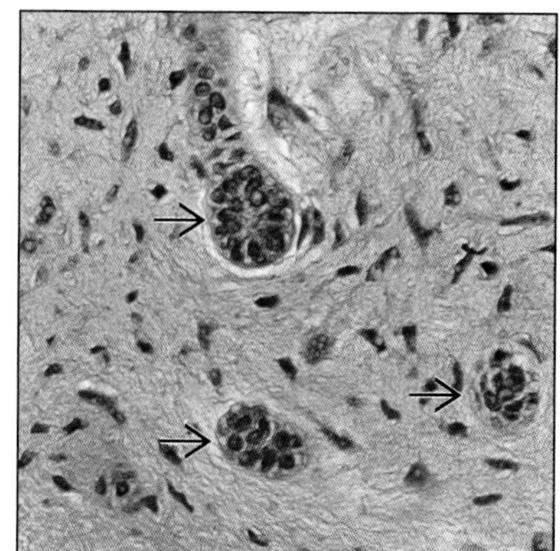

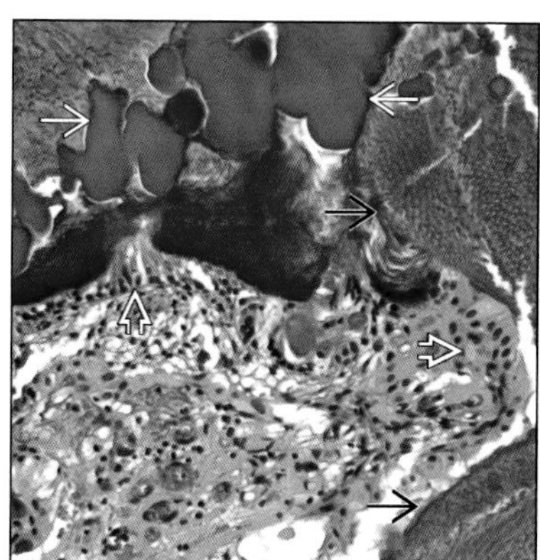

(Left) This ameloblastic fibro-odontoma is predominated by calcified material ➔ that is not easily distinguished as either dentin or enamel. Note the subtle odontogenic epithelium ➡. *(Center)* H&E shows ameloblastic fibroma with numerous small discrete islands of odontogenic epithelium ➔ in the slightly myxoid stroma. *(Right)* This ameloblastic fibro-odontoma shows mature dentin ➔ and calcified material ➡ in close relationship to odontogenic epithelium ➡.

ODONTOMA (COMPLEX AND COMPOUND)

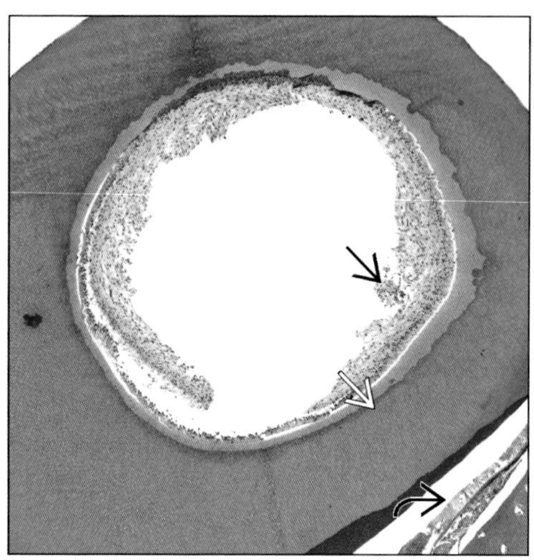

Hematoxylin & eosin shows a compound odontoma with central pulp tissue ➙ surrounded by dentin ➙ and a focus of enamel matrix ➙. This relationship is reminiscent of a normal tooth.

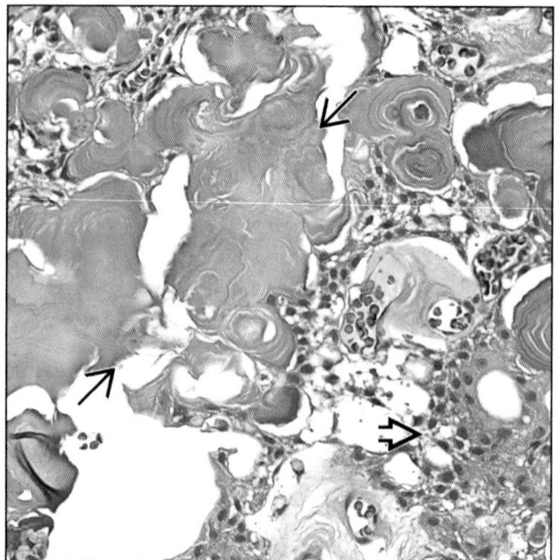

Hematoxylin & eosin shows a focus of disorganized enamel matrix ➙ and odontogenic epithelium ➙.

TERMINOLOGY

Definitions

- Hamartomas of odontogenic epithelium and ectomesenchyme

ETIOLOGY/PATHOGENESIS

Developmental Anomaly

- Hamartoma
  - Compound odontoma
    - Small tooth-like structures
  - Complex
    - Haphazard aggregate of enamel and dentin
  - Combination

CLINICAL ISSUES

Epidemiology

- Age
  - Most occur during 1st 2 decades of life
- Gender
  - Equal gender distribution

Site

- Most common in maxilla
  - Compound odontomas are most frequent in anterior maxilla
  - Complex odontomas are most frequent in posterior mandible

Presentation

- Usually detected on routine dental radiographs
- Vast majority are asymptomatic
- May prevent eruption of normal dentition
- Rarely, may erupt
- Rarely, may cause bone expansion
- May be part of syndrome (Rubinstein-Taybi)

Treatment

- Simple surgical excision
  - Complete removal of associated soft tissue
    - Dental follicular tissue
    - Dentigerous cyst
- Orthodontics to correct malocclusion, if needed

Prognosis

- Excellent, without recurrence

IMAGE FINDINGS

Radiographic Findings

- Radiographic characteristics are considered diagnostic
  - Rarely, may be confused with osteoma
- Compound
  - Tooth-shaped structures
  - Surrounded by radiolucent zone
- Complex
  - Radiodense mass
  - Surrounded by radiolucent zone

MACROSCOPIC FEATURES

General Features

- Compound
  - Tooth-shaped hard tissues
  - Associated fibrous connective tissue
- Complex
  - Disorganized mass of white-yellow hard tissues
  - Associated fibrous connective tissue

Size

- Generally do not exceed size of normal tooth
- Rarely, up to 6 cm

ODONTOMA (COMPLEX AND COMPOUND)

Key Facts

Terminology
- Hamartomas of odontogenic epithelium and ectomesenchyme

Clinical Issues
- Most occur during 1st 2 decades of life
- Most common in maxilla

Macroscopic Features
- Tooth-shaped hard tissues
- Disorganized mass of white-yellow hard tissues

Microscopic Pathology
- Dentin, enamel matrix, cementum, and pulp tissue
- Compound odontomas have organized architecture, recapitulating normal teeth
- Complex odontomas have haphazard arrangement

Top Differential Diagnoses
- Hyperdontia, root tip, or impacted tooth

MICROSCOPIC PATHOLOGY

Histologic Features
- Compound odontomas have architecture similar to normal tooth
  - Mature tubular dentin
  - Enamel matrix
    - Mature enamel is lost during decalcification process
  - Cementum
  - Pulp tissue
  - Dental follicular tissue
  - Occasional dentigerous cyst
- Complex odontomas have haphazard arrangement
  - Haphazardly arranged tubular dentin
  - Dentin often surrounds islands of enamel/matrix
  - Thin layer of cementum may surround mass
  - Epithelial ghost cells are frequently seen
  - Dental follicular tissue
  - Occasional dentigerous cyst
- May be found in conjunction with other odontogenic cysts or tumors
  - Odontoameloblastoma

DIFFERENTIAL DIAGNOSIS

Hyperdontia (Supernumerary Teeth)
- Complete, well-formed tooth, usually in males
- Rarely, syndrome associated
  - Gardner, Sturge-Weber, cleidocranial dysplasia

Root Tip
- History of incomplete tooth extraction
- May be symptomatic

Impacted Tooth
- Normal part of dentition

SELECTED REFERENCES

1. da Silva LF et al: Odontomas: a clinicopathologicstudy in a Portuguese population. Quintessence Int. 40(1):61-72, 2009
2. Ferrés-Padró E et al: A descriptive study of 113 unerupted supernumerary teeth in 79 pediatric patients in Barcelona. Med Oral Patol Oral Cir Bucal. 14(3):E146-52, 2009
3. Hidalgo-Sánchez O et al: Metaanalysis of the epidemiology and clinical manifestations of odontomas. Med Oral Patol Oral Cir Bucal. 13(11):E730-4, 2008
4. Yoon RK et al: Impacted maxillary anterior supernumerary teeth. A survey of forty-two cases. N Y State Dent J. 74(6):24-7, 2008
5. Fregnani ER et al: Odontomas and ameloblastomas: variable prevalences around the world? Oral Oncol. 38(8):807-8, 2002
6. de Oliveira BH et al: Compound odontoma--diagnosis and treatment: three case reports. Pediatr Dent. 23(2):151-7, 2001
7. Philipsen HP et al: Mixed odontogenic tumours and odontomas. Considerations on interrelationship. Review of the literature and presentation of 134 new cases of odontomas. Oral Oncol. 33(2):86-99, 1997
8. MacDonald-Jankowski DS: Odontomas in a Chinese population. Dentomaxillofac Radiol. 25(4):186-92, 1996

IMAGE GALLERY

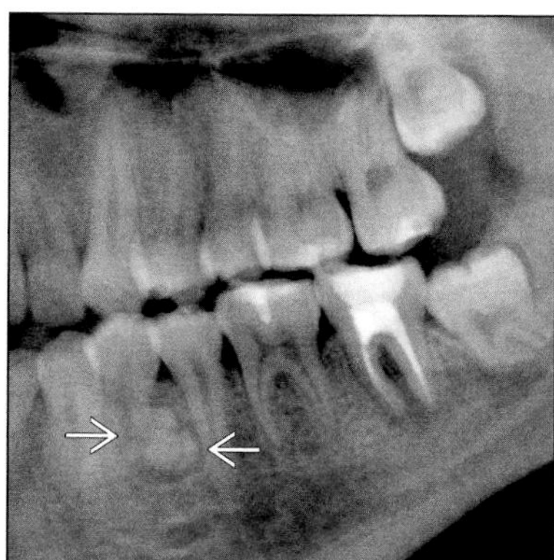
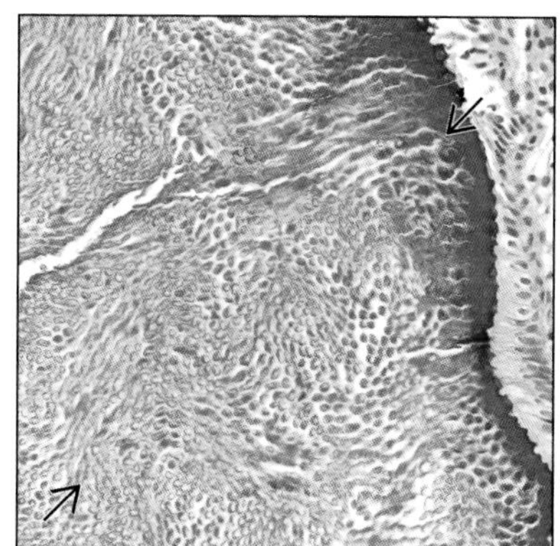
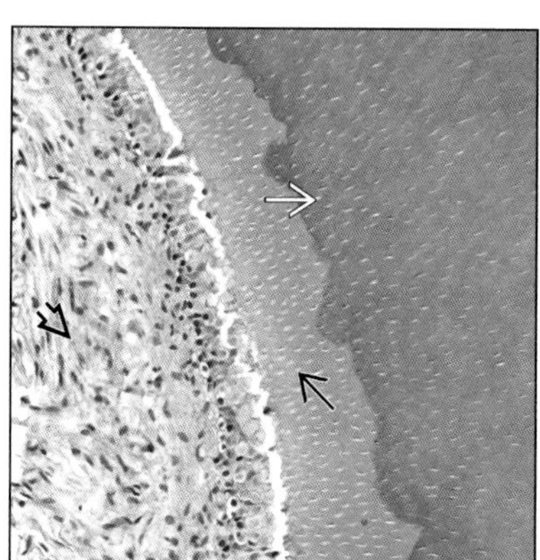

(Left) *Radiograph shows a compound odontoma ➔, resembling a small cluster of tooth-like structures. Note the radiolucent rim surrounding the calcifications; this may represent either a dentigerous cyst or a dental follicle.* ***(Center)*** *Hematoxylin & eosin shows a high-power view of decalcified enamel matrix ➔. Note the "fish scale" appearance. Mature enamel is completely lost during decalcification.* ***(Right)*** *Hematoxylin & eosin shows pulpal tissue ➔ immediately adjacent to predentin ➔ and mature mineralized dentin ➔.*

CENTRAL ODONTOGENIC FIBROMA

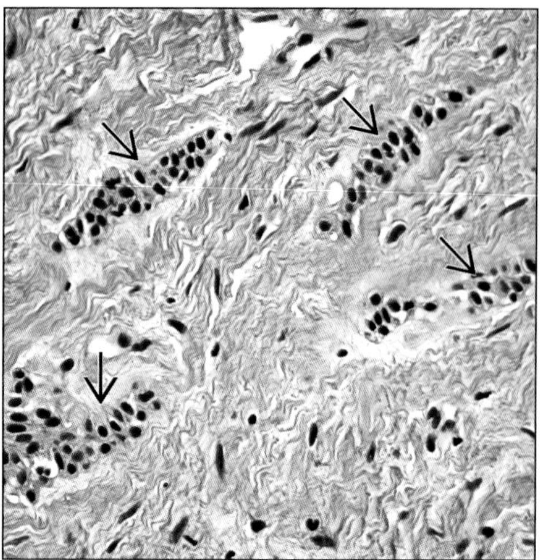

This central odontogenic fibroma has a loose stroma with fine collagen fibrils and small odontogenic epithelial rests ➔. Odontogenic rests are not always seen.

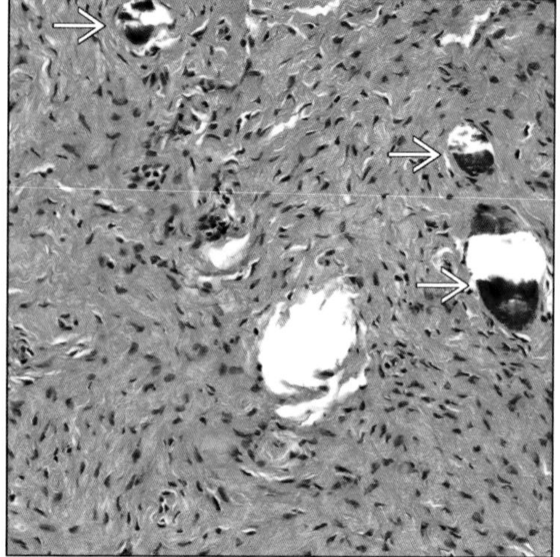

Dense fibrous stroma with a vague whorling pattern and focal calcifications ➔ are characteristic of the variant referred to as the WHO type. This subclassification is being phased out.

TERMINOLOGY

Abbreviations

- Central odontogenic fibroma (COF)

Definitions

- Benign odontogenic neoplasm showing varying amounts of inactive-appearing odontogenic epithelium embedded in mature fibrous stroma

ETIOLOGY/PATHOGENESIS

Pathogenesis

- Most are considered to be of periodontal ligament origin
- Dental follicle may be consideration
- Peripheral odontogenic fibroma is soft tissue counterpart

CLINICAL ISSUES

Epidemiology

- Incidence
  - Uncommon
- Age
  - Wide range
    - Mean: 40 years
- Gender
  - Female > Male (3:1)

Site

- Mandible
  - Usually posterior to 1st molar
- Maxilla
  - Usually anterior to 1st molar/premolar region

Presentation

- Asymptomatic
  - Detected on routine dental radiographs
- Symptomatic
  - Swelling
  - Loosening teeth
  - Mild pain to painless
  - Draining
  - Lesions of anterior maxilla
    - May have palatal boney depression
    - Occasionally creates characteristic cleft

Treatment

- Surgical approaches
  - Enucleation
  - Curettage

Prognosis

- Excellent
  - Few recurrences
  - Appears to have limited growth potential
    - Especially in anterior maxilla

IMAGE FINDINGS

Radiographic Findings

- Unilocular, radiolucent
  - Usually small lesions
- Multilocular, radiolucent
- Frequently associated with unerupted tooth
- Expansion of affected bone
- Root resorption
- Root divergence of associated teeth
- Occasional radiopaque flecks
- Sclerotic, well-defined border

MACROSCOPIC FEATURES

General Features

- Well circumscribed
- Firm, yellow-white, cut surface

CENTRAL ODONTOGENIC FIBROMA

Key Facts

Terminology
- Rare, benign, odontogenic neoplasm of inactive-appearing odontogenic epithelium embedded in mature fibrous stroma

Etiology/Pathogenesis
- Considered to be of periodontal ligament origin

Clinical Issues
- Wide age range
- Female > Male (3:1)

Microscopic Pathology
- Well-circumscribed, yellow-white cut surface
- Collagen stroma, dense to myxoid
- Odontogenic epithelium may or may not be present
- Cementum or dentin-like calcifications
- Dystrophic calcifications

Top Differential Diagnoses
- Dental follicle, desmoplastic fibroma, myxofibroma

MICROSCOPIC PATHOLOGY

Histologic Features
- Diverse
  - Simple
    - Fibroblasts
    - Collagen stroma, dense to myxoid
    - Odontogenic epithelium may or may not be present
    - Cementum or dentin-like calcifications
    - Dystrophic calcifications
    - Focal inflammation
  - WHO (World Health Organization) type
    - Subclassification term that is being phased out
    - Complex pattern of cellular fibrous tissue, dense to myxoid
    - Long cords or larger nests of odontogenic epithelium predominate
    - Dystrophic calcifications
    - Cementum or dentin-like calcifications
    - Focal inflammation
  - Granular cell odontogenic fibroma
    - Rare, composed of large, round granular cells

DIFFERENTIAL DIAGNOSIS

Dental Follicular Tissue
- Always associated with unerupted tooth
- Usually stroma is myxoid

Desmoplastic Fibroma
- More aggressive presentation
- Lacks odontogenic epithelial rests

Myxofibroma
- More acellular
- Myxoid
- Odontogenic epithelial rests rare

Fibrosarcoma
- Cellular neoplasm with uniform spindle cells in fascicular pattern
- Usually numerous mitoses
- More aggressive presentation

SELECTED REFERENCES

1. Lotay HS et al: Central odontogenic fibroma with features of central granular cell odontogenic tumor. Oral Surg Oral Med Oral Pathol Oral Radiol Endod. 109(2):e63-6, 2010
2. Lin CT et al: Peripheral odontogenic fibroma in a Taiwan chinese population: a retrospective analysis. Kaohsiung J Med Sci. 24(8):415-21, 2008
3. Ikeshima A et al: Case report of intra-osseous fibroma: a study on odontogenic and desmoplastic fibromas with a review of the literature. J Oral Sci. 47(3):149-57, 2005
4. Daniels JS: Central odontogenic fibroma of mandible: a case report and review of the literature. Oral Surg Oral Med Oral Pathol Oral Radiol Endod. 98(3):295-300, 2004
5. Ramer M et al: Central odontogenic fibroma--report of a case and review of the literature. Periodontal Clin Investig. 24(1):27-30, 2002

IMAGE GALLERY

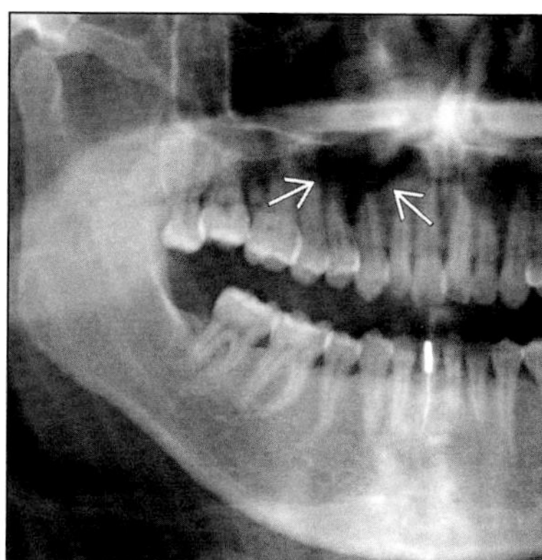

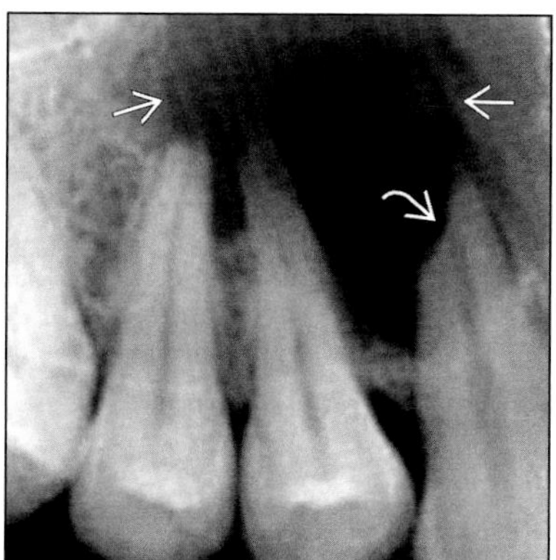

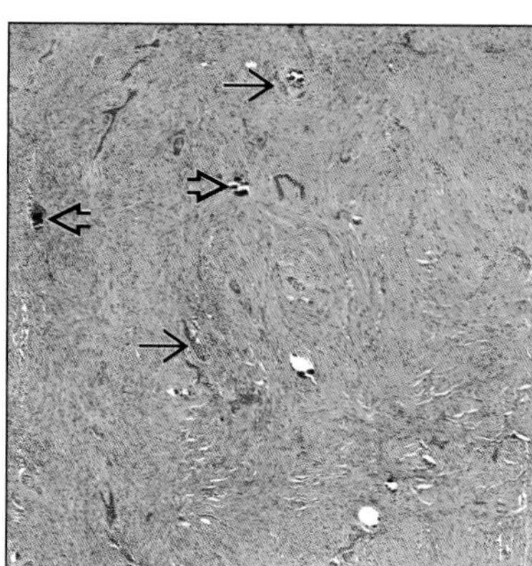

(Left) *Cropped panoramic radiograph reveals an expansile, radiolucent central odontogenic fibroma* ➔ *of the maxillary ridge. (Courtesy P. Sikorski, MD.)* ***(Center)*** *A radiograph shows a radiolucent, expansile lesion* ➔*. Root resorption of the #4 & #5 teeth is subtle, while #6 tooth root resorption is gross* ➔*. (Courtesy P. Sikorski, MD.)* ***(Right)*** *Low-power view shows isolated epithelial islands* ➔ *with calcification* ➔ *in a dense stroma.*

CALCIFYING CYSTIC ODONTOGENIC TUMOR

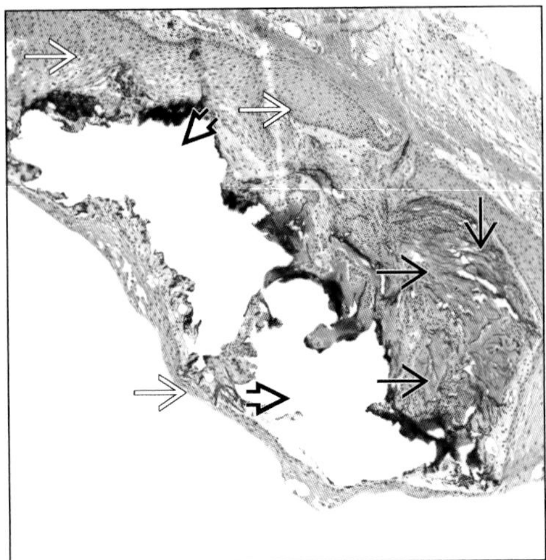

This low-power image shows typical odontogenic epithelium ➡, characteristic ghost cells ⇨, and areas of calcification ⇨, some of which may be lost during tissue processing.

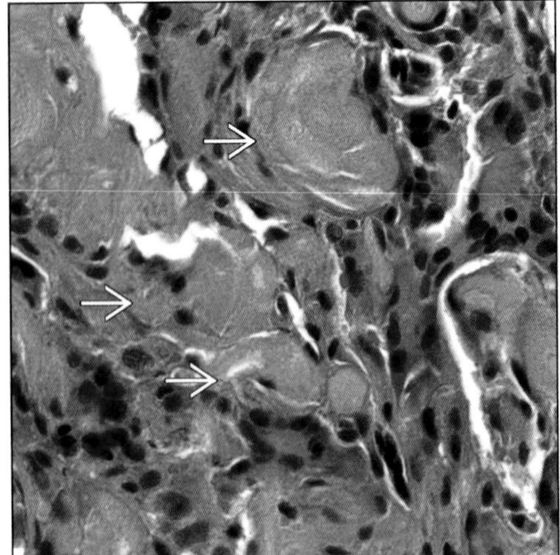

High-power image shows numerous large, eosinophilic ghost cells ➡. Ghost cells are found only in a few entities, narrowing the histologic differential diagnosis. No stellate reticulum is present.

TERMINOLOGY

Abbreviations

- Calcifying cystic odontogenic tumor (CCOT)
- Calcifying odontogenic cyst (COC)
- Peripheral calcifying odontogenic cyst (PCOC)

Synonyms

- Gorlin cyst
- Calcifying odontogenic cyst

Definitions

- Benign cystic neoplasm of odontogenic origin, characterized by ameloblastoma-like epithelium with ghost cells that may calcify
  - Separated into central (intraosseous) and peripheral (gingiva/alveolar mucosa)

ETIOLOGY/PATHOGENESIS

Pathogenesis

- Debate about developmental cyst vs. true neoplasm

CLINICAL ISSUES

Epidemiology

- Incidence
  - Uncommon
- Age
  - Wide range
    - 2nd and 3rd decades most common
  - If associated with odontoma: Younger age group
  - Aggressive variants: More common in older patients
- Gender
  - Slight male predilection

Site

- **Central**
  - Maxilla slightly more often
    - Anterior most frequently
    - Premolar and molar area
  - Anterior mandible
- **Peripheral**
  - Gingiva and alveolar mucosa
  - Up to 1/3 of tumors
  - Usually anterior to 1st molar: Incisor-canine area

Presentation

- Pain
- Bony expansion
- Asymptomatic, incidental finding on routine radiographs
- May be associated with other odontogenic tumors
- Peripheral lesions appear as nondescript gingival masses

Treatment

- Surgical approaches
  - Calcifying odontogenic cyst
    - Simple enucleation
  - Calcifying odontogenic cyst with other odontogenic tumor
    - Treat like more aggressive lesion
  - Peripheral cysts
    - Simple excision

Prognosis

- Excellent; few recurrences documented
- If associated with another tumor, prognosis reflects more aggressive tumor

IMAGE FINDINGS

Radiographic Findings

- **Central**
  - Unilocular or multilocular
  - Radiolucent with well-defined margin
    - Contains irregular internal calcifications, especially at periphery

CALCIFYING CYSTIC ODONTOGENIC TUMOR

Key Facts

Terminology

- Benign cystic neoplasm of odontogenic origin, characterized by ameloblastoma-like epithelium with ghost cells that may calcify

Clinical Issues

- Maxilla favored slightly, usually anterior
- Wide age range, slight male predominance
- May be associated with other odontogenic tumors
- Bone radiolucency, often with unerupted tooth

Microscopic Pathology

- Classified as central and peripheral
- Thin epithelium with columnar or cuboidal basal cells (ameloblast-like)
- Ghost cells: Most characteristic finding
- Calcified material

Top Differential Diagnoses

- Ameloblastoma, odontogenic cysts
- Peripheral ossifying fibroma, craniopharyngioma

  - May be associated with unerupted/impacted tooth
  - Root resorption and root divergence may be seen
- **Peripheral**
  - May show soft tissue calcification and cupping

MICROSCOPIC PATHOLOGY

Histologic Features

- Cysts may be nonproliferative (simple), proliferative, ameloblastomatous, combined with odontoma, or combined with other odontogenic tumors
- **Cysts**
  - May be unicystic (most common) or multicystic with daughter cysts
  - Thin epithelium with columnar or cuboidal basal cells (ameloblast-like) along fibrous wall
  - Lumen lined by tissue resembling stellate reticulum
- **Ghost cells**
  - Most characteristic finding (few entities have them)
  - Large epithelial cells with loss of nuclei
    - Develop as a result of coagulative necrosis
- **Calcified material**
  - May be associated with other odontogenic tumors
    - Most common is odontoma (compound)
    - Ameloblastoma, ghost cell odontogenic carcinoma

DIFFERENTIAL DIAGNOSIS

Ameloblastoma

- No ghost cells

Other Odontogenic or Developmental Cysts

- No ghost cells

Peripheral Ossifying Fibroma

- Gingival mass with bone, lacking ghost cells

Craniopharyngioma

- Histologically identical, affects children
- Pituitary gland involvement (unique anatomic site)

SELECTED REFERENCES

1. Li TJ et al: Clinicopathologic spectrum of the so-called calcifying odontogenic cysts: a study of 21 intraosseous cases with reconsideration of the terminology and classification. Am J Surg Pathol. 27(3):372-84, 2003
2. Toida M: So-called calcifying odontogenic cyst: review and discussion on the terminology and classification. J Oral Pathol Med. 27(2):49-52, 1998
3. Buchner A et al: Peripheral (extraosseous) calcifying odontogenic cyst. A review of forty-five cases. Oral Surg Oral Med Oral Pathol. 72(1):65-70, 1991
4. Buchner A: The central (intraosseous) calcifying odontogenic cyst: an analysis of 215 cases. J Oral Maxillofac Surg. 49(4):330-9, 1991
5. Hong SP et al: Calcifying odontogenic cyst. A review of ninety-two cases with reevaluation of their nature as cysts or neoplasms, the nature of ghost cells, and subclassification. Oral Surg Oral Med Oral Pathol. 72(1):56-64, 1991
6. Freedman PD et al: Calcifying odontogenic cyst. A review and analysis of seventy cases. Oral Surg Oral Med Oral Pathol. 40(1):93-106, 1975

IMAGE GALLERY

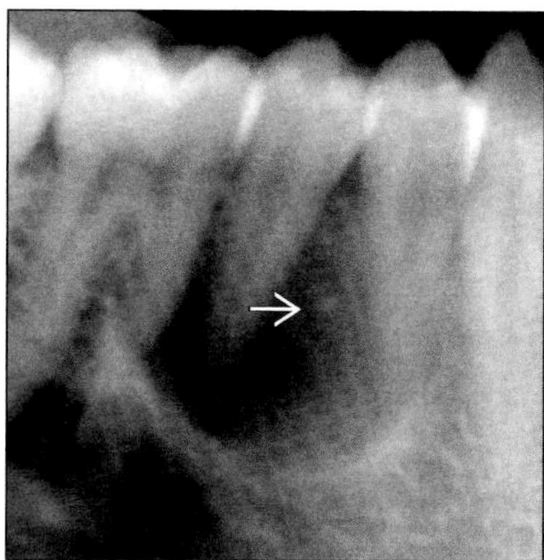

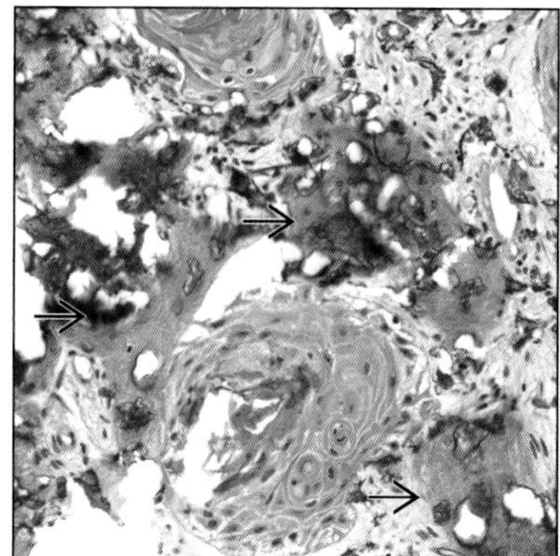

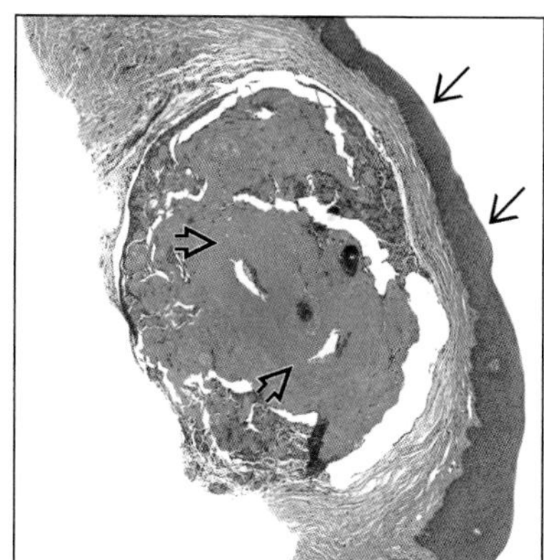

(Left) *This radiograph of a CCOT shows a mandibular radiolucency with irregular small calcifications ➡. (Courtesy J.T. Castle, DDS.)* ***(Center)*** *A CCOT with areas of calcification ➡ is shown. Mineralization usually starts within ghost cells and may result in large areas of calcification.* ***(Right)*** *This low-power image illustrates a peripheral CCOT, showing the overlying epithelium ➡. It is estimated that peripheral tumors make up about 1/3 of these neoplasms. Ghost cells predominate ➡.*

CEMENTOBLASTOMA

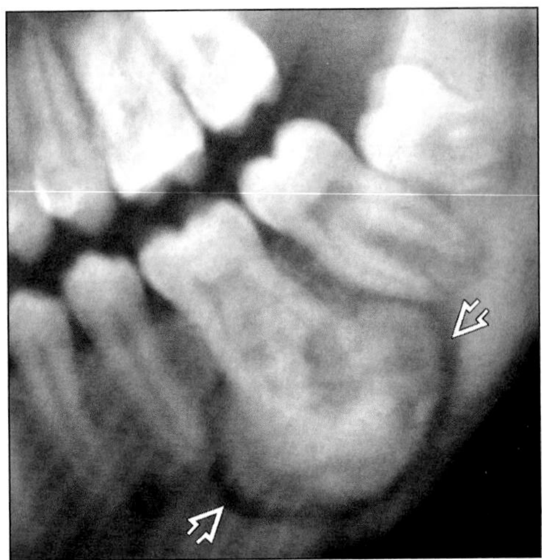

Radiograph shows a radiodensity intimately associated with the roots of the 1st mandibular molar. The periphery of the mass is surrounded by a characteristic radiolucent rim ➡.

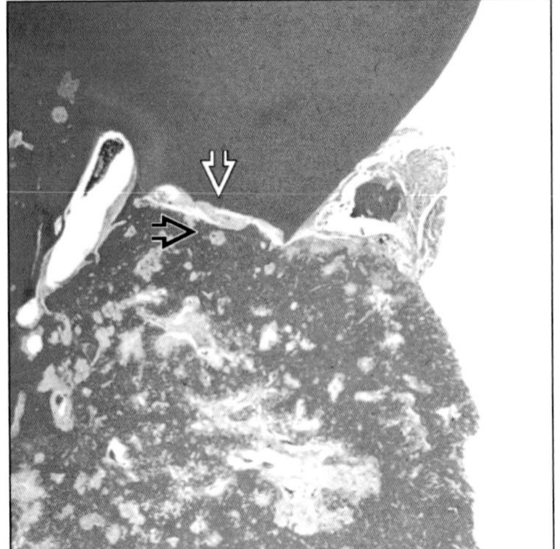

Hematoxylin & eosin shows the resorption of dentin ➡ and its replacement by cementoblastoma ➡.

TERMINOLOGY

Synonyms

- True cementoma
- Benign cementoblastoma

Definitions

- Neoplasm of cementum intimately involved with tooth root

CLINICAL ISSUES

Epidemiology

- Incidence
  - < 6% of odontogenic tumors
- Age
  - Most common in 2nd to 3rd decade
- Gender
  - Probably equal gender distribution
    - Series vary based on selection bias

Site

- Favors mandible
  - Premolar-molar region
- Maxilla
- Always intimately associated with tooth root
  - Erupted permanent teeth
  - Rarely impacted teeth
  - Rarely deciduous teeth

Presentation

- Asymptomatic
- Symptomatic
  - Pain
  - Swelling
- Associated tooth
  - Tooth may test vital
  - Vitality testing may be equivocal
- Rarely multiple

Treatment

- Surgical approaches
  - Removal of affected tooth and mass
    - Thorough curettage
    - Peripheral ostectomy
- Alternate treatment
  - Retention of tooth with prior endodontic treatment (root canal)
    - Surgical removal of mass
    - Partial root amputation
- Prosthetic replacement of affected tooth

Prognosis

- Recurrence is considered rare with complete removal
- Incomplete removal may result in recurrences
- Follow-up is indicated

IMAGE FINDINGS

Radiographic Findings

- Radiopaque mass
- Narrow radiolucent rim
- Intimate association with tooth root (pathognomonic)
- Rare perforation of cortex
- Root resorption may be seen

MACROSCOPIC FEATURES

General Features

- Yellow mineralized tissue
- Fused to root

MICROSCOPIC PATHOLOGY

Histologic Features

- Dense cementum-like tissue
  - Prominent basophilic reversal lines
  - Irregular lacunae

CEMENTOBLASTOMA

Key Facts

Terminology
- Neoplasm of cementum intimately involved with tooth root

Clinical Issues
- Favors mandible
  - Premolar-molar region
- Recurrence is considered rare with complete removal

Image Findings
- Intimately associated with tooth root (pathognomonic)
- Radiopaque mass
- Narrow radiolucent rim

Microscopic Pathology
- Dense cementum-like tissue
- Prominent basophilic reversal lines

  - Plump cementoblasts may line trabeculae
  - Cellular fibroblastic tissue between mineralized trabeculae
- Periphery of lesion
  - Uncalcified matrix
- Occasional giant cells
- Histologically vital pulp tissue

DIFFERENTIAL DIAGNOSIS

Osteoblastoma
- Does not have intimate relationship to tooth root
- Rare in jaw

Osteoid Osteoma
- Does not have intimate relationship to tooth root
- Rare in jaw
- Likely painful

Osteosarcoma
- Radiographically poorly circumscribed
- May demonstrate rapid growth
- Atypical histological proliferation

Reactive Lesions
- Periapical cyst
  - Almost always associated with non-vital tooth
  - Radiolucent lesion
  - Epithelial lining with inflammation
- Periapical granuloma
  - Almost always associated with non-vital tooth
  - Radiolucent lesion
  - Granulation type tissue reaction with inflammation

DIAGNOSTIC CHECKLIST

Clinically Relevant Pathologic Features
- Radiographic presentation is nearly pathognomonic

SELECTED REFERENCES

1. Sumer M et al: Benign cementoblastoma: a case report. Med Oral Patol Oral Cir Bucal. 11(6):E483-5, 2006
2. Ohki K et al: Benign cementoblastoma involving multiple maxillary teeth: report of a case with a review of the literature. Oral Surg Oral Med Oral Pathol Oral Radiol Endod. 97(1):53-8, 2004
3. Brannon RB et al: Cementoblastoma: an innocuous neoplasm? A clinicopathologic study of 44 cases and review of the literature with special emphasis on recurrence. Oral Surg Oral Med Oral Pathol Oral Radiol Endod. 93(3):311-20, 2002
4. El-Mofty SK: Cemento-ossifying fibroma and benign cementoblastoma. Semin Diagn Pathol. 16(4):302-7, 1999
5. Ulmansky M et al: Benign cementoblastoma. A review and five new cases. Oral Surg Oral Med Oral Pathol. 77(1):48-55, 1994
6. Slootweg PJ: Cementoblastoma and osteoblastoma: a comparison of histologic features. J Oral Pathol Med. 21(9):385-9, 1992
7. Goerig AC et al: Endodontic treatment of a cementoblastoma. Oral Surg Oral Med Oral Pathol. 58(2):133-6, 1984

IMAGE GALLERY

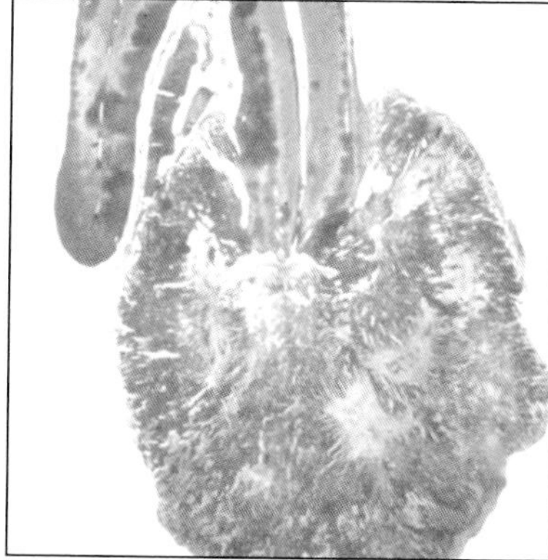

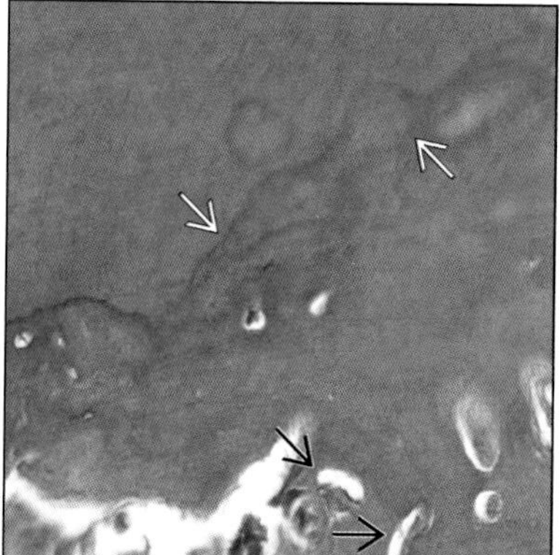

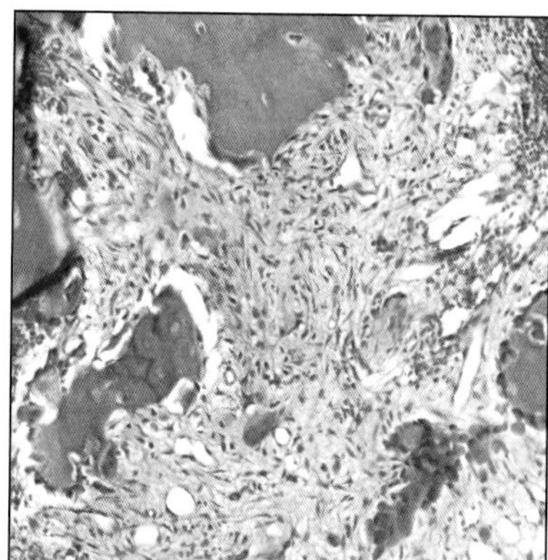

(Left) *Hematoxylin & eosin shows the relationship of the tumor to the root of this mandibular molar.* ***(Center)*** *Hematoxylin & eosin shows mineralized cementum with prominent basophilic reversal lines ➡. Lacunae with cementoblasts are readily seen ➡.* ***(Right)*** *Hematoxylin & eosin shows the cellular fibrovascular tissue seen between trabeculae.*

OSSIFYING FIBROMA

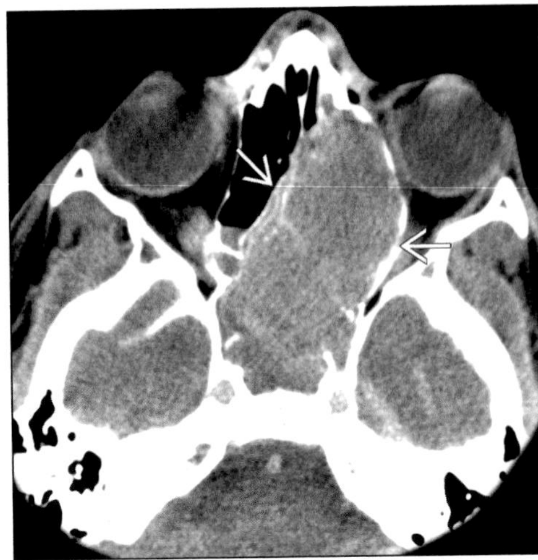

CT shows a large, well-delineated, expansile mass filling the left ethmoid and sphenoid sinuses. There is a periphery of ossified material ➡, a feature frequently seen in OF.

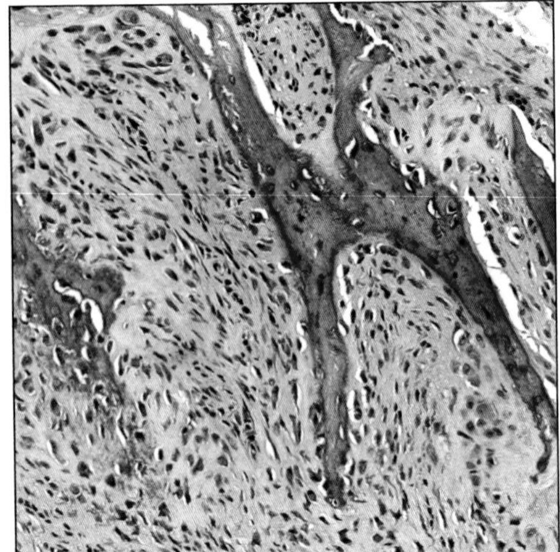

There are evenly spaced spicules of woven bone separated by a spindled cell proliferation. Note focal osteoblastic rimming around the spicules of bone. Osteoclasts can be present.

TERMINOLOGY

Abbreviations

- Ossifying fibroma (OF)

Definitions

- Benign neoplasm of bone with lamellar bone formation, osteoblastic rimming, and connective tissue stroma
- When cementum is present, cementifying fibroma or cemento-ossifying fibroma used

ETIOLOGY/PATHOGENESIS

Pathogenesis

- True neoplasm within fibro-osseous group, rather than a developmental anomaly
- Considered on spectrum with fibrous dysplasia and osseous dysplasia

CLINICAL ISSUES

Epidemiology

- Incidence
  - Rare
- Age
  - Peak: 2nd-4th decades
    - Mean: 31 years
- Gender
  - Female > > Male (5:1)

Site

- Mandible most commonly affected (up to 90%)
  - Posterior, pre-molar regions specifically

Presentation

- Vast majority are asymptomatic, identified by routine radiographic studies
- Slow growing but can have rapid increase in size
- Symptoms include facial asymmetry, swelling, neurosensory disturbances, pain, or hyperesthesia

Treatment

- Options, risks, complications
  - Small lesions can be managed with watchful waiting
  - Complications may develop if not completely removed
- Surgical approaches
  - Complete removal to avoid recurrence
- Radiation
  - Radiotherapy contraindicated, as it may induce malignant transformation

Prognosis

- Prognosis is excellent
- Recurrences develop if incompletely excised, resulting in morbidity

IMAGE FINDINGS

Radiographic Findings

- Best diagnostic clue is a well-demarcated, expansile monostotic mass with mixed soft tissue center surrounded by ossifying rim
- May cause teeth displacement, root divergence

CT Findings

- Sharply demarcated, expansile, mixed soft tissue and bone density lesion
  - Well-circumscribed margin, similar to other benign osseous lesions
  - Thick bony walls show remodeling and thickening

MACROSCOPIC FEATURES

General Features

- Well circumscribed, with definite boundaries, but not encapsulated

OSSIFYING FIBROMA

Key Facts

Terminology
- Benign bone neoplasm with lamellar bone formation, osteoblastic rimming, and connective tissue stroma

Clinical Issues
- Age range: 2nd-4th decades
- Female > > Male (5:1)
- Posterior mandible (up to 90%)
- Usually asymptomatic

Image Findings
- Well-demarcated, expansile, monostotic mass with mixed soft tissue center surrounded by ossifying rim

Microscopic Pathology
- Evenly spaced spicules of woven bone
- Osteoblasts and osteoclasts surround spicules
- Prominent calcified structures
- Cellular stellate stroma

- Cut surface: Tan-white, dry, avascular, smooth mass

Size
- Range: 0.5-10 cm

MICROSCOPIC PATHOLOGY

Histologic Features
- Composed of variable amounts of fibrous tissue proliferation and calcifications
- Evenly spaced spicules of woven bone
  - Lamellar transformation at periphery
  - Osteoblasts and osteoclasts surround spicules
    - Osteoblastic rimming is prominent
- Prominent calcified structures (ossicles, cementicles)
  - Eosinophilic or basophilic spherules of osteoid
- Cellular, spindled cell stroma
- Multinucleated giant cells can be seen

ANCILLARY TESTS

Immunohistochemistry
- Unnecessary
- Runx2: Nuclear reaction in spindled cells
- Osteocalcin: Distributed throughout calcified structures

Molecular Genetics
- Mutations in *HRPT2* gene reported
  - RT-PCR of *HRPT2* shows mutations

DIFFERENTIAL DIAGNOSIS

Fibrous Dysplasia
- Radiographic separation is difficult
  - Diffuse, poorly defined expansion, classic "ground-glass," with mixed patterns
- When polyostotic (30%), helps to exclude OF
- Irregularly shaped trabeculae of immature woven bone without osteoblastic rimming

Active Ossifying Fibroma
- a.k.a. psammomatoid ossifying fibroma, juvenile active ossifying fibroma
- Highly cellular stroma, mitoses, psammomatous calcifications

Cemento-osseous Dysplasia
- African-Americans commonly affected, involving periodontal ligament
- Sclerotic radiodensity, lacking osteoblastic rimming

SELECTED REFERENCES

1. Liu Y et al: Ossifying fibromas of the jaw bone: 20 cases. Dentomaxillofac Radiol. 39(1):57-63, 2010
2. MacDonald-Jankowski DS: Ossifying fibroma: a systematic review. Dentomaxillofac Radiol. 38(8):495-513, 2009
3. Mintz S et al: Central ossifying fibroma: an analysis of 20 cases and review of the literature. Quintessence Int. 38(3):221-7, 2007

IMAGE GALLERY

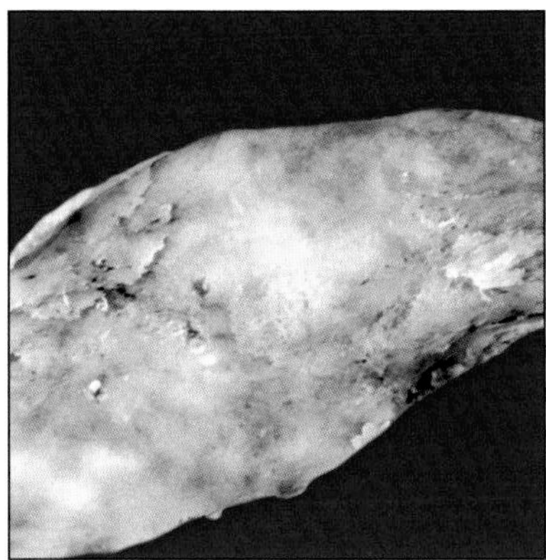

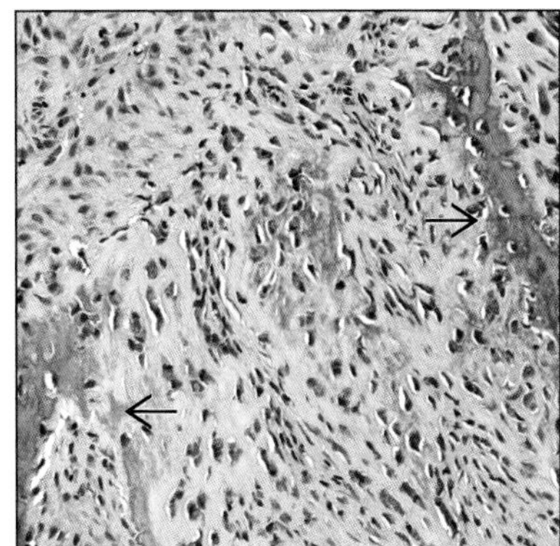

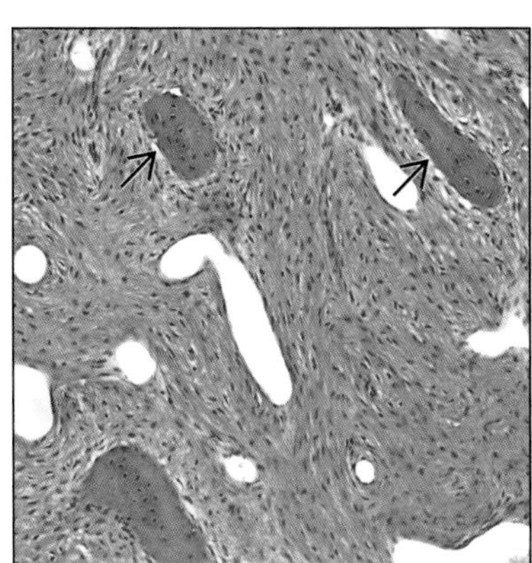

*(**Left**) There is a well-defined boundary to this lesion, which has a tan-white, dry, avascular, crumbly cut surface. Calcifications give a gritty appearance. (**Center**) Ossifying fibroma appears as islands and irregularly shaped spicules of woven bone ⇒ in the background of a bland fibrous stroma. (**Right**) As the lesion matures, the osseous spicules ⇒ mature to lamellar bone, particularly at the periphery. The background stroma becomes denser and more organized.*

JUVENILE ACTIVE OSSIFYING FIBROMA

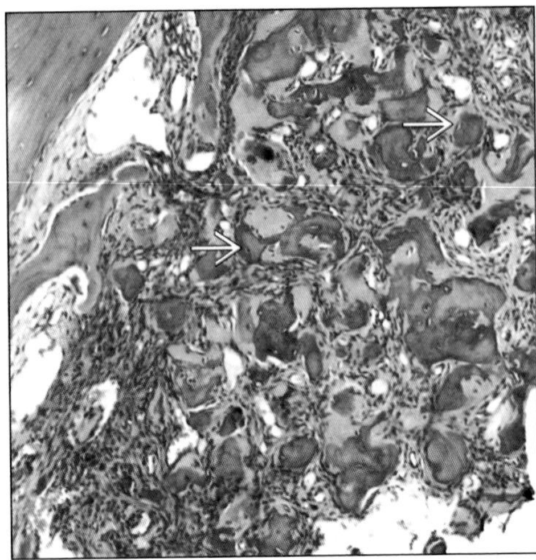

Lesions display cementicles ➡ that resemble true psammoma bodies. The background spindle cells are bland and without mitotic figures. Vessels are present but thin and delicate.

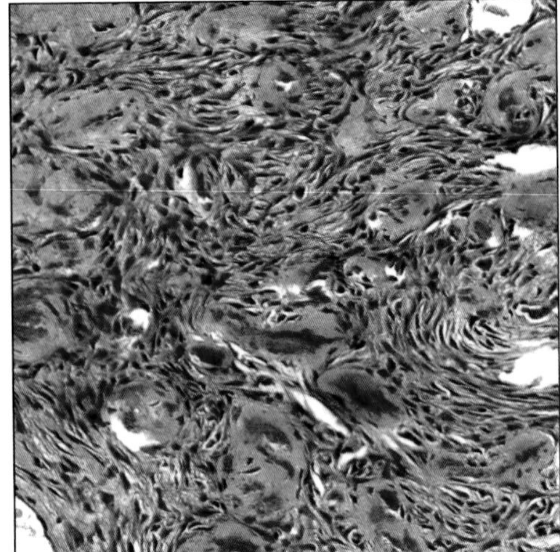

There is a spindled cellular stroma. The calcifications show a heavy collagenized collar around the calcifications. Psammoma-like bodies are not identified in this field.

TERMINOLOGY

Abbreviations

- Juvenile active ossifying fibroma (JAOF)
- Active ossifying fibroma (AOF)

Synonyms

- Aggressive psammomatoid ossifying fibroma

Definitions

- Benign fibro-osseous neoplasm composed of mixture of stroma and bone characterized by rapid and destructive growth

CLINICAL ISSUES

Epidemiology

- Incidence
  - Rare, much less common than conventional ossifying fibroma
- Age
  - Variable at presentation
    - Range: 3 months to 70 years, mean: < 15 years
- Gender
  - Equal gender distribution

Site

- Paranasal sinuses most common (~ 90%)
  - Ethmoid > frontal > maxillary > sphenoid
  - Can involve temporal bone
  - Occasional cases have soft tissue presentation
- Maxilla 2nd most common site
  - Mandible is infrequently involved
- Rarely involves calvaria or extracranial sites

Presentation

- Asymptomatic, discovered incidentally on routine radiographic exams
- If symptomatic
  - Chronic sinusitis, with rhinorrhea, obstruction, pain
  - Facial enlargement due to cortical expansion with displaced teeth
  - Proptosis, exophthalmos, diplopia, or visual acuity loss

Treatment

- Surgical approaches
  - Total removal at earliest possible stage
    - Complete endoscopic resection (may be difficult to achieve)

Prognosis

- Excellent prognosis after complete excision
- Increased recurrence rate if incompletely resected
  - 30-58%
  - Sinus > mandibular/maxillary tumors

IMAGE FINDINGS

Radiographic Findings

- Bone algorithm CT studies are best
- Well-demarcated (circumscribed), expansile mass
  - Mixed soft tissue density central areas surrounded by ossified rim

MR Findings

- Mixed low and high signals (T1 or T2WI)
- **T1WI**: Fibrous areas have intermediate signal, while ossified areas are hypointense
- **T2WI**: Fibrous areas are hyperintense (usually center and cystic areas), while ossified areas are hypointense

CT Findings

- Well-circumscribed, expansile, mixed soft tissue and bony density mass
- Usually unilocular
- Thick bony wall surrounds low-attenuation fibrous center
  - May have thin, "eggshell" periphery of bone
- Indistinguishable from fibrous dysplasia by CT

JUVENILE ACTIVE OSSIFYING FIBROMA

Key Facts

Terminology
- Neoplasm composed of mixture of stroma and bone characterized by rapid and destructive growth

Clinical Issues
- Mean age: < 15 years
- Paranasal sinuses most common location (~ 90%)

Image Findings
- Bone algorithm CT studies are best
- Well-demarcated (circumscribed), expansile mass

Microscopic Pathology
- Composed of variable amounts of fibrous tissue proliferation and calcifications
- Numerous psammomatous ossicles, with thick, irregular collagenous rim
- May show distinct osteoblastic rimming

Top Differential Diagnoses
- Fibrous dysplasia, meningioma, cementoma

MACROSCOPIC FEATURES

General Features
- Well-circumscribed, smooth surface, although infiltration may be seen
- Tumor "shelling out" is common
- Cut surface: Tan-white, rubbery, homogeneous mass with firm-to-gritty consistency

Size
- Range: 0.5-10 cm

MICROSCOPIC PATHOLOGY

Histologic Features
- Composed of variable amounts of fibrous tissue proliferation and calcifications
- Cellular stroma of small uniform stellate and spindle-shaped fibroblast-like cells
- Numerous small, rounded, mineralized collagenous ossicles and immature osteoid
  - Curved bodies with thick, irregular collagenous rim
  - Ossicles may fuse to form larger structures
  - Collagenous chondricles, cementum-like psammomatous bodies (cementicles)
- May show distinct osteoblastic rimming
- Multinucleated giant cells and scattered mitotic figures

DIFFERENTIAL DIAGNOSIS

Fibrous Dysplasia
- Radiographic separation is difficult
  - Poorly defined expansion, classic "ground-glass" appearance, mixed patterns
- Most are monostotic (70%), but when polyostotic, helps to exclude AOF

Meningioma
- Epithelial appearance arranged in whorled architecture with psammoma bodies
- Immunohistochemistry shows EMA or CK7 and vimentin

Cementoblastoma
- Dense mass associated with tooth root, arising from periodontal ligament region
- "Cementicles" can mimic calcifications or cementicle-like deposits in JAOF

SELECTED REFERENCES

1. Zama M et al: Juvenile active ossifying fibroma with massive involvement of the mandible. Plast Reconstr Surg. 113(3):970-4, 2004
2. Brannon RB et al: Benign fibro-osseous lesions: a review of current concepts. Adv Anat Pathol. 8(3):126-43, 2001
3. Wenig BM et al: Aggressive psammomatoid ossifying fibromas of the sinonasal region: a clinicopathologic study of a distinct group of fibro-osseous lesions. Cancer. 76(7):1155-65, 1995

IMAGE GALLERY

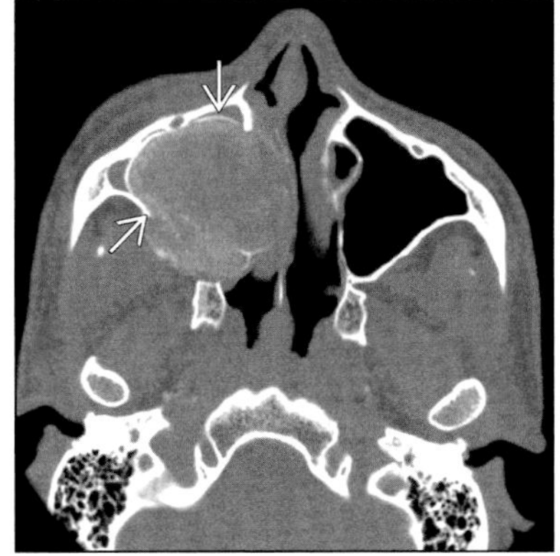
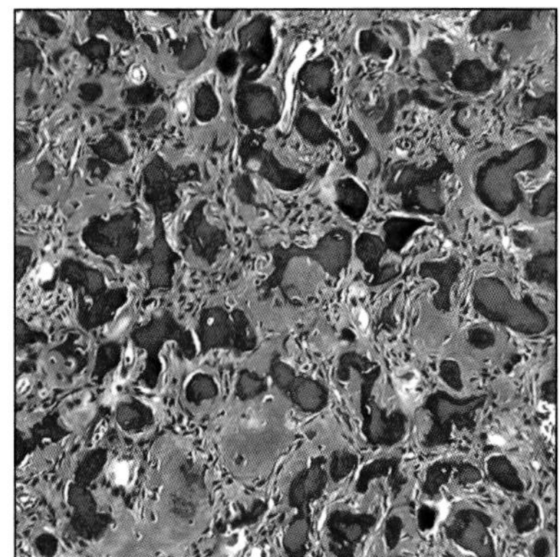
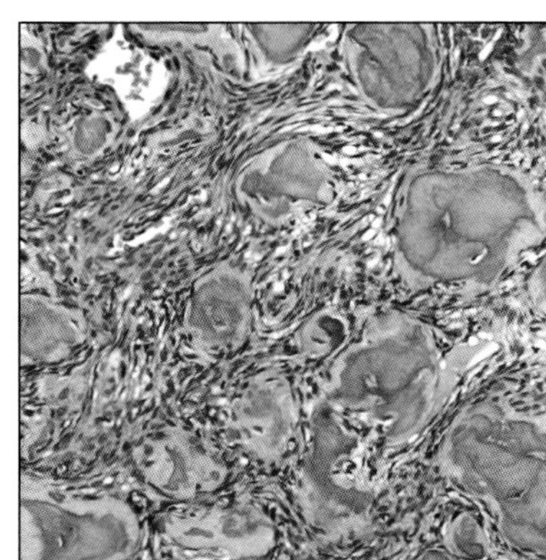

(Left) *Axial bone CT shows the maxillary sinus filled with an ossifying fibroma with the expected increased ossification along the superficial lesion margin ➡.* ***(Center)*** *A cellular stroma is filled with small, rounded to curved, mineralized collagenous ossicles. The collagenous rim is thick and irregular. The ossicles are focally fused.* ***(Right)*** *The ossicles or cementicles show varying degrees of mineralization. The material appears bony. Giant cells may be present.*

OSTEOMA

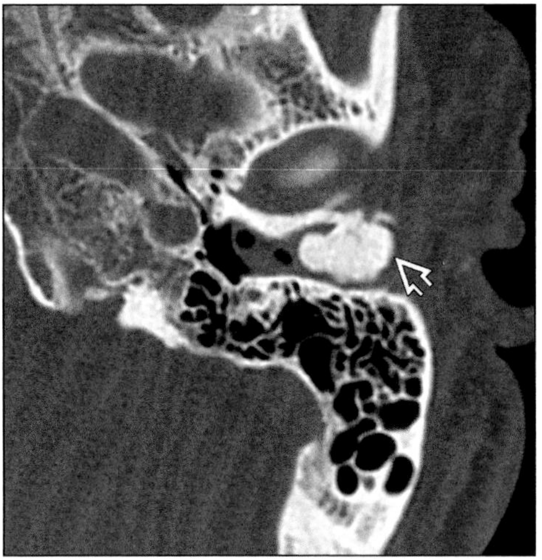

Hyperdense osteoma is seen filling the lateral external auditory canal ➡. The intensity of the signal and lack of lucencies give a clue to the diagnosis.

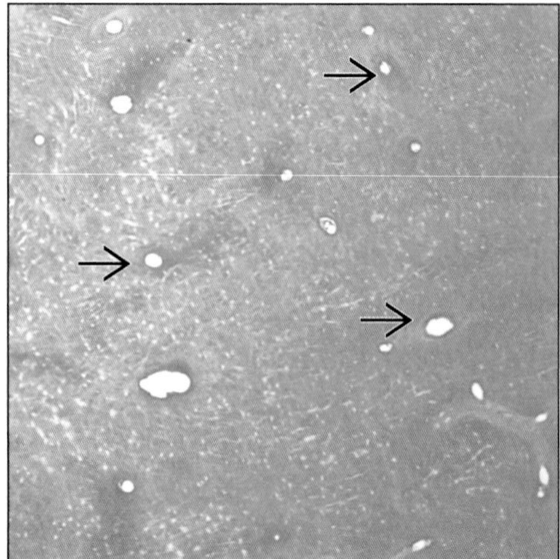

Dense lamellar bone with Haversian-like systems ➡ is the histologic hallmark of this lesion. There is a spectrum that includes higher portions of fibrous tissues.

TERMINOLOGY

Synonyms

- Cancellous bone osteomas: Osteoma spongiosum
- Compact osteomas: Osteoma durum

Definitions

- Osteoma is benign osteogenic lesion characterized by proliferation of compact or cancellous bone
  - Also referred to as cancellous or ivory
- Separated based on specific location
  - **Central**: Arises from endosteum
  - **Peripheral**: Arises from periosteum
  - **Extraskeletal**: Arises within a muscle

ETIOLOGY/PATHOGENESIS

Pathogenesis

- Unclear
  - Some investigators consider it a true neoplasm
  - Others classify it as developmental anomaly

CLINICAL ISSUES

Epidemiology

- Incidence
  - Uncommon
- Age
  - Peak during 2nd to 4th decades
- Gender
  - Equal gender distribution
    - Nasal osteomas show slight male predominance

Site

- May be single or multiple
- Most common head and neck sites as follows
  - **External auditory canal** (EAC) most common
  - **Temporal bone**
  - **Nasal**: Nasal and paranasal sinuses and bones
  - **Jaw**: Mandible most frequently affected
- **Cancellous** osteomas: Maxillary and ethmoidal sinuses most frequently
- **Compact** or **ivory** osteomas: Frontal sinus

Presentation

- Slow-growing lesions
- Clinical signs and symptoms depend on
  - Location, size, and growth direction
- Conductive hearing loss is most common symptom
  - Due to ossicular chain impingement
- Eustachian tube obstruction may cause otitis media with effusion
- Sinus ostium obstruction: Facial pain, nasal obstruction, sinusitis, or mucocele
- Nasolacrimal duct compression may cause epiphora
- Gardner syndrome
  - Should always be considered with osteoma diagnosis
  - Inherited as autosomal dominant syndrome
  - Gardner syndrome includes multiple osteomas
    - Polyposis of large bowel, epidermoid or sebaceous cysts, cutaneous fibromas

Treatment

- Options, risks, complications
  - Asymptomatic osteomas can be followed with periodic radiographic evaluation rather than surgical exploration
- Surgical approaches
  - Surgery for symptomatic lesions

Prognosis

- Excellent, without recurrence

IMAGE FINDINGS

Radiographic Findings

- Usually incidental findings on imaging
- 3D reconstruction of CT images achieves better resolution and more precise localization

OSTEOMA

Key Facts

Terminology

- Osteoma is benign osteogenic lesion characterized by proliferation of compact or cancellous bone

Clinical Issues

- Slow-growing lesions
- Peak during 2nd to 4th decades
- Conductive hearing loss for ear lesions
- Most important clinical aspect is relationship to Gardner syndrome
- Surgery for symptomatic lesions

Image Findings

- Usually incidental findings on imaging
- Bone scan can determine level of activity

Microscopic Pathology

- Dense lamellae with organized Haversian canals

Top Differential Diagnoses

- Osteochondroma, chondroma, exostoses

Bone Scan

- Identifies physiologic activity

MACROSCOPIC FEATURES

General Features

- Very dense, cortical bone, smooth surface

Size

- Varies greatly

MICROSCOPIC PATHOLOGY

Histologic Features

- Dense lamellae with organized Haversian canals
- Varying degrees of 3 tissue types
  - Peripheral area of compact bone
  - Underlying cancellous bone with networks of trabeculae within fibrovascular stroma
  - Central portion of loose fibrous stroma containing blood vessels and plump osteoblasts
- Intratrabecular stroma contains
  - Osteoblasts, fibroblasts, giant cells
  - Variable osteoblastic and osteoclastic activity
  - No hematopoietic cells
- Many fibrovascular channels surrounded by lamellated bone
- 3 histologic types of osteoma are described
  - Compact, spongiotic, mixed

DIFFERENTIAL DIAGNOSIS

Osteochondroma

- **Radiology findings**: Pedunculated or sessile lesion on bony stalk
  - Cartilage cap with or without mineralization
- **Pathology features**: Endochondral ossification similar to growth plate
  - Bony stalk with overlying cartilage cap

Chondroma

- **Radiology findings**: Lobular organization and calcification
- **Pathology features**: Lobules of hyaline-type cartilage

Exostoses

- **Radiology findings**: No underlying connection with marrow cavity
- **Pathology features**: Bony stalk with overlying cartilage cap

SELECTED REFERENCES

1. Kaplan I et al: Solitary central osteoma of the jaws: a diagnostic dilemma. Oral Surg Oral Med Oral Pathol Oral Radiol Endod. 106(3):e22-9, 2008
2. Davis TC et al: Osteomas of the internal auditory canal: a report of two cases. Am J Otol. 21(6):852-6, 2000
3. Roland PS et al: Disorders of the external auditory canal. J Am Acad Audiol. 8(6):367-78, 1997
4. Tran LP et al: Benign lesions of the external auditory canal. Otolaryngol Clin North Am. 29(5):807-25, 1996

IMAGE GALLERY

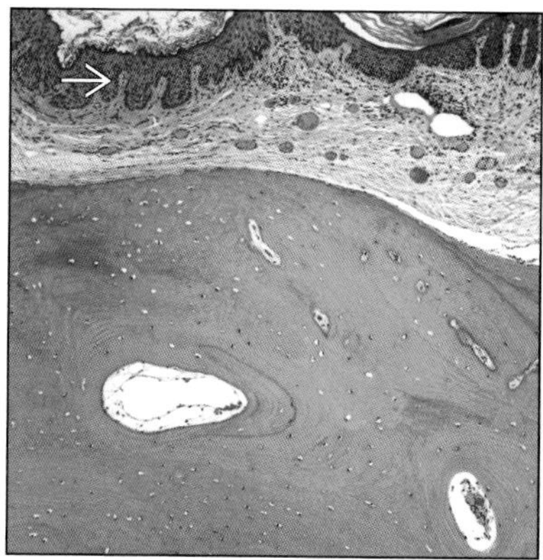

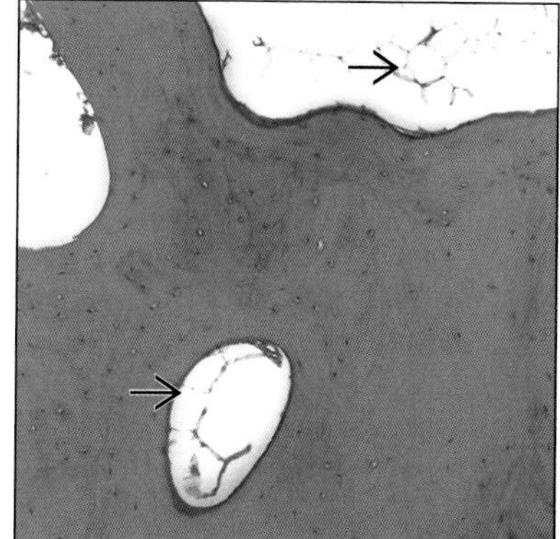

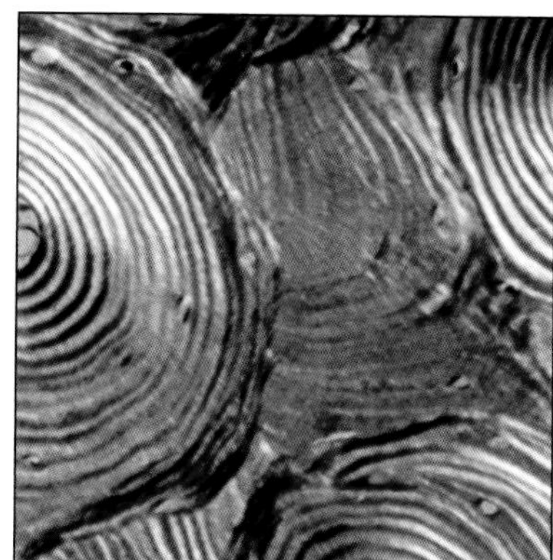

(Left) An ear osteoma demonstrates an intact squamous lining ➡, below which is an osteoma. The bone is mature with Haversian-like systems. A pushing border is noted. (Center) As the lesions mature, they can remodel to resemble thickened cortical and trabecular bone. Mature adipose tissue ➡ can be seen. (Right) Polarized light demonstrates both the Haversian-like arrangement of concentric rings of collagen layers, similar to a tree trunk seen in cross section.

OSTEOBLASTOMA

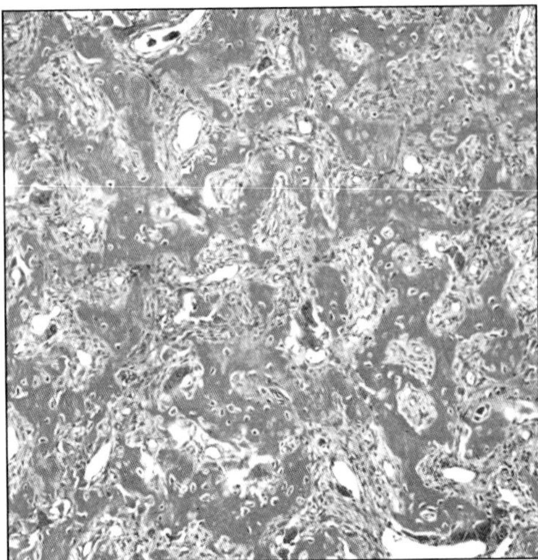

Islands of haphazardly arranged spicules of bone show plump osteoblasts and a number of multinucleated cells adjacent to the bone trabeculae. The stroma is slightly cellular.

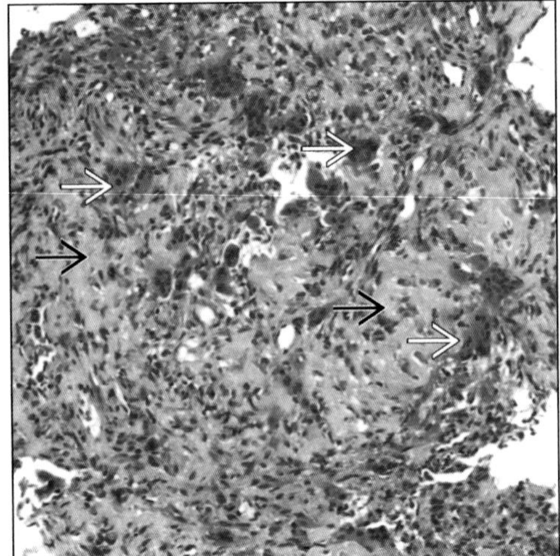

Islands and delicate fibrils of osteoid ⇒ and abundant giant cells ➡ characterize osteoblastoma. Background spindle cells are bland with plump nuclei.

TERMINOLOGY

Definitions

- Benign bone-forming neoplasm producing woven bone spicules bordered by prominent osteoblasts

CLINICAL ISSUES

Epidemiology

- Incidence
  - Rare, accounting for < 1% of all maxillofacial tumors
- Age
  - ~ 90% of cases within 1st 2 decades
- Gender
  - Male > Female (3:1)

Site

- < 10% of osteoblastomas develop in jaws and skull
  - Predilection for posterior mandible

Presentation

- Clinical manifestations depend on site and size of lesion, characterized by
  - Pain
  - Swelling
  - Soft tissue edema and erythema overlying tumor
  - Hearing loss if middle ear or ossicles affected
  - Facial paralysis and facial nerve compression
- Multifocal tumors are rare

Treatment

- Surgical approaches
  - Local conservative excision and thorough curettage usually adequate

Prognosis

- Benign behavior for vast majority
- Recurrences in ~ 10% of incompletely excised tumors
  - Mandibular tumors most likely to recur
  - Usually develop within 1 year of initial surgery
- Does not metastasize
- Spontaneous regression is reported
- Malignant transformation is extremely rare

IMAGE FINDINGS

Radiographic Findings

- Variable radiographic appearance
  - Depends on degree of calcification
  - May appear radiolucent or semiradiolucent with radiopaque mottling
  - Well-demarcated, narrow, radiolucent margin
- Well circumscribed but may expand bone
  - Cortical erosion and expansion/perforation is generally surrounded by thin shell of new bone
  - Younger lesions may appear more radiolucent but ossify as they mature

CT Findings

- CT is exam of choice for diagnosis
  - Great value in determining tumor extent
  - Assesses degree of calcification

MACROSCOPIC FEATURES

General Features

- Yellow to red, gritty or sandpaper-like due to mineralization
- Often cystic, with blood-filled spaces

Size

- Range: 2-10 cm
- Must be > 2 cm to distinguish from osteoid osteoma

MICROSCOPIC PATHOLOGY

Histologic Features

- Characterized by mixture of bone spicules, osteoblasts, and vascularized stroma

OSTEOBLASTOMA

Key Facts

Terminology
- Benign bone-forming neoplasm producing woven bone spicules bordered by prominent osteoblasts

Clinical Issues
- ~ 90% of cases within 1st 2 decades of life
- Male > Female (3:1)
- < 10% of osteoblastomas develop in jaws and skull
- Recurrences in ~ 10% of incompletely excised tumors

Microscopic Pathology
- Range: 2-10 cm
- Mixture of bone spicules, osteoblasts, and vascularized stroma
  - Osteoid islands variably calcified
  - Abundant, plump osteoblasts surrounding trabeculae of osteoid and immature bone

Top Differential Diagnoses
- Osteosarcoma, fibrous dysplasia, cementoblastoma

- Islands of haphazardly arranged spicules of bone undergoing varying degrees of calcification
  - Prominent basophilic reversal lines
  - Does not infiltrate preexisting lamellar bone
- Abundant, plump osteoblasts surrounding trabeculae of osteoid and immature bone
- Well-vascularized stroma
- Numerous multinucleated cells adjacent to bone
- Scant chronic inflammatory cells adjacent to vessels
- Absence of atypical mitoses and pleomorphism

ANCILLARY TESTS

Cytogenetics
- 3-way unbalanced translocation of chromosomes 15, 17, 20
- *MDM2* amplification reported

DIFFERENTIAL DIAGNOSIS

Osteosarcoma
- Ill-defined mass with destructive borders and cortical breakthrough and soft tissue extension
- Incorporation/destruction of peripheral lamellar bone
- Cellular pleomorphism, malignant osteoid, atypical mitoses, necrosis

Fibrous Dysplasia
- Poorly defined radiographically, multilocular radiolucency, with ground-glass appearance
- Immature and woven bone but in a distinctive "alphabet letter" distribution
- Spindled cell stroma more dense, with less vascularity than osteoblastoma

Cementoblastoma
- Found in association with or fused to teeth roots
- Consists of cementum-like tissue

Ossifying Fibroma
- Painless, more fibrous, less vascular, lacks large number of osteoblasts

Paget Disease
- Usually affects entire bone, with mixed lucent and sclerotic areas
- Islands of bone, extensive remodeling and reversal lines, large osteoclasts, osteoblasts
- Vascularity increased without spindle cell stroma

Chondroblastoma
- Rare in jaw, chondrocytes with cartilaginous matrix, no osteoblastic activity

SELECTED REFERENCES

1. Berry M et al: Osteoblastoma: a 30-year study of 99 cases. J Surg Oncol. 98(3):179-83, 2008
2. Saglik Y et al: Surgical treatment of osteoblastoma : a report of 20 cases. Acta Orthop Belg. 73(6):747-53, 2007
3. Rawal YB et al: Gnathic osteoblastoma: clinicopathologic review of seven cases with long-term follow-up. Oral Oncol. 42(2):123-30, 2006

IMAGE GALLERY

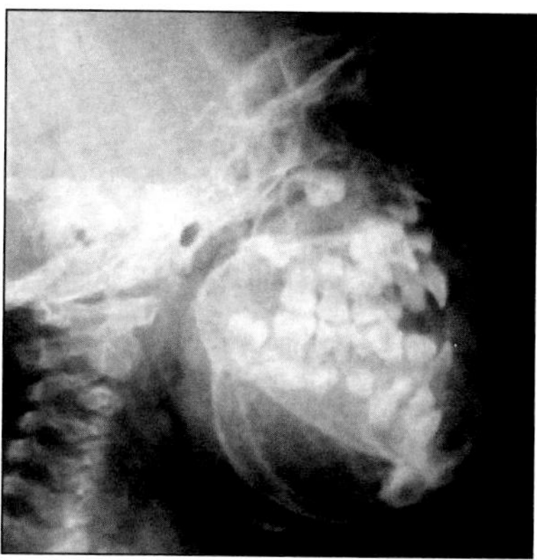

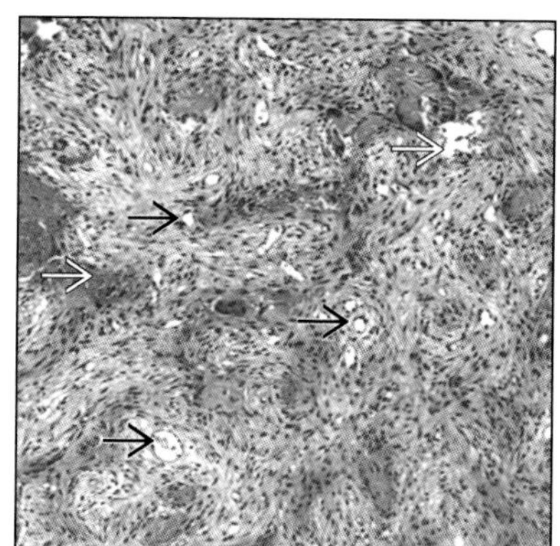

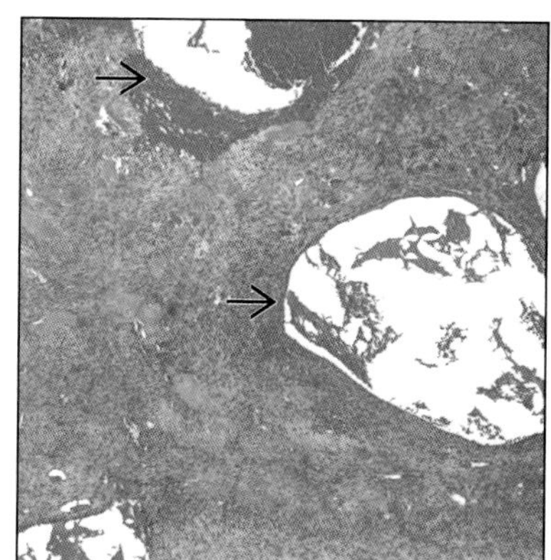

(Left) *A large mandibular lesion appears as a radiolucent mass with radiopaque mottling. There is a well-demarcated, narrow, radiolucent margin. Note the expanded bone with a thin shell of new bone.* **(Center)** *Smaller, delicate vessels are noted at higher power ➙, and occasional extravasated erythrocytes ➡ can be seen.* **(Right)** *As osteoblastomas mature, they often display secondary cystic change ➙ that mimics aneurysmal bone cysts on radiologic studies.*

MELANOTIC NEUROECTODERMAL TUMOR OF INFANCY

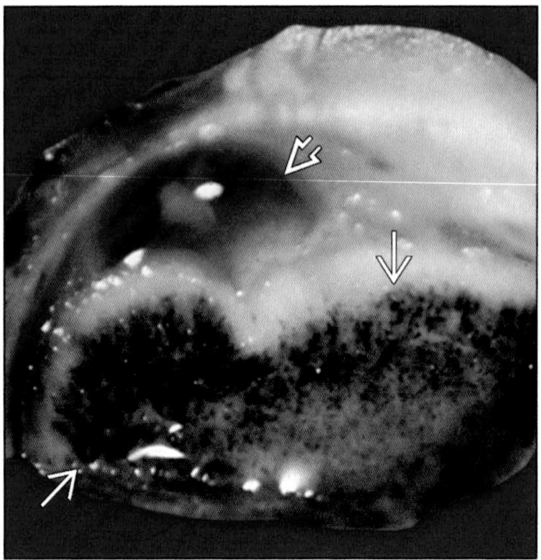

Gross photograph shows a dark, blue-black pigmented mass ➡ associated with an area of cystic change ➡. This is a tumor identified within the maxilla.

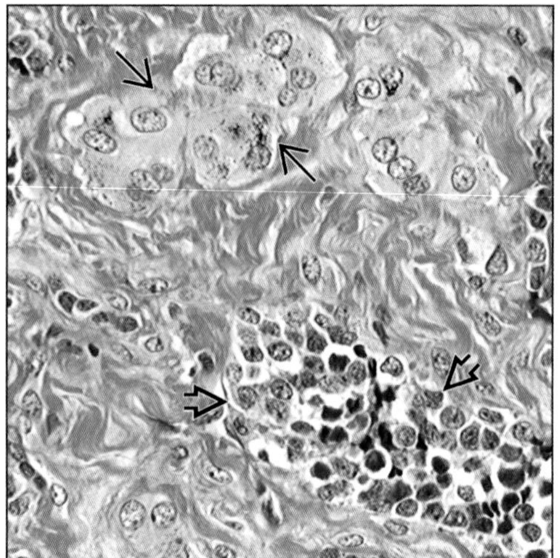

Hematoxylin & eosin shows a biphasic population with heavy desmoplastic stroma. The large, epithelioid cells contain pigment ➡. Nests of "small round blue cells" lack pigment ➡.

TERMINOLOGY

Abbreviations

- Melanotic neuroectodermal tumor of infancy (MNTI)

Definitions

- Rare, biphasic, neuroblastic, and pigmented epithelial neoplasm of craniofacial sites

ETIOLOGY/PATHOGENESIS

Developmental Anomaly

- Congenital presentation
- Neural crest origin
  - Expression of melanotransferrin (melanoma-specific peptide that may play a role in iron metabolism)

CLINICAL ISSUES

Epidemiology

- Incidence
  - Rare; < 500 reported cases
- Age
  - 95% of patients < 1 year; 80% < 6 months
- Gender
  - Female > Male (2:1)

Site

- Maxilla (70%)
- Mandible and skull (10% each)

Presentation

- Rapidly growing mass, with tooth displacement
  - Gives "bluish" appearance (pigment appears blue through mucosa)
- Usually maxillary anterior alveolar ridge

Laboratory Tests

- Elevated vanilmandelic acid levels

Treatment

- Options, risks, complications
  - Even though rapidly growing and destructive, tends to have benign clinical course
- Surgical approaches
  - Complete local excision (usually by partial maxillectomy) with clear margins
- Adjuvant therapy
  - Chemotherapy for recurrent or residual tumors

Prognosis

- Good, but capricious
  - No clinical or pathologic features predict behavior
- Recurrences are frequent (approximately 1/3)
- Metastases in < 10%

IMAGE FINDINGS

General Features

- Intrabony expansive areas of radiolucency, usually with poorly demarcated margins
- Extensive tumor calcification may be identified
- Teeth are usually displaced and appear within radiolucent area of tumor

MACROSCOPIC FEATURES

General Features

- Smooth, hard, firm mass
- Mottled white-gray to blue-black cut surfaces

Size

- Range: 1-10 cm; mean: 3.5 cm

MICROSCOPIC PATHOLOGY

Histologic Features

- Circumscribed but not encapsulated

Key Facts

Clinical Issues

- Usually involves maxillary anterior alveolar ridge
- Elevated vanilmandelic acid levels
- Maxilla (70%)
- 95% of patients < 1 year
- Even though rapidly growing and destructive, tends to have benign clinical course

Macroscopic Features

- Gray to blue-black

Microscopic Pathology

- Biphasic population
  - Centrally located, small, darkly staining cells
  - Larger, epithelioid polygonal pigmented cells
- Heavy, dense sclerotic stroma

Top Differential Diagnoses

- Rhabdomyosarcoma
- Ewing/PNET
- Lymphoma and immature teratoma

- Cells are arranged in alveolar or tubular configurations
- Biphasic population
  - Centrally located, small, darkly staining cells comprise majority of cells
    - "Neural" quality with scant, fibrillar cytoplasm
    - Round nuclei with coarse and heavy nuclear chromatin
  - Larger, epithelioid polygonal cells with vesicular nuclei
    - Much greater amount of opaque cytoplasm filled with granular melanin pigment
- Heavy, dense sclerotic vascularized fibrous connective tissue stroma
- Mitotic figures are absent
- Lacks hemorrhage and necrosis

ANCILLARY TESTS

Immunohistochemistry

- Polyphenotype: Neural, melanocytic, epithelial
  - Large cells: Keratin, vimentin, HMB-45, NSE, CD57
  - Small cells: Synaptophysin, GFAP, NSE, CD57
- Variable expression of EMA and S100 protein

DIFFERENTIAL DIAGNOSIS

Rhabdomyosarcoma

- Usually older age at presentation
- Strong muscle markers and unique translocations
- Rhabdomyoblastic differentiation can be seen in MNTI

Lymphoma

- Lacks biphasic appearance and pigment
- Positive immunohistochemical lymphoid markers

Ewing/PNET

- Sheet-like, nonpigmented small round blue cells
- Positive: CD99, chromogranin, S100 protein
- Diagnostic t(11;22) *EWS/FLI1* gene fusion product

Melanoma

- Very rare in infants, with S100 protein reaction and negative epithelial markers

Immature Teratoma

- Requires all 3 embryonic germ layers (neuroderm, ectoderm, mesoderm)

SELECTED REFERENCES

1. Fowler DJ et al: Melanotic neuroectodermal tumor of infancy: clinical, radiological, and pathological features. Fetal Pediatr Pathol. 25(2):59-72, 2006
2. Wenig BM et al: Aggressive psammomatoid ossifying fibromas of the sinonasal region: a clinicopathologic study of a distinct group of fibro-osseous lesions. Cancer. 76(7):1155-65, 1995
3. Kapadia SB et al: Melanotic neuroectodermal tumor of infancy. Clinicopathological, immunohistochemical, and flow cytometric study. Am J Surg Pathol. 17(6):566-73, 1993

IMAGE GALLERY

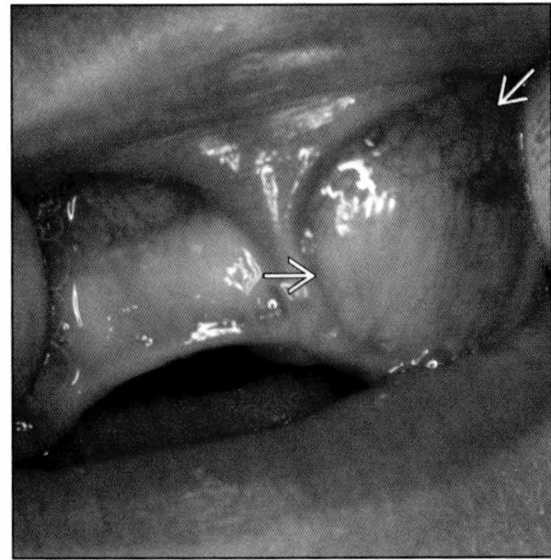

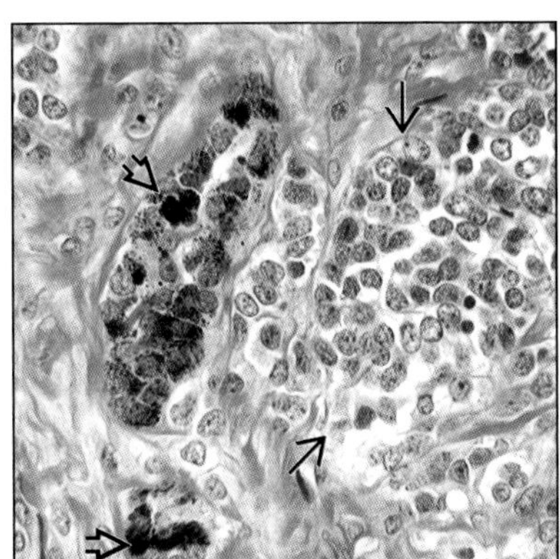

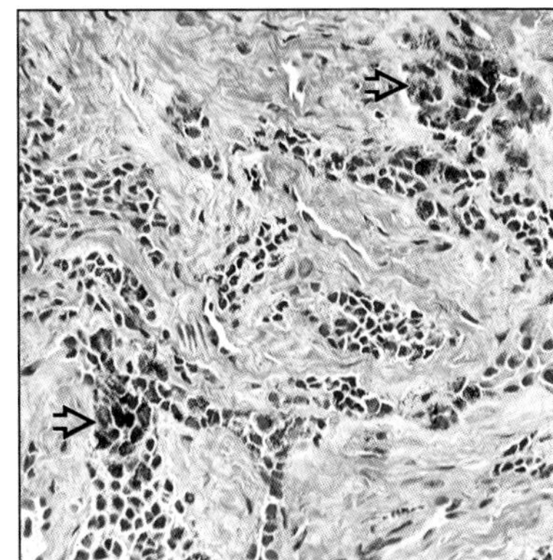

(Left) Clinical photograph shows a "bluish" swelling of the gum ➡ in an infant with an MNTI of the left maxilla. (Center) The neural-type cells have a very high nuclear to cytoplasmic ratio and delicate nuclear chromatin ➡. The larger cells are nearly obscured by cytoplasmic heavy, granular melanin pigment ➡. (Right) Interlaced nests of tumor cells show a biphasic appearance, separated by fibrous stroma. Pigmented larger epithelioid cells ➡ with smaller neural-like cells are visible.

AMELOBLASTIC CARCINOMA

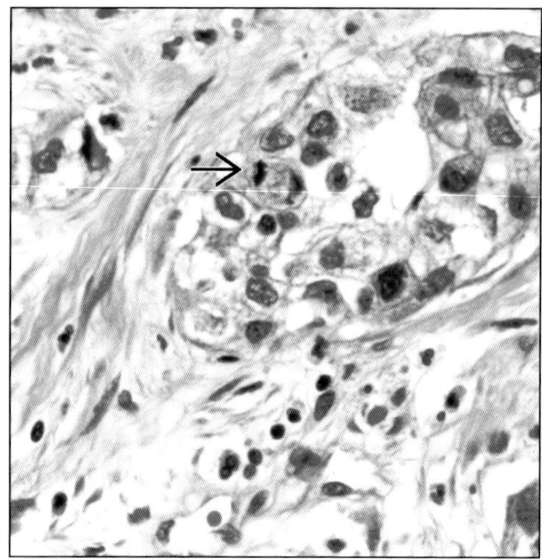

Ameloblastic carcinoma shows increased nuclear to cytoplasmic ratio, pleomorphism, and a mitotic figure ➔. This tumor shows few features of a benign ameloblastoma.

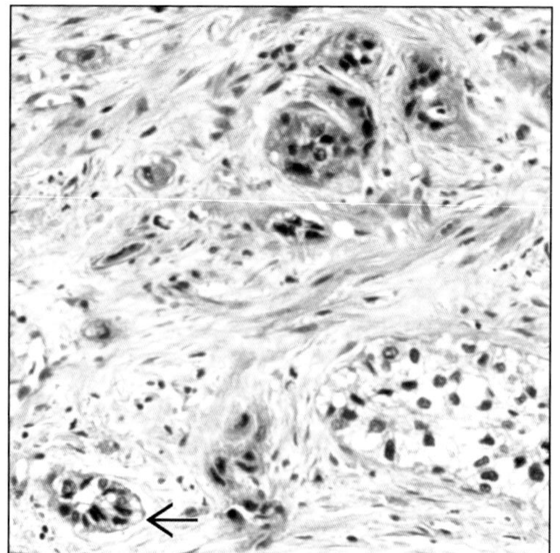

Areas of the tumor show features of a benign ameloblastoma including islands of epithelium with peripheral columnar cells and reverse polarity ➔, but note the pleomorphism and loss of cellular cohesion.

TERMINOLOGY

Definitions

- Odontogenic tumor that shows malignant histologic features within an ameloblastoma

ETIOLOGY/PATHOGENESIS

Types

- Ameloblastic carcinoma arising de novo
  - Primary tumor
- Ameloblastic carcinoma arising from intraosseous ameloblastoma
  - Secondary (dedifferentiated) or carcinoma ex intraosseous ameloblastoma
  - Far less common
- Ameloblastic carcinoma arising from a peripheral ameloblastoma
  - Exceedingly rare

CLINICAL ISSUES

Epidemiology

- Incidence
  - Extremely rare
- Age
  - Wide range
- Gender
  - Male > Female
- Ethnicity
  - May exhibit increased incidence in Chinese

Site

- Majority develop in mandible
  - Most frequently in posterior region
- Uncommon in maxilla
- Rarely involves other skull locations
  - Anterior skull base and paranasal sinuses

Presentation

- Painful swelling or mass
- Often associated with recent rapid growth
- Ulcer or fistula formation
- Paresthesia of lower lip
- Many present with metastatic disease
  - Regional lymph nodes, lung, bone

Treatment

- Options, risks, complications
  - Definitive management difficult to determine due to limited case reports
  - Long-term follow-up is essential
- Surgical approaches
  - All require radical resection
    - Partial or total mandibulectomy, maxillectomy
  - Enucleation or curettage not advocated
  - Neck dissection for clinically suspicious lymph nodes
- Drugs
  - Chemotherapy has limited application
- Radiation
  - Radiation therapy has limited effectiveness

Prognosis

- Generally poor prognosis
- High recurrence rate
  - Highest recurrences in patients treated by enucleation or curettage

IMAGE FINDINGS

Radiographic Findings

- Ill-defined or irregular radiolucent lesion
  - Multilocular
  - Unilocular
- Cortical expansion, frequently with perforation
  - May infiltrate into adjacent structures
- Well-defined borders

AMELOBLASTIC CARCINOMA

Key Facts

Terminology
- Odontogenic tumor that shows malignant histologic features within an ameloblastoma

Clinical Issues
- Extremely rare
- Most develop in mandible
- Definitive management difficult to determine due to limited case reports

Microscopic Pathology
- Features of ameloblastoma
  - Peripheral palisading, reverse polarization, central stellate reticulum, any histiologic subtype
- Epithelial atypia (malignancy)
  - Profound pleomorphism with hyperchromasia, increased N:C ratio, loss of adhesion
- Mitoses are increased, including atypical forms, necrosis, vascular and perineural invasion

MACROSCOPIC FEATURES

Sections to Be Submitted
- Must submit and evaluate epithelial and bony margins

MICROSCOPIC PATHOLOGY

Histologic Features
- Ameloblastoma features
  - Peripheral palisading
  - Reverse polarization
  - Central areas of stellate reticulum
  - Other features of any histological subtype of ameloblastoma
- Epithelial atypia (malignancy)
  - Profound pleomorphism with hyperchromasia
  - Increased nuclear to cytoplasmic ratio
  - Loss of cellular adhesion
  - Mitoses are increased, including atypical forms
- Necrosis
- Vascular &/or perineural invasion

ANCILLARY TESTS

Flow Cytometry
- Aneuploidy more frequently identified in ameloblastic carcinoma than in ameloblastoma

Molecular Genetics
- CGH has shown amplification of 5q13

DIFFERENTIAL DIAGNOSIS

Ameloblastoma
- Lacks cytologic atypia

Intraosseous Squamous Cell Carcinoma
- Lacks reverse polarity and basal palisading

Clear Cell Odontogenic Carcinoma
- Tumor cells are predominately clear
  - PAS-positive granules, degradable with diastase

Metastatic Disease
- Lacks reverse polarity
- Lacks basal palisading

SELECTED REFERENCES

1. Yoon HJ et al: Ameloblastic carcinoma: an analysis of 6 cases with review of the literature. Oral Surg Oral Med Oral Pathol Oral Radiol Endod. 108(6):904-13, 2009
2. Akrish S et al: Ameloblastic carcinoma: report of a new case, literature review, and comparison to ameloblastoma. J Oral Maxillofac Surg. 65(4):777-83, 2007
3. Infante-Cossio P et al: Ameloblastic carcinoma of the maxilla: a report of 3 cases. J Craniomaxillofac Surg. 26(3):159-62, 1998
4. Corio RL et al: Ameloblastic carcinoma: a clinicopathologic study and assessment of eight cases. Oral Surg Oral Med Oral Pathol. 64(5):570-6, 1987
5. Slootweg PJ et al: Malignant ameloblastoma or ameloblastic carcinoma. Oral Surg Oral Med Oral Pathol. 57(2):168-76, 1984

IMAGE GALLERY

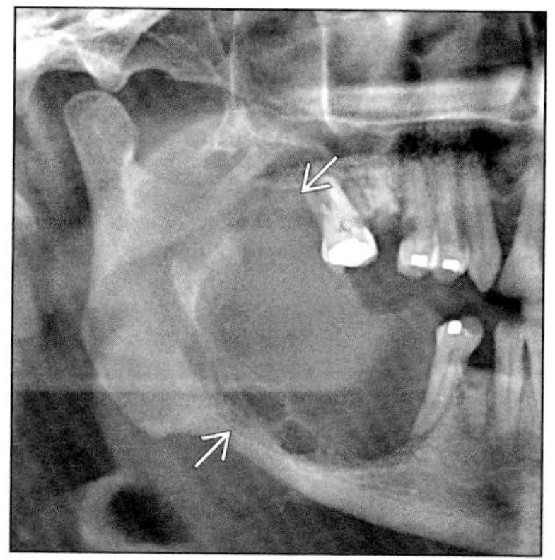

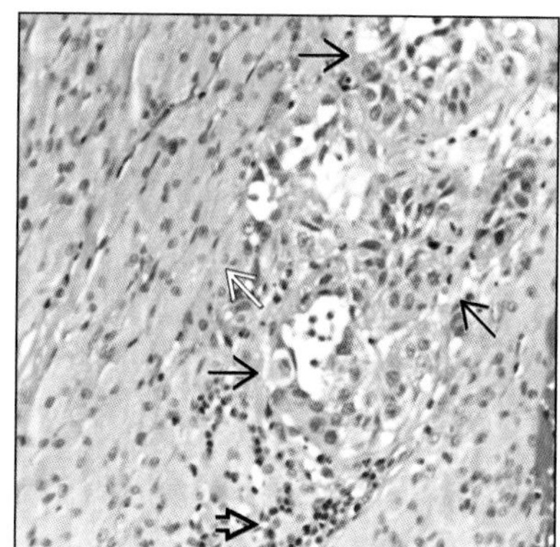

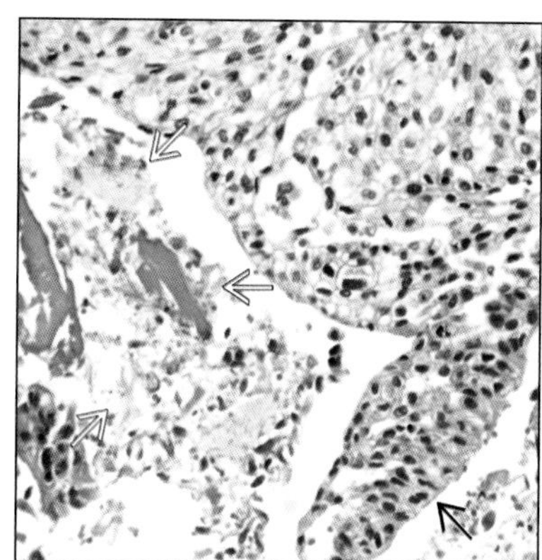

(Left) Radiograph shows destructive radiolucency ➡ of the posterior mandible. Biopsy later confirmed an ameloblastic carcinoma. (Center) This image shows invasion of the tumor ➡ into the skeletal muscle ➡ and the inflammatory reaction ➡ that resulted. (Right) Hematoxylin and eosin shows an ameloblastic carcinoma with a focus of preserved reverse polarity ➡ that has perforated the bone. Remnants of necrotic bone and debris are seen ➡ and are not uncommon in this tumor.

CLEAR CELL ODONTOGENIC CARCINOMA

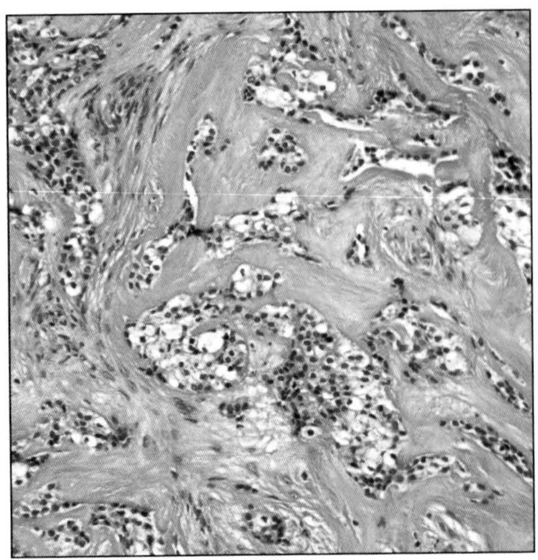

Hematoxylin & eosin shows islands of tumor cells demonstrating an invasive growth pattern. This invasive appearance is an indication of the tumor's malignancy despite it being cytologically bland.

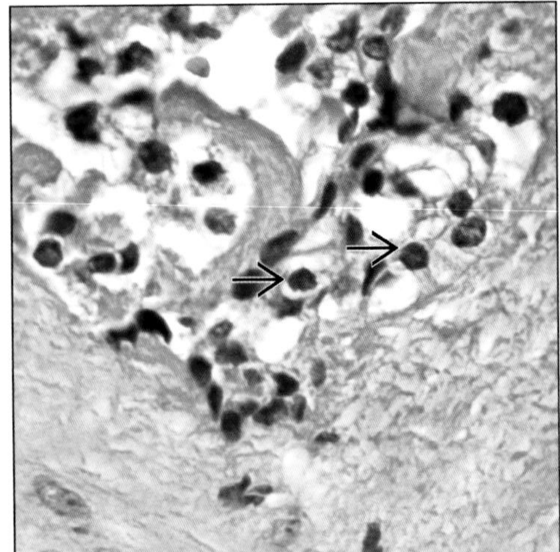

Hematoxylin & eosin shows optically clear cytoplasm and centrally placed uniform nuclei ⇒. The clear cells contain varying amounts of glycogen.

TERMINOLOGY

Abbreviations

- Clear cell odontogenic carcinoma (CCOC)

Synonyms

- Clear cell odontogenic tumor
  - Used to be called clear cell ameloblastoma

Definitions

- Malignant epithelial odontogenic neoplasm composed primarily of clear cells
  - Previously thought of as benign; change in terminology in recent WHO

CLINICAL ISSUES

Epidemiology

- Incidence
  - Rare, with < 100 reported cases
    - Initially described in 1985
- Age
  - Mean: 60 years old
  - Range: 17-90 years old
- Gender
  - Female > Male

Site

- 75% in mandible
  - Favor anterior mandible

Presentation

- Swelling
- Loosening of associated teeth
- Pain
- Destructive mass
- Asymptomatic

Treatment

- Surgical approaches
  - Aggressive resection
  - Elective neck dissection
  - Reconstruction
- Adjuvant therapy
  - Radiotherapy
    - Efficacy unknown
- Long-term follow-up

Prognosis

- High recurrence rate
- Frequent metastases
  - Lymphatic spread to lungs

IMAGE FINDINGS

Radiographic Findings

- Poorly defined radiolucency
- Bone destruction

MACROSCOPIC FEATURES

General Features

- Unencapsulated
- Invades medullary bone
- Cortical destruction
- May invade surrounding soft tissue

MICROSCOPIC PATHOLOGY

Histologic Features

- Biphasic tumor appearance
- Islands or cords of epithelial cells
  - Clear to finely granular, glycogen rich
  - Polygonal
  - Well-defined borders
  - Focal palisading of basal cells
  - Oval nuclei
  - Vesicular to hyperchromatic nuclei

CLEAR CELL ODONTOGENIC CARCINOMA

Key Facts

Terminology
- Malignant epithelial odontogenic neoplasm composed primarily of clear cells

Clinical Issues
- Rare
- 75% in mandible
- Aggressive resection
- High recurrence rate

Microscopic Pathology
- Small islands or nests
- Biphasic variant
- Islands or cords of epithelial cells
- Polygonal
- Focal palisading of basal cells
- Clear to finely granular, glycogen rich
- Fibrous stroma
- May have islands of other odontogenic tumors

- Fibrous stroma
  - Broad hyalinized bands
  - Some tumors may appear organoid
- May have islands of other odontogenic tumors
  - Ameloblastoma
  - Calcifying epithelial odontogenic tumor

ANCILLARY TESTS

Histochemistry
- PAS-diastase
  - Reactivity: Positive to equivocal
  - Staining pattern
    - Cytoplasm of clear cells (focal pattern)
- Alcian blue
  - Reactivity: Negative
- Mucicarmine
  - Reactivity: Negative

Immunohistochemistry
- Of little practical use
- Positive: Keratins (CK8, 18, 13, 14, 19); EMA weakly positive
- Negative: S100 protein, vimentin, SMA, HMB-45

DIFFERENTIAL DIAGNOSIS

Metastatic Renal Cell Carcinoma
- Rare; history of renal cell carcinoma
- Highly vascular
- IHCs may be useful (CD10, pax-2, RCC)

Intraosseous Mucoepidermoid Carcinoma
- Mucin-positive mucous cells
- Intermediate cells
- May be cytologically more atypical

Clear Cell Variant of Calcifying Epithelial Odontogenic Tumor
- Psammomatous calcifications
- Amyloid deposits

Ameloblastoma
- Rare cases may have clear cells

SELECTED REFERENCES

1. Avninder S et al: Clear cell odontogenic carcinoma: a diagnostic and therapeutic dilemma. World J Surg Oncol. 4:91, 2006
2. Ebert CS Jr et al: Clear cell odontogenic carcinoma: a comprehensive analysis of treatment strategies. Head Neck. 27(6):536-42, 2005
3. August M et al: Clear cell odontogenic carcinoma: evaluation of reported cases. J Oral Maxillofac Surg. 61(5):580-6, 2003
4. Brandwein M et al: Clear cell odontogenic carcinoma: report of a case and analysis of the literature. Arch Otolaryngol Head Neck Surg. 128(9):1089-95, 2002
5. Muramatsu T et al: Clear cell odontogenic carcinoma in the mandible: histochemical and immunohistochemical observations with a review of the literature. J Oral Pathol Med. 25(9):516-21, 1996

IMAGE GALLERY

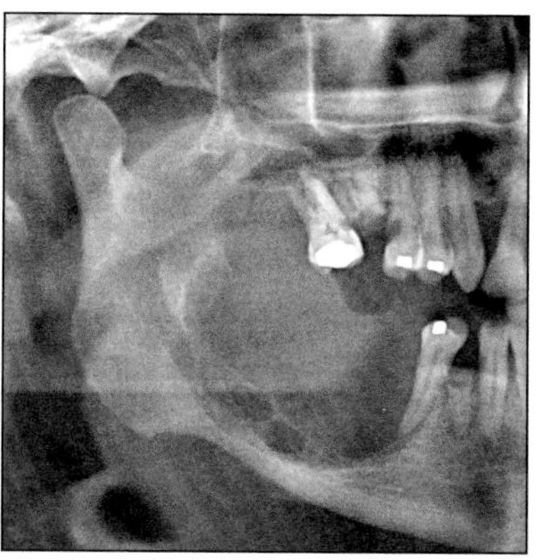

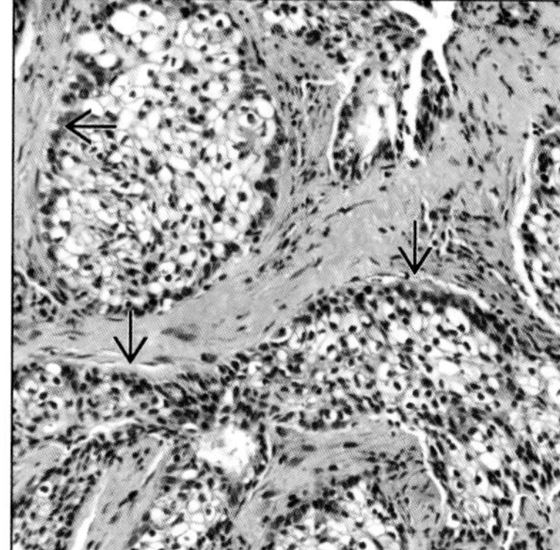

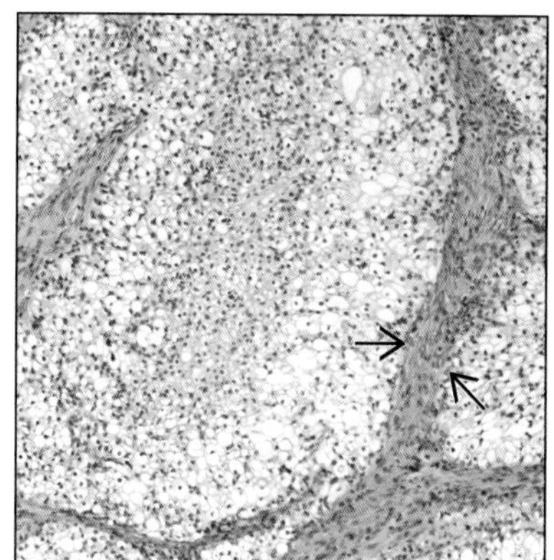

(Left) Radiograph shows a large radiolucency with focally irregular destructive borders. *(Center)* Hematoxylin & eosin shows tumor islands made up of clear cells with peripheral palisading ⇒. Because of the palisading, this tumor may be misdiagnosed as an ameloblastoma. A metastatic clear cell neoplasm must also be considered. *(Right)* Hematoxylin & eosin shows tumor islands of clear cells surrounded by a thickened hyalinized membrane ⇒.

AMELOBLASTIC FIBROSARCOMA

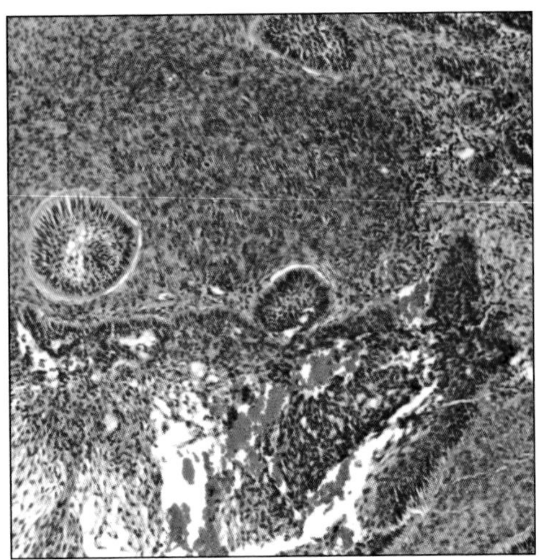

An ameloblastic fibrosarcoma resembles an ameloblastic fibroma except for the highly cellular, hyperchromatic, pleomorphic stroma. This feature is easily seen at low to medium magnification.

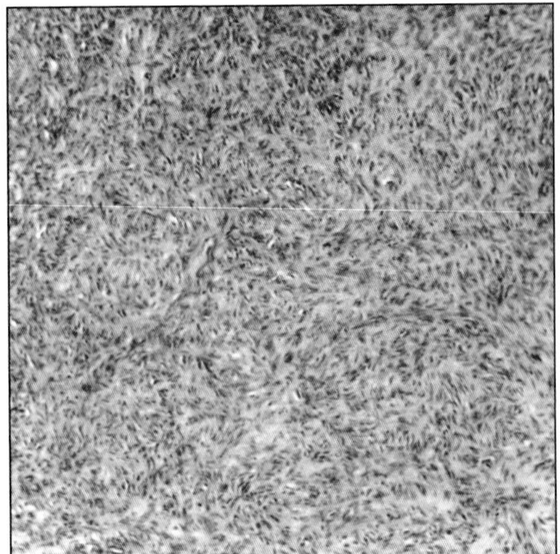

Hematoxylin & eosin shows an area of an AFS that lacks odontogenic epithelium. The stroma in this area of the tumor is looser and has a more storiform appearance.

TERMINOLOGY

Abbreviations

- Ameloblastic fibrosarcoma (AFS)
- Ameloblastic fibroma (AF)

Synonyms

- Ameloblastic sarcoma

Definitions

- Rare, malignant, odontogenic neoplasm; considered malignant counterpart to ameloblastic fibroma or fibro-odontoma

ETIOLOGY/PATHOGENESIS

Pathogenesis

- Many tumors (45%) arise from ameloblastic fibroma

CLINICAL ISSUES

Epidemiology

- Incidence
  - Extremely rare
- Age
  - Wide range at presentation
    - Mean: 3rd decade
    - Found in patients older than those affected by ameloblastic fibroma (14-25 years)
    - De novo tumors: Slightly younger average age

Site

- Mandible most commonly affected (80%)
  - Posterior specifically
- Maxilla
  - Often extends into sinus

Presentation

- Pain &/or swelling
- Ulceration of associated soft tissue

Treatment

- Surgical approaches
  - Radical resection (wide surgical margins required)
  - Neck dissection usually not indicated as sarcoma spread is generally hematogeneous
- Adjuvant therapy
  - Variably effective (radiation and chemotherapy)

Prognosis

- Overall prognosis is good, although unpredictable
- High recurrence rates
  - Up to 45%
  - Multiple recurrences are frequent
- Distant metastases generally do not develop
  - Lung, mediastinal lymph nodes, & liver (if present)
- Death is usually from direct extension into vital structures (base of skull)

IMAGE FINDINGS

Radiographic Findings

- Bone destruction with irregular borders
  - "Moth eaten"
- Expansive, multilocular radiolucencies
  - May demonstrate soft tissue expansion
- Perforation of cortical plate
- Maxillary tumors may erode into sinus
- Rarely, pathologic fracture

MACROSCOPIC FEATURES

General Features

- Large, osteolytic tumors spreading into soft tissues

AMELOBLASTIC FIBROSARCOMA

Key Facts

Terminology
- Rare odontogenic neoplasm, considered malignant counterpart to ameloblastic fibroma

Etiology/Pathogenesis
- Upward of 40% of tumors arise from ameloblastic fibroma

Clinical Issues
- Radical resection
- High recurrence rates

Microscopic Pathology
- Islands and cords of cuboidal to columnar epithelium
- Stroma is variably cellular
  - Pleomorphism
  - Hyperchromasia
  - Numerous mitotic figures
  - Storiform or herringbone pattern

MICROSCOPIC PATHOLOGY

Histologic Features
- Biphasic appearance is characteristic
  - Benign odontogenic epithelium within malignant mesenchymal fibrous stroma
- Islands & cords of bland cuboidal to columnar epithelium
  - Similar to ameloblastic fibroma
  - Epithelium decreases with successive recurrences
- Stroma made up of fibroblastic cells
  - Variably increased cellularity
  - Storiform or herringbone pattern
  - Pleomorphism and hyperchromasia
  - Numerous mitotic figures

ANCILLARY TESTS

Immunohistochemistry
- Stroma: Vimentin, muscle specific actin, smooth muscle actin, p53 positive; CD68 positive histiocytes
- AFS shows higher Ki-67 and PCNA labeling than AF (nearly 10x increase)

DIFFERENTIAL DIAGNOSIS

Ameloblastic Fibroma
- More ameloblastic epithelium
- Stroma less cellular, lacking pleomorphism & mitoses

Ameloblastic Fibro-odontoma
- Identical to AF, but with dental hard tissues

Ameloblastic Fibrodentinosarcoma
- Similar histologic findings with dental hard tissues
  - Dentin and enamel
- Prognosis essentially same

Ameloblastoma
- Mature, bland collagenous stroma
- More ameloblastic epithelium
  - Variable histologic subtypes

Fibrosarcoma
- Lacks ameloblastic epithelium

SELECTED REFERENCES

1. Kobayashi K et al: Malignant transformation of ameloblastic fibroma to ameloblastic fibrosarcoma: case report and review of the literature. J Craniomaxillofac Surg. 33(5):352-5, 2005
2. Müller S et al: Ameloblastic fibrosarcoma of the jaws. A clinicopathologic and DNA analysis of five cases and review of the literature with discussion of its relationship to ameloblastic fibroma. Oral Surg Oral Med Oral Pathol Oral Radiol Endod. 79(4):469-77, 1995
3. Dallera P et al: Ameloblastic fibrosarcoma of the jaw: report of five cases. J Craniomaxillofac Surg. 22(6):349-54, 1994
4. Takeda Y et al: Ameloblastic fibrosarcoma in the maxilla, malignant transformation of ameloblastic fibroma. Virchows Arch A Pathol Anat Histopathol. 404(3):253-63, 1984

IMAGE GALLERY

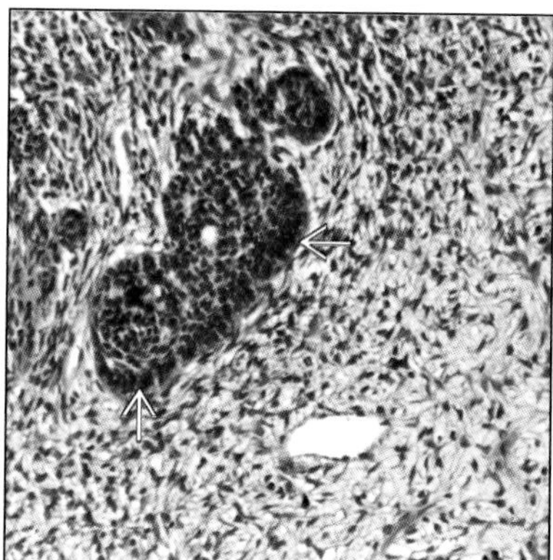

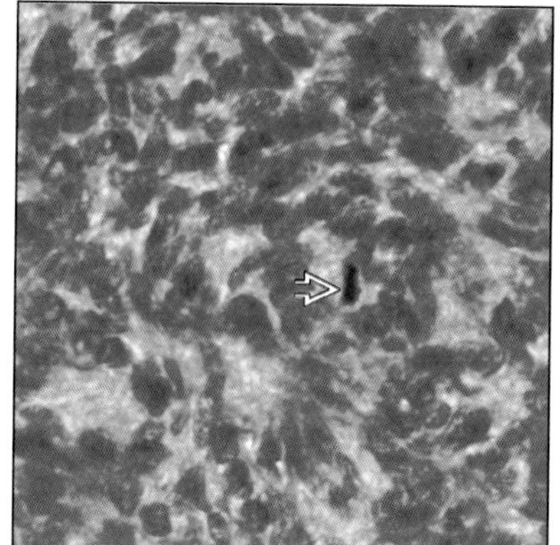

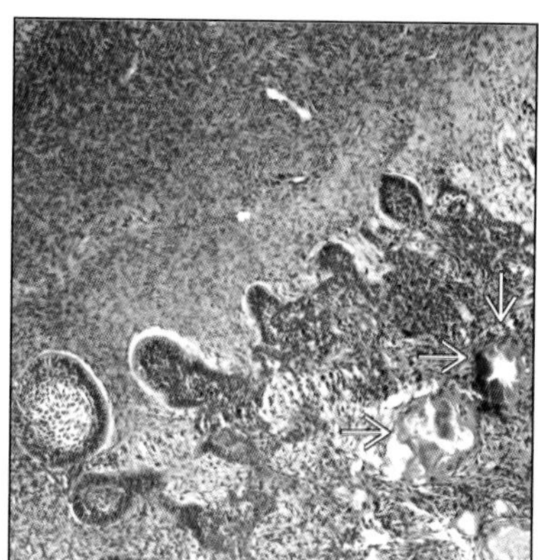

(Left) *High-power view shows an island of odontogenic epithelium with characteristic hyperchromatic columnar cells ➡ in a hypercellular stroma.* ***(Center)*** *AFS usually have numerous mitotic figures ➡, as shown here.* ***(Right)*** *This tumor has areas of dysplastic dentin ➡, making it an ameloblastic fibrodentinosarcoma. It is believed that the prognosis is essentially the same as a AFS. The WHO groups all these tumors under the broad category of "odontogenic sarcomas."*

OSTEOSARCOMA

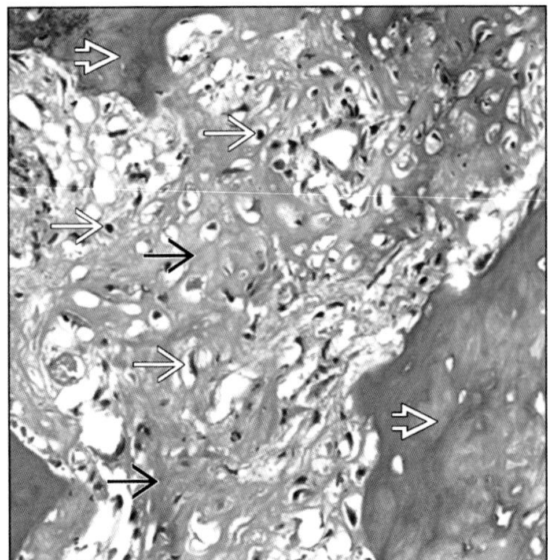

Osteosarcoma has a malignant mesenchymal lineage. Atypical osseous matrix ⇨ arises from the neoplastic osteoblasts ➡ infiltrating through the native trabeculae ⇨.

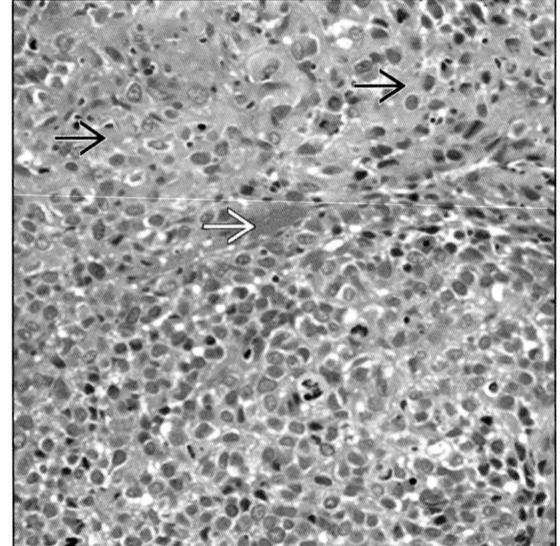

Histologically, osteosarcomas show a wide variety of patterns. Here, a delicate lace-like osseous matrix ⇨ arises around the pleomorphic osteoblasts. Delicate blood vessels ➡ are also noted.

TERMINOLOGY

Abbreviations

- Osteosarcoma (OS)

Definitions

- Primary intramedullary high-grade malignant tumor of mesenchymal origin in which neoplastic cells produce osteoid, even if only in small amounts

ETIOLOGY/PATHOGENESIS

Predisposing Factors

- May develop after radiation (or chemotherapy) for other neoplasms
  - Usually 5-15 years after therapy
  - Over 10% of jaw osteosarcomas are radiation induced
- Paget disease of bone and retinoblastoma
- History of trauma but probably just bringing underlying lesion to clinical attention

CLINICAL ISSUES

Epidemiology

- Incidence
  - OS is rare, even though it is the most common primary malignant bone tumor
    - Jaw incidence: 0.7 per million population
  - Craniofacial OSs are extremely rare
    - 7% of all osteosarcoma patients
- Age
  - Sinonasal OS: 3rd-4th decades
  - Gnathic OS: 3rd decade
  - Diagnosed about 10-20 years later than their long bone counterparts
- Gender
  - Male > Female (1.5:1)

Site

- Mandible and maxilla are equally affected
  - Angle of mandible and posterior region of mandibular body
  - Most are intramedullary rather than parosteal
  - Maxilla: Posterior alveolar ridge, antrum, sinus floor, and palate
- Much less common
  - Paranasal sinuses, zygoma, orbital ridge

Presentation

- Slow-growing mass or swelling
- Increasing pain with time
- Numbness and limitation of mouth opening
- Malocclusion and teeth loss
- Paresthesia or hypoesthesia less common
- Uncommonly present with trismus, nasal obstruction

Treatment

- Options, risks, complications
  - Treatment includes surgery, radiotherapy, &/or chemotherapy
- Surgical approaches
  - Surgery is mainstay of treatment
  - Single most important factor in curing OS is clear margins
    - Achieving clear margins is difficult due to anatomic constraints
- Adjuvant therapy
  - Adjuvant chemotherapy commonly recommended for high-grade OSs
    - Especially for close or positive margins
- Drugs
  - Chemotherapy has mixed results in jaw OS
    - Most OS of jaw are chondroblastic type, which fail to respond to chemotherapy
    - < 25% response for jaw OS
- Radiation
  - OS considered radioresistant
  - Postoperative radiotherapy is not well defined

OSTEOSARCOMA

Key Facts

Terminology

- Primary intramedullary high-grade malignant tumor of mesenchymal origin in which neoplastic cells produce osteoid, even if only in small amounts

Clinical Issues

- OS is rare, even though it is the most common primary malignant bone tumor
- Sinonasal and gnathic OS: 3rd-4th decades
- Slow-growing mass or swelling
- Treatment includes surgery, radiotherapy, &/or chemotherapy
  - Single most important factor in curing OS is clear margins
- Local recurrence rates up to 25%
- Metastatic risk is high
- Overall prognosis is guarded

Image Findings

- Best diagnostic clue: Bone destruction with aggressive periosteal reaction and tumor bone formation
  - Typical "sunray" (sunburst) appearance at tumor leading edge

Microscopic Pathology

- Hallmark is production of malignant bone or osteoid by atypical osteoblasts
  - Thin, lace-like eosinophilic strands interposed between sheets of malignant osteoblasts
- Moderate to high degree of pleomorphism

Top Differential Diagnoses

- Osteoblastoma, chondrosarcoma, fracture callus

  - 3D conformal radiotherapy and intensity-modulated radiation therapy may bypass these dose-limiting factors

Prognosis

- Local recurrence rates up to 25%
  - Main reason for treatment failure and mortality
  - Maxillary tumors particularly difficult to eradicate
- Metastatic risk is high
  - Micrometastases estimated to be 80%
    - Craniofacial osteosarcoma metastatic rate is lower
  - 20% of all OS patients have solid metastases when first diagnosed
  - Lung is most frequent site
    - Lung metastases have better prognosis than metastases in other organs
- Overall, prognosis is guarded
  - 80% survival with adequate margins
- Staging, to include chest and abdominal CT and bone scan, is required

IMAGE FINDINGS

General Features

- Best diagnostic clue: Bone destruction with aggressive periosteal reaction and tumor bone formation
  - Poorly defined, intramedullary mass with or without tumoral calcification, showing aggressive periosteal reaction

Radiographic Findings

- Widely variable from lytic, mottled to densely sclerotic destructive lesions
  - Most lesions have associated soft tissue mass
  - Might not be obvious on conventional radiographs due to anatomy
- Variable density based on degree of neoplastic bone formation
  - Typical "sunray" (sunburst) appearance at tumor leading edge due to cortical erosion
  - Higher grade lesions show higher degrees of lucency
  - "Moth-eaten" bone with ragged lytic areas
- Poorly defined borders with varying degrees of radiolucency and radiopacity
- Tumors adjacent to teeth may cause significant tooth resorption, widening of periodontal ligament, dissolution of lamina dura, and heightened interdental reactive or malignant bone deposition

MR Findings

- Useful for soft tissue extension, medullary bone involvement, and assessing marrow spread

CT Findings

- Noncontrast CT shows expansile lesion with increased density and aggressive periosteal reaction
- Contrast enhances solid components
- CT frequently shows unsuspected soft tissue mass

Bone Scan

- Increased uptake usually present
- Useful for staging, detection of metastases, and skip lesions

MACROSCOPIC FEATURES

General Features

- Irregular, poorly defined, firm tumor with gritty areas
- Tumors are of varying densities and compositions
  - Primarily osteoblastic tumors: Very hard & scirrhous
  - Chondroblastic OS: Pale blue-gray, glistening tissue areas
  - High-grade: Gelatinous and myxoid areas, hemorrhagic, necrotic
  - Soft tissue extension: Variable based on tumor type

Sections to Be Submitted

- 1 section per centimeter of tumor
- Adequate sampling of surgical margins

Size

- Range: 2-15 cm
- Majority: < 10 cm

OSTEOSARCOMA

MICROSCOPIC PATHOLOGY

Histologic Features

- Hallmark is production of malignant bone or osteoid by atypical osteoblasts
  - Moderate to high degree of pleomorphism
  - High nuclear to cytoplasmic ratio
  - Malignant osteoid must be present for diagnosis
    - Minimal and deposited as thin, lace-like eosinophilic strands interposed between sheets of malignant osteoblasts
    - Significant osteoid and bone production forming broad trabeculae with isolated single osteoblasts
- OS subclassified by most prominent histologic features
- Sarcomatous stroma varies in character based on tumor grade
- **Low grade**
  - Moderately cellular with minimal pleomorphism
  - Limited mitoses
  - Irregular bone and osteoid lacking lamellae
- **High grade (most jaw tumors)**
  - High cellular with closely packed spindled to polygonal cells
  - Significant pleomorphism, prominent nucleoli
  - High mitotic index, including atypical forms
  - Little to no bone formation

Histologic Subtypes

- **Osteoblastic**
  - Composed almost entirely of osseous matrix, with isolated atypical osteoblastic cells
- **Chondroblastic**
  - Most common type in head and neck
  - Cartilage must be malignant to qualify
    - Usually 5-50% of tumor is chondrosarcoma
- **Fibroblastic**
  - 5-50% of tumor composed of atypical spindle cells
- **Telangiectatic**
  - Large blood-filled spaces surrounded by pleomorphic cells and osseous matrix

ANCILLARY TESTS

Cytology

- Cytologic specimens are difficult to obtain
- Cellular smears
- Pleomorphic spindled and rounded tumor cells
- Basophilic cytoplasm with microvacuoles
- Large, hyperchromatic nuclei with indented membranes
- Multinucleated tumor cells often present
- Amorphous background "osteoid": Eosinophilic (alcohol fixed), magenta (air dried)

Cytogenetics

- High incidence of mutation in oncogenes *Rb*, *P53*, and *MDM-2*
- OS may be seen in familial cancer syndromes
  - Hereditary retinoblastoma; Li-Fraumeni, Rothmund-Thomson, Bloom syndromes

DIFFERENTIAL DIAGNOSIS

Osteoblastoma

- Radiology: Circumscribed mass with sclerotic margin of smaller lesion
- Remodeling of newly formed, thick bony trabeculae without pleomorphism or atypical mitoses
- Sheets of epithelioid osteoblasts with trabeculae rimming

Chondrosarcoma

- Chondroid and osteoid can be present in both tumors
- Lack of malignant osteoid or osteosarcoma

Fracture Callus

- Radiology is helpful in separation
- Bone formation during healing can be very reactive but has endochondral ossification and cartilage

Fibrous Dysplasia

- Radiology often very helpful in separation
- Malignant osteoid is absent

GRADING

Low Grade

- Moderately cellular with minimal pleomorphism and limited mitoses

Intermediate Grade

- Lace-like osteoid or seams of atypical osteoid infiltrating native trabeculae

High Grade

- Little to no osteoid present
- Significant pleomorphism, necrosis, and mitoses

SELECTED REFERENCES

1. Shao Z et al: Computed tomography findings in radiation-induced osteosarcoma of the jaws. Oral Surg Oral Med Oral Pathol Oral Radiol Endod. 109(3):e88-94, 2010
2. Guadagnolo BA et al: Osteosarcoma of the jaw/craniofacial region: outcomes after multimodality treatment. Cancer. 115(14):3262-70, 2009
3. Franco Gutiérrez V et al: Radiation-induced sarcomas of the head and neck. J Craniofac Surg. 19(5):1287-91, 2008
4. Huber GF et al: Head and neck osteosarcoma in adults: the province of alberta experience over 26 years. J Otolaryngol Head Neck Surg. 37(5):738-43, 2008
5. Laskar S et al: Osteosarcoma of the head and neck region: lessons learned from a single-institution experience of 50 patients. Head Neck. 30(8):1020-6, 2008
6. Fernandes R et al: Osteogenic sarcoma of the jaw: a 10-year experience. J Oral Maxillofac Surg. 65(7):1286-91, 2007
7. Gorsky M et al: Craniofacial osseous and chondromatous sarcomas in British Columbia--a review of 34 cases. Oral Oncol. 36(1):27-31, 2000
8. Smeele LE et al: Osteosarcoma of the head and neck: meta-analysis of the nonrandomized studies. Laryngoscope. 108(6):946, 1998
9. Odell PF: Head and neck sarcomas: a review. J Otolaryngol. 25(1):7-13, 1996

Imaging, Gross, and Microscopic Features

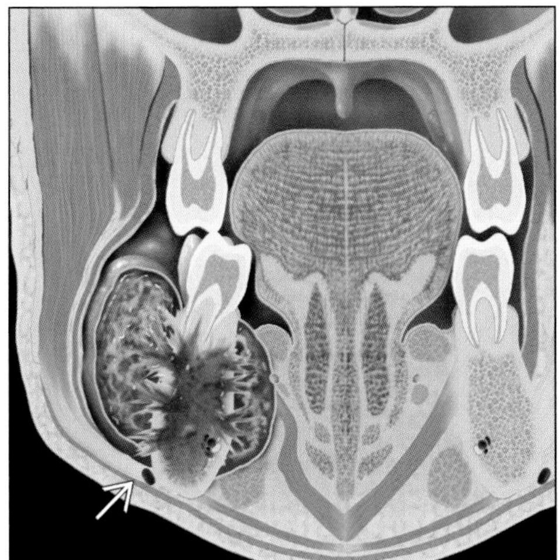

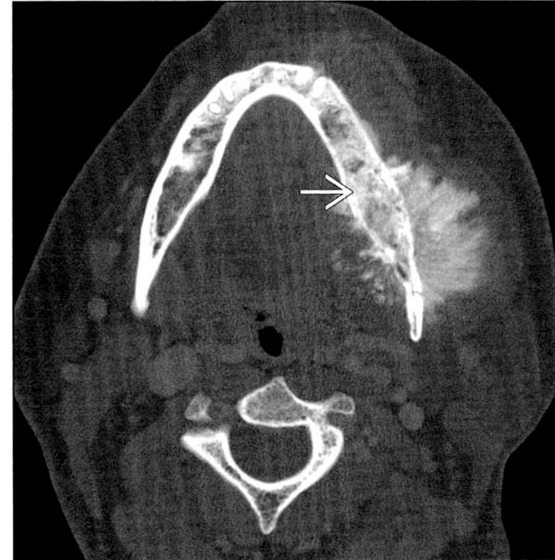

*(**Left**) A coronal graphic shows a right mandibular body osteosarcoma. There is destruction of the tooth root. This case has a soft tissue mass ➡. (**Right**) CT image (bone window) shows the classic periosteal reaction associated with osteosarcoma. This periosteal reaction is usually termed "sunburst" as the osseous matrix streams out perpendicular to the lesion. The marrow within the involved portion of the mandible is sclerotic ➡. There is an overlying soft tissue mass.*

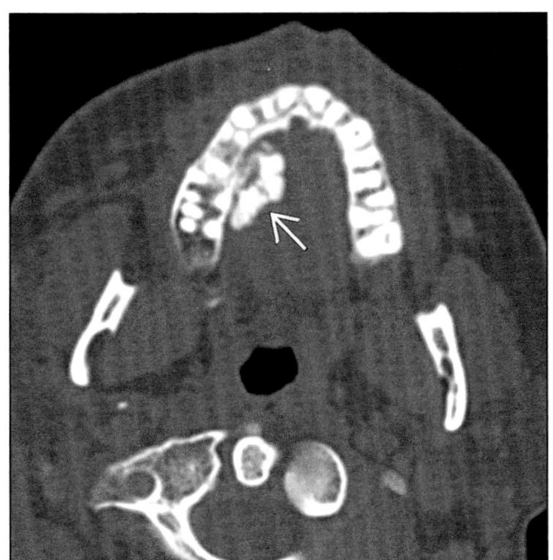

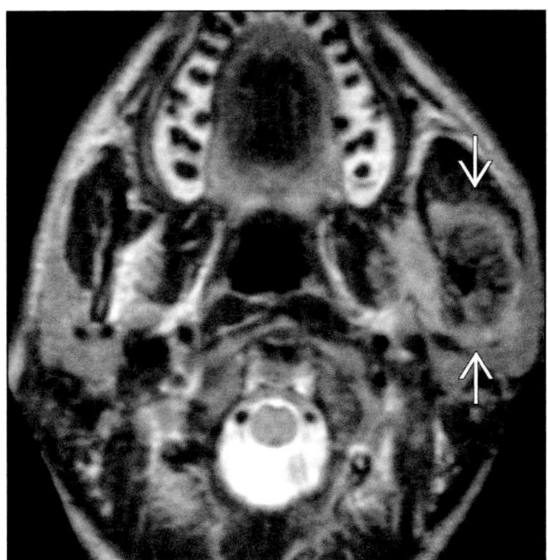

*(**Left**) Axial bone CT shows an exophytic mass with amorphous immature new bone, characteristic of osteosarcoma ➡. Osteosarcomas are heterogeneous in their radiologic appearance, and this case highlights a compact matrix formation. (**Right**) The "sunray" pattern of periosteal reaction ➡ surrounded by the hyperintense soft tissue mass is evident on an axial T2 image. MR is useful to delineate the extent of the lesions and marrow involvement.*

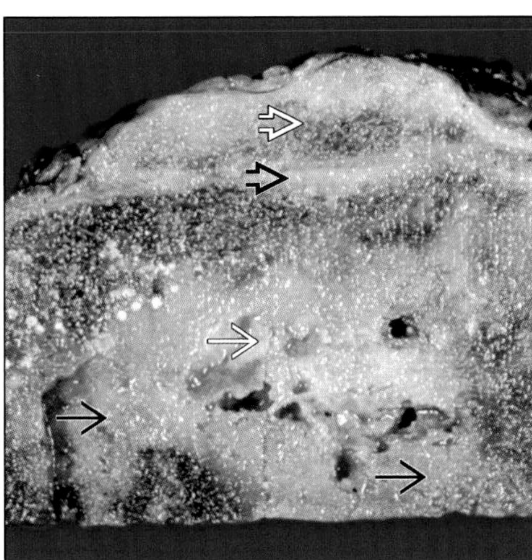

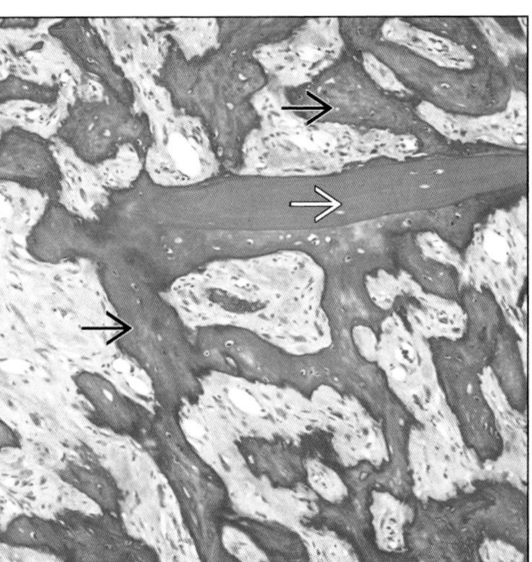

*(**Left**) Grossly these lesions can show dense sclerosis ➡ with areas of cystic change ➡. These tumors often break through the overlying cortex ➡ with the development of an associated soft tissue mass ➡. (**Right**) Moderately differentiated osteosarcoma will demonstrate struts and islands of atypical bone ➡ that infiltrate through and around the native trabeculae ➡. The background stroma is relatively bland in this tumor field.*

OSTEOSARCOMA

Microscopic Features

*(**Left**) The histologic features of a low-grade OS often present as large areas of fibrous-like tissue ➔ with islands of irregularly shaped bone and osseous matrix ➔ reminiscent of fibrous dysplasia. Careful search is necessary to find the scattered atypical cells. (**Right**) Native trabecular bone ➔ has been infiltrated and destroyed by the matrix-producing sarcoma. There are suggestions of cartilage-type tissue ➔, which can be seen even in nonchondroblastic OS.*

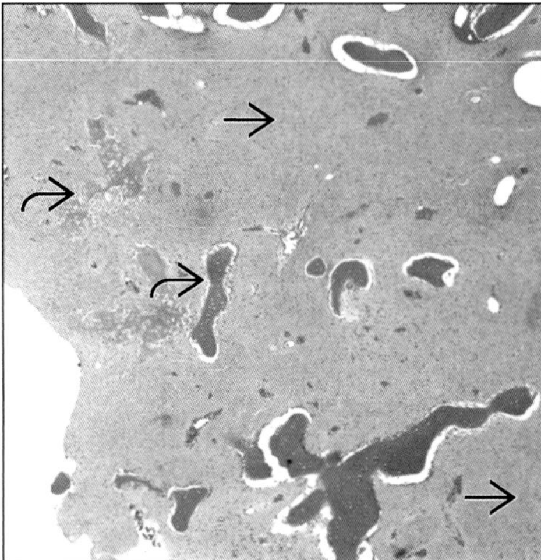

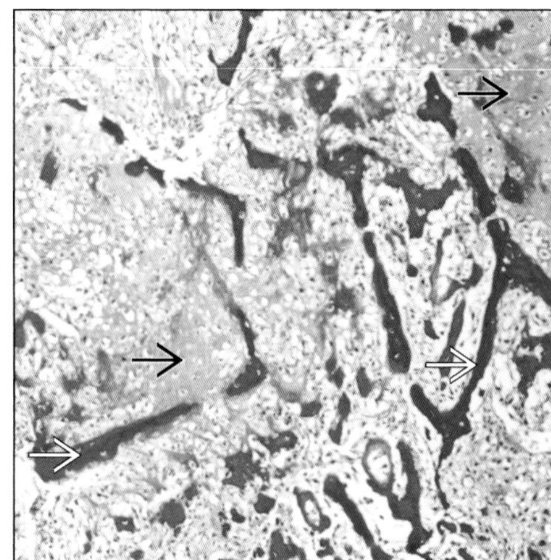

*(**Left**) High-grade lesions can have little to no osseous matrix. The pleomorphism can be striking and extensive enough to suggest pleomorphic sarcoma. There will be isolated foci of recognizable OS in most cases. Immunohistochemistry is usually of little use in these lesions, and correlation with radiology is necessary. (**Right**) Typical osteosarcoma demonstrates atypical cells of varying sizes with a readily identifiable osseous matrix. The bone lacks Haversian systems.*

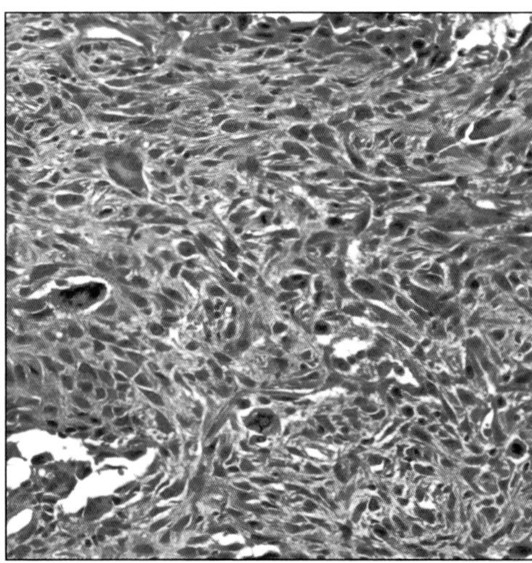

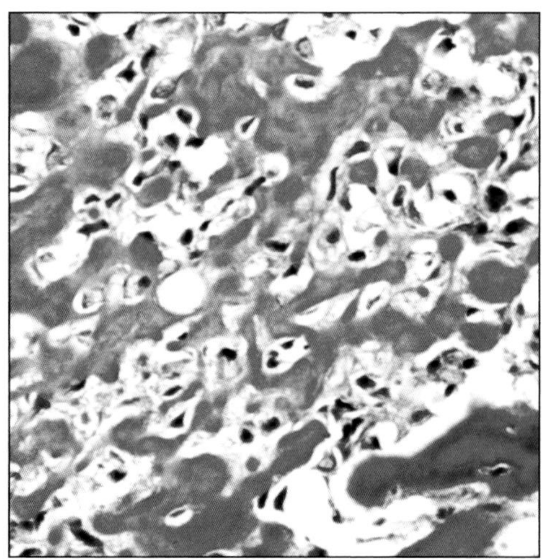

*(**Left**) Atypical cells are noted embedded within the osseous matrix ➔. Prominent nucleoli are noted, and apoptotic cells are abundant. The cells have a very high nuclear to cytoplasmic ratio, appearing plasmacytoid. (**Right**) Osteosarcoma shows atypical spindle cells with pleomorphism, increased nuclear to cytoplasmic ratio, and prominent nucleoli. Bone ➔ can be entrapped at the periphery or be new bone formation.*

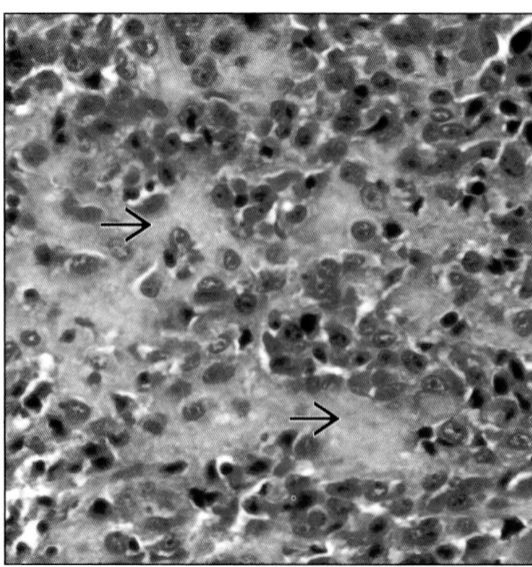

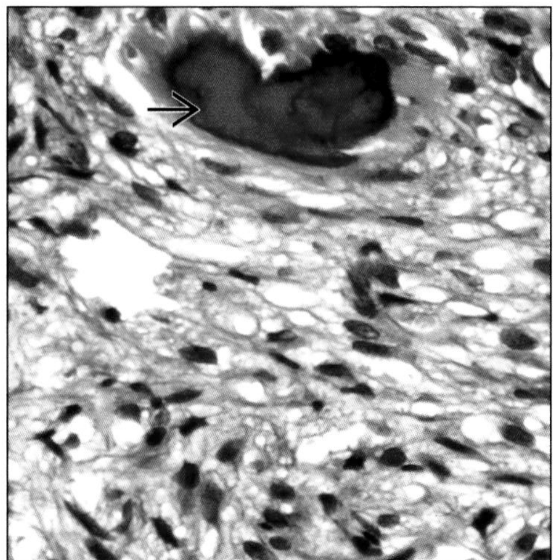

Microscopic and Molecular Features

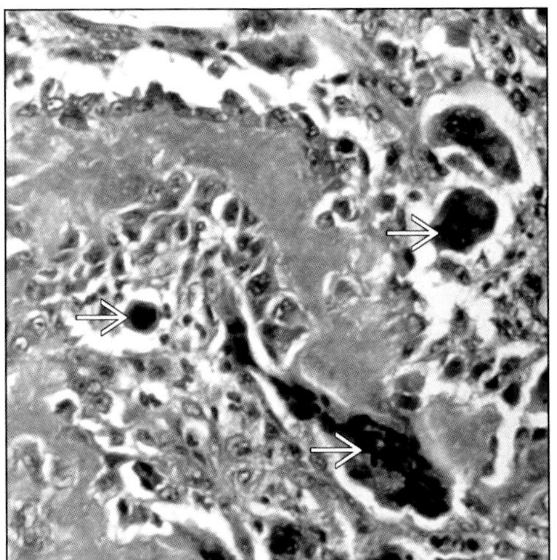

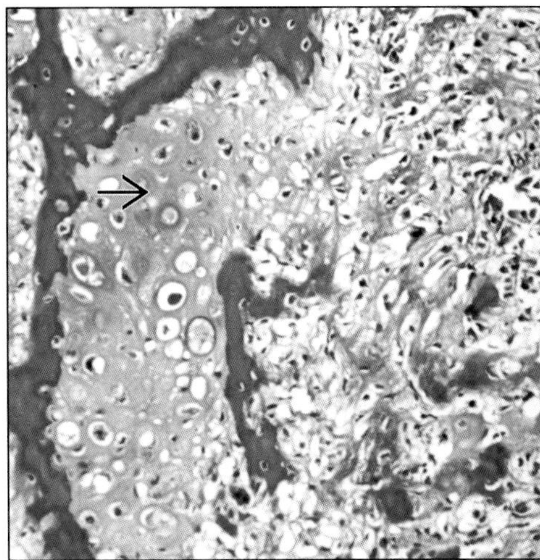

(Left) *Tumor giant cells* ➔ *can be seen in OS either in apposition to the neoplastic bone formation or within the stromal matrix.* ***(Right)*** *Chondroblastic OS will show features of typical OS with portions of malignant chondroid tissue* ➔*. Fracture callus can often make diagnosis difficult; however, the atypical features of the chondrosarcomatous elements can be readily identified in chondroblastic osteosarcoma. The key is to identify matrix infiltrating the other elements.*

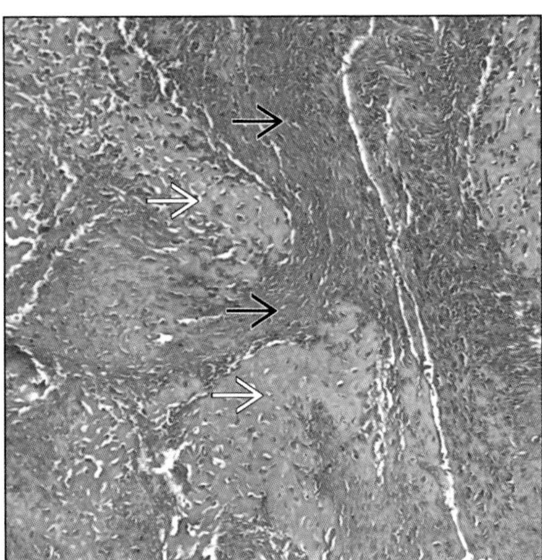

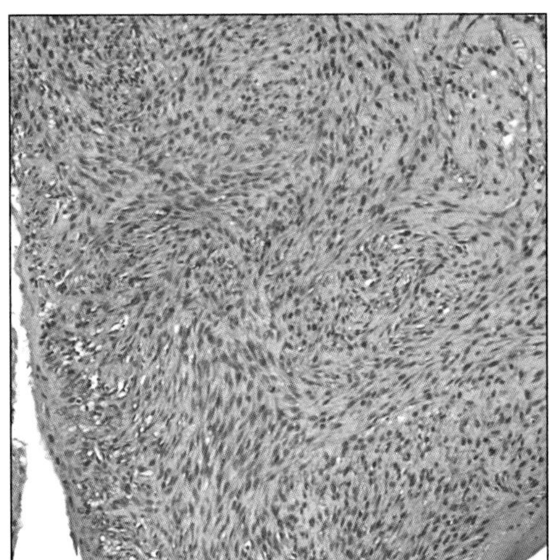

(Left) *Fibroblastic osteosarcoma, as its name implies, consists of spindle cell elements* ➔ *as part of the OS. Osteoid is easily identified throughout this field* ➔*.* ***(Right)*** *Fibroblastic osteosarcoma appears as a spindle cell neoplasm and can often have a paucity of matrix formation. In areas like this, the diagnosis can be difficult, necessitating adequate sampling of the lesion and correlation with the pertinent radiologic studies.*

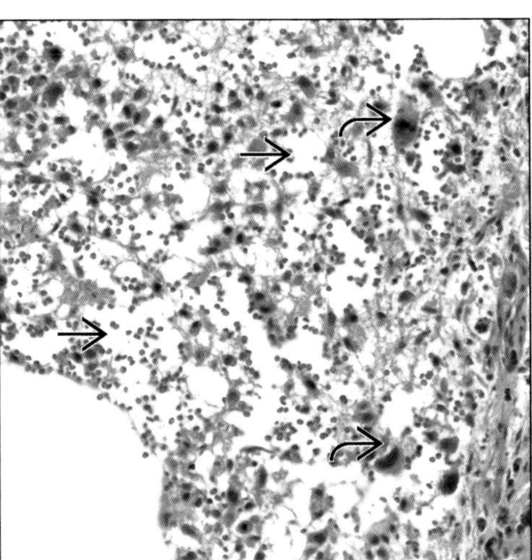

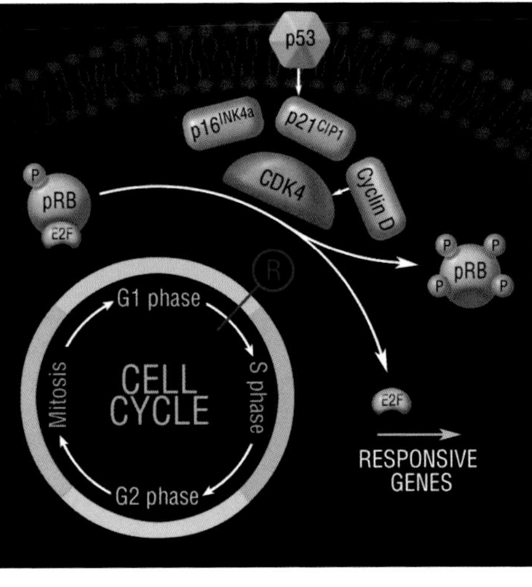

(Left) *Telangiectatic osteosarcoma often shows blood-filled spaces* ➔ *with varying amounts of blood &/or hemosiderin. Blood lakes are surrounded by large and atypical cells* ➔*, along with atypical mitoses.* ***(Right)*** *RB gene has A and B pocket-domains, which bind to E2F transcription factor, and binding of the hypophosphorylated pRB to these factors represses transcription of the genes. When phosphorylated, E2F is released, and responsive genes are expressed.*

CHONDROSARCOMA

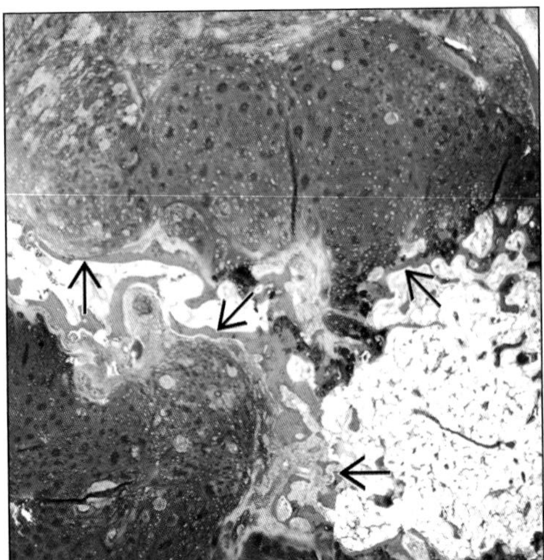

There is destruction of cortical bone by neoplastic chondrocytes, invading into the bone. The lobules of cellular cartilaginous matrix are separated by bone spicules ➔. The matrix has a dark blue appearance.

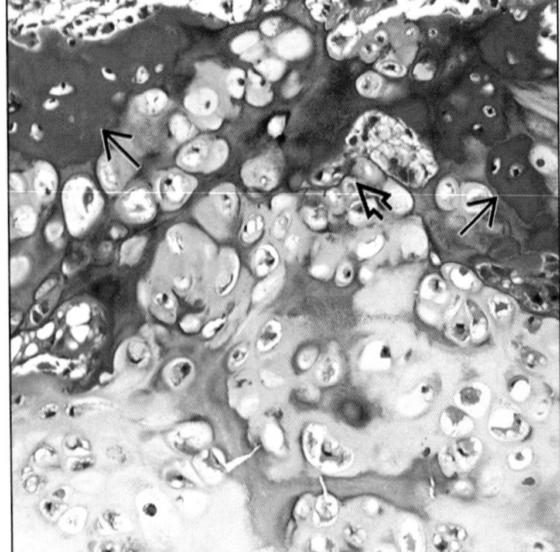

The highly atypical chondrocytes are within lacunae. There is destruction of bone tissue, which is noted at the periphery ➔. Native cartilage is also present, showing "abrupt" transition to the neoplastic foci ➔.

TERMINOLOGY

Definitions

- Malignant mesenchymal tumor with hyaline cartilage differentiation

ETIOLOGY/PATHOGENESIS

Developmental Anomaly

- May arise from cartilage or embryonal rests
  - Pluripotential mesenchymal cells

Inherited Syndromes

- Ollier disease: Enchondromas, but increased risk of chondrosarcoma
- Maffucci syndrome: Enchondromas and hemangiomas, but increased risk of chondrosarcoma

Predisposing Factors

- Ischemic change may contribute to development of chondrosarcoma

CLINICAL ISSUES

Epidemiology

- Incidence
  - 3rd most common primary bone tumor
    - About 25% of all bone tumors are chondrosarcoma
  - Very rare in head and neck, comprising < 10% of all chondrosarcomas
- Age
  - Broad range
  - Mean: 5th to 7th decades
- Gender
  - Male > Female (1.5:1)

Site

- Most often in maxilla and skull base
- Also seen in maxillary sinus, larynx, and nasal septum
- Uncommonly involves mastoid bone

Presentation

- Majority present with pain &/or swelling
- Loose teeth
- Cranial nerve dysfunction
- Symptoms are often present for long duration due to slow growth

Treatment

- Surgical approaches
  - Radical surgical resection is preferred treatment
    - Often requires 2-3 cm margin of normal tissue
    - Difficult to achieve in anatomic confines of jaws and sinuses

Prognosis

- Overall prognosis: ~ 70% 5-year survival
  - Grade 1: 90% 5-year survival
  - Grade 3: ~ 50% 5-year survival
- Vast majority of patients have grade 1 tumors
- Recurrences develop in up to 40% of cases
- Prognostic predictors
  - Adequacy of margins and resectability important in predicting biologic behavior
  - Tumor grade predicts biologic behavior
  - Pediatric patients have better prognosis than adult patients (independent of grade)
  - Dedifferentiated tumors have very poor prognosis
- Metastatic disease is uncommon, but grade dependent
  - Grade 1: < 5%, grade 2: ~ 20%, grade 3: 70%

IMAGE FINDINGS

General Features

- Best diagnostic studies: CT shows characteristic calcifications, but MR better delineates extent of tumor

CHONDROSARCOMA

Key Facts

Terminology

- Malignant mesenchymal tumor with hyaline cartilage differentiation

Clinical Issues

- Very rare in head and neck, comprising < 10% of all chondrosarcomas
- Mean age: 5th to 7th decades
- Most often in maxilla and skull base
- Majority present with pain &/or swelling
- Radical surgical resection is usual treatment
- Overall prognosis: ~ 70% 5-year survival
  - Adequacy of margins important prognostic factor

Image Findings

- Best diagnostic studies: CT shows characteristic calcifications, with MR delineating extent of tumor
  - Rings and crescents of calcium most characteristic

Macroscopic Features

- Cut surfaces have glassy to translucent, blue-white appearance, with myxoid areas

Microscopic Pathology

- Destruction of cancellous or cortical bone by neoplastic chondrocytes
- Lobules of cartilaginous matrix, showing variability in size and shape, with irregular maturation
- Lacunar spaces contain atypical chondrocytes

Top Differential Diagnoses

- Chondroma, chondroblastic osteosarcoma, chondromyxoid fibroma, spindle cell squamous cell carcinoma, true malignant mixed tumor, pleomorphic adenoma

---

- Soft tissue mass adjacent to or involving bone with variable calcification pattern
- Presence and degree of calcification depends on tumor grade
- Erosion of bone of origin and surrounding bones

MR Findings

- T1WI
  - Homogeneous intermediate signal
  - Calcifications make signal heterogeneous
- T2WI
  - High signal (due to high water content)
  - Homo- to heterogeneous, depending on degree of calcification

CT Findings

- Radiolucent mass with lobular borders and containing scattered calcifications
- Rings and crescents of calcium most characteristic of low-grade tumors

MACROSCOPIC FEATURES

General Features

- Appear as smooth, expansive, firm lesions
  - Erosion and cortical bone destruction may be seen
- Lobular appearance is common
- Cut surfaces are glassy to translucent
- Blue-white to gray
- Areas of myxoid or mucoid material are seen
- Cystic areas are infrequent
- Gritty calcifications appear as white, chalky areas

Sections to Be Submitted

- 1 section per linear cm of tumor

Size

- Range: 0.5-10 cm

MICROSCOPIC PATHOLOGY

Histologic Features

- Destruction of cancellous or cortical bone by neoplastic chondrocytes
  - Neoplastic cells invade into and replace bony tissue
  - **No** bone formation, only destruction or entrapment
- If native cartilage is present, there is abrupt transition from normal to neoplastic cartilage
- Lobules of cartilaginous matrix, showing variability in size and shape, with irregular maturation
- Fibrous bands or bone surround or separate lobules
- Increased cellularity
  - Variable from one field to the next, but overall increased cellularity
  - Matrix disarray
- Lacunar spaces contain atypical chondrocytes
  - Increased nuclear hyperchromasia
  - Stellate, spindled, or pleomorphic nuclei
- Bi- or multinucleation can be seen
- Mitoses are rare but can be seen in high-grade tumors
- Myxoid changes or liquefaction of cartilage is not uncommon
- Background of ischemic necrosis is frequently present
- Necrosis is seen in high-grade tumors
- Grading based on cellularity, nuclear size, nuclear hyperchromasia, mitoses, and necrosis
- Types
  - Periosteal (juxtacortical: Based on location)
  - Myxoid
  - Mesenchymal
  - Clear cell
  - Dedifferentiated

Margins

- Clear margins decrease risk of recurrence
  - 2-3 cm of uninvolved or normal tissue is considered adequate
  - Difficult to achieve in sinonasal tract and base of skull regions

CHONDROSARCOMA

Dedifferentiated Chondrosarcoma

- Dedifferentiated chondrosarcoma shows low- to intermediate-grade chondrosarcoma with high-grade spindle cell component (sarcoma)

ANCILLARY TESTS

Cytology

- Cellularity and cytology will depend on grade of tumor
- Cells are enlarged with increased nuclear to cytoplasmic ratio, vacuolated cytoplasm, and nuclear atypia
- Abundant chondromyxoid matrix material surrounding atypical chondrocytes
  - Cartilage matrix shows fibrillar matrix, deep magenta in air-dried preparations
  - Matrix difficult to detect on Pap-stained material

Immunohistochemistry

- Positive with S100 protein

Cytogenetics

- Complex numerical or structural chromosomal alterations
  - Loss of 13q associated with increased metastatic potential

DIFFERENTIAL DIAGNOSIS

Chondroma

- Radiographically, well marginated, ranging from radiolucent to densely sclerotic
- Lack bone invasion or destruction
- Less cellular than chondrosarcoma, lacking atypia
- No mitoses or necrosis

Chondroblastic Osteosarcoma

- Cartilaginous tissue in association with malignant osseous proliferation
- Osteoid is part of neoplasm (not entrapment)
- Radiology will show predominantly osteosarcomatous features

Chondromyxoid Fibroma

- May show bone "entrapment" at periphery
- Lobular neoplasm with spindled cells in myxoid matrix
- Cytoplasmic extensions create fusiform or bipolar appearance
- Hyaline cartilage is identified in about 20% of cases

Chondroblastoma

- Remarkably uniform, cellular tumor with strong cell borders
- Pseudolobulated growth or pavement pattern
- Usually clear to lightly eosinophilic cytoplasm
- Nuclei are often clefted or grooved, lacking atypia
- Scant to absent mature hyaline cartilage
- "Chicken wire" calcifications may be present

Odontogenic Myxoma

- Myxoid matrix is dominant finding
- Hypocellular tumor with isolated islands of odontogenic epithelium

Spindle Cell Squamous Cell Carcinoma

- Usually polypoid tumor with squamous and spindled differentiation
- Cartilaginous elements may be present (benign or malignant)
- Additional components must be present to confirm diagnosis (difficult on biopsy material)

True Malignant Mixed Tumor

- Presence of both carcinoma and sarcoma within salivary gland neoplasm
- Chondrosarcoma is most common sarcoma
- Usually has benign pleomorphic adenoma present

Pleomorphic Adenoma

- Usually easy to differentiate on histology sections
- Cytology may prove difficult

GRADING

Low Grade

- Resembles benign cartilage
- Relatively uniform, lobular histologic appearance
- Mild increase in cellularity
- Very rare mitotic figures

Intermediate Grade

- Often have myxoid type stroma as well as hyaline-type matrix
- Cellularity is increased and will often show binucleated cells
- Multiple cells within lacunae
- Occasional mitotic figures

High Grade

- High cellularity with pleomorphism
- High mitotic index
  - Atypical mitotic figures present
- May have tumor necrosis

SELECTED REFERENCES

1. Hong P et al: Chondrosarcoma of the head and neck: report of 11 cases and literature review. J Otolaryngol Head Neck Surg. 38(2):279-85, 2009
2. Prado FO et al: Head and neck chondrosarcoma: analysis of 16 cases. Br J Oral Maxillofac Surg. 47(7):555-7, 2009
3. Selz PA et al: Chondrosarcoma of the maxilla: a case report and review. Otolaryngol Head Neck Surg. 116(3):399-400, 1997
4. Watters GW et al: Chondrosarcoma of the temporal bone. Clin Otolaryngol Allied Sci. 20(1):53-8, 1995
5. Ruark DS et al: Chondrosarcomas of the head and neck. World J Surg. 16(5):1010-5; discussion 1015-6, 1992
6. Finn DG et al: Chondrosarcoma of the head and neck. Laryngoscope. 94(12 Pt 1):1539-44, 1984

Diagrammatic and Imaging Features

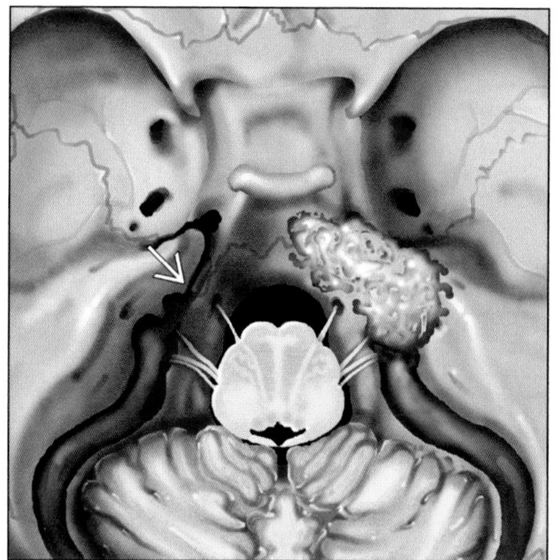

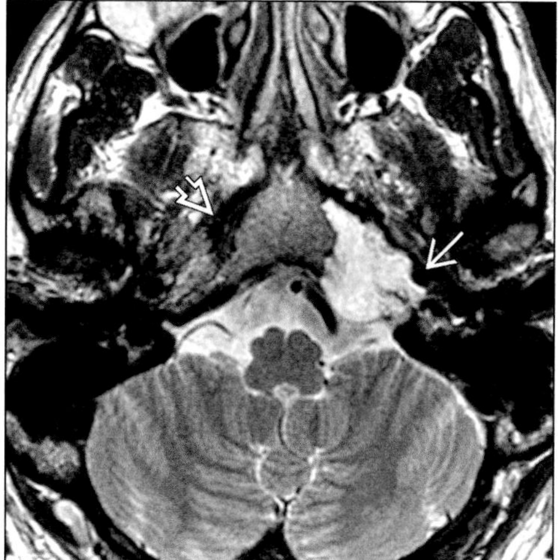

(Left) *Axial graphic shows a chondrosarcoma in the skull base, centered in the left petrooccipital fissure. Note the calcifications within the lesion. The normal right petrooccipital ➡ fissure is also shown.* ***(Right)*** *Axial T2WI MR reveals high signal chondrosarcoma of the petrooccipital fissure. Note that the vertical segment of petrous internal carotid artery is compressed ➡ and that the right petrooccipital fissure appears normal ➡.*

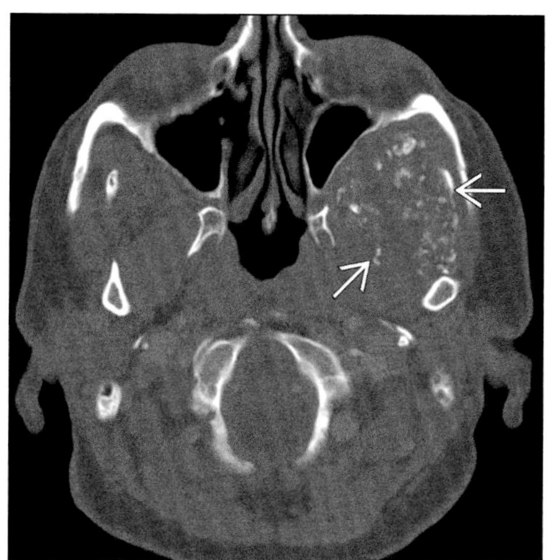

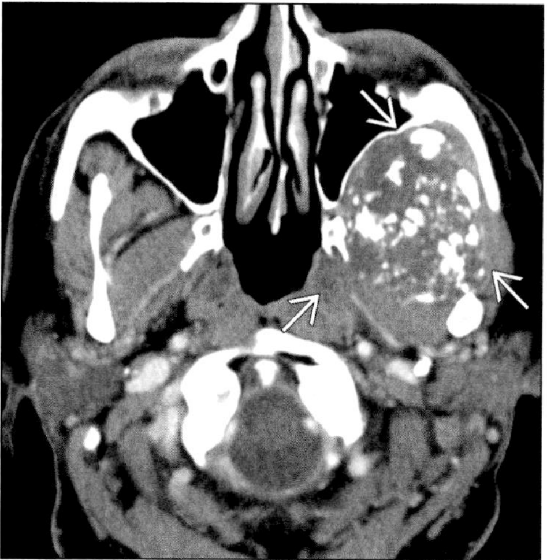

(Left) *Axial CECT image viewed with a bone window shows a soft tissue mass filling the masticator space. There are rings and crescents of calcification ➡, quite characteristic of chondrosarcoma.* ***(Right)*** *Axial CECT image on soft tissue window show an inherently low-density mass ➡ with intrinsic calcifications that fills the left infratemporal fossa. The calcifications are "fluffy," with rings and arcs. These changes are characteristic of a chondrosarcoma radiographically.*

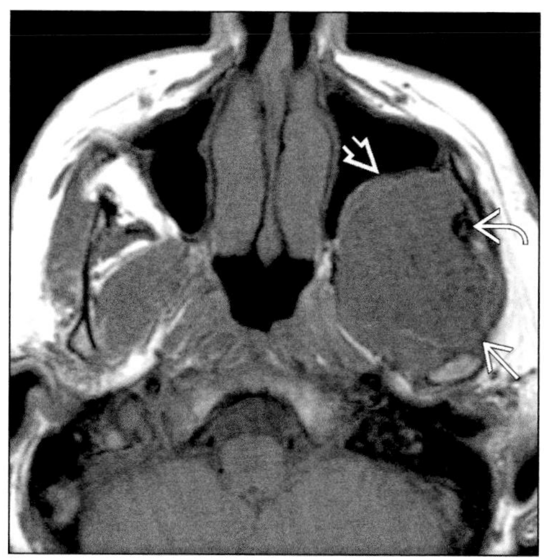

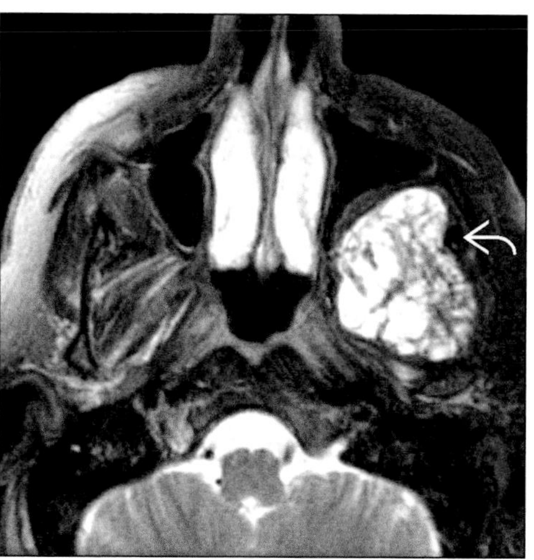

(Left) *T1WI MR demonstrates a mass ➡ distending the masticator space and bowing the posterior wall of the left maxillary sinus anteriorly ➡. A large focal calcification is seen as low signal intensity ➡.* ***(Right)*** *T2WI MR demonstrates the characteristically bright signal intensity of chondroid tumors. A large focal calcification is seen as low signal intensity ➡. The tumor is generally heterogeneous with intense enhancement with gadolinium.*

CHONDROSARCOMA

Clinical and Microscopic Features

(Left) There is a multilobular mass causing significant distortion of the mandible, resulting in teeth displacement. The surface epithelium is intact. This tumor proved to be a chondrosarcoma on histologic examination. ***(Right)*** A maxilla chondrosarcoma shows abutment against the tooth ➔. The tumor shows increased cellularity with nuclear atypia. There are multiple areas showing bi- and multinucleation. The chondroid matrix is easily identified.

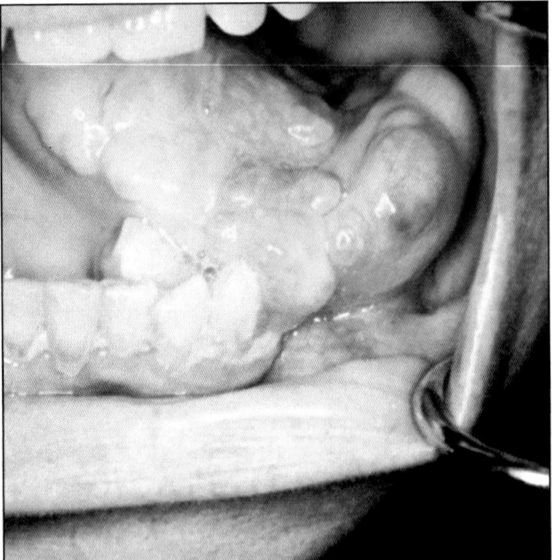

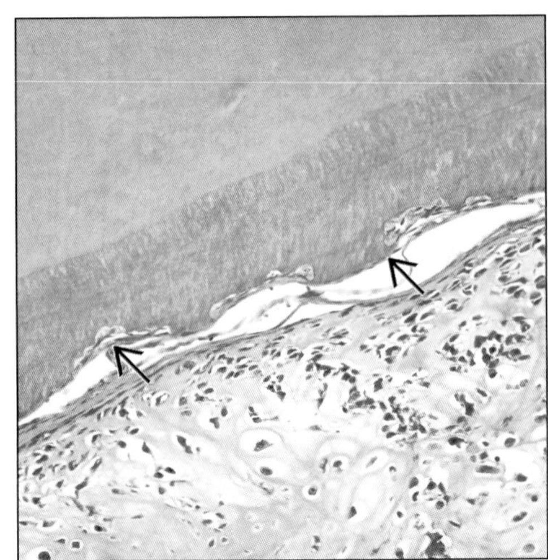

(Left) Atypical hyaline-like cartilage ➔ in lobules invade through and surround the existing trabecular bone ➔. Myxoid degeneration ➔ is often a component of these tumors. This would be considered a grade 1 lesion. ***(Right)*** There is increased cellularity with disarray of the lacunae. There is nuclear atypia, including nuclear hyperchromasia. This degree of atypia is consistent with a grade 1 tumor.

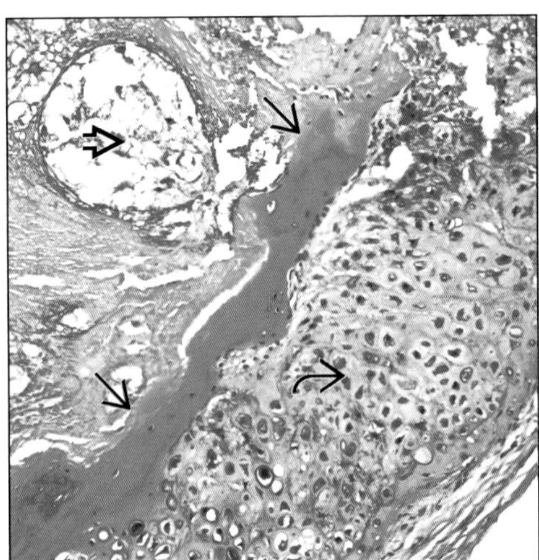

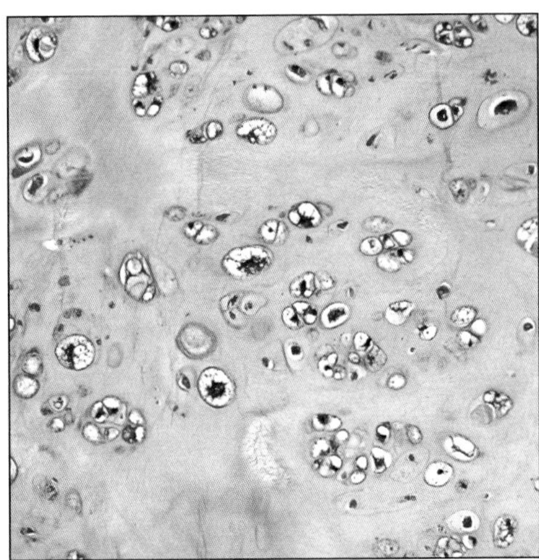

(Left) This neoplasm shows increased cellularity with cellular enlargement, filling the lacunae spaces. Bi- and multinucleation is present. A mitotic figure ➔ is noted within this tumor. This tumor would be interpreted as a grade 2 neoplasm. ***(Right)*** There is an abrupt juxtaposition between the chondrosarcoma and the native cartilage ➔. It is easy to see a difference in the size and shape of the nuclei. Increased nuclear to cytoplasmic ratio is present.

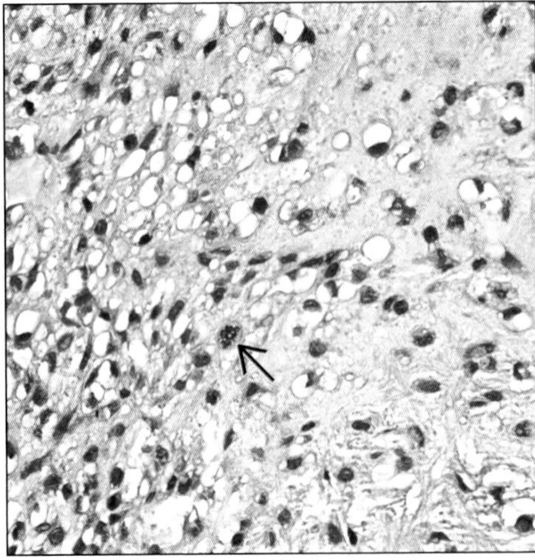

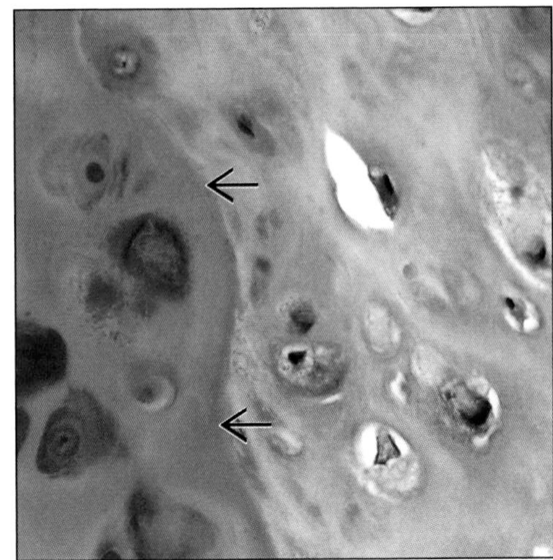

Microscopic and Cytologic Features

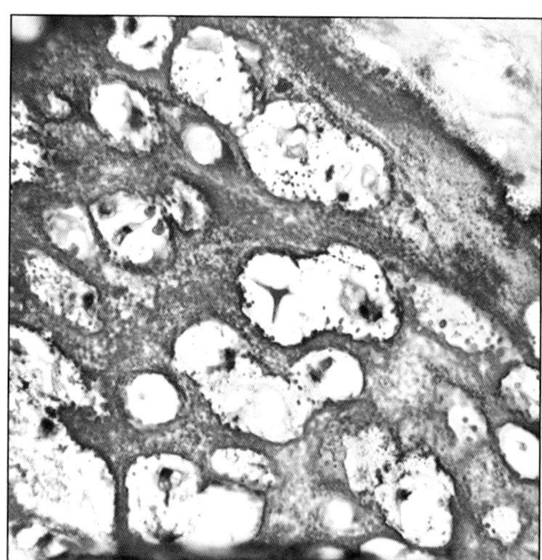

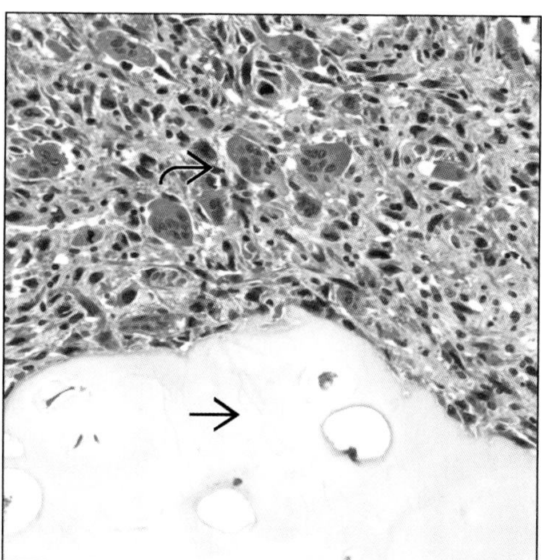

(Left) *It is quite common to see ischemic necrosis at the periphery of the tumor or within associated areas of chondroma. The cytoplasm is granular and darkly basophilic, with crenated nuclei. This is a characteristic appearance for ischemic necrosis within cartilage.* ***(Right)*** *Dedifferentiated chondrosarcoma can sometimes show giant cell tumor ⮫ in association with the low-grade chondrosarcomatous elements →. The tumor cell spindling is focally noted in this field.*

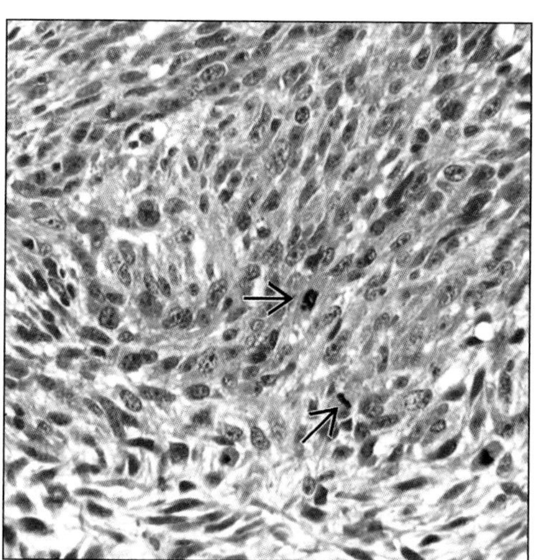

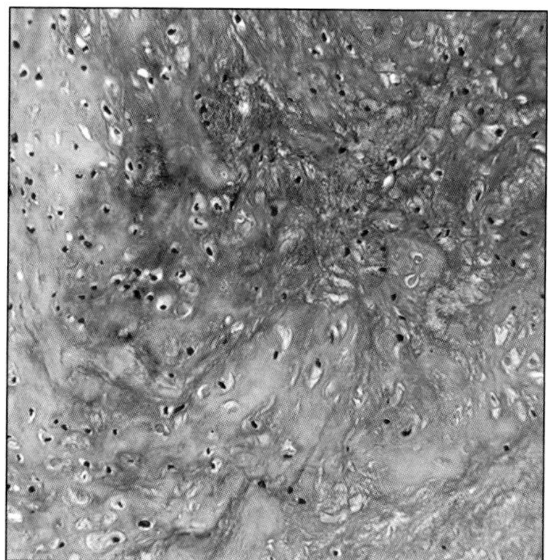

(Left) *Dedifferentiated chondrosarcoma is diagnosed when there is chondrosarcoma and a high-grade spindle cell component. The spindle cell component appears like malignant fibrous histiocytoma or fibrosarcoma. Pleomorphism is extensive. Mitotic figures, including atypical forms, can be seen →.* ***(Right)*** *A myxoid variant of chondrosarcoma shows a marked myxoid matrix in which the neoplastic chondrocytes are suspended.*

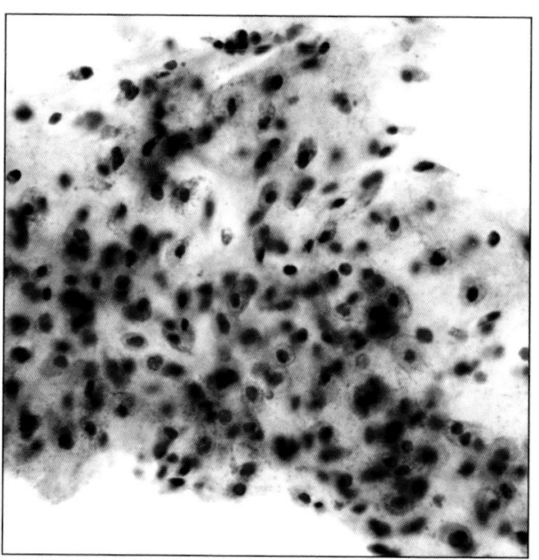

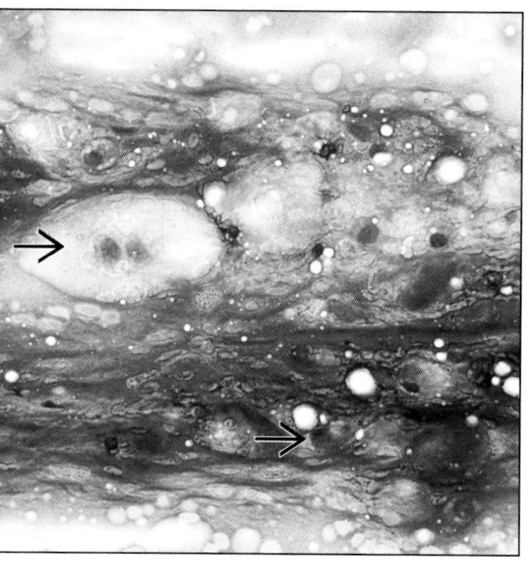

(Left) *Fine needle aspiration specimen of a jaw mass shows a highly cellular tumor with many lacunar spaces. Nuclear atypia is noted, including binucleation. Mitotic figures are not appreciated. These results can suggest a cartilage lesion, but correlation with radiology is necessary.* ***(Right)*** *Cytologic preparations often show a mucopolysaccharide background with isolated cells →. There is an increase in the nuclear to cytoplasmic ratio. The chondroid matrix is quite characteristic.*

FIBROSARCOMA

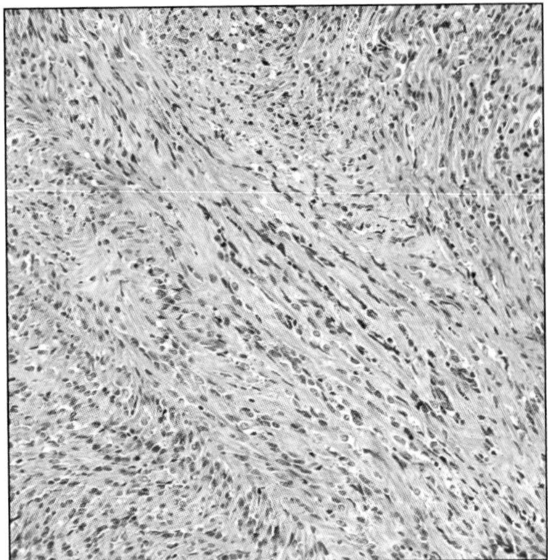

There are elongated fascicles of spindled to slightly epithelioid cells separated by dense, keloid-like collagen. This is a characteristic appearance of a low-grade fibrosarcoma.

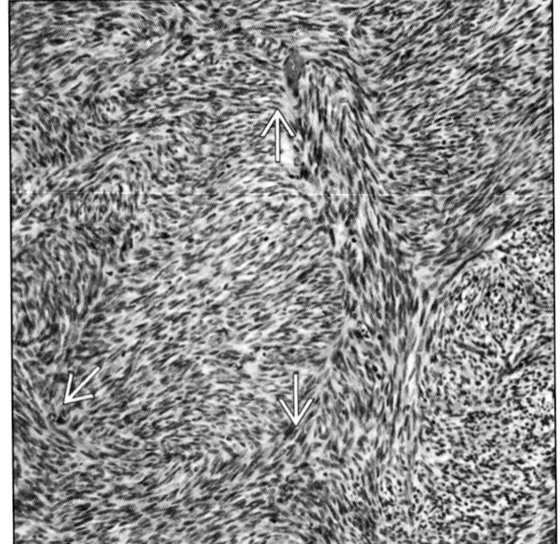

A "herringbone" ➡ pattern yields short, interlacing, acute-angle junctions to the fascicles of tumor cells. The nuclei are short, tapered, and hyperchromatic. There is a syncytial appearance.

TERMINOLOGY

Definitions

- Malignant mesenchymal tumor of fibroblasts

CLINICAL ISSUES

Epidemiology

- Incidence
  - Primary jaw lesions are rare
    - Up to 6% of all primary bone fibrosarcoma
- Age
  - Mean: 2nd to 6th decades
    - Rare before 3rd decade, except for infantile type
- Gender
  - Male > Female (1.6:1)

Site

- Most common in mandible (posterior) > > > maxilla

Presentation

- Swelling is most common symptom
- May be associated with
  - Pain, paresthesia, loose teeth, mucosal ulceration

Treatment

- Surgical approaches
  - Radical surgery is best treatment
    - Gnathic anatomy may complicate surgical technique
- Adjuvant therapy
  - Adjuvant radio- &/or chemotherapy is questionable
    - Often used in high-grade tumors
    - High-grade tumors may have subclinical or microscopic metastases at time of diagnosis
- Drugs
  - Chemotherapy is only palliative
- Radiation
  - Used for unresectable tumors

Prognosis

- Highly dependent on histologic grade and success of complete resection
- Local recurrences may develop and are a prognostic factor
- Overall survival
  - 83% at 10 years in low-grade tumors
  - 34% at 10 years in high-grade tumors

IMAGE FINDINGS

Radiographic Findings

- Radiolucent lesions
  - Geographical, "moth-eaten," or permeative pattern of bone destruction
  - No internal matrix production
  - Soft tissue invasion is detected in up to 86% of cases

MACROSCOPIC FEATURES

General Features

- Usually tan to grayish-white, rubbery, without matrix production

Sections to Be Submitted

- 1 section per cm of tumor, especially at margin

Size

- Range: 3-15 cm

MICROSCOPIC PATHOLOGY

Histologic Features

- Uniform spindle cells distributed in compact, interlacing fascicles
  - "Herringbone": Acute angle intersection of cell bundles
  - Cellularity between and within tumors is variable

FIBROSARCOMA

Key Facts

Terminology
- Malignant mesenchymal tumor of fibroblasts

Clinical Issues
- Mean age: 2nd to 6th decades
- Male > Female (1.6:1)
- Presents with swelling
- Most common in mandible (posterior) > > > maxilla
- Radical surgery is best treatment

Image Findings
- Radiolucent, geographical, "moth-eaten," or permeative bone destruction without matrix production

Microscopic Pathology
- Uniform spindle cells distributed in interlacing fascicles
  - "Herringbone" pattern
- Positive: Vimentin

  - Fusiform cells, centrally placed, hyperchromatic, needle-spaced nuclei
  - Tapered cytoplasm, creating syncytial appearance
- Delicate thin to dense keloid-like collagen deposition

ANCILLARY TESTS

Immunohistochemistry
- Positive: Vimentin
- Negative: Muscle markers
- May have focal immunoreactivity with
  - CD68, CD13, lysozyme, S100 protein, NSE, CD34, CD1, CD2, CD4, CD24, CD30, desmin, EMA

DIFFERENTIAL DIAGNOSIS

Fibromatosis
- Bland cytologic appearance, lacking herringbone pattern and mitoses, with abundant collagen production

Undifferentiated Pleomorphic Sarcoma
- High degree of pleomorphism, lacking herringbone pattern, with vimentin staining only

Leiomyosarcoma
- Interlacing fascicles, ovoid nuclei with "cigar" shape, perinuclear clearing, and muscle markers immunohistochemically

Mucosal Melanoma
- May be spindled, with or without pigment, prominent nucleoli, intranuclear cytoplasmic inclusions, and melanocytic markers

Spindle Cell Squamous Cell Carcinoma
- Direct extension from spindled cell carcinoma, may have epithelial areas and keratin immunoreactivity

GRADING

Low Grade
- Fascicles or herringbone arrangement of spindled cells
- Low to moderate cellularity with mild pleomorphism separated by collagenous stroma, rare mitoses

High Grade
- Increased cellularity, moderate to severe pleomorphism, atypical mitoses, and necrosis

SELECTED REFERENCES

1. Pereira CM et al: Primary intraosseous fibrosarcoma of jaw. Int J Oral Maxillofac Surg. 34(5):579-81, 2005
2. Yamaguchi S et al: Sarcomas of the oral and maxillofacial region: a review of 32 cases in 25 years. Clin Oral Investig. 8(2):52-5, 2004
3. Taconis WK et al: Fibrosarcoma of the jaws. Skeletal Radiol. 15(1):10-3, 1986
4. Slootweg PJ et al: Fibrosarcoma of the jaws. A study of 7 cases. J Maxillofac Surg. 12(4):157-62, 1984

IMAGE GALLERY

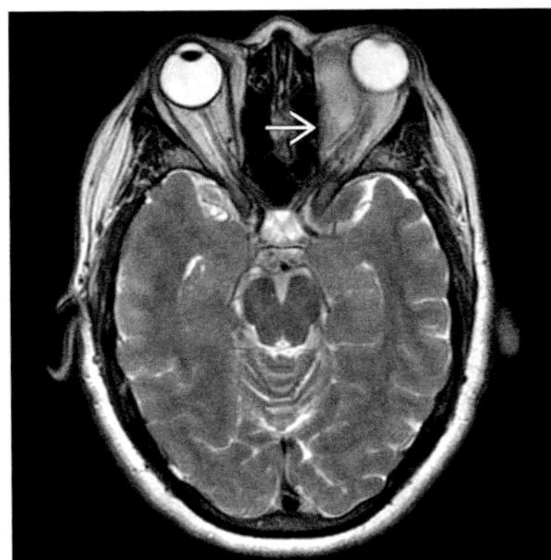

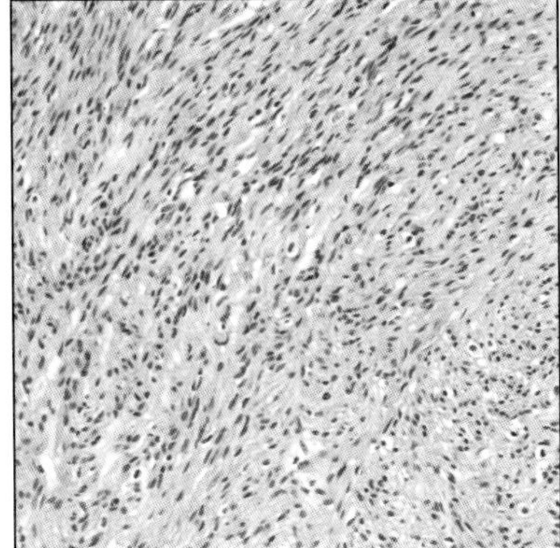

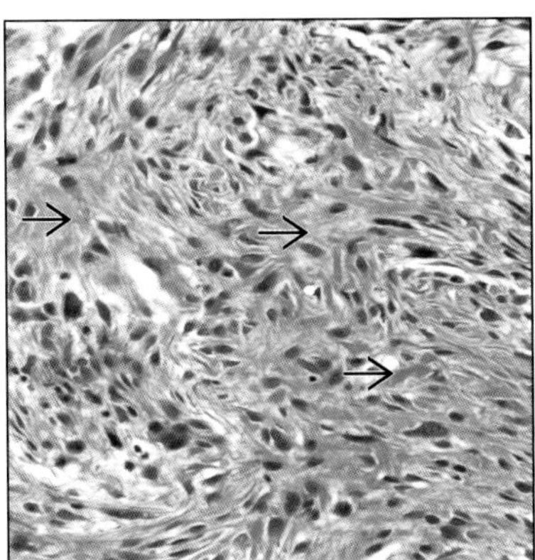

(Left) Axial T2WI MR shows increased heterogeneous signal of a periorbital mass with disruption of the paranasal sinuses ➡. (Center) Fascicles of spindle cells are arranged in a loose bundle. The nuclei are fusiform, surrounded by eosinophilic cytoplasm. The stroma contains collagen with small delicate vessels. (Right) In some fields, the collagen production ➡ can be more noticeable and give a clue as to cell of origin. Mitoses may be present but are often difficult to find; no mitoses are seen in this field.

PLASMA CELL MYELOMA

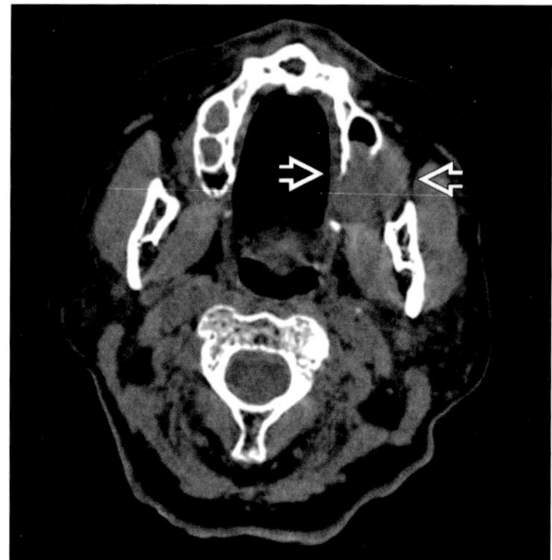

Axial CT image through the maxilla ➡ shows a patient with a recent history of an enlarging maxillary alveolus preventing denture placement. The patient had been treated for multiple myeloma 5 years prior.

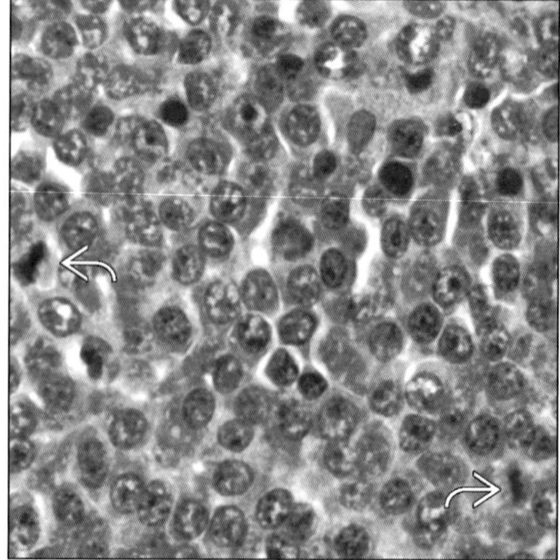

A maxillary soft tissue mass reveals sheets of mature and immature plasma cells characterized by eccentrically placed nuclei and stippled chromatin. Occasional mitoses are seen ➡.

TERMINOLOGY

Abbreviations

- Plasma cell myeloma (PCM)

Synonyms

- Multiple myeloma, plasma cell dyscrasia

Definitions

- Multifocal bone marrow-based plasma cell neoplasm associated with M-protein in serum &/or urine
  - Solitary plasmacytoma of bone (P-bone): Monoclonal population of plasma cells localized to 1 site without bone marrow involvement

CLINICAL ISSUES

Epidemiology

- Incidence
  - Accounts for ~ 1% of all malignant tumors (4/100,000 population/year)
    - Accounts for ~ 10-15% of hematologic malignancies
  - Solitary and extraosseous plasmacytoma each make up 3-5% of plasma cell neoplasms
- Age
  - Plasma cell myeloma: Median age: 70 years
    - Incidence increases with age (> 90% occur over 50 years)
  - P-bone and P-extraosseous: Median age: 55 years
- Gender
  - PCM: Male > Female (1.4:1)
  - P-bone: Male > > Female (3:1)
  - P-extraosseous: Male > > > Female (6:1)
- Ethnicity
  - Black > White (2:1)

Site

- PCM: Generalized bone marrow involvement
- P-bone: Spine, ribs, skull, pelvis
- P-extraosseous: 80% occur in upper respiratory tract (URT) (paranasal sinuses, oropharynx)

Presentation

- Bone pain is most common symptom
- Later symptoms include anemia, renal failure, weakness, headache, neuropathies, visual changes

Laboratory Tests

- M-protein in serum or urine (Bence-Jones protein)
  - Paraproteinemia with monoclonal protein
  - P-bone: M-protein in 24-72% of patients
  - P-extraosseous: M-protein in 20% of patients
- Hypercalcemia, elevated creatinine, hyperuricemia, hypoalbuminemia, high ESR

Natural History

- Up to 2/3 patients with P-bone develop additional lesions or evolve to generalized myeloma
- About 70% of patients with P-extraosseous remain disease free at 10 years

Treatment

- Surgical approaches
  - Debulking of solitary soft tissue disease in URT
- Adjuvant therapy
  - Different combination regimens are used depending on patient condition and tumor risk status
- Radiation
  - P-bone and P-extraosseous: Local radiation therapy
- Bone marrow transplant
  - Stem cell (autologous) transplant used in patients both as first-line treatment and for those who have failed chemotherapy

Prognosis

- Plasma cell myeloma is considered incurable
  - 5-year survival: 25%
- High rates of relapse due to treatment resistance

PLASMA CELL MYELOMA

Key Facts

Terminology
- Multifocal bone marrow-based plasma cell neoplasm associated with M-protein in serum &/or urine

Clinical Issues
- Accounts for 1% of all malignant tumors, 10-15% of hematologic malignancies
- Solitary and extraosseous plasmacytoma each make up 3-5% of plasma cell neoplasms

Microscopic Pathology
- Monotonous sheets of neoplastic plasma cells with little normal host tissue
- Plasma cell morphology generally recognizable unless cells are poorly differentiated (plasmablastic or anaplastic)

Ancillary Tests
- κ/λ light chain restriction to confirm monoclonal population of plasma cells

IMAGE FINDINGS

Radiographic Findings
- Multiple, "punched out" or ragged lytic lesions
- Soft tissue masses seen in P-extraosseous
- MR &/or PET to exclude multifocal lesions

MICROSCOPIC PATHOLOGY

Histologic Features
- Monotonous sheets of neoplastic plasma cells with little normal host tissue
  - Eccentric nuclear placement
  - Accentuated "hof" zone (Golgi apparatus)
  - "Clockface" chromatin distribution
- Plasma cell morphology generally recognizable unless cells are poorly differentiated (plasmablastic or anaplastic)
- Mitoses variable

ANCILLARY TESTS

Immunohistochemistry
- Positive: CD138 is most sensitive and specific plasma cell marker
  - CD79a and CD38 positive in most plasma cells
- κ/λ light chain restriction to confirm monoclonal plasma cell population

Flow Cytometry
- Useful for determining immunophenotype
  - Bone marrow aspirate, small biopsies, or fine needle aspirates can be used
- Ploidy analysis: Hypodiploid has worse prognosis

Cytogenetics
- t(4;14), t(14;16), and 17p- have worse prognosis

Molecular Genetics
- About 1/3 of cases exhibit chromosomal abnormalities, including deletions, trisomies, and translocations

DIFFERENTIAL DIAGNOSIS

Lymphomas with Plasmacytic Differentiation
- Includes MALT and B-cell lymphoma
- Flow cytometry, FISH, and cytogenetics may be required for diagnosis as well as clinical, laboratory, and radiographic correlation

SELECTED REFERENCES

1. Lae ME et al: Myeloma of the jaw bones: a clinicopathologic study of 33 cases. Head Neck. 25(5):373-81, 2003
2. Mendenhall WM et al: Solitary plasmacytoma of bone and soft tissues. Am J Otolaryngol. 24(6):395-9, 2003
3. Nofsinger YC et al: Head and neck manifestations of plasma cell neoplasms. Laryngoscope. 107(6):741-6, 1997

IMAGE GALLERY

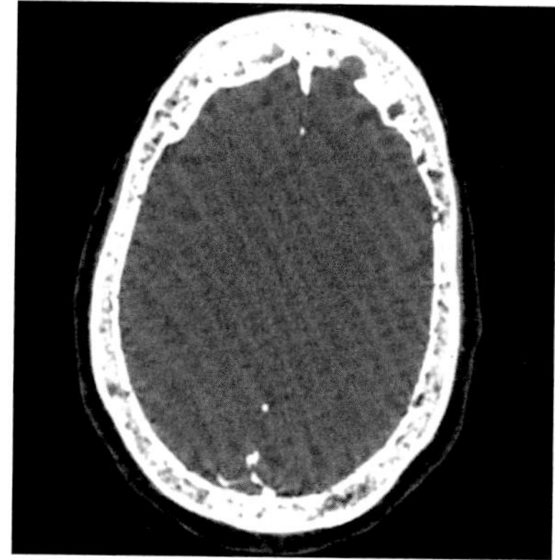

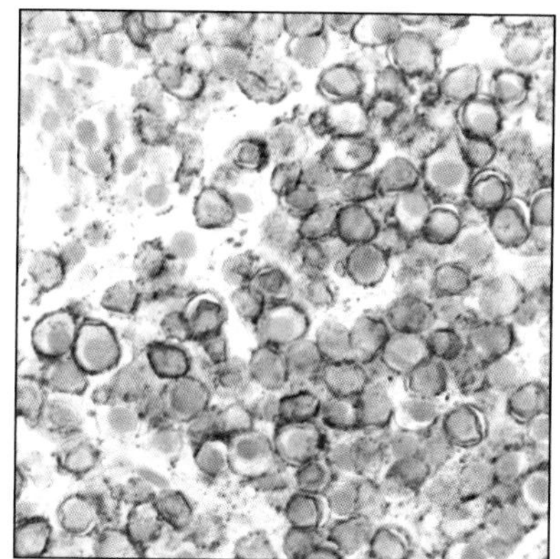

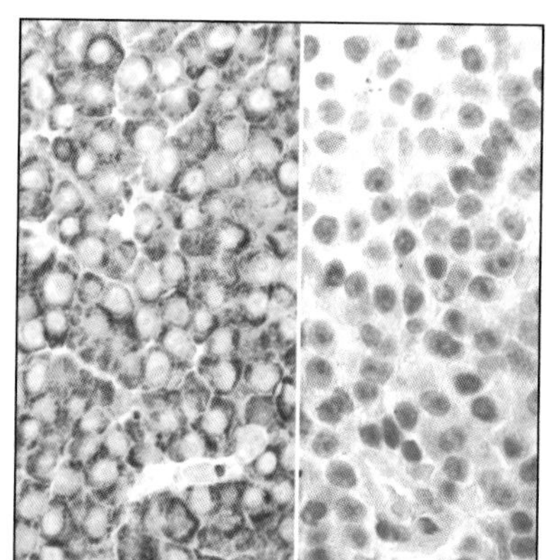

(Left) Axial CT of a skull from a patient with plasma cell myeloma shows multiple "punched out" radiolucencies. ***(Center)*** *CD138 is a highly specific marker for plasma cells and is used to quantitate and differentiate plasma cells. Both cell membrane and cytoplasmic staining can be seen.* ***(Right)*** *There is diffuse cytoplasmic κ light chain immunoreactivity (left) with absent λ light chain reaction (right) confirming the presence of a monoclonal plasma cell population.*

Ear and Temporal Bone

Congenital/Genetic/Hereditary

Infectious

Inflammatory-Immune Dysfunction

Degenerative

Metabolic

Reactive

Benign Neoplasm

Malignant Neoplasm

ACCESSORY TRAGUS

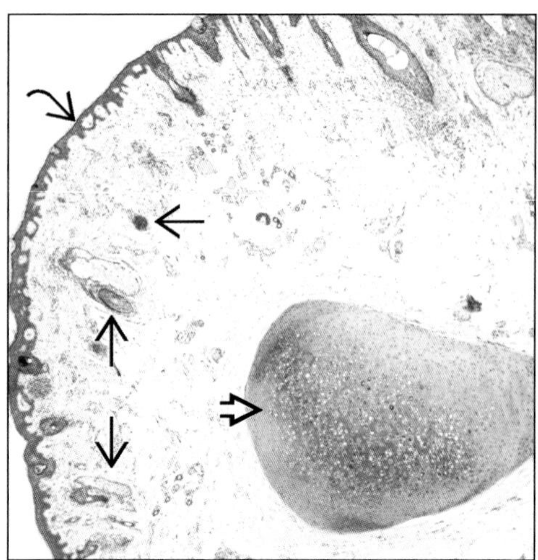

The histology of accessory tragi recapitulates that of the normal external auricle, including skin (squamous epithelium ⇗), cutaneous adnexal structures →, and central core of cartilage ⇨.

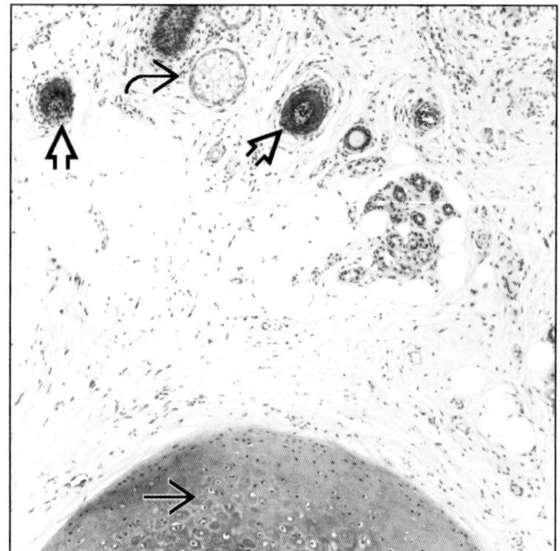

The diagnostic features of accessory tragus that differentiate it from squamous papilloma include cutaneous adnexal structures (sebaceous glands ⇗, hair follicles ⇨) and cartilage →.

TERMINOLOGY

Synonyms

- Supernumerary ears
- Accessory auricle
- Polyotia

Definitions

- Developmental anomaly resulting in presence of lesion recapitulating normal external ear

ETIOLOGY/PATHOGENESIS

Developmental Anomaly

- Thought to be 2nd branchial arch anomaly
  - May occur with other anomalies including
    - Cleft palate
    - Cleft lip
    - Mandibular hypoplasia
  - May occur in association with Goldenhar syndrome
    - Also known as oculo-auriculo-vertebral (OAV) syndrome
    - Term used interchangeably with hemifacial microsomia
    - Rare congenital defect
    - Characterized by incomplete development of ear, nose, soft palate, lip, mandible
    - Associated with anomalous development of 1st branchial arch and 2nd branchial arch
  - May also occur independent of other congenital anomalies

CLINICAL ISSUES

Epidemiology

- Age
  - Neonates
- Gender
  - Equal gender distribution

Site

- On skin surface, often anterior to auricle
- Unilateral or bilateral

Presentation

- Skin-covered nodules or papules

Treatment

- Surgical approaches
  - Simple surgical excision is curative

MACROSCOPIC FEATURES

General Features

- Nodules or papules
  - Sessile or pedunculated
  - Soft or cartilaginous

MICROSCOPIC PATHOLOGY

Histologic Features

- Recapitulation of normal external auricle
- Includes
  - Skin
  - Cutaneous adnexal structures
  - Central core of cartilage

DIFFERENTIAL DIAGNOSIS

Squamous Papilloma

- Benign tumor of squamous epithelium
- Exophytic proliferation of benign squamous epithelium with fibrovascular cores
- Lacks cutaneous adnexa and cartilage

ACCESSORY TRAGUS

Key Facts

Terminology
- Developmental anomaly resulting in presence of lesion recapitulating normal external ear

Etiology/Pathogenesis
- Thought to be 2nd branchial arch anomaly
- May occur with cleft palate or lip, mandibular hypoplasia, or other anomalies, such as oculo-auriculo-vertebral dysplasia (Goldenhar syndrome)
- May also occur independent of other congenital anomalies

Clinical Issues
- Simple surgical excision is curative

Microscopic Pathology
- Recapitulation of normal external auricle
  - Includes skin, cutaneous adnexal structures, and central core of cartilage

Teratoma
- Neoplasm characterized by tissue elements of all 3 germ layers including
  - Ectoderm
    - Cutaneous epithelium
    - Central and peripheral nervous system
    - Others
  - Endoderm may include
    - Columnar epithelium
    - Ciliated respiratory epithelium
    - Gastrointestinal epithelia, including glands
  - Mesoderm
    - Cartilage
    - Bone
    - Adipose tissue
    - Muscle
    - Others

DIAGNOSTIC CHECKLIST

Pathologic Interpretation Pearls
- Recapitulation of normal external auricle including
  - Skin
  - Cutaneous adnexal structures
  - Central core of cartilage
- In contrast to teratoma, lacks tissue elements of all 3 germ layers

SELECTED REFERENCES

1. Pan B et al: Surgical management of polyotia. J Plast Reconstr Aesthet Surg. 63(8):1283-8, 2010
2. Lam J et al: Multiple accessory tragi and hemifacial microsomia. Pediatr Dermatol. 24(6):657-8, 2007
3. Konaş E et al: Goldenhar complex with atypical associated anomalies: is the spectrum still widening? J Craniofac Surg. 17(4):669-72, 2006
4. Jansen T et al: Accessory tragus: report of two cases and review of the literature. Pediatr Dermatol. 17(5):391-4, 2000
5. Ban M et al: Hair follicle nevi and accessory tragi: variable quantity of adipose tissue in connective tissue framework. Pediatr Dermatol. 14(6):433-6, 1997
6. Heffner DK et al: Pharyngeal dermoids ("hairy polyps") as accessory auricles. Ann Otol Rhinol Laryngol. 105(10):819-24, 1996
7. Jones S et al: Accessory auricles: unusual sites and the preferred treatment option. Arch Pediatr Adolesc Med. 150(7):769-70, 1996
8. Cosman BC: Bilateral accessory tragus. Cutis. 51(3):199-200, 1993
9. Tadini G et al: Familial occurrence of isolated accessory tragi. Pediatr Dermatol. 10(1):26-8, 1993
10. Gao JZ et al: A survey of accessory auricle anomaly. Pedigree analysis of seven cases. Arch Otolaryngol Head Neck Surg. 116(10):1194-6, 1990
11. Resnick KI et al: Accessory tragi and associated syndromes involving the first branchial arch. J Dermatol Surg Oncol. 7(1):39-41, 1981
12. Brownstein MH et al: Accessory tragi. Arch Dermatol. 104(6):625-31, 1971

IMAGE GALLERY

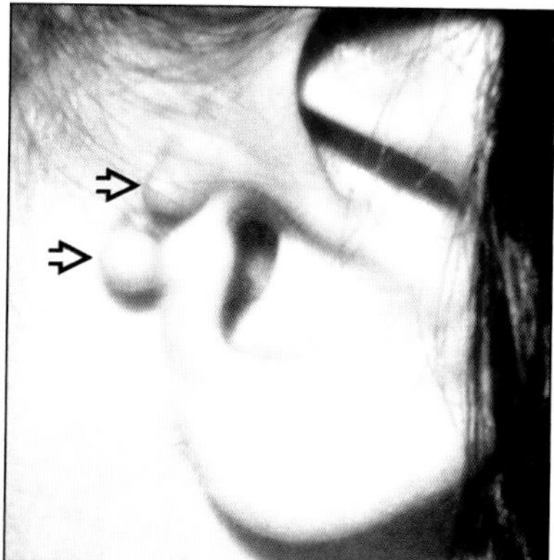

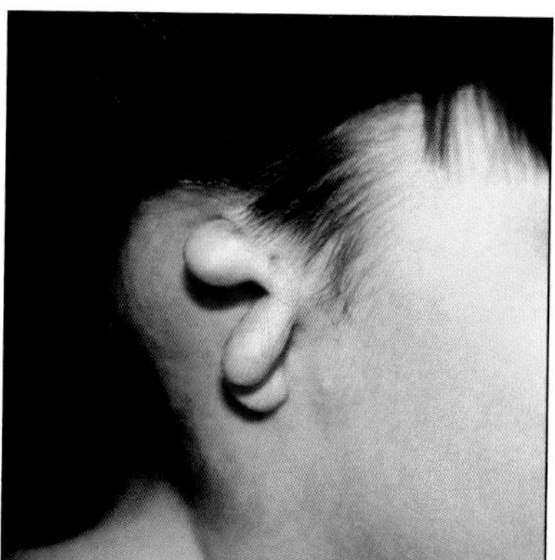

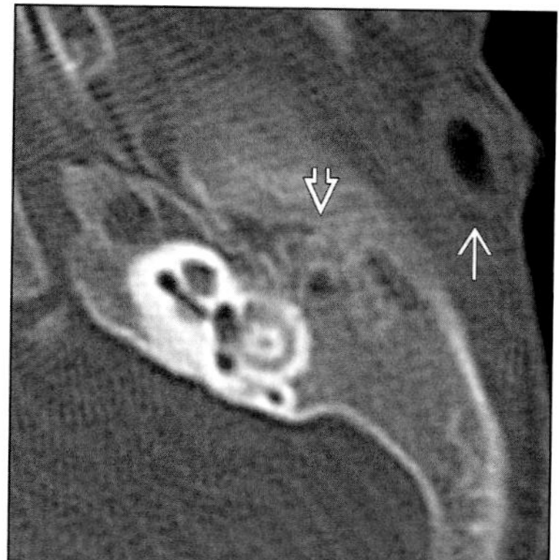

(Left) Accessory tragus appears as pedunculated, skin-covered papules ⇨ located on the skin surface anterior to the auricle. *(Center)* Accessory tragi may occur with other anomalies, including severe microtia. *(Right)* Axial temporal bone CT shows severe microtia ➡ and complete bony atresia ➡ with small rudimentary middle ear cavity, no identifiable ossicles, and normal inner ear structures.

ENCEPHALOCELE

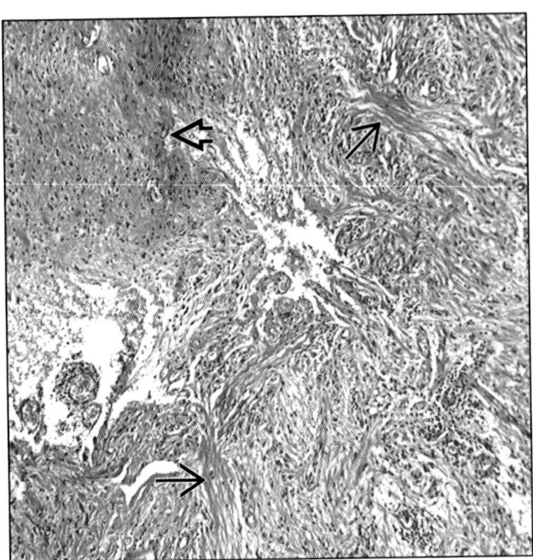

This encephalocele shows fibrosis ⇒ and intermixed gliosis ⇨. Inflammatory cells are sparse. Ear encephaloceles often have associated otitis media.

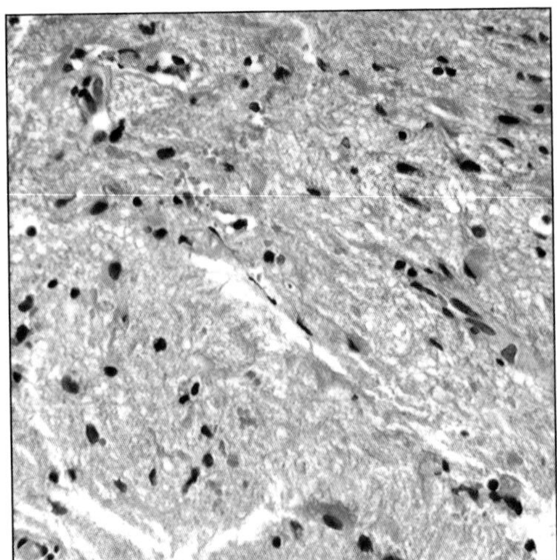

Hematoxylin & eosin shows the fibrillar neural matrix material and reactive fibroblasts. This appearance can sometimes mimic fibrosis. Careful evaluation shows the neural nature of the lesion.

TERMINOLOGY

Synonyms

- Neuroglial heterotopia, extracranial glioma, brain fungus, leptomeningeal neuroglial lesion
- Sequestered encephaloceles, glial choristomas, hamartoma, monodermal teratoma

Definitions

- Encephalocele represents herniation of brain tissue and leptomeninges through a bony defect of skull, maintaining continuity with cranial cavity
- Heterotopic neuroglial tissue defined as a mass of mature brain tissue isolated from cranial cavity or spinal canal

ETIOLOGY/PATHOGENESIS

Developmental Anomaly

- Defect in cranial bones or failure of cranial sutures to close
  - May be related to glial heterotopia if CNS connection has been resorbed

Iatrogenic or Acquired

- Surgery, trauma, postinfectious/inflammatory may result in encephalocele formation
- Most nonmidline lesions interpreted to be acquired

CLINICAL ISSUES

Epidemiology

- Incidence
  - Uncommon, but increased in postsurgical, traumatic, and infectious setting
- Age
  - Anatomic site of development associated with age
    - Nonmidline lesions develop in older patients (mean: 50 years)
    - Midline lesions develop at young age (< 2 years)

Site

- Nonmidline: Middle ear, mastoid bone, orbit, scalp, neck soft tissues
- Midline: Nasal cavity, nasopharynx, palate, tongue

Presentation

- Depends on anatomic site of involvement
- Ear lesions frequently associated with chronic otitis media &/or mastoiditis
  - Deafness, hearing loss, dizziness, tympanic membrane perforation, CSF otorrhea
- Nasal lesions frequently associated with rhinorrhea, obstruction, or difficulty breathing
- Previous surgery or trauma identified in many (especially older patients)

Laboratory Tests

- Test fluid for glucose and protein to exclude CSF

Treatment

- At surgery, CNS leak or bony abnormality documented to prove CNS connection
- Clinician and pathologist must communicate about exact location and relationship to dura or nerves

Prognosis

- Excellent outcome with surgery alone, although CNS connection needs to be documented to preclude postoperative CNS leak, infection, and herniation (increased intracranial pressure)

IMAGE FINDINGS

Radiographic Findings

- Must be done to identify relationship to CNS
- Even if "negative," CNS connection frequently identified at surgery

ENCEPHALOCELE

Key Facts

Terminology
- Encephalocele represents herniation of brain tissue

Clinical Issues
- Develops in ear and temporal bone as well as nasal cavity and nasopharynx
- Due to defect in cranial bones, failure of cranial sutures to close, surgery or trauma

Image Findings
- Must be performed to identify relationship to CNS

Microscopic Pathology
- Glial heterotopia indistinguishable pathologically from encephalocele
- Variable proportions of neurons and glia
- Chronic inflammatory cells (lymphocytes and macrophages) present

MICROSCOPIC PATHOLOGY

Histologic Features
- Glial heterotopia indistinguishable pathologically from encephalocele
- Variable proportions of neurons and glia
- Associated reactive gliosis
- Chronic inflammatory cells (lymphocytes and macrophages) present in nearly all cases
  - Encephalocele may be seen in association with otitis media
- Leptomeninges, ependyma, and choroid plexus nearly always absent
- Isolated glandular elements (apocrine, mucoserous glands native to regions), skin, and bone may be identified entrapped by process
- Keratin debris from concurrent cholesteatoma in middle ear lesions can be seen
- Tympanic membrane or eustachian tube epithelium must not be mistaken for teratomatous elements

ANCILLARY TESTS

Histochemistry
- Masson trichrome stains glial tissue red and collagen/fibrosis blue

Immunohistochemistry
- Positive
  - GFAP and S100 protein in glial tissue
  - Neurofilament protein in neuronal tissue
- Negative: Keratin

DIFFERENTIAL DIAGNOSIS

Teratoma
- Mature glial tissue may predominate, but tissue from all 3 germ cell primordia should be identified

Glioma
- Neoplastic proliferation with ↑ cellularity, disorganized growth, usually without fibrosis or inflammatory cells

Meningioma
- Epithelioid cells showing whorled and syncytial architecture, possible psammoma bodies
- Positive: EMA

Schwannoma
- Antoni A and B areas, spindle cell proliferation, elongated nuclei, palisading

SELECTED REFERENCES

1. Heffner DK: Brain in the middle ear or nasal cavity: heterotopia or encephalocele? Ann Diagn Pathol. 8(4):252-7, 2004
2. Gyure KA et al: A clinicopathological study of 15 patients with neuroglial heterotopias and encephaloceles of the middle ear and mastoid region. Laryngoscope. 110(10 Pt 1):1731-5, 2000

IMAGE GALLERY

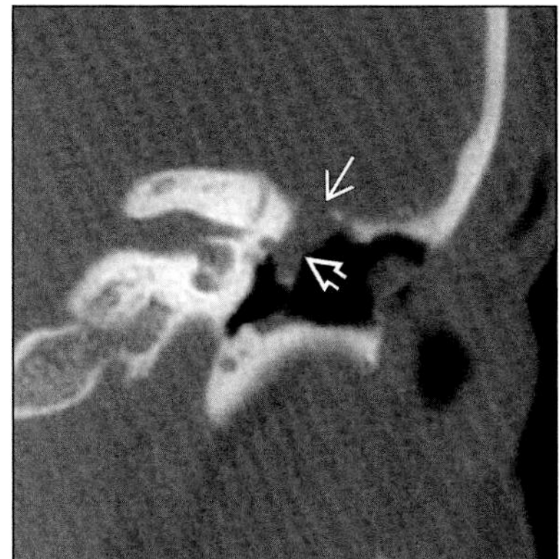

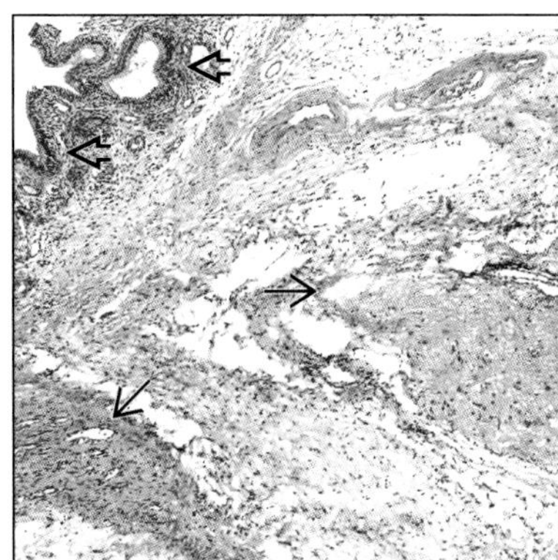

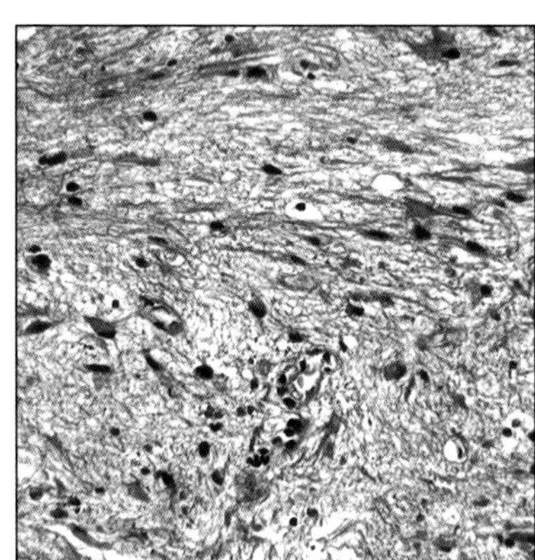

(Left) *A temporal bone CT reveals a pedunculated encephalocele ➡ hanging through a focal dehiscence of tegmen tympani ➡. This developed as a postoperative complication.* ***(Center)*** *A nasal cavity encephalocele demonstrates respiratory mucosa ⇨ and shows fibrosis → surrounding gliotic neural tissue. Glial heterotopia would be in the differential diagnosis.* ***(Right)*** *Masson trichrome stain shows very little fibrosis (blue) around the vessels or in the background tissue. The slightly eosinophilic population is glial tissue.*

FIRST BRANCHIAL CLEFT ANOMALY

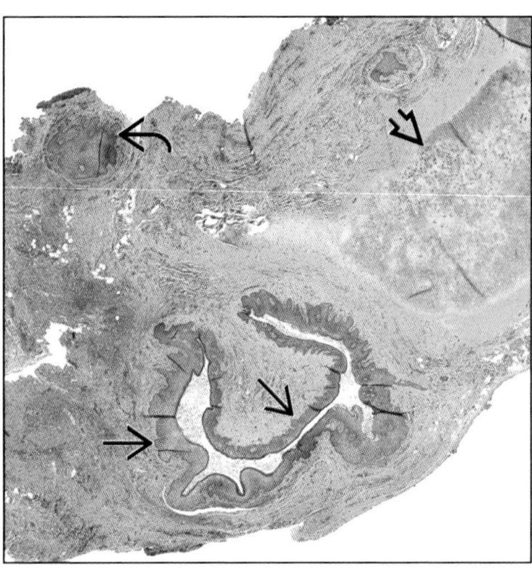

A fistula ➔ is lined by a keratinizing squamous lining, and cartilage ⇨ is identified in the immediately associated tissue. Note the "blind" ↗ ending of the fistula.

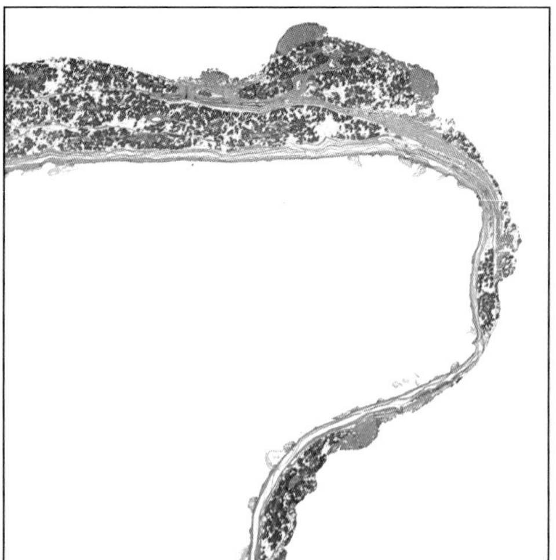

There is a cystic space within the superficial lobe of the parotid gland in a patient with a fistula extending to the external auditory canal. Histologically this could mimic a primary salivary gland lesion.

TERMINOLOGY

Abbreviations

- First branchial cleft cyst (1st BCC)

Synonyms

- Cervicoaural cyst
- 1st branchial apparatus remnant

Definitions

- Spectrum of benign, congenital lesions occurring in parotid, posterior submandibular space, or preauricular region as fistula, sinus, or cyst,
  - Results from incomplete fusion of 1st and 2nd branchial arches, with persistence of ventral component of 1st branchial cleft
  - This discussion excludes all other branchial apparatus (2nd to 4th) anomalies

ETIOLOGY/PATHOGENESIS

Developmental Anomaly

- Persistence of 1st branchial apparatus
  - 1st branchial cleft gives rise to external auditory canal (EAC)
  - 1st branchial arch gives rise to mandible, muscles of mastication, CN V, incus body, and head of malleus
  - 1st branchial pouch gives rise to eustachian tube, middle ear cavity, and mastoid air cells
- Branchial cleft cyst has no internal (pharyngeal) or external (cutaneous) communication (blind pouch)
- Branchial cleft fistula has internal and external connections from EAC to skin
- Branchial cleft sinus opens either internally (rare) or externally, with a closed-end blind pouch

CLINICAL ISSUES

Epidemiology

- Incidence
  - Uncommon
    - < 10% of all branchial cleft anomalies
    - About 2/3 of 1st branchial cleft remnants present as fistulas and sinuses rather than cysts
    - Type II > > Type I
  - Periauricular with sinuses/fistulas in anterolateral neck or external auditory canal
- Age
  - Most discovered in early childhood (< 10 years)
  - Type I anomalies usually seen in adults
    - Range: 13-81 years
  - Type II anomalies usually < 1 year of age
- Gender
  - Female > Male (2:1)

Site

- Periauricular: Preauricular and immediately postauricular, frequently involving parotid gland
- Not associated with **pretragal** cysts, pits, or sinuses

Presentation

- Painless cyst
- Soft, compressible mass
- Recurrent, preauricular or periparotid swelling
- Majority present as sinus or fistula rather than cyst
- Draining sinus tract on periauricular skin (type II)
- Chronic, unexplained otorrhea or purulent drainage from ear canal
- May have recurrent parotid gland abscess
- Rare association with congenital cholesteatoma
- Rare syndrome association: Branchiootorenal syndrome (Melnick-Fraser syndrome)

Natural History

- May wax and wane with upper respiratory tract infection

FIRST BRANCHIAL CLEFT ANOMALY

Key Facts

Terminology

- Spectrum of benign, congenital lesions occurring in parotid, posterior submandibular space, or preauricular region as fistula, sinus, or cyst, resulting from incomplete fusion of 1st and 2nd branchial arches, with persistence of ventral component of 1st branchial cleft

Clinical Issues

- < 10% of all branchial cleft anomalies
- Most discovered in early childhood (< 10 years)
- Recurrent, preauricular or periparotid swelling
- Draining sinus tract on periauricular skin (type II)
  - Chronic, unexplained otorrhea or purulent drainage from ear canal
- Complete excision of lesion(s); use antibiotic treatment prior to surgery (if infected)

Image Findings

- Cystic mass around pinna (type I) or extending from external auditory canal (EAC) to angle of mandible (type II: Using Arnot criteria)

Microscopic Pathology

- Cyst, sinus, or fistula lined by stratified squamous or ciliated respiratory epithelium
- Separated into 2 **histologic** types by Work
  - Type I: Epithelium only
  - Type II: Epithelium with cutaneous adnexal structures &/or cartilage

Top Differential Diagnoses

- Benign lymphoepithelial cyst, epidermal inclusion cyst, metastatic cystic squamous cell carcinoma, mucoepidermoid carcinoma

- May undergo repeat incision and drainage, with recurrence

Treatment

- Options, risks, complications
  - Recurrence if incompletely resected
  - Facial nerve at risk during surgery
    - Pay extra attention for young patients (< 6 months), those with fistulous tracts, and in patients with anomalous tract openings
  - Stenosis of external auditory canal or middle ear due to ear canal defect
- Surgical approaches
  - Complete excision of lesion(s) (cyst, sinus, &/or fistula); use antibiotic treatment prior to surgery (if infected)
  - Easily dissected
    - Except if there has been repeated infection
  - Must include termination of pouch at EAC between cartilaginous and bony portions
  - Type II
    - May split facial nerve trunk, with medial or lateral placement of CN VII
    - May be difficult to excise
    - Facial nerve monitoring suggested during surgery

Prognosis

- Completely benign without any malignant potential
- Secondary infection of cyst, sinus, or fistula
- Facial nerve injury must be avoided
- Recurrences if incompletely excised, or managed with incision and drainage procedures

IMAGE FINDINGS

General Features

- Best study is contrast-enhanced CT (high resolution) or MR
- Cystic mass around pinna (type I) or extending from external auditory canal (EAC) to angle of mandible (type II)
- Well-circumscribed, unilocular ovoid cyst
- Separated into **anatomic** sites based on Arnot
- Type I: Periauricular (less common)
  - Anterior, below or posterior to pinna
  - Most commonly preauricular
- Type II: Periparotid (most common)
  - Superficial parotid and parapharyngeal spaces

CT Findings

- Well-circumscribed, nonenhancing or rim-enhancing, low-density mass
- When infected may have thick enhancing rim
- Type I: Lesion may "beak" toward bony-cartilaginous junction of EAC
- Type II: Superficial, parotid, or parapharyngeal space with deep projection "beaking" to bony-cartilaginous junction of EAC

MACROSCOPIC FEATURES

General Features

- Discrete cysts, sinuses, or fistulas, or combination of these structures
- Cyst contents: Viscous, cloudy fluid to purulent and necrotic material (pus when infected)
- Cartilage may be identified
- Sinus tract extending from external auditory canal or periauricular skin

Size

- Variable; up to 4 cm

MICROSCOPIC PATHOLOGY

Histologic Features

- Cyst, sinus, or fistula lined by stratified squamous or ciliated respiratory epithelium
- Lymphoid aggregates may be present in cyst wall
- Separated into 2 **histologic** types by Work
  - Type I
    - Usually cyst rather than sinus or fistula

FIRST BRANCHIAL CLEFT ANOMALY

- Epithelium only, lined by either stratified squamous epithelium or ciliated respiratory epithelium
  - Type II
    - Cyst with sinus or fistula between neck and ear canal
    - Lined by either stratified squamous epithelium or ciliated respiratory epithelium
    - Contains **cutaneous adnexal structures &/or cartilage** (mesodermal component)
    - May need to do serial sections or deeper levels to identify cartilage or adnexal tissue
- Cyst wall may contain lymphoid aggregates, sometimes with germinal centers
- If infected, epithelium is largely denuded, replaced by heavily inflamed granulation tissue

ANCILLARY TESTS

Cytology

- Fine needle aspiration is recommended in evaluation of all neck cysts
  - Usually of residual cyst post antibiotic therapy
- Thick, yellow, pus-like material is aspirated
- Smears are generally cellular
- Comprised of anucleate squames and mature squamous epithelium
  - Columnar respiratory type cells are less common
- Amorphous debris often associated with macrophages
- Lymphoid infiltrate, including plasma cells
- Adnexal structures usually not aspirated

Immunohistochemistry

- p16(-)

Cytogenetics

- No known genetic predispositions

DIFFERENTIAL DIAGNOSIS

Benign Lymphoepithelial Cyst

- Intimate blending of epithelium with lymphoid tissue
- Parotid gland involvement primarily: HIV-associated if bilateral
- No sinus or fistula

Epidermal Inclusion Cyst

- Cyst containing keratin debris and lined by squamous epithelium
- Impossible to separate without clinical information, including exclusion of sinus or fistula

Folliculitis/Abscess

- Superficial dermis based
- Centered on hair or follicle structures
- Lacks sinus, fistula, or well-developed cyst

Metastatic Cystic Squamous Cell Carcinoma

- Jugulo-digastric lymph node most commonly affected
- Unilocular cyst
- Very thick, well-developed capsule
- Subcapsular sinus, medullary zone and interfollicular zones usually identified
- Ribbon-like distribution of atypical epithelium
- Lack of maturation, cellular enlargement, mitoses
- Pleomorphism is often limited and subtle
- Primary tumor usually identified in Waldeyer ring area
  - Tonsil, base of tongue, nasopharynx
  - Often nonkeratinizing and p16(+)
- For practical purposes, primary branchiogenic carcinoma does not exist!

Mucoepidermoid Carcinoma

- Multicystic malignancy of salivary gland (parotid in this setting)
- Epidermoid, transitional, and mucocytes blended together
- Invasion frequently present (capsule, vessel, nerve)
- Cytologic atypia usually easy to identify, although it does not have to be extensive
- Mitoses can be seen

STAGING

Arnot (Anatomic)

- Type I: Cyst or sinus in parotid gland; adulthood
- Type II: Cyst or sinus in anterior cervical triangle communicating with EAC; childhood

Work (Histology & Embryology)

- Type I: Ectodermal origin only; tend to be preauricular, parallel to EAC, with or without sinus tract
- Type II: Ectodermal and mesodermal origin; tend to be posterior and inferior to angle of mandible, with sinus tract to bone/cartilage junction of EAC (most common)

SELECTED REFERENCES

1. Martinez Del Pero M et al: Presentation of first branchial cleft anomalies: the Sheffield experience. J Laryngol Otol. 121(5):455-9, 2007
2. D'Souza AR et al: Updating concepts of first branchial cleft defects: a literature review. Int J Pediatr Otorhinolaryngol. 62(2):103-9, 2002
3. Triglia JM et al: First branchial cleft anomalies: a study of 39 cases and a review of the literature. Arch Otolaryngol Head Neck Surg. 124(3):291-5, 1998
4. Doi O et al: Branchial remnants: a review of 58 cases. J Pediatr Surg. 23(9):789-92, 1988
5. Harnsberger HR et al: Branchial cleft anomalies and their mimics: computed tomographic evaluation. Radiology. 152(3):739-48, 1984
6. Belenky WM et al: First branchial cleft anomalies. Laryngoscope. 90(1):28-39, 1980
7. Aronsohn RS et al: Anomalies of the first branchial cleft. Arch Otolaryngol. 102(12):737-40, 1976
8. Gaisford JC et al: First branchial cleft cysts and sinuses. Plast Reconstr Surg. 55(3):299-304, 1975
9. Work WP: Newer concepts of first branchial cleft defects. Laryngoscope. 82(9):1581-93, 1972
10. Arnot RS: Defects of the first branchial cleft. S Afr J Surg. 9(2):93-8, 1971

Clinical, Radiographic, and Microscopic Features

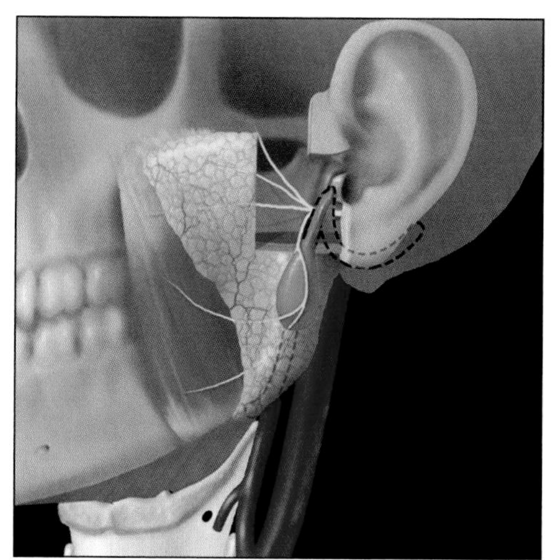

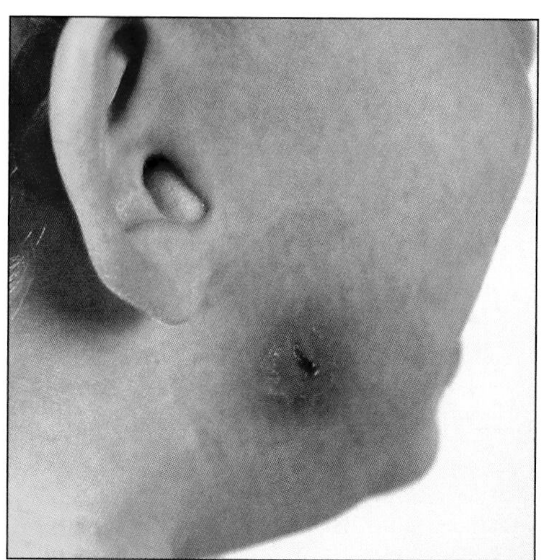

(Left) *Graphic shows the intimate association with the facial nerve (yellow) and the parotid gland with a 1st BCC. The tract of a sinus or fistula involves the EAC and can continue to the hyoid bone or show a retroauricular extension (dotted lines).* ***(Right)*** *This young person demonstrates a cutaneous opening at the angle of the mandible. The opening continued as a sinus, part of a type II 1st branchial cleft anomaly. Erythema suggests recurrent infection. (Courtesy J. Friendberg, MD.)*

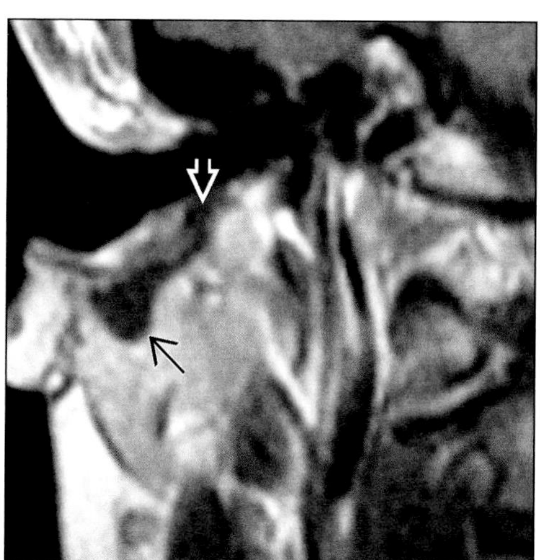

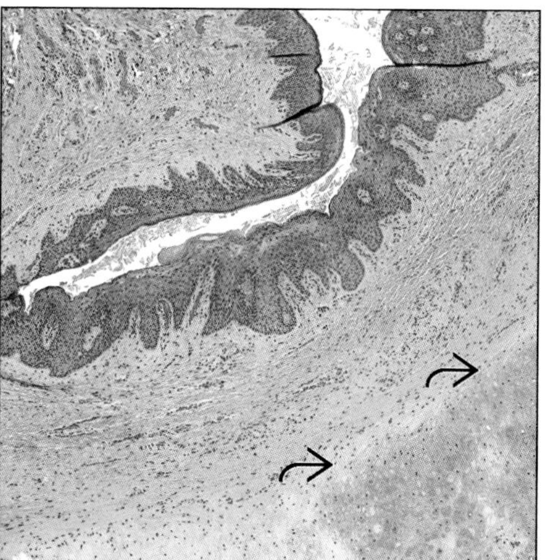

(Left) *Coronal T1WI MR with contrast shows a type I BCC ➙ immediately below and parallel to the EAC and superficial to CN VII, with a tract to the EAC at the confluence of the cartilaginous and bony portions ➙. This is a characteristic finding.* ***(Right)*** *The fistula or sinus is lined by either keratinizing squamous epithelium (as in this case) or by respiratory type epithelium. The presence of cartilage ➚ helps to confirm a Work type II lesion. There is no inflammation in this case.*

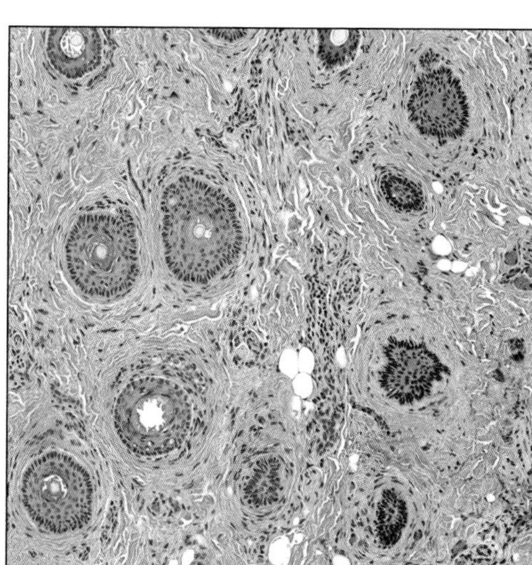

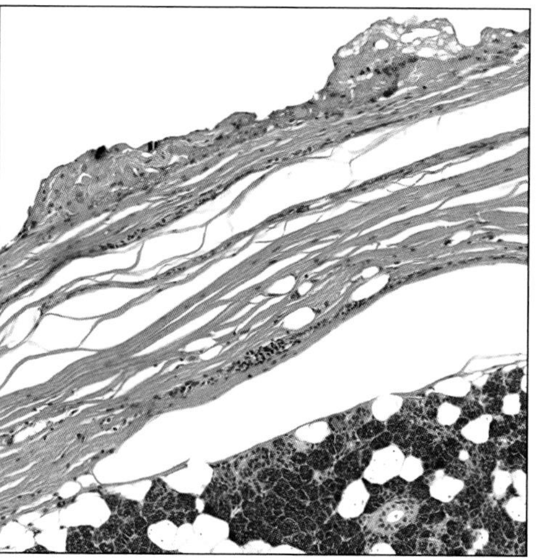

(Left) *The presence of skin adnexal structures in the form of hair shafts, follicular structures, or pilosebaceous units are frequently identified within the cyst wall or immediately adjacent to it in a Work type II anomaly.* ***(Right)*** *The parotid gland tissue is separated from the cyst by a capsule. The predominantly keratinized squamous epithelium is partially disrupted. There is no inflammation. These findings may mimic primary salivary gland cysts.*

OTITIS MEDIA

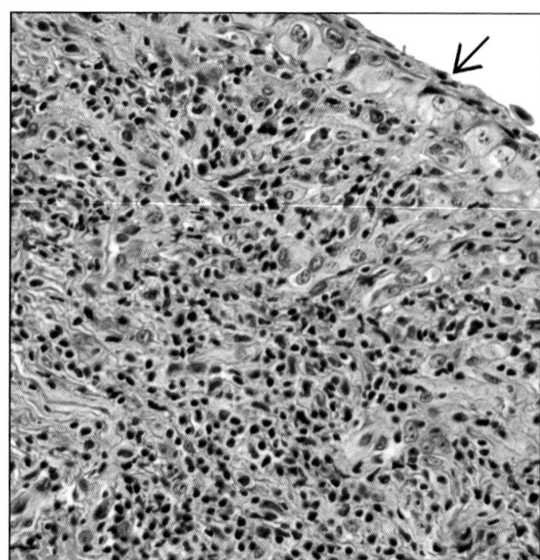

COM shows a low cuboidal surface epithelium ⇒ subtended by a rich inflammatory cell infiltrate of predominantly chronic inflammatory elements, including lymphocytes, plasma cells, and eosinophils.

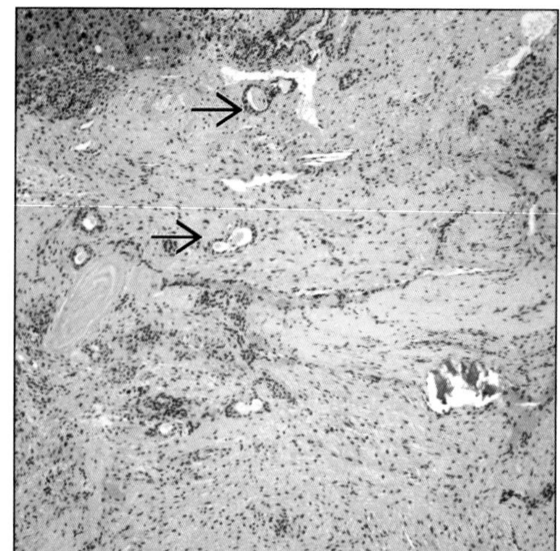

This case of COM shows very heavy and dense fibrosis, chronic inflammation, and epithelial inclusions ⇒. The epithelial inclusions are often misinterpreted as a tumor but are actually a metaplastic process.

TERMINOLOGY

Definitions

- Acute otitis media (AOM): Viral or bacterial infection of middle ear
- Chronic otitis media (COM): Persistent infection or inflammation of middle ear and mastoid air cells

ETIOLOGY/PATHOGENESIS

Environmental Exposure

- Environmental factors include
  - High moisture (swimming, sweating, humidity)
    - Macerates canal skin, elevates pH, removes protective cerumen layer
  - Trauma related to mechanical removal of cerumen yielding skin breakdown
    - Cotton buds, fingernails, hearing aids, ear plugs, paper clips, match sticks
  - Other factors: Frequent upper respiratory tract infections (URI), bottle-feeding, pacifier use, daycare attendance

Infectious Agents

- *Streptococcus pneumoniae* and *Haemophilus influenzae* most common cause of AOM (60-80%)
  - Penicillin-resistant *S. pneumoniae*: Most common cause of recurrent/persistent AOM
  - Spontaneous resolution more common with *H. influenzae* than *S. pneumoniae*
- *Moraxella catarrhalis*

Host Risk Factors

- Age, race, craniofacial abnormalities, gastroesophageal reflux, presence of adenoids, genetic predisposition

Pathogenesis

- Allergy or URI causes congestion
- Obstruction of eustachian tube results in accumulation of secretions
  - Due to swelling of nasal/nasopharynx mucosa
  - Eustachian tube dysfunction
- Secondary infection of effusion
  - Children with recurrent otitis media might lack sufficient secretory immunoglobulin A (IgA)
- Inflammation results in cytokine production
  - Cytokines can induce upregulation of mucin genes, increasing middle ear mucin production
  - Altered viscosity of middle ear effusion subsequently impairs mucociliary clearance

CLINICAL ISSUES

Epidemiology

- Incidence
  - High incidence: 30-35,000,000 cases/year
    - 3% of all patient visits
- Age
  - Peak: 6-12 months
    - Lower peak: 4-5 years
    - ~ 60% of children < 1 year old will have had AOM
  - Adults: < 20% of all AOM patients

Site

- Middle ear by definition
  - Tympanic membrane (TM) perforation may develop, extending into external auditory canal (EAC)

Presentation

- Symptoms are frequently nonspecific
  - Fever, irritability, pulling ears, headache, cough, rhinitis, listlessness, anorexia, vomiting, diarrhea
  - Similar to upper respiratory tract infection
- Otorrhea or middle ear effusion
  - Effusion detected by pneumatic otoscopy
    - Bulging, opaque, erythematous TM, possibly with perforation
- COM: Persistent or recurrent otorrhea through perforated tympanic membrane, thickened granular mucosa, cholesteatoma

OTITIS MEDIA

Key Facts

Terminology
- AOM: Viral or bacterial infection of middle ear
- COM: Persistent infection or inflammation of middle ear

Etiology/Pathogenesis
- High moisture (swimming, sweating, humidity) and skin trauma/breakdown
- *S. pneumoniae* and *H. influenzae* most common cause of AOM (60-80%)

Clinical Issues
- High incidence: 30-35,000,000 cases/year
- Peak age: 6-12 months
- Symptoms are frequently nonspecific
- 70-90% of AOMs resolve spontaneously within 14 days

Microscopic Pathology
- Chronic inflammation, dense fibrosis, epithelial inclusions (tunnel clusters)

- Adults: Present with otalgia, ear drainage, decreased acuity, sore throat

Treatment
- Options, risks, complications
  - 70-90% of AOMs resolve spontaneously within 14 days
    - Potential complications: TM perforation, otitis externa, mastoiditis, labyrinthitis, meningitis, vestibular dysfunction
- Surgical approaches
  - Tympanocentesis and culture in limited circumstances
    - Toxic patient, failed multiple courses of antibiotics, immune deficient
  - Myringotomy with or without ventilation tubes
  - Adenoidectomy
- Drugs
  - Wide variety used, but amoxicillin used most frequently (specific exclusions apply)

MICROSCOPIC PATHOLOGY

Histologic Features
- Arc of development: Edema, hyperemia, neutrophilic infiltrate, hemorrhage, periosteal thickening, cuboidal cell metaplasia
- Chronic inflammation
- Dense fibrosis
- Glandular metaplasia

ANCILLARY TESTS

Cytogenetics
- Recurrent OM associated with immunoglobulin markers, including allotype G2m-23 and HLA-A2

DIFFERENTIAL DIAGNOSIS

Middle Ear Adenoma
- a.k.a. neuroendocrine adenoma of middle ear (NAME)
- Infiltrating glandular neoplasm, biphasic epithelial appearance, no inflammation

Otic Polyp
- External auditory canal, polypoid mass, chronic inflammatory cells

SELECTED REFERENCES

1. Gould JM et al: Otitis media. Pediatr Rev. 31(3):102-16, 2010
2. Vergison A et al: Otitis media and its consequences: beyond the earache. Lancet Infect Dis. 10(3):195-203, 2010
3. Granström G: Middle ear infections. Periodontol 2000. 2009 Feb;49:179-93. Review. Retraction in: Periodontol 2000. 51:276, 2009
4. Morris PS et al: Acute and chronic otitis media. Pediatr Clin North Am. 56(6):1383-99, 2009
5. Vergison A: Microbiology of otitis media: a moving target. Vaccine. 26 Suppl 7:G5-10, 2008

IMAGE GALLERY

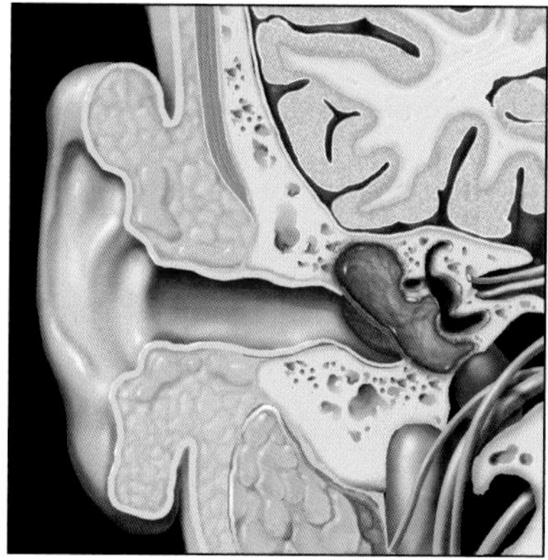

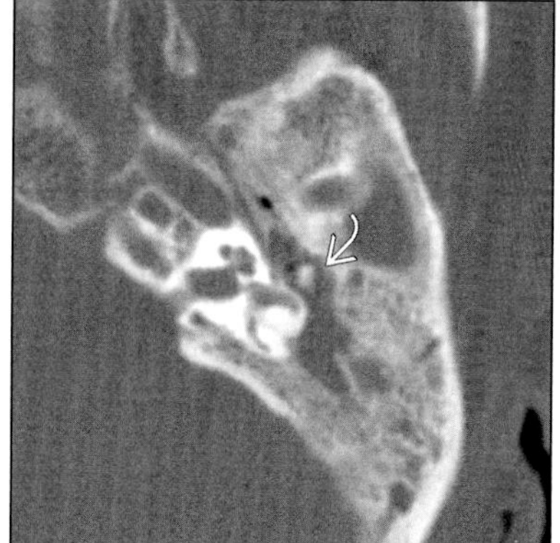

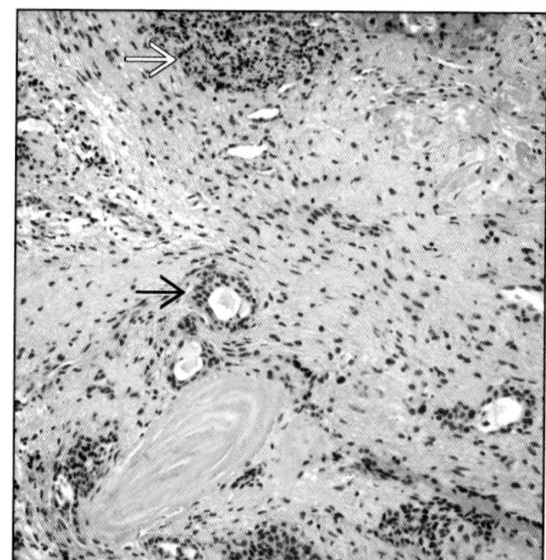

(Left) *This graphic highlights an infectious accumulation (green) within the middle ear.* ***(Center)*** *Axial bone CT shows complete opacification of the middle ear-mastoid, along with focal loss of the short process of the incus ➔. The loss of incus bony integrity indicates that acute infection is present.* ***(Right)*** *The fibrosis is cellular, and the epithelial inclusions ➔ are entrapped in the process. Hemosiderin is also noted ➔.*

NECROTIZING OTITIS EXTERNA

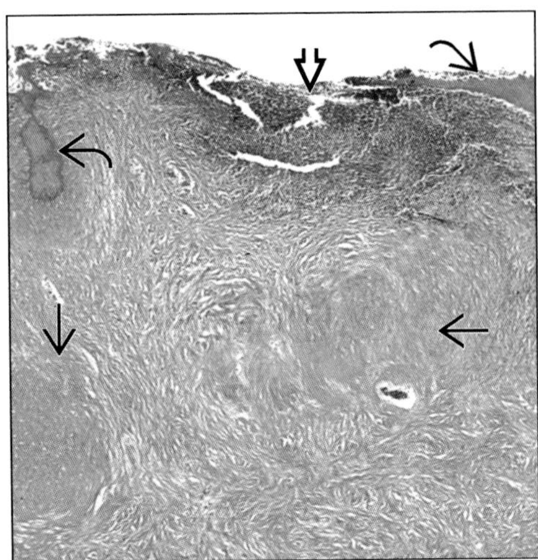

Epithelial ulceration is seen with a dense inflammatory cell infiltrate ➩ extending to bone ↗ and thick, acellular collagenous bands replacing the subcutis tissues →.

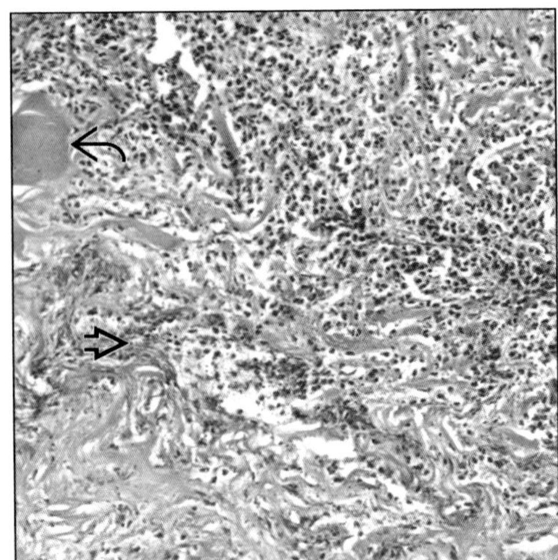

Necrosis ➩ and a dense acute and chronic inflammatory cell infiltrate extending to bone ↗ are identified. The histologic findings coupled to the clinical presentation are diagnostic for NEO.

TERMINOLOGY

Abbreviations

- Necrotizing external otitis (NEO)
- External auditory canal (EAC)

Synonyms

- "Malignant" external otitis
- Necrotizing granulomatous otitis

Definitions

- Virulent and potentially fatal form of external otitis related to *Pseudomonas aeruginosa* infection

ETIOLOGY/PATHOGENESIS

Infectious Agents

- *P. aeruginosa*
  - Produces endo- and exotoxins, neurotoxins, collagenases, and elastases, which cause tissue necrosis and necrotizing vasculitis

Pathogenesis

- Tissue ischemia secondary to underlying predisposing pathologic state (e.g., diabetic angiopathy)
- Migratory defect of polymorphonuclear leukocytes related to systemic disease
- Lethal potential of NEO attributed to these factors and destructive capacity of *P. aeruginosa*

CLINICAL ISSUES

Epidemiology

- Age
  - Primarily older patients; rarely occurs in children
- Gender
  - Equal gender distribution

Presentation

- Diabetic, chronically debilitated or immunologically deficient patients; may occur in nondebilitated patients
- Purulent otorrhea, swelling of ear, acute otitis externa
- Pain occurs with progression of disease
- Changes most pronounced in osseous portion of EAC where destruction begins
  - Skin ulceration leaves layer of thick granulation tissue covering exposed bone
- Fully developed NEO includes abundant necrotic tissue along with purulent exudate, which may obstruct EAC

Treatment

- Surgical approaches
  - Surgical debridement
- Adjuvant therapy
  - Hyperbaric oxygen therapy
- Drugs
  - Parenteral antibiotic therapy using 3rd generation cephalosporin and fluoroquinolones

Prognosis

- Mortality rates may exceed 75% if diagnosis and treatment are delayed
- Extensive spread of infection to adjacent structures, including cranial involvement, may result in death
- Cure can be achieved with early recognition and aggressive treatment
- Complications due to extension of infectious process include
  - Osteomyelitis, chondritis, cellulitis
  - Palsies, meningitis, intracranial venous thrombosis, brain abscess

NECROTIZING OTITIS EXTERNA

Key Facts

Etiology/Pathogenesis

- External otitis related to *Pseudomonas aeruginosa* infection

Clinical Issues

- Diabetic, chronically debilitated, or immunologically deficient patients
- Primarily affects older patients
- Mortality rates may exceed 75% if diagnosis and treatment are delayed

Microscopic Pathology

- Histology dominated by presence of necrotic material and exuberant granulation tissue
  - Diffuse heavy acute and chronic inflammation present in subcutis extending to bone
- Necrotizing vasculitis commonly present
- Thick, acellular collagen seen replacing most of subcutis
- Necrotic bone and cartilage

IMAGE FINDINGS

General Features

- CT preferred at initial diagnosis: Destructive osteomyelitis to bony EAC, especially affecting inferior portion
- MR imaging better for evaluation and follow-up of meningeal enhancement

MICROSCOPIC PATHOLOGY

Histologic Features

- Histology dominated by presence of necrotic material and exuberant granulation tissue
  - Intact epithelium may show pseudoepitheliomatous hyperplasia &/or atypical features
- Necrotizing vasculitis commonly present
- Diffuse heavy acute and chronic inflammation present in subcutis
- Thick, acellular collagen replaces dermis extending from cartilage to overlying dermis
- Necrosis of bone and cartilage with inflammatory cells infiltrating adjacent viable bone
- Sequestra of nonviable bone or cartilage may be seen

ANCILLARY TESTS

Histochemistry

- Presence of gram-negative bacilli readily identified

DIFFERENTIAL DIAGNOSIS

Squamous Cell Carcinoma (SCC)

- Clinical presentation of SCC of external auditory canal may mimic NEO or both may occur concurrently
  - Nests of squamous epithelium within dermis with atypical cytologic features
  - Radiographic evidence of destructive process
  - SCC associated with extensive necrosis may elude diagnosis in limited tissue sampling
- Infectious nature of NEO usually evident from clinical course and histologic findings

SELECTED REFERENCES

1. Hariga I et al: Necrotizing otitis externa: 19 cases' report. Eur Arch Otorhinolaryngol. 267(8):1193-8, 2010
2. Kaide CG et al: Hyperbaric oxygen: applications in infectious disease. Emerg Med Clin North Am. 26(2):571-95, xi, 2008
3. Franco-Vidal V et al: Necrotizing external otitis: a report of 46 cases. Otol Neurotol. 28(6):771-3, 2007
4. Kwon BJ et al: MRI findings and spreading patterns of necrotizing external otitis: is a poor outcome predictable? Clin Radiol. 61(6):495-504, 2006
5. Grandis JR et al: Necrotizing (malignant) external otitis: prospective comparison of CT and MR imaging in diagnosis and follow-up. Radiology. 196(2):499-504, 1995
6. Sobie S et al: Necrotizing external otitis in children: report of two cases and review of the literature. Laryngoscope. 97(5):598-601, 1987

IMAGE GALLERY

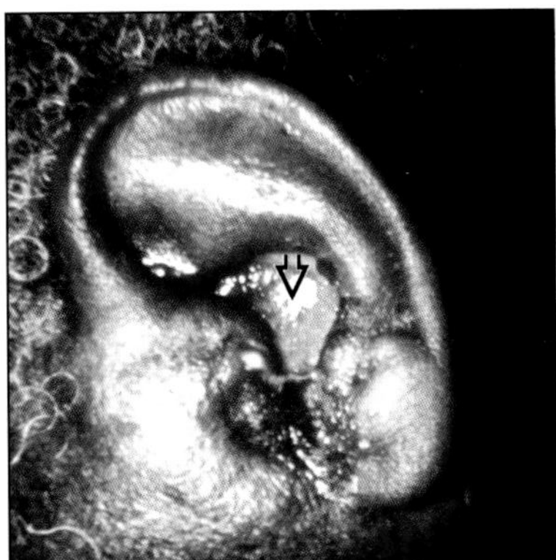

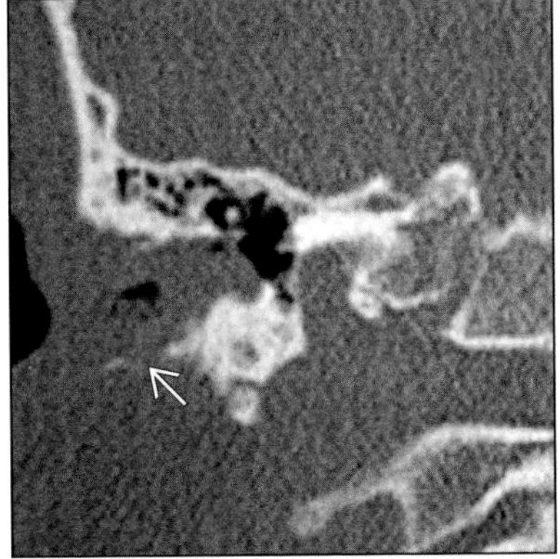

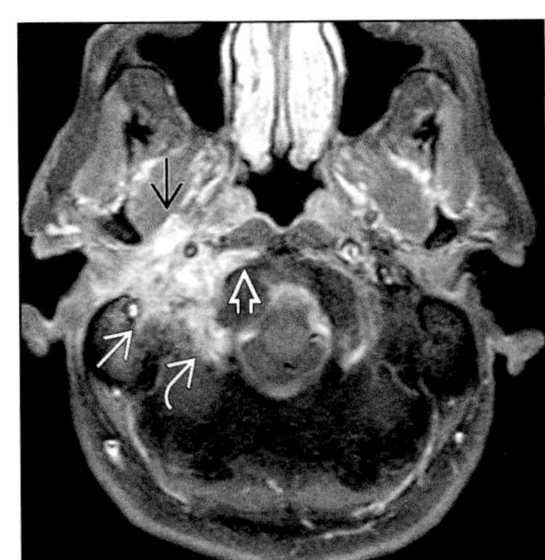

(Left) *A swollen ear with necrotic exudate in EAC ⇨ is shown.* ***(Center)*** *Temporal bone CT shows inflammatory changes in the region of the right external auditory canal. Destructive dehiscence ➡ of inferior bony EAC signals the beginning of associated osteomyelitis.* ***(Right)*** *Axial T1 C+ FS MR shows enhancing tissue extending from right EAC into parapharyngeal space →, prevertebral space ⇨, occipital bone ➡, and stylomastoid foramen ➡ in a patient with NEO.*

CHONDRODERMATITIS NODULARIS HELICIS

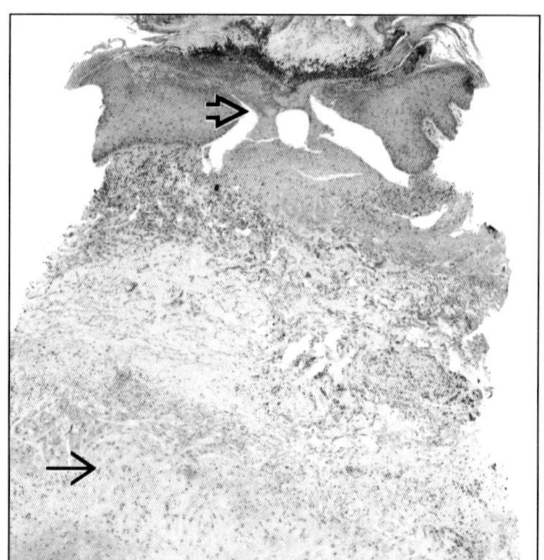

Surface crust overlies an area of ulceration ⮚. There is a necrobiosis of the collagen, extending down to the cartilage →, as well as mixed inflammation and solar elastosis.

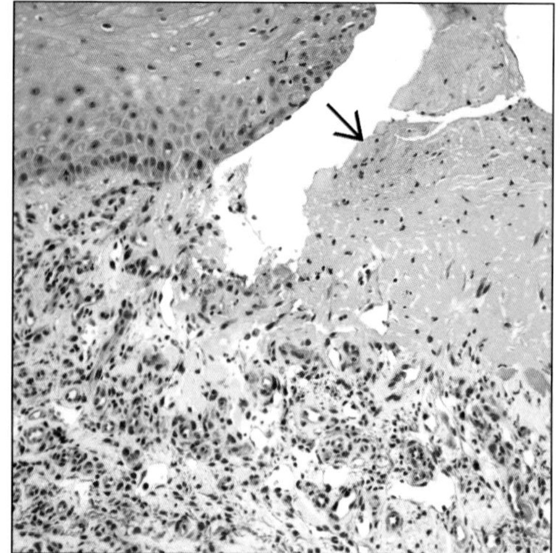

Fibrinoid necrosis is seen within the crater or ulceration →. A rich inflammatory infiltrate is noted within the dermis. A superficial biopsy specimen can sometimes be difficult to interpret.

TERMINOLOGY

Abbreviations

- Chondrodermatitis nodularis helicis (CDNH)

Synonyms

- Transepithelial elimination disorder
- Perforating dermatoses
- Winkler disease

Definitions

- Nonneoplastic inflammatory and degenerative process of auricle, characterized by necrobiotic changes in dermis that extend down to perichondrium

ETIOLOGY/PATHOGENESIS

Injury

- Dermal injury caused by combination of factors
  - Local trauma, such as rubbing or pressure (prurigo nodularis-like)
  - Actinic damage from long-term sun exposure
  - Relatively tenuous vascularity of auricle

Immune-Based

- Linked with granuloma annulare, dermatomyositis, and systemic sclerosis

CLINICAL ISSUES

Epidemiology

- Incidence
  - Relatively common
- Age
  - Mean: 6th decade
  - Patients older than 40 years
  - If patients are younger, may be marker of underlying systemic disease
- Gender
  - Male > Female (3:2)
- Ethnicity
  - Whites more commonly than other ethnicities

Site

- Helix of ear in men
- Antihelix of ear in women
- Rarely, antitragus may be involved

Presentation

- Painful, solitary nodule on external ear
- Exquisite tenderness
  - Often will interfere with sleep
- Discrete, gray to red mass
- Oval, with raised or rolled edges
- Central ulcer or depression with horny plug, with or without scale crust
- Clinically may simulate carcinoma (basal cell or squamous cell)
- May be marker of diseases with microvascular injury
  - Diabetes mellitus
  - Connective tissue disorders

Treatment

- Options, risks, complications
  - Needs to be shaved down to underlying cartilage to remove all inflammation
- Surgical approaches
  - Wide excision
    - Narrow skin ellipse with hydrodissection (injecting saline) to create cleavage plane
    - Greater amount of cartilage can then be removed
  - Deep shave
  - Smoothing of cartilage only

Prognosis

- Recurrences complicate treatment if areas of inflammation are not removed
  - Seen in up to 20% of patients

CHONDRODERMATITIS NODULARIS HELICIS

Key Facts

Terminology
- Nonneoplastic inflammatory and degenerative process of ear characterized by necrobiotic dermal changes
  - Etiologies include local trauma, actinic damage, and tenuous vascularity

Clinical Issues
- Male > Female (3:2)
- Mean age at presentation: 6th decade
- Exquisite tenderness/pain of helix of ear
- Central ulcer or depression with horny plug, often with scale crust

Microscopic Pathology
- Epidermal hyperplasia adjacent to keratinaceous plug
- Upper dermis displays fibrinoid necrosis
- Necrobiotic collagen (collagenolytic destruction)
- Sinus tract created from surface to underlying cartilage

MACROSCOPIC FEATURES

Size
- Mean: 4-7 mm

MICROSCOPIC PATHOLOGY

Histologic Features
- Epidermal hyperplasia adjacent to horny (keratinaceous) plug
  - Funnel-shaped defect in epidermis
- Transepidermal elimination of necrobiotic material
- Upper dermis displays fibrinoid necrosis or necrobiotic granuloma
- Necrobiotic collagen (collagenolytic destruction) in association with granulation tissue
  - Histiocytes, lymphocytes, and keratinous debris
- Sinus tract created from surface to underlying cartilage
- Eosinophilic degeneration of cartilage
  - Joined by slit-like spaces to central funnel
  - Perichondrium may show fibrosis and inflammation
- Nerve hyperplasia is frequently prominent
  - Suggested reason for exquisite tenderness clinically
- Solar elastosis and telangiectasia concurrently present in upper dermis

DIFFERENTIAL DIAGNOSIS

Relapsing Polychondritis
- Autoimmune disease affecting cartilage
- Eosinophilic cartilaginous destruction by inflammatory infiltrate
- No epidermal or dermal manifestations

Cystic Chondromalacia (Auricle Pseudocyst)
- No epidermal or dermal manifestations
- Central cystic degeneration of cartilage
- May undergo healing via granulation tissue and fibrosis

Squamous Cell Carcinoma
- Superficial biopsy makes separation difficult
- Epidermal changes with atypia, mitoses, and invasion

SELECTED REFERENCES

1. Thompson LD: Chondrodermatitis nodularis helicis. Ear Nose Throat J. 86(12):734-5, 2007
2. Zuber TJ et al: Chondrodermatitis nodularis chronica helicis. Arch Fam Med. 8(5):445-7, 1999
3. Bard JW: Chondrodermatitis nodularis chronica helicis. Dermatologica. 163(5):376-84, 1981
4. Weedon D: Elastotic nodules of the ear. J Cutan Pathol. 8(6):429-33, 1981
5. Santa Cruz DJ: Chondrodermatitis nodularis helicis: a transepidermal perforating disorder. J Cutan Pathol. 7(2):70-6, 1980

IMAGE GALLERY

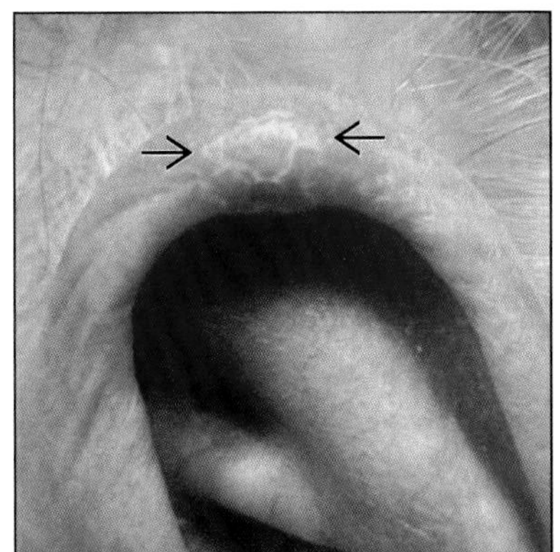
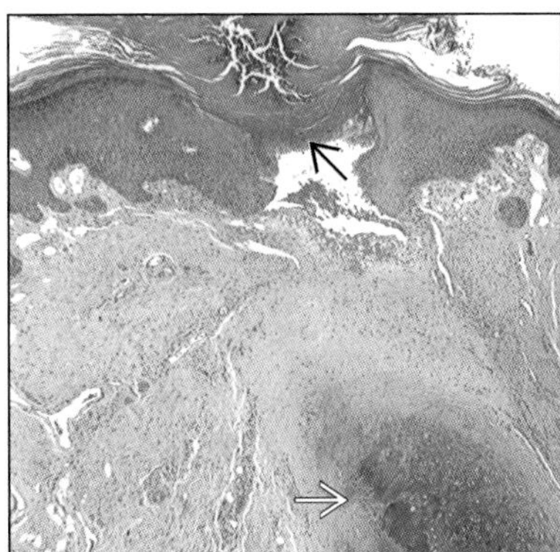
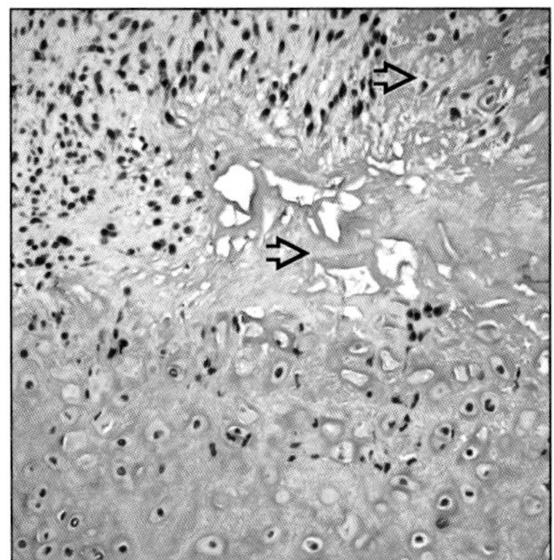

*(**Left**) There is a raised, erythematous nodule with slight scaling ➔ on the ear helix in a patient with chondrodermatitis nodularis helicis. (Courtesy M. Guralnick, MD.) (**Center**) A wedge biopsy specimen demonstrates the cartilage ➡ in the base of the ulcer. Note the degenerative changes in the dermis, with an overlying ulcer, showing a keratinaceous plug ➔. (**Right**) The cartilage has some fibrosis and an inflammatory infiltrate. There is fibrinoid necrosis ⇨ of the dermis.*

OTIC POLYP

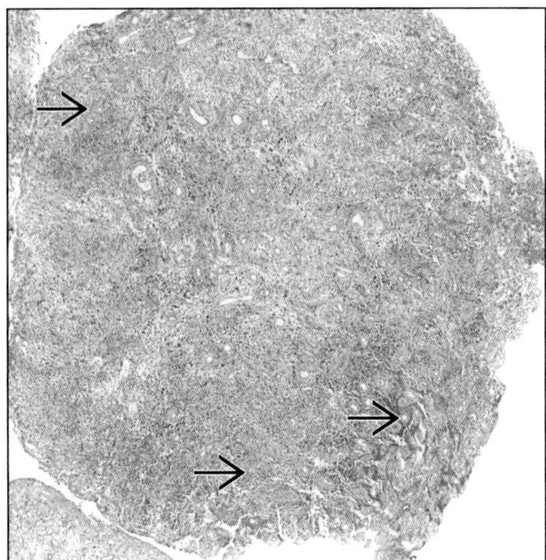

Hematoxylin & eosin shows a polypoid lesion composed of mixed inflammatory cells and vascular stroma. A number of "glandular" structures ⇒ can be seen, representing entrapped adnexal structures.

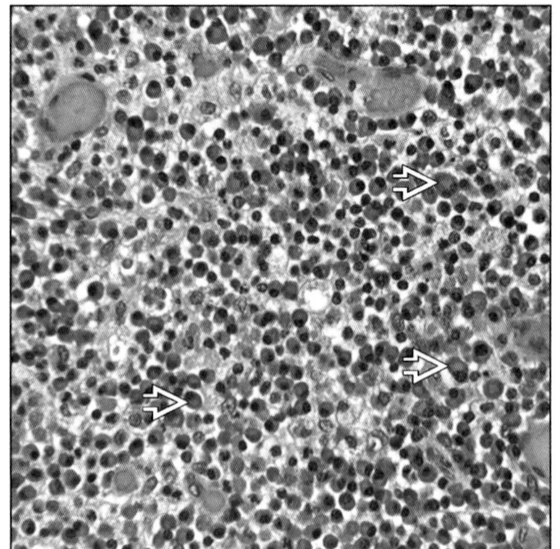

Hematoxylin & eosin shows sheets of plasma cells with a rich vascular tissue. The plasma cells are not atypical, showing eccentric cytoplasm and a "hof" zone ⇒.

TERMINOLOGY

Synonyms

- Aural polyp

Definitions

- Benign proliferation of chronic inflammatory cells and granulation tissue, usually lined by benign reactive epithelium, in response to longstanding inflammatory process of middle ear

ETIOLOGY/PATHOGENESIS

Infectious Agents

- Usually a complication of longstanding otitis

CLINICAL ISSUES

Epidemiology

- Incidence
  - Uncommon
- Age
  - Young
  - Mean: 30 years
- Gender
  - Male > Female (2:1)

Site

- Middle ear
- If tympanic membrane perforation is present, external auditory canal mass may be present

Presentation

- Otorrhea
- Conductive hearing loss
- Otalgia, bleeding, or sensation of mass

Treatment

- Options, risks, complications
  - Usually complication of longstanding otitis
- Surgical approaches
  - Second-line therapy for persistent disease after failed antibiotic therapy
  - Mastoid involvement may require more extensive surgery
  - Performed if cholesteatoma is identified in biopsy/curettage material
- Drugs
  - Antibiotics with appropriate sensitivity testing of causative bacterium

Prognosis

- Excellent, without bad outcome

IMAGE FINDINGS

Radiographic Findings

- Required to exclude possibility of concurrent cholesteatoma

MACROSCOPIC FEATURES

General Features

- Solitary, polypoid reddish mass
- Friable

Sections to Be Submitted

- All tissue submitted to exclude concurrent cholesteatoma

Size

- Usually < 2 cm

MICROSCOPIC PATHOLOGY

Histologic Features

- Polypoid architecture

OTIC POLYP

Key Facts

Terminology
- Benign proliferation of chronic inflammatory cells in response to longstanding otitis media

Image Findings
- Required to exclude possibility of concurrent cholesteatoma

Macroscopic Features
- Submit all tissue to exclude cholesteatoma
- Solitary, polypoid reddish mass

Microscopic Pathology
- Granulation-type tissue with edematous stroma and high density of capillaries
- Rich chronic inflammatory infiltrate

Top Differential Diagnoses
- Plasmacytoma
- Rhabdomyosarcoma

- Granulation-type tissue with edematous stroma and high density of capillaries
- Rich chronic inflammatory infiltrate
  - Lymphocytes, plasma cells, histiocytes, and eosinophils
- Plasma cells with Russell bodies and Mott cell formation
- Multinucleated giant cells and calcifications may be seen
- Cholesterol clefts (cholesterol granuloma) may be present
- "Glandular" inclusions within stroma (tunnel clusters) present in longstanding cases
- Concurrent cholesteatoma may be present
  - Stratified squamous epithelium, prominent granular layer, acellular keratinaceous debris

ANCILLARY TESTS

Immunohistochemistry
- Lymphoid and plasma cell population show mixture of B- and T-cells without light chain restriction
- Myoid markers are negative

DIFFERENTIAL DIAGNOSIS

Plasmacytoma
- Monoclonal proliferation of atypical, binucleated plasma cells, showing light chain restriction

Rhabdomyosarcoma
- "Small round blue cell" neoplasm pattern of embryonal rhabdomyosarcoma may mimic otic polyp
- Strap cells, destructive growth, and muscle immunophenotype

Middle Ear Adenoma
- a.k.a. neuroendocrine adenoma of middle ear (NAME)
- Biphasic glandular proliferation with pseudoinfiltrative pattern
- Nuclei showing neuroendocrine differentiation
- Epithelial and neuroendocrine immunohistochemistry

SELECTED REFERENCES

1. Nair S et al: Fibroblast growth factor receptor expression in aural polyps: predictor of cholesteatoma? J Laryngol Otol. 118(5):338-42, 2004
2. Prasannaraj T et al: Aural polyps: safe or unsafe disease? Am J Otolaryngol. 24(3):155-8, 2003
3. Hussain SS et al: Mast cells in aural polyps: a preliminary report. J Laryngol Otol. 109(6):491-4, 1995
4. Gliklich RE et al: The cause of aural polyps in children. Arch Otolaryngol Head Neck Surg. 119(6):669-71, 1993
5. Kurihara A et al: Bone destruction mechanisms in chronic otitis media with cholesteatoma: specific production by cholesteatoma tissue in culture of bone-resorbing activity attributable to interleukin-1 alpha. Ann Otol Rhinol Laryngol. 100(12):989-98, 1991
6. Friedmann I: Pathological lesions of the external auditory meatus: a review. J R Soc Med. 83(1):34-7, 1990

IMAGE GALLERY

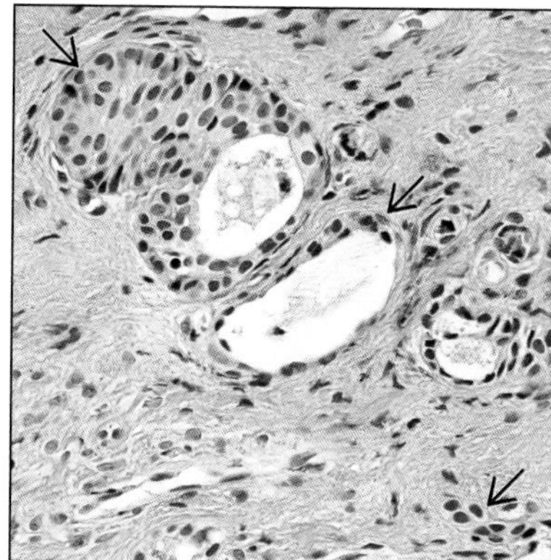

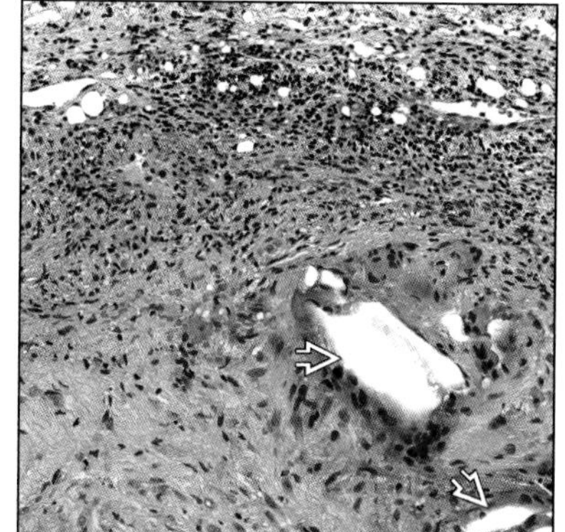

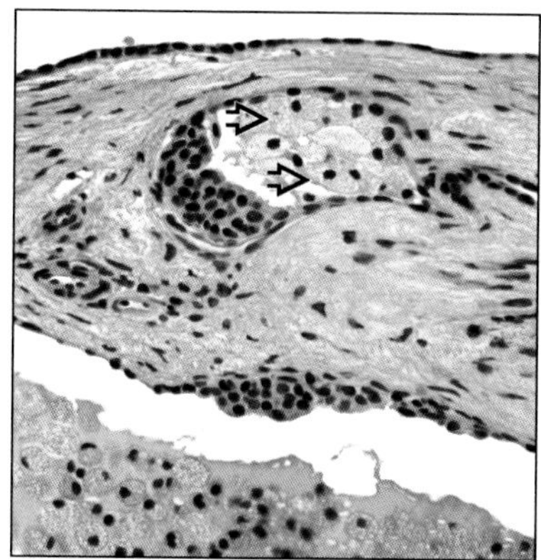

(Left) *This H&E shows fibrosis and entrapped surface epithelium ⇒, referred to as tunnel clusters.* ***(Center)*** *If an inflammatory polyp has been present for some time, cholesterol clefts ⇒ will be seen within the inflammatory background. These appear as empty spaces due to processing artifacts. There is fibrosis and mixed inflammation with blood.* ***(Right)*** *The surface epithelium of the polyp is entrapped below the surface, associated with foamy histiocytes ⇒.*

RELAPSING POLYCHONDRITIS

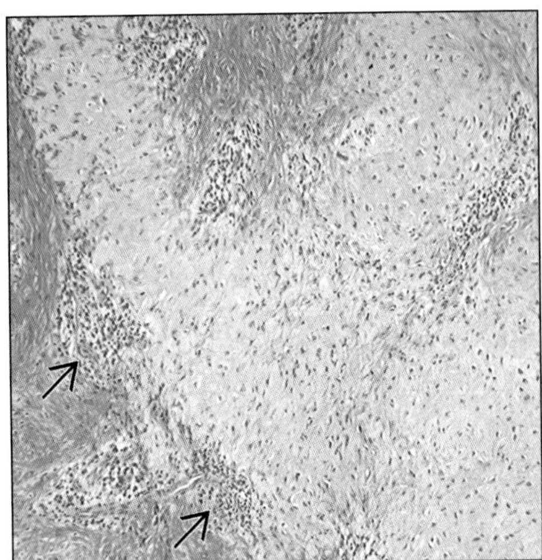

Hematoxylin & eosin shows mixed inflammatory cells destroying the cartilaginous plates, extending from the external surface ➔ in toward the center of the cartilage.

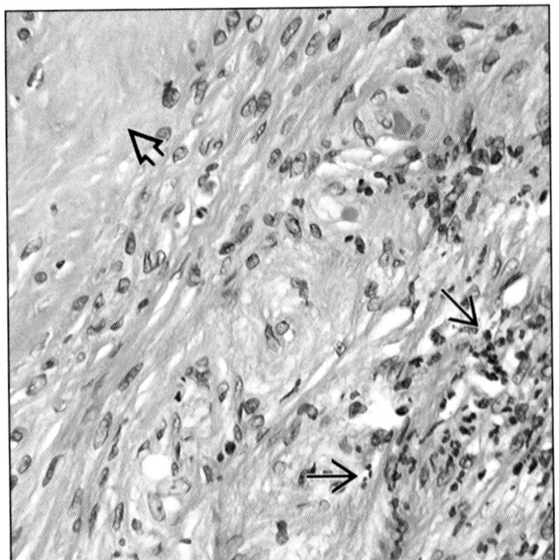

Hematoxylin & eosin shows scattered mixed inflammatory cells ➔ and destroyed cartilage in this example of relapsing polychondritis. Note the pink cartilage ➢ (loss of basophilia).

TERMINOLOGY

Definitions

- Inflammatory, autoimmune disorder against type II collagen, leading to destruction of cartilaginous or proteoglycan-rich tissues

ETIOLOGY/PATHOGENESIS

Pathogenesis

- Autoimmune inflammatory disorder with antibodies against type II collagen
- Susceptibility significantly associated with *HLA-DR4*

CLINICAL ISSUES

Epidemiology

- Incidence
  - Very rare
- Age
  - Mean: 5th-6th decades
- Gender
  - Female > Male (2:1)

Site

- Auricle most commonly affected site (85%)
  - Bilateral involvement in nearly all patients
- Others sites (order of frequency): Nose, joints, tracheobronchial tree, eye, heart, blood vessels

Presentation

- Acute vs. chronic phase
- Acute phase: Ears are red-purple, edematous (swollen), and tender
  - Noncartilaginous lobule is spared
- Chronic phase: Floppy ears
  - Identified after repeated bouts of acute disease
- Other symptoms relate to other anatomic sites
  - Nasal chondritis leads to saddle nose deformity (25-50%)
  - Laryngotracheal disease causes obstruction, laryngeal collapse, and predisposition to pulmonary infections (up to 50%)
  - Nonerosive arthritis: 2nd most common clinical site, affecting knees and small joints of hand
  - Cardiovascular disease: Shows up as vasculitis (up to 50%)
- Associated autoimmune disorder (up to 35%)
  - Rheumatoid arthritis, Hashimoto thyroiditis, systemic lupus erythematosus, Sjögren syndrome, inflammatory bowel disease, diabetes mellitus, primary biliary cirrhosis, myelodysplastic syndromes, Sweet syndrome

Laboratory Tests

- Elevated erythrocyte sedimentation rate; mild anemia
- Anti-type II collagen antibodies

Treatment

- Options, risks, complications
  - Airway must be secured
  - Frequently associated with myelodysplasia/leukemia
  - Autologous stem cell transplantation shows promise
- Surgical approaches
  - May be required to maintain a patent airway (reconstructive, rib interposition)
- Drugs
  - Variable success dependent on extent of disease
    - May decrease frequency, duration, and severity of flares, but fails to halt progression
  - Corticosteroid, nonsteroidal anti-inflammatory drugs, and immunomodulators

Prognosis

- Leading cause of death is airway compromise due to tracheobronchial damage
  - Less frequent complications and causes of death: Secondary infections, cardiovascular disease
- 10-year survival (55-95%)

Key Facts

Terminology

- Rare autoimmune disorder against type II collagen, resulting in cartilage destruction

Clinical Issues

- Bilateral auricles are most common sites affected
- Acute and chronic phases: Swollen to floppy ears
- Associated autoimmune disorders in up to 35%
- Frequently associated with myelodysplasia/leukemia
- Anti-type II collagen antibodies
- Leading cause of death is airway damage

Microscopic Pathology

- Loss of basophilia in cartilaginous plate
  - Damaged cartilage has moth-eaten appearance
- Perichondrium infiltrated by mixed inflammatory cell infiltrate (outside in)

Top Differential Diagnoses

- Necrotizing otitis externa, Wegener granulomatosis, cystic chondromalacia

---

  - Depends on disease severity and number of anatomic sites affected
- Negative prognostic factors: Advanced age at diagnosis, anemia, tracheobronchial stricture

MICROSCOPIC PATHOLOGY

Histologic Features

- Loss of basophilia in cartilaginous plate (earliest change)
- Perichondrium infiltrated by mixed inflammatory infiltrate
  - Neutrophils, lymphocytes, plasma cells, and eosinophils
  - Blurred (instead of sharp) interface between cartilaginous plate and surrounding soft tissues
- Damaged cartilage has moth-eaten appearance
  - Areas are replaced by granulation tissue
  - Eventually, fibrosis replaces granulation tissue

ANCILLARY TESTS

Immunofluorescence

- Granular immunoglobulins and C3 at chondrofibrous junction and within perichondral vessel walls

Electron Microscopy

- Chondrocytes surrounded by large numbers of dense granules and vesicles

DIFFERENTIAL DIAGNOSIS

Necrotizing Otitis Externa

- Infection due to *Pseudomonas aeruginosa*
- Usually rapidly progressive, but not cartilage specific

Wegener Granulomatosis

- Although there can be histologic overlap, in ear, Wegener is not usually a consideration
- In sinonasal tract, there is biocollagenolytic, blue, granular necrosis, frequently geographic

Extranodal NK-/T-cell Lymphoma

- Highly atypical lymphoid infiltrate
- Significant necrosis and vascular invasion
- Does not typically affect ear

Cystic Chondromalacia

- Pseudocyst within center of cartilage
- Granulation tissue seen with time
- Tends to develop from "inside out"

SELECTED REFERENCES

1. Bachor E et al: Otologic manifestations of relapsing polychondritis. Review of literature and report of nine cases. Auris Nasus Larynx. 33(2):135-41, 2006
2. Gergely P Jr et al: Relapsing polychondritis. Best Pract Res Clin Rheumatol. 18(5):723-38, 2004
3. Zeuner M et al: Relapsing polychondritis: clinical and immunogenetic analysis of 62 patients. J Rheumatol. 24(1):96-101, 1997

IMAGE GALLERY

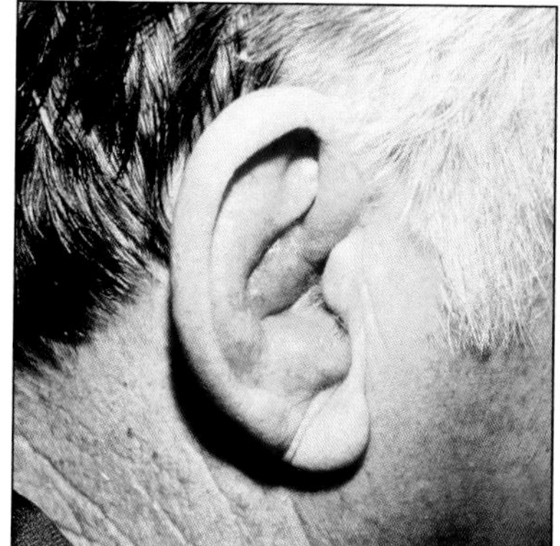

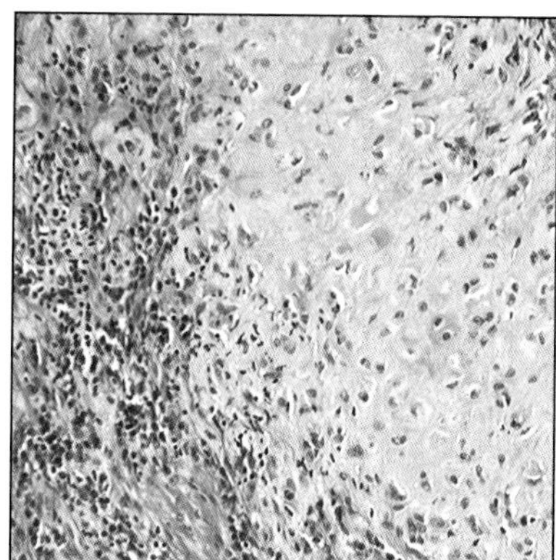

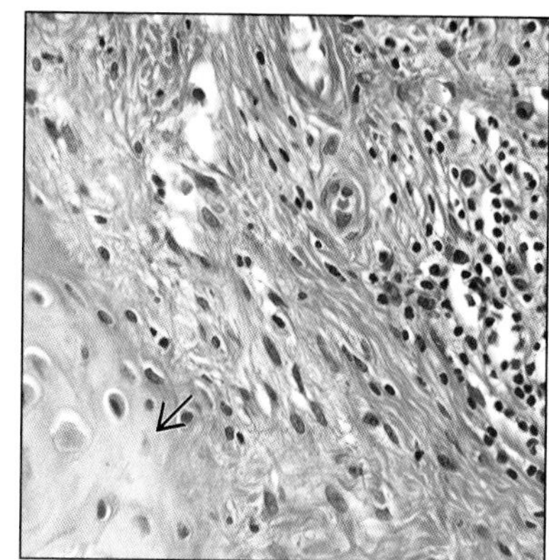

*(**Left**) Clinical photograph shows erythema and distortion of the cartilaginous portion of the pinna and scaphoid regions. (Courtesy V. Hyams, MD.) (**Center**) Hematoxylin & eosin shows a loss of cartilaginous structure, demonstrating slightly bluish appearance with inflammatory cells destroying the periphery, creating an interface chondritis. (**Right**) Hematoxylin & eosin shows a small collection of inflammatory cells associated with fibrosis adjacent to destroyed cartilage ⇒.*

CYSTIC CHONDROMALACIA (AURICULAR PSEUDOCYST)

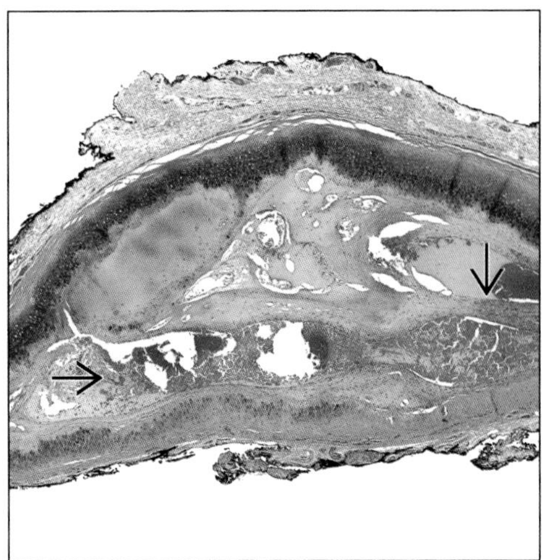

The plates of the ear cartilage are separated by a cystic cavity. The cavity shows no epithelial lining, but there is granulation-type tissue and blood ⇒.

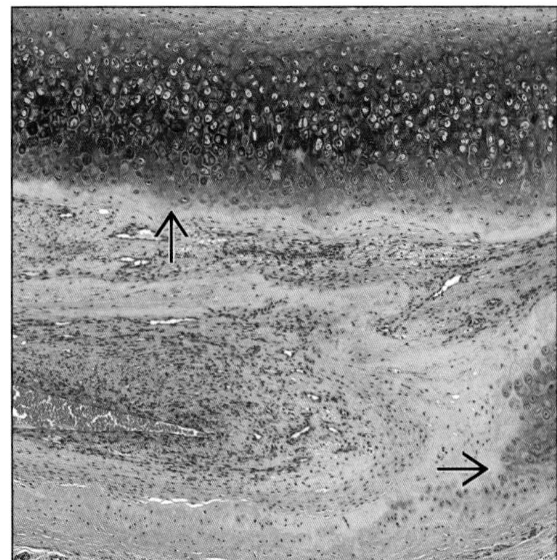

The central cavity is filled with a granulation tissue and fibrous connective tissue. There is slight degeneration of the cartilage plates ⇒, visible at the top and bottom of the field.

TERMINOLOGY

Synonyms

- Pseudocyst of the auricle (auricular pseudocyst)
- Idiopathic cystic chondromalacia
- Otoseroma

Definitions

- Degenerative cystic lesion of ear cartilage

ETIOLOGY/PATHOGENESIS

Developmental Anomaly

- Embryologic fusion defect is possible

Inflammatory

- Cytokine abnormalities
  - Interleukin-1 (IL-1, a mediator of inflammation) induces IL-6 (stimulates chondrocyte proliferation) and stimulates proteases and prostaglandin E2 production by chondrocytes, leading to decreased extracellular matrix formation

Trauma: Ischemic Necrosis

- Perhaps related to minor trauma
  - Rubbing, using hard pillows, earphones, cell phones, or helmets
- Abnormal release of lysosomal enzymes
  - Markedly elevated activity of lactate dehydrogenase, specifically LDH-4 and LDH-5

CLINICAL ISSUES

Epidemiology

- Incidence
  - Uncommon
- Age
  - Young usually
  - Mean: 35 years
- Gender
  - Male > > > Female (9:1)
- Ethnicity
  - Increased incidence in Chinese and Malay men

Site

- Helix or antihelix most common
  - Scaphoid fossa is most common subsite

Presentation

- Unilateral in almost all patients
- Usually painless
- Fusiform, fluctuant swelling of helix or antihelix
- Patients usually seek treatment early in disease development
- Overlying skin is unremarkable
- Possible association with patients who have atopic dermatitis

Treatment

- Options, risks, complications
  - Usually treated for cosmetic reasons only
  - Must preserve ear architecture
  - Incision and drainage with curettage is variably successful
  - Needle aspiration with suture compression is effective
- Surgical approaches
  - Unroofing of pseudocyst with insertion of sclerosing agent
    - Tincture of iodine or minocycline are effective

Prognosis

- Excellent
- Cosmetic deformity is possible

MACROSCOPIC FEATURES

General Features

- Central, slit-like cleft

CYSTIC CHONDROMALACIA (AURICULAR PSEUDOCYST)

Key Facts

Terminology
- Degenerative cystic lesion of ear cartilage

Clinical Issues
- Usually young patients
- Male > > > Female
- Unilateral
- Scaphoid fossa is most common site
- Usually treated for cosmetic reasons only
- Unroofing of pseudocyst with sclerosing agent

Microscopic Pathology
- Central cystic space within cartilage
- No epithelial lining (pseudocyst)
- Lined by granulation tissue with plump fibroblasts
- Hemosiderin deposits are often present
- Fibrous connective tissue obliterates lumen

Top Differential Diagnoses
- Relapsing polychondritis
- Chondrodermatitis nodularis helicis

- Cyst is filled with viscous clear to olive-oil fluid
- Usually < 2 cc of fluid
- If cyst is longstanding, granulation tissue within cavity

Sections to Be Submitted
- Must include cartilage and contents
  - Must know clinical appearance if only an unroofing is performed

Size
- Range: Up to 3 cm

MICROSCOPIC PATHOLOGY

Histologic Features
- Central cystic space within cartilage
- No epithelial lining (pseudocyst)
- Irregular contour of inner cystic space
  - Lined by granulation tissue with plump fibroblasts
  - Inflammatory cells present
- Hemosiderin deposits are often present
- Fibrous connective tissue replacement obliterates lumen in longstanding cases

DIFFERENTIAL DIAGNOSIS

Relapsing Polychondritis
- Painful lesion with rich inflammatory infiltrate that destroys cartilage
- Cartilages all over the body affected (autoimmune disorder)

Chondrodermatitis Nodularis Helicis
- Painful lesion with surface ulceration and extrusion of necrobiotic dermal collagen
- No cyst formation

Traumatic Perichondritis
- Acute infection (pseudomonas or proteus)
- No cyst formation

SELECTED REFERENCES

1. Lim CM et al: Pseudocyst of the auricle: a histologic perspective. Laryngoscope. 2004 Jul;114(7):1281-4. Erratum in: Laryngoscope. 115(4):759, 2005
2. Chang CH et al: Deroofing surgical treatment for pseudocyst of the auricle. J Otolaryngol. 33(3):177-80, 2004
3. Nelson BL et al: Cystic chondromalacia of the ear. Ear Nose Throat J. 82(2):104-5, 2003
4. Kopera D et al: "Pseudocyst of the auricle", othematoma and otoseroma: three faces of the same coin? Eur J Dermatol. 10(6):451-4, 2000
5. Heffner DK et al: Cystic chondromalacia (endochondral pseudocyst) of the auricle. Arch Pathol Lab Med. 110(8):740-3, 1986
6. Lazar RH et al: Pseudocyst of the auricle: a review of 21 cases. Otolaryngol Head Neck Surg. 94(3):360-1, 1986
7. Engel D: Pseudocysts of the auricle in Chinese. Arch Otolaryngol. 83(3):197-202, 1966

IMAGE GALLERY

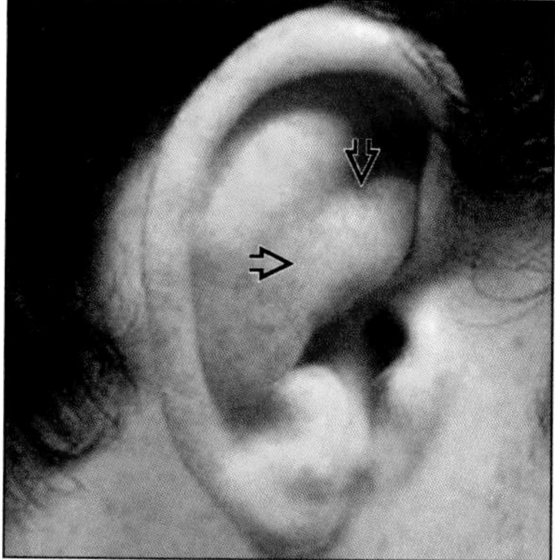

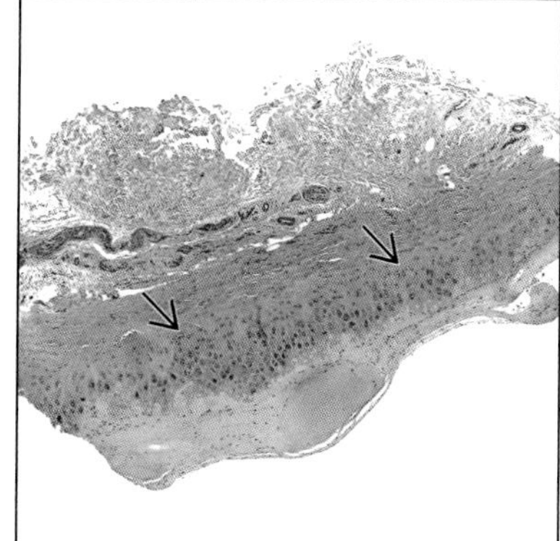

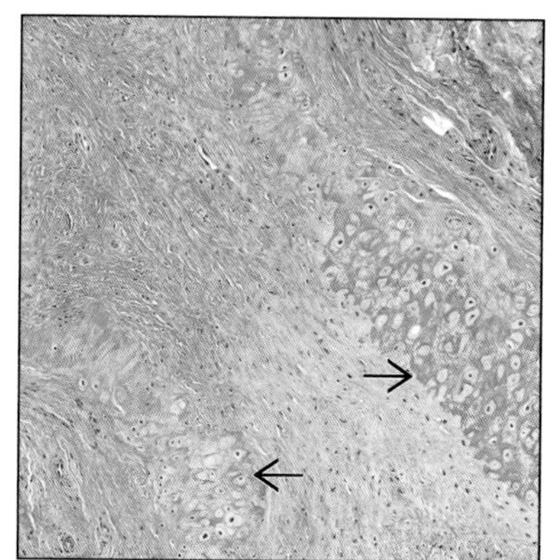

(Left) *Clinical photograph of a 20-year-old wrestler with a 1-week history of a painless swelling in the right ear shows a fluctuant but not inflamed area ⇨. (Courtesy D. Elpern, MD.)* ***(Center)*** *An unroofing procedure will only yield one of the cartilaginous plates ⇨. In this setting, the fluid in the cystic cavity will not be seen. Instead, there is a nonepithelial lining with edema and fibrosis.* ***(Right)*** *End-stage cases will show heavy fibrous connective tissue obliterating the potential lumen between the cartilaginous plates ⇨.*

OTOSCLEROSIS

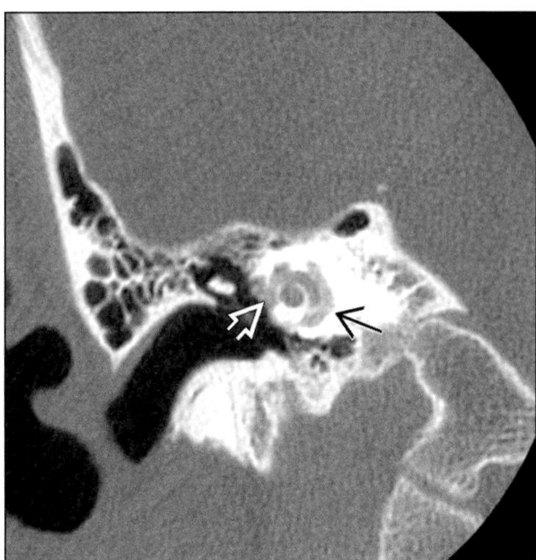

Coronal right temporal bone image reveals the cochlear disease ⇨ as well as the fenestral disease ➡. The increased signal is due to the sclerosis. CT is preferable to plain films for this condition.

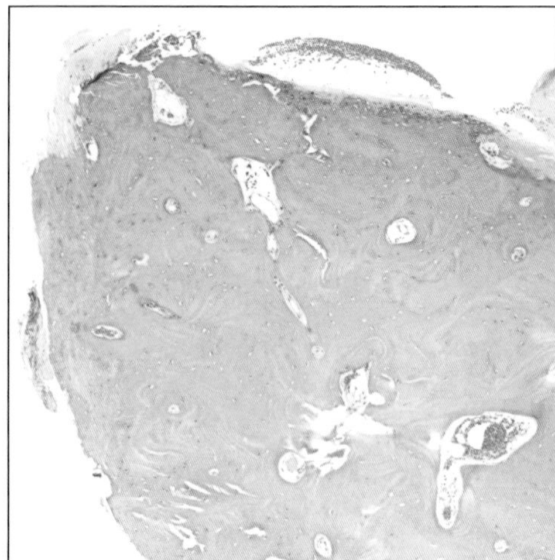

Otosclerosis is recognized histologically by increased density and thickness of bone distorting the affected areas. The resultant bone can appear similar to cortical bone.

TERMINOLOGY

Definitions

- Acquired abnormal bony growth resulting in fixation of stapes or lateral ossicular chain

ETIOLOGY/PATHOGENESIS

Environmental Exposure

- Increased in areas with low fluoride content in drinking water
- Cells from otosclerotic stapes in cell culture show abnormally high sulfation of bone matrix glycosaminoglycans (GAG)

Infectious Agents

- Measles virus may play a role in disease development

Inherited

- Otosclerosis shows several genetic linkages, with variable penetrance and expression

Pathophysiology

- Otosclerosis only affects bone derived from otic capsule
- Otosclerosis is characterized by increased rate of bone remodeling in otic capsule
- Disease development in 4 stages

CLINICAL ISSUES

Epidemiology

- Incidence
  - ~ 0.5% of population develops clinical otosclerosis
    - Much higher (10%) in autopsy series
- Age
  - Mean: Middle age (90% < 50 years)
    - Younger in inherited cases
- Gender
  - Female > Male (1.4-2:1) (reflects inheritance pattern differences)
- Ethnicity
  - Caucasians (whites) > > Asians, blacks, South American Indians (10-20:1)

Site

- Foci of abnormal bone deposition include oval and round windows (cochlea)
  - Results in fixation of stapes footplate to oval window of cochlea

Presentation

- Most patients are asymptomatic
- Symptom triad: Progressive conductive hearing loss, normal tympanic membrane, no otitis media
  - Faint pink tinge to cochlear promontory: Schwartze sign
- If symptomatic, hearing loss is most common symptom
  - Conductive hearing loss most common (low frequencies) (Rinne &/or Weber tests)
  - Sensorineural loss (high frequency) less frequent (10%) and a late manifestation
- Often unilateral initially but nearly always bilateral
- 3 major categories
  - **Classic**: Conductive hearing loss due to stapes fixation
  - **Mixed**: Stapes fixation and cochlear involvement resulting in mixed hearing loss
  - **Sensorineural**: Cochlear damage without stapes fixation
- Tinnitus
- Vestibular findings (imbalance, vertigo) in ~ 10%

Treatment

- Options, risks, complications
  - Medical management or surgery can be used
- Surgical approaches
  - Stapedectomy or stapedotomy (microdrill or laser) can restore conductive hearing loss

OTOSCLEROSIS

Key Facts

Terminology
- Acquired abnormal bony growth resulting in fixation of stapes or lateral ossicular chain

Clinical Issues
- ~ 0.5% of population develops clinical otosclerosis
  - Caucasians (whites) > > Asians, blacks
- Symptom triad: Conductive hearing loss, normal TM, no otitis media

Microscopic Pathology
- Abnormal bone deposition: Oval & round windows
- **Spongiotic**: Endochondral bone layer resorption, replaced by highly vascular and fibrous tissue
- **Sclerotic**: Production of immature basophilic bone and collagen fibrils deposition
- **Fibrotic**: Mature acidophilic woven bone

Top Differential Diagnoses
- Osteogenesis imperfecta, osteopetrosis, Paget disease

    - Cochlear implantation of prosthesis
- Medical
  - Hearing aids: Early in disease management
  - Fluoride additive: Slows disease progression

IMAGE FINDINGS

General Features
- Only employed in atypical cases, including sensorineural hearing loss
- High-resolution CT shows characteristic findings
  - Separated into 2 types
    - Fenestral otosclerosis
    - Cochlear otosclerosis

MICROSCOPIC PATHOLOGY

Histologic Features
- Fibrosis/sclerosis within middle ear bones
- 3 histologic phases
  - **Spongiotic**: Endochondral bone layer resorption by osteoclasts and replaced with highly vascular cellular and fibrous tissue
    - Bone resorption around existing vessels, resulting in dilated vascular spaces
  - **Sclerotic**: Production of immature basophilic bone and filling vascular spaces with collagen fibrils
    - Blue mantles of Manasse
  - **Fibrotic**: Mature acidophilic woven bone

ANCILLARY TESTS

Cytogenetics
- Up-regulation of *PF4* (platelet factor 4)
- Increased expression of *IBSP*
- Variation of *RELN* gene (reelin; chromosome 7)

DIFFERENTIAL DIAGNOSIS

Osteogenesis Imperfecta
- All layers of otic capsule affected
- Greater degree of structural disorganization and larger resorption spaces

Osteopetrosis
- Increased density of bone throughout entire body

Paget Disease
- Excessive bone resorption and formation due to activated osteoclasts
- "Moth-eaten" appearance eroding otic capsule from periphery

SELECTED REFERENCES

1. Markou K et al: An overview of the etiology of otosclerosis. Eur Arch Otorhinolaryngol. 266(1):25-35, 2009
2. Uppal S et al: Otosclerosis 1: the aetiopathogenesis of otosclerosis. Int J Clin Pract. 63(10):1526-30, 2009
3. Marshall AH et al: Cochlear implantation in cochlear otosclerosis. Laryngoscope. 115(10):1728-33, 2005

IMAGE GALLERY

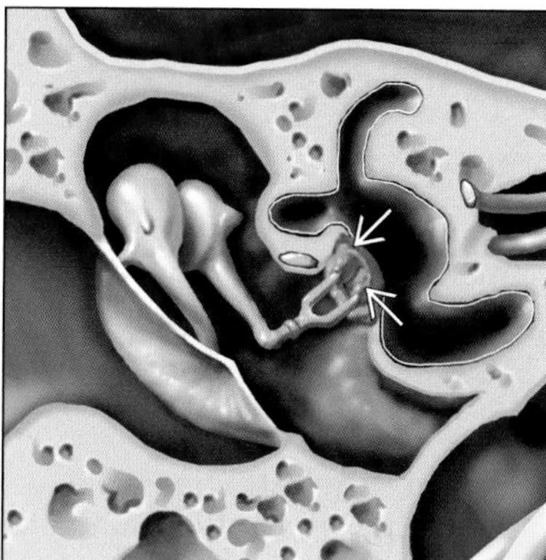

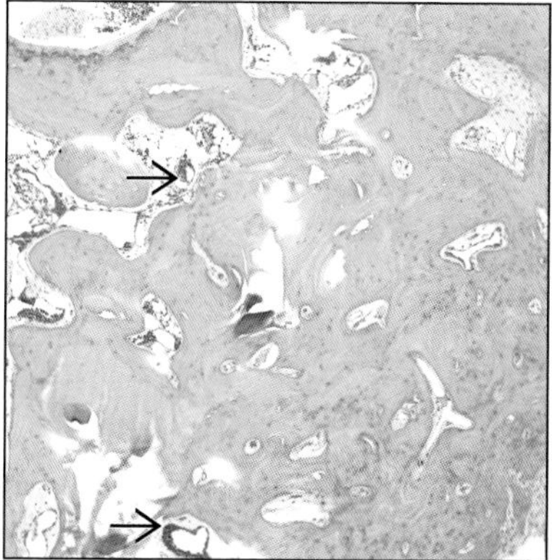

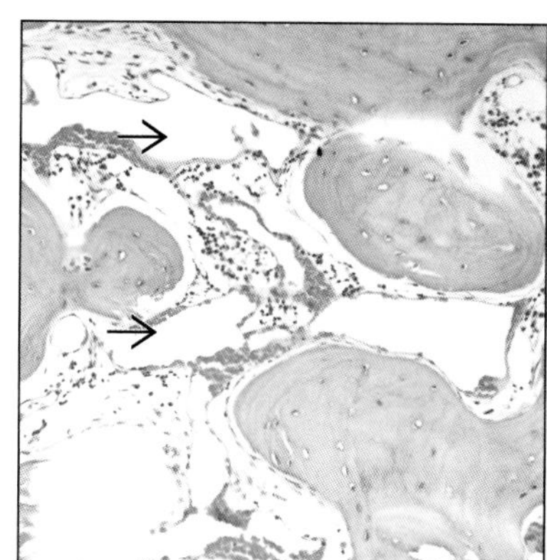

(Left) *Coronal graphic illustrates findings of fenestral otosclerosis, with a "donut" otospongiotic plaque ➡ surrounding the stapes footplate in the oval window. The crisp margins of the oval window are obscured by plaque. The ossicles are normal.* ***(Center)*** *Dense bone formation is accompanied by a vascular proliferation ➡ with increased osteocytes. The bone may be lamellar, woven or semi-woven.* ***(Right)*** *Vascular channels ➡ can be prominent, associated with bone deposition (mature acidophilic woven bone).*

GOUT

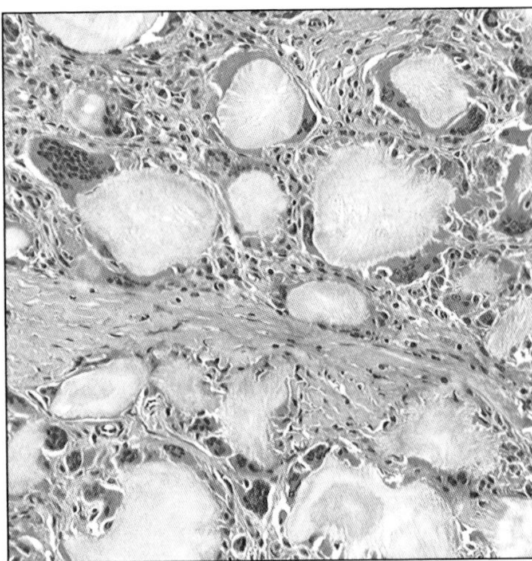

The foreign body giant cell reaction is remarkable, with crystal outlines easily identified in each collection. This is a characteristic appearance for a gouty tophus.

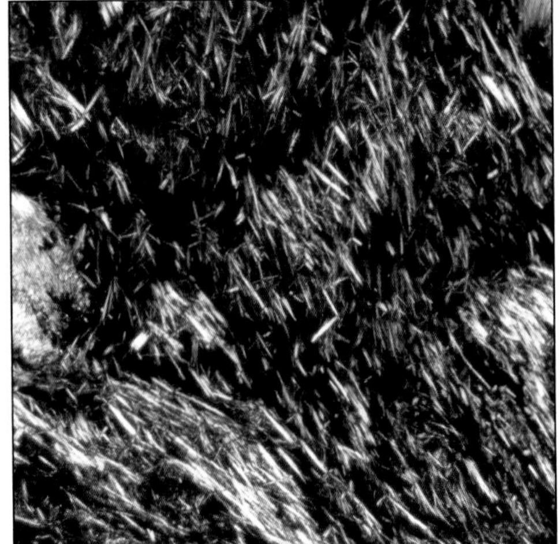

Unstained crystals examined under polarized light show needle-shaped crystals that appear very bright against the dark background. Examination should be done quickly to avoid degradation.

TERMINOLOGY

Definitions

- Inflammatory process initiated by soft tissue deposition of monosodium urate (MSU) crystals

ETIOLOGY/PATHOGENESIS

Pathogenesis

- Purine metabolism results in end product of uric acid by conversion of xanthine by xanthine oxidase
- Hyperuricemia is main factor facilitating MSU crystal formation
  - Urate is filtered by kidney, with > 90% resorbed
    - Main reason for increased urate is impaired renal function
  - Urate controlled by purine ingestion, liver production, recycling, degradation
  - Overproduction associated with excessive alcohol intake, fructose consumption
- Urate crystals provoke inflammatory response from leukocytes and synovial cells
  - Phagocytosed by monocytes as particles

CLINICAL ISSUES

Epidemiology

- Incidence
  - Gout is most prevalent inflammatory arthritis in developed countries
    - Incidence: 1-3/1,000 men/year, 1/5,000 women/year
  - Increasing, especially in older population
    - Increased in patient with high meat, seafood, and fructose consumption; high beer &/or alcohol intake
- Age
  - Older patients
- Gender
  - Male > Female (3:1)
    - Females increased in postmenopausal years (decreased estrogen is uricosuric)
- Ethnicity
  - Lower incidence in blacks, Japanese, Native Americans

Site

- Ear is most common site of tophus formation in head and neck
  - Larynx, thyroid cartilages, nasal septum, temporomandibular joint

Presentation

- Initial symptoms of gout are usually
  - Monoarticular arthritis and pain, usually of 1st toe
- **Ear**: Irregular, painful deposits in skin
- **Larynx**: Airway compromise and mucosal changes that mimic squamous cell carcinoma
- Drugs can also precipitate acute gout through altered uric acid concentrations
- Solid organ transplant patients develop hyperuricemia, with about 10% developing gout

Laboratory Tests

- Normal plasma urate levels: 200-410 μmol/L (3.3-6.9 mg/dL), with gout patients showing elevation

Natural History

- Natural history of gout
  - Asymptomatic hyperuricemia
  - Episodes of acute attacks of gout with asymptomatic intervals
  - Chronic tophaceous arthritis

Treatment

- Options, risks, complications
  - Acute attacks managed with rest, immediate treatment with colchicine, and anti-inflammatory agents

GOUT

Key Facts

Terminology
- Definition: Inflammatory process initiated by soft tissue deposition of monosodium urate crystals

Clinical Issues
- Gout is most prevalent inflammatory arthritis in developed countries
- Older male patients (Male > Female [3:1])
- Progression: Asymptomatic hyperuricemia, acute attacks, tophaceous deposits
- Ear: Irregular, painful deposits in skin
- Acute attacks managed with rest, immediate treatment with colchicine, and anti-inflammatory agents

Microscopic Pathology
- Tophi: Urate crystals surrounded by chronic mononuclear and giant cell reactions in soft tissues

Top Differential Diagnoses
- Rheumatoid nodules

  - Aim to maintain urate concentration below saturation point for MSU
- Drugs
  - Wide armamentarium of drugs to treat hyperuricemia and effects

Prognosis
- Disease waxes and wanes
- Polyarticular arthritis, renal injury, and nephrolithiasis are complications

MACROSCOPIC FEATURES

General Features
- Most specimens arrive as fluids for crystal examination
- Tophi will show white, chalky consistency when cut

Size
- Tophi range: 1-6 cm

MICROSCOPIC PATHOLOGY

Histologic Features
- Tophi: Urate crystals surrounded by chronic mononuclear and giant cell reactions in soft tissues
- Skin overlying the tophus ulcerates
  - MSU crystals are dissolved by formalin-based preservatives
    - Leave basophilic granular deposits on light microscopy when dissolved
    - Specimens should be submitted in ethanol
- Fluid should be examined rapidly at room temperature
  - Formation and solubility of crystals are affected by temperature and pH
  - Under direct polarized light
    - Crystals are strongly birefringent
    - Yellow when aligned parallel to light
    - Blue when aligned perpendicular to light
    - Bright against black background

DIFFERENTIAL DIAGNOSIS

Rheumatoid Nodules
- Necrotizing granulomatous inflammation with peripherally palisaded epithelioid histiocytes
- Vasculitis may be present

SELECTED REFERENCES

1. Kalish LH et al: Pseudogout mimicking an infratemporal fossa tumor. Head Neck. 32(1):127-32, 2010
2. Griffin GR et al: Auricular tophi as the initial presentation of gout. Otolaryngol Head Neck Surg. 141(1):153-4, 2009
3. Hollowell M et al: Gout. Ear Nose Throat J. 87(3):132, 134, 2008
4. Guttenplan MD et al: Laryngeal manifestations of gout. Ann Otol Rhinol Laryngol. 100(11):899-902, 1991
5. Stark TW et al: Gout and its manifestations in the head and neck. Otolaryngol Clin North Am. 15(3):659-64, 1982

IMAGE GALLERY

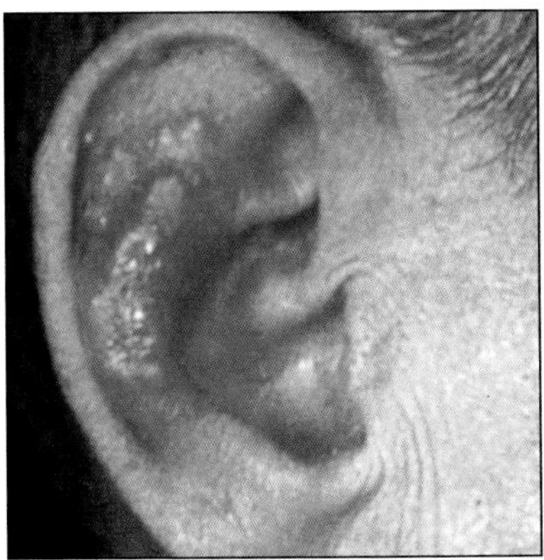

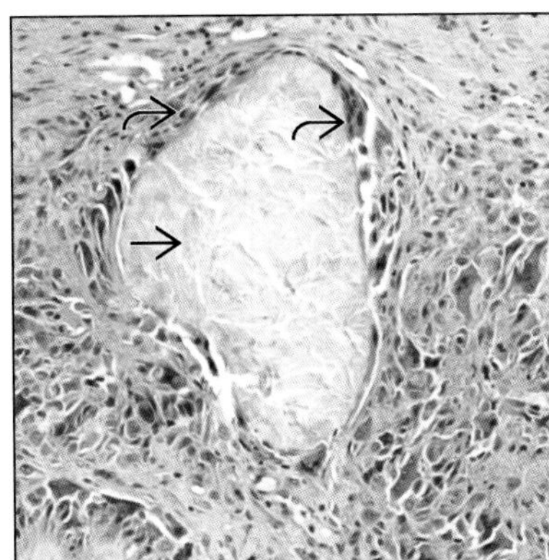

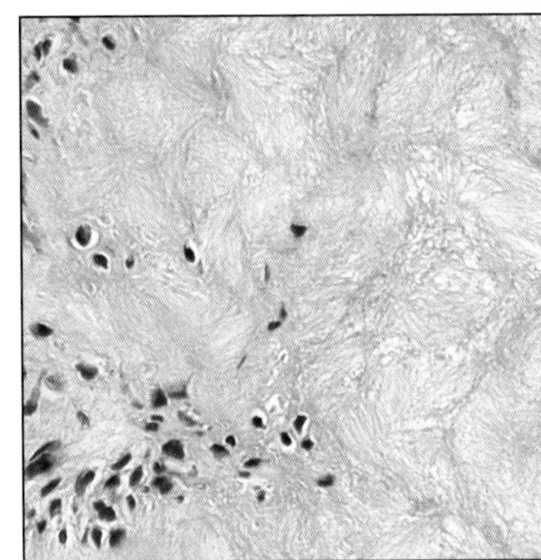

(Left) Tophaceous gout presents as irregularly shaped deposits under the skin and often present on the ear. Cut surfaces will have a white, chalky appearance. (Center) Gouty deposits show amorphous collections of crystals ➔ surrounded by foreign body giant cells ➚ and scattered inflammatory cells. (Right) Characteristic needle-like crystals will not polarize effectively if they have been fixed in formalin, as the crystals are water soluble. Ethanol tissue fixation will preserve the crystal polarization.

CHOLESTEATOMA

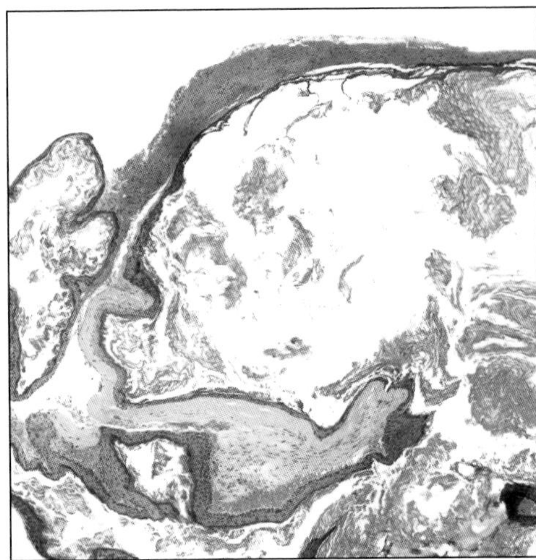

Hematoxylin & eosin shows squamous epithelium with keratin debris and fibrous connective tissue. The squamous epithelium is not thickened and shows no atypia.

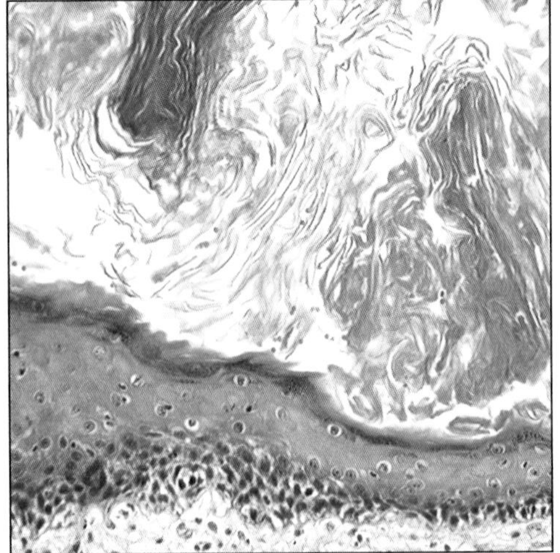

Hematoxylin & eosin shows squamous epithelium with keratin debris and fibrous connective tissue. There is a slightly prominent granular cell layer, although this is not always the case.

TERMINOLOGY

Synonyms

- Glue ear
- Mastoiditis
- Keratosis obturans (incorrect)
  - Acute, severe pain secondary to accumulation of large plugs of desquamated keratin in **ear canal**, not **middle ear**

Definitions

- Nonneoplastic, cystic keratinizing lesion of temporal bone, resulting in destruction of ossicular chain
- Congenital type
  - Develops behind normal and intact tympanic membrane
  - Lacks eustachian tube dysfunction and otitis media
  - Arises from fetal epidermoid formations
- Acquired type
  - Defect (perforation) in tympanic membrane
  - Associated with inflammation
  - Results in proliferation of keratinizing epithelium
    - Via migration, basal hyperplasia, retraction pocket, &/or trauma

ETIOLOGY/PATHOGENESIS

Infectious Agents

- Chronic inflammation (usually from bacterial infection)
  - Plays critical role in stimulating epithelium to proliferate
  - Releases cytokines (tumor necrosis factor-alpha [TNF-α] specifically but also RANKL and IL-1), producing collagenases, which results in osteolysis of bone

Congenital

- Small epidermoid formations occasionally develop during embryologic development
  - Found within anterosuperior quadrant of middle ear cleft epithelium
  - These give rise to congenital cholesteatoma if not resorbed (usually by end of 2nd year)

CLINICAL ISSUES

Epidemiology

- Incidence
  - Common
- Age
  - Wide age range
  - Propensity for older children and young adults (up to 4th decade)
- Gender
  - Equal gender distribution

Site

- Usually unilateral
- Superior, posterior middle ear (acquired); anterior, superior middle ear (congenital)
- Petrous apex
- May expand into adjacent structures

Presentation

- Long history of severe chronic otitis media, often refractory to therapy
- Hearing loss due to destruction of ossicular chain
  - Conductive loss rather than sensorineural
- Otalgia and otorrhea
- Foul smelling aural discharge
- Perforation of tympanic membrane (acquired form)
- Vestibular dysfunction, vomiting, vertigo, and tinnitus
- Facial paralysis
- Headaches

CHOLESTEATOMA

Key Facts

Terminology

- Cholesteatoma, whether congenital or acquired, is nonneoplastic, cystic keratinizing lesion of temporal bone, resulting in destruction of ossicular chain

Etiology/Pathogenesis

- Chronic inflammation plays critical role in stimulating epithelium to proliferate
- Releases cytokines, resulting in osteolysis of bone

Clinical Issues

- Propensity for older children and young adults (up to 4th decade)
- Superior, posterior middle ear and petrous apex
- Severe chronic otitis media, foul smelling discharge, hearing loss
- Complete surgical removal is treatment of choice, although recurrences develop in ~ 20%

Macroscopic Features

- Multiple fragments of flaky, keratinaceous debris, associated with foul odor

Microscopic Pathology

- 3 components required for diagnosis
  - Keratinous material (keratin flakes, anucleate squames)
  - Stratified squamous epithelium with granular layer
  - Inflamed stroma with fibrous connective tissue

Top Differential Diagnoses

- Cholesterol granuloma
- Squamous cell carcinoma

- Rarely, intracranial complications; when present, emergent management required
- Congenital cholesteatoma patients tend not to have otitis media or hearing loss

Treatment

- Options, risks, complications
  - Cholesteatoma are invasive, aggressive, and recurrent lesions, resulting in considerable morbidity if not managed correctly
  - Optimal treatment is controversial but needs to be highly individualized
    - Surgery with intact canal wall vs. open cavity technique
    - If 2nd look procedure is required, perhaps there is posterior mesotympanum involvement, ossicular chain interruption, or incomplete removal
    - Staging ossicular reconstruction, including prosthetics
  - Urgent surgery necessary if facial nerve dysfunction, vertigo, or severe headaches are present
  - Complications include fistula, sigmoid sinus erosion, cranial nerve dysfunction, meningitis, and epidural or brain abscess
- Surgical approaches
  - Complete surgical removal
    - Modified radical (ossicles left) or radical (stapes left) mastoidectomy
  - Attic compartments require adequate aeration
    - Achieved by removal of tensor and lateral incudomalleal folds
    - Different techniques depending on whether ossicular chain is intact or discontinuous
- Drugs
  - Early antibiotic treatment of otitis media and associated inflammatory conditions may decrease chance of developing cholesteatoma

Prognosis

- This reactive and osteolytic process can be aggressive and recidivistic
  - Recurrences in about 20% of cases
  - Increased risk of recurrence if < 20 years of age, marked ossicular chain erosion/destruction, polypoid mucosal disease, and extensive disease
- Congenital cholesteatoma patients tend to do better
  - Require early detection to achieve best result
  - Tend not to develop complications or recurrences postoperatively

IMAGE FINDINGS

Radiographic Findings

- Preoperative radiology essential to identify landmarks and extent of disease
- Soft tissue mass displacing ossicles medially
- Bone destruction usually present

MR Findings

- Best in characterizing expansile and destructive lesions of petrous apex
- High-resolution scanning techniques can define precise spatial relationships of middle and inner ear structures
  - Specifically, relationship to internal carotid artery and jugular vein
- Excellent in postoperative evaluation of completeness of removal, development of complications or recurrence
- Detects involvement of meninges and veins (sigmoid sinus, jugular)
- Prolongation of both T1 and T2 signals
  - T1 signal has low intensity
  - T2 signal has high intensity

CT Findings

- Highlights small abnormalities of thin and complex bony structures
- Precise extent of bone erosion
- Identifies fistulization through tegmen tympani or posterior wall of temporal bone

CHOLESTEATOMA

MACROSCOPIC FEATURES

General Features

- Gray-white to yellow irregular mass behind tympanic membrane
- Multiple fragments of flaky, keratinaceous debris
- Foul odor
- Bony fragments often identified macroscopically

Sections to Be Submitted

- Submit all tissue to confirm diagnosis

MICROSCOPIC PATHOLOGY

Histologic Features

- Epithelium behaves like wound-healing process without any inherent genetic instability
- Name is misnomer because it is not a neoplasm and does not contain cholesterol
  - However, it destroys local tissues and can recur
- Normal middle ear epithelium is cuboidal or columnar glandular epithelium: Squamous epithelium is abnormal
- 3 components required for diagnosis
  - Keratinous material (keratin flakes; dead, anucleate keratin squames)
  - Stratified squamous epithelium with granular layer (derived from external auditory canal)
  - Inflamed stroma with fibrous connective tissue
- Epithelium is keratinizing, stratified squamous epithelium without atypia, tends to be atrophic, and lacks rete pegs
- Epithelium lines cystic space filled with exfoliated anucleated squames
- Inflammatory component is usually lymphocytes, plasma cells, histiocytes, and mast cells
- Concurrent disorders include cholesterol granuloma, otic polyp, tympanosclerosis, acquired encephalocele, and middle ear adenoma (NAME)

ANCILLARY TESTS

Immunohistochemistry

- Ki-67 (MIB-1) and ErbB-2 are increased in cases that are more biologically aggressive
- Keratin 16 (K16) strong expression (marker of hyperproliferative keratinocytes)

In Situ Hybridization

- FISH shows extra copy of chromosome 7
  - Correlates with proliferation activity and is seen in cases that are more clinically aggressive

DIFFERENTIAL DIAGNOSIS

Cholesterol Granuloma

- Elongated clefts (spaces) left by cholesterol crystals dissolved in processing
- Foreign body giant cell reaction with inflammation
- Hemosiderin-laden macrophages
- Granulation-type tissue identified
- May be identified concurrently with cholesteatoma

Squamous Cell Carcinoma

- Squamous epithelial cells are pleomorphic/atypical
- Lack of maturation or polarity
- Have dyskeratosis and keratin pearl formation
- Increased mitotic figures, including atypical forms

Otitis Media

- Lacks proliferative squamous epithelium and anucleated squames

SELECTED REFERENCES

1. Louw L: Acquired cholesteatoma pathogenesis: stepwise explanations. J Laryngol Otol. 124(6):587-93, 2010
2. Vercruysse JP et al: Magnetic resonance imaging of cholesteatoma: an update. B-ENT. 5(4):233-40, 2009
3. Isaacson G: Diagnosis of pediatric cholesteatoma. Pediatrics. 120(3):603-8, 2007
4. Persaud R et al: Evidence-based review of aetiopathogenic theories of congenital and acquired cholesteatoma. J Laryngol Otol. 121(11):1013-9, 2007
5. Vitale RF et al: The role of tumor necrosis factor-alpha (TNF-alpha) in bone resorption present in middle ear cholesteatoma. Braz J Otorhinolaryngol. 73(1):117-21, 2007
6. Bennett M et al: Congenital cholesteatoma: theories, facts, and 53 patients. Otolaryngol Clin North Am. 39(6):1081-94, 2006
7. Schraff SA et al: Pediatric cholesteatoma: a retrospective review. Int J Pediatr Otorhinolaryngol. 70(3):385-93, 2006
8. Semaan MT et al: The pathophysiology of cholesteatoma. Otolaryngol Clin North Am. 39(6):1143-59, 2006
9. Ryan AF et al: Recent advances in otitis media. 4B. Biochemistry. Ann Otol Rhinol Laryngol Suppl. 194:50-5, 2005
10. Olszewska E et al: Etiopathogenesis of cholesteatoma. Eur Arch Otorhinolaryngol. 261(1):6-24, 2004
11. Maroldi R et al: Computed tomography and magnetic resonance imaging of pathologic conditions of the middle ear. Eur J Radiol. 40(2):78-93, 2001
12. Pisaneschi MJ et al: Congenital cholesteatoma and cholesterol granuloma of the temporal bone: role of magnetic resonance imaging. Top Magn Reson Imaging. 11(2):87-97, 2000
13. Watts S et al: A systematic approach to interpretation of computed tomography scans prior to surgery of middle ear cholesteatoma. J Laryngol Otol. 114(4):248-53, 2000
14. Palva T et al: Chronic inflammatory ear disease and cholesteatoma: creation of auxiliary attic aeration pathways by microdissection. Am J Otol. 20(2):145-51, 1999
15. Albino AP et al: Cholesteatoma: a molecular and cellular puzzle. Am J Otol. 19(1):7-19, 1998
16. Karmody CS et al: The origin of congenital cholesteatoma. Am J Otol. 19(3):292-7, 1998
17. Ferlito A et al: Clinicopathological consultation. Ear cholesteatoma versus cholesterol granuloma. Ann Otol Rhinol Laryngol. 106(1):79-85, 1997
18. Roger G et al: Predictive risk factors of residual cholesteatoma in children: a study of 256 cases. Am J Otol. 18(5):550-8, 1997
19. Corbridge RJ et al: Epithelial migration in keratosis obturans. Am J Otolaryngol. 17(6):411-4, 1996

Embryologic, Radiographic, and Microscopic Features

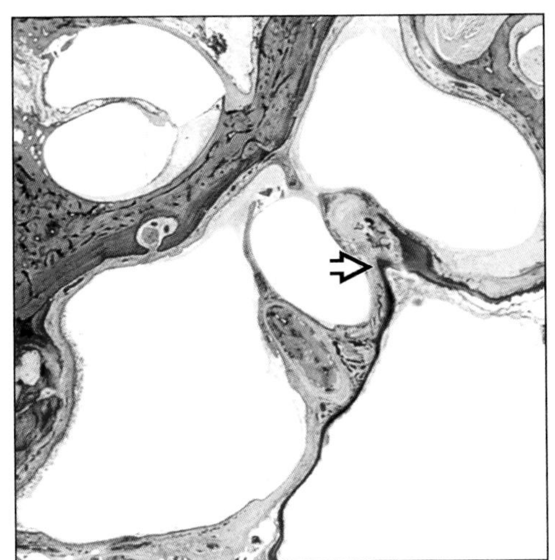

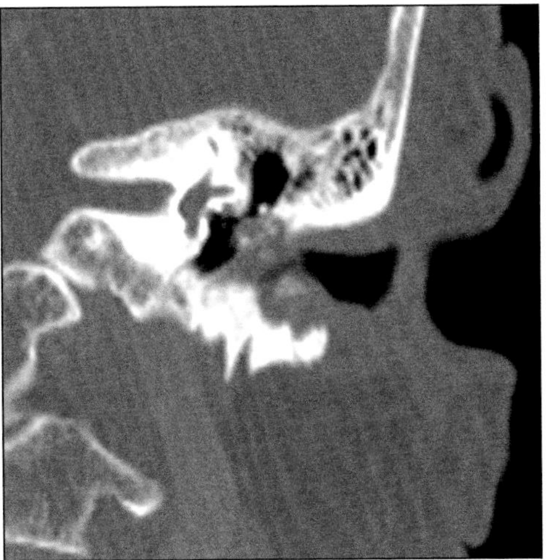

(Left) *Hematoxylin & eosin of a fetus temporal bone shows an area of retraction pocket formation ➯. (Courtesy L. Michaels, MD.)* ***(Right)*** *This image from a computed tomography scan demonstrates inflammatory debris associated with bone destruction of the middle ear. The ossicular chain is uninvolved.*

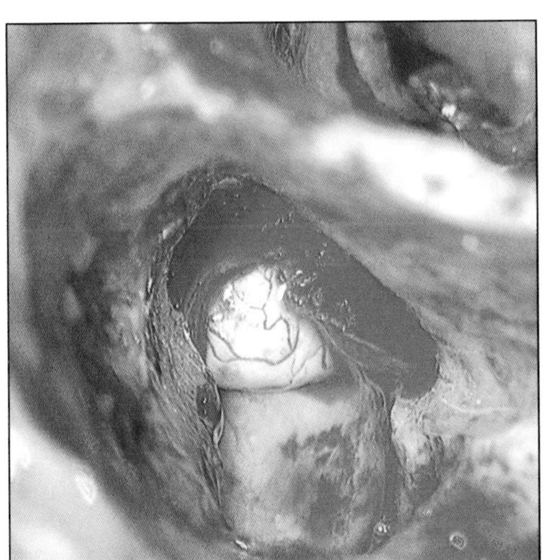

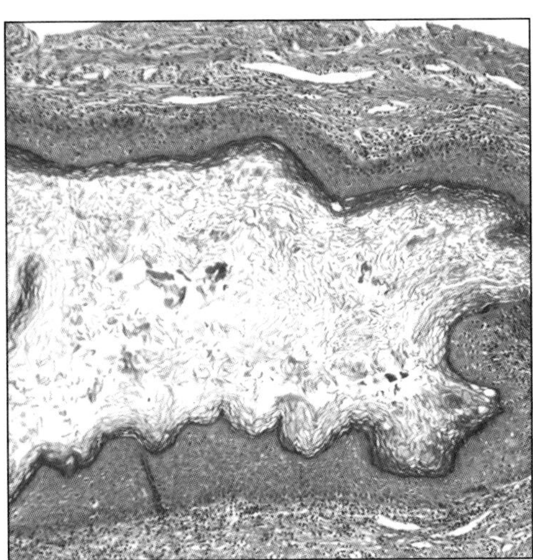

(Left) *An intraoperative photograph demonstrates the collection of debris within the cavity. (Courtesy D. Cua, MD.)* ***(Right)*** *Hematoxylin & eosin shows a proliferation of squamous epithelium with associated inflammation and keratin debris. The epithelium is sometimes corrugated or verruciform.*

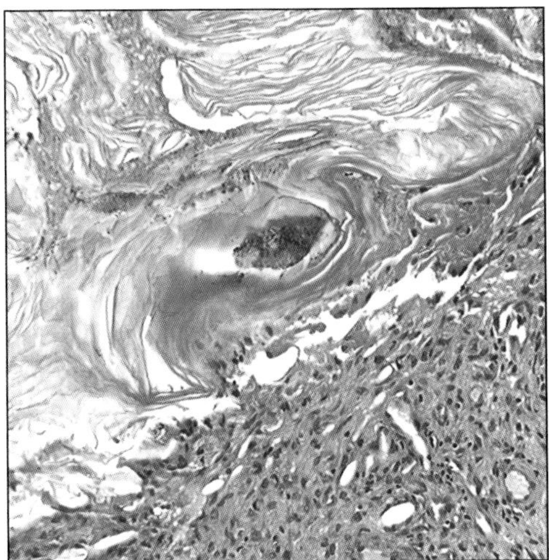

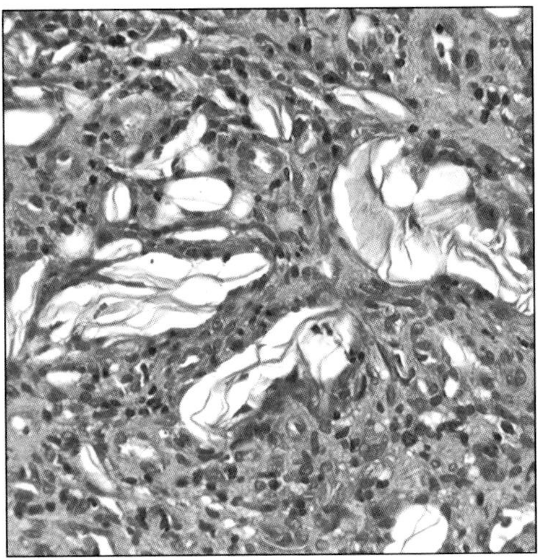

(Left) *Hematoxylin & eosin shows inflammation and keratin debris. There is no epithelium within this field, highlighting the necessity to review all material in cholesteatoma samples.* ***(Right)*** *Keratin flakes are frequently identified in association with inflammation and foreign body giant cell reaction. This is not a cholesterol granuloma; however, the lesions can sometimes be concurrent.*

EXOSTOSIS

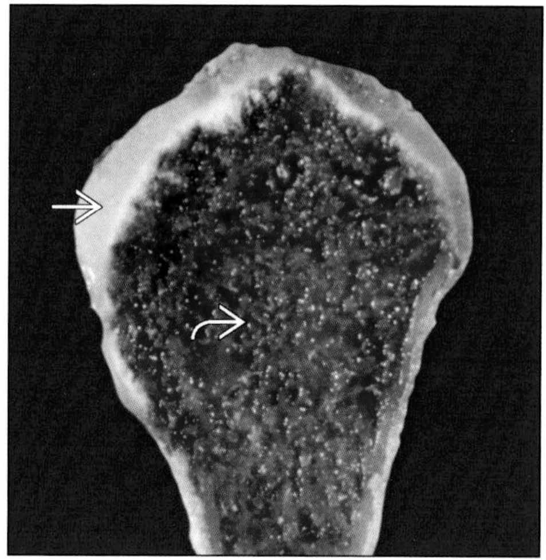

Grossly, exostoses are composed of a bony stalk ➔ with red and yellow marrow and an overlying bluish-gray cartilage cap ➔. Exostoses can be pedunculated or broad based.

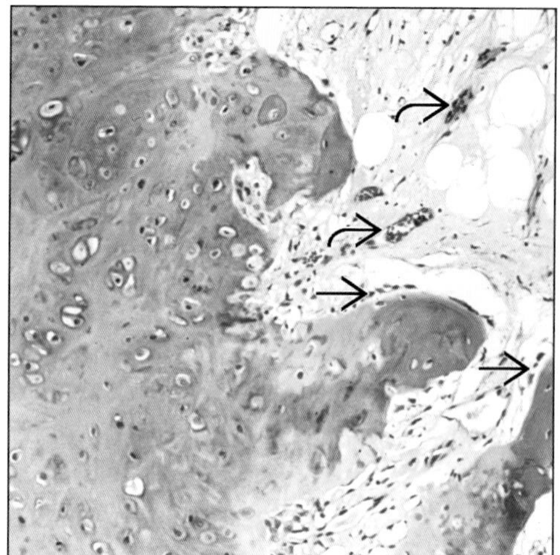

Cartilage merges seamlessly with bone. Prominent osteoblasts are noted, forming bone ➔ with associated intervening vessels ➔. These are features of endochondral ossification.

TERMINOLOGY

Abbreviations

- External auditory canal (EAC)

Synonyms

- Surfer's ear
- Cold water ear

Definitions

- Benign hyperostotic outgrowths of bony external auditory canal

ETIOLOGY/PATHOGENESIS

Environmental Exposure

- Cold water exposure causes more severe external auditory exostosis, possibly by 2 methods
  - Irritation of EAC
  - Increased vascular flow
- Other environmental factors may play a role
  - Climatologic factors
    - West coast surfers have more severe exostoses in right vs. left ear
    - Probably due to northerly wind in coldest months as surfers face west
    - Evaporative cooling is greater in wind-exposed ear

CLINICAL ISSUES

Epidemiology

- Incidence
  - While uncommon, incidence is related to patients with prolonged cold water exposure
    - Prevalence in **surfers**: 70-80%
    - Incidence in **saltwater** swimmers: 6%
    - Incidence in **freshwater** swimmers: 5%
- Age
  - Usually young patients
- Gender
  - Male > > > Female
- Ethnicity
  - Very low to absent in blacks (reason unknown)

Site

- Almost always bilateral
- Lesion usually present medial to isthmus of EAC
  - Both anterior and posterior for vast majority
  - Begins at medial osseous EAC

Presentation

- Conductive hearing loss
  - Although a bilateral disorder, 80% of patients present with unilateral symptoms
- Chronic history of prolonged cold water exposures
  - Swimmers, cold water surfers, divers (SCUBA), white-water kayakers
- Otitis externa, tinnitus, otalgia

Endoscopic Findings

- Otoscopic view shows circumferential submucosal narrowing

Treatment

- Options, risks, complications
  - Typically benign lesion, requiring no treatment
    - Ear plugs may decrease progression
  - If surgery is used, postsurgical complications can be seen in 5% and include
    - Canal stenosis, temporal-mandibular joint prolapse, sensorineural hearing loss, persistent tympanic membrane perforation
- Surgical approaches
  - EAC drilling is surgical management of choice, if patients are symptomatic
  - Potential surgical problems include
    - Skin over exostosis is frequently traumatized by drill

EXOSTOSIS

Key Facts

Terminology
- Benign hyperostotic outgrowths of bony external auditory canal

Clinical Issues
- Incidence is related to patients with chronic history of prolonged cold water exposure
  - Swimmers, cold water surfers, SCUBA divers
  - Prevalence in **surfers**: 70-80%
- Male > > > Female
- Almost always bilateral
- Conductive hearing loss
- Typically benign lesion, requiring no treatment

Microscopic Pathology
- Histologically composed of broad-based lamellar bone

Top Differential Diagnoses
- Osteoma

    - Tympanic membrane may be perforated, potentially damaging ossicular chain &/or chorda tympani nerve
    - Temporomandibular joint dehiscence

IMAGE FINDINGS

General Features
- Benign, broad-based, bilateral, circumferential overgrowth of osseous EAC with normal overlying soft tissues
- Noncontrast CT with bone algorithm of temporal bone

MACROSCOPIC FEATURES

General Features
- Identified near tympanic annulus, at tympanomastoid and tympanosquamous sutures

MICROSCOPIC PATHOLOGY

Histologic Features
- Bony stalk and overlying cartilage cap
  - Similar to normal epiphyseal growth
  - Cartilage cap may be very thinned or have matured fully to bone
- Histologically composed of broad-based lamellar bone
  - In many cases, exostoses and osteomata cannot be reliably separated without radiographic/clinical information

DIFFERENTIAL DIAGNOSIS

Osteoma
- Location (lateral to isthmus) and clinical symptoms different from exostoses

SELECTED REFERENCES

1. Kroon DF et al: Surfer's ear: external auditory exostoses are more prevalent in cold water surfers. Otolaryngol Head Neck Surg. 126(5):499-504, 2002
2. Longridge NS: Exostosis of the external auditory canal: a technical note. Otol Neurotol. 23(3):260-1, 2002
3. Agarwal A et al: Exostoses of the external auditory canal. Am J Otol. 20(6):807-8, 1999
4. Wong BJ et al: Prevalence of external auditory canal exostoses in surfers. Arch Otolaryngol Head Neck Surg. 125(9):969-72, 1999
5. Chaplin JM et al: The prevalence of exostoses in the external auditory meatus of surfers. Clin Otolaryngol Allied Sci. 23(4):326-30, 1998
6. Whitaker SR et al: Treatment of external auditory canal exostoses. Laryngoscope. 108(2):195-9, 1998
7. Fenton JE et al: A histopathologic review of temporal bone exostoses and osteomata. Laryngoscope. 106(5 Pt 1):624-8, 1996

IMAGE GALLERY

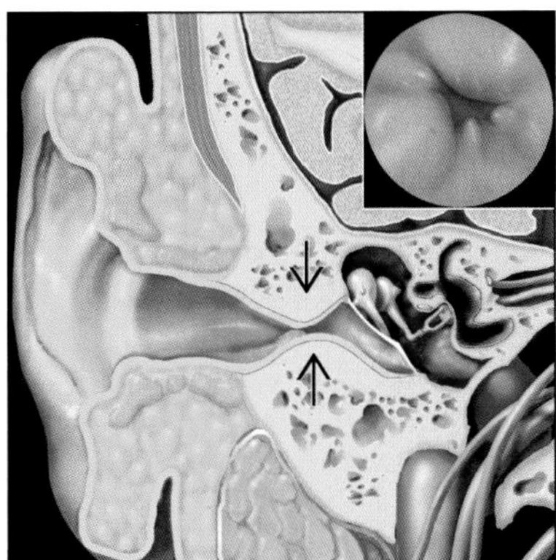

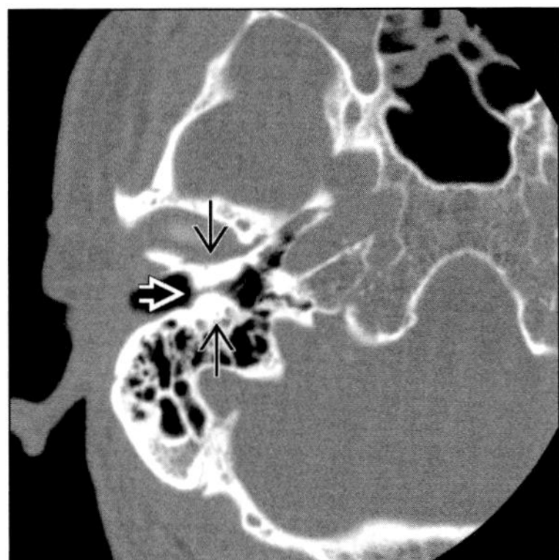

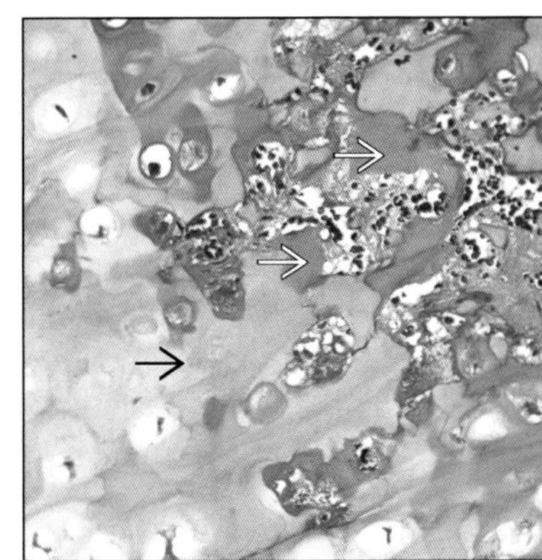

(Left) *Coronal graphic shows benign-appearing bony overgrowth of the right EAC ⇒ in a case of EAC exostoses. Insert shows otoscopic view of circumferential submucosal EAC narrowing.* ***(Center)*** *Right axial noncontrast bone CT shows osseous encroachment ⇒ of the EAC. It also demonstrates minimal soft tissue within the EAC, just lateral to the stenosis ➡.* ***(Right)*** *Endochondral ossification is similar to a growth plate. The cartilage ⇒ matures to bone ➡.*

KELOID

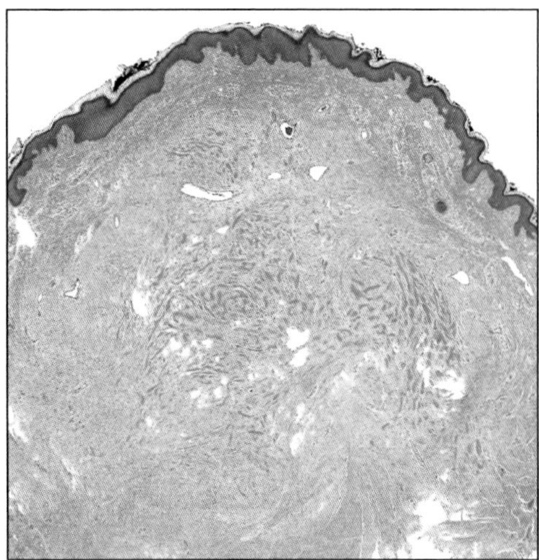

Low-power magnification shows a polypoid skin lesion with dense dermal collagen.

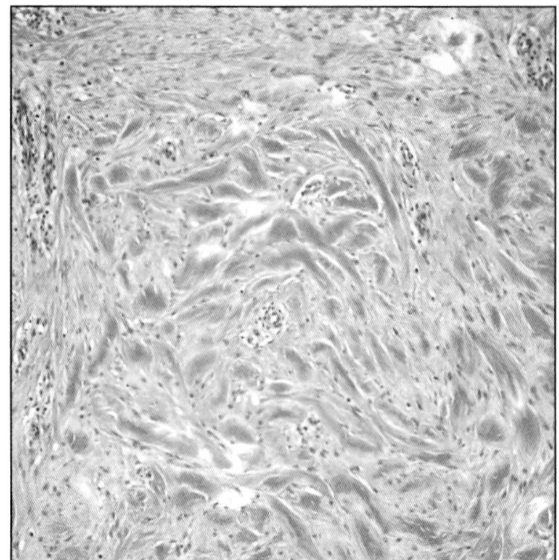

High-power magnification shows a proliferation of thickened, hyalinized eosinophilic collagen bundles with increased numbers of stromal fibroblasts and scattered lymphocytes.

TERMINOLOGY

Synonyms

- Scar with keloidal collagen

Definitions

- Scar with prominent thickened and eosinophilic bundles of collagen extending beyond original wound

ETIOLOGY/PATHOGENESIS

Idiopathic

- Fibroblasts from keloids show decreased apoptosis
- Many cytokines implicated in stimulating fibroblasts, including TGF-β and IL-15
- Genetic influence is likely

CLINICAL ISSUES

Epidemiology

- Age
  - Most common in patients < 30 years
- Ethnicity
  - More common in black patients
  - Least common in white patients

Site

- Earlobe is most common site
  - Typically follows ear piercing or other trauma
  - Usually develops within a few months

Presentation

- Mass is most common
- Scar growing beyond confines of original wound
- Often erythematous, pruritic lesions with predilection for earlobe in black patients

Treatment

- Options, risks, complications
  - Potentially disfiguring with high recurrence risk
- Surgical approaches
  - Complete excision, accompanied by concurrent steroid injections or radiotherapy to decrease risk of recurrence
- Drugs
  - Direct injection of steroids is often first-line treatment

Prognosis

- Persistence and recurrence are common
- No increased risk of malignancy

MACROSCOPIC FEATURES

General Features

- Large, nodular, dermal-based lesion
- Firm, white cut surface

MICROSCOPIC PATHOLOGY

Histologic Features

- Dense proliferation of thickened, hyalinized collagen bundles in dermis
- May be background of conventional or hypertrophic scar
  - Contains smaller collagen bundles and perpendicular vessels
- Decreased vessels compared to conventional and hypertrophic scars
  - Superficial telangiectatic vessels often present
  - Associated with mild chronic inflammation
- Overlying epidermis may show atrophy
- Increased fibroblasts, lymphocytes, and mast cells are usually present

KELOID

Key Facts

Terminology
- Scar with prominent thickened and eosinophilic bundles of collagen

Clinical Issues
- Persistence and recurrence are common, but no increased risk of malignancy
- Scar growing beyond original wound
- Often erythematous, pruritic lesions with predilection for earlobe in black patients

Microscopic Pathology
- Dense proliferation of thickened, hyalinized collagen bundles in dermis
- Decreased vessels compared to conventional and hypertrophic scars
- Increased fibroblasts, lymphocytes, and mast cells are usually present

Top Differential Diagnoses
- Hypertrophic scar

DIFFERENTIAL DIAGNOSIS

Hypertrophic Scar
- Lacks characteristic hyalinized collagen bundles of keloid
- More small, perpendicularly oriented vessels
- Lacks telangiectasia
- Overlapping cases may be seen; may be diagnosed as "hypertrophic scar with focal keloidal collagen"
- Not as clinically elevated as keloid

Desmoplastic Melanoma
- Unlikely, but rarely may enter differential diagnosis if no history of trauma or previous treatment (biopsy or excision)
- Re-excision specimens of desmoplastic melanoma may show keloidal collagen
- S100 protein immunohistochemical stains should be positive
  - Increased numbers of dermal dendritic cells may be seen in scars
  - Should not show spindled morphology of desmoplastic melanoma cells

Nodular Fasciitis
- May show focal keloidal collagen
- Background shows classic features of nodular fasciitis with loose, tissue culture appearance

DIAGNOSTIC CHECKLIST

Pathologic Interpretation Pearls
- Nodular, elevated lesion compared to adjacent skin
- Thickened, hyalinized eosinophilic collagen bundles
- Often see background of hypertrophic scar

SELECTED REFERENCES

1. Wolfram D et al: Hypertrophic scars and keloids--a review of their pathophysiology, risk factors, and therapeutic management. Dermatol Surg. 35(2):171-81, 2009
2. Butler PD et al: Current progress in keloid research and treatment. J Am Coll Surg. 206(4):731-41, 2008
3. Köse O et al: Keloids and hypertrophic scars: are they two different sides of the same coin? Dermatol Surg. 34(3):336-46, 2008
4. Froelich K et al: Therapy of auricular keloids: review of different treatment modalities and proposal for a therapeutic algorithm. Eur Arch Otorhinolaryngol. 264(12):1497-508, 2007
5. Rosen DJ et al: A primary protocol for the management of ear keloids: results of excision combined with intraoperative and postoperative steroid injections. Plast Reconstr Surg. 120(5):1395-400, 2007
6. Thompson LD: Skin keloid. Ear Nose Throat J. 83(8):519, 2004
7. Thompson LD et al: Nodular fasciitis of the external ear region: a clinicopathologic study of 50 cases. Ann Diagn Pathol. 5(4):191-8, 2001
8. Tuan TL et al: The molecular basis of keloid and hypertrophic scar formation. Mol Med Today. 4(1):19-24, 1998

IMAGE GALLERY

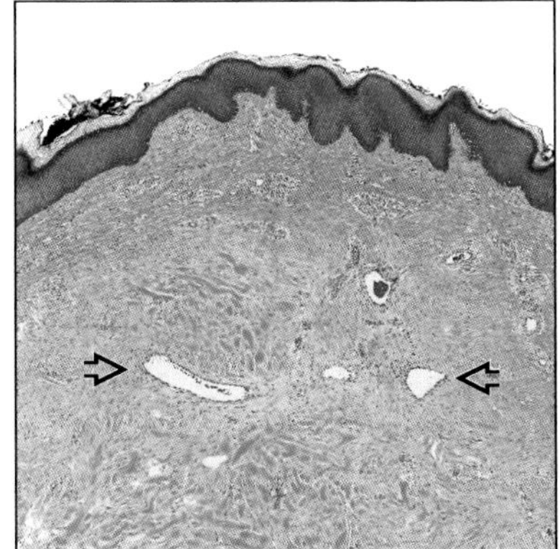

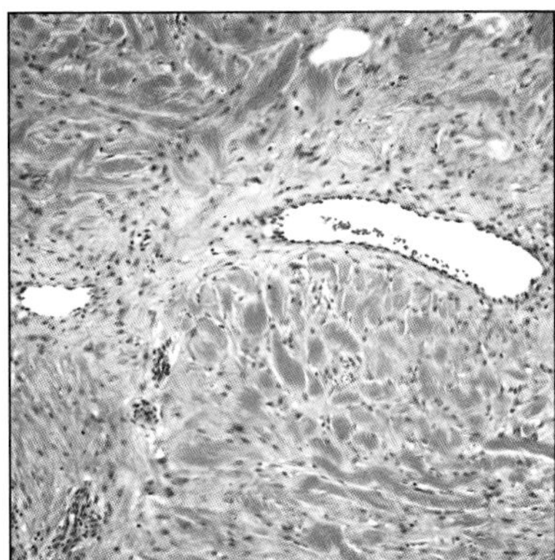

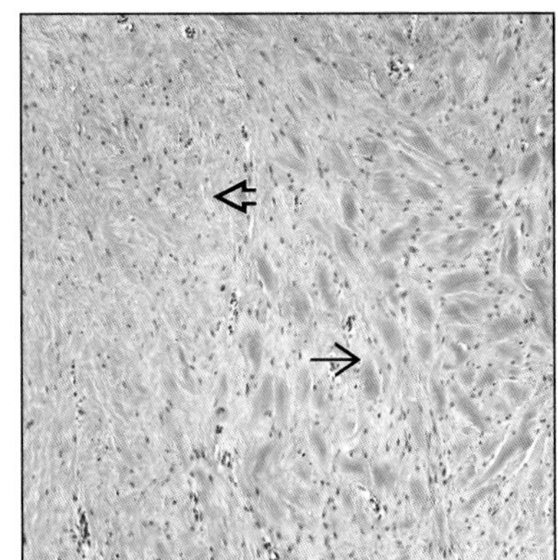

(Left) *Superficial aspect of the lesion shows scarring, telangiectasia ⇨, and prominent hyalinized collagen bundles.* ***(Center)*** *Superficial portion of a keloid shows telangiectatic vessels surrounded by thickened collagen bundles.* ***(Right)*** *Comparison between an area of hypertrophic scar ⇨ and a keloid → is shown.*

LANGERHANS CELL HISTIOCYTOSIS

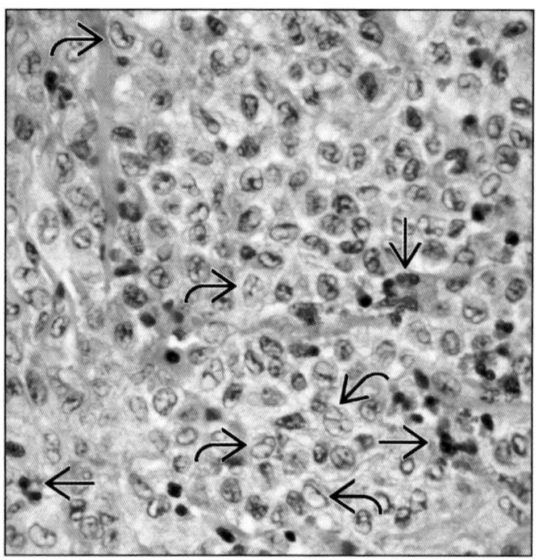

Sheet-like proliferation of Langerhans cells is characterized by vesicular nuclei, lobation of the nuclear membrane ↗, and admixed inflammatory cells, including eosinophils →.

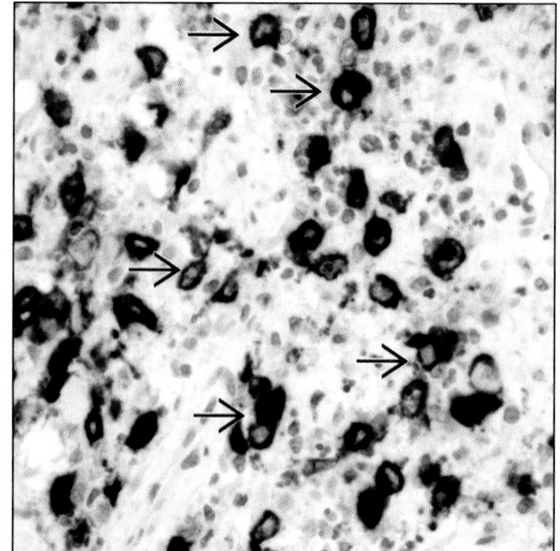

Langerhans cells show Langerin immunoreactivity → that, in conjunction with the light microscopic features and immunoreactivity for S100 protein and CD1a, confirms the diagnosis of Langerhans cell histiocytosis.

TERMINOLOGY

Abbreviations

- Langerhans cell histiocytosis (LCH)

Synonyms

- Langerhans cell (eosinophilic) granulomatosis
- Eosinophilic granuloma
- Histiocytosis X disease group including
  - Eosinophilic granuloma, Letterer-Siwe syndrome, and Hand-Schüller-Christian
  - Designation of LCH replaced histiocytosis X

Definitions

- Clonal proliferation of Langerhans cells (component of dendritic cell system) occurring as isolated lesion or part of systemic (multifocal) proliferation

CLINICAL ISSUES

Epidemiology

- Age
  - Most common in 2nd-3rd decades
- Gender
  - Male > Female

Presentation

- In patients with middle ear and temporal bone involvement
  - Aural discharge
  - Swelling of temporal bone area
  - Otitis media
  - Bone pain, otalgia
  - Hearing loss, vertigo

Treatment

- Options, risks, complications
  - Surgical excision and low-dose radiotherapy considered treatment of choice
- Surgical approaches
  - Surgical excision (curettage)
- Adjuvant therapy
  - Chemotherapy used for multifocal and systemic disease
- Radiation
  - 500-1,500 rads

Prognosis

- Considered very good
  - Failure of new bone lesion to occur within 1 year of diagnosis considered cure
  - Adverse prognostic findings
    - Younger age at onset
    - More extensive involvement (multiple sites, including bone and viscera)
- Recurrence may be part of systemic or multifocal process
  - Generally occurs within 6 months of diagnosis

IMAGE FINDINGS

General Features

- Single or multiple, sharply circumscribed, osteolytic lesions

MICROSCOPIC PATHOLOGY

Histologic Features

- Langerhans cells
  - Enlarged nuclei with vesicular chromatin, inconspicuous to small centrally located basophilic nucleoli, eosinophilic cytoplasm
  - Characteristic reniform nuclei showing nuclear membrane lobations or indentations
  - Nuclear pleomorphism, mitotic figures uncommonly seen
  - Foamy histiocytes and multinucleated giant cells may also be present
    - May show phagocytosis of mononuclear cells

LANGERHANS CELL HISTIOCYTOSIS

Key Facts

Terminology
- Clonal proliferation of Langerhans cells
  - Occurs as isolated lesion or part of systemic (multifocal) proliferation

Clinical Issues
- Most common in 2nd-3rd decades
- Surgical excision and low-dose radiotherapy considered treatment of choice

Image Findings
- Single or multiple, circumscribed, osteolytic lesions

Microscopic Pathology
- Langerhans cells
  - Enlarged vesicular nuclei with reniform nuclei
  - Typically accompanied by eosinophilic infiltrate

Ancillary Tests
- S100 protein, CD1a, Langerin positive

- Accompanied by inflammatory cell infiltrate
  - Primarily eosinophils but may include lymphocytes, plasma cells, neutrophils

ANCILLARY TESTS

Immunohistochemistry
- S100 protein, CD1a, Langerin positive
  - CD163 may be identified

Molecular Genetics
- Oncogenic *BRAF* V600E mutation identified

Electron Microscopy
- Elongated cytoplasmic granules (Langerhans or Birbeck granules) may be seen

DIFFERENTIAL DIAGNOSIS

Extranodal Sinus Histiocytosis with Massive Lymphadenopathy (Rosai-Dorfman)
- S100 protein, CD68 positive
- Negative for CD1a, Langerin

Non-Hodgkin Malignant Lymphoma
- Differentiation from LCH by light microscopy usually not problematic
  - Lymphoma cells show lineage specificity (B- or T-cell), lack S100 protein, CD1a, Langerin

SELECTED REFERENCES

1. Abla O et al: Langerhans cell histiocytosis: Current concepts and treatments. Cancer Treat Rev. 36(4):354-9, 2010
2. Badalian-Very G et al: Recurrent BRAF mutations in Langerhans cell histiocytosis. Blood. 116(11):1919-23, 2010
3. Nicollas R et al: Head and neck manifestation and prognosis of Langerhans' cell histiocytosis in children. Int J Pediatr Otorhinolaryngol. 74(6):669-73, 2010
4. Sachdev R et al: CD163 expression is present in cutaneous histiocytomas but not in atypical fibroxanthomas. Am J Clin Pathol. 133(6):915-21, 2010
5. Wang J et al: Langerhans cell histiocytosis of bone in children: a clinicopathologic study of 108 cases. World J Pediatr. 6(3):255-9, 2010
6. Imashuku S et al: Langerhans cell histiocytosis with multifocal bone lesions: comparative clinical features between single and multi-systems. Int J Hematol. 90(4):506-12, 2009
7. Lau SK et al: Immunohistochemical expression of Langerin in Langerhans cell histiocytosis and non-Langerhans cell histiocytic disorders. Am J Surg Pathol. 32(4):615-9, 2008
8. Lieberman PH et al: Langerhans cell (eosinophilic) granulomatosis. A clinicopathologic study encompassing 50 years. Am J Surg Pathol. 20(5):519-52, 1996
9. Willman CL et al: Langerhans'-cell histiocytosis (histiocytosis X)--a clonal proliferative disease. N Engl J Med. 331(3):154-60, 1994
10. Willman CL: Detection of clonal histiocytes in Langerhans cell histiocytosis: biology and clinical significance. Br J Cancer Suppl. 23:S29-33, 1994

IMAGE GALLERY

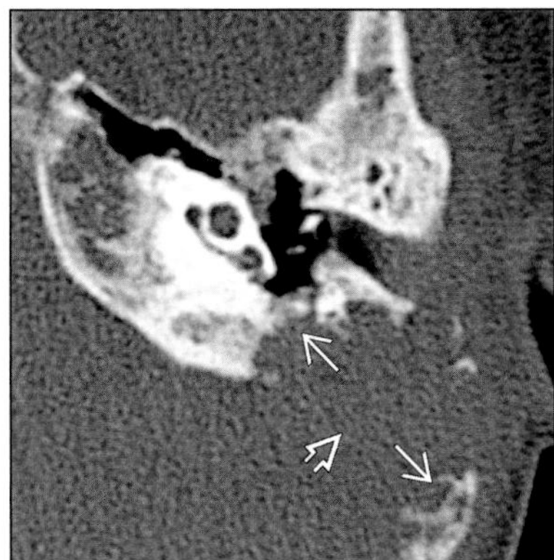
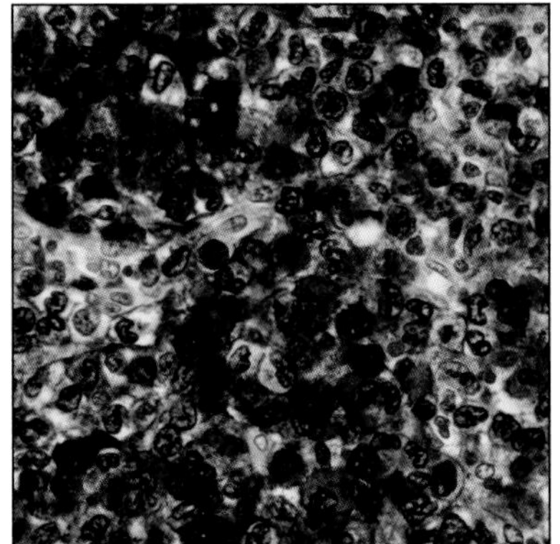
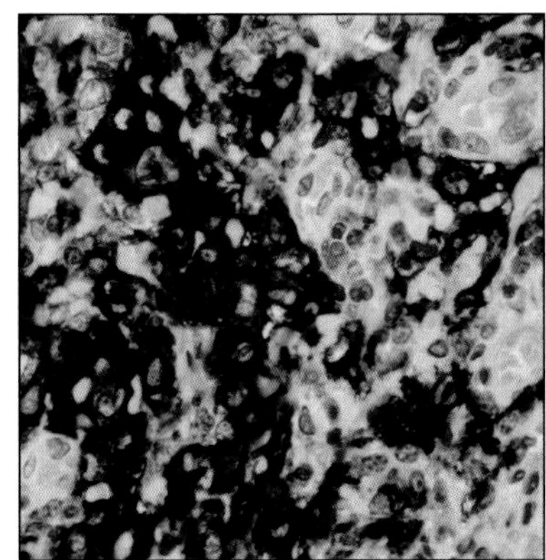

(Left) *Bone CT shows destruction of left mastoid complex. Transition between Langerhans cell histiocytosis lesion and normal temporal bone is abrupt ➡. Note sigmoid plate is completely eroded ⇨.* ***(Center)*** *Langerhans cells are diffusely immunoreactive for S100 protein (nuclear and cytoplasmic).* ***(Right)*** *Langerhans cells are immunoreactive for CD1a (cytoplasmic).*

ANGIOLYMPHOID HYPERPLASIA WITH EOSINOPHILIA

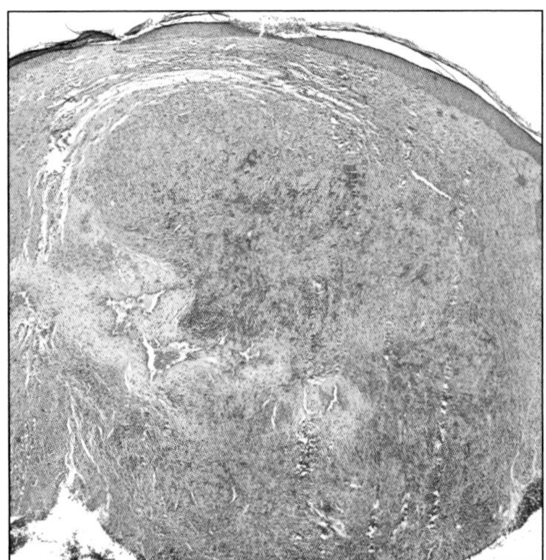

Hematoxylin & eosin shows an intact surface epithelium with a richly vascularized stroma containing lymphoid elements.

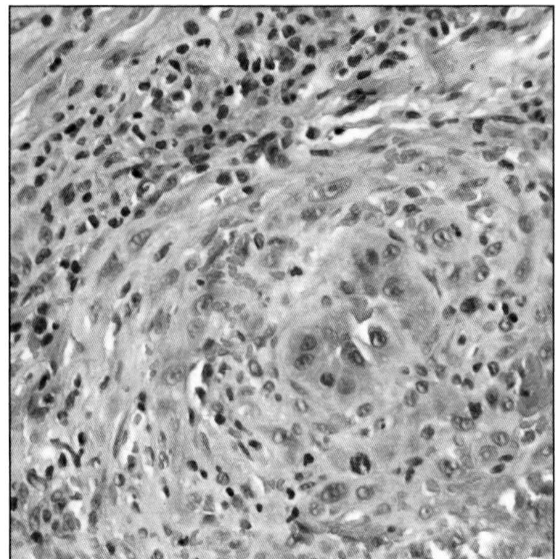

Hematoxylin & eosin shows endothelial hyperplasia with a thickened vessel wall, showing increased inflammatory cells, including eosinophils, in the surrounding tissue. Note the extravasated erythrocytes.

TERMINOLOGY

Abbreviations

- Angiolymphoid hyperplasia with eosinophilia (ALHE)

Synonyms

- Epithelioid hemangioma
- Nodular, angioblastic hyperplasia with eosinophilia and lymphofolliculosis

Definitions

- Benign vascular tumor with well-formed, immature blood vessels, most of which are lined by plump, epithelioid (histiocytoid) endothelial cells
- Most cases have prominent inflammatory component in which eosinophils are conspicuous feature

ETIOLOGY/PATHOGENESIS

Reactive

- History of trauma; larger vessels show damage with prominent inflammatory component

Neoplastic

- May represent benign neoplasm

CLINICAL ISSUES

Epidemiology

- Age
  - Wide range; mean: 3rd to 5th decades
- Gender
  - Female > Male
- Ethnicity
  - **Not** increased in Asian patients
    - This is **not** Kimura disease

Site

- Head (scalp, ears) most commonly affected
  - Digits next most common
  - Mucous membranes rare

Presentation

- Nodule or mass in subcutaneous tissues (**not** lymph nodes), present for up to 12 months
- Pain &/or pruritus; easily excoriate or bleed
- Pink to red-brown (hyperpigmented), dome-shaped papules or nodules
- Nodules may be multiple, ultimately coalescing
- Rarely may spontaneously regress/involute

Laboratory Tests

- Peripheral blood eosinophilia in some patients
- Absent raised IgE levels

Treatment

- Excision, but recurrences, regrowth, or persistence after surgery requires follow-up

Prognosis

- Excellent, although with frequent recurrence

MACROSCOPIC FEATURES

General Features

- May resemble lymph node due to circumscription and peripheral inflammation

Size

- Mean: 0.5-2 cm; rarely > 5 cm

MICROSCOPIC PATHOLOGY

Histologic Features

- Multiple lobules of inflammatory elements with increased vascularity on low power
- Surface usually intact, but can be excoriated
- Proliferation of small immature capillary type to medium vessels usually without lumina

ANGIOLYMPHOID HYPERPLASIA WITH EOSINOPHILIA

Key Facts

Terminology

- Benign vascular tumor with well-formed, immature blood vessels associated with prominent inflammatory component, rich in eosinophils

Clinical Issues

- Head is most commonly affected by nodules in subcutaneous tissues
- Nodules may be multiple, ultimately coalescing

Microscopic Pathology

- Multiple lobules composed of inflammatory cells within rich vascularity
- Proliferation of small immature capillary type vessels, lined by enlarged endothelial cells
- Endothelial cells are epithelioid or histiocytic with cytoplasmic vacuolization

Top Differential Diagnoses

- Papillary endothelial hyperplasia, Kimura disease

- May be attached to or associated with larger vessels
- May have solid appearance
- Endothelial cells are enlarged with epithelioid or histiocytic appearance
- Endothelial cells may have cytoplasmic vacuolization
- Endothelial nuclei are enlarged
- Many eosinophils, lymphocytes, and mast cells, although eosinophil number can vary greatly
- Lymphoid follicles sparse and poorly formed

ANCILLARY TESTS

Immunohistochemistry

- Endothelial cells positive for CD31, CD34, FVIIIRAg
- Actin(+) vascular muscle walls
- IgE(+) mast cells, but no IgE on follicular dendritic cells
  - Mast cells have IgE receptors but distinct from follicular dendritic cells

DIFFERENTIAL DIAGNOSIS

Papillary Endothelial Hyperplasia

- Reactive process limited to intravascular space(s)
- Papillary projections of enlarged endothelial cells

Kimura Disease

- Asian men with large disfiguring preauricular lymph node masses
- Peripheral eosinophilia
- Reactive lymphoid follicles with follicular lysis, eosinophilic abscesses, polykaryocytes, and IgE deposition

Angiosarcoma

- Highly atypical, mitotically active, freely anastomosing endothelial proliferation
- Usually shows necrosis and hemorrhage

Metastatic Papillary Thyroid Carcinoma

- Epithelioid cells with intranuclear cytoplasmic inclusions in lymphoid stroma
- TTF-1 &/or thyroglobulin positivity

SELECTED REFERENCES

1. Effat KG: Angiolymphoid hyperplasia with eosinophilia of the auricle: progression of histopathological changes. J Laryngol Otol. 120(5):411-3, 2006
2. Sun ZJ et al: Epithelioid hemangioma in the oral mucosa: a clinicopathological study of seven cases and review of the literature. Oral Oncol. 42(5):441-7, 2006
3. Martín-Granizo R et al: Epithelioid hemangiomas of the maxillofacial area. A report of three cases and a review of the literature. Int J Oral Maxillofac Surg. 26(3):212-4, 1997
4. Tosios K et al: Intravascular papillary endothelial hyperplasia of the oral soft tissues: report of 18 cases and review of the literature. J Oral Maxillofac Surg. 52(12):1263-8, 1994
5. Sharp JF et al: Angiolymphoid hyperplasia with eosinophilia. J Laryngol Otol. 104(12):977-9, 1990

IMAGE GALLERY

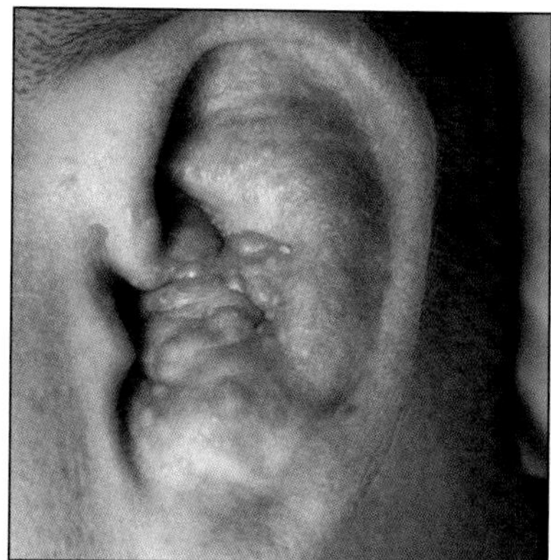

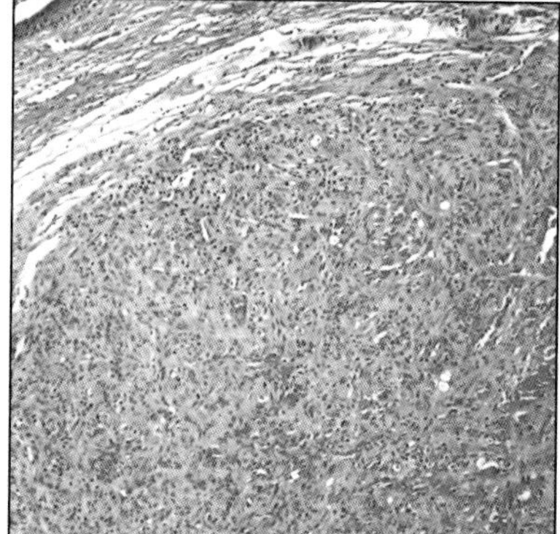

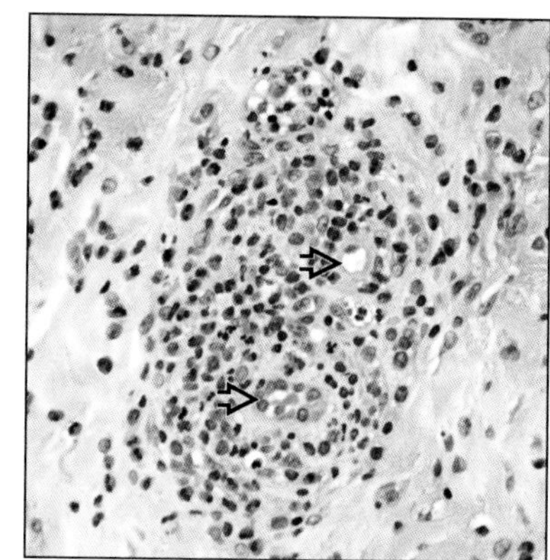

(Left) *This clinical photograph of the ear shows the characteristic multiple, superficial papules, focally coalescing to form plaque-like lesions of ALHE. (Courtesy M. Guralnick, MD.)* ***(Center)*** *Hematoxylin & eosin shows rich vascular proliferation, increased endothelial cells with extravasated erythrocytes and eosinophils with lymphocytes.* ***(Right)*** *Hematoxylin & eosin highlights the mixture of eosinophils and lymphocytes around 2 vessels ⇨ with high endothelial cells.*

MALAKOPLAKIA

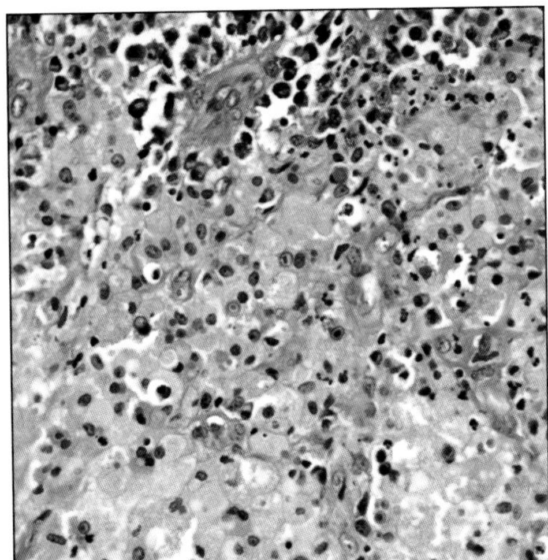

Hematoxylin & eosin shows sheets of histiocytes with mixed inflammatory infiltrate and targetoid bodies.

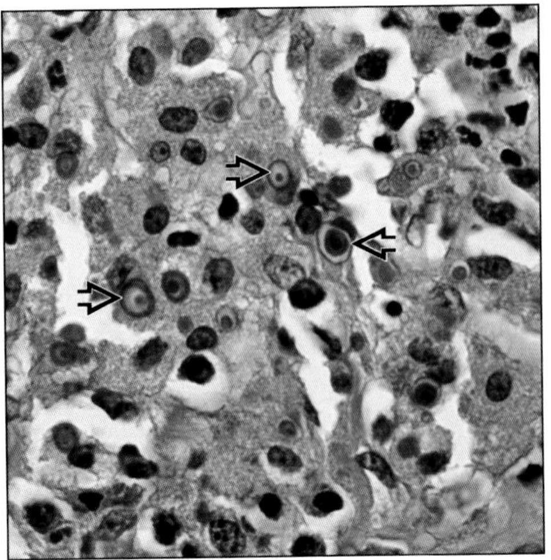

Foamy histiocytes have eosinophilic cytoplasm and the characteristic intracytoplasmic calcific inclusions (Michaelis-Gutmann bodies ➢) diagnostic for this entity.

TERMINOLOGY

Definitions

- Word origin: Malacos: Soft; Placos: Plaques
- Rare granulomatous disease often associated with abnormal reaction to infectious organisms
- Michaelis and Gutmann initially described the disease, which was further clarified by von Hansemann
- Usually develops in postoperative site or areas with inflammation or infection

ETIOLOGY/PATHOGENESIS

Infectious Agents

- End stage of inability of macrophages to destroy phagocytized bacteria
- Phagolysosomes that are unable to digest their contents yield Michaelis-Gutmann bodies
- *E. coli* is most common, but many bacteria and viruses reported

Immunocompromise

- Organ transplantation, malignancy, diabetes mellitus, acquired immunodeficiency syndrome (AIDS), tuberculosis, malnutrition
- Sarcoidosis, allergic conditions, and immunosuppressive medicines (chemotherapy and steroids)

CLINICAL ISSUES

Epidemiology

- Incidence
  - Rare
- Age
  - Usually adults, but can be any age
- Gender
  - Male > Female
    - Opposite from genitourinary and gastrointestinal sites

Site

- Most common in genitourinary and gastrointestinal tract
- While rare in head and neck, most commonly affects ear, oral cavity, and larynx

Presentation

- Nonspecific clinical presentation
- Mass with discharge
- Changes in hearing
- Fever, chills, night sweats

Treatment

- Options, risks, complications
  - Prolonged antibiotic therapy
- Surgical approaches
  - Excision of "mass"
- Must culture to identify causative organism

Prognosis

- High mortality when identified within vital organs
- Usually excellent when debrided with underlying infection treated

MACROSCOPIC FEATURES

General Features

- Yellow-brown soft plaques characterized by central navel or ulcer, hyperemic at edge
- Up to 3 cm

MICROSCOPIC PATHOLOGY

Histologic Features

- Marked pseudoepitheliomatous hyperplasia of surface epithelium

MALAKOPLAKIA

Key Facts

Terminology
- Rare granulomatous disease often associated with abnormal reaction to infectious organisms

Etiology/Pathogenesis
- End stage of inability of macrophages to destroy phagocytized bacteria

Clinical Issues
- Rare; ear most commonly affected head & neck site

Microscopic Pathology
- Marked pseudoepitheliomatous hyperplasia
- Large, granular, or foamy histiocytes with low nuclear to cytoplasm ratio (no atypia)
- Michaelis-Gutmann bodies are well-formed blue, calcific bodies, both intracytoplasmic and stromal
  - Targetoid and concentrically laminated
  - Black stain with von Kossa (calcium stain)
  - Blue stain with Prussian blue (iron stain)

- Subepithelial spaces filled with sheets of eosinophilic histiocytes, most of which contain granular cytoplasmic material
- Large, granular, or foamy histiocytes with low nuclear to cytoplasm ratio (no atypia)
- Heavy mixed inflammatory infiltrate
- Well-formed blue, calcific bodies, both intracytoplasmic and stromal: Michaelis-Gutmann bodies
  - Targetoid and concentrically laminated

ANCILLARY TESTS

Histochemistry
- von Kossa (calcium stain): Strongly black (positive)
- Prussian blue (iron): Strongly blue (positive)
- PAS: May highlight organisms

Immunohistochemistry
- CD68(+) histiocytes
- S100 protein, keratin, CD1a, and CD20 negative

DIFFERENTIAL DIAGNOSIS

Granular Cell Tumor
- Has pseudoepitheliomatous hyperplasia but lacks inflammation
- Granular cytoplasm of polygonal cells reactive with S100 protein

Poorly Differentiated Carcinoma
- Cytologic atypia, invasion, generally no calcific bodies, positive with keratin

Langerhans Histiocytosis
- Histiocytes with coffee bean-shaped nuclei with grooves, prominent background eosinophils, and immunoreactivity with CD1a

Lymphoma
- Monotypic, atypical lymphoid infiltrate

SELECTED REFERENCES

1. Pang LC: Malacoplakia manifesting as a chronic inflammatory mass at the site of a nonhealing surgical wound. Ear Nose Throat J. 82(11):876-8, 880, 2003
2. Schmerber S et al: Malakoplakia of the neck. Arch Otolaryngol Head Neck Surg. 129(11):1240-2, 2003
3. Puente López G et al: [Case presentation of malacoplakia of the middle ear.] Acta Otorrinolaringol Esp. 46(4):315-6, 1995
4. Douglas-Jones AG et al: Prediagnostic malakoplakia presenting as a chronic inflammatory mass in the soft tissues of the neck. J Laryngol Otol. 106(2):173-7, 1992
5. Azadeh B et al: Malakoplakia of the middle ear. Histopathology. 19(3):276-8, 1991
6. Nayar RC et al: Malakoplakia of the temporal bone in a nine-month-old infant. J Laryngol Otol. 105(7):568-70, 1991
7. Azadeh B et al: Malakoplakia of middle ear: a case report. Histopathology. 7(1):129-34, 1983

IMAGE GALLERY

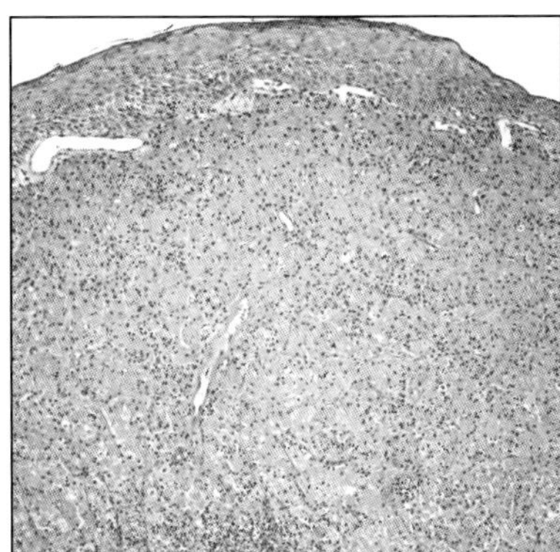

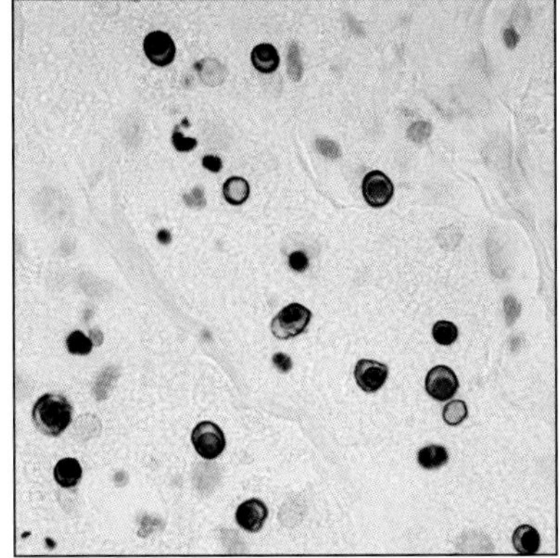

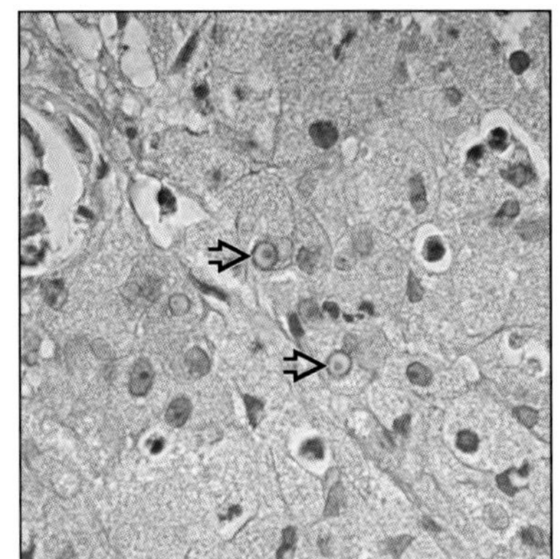

*(**Left**) Hematoxylin & eosin shows squamous epithelium overlying a mixed inflammatory infiltrate with sheets of histiocytes. (**Center**) von Kossa (calcium stain) highlights the Michaelis-Gutmann bodies by yielding a black stain. This is distinctive, as there is a "targetoid" appearance, different from usual calcium staining in other disorders. (**Right**) Iron (Prussian blue) stains the Michaelis-Gutmann bodies blue ⇨. Note the "targetoid" appearance, showing a central dark blue dot surrounded by a halo and an accentuated outer membrane.*

SYNOVIAL CHONDROMATOSIS (TEMPOROMANDIBULAR JOINT)

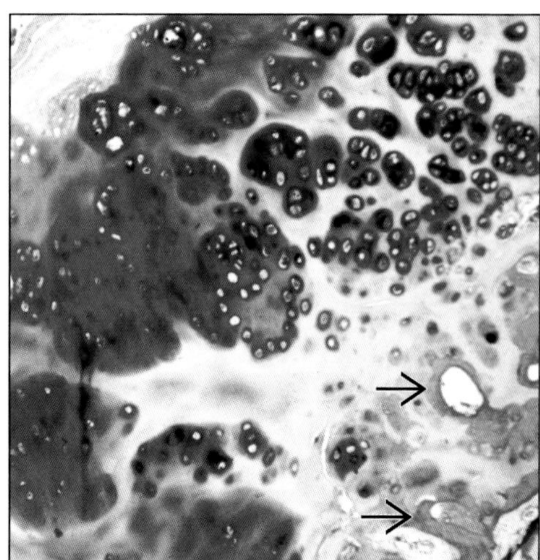

Foci within the lobules can show endochondral ossification ⇒ as a result of the normal evolution of cartilage. Review of the radiographs and clinical features will help confirm this impression.

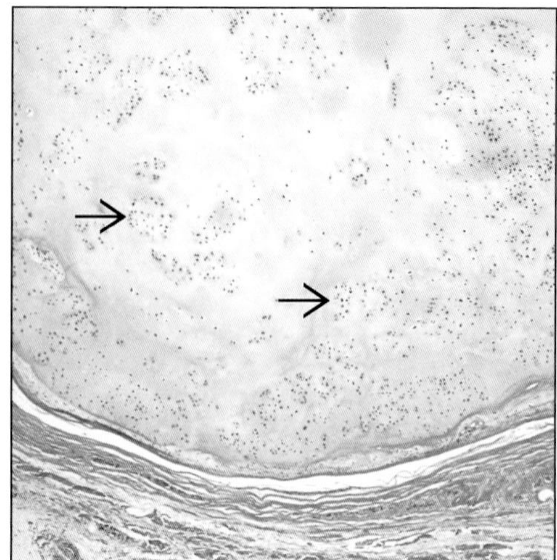

A lobule of cartilage is noted in apposition to surrounding soft tissue. There is increased cellularity ⇒ in the matrix, which can appear pink rather than blue. Radiographs and clinical features help confirm the diagnosis.

TERMINOLOGY

Abbreviations

- Synovial chondromatosis (SC)

Definitions

- Benign, nodular, progressive, metaplastic cartilaginous proliferation within joints

ETIOLOGY/PATHOGENESIS

Idiopathic

- **Primary** SC: No known etiologic factors
  - Thought to be more aggressive in behavior
- **Secondary** SC: More common and associated with
  - Inflammatory joint disease, noninflammatory arthropathy, joint overuse

CLINICAL ISSUES

Epidemiology

- Incidence
  - Rare in temporomandibular joint (TMJ) (< 0.5% of TMJ pain patients)
- Age
  - Mean: 45-47 years
- Gender
  - Female > Male (2.5:1)

Site

- May extend into and destroy floor of middle cranial fossa, ear, mandibular condyle

Presentation

- Symptoms are nonspecific, mimicking other disorders
  - Pain and swelling
  - Limited opening or movement of mouth/jaw
  - Occlusal changes &/or clicking
  - Crepitus
- Symptoms usually present for > 2 years

Treatment

- Surgical approaches
  - Complete removal of all tissue
  - Synovectomy sometimes necessary

Prognosis

- Excellent, although recurrences may be seen

IMAGE FINDINGS

MR Findings

- MR excellent for visualizing loose bodies, disc position, extraarticular tissues, and condyle displacement, while T2WI highlights fluid

CT Findings

- Define size, shape, and locations of loose, **calcified** bodies (must be calcified to be detected)

MACROSCOPIC FEATURES

General Features

- Synovial bodies are round to oval, hard
- Bluish gray, glistening surfaces
- Cut surface is gritty

Size

- Wide variability (usually < 1 cm)

MICROSCOPIC PATHOLOGY

Histologic Features

- Development of cartilaginous nodules within subsynovial connective tissue
  - Subsequently may detach, calcify, and form loose, free-floating bodies in joint

SYNOVIAL CHONDROMATOSIS (TEMPOROMANDIBULAR JOINT)

Key Facts

Terminology
- Benign, nodular, progressive, metaplastic cartilaginous proliferation within joints

Clinical Issues
- Mean age: 45-47 years
- Female > Male (2.5:1)
- Symptoms include pain and swelling
- Treatment: Complete removal of all tissue

Image Findings
- MR: Visualizes loose bodies, extraarticular tissues, and condyle displacement

Microscopic Pathology
- Nodules of variably cellular hyaline cartilage (blue-gray on H&E)
- Chondrocytes are usually clustered
- **3 phases** of development

- Nodules of variably cellular hyaline cartilage (blue-gray on H&E)
  - Within synovium or floating freely in joint space
- Lined by fine fibrous layer with/without synovial lining cells
- Chondrocytes are usually clustered
  - Lobules can be moderately to highly cellular
  - May have plump nuclei and moderate pleomorphism
  - Binucleate cells are frequent
- Mitoses are uncommon
- Endochondral ossification may be seen
- **3 phases** of development
  - **Early**: Intrasynovial disease without presence of loose bodies; islands of cartilage confined to hyperemic and edematous subsynovial connective tissue
  - **Intermediate**: Hyperemic synovial connective tissue and loose bodies
  - **Late**: Loose bodies only

DIFFERENTIAL DIAGNOSIS

Degenerative Joint Disease
- Fragments of articular-type cartilage and bone embedded within synovium
- Can progress to secondary synovial chondromatosis
- Radiologic studies will show degenerative changes
  - Joint space narrowing, subchondral sclerosis, subchondral cysts, osteophyte formation

Rheumatoid Arthritis
- Fragments of articular-type cartilage in synovium
- Synovial proliferation associated with acute and chronic inflammation
- Clinical symptoms and laboratory studies (rheumatoid factor) help

Chondrosarcoma
- Cartilage will surround, invade, and destroy bone

STAGING

Milgram Staging
- 1: Metaplastic synovia **without** loose bodies
- 2: Metaplastic synovia **with** loose bodies
- 3: Only loose bodies

SELECTED REFERENCES

1. Boffano P et al: Diagnosis and surgical management of synovial chondromatosis of the temporomandibular joint. J Craniofac Surg. 21(1):157-9, 2010
2. Guarda-Nardini L et al: Synovial chondromatosis of the temporomandibular joint: a case description with systematic literature review. Int J Oral Maxillofac Surg. 39(8):745-55, 2010
3. Ida M et al: An investigation of magnetic resonance imaging features in 14 patients with synovial chondromatosis of the temporomandibular joint. Dentomaxillofac Radiol. 37(4):213-9, 2008

IMAGE GALLERY

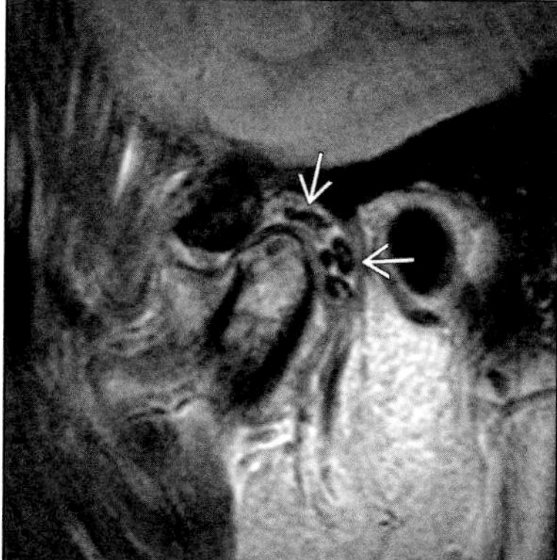

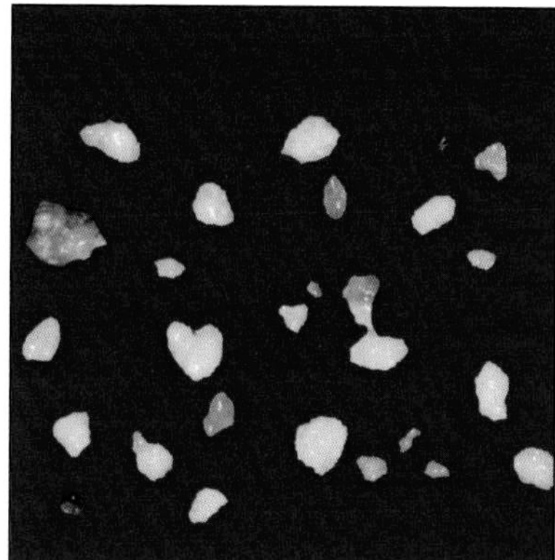

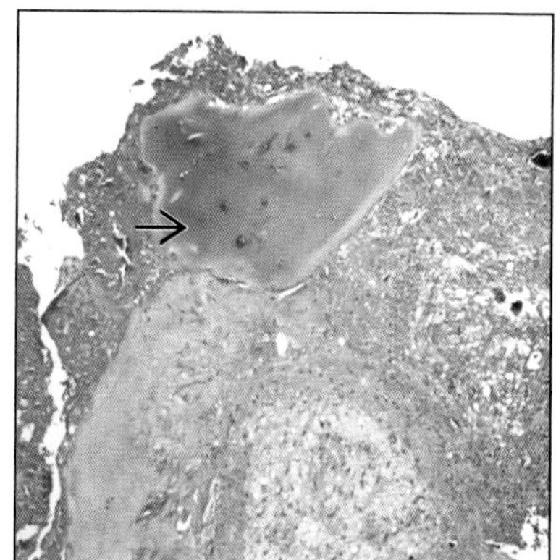

*(**Left**) Sagittal T2WI MR shows hyperintense fluid surrounding the low signal calcified loose bodies ➡. (**Center**) This gross photograph shows the lobular, glistening, white-blue calcified bodies of synovial chondromatosis. (**Right**) In this differential, osteoarthritis shows articular cartilage ➡ embedded in synovium within the joint space. However, the cartilage fragments have an irregular shape and associated inflammation.*

CERUMINOUS ADENOMA

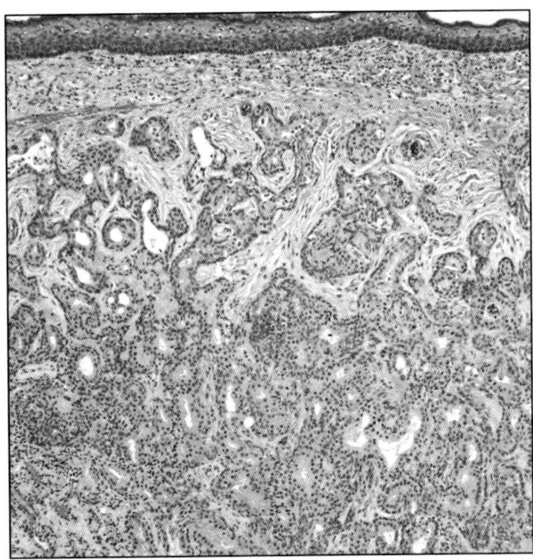

Hematoxylin & eosin shows intact surface epithelium with glandular neoplastic proliferation in the stroma.

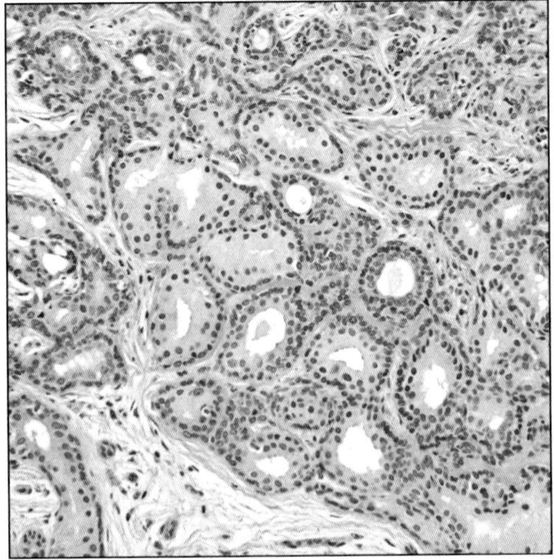

Hematoxylin & eosin shows a biphasic glandular proliferation with inner apocrine cells and basal myoepithelial cells, separated by fibrous connective tissue stroma.

TERMINOLOGY

Synonyms

- Ceruminoma, ceruminal adenoma
- Apocrine adenoma, cylindroma
- Chondroid syringoma (mixed tumor)

Definitions

- Benign glandular neoplasm of ceruminous glands of external auditory canal

CLINICAL ISSUES

Epidemiology

- Incidence
  - Rare neoplasm, < 1% of all external ear tumors
- Age
  - Mean: 55 years
  - Range: 12-85 years
- Gender
  - Equal gender distribution

Site

- Must involve outer 1/3 to 1/2 of external auditory canal
- Posterior region affected slightly more commonly

Presentation

- Mass
- May have associated pain
- Hearing loss (sensorineural and conductive), tinnitus
- Paralysis of nerves
- Asymptomatic

Treatment

- Surgical approaches
  - Complete surgical excision

Prognosis

- Excellent, although may have recurrences if incompletely excised

MACROSCOPIC FEATURES

Size

- Mean: 1.2 cm
- Range: 0.5-2 cm

MICROSCOPIC PATHOLOGY

Histologic Features

- Tumors are separated into 3 histologic types
  - Ceruminous adenoma
  - Ceruminous pleomorphic adenoma
  - Ceruminous syringocystadenoma papilliferum
- Well circumscribed but unencapsulated
- Surface intact but may be "involved" rather than origin
- Glandular and cystic patterns
- Dual-cell population
  - Inner luminal secretory cells with abundant granular, eosinophilic cytoplasm
  - Yellow-brown, ceroid, lipofuscin-like (cerumen) pigment granules in cytoplasm of luminal cells
  - Basal, myoepithelial cells at periphery adjacent to basement membrane
  - Luminal cells have decapitation (apocrine) blebbing or secretions
- Low to moderate cellularity
- Limited pleomorphism
- Lack necrosis
- Ceruminous pleomorphic adenoma
  - Chondromyxoid matrix material juxtaposed to epithelium and blended with it
- Ceruminous papillary cystadenoma papilliferum
  - Papillary projections lined by cuboidal to columnar cells

CERUMINOUS ADENOMA

Key Facts

Clinical Issues

- Must involve outer 1/3 to 1/2 of external auditory canal
- Mass and hearing changes
- Mass, rarely painful
- Hearing loss (sensorineural and conductive), tinnitus

Microscopic Pathology

- Separated into 3 histologic types
- Well circumscribed but unencapsulated
- Dual cell population
- Inner luminal secretory cells with abundant granular, eosinophilic cytoplasm
  - Luminal cells have decapitation (apocrine) blebbing or secretions
- Basal, myoepithelial cells at periphery adjacent to basement membrane
- Yellow-brown, ceroid, lipofuscin-like (cerumen) pigment granules in cytoplasm of luminal cells
- Background of dense, sclerotic fibrosis in some cases

Ancillary Tests

- Immunohistochemistry highlights dual cell population
- Positive luminal cells only: CK7
- Positive basal cells only: CK5/6, p63, S100 protein, and CD117 (predominantly)

Top Differential Diagnoses

- Neuroendocrine adenoma of middle ear (middle ear adenoma)
- Paraganglioma
- Endolymphatic sac tumor
- Ceruminous adenocarcinoma

  - Heavy plasma cell investment
- Background of dense, sclerotic fibrosis in some cases
- Limited mitotic figures, if any, and never atypical forms

ANCILLARY TESTS

Immunohistochemistry

- Highlights biphasic tumor cells
  - Positive luminal and basal cells: Pankeratin, EMA
  - Positive luminal cells only: CK7
  - Positive basal cells only: CK5/6, p63, S100 protein, and CD117 (predominantly)
  - Negative: CK20 and chromogranin

DIFFERENTIAL DIAGNOSIS

Ceruminous Adenocarcinoma

- Infiltrative, destructive growth
- Pleomorphism, including nucleoli
- Increased mitotic activity
- Lacks ceroid pigment
- Necrosis, when present, helps with diagnosis

Middle Ear Adenoma

- a.k.a. neuroendocrine adenoma of middle ear (NAME)
- Neuroendocrine tumor with "salt and pepper" nuclear chromatin distribution
- Involves middle ear as primary site
- Biphasic appearance
- Lacks decapitation secretions
- No ceroid granules in cytoplasm
- Positive with neuroendocrine markers (chromogranin, synaptophysin)

Paraganglioma

- Zellballen (nested) architecture
- Basophilic, slightly granular cytoplasm
- Nuclear pleomorphism
- Immunoreactions
  - Chromogranin or synaptophysin positive paraganglia cells
  - S100 protein positive supporting sustentacular cells

Endolymphatic Sac Tumor

- Specific region in temporal bone
- Papillary architecture with cystic spaces
- Low cuboidal cells with pale to clear cytoplasm

SELECTED REFERENCES

1. Magliulo G et al: Adenoma of the ceruminous gland. Otolaryngol Head Neck Surg. 143(3):459-60, 2010
2. Markou K et al: Primary pleomorphic adenoma of the external ear canal. Report of a case and literature review. Am J Otolaryngol. 29(2):142-6, 2008
3. Orendorz-Fraczkowska K et al: Middle-ear ceruminous adenoma as a rare cause of hearing loss and vertigo: case reports. Auris Nasus Larynx. 32(4):393-7, 2005
4. Thompson LD et al: Ceruminous adenomas: a clinicopathologic study of 41 cases with a review of the literature. Am J Surg Pathol. 28(3):308-18, 2004
5. Durko T et al: [Glandular neoplasms of the external auditory canal--clinical and morphologic observations] Otolaryngol Pol. 57(1):51-7, 2003
6. Lassaletta L et al: Avoiding misdiagnosis in ceruminous gland tumours. Auris Nasus Larynx. 30(3):287-90, 2003
7. Schenk P et al: Ultrastructural morphology of a middle ear ceruminoma. ORL J Otorhinolaryngol Relat Spec. 64(5):358-63, 2002
8. Torske KR et al: Adenoma versus carcinoid tumor of the middle ear: a study of 48 cases and review of the literature. Mod Pathol. 15(5):543-55, 2002
9. Mills RG et al: 'Ceruminoma'--a defunct diagnosis. J Laryngol Otol. 109(3):180-8, 1995
10. Mansour P et al: Ceruminous gland tumours: a reappraisal. J Laryngol Otol. 106(8):727-32, 1992
11. Lynde CW et al: Tumors of ceruminous glands. J Am Acad Dermatol. 11(5 Pt 1):841-7, 1984
12. Hicks GW: Tumors arising from the glandular structures of the external auditory canal. Laryngoscope. 93(3):326-40, 1983
13. Dehner LP et al: Primary tumors of the external and middle ear. Benign and malignant glandular neoplasms. Arch Otolaryngol. 106(1):13-9, 1980

CERUMINOUS ADENOMA

Imaging and Microscopic Features

*(**Left**) A computed tomography image demonstrates a mass within the external auditory canal ➩ that is filling the space. The middle ear is not involved. (**Right**) Hematoxylin & eosin shows the glandular neoplasm abutting the surface but not arising from it. Note the biphasic appearance with inner glandular and outer myoepithelial cells. There is a significant desmoplastic stromal response.*

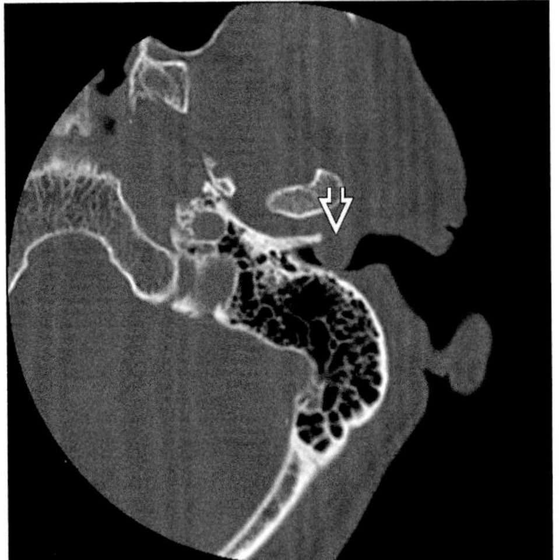

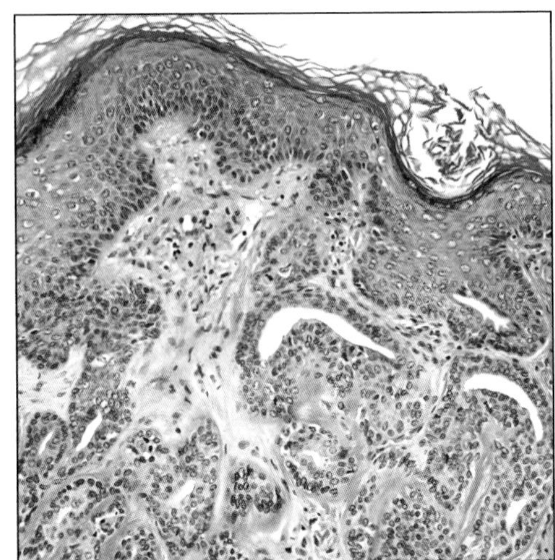

*(**Left**) Hematoxylin & eosin shows a biphasic glandular proliferation with inner secretory cells. There is a heavy fibrous connective tissue stroma. (**Right**) Hematoxylin & eosin shows brightly eosinophilic inner apocrine cells subtended by a basal cell proliferation, creating the biphasic appearance of a ceruminous adenoma.*

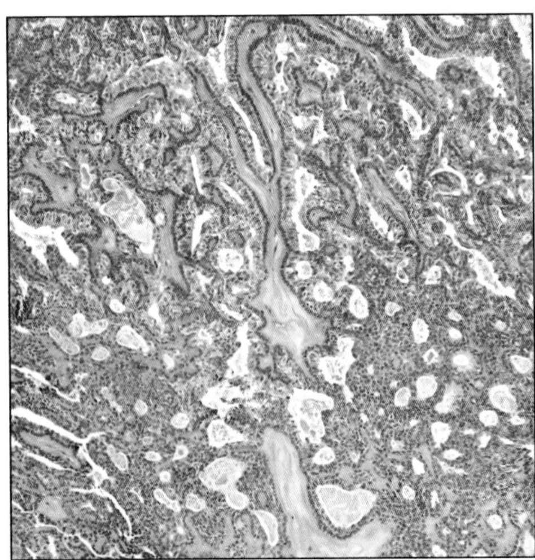

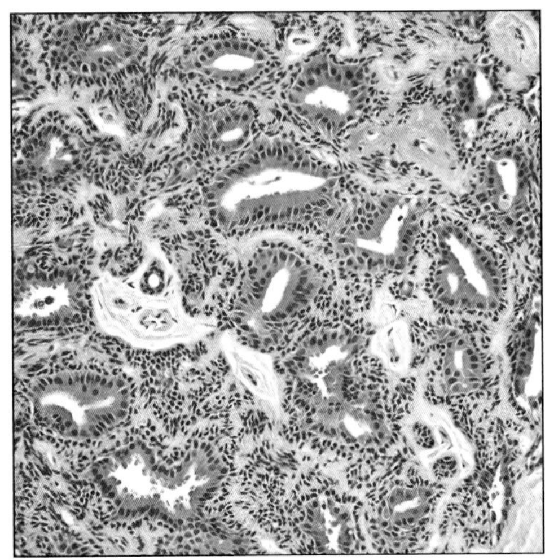

*(**Left**) Hematoxylin & eosin shows a pseudoinfiltrative appearance of ceruminous adenoma. This haphazard arrangement of cells is quite common in this benign tumor. (**Right**) High-power mangification shows tall columnar secretory cells with apocrine-type "snouts" subtended by basal myoepithelial cells. Heavy stroma separates the glands.*

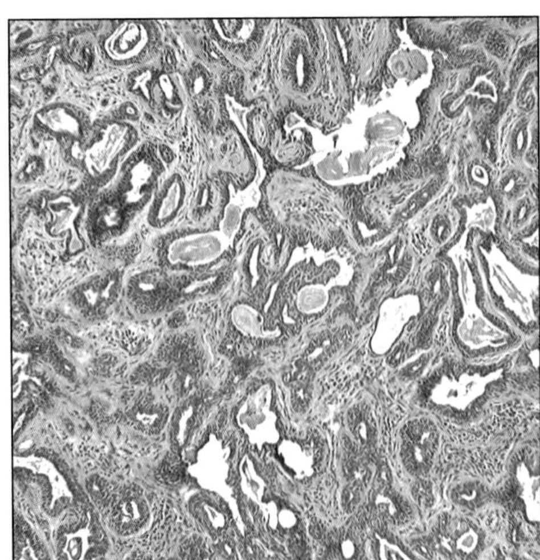

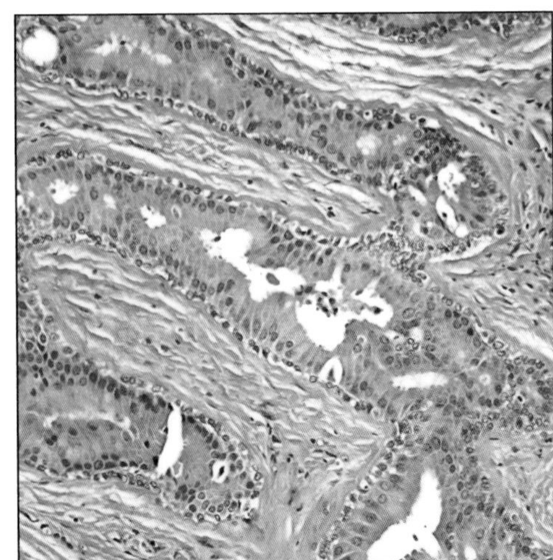

Microscopic and Immunohistochemical Features

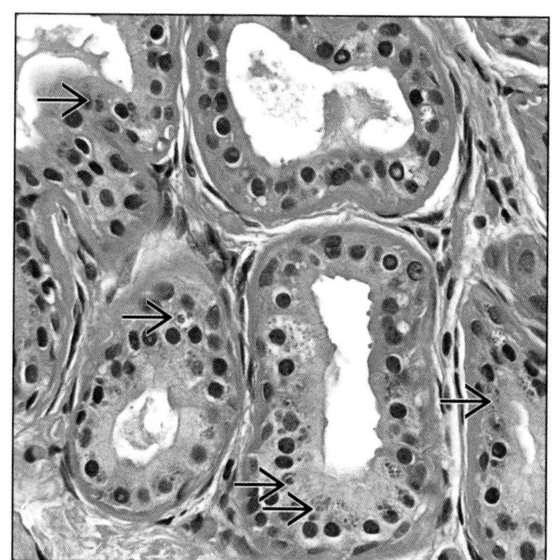

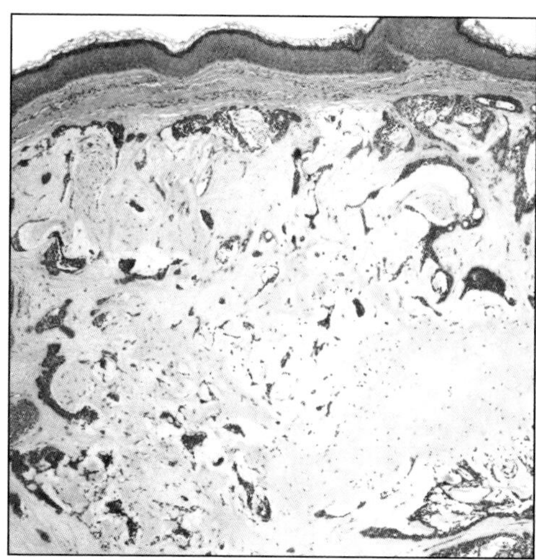

***(Left)** Hematoxylin & eosin shows numerous cerumen granules as yellow bodies* ➔ *within the cytoplasm of the luminal cells. There are only isolated basaloid cells in this proliferation. **(Right)** Hematoxylin & eosin shows myxochondroid matrix material with glandular cells below an intact surface in this ceruminous pleomorphic adenoma.*

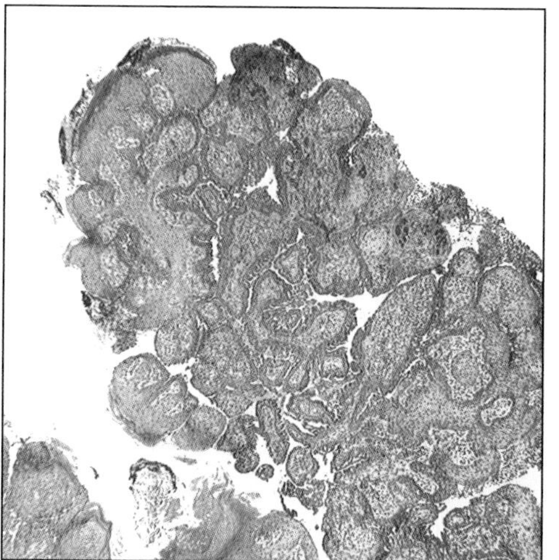

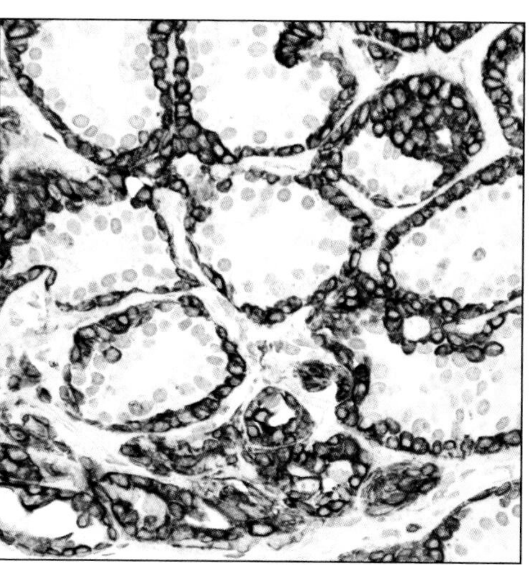

***(Left)** Hematoxylin & eosin shows papillary projections and columnar epithelium adjacent to the surface squamous mucosa. There are numerous plasma cells within the cores of this ceruminous syringocystadenoma papilliferum. **(Right)** CK5/6 shows basal staining, highlighting the biphasic appearance of the tumor.*

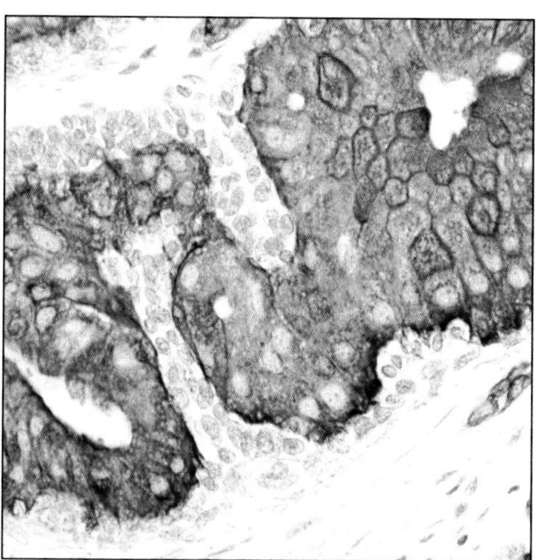

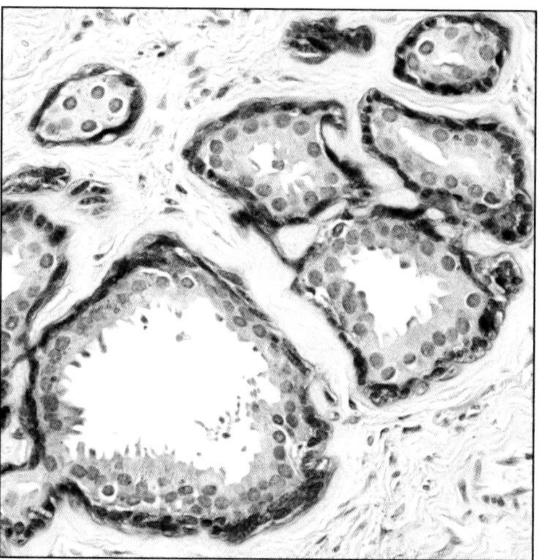

***(Left)** CK7 shows strong cytoplasmic immunoreactivity of the luminal secretory cells and a lack of staining in the basal cells. **(Right)** S100 protein shows nuclear and cytoplasmic immunoreactivity predominantly of the basal cells, although there is background nonspecific staining ("blush" or "tea" staining) of the luminal secretory cells (perhaps related to endogenous biotin in these secretory cells).*

MIDDLE EAR ADENOMA

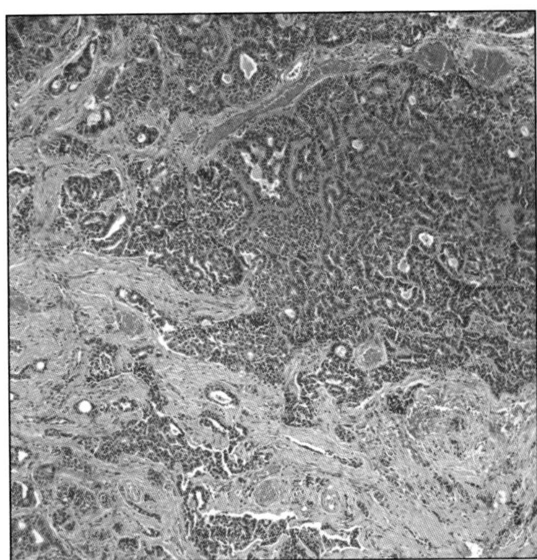

In general, middle ear adenomas are unencapsulated and infiltrative tumors, showing a variety of architectures, as seen in this low magnification: Glandular, tubular, trabecular, cords, and single cell architecture.

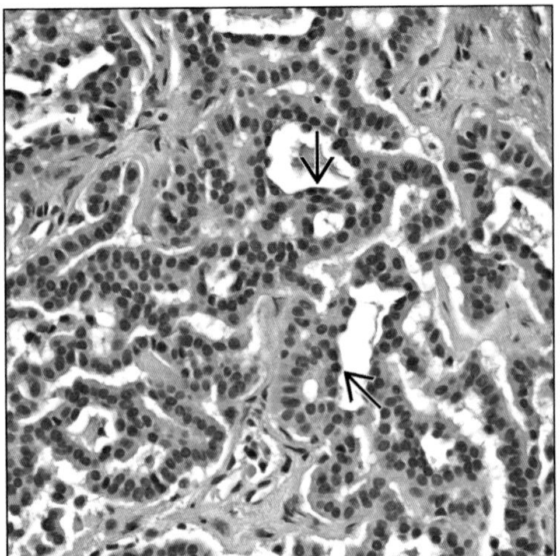

Duct-like structures show back to back configuration, with a dual population of inner, luminal, flattened eosinophilic cells ⇒ and basal, cuboidal-columnar cells with finely granular cytoplasm.

TERMINOLOGY

Abbreviations

- Middle ear adenoma (MEA)

Synonyms

- Neuroendocrine adenoma of middle ear (NAME)
- Carcinoid tumor
- Amphicrine adenoma
- Amphicrine tumor
- Adenocarcinoid
- Adenomatoid tumor of middle ear

Definitions

- Benign glandular neoplasm of middle ear showing both cytomorphologic and immunohistochemical neuroendocrine and mucin-secreting differentiation

CLINICAL ISSUES

Epidemiology

- Incidence
  - Uncommon (< 2% of ear tumors)
- Age
  - Average: 45 years (5th decade)
  - Range: 20-80 years
- Gender
  - Equal gender distribution

Site

- Middle ear cavity
- May extend into adjacent structures
  - External auditory canal (via tympanic membrane)
  - Mastoid bone
  - Eustachian tube

Presentation

- Unilateral hearing loss
  - Conductive hearing loss if ossicular chain involved
  - Muffled or decreased acuity
- Ear pressure or fullness
- Tinnitus
- Discharge
- Otitis media
- Bleeding
- Otoscopic exam
  - Pink soft tissue mass behind intact tympanic membrane
  - Dark brown-reddish fluid behind ear drum
- No serologic evidence of neuroendocrine function

Treatment

- Options, risks, complications
  - Facial nerve paralysis &/or paresthesias may be due to mass effect rather than invasion of nerves
- Surgical approaches
  - Complete surgical excision
    - Must include ossicular chain to prevent recurrence
  - Reconstruction required
- Radiation
  - No role for radiation in treatment of this benign tumor

Prognosis

- Excellent long-term clinical outcome
- Recurrences develop if incompletely excised
  - Approximately 15% of patients
  - Specifically if ossicular chain is not removed with tumor
- No metastatic potential

IMAGE FINDINGS

General Features

- Best study is axial and coronal bone CT without contrast
- Soft tissue mass within well-pneumatized mastoid
  - No chronic otitis media findings
- Nondestructive mass lesion within middle ear
  - Involves middle ear cavity proper (mesotympanum)

MIDDLE EAR ADENOMA

Key Facts

Terminology
- Benign neoplasm of middle ear showing both cytomorphologic and immunohistochemical neuroendocrine differentiation, mucin-secreting differentiation

Clinical Issues
- Most common tumor of middle ear
- Average patient age: 45 years
- Unilateral conductive hearing loss is most common presenting symptom
  - Tinnitus, discharge
- Complete excision (including ossicles) is treatment of choice

Image Findings
- Mass in middle ear with intact tympanic membrane
- No findings of chronic otitis media

Microscopic Pathology
- Unencapsulated and "infiltrative" growth
- Variable architectural patterns: Glandular, trabecular, cords, festoons, single cells
- Ducts show dual cell population
  - Inner, luminal, flattened eosinophilic cells
  - Basal, cuboidal-columnar cells
- Delicate, fine, "salt and pepper" nuclear chromatin

Ancillary Tests
- Both epithelial and neuroendocrine markers positive
  - Keratin, CK7, chromogranin, synaptophysin, HPP

Top Differential Diagnoses
- Paraganglioma, ceruminous adenoma, metastatic adenocarcinoma, meningioma

---

  - No bone invasion, but ossicular encasement
  - Usually shows irregular margination
  - Tympanic membrane is intact
- Bone remodeling can be seen if lesion is large or has been present for long duration

CT Findings
- Mass within middle ear behind intact tympanic membrane
- No findings of chronic otitis media
- May appear indistinguishable from cholesteatoma

MACROSCOPIC FEATURES

General Features
- Ossicular chain is usually affected
  - Tissue tends to "peel" away from bony structures
- Soft, rubbery, and unencapsulated
- Usually multiple white, yellow, gray-tan to reddish tissue fragments

Size
- Tumor generally limited by anatomic confines
- Usually < 1 cm

MICROSCOPIC PATHOLOGY

Histologic Features
- Surface origin is absent
- Unencapsulated and infiltrative growth
- Moderate cellularity
- Variable architectures
  - Glandular, trabecular, cords, festoons, single cells
- Duct-like structures with back to back configuration
- Ducts show dual cell population
  - Inner, luminal, flattened eosinophilic cells
  - Basal, cuboidal-columnar cells with finely granular cytoplasm
  - No myoepithelial cell layer
- Eccentrically placed (plasmacytoid) round to oval nuclei
- Delicate, fine, "salt and pepper" nuclear chromatin distribution
- Small nucleoli
- Mitotic figures absent to infrequent
- Gland lumen may have secretions
- Desmoplastic stroma is common
- Pleomorphism, necrosis, bone, and perineural/lymph-vascular space invasion all absent
- Cholesteatoma may be concurrently present but is not etiologically related

ANCILLARY TESTS

Histochemistry
- Mucinous material identified in gland lumen (or rarely intracytoplasmic) with PAS and Alcian blue

Immunohistochemistry
- Both epithelial and neuroendocrine markers positive
  - Keratin
  - CK7
  - CAM5.2
  - Chromogranin
  - Synaptophysin
  - Human pancreatic polypeptide (HPP)
- Differential staining can be seen
  - Inner luminal cells with CK7
  - Outer basal cells with neuroendocrine markers
- Peptides can also be reactive

Electron Microscopy
- Scanning
  - 2 distinct cell types
    - Type A: Apical dark cells with elongated microvilli and secretory mucus granules
    - Type B: Basal cells with cytoplasmic, solid, dense-core neurosecretory granules
  - Transitional forms with features of both cell types uncommon

MIDDLE EAR ADENOMA

Immunohistochemistry

Antibody	Reactivity	Staining Pattern	Comment
CK-PAN	Positive	Cytoplasmic	All tumor cells
CK7	Positive	Cytoplasmic	Highlights inner (luminal) cells within glandular spaces
CK8/18/CAM5.2	Positive	Cytoplasmic	All tumor cells
Chromogranin-A	Positive	Granular	Tends to be greater in basal layer
Synaptophysin	Positive	Cytoplasmic	Tends to be greater in basal layer
NSE	Positive	Granular	
CD56	Positive	Cytoplasmic	
HPP	Positive	Granular	Usually basal cells
Serotonin	Positive	Granular	
Glucagon	Positive	Granular	
EMA	Negative		
S100	Negative		
GFAP	Negative		
TTF-1	Negative		

DIFFERENTIAL DIAGNOSIS

Paraganglioma

- Zellballen architecture, although sometimes cells are compressed
- Isolated nuclear pleomorphism
- Basophilic, granular cytoplasm
- Paraganglia positive with chromogranin, synaptophysin, CD56
- Sustentacular cells positive with S100 protein

Ceruminous Adenoma

- Involves outer ear canal
- Has biphasic appearance
  - Inner luminal and outer basaloid cells
- Decapitation apocrine secretions and cerumen
- Epithelial markers positive
- Lacks neuroendocrine markers

Metastatic Adenocarcinoma

- Tumors tend to be destructively infiltrative
- Moderate to marked pleomorphism
- Usually increased mitotic count
- Clinical history combined with targeted immunohistochemistry helps differentiate

Meningioma

- Whorled, meningothelial pattern
- Psammoma bodies are frequently present
- Intranuclear cytoplasmic inclusions
- Delicate, sparse positive EMA reaction
- Lacks neuroendocrine markers

DIAGNOSTIC CHECKLIST

Pathologic Interpretation Pearls

- "Pseudoinfiltrative" pattern of tumor is characteristic
- Gland and duct-like pattern with secretions are common
- "Salt and pepper" nuclear chromatin distribution helpful
- Keratin and neuroendocrine markers concurrently positive

SELECTED REFERENCES

1. Leong K et al: Neuroendocrine adenoma of the middle ear (NAME). Ear Nose Throat J. 88(4):874-9, 2009
2. Berns S et al: Middle ear adenoma. Arch Pathol Lab Med. 130(7):1067-9, 2006
3. Ramsey MJ et al: Carcinoid tumor of the middle ear: clinical features, recurrences, and metastases. Laryngoscope. 115(9):1660-6, 2005
4. Thompson LD: Neuroendocrine adenoma of the middle ear. Ear Nose Throat J. 84(9):560-1, 2005
5. Devaney KO et al: Epithelial tumors of the middle ear--are middle ear carcinoids really distinct from middle ear adenomas? Acta Otolaryngol. 123(6):678-82, 2003
6. Torske KR et al: Adenoma versus carcinoid tumor of the middle ear: a study of 48 cases and review of the literature. Mod Pathol. 15(5):543-55, 2002
7. Ketabchi S et al: Middle ear adenoma is an amphicrine tumor: why call it adenoma? Ultrastruct Pathol. 25(1):73-8, 2001
8. Bold EL et al: Adenomatous lesions of the temporal bone immunohistochemical analysis and theories of histogenesis. Am J Otol. 16(2):146-52, 1995
9. Amble FR et al: Middle ear adenoma and adenocarcinoma. Otolaryngol Head Neck Surg. 109(5):871-6, 1993
10. Hale RJ et al: Middle ear adenoma: tumour of mixed mucinous and neuroendocrine differentiation. J Clin Pathol. 44(8):652-4, 1991
11. Davies JE et al: Middle ear neoplasms showing adenomatous and neuroendocrine components. J Laryngol Otol. 103(4):404-7, 1989
12. Wassef M et al: Middle ear adenoma. A tumor displaying mucinous and neuroendocrine differentiation. Am J Surg Pathol. 13(10):838-47, 1989
13. Stanley MW et al: Carcinoid tumors of the middle ear. Am J Clin Pathol. 87(5):592-600, 1987
14. McNutt MA et al: Adenomatous tumor of the middle ear. An ultrastructural and immunocytochemical study. Am J Clin Pathol. 84(4):541-7, 1985

Imaging and Microscopic Features

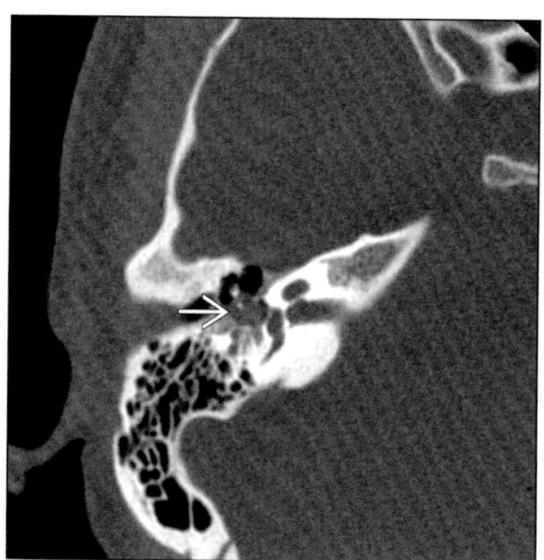

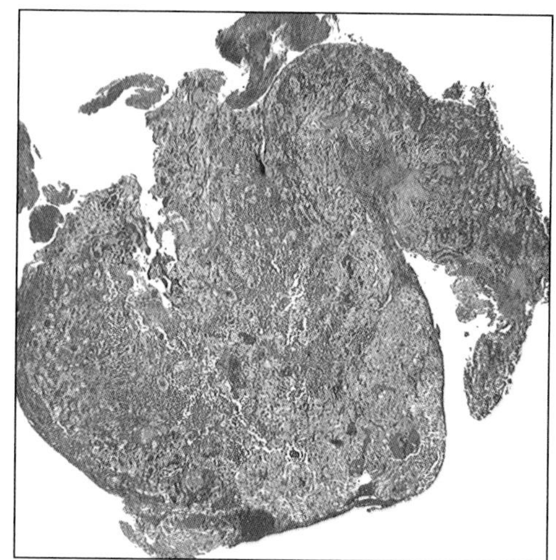

(Left) *Axial temporal bone CT shows a soft tissue mass ➡ in the middle ear that wraps around the ossicles without causing significant destruction.* ***(Right)*** *Hematoxylin & eosin shows a polypoid fragment of tissue and an infiltrate within the stroma. This low-power pattern can simulate an adenocarcinoma due to the "infiltrative" pattern of growth. However, careful high-power histologic examination will help make the correct diagnosis.*

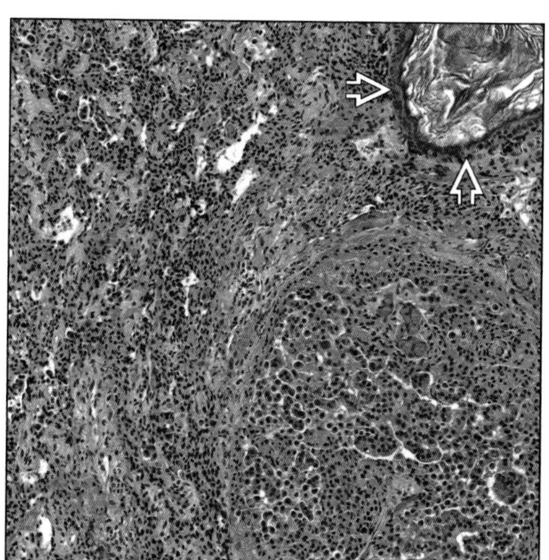

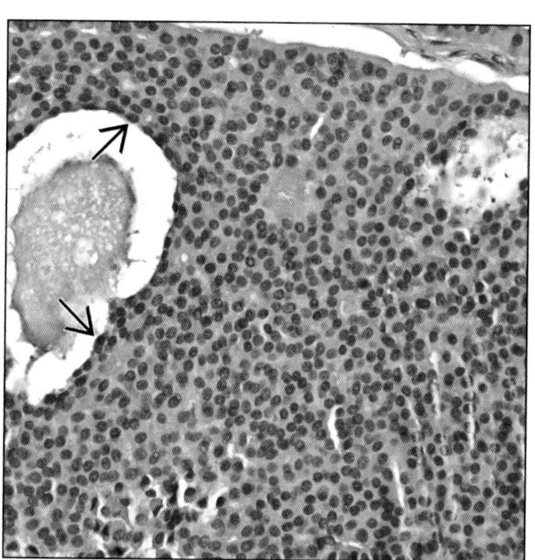

(Left) *This tumor shows a large number of different patterns within a single low-power field. A solid pattern shows pseudopapillary degenerative-type changes. There is a concurrent cholesteatoma ➡. This is not an uncommon associated finding.* ***(Right)*** *There is a solid pattern of growth in this part of a middle ear adenoma. However, open cystic spaces are present ➡, frequently lined by attenuated epithelial cells (which can be highlighted with CK7).*

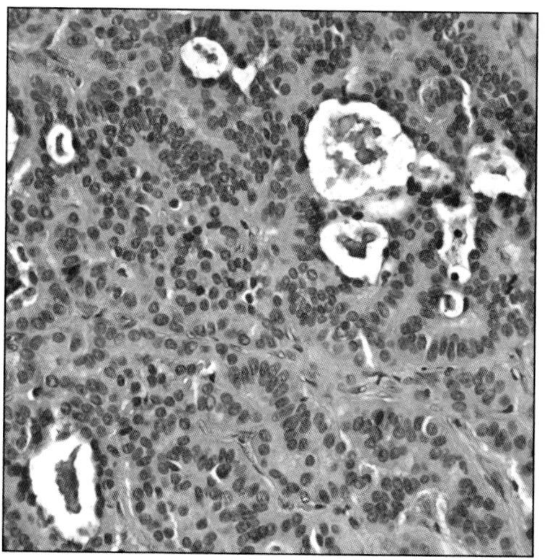

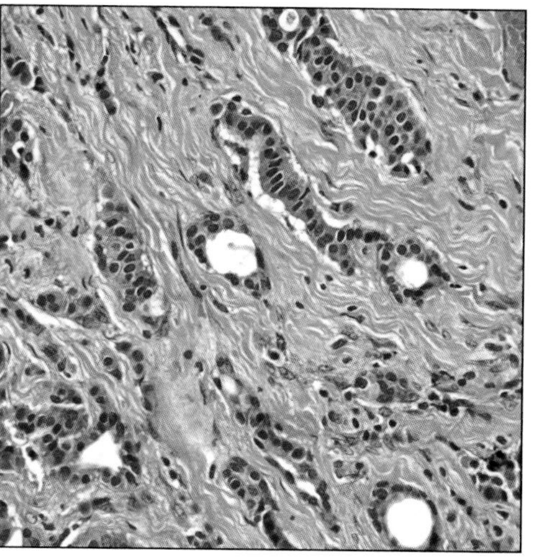

(Left) *Hematoxylin & eosin shows a glandular pattern blended with a festoon-ribbon pattern. There are concretions within the glandular lumen. The nuclei show the delicate "salt and pepper" nuclear chromatin distribution.* ***(Right)*** *The infiltrative pattern of small cells in single file or small nests to glandular patterns can mimic or simulate an infiltrating adenocarcinoma. The stroma is fibrotic and collagenized but is not desmoplastic.*

MIDDLE EAR ADENOMA

Tumor Patterns

(Left) There is a moderate cellularity to this tumor, immediately below an intact surface epithelium ⇨ that is not associated with the tumor. A number of different patterns are seen. *(Right)* Glandular or cribriform patterns can be seen in middle ear adenomas. The stroma surrounds the structures. There are concretions within the lumen of many of the glandular profiles. The cells are monotonous in this field, with delicate, "salt and pepper" nuclear chromatin distribution. A mitotic figure is noted ➡.

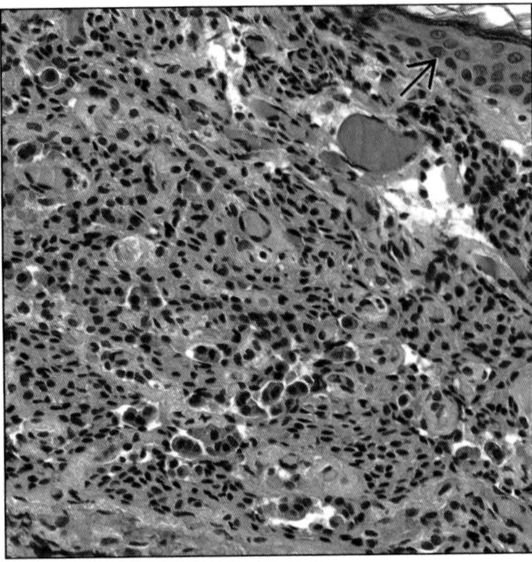

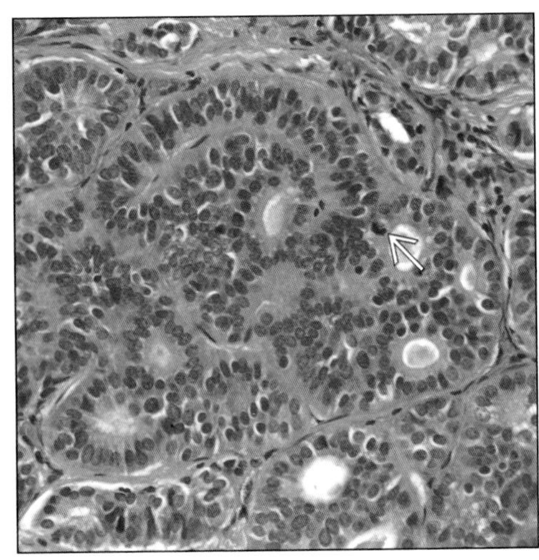

(Left) A biphasic glandular profile is seen in this tumor. There is an attenuated inner luminal layer with surrounding basal, cuboidal epithelial elements. This biphasic appearance is easily highlighted with immunohistochemistry. *(Right)* A certain degree of variability is often present in these tumors. Here, the cytoplasm surrounds eccentrically placed round to oval nuclei with hyperchromatic chromatin distribution. These cells have a plasmacytoid appearance.

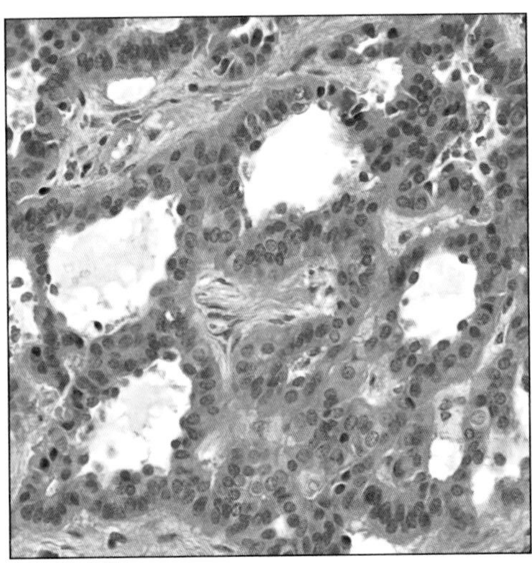

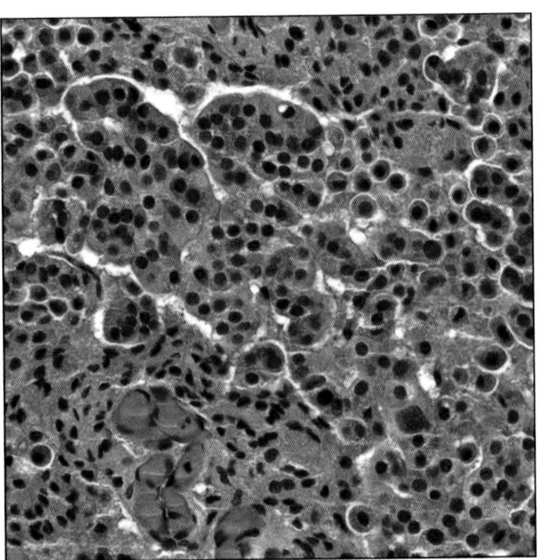

(Left) Abrupt transitions between various patterns is the norm for this tumor type. A solid pattern ⇨ is immediately adjacent to a more infiltrative, single cell pattern ➡. *(Right)* This cellular tumor shows a glandular pattern, but a festoon arrangement is noted throughout. The nuclei are round and regular with delicate chromatin distribution. Extravasated erythrocytes are focally noted in this tumor.

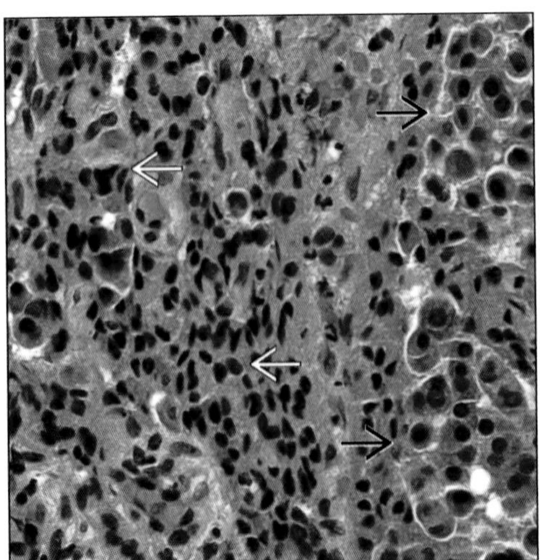

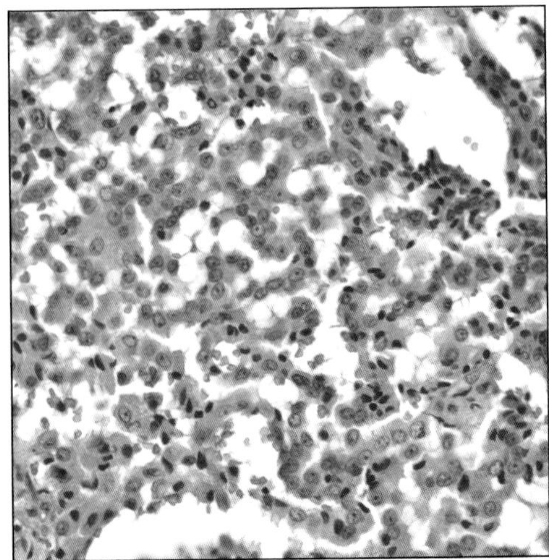

Immunohistochemical Features

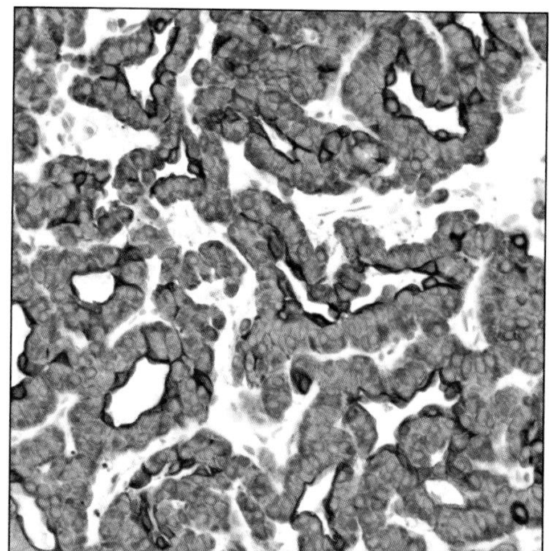

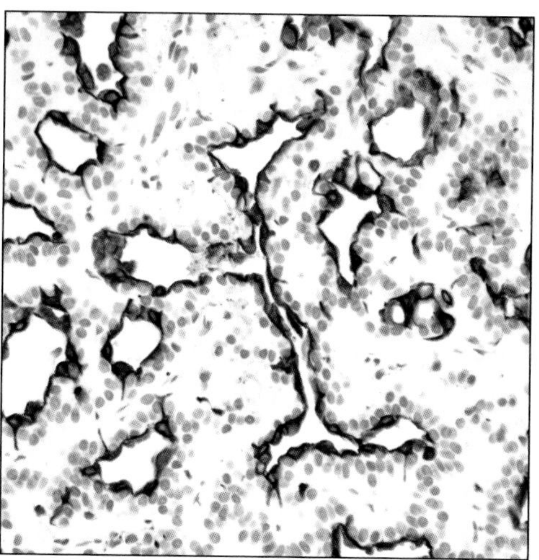

(Left) *Immunohistochemical evaluation is helpful in confirming the diagnosis. In this case, there is strong and diffuse keratin immunoreactivity. However, the "inner" lining cells are highlighted with a darker, heavier chromogen deposition.* ***(Right)*** *CK7 preferentially reacts with the inner lining cells of the glandular profiles. This marker can be useful in highlighting the biphasic nature of the neoplasm, with the basal cells staining more strongly with neuroendocrine markers.*

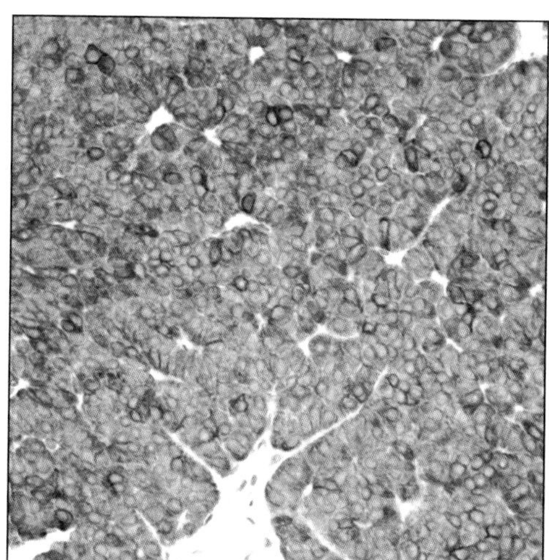

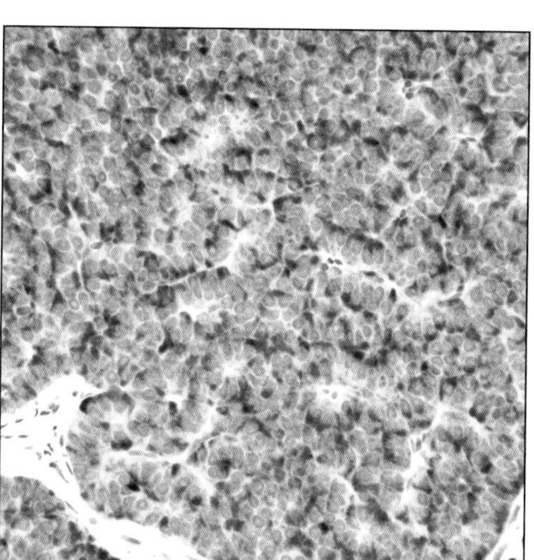

(Left) *There is strong and diffuse reaction with keratin in this tumor, even though this is in a solid region of the tumor. There are still isolated cells, which show an even stronger reaction.* ***(Right)*** *Neuroendocrine-type markers are positive in middle ear adenomas, although showing differential staining of the neoplastic population. There is a greater basal reactivity with synaptophysin, a finding seen with all of the neuroendocrine markers.*

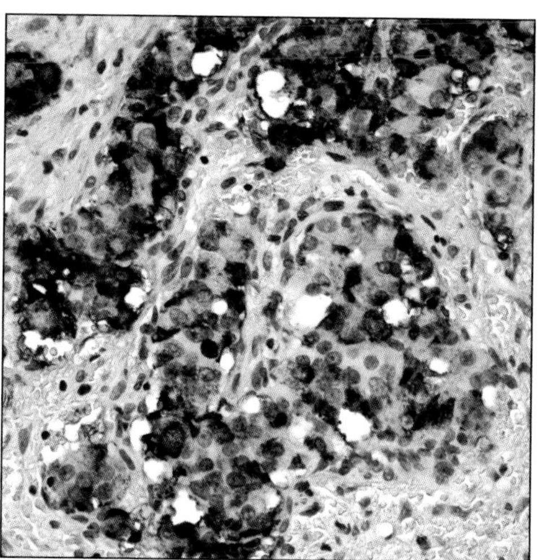

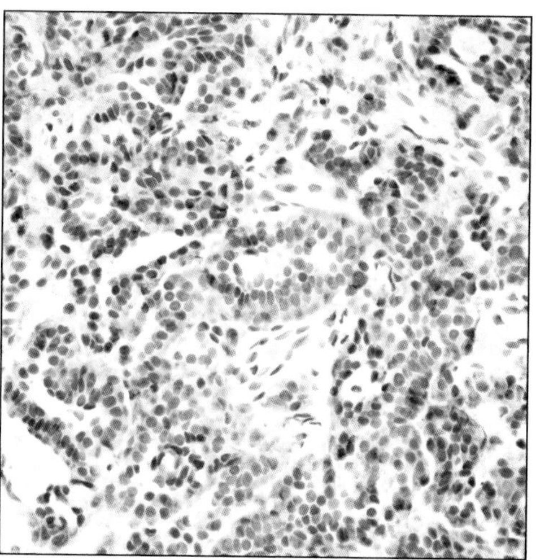

(Left) *Chromogranin highlights many neoplastic cells, but a number of cells are nonreactive, representing the inner, luminal, or glandular cells. There is a more granular reaction with chromogranin when compared to synaptophysin or CD56.* ***(Right)*** *Human pancreatic polypeptide shows strong and diffuse reaction in the basal cells of the glandular units. A variety of peptide markers can be positive, highlighting the neuroendocrine nature of the tumor.*

PARAGANGLIOMA (GLOMUS JUGULARE/TYMPANICUM)

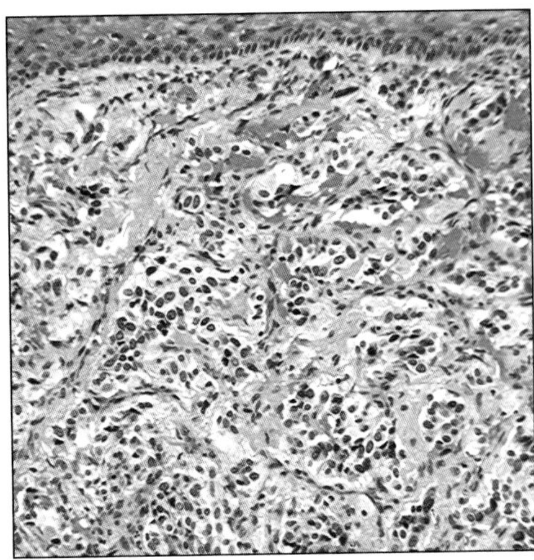

Hematoxylin & eosin shows an intact squamous epithelium (from the EAC) subtended by a nested neoplastic proliferation associated with a rich vascularized network and fibrous connective tissue.

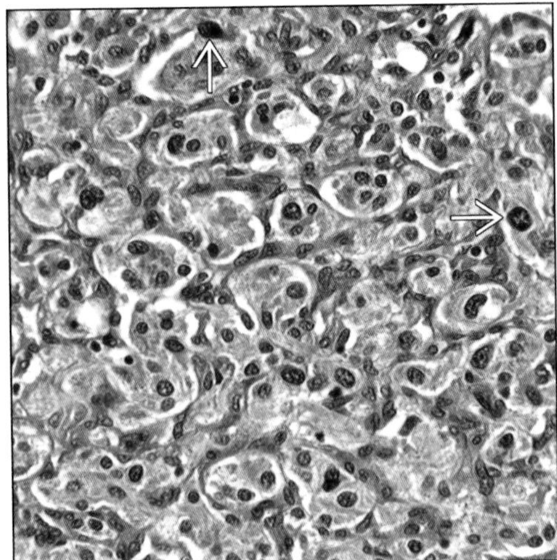

The zellballen arrangement gives a characteristic nesting or alveolar appearance to the neoplasm. There is focal nuclear pleomorphism ➡. The neoplasm is supported by a delicate vascular plexus.

TERMINOLOGY

Abbreviations

- Glomus tympanicum paraganglioma (GTP)
- Glomus jugulotympanicum paraganglioma (GJP)

Synonyms

- Glomus tympanicum
- Glomus jugulotympanicum
- Jugulotympanic chemodectoma
- Glomus jugulare
- Jugular glomus tumor
- Tympanic glomus tumor
- "Glomus" is usually applied to smooth muscle vascular tumor of nail bed soft tissue

Definitions

- Neoplasm arising from paraganglia in vicinity of jugular bulb or medial cochlea promontory
  - Radiographically and surgically "glomus tympanicum" (GTP) and "glomus jugulotympanicum" (GJP) paragangliomas are distinctive and unique
  - However, they are identical by pathology parameters; these clinical terms will be used for nonpathology findings

ETIOLOGY/PATHOGENESIS

Cell of Origin

- Arises from paraganglia
  - Along inferior tympanic nerve (Jacobson nerve)
  - Around jugular foramen
  - Auricular branch of CNX (Arnold nerve)
- Chemoreceptor cells are derived from neural crest
  - Respond to changes in blood oxygen and carbon dioxide levels

CLINICAL ISSUES

Epidemiology

- Incidence
  - Most common tumor of middle ear (GTP)
  - Most common tumor of jugular foramen (GJP) (~ 90%)
    - Together GTP and GJP account for 80% of head and neck paragangliomas
  - 10% multicentric
  - 10% bilateral
  - 10% familial
  - 10% pediatric
  - 10% malignant
  - May coexist with pheochromocytoma (adrenal gland) and carotid body tumors
- Age
  - Range: 10-85 years
  - Mean: 6th decade
- Gender
  - Female > > Male (5:1) for sporadic tumors
  - Male > Female for inherited/familial tumors

Site

- GTP: Middle ear surface of promontory
  - Anterior inferior quadrant of tympanic membrane
- GJP: Jugular foramen
  - Wall of jugular bulb

Presentation

- Pulsatile tinnitus (~ 90% of patients)
- Hearing loss (~ 50% of patients)
  - Conductive rather than sensorineural
- Vascular retrotympanic mass
- Pain
- Facial nerve paralysis
- Catecholamine function is rare
- If familial or syndrome: Autosomal dominant trait with genomic imprinting

PARAGANGLIOMA (GLOMUS JUGULARE/TYMPANICUM)

Key Facts

Terminology
- Synonyms: Glomus jugulare, glomus tympanicum
- Neoplasm arising from paraganglia in vicinity of jugular bulb or medial cochlea promontory

Clinical Issues
- 10% multicentric, 10% bilateral, 10% familial
- Female > > Male (5:1) in sporadic tumors
- 90% of tumors of jugular foramen are paraganglioma
- Pulsatile tinnitus
- Hearing loss (conductive)
- Do not biopsy: Very vascularized and will bleed
- Presurgical embolization for reduced bleeding
- 15% mortality due to proximity of vital anatomic structures

Image Findings
- CT: Bone only without contrast shows a mass with flat base on cochlear promontory
- MR T1WI: Multiple black dots in tumor indicate high-velocity flow voids
- Octreotide or MIBG scintigraphy helps with occult or familial tumors

Microscopic Pathology
- Clustered, zellballen architecture
- Richly vascularized stroma, sometimes with fibrosis
- Small to intermediate cells with ample granular, basophilic cytoplasm

Ancillary Tests
- Neuroendocrine markers

Treatment
- Options, risks, complications
  - Do not biopsy; very vascularized and will bleed
  - Slow growing but locally destructive tumor
    - Can be "watched" in older patients
  - Presurgical embolization for reduced bleeding
  - About 2/3 of patients experience postoperative cranial neuropathy
- Surgical approaches
  - GTP
    - Tympanotomy for small lesions
    - Mastoidectomy for larger lesions
  - GJP
    - Infratemporal fossa approach (Fisch type A)
- Radiation
  - May work for localized tumors
  - May be needed in combination with surgery for larger tumors
  - Palliative in poor surgical candidates or older patients

Prognosis
- Excellent overall outcome
- Aggressive clinical behavior is seen in ~ 8-10% of cases
- 15% mortality due to proximity of vital anatomic structures
- Distant metastases are rare

IMAGE FINDINGS

General Features
- Radiographs accurately define location, size, extent
- Glomus tympanicum
  - CT: Bone only without contrast shows a mass with flat base on cochlear promontory
  - MR: Enhancing mass with flat base on cochlear promontory
    - Performed after bone CT yields suspicious result
- Glomus jugulare
  - CT: Bone only shows a mass in jugular foramen with **permeative-destructive** change in adjacent bone
  - MR T1WI: Multiple black dots in tumor indicate high-velocity flow voids from feeder arterial branches
- Angiography: Allows for preoperative embolization
  - Demonstrates blood supply from ascending pharyngeal artery and its branches
- Octreotide or MIBG scintigraphy helps with occult or familial tumors
- PET with F18 FDG: Avid uptake by tumor cells

MACROSCOPIC FEATURES

General Features
- Fragmented due to anatomic restrictions
- Irregular, reddish masses
- Firm mass
- Variegated cut surface with blood and degeneration
- Tympanic membrane usually intact
- Can be widely invasive
  - Filling apical portion of petrous temporal bone and middle ear

Size
- Variable, but difficult to measure due to fragmentation
- GTP: Range: 0.3-2.5 cm
- GJP: Range: 2-6 cm

MICROSCOPIC PATHOLOGY

Histologic Features
- Clustered, zellballen architecture
- Richly vascularized stroma, sometimes with fibrosis
- Poorly encapsulated or circumscribed, often infiltrative
- Moderately cellular
- Cyst formation, hemorrhage, and hemosiderin-laden macrophages common
- Small to intermediate cells with ample granular, basophilic cytoplasm
- Nuclei are round to focally irregular and enlarged
- Delicate to coarse nuclear chromatin
- Multinucleated cells are uncommon

PARAGANGLIOMA (GLOMUS JUGULARE/TYMPANICUM)

Immunohistochemistry

Antibody	Reactivity	Staining Pattern	Comment
Chromogranin-A	Positive	Cytoplasmic	Paraganglia cells
Synaptophysin	Positive	Cytoplasmic	Paraganglia cells
NSE	Positive	Cytoplasmic	Paraganglia cells
CD56	Positive	Cell membrane	Paraganglia cells
S100	Positive	Nuclear & cytoplasmic	Sustentacular supporting cells
GFAP	Positive	Cytoplasmic	Sustentacular supporting cells
CK-PAN	Negative		
CEA-M	Negative		
HPP	Negative		

- Mitotic figures vanishingly rare

ANCILLARY TESTS

Cytology

- Fine needle aspiration is usually contraindicated as procedure may provoke hypertensive crisis or result in significant bleeding
- Smears are usually hypercellular, with cells arranged singly or in small groups, often creating a "pseudorosette"
- 3 cell types are interspersed throughout smear
  - Cells are small to moderate-sized polygonal-shaped with delicate, granular cytoplasm
  - Spindle cells with ample cytoplasm and elongated nuclei
  - Large, strap-like cells with large, eccentric nuclei with prominent nucleoli

Immunohistochemistry

- Neuroendocrine markers

Cytogenetics

- Germline mutations in several genes encoding various subunits of succinate-ubiquinone oxidoreductase gene (SDH)
  - These enzymes are in mitochondrial respiratory chain complex II
  - *PGL1-PLG4* encodes SDH subunits A-D on 11q, 1q, and 1p
- Inactivating mutations in *SDHB*, *SDHC*, and *SDHD* genes cause hereditary paraganglioma
- Genetic counseling and testing for *SDHX*, *VHL*, *NF1*, and *RET* genes should be offered to all patients with paraganglioma

Electron Microscopy

- Membrane-bound, electron-dense neurosecretory granules (150-250 nm) in cytoplasm

DIFFERENTIAL DIAGNOSIS

Schwannoma

- Spindle cells with alternating cellular and hypocellular areas
- Diffuse, strong S100 protein immunoreactivity

Meningioma

- Whorled, epithelioid proliferation with intranuclear cytoplasmic inclusions
- Psammoma bodies
- EMA immunoreactivity

Middle Ear Adenoma

- a.k.a. neuroendocrine adenoma of middle ear (NAME)
- Multiple growth patterns, with glandular appearance
- "Salt and pepper" nuclear chromatin distribution
- Immunoreactive with keratin and neuroendocrine markers

STAGING

Glasscock-Jackson Classification

- Type I: Tumor limited to cochlear promontory
- Type II: Tumor filling middle ear space
- Type III: Tumor filling middle ear and extending into mastoid air cells
- Type IV: Tumor filling middle ear, extending into mastoid bone &/or external auditory canal, or extending anterior to carotid artery

SELECTED REFERENCES

1. Suárez C et al: Temporal paragangliomas. Eur Arch Otorhinolaryngol. 264(7):719-31, 2007
2. Ramina R et al: Tumors of the jugular foramen: diagnosis and management. Neurosurgery. 57(1 Suppl):59-68; discussion 59-68, 2005
3. Pellitteri PK et al: Paragangliomas of the head and neck. Oral Oncol. 40(6):563-75, 2004
4. Tasar M et al: Glomus tumors: therapeutic role of selective embolization. J Craniofac Surg. 15(3):497-505, 2004
5. Al-Mefty O et al: Complex tumors of the glomus jugulare: criteria, treatment, and outcome. J Neurosurg. 97(6):1356-66, 2002
6. Myssiorek D: Head and neck paragangliomas: an overview. Otolaryngol Clin North Am. 34(5):829-36, v, 2001
7. Weber PC et al: Jugulotympanic paragangliomas. Otolaryngol Clin North Am. 34(6):1231-40, x, 2001
8. Somasundar P et al: Paragangliomas-- a decade of clinical experience. J Surg Oncol. 74(4):286-90, 2000
9. Rao AB et al: From the archives of the AFIP. Paragangliomas of the head and neck: radiologic-pathologic correlation. Armed Forces Institute of Pathology. Radiographics. 19(6):1605-32, 1999

Diagrammatic, Radiographic, and Microscopic Features

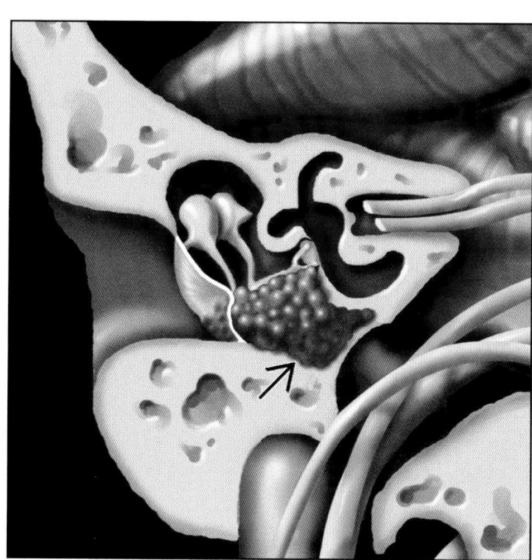

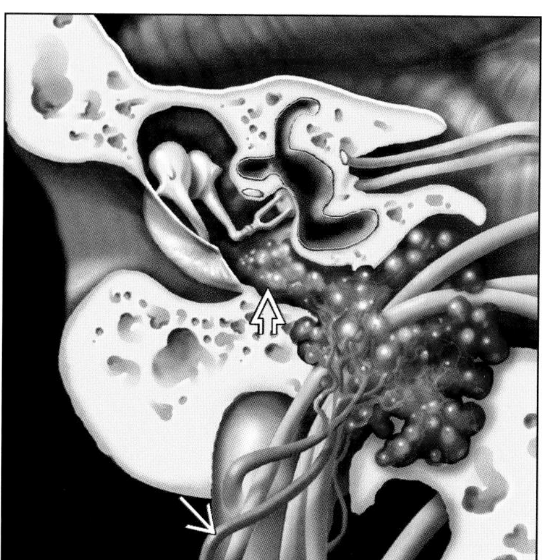

(Left) *This coronal graphic shows a highly vascular glomus tympanicum paraganglioma expanding off the cochlear promontory, filling the middle ear cavity, and subtly expanding into the bony floor ➔.* ***(Right)*** *This coronal graphic shows a glomus jugulare paraganglioma centered in the jugular foramen with superolateral extension into the middle ear ➔. The ascending pharyngeal artery ➔ is feeding this tumor and could be used for embolization during angiography.*

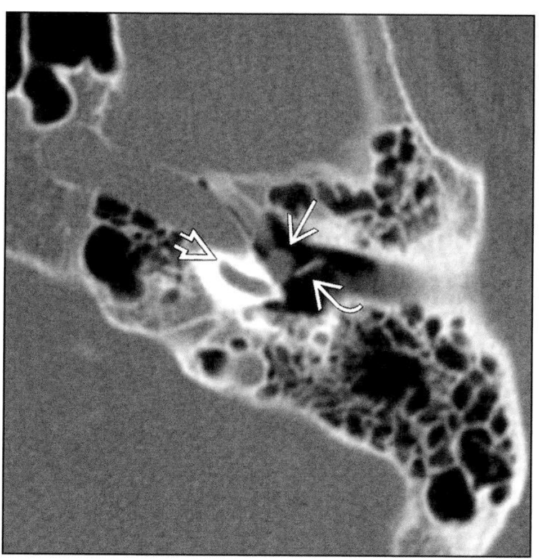

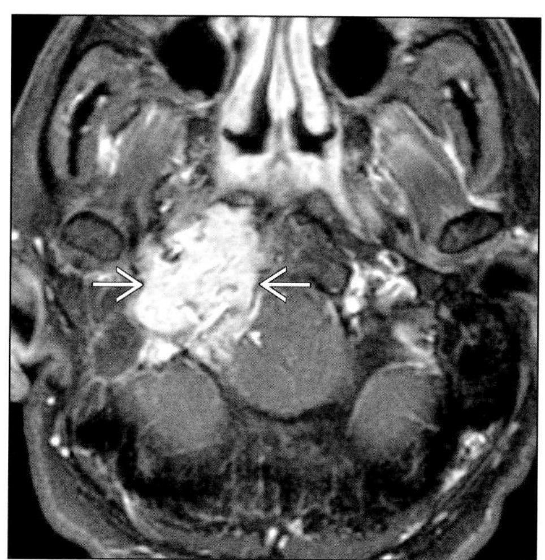

(Left) *An axial temporal bone CT of the left ear shows a very characteristic appearance of a tympanic paraganglioma. There is an ovoid mass on the low cochlear promontory ➔ abutting the manubrium of the malleus ➔. The basal turn of the cochlea is shown ➔.* ***(Right)*** *Axial T1WI FS MR with intravenous gadolinium shows a large enhancing mass ➔ centered in the right jugular foramen. This appearance is quite characteristic for a jugular paraganglioma.*

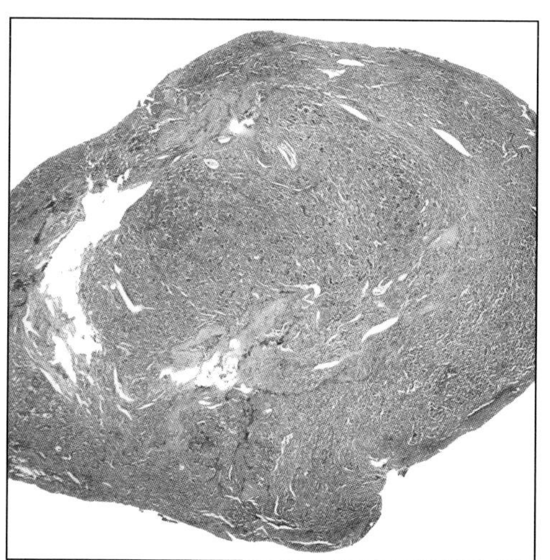

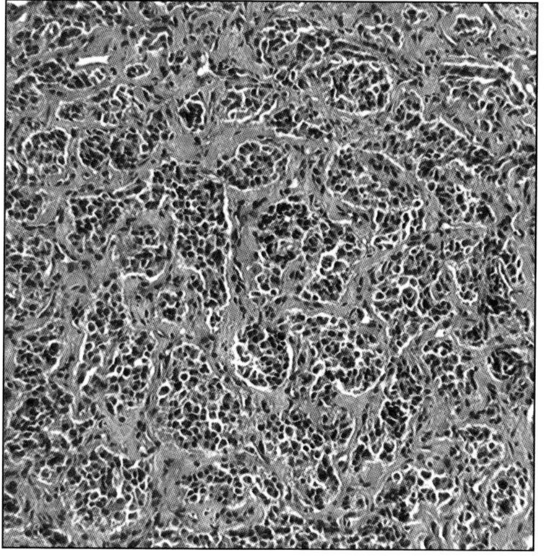

(Left) *Paraganglioma are usually a polypoid or pedunculated mass (if not fragmented). They are poorly encapsulated or circumscribed. Areas of degeneration and erythrocyte extravasation are present throughout the tumor.* ***(Right)*** *The fibrovascular stroma can be more fibrotic, especially in paraganglioma of the ear and temporal bone region. The cells in this tumor have a high nuclear to cytoplasmic ratio, with nuclear hyperchromasia, mimicking lymphocytes.*

PARAGANGLIOMA (GLOMUS JUGULARE/TYMPANICUM)

Microscopic Features

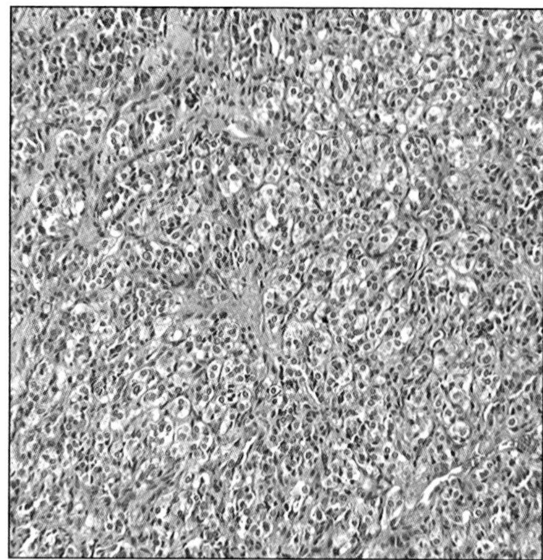

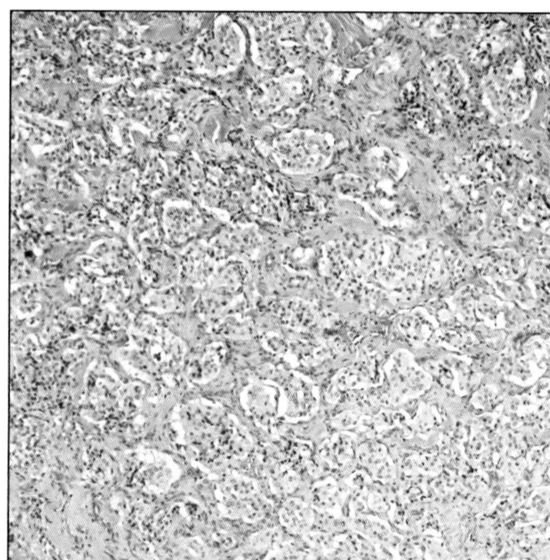

(Left) *There is a clustering and a zellballen architecture to this paraganglioma. Note the richly vascularized stroma, focally associated with fibrosis. The tumor is cellular.* ***(Right)*** *Paraganglioma have similar features but show quite significant variability between cases. Here the zellballen architecture is highlighted by a more well-developed fibrotic stroma. The cells show abundant cytoplasm.*

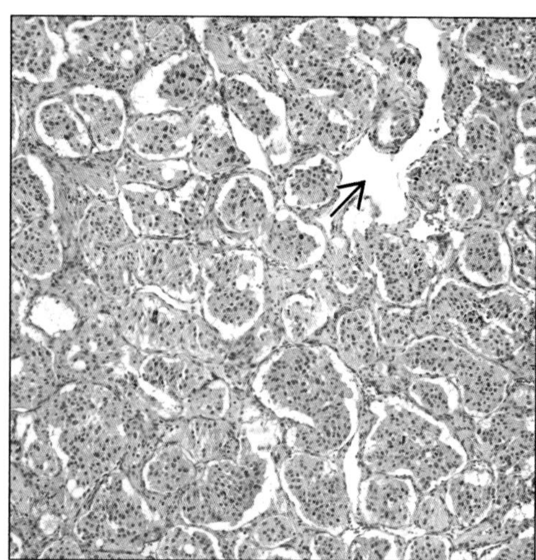

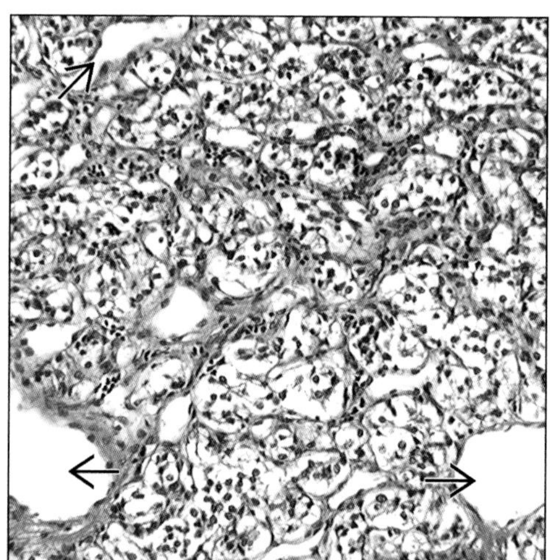

(Left) *This cellular tumor shows a nested to focally trabecular architecture. There is focal cyst formation ➔. The cells are small with a syncytial architecture. The cytoplasm is granular and eosinophilic.* ***(Right)*** *Hematoxylin & eosin shows a rich vascular plexus with associated nests of tumor. The cytoplasm is difficult to appreciate and appears cleared in this tumor. There are many larger vessels ➔ in this neoplasm.*

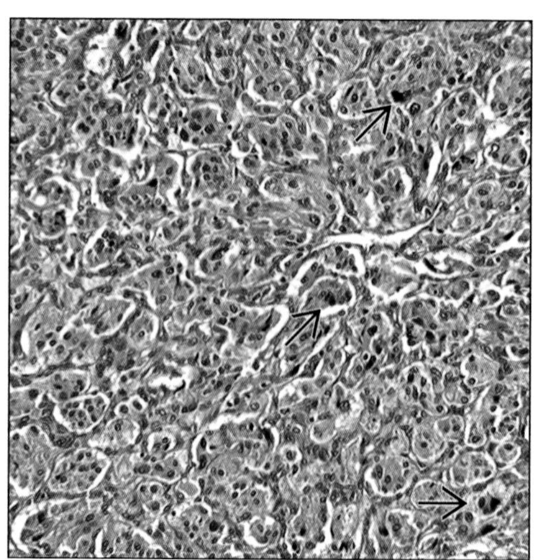

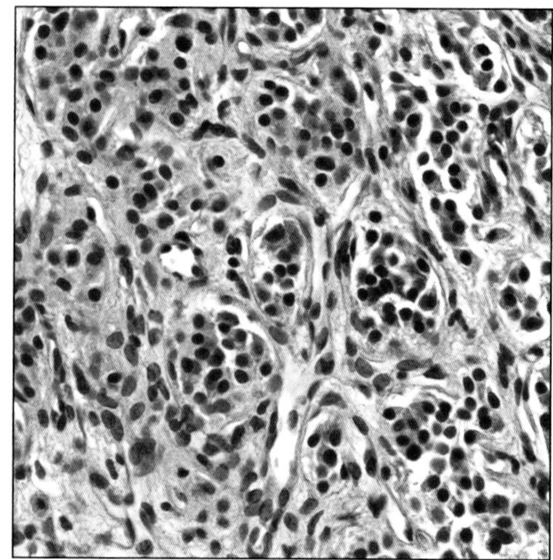

(Left) *The clustered growth of this tumor shows a vague meningothelial-type growth pattern. The sustentacular supporting framework is limited as is the fibrosis. There is still focal nuclear pleomorphism ➔.* ***(Right)*** *The neoplastic cells have a syncytial appearance, with small round nuclei with coarse nuclear chromatin. The cytoplasm is slightly basophilic. The sustentacular supporting framework cannot be detected with standard H&E stained slides. Mitoses are usually limited.*

Ancillary Techniques and Molecular Features

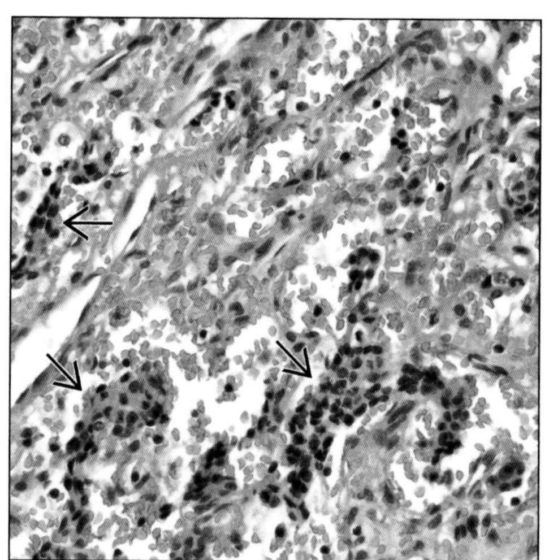

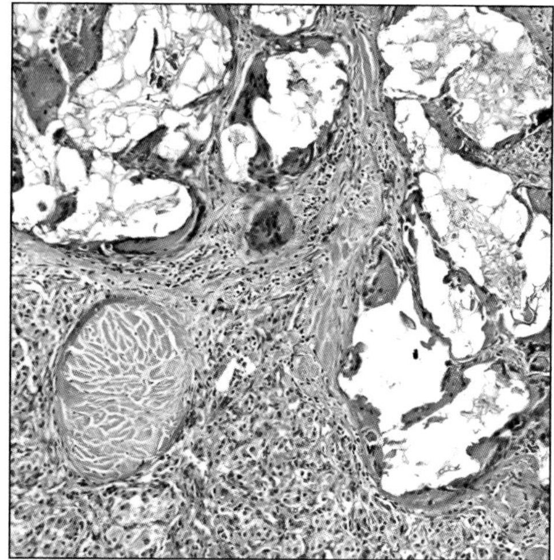

(Left) *The tumors are richly vascularized, and so it is not uncommon to have hemorrhage or bleeding into the tumor. In this case, there are only small isolated nests of neoplastic cells ➔, while the dominant finding is the hemorrhage or degeneration.* ***(Right)*** *Angiography is used to identify the feeder vessel to the tumor, allowing for embolization, which results in decreased hemorrhage during surgery and possible tumor infarction. Note the foreign embolic material.*

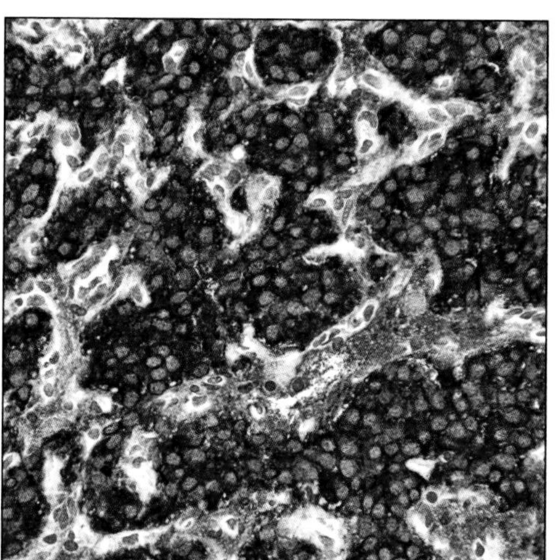

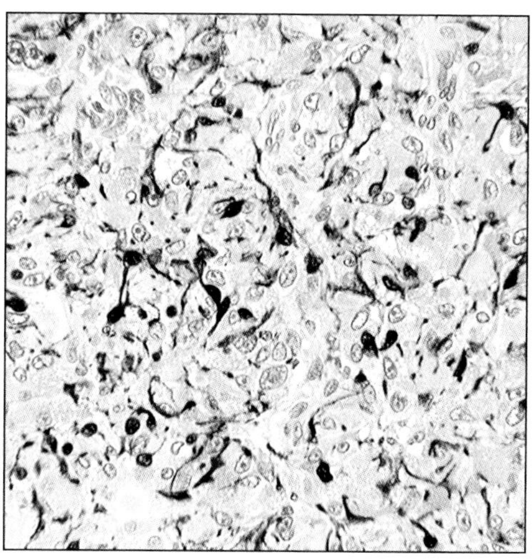

(Left) *Neuroendocrine markers will highlight the paraganglia cells. These include chromogranin (shown), synaptophysin, CD56, NSE, among others.* ***(Right)*** *The supporting sustentacular framework is highlighted with S100 protein. It is a discontinuous staining on a 2-dimensional section. Both the nucleus and the delicate wisps of cytoplasm will be highlighted with the stain.*

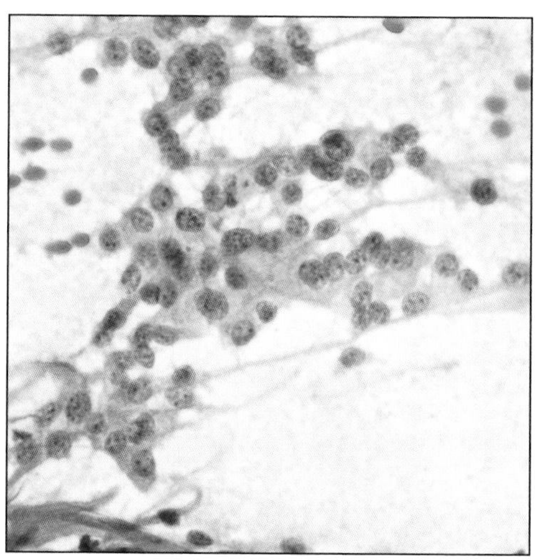

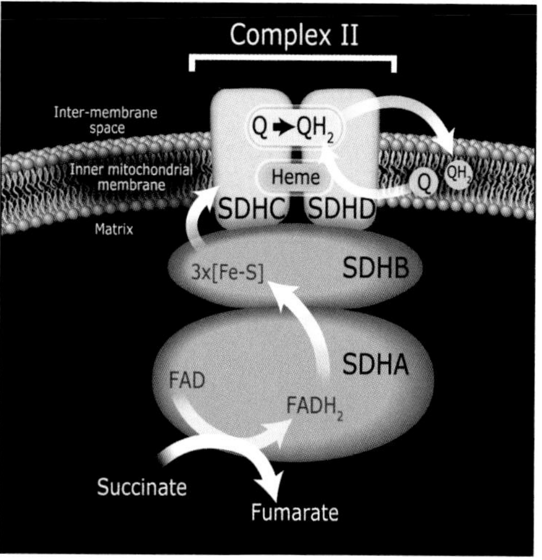

(Left) *This is a cellular smear, showing cells arranged in small groups. Usually 3 cell types are present in varying degree. Here, there are small to moderate-sized polygonal-shaped cells with delicate, granular cytoplasm. (Courtesy L. Layfield, MD.)* ***(Right)*** *Graphic of part of the mitochondrial respiratory chain complex II shows the relationship between the succinate-ubiquinone oxidoreductase subunits (SDHA-SDHD). Inactivating mutations result in hereditary paraganglioma.*

SCHWANNOMA (ACOUSTIC NEUROMA)

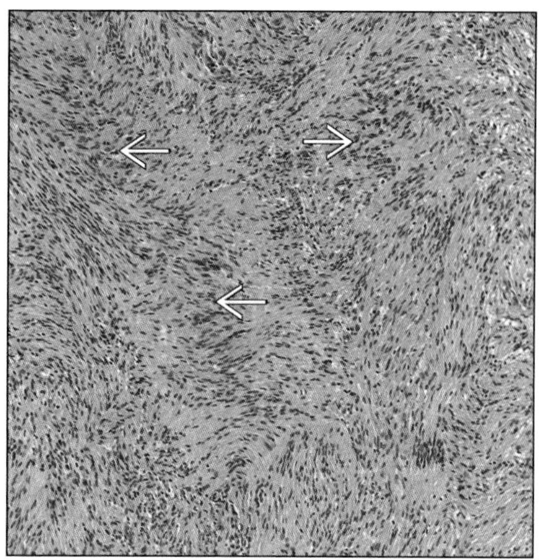

A low-power view demonstrates the interlacing short fascicles of spindled cells. There is palisading to the nuclei ➡, a feature quite characteristic of schwannoma.

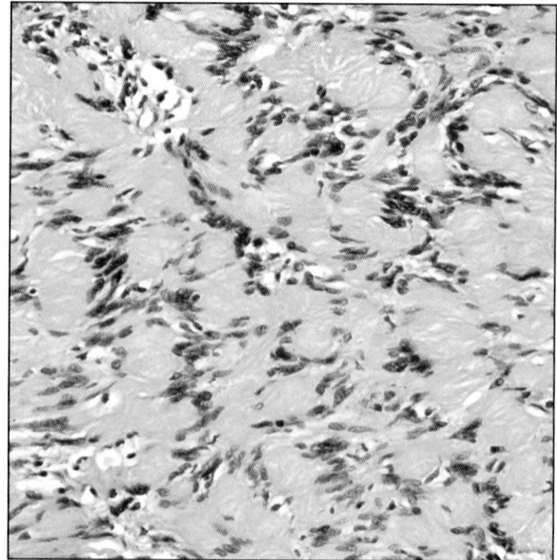

Hematoxylin & eosin shows spindled nuclei in a palisaded arrangement. There are abundant cellular processes between the nuclei (eosinophilic), creating a fibrillar material.

TERMINOLOGY

Synonyms

- Peripheral nerve sheath tumor (PNST)
- Neurilemmoma
- Acoustic neuroma
- Acoustic schwannoma
- Acoustic neurinoma
- Vestibular neurilemoma

Definitions

- Benign nerve sheath tumor arising within internal auditory canal (IAC)

ETIOLOGY/PATHOGENESIS

Cell of Origin

- Schwann cell (myelin-forming) derived neoplasm
- Most arise from vestibular portion of vestibulocochlear cranial nerve (CN VIII)

Etiology

- Unknown for majority of cases
- Occupational exposure to extremely loud noise trauma, especially when sustained (20 years), may be a risk factor in tumor development

CLINICAL ISSUES

Epidemiology

- Incidence
    - Accounts for 5-10% of all intracranial tumors
    - Most common neoplasm of temporal bone
        - Accounts for 80-90% of cerebellopontine angle (CPA) tumors
    - 95% of tumors are unilateral and sporadic
    - Identified in about 1 per 100,000 population worldwide
- Age
    - Most common in 5th to 6th decades
    - Tend to be younger (< 21 years) when associated with neurofibromatosis 2 (NF2)

Site

- Cerebellopontine angle
- If bilateral, consider NF2
- Internal auditory meatus
- No laterality (right = left)

Presentation

- Hearing loss
    - Unilateral progressive hearing loss in 90% of patients
    - Sensorineural loss, **not** conductive
- Tinnitus (80% of patients)
    - High-pitched ringing or steam-kettle-type hissing
- Headache
- Vertigo, often with nausea and vomiting
- Altered balance, with unsteady gait
- Facial pain, weakness or loss of taste
    - Development of tumor compresses the brainstem and so facial nerve (CN VII) is affected
- Symptoms are frequently present for years
- If present for a long duration, tumor may cause compression of pons and medulla, resulting in obstruction to flow of cerebrospinal fluid with increased intracranial pressure

Treatment

- Options, risks, complications
    - If tumor is small: Watchful waiting, monitoring by MR scanning, and using hearing aids (as required)
        - Tumors tend to grow slowly
        - Especially advocated in older patients (> 70 years)
    - Nerve preservation more difficult in NF2 patients (tumors infiltrate nerves)
        - Attempt to maintain hearing and vestibular function
    - Meningitis is potential postoperative complication
- Surgical approaches

SCHWANNOMA (ACOUSTIC NEUROMA)

Key Facts

Terminology
- Benign nerve sheath tumor arising within internal auditory canal (IAC)

Clinical Issues
- Most common neoplasm of temporal bone
- Involves the cerebropontine angle
  - If tumors are bilateral, consider NF2
- Patients present with hearing loss
  - Unilateral loss in 90% of patients
  - Sensorineural loss, **not** conductive
- Low recurrence potential

Image Findings
- Cerebropontine angle mass
- Funnel-shaped widening of internal auditory canal or small indentation of bone
- Intense enhancement into porus acusticus
- Cerebropontine angle; posterior fossa intracanalicular mass

Microscopic Pathology
- Cellular (Antoni A) closely packed spindle cells
- Microcystic or loosely reticular Antoni B areas
- Palisaded nuclei (Verocay body)
- Cells are fusiform, buckled nuclei, with fibrillary cytoplasm
- Medium-sized vessels with perivascular hyalinization

Ancillary Tests
- Strong and diffuse S100 protein immunoreactivity

Top Differential Diagnoses
- Meningioma
- Neurofibroma

  - Translabyrinthine
  - Craniotomy with middle fossa or suboccipital approach to internal auditory canal
    - Posterior petrosal
  - Postoperative reconstruction for surgical defects
- Radiation
  - Major methods
    - Stereotactic-guided gamma knife radiosurgery
    - Fractionated stereotactic radiotherapy
    - Proton therapy (infrequently used)
  - May have failure rates up to 15%
  - Development of 2nd malignancy is a risk

Prognosis
- Excellent overall prognosis
- Low recurrence potential
  - If radiated, tumors may be more difficult to remove

IMAGE FINDINGS

General Features
- Best diagnostic clue
  - Cerebropontine angle mass
- Location
  - Cerebropontine angle
  - Posterior fossa intracanalicular mass
- Morphology
  - Funnel-shaped widening of internal auditory canal or small indentation of bone
  - Mushroom shape: Stalk within canal; flange within CPA
- Virtual endoscopy shows promise as reconstructed views can create images used in surgical planning

MR Findings
- Iso- to hypointense mass on T1-weighted images
- Hyperintense mass on T2-weighted images (with gadolinium)
- Intense enhancement into porus acusticus

CT Findings
- Isodense to cerebellum and IAC widening
- Calcifications and blood may be seen

MACROSCOPIC FEATURES

General Features
- Eccentric, globular mass
- Frequently attached to vestibular division of 8th (vestibulocochlear) cranial nerve
  - If associated with cochlear division, nerve is stretched rather than attached
- Smooth, lobulated tumor surface
- Firm, yellowish-tan, solid to cystic mass
- Intratumoral hemorrhage is common

Size
- Variable, usually < 2 cm
  - Tumors > 1.8 cm more likely to recur

MICROSCOPIC PATHOLOGY

Histologic Features
- Schwann cell derivation gives histologic features
- Cellular (Antoni A) closely packed spindle cells
- Palisaded nuclei (Verocay body)
- Microcystic or loosely reticular Antoni B areas
- Cells are fusiform
- Buckled nuclei
- Fibrillary cytoplasm
- Mitotic figures are uncommon
- Medium-sized vessels with perivascular hyalinization
- Extensive degeneration results in only isolated tumor cells
- Necrosis is usually absent
- Lymphoid cuffing or peripheral infiltrate is absent in this location
- Extensive pleomorphism may suggest malignancy
  - Ancient change can be seen but in isolated cells
- Hydrops of endolymphatic system with atrophy of spiral ganglion cells in large tumors

SCHWANNOMA (ACOUSTIC NEUROMA)

Immunohistochemistry

Antibody	Reactivity	Staining Pattern	Comment
S100	Positive	Nuclear & cytoplasmic	Strong and diffuse
Vimentin	Positive	Cytoplasmic	Strong but nonspecific
GFAP	Positive	Cytoplasmic	Occasionally positive
NSE	Positive	Cytoplasmic	Occasionally positive
Ki-67	Positive	Nuclear	Higher rates in NF2-associated tumors
CK-PAN	Negative		
EMA	Negative		
NFP	Negative		
Desmin	Negative		
Actin-sm	Negative		
Actin-HHF-35	Negative		
CD34	Equivocal	Cytoplasmic	Only stains isolated, slender cells in degenerated areas

ANCILLARY TESTS

Immunohistochemistry

- Strong and diffuse S100 protein immunoreactivity

Cytogenetics

- Neurofibromatosis is autosomal dominant
- *NF2* is suppressor gene on long arm of chromosome 22 (22q12)
- 90% of mutations coded by merlin or schwannomin result in loss of protein function

Electron Microscopy

- Interdigitating slender cytoplasmic processes covered by continuous basal lamina
- Long spacing collagen with distinct periodicity (Luse body)

DIFFERENTIAL DIAGNOSIS

Meningioma

- Whorled appearance
- Psammoma bodies
- Intranuclear cytoplasmic inclusions
- EMA or focal keratin immunoreactivity

Neurofibroma

- Lacks Antoni A and B areas
- Lacks perivascular hyalinization
- Very rare in this anatomic site
- NFP may be immunoreactive

Solitary Fibrous Tumor

- Cellular neoplasm
- Rich collagen investment
- Spindle cells arranged in short fascicles
- CD34 and Bcl-2 immunoreactive

SELECTED REFERENCES

1. Abram S et al: Stereotactic radiation techniques in the treatment of acoustic schwannomas. Otolaryngol Clin North Am. 40(3):571-88, ix, 2007
2. Bennett M et al: Surgical approaches and complications in the removal of vestibular schwannomas. Otolaryngol Clin North Am. 40(3):589-609, ix-x, 2007
3. Mirzayan MJ et al: Management of vestibular schwannomas in young patients-comparison of clinical features and outcome with adult patients. Childs Nerv Syst. 23(8):891-5, 2007
4. Régis J et al: Modern management of vestibular schwannomas. Prog Neurol Surg. 20:129-41, 2007
5. Sanna M et al: Surgical management of jugular foramen schwannomas with hearing and facial nerve function preservation: a series of 23 cases and review of the literature. Laryngoscope. 116(12):2191-204, 2006
6. Thompson L: Temporal bone schwannoma. Ear Nose Throat J. 85(11):704, 2006
7. Swartz JD: Lesions of the cerebellopontine angle and internal auditory canal: diagnosis and differential diagnosis. Semin Ultrasound CT MR. 25(4):332-52, 2004
8. Huang MY et al: Clinical perspectives regarding patients with internal auditory canal or cerebellopontine angle lesions: surgical and radiation oncology perspectives. Semin Ultrasound CT MR. 24(3):124-32, 2003
9. Neff BA et al: Intralabyrinthine schwannomas. Otol Neurotol. 24(2):299-307, 2003
10. Brackmann DE et al: Prognostic factors for hearing preservation in vestibular schwannoma surgery. Am J Otol. 21(3):417-24, 2000
11. Lim DJ et al: Advances in neurofibromatosis 2 (NF2): a workshop report. J Neurogenet. 14(2):63-106, 2000
12. Rosenberg SI: Natural history of acoustic neuromas. Laryngoscope. 110(4):497-508, 2000
13. Sekiya T et al: A comprehensive classification system of vestibular schwannomas. J Clin Neurosci. 7(2):129-33, 2000
14. Gusella JF et al: Merlin: the neurofibromatosis 2 tumor suppressor. Biochim Biophys Acta. 1423(2):M29-36, 1999
15. Charabi S: Acoustic neuroma/vestibular schwannoma in vivo and in vitro growth models. A clinical and experimental study. Acta Otolaryngol Suppl. 530:1-27, 1997
16. Brackmann DE: A review of acoustic tumors: 1979-1982. Am J Otol. 5(3):233-44, 1984

Radiographic and Microscopic Features

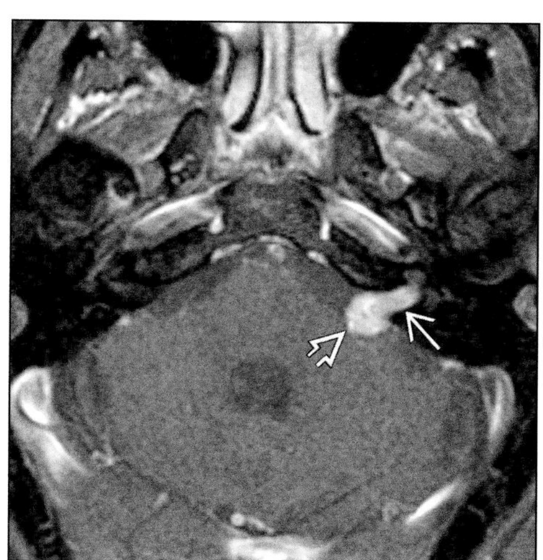

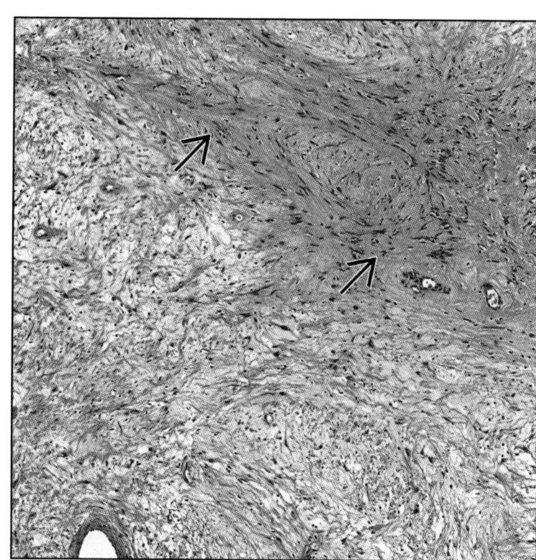

(Left) *Axial contrast-enhanced T1 MR image shows an enhancing acoustic neuroma filling the left internal auditory canal (IAC ➔) and extending out into the cerebellopontine angle (CPA ➔). Note the typical "ice cream cone" (IAC portion) and "ice cream" (CPA portion) morphology.* ***(Right)*** *The hypocellular appearance of spindled cells associated with myxoid and edematous Antoni B area is adjacent to an Antoni A ➔ cellular area. The nuclei are not atypical. Mitoses are absent.*

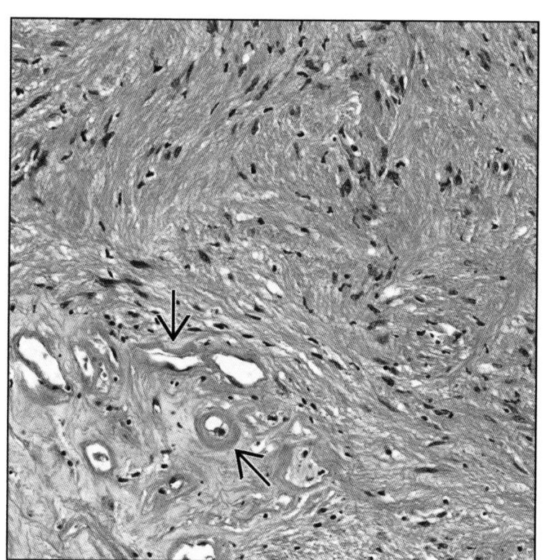

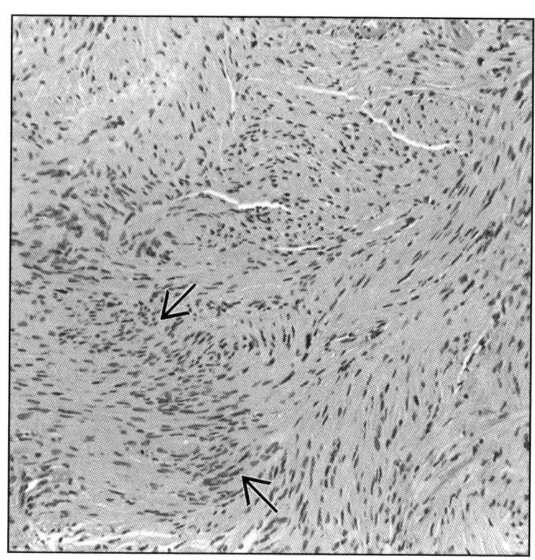

(Left) *Perivascular hyalinization ➔ is noted around a number of vessels in this schwannoma. There is hypocellularity with spindled cells arranged in interconnecting fascicles.* ***(Right)*** *Short fascicles of spindled cells with well-developed palisaded nuclei ➔ are seen. There is slight variability in cellularity, but all of the tissue in this field is from an Antoni A area.*

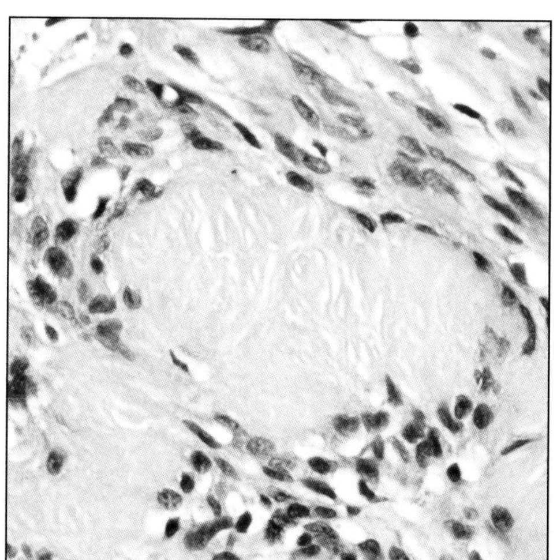

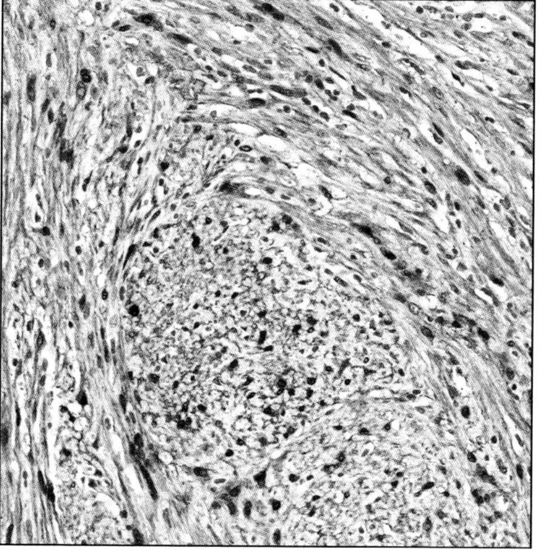

(Left) *Hematoxylin & eosin shows a well-formed Verocay body, creating palisaded nuclei around an eosinophilic acellular center.* ***(Right)*** *The spindled cells of schwannoma are highlighted with nuclear and cytoplasmic reactivity with S100 protein. The staining highlights the growth pattern of the tumor. This reaction is neither specific nor sensitive for schwannoma but does help separate it from other mesenchymal spindle cell lesions in the ear/temporal bone.*

MENINGIOMA

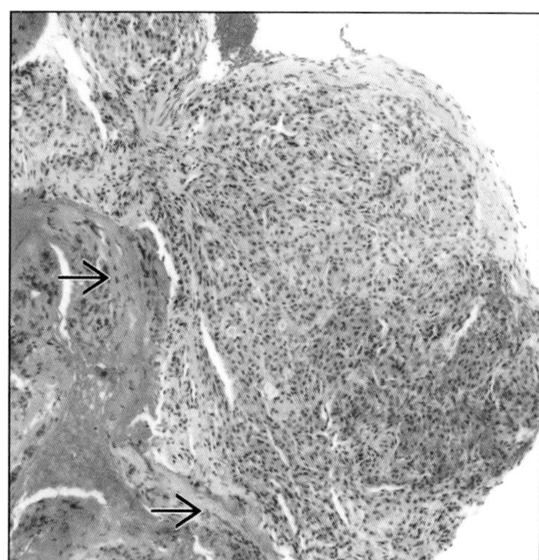

Hematoxylin & eosin shows a polypoid mass adjacent to bone ⇒. Note the vague "whorled" pattern. There is fibrous connective tissue at the edge, but it is not forming a capsule.

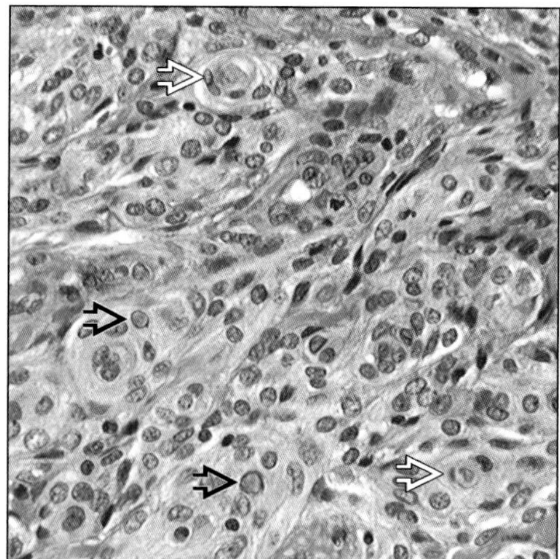

Hematoxylin & eosin shows a meningothelial and whorled pattern ➡ with syncytial cells. Nuclei are round to oval and bland, containing a number of intranuclear cytoplasmic inclusions ⇒.

TERMINOLOGY

Definitions

- Benign neoplasm of meningothelial cells within ear and temporal bone

CLINICAL ISSUES

Epidemiology

- Incidence
  - Approximately 10% of ear and temporal bone tumors
- Age
  - Mean: 50 years old
  - Range: 10-90 years old
  - Women tend to be older than men at presentation
- Gender
  - Female > Male (2:1)

Site

- Internal auditory meatus
- Jugular foramen, middle ear
- Eustachian tube roof

Presentation

- Hearing loss, tinnitus
- Otitis, pain
- Headaches, dizziness, vertigo

Treatment

- Options, risks, complications
  - Involvement of skull base makes treatment more complex
- Surgical approaches
  - Wide excision with clear margins
- Radiation
  - Used for patients who are poor surgical candidates

Prognosis

- Good: 80% 5-year survival
- Recurrences in approximately 20% of patients (but may be "residual" disease)
- Patients die from complications of CNS involvement (mastoiditis and meningitis), including sepsis

IMAGE FINDINGS

General Features

- Must exclude direct CNS extension
- En plaque lesions must be actively sought and excluded
- Temporal air cell opacification
- Bone erosion, sclerosis, or hyperostosis

MR Findings

- Isointense to gray matter on T1-weighted images
- Iso- to hyperintense on T2-weighted images

MACROSCOPIC FEATURES

General Features

- Infiltrative lesion into bone
- Skin/mucosa is intact
- Granular, gritty material with calcifications

Size

- Mean: < 1.5 cm

MICROSCOPIC PATHOLOGY

Histologic Features

- Tumor cell infiltration into bone, skin/mucosa, or soft tissues
  - Infiltration does not alter patient outcome or management
- Meningothelial and whorled architecture
- Lobules and nests of tumor cells
- Epithelioid cells with syncytial architecture

MENINGIOMA

Key Facts

Clinical Issues
- Female > Male (2:1)
- Patients present with hearing loss

Image Findings
- Must exclude direct CNS extension

Macroscopic Features
- Infiltrative lesion into bone

Microscopic Pathology
- Meningothelial and whorled architecture
- Psammoma bodies or "pre-psammoma" bodies

Ancillary Tests
- Positive: EMA, keratin, CAM5.2, weak S100 protein

Top Differential Diagnoses
- Paraganglioma
- Meningocele

- Bland, round to oval nuclei with delicate nuclear chromatin
- Intranuclear cytoplasmic inclusions
- Psammoma bodies or "pre-psammoma" bodies

ANCILLARY TESTS

Immunohistochemistry
- Positive: EMA, keratin (pre-psammoma-body pattern), CAM5.2
- Weak positive: S100 protein
- Negative: Chromogranin, synaptophysin
- Proliferation: < 5% Ki-67 labeling

DIFFERENTIAL DIAGNOSIS

Schwannoma
- Alternating cellular and hypocellular regions
- Cystic and degenerative changes, with perivascular hyalinization
- Usually very strong S100 protein immunoreactivity

Paraganglioma
- Zellballen, organoid, or nested architecture
- Prominent but isolated cytologic atypia
- Chromogranin reaction with supporting S100 protein positive sustentacular reactions

Middle Ear Adenoma
- a.k.a. neuroendocrine adenoma of middle ear (NAME)
- Organoid growth, middle ear tumor with "salt and pepper" nuclear chromatin and neuroendocrine immunohistochemistry

Meningocele
- Usually cystic with direct extension from CNS
- Acquired (postsurgical, infectious, or traumatic) or congenital

Ceruminal Adenoma
- External auditory canal
- Biphasic tumor with ceruminous differentiation (apocrine snouting)
- Strong keratin immunoreactions with myoepithelial/basal phenotype

SELECTED REFERENCES

1. Sanna M et al: Surgical management of jugular foramen meningiomas: a series of 13 cases and review of the literature. Laryngoscope. 117(10):1710-9, 2007
2. Wu ZB et al: Posterior petrous meningiomas: 82 cases. J Neurosurg. 102(2):284-9, 2005
3. Nakamura M et al: Meningiomas of the internal auditory canal. Neurosurgery. 55(1):119-27; discussion 127-8, 2004
4. Thompson LD et al: Primary ear and temporal bone meningiomas: a clinicopathologic study of 36 cases with a review of the literature. Mod Pathol. 16(3):236-45, 2003
5. Prayson RA: Middle ear meningiomas. Ann Diagn Pathol. 4(3):149-53, 2000

IMAGE GALLERY

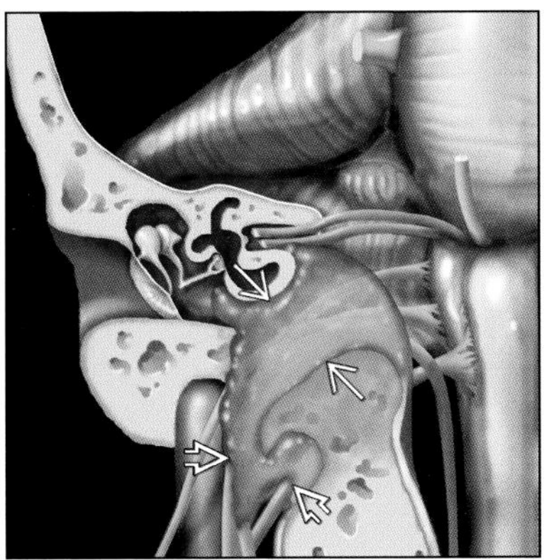

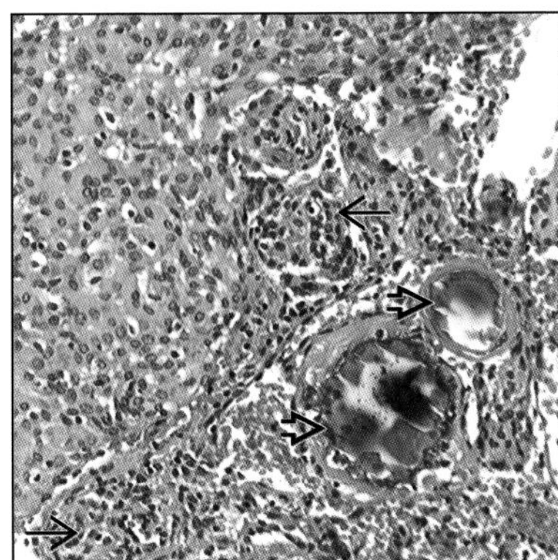

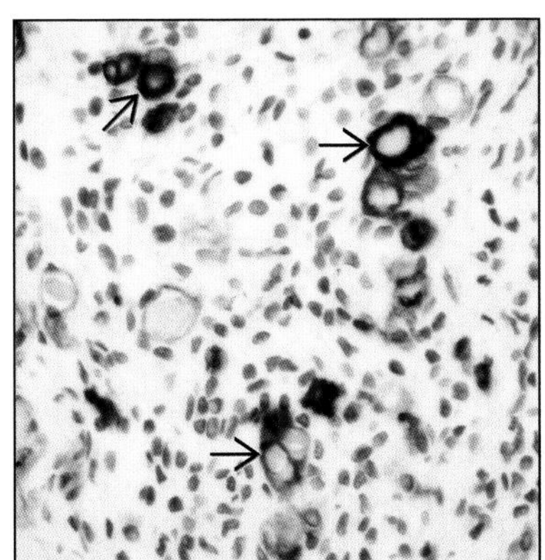

(Left) This is a graphic of a meningioma expanding into the middle ear ➡ and extending along the nerve roots ➡. *(Center)* Hematoxylin & eosin shows psammoma body-like calcifications ⇨ within the neoplastic tissue. An inflammatory infiltrate is also noted ⇨, although this is not a common finding. *(Right)* Cytokeratin shows the peculiar keratin immunoreactivity in a "pre-psammoma" body-like accentuation ⇨. The reaction is unique to this tumor in the head and neck.

ENDOLYMPHATIC SAC TUMOR

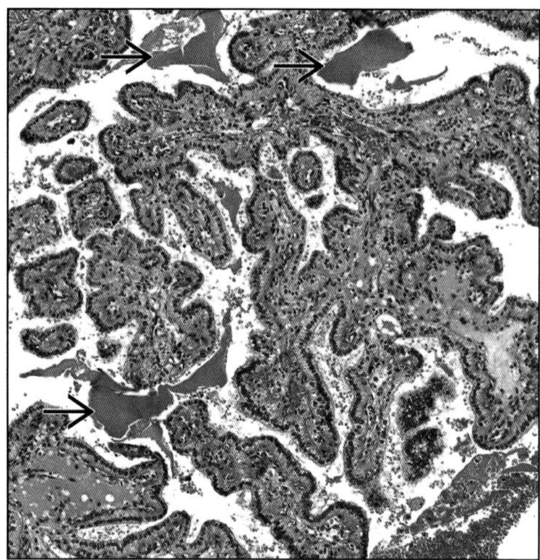

The tumor cells are arranged in broad but simple papillary projections. The stalks are frequently wide, filled with blood or fibrous connective tissue. Secretions ➔ may be present.

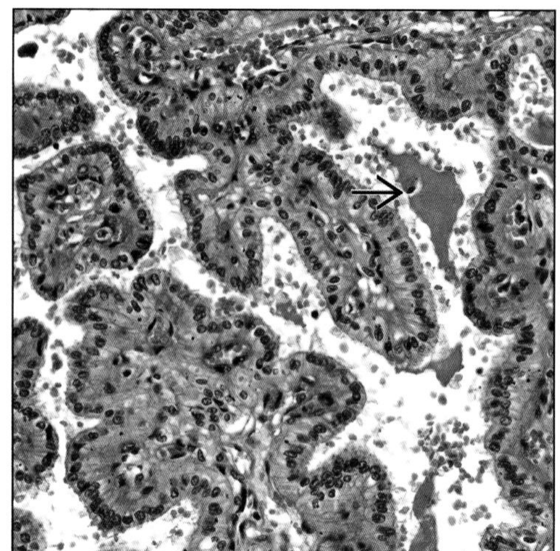

High-power view shows cuboidal to low columnar cells lining the broad papillary projections. The nuclei are regular with coarse nuclear chromatin distribution. Inspissated material is seen ➔.

TERMINOLOGY

Synonyms

- Papillary neoplasm of endolymphatic sac
- Aggressive adenomatous tumor
- Papillary adenomatous tumors
- Aggressive papillary adenoma
- Aggressive papillary tumor
- Invasive papillary cystadenoma
- Endolymphatic sac papillary tumor
- Papillary tumor of temporal bone
- Endolymphatic sac carcinoma
- Adenocarcinoma of endolymphatic sac
- Heffner tumor

Definitions

- Papillary epithelial neoplasm arising within endolymphatic sac/duct, showing high association with von Hippel-Lindau syndrome (VHL)

ETIOLOGY/PATHOGENESIS

Developmental Anomaly

- *VHL* germline mutation
  - Autosomal dominant inheritance pattern
    - About 20% of cases reflect new mutations
  - von Hippel-Lindau tumor suppressor gene (*VHL*)
    - Also called elongin binding protein and G7 protein
  - *VHL* protein is involved in up-regulation of hypoxic response (via *hypoxia inducible factor [HIF]-1 alpha*)
    - Mutations: Prevent production of any functional VHL protein or result in a change of structure of VHL protein
  - Also involved in tumor formation
    - Central nervous system, kidneys, pancreas, adrenal glands, epididymis, broad ligament, and endolymphatic sac
    - Microscopically, there are morphologically similar changes in adjacent epithelium
- Vast majority of cases develop in patients with von Hippel-Lindau syndrome

CLINICAL ISSUES

Epidemiology

- Incidence
  - Rare
  - Approximately 1 in 35,000 to 40,000 people have VHL
    - Approximately 10% have endolymphatic sac tumors
- Age
  - Mean: 30-40 years
  - Range: Wide age range at initial presentation
- Gender
  - Equal gender distribution

Site

- Posterior petrous bone
  - Intraosseous-vestibular aqueduct portion or operculum of endolymphatic duct/sac system
- Endolymphatic sac or endolymphatic duct, retrolabyrinthine

Presentation

- Hearing abnormality
  - Progressive, ipsilateral hearing loss
    - Sensorineural > > conductive usually
  - Tinnitus
- Vertigo
- Ataxia
- Vestibular dysfunction
- Facial nerve palsy
- May show stigmata of von Hippel-Lindau in other anatomic sites
  - Kidney, pancreas, cerebellum

ENDOLYMPHATIC SAC TUMOR

Key Facts

Terminology
- Papillary epithelial neoplasm arising within endolymphatic sac associated with von Hippel-Lindau syndrome

Clinical Issues
- Endolymphatic sac or endolymphatic duct
- Symptoms usually present for years, suggesting slow tumor growth
- Mean: 30-40 years (wide age range)
- Stigmata of von Hippel-Lindau in other organs: Kidney, pancreas, cerebellum

Image Findings
- T1-weighted images show hyperintensity (hypervascularity) of heterogeneous mass

Microscopic Pathology
- Up to 10 cm
- Bone invasion and "remodeling"
- Simple, coarse, broad papillary projections within cystic spaces
- Single layer of low cuboidal to columnar cells
- Clear to slightly eosinophilic, granular cytoplasm with indistinct cell borders/membranes

Ancillary Tests
- Epithelial markers are usually positive

Top Differential Diagnoses
- Paraganglioma
- Metastatic renal cell carcinoma
- Metastatic papillary thyroid carcinoma

- Symptoms usually present for years, suggesting slow tumor growth

Treatment
- Surgical approaches
  - Wide excision
  - Attempt at hearing preservation

Prognosis
- Good
  - Dependent on extent of tumor (difficult to eradicate based on size)
  - Dependent on other disease(s) present
    - Hemangioblastoma, renal cell carcinoma, pancreatic serous cystadenoma
  - Anatomic complexity may explain distinct difficulties in removal
- Recurrences develop if incompletely excised
- No metastatic potential

IMAGE FINDINGS

MR Findings
- T1-weighted images show hyperintensity (hypervascularity) of heterogeneous mass

CT Findings
- Lytic lesion with bone destruction
- Multilocular
- Centered on endolymphatic sac (between internal auditory canal and sigmoid sinus)
- Tumor may expand to involve cerebellopontine angle, cranial fossa and middle ear

MACROSCOPIC FEATURES

General Features
- Bilateral tumors are almost always associated with VHL
- Destruction of mastoid air spaces and extending into middle ear
- Frequently extends into posterior cranial fossa (cerebellum)

Size
- Depends on patient age
  - Larger lesions in older age patients
- Range up to 10 cm

MICROSCOPIC PATHOLOGY

Histologic Features
- Unencapsulated, destructive lesions
- Bone invasion and "remodeling"
- Simple, coarse, broad papillary projections
- Cystic spaces often filled with fluid or extravasated erythrocytes
- Acinar-follicular spaces filled with inspissated material may simulate thyroid-like differentiation
- Single layer of low cuboidal to columnar epithelial cells
- Clear to slightly eosinophilic, granular cytoplasm with indistinct cell borders/membranes
- Small, round, hyperchromatic nuclei
- Fibrovascular cores within papillary structures

ANCILLARY TESTS

Cytology
- Cyst fluid aspiration contains rare papillary groups
- Evenly placed cells with bland nuclei
- Lightly eosinophilic to vacuolated cytoplasm
- Foamy macrophages and blood may be present

Immunohistochemistry
- Epithelial markers are usually positive

Cytogenetics
- Germline mutations of *VHL* tumor suppressor gene
  - 3p25-26 (short arm of chromosome 3) gene mutations
    - Between base pair 10,158,318 to base pair 10,168,761 on chromosome 3

ENDOLYMPHATIC SAC TUMOR

Immunohistochemistry

Antibody	Reactivity	Staining Pattern	Comment
CK-PAN	Positive	Cytoplasmic	Often weak
CK7	Positive	Cytoplasmic	
CK8/18/CAM5.2	Positive	Cytoplasmic	
EMA	Positive	Cell membrane & cytoplasm	Often weak
S100	Positive	Nuclear & cytoplasmic	Often weak
Vimentin	Positive	Cytoplasmic	
NSE	Positive	Cytoplasmic	Weak and focal
GFAP	Positive	Cytoplasmic	Weak and focal
TTF-1	Negative		
Thyroglobulin	Negative		

DIFFERENTIAL DIAGNOSIS

Middle Ear Adenocarcinoma

- Difficult and uncommon diagnosis
- Nuclear pleomorphism
- Must exclude direct extension from adjacent organs

Middle Ear Adenoma

- a.k.a. neuroendocrine adenoma of middle ear (NAME)
- Involves middle ear
- Infiltrative, glandular pattern with biphasic appearance
- Delicate, "salt and pepper" nuclear features
- Positive immunohistochemistry for neuroendocrine markers

Paraganglioma

- Nested, zellballen appearance
- Isolated nuclear pleomorphism
- Granular, coarse to "salt and pepper" nuclear chromatin distribution
- Immunohistochemistry
  - Positive: Chromogranin and synaptophysin paraganglia cells; S100 protein sustentacular cells

Choroid Plexus Papilloma

- Usually midline without temporal bone destruction

Metastatic Renal Cell Carcinoma

- Not usually papillary
- Cytologic atypia is greater and extravasated erythrocytes more common in pseudoalveolar pattern
- Immunohistochemistry
  - CD10 and RCC positive reactions may help

Metastatic Papillary Thyroid Carcinoma

- Nuclear contour irregularities, cleared nuclear chromatin, and nuclear overlapping
- Positive TTF-1 and thyroglobulin immunohistochemistry

Ceruminous Adenoma

- External auditory canal
- Biphasic appearance with inner cuboidal and outer basal cells
- Apocrine decapitation secretions and cerumen
- Immunohistochemistry: Basal cells positive with p63, CK903, and smooth muscle actin

SELECTED REFERENCES

1. Connor SE et al: Imaging of the petrous apex: a pictorial review. Br J Radiol. 81(965):427-35, 2008
2. Leung RS et al: Imaging features of von Hippel-Lindau disease. Radiographics. 28(1):65-79; quiz 323, 2008
3. Doherty JK et al: Endolymphatic sac tumor: a report of 3 cases and discussion of management. Ear Nose Throat J. 86(1):30-5, 2007
4. Megerian CA et al: Evaluation and management of endolymphatic sac and duct tumors. Otolaryngol Clin North Am. 40(3):463-78, viii, 2007
5. Patel NP et al: The radiologic diagnosis of endolymphatic sac tumors. Laryngoscope. 116(1):40-6, 2006
6. Glasker S et al: Effects of VHL deficiency on endolymphatic duct and sac. Cancer Res. 65(23):10847-53, 2005
7. Rodrigues S et al: Endolymphatic sac tumors: a review of the St. Vincent's hospital experience. Otol Neurotol. 25(4):599-603, 2004
8. Devaney KO et al: Endolymphatic sac tumor (low-grade papillary adenocarcinoma) of the temporal bone. Acta Otolaryngol. 123(9):1022-6, 2003
9. Horiguchi H et al: Endolymphatic sac tumor associated with a von Hippel-Lindau disease patient: an immunohistochemical study. Mod Pathol. 14(7):727-32, 2001
10. Murphy BA et al: Cytology of endolymphatic sac tumor. Mod Pathol. 14(9):920-4, 2001
11. Richard S et al: Central nervous system hemangioblastomas, endolymphatic sac tumors, and von Hippel-Lindau disease. Neurosurg Rev. 23(1):1-22; discussion 23-4, 2000
12. Kempermann G et al: Endolymphatic sac tumours. Histopathology. 33(1):2-10, 1998
13. Richards FM et al: Molecular genetic analysis of von Hippel-Lindau disease. J Intern Med. 243(6):527-33, 1998
14. Roche PH et al: Endolymphatic sac tumors: report of three cases. Neurosurgery. 42(4):927-32, 1998
15. Batsakis JG et al: Papillary neoplasms (Heffner's tumors) of the endolymphatic sac. Ann Otol Rhinol Laryngol. 102(8 Pt 1):648-51, 1993
16. Heffner DK: Low-grade adenocarcinoma of probable endolymphatic sac origin A clinicopathologic study of 20 cases. Cancer. 64(11):2292-302, 1989

Radiographic and Microscopic Features

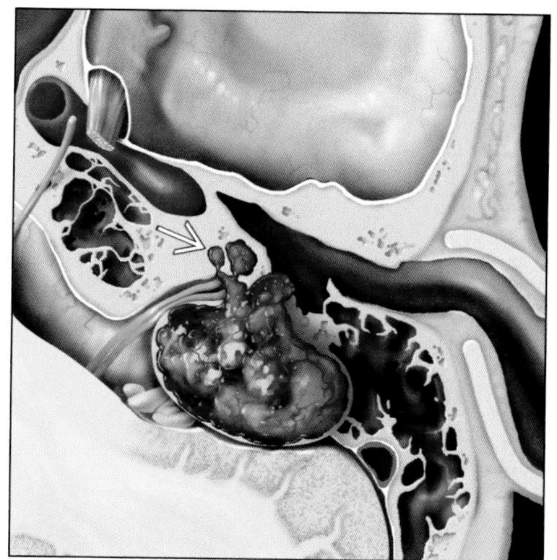

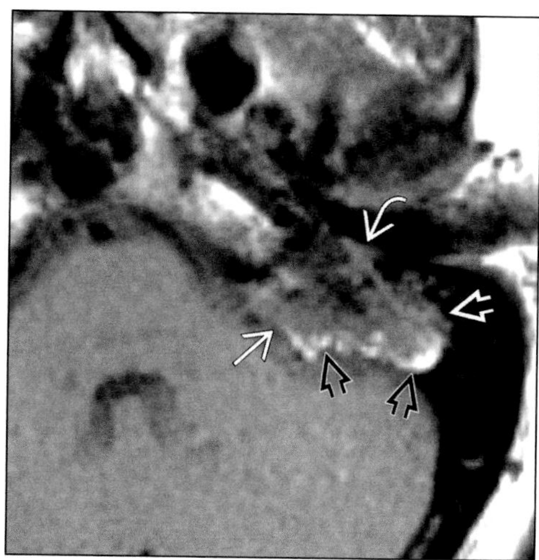

(Left) *Axial graphic of temporal bone shows the typical appearance of endolymphatic sac tumor. The tumor is vascular, shows a tendency to fistulize the inner ear →, and contains bone fragments within the tumor matrix.* ***(Right)*** *Axial T1 unenhanced MR demonstrates an invasive tumor → of the posterior wall of the left temporal bone that has reached the mastoid air cells → and middle ear →. The high signal (white) material represents methemoglobin within the tumor matrix →.*

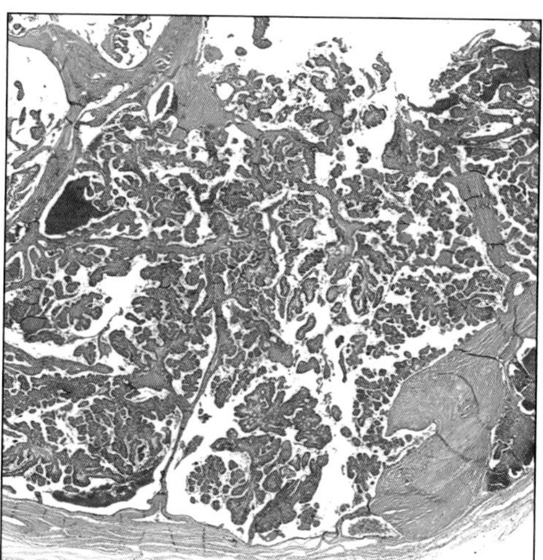

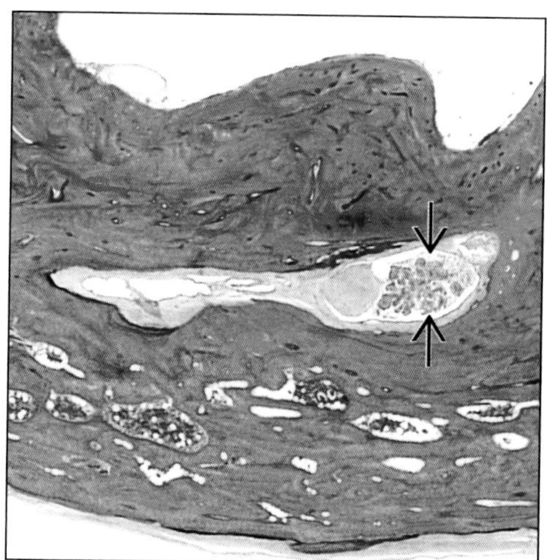

(Left) *Low-power view demonstrates the fibrous connective tissue stroma separating the numerous papillary projections. They appear complex at low power. Blood and secretions are frequently identified.* ***(Right)*** *This portion of the temporal bone demonstrates a small papillary projection →, an early development of an endolymphatic sac tumor. This was in a patient with von Hippel-Lindau. (Courtesy L. Michaels, MD.)*

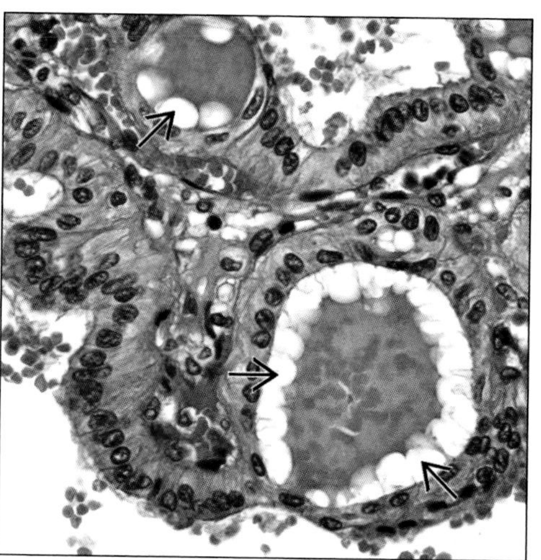

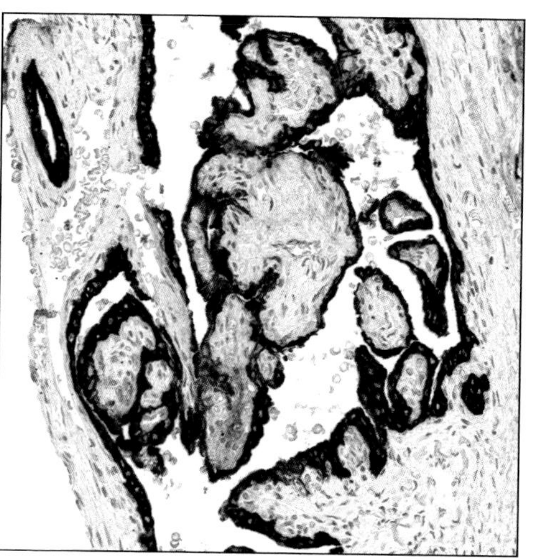

(Left) *The bland morphologic appearance and cuboidal-columnar pattern can sometimes mimic metastatic thyroid papillary carcinoma. Note the secretions creating a scalloping within the lumen →.* ***(Right)*** *The neoplastic cells are strongly and diffusely positive for a variety of epithelial immunohistochemistry markers. In this case the cells are stained with CK7, but keratin, CAM5.2, CK8/18, or EMA would also be positive in this tumor.*

ATYPICAL FIBROXANTHOMA

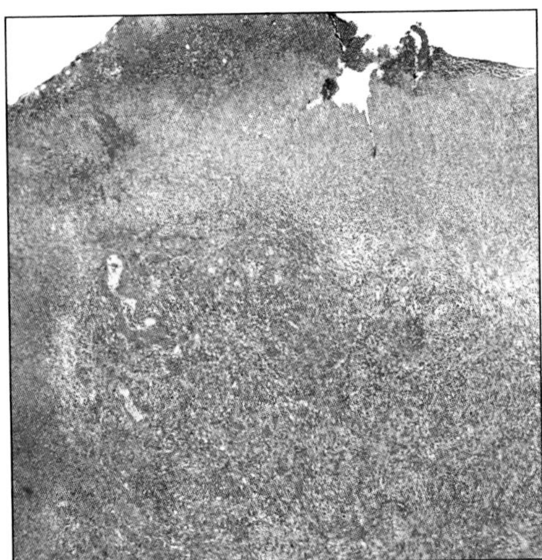

Low-power magnification shows a large, dermal-based nodular tumor with overlying ulceration and serum crusting.

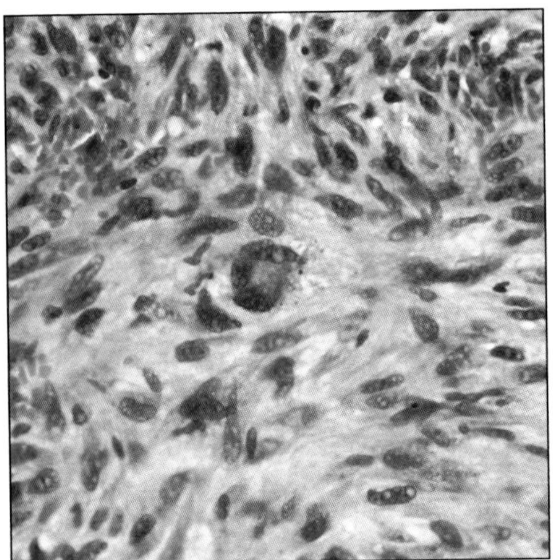

High-power magnification shows a proliferation of highly pleomorphic spindled and multinucleated tumor cells.

TERMINOLOGY

Abbreviations

- Atypical fibroxanthoma (AFX)
- Malignant fibrous histiocytoma (MFH)

Synonyms

- Superficial MFH/undifferentiated pleomorphic sarcoma

Definitions

- Dermal-based, low-grade mesenchymal neoplasm showing no specific lineage of differentiation

ETIOLOGY/PATHOGENESIS

Environmental Exposure

- Likely related to UV exposure, as most cases occur in sun-damaged skin

CLINICAL ISSUES

Epidemiology

- Age
  - Typically occurs in elderly patients
- Gender
  - Slight male predilection

Site

- Pinna of ear
  - Head and neck in general is commonly affected
  - Scalp is most common location

Presentation

- Skin nodule, asymptomatic in most cases
  - Dermal-based lesion
  - May show overlying ulceration or bleeding/crusting
- Regional lymph node metastases may be found in small number of cases

Treatment

- Surgical approaches
  - Complete and wide surgical excision
    - Mohs surgery is also effective
  - Unresectable or metastatic cases may be treated with chemoradiation

Prognosis

- Good; rate of local recurrence is low (< 10%)
- Majority of cases do not metastasize
  - Cases with subcutaneous involvement are considered MFH and can metastasize

MACROSCOPIC FEATURES

General Features

- Large, nodular, unencapsulated, dermal-based tumor

MICROSCOPIC PATHOLOGY

Histologic Features

- Proliferation of markedly atypical and pleomorphic spindled and epithelioid-appearing cells
  - Variants include spindle cell, clear cell, granular, chondroid, and osteoid
  - Cytoplasm of tumor cells is abundant, eosinophilic, and sometimes foamy
- Scattered large, bizarre-appearing multinucleated giant cells
- Numerous mitoses, including highly atypical forms

ANCILLARY TESTS

Immunohistochemistry

- IHC is key in confirming diagnosis
  - Essentially excluding specific diagnoses
- Positive for nonspecific markers, including CD68, CD10, CD99, and vimentin

ATYPICAL FIBROXANTHOMA

Key Facts

Terminology
- Atypical fibroxanthoma (AFX)
- Dermal-based, low-grade mesenchymal neoplasm showing no specific lineage of differentiation

Clinical Issues
- Mass lesion, may be ulcerated or bleeding

Microscopic Pathology
- Highly atypical and pleomorphic proliferation of spindled to epithelioid-appearing cells
- Scattered large, bizarre-appearing multinucleated cells

Ancillary Tests
- IHC is key in confirming diagnosis
  - Essentially excluding specific diagnoses
- Negative for melanocytic markers, cytokeratins (especially HMWCKs), p63, muscle and vascular markers
- Positive for nonspecific markers including CD68, CD10, CD99, and vimentin

Top Differential Diagnoses
- Sarcomatoid carcinoma (typically SCC)
  - Metastatic carcinoma should be considered
- Spindle cell melanoma
- Leiomyosarcoma

Diagnostic Checklist
- Depth of involvement: Subcutaneous extension implies more aggressive behavior
- Poorly differentiated malignancies often showing bizarre tumor cells and nonspecific IHC findings

- Negative for melanocytic markers, cytokeratins (especially HMWCKs), p63, muscle and vascular markers

Electron Microscopy
- Transitional forms from fibroblasts to large giant cells, with intermediate forms exhibiting features of both

DIFFERENTIAL DIAGNOSIS

Sarcomatoid Carcinoma
- Usually a spindle cell SCC, although spindled basal cell carcinoma, adnexal carcinomas, and sebaceous carcinomas may be considered
  - Surface origin may be identified; usually cellular; opacified cytoplasm, hyperchromatic nuclei, atypical mitoses
- Positive: High molecular weight cytokeratins (CK5/6, CK903), p63 (especially primary cutaneous), ± pankeratin (AE1/AE3), EMA, CAM5.2

Spindle Cell and Desmoplastic Melanoma
- Junctional component may be present in some cases
- Positive: S100 protein, ± Melan-A, HMB-45, Tyrosinase, MITF

Leiomyosarcoma
- Positive: SMA, MSA, desmin (most cases)
  - Focal SMA in some AFXs, likely indicating myofibroblastic differentiation

Other Sarcomas
- Much less likely, including metastatic sarcoma
- Angiosarcoma: CD31(+), CD34(+)
  - Other vascular neoplasms are less likely
- Malignant peripheral nerve sheath tumor
  - Usually deep-seated lesions
  - Focal to weak S100 protein(+) in 50-70% of cases

DIAGNOSTIC CHECKLIST

Clinically Relevant Pathologic Features
- Depth of involvement (subcutaneous extension implies more aggressive behavior)

Pathologic Interpretation Pearls
- Poorly differentiated malignancy often shows bizarre tumor cells and nonspecific IHC findings

SELECTED REFERENCES

1. Luzar B et al: Cutaneous fibrohistiocytic tumours - an update. Histopathology. 56(1):148-65, 2010
2. Ang GC et al: More than 2 decades of treating atypical fibroxanthoma at mayo clinic: what have we learned from 91 patients? Dermatol Surg. 35(5):765-72, 2009
3. Gleason BC et al: Utility of p63 in the differential diagnosis of atypical fibroxanthoma and spindle cell squamous cell carcinoma. J Cutan Pathol. 36(5):543-7, 2009
4. González-García R et al: Atypical fibroxanthoma of the head and neck: report of 5 cases. J Oral Maxillofac Surg. 65(3):526-31, 2007
5. Hultgren TL et al: Immunohistochemical staining of CD10 in atypical fibroxanthomas. J Cutan Pathol. 34(5):415-9, 2007
6. Ríos-Martín JJ et al: Granular cell atypical fibroxanthoma: report of two cases. Am J Dermatopathol. 29(1):84-7, 2007
7. Farley R et al: Diagnosis and management of atypical fibroxanthoma. Skinmed. 5(2):83-6, 2006
8. Hartel PH et al: CD99 immunoreactivity in atypical fibroxanthoma and pleomorphic malignant fibrous histiocytoma: a useful diagnostic marker. J Cutan Pathol. 33 Suppl 2:24-8, 2006
9. Murali R et al: Clear cell atypical fibroxanthoma - report of a case with review of the literature. J Cutan Pathol. 33(5):343-8, 2006
10. Seavolt M et al: Atypical fibroxanthoma: review of the literature and summary of 13 patients treated with mohs micrographic surgery. Dermatol Surg. 32(3):435-41; discussion 439-41, 2006
11. Rudisaile SN et al: Granular cell atypical fibroxanthoma. J Cutan Pathol. 32(4):314-7, 2005

ATYPICAL FIBROXANTHOMA

Microscopic Features

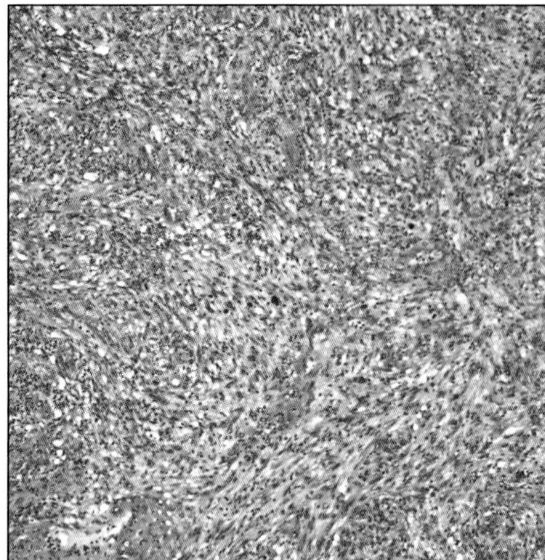

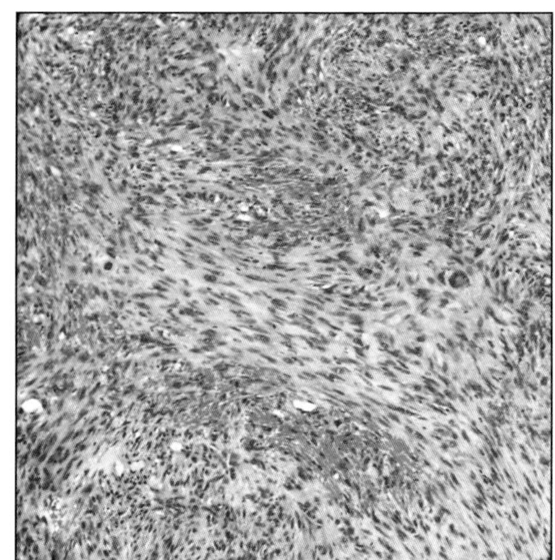

(Left) *Histiologic examination shows a cellular proliferation composed of sheet-like and haphazard fascicles of tumor cells associated with an inflamed and edematous stroma.* ***(Right)*** *Higher power histologic examination shows areas of spindle cells forming dense, short fascicles.*

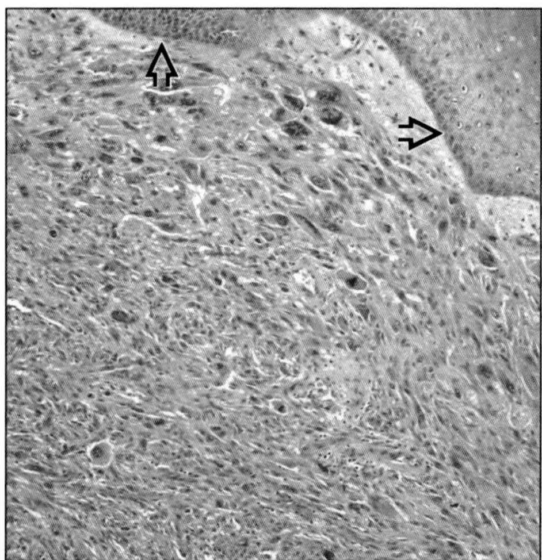

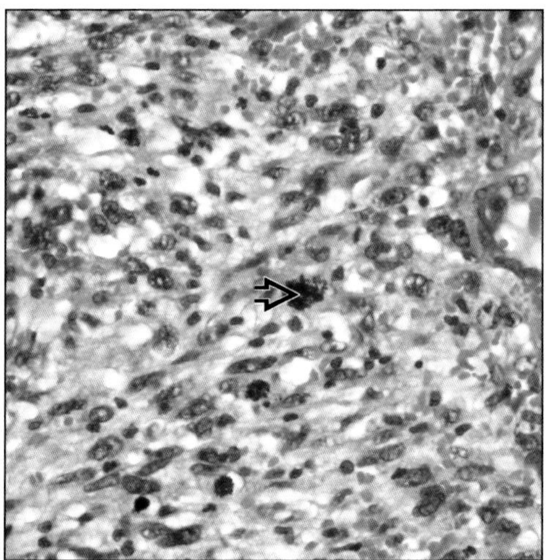

(Left) *Histologic examination shows a superficial portion of the tumor with a proliferation of markedly atypical spindled cells, epithelioid cells, and many multinucleated tumor cells. The tumor closely abuts, but does not involve, the overlying epidermis* ⇨*.* ***(Right)*** *High-power magnification shows highly atypical cells with numerous mitoses, including atypical forms* ⇨*.*

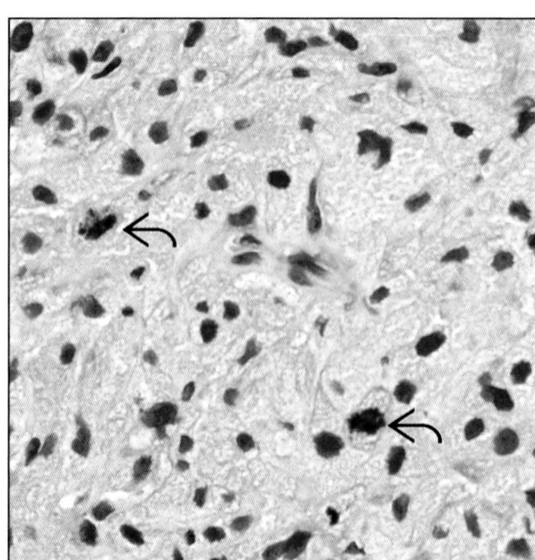

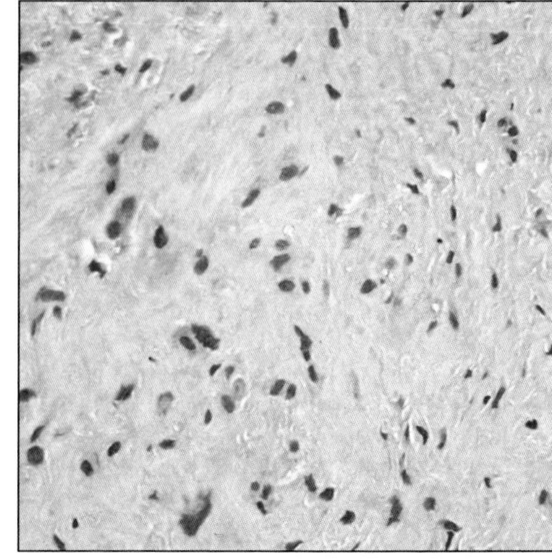

(Left) *An example of the granular cell variant of AFX shows large, bizarre-appearing histiocytoid cells containing abundant granular cytoplasm, similar to a malignant granular cell tumor. Mitoses are easily found* ↩*.* ***(Right)*** *High-power view shows an example of an unusual hypocellular AFX case with a chondromyxoid-appearing stroma (chondroid AFX).*

Immunohistochemical Features

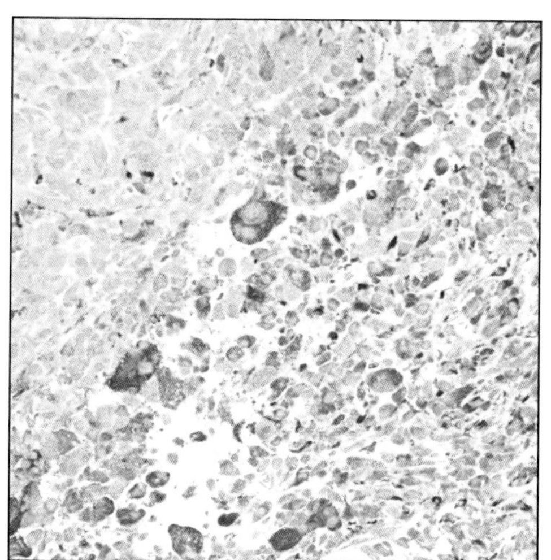

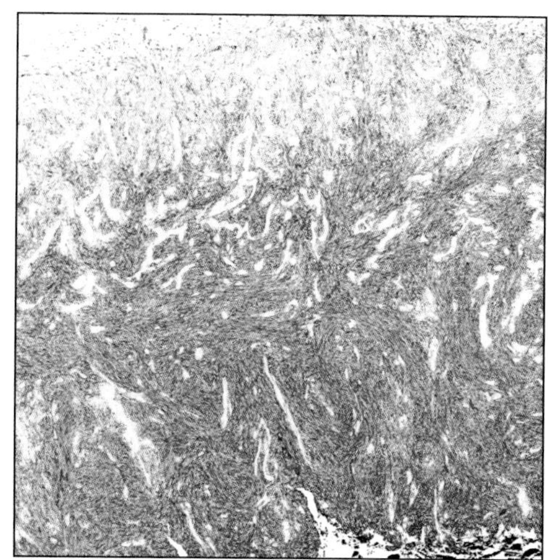

(Left) *CD68 stain shows moderate to strong cytoplasmic staining of most of the tumor cells, especially the large multinucleated tumor giant cells.* ***(Right)*** *CD10 stain shows strong and diffuse staining of the tumor cells, a finding which is not specific but is helpful as it is typically seen in AFX.*

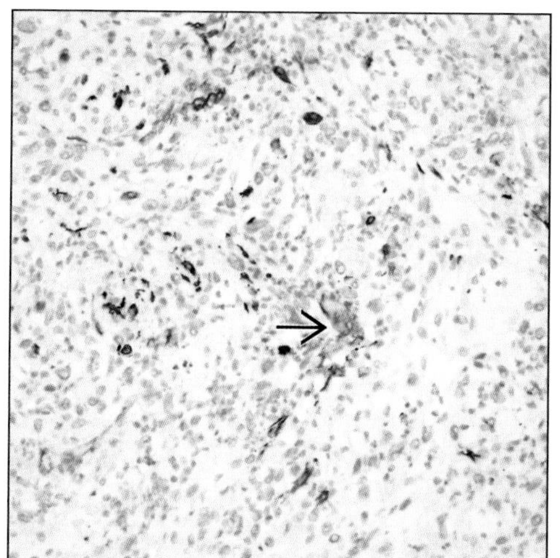

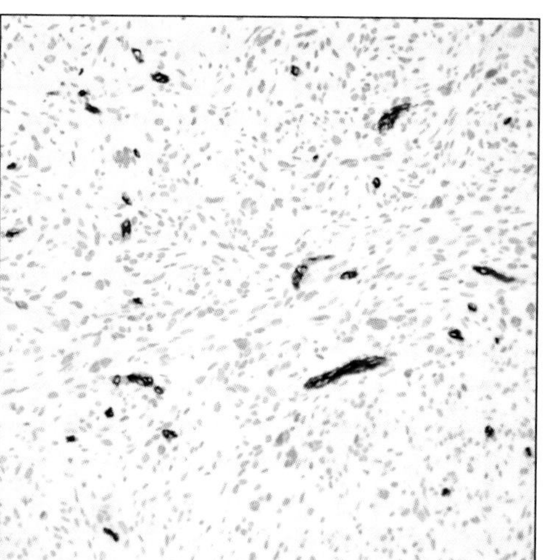

(Left) *Smooth muscle actin stain shows scattered weakly positive cells ⇒, likely indicating myofibroblastic differentiation.* ***(Right)*** *CD34 immunohistochemical stain shows strong positive staining of vessels but is negative within the tumor cells.*

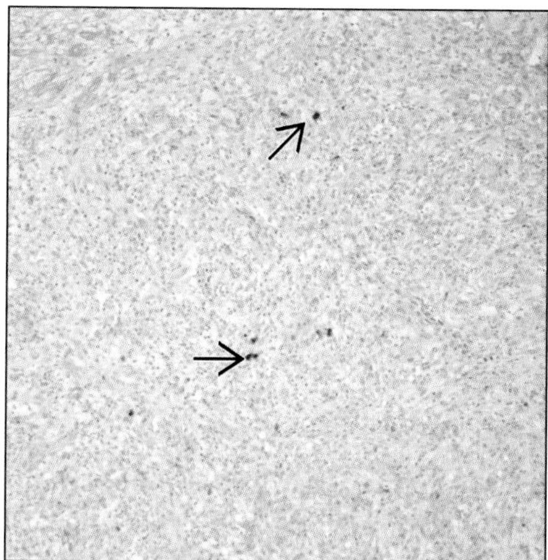

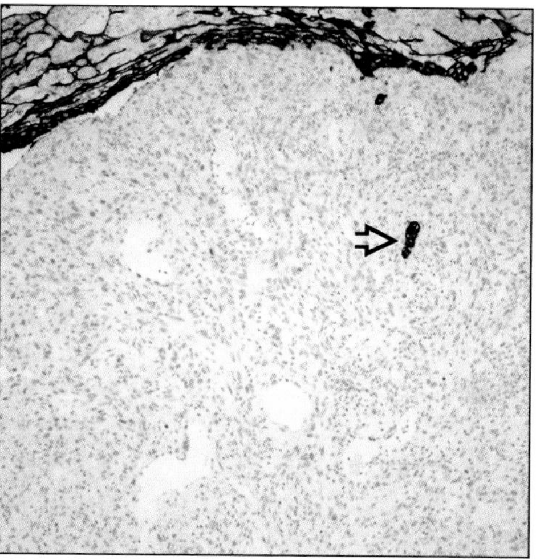

(Left) *S100 protein immunohistochemical stained section shows no staining of the tumor cells but highlights a few intradermal dendritic cells ⇒.* ***(Right)*** *High molecular weight cytokeratin stain shows positivity within the epidermis and a few adnexal ducts ⇨ but is negative within the tumor cells.*

SQUAMOUS CELL CARCINOMA

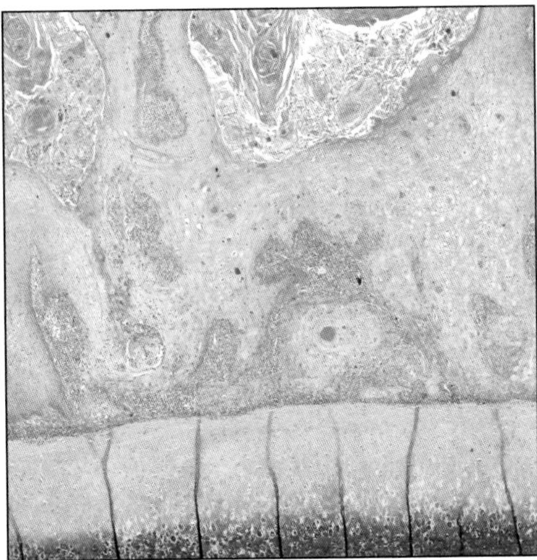

Invasive, well-differentiated squamous cell carcinoma of the ear is seen invading to the edge of the auricular cartilage.

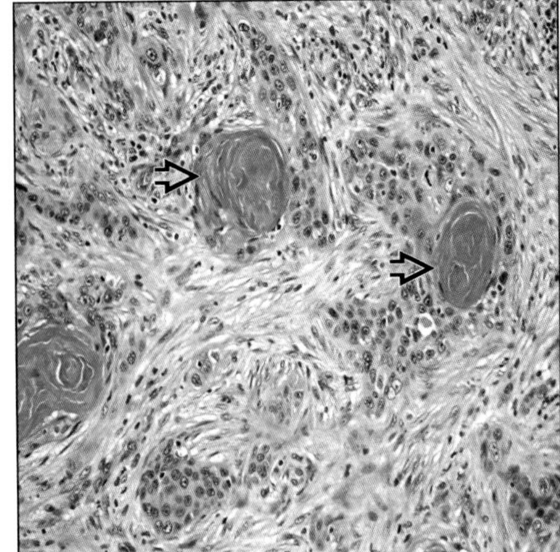

Moderately differentiated invasive SCC shows prominent keratin pearls ➡ and a sclerotic stroma with scattered inflammatory cells.

TERMINOLOGY

Abbreviations

- Squamous cell carcinoma (SCC)

Synonyms

- Epidermoid carcinoma
- Sarcomatoid carcinoma/spindle cell carcinoma/ carcinosarcoma/metaplastic carcinoma (poorly differentiated variants)
- Adenoid/pseudoglandular SCC (acantholytic SCC)
- Verrucous carcinoma (well-differentiated variant)
- Keratoacanthoma (very well-differentiated variant)
- Lymphoepithelioma-like carcinoma of the skin (LELCS) variant

Definitions

- Malignant tumor of squamous keratinocytes

ETIOLOGY/PATHOGENESIS

Environmental Exposure

- Most cases are related to UV radiation (external ear)
- Middle ear cases likely related to chronic inflammation
- Previous radiation therapy implicated in some cases, usually associated with more aggressive SCC
- Chronic wounds and burn scars also can be associated with high-risk SCC
- HPV is associated with some cases
  - Especially verrucous carcinoma (low grade) and SCC in immunosuppressed patients (high grade)

CLINICAL ISSUES

Epidemiology

- Age
  - Usually elderly, especially pinna lesions
  - Middle ear tumors show wide age range (34-85 years)
- Gender
  - Pinna lesions more common in males
  - External canal tumors more common in females
  - Middle ear lesions have equal gender distribution

Presentation

- Slow-growing papular, nodular, or plaque lesion
- Often arise in sun-damaged skin (external ear tumors)
  - Vast majority of cases associated with preexisting actinic keratosis (AK)
- May be ulcerated or bleeding
- Ear canal and middle ear tumors may present with pain, hearing loss, and discharge
  - Middle ear tumors often very advanced at presentation, with bone invasion and extension into internal auditory meatus
  - External canal tumor also may be present with stage showing invasion into middle ear and surrounding tissues

Treatment

- Surgical approaches
  - Complete surgical excision is optimal and definitive therapy
    - Mohs surgery has been shown to be highly effective for external ear tumors
- Drugs
  - If patients are not surgical candidates, topical chemotherapeutics or immunomodulators may be used for external ear lesions
- Radiation
  - May be used for very advanced cases where surgical therapy is not curative

Prognosis

- Usually excellent in most cases
- Worse prognosis with poorly differentiated, deeply invasive, or unusual aggressive subtypes
- Location of tumor is important for prognosis

SQUAMOUS CELL CARCINOMA

Key Facts

Terminology
- Squamous cell carcinoma (SCC)
  - Malignant epithelial tumor of squamous keratinocytes

Etiology/Pathogenesis
- Most cases are related to UV radiation (external ear)
- Previous radiation therapy implicated in some cases, usually associated with more aggressive SCC

Clinical Issues
- Often arise in sun-damaged skin of elderly patients (external ear cases)
  - Vast majority of cases associated with preexisting actinic keratosis (AK)
- Complete surgical excision is optimal and definitive therapy
- Prognosis usually good in external ear cases, poor in canal and middle ear tumors
- Worse prognosis with poorly differentiated, deeply invasive, or unusually aggressive subtypes

Microscopic Pathology
- Proliferation of invasive atypical keratinocytes, often with areas of keratinization (keratin pearls) and squamous eddies
- Cells are present in nests, sheets, and cords
- Cytologically, cells show abundant eosinophilic cytoplasm, and large nucleus with vesicular chromatin and prominent nucleoli
- Degree of differentiation is variable, ranges from well to moderately to poorly differentiated
- Multiple variants of differing malignant potential described

  - Middle ear tumors show very poor prognosis, regardless of degree of differentiation
  - External canal tumors have better prognosis but worse than external ear tumors

MACROSCOPIC FEATURES

General Features
- Papular to nodular or plaque-like lesion; can be exophytic
  - May be ulcerated or hemorrhagic

Size
- Variable; can be small or large lesions

MICROSCOPIC PATHOLOGY

Histologic Features
- Proliferation of invasive atypical keratinocytes
  - Cells are present in nests, sheets, and infiltrative cords
  - Often show areas of keratinization (keratin pearls) and squamous eddies
  - Attachments to overlying epidermis present in most cases
  - Associated AK is very common (external ear); less frequently, may be associated with SCC in situ (Bowen disease)
  - Cytologically, cells show abundant eosinophilic cytoplasm and large nucleus with vesicular chromatin and prominent nucleoli
  - Intercellular bridges (desmosomes) should be present on high-power examination
  - Presence of dyskeratotic cells (apoptotic keratinocytes) is reliable sign of squamous differentiation
  - If no definite squamous differentiation is present, immunohistochemistry (IHC) should be used to confirm diagnosis
- Degree of differentiation is variable, ranging from well to moderately to poorly differentiated
  - Amount of keratinization typically decreases, and cytologic atypia increases, with higher grades
  - Mitotic figures are usually numerous, and atypical forms are found especially in moderately to poorly differentiated cases
- Multiple variants of differing malignant potential described:
  - Low risk variants include well-differentiated SCC arising in AK, keratoacanthoma, verrucous carcinoma, and clear cell (trichilemmal) carcinoma
  - Intermediate risk variants include acantholytic (adenoid/pseudoglandular) and lymphoepithelioma-like carcinoma (LELC)
  - High risk variants include spindle cell/sarcomatoid, basaloid, adenosquamous, desmoplastic, and radiation, burn scar and immunosuppression-related SCCs
  - Variants of uncertain malignant potential include signet ring cell SCC, follicular SCC, papillary SCC, pigmented SCC, and SCC arising from adnexal ducts or cysts

Cytologic Features
- Dense eosinophilic cytoplasm, large nucleus with vesicular chromatin and prominent nucleoli

Predominant Pattern/Injury Type
- Epithelioid/squamoid

Predominant Cell/Compartment Type
- Squamous cell

ANCILLARY TESTS

Immunohistochemistry
- IHC is not necessary in well-/moderately differentiated cases, but may be needed in poorly differentiated and spindle cell cases
- Cytokeratins are most important markers, especially high molecular weight cytokeratin (HMWCK)

SQUAMOUS CELL CARCINOMA

- HMWCKs (including CK5/6 and CK903) are most sensitive markers for poorly differentiated and spindle cell/sarcomatoid SCC
  - Pankeratin and CK AE1/AE3 can be lost in poorly differentiated and spindle cell cases
- p63 is also a very sensitive marker, and can be used in addition to HMWCK to confirm diagnosis
- Vimentin may be positive in spindle cell/sarcomatoid cases
- Negative staining for markers, such as
  - S100 protein, Melan-A, and HMB-45 (positive in melanoma)
  - CD10 and CD68 (AFX)
  - Actin-sm and desmin (leiomyosarcoma)
  - BER-EP4 and androgen receptor (BCC)

DIFFERENTIAL DIAGNOSIS

Basal Cell Carcinoma (BCC)

- Cells are typically smaller, more hyperchromatic, and show areas of peripheral palisading, mucinous stroma, and retraction artifact
- Cytokeratins do not distinguish BCC from SCC, but BER-EP4 is almost always positive in BCC and negative in SCC

Atypical Fibroxanthoma (AFX)

- Usually a large, nodular lesion in heavily sun-damaged skin
- Immunohistochemistry is essential in excluding poorly differentiated SCC
  - SCC is typically positive for HMWCK and p63; AFX is negative for these markers, and often CD10(+) and CD68(+)

Poorly Differentiated Carcinoma (Includes Metastatic)

- Clinical history and imaging studies are paramount, as immunohistochemistry may not be able to distinguish some cases from primary SCC
- Adenocarcinomas may show varying degree of ductal/glandular differentiation
  - If present, ductal spaces can be highlighted with markers, such as EMA and CEA

Pseudoepitheliomatous Hyperplasia

- Can mimic SCC, especially SCC in situ, but does not show infiltrative features or high-grade cytologic atypia
- Mitotic figures can be numerous but should be in basilar keratinocytes and nonatypical

DIAGNOSTIC CHECKLIST

Clinically Relevant Pathologic Features

- Degree of differentiation
- Depth of invasion
  - Deeply invasive tumors have much higher rates of recurrence and metastasis
- Perineural invasion
  - Tumors with perineural invasion have high rates of local recurrence and increased risk of metastasis
- Location of tumor important (i.e., external vs. middle ear tumors)

Pathologic Interpretation Pearls

- Invasive proliferation of epithelioid cells, with areas of keratinization (keratin pearls) and squamous eddies
  - Intercellular bridges (desmosomes) and dyskeratotic cells confirm squamous differentiation in poorly differentiated cases
- Adjacent or overlying AK often present in external ear cases

SELECTED REFERENCES

1. Bridges MN et al: Cutaneous squamous cell carcinoma of the external auditory canal. Dermatol Online J. 15(2):13, 2009
2. McGuire JF et al: Nonmelanoma skin cancer of the head and neck I: histopathology and clinical behavior. Am J Otolaryngol. 30(2):121-33, 2009
3. Garcia-Zuazaga J et al: Cutaneous squamous cell carcinoma. Adv Dermatol. 24:33-57, 2008
4. Ulrich C et al: Skin cancer in organ transplant recipients--where do we stand today? Am J Transplant. 8(11):2192-8, 2008
5. Renzi C et al: Sentinel lymph node biopsy for high risk cutaneous squamous cell carcinoma: case series and review of the literature. Eur J Surg Oncol. 33(3):364-9, 2007
6. Weinberg AS et al: Metastatic cutaneous squamous cell carcinoma: an update. Dermatol Surg. 33(8):885-99, 2007
7. Cassarino DS et al: Cutaneous squamous cell carcinoma: a comprehensive clinicopathologic classification--part two. J Cutan Pathol. 33(4):261-79, 2006
8. Cassarino DS et al: Cutaneous squamous cell carcinoma: a comprehensive clinicopathologic classification. Part one. J Cutan Pathol. 33(3):191-206, 2006
9. Mizuno H et al: Squamous cell carcinoma of the auricle arising from keloid after radium needle therapy. J Craniofac Surg. 17(2):360-2, 2006
10. Veness MJ et al: High-risk cutaneous squamous cell carcinoma of the head and neck: results from 266 treated patients with metastatic lymph node disease. Cancer. 106(11):2389-96, 2006
11. Leibovitch I et al: Cutaneous squamous cell carcinoma treated with Mohs micrographic surgery in Australia I. Experience over 10 years. J Am Acad Dermatol. 53(2):253-60, 2005
12. Lindelöf B et al: Cutaneous squamous cell carcinoma in organ transplant recipients: a study of the Swedish cohort with regard to tumor site. Arch Dermatol. 141(4):447-51, 2005
13. Silapunt S et al: Squamous cell carcinoma of the auricle and Mohs micrographic surgery. Dermatol Surg. 31(11 Pt 1):1423-7, 2005
14. Ahmad I et al: Epidemiology of basal cell carcinoma and squamous cell carcinoma of the pinna. J Laryngol Otol. 115(2):85-6, 2001
15. Baker NJ et al: Surgical management of cutaneous squamous cell carcinoma of the head and neck. Br J Oral Maxillofac Surg. 39(2):87-90, 2001
16. Weinstock MA: Epidemiologic investigation of nonmelanoma skin cancer mortality: the Rhode Island Follow-Back Study. J Invest Dermatol. 102(6):6S-9S, 1994

Clinical and Microscopic Features

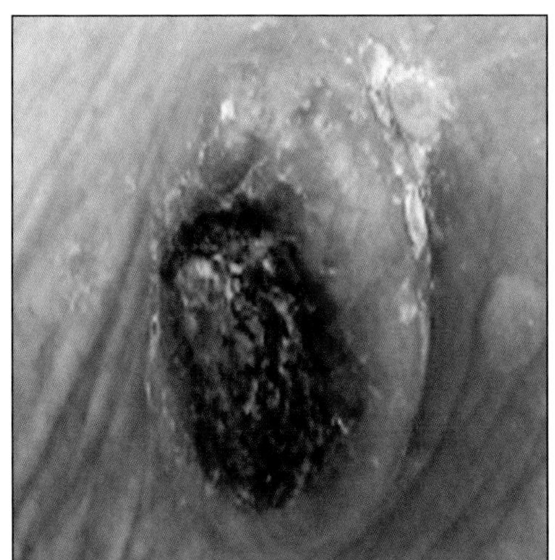
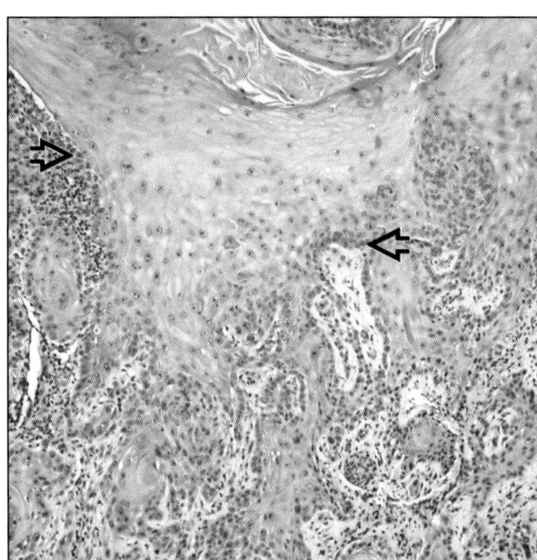

(Left) *Clinical photograph shows a squamous cell carcinoma with raised borders and a central, crateriform keratin-filled defect, suggestive of keratoacanthoma type. (Courtesy S. Yashar, MD.)* **(Right)** *Invasive, well-differentiated SCC is seen arising in association with an actinic keratosis ⇨.*

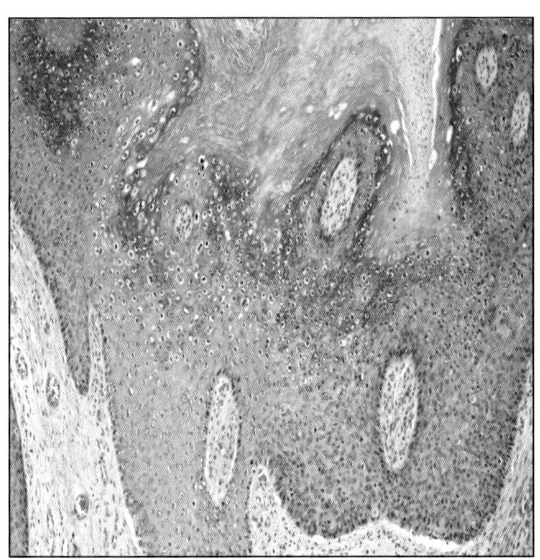
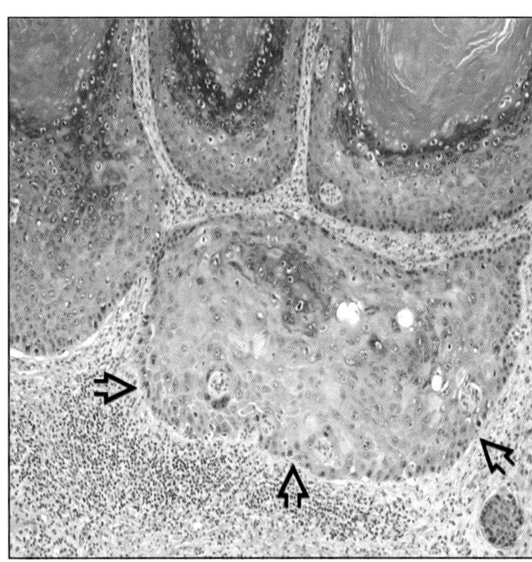

(Left) *SCC in situ (Bowen disease) is seen arising in a longstanding large verruca vulgaris.* **(Right)** *Higher power view of the base of the lesion shows tangentially sectioned SCC in situ with smooth borders ⇨ and lack of an infiltrative growth pattern. There is an associated inflammatory cell infiltrate.*

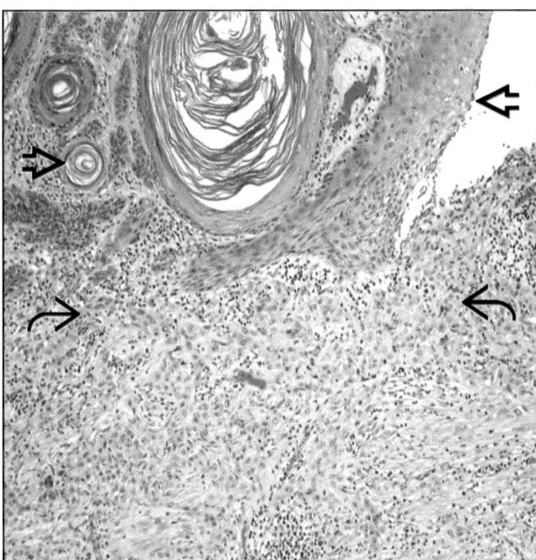
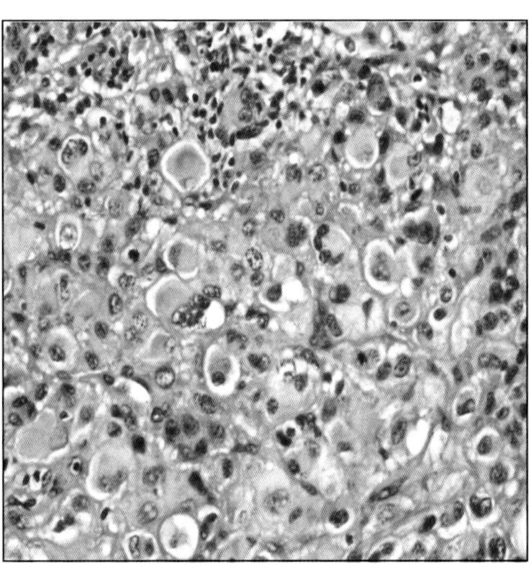

(Left) *High-power view of invasive SCC arising in association with a seborrheic keratosis shows sheets of poorly differentiated infiltrating squamous cells ↷ with overlying seborrheic keratosis ⇨.* **(Right)** *High-grade SCC shows a sheet-like proliferation of atypical and pleomorphic epithelioid and multinucleated cells with hyperchromatic nuclei, prominent nucleoli, and abundant glassy appearing eosinophilic cytoplasm.*

SQUAMOUS CELL CARCINOMA

Microscopic Features

*(**Left**) Acantholytic type of invasive squamous cell carcinoma with central cystic spaces ➪ contains dyscohesive squamous cells →. (**Right**) High-power view of acantholytic SCC shows large epithelioid cells with dense eosinophilic cytoplasm and scattered dyskeratotic (apoptotic) cells →. There is an associated heavy inflammatory cell infiltrate.*

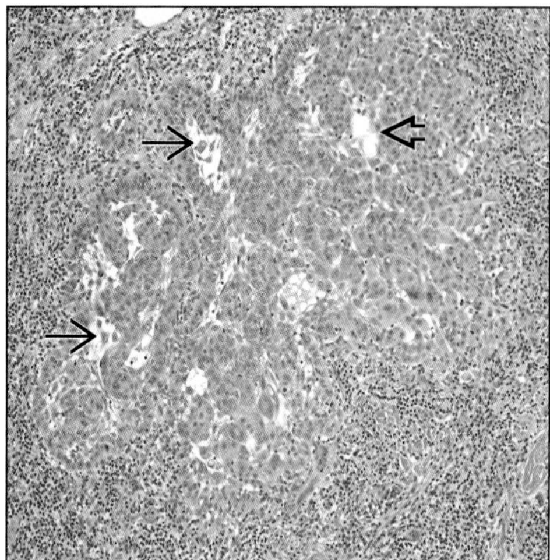

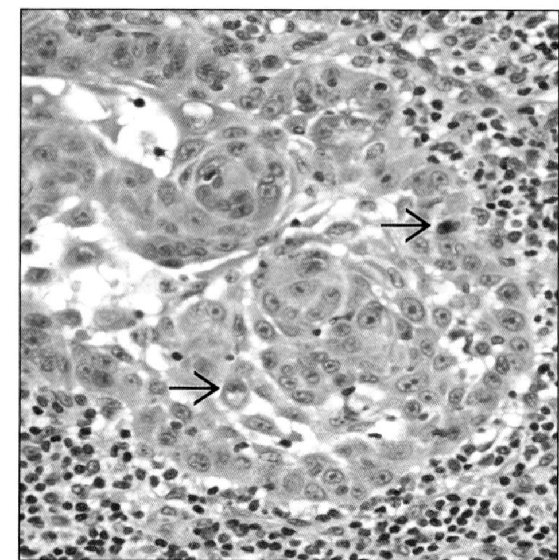

*(**Left**) Poorly differentiated invasive SCC is shown with signet ring cell-like features and focal myxoid stroma ➪. (**Right**) Higher power view of poorly differentiated SCC shows epithelioid to signet ring-like eosinophilic-staining cells ➪ with focal extracellular mucin.*

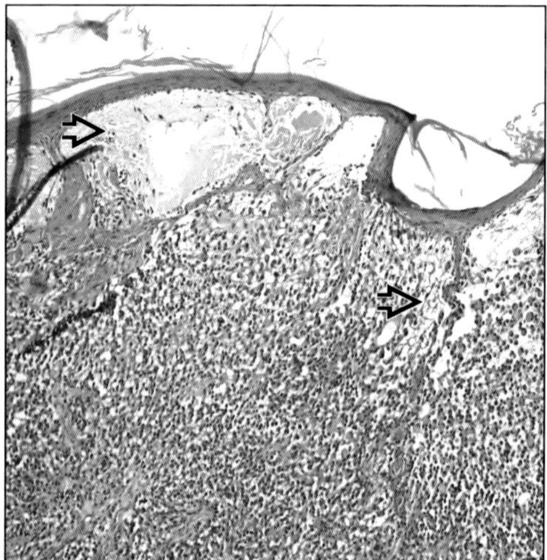

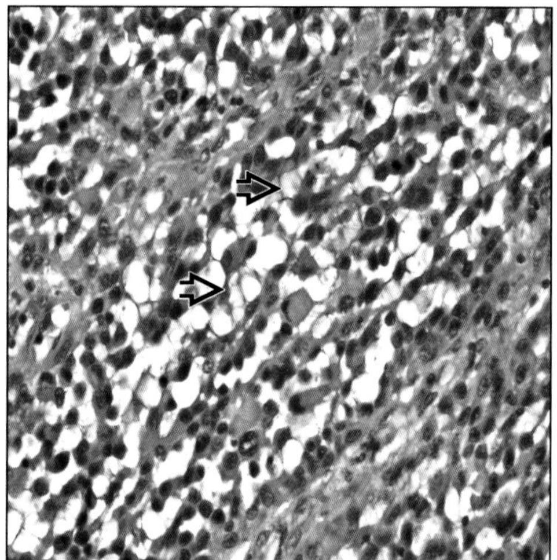

*(**Left**) Poorly differentiated infiltrating squamous cell carcinoma is seen forming cords mimicking ductal structures ➪. There is an associated dense desmoplastic stroma. (**Right**) Heavily inflamed invasive SCC with moderately differentiated tumor islands ➪ is surrounded by a sea of inflammatory cells, features suggestive of the lymphoepithelioma-like carcinoma (LELC) variant.*

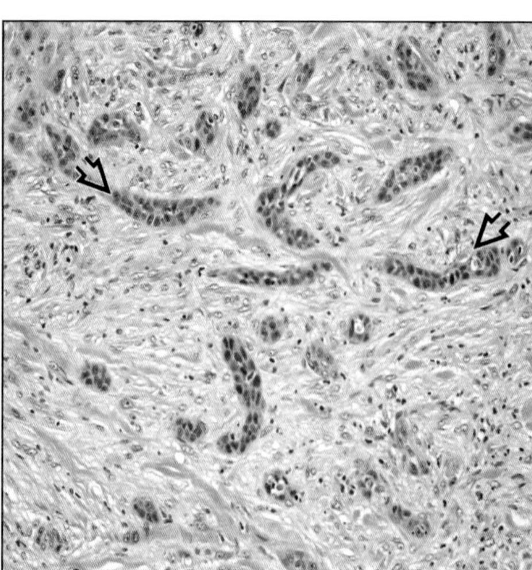

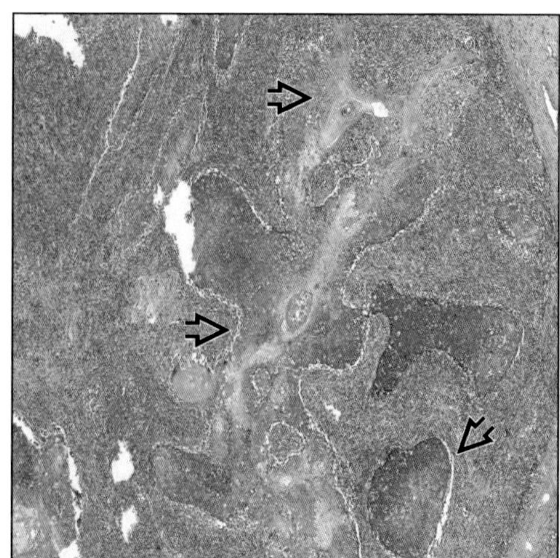

Microscopic and Immunohistochemical Features

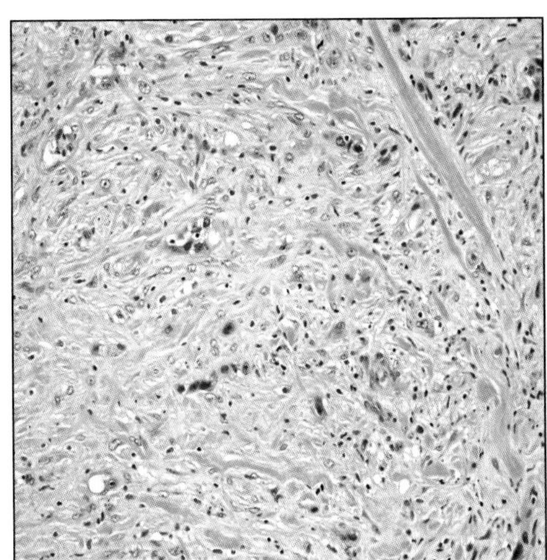

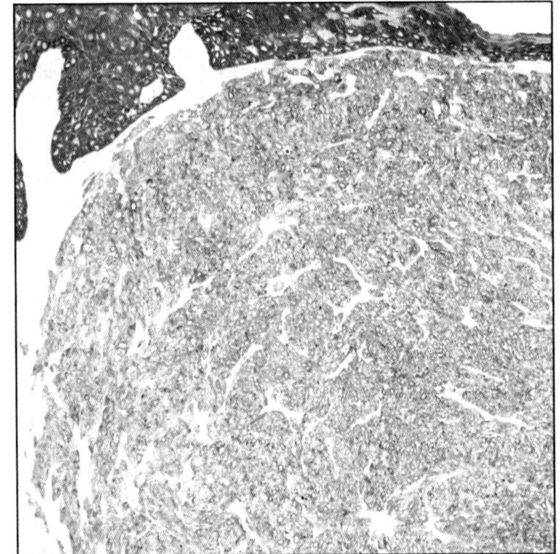

(Left) *Poorly differentiated infiltrating SCC associated with a sclerotic (desmoplastic) stroma is shown.* ***(Right)*** *CK903 shows strong staining of an invasive, poorly invasive SCC and the overlying epidermis.*

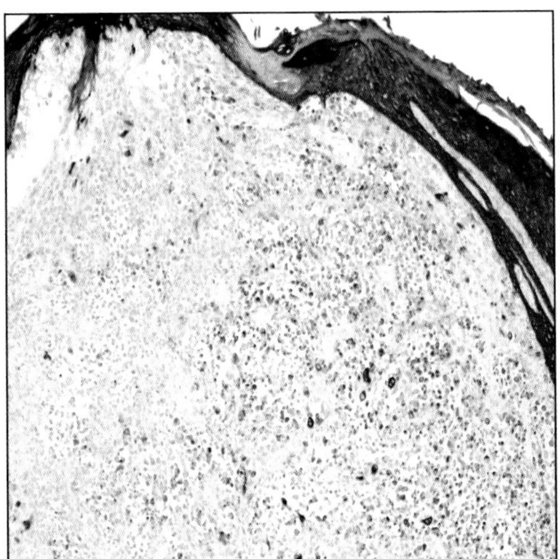

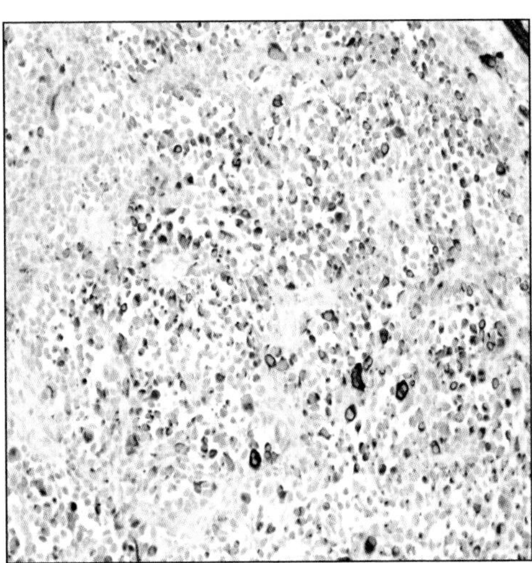

(Left) *CK5/6 (HMWCK) shows strong staining of the poorly differentiated squamous cells.* ***(Right)*** *High-power view of CK5/6 shows strong cytoplasmic staining of many of the tumor cells. Note the acantholytic appearance of the proliferation.*

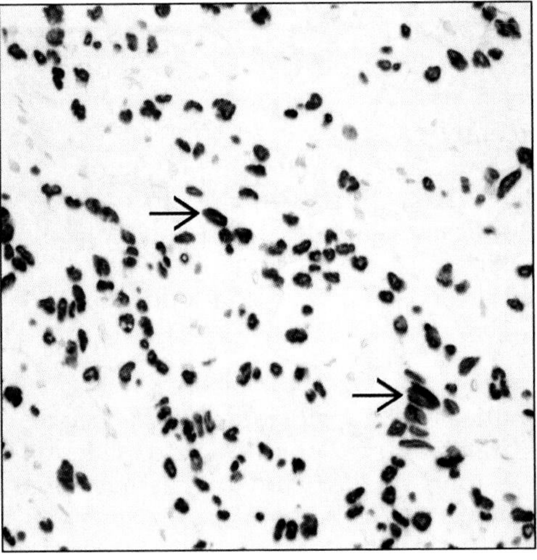

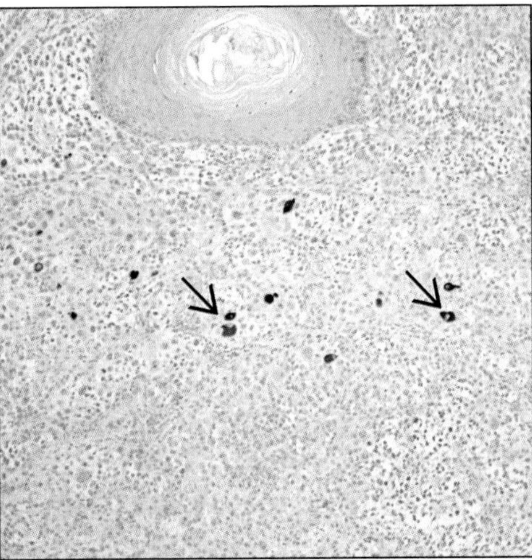

(Left) *IHC stain for p63 shows strong and diffuse nuclear staining → in a poorly differentiated infiltrating SCC.* ***(Right)*** *CK-PAN shows only focal staining of a few cells → in a case of poorly differentiated SCC. CK-PAN is much less sensitive than CK5/6 and p63 in cases of poorly differentiated and sarcomatoid SCC.*

BASAL CELL CARCINOMA

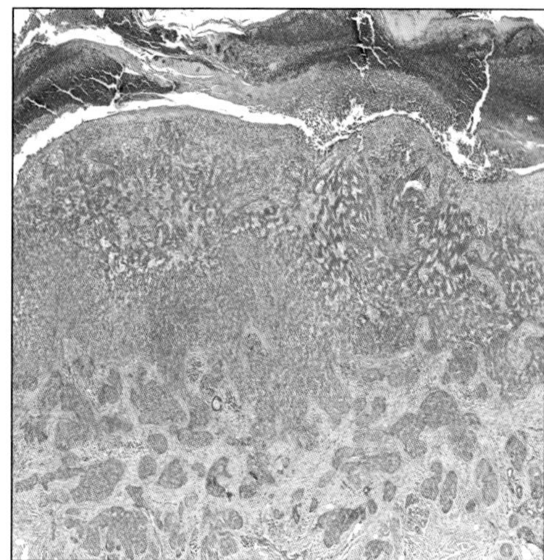

Hematoxylin & eosin shows a large, nodular and micronodular type BCC with overlying ulceration and serum crusting.

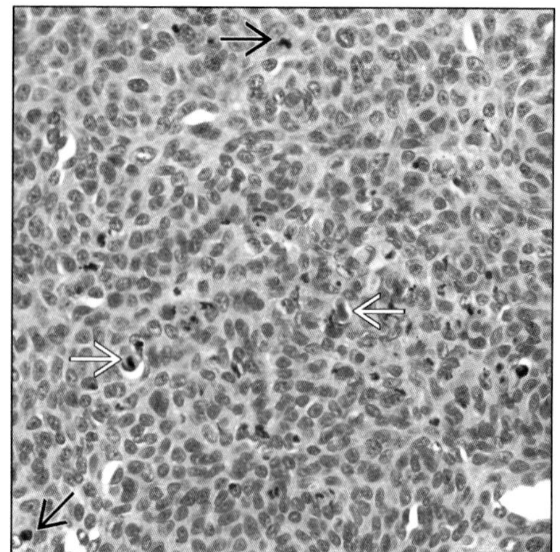

High magnification of nodular BCC shows a sheet-like proliferation of atypical basaloid cells with high nuclear to cytoplasmic ratios and numerous apoptotic ➔ and mitotic figures ⇒.

TERMINOLOGY

Abbreviations

- Basal cell carcinoma (BCC)

Synonyms

- Basal cell epithelioma (BCE)

Definitions

- Low-grade malignancy of basal keratinocytes

ETIOLOGY/PATHOGENESIS

Multifactorial

- Related to sun exposure, radiation, immunosuppression
- May be derived from follicular stem cells

CLINICAL ISSUES

Epidemiology

- Incidence
  - Very common: Most common cancer in humans
- Age
  - Typically older adults; few cases in young adults
- Gender
  - Slight male predilection
- Ethnicity
  - Caucasian/light-skinned individuals

Presentation

- Typically papular, plaque-like, or nodular lesion in head and neck region
  - Often ulcerated with overlying crusting

Treatment

- Surgical approaches
  - Complete excision or electrodessication and curettage
  - Mohs micrographic surgery often used in cosmetically sensitive locations, such as face

Prognosis

- Usually excellent, cured by local excision
- More aggressive subtypes, including micronodular, infiltrative, desmoplastic, and basosquamous, have higher rate of recurrence and low risk of metastasis

MACROSCOPIC FEATURES

Size

- Variable, small (few mm) to large (several cm)

MICROSCOPIC PATHOLOGY

Histologic Features

- Tumor is comprised of nodules, nests, &/or infiltrative cords
  - Overlying ulceration and serum crusting often present in large tumors
- Proliferation of small basaloid cells with peripheral palisading
- Stromal retraction artifact
  - Between tumor cells and stroma
- Mucinous material may be present
- Numerous mitotic and apoptotic figures present
- Cells show enlarged hyperchromatic nuclei with inconspicuous nucleoli and scant eosinophilic cytoplasm

Variants

- Superficial-multicentric: Superficial nests attached to epidermis separated by areas of uninvolved epidermis
- Nodular: Large, rounded predominantly dermal-based nests with prominent peripheral palisading
- Micronodular: Predominantly dermal-based infiltrative proliferation of small nests

BASAL CELL CARCINOMA

Key Facts

Terminology
- Low-grade malignancy of basal keratinocytes

Etiology/Pathogenesis
- Related to sun exposure, radiation, immunosuppression
- May be derived from follicular stem cells

Clinical Issues
- Very common: Most common cancer in humans
- Prognosis usually excellent, most cases cured by excision
- More aggressive subtypes, including infiltrative, micronodular, desmoplastic, and basosquamous, have higher rate of recurrence and low risk of metastasis
- Treated by complete excision or electrodessication and curettage

Microscopic Pathology
- Proliferation of nodules, nests, and cords of small basaloid cells with peripheral palisading, stromal retraction artifact, and mucinous material
- Numerous mitotic and apoptotic figures typically present
- Cells show enlarged hyperchromatic nuclei with inconspicuous nucleoli and scant amounts of eosinophilic cytoplasm

Top Differential Diagnoses
- Squamous cell carcinoma (SCC)
- Actinic keratosis (AK)
- Follicular neoplasms (trichoepithelioma and trichoblastoma)
- Merkel cell carcinoma

- Infiltrative: Small cords and nests, often deeply invasive
- Desmoplastic/morpheaform: Infiltrative strands and nests associated with dense sclerotic stroma
- Infundibulocystic: Mature folliculocystic spaces containing keratinous material
- Basosquamous/metatypical: Prominent squamous differentiation, less peripheral palisading present
- Rare variants include adenoid, clear cell, signet ring cell, plasmacytoid/myoepithelial, and fibroepithelioma of Pinkus

ANCILLARY TESTS

Immunohistochemistry
- Basal cell carcinoma vs. trichoepithelioma and trichoblastoma
  - BCC shows greater staining for Bcl-2, p53, and Ki-67
- BCC vs. SCC
  - BCC is positive for Ber-Ep4; SCC is almost always negative
  - Cytokeratins and p63 are not useful, as they are positive in both

DIFFERENTIAL DIAGNOSIS

Squamous Cell Carcinoma (SCC)
- Most cases are easily separated; however, basosquamous type of BCC shows prominent squamous differentiation
  - Usually, areas of more typical BCC are present, especially at periphery of tumor
  - Overlying AK or Bowen disease often seen in association with SCC

Actinic Keratosis (AK)
- Can be difficult to distinguish on very superficial shave biopsies
  - AK typically shows basilar budding and overlying parakeratosis
  - Numerous apoptotic and mitotic figures favor BCC

Follicular Neoplasms (Trichoepithelioma and Trichoblastoma)
- Typically lack degree of cytologic atypia, mitoses, and apoptotic figures of BCC
- Mucinous stroma and tumor-stromal retraction artifact typically lacking in benign follicular neoplasms

Merkel Cell Carcinoma
- Nodular to sheet-like proliferation of highly atypical basaloid cells
  - Mucinous stroma and tumor-stromal retraction artifact only rarely identified
- Nuclei typically show speckled ("salt and pepper") chromatin pattern or nuclear clearing

DIAGNOSTIC CHECKLIST

Pathologic Interpretation Pearls
- Proliferation of nodules, nests, and cords of small basaloid cells with peripheral palisading, stromal retraction artifact, and mucinous material

SELECTED REFERENCES

1. Ban JH et al: Basaloid squamous cell carcinoma of the external auditory canal: case report. Eur Arch Otorhinolaryngol. 264(6):697-9, 2007
2. Cohen PR et al: Basal cell carcinoma with mixed histology: a possible pathogenesis for recurrent skin cancer. Dermatol Surg. 32(4):542-51, 2006
3. Wadhera A et al: Metastatic basal cell carcinoma: a case report and literature review. How accurate is our incidence data? Dermatol Online J. 12(5):7, 2006
4. Vandeweyer E et al: Basal cell carcinoma of the external auditory canal. Acta Chir Belg. 102(2):137-40, 2002
5. Lim V et al: Primary basal cell carcinoma of the middle ear presenting as recurrent cholesteatoma. Am J Otol. 20(5):657-9, 1999
6. Lobo CJ et al: Basal cell carcinoma of the external auditory canal and Gorlin-Goltz syndrome: a case report. J Laryngol Otol. 111(9):850-1, 1997

BASAL CELL CARCINOMA

Microscopic Features

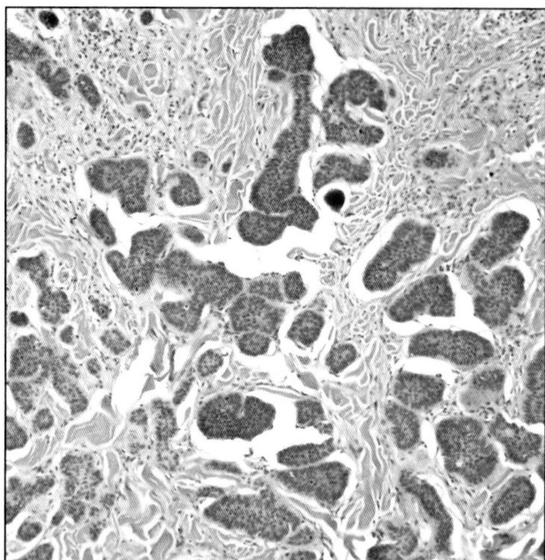
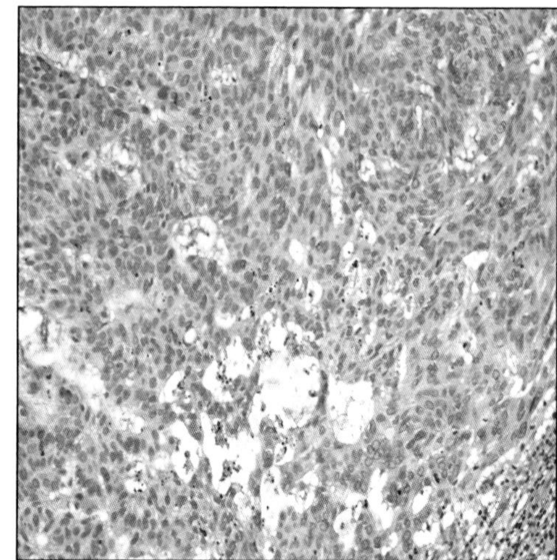

(Left) *Histologic section of a micronodular-type BCC shows a proliferation of small nests of basaloid cells in somewhat sclerotic-appearing stroma.* ***(Right)*** *Basosquamous-type BCC shows a proliferation of large, squamoid-appearing cells with abundant eosinophilic cytoplasm and focal mucin collections.*

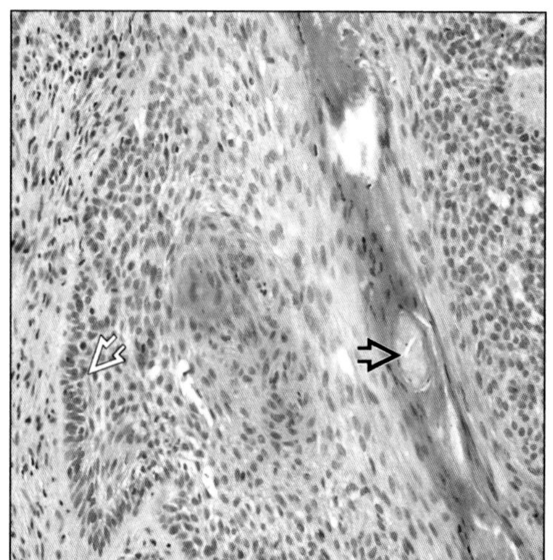
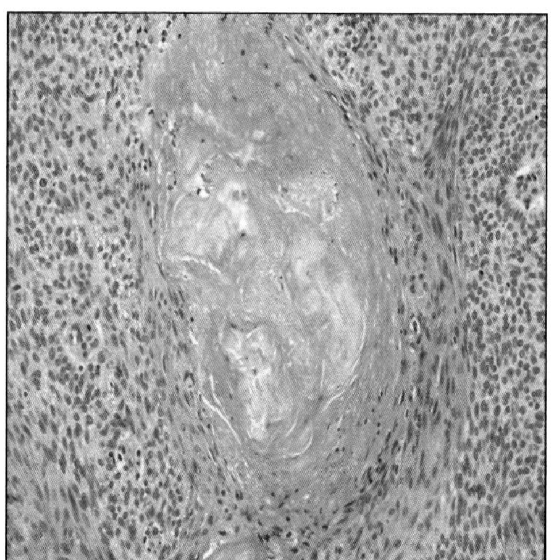

(Left) *Another example of basosquamous-type BCC shows traditional areas of BCC with peripheral palisading ⇨ surrounding collections of larger, squamoid-appearing cells associated with keratinization ➡.* ***(Right)*** *Hematoxylin & eosin shows a large area of central comedonecrosis in a basosquamous BCC.*

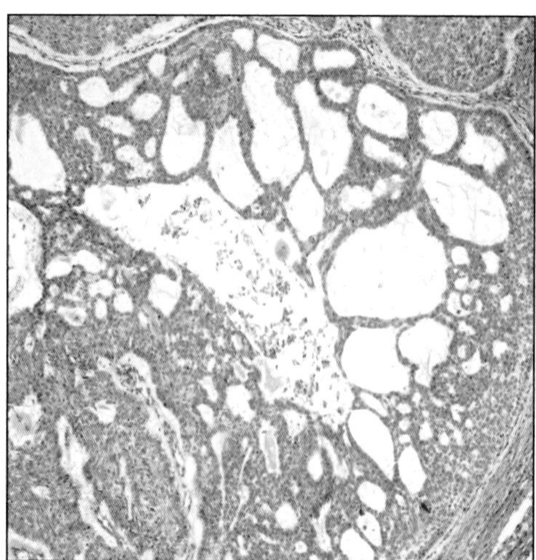
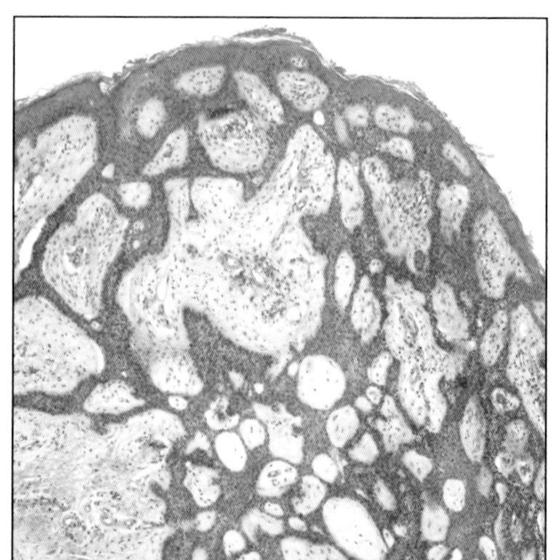

(Left) *Low-power view shows BCC with adenoid cystic features (adenoid BCC), characterized by numerous well-formed cystic spaces containing mucinous material.* ***(Right)*** *Scanning magnification shows a fibroepithelioma of Pinkus-type BCC, characterized by numerous small anastomosing cords of basaloid cells.*

Microscopic and Immunohistochemical Features

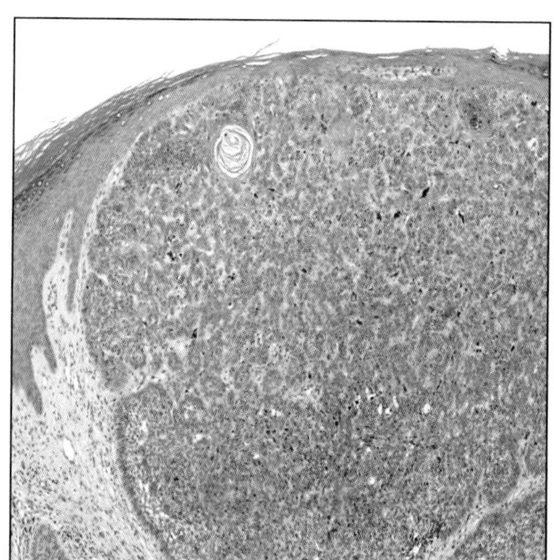

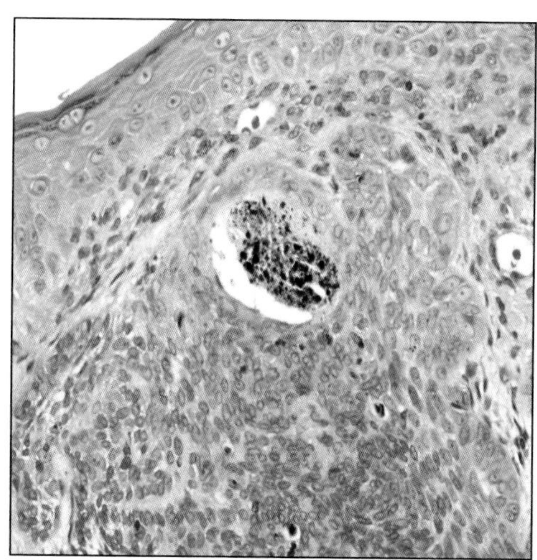

(Left) *Low-power view shows a large nodular BCC with prominent pigmentation throughout the nodule.* ***(Right)*** *High-power examination of pigmented BCC shows a large globule of pigment in a cystic structure.*

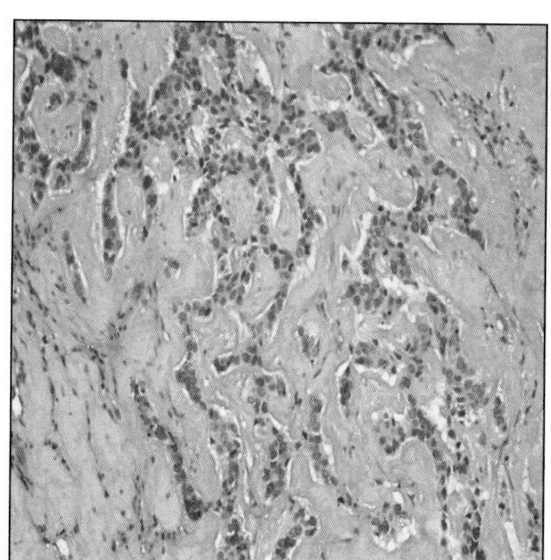

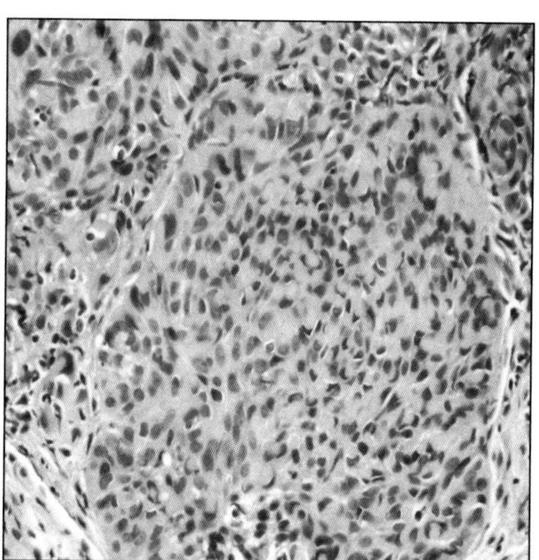

(Left) *Morpheaform (desmoplastic/sclerosing) BCC shows cords of atypical basaloid cells infiltrating a dense, desmoplastic stroma.* ***(Right)*** *High-power magnification shows a plasmacytoid or signet ring-like BCC, with dense eosinophilic cytoplasmic inclusions and displaced nuclei. These cases have been shown to exhibit myoepithelial differentiation.*

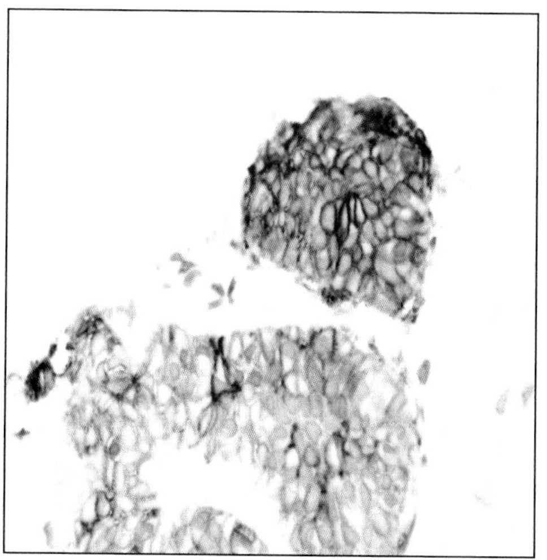

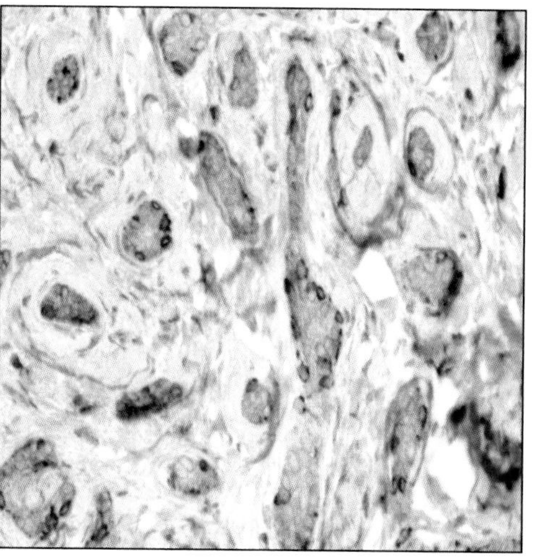

(Left) *Ber-Ep4 immunohistochemistry of a plasmacytoid BCC shows moderate to strong membranous staining of many cells.* ***(Right)*** *Bcl-2 immunohistochemistry of a micronodular BCC shows moderate to strong cytoplasmic staining of the tumor cells.*

MERKEL CELL CARCINOMA

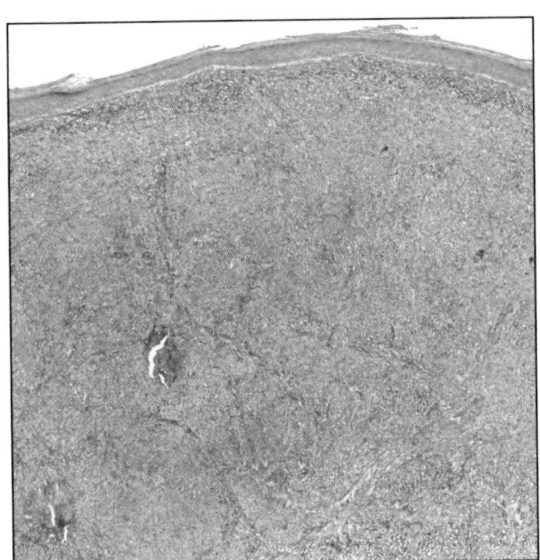

A low-power view shows diffuse dermal involvement by sheets and nodules of blue cells.

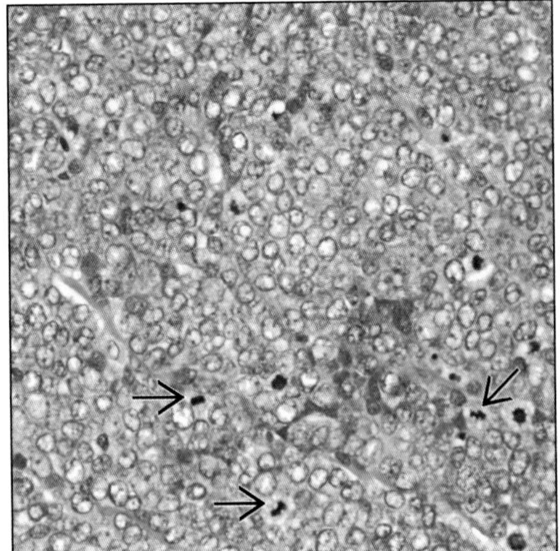

High magnification shows nuclear molding, hyperchromasia, and granular chromatin. There are also numerous apoptotic and mitotic figures ➔ easily identified.

TERMINOLOGY

Abbreviations

- Merkel cell carcinoma (MCC)

Synonyms

- Cutaneous neuroendocrine carcinoma
- Trabecular carcinoma
- Primary small cell carcinoma of skin

Definitions

- Malignant proliferation of cutaneous neuroendocrine cells

ETIOLOGY/PATHOGENESIS

Infectious Agents

- Recent studies have shown strong link to infection with polyomavirus
  - Merkel cell polyoma virus infection is found in up to 90% of cases
- Associated with immunosuppression
  - Organ transplant and HIV(+) patients have much higher incidence

Cell of Origin

- Postulated to represent malignant transformation of cutaneous neuroendocrine (Merkel) cells or pluripotent stem cells, but this remains speculative

CLINICAL ISSUES

Epidemiology

- Incidence
  - Rare
    - Approximately 500 cases/year in USA
- Age
  - Typically in elderly patients (> 65 years old)
- Gender
  - Male > Female (2.5:1)
- Ethnicity
  - Caucasians much more commonly than in other races

Site

- Sun-damaged skin
- Usually head and neck or extremities

Presentation

- Dermal nodular or plaque-like mass lesion
- Rapidly enlarging dermal mass lesion
  - May be ulcerated &/or hemorrhagic

Natural History

- Aggressive tumors with high incidence of local recurrence, lymph node and distant metastasis
- Clinical staging should include imaging studies, especially chest and abdominal CT scans

Treatment

- Surgical approaches
  - Complete and wide excision to ensure complete local removal
  - Consideration may be given to sentinel lymph node (SLN) biopsy
    - However, SLN positivity does not seem to be very sensitive for regional lymph node involvement, as many patients progress to distant metastases
- Adjuvant therapy
  - Radiotherapy is generally used and may lead to remission in some cases
  - Chemotherapy is less effective, and does not prolong overall survival

Prognosis

- High incidence of recurrence (up to 30%) and metastasis (up to 75%)
- Overall prognosis is poor
  - Death due to disease is high, even with treatment

MERKEL CELL CARCINOMA

Key Facts

Terminology
- Cutaneous neuroendocrine carcinoma
- Malignant proliferation of cutaneous neuroendocrine cells

Clinical Issues
- Highly aggressive tumors with greater metastatic potential than melanoma
- Rare (approximately 500 cases/year in USA)
- Typically occurs in sun-damaged skin of elderly (> 65 years old)
- Male > Female (2.5:1)
- Radiotherapy is generally used and may lead to remission

Microscopic Pathology
- Highly atypical basaloid neoplasm composed of infiltrative cords, trabeculae, and sheet-like areas
- Typically dermal-based but may show epidermal (pagetoid) involvement in 20% of cases
- Nuclear crush artifact and streaming may be seen, similar to small cell carcinomas

Ancillary Tests
- Immunohistochemistry is important in confirming diagnosis and excluding metastatic neuroendocrine carcinoma

Top Differential Diagnoses
- Basal cell carcinoma
- Metastatic small cell carcinoma (especially pulmonary origin)

  - Worse prognosis associated with advanced age, head and neck location, large size, and immunosuppression

MACROSCOPIC FEATURES

General Features
- Nodular tumor with blue or red appearance

Size
- Typically < 2 cm

MICROSCOPIC PATHOLOGY

Histologic Features
- Highly atypical invasive basaloid neoplasm
  - Composed of infiltrative cords, trabeculae, nests, and sheet-like areas
    - Associated dermal desmoplasia may be present
  - Enlarged, hyperchromatic basaloid tumor cells with high N:C ratio, scant cytoplasm, large nuclei, granular to clear chromatin, and indistinct nucleoli
  - Nuclear clearing is distinctive feature, which is often seen
    - This finding is not seen in BCC
  - Mitotic figures are abundant
  - Typically, numerous apoptotic cells
  - Areas of geographic necrosis often present, especially in larger tumors
  - Nuclear crush artifact and streaming may be seen, similar to small cell carcinoma
  - Angiolymphatic invasion identified in significant percentage of cases, often at periphery of tumor
  - Partial tumor regression may be present
- Typically dermal-based
  - May show epidermal (pagetoid) involvement in up to 20% of cases
  - Purely pagetoid (in situ) cases have been reported
- Areas of squamoid or adnexal (including follicular, ductal, or glandular) differentiation may be present in minority of cases
  - Rarely, melanocytic differentiation may be present
  - These findings suggest that MCC may arise from primitive pluripotential (stem) cell that can differentiate along multiple different lines, rather than specific neuroendocrine cell
- Rarely, spindle cell/sarcomatoid differentiation mimicking atypical fibroxanthoma (AFX), leiomyosarcoma, osteosarcoma, or rhabdomyosarcoma may be seen

ANCILLARY TESTS

Immunohistochemistry
- Important in confirming diagnosis and excluding metastatic neuroendocrine carcinoma
  - MCC is typically positive for keratins (pancytokeratin, CK20, CAM5.2), often with perinuclear dot-like staining
  - Putative prognostic markers include CD44, p53, and Bcl-2
  - Negative staining for melanocytic markers and lymphoid markers

Cytogenetics
- Trisomy 6 is identified in many cases of MCC, up to 50% in some studies
- Deletion of short arm of chromosome 1 (1p36) is also commonly identified

DIFFERENTIAL DIAGNOSIS

Basal Cell Carcinoma
- Less atypia and mitotic activity; most cases show areas of peripheral palisading, mucinous stroma, and retraction artifact
- MCC should always be considered in high-grade/pleomorphic-appearing cases of BCC
- Almost always positive for Ber-Ep4, but negative for CK20, chromogranin-A, synaptophysin

MERKEL CELL CARCINOMA

Immunohistochemistry

Antibody	Reactivity	Staining Pattern	Comment
CK-PAN	Positive	Dot positivity	May or may not show dot-like positivity but will be positive
CK20	Positive	Dot positivity	Rare cases may be negative
CK8/18/CAM5.2	Positive	Dot positivity	Most cases show dot reactivity
NSE	Positive	Cytoplasmic	Most cases are positive
Chromogranin-A	Positive	Cytoplasmic	Most cases are positive
Synaptophysin	Positive	Cytoplasmic	Most cases are positive
CK7	Positive	Dot positivity	Isolated cases may be CK7 positive when CK20 negative
S100	Negative		
melan-A103	Negative		
HMB-45	Negative		
TTF-1	Negative		
CD10	Negative		
CD45RB	Negative		
CD99	Negative		

Metastatic Small Cell Carcinoma

- Especially pulmonary origin, which are positive for TTF-1, negative for CK20
- Small cell carcinomas from others sites are TTF-1 negative
- Clinical history and complete examination important to exclude metastasis

Small Cell Melanoma

- Rare variant of melanoma; typically see areas of associated junctional nesting and overlying pagetoid spread
- Cells show more abundant cytoplasm, prominent nucleoli, and may see cytoplasmic pigmentation and intranuclear pseudoinclusions
- S100 protein, HMB-45, Melan-A typically positive; negative for cytokeratins, CK20, and neuroendocrine markers

Lymphoma

- Lymphomas are dyscohesive, lacking cord-like and trabecular growth pattern of MCC
- Various lymphoid markers will be positive, but CK20 and neuroendocrine markers negative

Small Round Blue Cell Tumors

- Include neuroblastoma, Ewing/primitive neuroectodermal tumor (PNET), rhabdomyosarcoma
- Very rare in skin (typically metastatic from other sites); most cases occur in children

DIAGNOSTIC CHECKLIST

Clinically Relevant Pathologic Features

- Mitotic rate
- Angiolymphatic invasion
- Large tumor size
- Small cell size

Pathologic Interpretation Pearls

- High-grade basaloid proliferation with neuroendocrine features
- Composed of infiltrative cords, trabeculae, nests, and sheet-like areas
  - Cells are hyperchromatic, with scant cytoplasm, granular-appearing chromatin, and indistinct nucleoli

SELECTED REFERENCES

1. Becker JC et al: Merkel cell carcinoma. Cell Mol Life Sci. 66(1):1-8, 2009
2. Sastre-Garau X et al: Merkel cell carcinoma of the skin: pathological and molecular evidence for a causative role of MCV in oncogenesis. J Pathol. 218(1):48-56, 2009
3. Feng H et al: Clonal integration of a polyomavirus in human Merkel cell carcinoma. Science. 319(5866):1096-100, 2008
4. Ball NJ et al: Merkel cell carcinoma frequently shows histologic features of basal cell carcinoma: a study of 30 cases. J Cutan Pathol. 34(8):612-9, 2007
5. Calder KB et al: A case series and immunophenotypic analysis of CK20-/CK7+ primary neuroendocrine carcinoma of the skin. J Cutan Pathol. 34(12):918-23, 2007
6. Eng TY et al: A comprehensive review of the treatment of Merkel cell carcinoma. Am J Clin Oncol. 30(6):624-36, 2007
7. Plaza JA et al: The Toker tumor: spectrum of morphologic features in primary neuroendocrine carcinomas of the skin (Merkel cell carcinoma). Ann Diagn Pathol. 10(6):376-85, 2006
8. Sandel HD 4th et al: Merkel cell carcinoma: does tumor size or depth of invasion correlate with recurrence, metastasis, or patient survival? Laryngoscope. 116(5):791-5, 2006
9. Yom SS et al: Merkel cell carcinoma of the tongue and head and neck oral mucosal sites. Oral Surg Oral Med Oral Pathol Oral Radiol Endod. 101(6):761-8, 2006
10. Gancberg D et al: Trisomy 6 in Merkel cell carcinoma: a recurrent chromosomal aberration. Histopathology. 37(5):445-51, 2000
11. Yanguas I et al: Spontaneous regression of Merkel cell carcinoma of the skin. Br J Dermatol. 137(2):296-8, 1997

Microscopic and Immunohistochemical Features

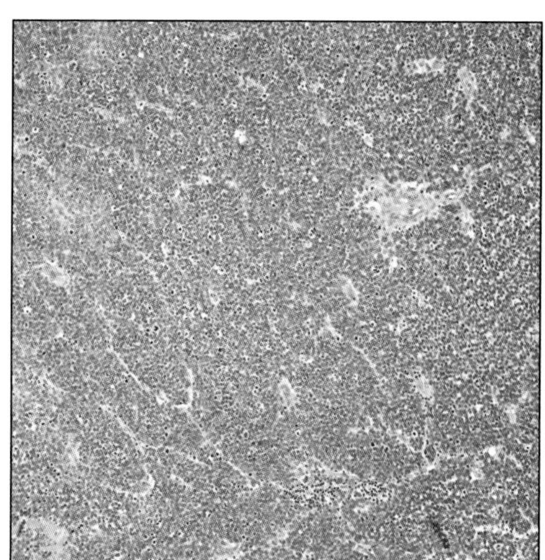

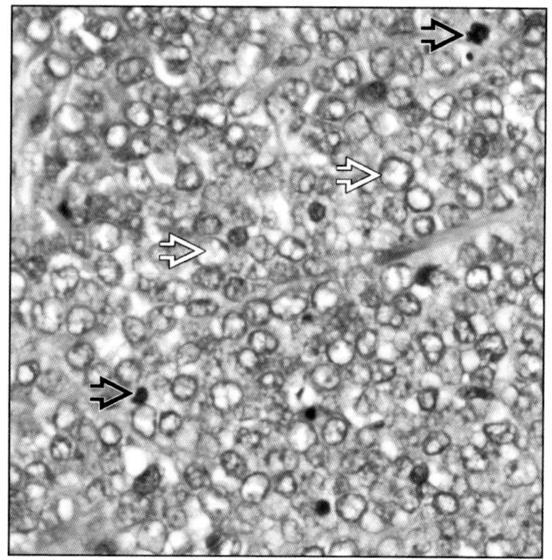

(Left) *The tumor is composed of broad cords and sheet-like collections of highly atypical basaloid cells. There is scant stroma intervening between the neoplastic cells.* ***(Right)*** *Nuclear clearing ➡ is often seen in Merkel cell carcinoma, a feature not seen in basal cell carcinoma. Note the apoptotic figures and mitotic figures ⇨.*

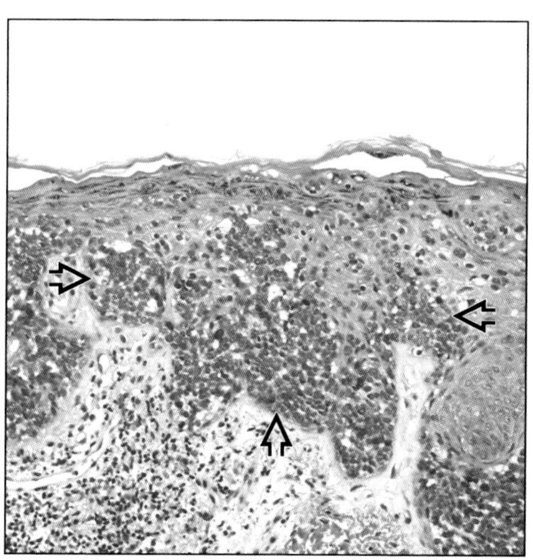

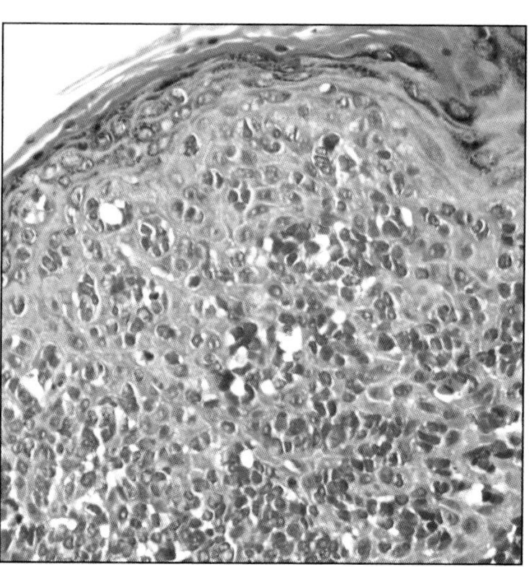

(Left) *Pagetoid intraepidermal spread of Merkel cell carcinoma ⇨ is rarely seen in a minority of cases. No dermal component is present in this image.* ***(Right)*** *High magnification of pagetoid intraepidermal spread of Merkel cells is shown.*

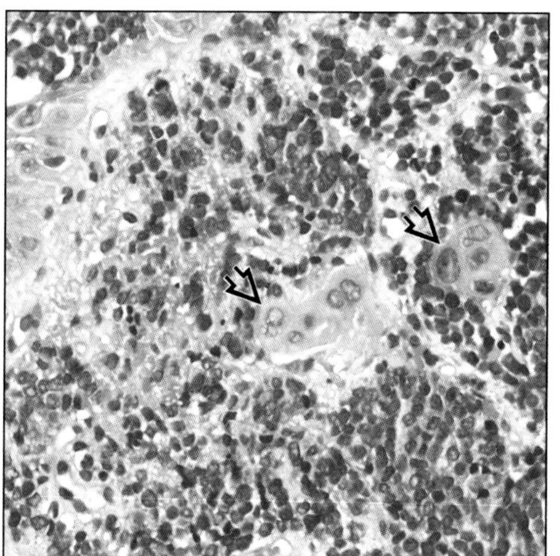

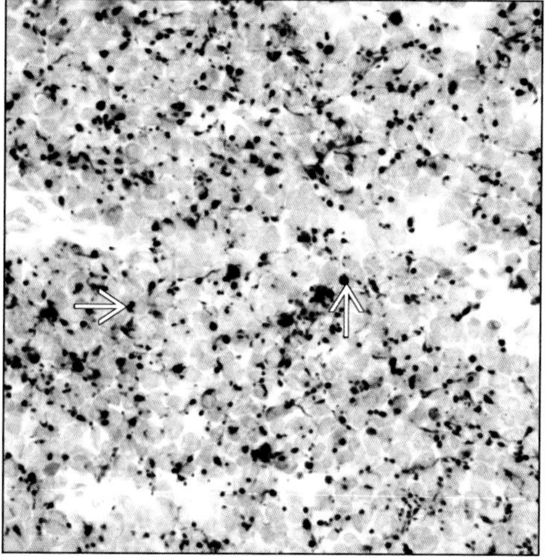

(Left) *Focal squamous differentiation ⇨ is seen in a Merkel cell carcinoma. The neoplastic cells are basophilic with a very high nuclear to cytoplasmic ratio. The nuclear chromatin is coarse and heavy, and nucleoli are not appreciated.* ***(Right)*** *CK20 immunohistochemistry shows cytoplasmic and perinuclear dot-like ➡ positivity. This pattern is not a feature identified in other basaloid tumor types, helping to confirm the diagnosis.*

DERMATOFIBROSARCOMA PROTUBERANS

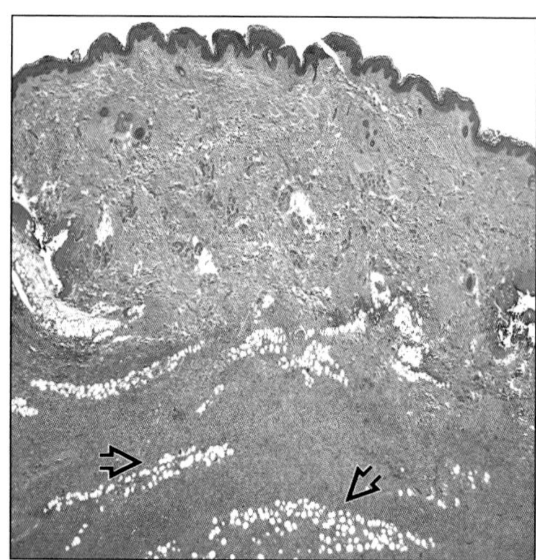

Low-power view of a DFSP shows deep dermal and subcutaneous involvement by a cellular spindle cell tumor with fat entrapping ⇨. The epidermis is unremarkable.

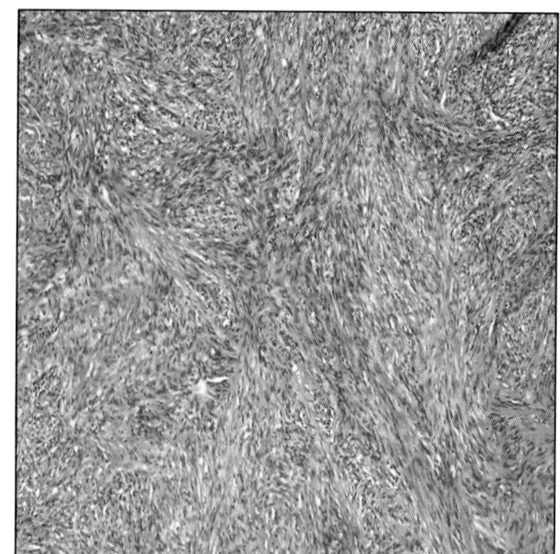

Higher power shows a cellular neoplastic proliferation arranged in a storiform pattern. The cells are monomorphous and spindled. Cellular pleomorphism is inconspicuous.

TERMINOLOGY

Abbreviations

- Dermatofibrosarcoma protuberans (DFSP)

Synonyms

- Bednar tumor (pigmented DFSP)

Definitions

- Low-grade malignant spindle cell tumor of skin characteristically showing prominent storiforming

ETIOLOGY/PATHOGENESIS

Unknown in Most Cases

- Rare cases reportedly associated with previous trauma, burns, or arsenic exposure

CLINICAL ISSUES

Epidemiology

- Incidence
  - Uncommon
- Age
  - Typically occurs in young adults
- Gender
  - Male > Female

Presentation

- Dermal and subcutaneous nodular or plaque-like mass
- Uncommon in head and neck region
  - Most often presents on trunk or extremities

Treatment

- Optimal treatment is complete surgical excision

Prognosis

- Excellent in most cases
- Recurrences in up to 30%
- Very low metastatic rates (only in cases with fibrosarcomatous transformation)

MACROSCOPIC FEATURES

General Features

- Polypoid, multinodular, or bosselated-appearing tumor
  - Rare cases may be atrophic-appearing
- Cut surface usually gray-white appearing
- May show hemorrhage and cystic changes

Size

- Range: 1-10 cm

MICROSCOPIC PATHOLOGY

Histologic Features

- Dermal and subcutaneous involvement
- Proliferation of monomorphic spindle-shaped cells
- Arrayed in storiform or cartwheel patterns
- Lesional cells typically lack significant pleomorphism
- Elongated spindle-shaped nuclei
- Mild nuclear hyperchromasia and small to inconspicuous nucleoli
- Moderate amounts of eosinophilic cytoplasm
- Mitoses are usually infrequent (< 4/10 HPF) and not atypical
  - Increased mitoses and atypical forms more common in fibrosarcomatous change
- Necrosis is usually absent
- Subcutaneous areas typically show "honeycomb" fat entrapment
- Myxoid stromal change may be prominent in some cases

DERMATOFIBROSARCOMA PROTUBERANS

Key Facts

Terminology
- Low-grade malignant spindle cell tumor of skin characteristically showing prominent storiforming
- Bednar tumor (pigmented DFSP)

Clinical Issues
- Typically occurs in young adults
- Excellent prognosis in most cases
- Relatively low recurrence rate
- Very low metastatic rates (usually only in cases with fibrosarcomatous transformation)

Microscopic Pathology
- Dermal and subcutaneous involvement
- Cells arrayed in storiform or cartwheel patterns
- Proliferation of monomorphic spindle-shaped cells
- Lesional cells lack significant pleomorphism
- Mitoses usually infrequent (less than 4/10 HPF)
  - Atypical mitoses usually absent

Ancillary Tests
- CD34 is most reliable marker, typically strongly and diffusely positive
  - May be weak and focal in some cases
- FXIIIA is typically negative
  - Focal staining, usually at periphery or in scattered dendritic cells

Top Differential Diagnoses
- Cellular dermatofibroma/fibrous histiocytoma
- Fibrosarcoma (including transformation in DFSP)
- Leiomyosarcoma

ANCILLARY TESTS

Immunohistochemistry
- Useful to confirm diagnosis, although not necessary in most cases
  - CD34 is most reliable marker
    - Typically, strong and diffuse reaction
    - May be weak and focal in some cases
  - FXIIIA is typically negative
    - May show focal staining, usually at periphery or in scattered dendritic cells
  - CD68, lysozyme, and chymotrypsin are typically negative
    - These antibodies are relatively nonspecific
  - S100 protein can rarely be positive in a few (dendritic) cells
    - It will also highlight pigmented cells in Bednar tumor

DIFFERENTIAL DIAGNOSIS

Cellular Dermatofibroma/Fibrous Histiocytoma
- More pleomorphic population of both small spindled fibroblastic-appearing cells and larger, histiocytoid-appearing cells
- No prominent storiforming and "honeycombing" fat entrapment
- FXIIIA(+) and CD34(-)
  - CD34 may be focally positive, usually at periphery

Fibrosarcoma (Includes Transformation in DFSP)
- Areas of increased cellularity and mitoses (> 5/10 HPF)
- Spindle cells typically arrayed in prominent fascicles with "herringbone" appearance

Leiomyosarcoma
- Usually shows more cytologic atypia and pleomorphism, and multiple mitoses
- Actin and desmin positive; CD34 negative

Spindle Cell/Desmoplastic Melanoma
- Typically shows greater atypia, pleomorphism, and nuclear hyperchromasia
- Lacks areas of storiforming
- Overlying melanoma in situ may be present
- S100 protein positive; other melanocytic markers often negative

DIAGNOSTIC CHECKLIST

Clinically Relevant Pathologic Features
- Fibrosarcomatous transformation
- Tumors with positive margins much more likely to recur

Pathologic Interpretation Pearls
- Dermal/subcutaneous proliferation of monomorphic spindle-shaped cells arrayed in storiform or cartwheel patterns

SELECTED REFERENCES

1. Heuvel ST et al: Dermatofibrosarcoma protuberans: recurrence is related to the adequacy of surgical margins. Eur J Surg Oncol. 36(1):89-94, 2010
2. Llombart B et al: Dermatofibrosarcoma protuberans: clinical, pathological, and genetic (COL1A1-PDGFB) study with therapeutic implications. Histopathology. 54(7):860-72, 2009
3. Sundram UN: Review: Dermatofibrosarcoma protuberans: histologic approach and updated treatment recommendations. Clin Adv Hematol Oncol. 7(6):406-8, 2009
4. Paradisi A et al: Dermatofibrosarcoma protuberans: wide local excision vs. Mohs micrographic surgery. Cancer Treat Rev. 34(8):728-36, 2008
5. Wang J et al: Detection of COL1A1-PDGFB fusion transcripts in dermatofibrosarcoma protuberans by reverse transcription-polymerase chain reaction using archival formalin-fixed, paraffin-embedded tissues. Diagn Mol Pathol. 8(3):113-9, 1999
6. Mopper C et al: Dermatofibrosarcoma protuberans. Am J Clin Pathol. 20(2):171-6, 1950

DERMATOFIBROSARCOMA PROTUBERANS

Microscopic Features

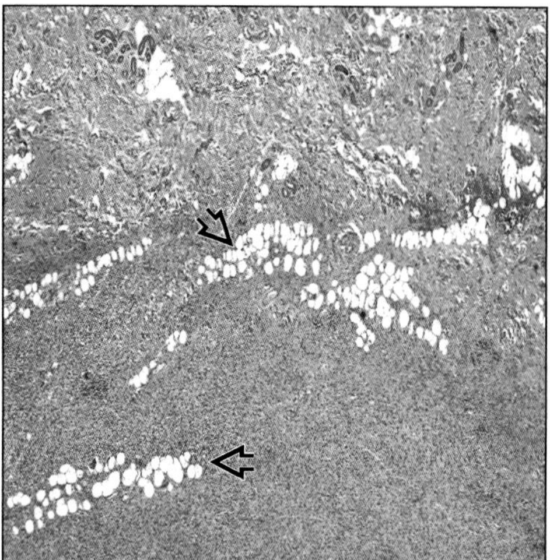

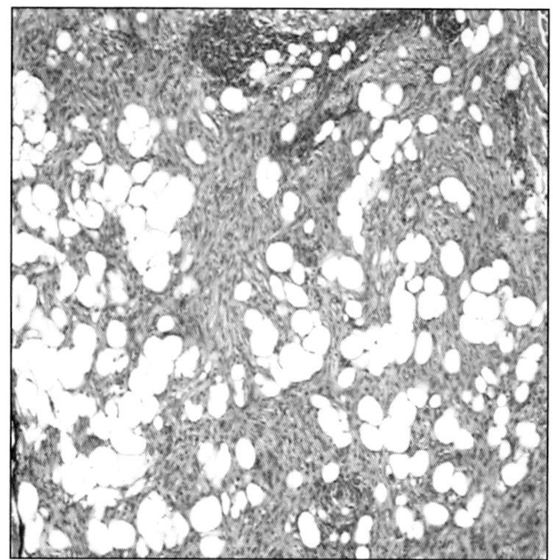

(Left) *There is deep dermal and subcutaneous involvement by a DFSP with prominent "honeycombing" ⊡ fat-trapping. The neoplasm is cellular, giving a "blue" appearance to the proliferation on low power. The borders of the tumor are irregular.* ***(Right)*** *The deep subcutaneous tissues of this DFSP highlight the significant fat entrapment or infiltration. The neoplastic cells are cytologically bland. Mitotic figures are not easily identified.*

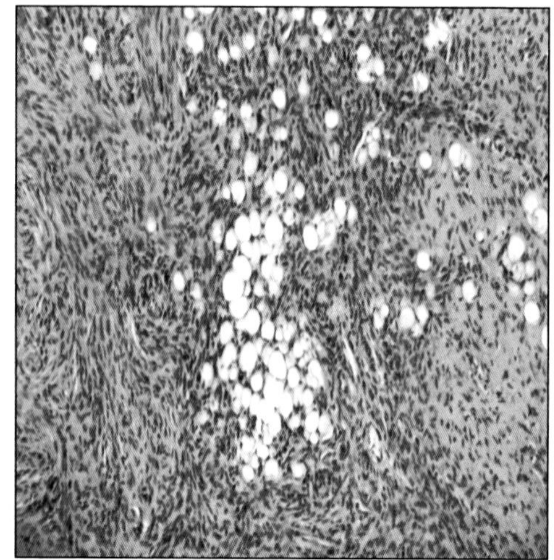

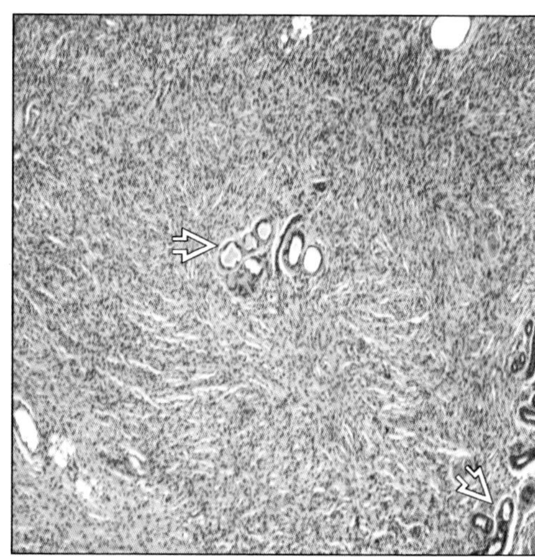

(Left) *In this area, the entrapped adipocytes have undergone atrophy. The proliferation is also more cellular in this area, and the cells show a more hyperchromatic spindled nucleus. Necrosis is absent.* ***(Right)*** *On low power, there are a number of adnexal glands, which are entrapped ⊡ by the cellular, vaguely storiform neoplastic proliferation. However, there is no destruction of these adnexal structures by the tumor.*

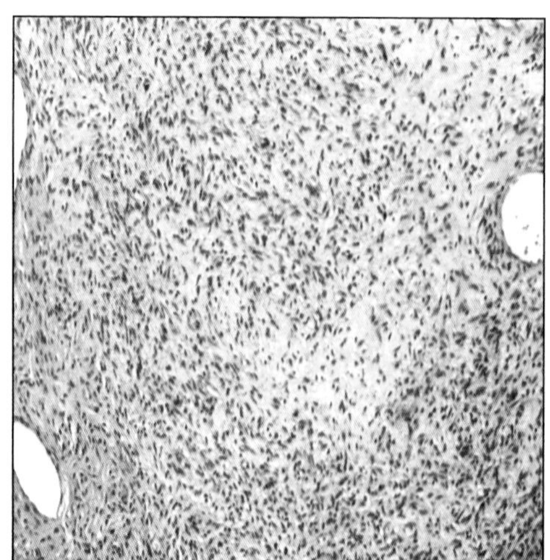

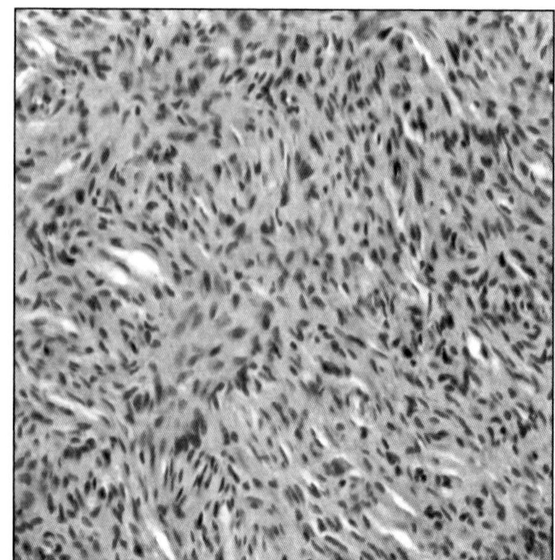

(Left) *Areas of myxoid stromal change may be seen in a minority of cases of DFSP. The myxoid changes gives a lighter stromal appearance to a tumor that is otherwise usually quite densely cellular.* ***(Right)*** *DFSP is a neoplasm that tends to be composed of bland cells, usually lacking in significant pleomorphism or anaplasia. Mitotic figures are often difficult to identify. Note the lack of necrosis.*

Microscopic and Immunohistochemical Features

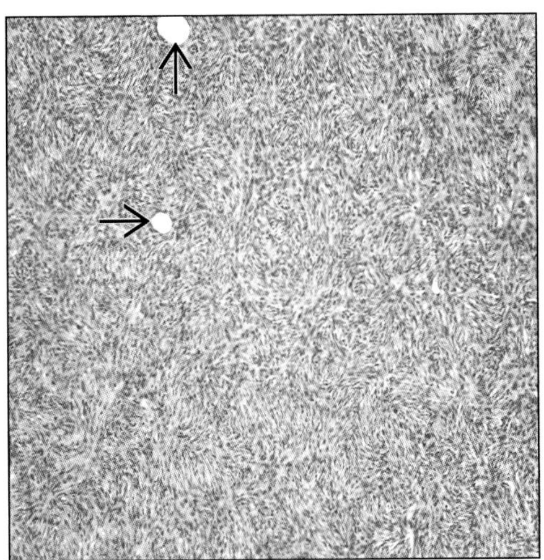

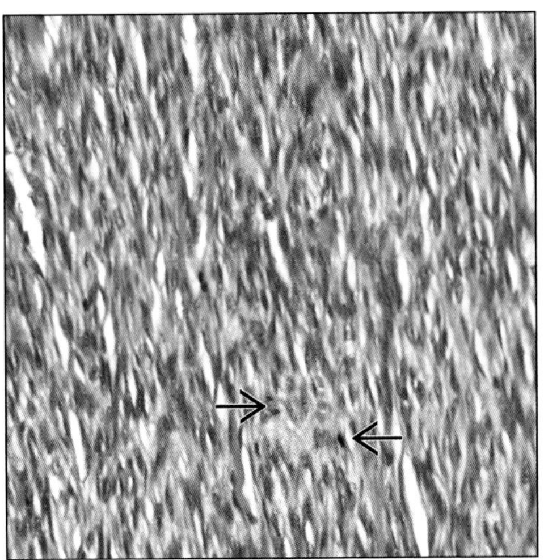

(Left) *Cellular area of DFSP shows a proliferation of densely packed atypical spindle cells with storiforming. A couple of adipocytes ⇨ are surrounded (entrapped) by the neoplastic population.* ***(Right)*** *Fibrosarcomatous transformation in a DFSP is diagnosed when there is increased cellularity, increased cytologic atypia, and multiple mitotic figures ⇨. The tumor is also arranged in a much more fascicular or "herringbone" architecture.*

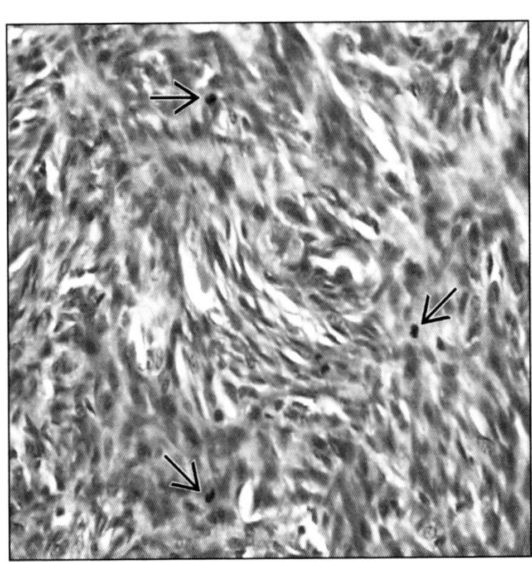

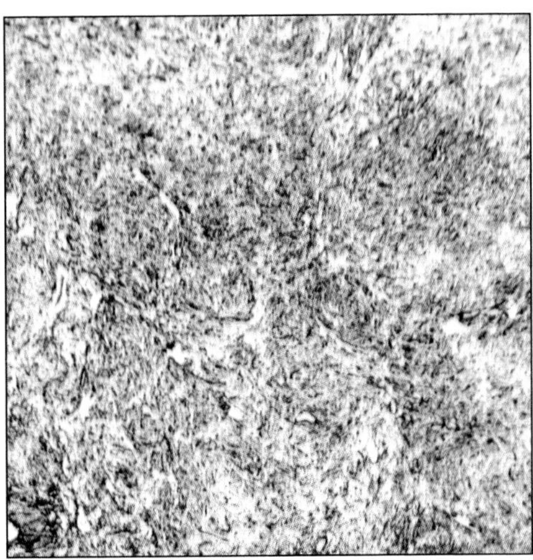

(Left) *Higher power view of fibrosarcomatous transformation in a DFSP shows vague storiforming by atypical spindle cells with numerous mitoses ⇨. This type of pattern tends to result in effacement of the usual pattern of growth seen in DFSP.* ***(Right)*** *Immunohistochemistry for CD34 typically shows strong and diffuse staining of the tumor cells, as well as background blood vessels. It is important to note that CD34 can be weak or absent in some cases.*

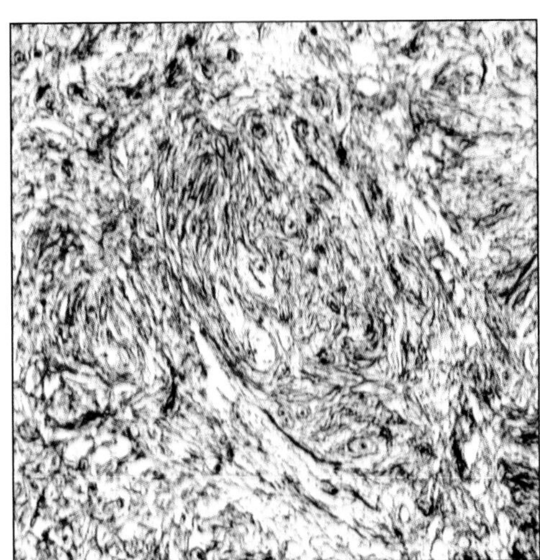

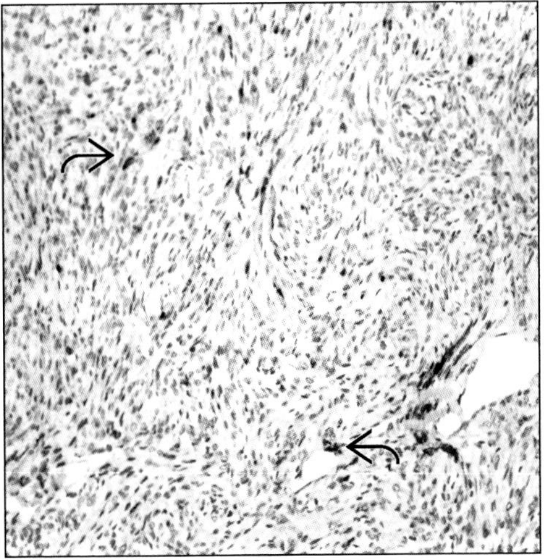

(Left) *Higher power view shows strong immunohistochemical staining for CD34 in nearly all of the tumor spindle cells. Tumor and nontumor vessels will also be highlighted with the stain, a good internal control.* ***(Right)*** *Immunohistochemistry for FXIIIA typically shows only scattered positive entrapped fibroblasts or dendritic cells ⇨, but the majority of the spindle cells are negative. The stain highlights the cytoplasm of these cells.*

CERUMINOUS ADENOCARCINOMA

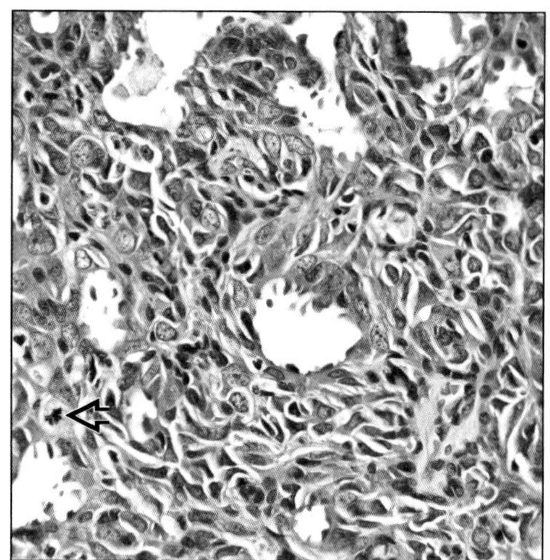

Hematoxylin & eosin shows markedly pleomorphic neoplastic proliferation with apocrine snouts, biphasic appearance, and mitotic figures ⇨ in this ceruminous adenocarcinoma, NOS.

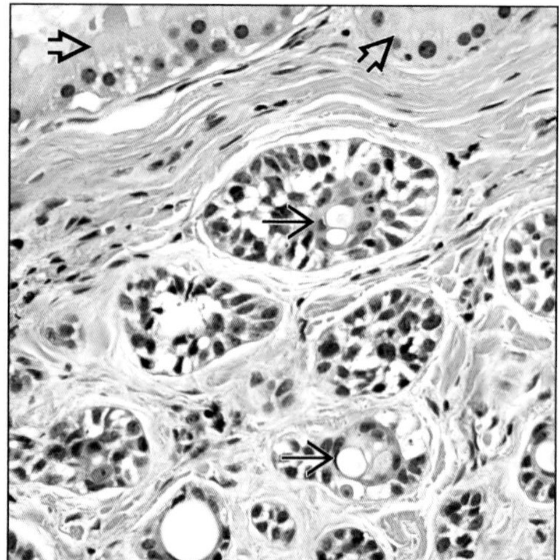

Hematoxylin & eosin shows native ceruminous glands ⇨ adjacent to neoplastic glands with ceruminous differentiation → in this ceruminous ACC.

TERMINOLOGY

Synonyms

- Ceruminal adenocarcinoma, cylindroma, ceruminoma
  - Ceruminous adenocarcinoma, not otherwise specified (NOS)
  - Ceruminous adenoid cystic carcinoma (ACC)
  - Ceruminous mucoepidermoid carcinoma

Definitions

- Malignant neoplasm derived from ceruminous glands of external auditory canal

CLINICAL ISSUES

Epidemiology

- Incidence
  - Rare neoplasm
    - Approximately 0.0003% of all tumors
    - < 2.5% of all external ear neoplasms
- Age
  - Mean: 49 years; range: 21-92 years
- Gender
  - Female > Male (1.5:1)

Site

- Outer 1/3 to 1/2 of external auditory canal

Presentation

- Pain is most common symptom
- Hearing loss (sensorineural or conductive)
- Tinnitus
- Slowly growing mass
- Drainage, discharge, or bleeding

Treatment

- Surgical approaches
  - Wide, radical complete surgical excision, especially when adenoid cystic carcinoma
- Radiation
  - Employed for ceruminous adenocarcinoma and mucoepidermoid carcinoma but usually only palliative

Prognosis

- Good, although approximately 50% of patients die from disease within 3-10 years of presentation
- Recurrences are common, especially if positive surgical margins or ceruminous adenoid cystic carcinoma

IMAGE FINDINGS

General Features

- Defines extent of tumor
- Excludes direct extension from parotid gland or nasopharyngeal tumor

MACROSCOPIC FEATURES

General Features

- Polypoid, often in posterior canal
- Surface ulceration can be seen

Size

- Mean: 1.4 cm
- Range: 0.5-3.0 cm

MICROSCOPIC PATHOLOGY

Histologic Features

- Separated into 3 tumor types
  - Ceruminous adenocarcinoma, NOS
  - Ceruminous adenoid cystic carcinoma
  - Ceruminous mucoepidermoid carcinoma
- Infiltrative into soft tissue, benign ceruminous glands, and bone
- Tumor may secondarily involve surface mucosa
- Cellular, arranged in solid, cystic, cribriform, glandular, and single cell patterns

CERUMINOUS ADENOCARCINOMA

Key Facts

Terminology
- Malignant neoplasm derived from ceruminous glands of external auditory canal

Clinical Issues
- Outer 1/3 to 1/2 of external auditory canal
- Painful mass
- Recurrences are common, especially if positive surgical margins or ceruminous adenoid cystic carcinoma

Microscopic Pathology
- Tumor necrosis (comedonecrosis) diagnostic of carcinoma
- Perineural invasion, if present, helps define malignancy
- Ceroid (cerumen) pigment absent in malignancies
- Separated into 3 tumor types
  - Ceruminous adenocarcinoma
  - Ceruminous adenoid cystic carcinoma
  - Ceruminous mucoepidermoid carcinoma

Ancillary Tests
- Immunohistochemistry highlights biphasic nature of tumor
  - Luminal cells: CK7, CD117
  - Basal cells: p63 (nuclear), S100 protein (cytoplasmic and nuclear), and CK5/6

Top Differential Diagnoses
- Parotid gland primary
- Ceruminous adenoma
- Neuroendocrine adenoma of middle ear

- Tumor necrosis (comedonecrosis) and perineural invasion diagnostic of carcinoma
- Nuclear pleomorphism with prominent nucleoli
- Easily identified mitotic figures, including atypical forms (3/10 HPF)
  - Adenoid cystic carcinoma tends to have fewer mitotic figures
- Desmoplastic stroma between neoplastic epithelial islands
- Ceroid (cerumen, wax) pigment absent in malignancies

Margins
- Must be free of tumor to achieve better long-term prognosis

ANCILLARY TESTS

Immunohistochemistry
- Highlights biphasic nature of tumor
  - Luminal cells: CK7, CD117
  - Basal cells: p63 (nuclear), S100 protein (cytoplasmic and nuclear), and CK5/6

DIFFERENTIAL DIAGNOSIS

Parotid Gland Primary
- Direct extension, especially by adenoid cystic carcinoma
- Must be excluded either clinically or radiographically

Ceruminous Adenoma
- Circumscribed, noninfiltrative, dual cell population with cerumen granules present

Middle Ear Adenoma
- a.k.a. neuroendocrine adenoma of middle ear (NAME)
- Neuroendocrine and epithelial neoplasm with multiple patterns, delicate "salt and pepper" nuclear chromatin, and chromogranin, synaptophysin, and HPP positive

SELECTED REFERENCES

1. Crain N et al: Ceruminous gland carcinomas: a clinicopathologic and immunophenotypic study of 17 cases. Head Neck Pathol. 3(1):1-17, 2009
2. Dong F et al: Adenoid cystic carcinoma of the external auditory canal. Laryngoscope. 118(9):1591-6, 2008
3. Jan JC et al: Ceruminous adenocarcinoma with extensive parotid, cervical, and distant metastases: case report and review of literature. Arch Otolaryngol Head Neck Surg. 134(6):663-6, 2008
4. Thompson LD et al: Ceruminous adenomas: a clinicopathologic study of 41 cases with a review of the literature. Am J Surg Pathol. 28(3):308-18, 2004
5. Iqbal A et al: Ceruminous gland neoplasia. Br J Plast Surg. 51(4):317-20, 1998
6. Aikawa H et al: Adenoid cystic carcinoma of the external auditory canal: correlation between histological features and MRI appearances. Br J Radiol. 70(833):530-2, 1997
7. Contreras A et al: [Adenocarcinoma of the ceruminous glands: report of three cases.] Acta Otorrinolaringol Esp. 45(1):49-51, 1994
8. Ito K et al: An immunohistochemical study of adenoid cystic carcinoma of the external auditory canal. Eur Arch Otorhinolaryngol. 250(4):240-4, 1993
9. Mansour P et al: Ceruminous gland tumours: a reappraisal. J Laryngol Otol. 106(8):727-32, 1992
10. Lynde CW et al: Tumors of ceruminous glands. J Am Acad Dermatol. 11(5 Pt 1):841-7, 1984
11. Hicks GW: Tumors arising from the glandular structures of the external auditory canal. Laryngoscope. 93(3):326-40, 1983
12. Perzin KH et al: Adenoid cystic carcinoma involving the external auditory canal. A clinicopathologic study of 16 cases. Cancer. 50(12):2873-83, 1982
13. Dehner LP et al: Primary tumors of the external and middle ear. Benign and malignant glandular neoplasms. Arch Otolaryngol. 106(1):13-9, 1980
14. Michel RG et al: Ceruminous gland adenocarcinoma: a light and electron microscopic study. Cancer. 41(2):545-53, 1978
15. Koopot R et al: Multiple pulmonary metastases from adenoid cystic carcinoma of ceruminous glands of external auditory canal. A case report and review of the literature. J Thorac Cardiovasc Surg. 65(6):909-13, 1973

CERUMINOUS ADENOCARCINOMA

Microscopic Features

*(**Left**) Hematoxylin & eosin shows uninvolved surface epithelium ⮚ with an infiltrative mixture of patterns in this ceruminous ACC. (**Right**) Hematoxylin & eosin shows invasion to the cartilage ⮚ by a glandular proliferation in this ceruminous adenocarcinoma, NOS.*

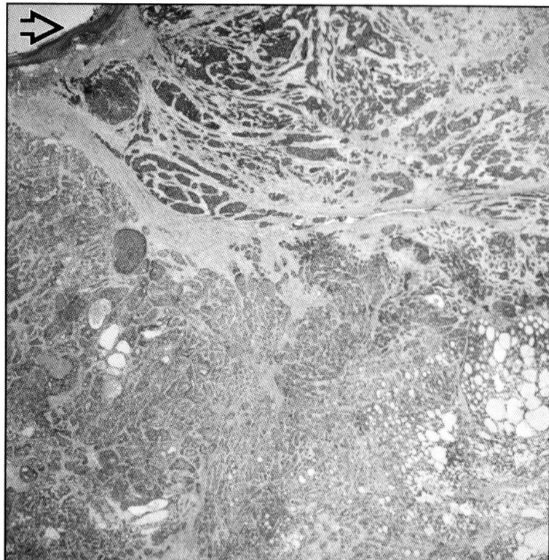

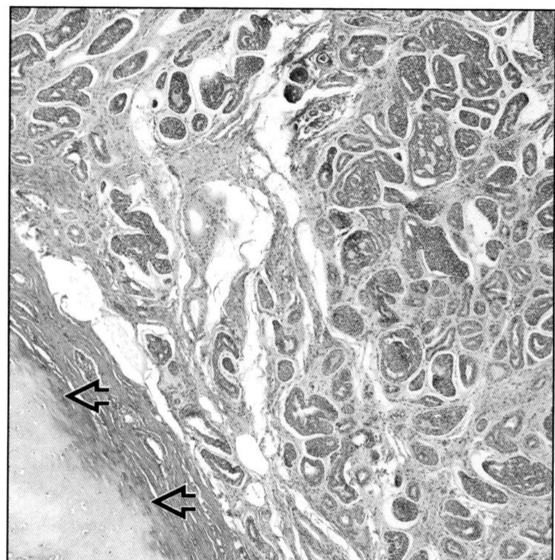

*(**Left**) Hematoxylin & eosin demonstrates a classic "Swiss cheese" cribriform pattern of ceruminous ACC. (**Right**) Hematoxylin & eosin demonstrates a cellular neoplasm, focally showing squamous differentiation and calcification ⮚ in this ceruminous adenocarcinoma, NOS.*

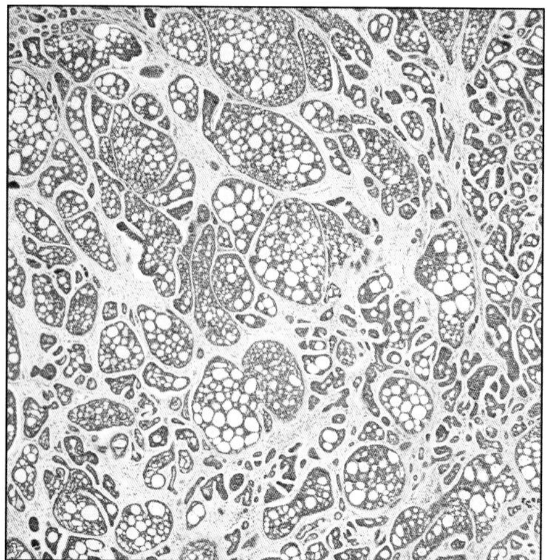

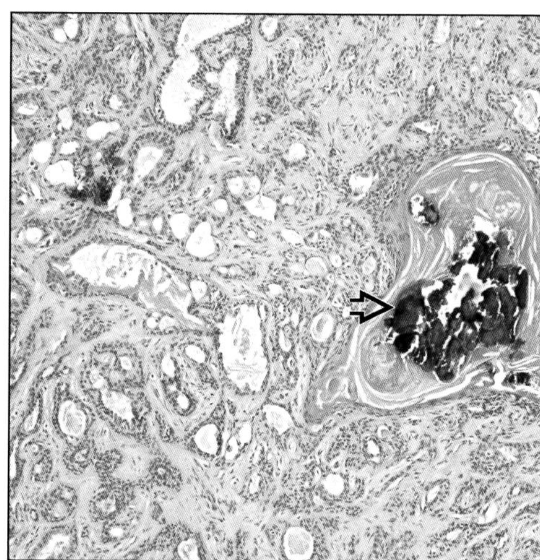

*(**Left**) Hematoxylin & eosin reveals desmoplastic stroma between epithelial cells that show a biphasic appearance in this ceruminous adenocarcinoma, NOS. (**Right**) There is remarkable pleomorphism of the cells with apocrine "snouting" in the glandular cells of this ceruminous adenocarcinoma, NOS.*

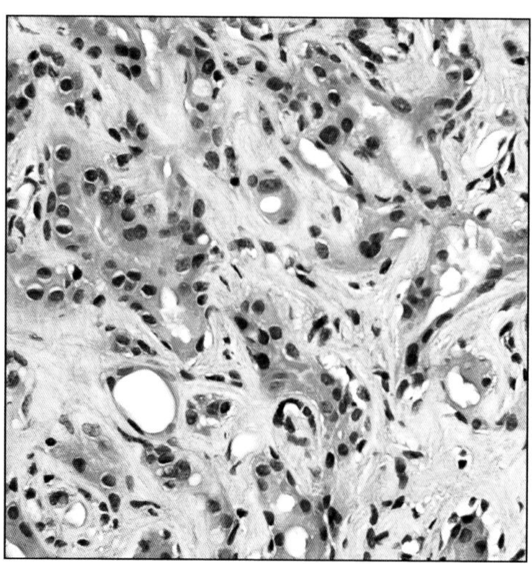

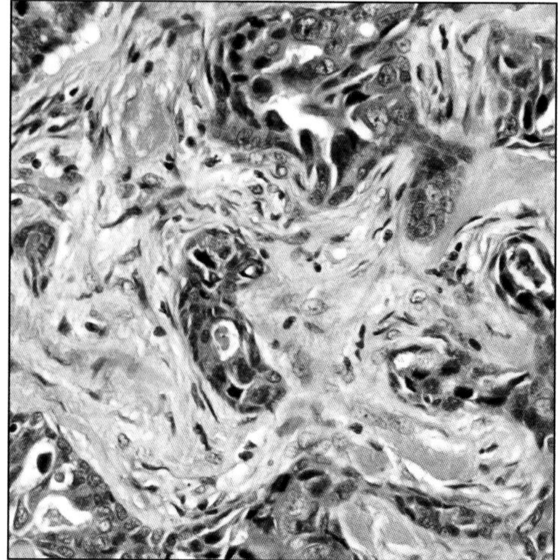

Microscopic and Immunohistochemical Features

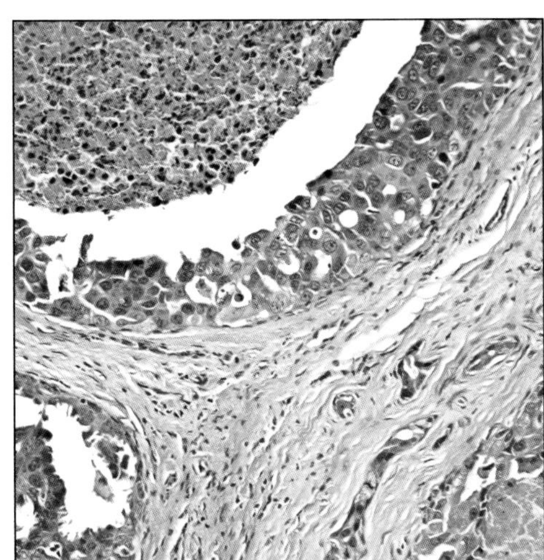

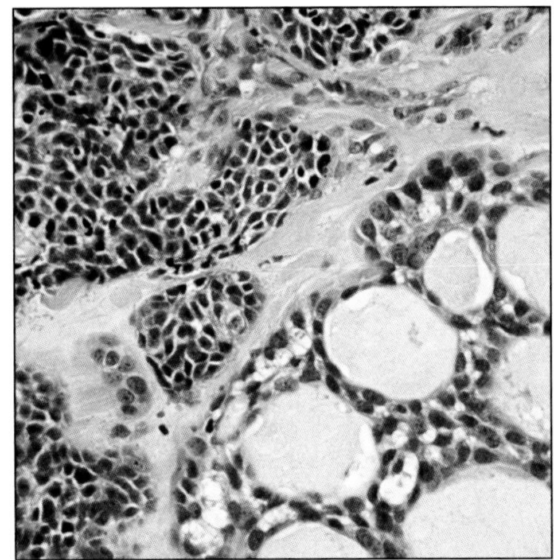

(Left) *A comedo-type necrosis is visible within a markedly pleomorphic epithelium. Comedonecrosis is not common, but when present, helps to define malignancy in ceruminous neoplasms.* ***(Right)*** *A solid pattern and a more characteristic cribriform pattern is seen in this ceruminous ACC. Basophilic material within the pseudocysts is glycosaminoglycans and reduplicated basement membrane material, which is in continuity with the stroma.*

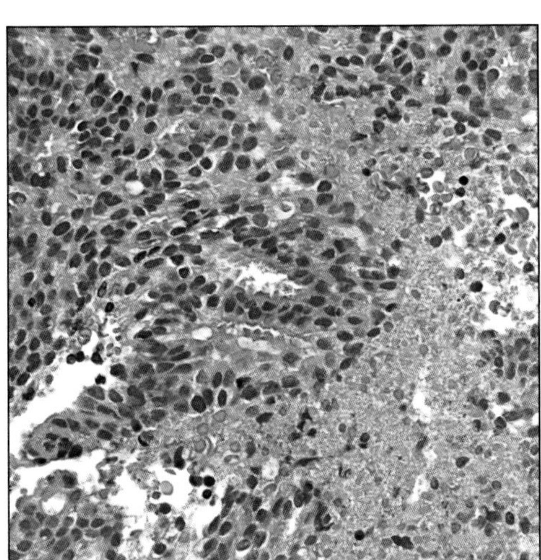

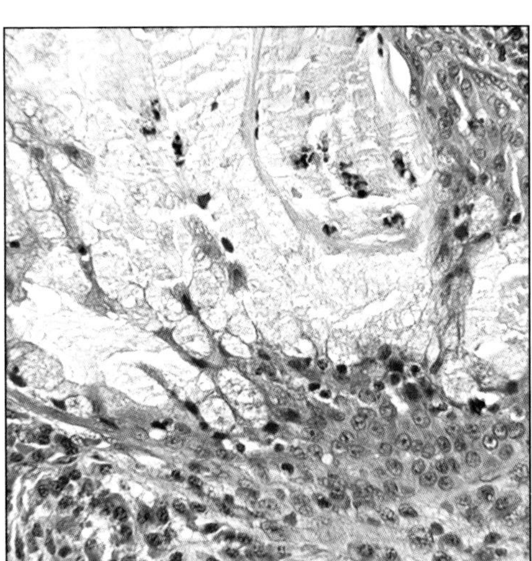

(Left) *Hematoxylin & eosin shows a glandular pattern with necrosis in this ceruminous adenocarcinoma, NOS.* ***(Right)*** *Hematoxylin & eosin reveals a mucoepidermoid carcinoma showing squamoid epithelium containing mucocytes.*

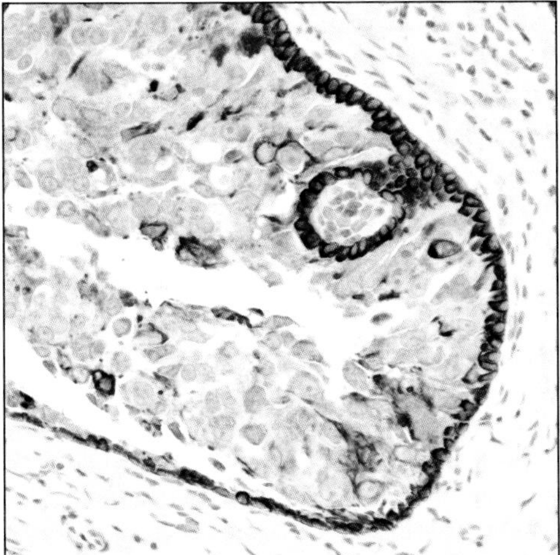

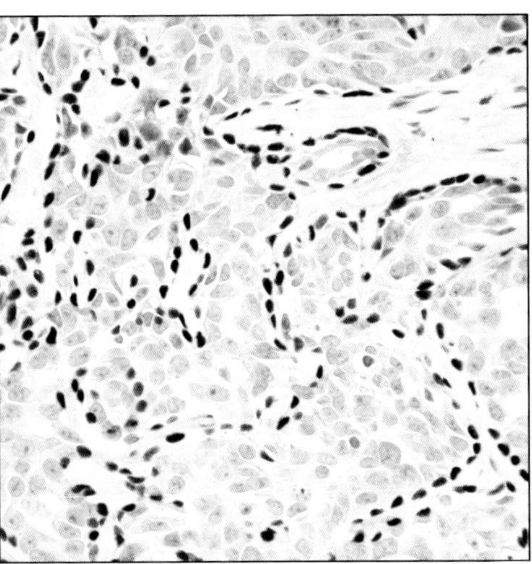

(Left) *CK5/6 shows basal immunoreactivity in this gland of a ceruminous adenocarcinoma.* ***(Right)*** *p63 shows basal immunoreactivity in this ceruminous adenocarcinoma, NOS.*

RHABDOMYOSARCOMA

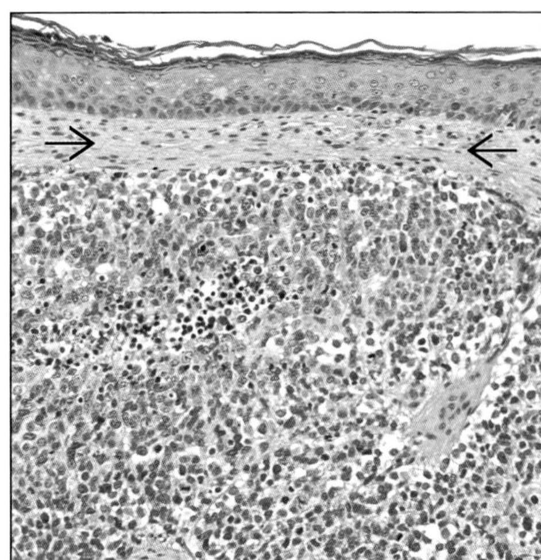

Aural RMS shows an intact surface squamous epithelium with a grenz zone ⇒ between the primitive mesenchymal cells and the surface. This "small round blue cell" pattern is common in embryonal RMS.

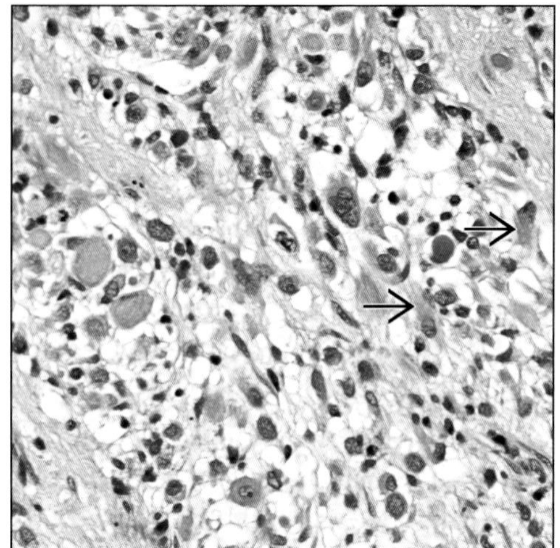

Embryonal RMS with rhabdomyoblasts shows primitive cells with eccentric, eosinophilic cytoplasm. Cytoplasmic extensions create elongated or tadpole cells ⇒. The stroma is myxoid to edematous.

TERMINOLOGY

Abbreviations

- Rhabdomyosarcoma (RMS)

Synonyms

- Embryonal rhabdomyosarcoma
  - Includes spindle, botryoid, and anaplastic variants
- Alveolar rhabdomyosarcoma
  - Includes anaplastic, botryoid, and spindle variants
- Myosarcoma
- Malignant rhabdomyoma
- Rhabdopoietic sarcoma
- Embryonal sarcoma

Definitions

- Primitive malignant soft tissue tumor with histologic and phenotypic features of embryonic skeletal muscle

CLINICAL ISSUES

Epidemiology

- Incidence
  - Most common soft tissue sarcoma in children and adolescents
  - Most common soft tissue sarcoma in head and neck
  - Embryonal RMS is most common in ear
  - Alveolar RMS is most common in sinonasal tract
- Age
  - Young people (usually < 20 years)
    - Embryonal subtype is most frequent
  - Adults may be affected, but less common
    - Alveolar subtype is most frequent
- Gender
  - Male > Female (1.2:1)

Site

- Sites affected (order of frequency)
  - **Head and neck**
    - Orbit and eyelid
    - Oropharynx
    - Parotid gland
    - Ear (auditory canal and middle ear): Botryoid type arises beneath mucosal membrane
    - Nasopharynx, nasal cavity, and paranasal sinuses
  - Urogenital tract
  - Extremities: Arms and legs

Presentation

- Unilateral, refractory otitis media
- Unilateral deafness
- Sanguinous or bloody discharge
- Otalgia
- Neurologic symptoms
- Mass, slowly enlarging

Treatment

- Options, risks, complications
  - Often mismanaged as infection or aural polyp initially
  - Diagnose early to prevent temporal bone destruction and meningeal involvement
  - Complications of treatment include
    - Facial growth retardation, intellectual retardation, neuroendocrine dysfunction
    - Visual changes, dental problems, hearing loss
    - Delayed effects of chondronecrosis
    - Hypothyroidism, esophageal stenosis
    - Second malignancy
    - Intracranial bleeds
- Surgical approaches
  - Wide local excision manages local disease
- Adjuvant therapy
  - Multiagent chemotherapy
    - Agents include: Vincristine, dactinomycin, cyclophosphamide, doxorubicin, melphalan, ifosfamide, etoposide
- Radiation
  - Used specifically to manage local disease
  - Combined with chemotherapy

RHABDOMYOSARCOMA

Key Facts

Terminology
- Primitive malignant tumor with histologic and phenotypic features of embryonic skeletal muscle

Clinical Issues
- Most common soft tissue sarcoma in children and adolescents
- Young people (usually < 20 years)
- Male > Female (1.2:1)
- Unilateral, refractory otitis media
- Embryonal RMS is most common in ear
- Often mismanaged as infection or aural polyp initially
- Relative good prognosis: 60% 5-year survival overall
  - Age, stage, anatomic site, and histologic subtype dependent

Macroscopic Features
- Polypoid mass, often with intact epithelial surface

Microscopic Pathology
- Primitive mesenchymal cells
- Rhabdomyoblasts: Eccentric, eosinophilic cytoplasm
- Cytoplasmic eosinophilia with tadpole, elongated cytoplasmic extensions

Ancillary Tests
- Translocations generate *PAX3-FKHR* (t(2;13)(q35;q14) and *PAX7-FKHR* (t(1;13)(p36;q14) gene fusions

Top Differential Diagnoses
- Aural polyp
- Fetal rhabdomyoma
- Lymphoma

  - May not be necessary for group I patients

Prognosis
- Considered systemic disease by definition
- Relatively good: ~ 60% 5-year survival overall
  - Depends on age, stage, anatomic site, and histologic subtype
    - 80% 5-year survival for group I patients
    - Anatomic site prognosis: Head and neck > genitourinary > extremities > retroperitoneum
- Highly aggressive neoplasm with rapid expansion into pharynx and cranial cavity
- Most tumors present as pT2 lesions
- Smaller tumors tend to behave better
- *PAX7-FKHR* tumors: Younger patients, less locally aggressive, seem to have better prognosis than *PAX3-FKHR* tumors

IMAGE FINDINGS

General Features
- Used to delineate extent of disease for staging purposes
  - May include chest and abdomen CT and bone scan for metastatic disease
- Expansile soft tissue mass
- Heterogeneous signals showing mixture of stroma, necrosis, and vascularity

MACROSCOPIC FEATURES

General Features
- Polypoid mass, often with intact epithelial surface
- Poorly circumscribed
- Fleshy, pale tan mass
- Spindle cell tumors are more fibrous and firm with whorled cut surface

Size
- Usually small (anatomic site dependent)
- Usually < 2.5 cm

MICROSCOPIC PATHOLOGY

Histologic Features
- Usually intact surface epithelium
- Primitive mesenchymal cells
- Fascicles and whorls of spindle cells
- Rhabdomyoblasts (eccentric, eosinophilic cytoplasm) may be seen
- Stellate cells with round nuclei
- Cytoplasmic eosinophilia with tadpole, elongated cytoplasmic extensions
- Cross striations are uncommon and difficult to identify
- Multinucleation may be seen
- Myxoid background stroma is common
- Necrosis may be noted
- Botryoid variant has cambium layer
  - Increased cellularity immediately below intact surface
  - Then hypocellular deeper into stroma

ANCILLARY TESTS

Cytology
- Smears used as triage for ancillary studies (immunohistochemistry, molecular FISH analysis)
- Cellular smears with plasmacytoid rhabdomyoblasts
- Small blue round cell appearance
- Lacks lymphoglandular bodies and cellular cohesion

Histochemistry
- PAS-diastase highlights cytoplasmic glycogen

Immunohistochemistry
- Muscle markers positive

Cytogenetics
- Alterations in short arm of chromosome 11 (11p15)

In Situ Hybridization
- Alveolar RMS shows *FKHR* gene fusions with *PAX3* or *PAX7*

RHABDOMYOSARCOMA

Immunohistochemistry

Antibody	Reactivity	Staining Pattern	Comment
Vimentin	Positive	Cytoplasmic	All tumor cells
Myogenin	Positive	Nuclear	All tumor cells
MITF	Positive	Nuclear	All tumor cells
Desmin	Positive	Cytoplasmic	Most tumor cells (eccentric)
Actin-HHF-35	Positive	Cytoplasmic	Most tumor cells are positive
Actin-sm	Positive	Cytoplasmic	
MYOD1	Positive	Nuclear	Myoblast determination protein 1 (MYOD1)
Myoglobin	Positive	Cytoplasmic	
Myosin	Positive	Cytoplasmic	
CD56	Positive	Cytoplasmic	Many cases will have positive reaction
CK-PAN	Positive	Dot positivity	< 5% of cases with isolated cells
CD45RB	Negative		
Chromogranin-A	Negative		
HMB-45	Negative		
S100	Negative		

    - *FKHR*: Forkhead homolog 1 at chromosome 13q14.1
    - *PAX3*: Paired box homeotic gene 3 (2q35)
        - Mutations result in gain of function when fused with *FKHR* gene
    - *PAX7*: Paired box gene 7 (1p36.2-p36.12)
        - Variant translocation
    - Translocations generate *PAX3-FKHR* [t(2;13)(q35;q14)] and *PAX7-FKHR* [t(1;13)(p36;q14)] gene fusions
        - 5' *PAX3*-3' *FKHR* chimeric transcript produces fusion protein
        - Intact *PAX3* DNA binding domains, truncated *FKHR* DNA binding domain, and C-terminal *FKHR* regions
- FISH break apart probe most easily detects *FKHR* fusion

DIFFERENTIAL DIAGNOSIS

Aural Polyp

- Plasma cells and lymphocytes within stroma

Lymphoma

- Atypical lymphoid cells with B- or T-cell monoclonal population

Melanoma

- Surface involvement, pigment, S100 protein and HMB-45 immunoreactivity

PNET/Ewing Sarcoma

- "Small round blue cell" tumor with necrosis, hyperchromatic nuclei, and lack of myogenic immunophenotype

Fetal Rhabdomyoma

- Young age, spindle cell proliferation with gradient of cellularity, lack of cytologic atypia, muscle differentiation

STAGING

Intergroup Rhabdomyosarcoma Study

- Group I
    - Local disease only
- Group II
    - Residual disease or local spread
- Group III
    - Incomplete resection with gross residual disease
- Group IV
    - Metastatic disease at onset

SELECTED REFERENCES

1. Raney B et al: Results in patients with cranial parameningeal sarcoma and metastases (Stage 4) treated on Intergroup Rhabdomyosarcoma Study Group (IRSG) Protocols II-IV, 1978-1997: report from the Children's Oncology Group. Pediatr Blood Cancer. 51(1):17-22, 2008
2. Durve DV et al: Paediatric rhabdomyosarcoma of the ear and temporal bone. Clin Otolaryngol Allied Sci. 29(1):32-7, 2004
3. Sautter NB et al: Embryonal rhabdomyosarcoma of the ear. Ear Nose Throat J. 83(5):316-7, 2004
4. Hawkins DS et al: Improved outcome for patients with middle ear rhabdomyosarcoma: a children's oncology group study. J Clin Oncol. 19(12):3073-9, 2001
5. Maroldi R et al: Computed tomography and magnetic resonance imaging of pathologic conditions of the middle ear. Eur J Radiol. 40(2):78-93, 2001
6. Paulino AC et al: Long-term effects in children treated with radiotherapy for head and neck rhabdomyosarcoma. Int J Radiat Oncol Biol Phys. 48(5):1489-95, 2000
7. Mehta S et al: Rhabdomyosarcoma of head and neck--an analysis of 24 cases. Indian J Cancer. 33(1):37-42, 1996
8. Wiener ES: Head and neck rhabdomyosarcoma. Semin Pediatr Surg. 3(3):203-6, 1994
9. Wiatrak BJ et al: Rhabdomyosarcoma of the ear and temporal bone. Laryngoscope. 99(11):1188-92, 1989

Diagrammatic, Radiographic, and Microscopic Features

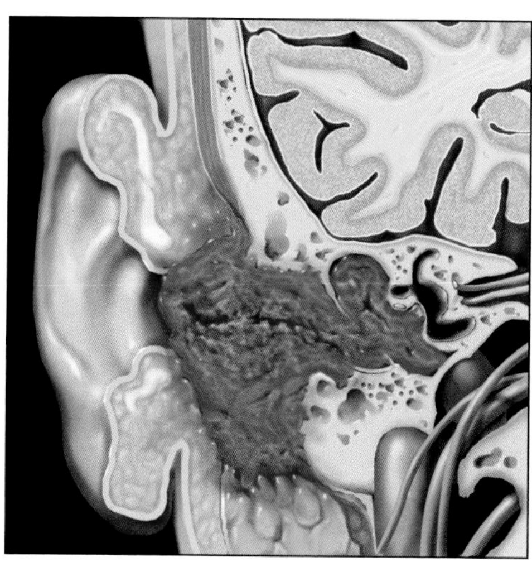

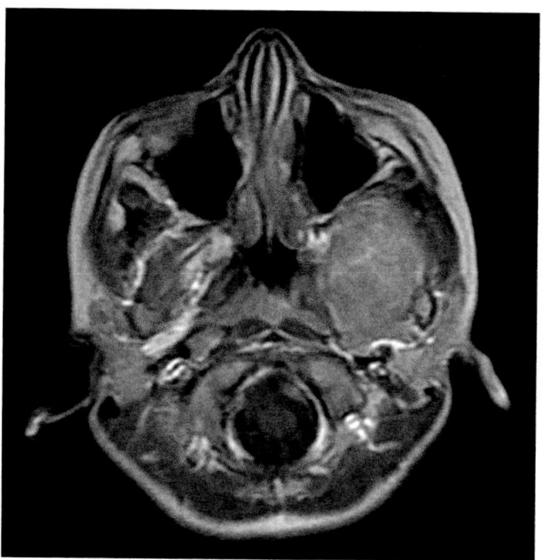

(Left) *This diagrammatic representation shows a rhabdomyosarcoma affecting the external auditory canal, temporal bone, middle ear, and expanding into the salivary gland. A "mass" in the external ear canal is frequently the presenting symptom.* ***(Right)*** *Axial MR T1-weighted image (post contrast) shows slightly heterogeneous enhancement of a rhabdomyosarcoma identified in the ear and masticator space. This finding is nonspecific but does delineate the extent of the tumor.*

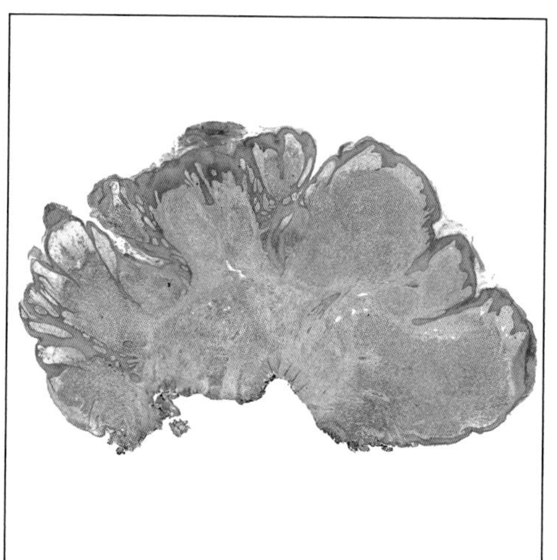

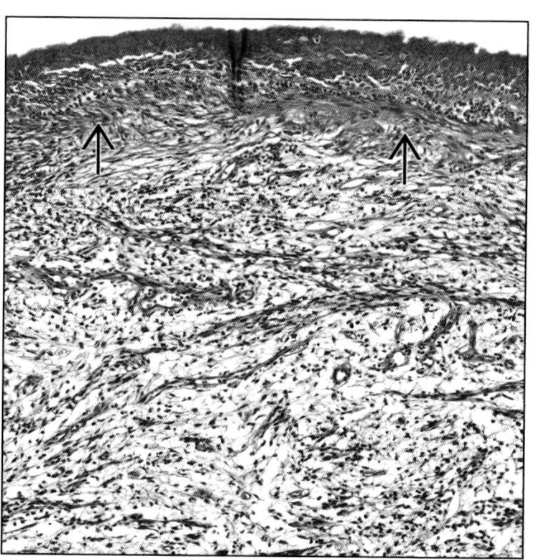

(Left) *Rhabdomyosarcoma are frequently polypoid masses, often with an intact epithelial surface. This was an aural "polyp" identified in the external auditory canal.* ***(Right)*** *The surface epithelium is intact overlying this botryoid variant of embryonal RMS. There is a cambium layer (increased cellularity ⇒ immediately below an intact surface), overlying a gradient of cellularity, which becomes more hypocellular as it goes deeper. The stroma is myxoid.*

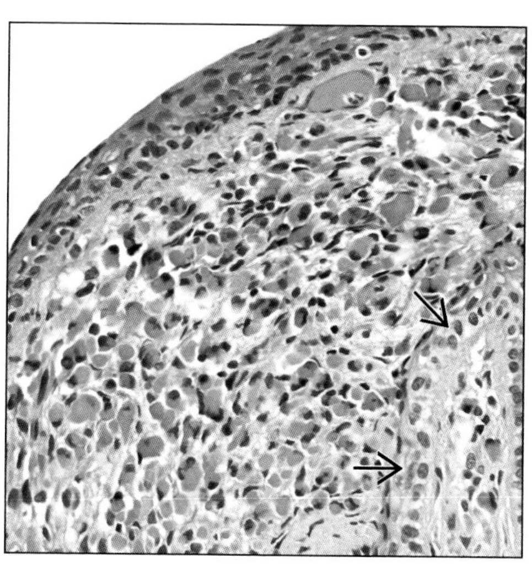

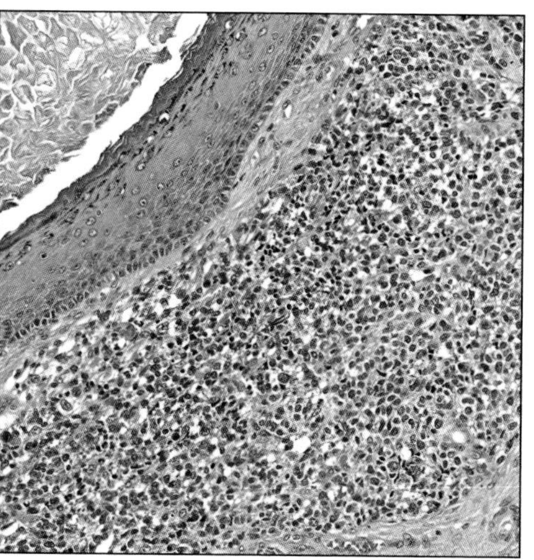

(Left) *The epidermis is intact, subtended by a sheet-like distribution of rhabdomyoblasts, showing eccentric, eosinophilic cytoplasm around dark nuclei. An uninvolved ceruminous gland ⇒ is present.* ***(Right)*** *The primitive "small round blue cell" pattern of this embryonal rhabdomyosarcoma can frequently be misinterpreted to represent chronic inflammation (otitis media). However, the atypia and destructive growth are tip-offs to the diagnosis.*

RHABDOMYOSARCOMA

Microscopic and Cytologic Features

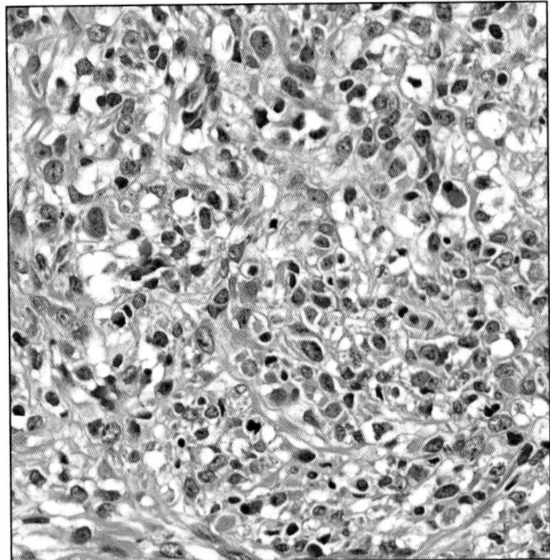

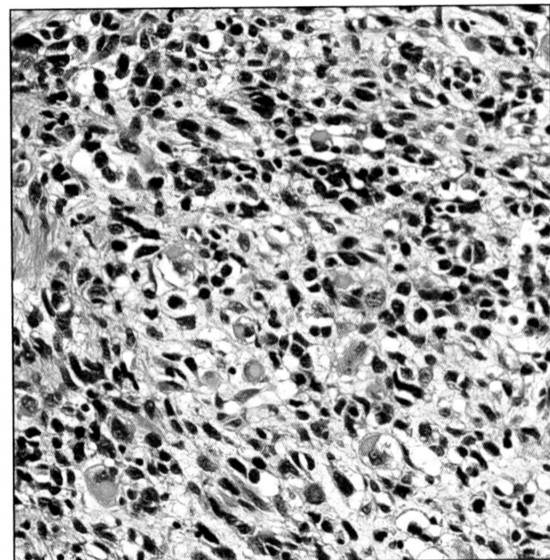

*(**Left**) These primitive mesenchymal cells are arranged in a haphazard pattern. However, there is pleomorphism and increased mitoses. This type of tumor benefits from immunohistochemistry studies. (**Right**) There are spindled cells and rhabdomyoblasts in this RMS. The nuclear chromatin is often coarse and heavy. Eosinophilic, eccentric cytoplasm is a helpful clue to the diagnosis.*

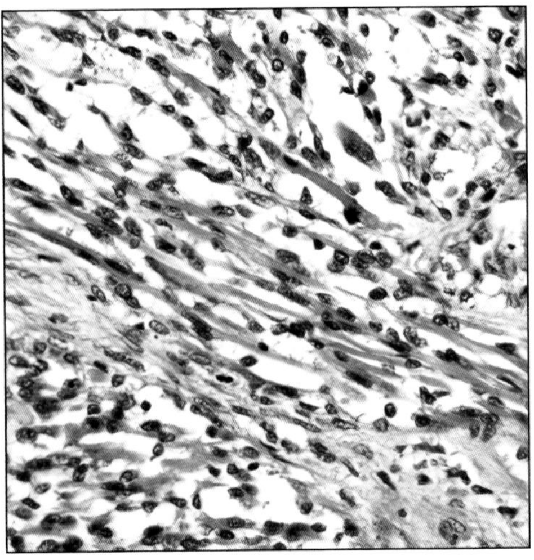

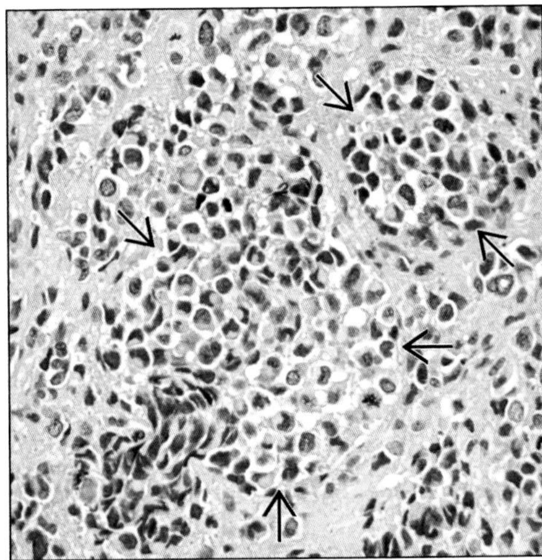

*(**Left**) There is a fascicular arrangement to this RMS. The cells are stellate, showing remarkably elongated cytoplasmic extension. A few cells have cross striations, but they are difficult to detect without special studies or oil magnification. (**Right**) An alveolar RMS shows a vague alveolus ⇒ with cells adherent at the periphery and then showing central degeneration or a dilapidated appearance. Note the remarkable eccentric, eosinophilic cytoplasm.*

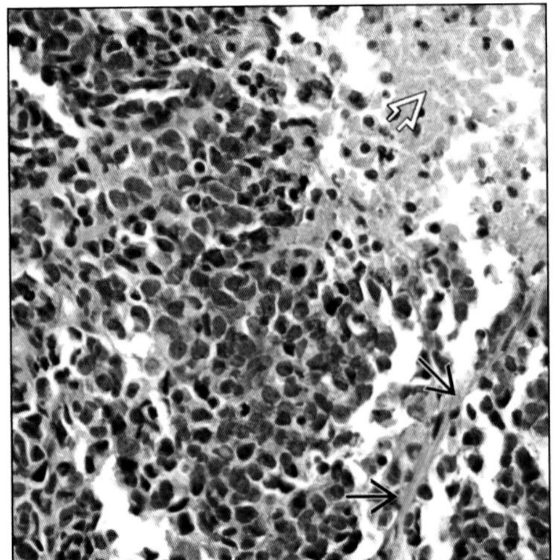

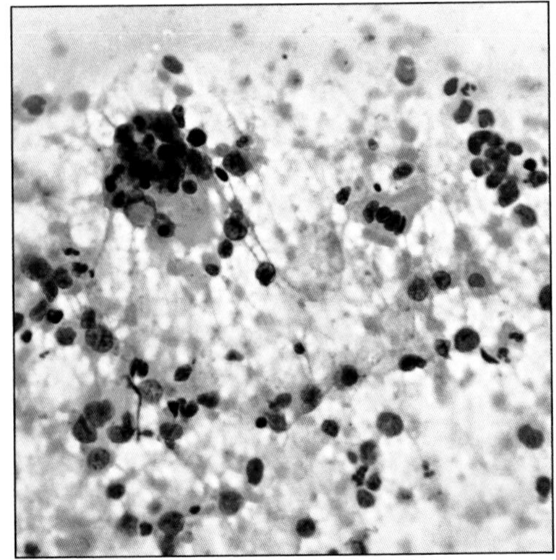

*(**Left**) This alveolar RMS is comprised of "small blue round cells" shown falling off the scaffolding ⇒ of the stroma. Tumor necrosis ➡ is present, a finding that is not common in head and neck tumors. (**Right**) FNA smears are cellular, showing small dyscohesive aggregates of "small blue round cells" and eccentric cytoplasm focally. The background is degenerated but lacks lymphoglandular bodies or lymphoid tangles.*

Ancillary Techniques

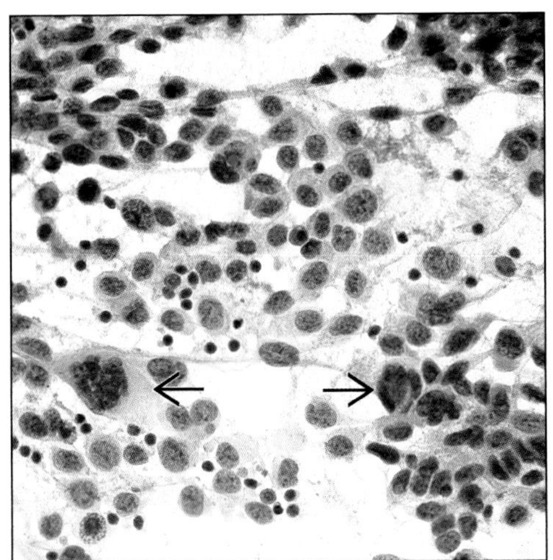

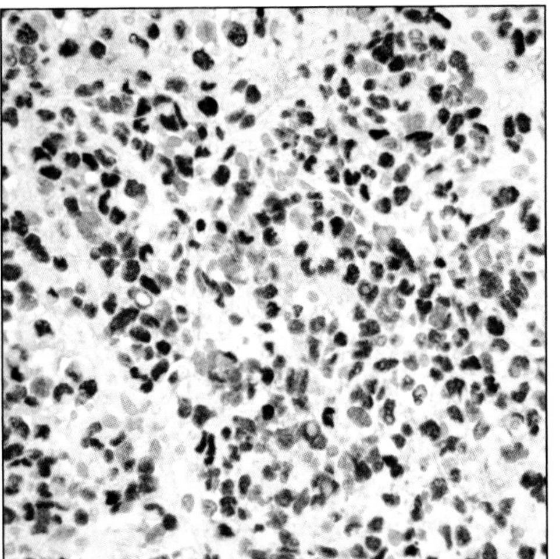

(Left) *The cellular smears show a small amount of cytoplasm surrounding round nuclei. A focally plasmacytoid appearance is noted. Focal degenerative changes are present. Multinucleated giant tumor cells* ➔ *are present.* ***(Right)*** *A variety of muscle markers are positive in RMS. Myogenin gives a strong, diffuse, nuclear reaction in nearly all of the tumor cells of a rhabdomyosarcoma.*

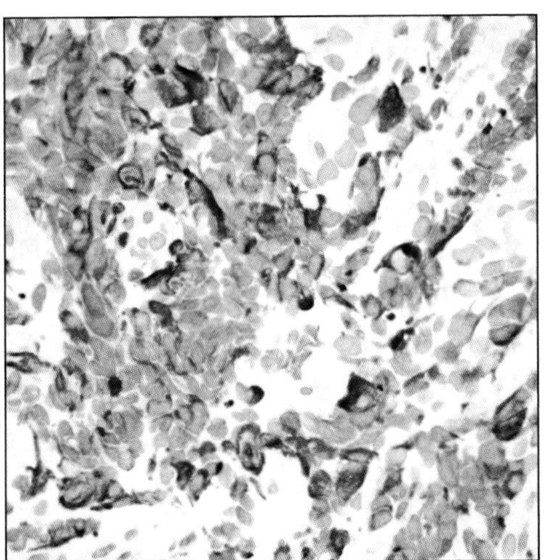

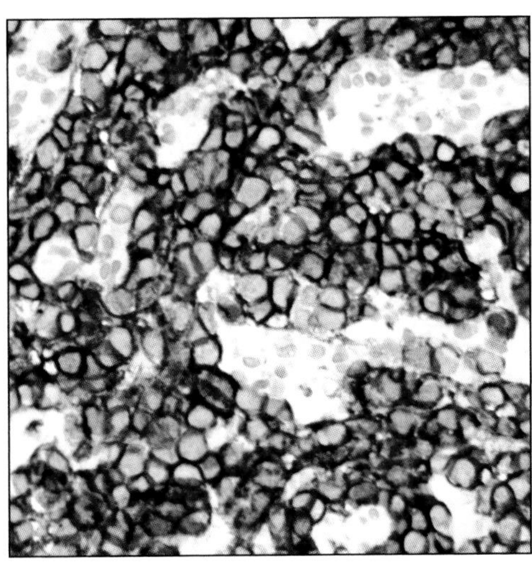

(Left) *There is frequent variability in reactivity with the muscle markers used to confirm the diagnosis of RMS. Note that not all of the tumor cells are reactive with desmin. However, the pattern of reaction highlights the eccentric or tadpole cytoplasm.* ***(Right)*** *A number of nonmyogenic markers are positive in rhabdomyosarcoma, including a strong and diffuse membranous reactivity with CD56 (pictured), and focal, dot-like keratin reactivity in about 5% of cases.*

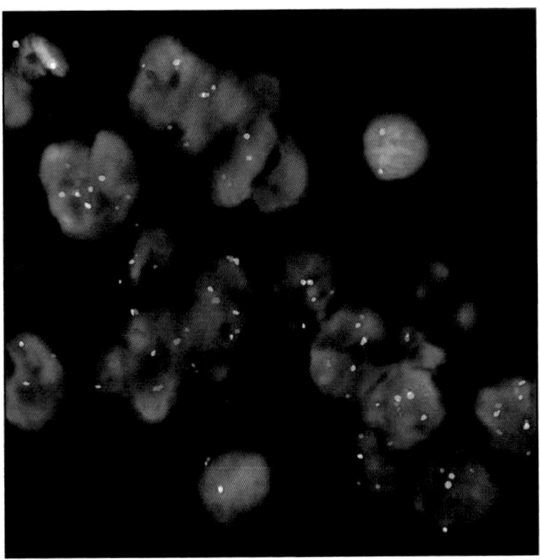

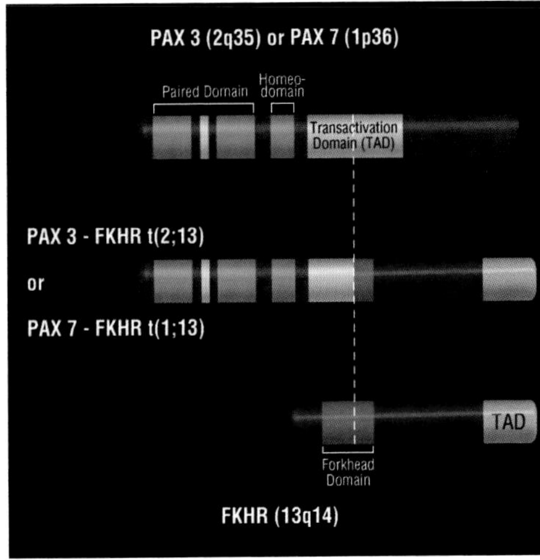

(Left) *FISH shows rearrangement of the FKHR (FOXO1) gene. Two probes (green and orange) in the Vysis LSI break apart probe show rearrangement is present by detecting green and orange signals, rather than the "yellow" signal identified in normal cells that lack the translocation.* ***(Right)*** *This diagrammatic representation shows the breakpoints and subsequent fusion sites between FKHR (13q14) forkhead region and either PAX3 (2q35) or PAX7 (1p36) transactivation domain region.*

METASTATIC/SECONDARY TUMORS

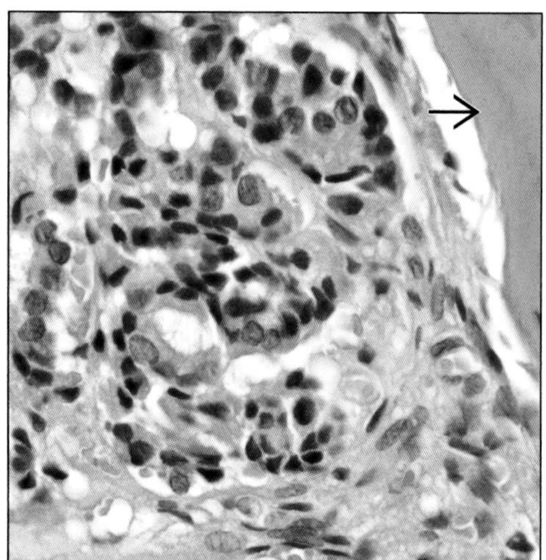

Hematoxylin & eosin shows back to back glands within a stroma adjacent to spicules of bone ⇒ as an example of metastatic breast carcinoma.

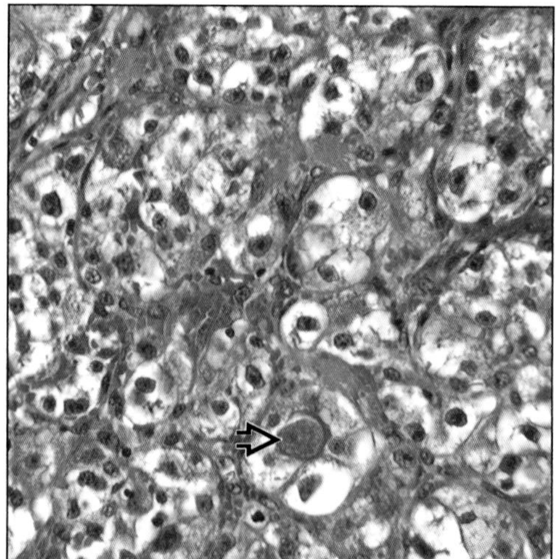

Hematoxylin & eosin shows glands with erythrocytes within pseudolumen ⇨, with a pseudoalveolar pattern of metastatic renal cell carcinoma.

TERMINOLOGY

Synonyms

- Secondary tumors

Definitions

- Tumors that secondarily involve ear &/or temporal bone, which originate from, but are not in continuity with, primary malignancies of other sites
  - Some include direct continuity in this definition
  - Lymphomas and leukemias are excluded by definition

CLINICAL ISSUES

Epidemiology

- Incidence
  - Uncommon (< 2% of all malignancies of ear and temporal bone) in surgical pathology
  - Up to 20% in autopsy studies performed on cancer patients with disseminated disease
- Age
  - Older ages, correlated with increased malignancies of other anatomic sites
- Gender
  - Female > Male (but tumor type dependent)

Site

- Usually bilateral, multiple, and include other bones
- Petrous apex most common site (~ 80%)
- Mastoid bone, internal auditory canal, and middle ear

Presentation

- Asymptomatic
  - Most common (about 1/3 of patients)
- Presentation is late in disease course
- Changes in hearing
- Dizziness, tinnitus
- Facial palsy and otalgia
- Otorrhea, mass

Treatment

- Options, risks, complications
  - Rarely, may be isolated metastases
- Surgical approaches
  - Excision is performed for symptomatic relief

Prognosis

- Matches underlying disease but usually part of disseminated disease

MACROSCOPIC FEATURES

General Features

- Lytic or blastic lesion depending on tumor type

Size

- Variable but may be quite large

MICROSCOPIC PATHOLOGY

Histologic Features

- Vascular-lymphatic metastases have different profile than direct extension
- Specific tumor type dictates histology
- Most common tumors are carcinomas
  - Breast (~ 25%)
  - Lung (~ 10%)
  - Prostate (~ 10%)
- Melanoma (~ 6%)
- Mesenchymal tumors rarely metastasize to ear and temporal bone
- Direct extension via eustachian tube, posterior fossa of skull, and external ear from parotid gland area
  - Upper aerodigestive tumors most common

METASTATIC/SECONDARY TUMORS

Key Facts

Clinical Issues

- Middle ear most frequently
- Petrous apex most common site (~ 80%)
- Mastoid bone, internal auditory canal, middle ear
- Usually bilateral, multiple, and include other bones
- Mastoid bone, internal auditory canal, middle ear
- Excision is performed for symptomatic relief
- Matches underlying disease but usually part of disseminated disease
- Uncommon (< 2% of all malignancies of ear and temporal bone) in surgical pathology

Microscopic Pathology

- Most common tumors are carcinomas
  - Breast (~ 25%)
  - Lung (~ 10%)
  - Prostate (~ 10%)
- Direct extension must be excluded (eustachian tube, posterior fossa of skull, parotid gland)

ANCILLARY TESTS

Immunohistochemistry

- Pertinent and targeted antibodies used to confirm metastatic disease

DIFFERENTIAL DIAGNOSIS

Direct Extension

- Direct extension from salivary gland, nasopharynx, brain or skin needs to be excluded
  - In general, this can be achieved by
    - Clinical history
    - Radiographic studies
    - Architectural and histologic features
    - Immunohistochemistry
    - Molecular studies

Primary Tumor

- Poorly differentiated ear primaries may mimic metastatic tumors
  - Middle ear adenoma
  - Squamous cell carcinoma
  - Primary middle ear adenocarcinoma

SELECTED REFERENCES

1. Shrivastava V et al: Prostate cancer metastatic to the external auditory canals. Clin Genitourin Cancer. 5(5):341-3, 2007
2. Yasumatsu R et al: Metastatic hepatocellular carcinoma of the external auditory canal. World J Gastroenterol. 13(47):6436-8, 2007
3. Suzuki T et al: Sudden hearing loss due to meningeal carcinomatosis from rectal carcinoma. Auris Nasus Larynx. 33(3):315-9, 2006
4. Carson HJ et al: Metastasis of colonic adenocarcinoma to the external ear canal: an unusual case with a complex-pattern of disease progression. Ear Nose Throat J. 84(1):36-8, 2005
5. Michaelson PG et al: Metastatic renal cell carcinoma presenting in the external auditory canal. Otolaryngol Head Neck Surg. 133(6):979-80, 2005
6. Ueyama H et al: Solitary metastasis of prostatic cancer to the internal auditory canal. Clin Neurol Neurosurg. 105(3):180-2, 2003
7. Kundu S et al: Extensive metastatic renal cell carcinoma presenting as facial nerve palsy. J Laryngol Otol. 115(6):488-90, 2001
8. Ziegler EA et al: [Bilateral progressive hearing loss as the first manifestation of metastatic carcinoma of the head of the pancreas. Case report] Laryngorhinootologie. 80(8):436-8, 2001
9. Ferri GG et al: [Metastasis in the inner auditory canal] Acta Otorhinolaryngol Ital. 18(4):269-75, 1998
10. Ingelaere PP et al: Metastatic renal cell carcinoma presenting as an aural polyp. J Laryngol Otol. 111(11):1066-8, 1997
11. Suzuki Y et al: Sudden bilateral hearing loss due to gastric carcinoma and its histological evidence. J Laryngol Otol. 111(12):1142-6, 1997
12. Cumberworth VL et al: Late metastasis of breast carcinoma to the external auditory canal. J Laryngol Otol. 108(9):808-10, 1994

IMAGE GALLERY

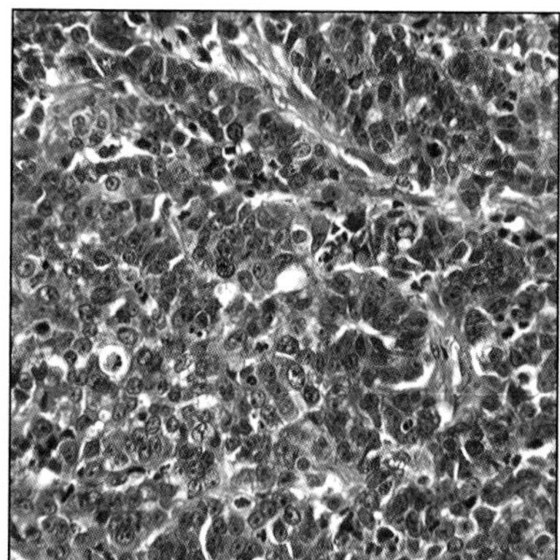
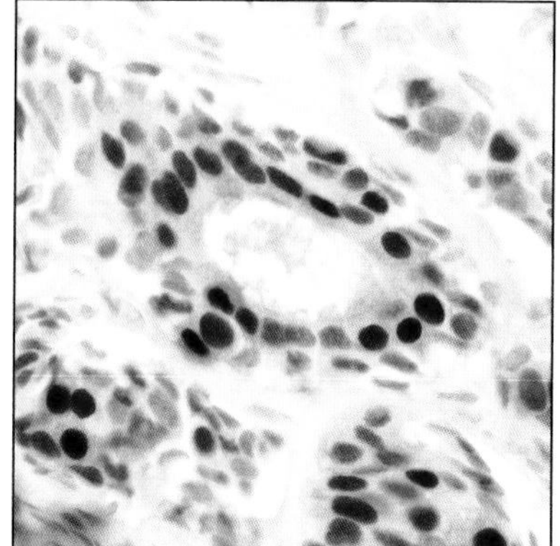
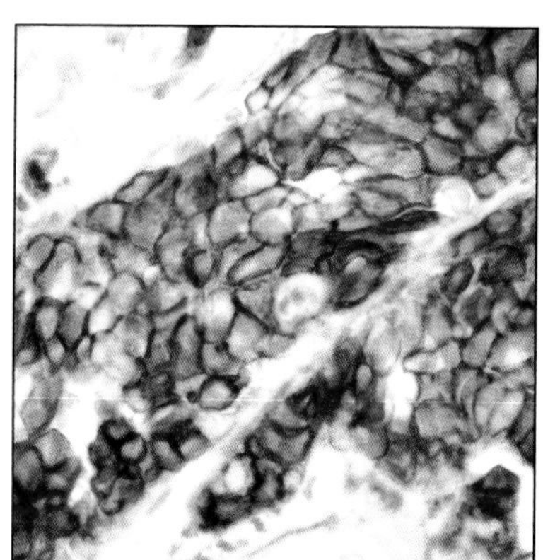

(Left) *There are back to back glands lined by columnar cells in a metastatic colon adenocarcinoma. Further positive reactivity with CDX-2 and CK20 would help to confirm the diagnosis.* ***(Center)*** *The estrogen receptor shows shows strong and diffuse nuclear reactivity within glandular profiles. This helps to support a diagnosis of metastatic breast carcinoma.* ***(Right)*** *There is strong, circumferential membrane reactivity with HER-2/neu in this metastatic breast carcinoma.*

Neck (Soft Tissue and Lymph Nodes)

Congenital/Genetic/Hereditary

Infectious

Inflammatory-Immune Dysfunction

Reactive

Benign Neoplasm

Malignant Neoplasm

BRANCHIAL CLEFT CYST

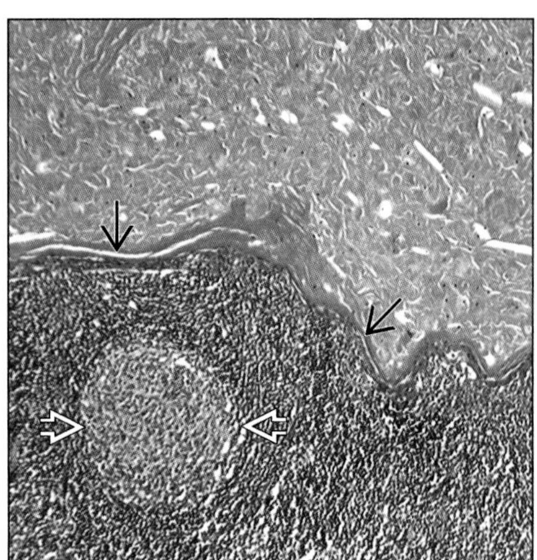

The lumen of this BCC is filled with keratinaceous debris. There is a thin, squamous epithelium ⇨ without any atypia. There is a germinal center ➡ within the associated lymphoid tissue.

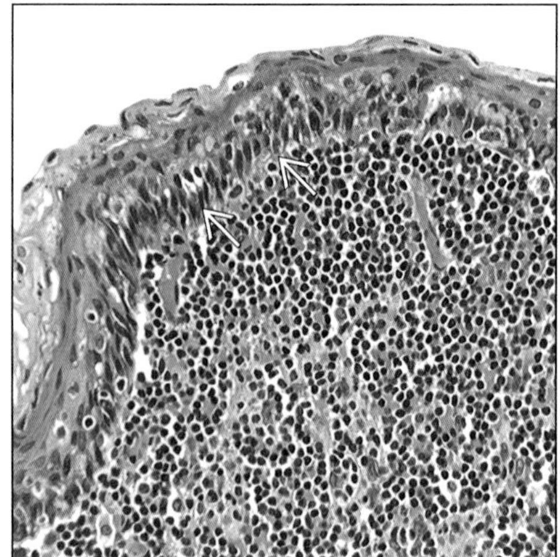

The cyst is lined by metaplastic squamous epithelium, although a residuum of columnar epithelium is still present ➡. There is a very thin basement membrane between the epithelium and lymphoid tissue.

TERMINOLOGY

Abbreviations

- Branchial cleft cyst (BCC)

Synonyms

- Lateral neck cyst
- Cervical lymphoepithelial cyst

Definitions

- By convention, "branchial cleft cyst" refers to congenital developmental lateral cervical cyst derived from remnants of 2nd branchial apparatus
  - ~ 80-90% of all branchial anomalies arise from 2nd branchial apparatus
  - Encompasses branchial cyst, sinus, or fistula

ETIOLOGY/PATHOGENESIS

Branchial Apparatus

- Precursor of many head and neck structures
- 2nd branchial arch overgrows 2nd, 3rd, and 4th clefts
- This overgrowth forms "cervical sinus"
- Embryogenesis usually complete by 6-7 weeks of gestation
- Failure of obliteration of cervical sinus results in 2nd branchial cleft remnant (cyst, sinus, or fistula)
  - Respiratory epithelium lined pharyngeal tonsils while not native to salivary glands
  - Squamous metaplasia and lymphoid hyperplasia develop as consequence of immunologic stimulation during infection
- 2nd branchial cleft fistula extends from skin anterior to sternocleidomastoid muscle (SCM), through carotid artery bifurcation to terminate in tonsillar fossa
- 3rd and 4th branchial cleft cysts are very uncommon (< 5%)
  - Recurrent neck abscess or acute suppurative thyroiditis
  - Vast majority on left side (90-95%)
- Some posit cystic transformation of cervical lymph nodes
  - Especially in adults

CLINICAL ISSUES

Epidemiology

- Incidence
  - Uncommon
    - Still, BCC are one of the most commonly encountered congenital anomalies in pediatric otolaryngic practice
    - Thyroglossal duct cysts are most common
  - BCC accounts for ~ 20% of all congenital cervical cysts
    - Cysts > > sinuses (3:1)
  - About 80-90% of all branchial cleft anomalies are 2nd branchial cleft cysts
  - 4th branchial cleft anomalies are rare and involve larynx (neonatal stridor and recurrent deep neck infection)
- Age
  - Bimodal presentation
    - < 5 years old
    - 20-40 years old (75%)
    - ~ 1% in > 50 years
- Gender
  - Equal gender distribution

Site

- Lateral neck near mandibular angle
- Along anterior border of SCM
  - Anywhere from hyoid bone to suprasternal notch
- Curiously, left-sided predominance for 4th branchial anomalies (> 90%)

Presentation

- Painless cervical swelling
  - Along anterior border of SCM

BRANCHIAL CLEFT CYST

Key Facts

Terminology

- Branchial cleft cyst refers to congenital developmental lateral cervical cyst derived from remnants of 2nd branchial apparatus

Etiology/Pathogenesis

- Failure of obliteration of cervical sinus results in 2nd branchial cleft remnant (cyst, sinus, or fistula)

Clinical Issues

- BCC: ~ 20% of all congenital cervical cysts
- Bimodal presentation (< 5 years; 20-40 years)
- Waxing and waning, painless, compressible, cervical swelling
  - Enlarges after upper respiratory tract infection
- Along anterior border of sternocleidomastoid muscle
- Initial work-up of suspected branchial cleft anomaly (in order)
  - Intravenous or oral antibiotics (if infected), FNA, endoscopy &/or radiographic studies, surgery
- Complete surgical excision yields a low recurrence risk

Microscopic Pathology

- Usually a unilocular cyst
- Cyst lined by various types of epithelium (90% stratified squamous)
- Lymphoid aggregates in cyst wall

Top Differential Diagnoses

- Metastatic cystic squamous cell carcinoma, bronchial cyst, cervical thymic cyst, metastatic thyroid papillary carcinoma

  - Often present for long duration
  - May be painful (if infected)
- Waxing and waning lesion
  - Frequently enlarges in concert with upper respiratory tract infection
  - Patients present during phase of recent enlargement
  - May lie dormant (clinically silent) for years
- Compressible, fluctuant
- Mucoid or pus-like secretions from sinus tract skin opening (when opening is present)
  - Patients present with external fistulae ± internal opening
- Clinically, some lesions may mimic parotid mass or odontogenic infection
- Bilateral lesions are usually identified in syndromic or familial association
- Clinically, 1st or 4th BCC more likely to have incision and drainage procedures, resulting in "recurrence"
- **Important**: Must consider metastatic cystic squamous cell carcinoma in adults

Endoscopic Findings

- Advocated as part of initial assessment of neck cyst
  - Assess internal opening or draining sinus/fistula

Natural History

- Repeated infections and inflammation

Treatment

- Options, risks, complications
  - Initial work-up of suspected branchial cleft anomaly (in order)
    - Intravenous or oral antibiotics (if infected)
    - Fine needle aspiration
    - Endoscopy (concurrent with surgery in some cases)
    - Radiographic studies
    - Surgery in nonresolving cases
  - Avoid repeated incision and drainage
    - Yields high recurrence rate
  - Noninfected lesions are more easily removed than infected lesions
  - Entire fistula tract must be removed to prevent recurrence
  - Complications include
    - Possible wound infection
    - Cranial nerve paresis
- Surgical approaches
  - Combined, simultaneous endoscopic identification of sinus tract with lateral external cervical dissection
    - Cauterization of fistula used by some
    - Endoscopic placement of catheter into sinus lumen before surgical exploration
  - Complete surgical excision
    - May be difficult in recurrent cases due to scarring
    - Excision performed during quiescent phase (no active infection; 6-8 weeks after antibiotics)
    - May need to include thyroid lobectomy to decrease recurrences
  - Must dissect around cyst bed to exclude fistula
    - If superomedial tract: Usually ends in faucial tonsil
    - If inferior tract: Travels down carotid space, exiting in supraclavicular area skin

Prognosis

- Lesions are benign without malignant potential
- Recurrence rate is variable
  - < 3% if not infected before surgery
  - ~ 20% if infected or previously incised/drained or incompletely removed

IMAGE FINDINGS

Radiographic Findings

- Combination of radiographic studies and endoscopy greatly improve surgical management and outcome
- Contrast CT (or MR) will easily suggest this diagnosis and differentiate it from a solid mass
- Well-circumscribed nonenhancing low-density cystic mass with smooth cavity and thin wall (unless infected)
  - If infected, wall is thicker and enhances (cellulitis)

BRANCHIAL CLEFT CYST

- Cystic, ovoid to rounded mucoid density mass in characteristic location is diagnostic
- Location
  - Posterolateral to submandibular gland
  - Lateral to carotid space
  - Anteromedial to sternocleidomastoid muscle
  - Most are at or immediately caudal to mandibular angle
- Focal rim of cyst extending to carotid bifurcation
  - "Notch" sign is pathognomonic for 2nd BCC

MACROSCOPIC FEATURES

General Features

- Unilocular
- Contain clear to grumous material

Size

- Wide range, up to 10 cm

MICROSCOPIC PATHOLOGY

Histologic Features

- Usually a unilocular cyst
- Cyst lined by various types of epithelium
  - Stratified squamous (90%)
  - Respiratory epithelium (~ 8%)
    - Considered native lining in uninflamed cyst
  - Transitions or both (2%)
- Lumen is filled with keratinaceous debris in many cases
- Lymphoid aggregates usually subtend epithelial lining
  - Basement membrane frequently seen between epithelium and lymphoid elements
- Reactive germinal centers commonly present (~ 80%)
- Lymph node architecture is not present
  - No subcapsular sinus formation
  - No medullary region
  - No interfollicular zone
- Acute and chronic inflammation frequently present
- Foreign body giant cell reaction within wall of cyst
- Fibrosis is frequently seen
  - Not heavy, thick "capsule" formation seen in metastatic cystic squamous cell carcinoma (SCC)
- Salivary gland tissue may be detected in wall
- Adnexa and cartilage are not seen in this type of BCC
  - Only seen in 1st branchial cleft cysts/sinuses
- Absence of
  - Dysplasia
  - Pleomorphism
  - Carcinoma

ANCILLARY TESTS

Cytology

- Fine needle aspiration is recommended in evaluation of all neck cysts
  - Usually of residual cyst post-antibiotic therapy
- Thick, yellow, pus-like material is aspirated
- Smears are generally cellular
- Comprised of anucleate squames and mature squamous epithelium
  - Columnar respiratory type cells are less common
- Amorphous debris often associated with macrophages
- Lymphoid infiltrate, including plasma cells

Immunohistochemistry

- Variety of keratins are positive, depending on type of lining
  - Pseudostratified respiratory, transitional, stratified keratinizing, or nonkeratinizing squamous epithelium
- p16 negative in BCC but positive in metastatic SCC of oropharyngeal origin
- Glucose transporter 1 (*GLUT-1*) negative in BCC but positive in metastatic cystic SCC

DIFFERENTIAL DIAGNOSIS

Metastatic Cystic Squamous Cell Carcinoma

- Jugulo-digastric lymph node most commonly affected
- Unilocular cyst
- Very thick and well-developed capsule
- Subcapsular sinus, medullary zone, and interfollicular zones usually identified
- Ribbon-like distribution of atypical epithelium
- Lack of maturation, cellular enlargement, mitoses
- Pleomorphism is often limited and subtle
- Primary usually identified in
  - Tonsil and base of tongue
    - Often p16 positive
  - Nasopharynx
    - Often EBER positive
- For practical purposes: Primary branchiogenic carcinoma does not exist!

Bronchogenic Cyst

- Identified in subcutaneous tissue of supraclavicular region
- Radiographic appearance is different from BCC: Low in neck
- Cyst is lined by respiratory mucosa
- Cyst wall containing smooth muscle and bronchial glands

Metastatic Cystic Thyroid Papillary Carcinoma

- Lymph node architecture is easily identified
- May be unilocular lesion, with only serum or clear fluid in lumen
- Lining shows characteristic features of thyroid papillary carcinoma
  - Large cuboidal to columnar cells
  - Cellular crowding and overlapping
  - Cells have high nuclear to cytoplasmic ratio
  - Nuclear features of papillary carcinoma
    - Nuclear grooves
    - Nuclear contour irregularities
    - Intranuclear cytoplasmic inclusions
    - Nuclear chromatin clearing
  - Papillary architecture is frequently absent
  - Thyroglobulin and TTF-1 immunoreactive

Cervical Thymic Cyst
- Often develop in children
- Affecting lateral cervical region
  - Angle of mandible to sternum, although usually lower neck
- Thymic tissue is present in cyst wall
  - Hassall corpuscles (squamous eddies)
  - Calcifications
  - Lymphoid elements

Lymphangioma
- Generally a clinical consideration
- Usually involves posterior cervical space
- Endothelial-lined spaces with serum, lymphocytes, and smooth muscle wall

Thyroglossal Duct Cyst
- Midline location
- Associated with thyroid tissue
- Hyoid bone involved

Dermoid Cyst
- Sequestration of ectodermal tissue only
- Floor of mouth is most common location
- Squamous lining without lymphoid elements
- **No** other components
  - Muscle
  - Nerve
  - Cartilage

Laryngocele
- Midline lesion, seldom confused with BCC
- Clinically classified into internal, external, and mixed types
- Lacks lymphoid stroma

SELECTED REFERENCES

1. Nicoucar K et al: Management of congenital fourth branchial arch anomalies: a review and analysis of published cases. J Pediatr Surg. 44(7):1432-9, 2009
2. Ozolek JA: Selective pathologies of the head and neck in children: a developmental perspective. Adv Anat Pathol. 16(5):332-58, 2009
3. Doshi J et al: Branchial cyst side predilection: fact or fiction? Ann Otol Rhinol Laryngol. 116(2):112-4, 2007
4. Kadhim AL et al: Pearls and pitfalls in the management of branchial cyst. J Laryngol Otol. 118(12):946-50, 2004
5. Thompson LD: Branchial cleft cyst. Ear Nose Throat J. 83(11):740, 2004
6. Weiner MF et al: Diagnostic value of GLUT-1 immunoreactivity to distinguish benign from malignant cystic squamous lesions of the head and neck in fine-needle aspiration biopsy material. Diagn Cytopathol. 31(5):294-9, 2004
7. Glosser JW et al: Branchial cleft or cervical lymphoepithelial cysts: etiology and management. J Am Dent Assoc. 134(1):81-6, 2003
8. Prasad KK et al: Cervical thymic cyst: report of a case and review of the literature. Indian J Pathol Microbiol. 44(4):483-5, 2001
9. Koeller KK et al: Congenital cystic masses of the neck: radiologic-pathologic correlation. Radiographics. 19(1):121-46; quiz 152-3, 1999
10. Edmonds JL et al: Third branchial anomalies. Avoiding recurrences. Arch Otolaryngol Head Neck Surg. 123(4):438-41, 1997
11. Regauer S et al: Lateral neck cysts--the branchial theory revisited. A critical review and clinicopathological study of 97 cases with special emphasis on cytokeratin expression. APMIS. 105(8):623-30, 1997
12. Thompson LD: Diagnostically challenging lesions in head and neck pathology. Eur Arch Otorhinolaryngol. 254(8):357-66, 1997
13. Choi SS et al: Branchial anomalies: a review of 52 cases. Laryngoscope. 105(9 Pt 1):909-13, 1995
14. Clevens RA et al: Familial bilateral branchial cleft cysts. Ear Nose Throat J. 74(6):419-21, 1995
15. Blackwell KE et al: Functional neck dissection for treatment of recurrent branchial remnants. Arch Otolaryngol Head Neck Surg. 120(4):417-21, 1994
16. Golledge J et al: The aetiology of lateral cervical (branchial) cysts: past and present theories. J Laryngol Otol. 108(8):653-9, 1994
17. Todd NW: Common congenital anomalies of the neck. Embryology and surgical anatomy. Surg Clin North Am. 73(4):599-610, 1993
18. Rosenfeld RM et al: Fourth branchial pouch sinus: diagnosis and treatment. Otolaryngol Head Neck Surg. 105(1):44-50, 1991
19. Takimoto T et al: Branchial cleft (pouch) anomalies: a review of 42 cases. Auris Nasus Larynx. 18(1):87-92, 1991
20. Godin MS et al: Fourth branchial pouch sinus: principles of diagnosis and management. Laryngoscope. 100(2 Pt 1):174-8, 1990
21. Kenealy JF et al: Branchial cleft anomalies: a five-year retrospective review. Trans Pa Acad Ophthalmol Otolaryngol. 42:1022-5, 1990
22. Doi O et al: Branchial remnants: a review of 58 cases. J Pediatr Surg. 23(9):789-92, 1988
23. Harnsberger HR et al: Branchial cleft anomalies and their mimics: computed tomographic evaluation. Radiology. 152(3):739-48, 1984

BRANCHIAL CLEFT CYST

Diagrammatic and Imaging Features

__(Left)__ The failure of a branchial apparatus cleft (c) or pouch (p) to involute or fuse during embryologic development results in the development of 2nd, 3rd, and 4th branchial cleft anomalies. __(Right)__ A 2nd branchial cleft cyst/ sinus/fistula can develop anywhere along the normal development of the branchial pouches and arches. The opening in the tonsil may be associated with a tract along the anterior border of the SCM, which extends to a supraclavicular skin opening .

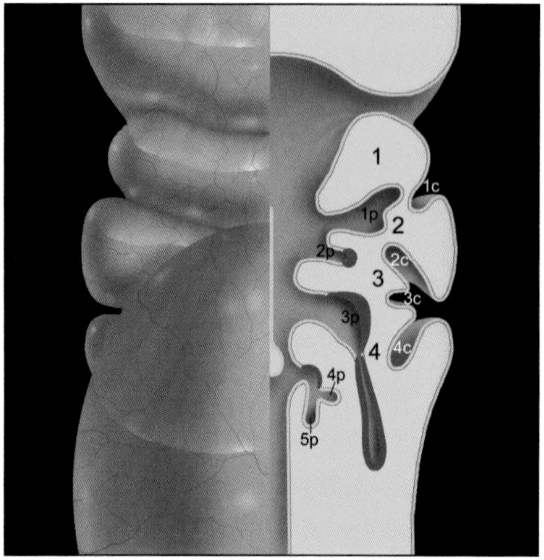

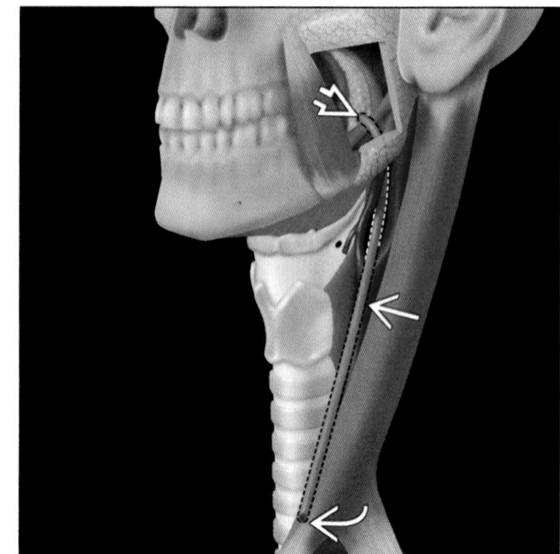

__(Left)__ This clinical photograph shows a compressible lateral neck mass in a young adult male, quite characteristic for a 2nd branchial cleft cyst. The patient came to clinical attention after an upper respiratory tract viral infection. __(Right)__ CT shows a low-attenuation nonenhancing right branchial cleft cyst anterolateral to the carotid sheath , anteromedial to SCM , and posterolateral to the submandibular gland . This is characteristic of a noninflamed branchial cleft cyst.

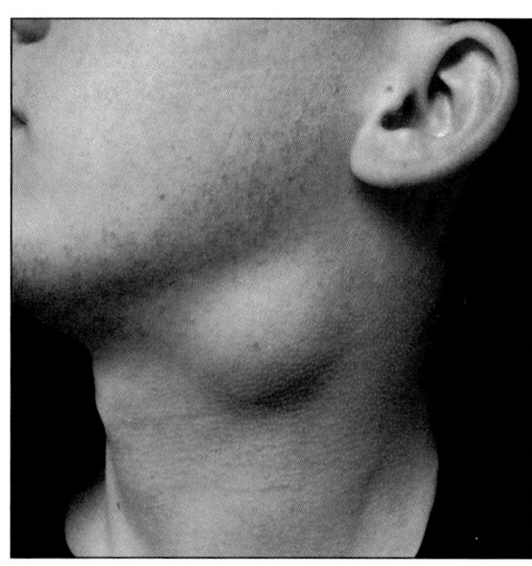

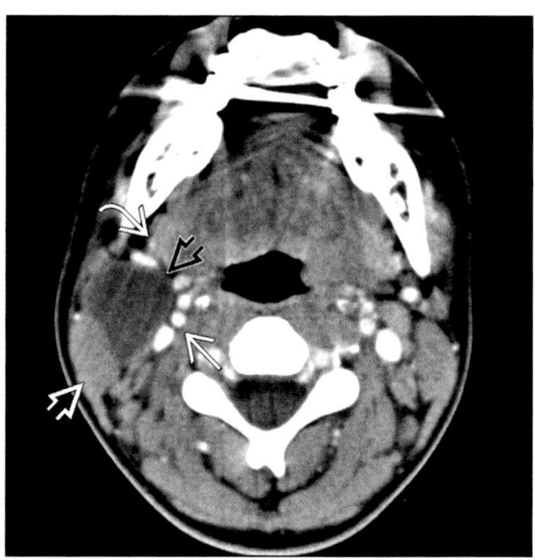

__(Left)__ Axial contrast CT reveals a typical 2nd branchial cleft cyst located posterior to submandibular gland , lateral to carotid space , and anterior to sternomastoid muscle . There is slight thickening of the capsule to suggest infection or inflammation. __(Right)__ Plain film image from a lipiodol fistulogram demonstrates the presence of a complete fistulous tract extending from the tonsillar fossa in the oropharynx to the right supraclavicular fossa skin opening.

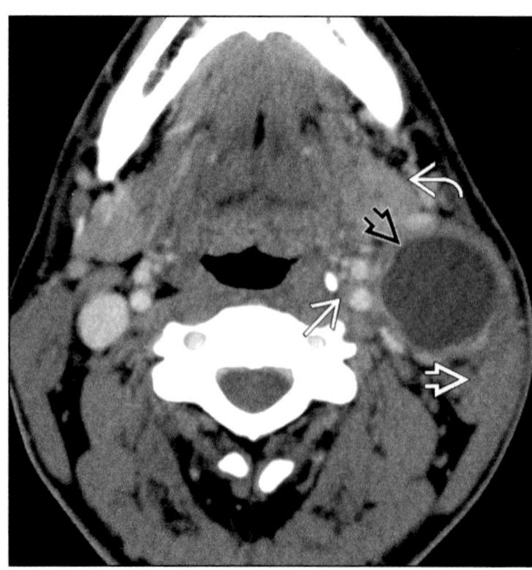

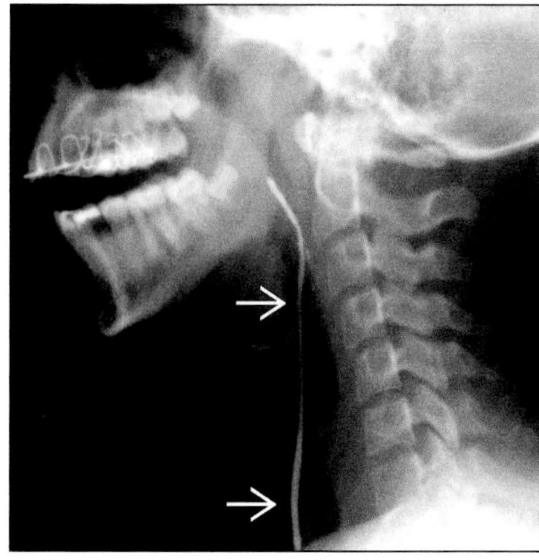

BRANCHIAL CLEFT CYST

Macroscopic and Microscopic Features

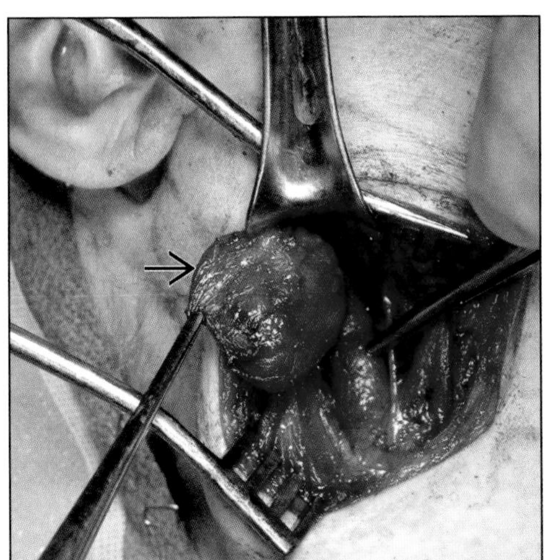

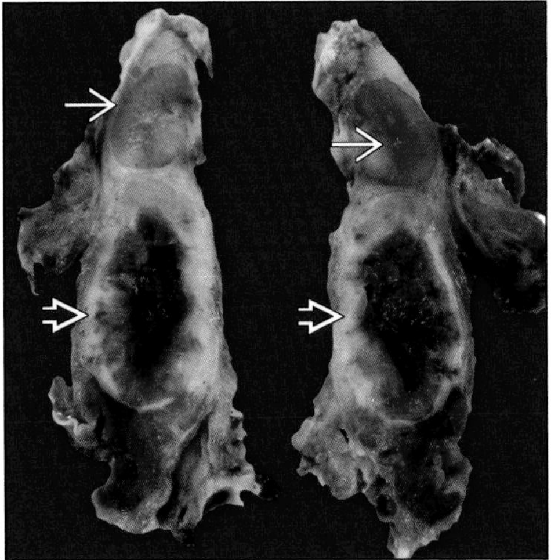

(Left) *The cyst ➔ has been retracted out of the operative field, highlighting the intimate association with the muscles, veins, arteries, and nerves of the neck.* ***(Right)*** *The resection specimen includes a benign lymph node ➔, completely separate from the cyst immediately below. Note the thick, fibrous connective tissue wall ➔ surrounding the cyst, which is filled with hemorrhagic and keratinaceous material. This gross appearance can also be seen in a metastatic cystic SCC.*

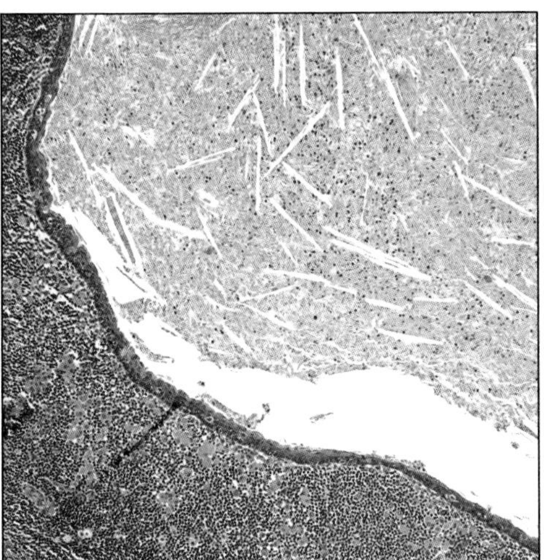

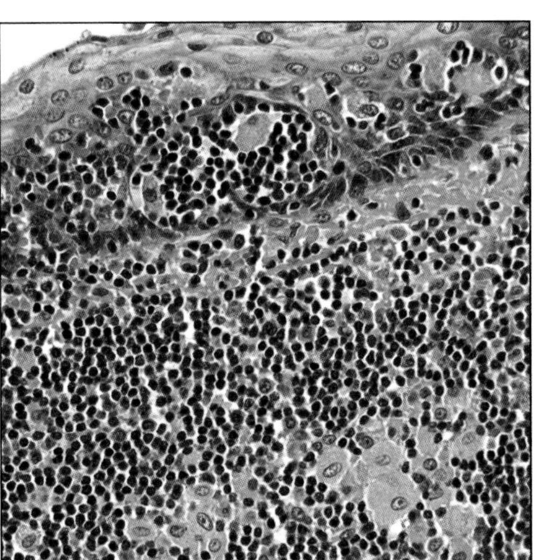

(Left) *There is a very thin, mature squamous epithelium lining the unilocular cyst. There is keratinaceous debris with cholesterol clefts. The stroma contains lymphoid elements.* ***(Right)*** *The squamous epithelium is mature and lacks cytologic atypia. A well-developed basement membrane is seen, separating the epithelium from the stroma. Histiocytes are also present within the lymphoid background.*

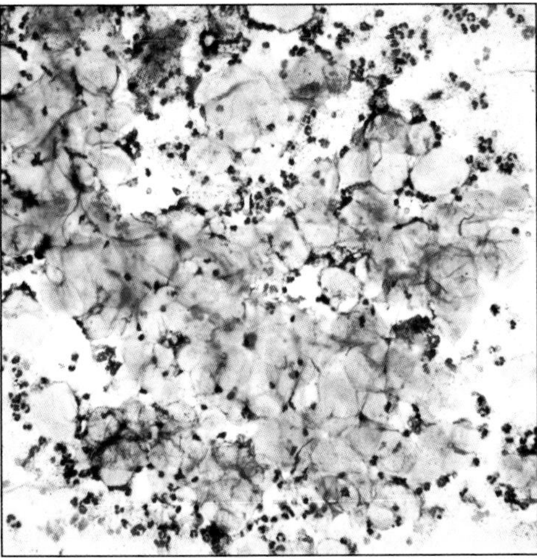

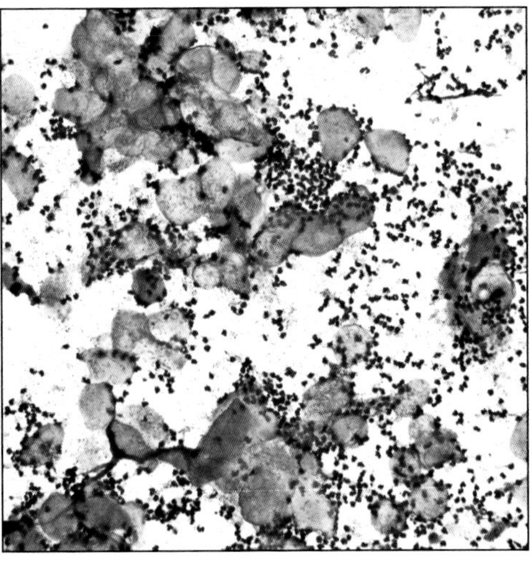

(Left) *Numerous acute inflammatory cells are seen in direct association with the anucleated squamous cells. Keratin debris like this is quite characteristic of a branchial cleft cyst. There is no cytologic atypia and no irregular cell shapes.* ***(Right)*** *There are many neutrophils intimately associated with squamous and anucleated squames in this smear from a BCC. There is no pleomorphism, no irregular shapes, and no mitotic figures. Necrosis is absent, although debris is present.*

CERVICAL THYMIC CYST

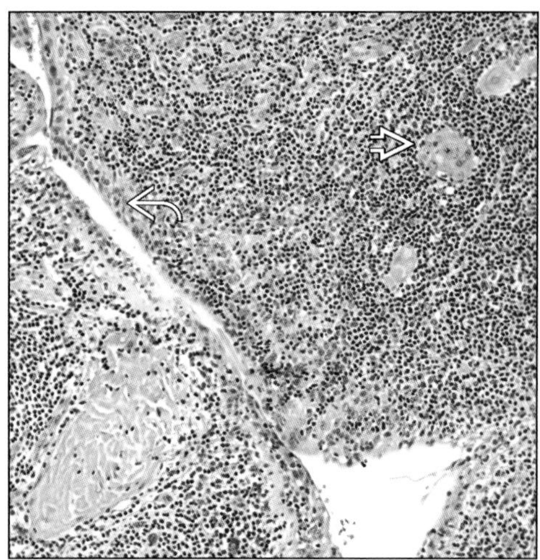

Epithelial-lined cyst ➡ with a dense mixed inflammatory cell infiltrate and a Hassall corpuscle ➡ in the cyst wall are shown; these findings are diagnostic of a thymic cyst.

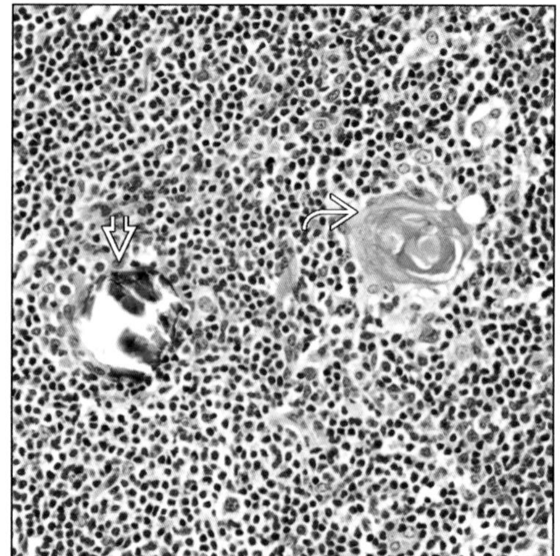

The wall of the cyst includes an identifiable Hassall corpuscle ➡ characterized by a concentric island of squamous cells with central keratinization; microcalcification ➡ is focally present.

TERMINOLOGY

Definitions

- Congential cyst that develops within embryonic remnants of thymus

ETIOLOGY/PATHOGENESIS

Embryogenesis

- Thymus develops in 6th week of gestation, arising primarily from 3rd branchial pouch (mesoderm)
  - Failure of descent or failure to involute results in thymic abnormalities, including cervical thymic cyst

CLINICAL ISSUES

Epidemiology

- Incidence
  - Rare
- Age
  - Most common in pediatric population
    - Majority occur during 1st decade of life
    - Remainder occur in 2nd-3rd decades
    - Rarely occurs in adults
- Gender
  - Male > Female

Site

- Found anywhere between angle of mandible and sternum, including lateral and midline neck
  - Most common location is anterior cervical triangle
  - May extend into mediastinum or may be in continuity with intrathoracic thymus gland

Presentation

- Slow-growing, painless, unilateral neck mass
  - May transiently increase in size during Valsalva movement
- Uncommonly, presentation may include
  - Dyspnea, dysphagia, hoarseness, or pain
  - Vocal cord paralysis, stridor, odynophagia
  - Life-threatening airway obstruction
- Rarely (if ever) associated with sinus or fistula

Treatment

- Surgical approaches
  - Simple excision

Prognosis

- Cured following excision
  - No recurrences with complete excision
  - No potential to undergo malignant transformation
  - No association with myasthenia gravis

IMAGE FINDINGS

CT Findings

- Shows cystic nature of lesion
- Demonstrates association with large vessels (e.g., intimate relationship to carotid sheath)

MACROSCOPIC FEATURES

General Features

- Unilocular or multilocular
- Cyst lining smooth or trabeculated
- Cyst wall varies in thickness
- Cystic content may include clear serous or hemorrhagic fluid, semi-solid debris

Size

- 1.4-17.0 cm

MICROSCOPIC PATHOLOGY

Histologic Features

- Cystic lesion variably lined by cuboidal, columnar, &/ or squamous epithelium

Key Facts

Terminology
- Congential cyst that develops within embryonic remnants of thymus

Clinical Issues
- Majority (67%) occur during 1st decade of life
- Most common location anterior cervical triangle
- Majority of patients present with slow-growing, painless, unilateral neck mass
- Simple excision is curative

Microscopic Pathology
- Cystic lesion variably lined by cuboidal, columnar, &/ or squamous epithelium
- By definition, wall contains thymic tissue including Hassall corpuscles
  - Concentric islands/aggregates of squamous cells often with central keratinization
- Foreign body giant cell reaction &/or cholesterol granulomas commonly seen

---

  - When infected, lining epithelium may be replaced by fibrous tissue
- By definition, wall contains thymic tissue, including
  - Hassall corpuscles: Concentric islands/aggregates of squamous cells often with central keratinization
  - Lymphoid follicles
  - Identification of thymic tissue may require extensive sampling
- Foreign body giant cell reaction &/or cholesterol granulomas commonly seen
- Parathyroid parenchyma may be found in thymic cysts

DIFFERENTIAL DIAGNOSIS

Branchial Cleft Cyst
- Tend to occur in 3rd decade of life
- Lymphoid tissue in wall without thymic tissue
- Commonly associated with cysts and fistulas

Cystic Hygroma (Lymphangioma)
- Majority identified in lateral neck (posterior and anterior triangles)
- Histology includes endothelial cell-lined spaces containing proteinaceous fluid and lymphocytes
- Intervening stroma contains small amounts of fibrous connective tissue and muscle with lymphoid aggregates
- Stroma may become inflamed and fibrotic following repeated infections

Dermoid Cyst
- Cyst wall contains cutaneous adnexal structures (hair follicles, sebaceous, eccrine, or apocrine glands)

Thyroglossal Duct Cyst
- Usually midline neck above thyroid isthmus but below level of hyoid bone
  - Nearly always connected to hyoid bone
  - Uncommonly may occur lateral to midline but does not occur in lateral portion of neck (i.e., lateral to jugular vein)
- May have thyroid follicular epithelium in wall

SELECTED REFERENCES

1. Komura M et al: A pediatric case of life-threatening airway obstruction caused by a cervicomediastinal thymic cyst. Pediatr Radiol. 40(9):1569-71, 2010
2. Sturm-O'Brien AK et al: Cervical thymic anomalies--the Texas Children's Hospital experience. Laryngoscope. 119(10):1988-93, 2009
3. Cigliano B et al: Cervical thymic cysts. Pediatr Surg Int. 23(12):1219-25, 2007
4. Petropoulos I et al: Thymic cyst in the differential diagnosis of paediatric cervical masses. B-ENT. 2(1):35-7, 2006
5. Ridder GJ et al: Multilocular cervical thymic cysts in adults. A report of two cases and review of the literature. Eur Arch Otorhinolaryngol. 260(5):261-5, 2003
6. Burton EM et al: Cervical thymic cysts: CT appearance of two cases including a persistent thymopharyngeal duct cyst. Pediatr Radiol. 25(5):363-5, 1995

IMAGE GALLERY

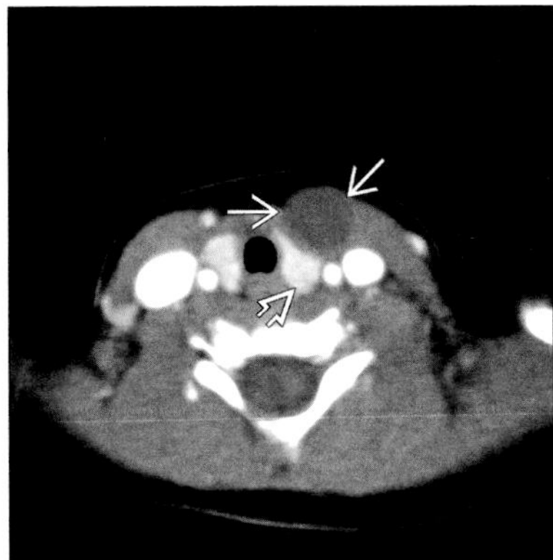
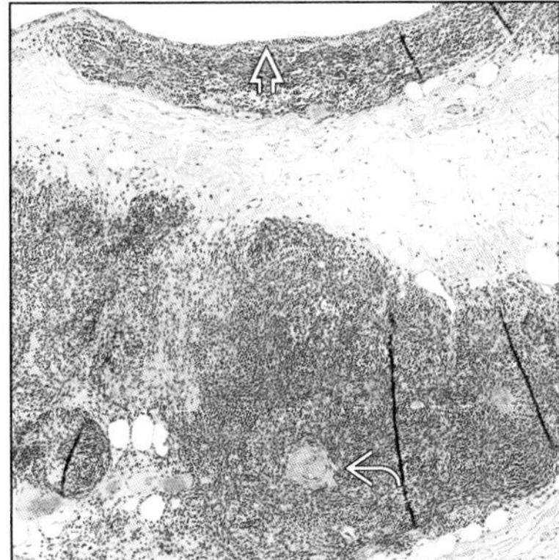
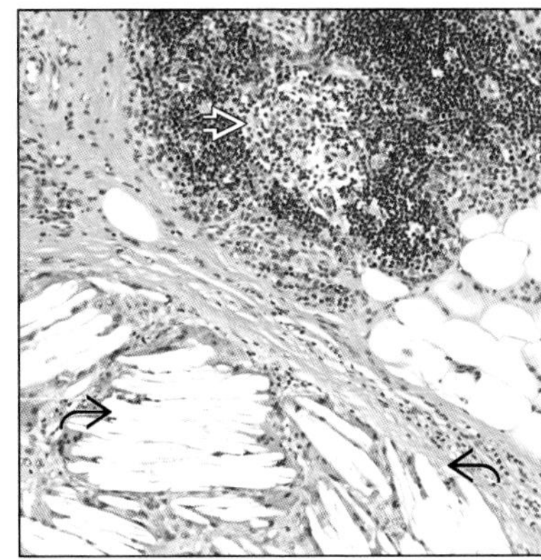

(Left) *Axial CECT shows a well-defined cystic mass ➡ closely applied to the anterior aspect of the carotid sheath and anterolateral to the left thyroid lobe ➡.* ***(Center)*** *Unilocular cyst with epithelial lining ➡ and cyst wall is comprised of lymphoid aggregates containing a Hassall corpuscle ➡.* ***(Right)*** *A common finding is the presence of cholesterol granulomas in the cyst wall ➡, which may also include lymphoid follicles, including germinal centers ➡.*

BRONCHOGENIC CYST

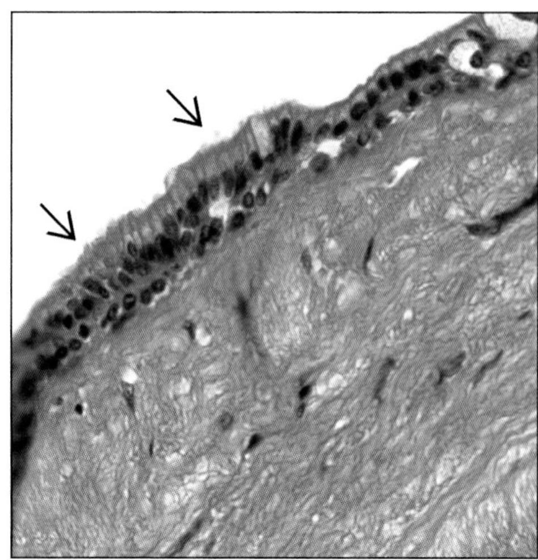

A cervical bronchogenic cyst from the lateral neck of a 2-month-old male child is shown. Clinically it was thought to be a branchial cleft cyst. Note the ciliated respiratory epithelium ⇒.

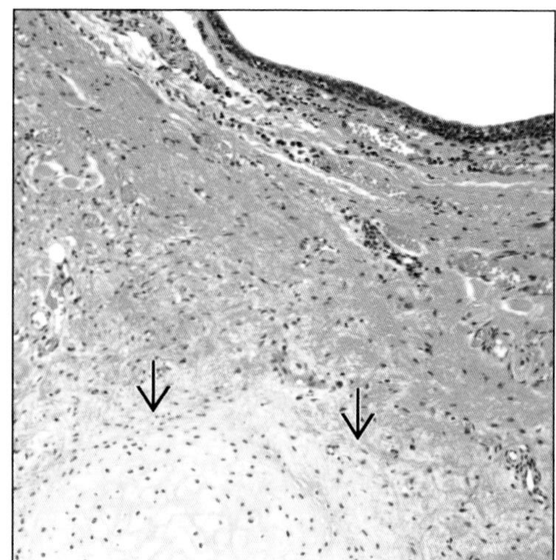

While hyaline cartilage ⇒ is readily seen in intrathoracic bronchogenic cysts, it may be more difficult to identify the cervical variant. Multiple recuts may be required.

TERMINOLOGY

Synonyms

- Bronchial cyst

Definitions

- Rare congenital malformation of ventral foregut
  - Enteric cyst, neurenteric cysts are part of same family

ETIOLOGY/PATHOGENESIS

Embryogenesis

- Derived from small buds of diverticula that separate from foregut during formation of tracheobronchial tree
- Usually between 26th and 40th days of gestation

CLINICAL ISSUES

Epidemiology

- Incidence
  - Rare
- Age
  - Pediatric population; rare in adults
- Gender
  - Male > Female (4:1)

Site

- **Cervical**
  - Midline superficial presternal or suprasternal is most common location
  - Less commonly
    - Lateral
    - Thyroid
    - Subcutaneous
- **Noncervical**
  - Mediastinum
  - Around hilum

Presentation

- Compression of airway
  - Respiratory distress
  - Cough
  - Dyspnea
- Dysphagia
- Infection may be uncommon
  - Drainage associated with sinus tract
  - Fever
- Asymptomatic presentation is uncommon

Endoscopic Findings

- May show compression of laryngotracheal axis

Treatment

- Options, risks, complications
  - Drainage and infection are possible complications
- Surgical approaches
  - Complete surgical excision is treatment of choice
    - Neck exploration and selective dissection via transcervical approach
    - Great vessels and the recurrent laryngeal nerve are at risk
    - If sinus tract is present, it should be removed with cyst
  - Drainage and ablation
    - Indicated for only high-risk adults

Prognosis

- Excellent long-term clinical prognosis
- Recurrence develops if incompletely excised
- Rare cases of carcinoma arising from bronchogenic cyst

IMAGE FINDINGS

Radiographic Findings

- Best study: Contrast-enhanced T1WI or T2WI MR to show homogeneously increased signal
- Well-defined, solitary, smooth-bordered mass

BRONCHOGENIC CYST

Key Facts

Terminology
- Rare congenital malformation of ventral foregut

Clinical Issues
- Pediatric population; rare in adults
- Midline superficial presternal or suprasternal is most common neck location
- Male > Female (4:1)
- Presents with airway compression, dysphagia, infection, or may be asymptomatic
- Complete surgical excision is treatment of choice

Image Findings
- Best study: Contrast-enhanced MR T1WI or T2WI to show well-defined, solitary, smooth-bordered mass

Microscopic Pathology
- Cyst lined by respiratory-type epithelium
- Cyst wall with mucoserous glands, hyaline cartilage, and smooth muscle

MACROSCOPIC FEATURES

General Features
- Grossly tubular, altered by infection
- Cut sections show clear serous to mucoid material

MICROSCOPIC PATHOLOGY

Histologic Features
- Cyst lined by respiratory-type epithelium
  - Ciliated
  - Pseudostratified
  - Columnar
  - Epithelium may be altered by infection: Stratified squamous
- Cyst wall contains
  - Mucoserous glands
  - Hyaline cartilage
  - Haphazard smooth muscle
  - Scant lymphoid tissue

ANCILLARY TESTS

Cytology
- Normal ciliated columnar cells
- Serous or mucinous material

DIFFERENTIAL DIAGNOSIS

Teratoma
- Tissues from sites other than respiratory tract

Dermoid Cyst
- Hair and skin appendages
- Squamous epithelium

Branchial Cleft Cyst
- Lymphoid tissue arranged in germinal centers
- Typically has stratified squamous epithelium
- Lacks smooth muscle and cartilage
- Clinically, usually found laterally

Thyroglossal Duct Cyst
- Usually has thyroid follicles
- Lacks smooth muscle and cartilage

Cystic Hygroma (Lymphangioma)
- Variably sized lymphatic vessels

SELECTED REFERENCES

1. Moz U et al: Bronchogenic cysts of the neck: a rare localization and review of the literature. Acta Otorhinolaryngol Ital. 29(1):36-40, 2009
2. Teissier N et al: Cervical bronchogenic cysts: usual and unusual clinical presentations. Arch Otolaryngol Head Neck Surg. 134(11):1165-9, 2008
3. Newkirk KA et al: Bronchogenic cysts of the neck in adults. Ann Otol Rhinol Laryngol. 113(9):691-5, 2004

IMAGE GALLERY

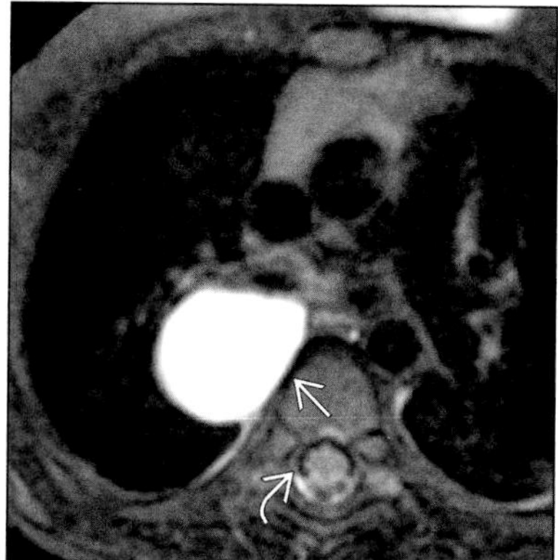

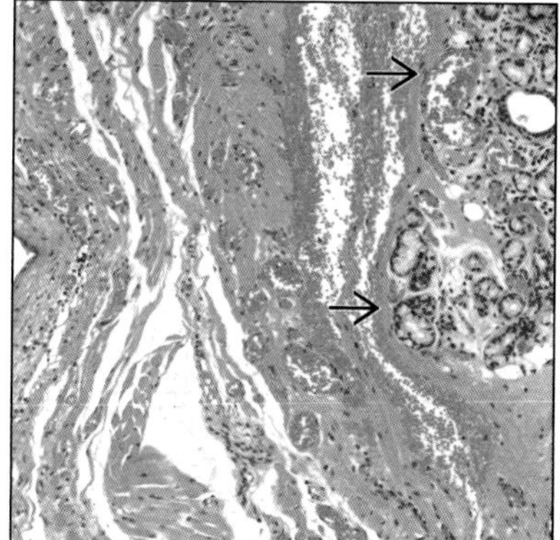

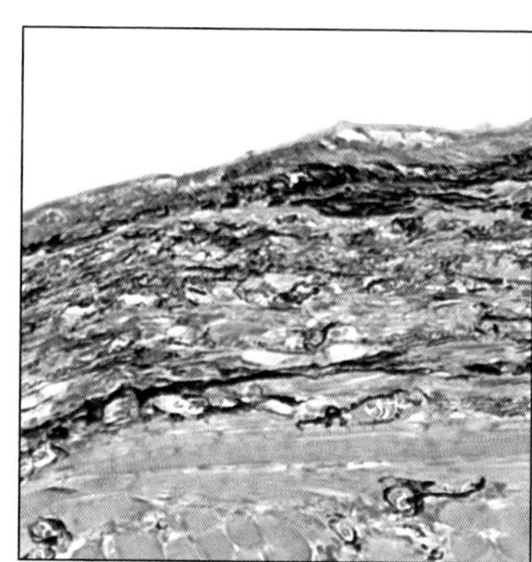

***(Left)** Axial T2WI MR shows homogeneous, well-circumscribed ovoid mass ➡ with signal greater than CSF ➡. This lesion extended into the lower neck. **(Center)** Hematoxylin and eosin shows the fibrous wall of a bronchogenic cyst. Seromucinous glands ➡ are found throughout the wall and may contribute to the mucoid material found within the cyst. **(Right)** Smooth muscle, highlighted with smooth muscle actin, is characteristic within the wall of a bronchogenic cyst.*

CAT SCRATCH DISEASE

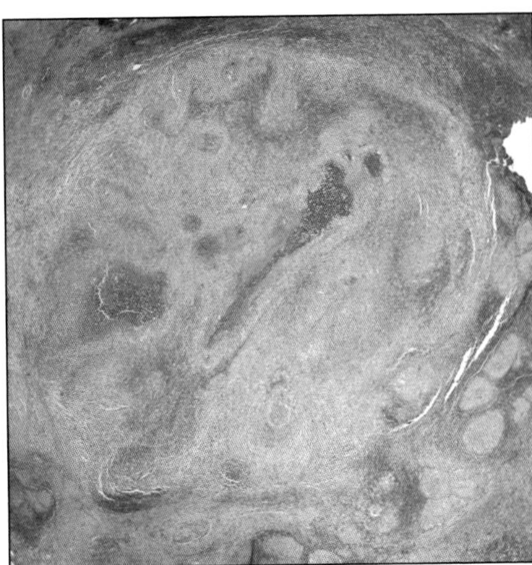

A low-power micrograph demonstrates stellate areas of central necrosis within this lymph node. The necrotic material is granular and blue, surrounded by histiocytes.

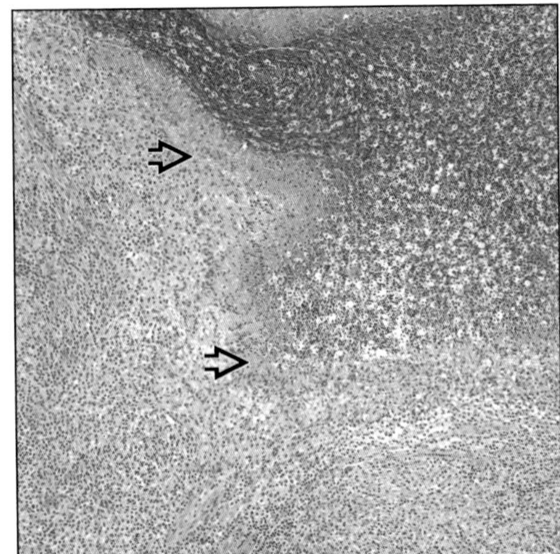

The stellate abscesses are formed by debris and neutrophils filling in central areas within the lymph node. There is a palisade of histiocytes ➩ at the border with the surrounding parenchyma.

TERMINOLOGY

Abbreviations

- Cat scratch disease (CSD)

Synonyms

- Cat scratch fever
- Cat scratch adenitis
- Inoculation lymphoreticulosis
- Debre syndrome
- Foshay-Mollaret syndrome
- Subacute regional lymphadenitis
- Oculoglandular syndrome

Definitions

- Benign infectious disease caused by *Bartonella* organism introduced into humans via scratch or bite from cat, resulting in necrotizing granulomatous lymphadenitis

ETIOLOGY/PATHOGENESIS

Transmission

- Causative organism is *Bartonella henselae* bacillus, a gram-negative pleomorphic rod-shaped bacteria
    - Organism originally classified as *Afipia felis*
    - Rarely caused by *Bartonella clarridgeiae*
    - Cat fleas may serve as vector for cat-cat transmission or via feces-wound contact in humans
    - Kittens transmit disease more frequently than adult cats due to higher bacteremia
- Cat scratch or bite, causing skin erythema within 3-10 days
- Acute regional lymphadenopathy proximal to inoculation site developing after 1-3 weeks
- Most cases show gradual involution (self-limited) in 3-4 months

CLINICAL ISSUES

Epidemiology

- Incidence
    - Uncommon
        - ~ 10-12% of patients with cervical lymphadenopathy
    - Most cases develop in fall and winter
- Age
    - Wide age range, but generally children/young adults
- Gender
    - Equal gender distribution

Site

- Lymph node enlargement: Cervical ~ axillary > epitrochlear > supraclavicular ~ submandibular

Presentation

- Skin inoculation site &/or regional lymphadenitis most common
- Separated into classical and atypical presentations
    - **Classic**: Immunocompetent patients
        - Scratch, bite, or papule at site of initial injury/ inoculation (3-10 days), pustular or crusted with time
        - 7-60 days for additional symptoms to develop
        - Tender, painful, and swollen proximal regional lymph nodes with overlying erythematous skin
        - Matted nodes may suppurate (10-15% of patients)
        - Some patients may have concurrent fever, chills, malaise, headache, backache, arthralgia, abdominal pain
        - Resolves spontaneously in about 30-120 days
    - **Atypical (~ 10%)**: Ocular, neurologic, &/or visceral organ involvement
        - Granulomatous conjunctivitis (Parinaud oculoglandular syndrome)
        - Optic neuritis, involvement of retina, and neuropathy

CAT SCRATCH DISEASE

Key Facts

Terminology
- Benign infectious disease caused by *Bartonella* organism introduced into humans via scratch or bite from cat, resulting in necrotizing granulomatous lymphadenitis

Etiology/Pathogenesis
- Causative organism is *Bartonella henselae* bacillus, a pleomorphic 1-3 μm rod, coccus or L-shaped bacteria
- Acute regional lymphadenopathy proximal to inoculation site developing after 1-3 weeks

Clinical Issues
- Wide age range, but generally children/young adults
- Lymph node enlargement: Cervical ~ axillary > epitrochlear > supraclavicular ~ submandibular
  - Tender, painful, and swollen regional lymph nodes
- Benign and self-limited in vast majority of patients

Microscopic Pathology
- Follicular hyperplasia
- Central stellate necrosis
- Palisading epithelioid histiocytes create granulomas
- Multinucleated foreign body-type giant cells

Ancillary Tests
- Warthin-Starry stain highlights focal and scant organisms

Top Differential Diagnoses
- Suppurative granulomatous inflammation, metastatic disease, branchial cleft cyst, sarcoid

---

    - Immunocompromised patients may develop life-threatening systemic disease with severe complications
    - Enlarged spleen (abscess), swollen parotid gland (granuloma), liver enlargement (granuloma)
    - Neck stiffness, sore throat, respiratory distress, and trismus if abscess develops
    - Rare development of erythema nodosum (2% of patients)
    - Lymphadenitis may persist for years

Laboratory Tests
- Specific tests
  - Serology for *B. henselae* antibodies (immunofluorescence assay, enzyme immunoassay) has poor sensitivity/specificity
  - Polymerase chain reaction (PCR) assay for organism is only performed at specialty laboratories
  - Culture is difficult to perform as organism is fastidious and slow-growing
- Elevated WBC: Mild neutrophilia or eosinophilia
- Elevated ESR

Treatment
- Options, risks, complications
  - Full resolution without treatment for most patients (< 1 month)
  - Excision, drainage, and antibiotic therapy
- Surgical approaches
  - Lymph node biopsy since organisms are difficult to culture and organisms are sparse
- Drugs
  - Wide variety of antibiotics are employed; azithromycin usually most frequently
    - Oral or intravenous antibiotics, latter for systemic disease

Prognosis
- Prognosis is generally excellent
  - Benign and self-limited in vast majority of patients
  - Rarely, persistent lymphadenopathy for months

IMAGE FINDINGS

Radiographic Findings
- Contrast-enhanced CT is first-line tool for neck adenopathy evaluation
- Conglomeration of lymph nodes with well-defined, thick, enhancing walls with low-attenuation centers (suppuration) and surrounding cellulitis

MACROSCOPIC FEATURES

General Features
- Confluent or matted lymph nodes with central pus/ abscess

Size
- Range: Up to 10 cm

MICROSCOPIC PATHOLOGY

Histologic Features
- Lymph node biopsy performed due to failure of other methods to diagnose disease and slow resolution
- Lymph node changes vary according to disease stage
  - Follicular hyperplasia (early stage)
    - Focal areas of necrosis with neutrophils
    - Subcapsular sinuses packed with monocytoid B-cells
  - Central stellate necrosis (middle stage)
    - Debris and neutrophils fill central necrotic areas: Microabscesses
    - Fibrin usually easily identified
  - Palisading epithelioid histiocytes create granulomas (late stage)
    - Lymphocytes blend with epithelioid histiocytes
    - Multinucleated foreign body-type giant cells
  - Granuloma may be scattered throughout lymph node
  - Plasmacytoid dendritic cells are increased

CAT SCRATCH DISEASE

ANCILLARY TESTS

Cytology

- FNA used to diagnose granulomatous inflammation and to obtain culture material
- Necrotic debris in background, epithelioid histiocytes, possible palisading, giant cells

Histochemistry

- Warthin-Starry silver impregnation stain highlights focal and scant organisms
  - Intracellular, 1-3 μm rods, cocci or L-shaped bacteria (pleomorphic rod)
  - Difficult to interpret due to high background silver precipitate in necrotic debris and macrophages
- **Weak reaction**: Red with Brown-Hopps tissue Gram stain; **negative**: Ziehl-Neelsen

Immunohistochemistry

- Positive: Monoclonal antibody to *B. henselae* (more sensitive and specific than histochemistry stains, but fastidious and capricious to perform)

PCR

- Polymerase chain reaction (PCR) targeting *B. henselae* and *B. quintana* is both sensitive and specific, but not widely performed
  - May only be detected during initial disease development (1st 6 weeks)

DIFFERENTIAL DIAGNOSIS

Suppurative Granulomatous Inflammation

- Mycobacterial infections (*Mycobacteria tuberculosis, M. avium-intracellulare, M. kansasii, M. scrofulaceum*): Caseating but usually not stellate; many giant cells; positive with acid-fast stains
- Fungal infections: Necrotizing granulomas, but not usually stellate; fungi identified by special stains
- Staphylococcal and streptococcal infections: Begin as pharyngitis, dental caries, or osteomyelitis, then expand to cervical lymph nodes
- Toxoplasmosis (*Toxoplasma gondii*): Cat vector; parasitic infection; may have granulomas
- Tularemia (*Francisella tularensis*): Lymph node enlargement with possible necrotizing granulomas
- Brucellosis (*Brucella* species): Human disease after exposure to contaminated dairy products; noncaseating granulomas; gram-negative coccobacilli
- Leishmaniasis (*Leishmania donovani*): Protozoan infection; obligate intracellular organisms (amastigote) identified by Giemsa
- Chancroid (*Haemophilus ducreyi*): Very rare in head and neck; lacks stellate microabscesses and shows capsular edema and sinus tract formation
- Lymphogranuloma venereum (*Chlamydia trachomatis*): Very rare in head and neck; histologically identical findings; cultures and special stains are diagnostic
- Granuloma inguinale (*Calymmatobacterium granulomatis*): Ulcerated, necrotizing skin lesions; suppuration and granulomas of lymph nodes late in disease; organisms found in clusters with Gram or Giemsa stains

Metastatic Disease

- Painless, hard lymph nodes without skin erythema
- Metastatic squamous cell carcinoma, nasopharyngeal carcinoma, thyroid carcinoma
- Lymphoma, including Hodgkin lymphoma, may show extensive necrosis
- Extensive necrosis and granulomas, but malignant cells are easily identified
- Immunohistochemistry (keratin) highlights epithelium within lymph node; specific lymphoid markers will help exclude lymphoma

Branchial Cleft Cyst

- Usually single, unilateral mass without granulomatous inflammation or suppurative necrosis

Sarcoid

- Serologic and clinical evaluation is different
- Tight, well-formed, small granuloma
- Necrosis or caseation is uncommon
- Frequently have asteroid bodies or Schaumann bodies
- Infectious disease work-up (culture &/or special studies) negative

Kikuchi-Fujimoto Disease

- Histiocytic necrotizing lymphadenitis: Localized lymphadenopathy
- Well-defined, paracortical zones of necrosis with karyorrhectic debris
- No acute inflammatory cells (**absent** neutrophils)
- Granulomatous inflammation is present (palisading epithelioid histiocytes), with large, activated lymphocytes

Kawasaki Disease

- Acute, nonsuppurative lymphadenopathy
- Effaced architecture with expanded interfollicular zones
- Zones of necrosis, often becoming confluent
- Nuclear debris and microthrombi of vessels
- No granuloma or suppurative necrosis (per se)

SELECTED REFERENCES

1. Caponetti GC et al: Evaluation of immunohistochemistry in identifying Bartonella henselae in cat-scratch disease. Am J Clin Pathol. 131(2):250-6, 2009
2. Caponetti G et al: Cat-scratch disease lymphadenitis. Ear Nose Throat J. 86(8):449-50, 2007
3. Cheuk W et al: Confirmation of diagnosis of cat scratch disease by immunohistochemistry. Am J Surg Pathol. 30(2):274-5, 2006
4. Ridder GJ et al: Cat-scratch disease: Otolaryngologic manifestations and management. Otolaryngol Head Neck Surg. 132(3):353-8, 2005
5. Lamps LW et al: Cat-scratch disease: historic, clinical, and pathologic perspectives. Am J Clin Pathol. 121 Suppl:S71-80, 2004
6. Chomel BB: Cat-scratch disease. Rev Sci Tech. 19(1):136-50, 2000

Clinical, Imaging, and Microscopic Features

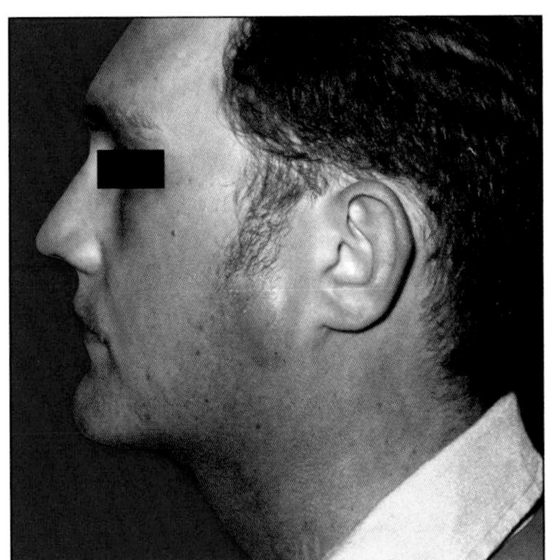

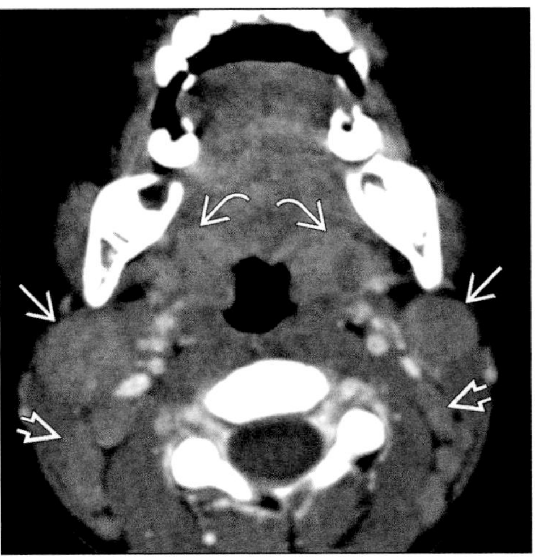

(Left) *This man had been bitten on the arm by a feral cat about 3 weeks earlier. There is significant enlargement of the left preauricular/parotid gland region, with shiny, erythematous, warm skin covering the mass.* ***(Right)*** *Contrast-enhanced CT shows bilateral jugulodigastric* ➔*, spinal accessory* ➔ *lymphadenopathy, and tonsillar hypertrophy* ➔ *in a patient who was bitten on her tongue by a cat. Imaging findings are not specific for CSD. (Courtesy R. Harnsberger, MD.)*

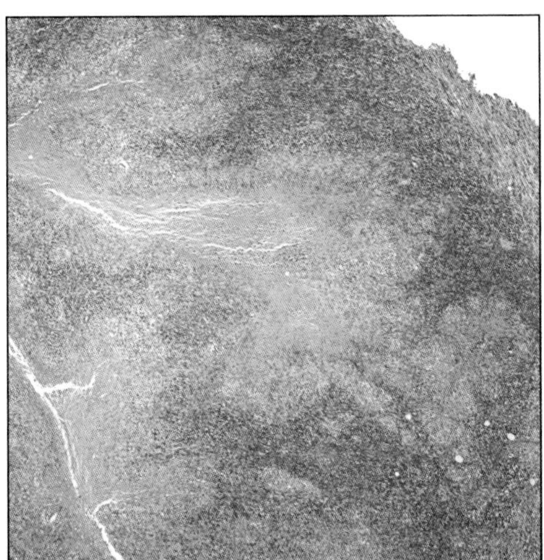

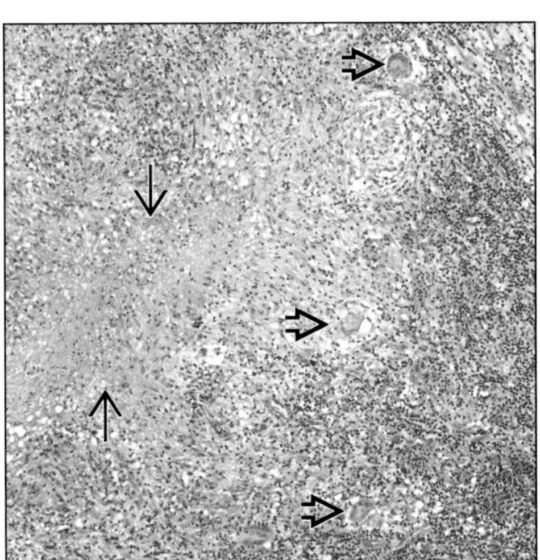

(Left) *There is a background of follicular hyperplasia with stellate abscess formation within the lymph node. The brightly eosinophilic necrotic areas are surrounded by a palisade of epithelioid histiocytes and monocytoid cells.* ***(Right)*** *The necrotic material* ➔ *is surrounded by a well-developed layer of histiocytes. A number of foreign body-type giant cells* ➔ *are seen at the interface with the remaining lymphoid parenchyma. These features, while characteristic of CSD, are not specific.*

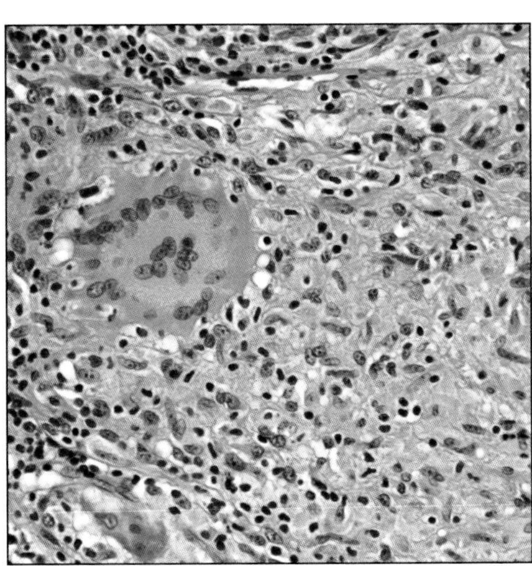

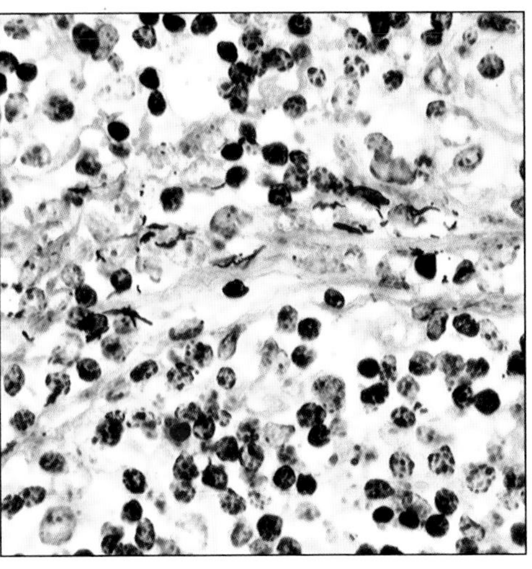

(Left) *A multinucleated foreign body-type giant cell is seen immediately adjacent to epithelioid histiocytes in this example of CSD. Again, isolated elements alone are nondiagnostic of CSD.* ***(Right)*** *There are multiple pleomorphic rod-shaped bacteria in this oil immersion photomicrograph stained with Warthin-Starry stain. The organisms are usually intracellular, 1-3 μm rods, cocci or L-shaped bacteria. They are usually not this abundant, requiring careful oil examination to identify them.*

BACILLARY ANGIOMATOSIS

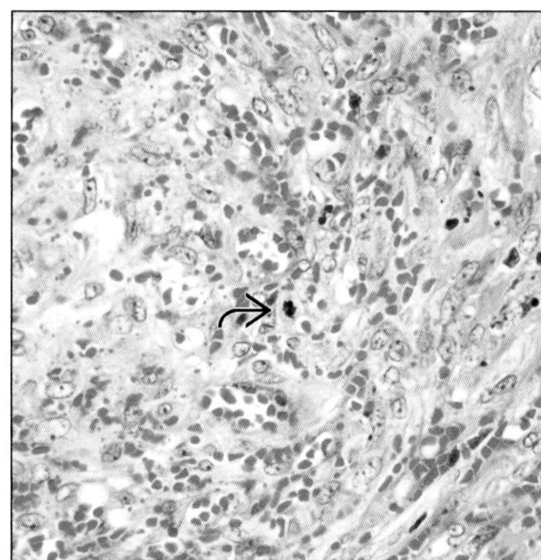

Part of a circumscribed submucosal lesion shows vascular proliferation comprised of ectatic vessels lined by prominent-appearing endothelial cells; mitotic figures can be identified ➦.

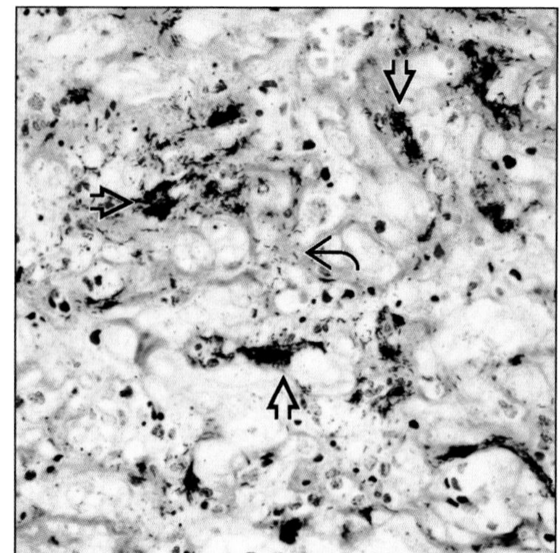

Warthin-Starry staining shows the presence of slender-appearing bacilli ➦ representing Bartonella henselae (formerly R. henselae). Bacilli form the darker staining clumps ➪.

TERMINOLOGY

Abbreviations

- Bacillary angiomatosis (BA)

Synonyms

- Epithelioid angiomatosis
- Epithelioid hemangioma-like vascular proliferation

Definitions

- Pseudoneoplastic capillary proliferative lesion caused by opportunistic bacterial infection

ETIOLOGY/PATHOGENESIS

Infectious Agents

- Caused by
  - *Bartonella henselae* (formerly *Rochalimaea henselae*)
  - *Bartonella quintana* (trench fever)
- Acquired through exposure to cats, soil, or waste
- Occurs as complication of HIV infection
  - May occur in association with Kaposi sarcoma
- May occur in immunocompetent patients

CLINICAL ISSUES

Epidemiology

- Age
  - Occurs over wide age range (from young to old)
- Gender
  - Equal gender distribution

Site

- Most commonly presents as cutaneous or mucocutaneous lesion
  - Mucosal sites of upper respiratory tract
    - Nasal cavity, oral cavity, pharynx
- May involve other organs sites including
  - Lymph nodes, spleen, liver
  - Bone, brain, lungs, heart, conjunctiva

Presentation

- Commonly associated with systemic symptoms including
  - Fever, chills, weight loss, night sweats
- Multiple erythematous papules ± crusting

Treatment

- Options, risks, complications
  - Full-dose erythromycin is 1st drug of choice
    - Doxycycline effective for patients who do not tolerate erythromycin

Prognosis

- Antibiotic therapy is effective, often resulting in resolution of lesions
- If left untreated, may be progressive and potentially life threatening

MACROSCOPIC FEATURES

General Features

- Skin lesions appear as red to violet papules or nodules
  - Deep-seated lesions similar in appearance to cellulitis and may erode into bone
  - Mucosal-based mass appears as erythematous nodular lesion

Size

- 0.5-4 cm

MICROSCOPIC PATHOLOGY

Histologic Features

- Well-circumscribed lobular capillary proliferation
  - Small capillaries arranged around ectatic vessels lined by prominent endothelial cells
    - Endothelial cells appear hyperchromatic and pleomorphic

BACILLARY ANGIOMATOSIS

Key Facts

Clinical Issues

- Pseudoneoplastic capillary proliferative lesion caused by *Bartonella henselae* (formerly *R. henselae*), *Bartonella quintana* (trench fever)
- Full-dose erythromycin is 1st drug of choice

Microscopic Pathology

- Small capillaries arranged around ectatic vessels lined by prominent endothelial cells
  - Endothelial cells appear hyperchromatic and pleomorphic
- Presence of neutrophils and neutrophilic debris adjacent to capillary proliferation with granular clumps that contain masses of bacilli

Ancillary Tests

- Warthin-Starry staining shows granular material to contain bacilli located interstitially

---

  - Mitotic figures, including atypical forms and necrosis, may be present
- Presence of neutrophils and neutrophilic debris adjacent to capillary proliferation
  - Granular clumps associated with neutrophils correspond to masses of bacilli
- Overlying epithelium may be ulcerated or thinned or show pseudoepitheliomatous hyperplasia
- Solid areas may be present and may obscure vascular proliferation

ANCILLARY TESTS

Histochemistry

- Warthin-Starry staining shows granular material to contain bacilli
  - Bacilli appear slender, located interstitially

Immunohistochemistry

- Human herpesvirus 8 (HHV8) negative

Molecular Genetics

- PCR used to confirm diagnosis as routine cultures inadequate for isolating bacilli

DIFFERENTIAL DIAGNOSIS

Hemangioma (Lobular Capillary, Epithelioid)

- Lacks clusters of bacilli

Angiosarcoma

- Interconnecting, ramifying vascular channels with vascular tufting, atypical endothelial cells, increased mitoses

Kaposi Sarcoma

- Spindled cells, interconnecting vascular channels, extravasated red cells, hyaline globules
- HHV8 positive

Verruga Peruana

- Vascular proliferation caused by infectious agent *Bartonella bacilliformis,* endemic to Peru
- Presence of characteristic Rocha-Lima inclusions

SELECTED REFERENCES

1. Maguiña C et al: Bartonellosis. Clin Dermatol. 27(3):271-80, 2009
2. Koehler JE et al: Molecular epidemiology of bartonella infections in patients with bacillary angiomatosis-peliosis. N Engl J Med. 337(26):1876-83, 1997
3. Cáceres-Ríos H et al: Verruga peruana: an infectious endemic angiomatosis. Crit Rev Oncog. 6(1):47-56, 1995
4. Webster GF et al: The clinical spectrum of bacillary angiomatosis. Br J Dermatol. 126(6):535-41, 1992
5. Chan JK et al: Histopathology of bacillary angiomatosis of lymph node. Am J Surg Pathol. 15(5):430-7, 1991
6. LeBoit PE et al: Bacillary angiomatosis. The histopathology and differential diagnosis of a pseudoneoplastic infection in patients with human immunodeficiency virus disease. Am J Surg Pathol. 13(11):909-20, 1989

IMAGE GALLERY

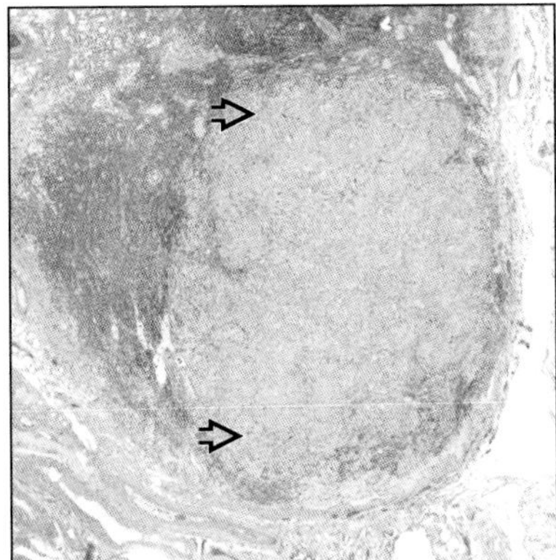

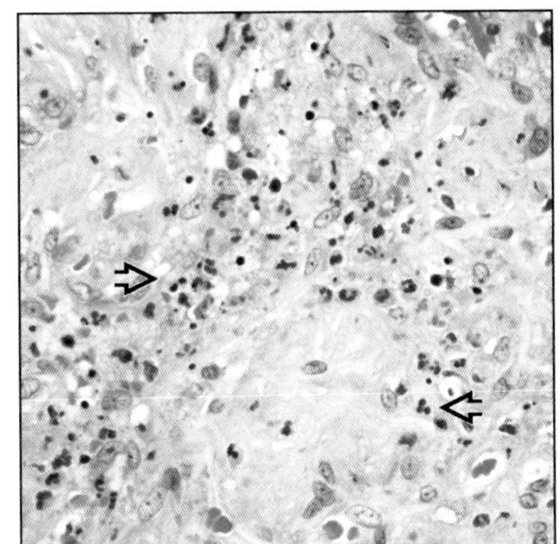

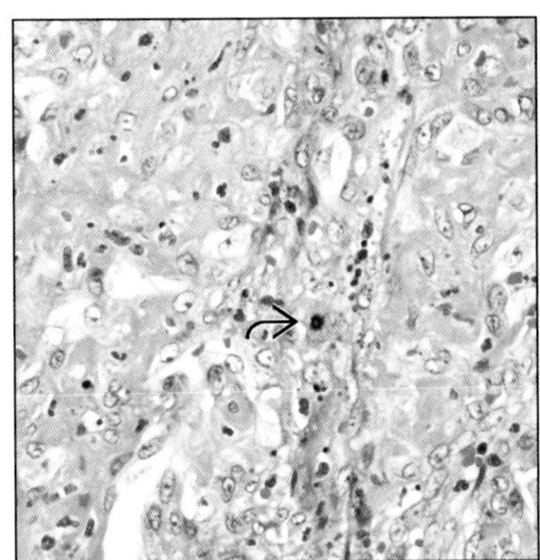

(Left) *A lymph node shows partial replacement by a well-circumscribed lobular proliferation* ➢. ***(Center)*** *The presence of neutrophils* ➢ *and neutrophilic debris seen adjacent to the capillary proliferation is a key histologic clue to the diagnosis of BA.* ***(Right)*** *Solid areas may be present, obscuring the vascular proliferation. The presence of pleomorphic nuclei and mitotic figures* ↪ *in BA may raise concern for a possible diagnosis of a malignant vascular neoplasm.*

MYCOBACTERIAL SPINDLE CELL PSEUDOTUMOR

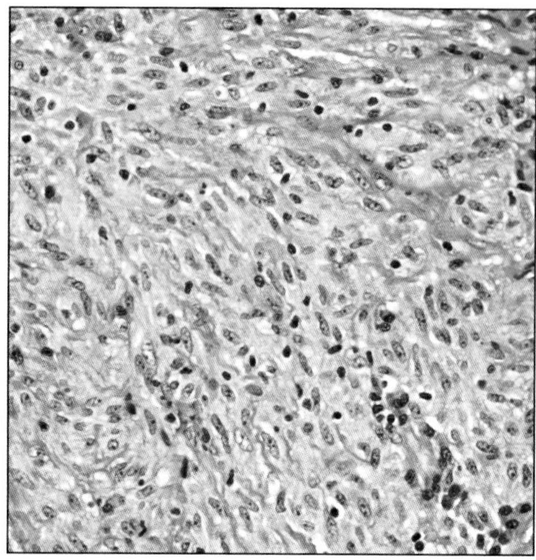

This immunocompromised patient presented with lymphadenopathy. Histologically, the lymph node is replaced by a bland spindle cell proliferation without features of a possible mycobacterial infection.

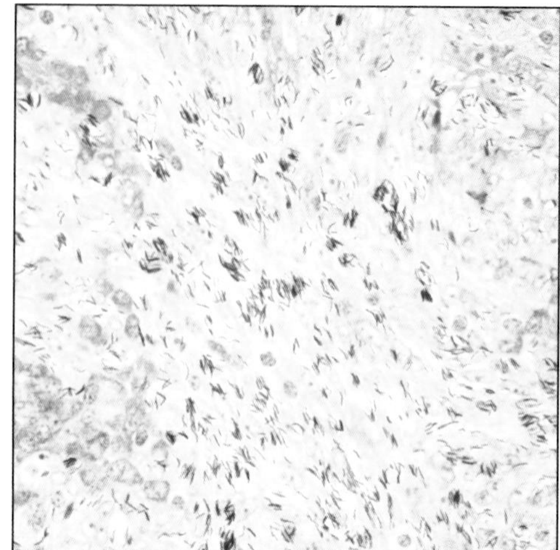

Ziehl-Neelsen stain shows the presence of numerous positive (red) mycobacteria in the cytoplasm of the spindled cells. The main diagnostic clue is the history of immunosuppression.

TERMINOLOGY

Abbreviations

- Mycobacteria other than tuberculosis (MOTT)

Synonyms

- Mycobacterial pseudotumor
- *M. avium-intracellulare* pseudotumor
- Spindled nontuberculous mycobacteriosis
- Histoid mycobacteriosis

Definitions

- Pseudoneoplastic spindle cell proliferation caused by *M. avium-intracellulare* and almost exclusively occurring in HIV-infected patients

ETIOLOGY/PATHOGENESIS

Infectious Agents

- Causative microorganism is *M. avium-intracellulare*
  - Almost always found in immune-compromised individuals
    - AIDS/HIV-positive patients
    - Patients receiving immunosuppressive therapy, including steroids

CLINICAL ISSUES

Epidemiology

- Incidence
  - Uncommon
- Age
  - Occurs over wide age range
- Gender
  - Equal gender distribution

Site

- Lymph nodes
- Extranodal sites
  - Skin, spleen, brain, bone marrow
  - Rarely occur in mucosal sites of upper aerodigestive tract (nasal septum)

Presentation

- Subcutaneous or submucosal firm nodule
- Lymphadenopathy

Treatment

- Options, risks, complications
  - Treatment guidelines are based on species of mycobacteria and susceptibility testing of the isolate
    - In some cases would be modified because of immune status of patient or other concurrent therapy
  - MOTT less sensitive to standard anti-*M. tuberculosis* drugs
    - Clarithromycin and azithromycin more effective in MOTT than standard anti-*M. tuberculosis* drugs

MICROSCOPIC PATHOLOGY

Histologic Features

- Cellular proliferation composed of bland-appearing spindle-shaped cells in storiform pattern
  - Spindle cells represent histiocytes
- Absent granuloma formation
  - Multinucleated giant cells and foamy histiocytes typically not present
  - Necrotic foci may be present
- Associated lymphocytes and plasma cells present
- Partial or complete effacement of nodal or mucosal architecture

ANCILLARY TESTS

Histochemistry

- Acid-fast bacilli (AFB) or Ziehl-Neelsen stain

MYCOBACTERIAL SPINDLE CELL PSEUDOTUMOR

Key Facts

Terminology

- Pseudoneoplastic spindle cell proliferation caused by *M. avium-intracellulare* and almost exclusively occurring in HIV-infected patients

Clinical Issues

- Treatment guidelines are based on species of mycobacteria and susceptibility testing of isolate

Microscopic Pathology

- Cellular proliferation of bland spindle-shaped cells in storiform pattern
- Multinucleated giant cells and foamy histiocytes are not present

Ancillary Tests

- Acid-fast bacilli (AFB) and Ziehl-Neelsen
- Presence of numerous AFB-positive organisms within cytoplasm of spindle cells

  - Presence of numerous AFB-positive organisms within cytoplasm of spindle cells
    - Spindle cells engulf (phagocytize) organisms acting as facultative histiocytes

Immunohistochemistry

- Spindle cells are CD68, lysozyme, α-1-antichymotrypsin, vimentin positive
- S100 protein, desmin, and muscle specific actin may be positive
- CD31 and CD34 negative

Molecular Genetics

- PCR used in identification of mycobacteria

DIFFERENTIAL DIAGNOSIS

Kaposi Sarcoma

- May occur concomitantly (in same lymph node) as mycobacterial spindle cell tumor
- Morphologic features include
  - Prominent fascicular arrangement of spindle cells with slit-like spaces
  - Extravasated red cells, hyaline globules, increased mitoses
  - CD34, Podoplanin, HHV8(+); CD68(-)

Fibrohistiocytic Neoplasm

- Typically include multinucleated cells
- Absence of MOTT

Hodgkin Lymphoma, Nodular Sclerosing

- CD30, CD15 immunoreactivity; EBV(+) (10-40%)
- Absence of MOTT

SELECTED REFERENCES

1. Gunia S et al: Mycobacterial spindle cell pseudotumor (MSP) of the nasal septum clinically mimicking Kaposi's sarcoma: case report. Rhinology. 43(1):70-1, 2005
2. Logani S et al: Spindle cell tumors associated with mycobacteria in lymph nodes of HIV-positive patients: 'Kaposi sarcoma with mycobacteria' and 'mycobacterial pseudotumor'. Am J Surg Pathol. 23(6):656-61, 1999
3. Morrison A et al: Mycobacterial spindle cell pseudotumor of the brain: a case report and review of the literature. Am J Surg Pathol. 23(10):1294-9, 1999
4. Chen KT: Mycobacterial spindle cell pseudotumor of lymph nodes. Am J Surg Pathol. 16(3):276-81, 1992
5. Umlas J et al: Spindle cell pseudotumor due to Mycobacterium avium-intracellulare in patients with acquired immunodeficiency syndrome (AIDS). Positive staining of mycobacteria for cytoskeleton filaments. Am J Surg Pathol. 15(12):1181-7, 1991
6. Brandwein M et al: Spindle cell reaction to nontuberculous mycobacteriosis in AIDS mimicking a spindle cell neoplasm. Evidence for dual histiocytic and fibroblast-like characteristics of spindle cells. Virchows Arch A Pathol Anat Histopathol. 416(4):281-6, 1990
7. Wood C et al: Pseudotumor resulting from atypical mycobacterial infection: a "histoid" variety of Mycobacterium avium-intracellulare complex infection. Am J Clin Pathol. 83(4):524-7, 1985

IMAGE GALLERY

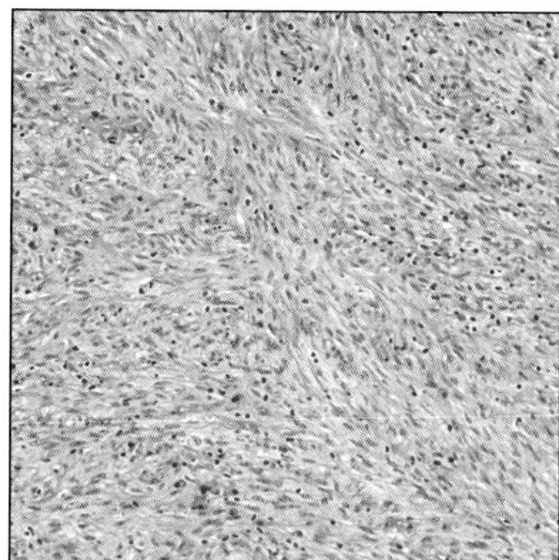

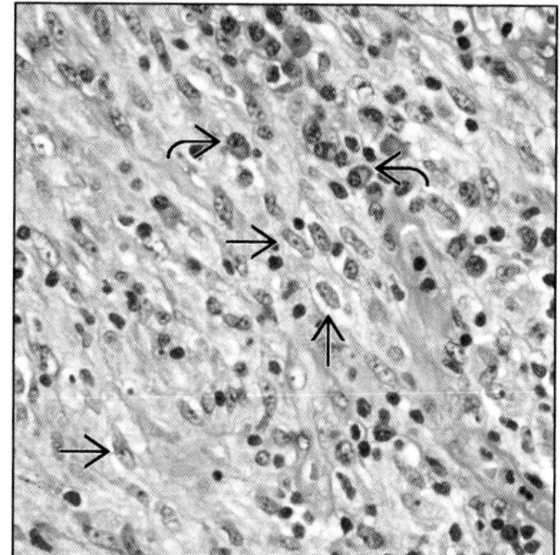

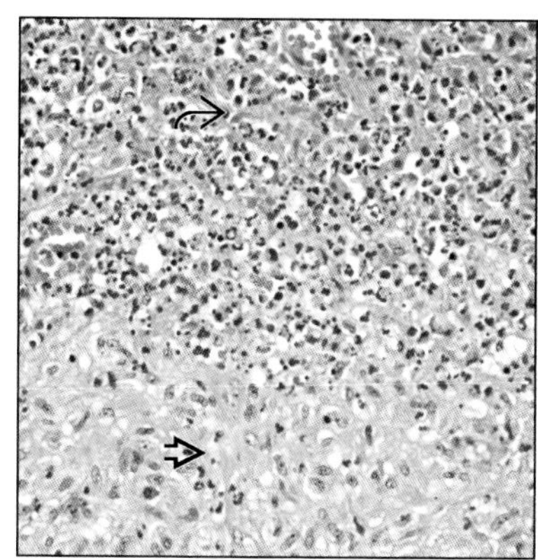

(Left) *The storiform pattern of growth is evident, comprised of short interconnecting fascicles reminiscent of the growth pattern seen in fibrohistiocytic tumors.* ***(Center)*** *The cellular proliferation is composed of bland spindle-shaped cells ⇒. There is an absence of granuloma formation and multinucleated giant cells. Scattered lymphocytes and plasma cells ⇗ are present.* ***(Right)*** *Foci of necrosis ⇗ are seen adjacent to the spindle cell proliferation ⇨.*

SARCOIDOSIS

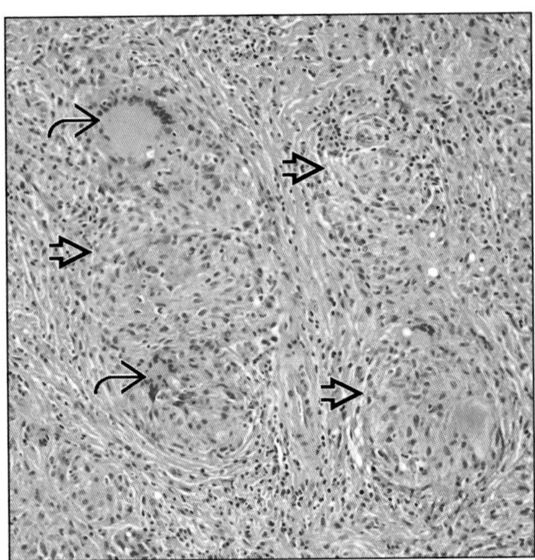

Multiple well-formed, noncaseating granulomas ➩ comprised of nodules of epithelioid histiocytes are shown surrounded by a mixed inflammatory infiltrate; Langhans-type giant cells are seen ↗.

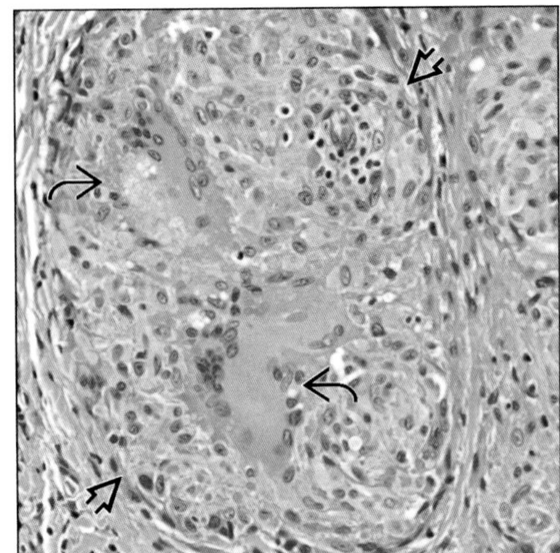

This is a well-formed, noncaseating granuloma ➩ consisting of epithelioid histiocytes, including Langhans-type giant cells ↗. Special stains for microorganisms were negative (not shown).

TERMINOLOGY

Definitions

- Multisystem granulomatous disorder of unknown etiology
  - Diagnosis of sarcoidosis is generally one of exclusion made by correlation of clinical, radiologic, and pathologic findings
  - Pathologic features are characteristic but not specific for diagnosis
  - Diagnosis can only be suggested once an infectious etiology is excluded

ETIOLOGY/PATHOGENESIS

Etiology

- Remains unknown
  - Evidence of finding mycobacterial DNA by polymerase chain reaction in sarcoid granulomas
  - Foreign particulates suggested as causative

CLINICAL ISSUES

Epidemiology

- Incidence
  - Uncommon
- Age
  - Occurs in all age groups but most commonly seen in young adults
    - Peak incidence: 2nd-4th decades
- Gender
  - Female predominance (slight)
- Ethnicity
  - Blacks > > > Caucasians (12:1)

Site

- Any organ may be affected but most commonly lung, lymph nodes, skin
- Isolated extranodal head and neck involvement only occurs in small percentage of cases and includes
  - Pharynx, tonsils, sinonasal tract, larynx, salivary glands
    - Salivary gland involvement referred to as Heerfordt syndrome or uveoparotid fever
  - Ear and temporal bones
  - Thyroid gland, parathyroid glands

Presentation

- Most common clinical presentation includes fever, weight loss and hilar adenopathy
- Otolaryngic symptoms vary according to site and include
  - Cervical adenopathy, pharyngotonsillitis with tonsillar enlargement, nasal obstruction, nasal discharge, epistaxis, septal perforation
  - Salivary gland involvement may
    - Clinically simulate Sjögren syndrome with enlargement, xerostomia and xerophthalmia
    - Present with facial nerve paralysis
- May occur in association with head and neck cancer

Laboratory Tests

- Elevated angiotensin-converting enzyme (ACE) levels
- Cutaneous anergy to skin test antigens (Kveim test) positive in 60-85% of patients

Treatment

- Options, risks, complications
  - Treatment for symptomatic patients is with corticosteroid therapy
- Surgical approaches
  - May be necessary in presence of severe airway obstruction

Prognosis

- Prognosis generally good
  - Approximately 70% improve or remain stable following therapy
  - Approximately 10-20% do not respond to therapy

Key Facts

Clinical Issues

- Multisystem granulomatous disorder of unknown etiology
- Blacks > > > Caucasians (12:1)
- Most commonly affects lung, lymph nodes, skin
- Clinical presentation includes fever, weight loss and hilar adenopathy
- Elevated angiotensin-converting enzyme (ACE) levels
- Treatment for symptomatic patients with corticosteroid therapy

Microscopic Pathology

- Multiple well-formed noncaseating granulomas

Diagnostic Checklist

- Diagnosis generally one of excluding infectious disease; requires clinical, radiologic and pathologic correlation

- Advanced multisystem disease leading to extensive pulmonary involvement and respiratory failure may occur
  - Only seen in small percentage of cases
  - About 10% may die with disease as result of respiratory or central nervous system complications

MICROSCOPIC PATHOLOGY

Histologic Features

- Multiple well-formed noncaseating granulomas consisting of nodules of epithelioid histiocytes surrounded by mixed inflammatory infiltrate
  - Langhans-type giant cells may be present
  - Necrosis absent but some examples, especially extranodal, may have small central foci of necrosis
  - Intracytoplasmic star-shaped inclusions (asteroid bodies) may be seen
  - Intracytoplasmic calcific laminated bodies (Schaumann bodies or Hamazaki-Wesenberg inclusions) may be seen
  - Calcium oxylate crystals may be present in cytoplasm of giant cells

ANCILLARY TESTS

Histochemistry

- Special stains for microorganisms are negative

DIFFERENTIAL DIAGNOSIS

Infectious Diseases

- Noncaseating granulomatous inflammation can be seen in
  - Tuberculosis (typical and atypical), fungal diseases, leprosy, cat scratch disease, other infectious diseases
  - Identification of causative microorganism by one or more of the following
    - Microbiologic cultures
    - Histochemical stains
    - Molecular diagnostics (e.g., PCR, others)

SELECTED REFERENCES

1. Heffner DK: The cause of sarcoidosis: the Centurial enigma solved. Ann Diagn Pathol. 11(2):142-52, 2007
2. Schwartzbauer HR et al: Ear, nose, and throat manifestations of sarcoidosis. Otolaryngol Clin North Am. 36(4):673-84, 2003
3. Kardon DE et al: A clinicopathologic series of 22 cases of tonsillar granulomas. Laryngoscope. 110(3 Pt 1):476-81, 2000
4. Shah UK et al: Otolaryngologic manifestations of sarcoidosis: presentation and diagnosis. Laryngoscope. 107(1):67-75, 1997
5. Israel HL et al: 67Gallium scans in Löfgren's syndrome. Sarcoidosis. 12(1):58-60, 1995
6. Roger G et al: Sarcoidosis of the upper respiratory tract in children. Int J Pediatr Otorhinolaryngol. 30(3):233-40, 1994

IMAGE GALLERY

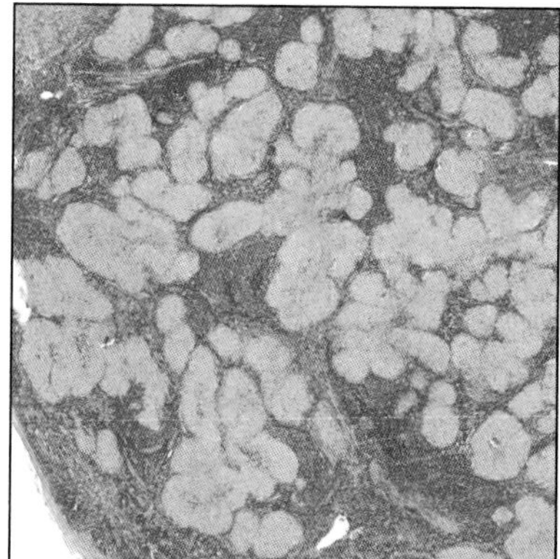

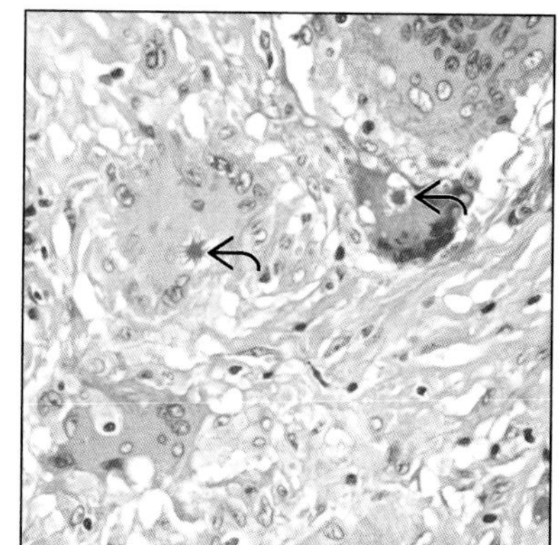

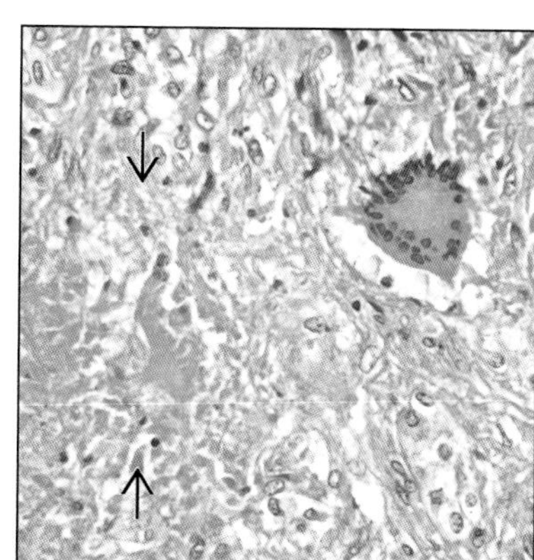

(Left) H&E shows a lymph node replaced by confluent-appearing well-formed granulomas. (Center) Star-shaped asteroid bodies ➔ are seen in the cytoplasm of Langhans giant cells, a finding supporting a diagnosis of sarcoidosis. (Right) Typically, the granulomas of sarcoidosis lack necrosis (caseation) but rarely necrosis ➔ may be present in association with sarcoid granulomas. An infectious etiology must be excluded by cultures, stains &/or molecular diagnostic testing.

NODULAR FASCIITIS

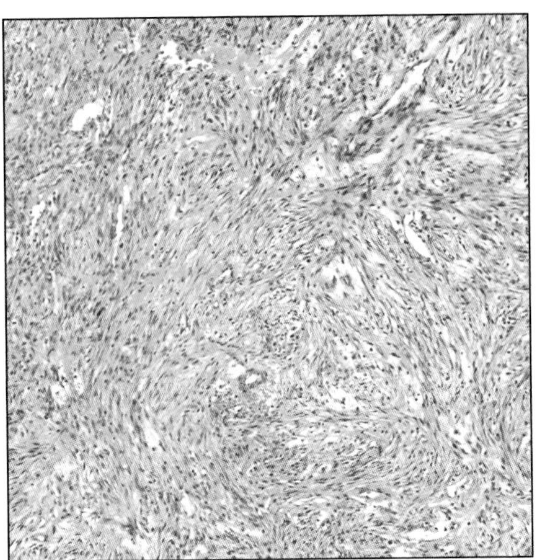

Hematoxylin & eosin shows interlacing short fascicles of spindled cells with extravasated erythrocytes and a rich vascular plexus.

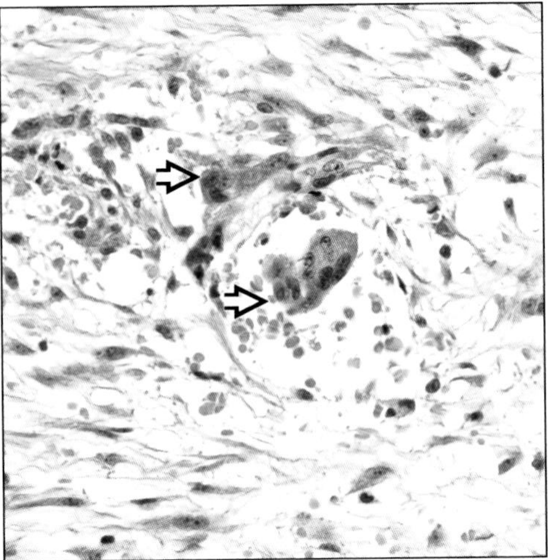

Hematoxylin & eosin shows fibroblasts with wispy cytoplasm. Giant cells ➪ are seen along with extravasated erythrocytes.

TERMINOLOGY

Synonyms

- Cranial fasciitis
- Intravascular fasciitis

Definitions

- Mass-forming myofibroblastic proliferation displaying a tissue culture-like growth pattern

ETIOLOGY/PATHOGENESIS

Trauma

- May be slight and limited, overlooked by patient

CLINICAL ISSUES

Epidemiology

- Incidence
    - Uncommon lesion
    - 30% of cases develop in head and neck
- Age
    - Children and young people (≤ 35 years)
    - Rare in elderly (> 60 years)
- Gender
    - Equal gender distribution

Site

- Upper extremities and neck
- Less frequently in face, orbit, and oral cavity

Presentation

- Rapidly growing mass
- Short duration (< 3 weeks)

Natural History

- Spontaneous involution with time

Treatment

- Simple excision

Prognosis

- Recurs in 2%, although potentially persistent
    - Usually within short duration after surgery

IMAGE FINDINGS

CT Findings

- Moderate to strong enhancement of soft tissue mass with smooth margins

MACROSCOPIC FEATURES

General Features

- Unencapsulated, round to oval, nodular mass, frequently attached to fascia
- Cut surfaces range from firm to soft and gelatinous, depending on duration
- Cystic areas common

Size

- Mean: < 3 cm, although up to 5 cm

MICROSCOPIC PATHOLOGY

Histologic Features

- Poorly circumscribed with irregular stellate appearance
- Plump myofibroblasts in tissue culture-like appearance
- Arranged in storiform, short, irregular interlacing fascicles and bundles
- Benign myofibroblasts with oval nuclei, pale chromatin, and prominent nucleoli
- Easily identified mitotic figures, but never atypical
- Background of extravasated erythrocytes, inflammatory cells, and giant cells
- Keloid-like collagen deposition
    - More collagen with lesions of longer duration

NODULAR FASCIITIS

Key Facts

Clinical Issues
- Rapidly growing mass
- Short duration (< 3 weeks)
- Children and young people (≤ 35 years)

Macroscopic Features
- Unencapsulated, round to oval, nodular mass, frequently attached to fascia

Microscopic Pathology
- Plump fibroblasts in tissue culture-like appearance
- Arranged in storiform, short, irregular interlacing fascicles and bundles
- Background of extravasated erythrocytes, inflammatory cells, and giant cells
- Keloid-like collagen deposition

ANCILLARY TESTS

Cytology
- Cellular smears with interlaced short, plump spindled fibroblasts in slightly myxoid background
- Fibroblasts with eccentric nuclear placement, occasionally binucleated
- Mitotic figures may be seen
- Clumps of collagen in background

Immunohistochemistry
- Although unnecessary, actins and vimentin immunoreactive and CD68(+) histiocytes

Electron Microscopy
- Elongated, bipolar fibroblastic cells, extensive rough endoplasmic reticulum and bundles of microfilaments

DIFFERENTIAL DIAGNOSIS

Fibrosarcoma
- More dense cellularity, herringbone configuration, with atypical mitotic figures

Rhabdomyosarcoma
- Pleomorphic cells, increased mitotic figures, with unique immunohistochemical and molecular profile

Fibromatosis
- Ill-defined, but slender, elongated fibroblasts arranged parallel to vessels and collagen

Fetal Rhabdomyoma
- Cellular tumor with gradient of cells showing striations

SELECTED REFERENCES

1. Abdel-Aziz M et al: Nodular fasciitis of the external auditory canal in six Egyptian children. Int J Pediatr Otorhinolaryngol. 72(5):643-6, 2008
2. Silva P et al: Nodular fasciitis of the head and neck. J Laryngol Otol. 119(1):8-11, 2005
3. Kong CS et al: Nodular fasciitis: diagnosis by fine needle aspiration biopsy. Acta Cytol. 48(4):473-7, 2004
4. Thompson LD et al: Nodular fasciitis of the external ear region: a clinicopathologic study of 50 cases. Ann Diagn Pathol. 5(4):191-8, 2001
5. DiNardo LJ et al: Nodular fasciitis of the head and neck in children. A deceptive lesion. Arch Otolaryngol Head Neck Surg. 117(9):1001-2, 1991
6. Montgomery EA et al: Nodular fasciitis. Its morphologic spectrum and immunohistochemical profile. Am J Surg Pathol. 15(10):942-8, 1991
7. Davies HT et al: Oral nodular fasciitis. Br J Oral Maxillofac Surg. 27(2):147-51, 1989
8. Patterson JW et al: Cranial fasciitis. Arch Dermatol. 125(5):674-8, 1989
9. Batsakis JG et al: The pathology of head and neck tumors: spindle cell lesions (sarcomatoid carcinomas, nodular fasciitis, and fibrosarcoma) of the aerodigestive tracts, Part 14. Head Neck Surg. 4(6):499-513, 1982
10. Patchefsky AS et al: Intravascular fasciitis: a report of 17 cases. Am J Surg Pathol. 5(1):29-36, 1981

IMAGE GALLERY

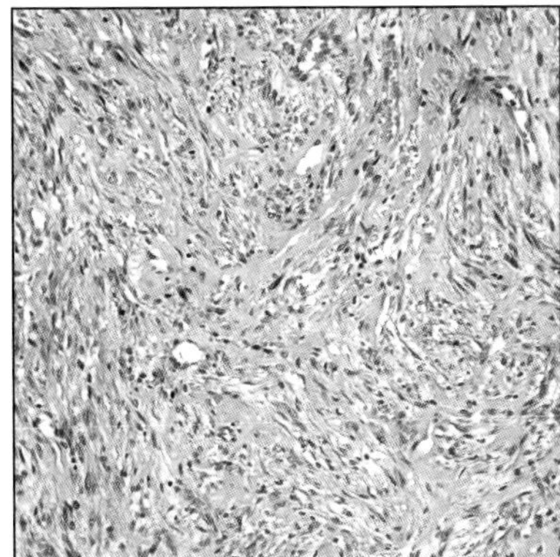

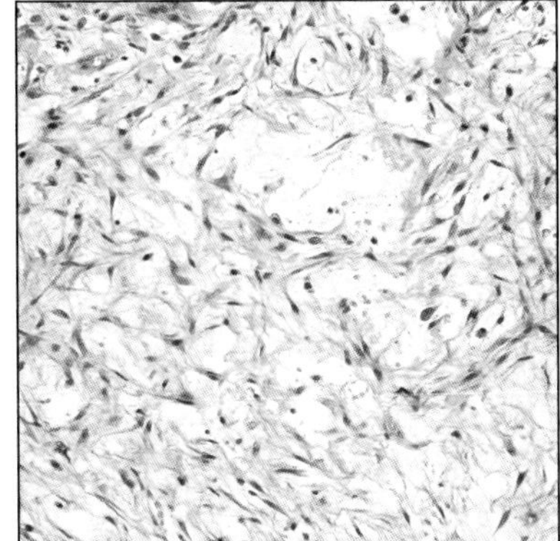

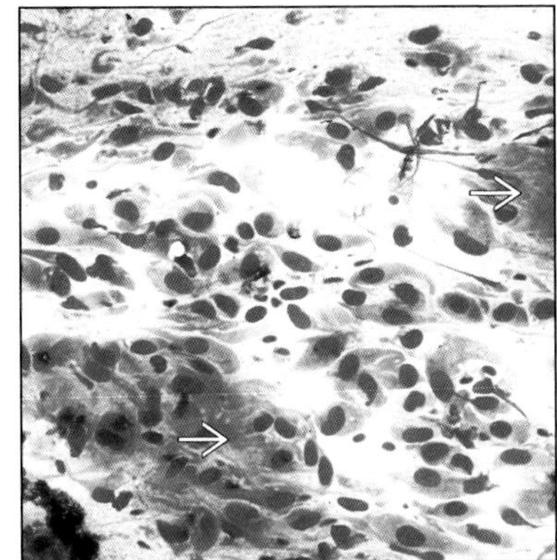

*(**Left**) Hematoxylin & eosin shows keloid-like collagen deposition within a proliferation of spindled fibroblasts. Erythrocytes are noted. (**Center**) Hematoxylin & eosin shows a myxoid background between the fibroblasts and erythrocytes. (**Right**) Diff-Quik shows bipolar fibroblasts with elongated cytoplasmic extensions. "Pink" collagen material ➡ is noted in the background.*

CAROTID BODY PARAGANGLIOMA

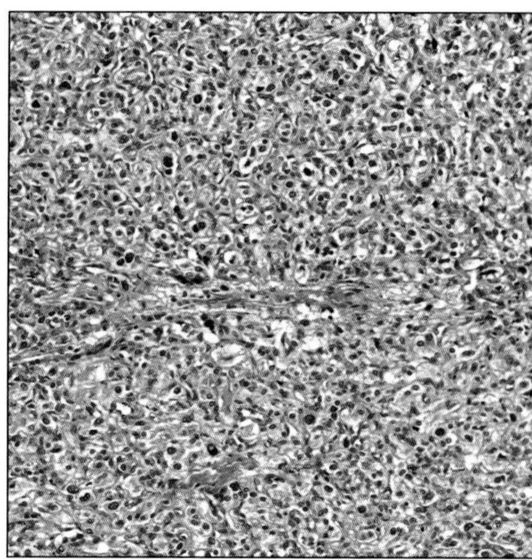

Clusters and small ball-like (zellballen) configurations are well represented in this paraganglioma. There is a well-developed fibrovascular stroma separating the tumor nests.

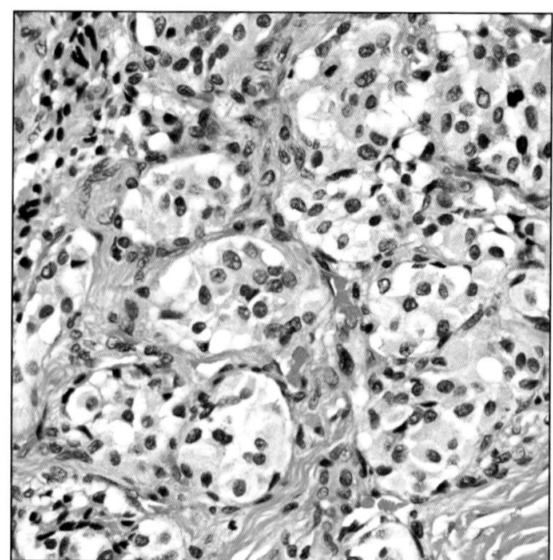

The small to medium-sized cells have slightly basophilic, delicately granular cytoplasm surrounding round to oval nuclei. The packeted arrangement with surrounding fibrosis is common.

TERMINOLOGY

Synonyms

- Chemodectoma, glomus tumor, non-chromaffin paraganglioma, neuroendocrine tumor, branchiomeric paraganglioma

Definitions

- Neuroendocrine neoplasm derived from **carotid body** paraganglia composed of chief and sustentacular cells arranged in characteristic (zellballen) pattern

ETIOLOGY/PATHOGENESIS

Etiology

- Familial inheritance
  - Part of MEN2A and 2B (Carney triad)
  - Patients have mutations in succinate dehydrogenase complex (*SDHD*, *PGL2*, *SDHC* genes)
- Chronic hypoxia is known risk factor
  - Tumors are increased in frequency in patients living at high altitudes
  - Women (presumably due to menstruation) show greater hypoxia at high altitudes
  - Athletic patients and patients with large lung capacity may overcome hypoxia

Pathogenesis

- Paraganglia are aggregates of specialized neuroendocrine tissue (glomus cells)
  - Arise from embryonic neural crest (part of sympathetic nervous system)
  - Found at bifurcation of common carotid artery
    - Posteromedial wall, either within or immediately external to adventitia
    - Paired and bilateral carotid bodies
    - Measure 3-7 mm and weigh 3-15 mg
  - Attached by a band of fibrovascular tissue to the artery (ligament of Mayer)
- Function as chemoreceptors
  - Respond to acute changes in oxygen tension, carbon dioxide levels, and hydrogen ion concentration

CLINICAL ISSUES

Epidemiology

- Incidence
  - ~ 3% of all paragangliomas develop in head and neck
    - Abdomen > > > chest > > head and neck
  - Carotid body > jugular, tympanic > vagal > > > larynx, paranasal sinuses > thyroid
  - Rule of 10s: 10% multicentric, bilateral, familial, pediatric, &/or malignant
- Age
  - Mean: 40-50 years
    - Rare in children, except if familial
- Gender
  - Female > > Male (4-8:1)
    - Menstrual blood loss may contribute to hypoxia
  - Male > Female for inherited/familial tumors

Site

- Crotch of common carotid artery bifurcation
  - Between external carotid artery (ECA) and internal carotid artery (ICA)
- Deep to anterior border of sternocleidomastoid muscle, below mandibular angle

Presentation

- Painless (asymptomatic), slowly enlarging neck mass
  - Shows easy side to side movement (Fontaine sign), but no vertical movement
- Cranial nerve paresis or paralysis with larger tumors
- Infrequently associated with dysphagia, hoarseness, headache, Horner syndrome, syncope
- Bruit or thrill may be present
- Catecholamine function is very rare
  - If present, hypertension is most common symptom

CAROTID BODY PARAGANGLIOMA

Key Facts

Terminology
- Neuroendocrine neoplasm derived from paraganglia composed of chief and sustentacular cells arranged in zellballen pattern

Clinical Issues
- ~ 3% of all paragangliomas develop in head and neck
  - Carotid body > jugular, tympanic > vagal > larynx
- Female > > Male (4-8:1)
- Crotch of common carotid artery bifurcation
- Painless, slowly enlarging neck mass
- Presurgical embolization for reduced bleeding
- Surgery is treatment of choice

Image Findings
- Studies show exact location and tumor extent, guide surgical approach, provide therapeutic alternatives

Microscopic Pathology
- Clustered, zellballen, alveolar, or whorled architecture
  - Chief cells: Small to intermediate, epithelioid cells with ample granular, basophilic cytoplasm
  - Nuclei are round to focally irregular and enlarged
  - Sustentacular supporting cells
- Highly vascularized stroma, sometimes with fibrosis
- Malignant tumors are uncommon (document metastases)

Ancillary Tests
- Chief cells **positive**: Neuroendocrine markers
- Sustentacular cells **positive**: S100 protein, GFAP

Top Differential Diagnoses
- Medullary thyroid carcinoma, schwannoma, undifferentiated carcinoma, metastatic melanoma

- If familial or syndromic cases
  - Autosomal dominant trait with genomic imprinting
  - More commonly bilateral (30%) &/or multifocal
  - Associated with thyroid medullary carcinoma, parathyroid disease, gastrointestinal neuromas
  - Rare association with clotting factor VII and X deficiencies

Laboratory Tests
- < 3% of tumors secrete catecholamines that result in clinical symptoms

Treatment
- Options, risks, complications
  - **Do not biopsy**: Very vascularized with heavy bleeding
  - Presurgical embolization for reduced bleeding
- Surgical approaches
  - Surgery, including one or more branches of carotid artery system, is treatment of choice
- Adjuvant therapy
  - Not used because it is presently ineffective
  - New molecular-based therapies show promise
- Radiation
  - Radiotherapy can be used for localized tumors
    - Stereotatic methods are safe
  - Combined with surgery for large tumors
  - Palliative in poor surgical candidates or older patients

Prognosis
- Excellent overall outcome
  - Slowly growing tumors (estimated 7 year doubling time)
- Up to 10% will recur (inadequate excision and regrowth)
- Mortality due to proximity with vital anatomic structures
- Malignant tumors are uncommon (~ 10%)
  - Cervical lymph nodes (90% of time), lung and bone (10%) metastases
  - 60% 5-year survival for malignant tumors
  - Patients managed with surgery **and** radiation have better outcome

IMAGE FINDINGS

Radiographic Findings
- Imaging studies show exact location and tumor extent, guide surgical approach, and provide therapeutic alternatives
- Avidly enhancing vascular mass splaying ECA and ICA, displacing ICA posterolaterally
- **Angiography**: Hypervascular mass at carotid artery bifurcation
  - Prolonged, intense tumor blush
  - Can be used to detect multicentric disease
  - Allows for presurgical embolization
  - Determines collaterals and vascular roadmap for surgery, especially if vessels need to be sacrificed
- Octreotide or MIBG scintigraphy helps with occult or familial tumors
- PET with 18F FDG: Avid uptake by tumor cells

Ultrasonographic Findings
- Solid, inhomogeneous mass; color Doppler flow shows extensive vascularity

MR Findings
- T1WI: "Salt and pepper" appearance when > 1.5 cm, hypointense punctate flow channels due to tumor vascularity
- T2WI with contrast: Intense enhancement, larger high velocity flow voids

MACROSCOPIC FEATURES

General Features
- Firm, rubbery, well-circumscribed, polypoid mass
- Reddish, firm mass
  - Variegated cut surface, yellow, tan, pink, or brown
- May be large and widely invasive

CAROTID BODY PARAGANGLIOMA

Size

- Range: 1-6 cm (mean: 4 cm)

MICROSCOPIC PATHOLOGY

Histologic Features

- Clustered, zellballen, alveolar, or whorled architecture
  - Zellballen is German for "cell balls"
- Highly vascularized stroma, sometimes with fibrosis
- Poorly encapsulated or circumscribed, often infiltrative
  - Vascular and perineural invasion uncommon but not prognostically significant
- Moderately cellular, biphasic tumor
- Cyst formation, hemorrhage, and hemosiderin-laden macrophages common
- Paraganglia (chief) cells (type I)
  - Small to intermediate, epithelioid cells with ample granular, basophilic cytoplasm
  - Nuclei are round to focally irregular and enlarged
  - Delicate to coarse nuclear chromatin
  - Multinucleated giant cells and spindled cells are uncommon
- Sustentacular supporting cells (type II)
  - Create net or supporting framework surrounding nests
  - Cannot be detected reliably without special stains (S100 protein, GFAP)
- Mitotic figures are very rare
- Malignant tumors are uncommon (up to 10%)
  - Malignant if documented metastases
  - Histology does not predict clinical behavior

ANCILLARY TESTS

Cytology

- Fine needle aspiration usually contraindicated as it may provoke hypertensive crisis or significant bleeding
- Smears have moderate to high cellularity with background of blood
- Cells arranged singly or in small groups, sometimes forming acinar or "pseudorosette"
- 3 cell types are interspersed throughout smear
  - Small to moderate-sized, polygon-shaped cells with delicate granular cytoplasm
  - Spindle cells with ample granulated cytoplasm and elongated nuclei
  - Large, "strap-like" cells with large eccentric nuclei with prominent nucleoli

Immunohistochemistry

- Chief cells **positive**: Synaptophysin, chromogranin-A, NSE, CD56
- Sustentacular cells **positive**: S100 protein, glial fibrillary acidic protein (GFAP)
- **Negative**: Cytokeratin, carcinoembryonic antigen

Cytogenetics

- Inactivating germline mutations in mitochondrial complex II subunits of succinate-ubiquinone oxidoreductase gene (*SDH*, subunits *SDHB*, *SDHC*, *SDHD*) are associated with hereditary paraganglioma
- Genetic counseling and testing for *SDHX*, *VHL*, *NF1*, and *RET* genes should be offered to all patients with paraganglioma

Electron Microscopy

- **Chief** cells: Cytoplasmic, membrane-bound, electron-dense, catecholamine-bound neurosecretory granules

DIFFERENTIAL DIAGNOSIS

Medullary Thyroid Carcinoma

- Thyroid mass, frequently with neck metastases
- Spindled epithelioid cells with round to irregular nuclei and "salt and pepper" nuclear chromatin distribution
- **Positive**: Calcitonin, neuroendocrine markers, keratin, TTF-1, CEA-M

Schwannoma

- Spindle cells, alternating cellular and hypocellular areas
- Diffuse, strong S100 protein immunoreactivity in all cells

Undifferentiated Carcinoma

- Specifically metastatic tumor to the neck
- **Positive**: Strong keratin; **negative**: S100 protein

Metastatic Melanoma

- Can be histologic mimic of any tumor; pigmented; intranuclear cytoplasmic inclusions
- **Positive**: Melanoma markers (S100 protein, HMB-45, Melan-A); **negative**: Keratin, neuroendocrine markers

SELECTED REFERENCES

1. Zeitler DM et al: Preoperative embolization in carotid body tumor surgery: is it required? Ann Otol Rhinol Laryngol. 119(5):279-83, 2010
2. Papaspyrou K et al: Management of head and neck paragangliomas: review of 120 patients. Head Neck. 31(3):381-7, 2009
3. Jani P et al: Familial carotid body tumours: is there a role for genetic screening? J Laryngol Otol. 122(9):978-82, 2008
4. Jech M et al: Genetic analysis of high altitude paragangliomas. Endocr Pathol. 17(2):201-2, 2006
5. Pellitteri PK et al: Paragangliomas of the head and neck. Oral Oncol. 40(6):563-75, 2004
6. Baysal BE et al: Etiopathogenesis and clinical presentation of carotid body tumors. Microsc Res Tech. 59(3):256-61, 2002
7. Lee JH et al: National Cancer Data Base report on malignant paragangliomas of the head and neck. Cancer. 94(3):730-7, 2002
8. Rao AB et al: From the archives of the AFIP. Paragangliomas of the head and neck: radiologic-pathologic correlation. Armed Forces Institute of Pathology. Radiographics. 19(6):1605-32, 1999
9. Layfield LJ: Fine-needle aspiration of the head and neck. Pathology (Phila). 4(2):409-38, 1996
10. Netterville JL et al: Carotid body tumors: a review of 30 patients with 46 tumors. Laryngoscope. 105(2):115-26, 1995

Diagrammatic, Imaging, Clinical, and Microscopic Features

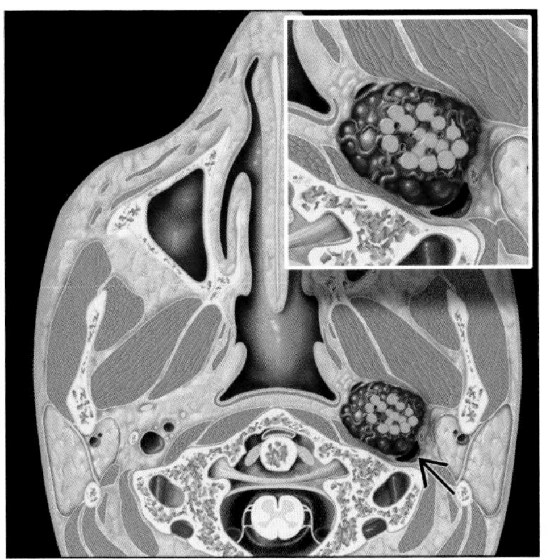

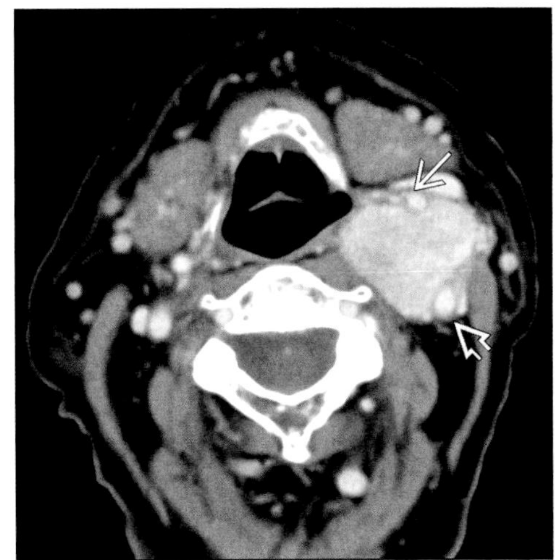

(Left) *Axial graphic of the nasopharyngeal bilateral carotid spaces shows a paraganglioma (inset) expanding the left carotid sheath and compressing the internal jugular vein* →*. The cranial nerves (9, 10, 11, and 12) are within the sheath and may be compressed by the tumor.* ***(Right)*** *Axial contrast-enhanced CT shows a classic example of carotid body paraganglioma as an avidly enhancing mass splaying external* ➡ *and internal* ➡ *carotid arteries at the carotid bifurcation.*

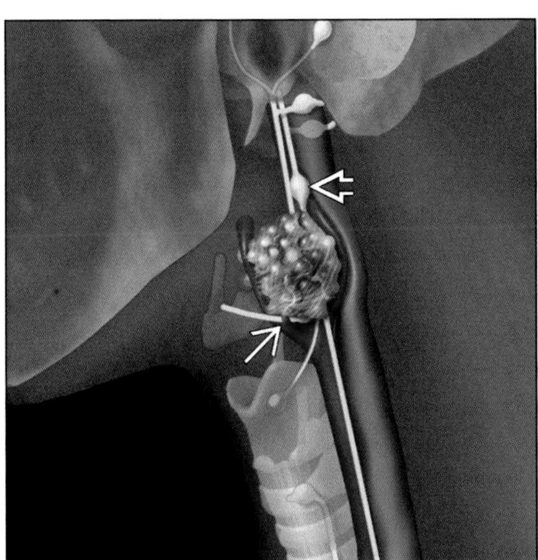

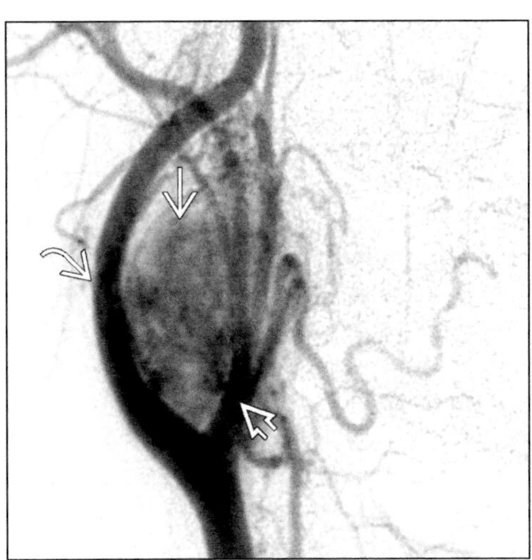

(Left) *Lateral graphic shows a carotid body paraganglioma splaying the external and internal carotid arteries. The main arterial feeder is the ascending pharyngeal artery* ➡*. The glomus bodies are illustrated in the nodose ganglion of CN10* ➡*.* ***(Right)*** *Lateral common carotid angiogram demonstrates intense carotid body paraganglioma tumor blush* ➡ *between the external* ➡ *and internal* ➡ *carotid arteries.*

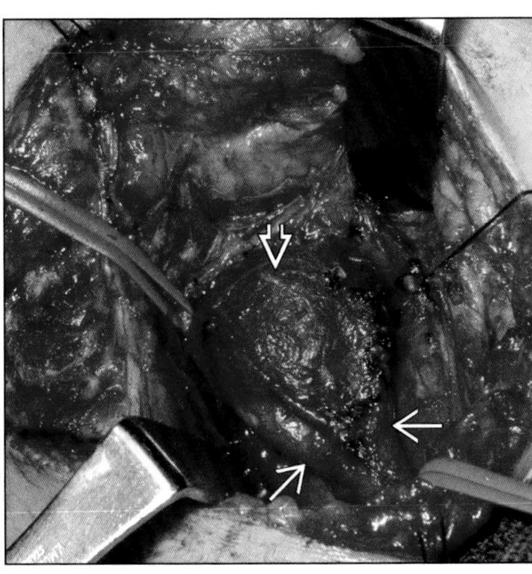

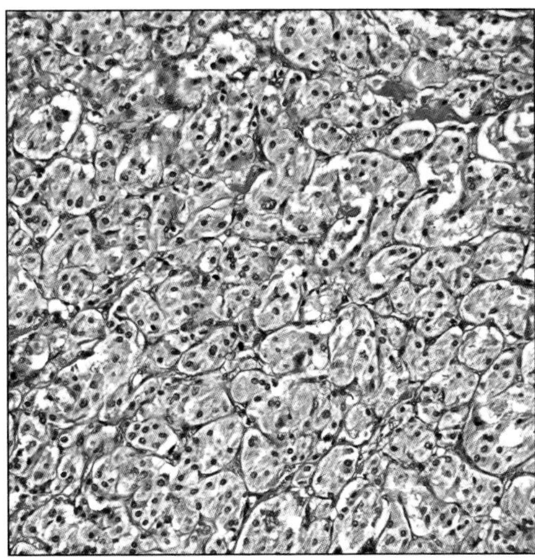

(Left) *Intraoperative photograph shows splaying of the internal and external carotid arteries* ➡*, as well as a large, richly vascularized tumor* ➡ *set in the crotch of the carotid artery bifurcation.* ***(Right)*** *The most characteristic pattern of a paraganglioma is the presence of zellballen. Small, well-formed balls of neoplastic cells are separated by a very delicate fibrovascular plexus.*

Microscopic Features

(Left) Cell nesting is one of the most characteristic appearances of paraganglioma. The cytoplasm of these tumor cells is abundant, showing a more eosinophilic appearance than usual. There are fibrovascular septa surrounding the paraganglia cells. ***(Right)*** Paraganglioma, especially within the carotid body, can have larger nests of cells ➾, separated by a fibrovascular plexus. Cellular pleomorphism is frequently present within these larger nests. They do not equate to malignancy, however.

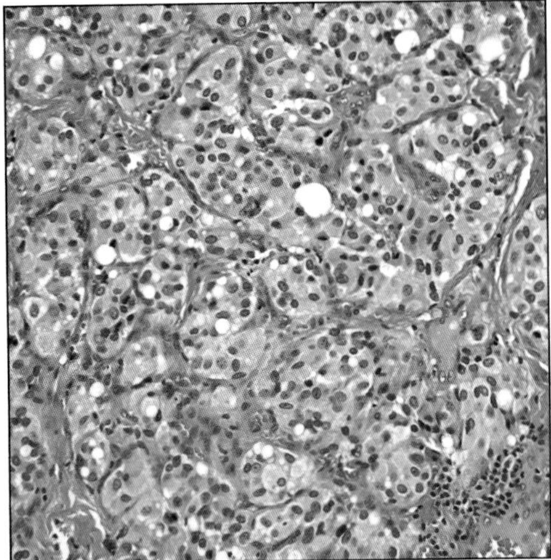

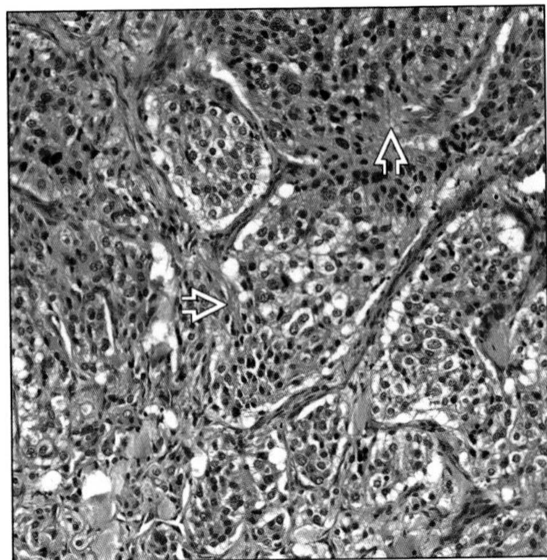

(Left) The nested pattern is composed of cells that have more of a spindled appearance. The cytoplasmic quality is similar, with hyperchromatic nuclear chromatin. ***(Right)*** In many tumors, the zellballen architecture can sometimes be subtle, instead showing a more sheet-like distribution. The nuclei show vague pleomorphism in a few cells. Tumors with subtle zellballen architecture generally benefit from an immunohistochemistry evaluation.

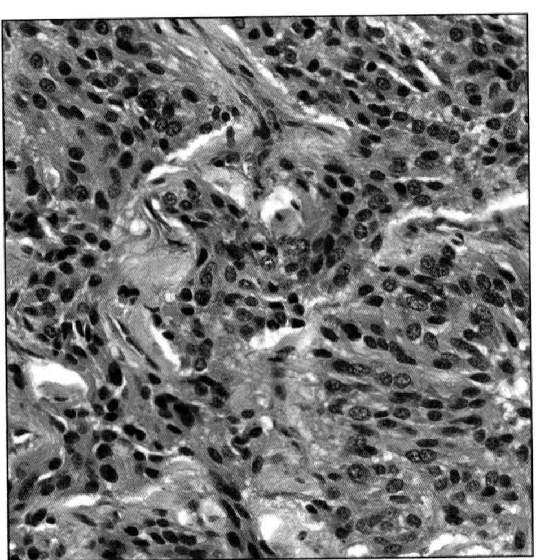

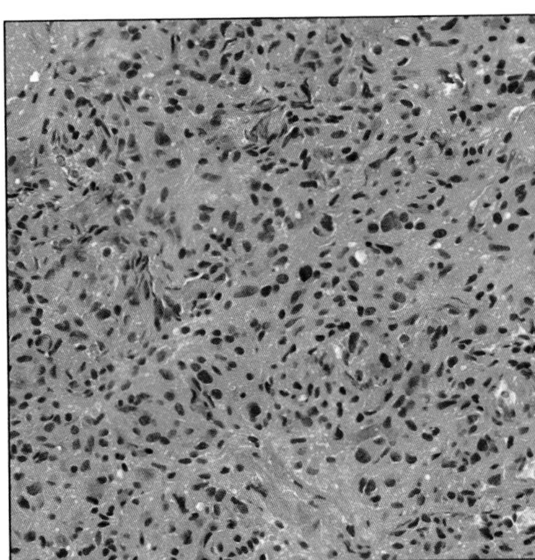

(Left) This high-power image demonstrates a syncytial arrangement of the neoplastic cells. There are delicate fibrovascular septa around the tumor nests. The nuclei show coarse but "salt and pepper" nuclear chromatin distribution. ***(Right)*** Most neoplastic cells have a bland appearance, with round to oval hyperchromatic nuclei. However, isolated neoplastic cells will show pleomorphism ➔.

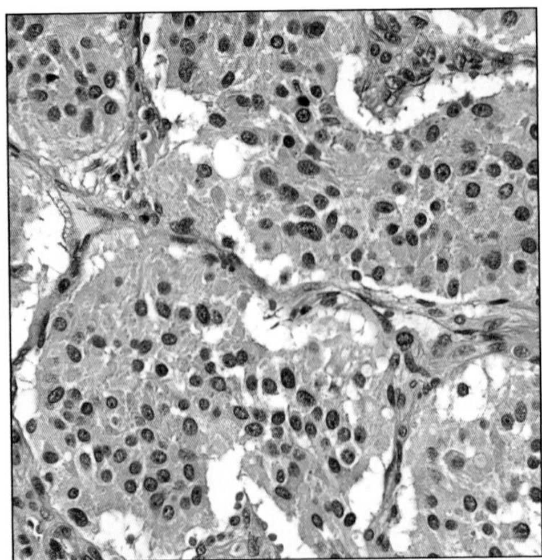

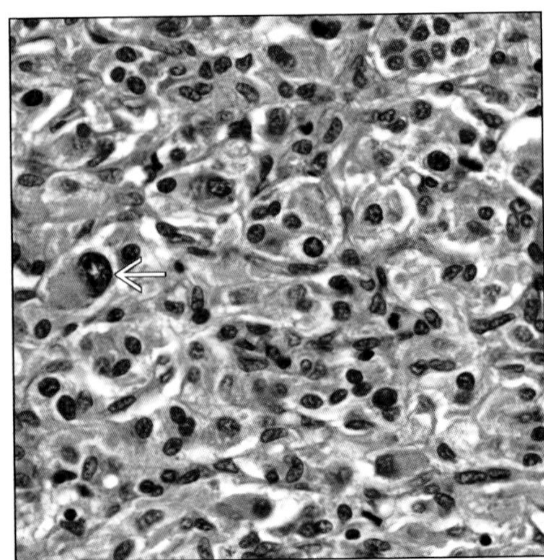

Microscopic Features and Ancillary Techniques

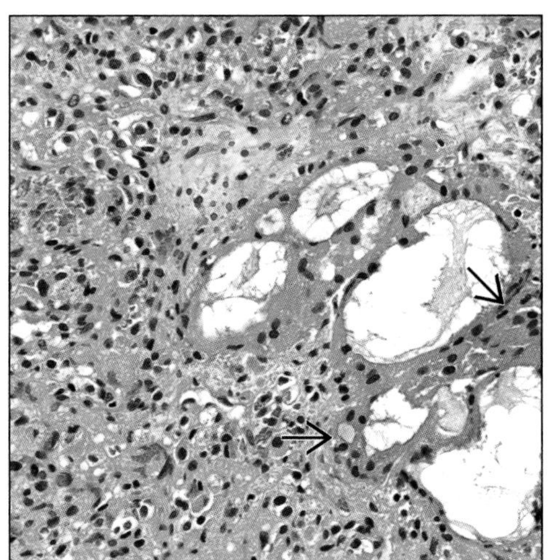

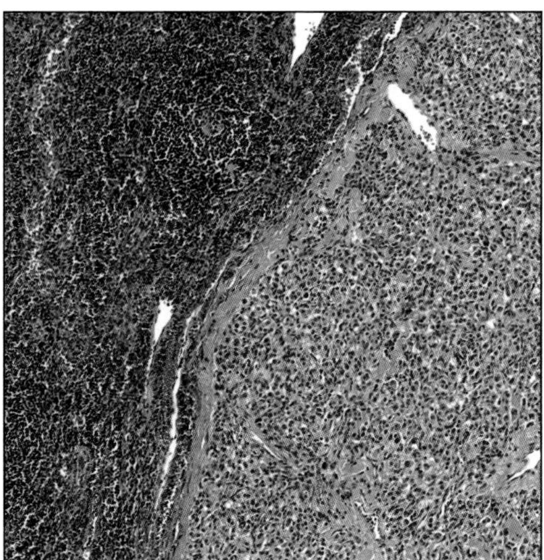

*(**Left**) Tumor architecture is very difficult to determine in this field. There is a foreign body giant cell reaction to the embolic material ➔ within this tumor, which was preoperatively embolized to decrease bleeding. (**Right**) Malignant paraganglioma is usually confirmed by the presence of lymph node metastasis or tumor in a space where paraganglia are normally not found. Histologic criteria of malignancy (barring metastases) are unreliable, so all paragangliomas are followed long term.*

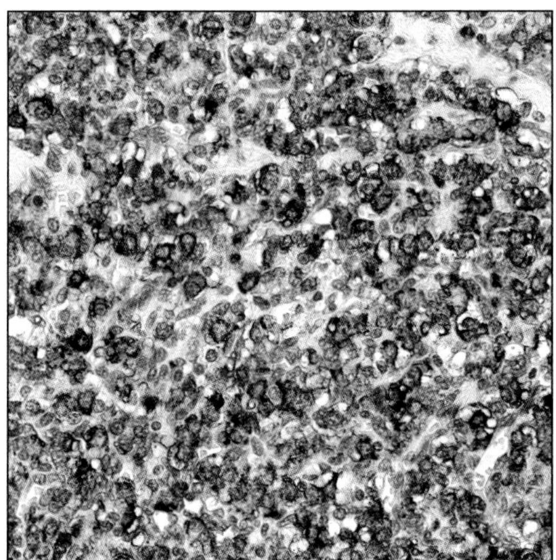

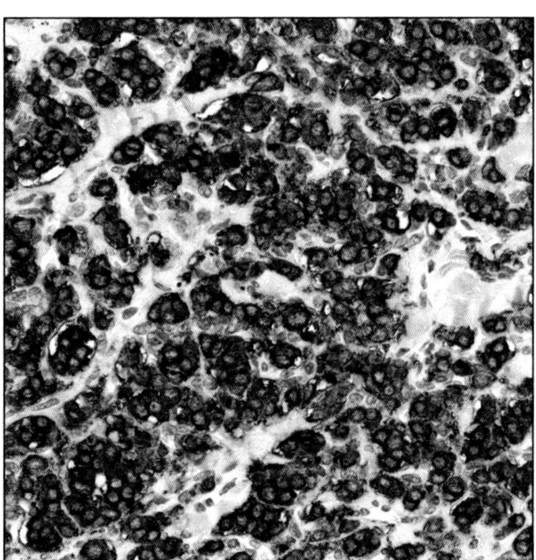

*(**Left**) A number of neuroendocrine markers are positive in the paraganglia cells, with chromogranin highlighting the cells of this tumor. Note the relative lack of zellballen architecture in this tumor. It is not uncommon to have variability in patterns within the same tumor. (**Right**) Synaptophysin is one of the positive neuroendocrine markers in the chief cells (paraganglia cells) of a paraganglioma. Others include chromogranin, CD56, and NSE.*

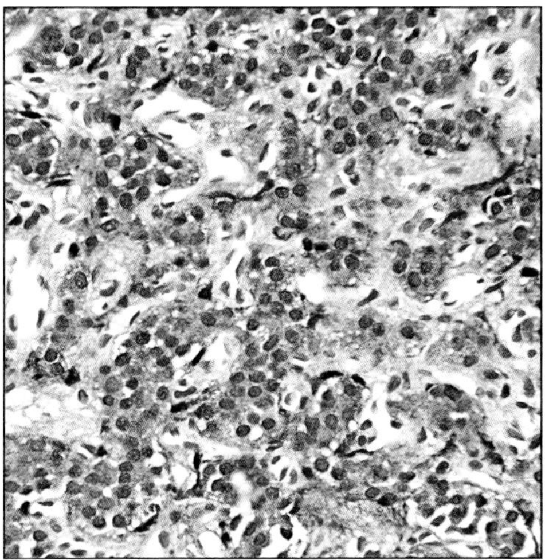

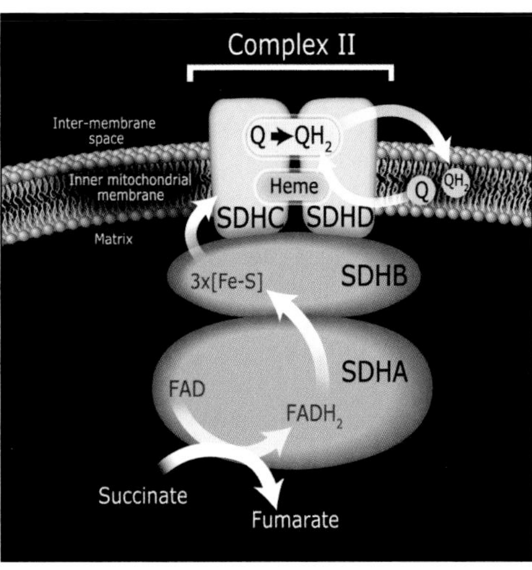

*(**Left**) S100 protein stains the nucleus and cytoplasm of the peripherally located sustentacular cells. There is often a "blush" or background cytoplasmic reaction that should not be interpreted as positive. (**Right**) A graphic of part of the mitochondrial respiratory chain complex II shows the relationship between the succinate ubiquinone oxidoreductase subunits (SDHA → SDHD). Inactivating mutations result in hereditary paraganglioma.*

ELASTOFIBROMA

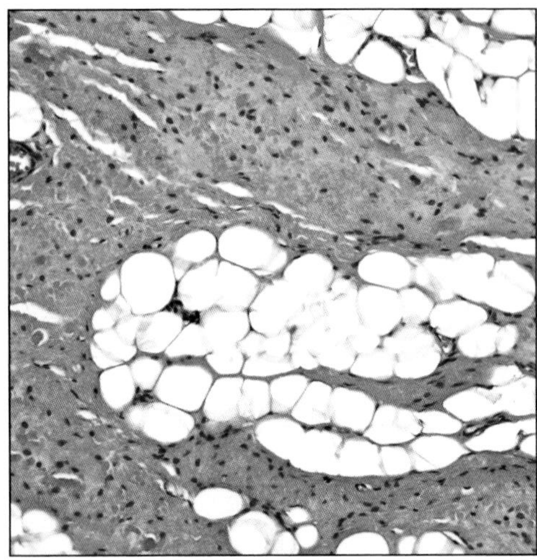

Hematoxylin & eosin shows heavy collagen deposition within adipose connective tissue. Degenerated collagen fibers are present.

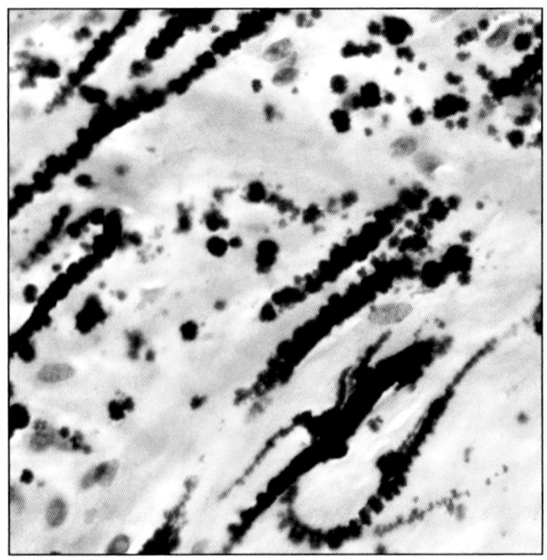

Elastic van Gieson shows a classic "pipe cleaner" appearance with degenerated globules of elastic fibers in the background.

TERMINOLOGY

Synonyms

- Elastofibroma dorsi

Definitions

- Ill-defined fibroelastic tumor-like condition comprised of enlarged and irregular elastic fibers

ETIOLOGY/PATHOGENESIS

Developmental Anomaly

- Support for genetic predisposition (alterations of short arm of chromosome 1)
- Multifocality may suggest systemic enzymatic defect, resulting in abnormal elastogenesis
- Repeated trauma or friction unlikely

CLINICAL ISSUES

Epidemiology

- Incidence
  - Uncommon, reported < 0.001% of soft tissue tumors
  - Pre-elastofibroma-like reactions can be seen in autopsies (up to 24% of patients)
- Age
  - Elderly patients, nearly exclusively > 50 years old
  - Peak at 60-70 years
- Gender
  - Female > > Male (5:1)
- Ethnicity
  - Increased frequency in Okinawa, Japan (but may be reporting bias)

Site

- Subscapular/infrascapular area, deep to muscle, sometimes attached to periosteum of ribs
- Between shoulder blades and lower neck
- Chest wall less common

Presentation

- Slow growing, deep-seated, firm mass, frequently bilateral
- Uncommonly presents with pain or tenderness

Treatment

- Surgical approaches
  - Simple excision in symptomatic patients
    - Postoperative hematoma or seroma is frequent complication

Prognosis

- Excellent; isolated recurrences reported

IMAGE FINDINGS

MR Findings

- Inhomogeneous soft tissue mass with contrast enhancement

CT Findings

- Poorly circumscribed, heterogeneous soft tissue mass
- Signal intensity/attenuation similar to skeletal muscle with fat
- Frequently bilateral: Removes sarcoma from consideration

MACROSCOPIC FEATURES

General Features

- Ill defined, nonencapsulated, rubbery, and firm
- White fibrous tissue with interposed yellow fat

Size

- Mean: 5 cm
- Range: Up to 20 cm

ELASTOFIBROMA

Key Facts

Clinical Issues
- Subscapular area
- Female > > Male
- Elderly patients, nearly exclusively > 50 years old
- High frequency of bilateral lesions

Microscopic Pathology
- Mixture of heavy dense bands of collagenous tissue dissected by fat and abnormal elastic fibers
- Fragmented into linearly arranged globules, simulating beads on string or pipe cleaners
- Weigert or von Gieson elastic stains highlight bead-like arrangement
- Large numbers of elastic fibers

Top Differential Diagnoses
- Spindle cell lipoma
- Nuchal fibroma

MICROSCOPIC PATHOLOGY

Histologic Features
- Mixture of heavy dense bands of collagenous tissue dissected by fat and abnormal elastic fibers
  - Fat is generally entrapped
- Large numbers of elastic fibers
  - Elastic fibers are large (hypertrophic), coarse, thick, and darkly eosinophilic
  - Fragmented into linearly arranged globules, simulating beads on string or pipe cleaners
  - Globules have serrated edge
  - Degenerated elastic fibers create eosinophilic globules or "balls" in stroma

Fine Needle Aspiration
- Cellular, braid-like, or fern leaf-like smears

Histochemistry
- Weigert or von Gieson elastic stains highlight bead-like arrangement

DIFFERENTIAL DIAGNOSIS

Spindle Cell Lipoma
- Spindle cells and adipose tissue but no degenerated collagen

Nuchal Fibroma
- Soft tissue at base of neck showing fat within fibrous connective tissue with entrapped nerves

Fibromatosis
- Heavily collagenized stroma with spindled fibroblasts arranged in single direction with parallel vessels

SELECTED REFERENCES

1. Parratt MT et al: Elastofibroma dorsi: management, outcome and review of the literature. J Bone Joint Surg Br. 92(2):262-6, 2010
2. Chandrasekar CR et al: Elastofibroma dorsi: an uncommon benign pseudotumour. Sarcoma. 2008:756565, 2008
3. Daigeler A et al: Elastofibroma dorsi--differential diagnosis in chest wall tumours. World J Surg Oncol. 5:15, 2007
4. Mortman KD et al: Elastofibroma dorsi: clinicopathologic review of 6 cases. Ann Thorac Surg. 83(5):1894-7, 2007
5. Muramatsu K et al: Elastofibroma dorsi: diagnosis and treatment. J Shoulder Elbow Surg. 16(5):591-5, 2007
6. Ochsner JE et al: Best cases from the AFIP: Elastofibroma dorsi. Radiographics. 26(6):1873-6, 2006
7. Schafmayer C et al: Elastofibroma dorsi as differential diagnosis in tumors of the thoracic wall. Ann Thorac Surg. 82(4):1501-4, 2006
8. Domanski HA et al: Elastofibroma dorsi has distinct cytomorphologic features, making diagnostic surgical biopsy unnecessary: cytomorphologic study with clinical, radiologic, and electron microscopic correlations. Diagn Cytopathol. 29(6):327-33, 2003
9. Briccoli A et al: Elastofibroma dorsi. Surg Today. 30(2):147-52, 2000
10. Nakamura Y et al: Elastofibroma dorsi. Cytologic, histologic, immunohistochemical and ultrastructural studies. Acta Cytol. 36(4):559-62, 1992

IMAGE GALLERY

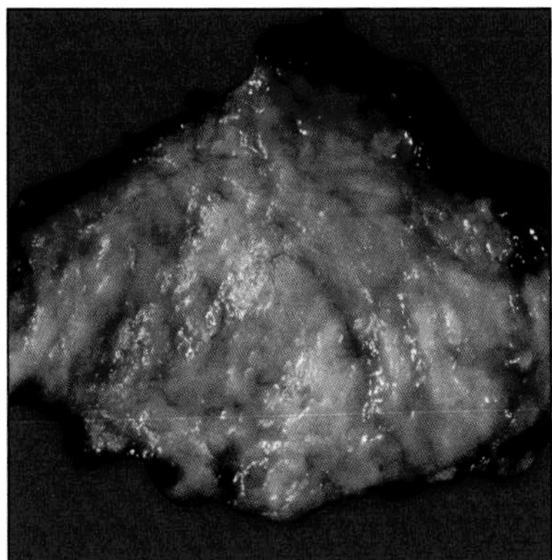

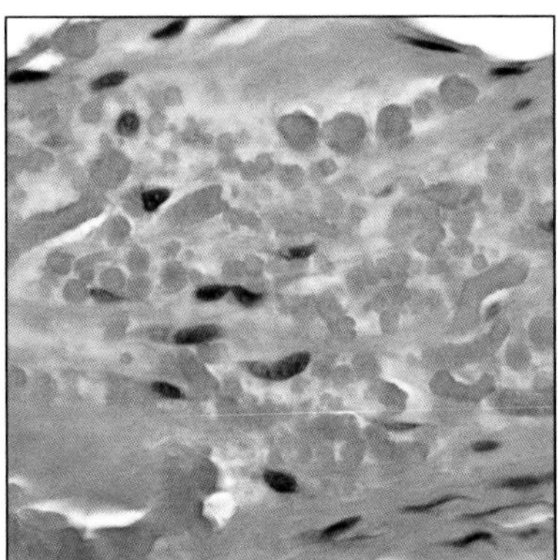

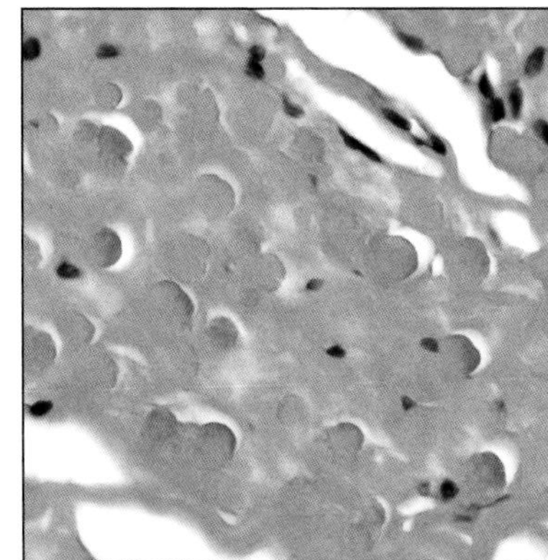

(Left) *Gross photograph shows bands of fibrosis dissecting between fat. There is an irregular periphery.* ***(Center)*** *Hematoxylin & eosin shows globules of degenerated elastic fibers with collagen.* ***(Right)*** *Hematoxylin & eosin shows the rounded globules of degenerated elastic fibers characteristic for elastofibroma.*

PERINEURIOMA

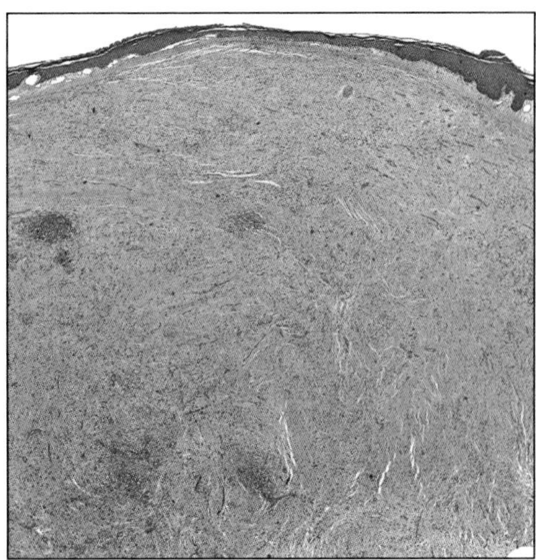

There is an intact surface epithelium overlying a proliferation of spindled cells arranged in a vaguely storiform pattern with focal small whorls. Collections of inflammatory cells are present.

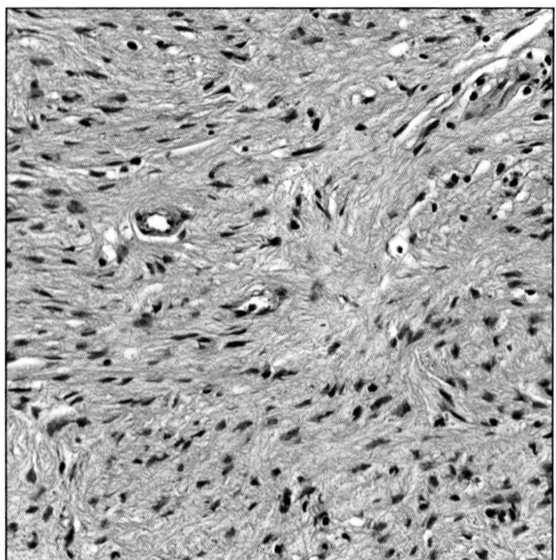

There is a haphazard spindle cell proliferation showing a syncytial appearance. The cells show slightly spindled nuclei with cytoplasmic processes. The background stroma is slightly loose to myxoid.

TERMINOLOGY

Abbreviations

- Soft tissue perineuriomas (STP)

Synonyms

- Storiform perineurial fibroma
- Perineurial cell tumors

Definitions

- Benign peripheral nerve sheath tumor, specifically of perineurial cell derivation that surrounds endoneurial connective tissue space of nerve fibers
  - Tumors are traditionally separated into intraneural, sclerosing, and soft tissue perineurioma
  - Perineurial cells can be seen in other tumors, such as neurofibroma and schwannoma

ETIOLOGY/PATHOGENESIS

Pathogenesis

- May be related to Schwann cells, fibroblasts, or arachnoid cap cells

CLINICAL ISSUES

Epidemiology

- Incidence
  - Exceedingly rare
  - Represents < 0.5% of peripheral nerve sheath tumors
- Age
  - Wide age range: 2-85 years
  - Majority: 2nd-5th decades
    - Mean: 45 years
- Gender
  - Slight female predilection
    - Female > Male (1.1-1.2:1)

Site

- Superficial subcutaneous soft tissues of head and neck
  - Approximately 15% of all perineuriomas affect head and neck sites
  - Most common in soft tissues of lower and upper extremities, followed by trunk
  - May rarely affect gnathic bones (mandible)
- Oral cavity is affected about 4% of the time

Presentation

- Most patients present with a solitary painless mass
- May have syndrome/familial association
  - Neurofibromatosis type 2 (NF2)
  - Nevoid basal cell carcinoma (Gorlin) syndrome
  - Interestingly, both have meningioma in common
    - Perineurium may be derived from arachnoid cap cells

Treatment

- Surgical approaches
  - Excision is treatment of choice
    - Wide excision to prevent recurrence

Prognosis

- Local recurrence is uncommon (< 5% of cases)
  - May develop late
  - Only seen if originally incompletely excised
- Metastases are not reported
- Pleomorphic cells and infiltrative margins do not affect clinical outcome

MACROSCOPIC FEATURES

General Features

- Usually discrete, but without easily detected capsule
  - Well circumscribed

Size

- Wide range: 0.3 cm up to 20 cm
- Mean: ~ 3 cm

PERINEURIOMA

Key Facts

Terminology
- Benign peripheral nerve sheath tumor, specifically of perineurial cell derivation that surrounds endoneurial connective tissue space of nerve fibers

Etiology/Pathogenesis
- May be related to Schwann cells, fibroblasts, or arachnoid cap cells

Clinical Issues
- Approximately 15% develop in superficial subcutaneous soft tissues of head and neck as solitary painless mass

Macroscopic Features
- Usually discrete but without easily detected capsule

Microscopic Pathology
- Superficial subcutaneous or dermal site, well circumscribed
- Spindled tumor cells organized in many patterns (fascicles, storiform, pinwheel, whorled, lamellar)
- Bipolar, bland, plump spindled cells with pale, eosinophilic cytoplasm
- Background stroma is collagenous, myxoid or a mixture, without vascular hyalinization

Ancillary Tests
- Variably positive with perineurial markers (EMA, Claudin-1, GLUT1, CD34) and collagen IV

Top Differential Diagnoses
- Neurofibroma, schwannoma, solitary fibrous tumor, meningioma

MICROSCOPIC PATHOLOGY

Histologic Features
- Superficial subcutaneous or dermal site
- Well circumscribed, focally showing changes suggesting a collagenous capsule
  - "Infiltrating" borders can be seen
  - Significant invasion is rare
- Spindled tumor cells organized in many patterns
  - Fascicles
  - Storiform or pinwheel
  - Whorled to concentrically stratified
  - Lamellar architecture
- Tumors are hypo- or hypercellular
  - Alternating zones can be seen
- Bipolar, bland, plump spindled cells with pale, eosinophilic cytoplasm
  - Indistinct cytoplasmic borders
- Nuclei vary
  - Oval, tapered, elongate, triangular, curved, compressed, twisted, or wavy
  - Intranuclear pseudoinclusions are rare
- Isolated pleomorphic cells ("ancient change") is unusual
- Background stroma is collagenous, myxoid, or a mixture
  - Sclerotic, round to elliptical collagen deposits may be present
  - Pericellular cracking or clefting between collagen and cells
- Mitoses are sparse
  - Most tumors have none
- Degeneration and hemorrhage may be present
- Calcifications (calcospherites or metaplastic bone) are exceptional
- Chronic inflammation is uncommon
- Peripheral nerve association is unique, usually "twigs" of nerves
- Vessel hyalinization is not present
- Sclerosing, reticular (retiform), granular and epithelioid subtypes are recognized, although very rare in head and neck
  - Reticular: Lace-like growth pattern of anastomosing cords of spindle cells
  - Sclerosing: Epithelioid and spindle cells in trabecular or whorled pattern within markedly dense sclerotic stroma

ANCILLARY TESTS

Cytology
- Cellular smears with sheets and clusters of spindle-shaped tumor cells
- Cells are bipolar with cytoplasmic extensions
- May have a "signet ring" appearance
- Prominent myxoid background

Immunohistochemistry
- Variably positive with perineurial markers
  - EMA: Strong and diffuse in all cases
  - Claudin-1: Distinctly particulate pattern along cell membrane in nearly all cases
  - GLUT1: Usually membranous to stippled
  - CD34: Up to 65% of tumors may be positive
  - May have smooth muscle actin (~ 20%) and S100 protein (~ 5%)
- Strong membranous staining with collagen IV

Cytogenetics
- Chromosome 22 abnormalities seen in conventional STP
- Chromosome 10 aberrations seen in sclerosing variants
  - Deletion of 10q
  - t(2;10)(p23;q24)
  - Monosomy 10

Electron Microscopy
- Long, thin, cytoplasmic processes with incomplete basal lamina (basement membrane) and pinocytotic vesicles

PERINEURIOMA

Immunohistochemistry

Antibody	Reactivity	Staining Pattern	Comment
EMA	Positive	Cytoplasmic	Strong and diffuse in all cases
Claudin-1	Positive	Cell membrane	Distinctly particulate pattern along cell membrane in nearly all cases
GLUT1-cytoplasm	Positive	Cell membrane	Usually membranous to stippled
CD34	Positive	Cytoplasmic	Seen in up to 65% of cases
Collagen IV	Positive	Stromal matrix	Strong membranous staining of cells
Actin-sm	Positive	Cytoplasmic	Up to 20% of cases
S100	Positive	Nuclear & cytoplasmic	Only in up to 5% of cases
CK-PAN	Negative		
GFAP	Negative		
NFP	Negative		Axons adjacent to tumor may be highlighted
Desmin	Negative		

- Tapering nuclei with condensed heterochromatin
- Axons absent

DIFFERENTIAL DIAGNOSIS

Neurofibroma and Schwannoma

- Benign peripheral nerve sheath tumors include neurofibromas, schwannomas, and perineuriomas
  - Hybrid combinations of schwannoma/neurofibroma and perineurioma are known
  - Show alternating layers of S100 protein- and EMA-positive cells layered adjacent to one another
- Has association with a nerve in many cases
- Wavy nuclei with background loose stroma
- Antoni A and Antoni B areas will be seen
- Perivascular hyalinization is usually found
- Preponderance of cases show S100 protein immunoreactivity

Solitary Fibrous Tumor

- Cellular tumors with spindled cells
- Much more heavily collagenized stroma
- Will have CD34, Bcl-2, and CD99 reactions
  - CD34 is limited, as it is positive in many perineurioma

Meningioma

- Central nervous system association is usual
  - Ectopic tumors may be seen
- Whorled architecture with psammoma bodies
- Lacks collagen IV immunoreactivity
- Will show EMA reactivity
  - Perineurial and arachnoidal cells may be related

SELECTED REFERENCES

1. Fang WS et al: An unusual sinonasal tumor: soft tissue perineurioma. AJNR Am J Neuroradiol. 30(2):437-9, 2009
2. Hornick JL et al: Hybrid schwannoma/perineurioma: clinicopathologic analysis of 42 distinctive benign nerve sheath tumors. Am J Surg Pathol. 33(10):1554-61, 2009
3. Kum YS et al: Intraneural reticular perineurioma of the hypoglossal nerve. Head Neck. 31(6):833-7, 2009
4. Hornick JL et al: Soft tissue perineurioma: clinicopathologic analysis of 81 cases including those with atypical histologic features. Am J Surg Pathol. 29(7):845-58, 2005
5. Ide F et al: Comparative ultrastructural and immunohistochemical study of perineurioma and neurofibroma of the oral mucosa. Oral Oncol. 40(9):948-53, 2004
6. de la Jarte-Thirouard AS et al: Intraneural reticular perineurioma of the neck. Ann Diagn Pathol. 7(2):120-3, 2003
7. Chrysomali E et al: Benign neural tumors of the oral cavity: a comparative immunohistochemical study. Oral Surg Oral Med Oral Pathol Oral Radiol Endod. 84(4):381-90, 1997
8. Li D et al: Intratemporal facial nerve perineurioma. Laryngoscope. 106(3 Pt 1):328-33, 1996
9. Tsang WY et al: Perineurioma: an uncommon soft tissue neoplasm distinct from localized hypertrophic neuropathy and neurofibroma. Am J Surg Pathol. 16(8):756-63, 1992
10. Housini I et al: Fine needle aspiration cytology of perineurioma. Report of a case with histologic, immunohistochemical and ultrastructural studies. Acta Cytol. 34(3):420-4, 1990

Microscopic and Immunohistochemical Features

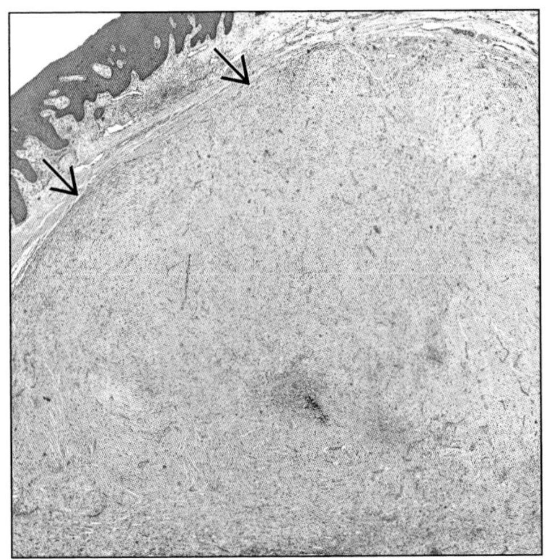

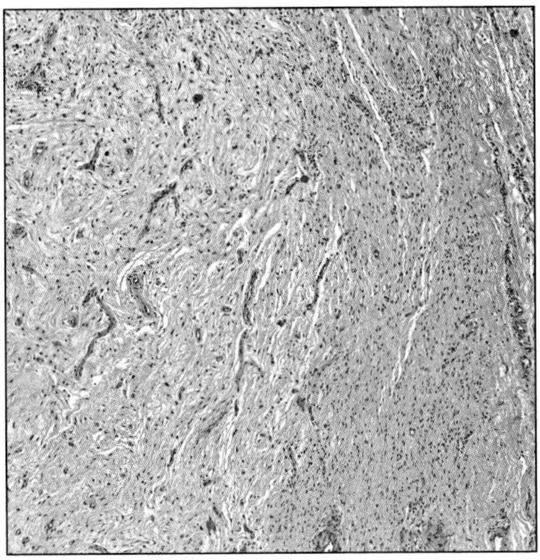

(Left) *The periphery of the tumor seems to be well circumscribed or encapsulated* ⇒*. The surface epithelium is intact, showing a slightly pseudoepitheliomatous appearance.* ***(Right)*** *The proliferation blends at the periphery with the densely collagenized stroma. There is a haphazard storiform appearance to the proliferation. The stroma is myxoid to edematous, perhaps having a vaguely tissue-culture-like appearance.*

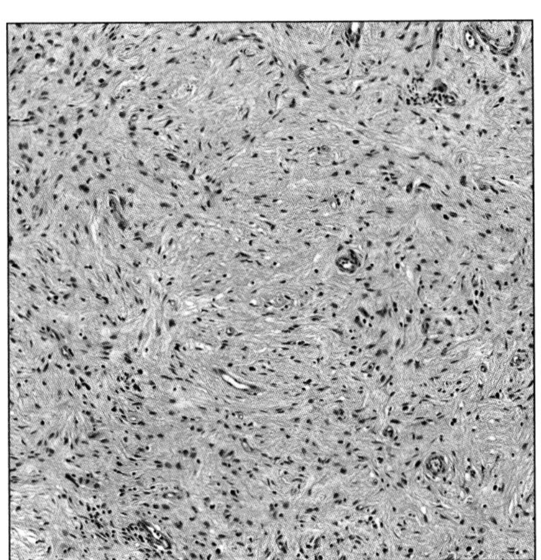

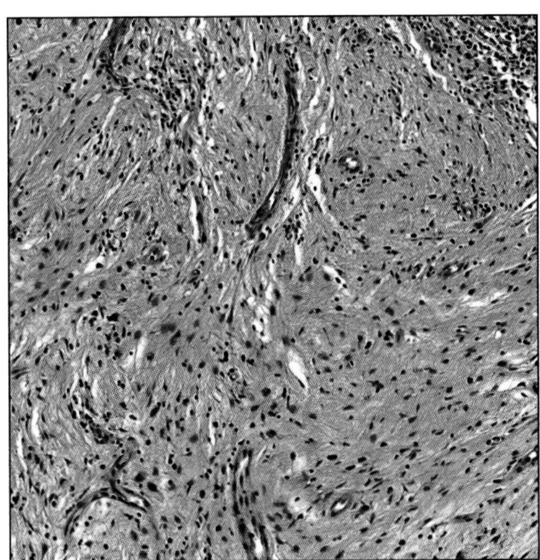

(Left) *The cells are arranged in a syncytial pattern, although the spindle cells are easily identified. There are vessels within the proliferation, but they do not show hyalinized walls.* ***(Right)*** *The proliferation is less cellular in this field, although the vessels are more prominent. There is still a lack of perivascular hyalinization. The nuclei are small and spindled. There is a lack of cytologic atypia and mitoses.*

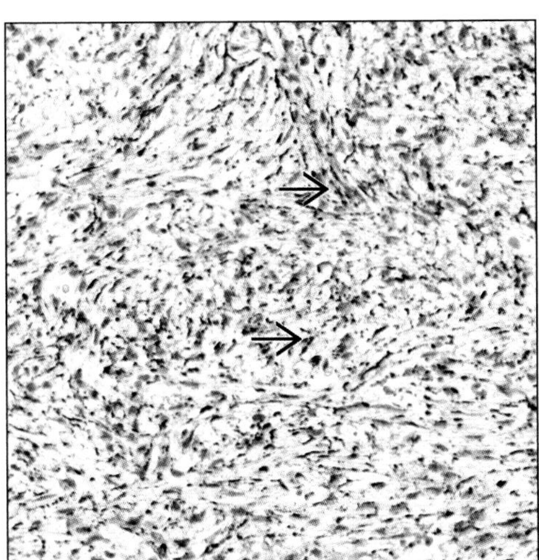

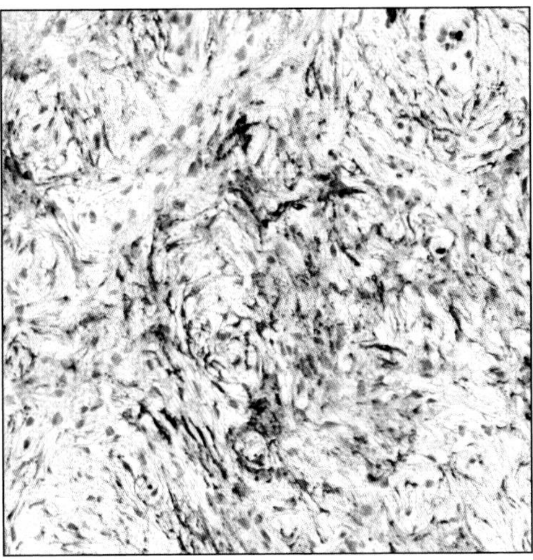

(Left) *Claudin-1 will frequently display a stippled, beaded or granular staining* ⇒*, while also highlighting the cell membranes. This staining pattern is quite unique to this tumor.* ***(Right)*** *The neoplastic spindle cells are highlighted by GLUT1, giving a slightly stippled to granular appearance. The wisps of cytoplasm are stained, creating a feathery appearance to the cells.*

LIPOMA

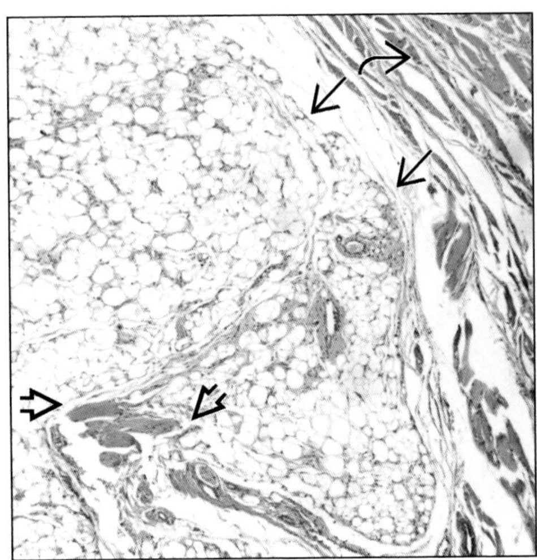

Intramuscular lipomas may have a well-defined interface ➔ with the surrounding skeletal muscle ➔ or may show infiltrative growth ➔. This lesion presented as a slow-growing neck mass.

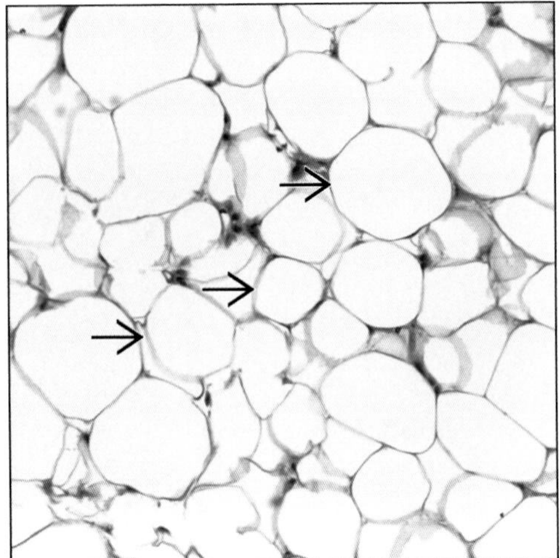

Hematoxylin and eosin shows mature adipocytes ➔ that vary slightly in size and shape. Clinical and radiographic correlation may be important in differentiating this from normal fat tissue.

TERMINOLOGY

Definitions

- Lipoma: Benign tumor of mature white fat
- Angiolipoma: Benign tumor of mature white fat cells with intermixed thin-walled vessels, often with thrombi
- Myolipoma (Lipomyoma): Benign tumor of mature fat and mature smooth muscle

CLINICAL ISSUES

Epidemiology

- Incidence
  - Common tumor, but relatively uncommon in head and neck
    - Myolipomas are extremely rare
- Age
  - Wide age range
    - Angiolipomas: Young adults and teenagers
- Gender
  - Equal gender distribution
    - Variant tumors have male predominance

Site

- Head and neck is not common primary site
  - Posterior cervical space
  - Submandibular space
  - Anterior cervical space and parotid gland
  - Scalp and forehead

Presentation

- Soft tissue mass with slow size increase
- Multiple tumors in 5-15% (familial)
- Angiolipomas: Distinctive for pain and tenderness

Treatment

- Complete surgical excision

Prognosis

- Excellent overall prognosis
- Infiltrative lipomas are more likely to recur
- Rare complications related to anatomic site

IMAGE FINDINGS

Radiographic Findings

- Well-circumscribed, homogeneous mass clearly demonstrated on CT or MR
- Thin capsule, with smooth, noninvasive, convex margins
- Majority have homogeneous fat content
  - Thin septae may be seen

MACROSCOPIC FEATURES

General Features

- Generally appear encapsulated or well circumscribed
- Yellow, greasy cut surface
- Angiolipoma: Yellow pink
- Myolipoma: Intermixed with firm white-tan tissue

Size

- Wide range: < 0.5-30 cm

MICROSCOPIC PATHOLOGY

Histologic Features

- **Lipoma**
  - Lobules of mature fat
  - Similar to normal fat with slight variation in size
  - Occasionally other types of tissue may be seen
    - Bone: Osteolipoma; cartilage: Chondrolipoma; fibrous tissue: Fibrolipoma
  - Intramuscular: May show infiltration
- **Angiolipoma**
  - Mature fat cells

Key Facts

Clinical Issues
- Common tumor but relatively uncommon in head and neck
- Soft tissue mass
- Gradual increase in size

Macroscopic Features
- Yellow, greasy cut surface
- Angiolipoma: Yellow pink
- Myolipoma: Intermixed with firm white-tan tissue

Microscopic Pathology
- Lipoma
  - Lobules of mature fat
  - Similar to normal fat with slight variation in size
- Angiolipoma
  - Capillaries of varying sizes with fibrin thrombi
- Myolipoma
  - Smooth muscle evenly distributed or in short fascicles

  - Capillaries of varying sizes with fibrin thrombi
  - Fibrous changes may be seen as lesion ages
- **Myolipoma**
  - Mature fat cells
  - Smooth muscle: Evenly distributed or short fascicles
  - Sclerosis and focal inflammation

ANCILLARY TESTS

Cytology
- Fatty/lipid droplets on slides
- Lobules of benign fibroadipose connective tissue

Immunohistochemistry
- Lipoma
  - Fat cells positive: Vimentin, S100 protein
- Myolipoma
  - Smooth muscle positive: SMA, desmin

Cytogenetics
- Aberrations are heterogeneous, 3 major groups
  - 12q13-15
  - 6p21-23
  - Loss of material from 13q

DIFFERENTIAL DIAGNOSIS

Lipoma
- Atypical lipomatous tumor (a.k.a. well-differentiated liposarcoma)
  - More variable cell size, irregular hyperchromatic nuclei, lipoblasts
- Lipoblastoma
  - Affects primarily children
  - Lobulated, thicker fibrous septae, lipoblasts
- Lipomatosis
  - Clinically, diffuse growth of fat tissue, possibly infiltrating other tissues
  - Associated with numerous genetic disorders

Angiolipoma
- Hemangioma: Vessels only, variable size
- Kaposi sarcoma: Infiltrative, cellular, eosinophilic globules, no thrombi
- Angiosarcoma: Infiltrative, necrosis, pleomorphism

Myolipoma
- Leiomyoma: Lacks fat
- Leiomyosarcoma: Lacks fat with distinctive pleomorphism

SELECTED REFERENCES

1. Arenaz Búa J et al: Angiolipoma in head and neck: report of two cases and review of the literature. Int J Oral Maxillofac Surg. 39(6):610-5, 2010
2. El-Monem MH et al: Lipomas of the head and neck: presentation variability and diagnostic work-up. J Laryngol Otol. 120(1):47-55, 2006
3. Murphey MD et al: From the archives of the AFIP: benign musculoskeletal lipomatous lesions. Radiographics. 24(5):1433-66, 2004

IMAGE GALLERY

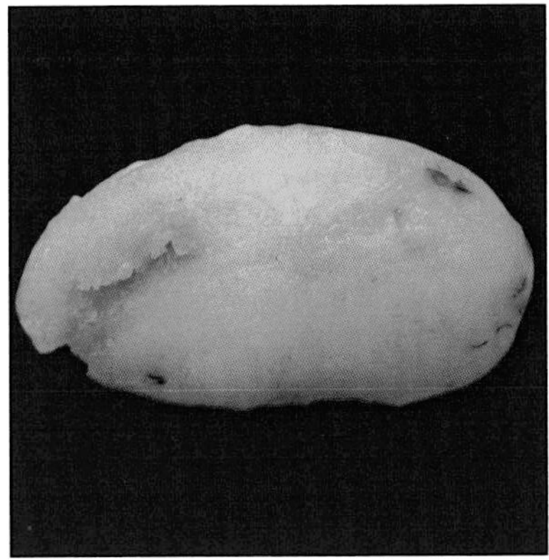

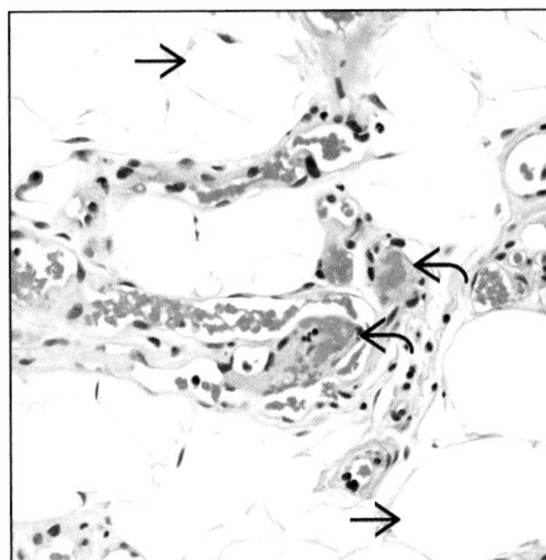

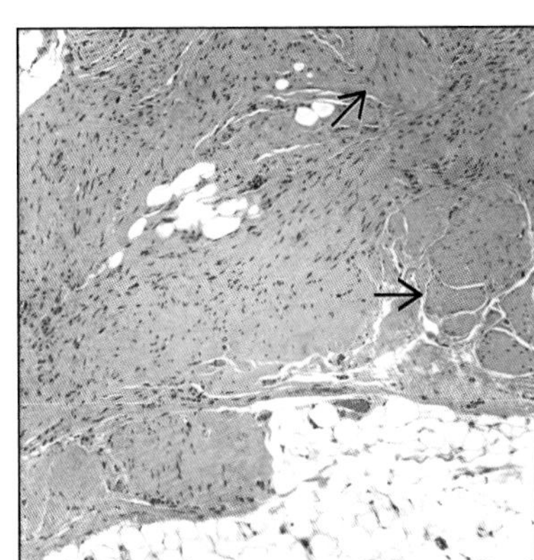

*(**Left**) The cut surfaces of this lipoma show a glistening cut surface of bright yellow lobules of fat, characteristic for this entity. (**Center**) Angiolipoma consists of a mixture of mature fat cells ⇨ and numerous narrow vascular channels, the latter containing characteristic fibrin thrombi ⬀. (**Right**) This example of myolipoma shows fat immediately associated with bundles of smooth muscle ⇨. The term "myolipoma" or "lipomyoma" is used for this lesion.*

SPINDLE CELL LIPOMA

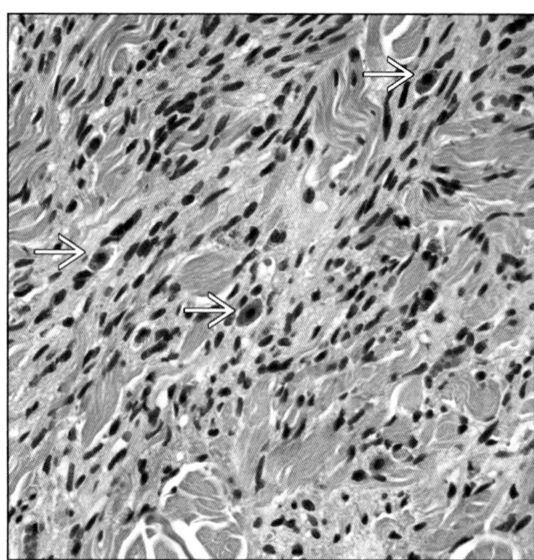

Hematoxylin & eosin shows a mixture of fibroblastic-like cells and heavy, birefringent collagen bundles. The fibroblasts are arranged in a parallel array. Mucinous-type degeneration is present and mast cells are seen ➔.

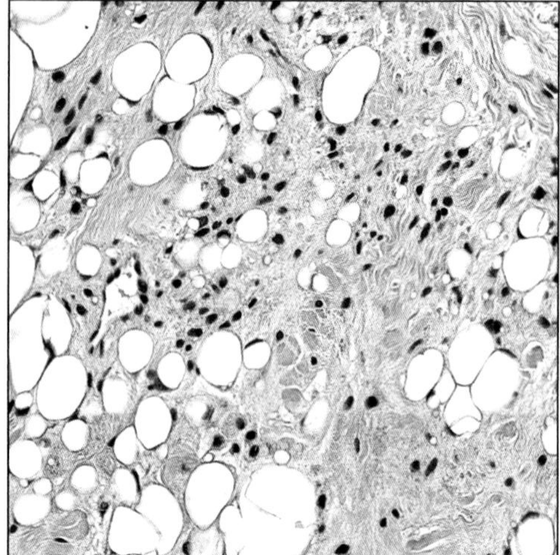

The mixture of fat cells and fibroblast-like spindle cells are seen in this field. There is a myxoid degeneration of the background material and focal pleomorphism of the nuclei.

TERMINOLOGY

Abbreviations

- Spindle cell lipoma (SCL)

Definitions

- Distinctive lipomatous tumor composed of admixture of bland spindled cells, hyperchromatic rounded cells, and multinucleate giant cells associated with ropey collagen
  - First described in 1975

ETIOLOGY/PATHOGENESIS

Pathogenesis

- Stellate mesenchymal cells of primitive fat lobule develop into spindled cells within tumor

CLINICAL ISSUES

Epidemiology

- Incidence
  - 1.5% of all adipocytic neoplasms
    - Lipoma: Spindle cell lipoma (60:1)
- Age
  - Mean: 55 years
  - Range: 40-70 years
- Gender
  - Male > > > Female (9:1)

Site

- Subcutaneous fat
- Posterior neck, upper back, shoulder girdle
- Parotid gland, oral cavity (lip specifically), and maxillofacial region are most common mucosal sites of involvement

Presentation

- Usually asymptomatic
- Circumscribed, mobile, smooth mass
- Most patients report mass present for years
- Familial cases are exceptional

Treatment

- Surgical approaches
  - Local excision is treatment of choice
  - Radical surgical procedures unnecessary

Prognosis

- Excellent
- Local recurrence reported very rarely

MACROSCOPIC FEATURES

General Features

- Yellow to pale, pink, occasionally mucoid
- Discoid to ovoid masses

Size

- Mean: 5 cm
  - Oral cavity lesions, mean: 2 cm
- Range: 0.5-12 cm

MICROSCOPIC PATHOLOGY

Histologic Features

- Develops within subcutaneous fat
- Mixture of fat cells and fibroblast-like spindle cells
- Fibroblastic-like cells often arranged in parallel array
- Matrix with variable amounts of birefringent collagen fibers and mucosubstances
  - Myxoid or mucinous type material
- Mast cells easily identified
- Profound, usually focal, nuclear pleomorphism
  - Considered ancient, retrogressive, or degenerative change (ancient spindle cell lipoma)
- Hyperchromatic, multinucleated cells, nuclei arranged in floret pattern

SPINDLE CELL LIPOMA

Key Facts

Terminology
- Distinctive lipomatous tumor composed of mixture of fat cells and fibroblast-like spindle cells

Clinical Issues
- 1.5% of all adipocytic neoplasms
- Male > > > Female (9:1)
- Posterior neck

Microscopic Pathology
- Mixture of fat cells and fibroblast-like spindle cells
- Matrix with variable amounts of birefringent collagen fibers and mucosubstances
- Marked, but focal, nuclear pleomorphism is possible

Ancillary Tests
- CD34 strongly positive
- S100 protein weakly positive (focal)

- Absence of mitotic activity
- Secondary changes can be seen
  - Fat necrosis, atrophy, hyalinization

ANCILLARY TESTS

Cytology
- Mixture of mature adipocytes, monotonous spindle cells, and collagen fibers in varying proportions
- Myxoid matrix and mast cells are seen

Immunohistochemistry
- CD34 strongly positive
- S100 protein weakly positive (focal)

Cytogenetics
- Loss from the region 16q13-qter
- 13q deletion: 13q12 and 13q14-q22

Electron Microscopy
- Spindled fibroblastic cells and mature lipocytes

DIFFERENTIAL DIAGNOSIS

Well-differentiated Liposarcoma
- Lipoblasts, chicken-wire vascular pattern, myxoid change

Schwannoma
- Antoni A cellular areas with buckled nuclei and Verocay bodies

Lipoma
- Vascular pattern of angiolipoma is absent in SCL
- Profound, isolated, atypical cells not a feature of lipoma

Chondroid Lipoma
- Chondroid material identified
- Lacks spindle cells and collagen bundles

Myxoma
- No fat, thick bundles of collagen are absent, and the tumor is hypocellular

SELECTED REFERENCES

1. Billings SD et al: Diagnostically challenging spindle cell lipomas: a report of 34 "low-fat" and "fat-free" variants. Am J Dermatopathol. 29(5):437-42, 2007
2. Mentzel T: Cutaneous lipomatous neoplasms. Semin Diagn Pathol. 18(4):250-7, 2001
3. Fanburg-Smith JC et al: Multiple spindle cell lipomas: a report of 7 familial and 11 nonfamilial cases. Am J Surg Pathol. 22(1):40-8, 1998
4. Weiss SW: Lipomatous tumors. Monogr Pathol. 38:207-39, 1996
5. Fletcher CD et al: Spindle cell lipoma: a clinicopathological study with some original observations. Histopathology. 11(8):803-17, 1987
6. Bolen JW et al: Spindle-cell lipoma. A clinical, light- and electron-microscopical study. Am J Surg Pathol. 5(5):435-41, 1981

IMAGE GALLERY

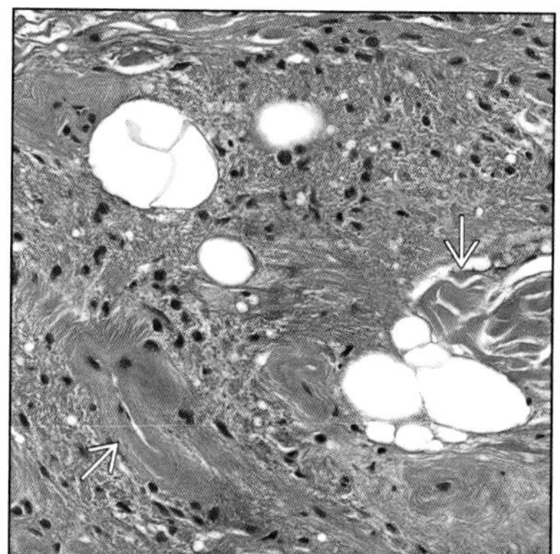

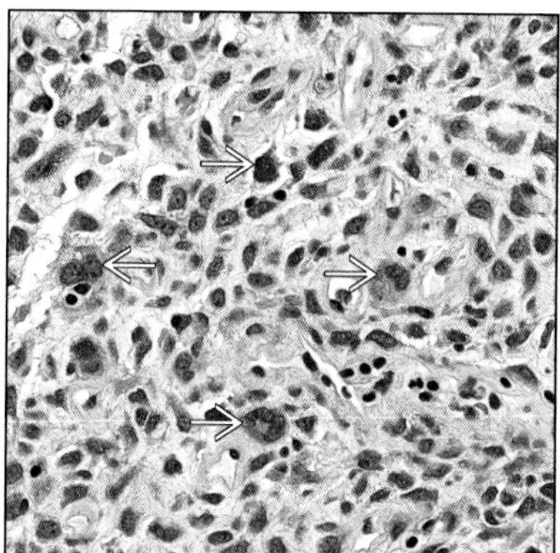

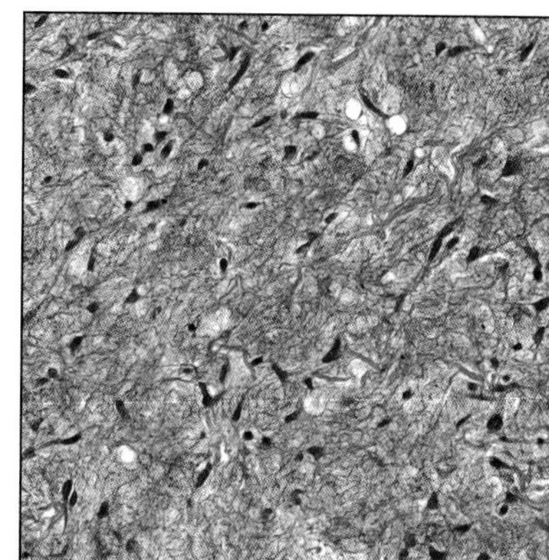

(Left) *There is hyalinization in the background, while collagen bundles ➡ and fat cells are set within the stroma. The spindle cell population is limited in this field.* ***(Center)*** *This field shows a number of profoundly pleomorphic nuclei, including multinucleated cells ➡. The pleomorphism is considered an ancient change.* ***(Right)*** *This case highlights the remarkably myxoid background matrix that can be present in a spindle cell lipoma. The fibroblasts have elongated cell processes.*

LIPOBLASTOMA

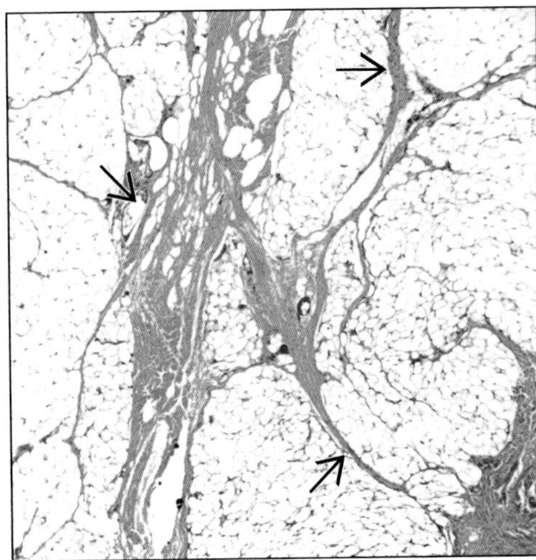

This image shows the characteristic lobulated appearance of a lipoblastoma. The connective tissue septa ⇒ separates the lobules, which are made up of mature adipose cells and lipoblasts.

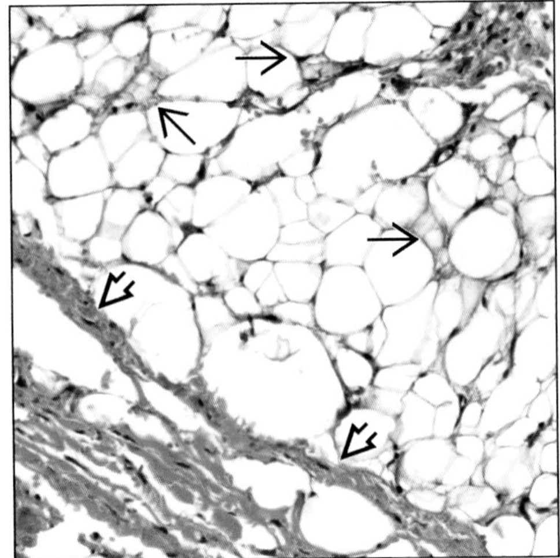

Hematoxylin and eosin shows an admixture of multivacuolated lipoblasts ⇒ and mature adipose cells abutting a fibrous connective tissue septum ⇨.

TERMINOLOGY

Definitions

- Benign tumor derived from embryonic white fat

CLINICAL ISSUES

Epidemiology

- Incidence
  - Exceedingly rare
- Age
  - Infancy and childhood
    - Mean: 2 years
    - Range: Newborn to 12 years
- Gender
  - Male > Female (2:1)

Site

- Neck is uncommon site
  - ~ 8% of tumors develop in head and neck
- Most common locations (order of frequency)
  - Extremities > axilla > mediastinum > retroperitoneum > prevertebral

Presentation

- Rapidly enlarging, painless mass (~ 50%)
- Compression of adjacent nerves or cervical structures
  - Respiratory distress
  - Dysphasia and odynophagia
  - Trismus, hoarseness, or respiratory compromise
  - Hemiparesis

Treatment

- Surgical approaches
  - Complete excision
    - Must preserve vital structures

Prognosis

- Excellent long-term outcome for this benign tumor
- Recurrences common (~ 30%)
  - Associated with incomplete excision
  - Recurrences more likely in lipoblastomatosis (diffuse)
- Metastasis has not been reported

IMAGE FINDINGS

Ultrasonographic Findings

- Shows solid, noncystic mass

MR Findings

- Well-circumscribed, heterogeneous mass
  - T1WI: Predominately high signal but shows lower intensity than mature fat
  - T2WI: Predominately high signal, caused by lipoblasts and myxoid stroma

MACROSCOPIC FEATURES

General Features

- Encapsulated
- Lobulated with fibrous bands
- White to yellow cut surface

Size

- Range: 1.2-15.5 cm

MICROSCOPIC PATHOLOGY

Histologic Features

- Lobulated adipose tissue
- Fibrous septa
- Entrapment of skeletal muscle fibers
- Mixture of mature fat cells and lipoblasts
  - Mature cells tend to be located centrally
  - Lipoblasts may be multivacuolated
  - Lipoblasts appear to be in various stages of differentiation
- Stroma may be focally myxoid

LIPOBLASTOMA

Key Facts

Terminology
- Rare benign tumor arising from embryonic white fat

Clinical Issues
- Infancy and childhood
- Rapidly enlarging, painless mass
- Complete excision, preserving vital structures

Microscopic Pathology
- Lobulated adipose tissue with fibrous septa
- Mixture of mature fat cells and lipoblasts
- Stroma may be focally myxoid

Ancillary Tests
- Rearrangements involving *PLAG1* gene (8q12.1)
  - Fusion proteins (*HAS2-PLAG1* or *COL1A2-PLAG1*) encode for *PLAG1* protein

Top Differential Diagnoses
- Lipoblastomatosis, myxoid liposarcoma, hibernoma

  - Stellate to spindled mesenchymal cells
- Rare mitoses (< 1/20 HPF)

ANCILLARY TESTS

Immunohistochemistry
- Neoplastic cells are positive with
  - S100 protein and CD34

Cytogenetics
- Gain of chromosome 8 in many cases

Molecular Genetics
- Rearrangements involving chromosome 8q11-q13 region
  - *PLAG1* gene (8q12.1)
  - Rearrangements cause promoter-swapping event, with other genes' promoters causing *PLAG1* transcriptional up-regulation
  - Fusion proteins (*HAS2-PLAG1* or *COL1A2-PLAG1*) encode for *PLAG1* protein
- Detected by metaphase or interphase FISH using *PLAG1* probes

DIFFERENTIAL DIAGNOSIS

Lipoblastomatosis
- Unencapsulated
- Diffuse growth
- Infiltrative into surrounding tissue

Myxoid Liposarcoma
- Occurs primarily in 3rd-6th decade
- Atypical lipoblasts
- Mitosis
- Mature adipose cells seen peripherally
- Characterized by t(12;16)(q13;p11)

Lipoma/Fibrolipoma/Angiolipoma
- Lack lipoblasts

Hibernoma
- Fat cells have eosinophilic, granular cytoplasm
- Rearrangement in chromosome 11q13

SELECTED REFERENCES

1. Pham NS et al: Pediatric lipoblastoma in the head and neck: a systematic review of 48 reported cases. Int J Pediatr Otorhinolaryngol. 74(7):723-8, 2010
2. Brodsky JR et al: Cervical lipoblastoma: case report, review of literature, and genetic analysis. Head Neck. 29(11):1055-60, 2007
3. Sakaida M et al: Lipoblastoma of the neck: a case report and literature review. Am J Otolaryngol. 25(4):266-9, 2004
4. Shah AR et al: Cervical lipoblastoma: an uncommon diagnosis of neck mass. Otolaryngol Head Neck Surg. 130(4):504-7, 2004
5. Hibbard MK et al: PLAG1 fusion oncogenes in lipoblastoma. Cancer Res. 60(17):4869-72, 2000
6. Chung EB et al: Benign lipoblastomatosis. An analysis of 35 cases. Cancer. 32(2):482-92, 1973

IMAGE GALLERY

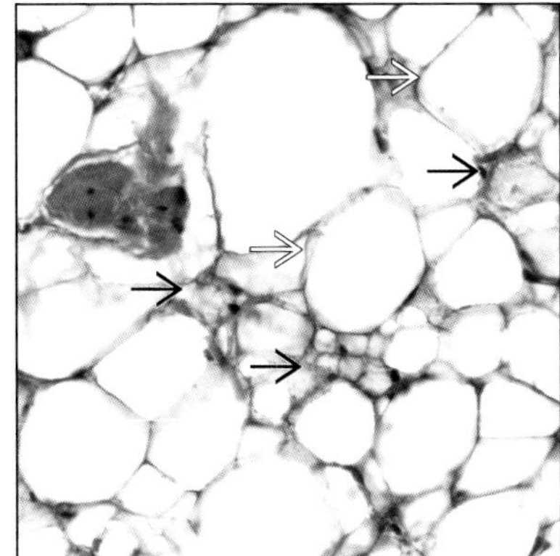
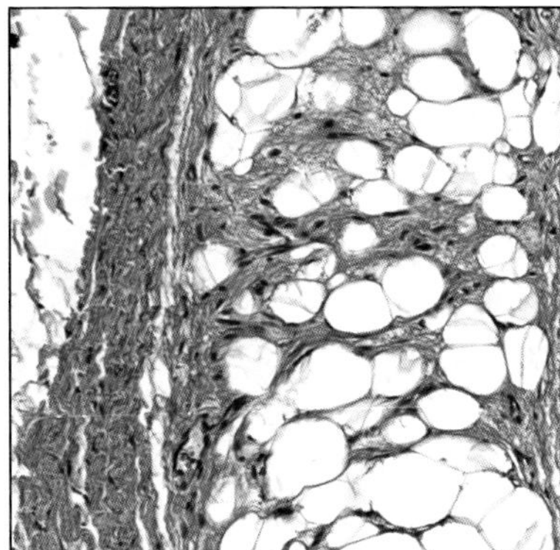
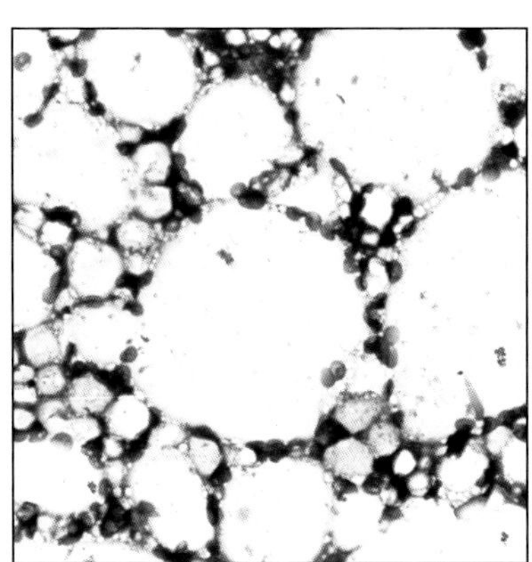

*(**Left**) A high-power image shows a lipoblastoma with mature fat cells ➡ and characteristic multivacuolated lipoblasts ⇨. (**Center**) An admixture of fat cells is shown in a myxoid stroma. This myxoid stroma is also a feature of myxoid liposarcoma. However, no atypia should be identified in a lipoblastoma. (**Right**) This cytology specimen is from the neck of a 1-year-old boy. Benign adipose tissue, in conjunction with the patient's age, may be suggestive of a lipoblastoma, although not diagnostic.*

HIBERNOMA

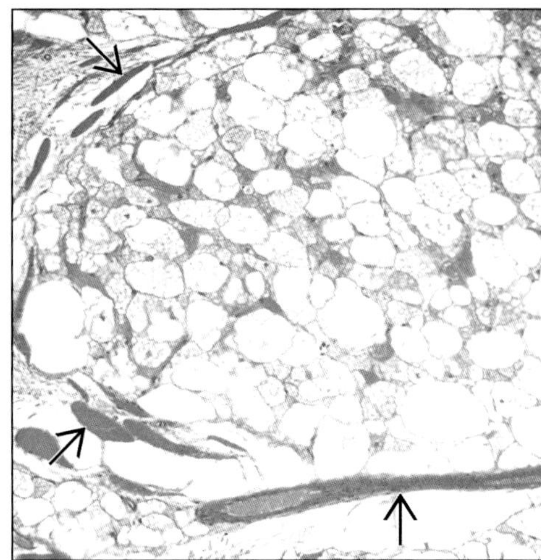

This hibernoma shows a predominance of vacuolated granular eosinophilic cells. There are bands of skeletal muscle ⇒ at the periphery of the nodule of tumor.

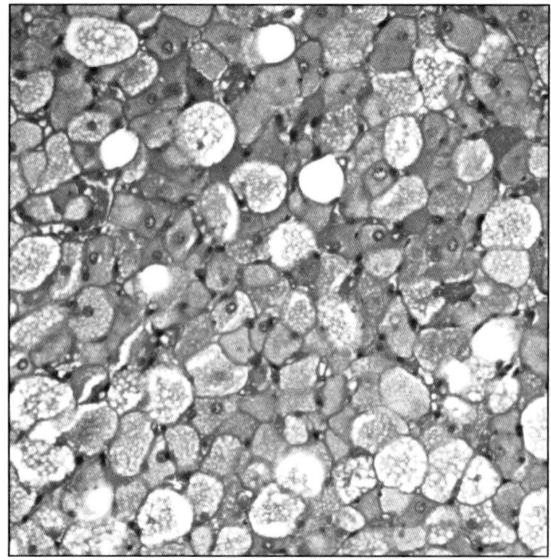

This intermediate power shows the characteristic appearance of granular, microvesicular and multivacuolated cells in a hibernoma. This is the typical appearance.

TERMINOLOGY

Synonyms

- Fetal lipoma
- Lipoma of embryonic fat
- Lipoma of immature adipose tissue

Definitions

- Benign neoplasm of vestigial brown fat
  - Term originally used by Gery in 1914

CLINICAL ISSUES

Epidemiology

- Incidence
  - Rare
- Age
  - Adults most frequently
    - Mean: 4th decade
  - Patients usually younger than patients with lipoma
- Gender
  - Slight male predominance

Site

- Head & neck: Shoulders, neck, scapular
  - Thigh, back, chest, abdomen, arms

Presentation

- Slow-growing painless solitary mass
- Subcutis most frequently
  - Uncommonly intramuscular
- Symptoms present for years

Treatment

- Surgical approaches
  - Complete surgical excision

Prognosis

- Excellent without recurrence or aggressive behavior
  - Even when incompletely excised

IMAGE FINDINGS

General Features

- Well-defined, heterogeneous mass
- MR T1-weighted images show a mass, which is diffusely although only slightly hypointense to subcutaneous fat
  - Serpentine, thin, low signal bands (septations or vessels) throughout tumor suggest diagnosis

MACROSCOPIC FEATURES

General Features

- Well-defined, encapsulated or circumscribed tumors
- Soft, yellow, tan to deep brown-red

Size

- Wide range: 1-27 cm; mean: 10 cm

MICROSCOPIC PATHOLOGY

Histologic Features

- Histologically, a mass resembling brown adipose tissue
- While 4 histologic types are recognized, 1 is most common (typical)
- Background of rich vascularity
- **Lobular type**
  - Variable degrees of differentiation
    - Uniform, round to oval cells
    - Granular eosinophilic cells with prominent borders
    - Coarsely multivacuolated fat cells (pale cells)
    - Centrally placed small nuclei lacking atypia
    - Cells with large cytoplasmic lipid droplets interspersed

Variants

- **Myxoid variant**

HIBERNOMA

Key Facts

Terminology
- Benign neoplasm of vestigial brown fat

Microscopic Pathology
- Wide range: 1-27 cm, mean: 10 cm
- Uniform, round to oval cells
- Granular eosinophilic cells with prominent borders
- Coarsely multivacuolated fat cells (pale cells)
- Centrally placed small nuclei lacking atypia
- Background of rich vascularity
- **Variants**: Myxoid, lipoma-like, spindle cell

Ancillary Tests
- Oil red O positive droplets of cytoplasmic lipid
- S100 protein and CD31 (membrane and vacuoles)
- Structural rearrangements of 11q13-21

Top Differential Diagnoses
- Adult rhabdomyoma, granular cell tumor, liposarcoma

  - Loose, basophilic matrix, thick fibrous septa, foamy histiocytes
- **Lipoma-like variant**
  - Univacuolated lipocytes, with only isolated hibernoma cells
- **Spindle cell variant**
  - Spindle cell lipoma combined with hibernoma; neck or scalp affected; CD34 positive

ANCILLARY TESTS

Cytology
- Smears of small, round, brown fat-like cells
  - Uniform, small cytoplasmic vacuoles
  - Regular, small, round nuclei
- Small, branching capillaries
- Mature fat cells are also present

Histochemistry
- Oil red O-positive droplets of cytoplasmic lipid

Immunohistochemistry
- **Positive**
  - S100 protein (approximately 80%)
  - AP2 protein strongly (but also positive in lipoblasts)
  - CD31 intensely and diffusely: Membrane and vacuoles
  - Multilocular cells express uncoupling protein 1 (UCP1), a unique brown fat mitochondrial protein

Cytogenetics
- Structural rearrangements of 11q13-21 most characteristic
  - Complex rearrangement usually detected by metaphase fluorescence in situ hybridization (FISH)
  - *MEN1* gene (11q13.1) is most frequently deleted
  - *GARP* gene (11q13.5) may be involved

DIFFERENTIAL DIAGNOSIS

Adult Rhabdomyoma
- Polygonal cells, with granular not vesicular cytoplasm
- Cross-striations, "spiderweb" cells, and crystals
- Large amounts of glycogen

Granular Cell Tumor
- Eosinophilic, granular cytoplasm, with round nuclei
- Nerve association; strong S100 protein and CD68 positive

Liposarcoma
- True lipoblasts: Nuclear notches and pleomorphism
- Different stroma and vascularity

SELECTED REFERENCES

1. Furlong MA et al: The morphologic spectrum of hibernoma: a clinicopathologic study of 170 cases. Am J Surg Pathol. 25(6):809-14, 2001
2. Paul MA et al: Hibernoma, a brown fat tumour. Neth J Surg. 41(4):85-7, 1989

IMAGE GALLERY

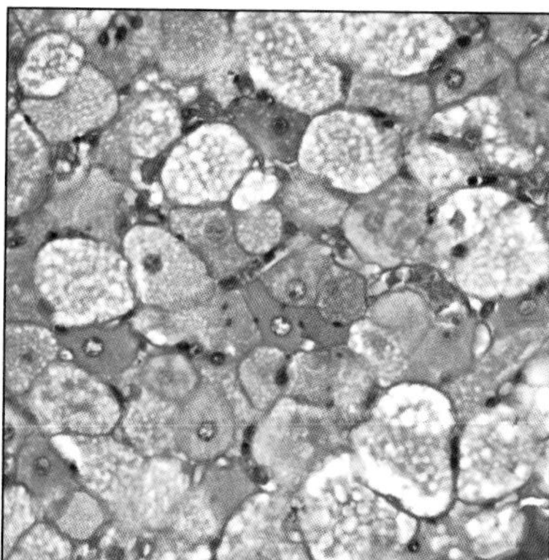

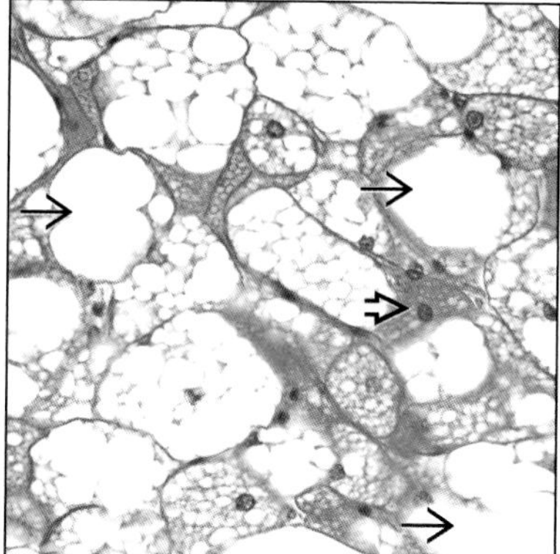

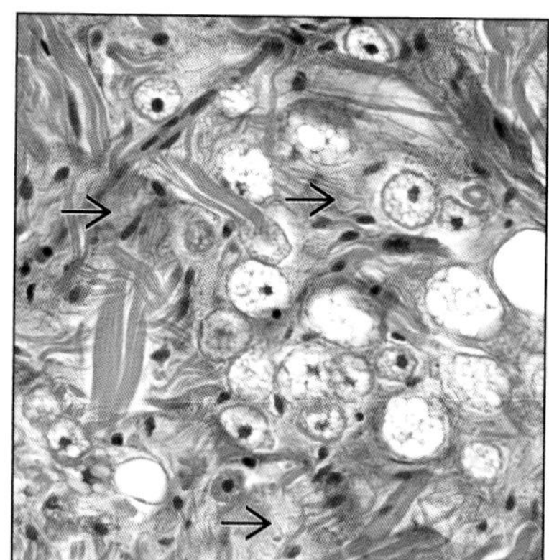

(Left) *High power shows microvacuolation of many of the cells but a more solid and granular appearance in others.* ***(Center)*** *This hibernoma shows a much more prominent cytoplasmic vacuole formation. Single large vacuoles ⇒ within cells are juxtaposed to microvacuolated cells. Isolated granular cells are present ⇒.* ***(Right)*** *The myxoid variant has myxoid change in the stroma ⇒ immediately surrounding the granular microvesicular cells. Fat is also present in the background.*

NUCHAL-TYPE FIBROMA

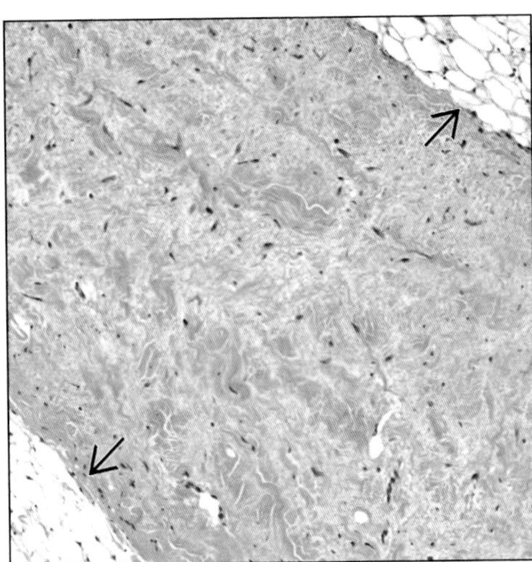

Hematoxylin & eosin shows a nuchal-type fibroma with thick, haphazardly arranged collagen fibers. Fat entrapment ⇒ is a highly reproducible and characteristic feature of NTFs.

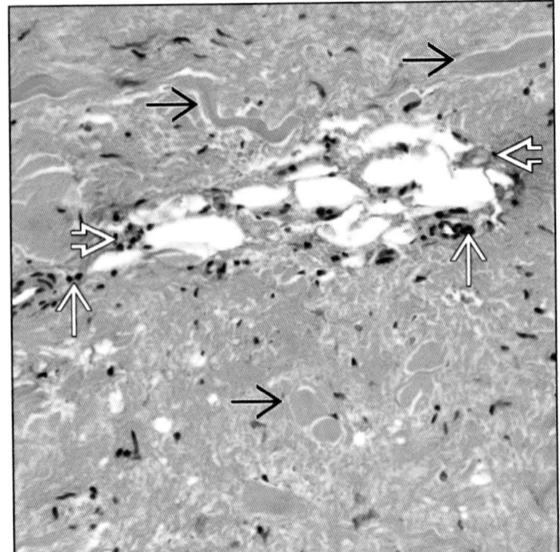

This medium-power image shows a NTF with entrapment of adipose tissue ➡ by the hypocellular fibrous stroma containing dense collagen bundles ⇒. Note the scattered lymphocytes ➡.

TERMINOLOGY

Abbreviations

- Nuchal-type fibroma (NTF)

Synonyms

- Nuchal fibroma
  - Terminology no longer technically correct since lesions may be found in areas other than posterior neck (though rarely)

Definitions

- Benign, hyalinized, fibroblastic proliferation involving dermis and subcutis

ETIOLOGY/PATHOGENESIS

Pathogenesis

- Unknown; may be related to local or systemic factors

CLINICAL ISSUES

Epidemiology

- Incidence
  - Rare
- Age
  - Wide age range
  - Peak: 3rd-5th decades
- Gender
  - Male > Female
    - Syndrome-associated lesions have equal gender distribution

Site

- Most common location is posterior neck
- Other sites
  - Extremities
  - Lumbosacral area and buttock
  - Head, neck, face

Presentation

- Generally asymptomatic
- Long history of superficial mass
- Solitary lesion
- Strong association with diabetes mellitus and Gardner syndrome
  - May be sentinel presentation of Gardner syndrome

Treatment

- Options, risks, complications
  - In patients with Gardner syndrome, up to 45% will develop desmoid-type fibromatosis at other sites
- Surgical approaches
  - Excision

Prognosis

- Excellent outcome, without functional compromise
- Due to frequent recurrences, follow-up is indicated

MACROSCOPIC FEATURES

General Features

- Poorly circumscribed and unencapsulated
- Firm, white
- May extend into deep dermis or skeletal muscle

Size

- Range: Up to 8 cm
- Mean: 3.5 cm

MICROSCOPIC PATHOLOGY

Histologic Features

- Unencapsulated and ill-defined
- Thick, haphazardly arranged collagen fibers
- Low cellularity, overall bland appearance
- Vague lobular pattern
- Entrapped
  - Adipose tissue within collagen bundles

NUCHAL-TYPE FIBROMA

Key Facts

Terminology
- Benign, hyalinized, fibroblastic proliferation involving dermis and subcutis

Clinical Issues
- Most common in posterior neck
- Long history of superficial mass

Microscopic Pathology
- Thick, haphazardly arranged collagen fibers
- Unencapsulated with low cellularity
- Entrapped adipose and skeletal muscle
- Proliferation of peripheral nerves

Ancillary Tests
- Positive: Vimentin, CD34, nuclear β-catenin

Top Differential Diagnoses
- Elastofibroma, fibrolipoma, desmoid-type fibromatoses, nuchal fibrocartilaginous pseudotumor

  - Skeletal muscle
  - Proliferation of peripheral nerves
    - Similar to traumatic neuroma
    - Perineural fibrosis
  - May see scattered lymphocytes
  - May see encasement of adnexa from associated skin
- Elastic fibers may occasionally be altered

ANCILLARY TESTS

Immunohistochemistry
- Positive
  - Vimentin
  - CD34
  - CD99 (a few cases)
  - Nuclear β-catenin (up to 2/3 of cases)
- Negative
  - Desmin and smooth muscle actin
- CD34 highlights vessels

DIFFERENTIAL DIAGNOSIS

Elastofibroma
- Abundant and abnormal elastic fibers
- Generally more cellular

Fibrolipoma
- Well circumscribed and encapsulated
- Much more adipose tissue, lacking entrapped nerves

Desmoid-type Fibromatoses
- More cellular, but not in subcutaneous tissues
- Can demonstrate aggressive behavior

Nuchal Fibrocartilaginous Pseudotumor
- Deep to fascia, at base of skull
- Cartilaginous metaplasia

Lipomatosis
- Sheets of adipocytes infiltrating skeletal muscle and other tissues
- Associated with numerous systemic diseases

DIAGNOSTIC CHECKLIST

Clinically Relevant Pathologic Features
- Should exclude Gardner syndrome

SELECTED REFERENCES

1. Dawes LC et al: Nuchal fibroma should be recognized as a new extracolonic manifestation of Gardner-variant familial adenomatous polyposis. Aust N Z J Surg. 70(11):824-6, 2000
2. Samadi DS et al: Nuchal fibroma: a clinicopathological review. Ann Otol Rhinol Laryngol. 109(1):52-5, 2000
3. Michal M et al: Nuchal-type fibroma: a clinicopathologic study of 52 cases. Cancer. 85(1):156-63, 1999
4. Balachandran K et al: Nuchal fibroma. A clinicopathological study of nine cases. Am J Surg Pathol. 19(3):313-7, 1995

IMAGE GALLERY

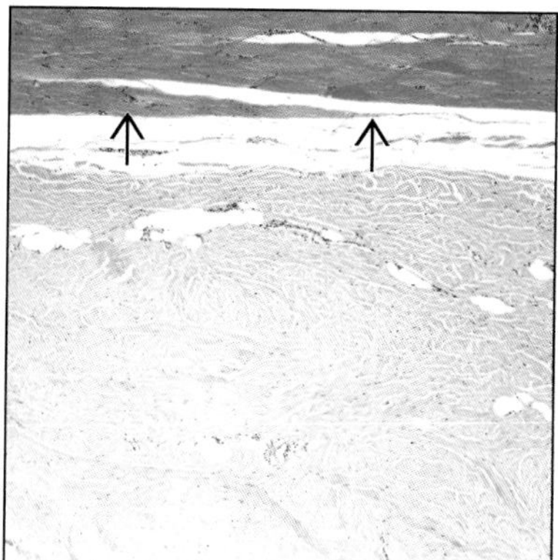

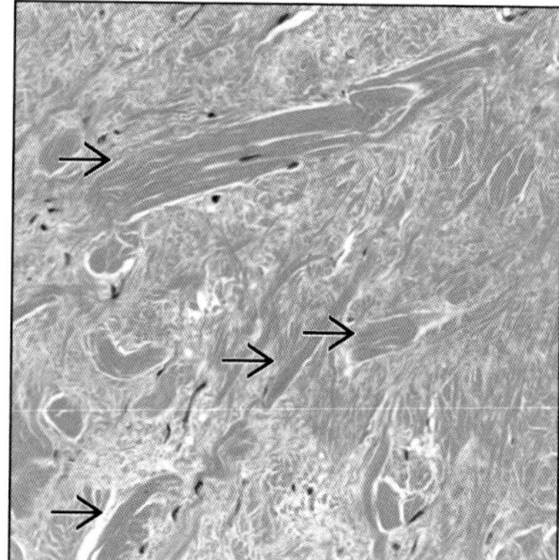

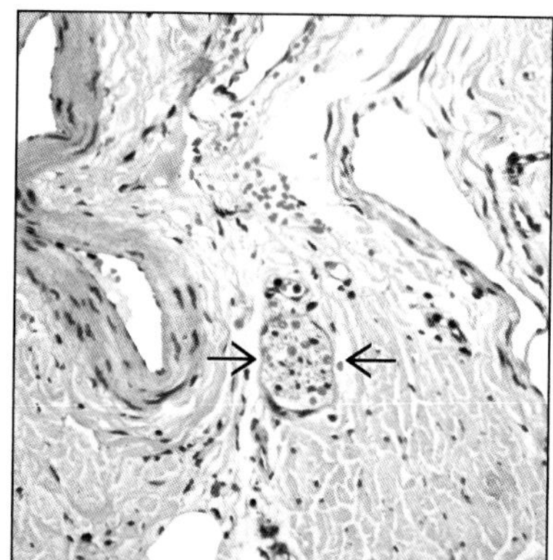

(Left) *The skeletal muscle ⇒ is seen overlying a very heavily collagenized soft tissue lesion. Note the number of adipocytes present at the periphery but also entrapped within the lesion.* ***(Center)*** *Hematoxylin & eosin shows thick collagen bundles ⇒. These bundles may intersect to create a lobular architecture.* ***(Right)*** *Nuchal-type fibromas frequently have proliferations of nerve twigs ⇒ that are surrounded by dense collagen fibers. Nerves are helpful in the differential diagnosis.*

LYMPHANGIOMA

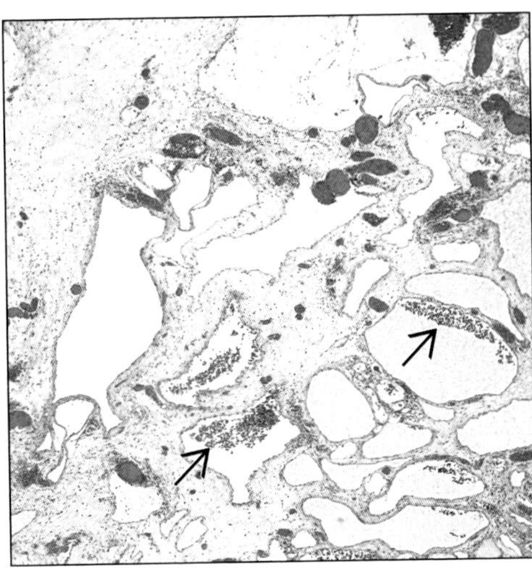

There are multiple endothelial-lined channels in this lymphangioma. There are small collections of lymphocytes ➔ within the lumen along with lymph. Erythrocytes are also focally present.

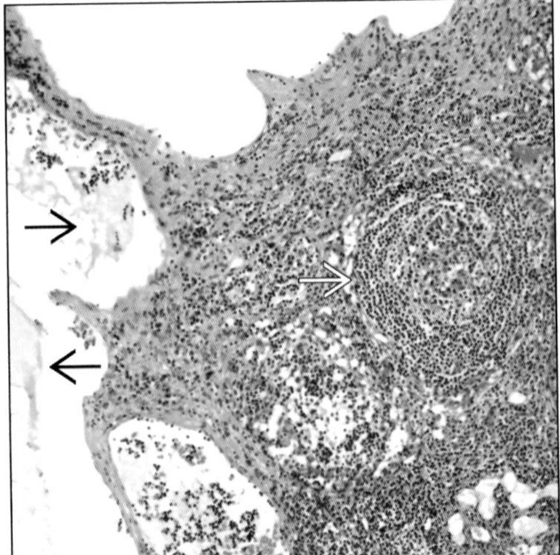

The lumen is lined by flattened endothelium and contains proteinaceous fluid ➔. Note the lymphocytic aggregate with a germinal center ➔ in the connective tissue. Smooth muscle may sometimes be seen.

TERMINOLOGY

Synonyms

- Cystic hygroma

Definitions

- Malformation of lymphatic system, generally considered congenital
  - Cavernous/cystic mass composed of dilated lymph channels
  - Capillary lesion are composed of small vessels
    - Usually associated with skin

ETIOLOGY/PATHOGENESIS

Etiology

- Congenital
  - Associated with chromosomal abnormalities
    - Turner syndrome: 45, XO
    - Noonan syndrome
    - Trisomies: 13, 18, & 21
    - Others
  - Environmental factors
    - Maternal viral infection
    - Substance abuse
- Rare adult lesions likely associated with infection or trauma

CLINICAL ISSUES

Epidemiology

- Incidence
  - 6% of benign tumors of childhood
- Age
  - Often present at birth
  - Usually diagnosed in the first 2 years of life
    - 80-90%
  - Exceedingly rare in adults

Site

- Head and neck most common location
  - Cervical lesions
    - Most common in posterior triangle
    - Less commonly seen in anterior triangle, but associated with more symptoms
    - Occasionally extend into mediastinum or oral cavity
- Axilla
- Groin
- Abdominal cavity
- Limbs
- Others

Natural History

- Large, congenital lesions may be diagnosed prenatally or may result in spontaneous abortion
- Slowly enlarging mass
- Generally painless
- Large lesions
  - Respiratory distress
  - Difficulty swallowing

Treatment

- Surgical approaches
  - Complete resection
    - May be difficult if lesion abuts vital structures
- Drugs
  - Intralesional injections of sclerosing agents
    - Bleomycin (BLM)
    - OK-432

Prognosis

- Recurrence rate high when associated with incomplete removal
- Airway obstruction may result in death
- Malignant transformation does not occur

LYMPHANGIOMA

Key Facts

Terminology
- Cystic hygroma
- Malformation of lymphatic system, generally considered congenital

Etiology/Pathogenesis
- Associated with chromosomal abnormalities

Clinical Issues
- Head and neck is most common location
- Complete resection is treatment of choice

Microscopic Pathology
- Variably sized lymphatic spaces lined by endothelial cells
- Lumina contain
  - Lymph
  - Lymphocytes
  - Red blood cells

IMAGE FINDINGS

Ultrasonographic Findings
- Used prenatally
- Shows cystic lesion

CT Findings
- Multiple homogeneous cavities
- Nonenhancing

MACROSCOPIC FEATURES

General Features
- Variably sized cavities with clear to white fluid

MICROSCOPIC PATHOLOGY

Histologic Features
- Variably sized lymphatic spaces lined by endothelial cells
- Lumina contain
  - Lymph
  - Lymphocytes
  - Red blood cells
- Large vessels may have smooth muscle layer
- Longstanding lesions
  - Fibrous
  - Inflammation

ANCILLARY TESTS

Immunohistochemistry
- **Positive**
  - FVIIIRAg
  - CD31
  - CD34
  - D2-40 (Podoplanin)

DIFFERENTIAL DIAGNOSIS

Hemangioma
- May be a difficult distinction
- Lacks copious lymph
- Clinical correlation is helpful

SELECTED REFERENCES

1. Kraus J et al: Cystic lymphangioma of the neck in adults: a report of three cases. Wien Klin Wochenschr. 120(7-8):242-5, 2008
2. Mosca RC et al: Cystic hygroma: characterization by computerized tomography. Oral Surg Oral Med Oral Pathol Oral Radiol Endod. 105(5):e65-9, 2008
3. Gedikbasi A et al: Cystic hygroma and lymphangioma: associated findings, perinatal outcome and prognostic factors in live-born infants. Arch Gynecol Obstet. 276(5):491-8, 2007
4. Okazaki T et al: Treatment of lymphangioma in children: our experience of 128 cases. J Pediatr Surg. 42(2):386-9, 2007

IMAGE GALLERY

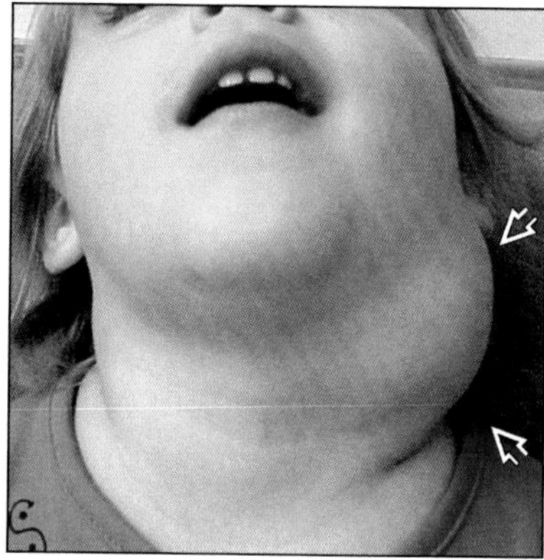

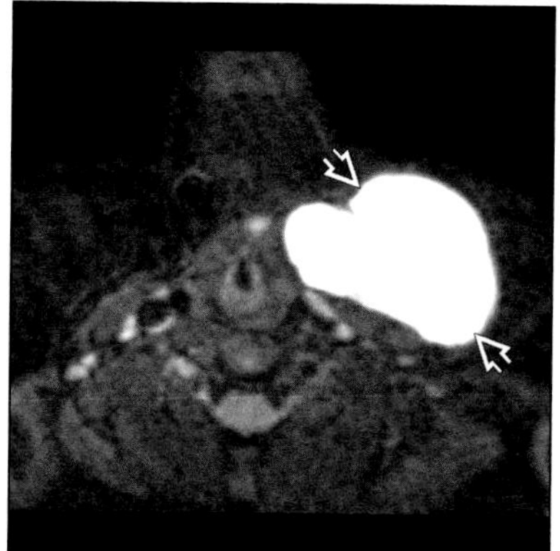

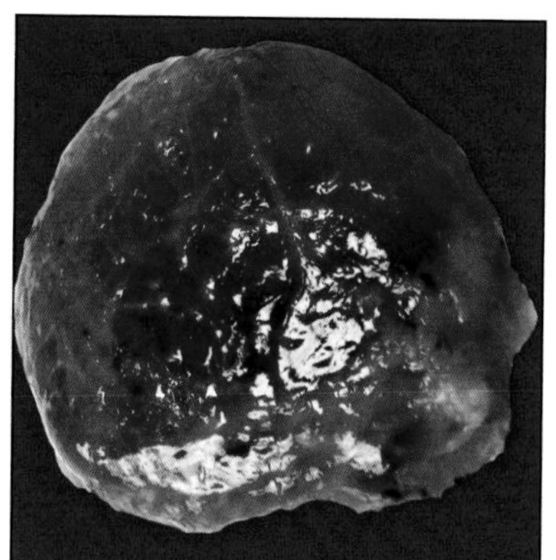

*(**Left**) The large, soft, ballotable left neck mass ➡ in this young girl proved to be a lymphangioma. (**Center**) Axial T2WI MR shows a large, high signal, cystic structure ➡ with septation in the lateral neck. This is diagnostic of a cyst, although the exact type requires histology. (**Right**) This macroscopic view of a lymphangioma shows a very translucent mass. Small vessels are noted within the lining. The cyst was filled with clear, watery type fluid.*

METASTATIC CYSTIC SQUAMOUS CELL CARCINOMA

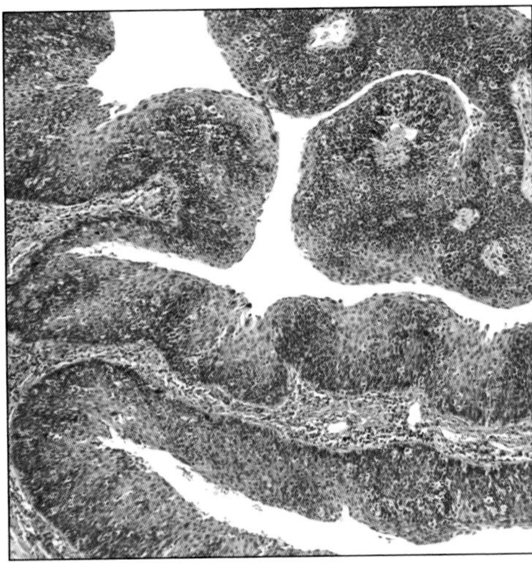

There is a ribbon-like or band-like uniformly thick epithelium lining the cystic space. From low power, pleomorphism is difficult to detect. The papillary projections can be complex.

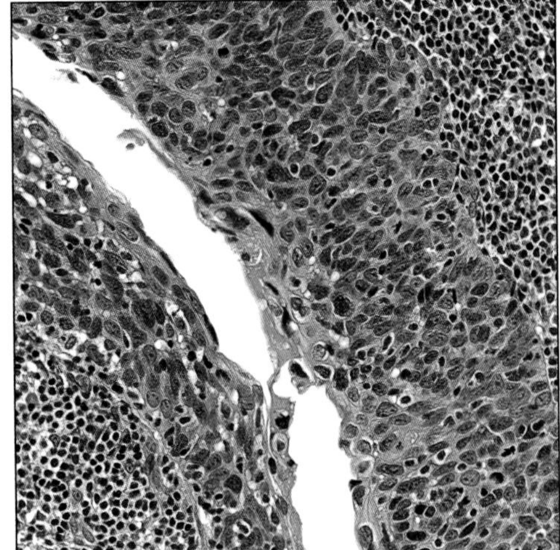

The epithelium lining the cystic spaces lacks maturation toward the lumen, shows focal keratinization at the surface, and shows pleomorphism that is beyond what would be seen in a branchial cleft cyst.

TERMINOLOGY

Abbreviations

- Squamous cell carcinoma (SCC)

Synonyms

- Metastatic cancer to the neck from an unknown primary site (MCCUP)
- Carcinoma of unknown primary (CUP)

Definitions

- Predominantly cystic SCC metastatic to neck lymph nodes
  - Histomorphology of metastases may be divided into
    - Keratinizing SCC
    - Nonkeratinizing carcinoma
    - Undifferentiated carcinoma
- MCCUP
  - Histologic diagnosis of metastatic carcinoma without a diagnosis of a primary tumor

ETIOLOGY/PATHOGENESIS

Etiology

- Tobacco and alcohol abuse
  - Often linked to a primary SCC, keratinizing type
  - Primary carcinoma may originate in various mucosal sites of the upper aerodigestive tract
    - Histomorphology not specifically linked to any primary site
- Viral-related
  - Human papillomavirus (HPV)
    - May be referred to as HPV-associated SCC
    - Linked to primary SCC, nonkeratinizing type
    - p16 positive by immunohistochemistry, in situ hybridization (ISH), or polymerase chain react (PCR)
    - p16 positive SCC represents reliable predictor of origin from oropharynx (tonsil, base of tongue)
    - Patients typically are nonsmokers and do not abuse alcohol
  - Epstein Barr virus (EBV)
    - May be referred to as EBV-associated SCC
    - Linked to primary SCC, nonkeratinizing and undifferentiated types
    - Primary cancer may be localized to nasopharynx or other Waldeyer ring sites (tonsil, base of tongue)
    - Positive ISH for Epstein Barr encoded RNA (EBER)

Origin

- Dedicated lymphatic drainage of neck lymph nodes often (but not always) allows for determination of primary carcinoma site
- Aside from oropharynx and nasopharynx, metastatic SCC to neck lymph nodes may originate from any site mucosal site in head and neck
- Metastatic thyroid papillary carcinoma may be incidentally identified in neck dissections performed for metastatic SCC
  - Primary thyroid-based papillary carcinoma
    - Usually is in ipsilateral thyroid lobe
    - May be a papillary microcarcinoma (defined as measuring < 1 cm) and clinically difficult to detect

CLINICAL ISSUES

Epidemiology

- Incidence
  - MCCUP
    - Constitutes approximately 3% of all malignant neoplasms
    - As a distinct subgroup, represents 2-9% of all H&N cancers
- Age
  - Most frequently diagnosed between 5th-7th decades
    - Peak: 6th decade
  - HPV-associated

METASTATIC CYSTIC SQUAMOUS CELL CARCINOMA

Key Facts

Terminology

- MCCUP: Histologic diagnosis of metastatic carcinoma without diagnosis of a primary tumor

Etiology/Pathogenesis

- Tobacco and alcohol abuse
- Viral-associated (HPV, EBV)

Clinical Issues

- Painless mass in upper neck
- Jugulodigastric lymph node chain
- 30% of patients never have primary identified
- Radiation is mainstay of therapy
- MCCUP: 5-year survival rates range from 18-48%
- HPV-associated SCC: Better outcome than non-HPV-associated SCC
- EBV-associated SCC: 65% 5-year survival

Microscopic Pathology

- **Metastatic keratinizing SCC**
  - Presence of keratinization in majority of carcinoma
- **Metastatic nonkeratinizing SCC**
  - Often appears as cystic metastasis with central necrotic material
  - Recapitulates histomorphology of primary oropharyngeal carcinoma
  - Primary tumor may be small and localized deep in tonsillar crypts making clinical detection difficult
- **Metastatic undifferentiated SCC**
  - May appear as cystic metastasis with central necrotic material
  - Histomorphology similar to that of nasopharyngeal carcinoma, undifferentiated type

    - Occurs in younger patients than non-HPV-associated SCC
- Gender
  - Male > > Female (4:1)

Site

- Jugulodigastric lymph node chain
  - Rich lymphatic plexus of Waldeyer ring results in early metastatic disease from small, clinically inapparent tumors
- Can present anywhere within neck, but jugulodigastric lymph node group is most common
  - Level II most common followed by level I and III
- Isolated nodal mass in submental triangle is rarely carcinoma
  - Typically are inflammatory or related to benign conditions of salivary glands
- Posterior palpable nodes in young patient are usually benign (e.g., inflammatory)

Presentation

- Painless neck mass that has enlarged over recent months
  - Often fixed
  - Usually < 6 months duration
- May have bilateral enlargement in 10% of patients
- When metastasis is diagnosed, primary can be sought
  - Panendoscopy (nasal cavity, nasopharynx, oral cavity, oropharynx, esophagus, larynx)
  - High-resolution PET/CT scans to determine biopsy sites
  - "Blind" biopsies of various mucosal sites but oropharynx and nasopharynx, specifically
  - Tonsillectomy if biopsies are negative
  - Primaries include base of tongue, lingual or faucial tonsils (Waldeyer ring), nasopharynx, esophagus, and larynx
- 30% of patients never have primary identified
- About 30% of patients with metastatic squamous cell carcinoma show exclusively cystic metastases
- Primaries within tonsil or base of tongue may be very small (< 0.1 cm), making diagnosis difficult

Treatment

- Options, risks, complications
  - Misdiagnosed as "primary branchial cleft carcinoma"; means that primary is never discovered and continues to grow and metastasize
  - Must do extensive work-up to find primary
    - Panendoscopy, high-resolution PET/CT, and multiple biopsies, including tonsillectomy if needed
- Surgical approaches
  - Excision of lymph nodes
  - Multiple "blind" biopsies of mucosal sites of upper aerodigestive tract
    - Performed in an attempt to find primary carcinoma
  - Tonsillectomy performed in biopsies negative for carcinoma
    - Ipsilateral tonsillectomy in presence of unilateral neck disease
    - Bilateral tonsillectomy in presence of bilateral neck disease
- Radiation
  - Mainstay of therapy
  - When primary is identified, intensity modulated radiation therapy (IMRT) can be used
    - Delivers treatment dose to areas at risk while limiting dose given to normal structures
    - Main advantage is that it spares normal structures (e.g., larynx, parotid) while delivering sufficient radiation does to areas of gross or clinical disease
  - Brachytherapy
    - Form of radiotherapy where radiation source is placed inside or next to area requiring treatment
    - Can be used alone or in combination with other therapies such as surgery, external beam radiotherapy, and chemotherapy
    - Can be used in treatment of variety of SCC of H&N including HPV-associated SCC

Prognosis

- MCCUP
  - 5-year survival rates range from 18-48%

METASTATIC CYSTIC SQUAMOUS CELL CARCINOMA

- Dependent on patient and tumor characteristics
- Prognostic factors include
  - Clinical stage of neck
    - Most reliable clinical prognostic indicator
    - Higher clinical stage associated with worse prognosis (decreased survival)
  - Presence of extracapsular spread (ECS)
    - Single most important histologic prognostic factor in recurrent disease, distant metastases, and overall survival
  - Histologic type of metastatic carcinoma
    - HPV-associated and EBV-associated SCC associated with better overall survival than non-viral associated SCC
    - Metastatic adenocarcinoma associated with worse prognosis than metastatic SCC
  - Location of largest lymph node
    - Metastatic carcinoma to supraclavicular or in low cervical lymph nodes rarely cured by any treatment modality
- HPV-associated SCC
  - Radioresponsive cancers
  - Associated with better outcome (better overall- and disease-specific survival) than non-HPV-associated SCC possible due to
    - Absence of field cancerization
    - Enhanced radiation sensitivity
  - Highly curable even in presence of advanced disease
- EBV-associated SCC
  - Radioresponsive cancers
  - Approximately 65% 5-year survival

IMAGE FINDINGS

General Features

- High-resolution PET/CT to document cystic mass
- Used to identify possible primary location

MACROSCOPIC FEATURES

General Features

- Unilocular cyst with thick capsule
- Cyst is filled with grumous, thick, tenacious, purulent yellow to hemorrhagic material
  - May simulate pus or infection

Size

- Mean: 4 cm

MICROSCOPIC PATHOLOGY

Histologic Features

- **Nodal metastasis**
  - Predominantly cystic
  - Viable cancer may include
    - Keratinizing SCC
    - Nonkeratinizing SCC
    - Undifferentiated SCC
  - Thick, dense, fibrous connective tissue capsule
  - Presence of subcapsular sinus defines structure as a lymph node
  - Lymphoid tissue immediately below capsule
  - Often zone of separation between lymphoid stroma and tumor
- **Metastatic keratinizing SCC**
  - Histologic grades include well-, moderately and poorly-differentiated
  - Presence of keratinization in majority of carcinoma
    - In poorly-differentiated SCC evidence of keratinization may be minimal
  - Typically associated with desmoplastic tissue response
  - Pattern of carcinoma and presence of desmoplasia contrast to features seen in nonkeratinizing and undifferentiated SCC
- **Metastatic nonkeratinizing carcinoma**
  - Often appears as cystic metastasis with central necrotic material
    - Recapitulates histomorphology of primary oropharyngeal carcinoma
  - Ribbon-like or band-like, uniformly thick epithelium lining cystic spaces, frequently thrown into papillary folds or projections
  - Endophytic pattern can be seen with budding into lymphoid stroma
  - Lacks maturation toward cyst lumen
  - Shows loss of polarity, disorganization and enlarged cells with high nuclear to cytoplasmic ratio
    - May have significant pleomorphism focally or diffusely
  - Limited keratinization
    - Presence of keratinization does not exclude diagnosis of nonkeratinizing SCC
  - Transitional-like epithelium with limited atypia may be present
    - Remarkably bland epithelium
    - Such benign-appearing epithelium suggests branchial cleft cyst
  - Primary tumor may be small and localized deep in tonsillar crypts making clinical detection difficult
- **Metastatic undifferentiated carcinoma**
  - May appear as cystic metastasis with central necrotic material
  - Syncytial growth in form of cohesive nests
  - Neoplastic cells characterized by enlarged nuclei with vesicular chromatin and prominent nucleoli
  - Limited keratinization
    - Presence of keratinization does not exclude diagnosis of undifferentiated SCC
  - Desmoplastic response may be absent
    - Neoplastic cells may be overrun and obscured by benign lymphocytes
- **Post-treatment (irradiation, chemotherapy) metastatic SCC**
  - Early alterations
    - Increase in abnormal nuclear types (macronucleoli, double or multiple nuclei)
    - Increased apoptosis
    - Hyperkeratinization
  - Late alterations
    - Necrosis and calcifications
    - Keratin granuloma formation

- Viable tumor cells may be completely absent or be focally present in association with small islands of residual intact tumor
- In absence of malignant cells, keratin granuloma may be replaced by fibrotic acellular nodules

ANCILLARY TESTS

Cytology

- Smears quite cellular, dominated by anucleate squamous and debris
- Rare fragments of atypical squamous epithelium
- Isolated, individual atypical keratinocytes with nuclear atypia, increased nuclear to cytoplasm ratio, "hard" keratinization, and irregular cell shape (tadpole cells)
- Must have more than just isolated atypical cells to confirm diagnosis

Immunohistochemistry

- **Positive**: CK-PAN, CAM5.2, CK5/6, CK8, CK14, CK19, p63
- **Negative**: CK7, CK20, EMA
- **HPV-associated SCC**
  - p16 positive
    - Represents surrogate marker for HPV-associated carcinomas
    - Nuclear and cytoplasmic staining
    - Reliable reliable predictor of origin from oropharynx
    - Can be performed on cytologic &/or surgical resection material
  - Oropharyngeal carcinomas with morphology of undifferentiated SCC may be p16-positive and EBER-negative
    - Such carcinomas may metastasize as MCCUP so work-up should include **both** p16 and EBER staining
- **EBV-associated SCC**
  - EBER-positive
    - Nuclear staining
  - Carcinomas with morphology of nasopharyngeal nonkeratinizing carcinoma, differentiated and undifferentiated types may be p16-positive and EBER-negative
    - Such carcinomas may metastasize as MCCUP so work-up should include **both** EBER and p16 staining
- **Post-treatment metastatic SCC**
  - Cytokeratin staining (CK-PAN, CAM5.2, CK5/6) may assist in identification of
    - Viable malignant cells
    - Keratin granuloma formation

DIFFERENTIAL DIAGNOSIS

Branchial Cleft Cyst

- Benign epithelium lining cystic spaces, usually showing intimate admixture of epithelium with stroma
- Maturation is noted without atypia or mitotic figures
- Lacks desmoplastic or thickened fibrous capsule
- p16 and EBER negative

Primary Branchiogenic Carcinoma

- Does not exist

SELECTED REFERENCES

1. Ang KK et al: Human papillomavirus and survival of patients with oropharyngeal cancer. N Engl J Med. 363(1):24-35, 2010
2. Cao D et al: Expression of p16 in benign and malignant cystic squamous lesions of the neck. Hum Pathol. 41(4):535-9, 2010
3. Singhi AD et al: Comparison of human papillomavirus in situ hybridization and p16 immunohistochemistry in the detection of human papillomavirus-associated head and neck cancer based on a prospective clinical experience. Cancer. 116(9):2166-73, 2010
4. Singhi AD et al: Lymphoepithelial-like carcinoma of the oropharynx: a morphologic variant of HPV-related head and neck carcinoma. Am J Surg Pathol. 34(6):800-5, 2010
5. Nichols AC et al: HPV-16 infection predicts treatment outcome in oropharyngeal squamous cell carcinoma. Otolaryngol Head Neck Surg. 140(2):228-34, 2009
6. Goldenberg D et al: Cystic lymph node metastasis in patients with head and neck cancer: An HPV-associated phenomenon. Head Neck. 30(7):898-903, 2008
7. Begum S et al: Detection of human papillomavirus-16 in fine-needle aspirates to determine tumor origin in patients with metastatic squamous cell carcinoma of the head and neck. Clin Cancer Res. 13(4):1186-91, 2007
8. Begum S et al: Tissue distribution of human papillomavirus 16 DNA integration in patients with tonsillar carcinoma. Clin Cancer Res. 11(16):5694-9, 2005
9. Iganej S et al: Metastatic squamous cell carcinoma of the neck from an unknown primary: management options and patterns of relapse. Head Neck. 24(3):236-46, 2002
10. Gillison ML et al: Human papillomavirus-associated head and neck squamous cell carcinoma: mounting evidence for an etiologic role for human papillomavirus in a subset of head and neck cancers. Curr Opin Oncol. 13(3):183-8, 2001
11. Hamakawa H et al: Histological effects and predictive biomarkers of TPP induction chemotherapy for oral carcinoma. J Oral Pathol Med. 27(2):87-94, 1998
12. Thompson LD et al: The clinical importance of cystic squamous cell carcinomas in the neck: a study of 136 cases. Cancer. 82(5):944-56, 1998
13. Carter RL et al: Radical neck dissections for squamous carcinomas: pathological findings and their clinical implications with particular reference to transcapsular spread. Int J Radiat Oncol Biol Phys. 13(6):825-32, 1987
14. Tanner NS et al: The irradiated radical neck dissection in squamous carcinoma: a clinico-pathological study. Clin Otolaryngol Allied Sci. 5(4):259-71, 1980

METASTATIC CYSTIC SQUAMOUS CELL CARCINOMA

Anatomic, Imaging, and Microscopic Features

(Left) There is a small but well-defined carcinoma ➔ at the base of the tongue that has developed a lymph node metastasis to the jugulodigastric lymph node ➔. This is a characteristic metastatic location. *(Right)* The primary site for the metastatic tumors to the neck most frequently encompasses Waldeyer ring: Lingual and faucial tonsils ➔, base of tongue, and nasopharynx. The larynx and esophagus can also present with neck metastatic disease, but it is usually not cystic.

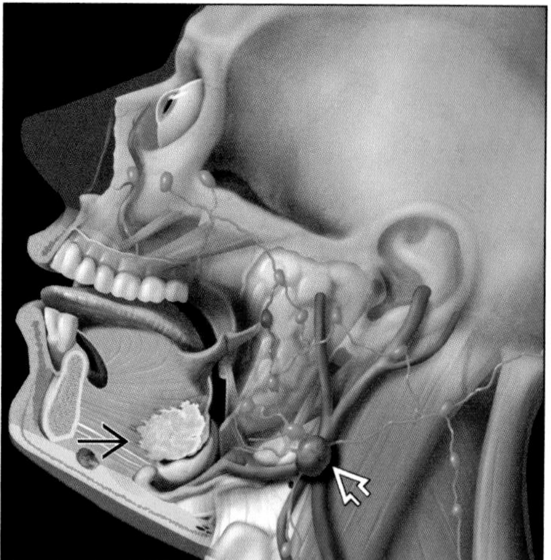

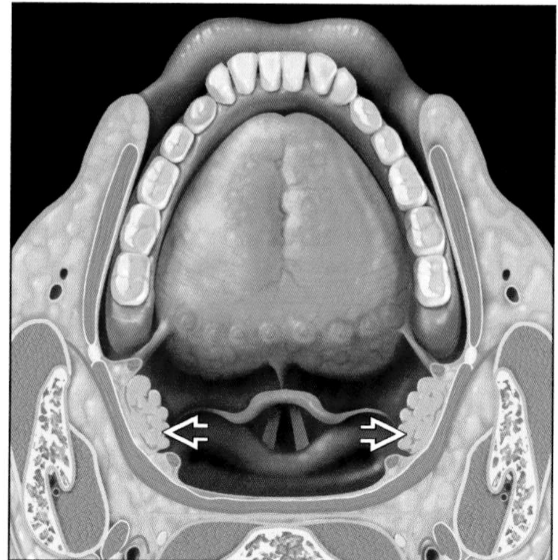

(Left) Axial CECT shows subtle asymmetrical fullness ➔ in the left floor of the mouth. This patient was recently diagnosed with metastatic cystic squamous cell carcinoma in a left neck lymph node without an identifiable primary lesion. *(Right)* Axial fused PET/CT shows intense FDG activity ➔ in the area of questionable fullness on the CT portion of the exam, confirming the presence of malignancy. This was the site of the primary, which had resulted in neck lymph node metastases.

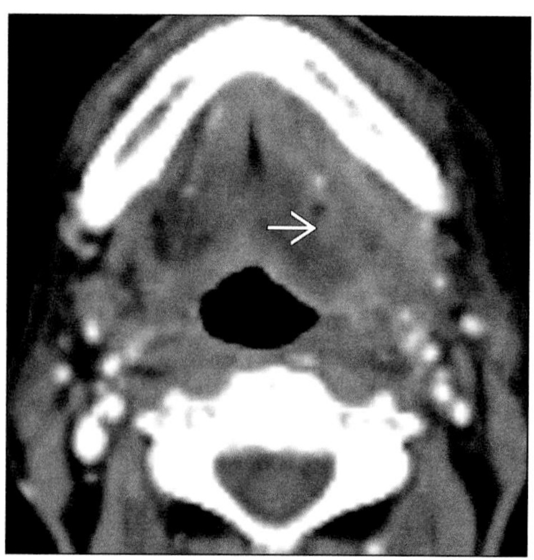

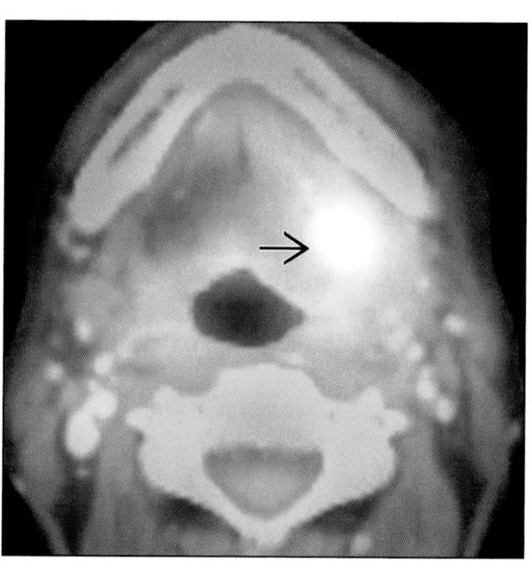

(Left) There is a very thick fibrous connective tissue capsule in this lymph node ➔. There is a large, debris-filled cystic space lined by a ribbon-like epithelium. This is a characteristic appearance for this type of metastatic tumor. *(Right)* In this example, there is a "lining" epithelium that plunges down into the lymphoid stroma of the lymph node, creating islands and nests of tumor. However, they still show a ribbon-like appearance, focally showing necrosis ➔.

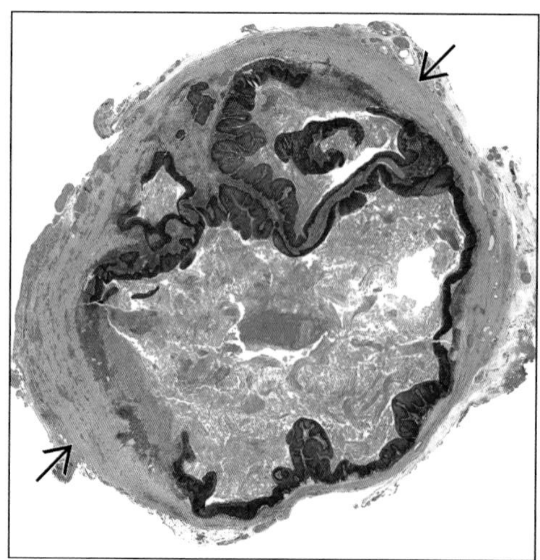

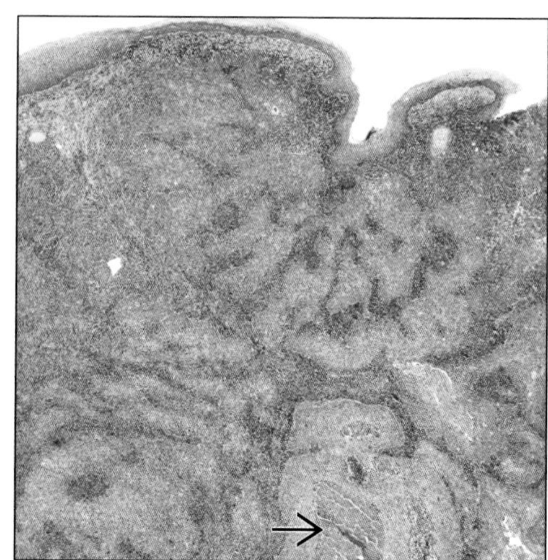

Microscopic and Immunohistochemical Features

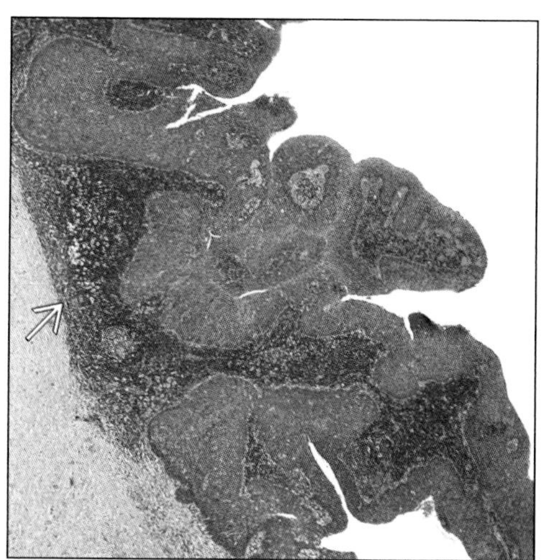

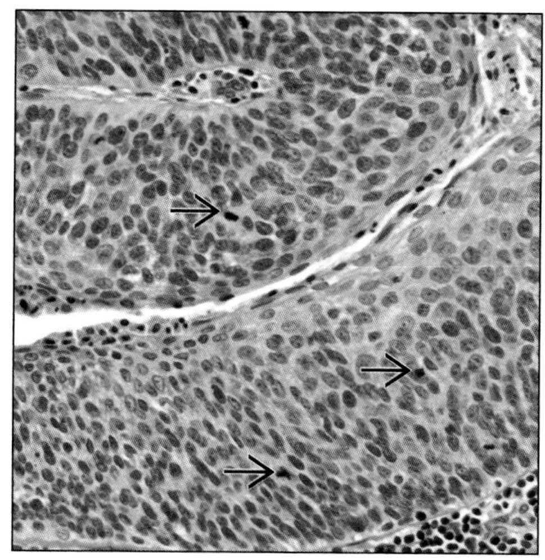

(Left) *One of the most histologically reproducible features on low power is the uniformly thick band-like epithelium lining the cystic spaces within the lymph node. There are papillary projections into the lumen. Note the lymphoid remnants ➔ of the lymph node.* ***(Right)*** *The epithelium shows a subtle increased cellularity, lacking significant maturation toward the surface, and including a number of mitoses →. This would be exceptional in a branchial cleft cyst.*

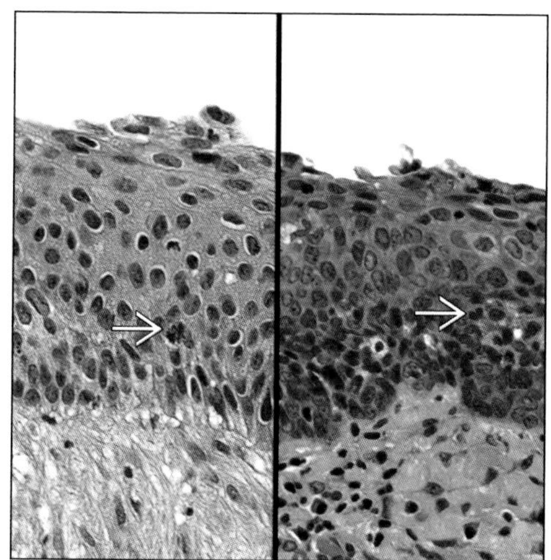

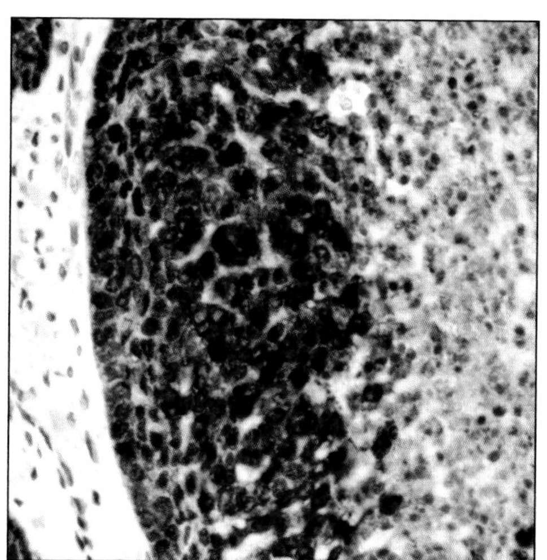

(Left) *A split field demonstrates very subtle cellular features of a metastatic cystic SCC. There is slight pleomorphism, increased cellularity, and isolated mitotic figures ➔ that help to confirm the diagnosis.* ***(Right)*** *Metastatic nonkeratinizing SCC shows diffuse nuclear and cytoplasmic p16 immunoreactivity. This finding represents a reliable indicator of a primary oropharyngeal carcinoma. The primary carcinoma may be small and difficult to detect.*

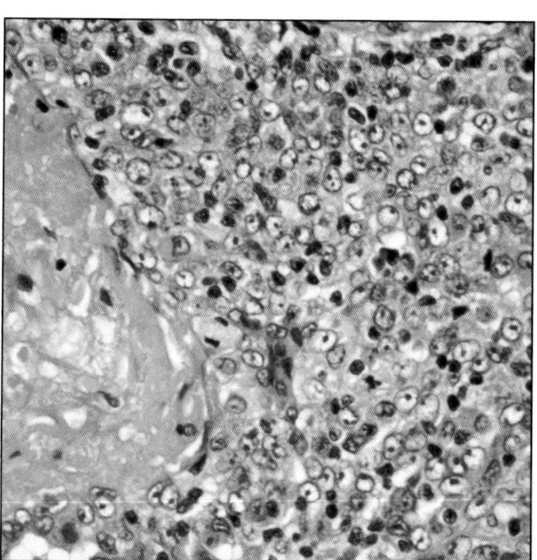

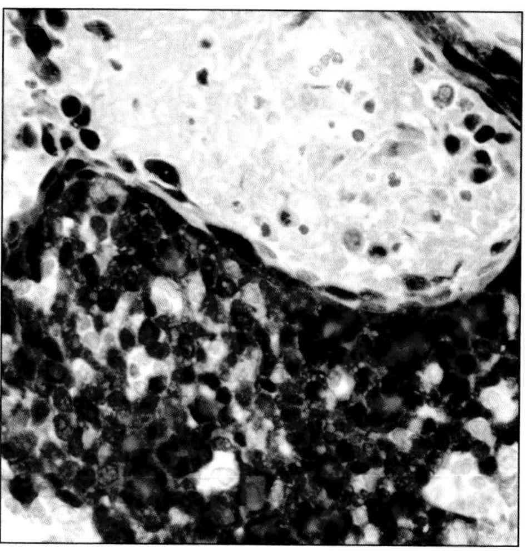

(Left) *MCCUP with histologic features suggesting origin from a nasopharyngeal undifferentiated carcinoma is shown, including cells with enlarged nuclei, vesicular chromatin, and prominent nucleoli.* ***(Right)*** *The neoplastic cells are p16 immunoreactive and were EBER negative. In spite of showing histologic features similar to those of nasopharyngeal undifferentiated carcinoma, the origin for this metastasis was located in the oropharynx (tonsillar crypt).*

METASTATIC CYSTIC SQUAMOUS CELL CARCINOMA

Microscopic Features and Ancillary Techniques

(Left) MCCUP with histologic features suggesting origin from a nasopharyngeal undifferentiated carcinoma is shown, including cells with enlarged nuclei, vesicular chromatin, and prominent nucleoli. ***(Right)*** The neoplastic cells are EBER positive (nuclear staining) and were p16 negative. The histologic features coupled with EBER-positive staining support origin for this MCCUP from the nasopharynx. The primary carcinoma may be small and clinically difficult to detect.

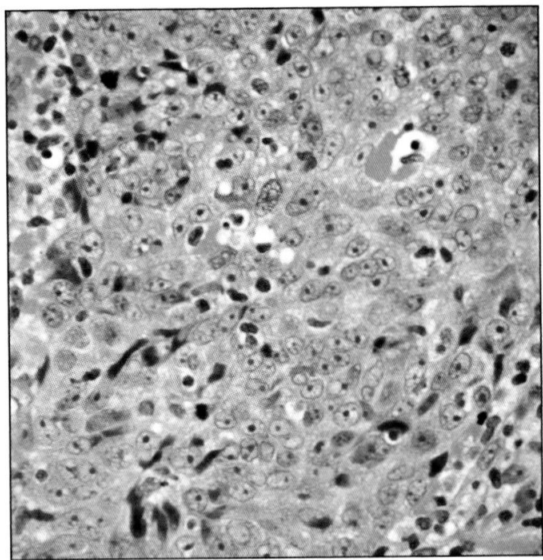

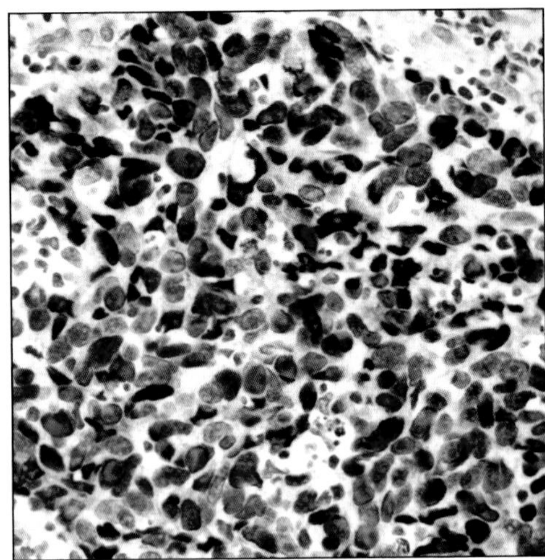

(Left) Metastatic cystic keratinizing squamous cell carcinoma to a cervical lymph node is seen. The metastasis is confined to the lymph node without extranodal extension. ***(Right)*** In some cases, the epithelium is associated with significant keratin debris, which is sloughed into the lumen of the cystic metastasis ⇨. A prominent neutrophilic response is present. The epithelium is atypical in the basal zone, including hyperchromasia, nuclear pleomorphism, and dyskeratotic cells ↪.

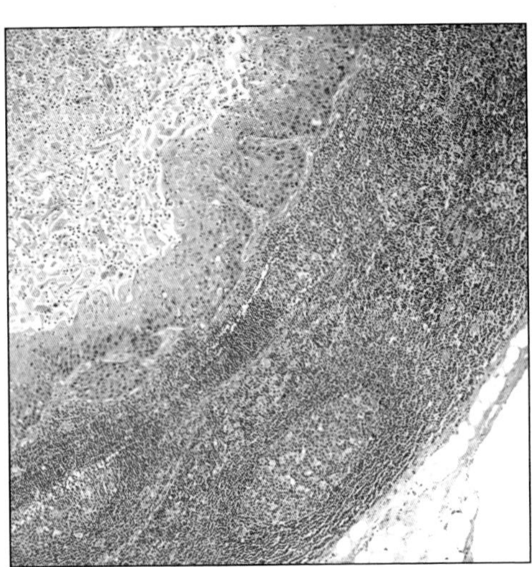

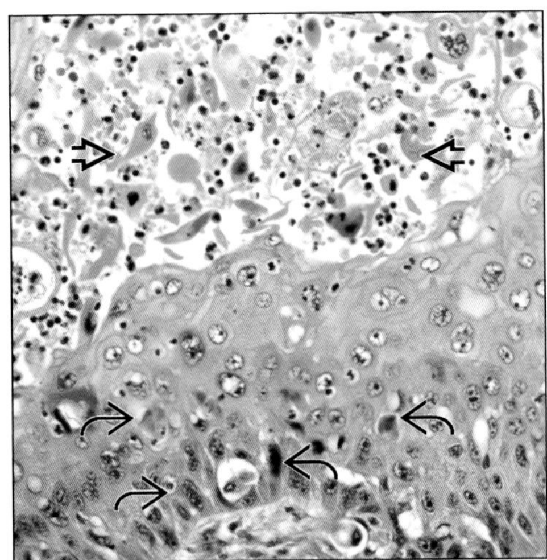

(Left) Cystic metastatic squamous cell carcinoma is usually not associated with profoundly pleomorphic cells, but as shown in this case, it can be seen. Atypical mitoses are also present →. ***(Right)*** Anucleate squames and inflammatory debris are the dominant findings in cytology aspirates from the lymph nodes of metastatic cystic SCC. This field shows atypical keratinocytes with "hard" keratinization ➔ and irregular cell shapes.

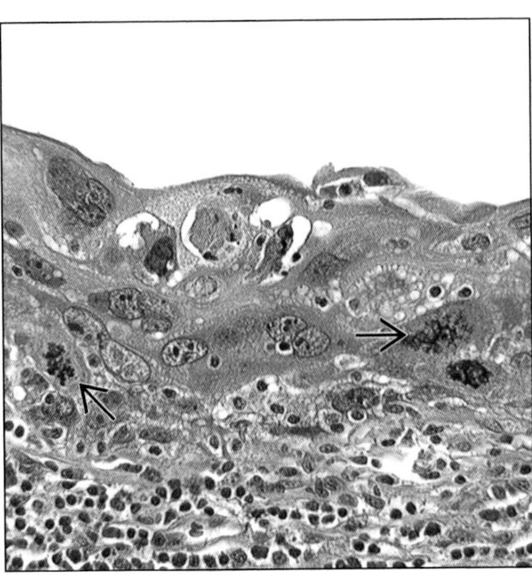

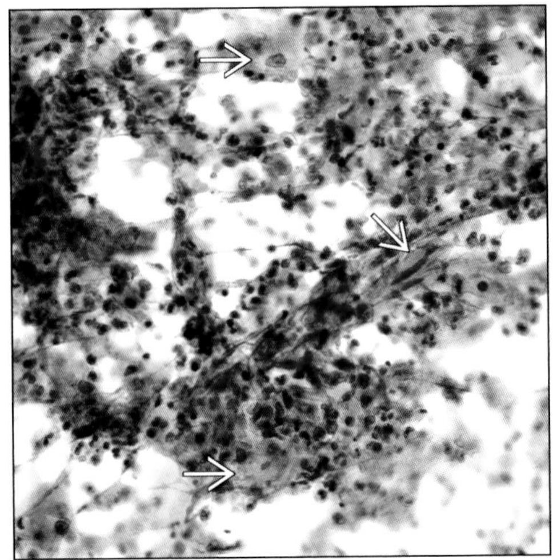

Microscopic Features

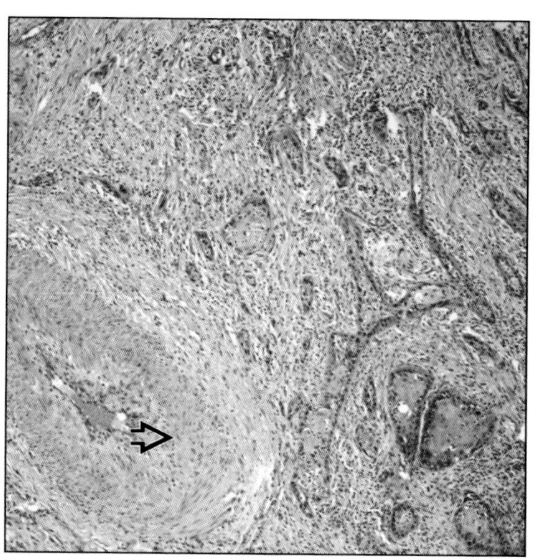

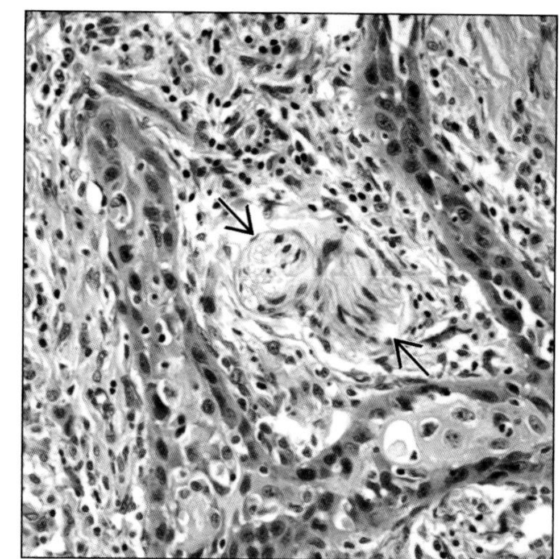

(Left) *Metastatic SCC to a cervical lymph node shows the presence of extracapsular spread with extension of the carcinoma to perinodal soft tissues, including a thick-walled blood vessel ⇨.* ***(Right)*** *In addition to the perivascular invasion, extracapsular spread includes perineural invasion →. The presence of extracapsular spread represents the single most important histologic prognostic factor in recurrent disease, distant metastases, and overall survival.*

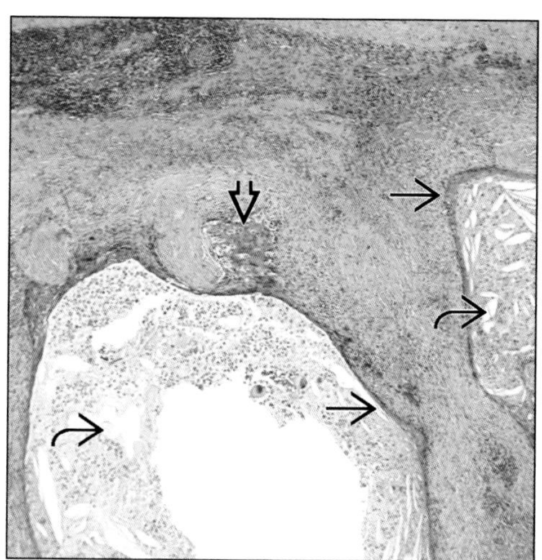

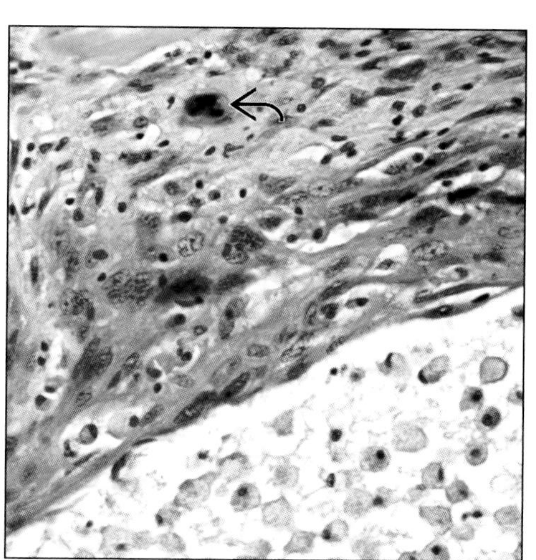

(Left) *Post-irradiated radical neck dissection shows foci of cystic metastatic SCC ↪ surrounded by fibrotic areas. Even at this magnification, lining epithelium can be seen → as well as a more solid-appearing tumor foci ⇨.* ***(Right)*** *In spite of the radiation therapy, residual viable metastatic SCC is identified including malignant cells lining the cyst as well as isolated malignant cells in the wall of the cyst ↪.*

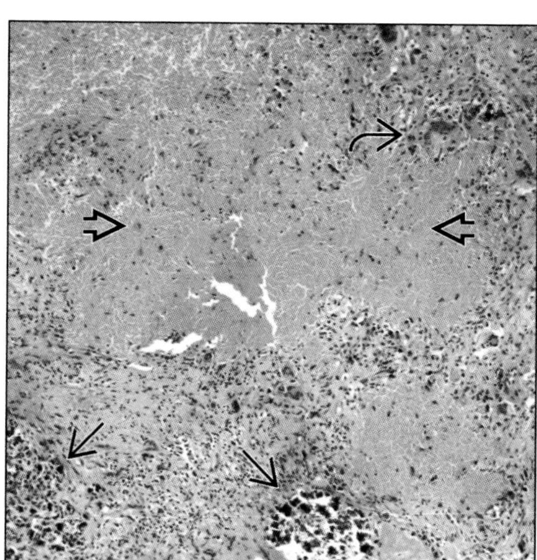

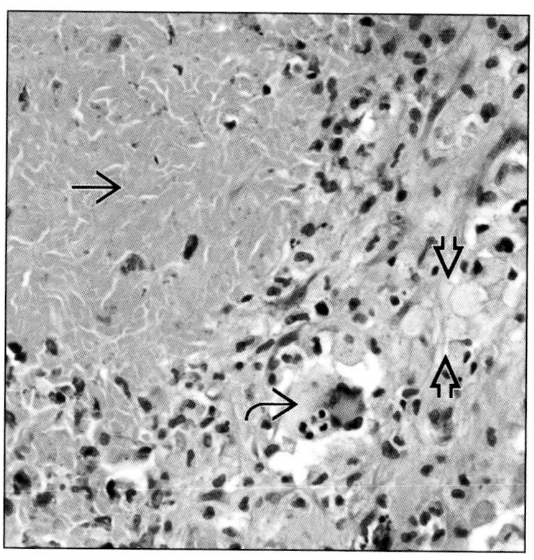

(Left) *Later stage following radiation therapy shows a lymph node with broad areas of necrosis ⇨ and calcifications →. Scattered multinucleated giant cells are present ↪.* ***(Right)*** *Viable tumor cells are completely absent, replaced by fibrotic acellular nodule →. Additional findings include the presence of multinucleated giant cell ↪ and foamy histiocytes ⇨ indicative of granuloma formation.*

SYNOVIAL SARCOMA

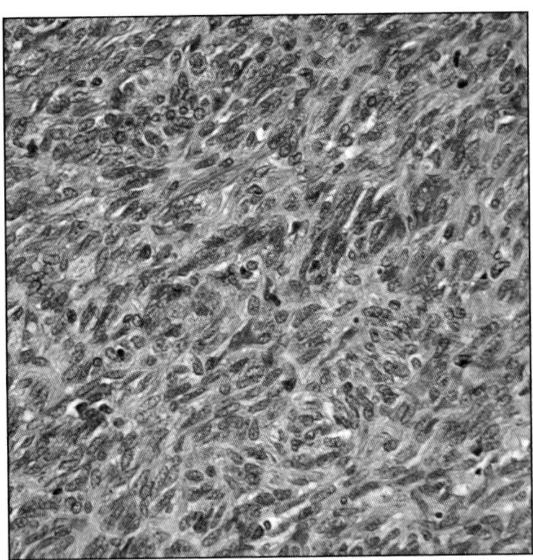

This monophasic SS shows a densely packed, interlacing spindled cell proliferation with monotonous cells arranged in a syncytium. The nuclei are ovoid, pale staining with small nucleoli. There is a rich vascularity.

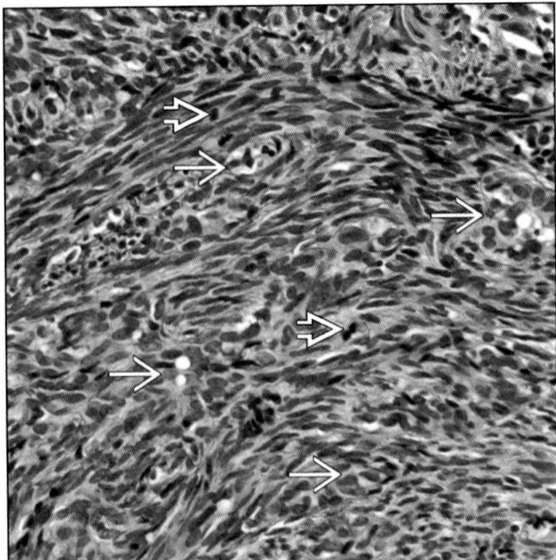

A biphasic SS shows an admixture of epithelial ➡ and spindle cell components. The epithelial cells have abundant cytoplasm, creating a glandular appearance with lumina. Mitotic figures are identified ➡.

TERMINOLOGY

Abbreviations

- Synovial sarcoma (SS)

Synonyms

- Tendosynovial sarcoma
- Synovial cell sarcoma
- Malignant synovioma
- Synovioblastic sarcoma

Definitions

- Mesenchymal spindled cell neoplasm with variable epithelial differentiation and specific chromosomal translocation: t(X;18)(p11;q11)

CLINICAL ISSUES

Epidemiology

- Incidence
  - Up to 10% of soft tissue sarcomas
    - About 10% develop in head and neck
- Age
  - Bimodal presentation
    - Young adults (15-35 years; mean: 25 years)
    - Older age (around 50 years)
- Gender
  - Male > Female (3:1)

Site

- No association with synovium or bursa
- Neck, oropharynx and hypopharynx/larynx
- Direct extension into larynx may be initial presentation

Presentation

- Nonspecific, usually related to anatomic site
- Mass
- Hoarseness and dysphasia
- Pain may be present

Treatment

- Options, risks, complications
  - Need aggressive local excision
  - Presence of calcifications associated with improved prognosis
- Surgical approaches
  - Meticulous attention to surgical margins during wide surgical resection
- Adjuvant therapy
  - Combined with radiation
- Radiation
  - Combined with chemotherapy

Prognosis

- Head and neck mucosal tumors tend to have better prognosis than soft tissue counterparts
- Recurrences in about 25% of patients
- Metastatic disease in about 25% of patients (lung)
- About 1/3 of patients die from disease
- Best outcomes for small tumors, pediatric patients, and mitotically inactive tumors
- Patients with *SSX2* gene tend to have a better prognosis

IMAGE FINDINGS

General Features

- Soft tissue mass, frequently with calcifications
- Frequently multilobulated with heterogeneity
  - Hemorrhage, fluid levels, and septa
- May have well-defined margins

CT Findings

- Gives information about site of origin and size/extent
- Spiculated, irregular calcifications in about 20% of cases

SYNOVIAL SARCOMA

Key Facts

Terminology
- Mesenchymal spindle cell neoplasm with variable epithelial differentiation and specific chromosomal translocation: t(X;18)(p11;q11)

Clinical Issues
- No association with synovium or bursa
- Bimodal presentation
- About 10% develop in head and neck
- Male > Female (3:1)
- Head and neck mucosal tumors tend to have better prognosis than soft tissue counterparts

Image Findings
- Soft tissue mass, frequently with calcifications
- Spiculated, irregular calcifications in about 20% of cases

Macroscopic Features
- Usually < 5 cm

Microscopic Pathology
- Separated into monophasic and biphasic
  - Epithelial &/or spindle cell components
- May be marbled

Ancillary Tests
- Classically show t(X;18)(p11.2;q11.2)
- Epithelial markers within spindled and epithelial components

Top Differential Diagnoses
- Spindle cell (sarcomatoid) squamous cell carcinoma, malignant peripheral nerve sheath tumor

MACROSCOPIC FEATURES

General Features
- Pedunculated or polypoid within mucosal sites
- Mass is usually circumscribed, but can be infiltrative
- Multinodular and may be multicystic
- Cut surface yellow, gray, gritty to boggy
- May have mucoid or hemorrhagic degeneration

Size
- Range: 1-12 cm
  - Usually < 5 cm

MICROSCOPIC PATHOLOGY

Histologic Features
- Separated into monophasic and biphasic
  - In head and neck, monophasic spindled is most common type
- Biphasic
  - Has epithelial and spindled cell components
  - Variable proportions
  - Epithelial cells have abundant cytoplasm
  - Creates glandular appearance with lumina
  - May have papillary projections or pseudoglandular spaces
  - Epithelial component may predominate
- Densely packed, short fascicles
  - May be marbled: Alternating light and dark areas
- Hemangiopericytoma-like vasculature may be seen
- Spindled cells are uniform with indistinct cell boundaries
- Nuclei are ovoid, pale staining with small nucleoli
- Mitotic figures are identified, but not increased
- Stromal collagen is wiry and scant
- Myxoid change may be seen
- Calcifications are noted
- Mast cells are usually easy to identify
- Rich vascularity is noted

ANCILLARY TESTS

Cytology
- Yield is usually high, with cellular smears
- 3-dimensional, densely cellular tumor tissue fragments with irregular borders in almost all cases
  - Vascular plexus or network within tissue fragments
  - Pericapillary arrangement is common
- Dispersed cells in background, often with naked (striped) nuclei
- Tumor cells are small to medium, monomorphic and bland
- Cells are spindled to club-shaped, arranged in fascicles or whorls
  - Nuclei are fusiform, ovoid to rounded
  - Nuclear chromatin is bland
  - Nucleoli may occasionally be present
- Small gland-like structures can be seen (only in epithelioid-biphasic type)
  - Polygonal cells separated from spindle cells
- Amorphous, hyaline matrix material may be mixed with cells
  - Collagenous stroma, hyalinized to fibrillar
  - May yield a rosette-like structure with cells surrounding central pink material
- Mast cells may be present
- Poorly differentiated and myxoid variants may be difficult to diagnose on cytology
- FISH for translocation can be performed on FNA material

Histochemistry
- Mucicarmine found within epithelial cells, glandular lumens, and intracellular areas
- Alcian blue identified in spindle cell and myxoid areas (similar to colloidal iron)

Immunohistochemistry
- Epithelial markers within spindled and epithelial components

SYNOVIAL SARCOMA

Immunohistochemistry

Antibody	Reactivity	Staining Pattern	Comment
TLE1	Positive	Nuclear	Nearly all tumor cells
CK-PAN	Positive	Cytoplasmic	Epithelial cells; isolated spindle cells
CK7	Positive	Cytoplasmic	Epithelial and spindle cells
CK19	Positive	Cytoplasmic	Epithelial and spindle cells
EMA	Positive	Cytoplasmic	Glandular lumens and slit-like spaces
S100	Positive	Nuclear & cytoplasmic	About 30% of cases
CD99	Positive	Cytoplasmic	About 60% of cases
Bcl-2	Positive	Cytoplasmic	Especially spindle cells
Vimentin	Positive	Cytoplasmic	Especially spindle cells
CD34	Negative		
Desmin	Negative		

Cytogenetics

- *SSX1*, *SSX2*, *SSX4* from X chromosome
  - Vast majority accounted for by *SSX1*
- *SYT* from chromosome 18

In Situ Hybridization

- Classic t(X;18)(p11.2;q11.2) (required for diagnosis)
  - FISH break apart probe is best

Electron Microscopy

- Epithelial cells with hemidesmosomes, microvilli, tonofilaments, and basal lamina

DIFFERENTIAL DIAGNOSIS

Spindle Cell "Sarcomatoid" Squamous Cell Carcinoma

- Tends to be mucosal primary
- Will have positive epithelial markers (keratin, EMA, CK1, CK5/6)
- Lacks characteristic translocation of SS

Fibrosarcoma

- Herringbone, long fascicles
- Only reactive with vimentin
- Lacks characteristic translocation of SS

Malignant Peripheral Nerve Sheath Tumor

- Can be almost indistinguishable
- Both have marbling pattern
- S100 protein positive, but weak in high-grade tumors
- Lacks characteristic translocation of SS

Leiomyosarcoma

- More of a whorled appearance
- Blunted nuclei with perinuclear cytoplasmic clearing
- Positive for muscle markers (desmin, SMA, MSA)

Mucosal Malignant Melanoma

- Can be a histologic mimic
- Will also be S100 protein positive
- Additional melanoma markers will help
- Lacks characteristic translocation of SS

Hemangiopericytoma ↔ Solitary Fibrous Tumor

- HPC will have patternless appearance
- Vascularity may be similar
- Will have CD34, Bcl-2, &/or CD99 immunoreactivity

Epithelioid Sarcoma

- Does not usually develop in head and neck locations
- Will have biphasic appearance
- Similar immunohistochemistry
- Lacks characteristic translocation of SS

SELECTED REFERENCES

1. Wang H et al: Synovial sarcoma in the oral and maxillofacial region: report of 4 cases and review of the literature. J Oral Maxillofac Surg. 66(1):161-7, 2008
2. Miettinen M: From morphological to molecular diagnosis of soft tissue tumors. Adv Exp Med Biol. 587:99-113, 2006
3. Murphey MD et al: From the archives of the AFIP: Imaging of synovial sarcoma with radiologic-pathologic correlation. Radiographics. 26(5):1543-65, 2006
4. Randall RL et al: Diagnosis and management of synovial sarcoma. Curr Treat Options Oncol. 6(6):449-59, 2005
5. Artico R et al: Monophasic synovial sarcoma of hypopharynx: case report and review of the literature. Acta Otorhinolaryngol Ital. 24(1):33-6, 2004
6. Meer S et al: Oral synovial sarcoma: a report of 2 cases and a review of the literature. Oral Surg Oral Med Oral Pathol Oral Radiol Endod. 96(3):306-15, 2003
7. Potter BO et al: Sarcomas of the head and neck. Surg Oncol Clin N Am. 12(2):379-417, 2003
8. Grayson W et al: Synovial sarcoma of the parotid gland. A case report with clinicopathological analysis and review of the literature. S Afr J Surg. 36(1):32-4; discussion 34-5, 1998
9. Odell PF: Head and neck sarcomas: a review. J Otolaryngol. 25(1):7-13, 1996
10. Miloro M et al: Monophasic spindle cell synovial sarcoma of the head and neck: report of two cases an review of the literature. J Oral Maxillofac Surg. 52(3):309-13, 1994
11. Robinson DL et al: Synovial sarcoma of the neck: radiographic findings with a review of the literature. Am J Otolaryngol. 15(1):46-53, 1994
12. Ferlito A et al: Endolaryngeal synovial sarcoma. An update on diagnosis and treatment. ORL J Otorhinolaryngol Relat Spec. 53(2):116-9, 1991
13. Quinn HJ Jr: Synovial sarcoma of the larynx treated by partial laryngectomy. Laryngoscope. 94(9):1158-61, 1984

Imaging, Gross, and Microscopic Features

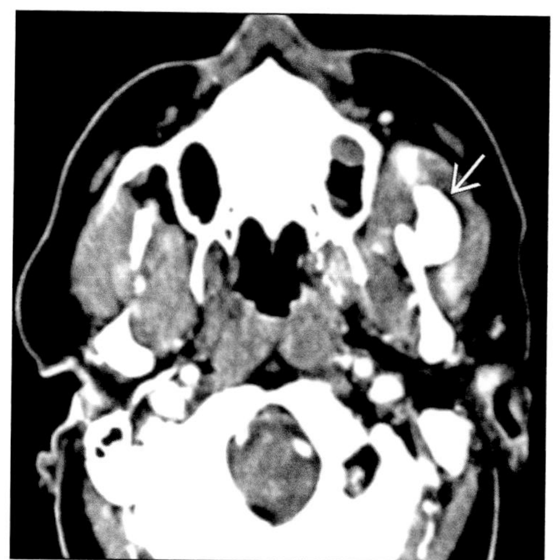

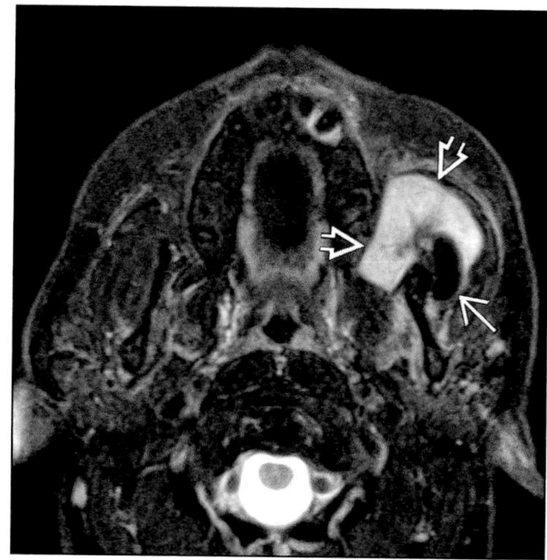

(Left) Axial CECT demonstrates a left masticator space lesion with a central crescentic bony center lateral to the mandible ➔. White bizarre lesions seen on imaging in the masticator space are often sarcomas. **(Right)** Axial T2 MR image shows the soft tissue extent ➔ of the masticator space synovial sarcoma. The bony central area ➔ is visible as a very low-signal component of the tumor. There are no "specific" features on imaging.

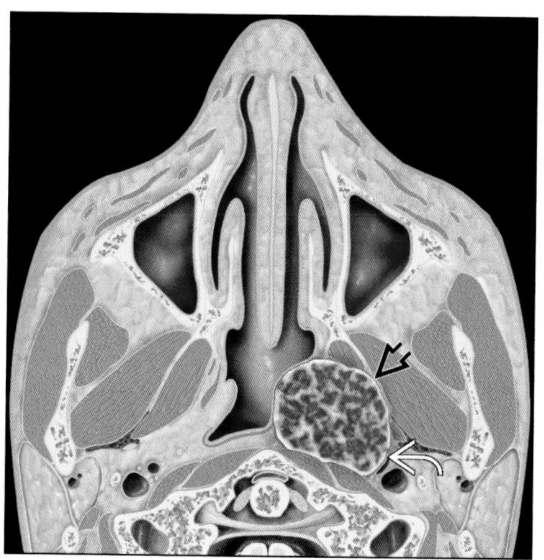

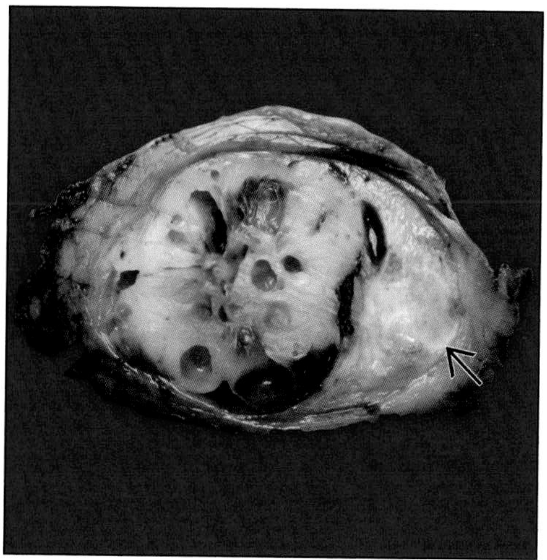

(Left) This graphic shows a synovial sarcoma within the naso- and oropharynx region. The tumor compresses and displaces the muscle ➔ outward, and compresses the carotid sheath, impinging on the carotid artery ➔ but not invading it. **(Right)** The neck mass is circumscribed, showing a slightly nodular appearance, with several cysts. The cut surface shows bright yellow areas ➔ and gray areas. This tumor was approximately 4 cm.

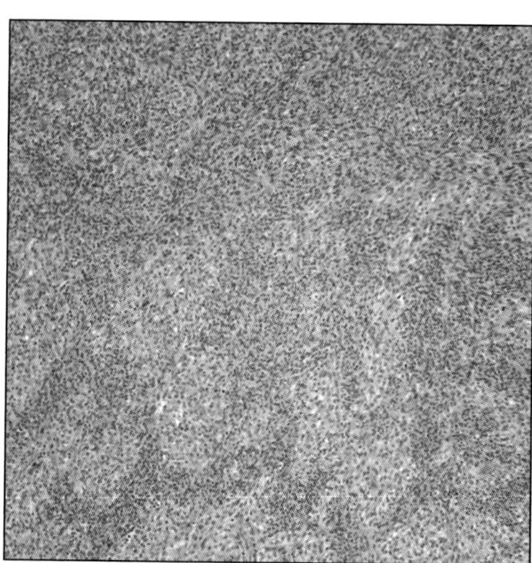

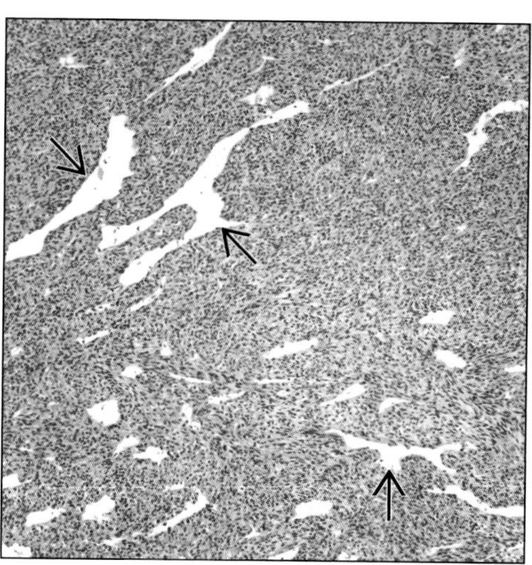

(Left) One of the characteristic features for a synovial sarcoma is a "marbled" appearance, with alternating light and dark areas created by the short fascicles. The spindled cells are uniform. **(Right)** This monophasic SS shows the spindled cells arranged around hemangiopericytoma-like vasculature ➔. This pattern is seen in many different tumor types and is not specific. However, SS usually has a rich vascularity as seen here.

SYNOVIAL SARCOMA

Microscopic Features

(Left) *A monophasic spindled SS shows high cellularity, along with numerous inflammatory cells ➡. Inflammatory cells are uncommon, although mast cells are frequently seen.* ***(Right)*** *The spindled cell population can show a variety of different patterns of growth. Here, a whorled appearance predominates. There is also a rich vascular plexus, easily identified throughout this image.*

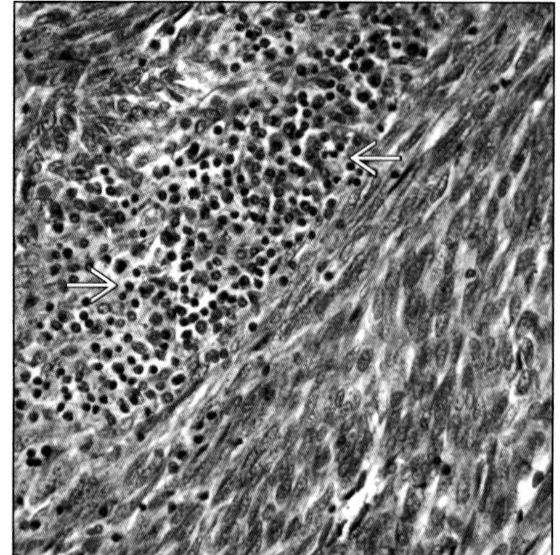

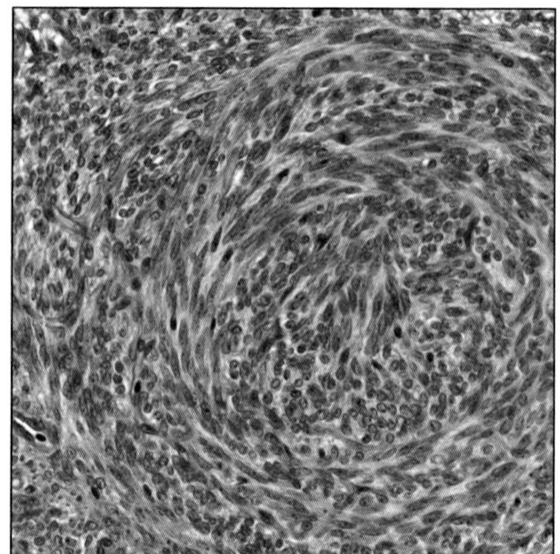

(Left) *The densely packed, short, interlacing fascicles of this monophasic SS blend with wiry stromal collagen. Mitoses ➡ are usually easy to find, although they are not usually increased.* ***(Right)*** *The interlaced fascicles can give an end-on or longitudinal appearance, simulating neural or smooth muscle tumors. There is a patulous vessel ➡ in this tumor, a frequent finding in SS.*

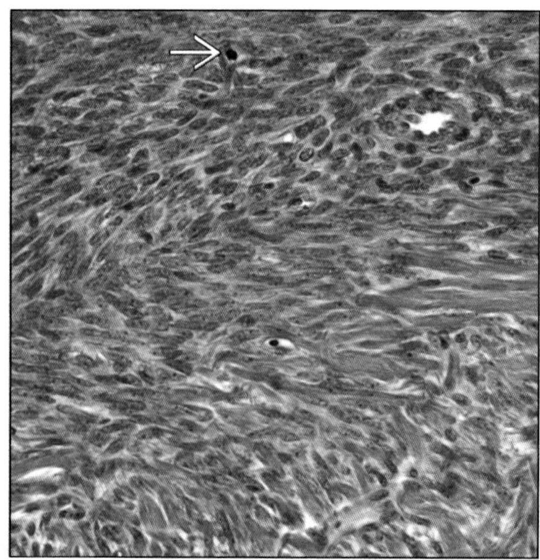

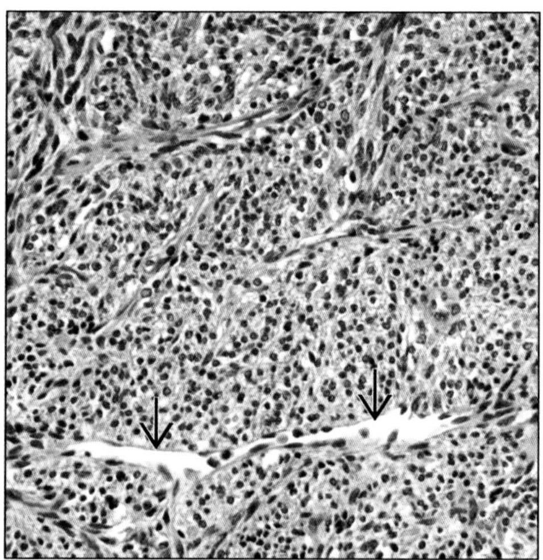

(Left) *Monophasic spindled SS may undergo myxoid change and degeneration. True tumor necrosis is rarely seen. This appearance can simulate Antoni B areas of a peripheral nerve sheath tumor.* ***(Right)*** *Cellular pleomorphism is uncommon in SS, and tends to be a localized phenomenon. This photograph shows a small collection of highly pleomorphic tumor cells. This was an isolated finding within a biphasic SS. Some view this as an "ancient" change phenomenon.*

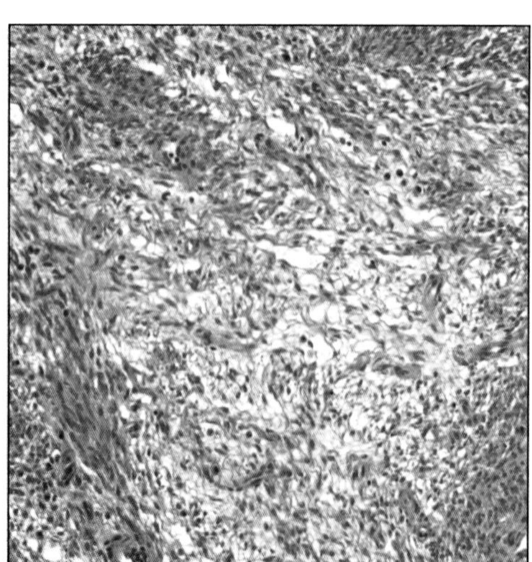

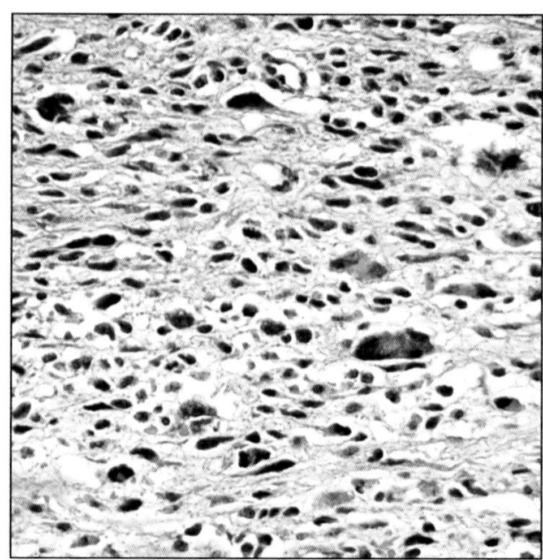

Ancillary Techniques

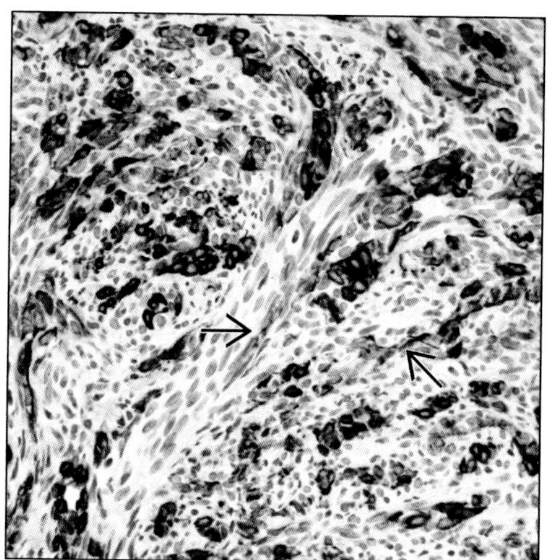

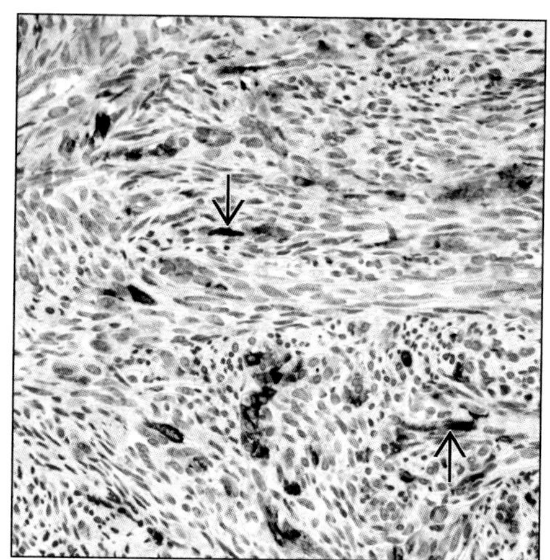

(Left) *In this biphasic SS, the keratin decorates the cytoplasm of epithelial cells, while only a few of the spindled cells are positive ⇒. Each of the keratins (CK7, CK19, EMA) has a slightly different reaction pattern.* ***(Right)*** *This biphasic SS demonstrates a positive cytoplasmic reaction in the glandular lumens with EMA, while also showing focal decoration of slit-like spaces ⇒ within the spindled cell population.*

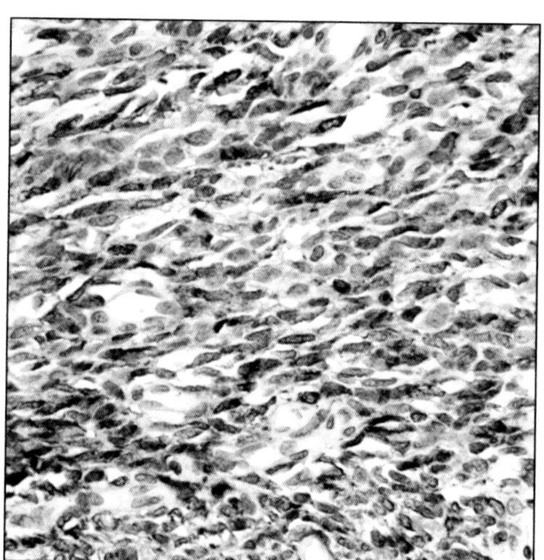

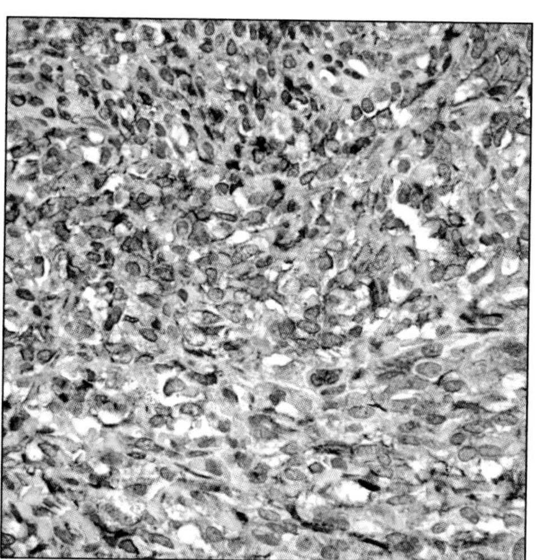

(Left) *Bcl-2 is not a specific or sensitive marker for SS, but shows a strong and diffuse cytoplasmic reaction within the spindled cells specifically. Vimentin shows a similar reaction profile.* ***(Right)*** *CD99 is identified in approximately 60% of SS cases. There is a delicate cytoplasmic reaction. This marker is neither specific nor sensitive for synovial carcinoma.*

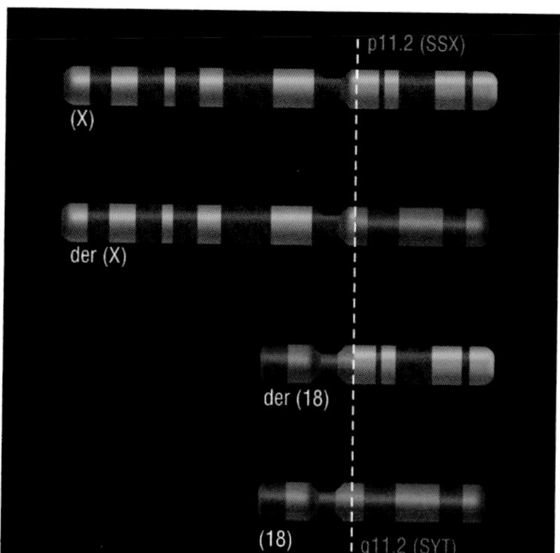

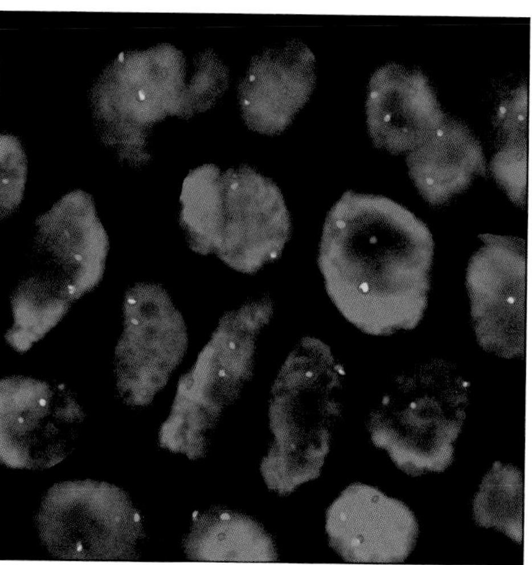

(Left) *The characteristic translocation t(X;18)(p11.2;q11.2) of the SSX gene (chromosome X, green) and SYT gene (chromosome 18, red) is present in > 95% of synovial sarcomas (translocation shown in the center). The fusion protein can be detected by a FISH probe.* ***(Right)*** *A FISH break apart probe can be performed on paraffin embedded material to highlight the translocation between SSX and SYT. Single red and green signals in each cell confirm the break apart (yellow signal is normal).*

CHORDOMA

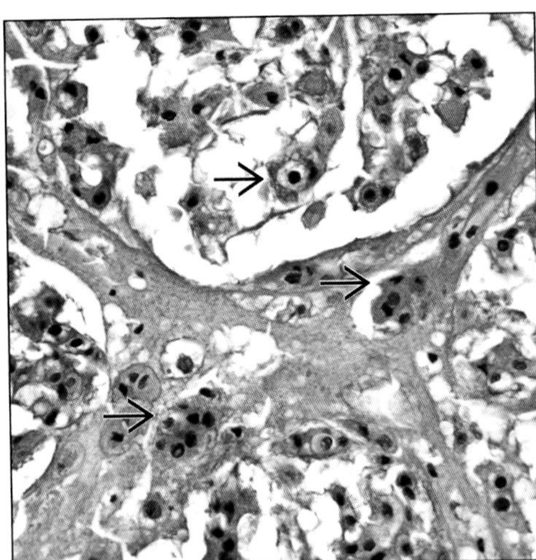

Histologically, chordomas are composed of 2 cells types, eosinophilic chief cells ⇒ and physaliferous cells set within a myxoid background matrix. The cells are arranged in nests and cords.

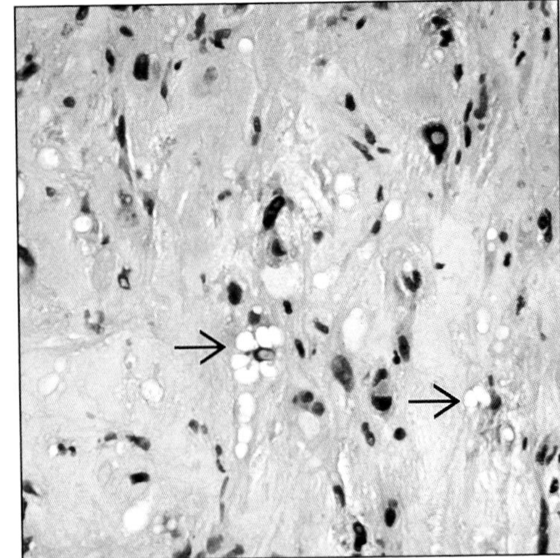

There is a rich myxoid background surrounding atypical epithelioid polygonal cells. Intranuclear inclusions are seen. Physaliphorous cells ⇒ with vacuolated cytoplasm are noted.

TERMINOLOGY

Definitions

- Low- to intermediate-grade malignant tumor that recapitulates embryonic notochord
  - Divided into 3 broad groups
    - Sacrococcygeal (60%)
    - Craniocervical (sphenooccipital) (25%)
    - Vertebral (15%)

ETIOLOGY/PATHOGENESIS

Developmental Anomaly

- Neoplastic transformation from vestigial remnants of embryonic notochord tissue
- Notogenesis begins by 3rd gestational week
  - Superior notochord limit: Rathke pouch
    - Lies at level of sphenoid
    - If persistent notochord canal, may result in Tornwaldt cyst
  - Inferior notochord limit: Coccyx
    - Extends entire length of future vertebral column
    - Becomes enveloped by developing vertebral bodies derived from mesoderm
- Notochord involutes during 8th week of development
  - Vestiges form nucleus pulposus within intervertebral discs
- Incomplete regression of notochordal tissue can result in chordoma

Familial

- Limited number with familial association
  - Autosomal dominant trait

CLINICAL ISSUES

Epidemiology

- Incidence
  - Approximately 0.05/100,000 population/year
  - Represents ~ 2% of all malignant bone tumors
  - Represents < 1% of central nervous system tumors
  - Represents 0.2% of all nasopharyngeal tumors
  - Dedifferentiated chordoma comprises 1-6% of chordoma
- Age
  - May occur at any age
  - Predominance for head and neck in 4th decade
  - Clivus-based tumors: Peak between 20 and 40 years
  - Spinal tumors: 5th to 6th decades most frequently
- Gender
  - Male > Female (5:3)
- Ethnicity
  - No racial or ethnic differences

Site

- Within craniocervical sites
  - Dorsum sellae
  - Clivus
  - Retropharyngeal regions
  - Nuclei pulposi of cervical vertebrae
  - Ectopic
    - Frontal sinuses
    - Other paranasal sinuses
    - Mandible

Presentation

- Symptoms are usually nonspecific
  - Headaches
  - Diplopia (abducens nerve, often left-sided)
    - Visual loss, visual field defects
  - Pain (type depends on tumor location)
  - Neurologic symptoms from local compression (nerve impingement)
    - Cranial nerve deficits (most commonly 3rd and 6th cranial nerves)
    - Hydrocephalus
    - Sensorimotor deficits
  - Mass, especially if in parapharyngeal space

CHORDOMA

Key Facts

Terminology
- Low- to intermediate-grade malignant tumor that recapitulates embryonic notochord
- Divided into 3 broad groups: Sacrococcygeal, craniocervical, vertebral

Clinical Issues
- Predominance for head and neck in 4th decade
- Male > Female (5:3)
- Symptoms are usually nonspecific
- Surgery is treatment of choice
- Postoperative radiotherapy is frequently employed

Image Findings
- Destructive mass with osseous erosion and expansion, frequently associated with soft tissue mass

Microscopic Pathology
- Histologically stratified into classic, chondroid, and dedifferentiated
- Lobular growth, arranged in cords, clusters, islands
- Epithelioid polygonal cells, which may be slightly elongated
- Large physaliphorous cells with multivacuolated cytoplasm
- Abundant intercellular mucinous matrix

Ancillary Tests
- Positive with CK-PAN, EMA, S100 protein

Top Differential Diagnoses
- Chondrosarcoma, mucinous adenocarcinoma, chordoid glioma, liposarcoma, chordoid meningioma

- Tumors are slow growing, resulting in local spread
  - Locally destructive
  - Rarely exhibit lymphatic &/or hematogenous dissemination
- May present with endocrinopathies
  - Result of invasion of sella turcica
- Other symptoms may include
  - Nasal obstruction, discharge, anosmia, nasal speech, epistaxis
  - Dysphagia, dyspnea, dysphonia
  - Hearing loss, tinnitus, dizziness, ataxia

Treatment
- Options, risks, complications
  - Transient complications may include
    - Cerebrospinal fluid leak with meningitis
    - Nerve paralysis/paresis: 5th, 6th, and 7th nerves
    - Oronasal fistula
    - Epistaxis
- Surgical approaches
  - Surgery is treatment of choice
    - Because of anatomic location, complete resection is difficult
    - Approaches based on anatomic site
    - Transnasal-transsphenoidal approach for small cranial cases
    - Midfacial degloving and pterygomaxillotomy approach
    - Transoral-transpharyngeal approach
    - Middle fossa approach
- Drugs
  - Chemo-resistant tumors, usually lacking even palliative response
- Radiation
  - Postoperative radiotherapy is frequently employed
    - Linear accelerator or proton therapy
  - Tends to be radioresistant, requiring high dose for good response
  - Complications include
    - Hypopituitarism, memory impairment, oculomotor impairment, severe hearing loss, bilateral visual loss

Prognosis
- Prognosis based on site, completeness of resection, age, gender, and whether radiation is employed
  - Aggressive surgery & radiation: 50-75% 5-year survival; 45-65% 10-year survival
  - Incomplete excision with conventional radiation: 20% 5-year survival
  - Radiation therapy alone: 30% survival
  - Up to 60% of patients ultimately die from disease
- Recurrences may be observed many years after treatment
  - Patients may survive for years after recurrence
- Metastases are uncommon (< 10% of cases)
  - Lung, bone, liver, soft tissue
- Prognostic indicators
  - Tumor location, size, resectability, gender, age
  - Chondroid variant has slightly better prognosis
- When genetic abnormalities are present, there is increased incidence of recurrence, disease progression, and poor survival

IMAGE FINDINGS

General Features
- Best studies: CT & MR are complementary
  - MR for soft tissue extent
  - Bone CT for bone changes
- Destructive lesion with large, well-defined, T2 hyperintense, enhancing soft tissue mass on MR
- Most common locations
  - Sacrococcygeal > > sphenooccipital > > vertebral (C2-5 and lumbar)
- Extension into epidural and perivertebral space, along with vertebral artery encasement
- May extend along nerve roots
- May enlarge neural foramina (mimic of peripheral nerve sheath tumors)

Radiographic Findings
- Expansile, lytic, destructive mass with extensive bony erosion including into sella turcica

CHORDOMA

- Destructive vertebral body mass with osseous erosion and expansion, sparing posterior elements
- Large soft tissue mass (may be dominant finding)
- Osteolysis is well circumscribed, without osteosclerotic rim
  - Sclerosis of vertebral body is usually seen
- Coarse, amorphous tumor calcifications (site specific)
  - Sacrococcygeal (90%)
  - Clival (50-60%)
  - Vertebral (30%)

MR Findings

- Homogeneously isointense with muscle on T1-weighted studies
  - Moderate enhancement after gadolinium injection
- Hyperintense on T2-weighted studies (same intensity as CSF)
  - Similar to nucleus pulposus

CT Findings

- Heterogeneous mass
- Similar signal to adjacent muscle
- Tumor calcifications are highlighted

Bone Scan

- Cold lesion usually

MACROSCOPIC FEATURES

General Features

- Expansive, lobulated tumors
- Cut surface is gelatinous, slippery, mucoid to myxoid
- Gritty areas due to calcifications

Sections to Be Submitted

- 1 section per cm

Size

- Range: 1.5-15.0 cm
  - Median: 4 cm
- Tumor volume: 2-125 cm^3
  - Median: 21 cm^3

MICROSCOPIC PATHOLOGY

Histologic Features

- Histologically stratified into classic, chondroid, and dedifferentiated
- 4 major histologic features
  - Lobular growth
  - Arranged in cords, clusters, islands, "hepatoid" columns
  - Epithelioid polygonal cells, which may be slightly elongated
    - Nuclei are round and uniform
    - Pleomorphism can be considerable
  - Large physaliphorous cells
    - Characteristic vacuolated cells
    - Cytoplasm filled with mucin
  - Abundant intercellular mucinous matrix surrounds epithelioid cells

Chondroid Chordoma

- Hyaline-type chondroid or cartilaginous tissue
- Only seen in about 5% of chordomas
- More common in women and younger patients

Dedifferentiated Chordoma

- Conventional chordoma in association with sarcomatous elements
  - Malignant fibrous histiocytoma
  - Fibrosarcoma
  - High-grade chondrosarcoma
  - Osteosarcoma
- Seen in ~ 5% of chordomas

ANCILLARY TESTS

Cytology

- Smears are usually moderately to highly cellular
  - Physaliferous cells are usually easily identified
    - Finely bubbled cytoplasm
    - Larger than chief cells
  - Epithelioid cells
    - Eosinophilic cytoplasm
    - Regular chromatin distribution
    - Intranuclear cytoplasmic inclusions
- Myxoid or chondromyxoid background matrix
- Mitotic figures are rarely identified

Histochemistry

- Mucin positive with mucicarmine and periodic acid-Schiff

Immunohistochemistry

- Standard positive immunohistochemical panel includes
  - Cytokeratin
  - Epithelial membrane antigen (EMA)
  - S100 protein and brachyury
- GFAP negative

Cytogenetics

- Up to 70% of patients have normal karyotype
- There is wide variety of complex karyotypic abnormalities
  - Alterations of chromosomes 3, 4, 12, 13, 14, and 21
  - Breakpoint of 1q21
  - Frequent 7q gain

Molecular Genetics

- Loss of heterozygosity of region 1p36
- Suggested **genesis** or **progression** candidates on chromosome 7q33
  - Sonic hedgehog homolog (SHH) protein is key in regulating notochord and vertebral body development gene, found on chromosome 7

Electron Microscopy

- Large cells with abundant cytoplasm and variably sized vacuoles
  - Vacuoles may be empty, contain glycogen granules or amorphous mucin
- Mitochondria-rough endoplasmic reticulum (RER) complexes

CHORDOMA

Immunohistochemistry

Antibody	Reactivity	Staining Pattern	Comment
AE1/AE3	Positive	Cytoplasmic	All tumor cells
CK-PAN	Positive	Cytoplasmic	All tumor cells
CK8/18/CAM5.2	Positive	Cytoplasmic	All tumor cells
Brachyury	Positive	Nuclear	Approximately 95% of cases
HBME-1	Positive	Cytoplasmic	Nearly all tumor cells
Vimentin	Positive	Cytoplasmic	Nearly all tumor cells
CK19	Positive	Cytoplasmic	Nearly all tumor cells
EMA	Positive	Cell membrane & cytoplasm	Nearly all tumor cells
NSE	Positive	Cytoplasmic	Nearly all tumor cells; however, it is nonspecific
S100	Positive	Nuclear & cytoplasmic	About 40-50% of tumor cells, strong but focal
34bE12	Positive	Cytoplasmic	Approximately 60% of cases
CD24	Positive	Cytoplasmic	Approximately 50% of cases
HMB-45	Positive	Cytoplasmic	Approximately 45% of cases
CEA-P	Positive	Cytoplasmic	Approximately 40% of cases
Podoplanin	Positive	Cytoplasmic	Same as D2-40; approximately 15% of cases
CK7	Positive	Cytoplasmic	Only about 10% of cases
CEA-M	Negative		
GFAP	Negative		

  - Single cisternae of RER surround mitochondria
- Intracytoplasmic lumens with scant, small, immature microvilli
- Desmosomes, primitive cell junctions, intermediate filaments, and tonofibrils
- Fragmented basal lamina

DIFFERENTIAL DIAGNOSIS

Chondrosarcoma

- Rare cartilaginous malignancies comprising 6-15% of all skull base tumors
- Majority of skull base chondrosarcomas are well differentiated
- Tumor produces cartilage matrix and very rarely myxoid matrix
- No chief cells or physaliferous cells present
- Not brachyury positive

Mucinous Adenocarcinoma

- Salivary gland or metastatic
- Atypical epithelial cells present in glandular arrangement
- Matrix is mucinous rather than myxoid
- S100 protein and brachyury are not positive

Chordoid Glioma

- Benign neoplasm, 3rd ventricle
- Positive glial markers

Liposarcoma

- Lipoblasts have multivacuolated cells with nuclear compression
- Fat in background, which can be myxoid
- May be reactive with S100 protein, but negative with keratin, EMA, and brachyury

Chordoid Meningioma

- Rare, frequently with peritumoral lymphoid infiltrate
- Nearly always supratentorial
- Spindled, epithelioid cells with myxoid matrix
- Shows EMA, but not S100 protein or brachyury immunoreactivity

STAGING

AJCC Bone Staging (2010)

- T1: Tumor 8 cm or less in greatest dimension
- T2: Tumor more than 8 cm in greatest dimension
- T3: Discontinuous tumors in primary bone site

SELECTED REFERENCES

1. Amichetti M et al: Proton therapy in chordoma of the base of the skull: a systematic review. Neurosurg Rev. 32(4):403-16, 2009
2. Oakley GJ et al: Brachyury, SOX-9, and podoplanin, new markers in the skull base chordoma vs chondrosarcoma differential: a tissue microarray-based comparative analysis. Mod Pathol. 21(12):1461-9, 2008
3. Chugh R et al: Chordoma: the nonsarcoma primary bone tumor. Oncologist. 12(11):1344-50, 2007
4. Mendenhall WM et al: Skull base chordoma. Head Neck. 27(2):159-65, 2005
5. Yamaguchi T et al: Benign notochordal cell tumors: A comparative histological study of benign notochordal cell tumors, classic chordomas, and notochordal vestiges of fetal intervertebral discs. Am J Surg Pathol. 28(6):756-61, 2004
6. Kay PA et al: Chordoma. Cytomorphologic findings in 14 cases diagnosed by fine needle aspiration. Acta Cytol. 47(2):202-8, 2003
7. St Martin M et al: Chordomas of the skull base: manifestations and management. Curr Opin Otolaryngol Head Neck Surg. 11(5):324-7, 2003

CHORDOMA

Imaging and Microscopic Features

(Left) Sagittal graphic shows an expansile, destructive mass originating from the clivus, "thumbing" the pons ➔, and elevating the pituitary gland ➔. Note bone fragments within the chordoma. *(Right)* Sagittal MR T1WI with contrast reveals near total replacement of the clivus by a heterogeneously enhancing, destructive mass. There is invasion into the sphenoid ➔ and basiocciput ➔. The mass shows "thumbing" of the pons posteriorly ➔.

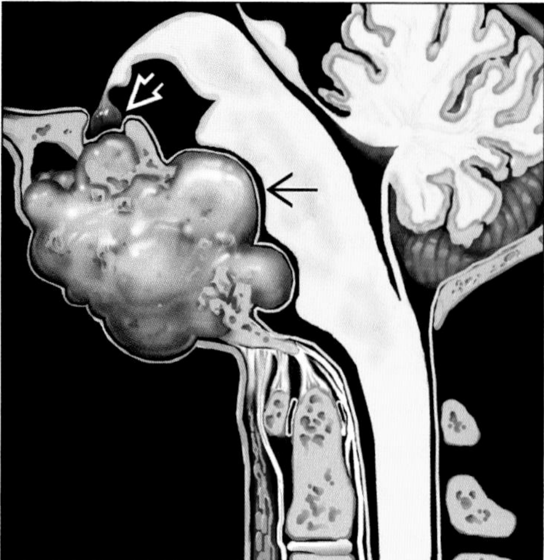

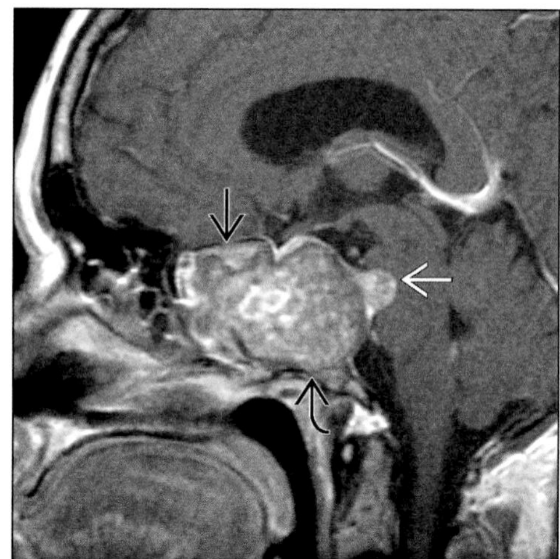

(Left) Axial contrast-enhanced CT shows an unenhancing clival chordoma with significant myxoid content engulfing and encasing the right ICA circumferentially and abutting the left ICA ➔. Bony fragments ➔ are seen in the anterior margins. *(Right)* At medium power the distribution of matrix and nests of cells can resemble a number of entities, including salivary gland tumors and metastases. Correlation with radiology and immunohistochemistry helps make the separation.

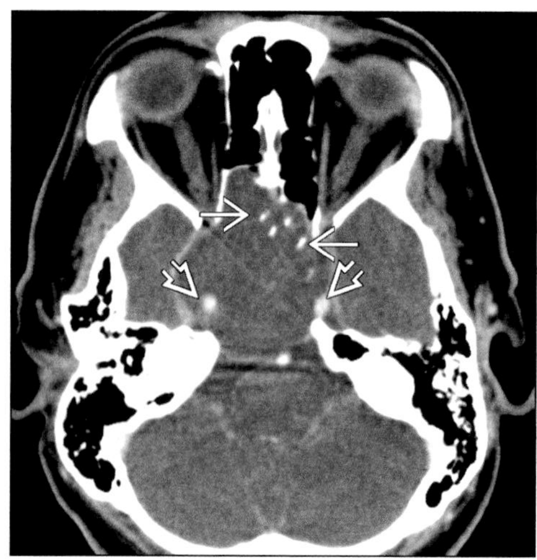

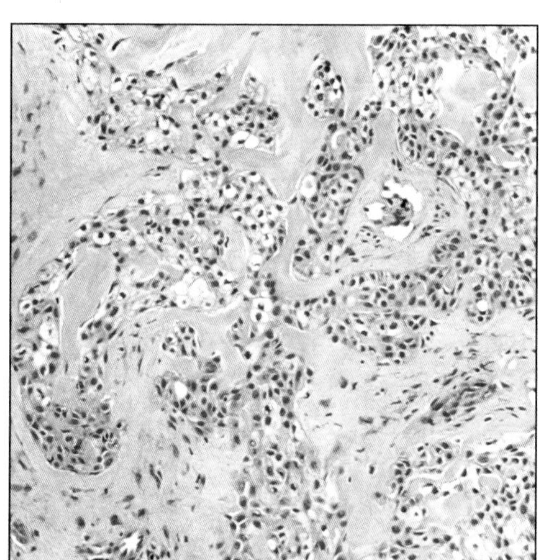

(Left) Physaliferous cells ➔ are characteristic of chordoma, showing "bubbly" cytoplasm and eccentric nuclei. Short cords of epithelioid polygonal cells ➔ are set in a myxoid to mucinous matrix ➔. *(Right)* Occasionally, foci of chordomas can have a background matrix that is solid to the point of resembling hyaline-like cartilage matrix. This is an example of a chondroid chordoma. Immunohistochemistry can be useful in separating this tumor from others in the differential.

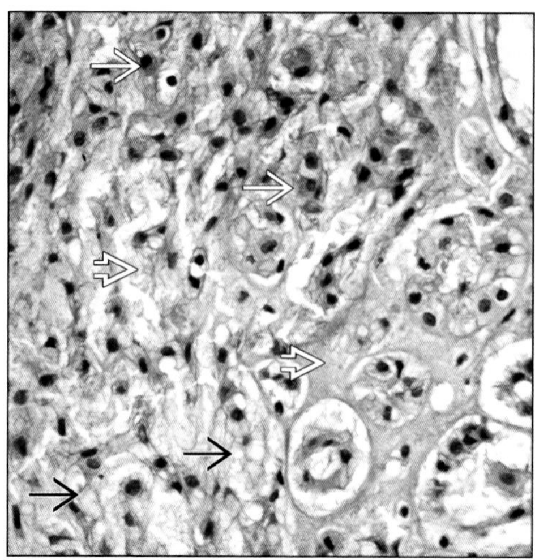

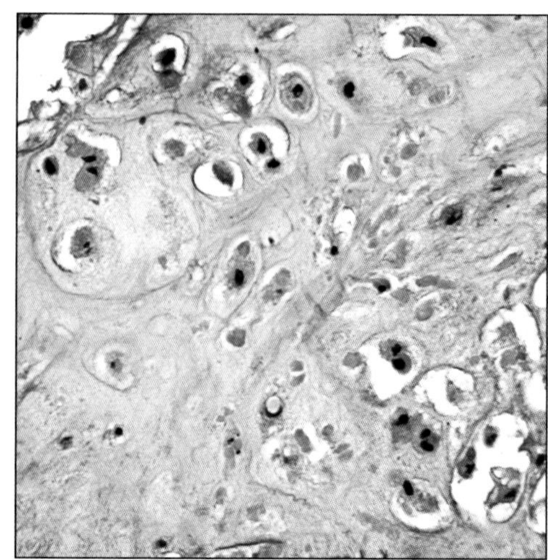

Ancillary Techniques

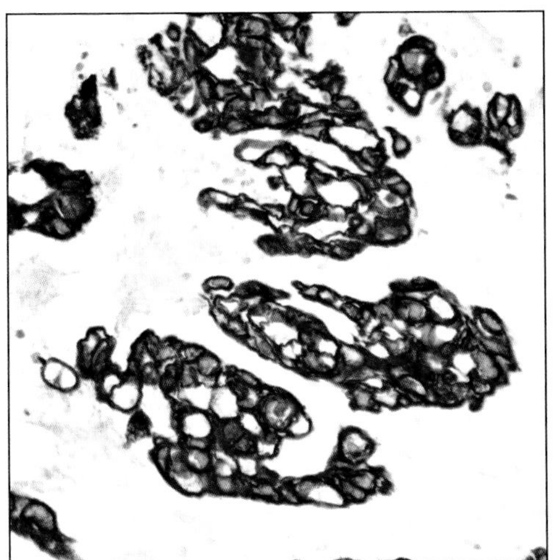

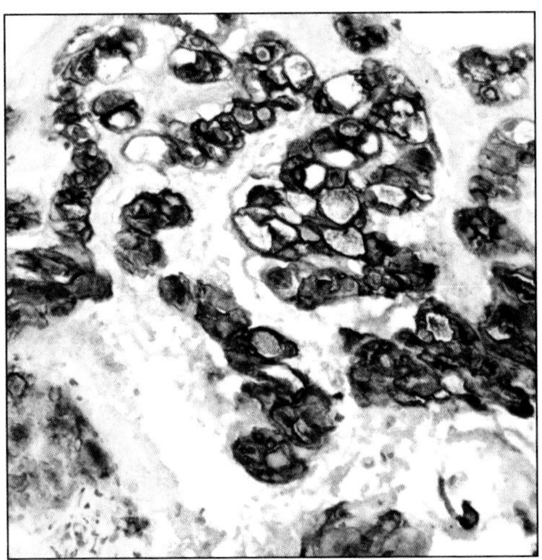

(Left) *Immunohistochemistry for cytokeratin results in a strong, diffuse cytoplasmic reaction in chordoma, a reliable way to help separate chordoma from chondrosarcoma.* ***(Right)*** *Immunohistochemistry for epithelial membrane antigen (EMA) is strongly positive in chordomas and is especially helpful on needle core biopsy specimens or in cytologic preparation. EMA is not positive in chondrosarcomas and is helpful in distinguishing between the 2 tumors.*

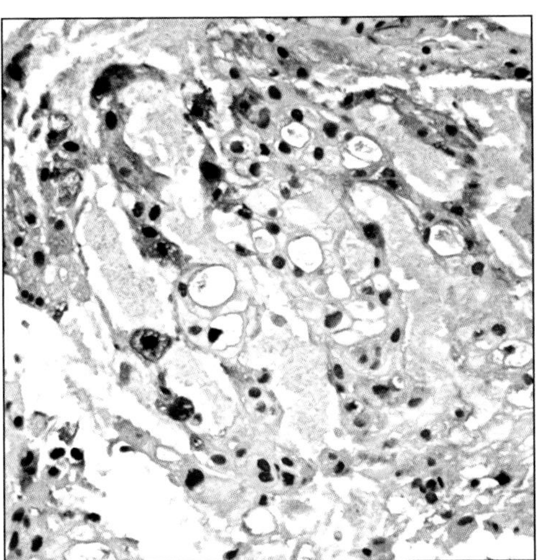

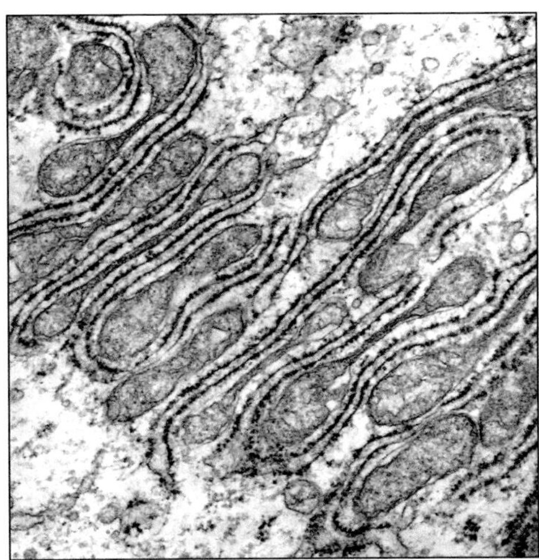

(Left) *S100 protein is usually focally, although strongly positive in the nucleus and cytoplasm of chordoma.* ***(Right)*** *Clusters of mitochondria are nearly completely surrounded by a single rough endoplasmic reticulum (RER) cisternae, forming a mitochondria-RER complex. This complex is quite characteristic for chordoma. Glycogen, microvilli, and intermediate filaments were present elsewhere in the cells of this case. (Courtesy S. Bhuta, MD.)*

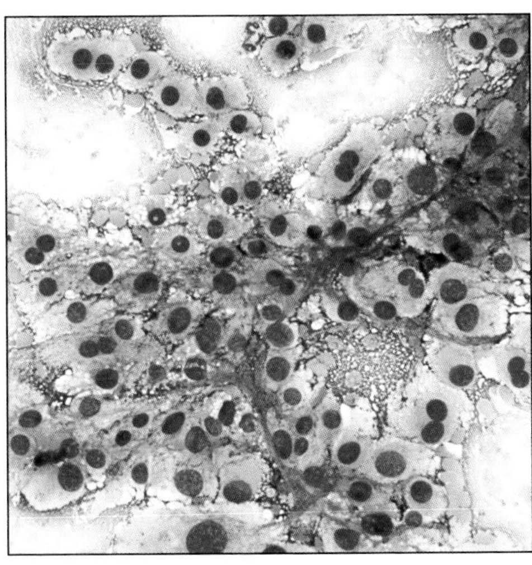

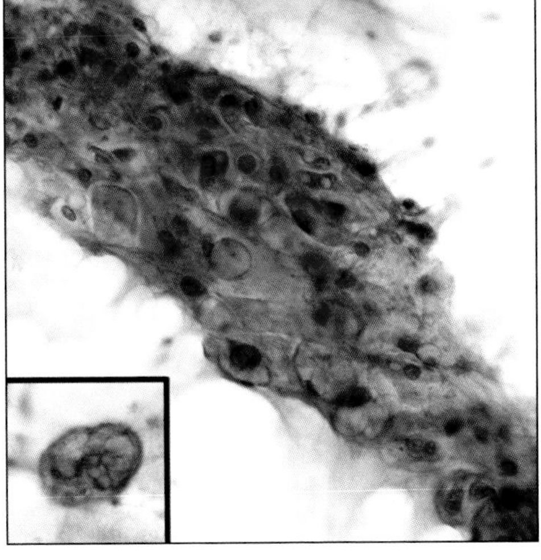

(Left) *Fine needle aspiration will often show cords and nests of cells with a regular polygonal shape, amphophilic cytoplasm, and nuclei with finely dispersed chromatin. The cells can be arranged around vascular cores and make definitive diagnosis difficult.* ***(Right)*** *There are 2 cell types noted in chordomas, the chief cells and the physaliferous cells. Physaliferous cells (inset) show a finely bubbled cytoplasm and are distinctive in these tumors.*

LIPOSARCOMA

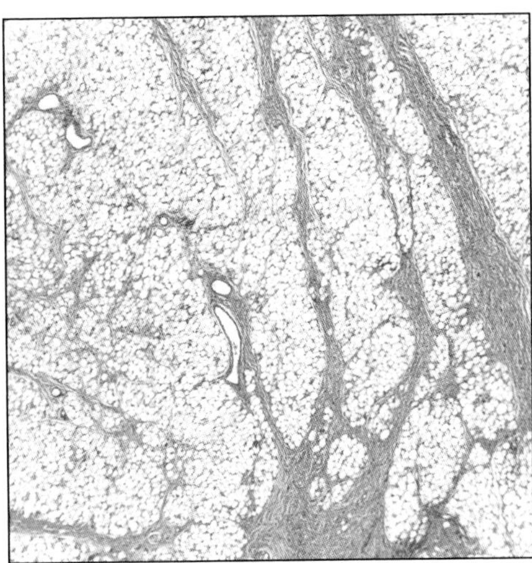

Cervical neck well-differentiated (lipoma-like) liposarcoma shows an unencapsulated adipose tissue proliferation composed of nests of fat cells separated by fibrous septa.

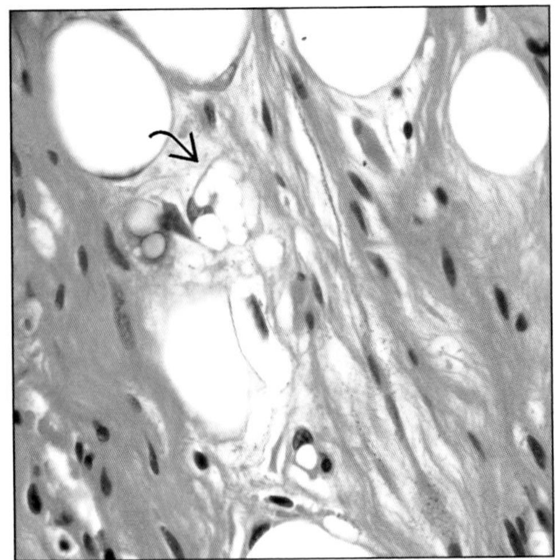

A multivacuolated lipoblast ➔ is identified representing a feature supportive of the diagnosis of a liposarcoma.

TERMINOLOGY

Abbreviations

- Liposarcoma (LPS)

Synonyms

- Lipoma-like liposarcoma
- Well-differentiated liposarcoma (WDLPS)
- Atypical lipoma or atypical lipomatous tumor (ALT)
  - Terms utilized for superficial (cutaneous or subcutaneous) lipogenic tumors with histologic appearance of well-differentiated liposarcomas with tendency to recur
  - Terminology should be used with caution in relation to lesions occurring in vital areas (deep neck, nasopharynx, sinonasal cavity, larynx and hypopharynx)
    - Inadequate excision and subsequent recurrence may result in increased morbidity and mortality
    - Use of well-differentiated liposarcoma rather than atypical lipoma conveys to surgeon need for complete resection as conservatively as possible to ensure tumor-free margins

Definitions

- Malignant neoplasm of adipose tissue (adipocytes)
- Histologic types include
  - Well differentiated
    - Lipoma-like subtype
    - Sclerosing subtype
    - Inflammatory subtype
    - Spindle cell subtype
  - Myxoid
  - Round cell
  - Pleomorphic
  - Dedifferentiated

ETIOLOGY/PATHOGENESIS

Idiopathic

- No known associated etiologic factors
- Arise de novo
  - Rarely may originate from preexisting lipoma

Histogenesis

- Arise from primitive mesenchymal cells rather than mature adipose tissue
  - Accounts for occurrence in areas relatively devoid of fat (i.e., mucosal sites of head and neck)

CLINICAL ISSUES

Epidemiology

- Incidence
  - Represent up to 18% of all soft tissue sarcomas
    - Approximately 3-6% of liposarcomas occur in head and neck
- Age
  - Laryngeal and hypopharyngeal liposarcoma
    - Occurs over wide age range but most common in 6th and 7th decades of life
  - Neck liposarcomas
    - Occur over wide age range, usually at younger ages (approximately a decade younger) than non-head and neck liposarcomas
- Gender
  - For laryngeal and hypopharyngeal liposarcoma
    - Male > Female
  - Neck liposarcomas
    - Equal gender distribution

Site

- In head and neck, most common sites of occurrence include larynx and hypopharynx followed by neck

Presentation

- Symptoms vary per site of involvement and tumor size

LIPOSARCOMA

Key Facts

Terminology
- Malignant neoplasm of adipose tissue (adipocytes)

Clinical Issues
- Represent up to 18% of all soft tissue sarcomas
  - Approximately 3-6% occur in head and neck
- Most common sites in head and neck include larynx/hypopharynx, followed by neck
- Wide local surgical excision to include tumor-free margins is treatment of choice
- More aggressive surgical procedures may be indicated for higher grade histologic variants

Microscopic Pathology
- Lipoblasts represent key diagnostic finding
- Histologic types include
  - Well differentiated
  - Myxoid
  - Round cell
  - Pleomorphic
  - Dedifferentiated

Ancillary Tests
- MDM2 and CDK4 immunoreactivity and fluorescent in situ hybridization (FISH)
  - Relatively sensitive and specific markers for ALT/WDLPS and dedifferentiated LPS
- p16
  - Valuable marker to differentiate ALT/WDLPS from deep-seated lipomas
  - Detected in > 80% of ALT/WDLPS
  - Not present in lipomas

- Larynx
  - Hoarseness, dysphonia, dysphagia, airway obstruction
- Pharynx
  - Dysphagia, airway obstruction
- Neck
  - Slowly growing painless mass

Treatment
- Surgical approaches
  - Wide local surgical excision to include tumor-free margins is treatment of choice
    - More aggressive surgical procedures may be indicated for higher grade histologic variants
- Radiation
  - Utility of radiotherapy remains controversial
  - Evidence supports use of postoperative radiotherapy as adjunct to surgery in cases where
    - Tumor cannot be completely resected
    - Tumor is close to surgical margins

Prognosis
- Recurrence common
  - In particular for WDLPS, which initially may be diagnosed as lipoma
    - Molecular testing for "relapsing lipomas" may assist in diagnosing WDLPS by presence of *MDM2/CPM* amplification
  - Generally occurs within 3 years following initial treatment
  - Usually is of same histology as primary tumor
  - May rarely "dedifferentiate"
    - Histologic appearance less differentiated
    - Associated with more aggressive biology than primary ("differentiated") tumor
- Nodal metastasis rare
  - Neck dissection generally not indicated
- Distant metastasis may occur
  - More common with higher grade histologic variants
  - Metastases occur to lungs, bone, liver
- 5-year survival rates similar to liposarcomas occurring in non-H&N sites
  - Influenced by histologic type
  - 5-year survival rate
    - For all head and neck liposarcomas: Approximately 67%
    - Well-differentiated LPS: 85-100%
    - Myxoid liposarcoma: 71-95%
    - Round cell liposarcoma: 12.5-55%
    - Pleomorphic liposarcoma: 45%
- In addition to histologic type, other important prognostic factors include
  - Size of tumor
  - Location of tumor
    - Laryngeal/hypopharyngeal, facial tumors have best prognosis
    - Oral and pharyngeal tumors have worst prognosis
  - Controversy exists as to issue of multicentric liposarcomas vs. metastatic liposarcoma

MACROSCOPIC FEATURES

General Features
- Circumscribed &/or encapsulated, lobulated mass
- Vary in appearance from yellow to tan-white in color
  - Myxoid or gelatinous appearance

Size
- Can attain very large sizes especially relative to soft tissue sites (e.g., neck)
- Mucosal-based lesions rarely exceed 10 cm and generally measure < 5 cm in greatest dimension

MICROSCOPIC PATHOLOGY

Histologic Features
- Lipoblasts represent key diagnostic finding
  - Range from primitive appearing cells demonstrating little if any detectable lipid to signet ring cells in which cytoplasm filled with lipid displaces nucleus peripherally

- Lipoblasts must be distinguished from vacuolated cells closely simulating appearance of lipoblasts and identified in other soft tissue sarcomas
- Identifying lipoblasts often require diligence and ample sections for detection

- Classic appearing lipoblasts have
  - Sharply defined lipid droplets causing scalloping or distortion of nucleus
  - Nucleus either centrally or peripherally located in cell
  - Large and hyperchromatic nuclei
- Mitoses, necrosis, and hemorrhage can be identified in all histologic variants
  - Generally correlate to amount of cellular pleomorphism
  - Mitoses are particularly prominent in pleomorphic variant

Well-differentiated LPS

- **Lipoma-like subtype** histologically resembles lipoma except for
  - Greater variation in size and shape of adipocytes
  - Presence of scattered lipoblasts (absence of lipoblasts does not preclude diagnosis)
  - Absence of encapsulation
  - Most common morphologic type in relationship to upper aerodigestive tract (mucosal-based) liposarcomas
  - Often diagnosed as lipoma due to bland histology
    - Only following one or more recurrences will diagnosis of liposarcoma be considered/rendered
- **Sclerosing subtype**
  - Composed of broad, dense fibrous bands containing atypical or bizarre-appearing cells characterized by hyperchromatic nuclei and lipoblasts alternating with areas of lipomatous proliferation
  - Sclerotic foci may represent majority of tumor and lipogenic areas may be limited and easily overlooked
- **Inflammatory subtype**
  - Occurs most often in retroperitoneum
  - Chronic inflammatory cell infiltrate including mature lymphocytic and plasma cells predominance
  - Presence of bizarre multinucleated stromal cells represent important diagnostic clue
- **Spindle cell subtype**
  - Composed of morphologically bland-appearing neural-like spindle cells in fibrous &/or myxoid background
  - Associated with atypical lipomatous proliferation that includes lipoblasts

Myxoid LPS

- Represent most common type in soft tissue sites, accounting for approximately 50% of all cases
- Characterized by presence of
  - Lobular or nodular growth
  - Uniform round to oval-shaped mesenchymal (nonlipogenic appearing) cells
  - Variable numbers of signet ring lipoblasts
  - Prominent myxoid stroma
  - Associated plexiform vascularity with delicate arborizing (capillary-like) pattern
  - Cellular component typically lacks nuclear pleomorphism, significant mitotic activity, or tumor giant cells
  - Extracellular mucin pools or lakes creating a lymphangioma-like appearance can be identified

Round Cell LPS

- Represents poorly differentiated form of myxoid liposarcoma
- Characterized by presence of
  - Densely cellular solid sheets of back to back primitive round cells with hyperchromatic nuclei, prominent nucleoli, increased nuclear to cytoplasmic ratio, granular to vacuolated appearing cytoplasm
  - Increased mitotic activity as well as necrosis and hemorrhage are present
  - Sparse to absent intervening myxoid, fibrillar or myxomucinous stroma
  - Vascular pattern present but generally compressed by cellular proliferation
  - Presence of transitional areas from myxoid to hypercellular round cell supports contention that myxoid and round cell liposarcomas represent histological continuum of myxoid LPS
  - Notion that myxoid and round cell LPS represent histological continuum further supported by presence of shared chromosomal aberrations

Pleomorphic LPS

- Pleomorphic high-grade sarcoma composed of
  - Variable numbers of pleomorphic lipoblasts characterized by spindle and giant cells with one or more enlarged hyperchromatic nuclei scalloped by cytoplasmic vacuoles
  - Cytoplasmic vacuoles contain lipid droplets
  - Majority have fascicles of spindle-shaped cells and smaller, round cells admixed with multinucleated giant cells as well as pleomorphic lipoblasts
  - May resemble other sarcomas (e.g., malignant fibrous histiocytoma)
  - Limited lipoblastic features may be present
  - Prominent cytoplasmic eosinophilia may be present and in presence of limited lipoblastic findings may suggest diagnosis of rhabdomyosarcoma
  - Extra- and intracellular eosinophilic hyaline globules may be identified (likely represent lysosomal structures)
  - Tumor necrosis present
- Epithelioid variant of pleomorphic liposarcoma
  - Predominantly composed of solid, cohesive sheets and clusters of epithelioid cells with round to oval nuclei, prominent nucleoli, eosinophilic cytoplasm, and distinct cell borders
  - Lipogenic differentiation in form of pleomorphic lipoblasts focally present
  - Often associated with higher mitotic rate than seen in association with pleomorphic (nonepithelioid) liposarcoma
  - Tumor necrosis present

Dedifferentiated LPS

- Histologic hallmark is presence of transition either in primary tumor or in recurrent tumor from well-differentiated liposarcoma to nonlipogenic sarcoma
  - Nonlipogenic sarcoma resembles fibrosarcoma or malignant fibrous histiocytoma
  - Can show lipoblastic differentiation in high-grade component resulting in areas indistinguishable from pleomorphic LPS
- Areas of dedifferentiation often (but not always) histologically high-grade sarcoma but may be low-grade sarcomas
- Heterologous differentiation may be present in up to 10% usually with myogenic or osteo/chondrosarcomatous elements

Mixed-type LPS

- Extremely rare
- Histologically defined by presence of combined histologic types including
  - Myxoid/round cell and well-differentiated/dedifferentiated liposarcoma
  - Myxoid/round cell and pleomorphic liposarcoma

ANCILLARY TESTS

Cytology

- Smears may include mixture of mature-appearing fat traversed by bands of fibrous collagen and vessels
- Nuclei within fat and fibrous bands mildly irregular, hyperchromatic, and enlarged, with 1 or 2 small nucleoli
- Infrequently lipoblasts may be identified

Histochemistry

- Prominent myxoid stroma rich in
  - Glycosaminoglycans or hyaluronidase-sensitive acid
  - Mucopolysaccharides
- In general, special stains are of little if any assistance in diagnosis

Immunohistochemistry

- Adipocytes and lipoblasts
  - Variable S100 protein immunoreactivity
  - Vimentin positive
  - All other markers essentially negative
- MDM2 immunoreactivity and fluorescent in situ hybridization (FISH)
  - Relatively sensitive and specific markers for ALT/WDLPS and dedifferentiated LPS
    - Nuclear reactivity
    - Present in high percentage of ALT/WDLPS
    - Absent in majority of benign lipomatous tumors, in particular deep-seated lipomas
    - Can be present in small percentage of spindle cell/pleomorphic lipomas
    - Can be present in nonlipomatous sarcomas (e.g., malignant peripheral nerve sheath tumor)
  - MDM2/chromosome 12 FISH
    - Sensitive and specific (both 100%) in low-grade lipomatous neoplasms
    - Specificity decreases in high-grade sarcomas as MDM2 amplification present in small portion of pleomorphic sarcomas and high-grade sarcomas other than dedifferentiated LPS
    - Benign lipomatous lesions not MDM2 amplified
- p16
  - Valuable marker to differentiate ALT/WDLPS from deep-seated lipomas
  - Detected in > 80% of ALT/WDLPS
  - Not present in lipomas
- HMGA2
  - Immunohistochemical detection of HMGA2 protein helpful for distinction of normal adipose tissue from well-differentiated lesions
    - Normal adipose tissue always negative for HMGA2
    - Less sensitive than MDM2 for dedifferentiated LPS diagnosis
    - Appears more specific to distinguish dedifferentiated LPS from other poorly differentiated sarcomas

Cytogenetics

- Ring and giant chromosomes composed of 12q13-15 amplicons including *MDM2* gene

Molecular Genetics

- ALT/WDLPS, dedifferentiated LPS characterized by 12q13-15 region amplification
  - Molecular event not reported in benign lipomas
  - *MDM2, CPM, HMGA2, CDK4, SAS* genes most frequent targets of amplification
  - Co-amplification of 2 genes as well as higher-level amplification more frequent in dedifferentiated liposarcomas than in well-differentiated liposarcomas
  - Indications for molecular analysis for lipomatous tumors include
    - Presence of equivocal cytologic atypia
    - Recurrent "lipomas"
    - Deep-seated tumors without cytologic atypia > 15 cm
    - Retroperitoneal or intraabdominal tumors without cytologic atypia

DIFFERENTIAL DIAGNOSIS

Lipoma

- Typically encapsulated
- Lipoblasts not present
- Majority negative for MDM2 and CDK4

Nodular Fasciitis

- Rapidly enlarging mass over short time period
- Characteristic "tissue culture" type growth
- Myofibroblastic dominant lesion with
  - Minimal cytologic atypia
  - Increased mitotic activity
  - Extravasated red cells
  - Absence of lipoblasts
  - Negative for MDM2 and CDK4

Myxoma

- Generally hypo- or paucicellular proliferation

LIPOSARCOMA

- Absence of lipoblasts
- Absence of plexiform vascularity with delicate arborizing (capillary-like) pattern
- Negative for MDM2 and CDK4

Other Sarcomas

- Potentially overlapping histologic features especially in higher grade sarcomas
- May have "lipoblastic" appearing cells
- Unique immunohistochemical &/or cytogenetics relative to some sarcomas (e.g., rhabdomyosarcoma, leiomyosarcoma, synovial sarcoma)

Carcinoma

- Presence of epithelial immunomarkers (cytokeratins, p63, others)
- Absence of lipoblasts
- Negative for MDM2 and CDK4

Malignant Lymphoma

- Presence of hematolymphoid immunomarkers (leucocyte common antigen, B-cell or T-cell markers)
- Absence of lipoblasts
- Negative for MDM2 and CDK4

Malignant Melanoma

- Presence of melanocytic immunomarkers (e.g., HMB-45, Melan-A, tyrosinase)
- Absence of lipoblasts
- Negative for MDM2 and CDK4

SELECTED REFERENCES

1. Dreux N et al: Value and limitation of immunohistochemical expression of HMGA2 in mesenchymal tumors: about a series of 1052 cases. Mod Pathol. 23(12):1657-66, 2010
2. Makeieff M et al: Laryngeal dedifferentiated liposarcoma. Eur Arch Otorhinolaryngol. 267(6):991-4, 2010
3. Mariño-Enríquez A et al: Dedifferentiated liposarcoma with "homologous" lipoblastic (pleomorphic liposarcoma-like) differentiation: clinicopathologic and molecular analysis of a series suggesting revised diagnostic criteria. Am J Surg Pathol. 34(8):1122-31, 2010
4. Mentzel T et al: Well-differentiated spindle cell liposarcoma ('atypical spindle cell lipomatous tumor') does not belong to the spectrum of atypical lipomatous tumor but has a close relationship to spindle cell lipoma: clinicopathologic, immunohistochemical, and molecular analysis of six cases. Mod Pathol. 23(5):729-36, 2010
5. Zhang H et al: Molecular testing for lipomatous tumors: critical analysis and test recommendations based on the analysis of 405 extremity-based tumors. Am J Surg Pathol. 34(9):1304-11, 2010
6. Chung L et al: Overlapping features between dedifferentiated liposarcoma and undifferentiated high-grade pleomorphic sarcoma. Am J Surg Pathol. 33(11):1594-600, 2009
7. Davis EC et al: Liposarcoma of the head and neck: The University of Texas M. D. Anderson Cancer Center experience. Head Neck. 31(1):28-36, 2009
8. He M et al: p16 immunohistochemistry as an alternative marker to distinguish atypical lipomatous tumor from deep-seated lipoma. Appl Immunohistochem Mol Morphol. 17(1):51-6, 2009
9. Macarenco RS et al: Retroperitoneal lipomatous tumors without cytologic atypia: are they lipomas? A clinicopathologic and molecular study of 19 cases. Am J Surg Pathol. 33(10):1470-6, 2009
10. Mahmood U et al: Atypical lipomatous tumor/well-differentiated liposarcoma of the parotid gland: case report and literature review. Ear Nose Throat J. 88(10):E10-6, 2009
11. Weaver J et al: Fluorescence in situ hybridization for MDM2 gene amplification as a diagnostic tool in lipomatous neoplasms. Mod Pathol. 21(8):943-9, 2008
12. Sirvent N et al: Detection of MDM2-CDK4 amplification by fluorescence in situ hybridization in 200 paraffin-embedded tumor samples: utility in diagnosing adipocytic lesions and comparison with immunohistochemistry and real-time PCR. Am J Surg Pathol. 31(10):1476-89, 2007
13. Binh MB et al: MDM2 and CDK4 immunostainings are useful adjuncts in diagnosing well-differentiated and dedifferentiated liposarcoma subtypes: a comparative analysis of 559 soft tissue neoplasms with genetic data. Am J Surg Pathol. 29(10):1340-7, 2005
14. Hornick JL et al: Pleomorphic liposarcoma: clinicopathologic analysis of 57 cases. Am J Surg Pathol. 28(10):1257-67, 2004
15. Hostein I et al: Evaluation of MDM2 and CDK4 amplification by real-time PCR on paraffin wax-embedded material: a potential tool for the diagnosis of atypical lipomatous tumours/well-differentiated liposarcomas. J Pathol. 202(1):95-102, 2004
16. Collins BT et al: Fine needle aspiration biopsy of well-differentiated liposarcoma of the neck in a young female. A case report. Acta Cytol. 43(3):452-6, 1999
17. Mandell DL et al: Upper aerodigestive tract liposarcoma: report on four cases and literature review. Laryngoscope. 109(8):1245-52, 1999
18. Golledge J et al: Head and neck liposarcoma. Cancer. 76(6):1051-8, 1995
19. Wenig BM et al: Liposarcomas of the larynx and hypopharynx: a clinicopathologic study of eight new cases and a review of the literature. Laryngoscope. 105(7 Pt 1):747-56, 1995
20. McCormick D et al: Dedifferentiated liposarcoma. Clinicopathologic analysis of 32 cases suggesting a better prognostic subgroup among pleomorphic sarcomas. Am J Surg Pathol. 18(12):1213-23, 1994
21. Stewart MG et al: Atypical and malignant lipomatous lesions of the head and neck. Arch Otolaryngol Head Neck Surg. 120(10):1151-5, 1994
22. Dal Cin P et al: Cytogenetic and fluorescence in situ hybridization investigation of ring chromosomes characterizing a specific pathologic subgroup of adipose tissue tumors. Cancer Genet Cytogenet. 68(2):85-90, 1993
23. Wenig BM et al: Laryngeal and hypopharyngeal liposarcoma. A clinicopathologic study of 10 cases with a comparison to soft-tissue counterparts. Am J Surg Pathol. 14(2):134-41, 1990
24. Evans HL et al: Atypical lipoma, atypical intramuscular lipoma, and well differentiated retroperitoneal liposarcoma: a reappraisal of 30 cases formerly classified as well differentiated liposarcoma. Cancer. 43(2):574-84, 1979
25. Saunders JR et al: Liposarcomas of the head and neck: a review of the literature and addition of four cases. Cancer. 43(1):162-8, 1979
26. Kindblom LG et al: Liposarcoma of the neck: a clinicopathologic study of 4 cases. Cancer. 42(2):774-80, 1978

Microscopic Features and Ancillary Techniques

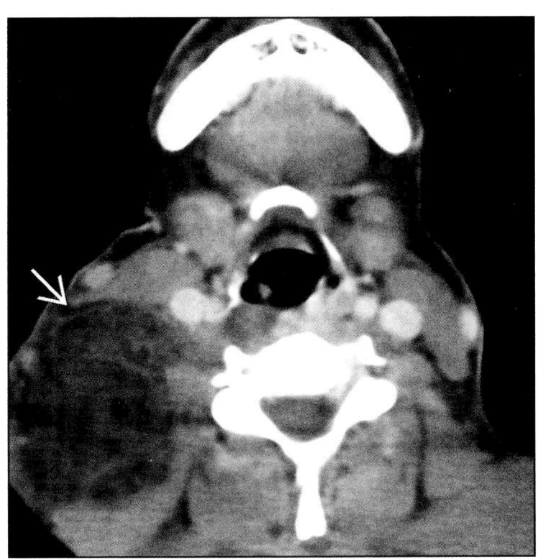

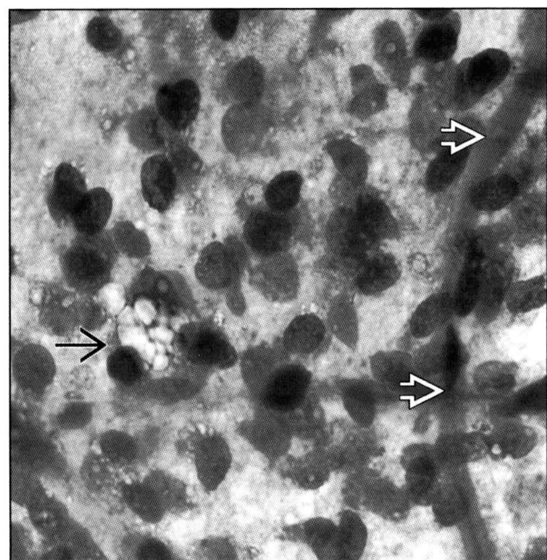

(Left) *CT scan demonstrates a typical head & neck liposarcoma ➡ in the right posterior cervical space in which the mass is predominantly composed of fat with diffuse thin stranding throughout the tumor matrix.* ***(Right)*** *A lipoblast ➡ is identified within a very cellular smear taken from the anterior neck/base of tongue region. There is compression of the nucleus by a multivacuolated cytoplasm. Note the endothelium ➡ within the proliferation.*

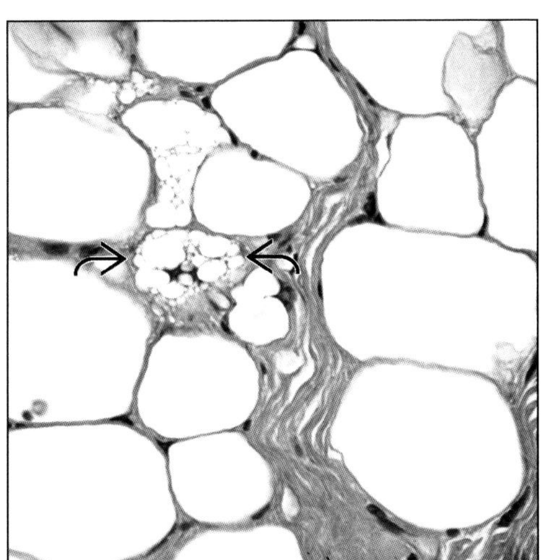

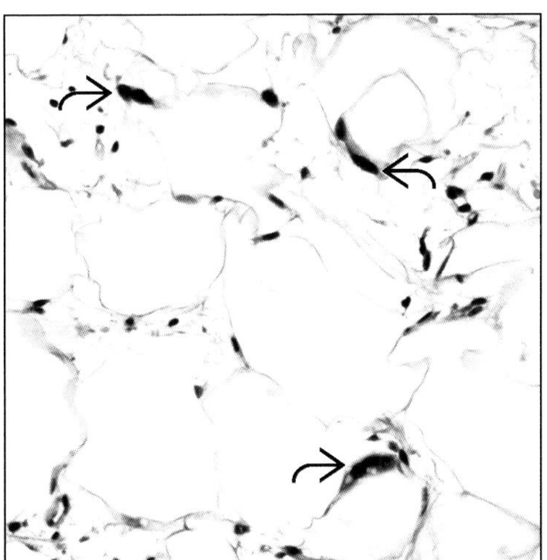

(Left) *Adipose tissue proliferation composed of nests of fat cells (adipocytes) with a multivacuolated lipoblast ➡ (characterized by sharply defined lipid droplets causing scalloping or distortion of nucleus), centrally or peripherally located nucleus, and nuclear enlargement with hyperchromasia.* ***(Right)*** *In addition to variation in size and shape of lipoblasts, nuclear pleomorphism and hyperchromasia ➡ of adipocyte nuclei may be present in well-differentiated liposarcomas.*

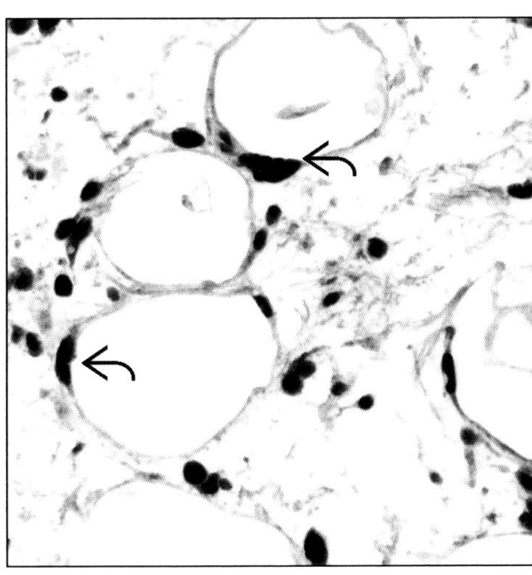

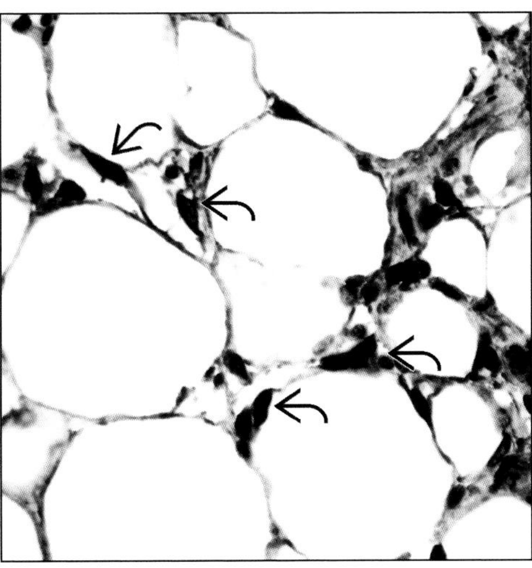

(Left) *MDM2 nuclear immunoreactivity ➡ is present in WDLPS. MDM2 represents a relatively sensitive and specific marker for WDLPS (and dedifferentiated LPS). MDM2 reactivity is absent in the majority of benign lipomatous tumors, in particular deep-seated lipomas.* ***(Right)*** *p16 nuclear immunoreactivity ➡ is another valuable marker in the diagnosis of WDLPS. p16 is present in the majority (> 80%) of WDLPS and is absent in lipomas, especially deep-seated lipomas.*

Microscopic Features and Ancillary Techniques

*(**Left**) Axial enhanced CT shows a well-circumscribed retropharyngeal space mass with its right side showing nodular enhancement ➡ and its left side primarily of fatty density ➡. The left side of the mass protrudes anteriorly ➡ into the submandibular space, elevating the submandibular gland. The anterolateral margin of the right-sided enhancing nodule shows invasive growth ➡. (**Right**) Cellular smear shows delicately arborizing vascular plexus ➡, a feature seen in myxoid LPS.*

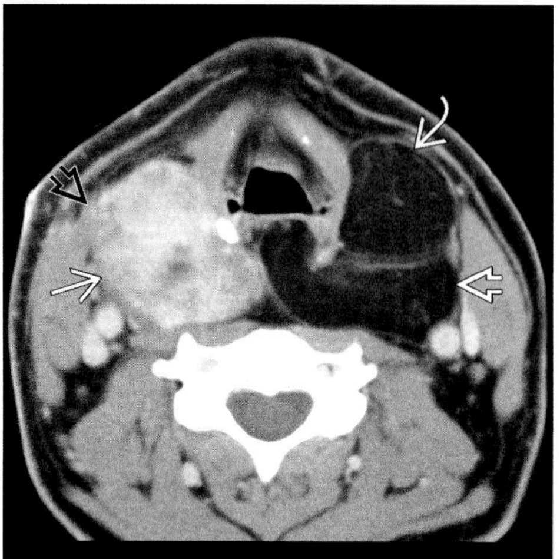

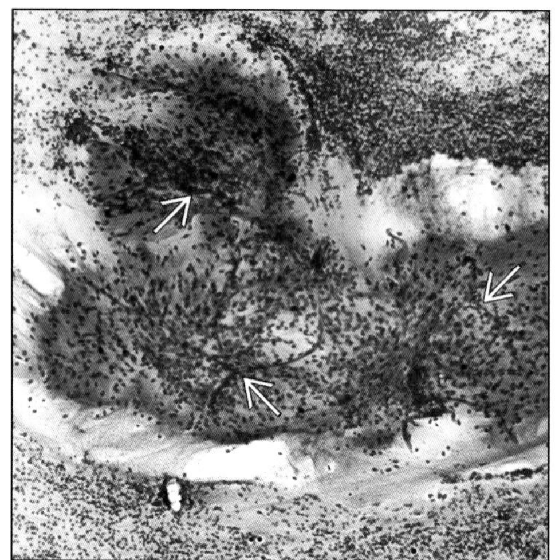

*(**Left**) Variably cellular myxoid lesion is shown with plexiform capillary pattern vascularity characterized by a delicate arborizing (capillary-like) pattern ➡. This vascular pattern is typically not present in reactive &/or benign lesions. (**Right**) Plexiform capillary pattern vascularity with arborizing pattern ➡ is a feature seen in several types of sarcomas including myxoid LPS. Lipoblasts in varying stages of development, including signet ring ➡ forms, are present.*

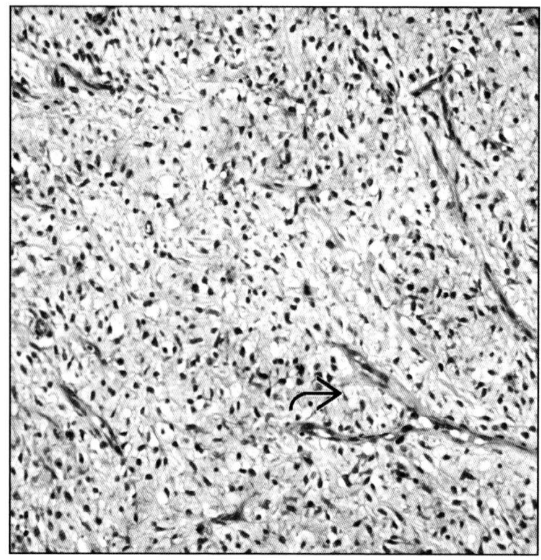

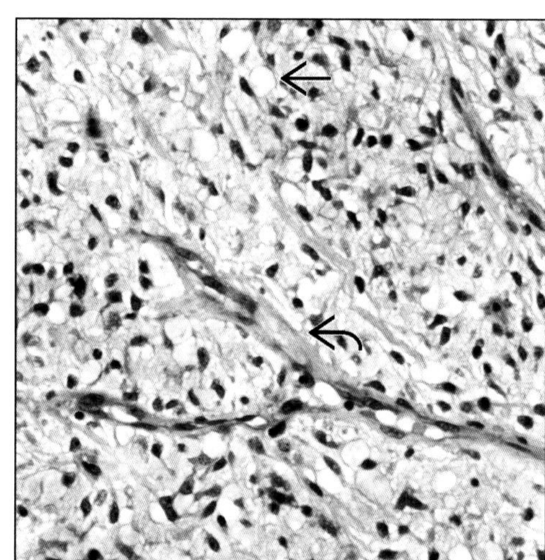

*(**Left**) Less cellular lipogenic neoplasm with myxoid stroma shows relatively bland appearing adipocytes without nuclear atypia &/or lipoblasts. However, the delicate arborizing capillary vascular network ➡ supports the consideration of a LPS. (**Right**) p16 nuclear immunoreactivity ➡ is a valuable marker in the diagnosis of LPS and assists in differentiating WDLPS from lipomas and other sarcomas with myxoid features and a delicate arborizing capillary vascular network.*

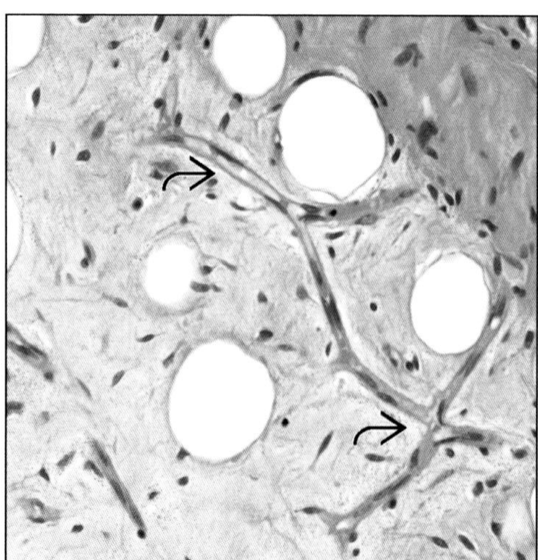

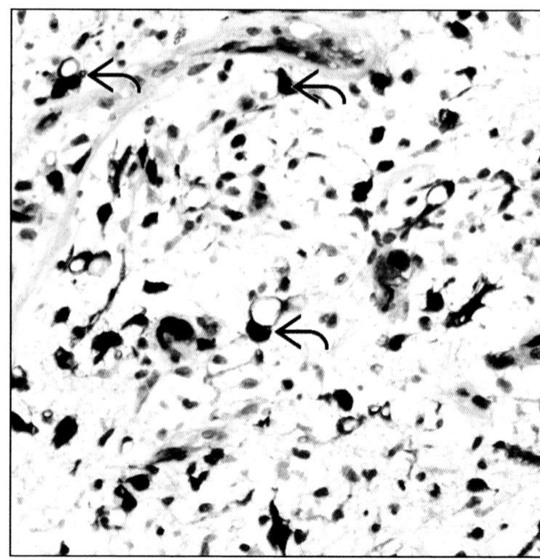

Microscopic and Immunohistochemical Features

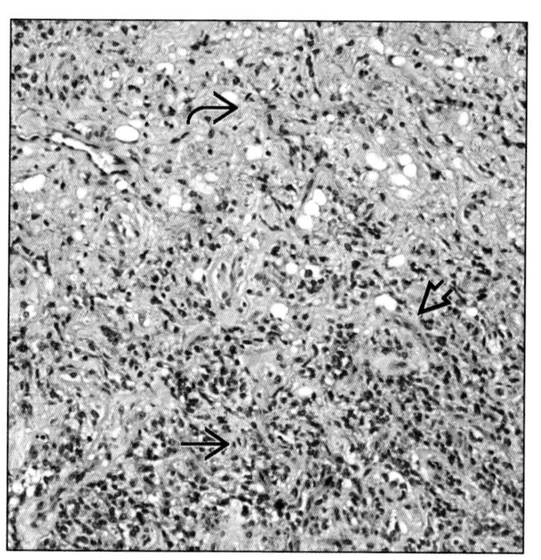

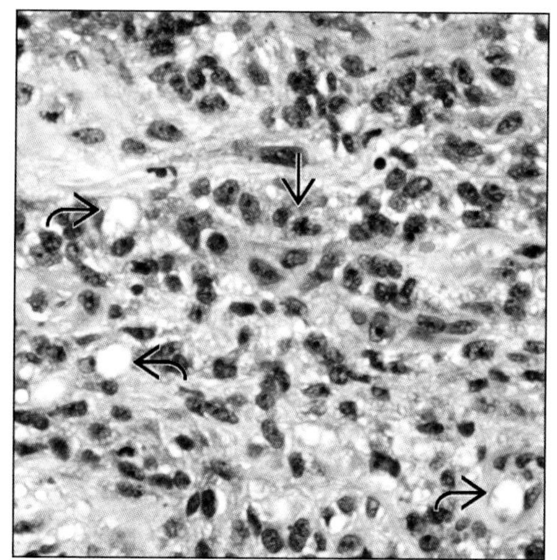

(Left) *Myxoid LPS ⇾ transitions to cellular round cell LPS →. Round cell LPS represents a poorly differentiated form of myxoid liposarcoma. A vascular pattern is present ⇨ but is generally compressed by the cellular proliferation.* ***(Right)*** *Round cell LPS is characterized by densely cellular solid sheets of primitive round cells with hyperchromatic nuclei, prominent nucleoli, and granular to vacuolated-appearing cytoplasm ⇾. Increased mitotic activity is present →.*

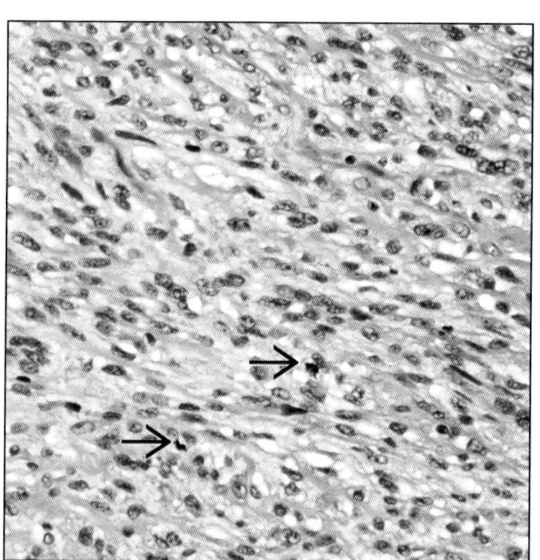

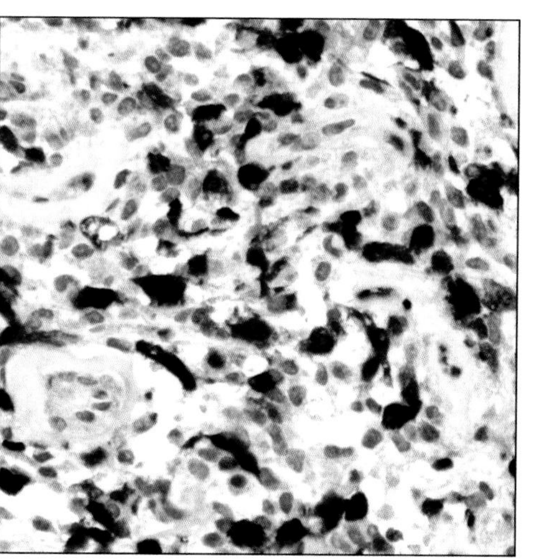

(Left) *Dedifferentiated LPS shows the presence of a histologically high-grade sarcoma including increased mitotic figures → characterized by features similar to nonlipogenic sarcomas. A histologic hallmark (not shown) is the presence of transition either in primary tumor or in recurrent tumor from well-differentiated LPS to nonlipogenic sarcoma.* ***(Right)*** *Dedifferentiated LPS shows MDM2 nuclear immunoreactivity assisting in differentiating it from nonlipogenic sarcomas.*

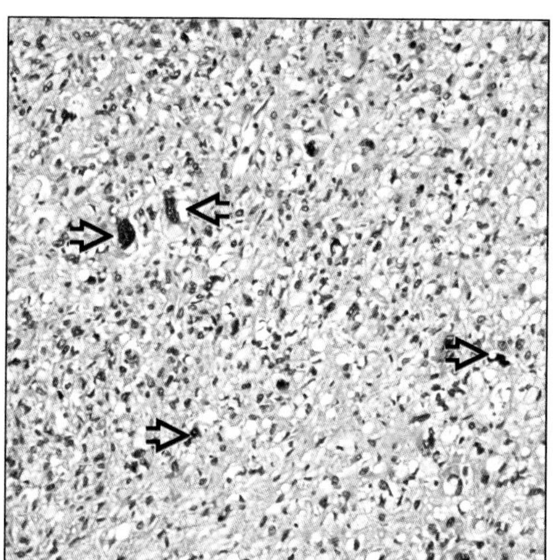

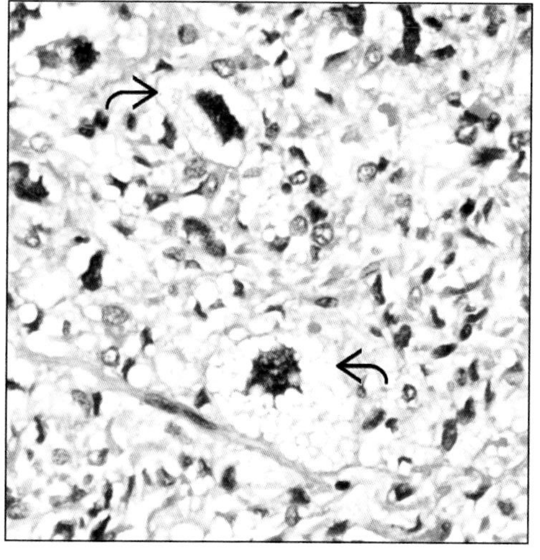

(Left) *Pleomorphic LPS is a hypercellular lesion composed of spindle-shaped cells with vacuolated cytoplasm and markedly pleomorphic and hyperchromatic nuclei ⇨.* ***(Right)*** *Multivacuolated lipoblasts ⇾ are characterized by 1 (or more) enlarged hyperchromatic nuclei scalloped by cytoplasmic vacuoles. Pleomorphic LPS resembles other sarcomas but the presence of lipoblasts is a differentiating finding supporting the diagnosis of LPS.*

Thyroid Gland

Congenital/Genetic/Hereditary

Infectious

Inflammatory-Immune Dysfunction

Reactive

Benign Neoplasm

Malignant Neoplasm

Specimen Examination, Thyroid

THYROGLOSSAL DUCT CYST

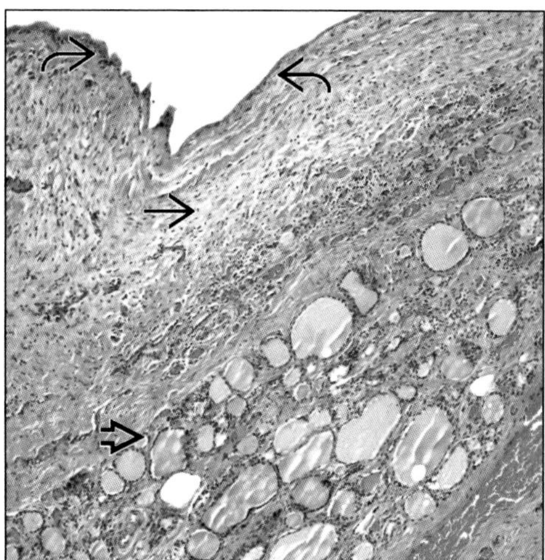

Resection of midline neck mass in the area of hyoid bone shows a cyst with cuboidal to columnar epithelial lining ➔, fibrous wall ➔, and benign thyroid tissue within the cyst wall ➔.

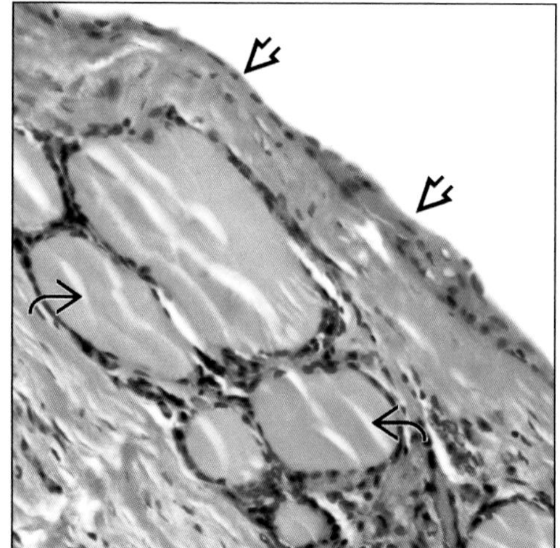

Benign colloid-filled thyroid follicular epithelium ➔ lies immediately below a cuboidal to stratified epithelial lined cyst ➔. Thyroid parenchyma can be found in approximately 25% of cases.

TERMINOLOGY

Abbreviations

- Thyroglossal duct cyst (TGDC)

Definitions

- Persistence and cystic dilatation of thyroglossal duct in midline of neck

ETIOLOGY/PATHOGENESIS

Idiopathic

- No known etiology

Thyroid Embryogenesis

- Thyroid follicular epithelium develops from foramen cecum at base of tongue
  - Migration is in midline in caudad direction until situated in normal anatomic position in midline cervical neck
- TGDC develops along path of embryologic development of thyroid gland
- Thyroglossal duct
  - Normally undergoes obliteration by 6 weeks of gestation
  - Failure of thyroglossal duct obliteration results in potential for cyst to develop

CLINICAL ISSUES

Epidemiology

- Incidence
  - Approximately 5-7% of population have TGDC
  - Represent approximately 60-70% of congenital neck cysts
    - 2x as common as branchial cleft cysts
- Age
  - Occurs over wide age range
    - Majority occur prior to 4th decade of life
- Gender
  - Equal gender distribution

Site

- Majority (approximately 75%) occur in midline neck at or just below level of hyoid bone
  - Nearly always connected to hyoid bone
  - Approximately 25% are suprahyoid with 2-4% at base of tongue
  - Uncommonly may occur lateral to midline but
    - Lateral localization may occur in setting of significant inflammation and fibrosis or prior surgery
    - Do not occur in lateral portion of neck (i.e., lateral to jugular vein, carotid artery)
  - May be site of recurrent infections
    - Fistulas may develop secondary to infection and open into pharynx or skin

Presentation

- Asymptomatic midline neck mass
  - Typically moves upward on swallowing
  - Inflamed or infected TGDCs may be associated with tenderness and pain
  - Extrinsic airway compression in neonates may be associated with
    - Apnea
    - Cyanosis
    - Respiratory compromise

Treatment

- Surgical approaches
  - Surgery is treatment of choice (Sistrunk procedure)
  - Sistrunk procedure includes
    - En bloc surgical resection of cyst
    - Middle 1/3 of hyoid bone
    - Suprahyoid tract up to foramen cecum (at base of tongue)

Prognosis

- Adequate surgery results in cure

THYROGLOSSAL DUCT CYST

Key Facts

Terminology

- Persistence and cystic dilatation of thyroglossal duct in midline of neck

Clinical Issues

- Occurs over wide age range but majority occur prior to 4th decade of life
- Majority (approximately 75%) occur in midline neck at or just below level of hyoid bone
  - Nearly always connected to hyoid bone
- Asymptomatic midline neck mass
- Adequate surgery results in cure with low, if any, recurrence(s)
- Surgery (Sistrunk procedure) is treatment of choice
  - En bloc surgical resection of cyst
  - Middle 1/3 of hyoid bone
  - Suprahyoid tract up to foramen cecum (at base of tongue)

Microscopic Pathology

- In noninflamed cyst, lining is
  - Respiratory (columnar) epithelium but may also include squamous epithelium
- Inflamed cysts may undergo metaplasia and lined by
  - Squamous epithelium
- Presence of thyroid tissue in cyst wall varies
  - May be dependent on extent of specimen sampling
  - Generally, thyroid tissue found in > 60% of cases
- Development of carcinoma in TGDC is rare
  - Majority are thyroid papillary carcinomas
  - Papillary carcinoma can be diagnosed by fine needle aspiration
  - Diagnosis based on diagnostic nuclear alterations

  - Low, if any, recurrence(s)

IMAGE FINDINGS

Radiographic Findings

- Midline round or elongated cystic lesion
- Expansion &/or destruction of cartilaginous structure of hyoid bone may be seen
- Seldom contains enough thyroid follicular tissue to be seen on scintiscan

CT Findings

- Presence of nodular soft tissue excrescences in midline cystic neck mass
  - May suggest possibility of papillary carcinoma arising in TGDC

MACROSCOPIC FEATURES

General Features

- Smooth-walled cystic structures
- Cystic content includes clear mucinous fluid
  - Infected cysts contain purulent material

Size

- Usually measure < 2 cm

MICROSCOPIC PATHOLOGY

Histologic Features

- Cyst lining
  - In noninflamed cysts, lined by
    - Respiratory (columnar) epithelium but may also include squamous epithelium
  - In presence of inflammation, lined by
    - Squamous epithelium secondary to metaplastic change
- Presence of thyroid tissue in cyst wall varies
  - May be dependent on extent of specimen sampling
    - Generally, thyroid tissue found in approximately 25% of cases
    - Thyroid tissue may be normal, hyperplastic and nodular, or neoplastic
- Fibrosis and chronic inflammatory cell infiltrate seen in cyst wall
- Cholesterol granulomas rarely identified
- Benign and malignant neoplasms may occur in setting of TGDC
  - Benign neoplasms include
    - Follicular adenoma
  - Malignant neoplasms may include
    - Papillary carcinoma
    - Follicular carcinoma
    - Others
  - Development of carcinoma in TGDC is rare
    - Most carcinomas developing in TGDCs are thyroid papillary carcinoma
  - **Thyroid papillary carcinoma arising in TGDC**
    - Occur more commonly in women than men
    - Occur over wide age range (1st to 8th decades of life)
    - Are of usual morphologic type
    - Are treated similar to benign TGDCs
    - Have similar (excellent) prognosis to that of thyroid-based papillary carcinoma
    - May recur or metastasize
    - Rarely may be lethal
  - Other types of carcinomas in TGDCs are rare and may include
    - Squamous (epidermoid) carcinoma: In all probability arises from cyst lining rather than from thyroid component
    - Undifferentiated (anaplastic) thyroid carcinoma
  - C-cell related lesions including medullary carcinoma do not occur in TGDCs
    - Embryologic derivation of C-cells differs from follicular epithelial cells
    - C-cells develop from ultimobranchial apparatus via neural crest rather than from lingual-based foramen cecum
    - C-cells migrate to lateral thyroid lobes
    - C-cells do not migrate in midline as do follicular epithelial cells

- C-cell lesions including medullary carcinoma do not occur in isthmic portion of thyroid gland

ANCILLARY TESTS

Cytology

- Smears from TGDCs are
  - Low in cellularity
  - Inflammatory cells more numerous than epithelial cells
    - Inflammatory cells, especially mature lymphocytes, frequently present
  - Squamous or respiratory epithelium may be identified
- Presence of papillary carcinoma can be diagnosed by fine needle aspiration
  - Diagnosis based on diagnostic nuclear alterations, including
    - Nuclear enlargement
    - Variation in nuclear size and shape
    - Optically clear ("Orphan Annie") to dispersed (very fine) appearing nuclear chromatin
    - Nuclear crowding and overlapping
    - Nuclear grooves
    - Intranuclear inclusions

DIFFERENTIAL DIAGNOSIS

Branchial Cleft Cyst

- Generally located in lateral neck not in midline neck
- Lack connection to hyoid bone
- Absence of thyroid follicles

Cervical Thymic Cyst

- Generally not located &/or connected to hyoid bone
- Presence of thymic tissue
- Absence of thyroid follicles

Metastatic (Cystic) Thyroid Papillary Carcinoma

- Presence of papillary carcinoma associated with TGDC
  - Necessitates excluding possible metastasis from primary carcinoma in normally situated thyroid gland
- Transitional areas from benign TGDC lining cells to papillary carcinoma may be seen
  - Supports primary origin of papillary carcinoma in TGDC
  - Not a common finding
- Differentiation of primary carcinoma in TGDC from metastatic papillary carcinoma
  - Often predicated on
    - Clinical features
    - Radiologic evaluation
  - Histologic features of primary vs. metastatic papillary carcinoma are identical

SELECTED REFERENCES

1. Shvili I et al: Cholesterol granuloma in thyroglossal cysts: a clinicopathological study. Eur Arch Otorhinolaryngol. 266(11):1775-9, 2009
2. Ahuja AT et al: Imaging for thyroglossal duct cyst: the bare essentials. Clin Radiol. 60(2):141-8, 2005
3. Aluffi P et al: Papillary thyroid carcinoma identified after Sistrunk procedure: report of two cases and review of the literature. Tumori. 89(2):207-10, 2003
4. Dedivitis RA et al: Thyroglossal duct: a review of 55 cases. J Am Coll Surg. 194(3):274-7, 2002
5. Doshi SV et al: Thyroglossal duct carcinoma: a large case series. Ann Otol Rhinol Laryngol. 110(8):734-8, 2001
6. Josephson GD et al: Thyroglossal duct cyst: the New York Eye and Ear Infirmary experience and a literature review. Ear Nose Throat J. 77(8):642-4, 646-7, 651, 1998
7. Hama Y et al: Squamous cell carcinoma arising from thyroglossal duct remnants: report of a case and results of immunohistochemical studies. Surg Today. 27(11):1077-81, 1997
8. Batsakis JG et al: Thyroid gland ectopias. Ann Otol Rhinol Laryngol. 105(12):996-1000, 1996
9. Deshpande A et al: Squamous cell carcinoma in thyroglossal duct cyst. J Laryngol Otol. 109(10):1001-4, 1995
10. Chen KT: Cytology of thyroglossal cyst papillary carcinoma. Diagn Cytopathol. 9(3):318-21, 1993
11. Kashkari S: Identification of papillary carcinoma in a thyroglossal cyst by fine-needle aspiration biopsy. Diagn Cytopathol. 6(4):267-70, 1990
12. Pelausa ME et al: Sistrunk revisited: a 10-year review of revision thyroglossal duct surgery at Toronto's Hospital for Sick Children. J Otolaryngol. 18(7):325-33, 1989
13. Katz AD et al: Thyroglossal duct cysts. A thirty year experience with emphasis on occurrence in older patients. Am J Surg. 155(6):741-4, 1988
14. LiVolsi VA et al: Carcinoma arising in median ectopic thyroid (including thyroglossal duct tissue). Cancer. 34(4):1303-15, 1974
15. Jaques DA et al: Thyroglossal tract carcinoma. A review of the literature and addition of eighteen cases. Am J Surg. 120(4):439-46, 1970

Imaging and Variant Microscopic Features

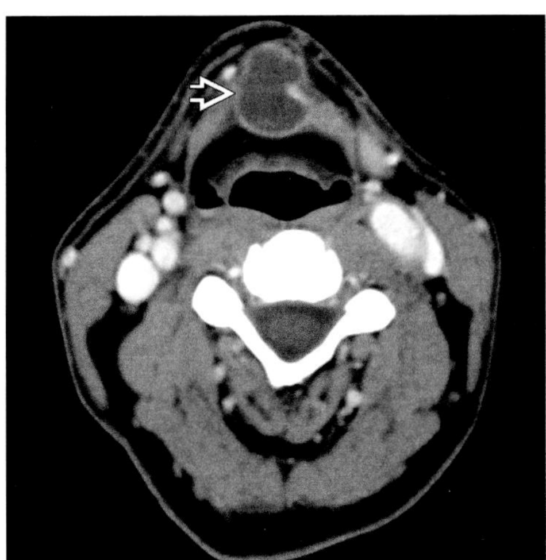

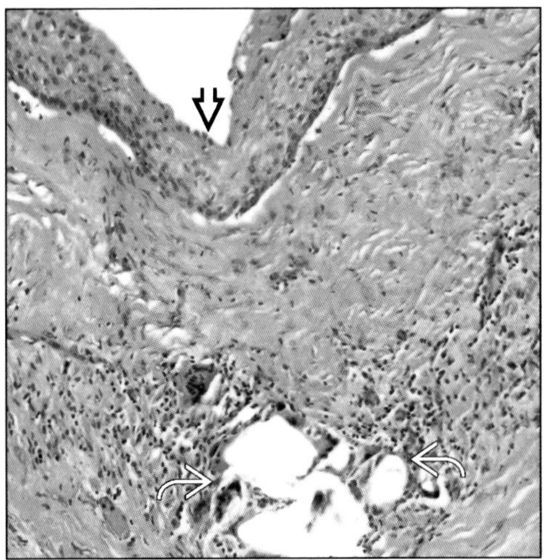

(Left) *Axial CT demonstrates a lobulated low-attenuation nonenhancing mass ➨ embedded within the strap muscles at the level of the hyoid bone, extending into the preepiglottic space without direct connection to the airway.* ***(Right)*** *TGDCs may be the site of recurrent infections resulting in squamous metaplasia ➨ of the cyst lining. The cyst wall is fibrotic with chronic inflammation and cholesterol granuloma formation ➨ but absent thyroid tissue. Identifying thyroid tissue may require extensive sampling.*

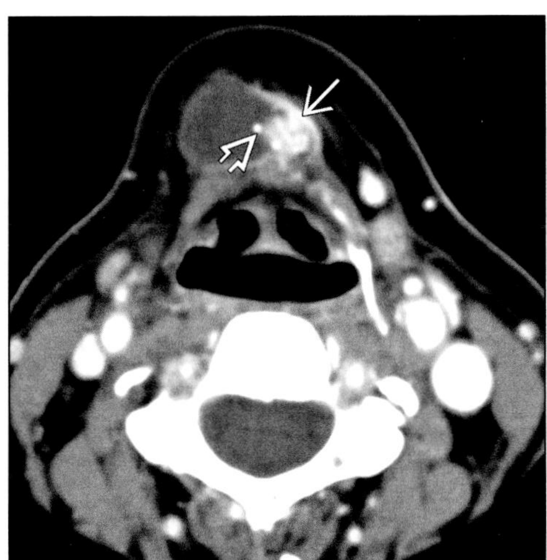

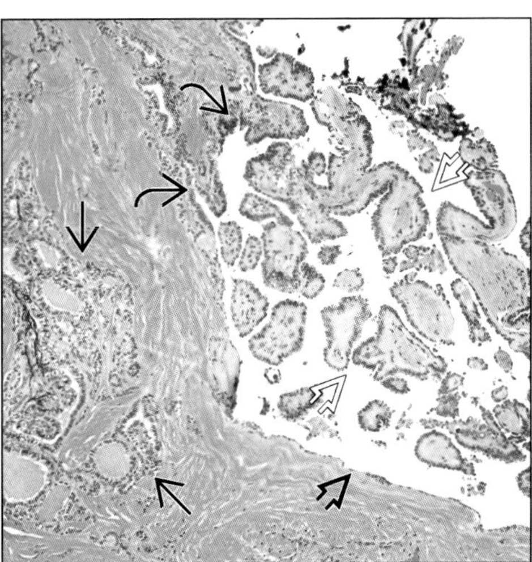

(Left) *Axial CT reveals a complex cystic and solid midline mass at hyoid bone level. Enhancing nodule ➨ with calcification ➨ highly suggestive of papillary carcinoma arising in TGDC.* ***(Right)*** *Thyroid papillary carcinoma arising in TGDC shows transition from nonneoplastic cyst lining ➨ to neoplastic proliferation of the cyst epithelial lining ➨ as well as intracystic papillary growth ➨. The carcinoma is also present in the cyst wall ➨.*

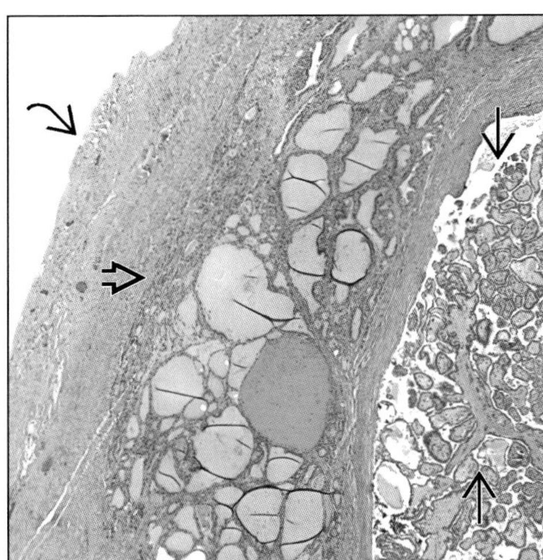

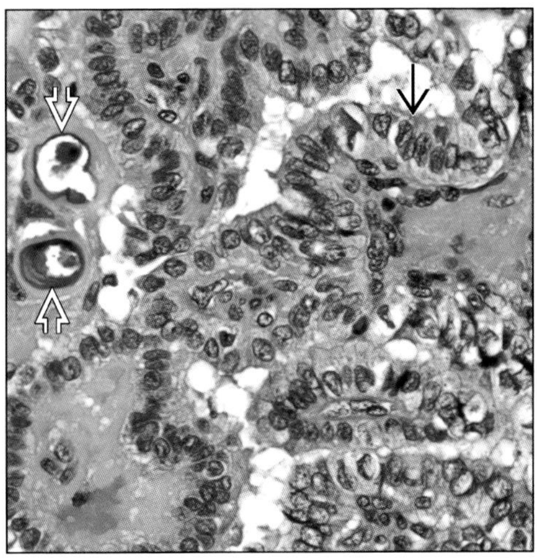

(Left) *Thyroid papillary carcinoma arising in a TGDC shows attenuated benign epithelial cyst lining ➨, benign thyroid tissue ➨ in the cyst wall, and thyroid papillary carcinoma lying deep in the cyst wall ➨.* ***(Right)*** *Diagnostic nuclear features of papillary carcinoma include nuclear enlargement with variation in size and shape, optically clear to dispersed nuclear chromatin, crowding and overlapping, and nuclear grooves ➨. In addition, psammoma bodies are present ➨.*

ECTOPIC THYROID

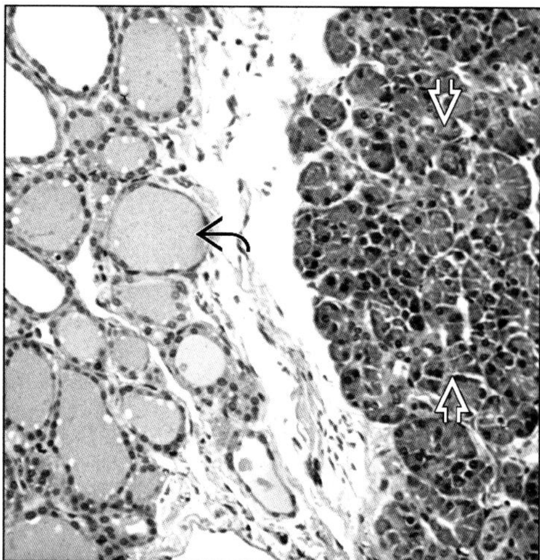

Intrapancreatic ➡ ectopic thyroid tissue ↷ lacks features for papillary carcinoma. The patient had a normally situated thyroid gland without identifiable lesions (e.g., follicular carcinoma).

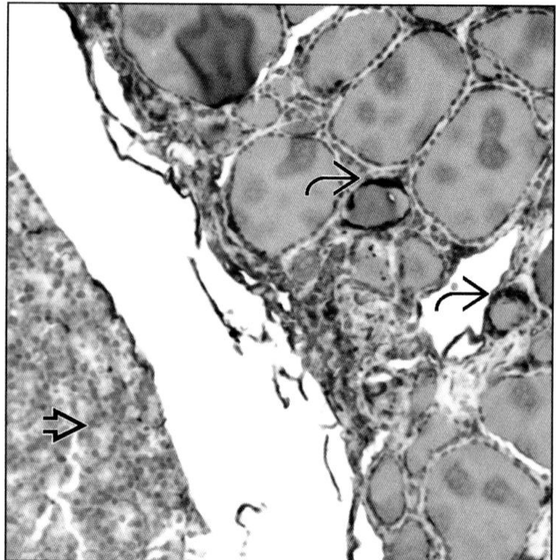

The intrapancreatic thyroid tissue is immunoreactive for thyroglobulin ↷, confirming the ectopia as definitively being thyroid tissue; the pancreatic parenchyma ➡ is negative for thyroglobulin.

TERMINOLOGY

Synonyms

- Aberrant rests
- Thyroid heterotopia
- Thyroid choristoma

Definitions

- Presence of otherwise normal thyroid parenchyma in any location other than its normal anatomic position

ETIOLOGY/PATHOGENESIS

Developmental Anomaly

- Ectopic thyroid tissue may represent failure of descent from foramen cecum (median anlage)
- Less likely, ectopia occurs via differentiation of thyroid tissue in abnormal locations
- Complete or partial agenesis of thyroid gland is extremely rare
- Rarely, familial thyroid ectopia may occur

Thyroid Embryogenesis

- Thyroid follicular epithelium develops from foramen cecum located at base of tongue
  - Migration is in midline in caudad direction until situated in normal anatomic position in midline cervical neck
  - Failure to migrate may result in ectopia anywhere along midline descent from foramen cecum to cervical neck
- Thyroid neuroendocrine cells (C-cells) develop from neural crest
  - Migrate to ultimobranchial apparatus located in 3rd-4th branchial arches
  - C-cells migrate only to lateral lobes of thyroid gland
  - C-cells do not migrate in midline fashion
    - C-cells not found in isthmic portion of thyroid gland

CLINICAL ISSUES

Epidemiology

- Incidence
  - Rare
- Age
  - Any age
- Gender
  - Equal gender distribution

Site

- Ectopic thyroid tissue seen in any location from tongue (foramen cecum at base of tongue) to suprasternal notch (site of normal gland)
- Excluding thyroglossal duct cyst, presence of ectopic thyroid tissue rare
  - Almost exclusively seen in suprahyoid locations usually located in or close to midline
  - Most common thyroid ectopia is at base of tongue (referred to as lingual thyroid)
  - Other sites include (from cranial to caudal direction)
    - Sella turcica
    - Submandibular region
    - Larynx, trachea
    - Mediastinum (superior > posterior)
    - Aortic arch, pericardium, and heart
    - Esophagus
  - More distant sites of ectopic thyroid tissue include
    - Hepatobiliary (liver, porta hepatis, gallbladder, common bile duct)
    - Pancreas
    - Adrenal gland
    - Retroperitoneum
    - Vagina and inguinal region
    - Ovarian thyroid tissue (referred to as struma ovarii)
  - Rarely, dual thyroid ectopia occurs, including separate ectopic sites occurring in same patient
  - Orthotopic thyroid gland usually present but may be absent

ECTOPIC THYROID

Key Facts

Terminology
- Presence of otherwise normal thyroid parenchyma in any location other than its normal anatomic position
- Ectopic thyroid tissue may represent failure of descent from the foramen cecum (median anlage)
- Thyroid follicular epithelium develops from foramen cecum located at base of tongue
- Migration is in midline in caudad direction until situated in normal anatomic position in midline cervical neck

Clinical Issues
- Ectopic thyroid tissue may be seen in any location from tongue (foramen cecum at base of tongue) to suprasternal notch (site of normal gland)
- Excluding thyroglossal duct cyst, presence of ectopic thyroid tissue rare and almost exclusively seen in suprahyoid locations usually located in or close to midline
- Most common thyroid ectopia is at base of tongue (referred to as lingual thyroid)
- Rarely, dual thyroid ectopia occurs including separate ectopic sites occurring in same patient
- In general, ectopic thyroid tissue is benign
  - Malignant neoplasms may arise in thyroid ectopia including papillary carcinoma and follicular carcinoma

Microscopic Pathology
- Normal-appearing thyroid tissue (i.e., colloid-filled follicles)
- Neuroendocrine C-cells not identified

      - Ectopic thyroid tissue may represent only thyroid tissue present

Presentation
- Excluding thyroglossal duct cyst and lingual thyroid, majority of thyroid ectopia are asymptomatic
- Depending on location, presentation may include
  - Local obstruction
  - Presence of mass lesion
  - Stridor
  - Hemorrhage
  - Heart murmur &/or voluminous cardiac mass resembling cardiac tumor

Laboratory Tests
- Ectopic thyroid may function abnormally including laboratory evidence of hypo- and hyperthyroidism

Prognosis
- In general, ectopic thyroid tissue is benign
  - Different types of malignant neoplasms may arise in thyroid ectopia, including thyroid papillary carcinoma and follicular carcinoma

MICROSCOPIC PATHOLOGY

Histologic Features
- Normal-appearing thyroid tissue (i.e., colloid-filled follicles)
- Neuroendocrine C-cells not identified
- Cytomorphologic features of thyroid papillary carcinoma absent
- **Thyroid inclusions in lymph nodes**
  - Controversial issue whether benign intranodal thyroid inclusions exist or whether all nodal-based thyroid tissue represents metastatic thyroid papillary carcinoma
  - Benign thyroid inclusions in lymph nodes may occur but require strict criteria including
    - Lymph node located in midline or medial to jugular vein
    - Thyroid tissue located in nodal capsule and not found in several lymph nodes &/or replace nodal parenchymal tissue
    - Inclusions are cytologically bland without histologic features of thyroid papillary carcinoma
    - Primary thyroid (papillary) carcinoma is not present
    - Of note, *BRAF* V600E point mutation, a highly specific biomarker for thyroid papillary carcinoma, has been identified in morphologically bland thyroid inclusions
  - Even if above criteria are met, diagnosis of benign thyroid inclusions in lymph nodes should be made with caution as these foci likely represent metastatic thyroid papillary carcinoma
- **Thyroid tissue in perithyroidal soft tissues**
  - Normal thyroid tissue can be found within skeletal muscle &/or fat of cervical neck
    - Reflects developmental abnormality and should not be mistaken for malignancy
    - Thyroid in skeletal muscle often seen in relation to isthmic portion of gland
    - Mature adipose tissue can be found in wide variety of intrathyroidal lesions

ANCILLARY TESTS

Immunohistochemistry
- Thyroglobulin, TTF-1 positive
- Cytokeratins positive
- Calcitonin and neuroendocrine markers negative

DIFFERENTIAL DIAGNOSIS

Metastatic Thyroid Papillary Carcinoma
- Demonstrate diagnostic nuclear features
- Any thyroid tissue found in lymph nodes lateral to great vessels (jugular vein, carotid artery) represents metastatic papillary carcinoma
  - Should be considered metastatic even in absence of unequivocal diagnostic nuclear features

ECTOPIC THYROID

- Nodal metastasis may be identified incidentally in neck dissection for other reasons
  - Staging neck dissection for other head and neck carcinomas (e.g., mucosal-based squamous cell carcinoma)
- In presence of papillary carcinoma in thyroid gland proper
  - Presence of thyroid tissue in "ectopic" sites, especially lymph nodes, in all probability represents metastatic disease

Mediastinal Thyroid (Substernal Goiter)

- Represents goitrous thyroid extending from thyroid gland proper into mediastinum (substernal or retrosternal)
- As multinodular goiter enlarges it has tendency to move inferiorly due to fascial planes favoring this migration
- Most mediastinal goiters are benign (adenomatoid nodules)
  - Thyroid malignancies (papillary carcinoma, follicular carcinoma, anaplastic carcinoma) can be seen in mediastinal thyroid tissue
- Mediastinal goiters generally do not respond to thyroid suppression and require surgical removal
  - Due to risk of sudden enlargement with possibility of airway compression or obstruction, intrathoracic goiters should be surgically removed

Parasitic Nodule (Lateral Aberrant Thyroid)

- Represents part of goitrous thyroid in which
  - Peripherally located nodule(s) anatomically separated from main gland in soft tissues of neck
    - Aberrant tissue may be connected to thyroid by thin fibrous strand that may or may not be appreciated by surgeon
    - May erroneously be considered malignant given localization away from thyroid gland
  - Pathologic findings may include adenomatoid nodule(s) &/or lymphocytic thyroiditis
    - Care should be taken not to interpret thyroid tissue in lymphocytic thyroiditis as within a lymph node
    - May lead to erroneous diagnosis of metastatic papillary carcinoma
    - Absence of subcapsular sinus, a feature of lymph nodes, in lymphocytic thyroiditis
- Stipulations for diagnosis include
  - Thyroid tissue not be identified in relationship to lymph node
  - Aberrant thyroid tissue should not demonstrate histomorphologic features of thyroid papillary carcinoma

Mechanical Implantation

- Thyroid tissue (normal or hyperplastic) unattached to thyroid gland in neck
  - May be result of prior surgery or accidental trauma
  - In such instances there is usually prominent fibrotic reaction &/or suture material seen in association with thyroid tissue

SELECTED REFERENCES

1. Chawla M et al: Dual ectopic thyroid: case series and review of the literature. Clin Nucl Med. 32(1):1-5, 2007
2. Huang TS et al: Dual thyroid ectopia with a normally located pretracheal thyroid gland: case report and literature review. Head Neck. 29(9):885-8, 2007
3. Mojica WD et al: Presence of the BRAF V600E point mutation in morphologically benign appearing thyroid inclusions of cervical lymph nodes. Endocr Pathol. 17(2):183-9, 2006
4. Shuno Y et al: Ectopic thyroid in the adrenal gland presenting as cystic lesion. Surgery. 139(4):580-2, 2006
5. Bowen-Wright HE et al: Ectopic intratracheal thyroid: an illustrative case report and literature review. Thyroid. 15(5):478-84, 2005
6. León X et al: Incidence and significance of clinically unsuspected thyroid tissue in lymph nodes found during neck dissection in head and neck carcinoma patients. Laryngoscope. 115(3):470-4, 2005
7. Maino K et al: Benign ectopic thyroid tissue in a cutaneous location: a case report and review. J Cutan Pathol. 31(2):195-8, 2004
8. Ghanem N et al: Ectopic thyroid gland in the porta hepatis and lingua. Thyroid. 13(5):503-7, 2003
9. Ihtiyar E et al: Ectopic thyroid in the gallbladder: report of a case. Surg Today. 33(10):777-80, 2003
10. Williams RJ et al: Ectopic thyroid tissue on the ascending aorta: an operative finding. Ann Thorac Surg. 73(5):1642-3, 2002
11. Eyüboğlu E et al: Ectopic thyroid in the abdomen: report of a case. Surg Today. 29(5):472-4, 1999
12. Shiraishi T et al: Ectopic thyroid in the adrenal gland. Hum Pathol. 30(1):105-8, 1999
13. Jamshidi M et al: Ectopic thyroid nodular goiter presenting as a porta hepatis mass. Am Surg. 64(4):305-6, 1998
14. Batsakis JG et al: Thyroid gland ectopias. Ann Otol Rhinol Laryngol. 105(12):996-1000, 1996
15. Bando T et al: Ectopic intrapulmonary thyroid. Chest. 103(4):1278-9, 1993
16. Salam MA: Ectopic thyroid mass adherent to the oesophagus. J Laryngol Otol. 106(8):746-7, 1992
17. al-Hajjaj MS: Ectopic intratracheal thyroid presenting as bronchial asthma. Respiration. 58(5-6):329-31, 1991
18. Carmi D et al: Ectopic thyroid in siblings. J Endocrinol Invest. 14(2):151, 1991
19. Ogden CW et al: Intratracheal thyroid tissue presenting with stridor. A case report. Eur J Cardiothorac Surg. 5(2):108-9, 1991
20. Takahashi T et al: Ectopic thyroid follicles in the submucosa of the duodenum. Virchows Arch A Pathol Anat Histopathol. 418(6):547-50, 1991
21. Richmond I et al: Intracardiac ectopic thyroid: a case report and review of published cases. Thorax. 45(4):293-4, 1990
22. Snyder RW et al: Spontaneous hemorrhage of an ectopic mediastinal thyroid. Chest. 98(6):1548, 1990
23. Hall TS et al: Substernal goiter versus intrathoracic aberrant thyroid: a critical difference. Ann Thorac Surg. 46(6):684-5, 1988
24. Kaplan M et al: Ectopic thyroid gland. A clinical study of 30 children and review. J Pediatr. 92(2):205-9, 1978
25. LiVolsi VA et al: Carcinoma arising in median ectopic thyroid (including thyroglossal duct tissue). Cancer. 34(4):1303-15, 1974

Microscopic Features and Differential Diagnosis

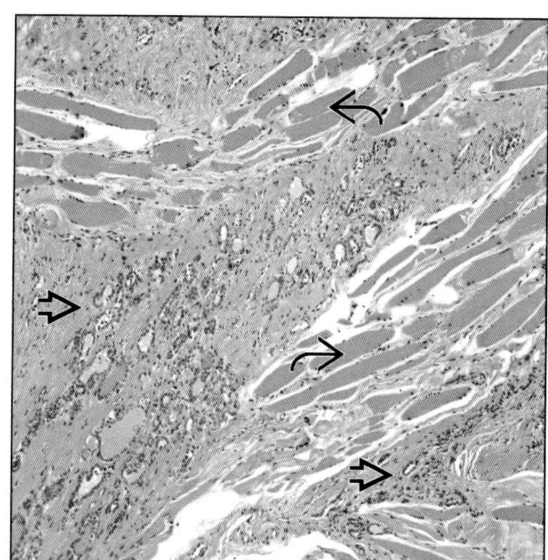

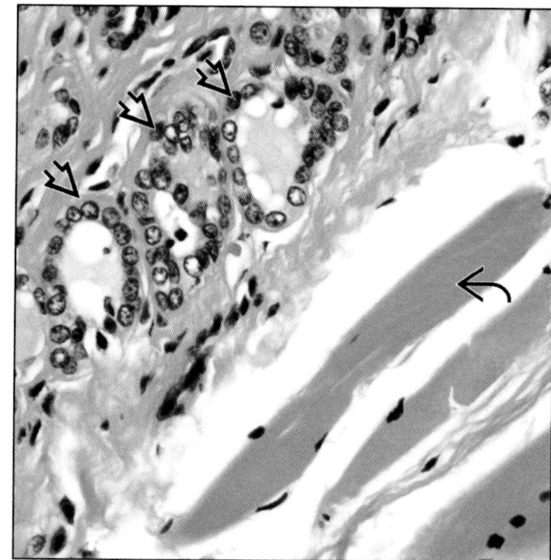

(Left) *Thyroid follicular epithelium* ➩ *in skeletal muscle* ➦ *lying outside the gland proper is a normal developmental finding typically seen in the isthmic portion of the gland.* ***(Right)*** *The thyroid follicular epithelium* ➩ *in skeletal muscle* ➦ *is within normal limits, lacking nuclear alterations associated with papillary carcinoma. Further, there was no evidence of a follicular carcinoma in the gland proper that might have included extrathyroidal extension.*

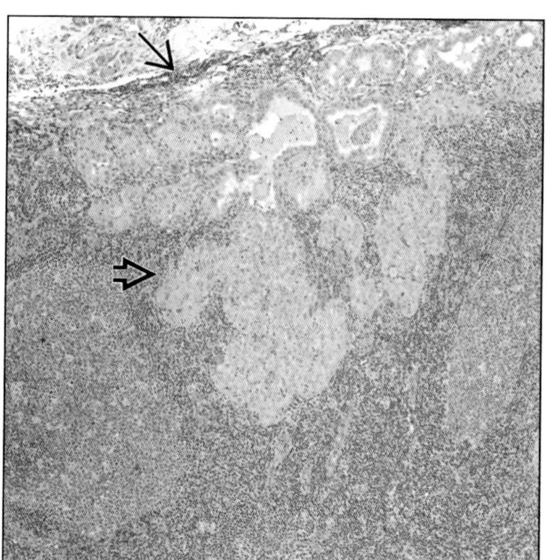

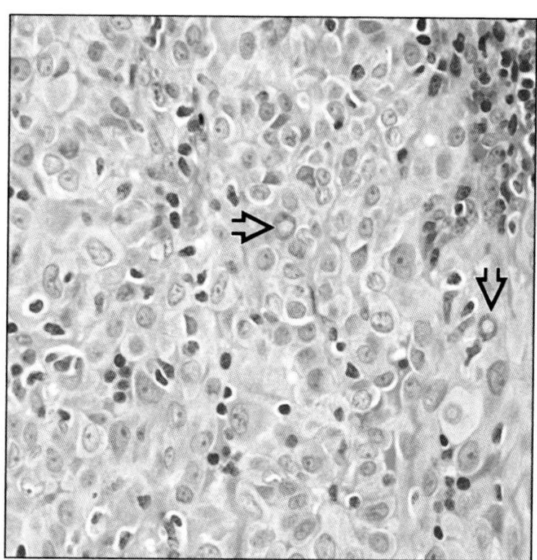

(Left) *Nodal metastatic thyroid papillary carcinoma shows subcapsular localization of the tumor* ➔*, a large volume of lesional tissue, and extension into the lymph node parenchyma* ➩*. These findings are well beyond the scope of criteria for nodal-based thyroid inclusions.* ***(Right)*** *The cells show nuclear features of papillary carcinoma with nuclear enlargement, variation in nuclear size and shape, dispersed (very fine) appearing nuclear chromatin, grooves, and inclusions* ➩*.*

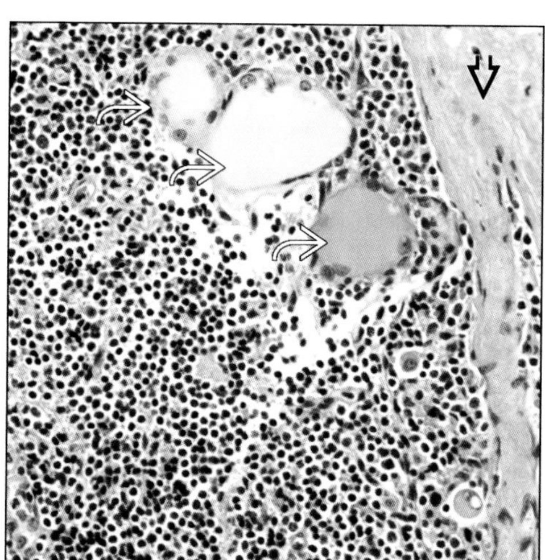

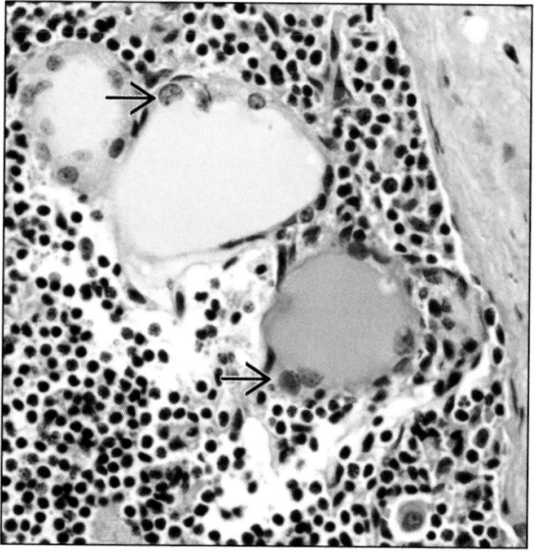

(Left) *Lymph node shows 3 colloid-filled thyroid follicles* ➦ *lying within the parenchyma and not in the capsule* ➩*.* ***(Right)*** *The nuclei* ➔ *are not diagnostic for papillary carcinoma. Nevertheless, metastatic papillary carcinoma is diagnosed based on the parenchymal involvement (rather than intracapsular localization) and in spite of the limited volume of lesion and absence of diagnostic nuclear features. A primary ipsilateral papillary carcinoma was present (not shown).*

SOLID CELL NEST

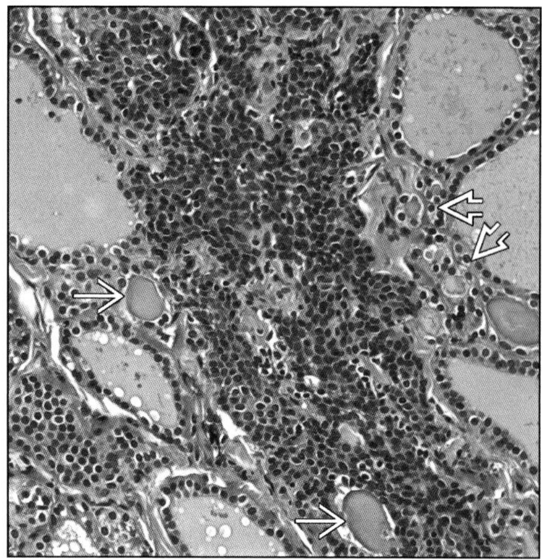

There is a well-demarcated collection of epithelial cells identified in an interfollicular distribution. Follicles are entrapped ➡ by the proliferation in a number of foci. C-cells are present ⇨.

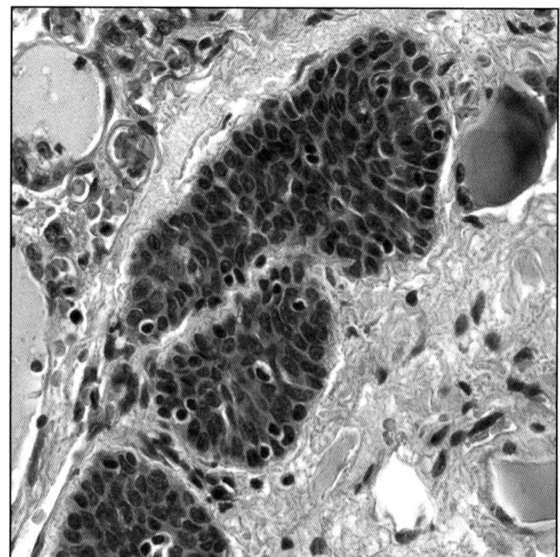

In many SCNs, the epithelial cells show a compact arrangement, surrounded by a basement membrane. Cytologic atypia is absent, as are mitoses.

TERMINOLOGY

Abbreviations

- Solid cell nests (SCNs)
- Ultimobranchial body (UBB)

Definitions

- Small remnant of ultimobranchial apparatus, associated with development of thyroid C-cells

ETIOLOGY/PATHOGENESIS

Pathogenesis

- May be derived from branchial pouch remnants
- May be derived from ultimobranchial body vestiges (endoderm)
  - High density of C-cells intermingled with SCNs

CLINICAL ISSUES

Epidemiology

- Incidence
  - Present in all thyroid glands if sought
  - Incidental finding in about 25% of thyroid specimens
- Age
  - All ages
- Gender
  - Equal gender distribution

Site

- Posteromedial and lateral area of bilateral middle to upper 1/3 of thyroid lobes

Presentation

- Incidental, discovered by extensive sampling
- Possibly increased frequency in patients with
  - Chronic lymphocytic thyroiditis

MACROSCOPIC FEATURES

Sections to Be Submitted

- Middle to upper 1/3 of thyroid lobes, outer to lateral-posterior area
- Multistep, serial sectioning method may be required to identify

Size

- < 0.1 cm (microscopic only)
  - 50 to 1,000 μm in greatest dimension

MICROSCOPIC PATHOLOGY

Histologic Features

- Interfollicular distribution of well-demarcated nests
  - Follicular epithelium frequently interspersed or trapped
- Irregular small nests, clusters, or lobulated compact aggregates
  - Distinct eosinophilic basement membrane surrounds groups
- Small epithelial cells, ovoid to polygonal; rarely spindled
  - Often there are C-cells within proliferation
  - These cells have granular-bluish cytoplasm
- Lesions may be partially cystic (up to 55%)
  - Oxymoronic nomenclature: Solid cell nests that are cystic
  - Larger cysts resemble branchial cleft cyst
- Nuclei are ovoid, with evenly distributed, finely granular chromatin
  - Frequent longitudinal nuclear groove
  - Nucleoli are absent to inconspicuous
- No keratinization or intercellular bridges
- Amphophilic cytoplasm
  - Occasional clear cells
- Degeneration may result in mucicarminophilic mucoid material or concretions

SOLID CELL NEST

Key Facts

Terminology
- Small remnant of ultimobranchial apparatus, associated with development of thyroid C-cells

Clinical Issues
- Posteromedial and lateral area of bilateral middle to upper 1/3 of thyroid lobes

Microscopic Pathology
- 50 to 1,000 µm in greatest dimension
- Interfollicular distribution of well-demarcated, irregular small nests
- Small epithelial cells, ovoid to polygonal
- Nuclei are ovoid, with evenly distributed chromatin
- Frequent longitudinal nuclear groove
- No keratinization or intercellular bridges
- High density of C-cells intermingled with SCNs

Ancillary Tests
- **Positive**: p63, pCEA; **negative**: Thyroglobulin, TTF-1

  - Goblet cells may be seen within epithelial nests
  - Ciliated columnar cells are uncommon
- Rarely, cartilage may be present

ANCILLARY TESTS

Immunohistochemistry
- Strongly positive: p63 (may be compartmentalized), carcinoembryonic antigen (pCEA), high and low molecular weight keratins, neurotensin, somatostatin, galactin 3
- Variably positive: Chromogranin-A, synaptophysin, calcitonin, calcitonin gene-related peptide, neuron-specific enolase
  - Highlights C-cells specifically within nests
- Negative: Thyroglobulin, TTF-1, HBME-1

Electron Microscopy
- Electron-dense secretory granules observed in C-cells only

DIFFERENTIAL DIAGNOSIS

Squamous Metaplasia
- Multifocal throughout gland, showing intercellular bridges, keratinization
- Usually associated with other disorders (chronic lymphocytic thyroiditis, carcinomas)

Papillary Carcinoma (Microscopic)
- Microscopic, solid or cystic
- Infiltrative pattern with heavy sclerosis/desmoplasia
- Enlarged, overlapping cells, with grooves, contour irregularities, intranuclear cytoplasmic inclusions
- Positive: Thyroglobulin, TTF-1

Inclusions
- Normal thymic tissue (Hassall corpuscles; lymphoid tissue), parathyroid gland (cleared cytoplasm, well-defined cell borders), and salivary gland tissue
- Histologically distinct and different from SCNs

Metastatic Squamous Cell Carcinoma
- Lymphatic location, marked pleomorphism, mitotic figures, keratinization, and intercellular bridges

SELECTED REFERENCES

1. Reis-Filho JS et al: p63 expression in solid cell nests of the thyroid: further evidence for a stem cell origin. Mod Pathol. 16(1):43-8, 2003
2. Cameselle-Teijeiro J et al: Solid cell nests of the thyroid: light microscopy and immunohistochemical profile. Hum Pathol. 25(7):684-93, 1994
3. Mizukami Y et al: Solid cell nests of the thyroid. A histologic and immunohistochemical study. Am J Clin Pathol. 101(2):186-91, 1994
4. Harach HR: Solid cell nests of the thyroid. J Pathol. 155(3):191-200, 1988

IMAGE GALLERY

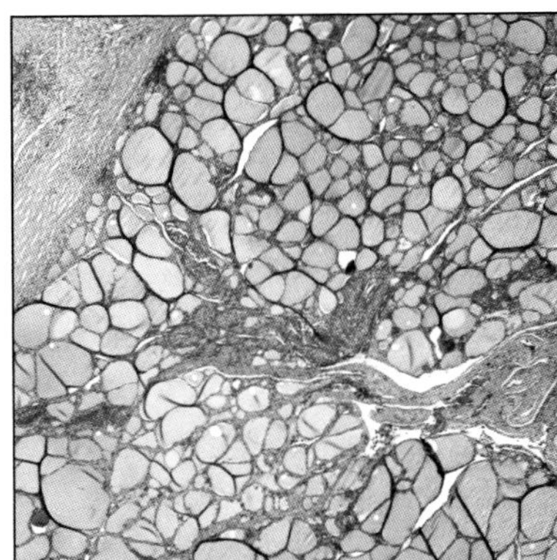
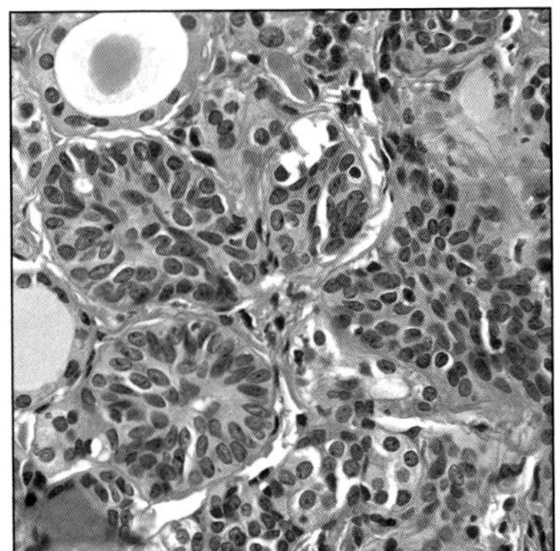
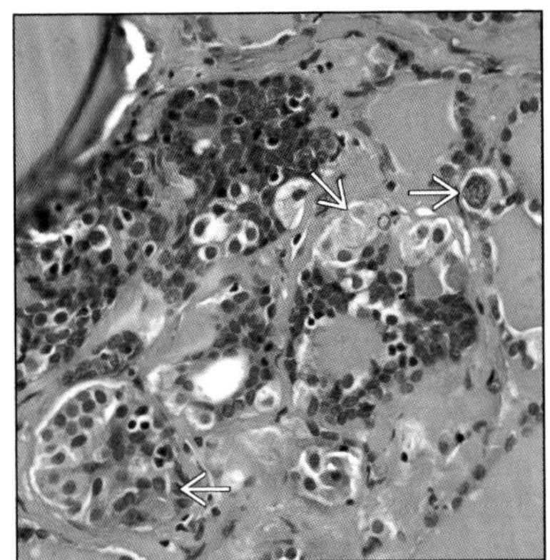

*(**Left**) At low power, the lobulated small nests are easily identified in the background thyroid follicular epithelium. However, squamous metaplasia can appear identical from low power. (**Center**) The cells are epithelial and oval, with oval nuclei. The nuclear chromatin is delicate and even, with a longitudinal nuclear groove. Intercellular bridges are absent. (**Right**) The SCNs are frequently associated with C-cells ➡. Note the basophilic cytoplasm and plasmacytoid appearance to the C-cells.*

DYSHORMONOGENETIC GOITER

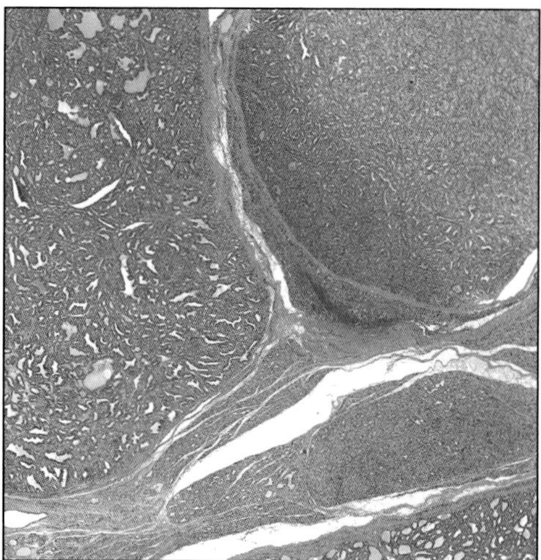

The thyroid gland is asymmetric and nodular, with the nodules resembling adenomatoid nodules. There is colloid present, although it is not prominent. The nodules are cellular.

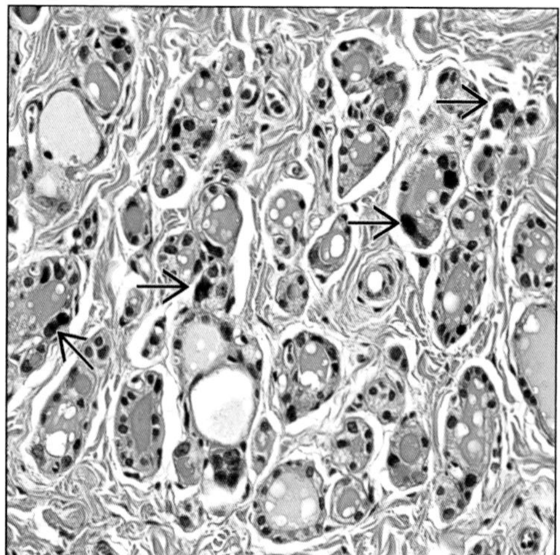

Within the septal regions of the gland, there are a number of isolated, highly atypical cells ➔. Note the variability in the colloid in this high-power field. There is also a background of fibrosis.

TERMINOLOGY

Synonyms

- Inherited goiter

Definitions

- Thyroid enlargement due to hereditary defect in thyroid hormone synthesis

ETIOLOGY/PATHOGENESIS

Developmental Anomaly

- Genetic defect in one of the biochemical steps of thyroid hormone synthesis
  - Usually autosomal recessive
  - Several major enzyme defects are known
    - Loss of any of genes involved in thyroglobulin synthesis, iodine transport, iodide oxidation and organification, coupling of MIT and DIT, proteolytic breakdown of thyroglobulin, and iodide recycling
    - Deficiency in thyroperoxidase (TPO) activity is most frequent cause of dyshormonogenetic goiter

CLINICAL ISSUES

Epidemiology

- Incidence
  - Very rare cause of permanent congenital hypothyroidism
    - 2nd most frequent cause of permanent congenital hypothyroidism
  - Congenital hypothyroidism (thyroid dysgenesis): 1 in 3,000-4,000 births
    - About 15% due to dyshormonogenetic goiter
  - Prevalence of dyshormonogenetic goiter: 1 in 30,000-50,000 population
- Age
  - Average age at presentation: 16 years
    - Majority manifest before age 25 years
  - Ranges from neonates to adults
- Gender
  - Female slightly > Male

Site

- Entire thyroid gland affected
  - Whenever "whole thyroid" is affected, must consider genetic or autoimmune etiologies

Presentation

- Absent or severely decreased thyroid hormone synthesis
  - Results in increased secretion of TSH due to functional hypothyroidism
    - Insufficient hormone production for feedback loop
  - Insufficient hormone production results in continuous TSH stimulation
  - Yields thyroid hyperplasia without thyroid function improvement
- Only patients with most severe impairment in thyroid hormone production present in infancy with cretinism
- Most patients (2/3) have known hypothyroidism prior to recognition of goiter
  - Thyroid enlargement (goiter) tends to develop later in life
- Family history of hypothyroidism &/or goiter is elicited in 20% of patients
- Pendred syndrome very rare (*SLC26A4* at 7q31)
  - Association of dyshormonogenetic goiter (impaired iodide organification) with familial deaf-mutism due to sensorineural deafness
  - Biallelic mutations in *SLC26A4* gene
    - *SLC26A4* gene encompasses 21 exons and contains open-reading frame of 2343 bp

Laboratory Tests

- Low to absent T4 and T3

DYSHORMONOGENETIC GOITER

Key Facts

Terminology
- Thyroid enlargement due to hereditary defect in thyroid hormone synthesis

Clinical Issues
- Usually autosomal recessive, enzyme defect in one of the biochemical steps of thyroid hormone synthesis
- Congenital hypothyroidism: 1 in 3,000-4,000 births
  - About 15% due to dyshormonogenetic goiter
- Average age at presentation: 16 years
- Absent or severely decreased thyroid hormone synthesis
  - Low to absent T4 and T3, with high TSH
- Treatment of hypothyroidism is primary goal, using surgery for symptomatic goiter

Macroscopic Features
- Thyroid is enlarged, asymmetric, and nodular, resembling adenomatoid nodules

Microscopic Pathology
- All thyroid tissue is abnormal
- Nodules vary considerably but hypercellular with scant/absent colloid
- Pleomorphism highlighted or accentuated in cells between nodules
  - In fibrous septae or internodular parenchyma

Top Differential Diagnoses
- Adenomatoid nodules, diffuse hyperplasia (Graves disease), radiation thyroiditis, follicular carcinoma, iatrogenic goiter

- High TSH

Natural History
- If severe or complete, cretinism at birth
- Death without replacement therapy

Treatment
- Options, risks, complications
  - Treatment of hypothyroidism is primary goal
- Surgical approaches
  - Total thyroidectomy for symptomatic goiter
- Drugs
  - Replacement hormone manages hypothyroidism
    - Synthroid

Prognosis
- Excellent outcome with thyroid hormone replacement therapy
- No increased risk of thyroid carcinoma
  - If carcinoma does develop, no difference in long-term prognosis

MACROSCOPIC FEATURES

General Features
- Thyroid is enlarged, asymmetric, and nodular
- Enlargement varies from mild to marked
- Nodules resemble adenomatoid nodules
  - But colloid is not seen on cut surface
  - Nodules tend to be more opaque instead of translucent (like adenomatoid nodules)

Sections to Be Submitted
- Junction of nodules to intervening parenchyma (fibrovascular septae)
- Must sample any encapsulated lesions thoroughly

Size
- Up to 600 grams
  - Usually between 50-250 grams

MICROSCOPIC PATHOLOGY

Histologic Features
- All thyroid tissue is abnormal
  - Distinctly different from relatively normal thyroid seen between adenomatoid nodules
- Nodules vary considerably
  - Due to different enzyme defects and duration of disease (age of patient) at time of diagnosis
  - Hypercellular nodules
  - Solid or microfollicular pattern
  - Papillary, trabecular, or insular patterns may be observed
- Colloid is usually scant to absent
  - When present, it has different color, quality, and quantity than normal colloid
  - Gives a "washed out," "thin" or "watery" appearance
  - Tends to be more easily identified within nodules
- Fibrosis is often a prominent finding
  - Sometimes so extensive it distorts architecture, suggesting invasion
- Cytologic atypia is usually present
  - Pleomorphism highlighted or accentuated in cells between nodules
    - In fibrous septae or internodular parenchyma
    - These regions tend to be solid or microfollicular
    - Enlarged, hyperchromatic nuclei
    - May have contour irregularities and grooves
  - Can be quite striking, similar to radiation thyroiditis

ANCILLARY TESTS

Cytology
- Cannot be used to exclude follicular neoplasm
- Aspirates are remarkably cellular
- Little or no colloid
- Often with prominent nuclear atypia
- May help exclude thyroid papillary carcinoma

Metabolic Workup
- Evaluation of thyroid function

DYSHORMONOGENETIC GOITER

Defects Associated with Dyshormonogenetic Goiter

Steps in Thyroid Hormone Synthesis	Related Gene
Thyroglobulin synthesis	Thyroglobulin (*TG*)
Iodine transport into follicular cell	Sodium-iodide symporter (*SIS*)
Iodine transport into lumen	Pendrin (*PDS*)
Oxidation of iodine	Thyroperoxidase (*TPO*)
	Dual oxidase genes (*DUOX1* and *DUOX2*); a.k.a. thyroid oxidase genes (*THOX1* and *THOX2*)
Organification of thyroglobulin	Thyroperoxidase (*TPO*)
Coupling of MIT and DIT	Thyroperoxidase (*TPO*)
Proteolytic breakdown of TG	Various lysosomal endopeptidases and exopeptidases
Dehalogenation of MIT and DIT	Dehalogenase 1 (*DEHAL1*)

DIT = di-iodotyrosine; MIT = mono-iodotyrosine.

- Evaluation of pituitary-thyroid axis

DIFFERENTIAL DIAGNOSIS

Adenomatoid Nodules

- Usually in middle-aged adults with asymmetric thyroid enlargement
- Hyperplasia is only present within nodules
- Easily identifiable colloid
- Secondary degenerative changes (cyst formation, hemosiderin-laden macrophages, hemorrhage, calcification, fibrosis) more common
- Lacks internodular cytologic atypia

Diffuse Hyperplasia (Graves Disease)

- Clinical hyperthyroidism
- Autoantibodies detected serologically
- Entire thyroid affected
- Usually has colloid present, although variable
- Papillary and follicular structures predominate
- Lacks pleomorphism or atypia
- Lymphoid aggregates (germinal centers) are common finding

Radiation Thyroiditis

- Clinical history of radiation and age of patient at presentation helps
- Frequently has cellular nodules
- Cytologic atypia is random throughout gland, not accentuated in internodular zones
- Increased fibrosis

Follicular Carcinoma

- Encapsulated tumor
  - Capsule is usually quite thick and well formed
  - Reticulin fibers within fibrosis help to define true capsule
  - Smooth muscle-walled vessels within fibrosis help define capsule
  - Remember that irregular perinodular fibrosis in dyshormonogenetic goiter can simulate capsular invasion
- Shows definitive capsular &/or vascular invasion
- Cellular atypia is not diagnostic criteria

Iatrogenic Goiter

- Due to antithyroidal drugs
- May have nodules with limited colloid
- Can be indistinguishable on histologic basis alone

DIAGNOSTIC CHECKLIST

Pathologic Interpretation Pearls

- All of thyroid gland is abnormal
- Bizarre, pleomorphic nuclei in parenchyma
- Limited or thin colloid

SELECTED REFERENCES

1. Francois A et al: Fetal treatment for early dyshormonogenetic goiter. Prenat Diagn. 29(5):543-5, 2009
2. Deshpande AH et al: Cytological features of dyshormonogenetic goiter: case report and review of the literature. Diagn Cytopathol. 33(4):252-4, 2005
3. Park SM et al: Genetics of congenital hypothyroidism. J Med Genet. 42(5):379-89, 2005
4. Thompson L: Dyshormonogenetic goiter of the thyroid gland. Ear Nose Throat J. 84(4):200, 2005
5. Camargo RY et al: Pathological Findings in Dyshormonogenetic Goiter with Defective Iodide Transport. Endocr Pathol. 9(3):225-233, 1998
6. Ghossein RA et al: Dyshormonogenetic Goiter: A Clinicopathologic Study of 56 Cases. Endocr Pathol. 8(4):283-292, 1997
7. Medeiros-Neto G et al: Prenatal diagnosis and treatment of dyshormonogenetic fetal goiter due to defective thyroglobulin synthesis. J Clin Endocrinol Metab. 82(12):4239-42, 1997
8. Matos PS et al: Dyshormonogenetic goiter: a morphological and immunohistochemical study. Endocr Pathol. 5:49-58, 1994
9. Medeiros-Neto GA et al: Defective organification of iodide causing hereditary goitrous hypothyroidism. Thyroid. 3(2):143-59, 1993
10. Yashiro T et al: Papillary carcinoma of the thyroid arising from dyshormonogenetic goiter. Endocrinol Jpn. 34(6):955-64, 1987
11. Lever EG et al: Inherited disorders of thyroid metabolism. Endocr Rev. 4(3):213-39, 1983
12. Kennedy JS: The pathology of dyshormonogenetic goitre. J Pathol. 99(3):251-64, 1969

Gross and Microscopic Features

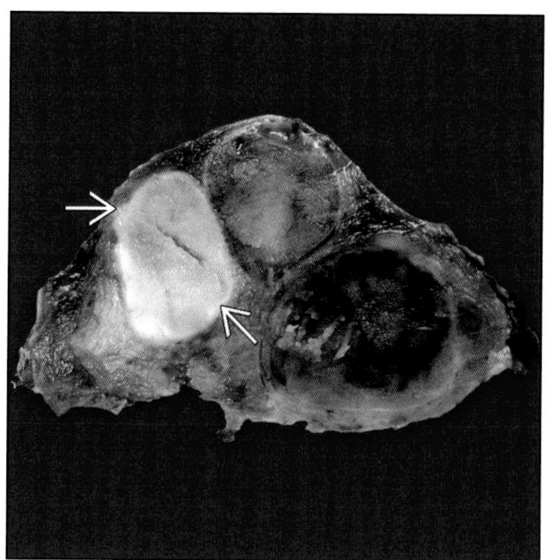

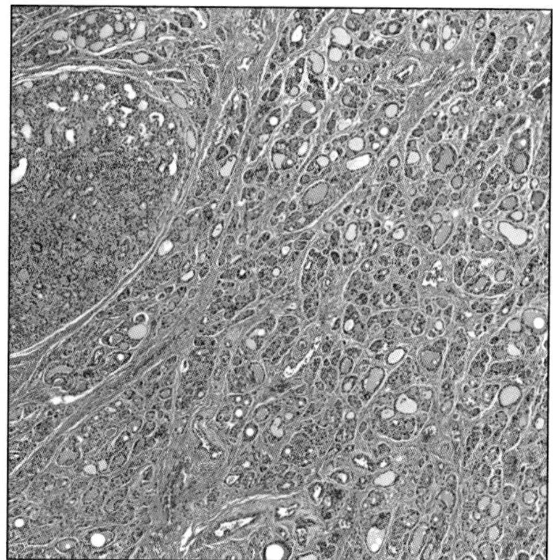

(Left) *The thyroid gland shows a multinodular appearance, with the nodules showing a variety of different appearances. The nodules have a different appearance from the remaining parenchyma. There is a suggestion of an encapsulated mass ➡.* ***(Right)*** *There is a vague nodularity to this thyroid section. Note the variable colloid appearance and overall increased cellularity and fibrosis.*

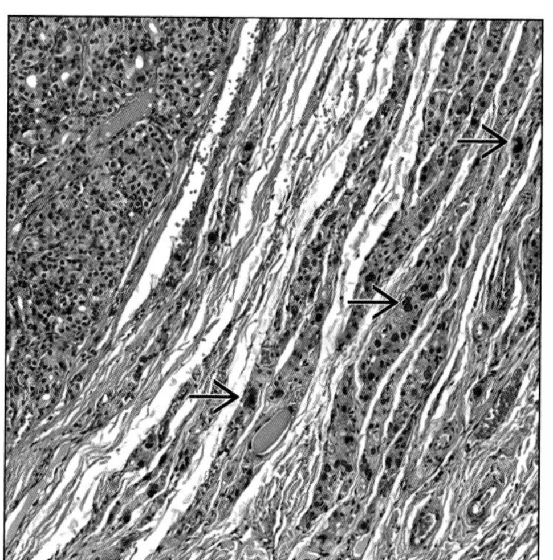

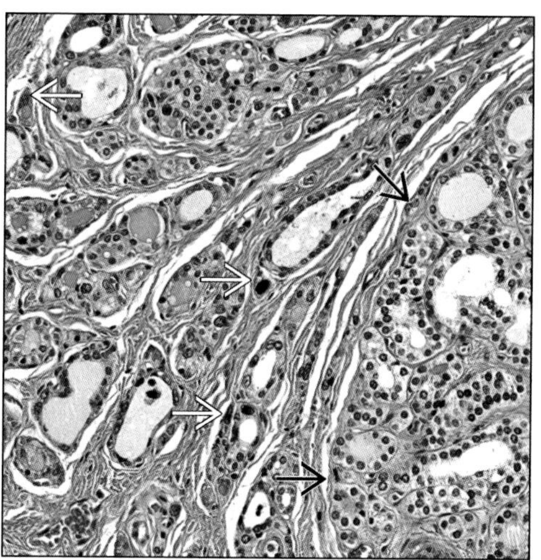

(Left) *Nodules are cellular, usually without colloid. The intervening septations show increased fibrosis and a number of isolated, remarkably atypical and hyperchromatic nuclei ⇨. The atypia is not usually seen within the nodules, only in the septal tissues.* ***(Right)*** *The nodule has colloid ⇨, although it is thin. There is heavy fibrosis surrounding the nodule, with isolated atypical follicular epithelial cells ➡.*

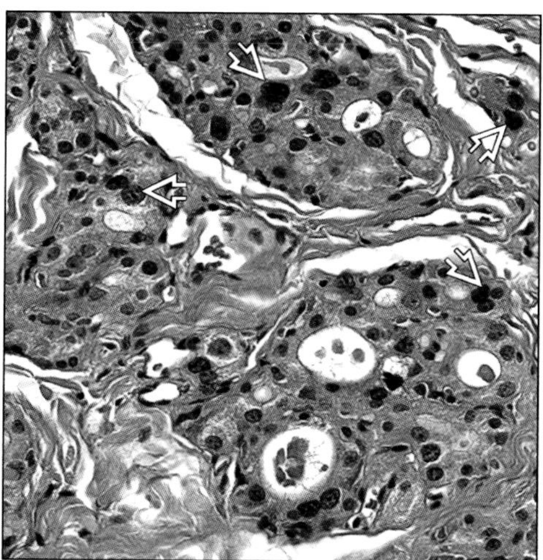

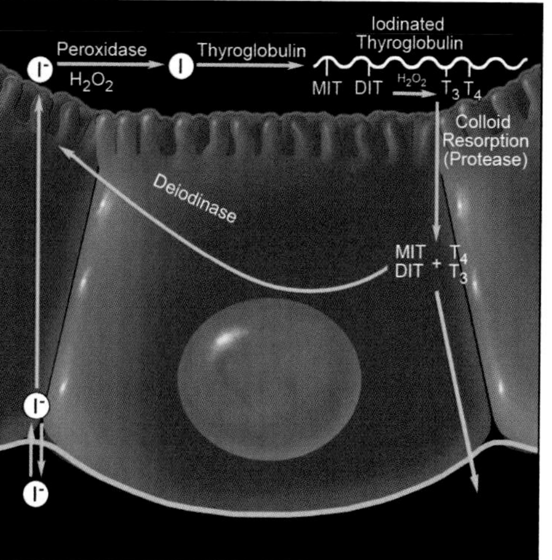

(Left) *On high power, it is important to note the atypia is within the epithelial cells ➡, not in the stromal cells (the latter seen in radiation thyroiditis). The atypical nuclei are not seen throughout the sample but only in isolation or small clusters.* ***(Right)*** *This graphic shows normal thyroid hormone production pathways. Several major enzyme defects are known, including loss of any of the genes involved in thyroglobulin synthesis, coupling of MIT and DIT, and iodide recycling.*

INFECTIOUS THYROIDITIS

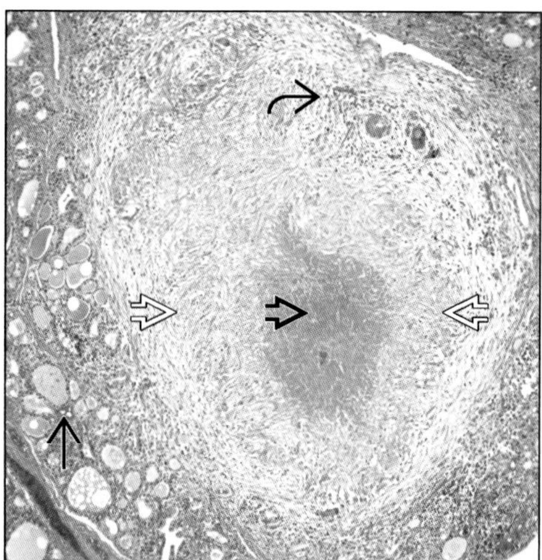

Intrathyroidal ⇒ M. tuberculosis infection shows caseating, well-formed granulomatous inflammation with central necrosis ⇒, palisading histiocytes ⇒, and multinucleated giant cells ⇒.

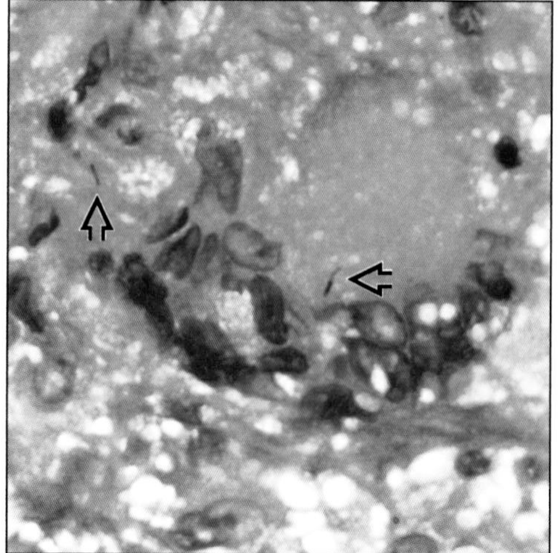

Under oil immersion, 2 AFB organisms ⇒, characterized by a beaded appearance and red color, are seen in multinucleated giant cells. These organisms can be difficult to find, even with special stains.

TERMINOLOGY

Synonyms

- Acute suppurative thyroiditis
- Acute mycotic thyroiditis

Definitions

- Infectious disease of thyroid with identifiable microorganism

ETIOLOGY/PATHOGENESIS

Infectious Agents

- Bacteria, mycobacteria, fungi, rarely viruses
- Causative bacteria include
  - *Streptococcus haemolyticus*
  - *Staphylococcus aureus*
  - *Pneumococcus*
  - *Actinomyces*
  - Less commonly gram-negative bacteria
- Mycobacteria
  - *M. tuberculosis*, *M. avium-intracellulare*
  - Mycobacterial infections are rare even in patients with miliary tuberculosis
- Causative fungi include
  - *Candida* species
  - *Pneumocystis jirovecii* (formerly *Pneumocystis carinii*)
  - Rarely, *Cryptococcus* or *Mucor*
- Causative viruses include
  - Cytomegalovirus
    - Occurs in patients with AIDS

CLINICAL ISSUES

Epidemiology

- Incidence
  - Uncommon
  - Tends to develop in immunocompromised, immunosuppressed, or malnourished patients
  - Not infrequently associated with
    - Concomitant localized infection
    - Part of systemic involvement
  - Spread of infection to thyroid gland via lymphatics and, less commonly, via hematogenous routes
- Age
  - Occurs in any age group
- Gender
  - Equal gender distribution

Site

- No specific localization

Presentation

- Fever with swelling and pain in neck region radiating or referred to jaw &/or ear region
- Additional symptoms may include fatigue, dyspnea, dysphagia, and hoarseness
- For acute thyroiditis
  - Not infrequently, history of antecedent or concomitant upper aerodigestive tract infection
- Thyroid glands are warm to hot on palpation

Laboratory Tests

- Patients are usually euthyroid but clinical evidence of hyper- or hypothyroidism may occur
- Cultures for microorganisms may be of assistance in diagnosis
  - Microbiologic analysis can be performed on material from fine needle aspiration

Treatment

- Options, risks, complications
  - Acute and granulomatous thyroiditis
    - Treatment is predicated on diagnosis and identification of causative microbe
    - Once microorganism identified, appropriate antimicrobial therapy can be initiated
- Surgical approaches

INFECTIOUS THYROIDITIS

Key Facts

Terminology

- Infectious disease of thyroid with identifiable microorganism including
  - Bacteria
  - Mycobacteria
  - Fungi
  - Viruses (rare)

Clinical Issues

- Tends to develop in immunocompromised, immunosuppressed, or malnourished patients
- Frequently associated with
  - Part of systemic involvement, concomitant localized infection
- Spread of infection to thyroid gland via lymphatics and, less commonly, via hematogenous routes
- Prognosis excellent for bacterial-related acute thyroiditis
- Prognosis poor for fungal-related infection

Microscopic Pathology

- **Acute thyroiditis**
  - Focal to diffuse acute inflammatory cell infiltrate (polymorphonuclear leukocytes) with destruction of follicular epithelial cell architecture
  - Areas of abscess formation characterized by dense pool of leukocytes can be seen
- **Granulomatous inflammation**
  - Classic caseating granulomas may be present
  - Include foci of central necrosis surrounded by histiocytic cell reaction with multinucleated giant cells

---

- Surgical intervention (drainage) may be required in presence of abscess formation

Prognosis

- For bacterial-related acute thyroiditis
  - Excellent prognosis with most patients experiencing recovery
  - Rarely, recurrence and even death may occur
  - Recurrent acute suppurative thyroiditis may occur secondary to piriform sinus fistula
    - Piriform sinus fistula identified by radiographic evaluation
    - In this setting, thyroiditis usually left-sided
    - Treatment for piriform sinus fistula includes fistulectomy
- Prognosis for fungal infection is poor
  - Generally terminal event in immunocompromised patient
- Prognosis for mycobacterial infection correlates with that of other organ system involvement

MACROSCOPIC FEATURES

General Features

- **Acute thyroiditis**
  - Gross appearance quite variable, includes focal or diffuse enlargement
  - In some instances, thyroid appears normal
  - Abscess formation can be seen by soft purulent areas
- **Granulomatous thyroiditis**
  - May include soft purulent (caseating) areas, abscess formation, or miliary tubercles

MICROSCOPIC PATHOLOGY

Histologic Features

- **Acute thyroiditis**
  - Pathologic process may be suppurative or nonsuppurative
  - Focal to diffuse acute inflammatory cell infiltrate (polymorphonuclear leukocytes) with destruction of follicular epithelial cell architecture
  - Areas of abscess formation characterized by dense pool of leukocytes can be seen
  - Areas of necrosis and leukocytic debris may be present
  - Depending on causative microorganism, offending agent may or may not be identifiable by light microscopy
- **Granulomatous inflammation**
  - Classic caseating granulomas may be present in either mycobacterial or fungal infection
    - Include foci of central necrosis surrounded by histiocytic cell reaction with scattered associated multinucleated giant cells
  - In immunocompromised patient
    - Typical granulomatous inflammatory process may not occur in face of mycobacterial or fungal infection
    - Changes of acute thyroiditis may be seen
- Irrespective of causative organism, histologic picture of mycobacterial infection is same

ANCILLARY TESTS

Cytology

- Fine needle aspiration represents primary diagnostic modality
  - Diagnostic findings include identification of microorganism by
    - Cytologic examination
    - Ancillary studies (e.g., histochemistry, immunohistochemistry)
  - Cytologic diagnosis may
    - Obviate need for surgical intervention
    - Allow for initiation of appropriate antimicrobial therapy

Histochemistry

- Histochemical stains may assist in identification of microorganism

- Fungal infections
  - GMS, PAS positive
  - Fluorostain is helpful
- Mycobacterial infection
  - Acid-fast bacilli (AFB) and Ziehl-Neelsen positive
  - May be difficult to identify and defy detection despite all efforts
  - When identified, they appear beaded, showing red or purple color
  - Fluorostain may be helpful

Immunohistochemistry

- Immunohistochemical stains may assist in identification of microorganism (e.g., CMV)

DIFFERENTIAL DIAGNOSIS

Sarcoidosis

- Multisystem chronic granulomatous disease of unknown etiology
- May involve thyroid as part of systemic process or, rarely, localized to thyroid
- Increased angiotensin-converting enzyme (ACE) levels
- Noncaseating granulomas consisting of epithelioid histiocytes surrounded by mixed inflammatory infiltrate and multinucleated giant cells
  - Intracytoplasmic star-shaped inclusions (asteroid bodies) &/or calcific laminated bodies (Schaumann bodies) can be seen
- All special stains for microorganisms are negative

Subacute (de Quervain) Thyroiditis

- Granulomatous inflammatory condition of thyroid gland with characteristic clinical and pathologic findings
- Etiology in all probability infectious with strong evidence supporting viral agent
- Autoimmunity may play role in development of subacute thyroiditis
  - Thyroid antibodies found in some patients transiently present and disappear following resolution of disease
- Histologic appearance varies
  - Early phase includes destruction of follicular epithelial cells with extravasation and depletion of colloid
    - Colloid may be identifiable "floating" within inflammatory cell infiltrate
    - Periodic acid-Schiff staining effective for identifying colloid
    - "Colonization" of follicles by polymorphonuclear leukocytes (including microabscesses) in initial stages
  - Later phase includes replacement of leukocytes by chronic inflammatory infiltrate composed of lymphocytes, histiocytes, giant cells, plasma cells

Palpation Thyroiditis

- Traumatically induced lesions caused by vigorous clinical palpation of thyroid gland
- Does not cause abnormalities in thyroid function (hypo- or hyperthyroidism)
- Incidental microscopic finding in thyroid glands resected for other reasons
  - Focal or multifocal lesion due to rupture of follicles with extrusion of colloid in area of manipulation
  - Isolated follicle or groups of follicles show replacement of follicular epithelial cells by mixed chronic inflammatory cell infiltrate
    - Predominantly comprised of histiocytes as well as lymphocytes and plasma cells, multinucleated (foreign body giant reaction)
    - Necrosis generally absent but occasionally may be present
  - Colloid may be present or absent
  - Special stains for microorganisms are negative

SELECTED REFERENCES

1. Paes JE et al: Acute bacterial suppurative thyroiditis: a clinical review and expert opinion. Thyroid. 20(3):247-55, 2010
2. Ozekinci S et al: Histopathologic diagnosis of thyroid tuberculosis. Thyroid. 19(9):983-6, 2009
3. Goel MM et al: Fine needle aspiration cytology and immunocytochemistry in tuberculous thyroiditis: a case report. Acta Cytol. 52(5):602-6, 2008
4. Smith SL et al: Suppurative thyroiditis in children: a management algorithm. Pediatr Emerg Care. 24(11):764-7, 2008
5. Zavascki AP et al: Pneumocystis jiroveci thyroiditis: report of 15 cases in the literature. Mycoses. 50(6):443-6, 2007
6. Bulbuloglu E et al: Tuberculosis of the thyroid gland: review of the literature. World J Surg. 30(2):149-55, 2006
7. Goldani LZ et al: Fungal thyroiditis: an overview. Mycopathologia. 161(3):129-39, 2006
8. Karatoprak N et al: Actinomycotic suppurative thyroiditis in a child. J Trop Pediatr. 51(6):383-5, 2005
9. Avram AM et al: Cryptococcal thyroiditis and hyperthyroidism. Thyroid. 14(6):471-4, 2004
10. Brook I: Microbiology and management of acute suppurative thyroiditis in children. Int J Pediatr Otorhinolaryngol. 67(5):447-51, 2003
11. Basílio-De-Oliveira CA: Infectious and neoplastic disorders of the thyroid in AIDS patients: an autopsy study. Braz J Infect Dis. 4(2):67-75, 2000
12. Shah SS et al: Diagnosis and Management of Infectious Thyroiditis. Curr Infect Dis Rep. 2(2):147-153, 2000
13. Danahey DG et al: HIV-related Pneumocystis carinii thyroiditis: a unique case and literature review. Otolaryngol Head Neck Surg. 114(1):158-61, 1996
14. Mondal A et al: Efficacy of fine needle aspiration cytology in the diagnosis of tuberculosis of the thyroid gland: a study of 18 cases. J Laryngol Otol. 109(1):36-8, 1995
15. Gandhi RT et al: Diagnosis of Candida thyroiditis by fine needle aspiration. J Infect. 28(1):77-81, 1994
16. Robillon JF et al: Mycobacterium avium intracellulare suppurative thyroiditis in a patient with Hashimoto's thyroiditis. J Endocrinol Invest. 17(2):133-4, 1994
17. Das DK et al: Fine needle aspiration cytology diagnosis of tuberculous thyroiditis. A report of eight cases. Acta Cytol. 36(4):517-22, 1992
18. Nieuwland Y et al: Miliary tuberculosis presenting with thyrotoxicosis. Postgrad Med J. 68(802):677-9, 1992
19. Frank TS et al: Cytomegalovirus infection of the thyroid in immunocompromised adults. Yale J Biol Med. 60(1):1-8, 1987

Microscopic Features and Ancillary Techniques

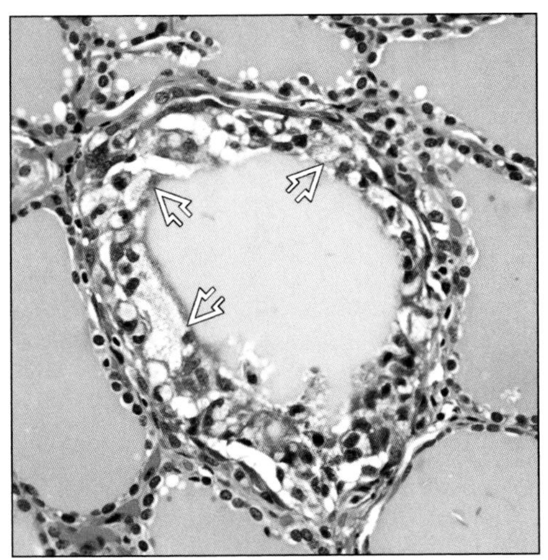

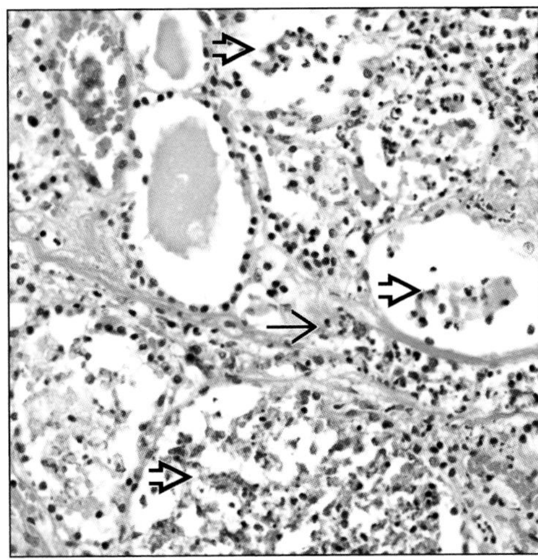

(Left) *Palpation thyroiditis, an incidental microscopic finding caused by vigorous palpation, shows replacement of follicular epithelial cells by histiocytes* ➡ *and chronic inflammatory cells.* ***(Right)*** *Acute suppurative thyroiditis shows marked inflammation dominated by polymorphonuclear leukocytes colonizing thyroid follicles* ➡ *as well as located within the intervening stroma* →*. Microorganisms that may be associated with acute thyroiditis include bacteria and fungi.*

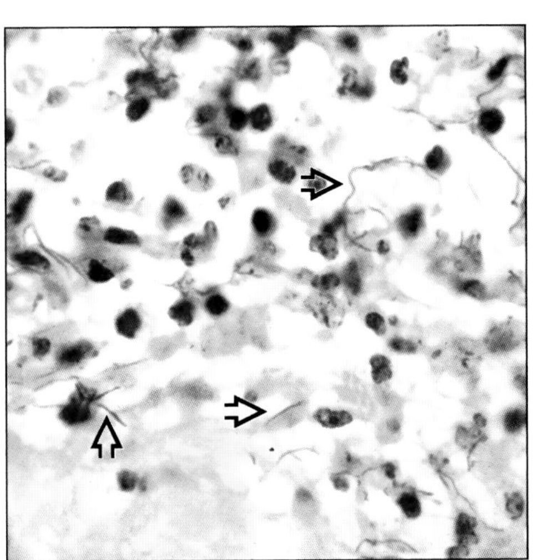

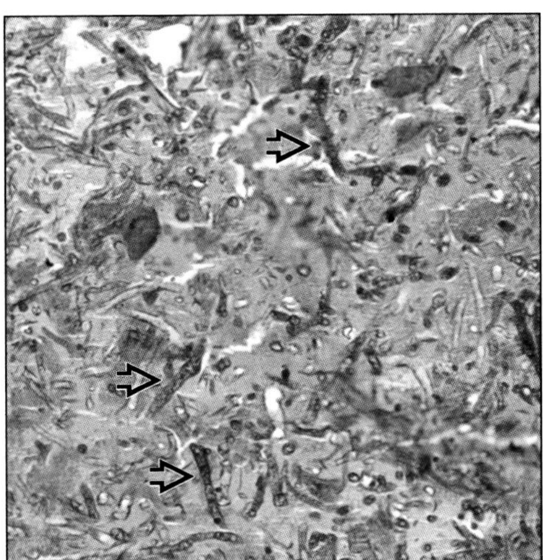

(Left) *Nocardia, an aerobic, branching, actinomycete, filamentous, gram-positive organism* ➡*, can infect the thyroid, causing suppurative lesions, characterized by a neutrophilic cell infiltrate.* ***(Right)*** *Mucormycosis may infect the thyroid causing acute thyroiditis. This fungus is identified by routine staining characterized by haphazardly branched hyphae* ➡ *that, in contrast to Aspergillus species, are broad, irregularly branched, and rarely septated.*

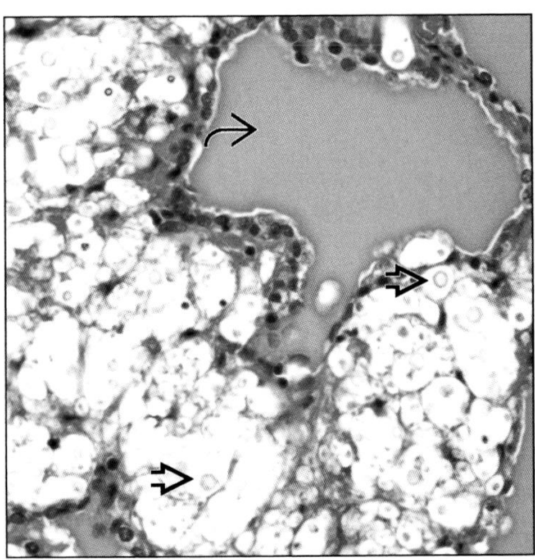

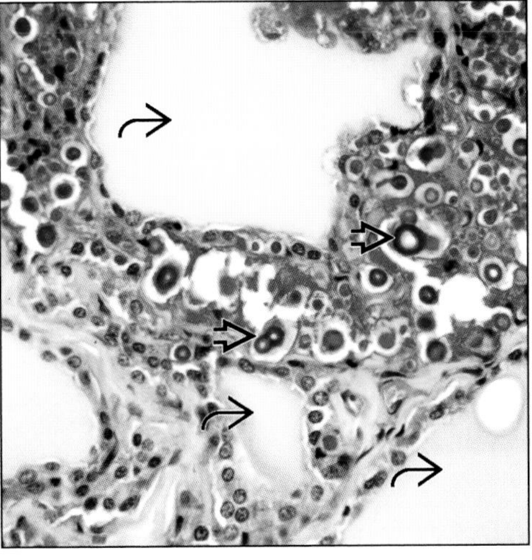

(Left) *Cryptococcus, a fungus, may rarely infect the thyroid gland* ↗*. The microorganisms are readily identified in routine staining and are characterized by spherical organisms with thickened capsule* ➡*.* ***(Right)*** *Thyroid follicles* ↗ *surrounded by organisms show characteristic mucicarminophilic cell walls* ➡*. Cryptococcal infection typically causes an acute inflammatory infiltrate but in immunocompromised hosts may be devoid of associated inflammation.*

PALPATION THYROIDITIS

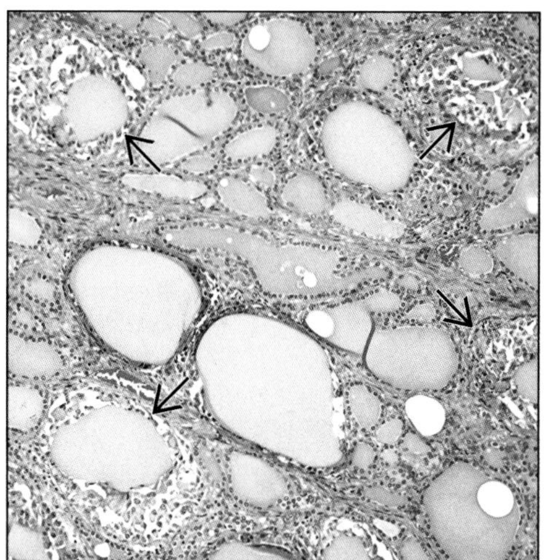

There are multiple separate "micro-granulomas" centered on a single follicle ➔ in this case of palpation thyroiditis. There are scattered, single follicles destroyed with the lumina filled with histiocytes.

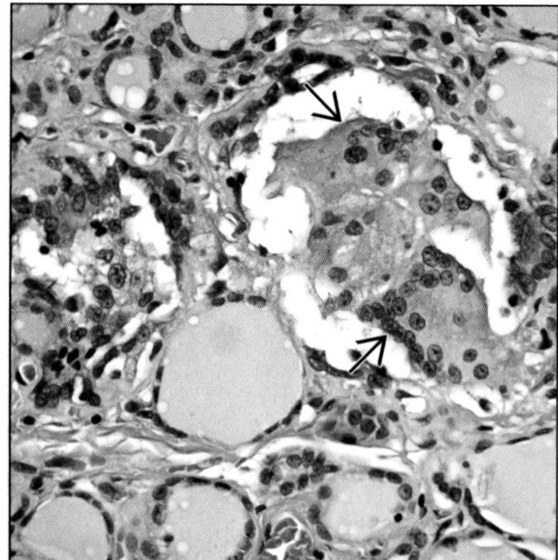

In this example of palpation thyroiditis, foreign-body type giant cells ➔ are noted within the single destroyed follicle. Histiocytes are present but follicular epithelium is absent.

TERMINOLOGY

Synonyms

- Multifocal granulomatous folliculitis

Definitions

- Microscopic granulomatous foci centered on thyroid follicles thought to result from rupture of follicles due to palpation

ETIOLOGY/PATHOGENESIS

Pathogenesis

- Pressure-induced damage and rupture of follicles by squeezing during manual examination
  - Palpation
    - Often vigorous, repeated manipulation of thyroid gland preoperatively
    - Identified in thyroids of patients who died while hospitalized versus patients who died at home
    - Identical findings produced experimentally in dogs whose thyroids were vigorously squeezed
  - Martial arts (karate, tang soo do, jiu-jitsu, judo)
- Possibly related to physiologic alterations in follicular basement membrane (similar to subacute granulomatous thyroiditis)

CLINICAL ISSUES

Epidemiology

- Incidence
  - Very common in surgically resected thyroid glands
- Age
  - All ages
- Gender
  - Equal gender distribution

Presentation

- No clinical presentation as signs and symptoms are subclinical if present at all
  - Usually a nodule present that precipitated palpation in the first place

Laboratory Tests

- No change in thyroid function tests

Natural History

- Resolves with time

Treatment

- Options, risks, complications
  - No treatment required
    - Decrease aggressive examination!

Prognosis

- Palpation thyroiditis is of no clinical significance
  - Outcome predicated on reason for palpation: Nodule, thyroiditis, neoplasm

MACROSCOPIC FEATURES

General Features

- No gross findings
  - Isolated foci of hemorrhage are occasionally seen
- Usually a nodule which prompted palpation

Size

- Microscopic only: 50-1,000 μm

MICROSCOPIC PATHOLOGY

Histologic Features

- Widely scattered throughout gland
- Small foci, centered on one or a few adjacent follicles
- Follicle contains aggregates of foamy histiocytes, a few lymphocytes/plasma cells, and occasional multinucleated giant cells

PALPATION THYROIDITIS

Key Facts

Terminology

- Microscopic granulomatous foci centered on thyroid follicles

Clinical Issues

- Likely caused by vigorous, repeated manipulation of thyroid gland preoperatively
  - Usually a nodule present that precipitated palpation in the first place
- Prominent in **completion thyroidectomy** specimens

Microscopic Pathology

- Widely scattered throughout gland
- Small foci, centered on one or a few adjacent follicles
- Follicle contains foamy histiocytes, lymphocytes/plasma cells, and multinucleated giant cells
  - Generally no follicular epithelium

Top Differential Diagnoses

- Hashimoto thyroiditis, subacute thyroiditis, infectious thyroiditis, sarcoidosis, FNA

  - Called "micro-granulomas"
  - No neutrophils
  - No necrosis
  - Generally no follicular epithelium
- Ruptured follicles, associated with minimal fibrosis
- Much more prominent in **completion thyroidectomy** specimens
- **Important**: Clinically significant disorders are usually present
  - Nodules, neoplasms

DIFFERENTIAL DIAGNOSIS

Chronic Lymphocytic (Hashimoto) Thyroiditis

- Affects entire gland
- Oncocytic epithelium within nodules
- Lymphocytes, plasma cells, germinal centers
- Generally no follicle destruction

Subacute Thyroiditis (de Quervain)

- Larger aggregates of follicle-centered granulomas
- Early phase: Neutrophils and histiocytes are present with large areas of involvement
  - Necrosis may be present, although not frequent
- Later stages: Fibrosis is prominent with foreign-body type giant cells

Infectious Thyroiditis

- Specifically tuberculosis, fungal organisms, syphilis
- Much more prominent granulomatous inflammation affecting more tissue
- May have necrosis (caseating granuloma)
- Organisms can be identified with special studies (histochemistry, immunofluorescence, immunohistochemistry)

Sarcoidosis

- Interstitial aggregates
- Small, tight, compact granulomas
- Asteroid bodies and Schaumann bodies
- Usually part of systemic disease

Fine Needle Aspiration Changes

- History of fine needle aspiration (FNA)
- Hemosiderin, erythrocytes, and reactive fibrosis
- Linear process, often centered on nodule/tumor

SELECTED REFERENCES

1. Mai VQ et al: Palpation thyroiditis causing new-onset atrial fibrillation. Thyroid. 18(5):571-3, 2008
2. Harach HR: Palpation thyroiditis resembling C cell hyperplasia. Usefulness of immunohistochemistry in their differential diagnosis. Pathol Res Pract. 189(4):488-90, 1993
3. Harach HR et al: The pathology of granulomatous diseases of the thyroid gland. Sarcoidosis. 7(1):19-27, 1990
4. Hwang TS et al: Histopathologic study of the so called 'palpation thyroiditis'. J Korean Med Sci. 3(1):27-9, 1988
5. Carney JA et al: Palpation thyroiditis (multifocal granulomatour folliculitis). Am J Clin Pathol. 64(5):639-47, 1975

IMAGE GALLERY

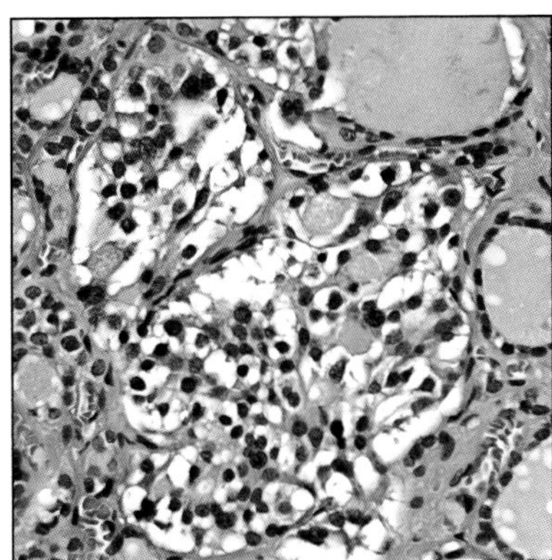

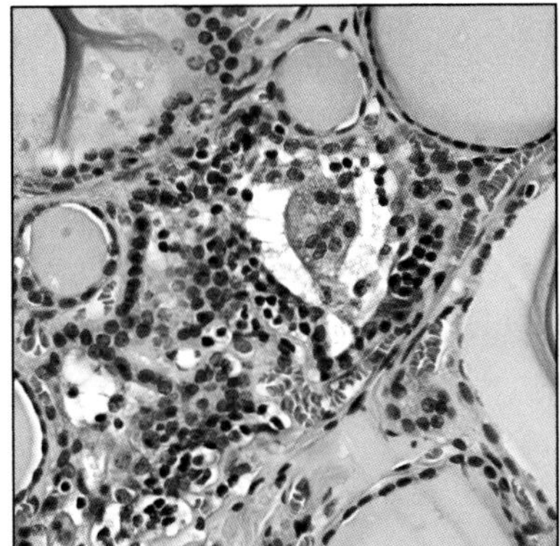

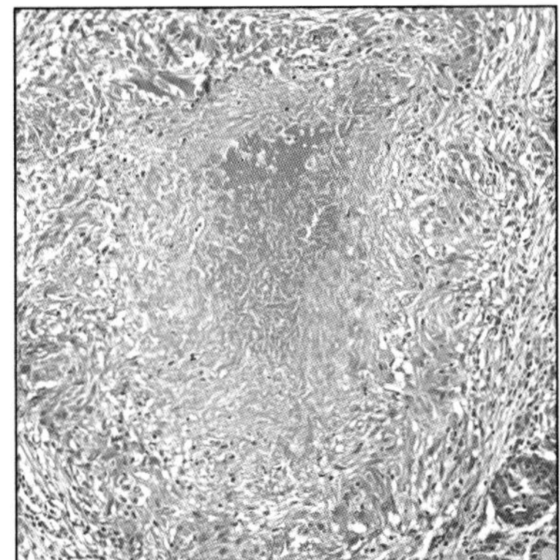

*(**Left**) Two adjacent follicles are destroyed and the follicle outline is now filled with lymphocytes and histiocytes. No residual follicular epithelium is present. (**Center**) These 2 follicles contain giant cells and lymphocytes, an isolated "micro-granuloma," commonly seen in palpation thyroiditis. (**Right**) Caseating granulomatous inflammation with a peripheral palisade of epithelioid histiocytes has completely effaced the follicular epithelium. This is an example of tuberculosis, one of the differential diagnostic considerations.*

SUBACUTE GRANULOMATOUS THYROIDITIS (DE QUERVAIN)

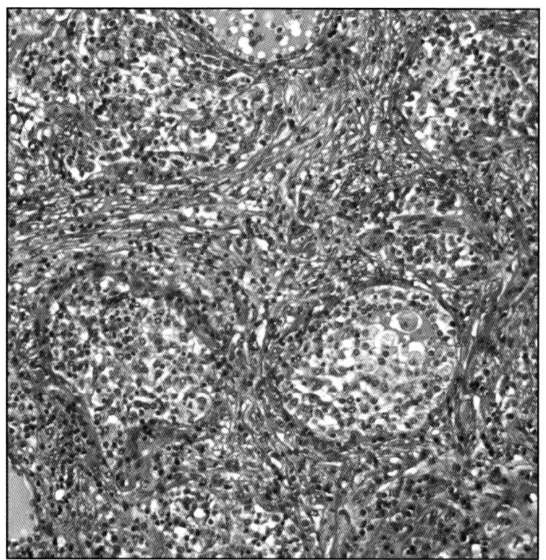

Multiple follicles are affected by a mixed inflammatory infiltrate, including histiocytes and neutrophils. There is a background of interfollicular fibrosis. This early stage shows the folliculocentric process.

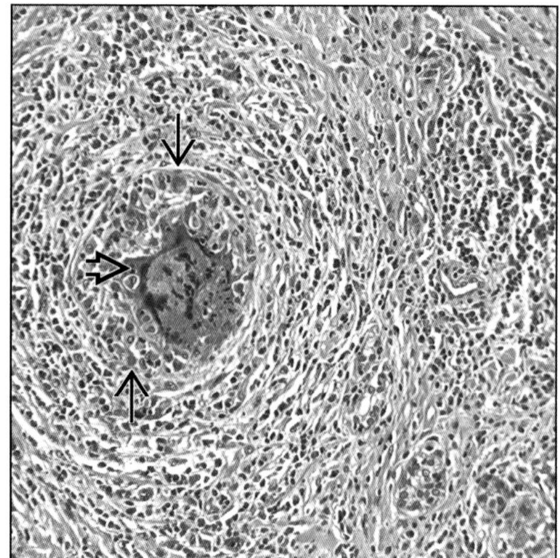

The mixed inflammatory infiltrate shows lymphocytes surrounding a destroyed follicle ➡, filled with epithelioid histiocytes and multinucleated giant cells ➡ with neutrophils. Fibrosis is also seen.

TERMINOLOGY

Abbreviations

- Subacute granulomatous thyroiditis (SGT)

Synonyms

- Subacute thyroiditis
- Granulomatous thyroiditis
- de Quervain thyroiditis
- Painful subacute thyroiditis
- Postviral thyroiditis
- Giant cell thyroiditis
- Subacute nonsuppurative thyroiditis
- Pseudotuberculous thyroiditis
- Struma granulomatosa

Definitions

- Self-limited inflammatory condition characterized by epithelioid histiocytes, multinucleated giant cells, and acute inflammatory cells (at certain times in disease development)
  - Requires clinicopathologic correlation with known systemic disease
  - Granulomatous inflammation can be seen in patients with tuberculosis, fungal infections, sarcoidosis

ETIOLOGY/PATHOGENESIS

Infectious

- Systemic viral infection most common
  - Common prodromal signs and symptoms
  - Intrathyroidal activated T-cytotoxic cells with interferon γ positive lymphocytes
  - Incidence highest in summer months, coincident with enteroviral infections
  - Associated with mumps, influenza, Coxsackie adenovirus, and measles epidemics
  - However, a significant number of patients do not have viral infection
- Develops after antiviral therapy, specifically interferon

Inherited

- Genetic predisposition suggested
  - Increased frequency in patients with HLA-B35 haplotype

Autoimmune

- Possible autoimmune component, as there are thyroid autoantibodies in a few patients

CLINICAL ISSUES

Epidemiology

- Incidence
  - Incidence approximately 5 per 100,000 population per year
  - Suggested seasonal increase in spring and summer
- Age
  - Wide range
    - Peak: 5th decade
  - Rare in children
- Gender
  - Female > > Male (3.5:1)

Site

- Entire gland usually involved
  - May be localized to 1 lobe or a distinct nodule

Presentation

- Prodrome heralds disease
  - Low-grade fever, myalgias, fatigue, sore throat
- Painful thyroid gland is most common symptom
  - SGT is most common cause of painful thyroid
  - May radiate to jaw
  - Tender to palpation
  - Some patients may not have pain or tenderness
- Frequently presents with hyperthyroidism

SUBACUTE GRANULOMATOUS THYROIDITIS (DE QUERVAIN)

Key Facts

Terminology
- Self-limited inflammatory condition characterized by epithelioid histiocytes, multinucleated giant cells, and acute inflammatory cells

Clinical Issues
- Female > > Male (3.5:1)
- Entire gland usually involved
- Painful thyroid gland is most common symptom
- Frequently presents with hyperthyroidism
- Spontaneous return to normal function in most patients within 12 months
- Thyroid function varies during disease arc
- Supportive therapy is treatment of choice

Microscopic Pathology
- Asymmetric enlargement with tan to yellow-white ill-defined nodules
- Inflammatory process unevenly affects entire gland
- Topographic and temporal variation of histology depending on stage
- **Acute stage**: Folliculocentric, follicular damage, loss of epithelium and colloid, replaced by neutrophils
- **Mid stage**: Chronic inflammation, epithelioid histiocytes, multinucleated giant cells, fibrosis
- **Resolution stage**: Follicular tissue is regenerated, restoring normal structure

Top Differential Diagnoses
- Subacute lymphocytic thyroiditis, granulomatous thyroiditis, sarcoidosis, palpation thyroiditis

---

  - Rarely, may present with thyroid storm
- Become hypothyroid in ensuing weeks to months
- Spontaneous return to normal function in most patients within 12 months
  - ~ 7% have persistent hypothyroidism
- May have other symptoms, including
  - Dysphagia, arthralgia, tremor, excessive sweating, weight loss

Laboratory Tests
- Thyroid function varies during disease arc
  - **Early phase**: May be hyperthyroid due to follicle destruction and release of hormone
    - TSH is suppressed; T4 and T3 are elevated
  - **Mid phase**: Become hypothyroid after follicles are destroyed
  - **Late phase**: Regain euthyroid after disease resolution
  - Few patients may have transient elevation of antibodies to thyroglobulin or thyroperoxidase
- C-reactive protein and erythrocyte sedimentation rate are usually elevated

Natural History
- Self-limited disease
- Resolves in several months
- Rarely, may recur years later

Treatment
- Options, risks, complications
  - Supportive therapy
    - Nonsteroidal anti-inflammatory drugs
    - Aspirin contraindicated as it displaces thyroid hormone from thyroid-binding globulin
    - Steroids (such as prednisone) for more severe symptoms
    - β-blocking agents (like propranolol) if thyrotoxicosis is present
  - Surgery is not necessary

Prognosis
- Self-limiting disease
  - Resolves within several months
- Infrequently (~ 2%), recurrence may develop, often years after initial episode
- Approximately 7% of patients remain permanently hypothyroid
- Rarely, chronic lymphocytic thyroiditis or Graves disease may develop

IMAGE FINDINGS

Radiographic Findings
- Best radiographic clue is very low thyroid radioactive iodine uptake in clinically hyperthyroid patient
  - Acute phase: Radioactive iodine uptake is very low (< 1% at 24 hours)
  - Uptake will improve with recovery

Ultrasonographic Findings
- Acute phase: Hypoechoic with nonechoic regions secondary to inflammation and tissue damage
- Recovery phase: Isoechoic with slightly increased vascularity

MACROSCOPIC FEATURES

General Features
- Asymmetric enlargement (usually 2x) with vague nodularity
- Tan to yellow-white ill-defined nodules
- Somewhat firm consistency

MICROSCOPIC PATHOLOGY

Histologic Features
- Inflammatory process unevenly affects entire gland
  - Nodular, even though whole gland is affected
  - Few cases have solitary nodule
- Topographic and temporal variation of histology depending on stage

SUBACUTE GRANULOMATOUS THYROIDITIS (DE QUERVAIN)

- Inflammatory infiltrate composed of lymphocytes, plasma cells, foamy histiocytes, epithelioid histiocytes, multinucleated giant cells, neutrophils
- Variable background of fibrosis
- Zones of active inflammation coexist with areas of fibrosis as inflammatory process migrates to previously unaffected parenchyma

- **Early stage** (acute; hyperthyroidism)
  - Folliculocentric, with follicular damage and loss of epithelium and colloid
  - Groups of follicles filled with mixed inflammatory cells
    - Neutrophils predominant, occasionally forming microabscesses
  - Inflammation (predominantly lymphohistiocytic) expands into adjacent interfollicular zones
- **Mid stage** (hypothyroidism)
  - Chronic inflammation
    - Lymphocytes, plasma cells
  - Epithelioid and nonepithelioid macrophages and multinucleated giant cells (histiocytic)
    - Giant cells adjacent to or within disrupted follicles
    - Giant cells may surround and engulf residual colloid
    - Well-formed granulomata are not seen
  - Variable degrees of fibrosis
  - Follicular epithelium may be difficult to detect, as it has been destroyed
- **Late stage** (resolution; recovery)
  - Fibrosis replaces destroyed follicles
  - Follicular tissue is regenerated, restoring normal structure
  - Fibrosis and inflammatory infiltrate resolves

ANCILLARY TESTS

Cytology

- FNA seldom requested, except in pain-free patients
- Mixture of lymphocytes, plasma cells, foamy and epithelioid histiocytes, multinucleated giant cells
- Neutrophils may be prominent in early phase
- Giant cells may contain colloid fragments
- Colloid and degenerated follicular epithelial cells usually scant (especially early phase)
  - Oncocytic follicular cells are absent

DIFFERENTIAL DIAGNOSIS

Subacute Lymphocytic Thyroiditis

- Also called postpartum lymphocytic thyroiditis
  - 1-6 months after delivery
- Painless and clinically silent
- Thought to be autoimmune mediated
  - Perhaps a variant of Hashimoto thyroiditis
- Lymphoid follicles with germinal centers
  - Not seen in SGT

Granulomatous Thyroiditis

- Well-formed granuloma
  - Ring of epithelioid histiocytes around area of central caseating necrosis
- Infectious agents should be excluded
  - Special studies for mycobacteria &/or fungi

Sarcoidosis

- Usually found in interstitium
  - Not folliculocentric
- Small, compact aggregates of epithelioid histiocytes
- Giant cells may be present
- Necrosis tends to be absent

Palpation Thyroiditis

- Affects one to a few follicles
  - May be distributed throughout gland
- No neutrophils
- Multinucleated giant cells a constant feature

SELECTED REFERENCES

1. Desailloud R et al: Viruses and thyroiditis: an update. Virol J. 6:5, 2009
2. Sarkar SD: Benign thyroid disease: what is the role of nuclear medicine? Semin Nucl Med. 36(3):185-93, 2006
3. Mori K et al: [Subacute thyroiditis and silent thyroiditis.] Nippon Rinsho. 63 Suppl 10:122-6, 2005
4. Cooper DS: Hyperthyroidism. Lancet. 362(9382):459-68, 2003
5. Ogawa E et al: Subacute thyroiditis in children: patient report and review of the literature. J Pediatr Endocrinol Metab. 16(6):897-900, 2003
6. Duininck TM et al: de Quervain's thyroiditis: surgical experience. Endocr Pract. 8(4):255-8, 2002
7. Slatosky J et al: Thyroiditis: differential diagnosis and management. Am Fam Physician. 61(4):1047-52, 1054, 2000
8. Summaria V et al: Diagnostic imaging in thyrotoxicosis. Rays. 24(2):273-300, 1999
9. Ross DS: Syndromes of thyrotoxicosis with low radioactive iodine uptake. Endocrinol Metab Clin North Am. 27(1):169-85, 1998
10. García Solano J et al: Fine-needle aspiration of subacute granulomatous thyroiditis (De Quervain's thyroiditis): a clinico-cytologic review of 36 cases. Diagn Cytopathol. 16(3):214-20, 1997
11. Walfish PG: Thyroiditis. Curr Ther Endocrinol Metab. 6:117-22, 1997
12. Farwell AP et al: Inflammatory thyroid disorders. Otolaryngol Clin North Am. 29(4):541-56, 1996
13. Schubert MF et al: Thyroiditis. A disease with many faces. Postgrad Med. 98(2):101-3, 107-8, 112, 1995
14. Volpé R: The management of subacute (DeQuervain's) thyroiditis. Thyroid. 3(3):253-5, 1993
15. Harach HR et al: The pathology of granulomatous diseases of the thyroid gland. Sarcoidosis. 7(1):19-27, 1990
16. Felicetta JV. Painful et al: Distinct entities or merely variants? Postgrad Med. 86(5):269-72, 277, 1989
17. Hwang SC et al: Subacute thyroiditis--61 cases review. Zhonghua Yi Xue Za Zhi (Taipei). 43(2):113-8, 1989
18. Hamburger JI: The various presentations of thyroiditis. Diagnostic considerations. Ann Intern Med. 104(2):219-24, 1986
19. Hay ID: Thyroiditis: a clinical update. Mayo Clin Proc. 60(12):836-43, 1985
20. Volpé R: Subacute (de Quervain's) thyroiditis. Clin Endocrinol Metab. 8(1):81-95, 1979
21. de Pauw BE et al: De Quervain's subacute thyroiditis. A report on 14 cases and a review of the literature. Neth J Med. 18(2):70-8, 1975

Radiographic and Microscopic Features

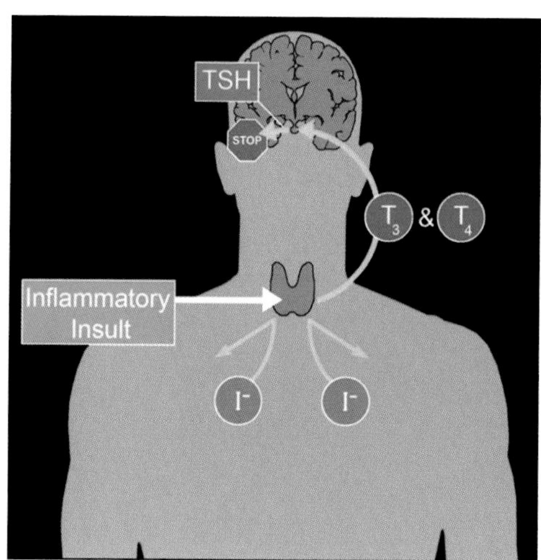

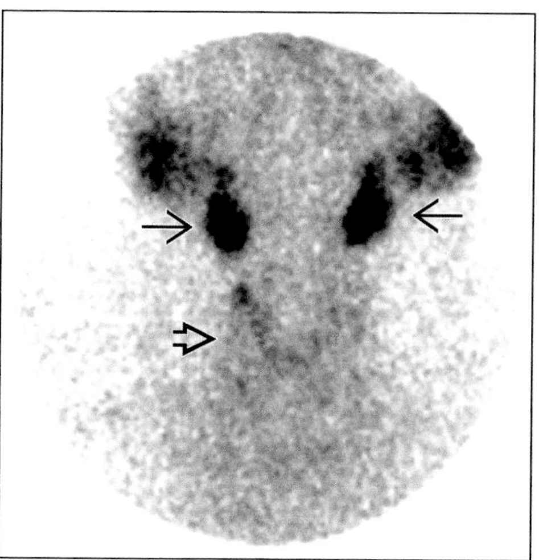

(Left) *This is a graphic representation of the biochemical pathway seen in subacute thyroiditis. The inflammatory insult results in a release of T4, which causes a negative feedback inhibition of pituitary TSH release.* ***(Right)*** *One of the best radiographic clues to the diagnosis is a very low thyroid radioactive iodine uptake (< 1% at 24 hours) in a clinically hyperthyroid patient (acute phase). This anterior thyroid scan shows nearly absent thyroid activity ⇨ with normal salivary activity →.*

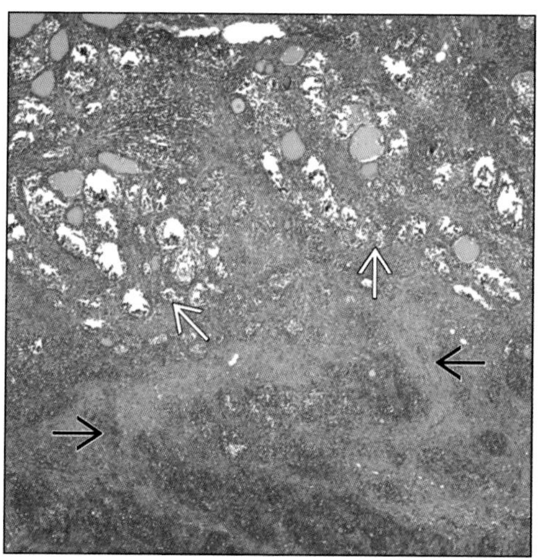

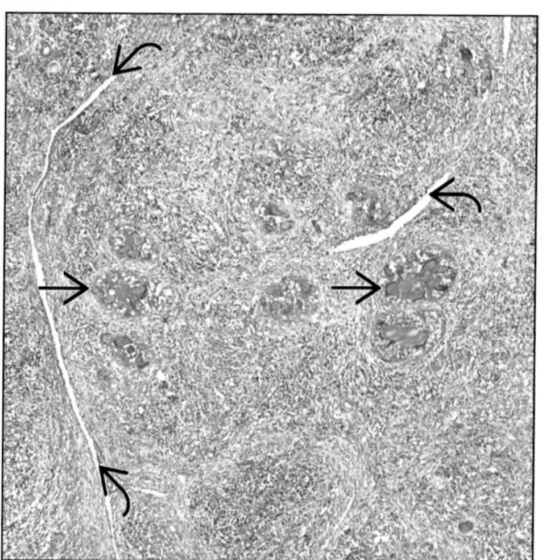

(Left) *A nodule of fibrosis → is immediately adjacent to a zone of active inflammation →. The coexistence of temporally different zones (fibrosis vs. active disease) is due to migration of the inflammatory process to previously unaffected regions.* ***(Right)*** *This whole area is affected by the inflammatory reaction. Fibrosis is noted, along with dilated lymphatics ↷. There are groups of histiocytes filling destroyed follicles, with multinucleated giant cells engulfing colloid →.*

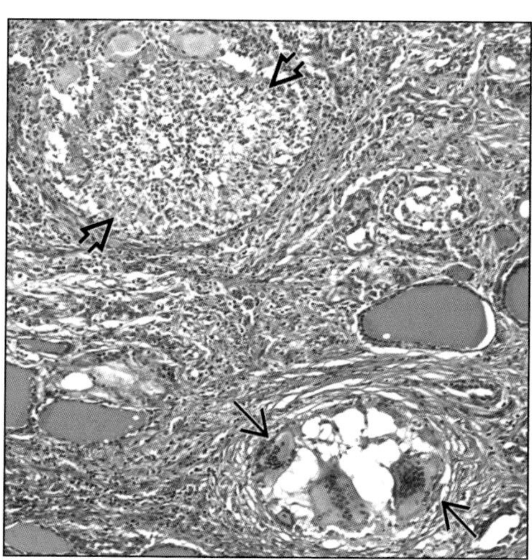

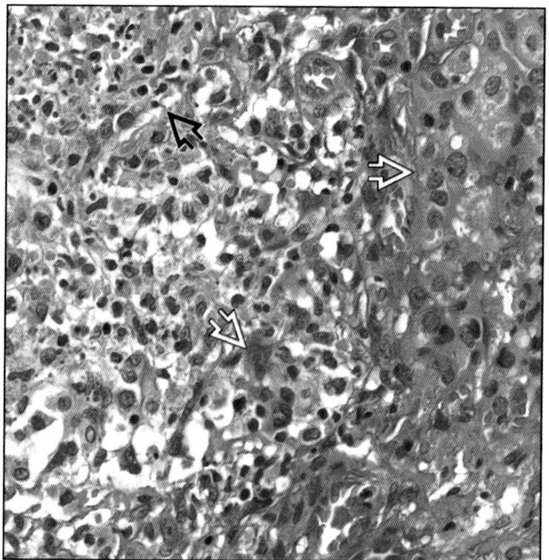

(Left) *A topographic separation of temporally distinctive processes is shown: Acute stage shows a destroyed follicle filled with neutrophils (microabscess ⇨); mid stage shows multinucleated giant cells within a follicle →. Fibrosis is noted between the 2 regions.* ***(Right)*** *High power shows a follicle with neutrophils and debris ⇨ surrounded by foamy histiocytes and epithelioid histiocytes ⇨. No colloid or follicular epithelium is present.*

CHRONIC LYMPHOCYTIC (HASHIMOTO) THYROIDITIS

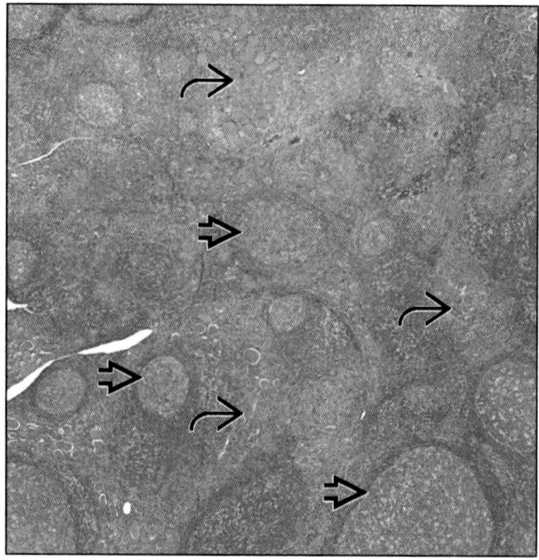

Diffuse involvement of the thyroid gland by a prominent lymphocytic infiltrate including associated germinal centers ➪ is seen in and around the residual thyroid parenchyma ↗.

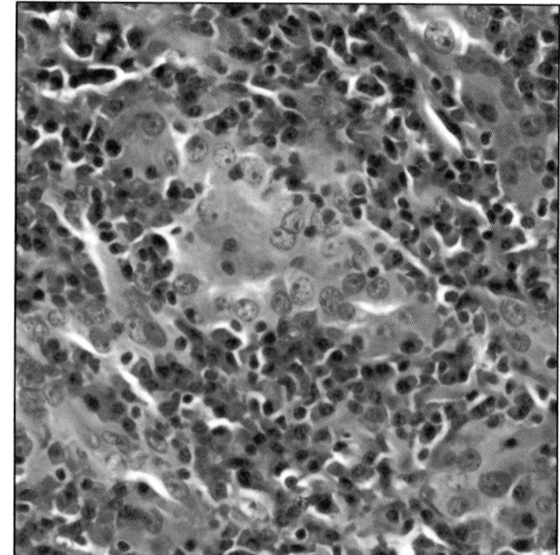

Oncocytic metaplasia may include nuclear atypia that can be misdiagnosed as papillary carcinoma. Nuclei are enlarged but lack the constellation of nuclear alterations seen in papillary carcinoma.

TERMINOLOGY

Abbreviations

- Hashimoto thyroiditis (HT)
- Lymphocytic thyroiditis (LT)

Synonyms

- Struma lymphomatosa
- Classic form of autoimmune thyroiditis
- Lymphadenoid goiter

Definitions

- Autoimmune thyroiditis characterized by
  - Infiltration by inflammatory cells
  - Production of autoantibodies to thyroid-specific antigens and thyroglobulin
  - Hypothyroidism due to destruction and eventual fibrous replacement of follicular epithelial cells

ETIOLOGY/PATHOGENESIS

Autoimmunity

- Autoimmune thyroid diseases (AITD) include HT and Graves disease
  - Complex diseases caused by interaction between susceptibility genes and environmental triggers
- Precise antigen(s) causing autosensitization are unknown
  - Presence of antithyroglobulin and antimicrosomal antibodies suggest these antigens are involved
- Patients with HT at greater risk of having other coexisting autoimmune diseases including
  - Endocrine disease
    - Insulin-dependent diabetes mellitus
    - Addison disease
    - Autoimmune oophoritis
    - Hypoparathyroidism and hypophysitis
  - Nonendocrine disease
    - Sjögren syndrome
    - Myasthenia gravis
    - Pernicious anemia
    - Thrombocytopenic purpura
  - Compared to matched controls, patients with AITD show higher prevalence of autoantibody against
    - Thyroid-specific antigens
    - Non-thyroid-specific antigens
- HT and Graves disease share common features including
  - Aggregation of both conditions in same families or within same thyroid gland
    - e.g., identical twins in which 1 twin has HT and other has Graves disease
  - Lymphocytic infiltration and various immunoglobulins found within thyroid in both disorders
  - Thymic enlargement and thyroid autoantibodies found in both diseases
  - Graves disease may evolve into Hashimoto thyroiditis with hypothyroidism
  - Rarely, HT (± hypothyroidism) may evolve into Graves disease with hyperthyroidism
- In spite of shared features, sufficient differences (genetic, clinical, immunologic, pathologic) to consider HT and Graves as distinctly different

CLINICAL ISSUES

Epidemiology

- Incidence
  - Primary hypothyroidism is common
    - Population-based surveys reveal presence in 5% of individuals
    - Most common cause is autoimmune (Hashimoto) thyroiditis
  - **Fibrous variant**
    - Occurs in approximately 10% of cases of HT
- Age
  - **"Classic" type**

CHRONIC LYMPHOCYTIC (HASHIMOTO) THYROIDITIS

Key Facts

Terminology
- Autoimmune thyroiditis characterized by
  - Infiltration by inflammatory cells
  - Production of autoantibodies to thyroid-specific antigens and thyroglobulin
  - Hypothyroidism due to destruction and eventual fibrous replacement of follicular epithelial cells

Clinical Issues
- "Classic" type: Wide variation in clinical features
  - Many patients present with no signs or symptoms with diagnosis made on basis of
  - Laboratory tests of thyroid function
  - Screening done for thyroid antibodies
  - Patients may present with mass lesion (goiter)
- **Fibrous variant**
  - Symptoms of large goiter that may produce dysphagia and dyspnea

Microscopic Pathology
- **"Classic" type**
  - Diffuse involvement of thyroid gland
  - Mature lymphocytic cell infiltrate ± germinal centers
  - Oncocytic cytoplasmic change of follicular epithelial cells
- **Fibrous variant**
  - Presence of nodular or lobular pattern of growth with associated dense fibrosis
  - Inflammatory cell infiltrate includes mature lymphocytes as well as plasma cells
  - Follicular epithelial changes include follicular atrophy, oncocytic cytoplasmic changes

    - Occurs over wide range
    - Frequency increases with age
    - Most common cause of goiter and acquired hypothyroidism in children and adolescents in iodine-replete areas
  - **Fibrous variant**
    - Occurs in older patients
- Gender
  - **"Classic" type**
    - Female > > > Male (10:1)
  - **Fibrous variant**
    - Male > Female

Site
- No specific localization or lateralization

Presentation
- **"Classic" type**
  - Wide variation in clinical features
    - In some patients, enlarged thyroid only clinical manifestation of autoimmune thyroiditis
    - In many patients, clinical evidence of hypothyroidism present
  - Many patients present with no signs or symptoms, with diagnosis made on basis of
    - Laboratory tests of thyroid function
    - Screening done for thyroid antibodies
    - Incidental finding in thyroid glands surgically excised for other reasons
  - Patients may present with mass (goiter)
    - Typically there is bilateral diffuse enlargement of thyroid
    - Infrequently, dominant mass lesion confined to 1 lobe of thyroid may be seen simulating neoplastic proliferation
- **Fibrous variant**
  - Patients present with symptoms of large goiter that may produce dysphagia and dyspnea

Laboratory Tests
- **"Classic" type**
  - Laboratory evidence of hypothyroidism may include
    - Decreased thyroxine (T4) and possibly decreased triiodothyronine (T3) (although latter may be normal)
  - Laboratory evidence of autoimmune thyroiditis includes circulating antibodies to
    - Thyroglobulin
    - Thyroid peroxidase (microsomal antigen)
    - Colloid antigen
    - Thyroid hormones
  - With progression of disease, patients who are not hypothyroid at presentation may develop evidence of hypothyroidism at later time
  - Patients may be euthyroid
  - Rarely patients are hyperthyroid
- **Fibrous variant**
  - Patients often present with severe hypothyroidism
    - High titers of antithyroglobulin antibodies

Treatment
- Options, risks, complications
  - T4 therapy is treatment of choice for all patients with hypothyroidism (overt or subclinical) as result of autoimmune thyroiditis
    - Treatment is generally lifelong, as hypothyroidism will recur with cessation of thyroxine
    - Proper response to T4 therapy will include decrease in levels of thyroid antibodies
  - Immunosuppressive (corticosteroid) therapy may result in regression of thyroid enlargement and decrease in thyroid antibody levels
    - Due to serious side effects of steroids and efficacy of thyroxine therapy, immunosuppressive therapy not indicated
  - Appropriate therapy for patients who are euthyroid but have enlarged glands (goiter) remains uncertain
    - T4 administration may result in decrease in size of gland
    - In other patients there may be progressive enlargement of thyroid
    - Further, up to 10-15% of patients may become hypothyroid

CHRONIC LYMPHOCYTIC (HASHIMOTO) THYROIDITIS

- Complications of thyroxine therapy limited to iatrogenic thyrotoxicosis
  - Patients with thyrotoxicosis should be treated accordingly
- Surgical approaches
  - Surgery can be used in patients
    - Who do not respond to thyroxine therapy
    - Who have continued enlargement (with or without local symptoms) of thyroid gland

Prognosis

- Generally considered to be good
- Complications include potential development of malignant neoplasm, including
  - Hematolymphoid malignancy (lymphoma or leukemia)
  - Follicular epithelial-derived tumors, including thyroid papillary carcinoma and follicular carcinoma
- No increased risk of developing thyroid neuroendocrine neoplasm (medullary carcinoma)

IMAGE FINDINGS

Radiographic Findings

- Normal glandular enlargement or diffuse abnormality with heterogeneous echogenicity
- MRI T2WI show areas of increased signal intensity
- In fibrous variant, gland may appear atrophied and fibrotic resulting in heterogeneous echotexture

MACROSCOPIC FEATURES

General Features

- **"Classic" type**
  - Symmetrically enlarged gland
    - Firm consistency, pale in color and characterized by prominent multilobulated appearance; lobules tend to bulge from cut surface and are separated by fibrous tissue
    - Diffuse thyroid enlargement, as compared to single dominant mass, assists in decreasing clinical suspicion for neoplastic proliferation
    - Thyroid not adherent to surrounding structures
- **Fibrous variant**
  - Diffusely enlarged, firm to hard, pale tan-appearing thyroid characterized by
    - Presence of fibrosis and prominent lobular appearance
  - Thyroid glands may weigh as much as 200 grams or more
  - Thyroid not adherent to surrounding structures

MICROSCOPIC PATHOLOGY

Histologic Features

- **"Classic" type**
  - Diffuse involvement of thyroid gland
  - Mature lymphocytic infiltrate ± germinal centers
  - Oncocytic cytoplasmic change of follicular epithelial cells characterized by
    - Eosinophilic granular-appearing cytoplasm
    - Nuclear enlargement
    - Clear to coarse-appearing chromatin
    - Nuclei retain round appearance
    - Prominent nucleoli
  - Squamous metaplasia and solid cell nests may be present
- **Lymphoepithelial cysts**
  - Part of spectrum of changes associated with chronic lymphocytic thyroiditis
  - Represent secondary changes (e.g., squamous metaplastic foci with cystic change)
  - Usually incidental findings
  - Occasionally may attain large sizes presenting as thyroid mass
  - Often multifocal and bilateral
  - Predominantly lined by squamous epithelium consisting of one or multiple layers of cells
  - Columnar cell (respiratory-type) epithelium can be seen, possibly containing goblet cells
- **Fibrous variant**
  - Also referred to as advanced lymphocytic thyroiditis
  - Presence of nodular or lobular pattern of growth with associated dense fibrosis
    - Fibrosis is keloid-like with irregular broad bands of acellular fibrous tissue coursing in and around remnant of thyroid parenchyma
    - Fibrosis does not extend outside gland
    - Chronic inflammatory cell infiltrate can be seen within fibrotic tissue
  - Mature lymphocytic infiltrate ± germinal centers
    - Inflammatory cell infiltrate includes mature lymphocytes as well as plasma cells
  - Follicular epithelial changes include
    - Follicular atrophy
    - Oncocytic cytoplasmic changes
    - Squamous metaplasia may be prominently seen

ANCILLARY TESTS

Cytology

- **"Classic" type**
  - Mixed inflammatory cell infiltrate including mature lymphocytes and plasma cells
  - Multinucleated giant cells may be present
  - Presence of germinal centers may be reflected by variety of lymphocytes and tingible body macrophages
  - Follicular epithelial cells may show oxyphilic cytoplasmic changes
    - Usually appear in cohesive clusters but may appear as single cells
  - Minimal to absent colloid
- **Fibrous variant**
  - Due to marked fibrosis, aspiration generally yields very little material

Immunohistochemistry

- Reactivity for both B-cell (CD20 [L26]) and T-cell (CD45RO [UCHL-1] or CD3) markers
- B-cells and plasma cells exhibit
  - κ and λ staining (i.e., lack light chain restriction)

- Exhibit IgG, IgM, and IgA heavy chains
- B-cells most often of IgG κ type

Cytogenetics

- Molecular studies show absence of *BRAF* point mutation
  - Present in 35-69% of thyroid papillary carcinoma
- Absence of gene rearrangements
- Reports of *RET/PTC* rearrangements, even in absence of morphologic findings diagnostic for thyroid papillary carcinoma
  - Coupled with reports showing purported immunohistochemical features of papillary carcinoma, suggest possibility of early focal premalignant transformation
  - Despite above findings, from practical perspective absence of nuclear features reaching diagnostic level for papillary carcinoma preclude diagnosis
  - Concept of early focal premalignant transformation remains unproven

DIFFERENTIAL DIAGNOSIS

Nonspecific Chronic Lymphocytic Thyroiditis

- Non-mass-forming
- Incidental finding in thyroid excised for other reasons
- Scattered but limited foci of lymphocytic infiltrate
- Typically, absence of oncocytic cytoplasmic changes of follicular cells
- Absence of laboratory evidence of abnormal thyroid function

Non-Hodgkin Malignant Lymphoma

- Effacement of thyroid parenchyma with
  - Destruction of follicular epithelium
  - Presence of lymphoepithelial lesions characterized by "packing" or "stuffing" of follicles with neoplastic cells
- Monomorphic malignant cellular infiltrate
  - Majority are of B-cell origin
- Malignant cellular infiltrate often "spills out" into perithyroidal soft tissues
  - Thyroid may be adherent to surrounding structures

Thyroid Papillary Carcinoma

- Alterations of follicular epithelium in HT may raise concern for diagnosis of papillary carcinoma
- Constellation of diagnostic nuclear features identified
- Presence of *BRAF* mutation present in 35-69% of cases of thyroid papillary carcinoma
  - Absence of *BRAF* point mutation in thyroid follicular epithelium in HT

Riedel Disease (Invasive Fibrous Thyroiditis)

- Differential diagnosis with fibrous variant of lymphocytic thyroiditis
- Fibrosis outside thyroid gland often adherent to surrounding structures
- Lacks high titers of antithyroglobulin antibodies
- Histology includes
  - Destruction and replacement of thyroid parenchyma by dense keloid-like fibrosis
    - Not confined to thyroid but also involves extrathyroidal soft tissues
    - Atrophic changes of follicular epithelium
    - Not associated with oxyphilic metaplasia of follicular epithelial cells
  - Chronic inflammatory infiltrate predominantly composed of lymphocytes and plasma cells
  - Vasculitis primarily involving veins (phlebitis)

Nodal Tissue

- Histology of HT may simulate appearance of nodal architecture
  - In this setting, presence of thyroid tissue may raise concern for metastatic thyroid carcinoma
- Lymph nodes characterized by
  - Presence of subcapsular sinuses
    - Subcapsular sinuses absent in HT
  - Nuclear features in HT not diagnostic for papillary carcinoma

SELECTED REFERENCES

1. Anil C et al: Hashimoto's thyroiditis is not associated with increased risk of thyroid cancer in patients with thyroid nodules: a single-center prospective study. Thyroid. 20(6):601-6, 2010
2. Sadow PM et al: Absence of BRAF, NRAS, KRAS, HRAS mutations, and RET/PTC gene rearrangements distinguishes dominant nodules in Hashimoto thyroiditis from papillary thyroid carcinomas. Endocr Pathol. 21(2):73-9, 2010
3. Haberal AN et al: Diagnostic pitfalls in the evaluation of fine needle aspiration cytology of the thyroid: correlation with histopathology in 260 cases. Cytopathology. 20(2):103-8, 2009
4. Nasr MR et al: Absence of the BRAF mutation in HBME1+ and CK19+ atypical cell clusters in Hashimoto thyroiditis: supportive evidence against preneoplastic change. Am J Clin Pathol. 132(6):906-12, 2009
5. Burek CL et al: Autoimmune thyroiditis and ROS. Autoimmun Rev. 7(7):530-7, 2008
6. Shih ML et al: Thyroidectomy for Hashimoto's thyroiditis: complications and associated cancers. Thyroid. 18(7):729-34, 2008
7. Caturegli P et al: Autoimmune thyroid diseases. Curr Opin Rheumatol. 19(1):44-8, 2007
8. Demirbilek H et al: Hashimoto's thyroiditis in children and adolescents: a retrospective study on clinical, epidemiological and laboratory properties of the disease. J Pediatr Endocrinol Metab. 20(11):1199-205, 2007
9. McLachlan SM et al: The link between Graves' disease and Hashimoto's thyroiditis: a role for regulatory T cells. Endocrinology. 148(12):5724-33, 2007
10. Aust G et al: Graves' disease and Hashimoto's thyroiditis in monozygotic twins: case study as well as transcriptomic and immunohistological analysis of thyroid tissues. Eur J Endocrinol. 154(1):13-20, 2006
11. Sargent R et al: BRAF mutation is unusual in chronic lymphocytic thyroiditis-associated papillary thyroid carcinomas and absent in non-neoplastic nuclear atypia of thyroiditis. Endocr Pathol. 17(3):235-41, 2006
12. MacDonald L et al: Fine needle aspiration biopsy of Hashimoto's thyroiditis. Sources of diagnostic error. Acta Cytol. 43(3):400-6, 1999

CHRONIC LYMPHOCYTIC (HASHIMOTO) THYROIDITIS

Imaging, Gross, and Microscopic Features

(Left) Axial CECT shows Hashimoto thyroiditis as diffuse enlargement of both thyroid lobes → and pyramidal lobe ⇨. **(Right)** Thyroid resection in patient with Hashimoto thyroiditis shows diffuse involvement of the gland with replacement of the normal thyroid parenchyma by tissue that appears light brown. Cut section shows a nodular appearance ⇨. Residual grossly normal-appearing thyroid tissue is present at the periphery →.

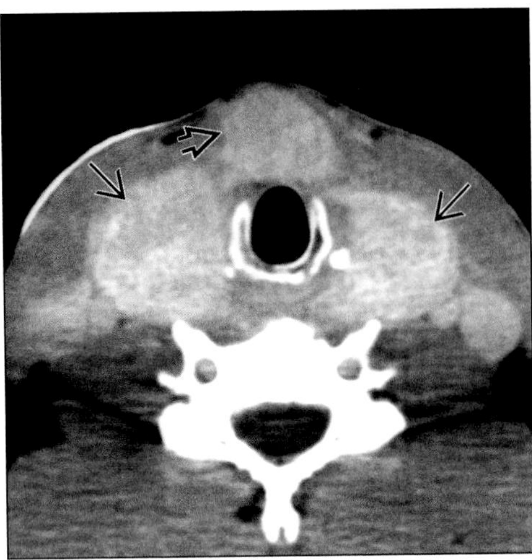

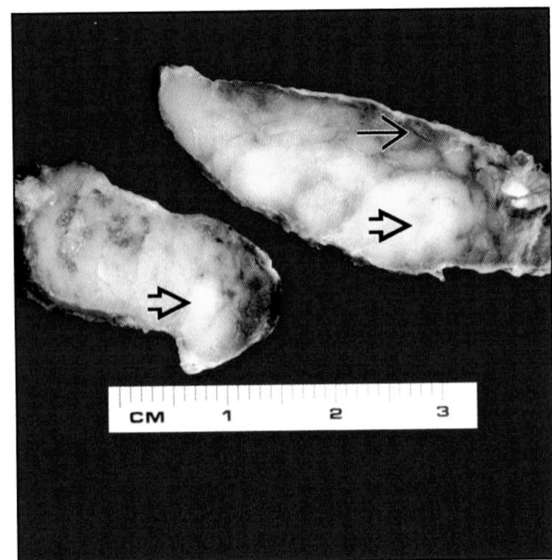

(Left) Fibrous variant of HT (advanced lymphocytic thyroiditis) shows a diffusely enlarged gland that is firm to hard with fibrosis and lobulated or nodular appearance. Due to marked fibrosis, aspiration generally yields very little material for diagnosis. **(Right)** Fibrous variant shows fibrous bands → creating a nodular appearance with lymphocytic infiltrate including germinal centers ⇨ overrunning the thyroid tissue. The fibrosis does not extend outside the gland.

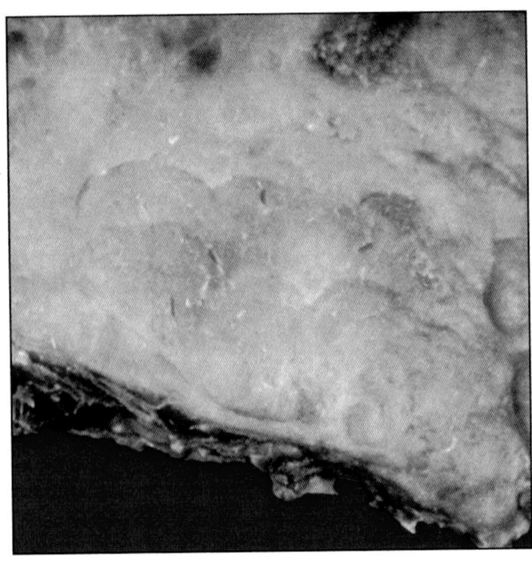

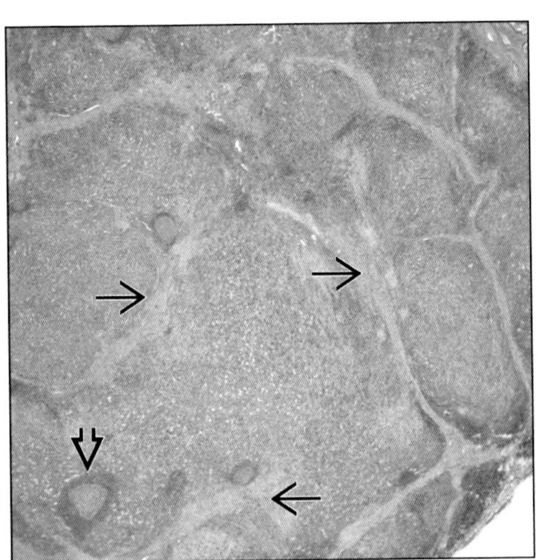

(Left) Cysts ⇨ may be present focally in the setting of HT. The cysts are usually incidental findings appearing small and indiscrete with associated lymphocytic infiltrate (lymphoepithelial cysts), but cysts occasionally may be large, representing a dominant lesion. **(Right)** The cyst is lined by columnar cell epithelium, including cilia ⇨. More often, the cysts seen in HT are predominantly lined by squamous epithelium composed of one or multiple layers of cells (not shown).

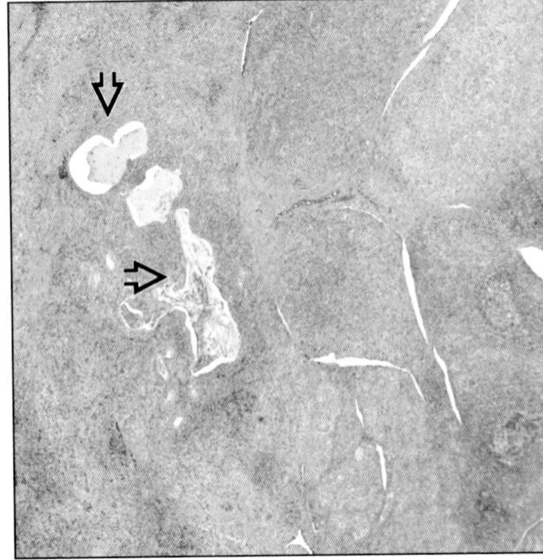

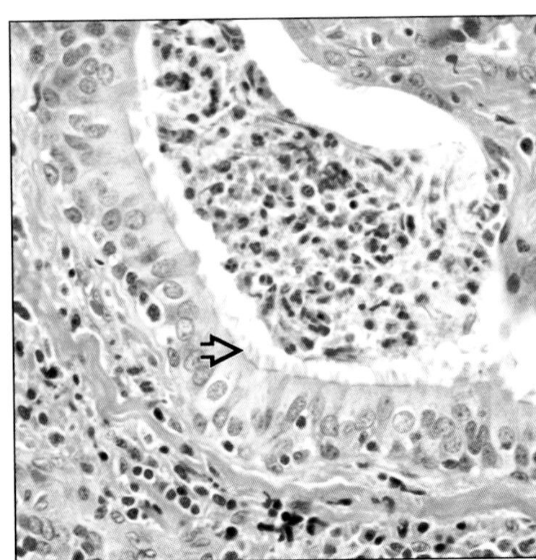

Microscopic and Cytologic Features

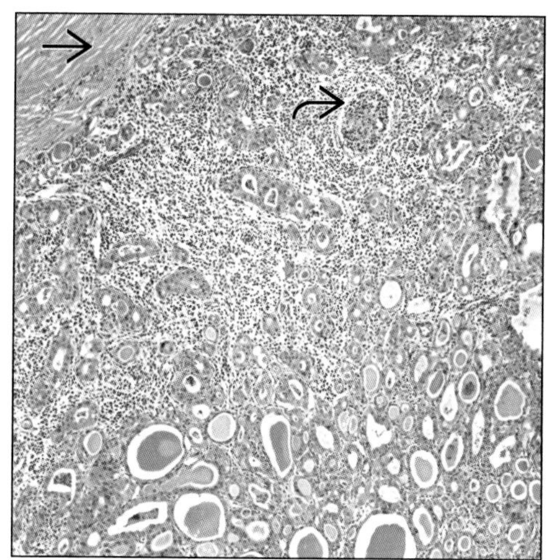

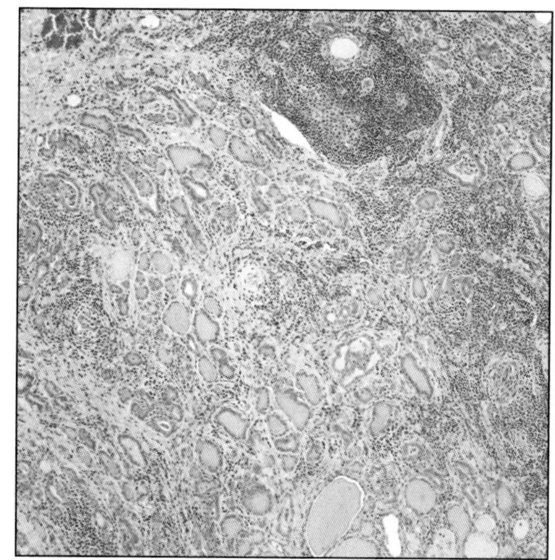

(Left) *A peripherally situated nodular focus composed of lymphocytic cells with germinal centers ⮳ surrounded by fibrous tissue → may simulate features of a lymph node. The absence of a subcapsular sinus and continuity/proximity to the gland proper should preclude misdiagnosis as metastatic carcinoma.* ***(Right)*** *Nonspecific lymphocytic thyroiditis, a rather common finding, shows limited (not diffuse) lymphocytic infiltrate without alterations of the follicular cells.*

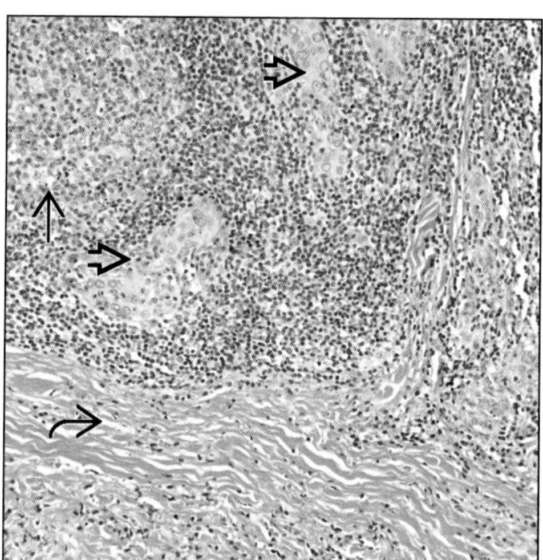

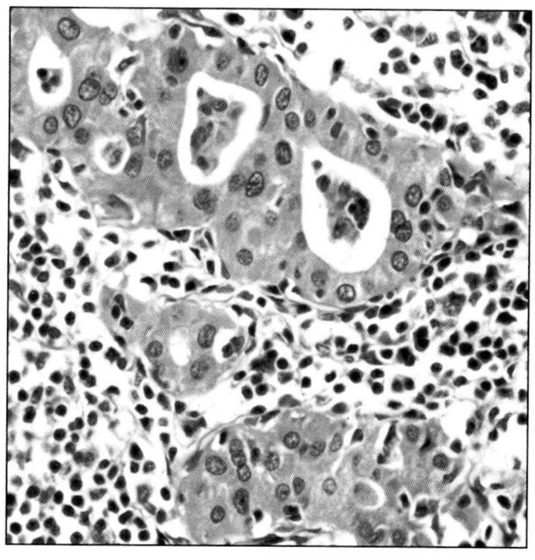

(Left) *Fibrous variant shows keloid-like fibrosis ⮳ with atrophic changes of follicular epithelium ⇨ overrun by a lymphocytic infiltrate; a portion of a germinal center is present →. In contrast to the fibrosis in Reidel disease, which extends outside the thyroid, the fibrosis in the fibrous variant of HT is confined within the thyroid.* ***(Right)*** *The follicular epithelial cells show brightly eosinophilic (oncocytic) cytoplasm with round and regular-appearing nuclei and coarse chromatin.*

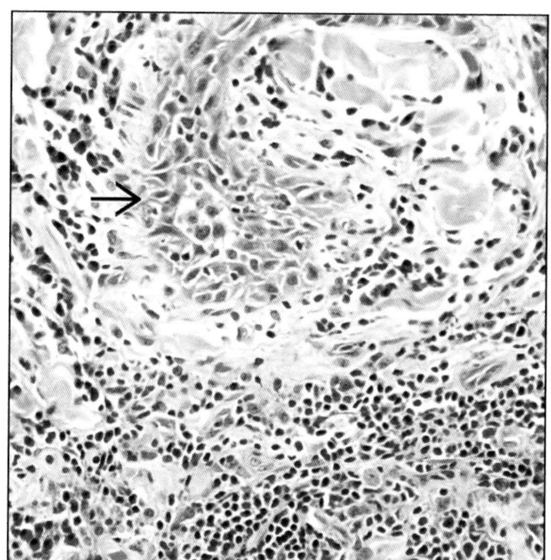

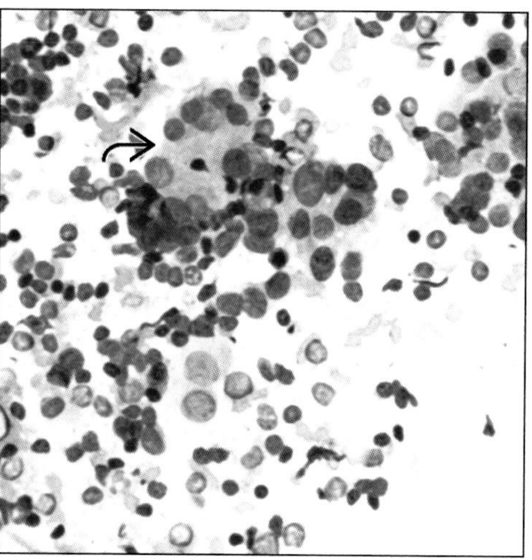

(Left) *Dense fibrosis with infiltration of the gland by a mature lymphoplasmacytic infiltrate with squamous metaplasia is shown →.* ***(Right)*** *Fine needle aspiration specimen of HT shows a mixed lymphoplasmacytic cell infiltrate surrounding and partially overrunning clusters of follicular epithelium ⮳ characterized by oncocytic cytoplasmic changes, nuclear enlargement, and variable nuclear pleomorphism.*

GRAVES DISEASE (DIFFUSE HYPERPLASIA)

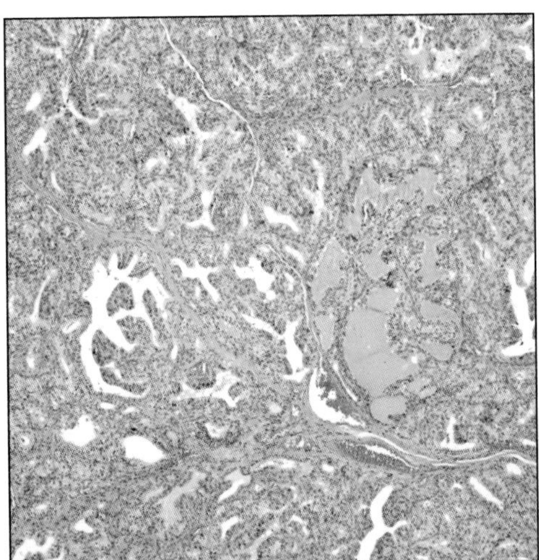

Hematoxylin & eosin shows that the entire gland is affected by a hyperplasia. Note that the right side of the image has colloid, but it is not seen throughout. There are delicate fibrovascular septae.

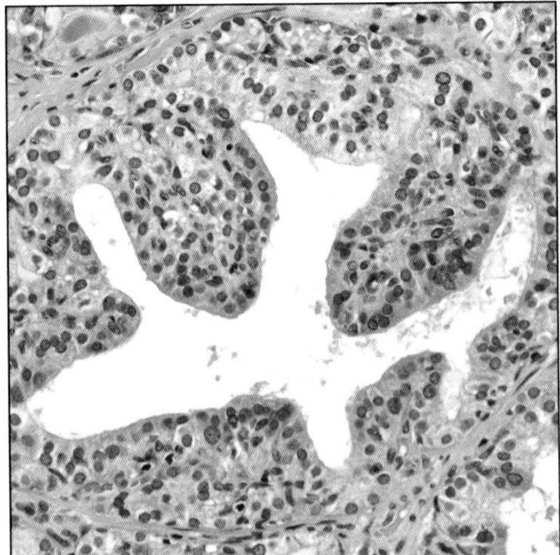

Hematoxylin & eosin shows blunt, simple papillary projections into a lumen without colloid. This is characteristic for a diffuse hyperplasia. Note the lack of atypia.

TERMINOLOGY

Synonyms

- Diffuse toxic goiter

Definitions

- Autoimmune disorder characterized by excessive production of thyroid hormone and diffuse enlargement of thyroid
- Eponymous for Irish physician Robert Graves who described cardiac palpitations, thyroid enlargement, and exophthalmos in 1835

ETIOLOGY/PATHOGENESIS

Environmental Exposure

- Iodine supplementation in previously deficient populations is associated with increased risk of hyperthyroidism (Jod-Basedow phenomenon)
  - Unmasks the underlying immune modulation abnormality
- Stress
- Smoking associated with increased risk (2-3x) but most significant for ophthalmopathy

Autoimmune

- Genetic susceptibility combined with environmental triggers that precipitate autoimmune response

Female Gender

- Interestingly, there is 6x increase risk of Graves postpartum
  - May be rebound of immunologic activity after immune tolerance for fetus
  - Fetal cells may accumulate in thyroid (fetal microchimerism), with development of autoimmunity

Genetic

- Concordance rate of 20-35% for monozygotic twins
- *HLA-DR3* associated with increased risk of 3-4x
- Polymorphisms of cytotoxic T-lymphocyte antigen 4 gene (*CLTA-4*)

Pathogenesis

- Hyperthyroidism is due to production of autoantibodies (immunoglobulin: Thyroid stimulating immunoglobulin [TSI])
  - Autoantibodies to extracellular domain of thyroid stimulating hormone receptor (*TSHR*) on follicular cells
  - Previously called long-acting thyroid stimulator (LATS)
    - Sera of patients with Graves disease stimulated the thyroids of test animals for a longer time than TSH
  - *TSHR* gene is on chromosome 14q31
- Disturbance of balance of immune response and inhibition results in a loss of self tolerance, basic feature of autoimmunity
- Autoantibodies activate receptor and stimulate thyroid hormone synthesis and secretion; also cause diffuse proliferation of follicular epithelium
  - There is complex interaction of T and B lymphocytes and thyroid follicular cells with T lymphocytes playing critical role
- Follicular cells may contribute to increased vascularity of thyroid by secreting vascular endothelial growth factor in response to stimulation by TSHR autoantibodies

CLINICAL ISSUES

Epidemiology

- Incidence
  - One of the most common autoimmune diseases
  - Prevalence: 0.4-1% (USA population)
  - Annual incidence: 20-25 per 100,000 population
- Age

GRAVES DISEASE (DIFFUSE HYPERPLASIA)

Key Facts

Terminology
- Autoimmune disorder characterized by excessive production of thyroid hormone and diffuse thyroid enlargement

Clinical Issues
- Female > > > Male (7-10:1)
- Generalized manifestations of hyperthyroidism
- Mild to moderate goiter
- Graves ophthalmopathy and pretibial myxedema
- Elevated free T4, low/absent TSH, antibodies to TSH receptors
- Methimazole, carbimazole, and propylthiouracil used medically, with radioactive iodine as alternate treatment
- Surgery only for symptomatic or unresponsive patients

Microscopic Pathology
- Entire gland affected by diffuse hyperplasia of follicular epithelium
- Follicles show simple, nonbranching papillary projections into lumen
- Colloid is scant (untreated cases), but most cases have been treated, so colloid is seen
- Nuclei are round to oval, regular, basally located with granular to coarse chromatin
- Lymphoid infiltrate, including germinal center formation, is common
- If carcinoma is present, nearly always thyroid papillary carcinoma

Top Differential Diagnoses
- Thyroid papillary carcinoma, lymphocytic thyroiditis

  - All ages but rare before adolescence
  - Peak incidence: 4th-6th decades
- Gender
  - Female > > > Male (7-10:1)
- Ethnicity
  - *HLA-B35* is associated with Graves among Japanese patients
  - *HLA-Bw46* is associated with Graves among Chinese populations

Presentation
- Generalized manifestations of hyperthyroidism
  - Patients present with nervousness, anxiety, fatigue, heat hypersensitivity, increased perspiration, palpitations, increased appetite but with loss of weight
  - Warm moist skin, tremor, tachycardia, hypertension
  - Muscle weakness
  - Personal or family history of autoimmune disease
- Mild to moderate goiter
- Inflammation of orbital tissues (Graves ophthalmopathy)
  - Lid lag and stare
  - Ophthalmopathy is most frequent and significant extrathyroidal manifestation
  - Extraocular muscles become inflamed and edematous
    - Bilateral in 90%, even if symptoms are unilateral
    - Symmetrical in 70%
    - Predilection: Inferior > medial > superior > lateral > oblique (I'M SLOW mnemonic)
  - Orbital fibroadipose tissue and lacrimal glands increase in volume
- Excessive accumulation of glycosaminoglycans in skin
  - Anterior region of leg (pretibial myxedema)

Laboratory Tests
- Elevated free T4
  - Normal free T4 is found in a limited number of cases
  - Elevated free T3 instead may prove elevated hormone production
- TSH is abnormally low or undetectable
- Antibodies to TSH receptors are identified in nearly all untreated cases
  - 2 assays: TSH binding inhibiting immunoglobulins (TBII), an immunoassay; thyroid stimulating immunoglobulin/antibodies (TSI), a bioassay
  - Assays are not comparable
  - TSHR autoantibodies are heterogeneous and can be agonistic, antagonistic, or neutral in their effects on receptor
  - Stimulating and blocking antibodies are found
- Alternative names for TBII test include thyroid receptor antibody (TRAb) and long-acting thyroid stimulator (LATS)
- Antibodies to thyroperoxidase (TPO) detected in majority of cases
- Antibodies to thyroglobulin present in about 1/2 of patients

Treatment
- Options, risks, complications
  - Low risk of recurrent hyperthyroidism
  - Low to moderate risk of hypothyroidism (post surgery)
- Surgical approaches
  - Total or subtotal thyroidectomy (diffuse and bilateral disease)
  - Only used for symptomatic hyperthyroid patients and ineffectively treated or unresponsive patients
  - Also used in children to reduce radiation-induced carcinoma risk
  - Nodule or malignancy is surgical indicator
- Drugs
  - Methimazole, carbimazole, and propylthiouracil are antithyroid drugs
    - Act by primarily inhibiting hormone synthesis through interference with peroxidase-mediated iodination of tyrosine residues
    - Withdrawal of medication may result in relapse of symptoms
  - Nonradioactive iodine inhibits release of thyroid hormones and peripheral conversion of T4 to T3

GRAVES DISEASE (DIFFUSE HYPERPLASIA)

- Reduces thyroid vascularity, increases colloid stores, and promotes involution of follicular epithelium
- Reduction of vascularity helps in presurgical preparation
  - β-adrenergic blockers (propanolol) relieves symptoms (cardiovascular and neurological) but does not affect thyroid gland (per se)
- Radiation
  - Radioactive iodine is alternate treatment to medical management
  - Ablates thyroid
  - Eliminates signs and symptoms of hyperthyroidism
  - After time, patients will require T4 replacement

Prognosis

- Usually excellent
- Post treatment hypothyroidism must be managed with replacement therapy

IMAGE FINDINGS

Radiographic Findings

- Diffuse enlargement of entire gland
- Scintigraphic imaging studies with radioiodine reveal diffusely elevated uptake

MACROSCOPIC FEATURES

General Features

- Diffuse symmetrical enlargement, vaguely nodular
- Variable colors of cut surface depending on vascularity
  - Untreated cases have high vascularity and dark red color
  - Treated cases have decreased vascularity and lighter cut surface
- Spongy to firm
- Resembles skeletal muscle

Size

- 50-150 grams

MICROSCOPIC PATHOLOGY

Histologic Features

- Entire gland is affected, although sometimes unevenly
- Diffuse hyperplasia of follicular epithelium
- Follicles show simple, nonbranching papillary projections into lumen
  - When untreated, papillae are more prominent
- Colloid is scant (untreated cases), but most cases have been treated, so colloid is seen
  - Colloid appears lighter/pale compared to normal thyroids
  - Scalloping is usually prominent, especially at epithelial junction with hyperplastic papillae
- Tall columnar cells with eosinophilic to amphophilic cytoplasm
- Nuclei are round to oval, regular, basally located with granular to coarse chromatin
- Nuclei may be atypical, especially after radioiodine ablative therapy
- Lymphoid infiltrate, including germinal center formation, is common
  - Oncocytic metaplasia adjacent to lymphocytes is not seen
- Fibrosis is limited, although accentuated along septae
  - Heavier in longstanding cases or those treated with radioactive iodine
- Extraocular muscles and soft tissue infiltrated by predominantly T lymphocytes
  - Accumulation of excessive amounts of hydrophilic glycosaminoglycans
  - After time, extraocular muscles become atrophic with associated fibrosis

Therapy Effects

- Hyperplastic changes are decreased/regressed but are not uniformly altered
- Hyperplastic areas are still identified
- Colloid is increased
- Radioactive iodine therapy causes follicular atrophy, fibrosis, oncocytic metaplasia, nuclear atypia, hyperplastic nodules, and persistence of lymphocytic infiltrates

Concurrent Carcinoma

- Nodules can be found, up to 25% of which will contain carcinoma (about 1-4% overall incidence)
- Nearly all carcinomas are thyroid papillary carcinoma
  - Most are incidental/microscopic tumors

ANCILLARY TESTS

Cytology

- Aspiration is seldom needed, as diagnosis is usually based on clinical findings and laboratory tests
- Scant, bloody material
- Low to moderate cellularity
- Colloid is scant, thin, or pale (especially with Papanicolaou-stained material)
- Follicular cells in flat sheets or microfollicles
- Cytoplasm is increased with pale, finely granular appearance
  - Marginal cytoplasmic vacuolization (clear with Papanicolaou stained material; pink with Diff-Quik stained material) called flame or flare cells
- Nuclei are slightly enlarged but round with small nucleoli
- Lymphocytes and oncocytic cells can be seen
- Post-treatment aspirates can show atypia

Immunohistochemistry

- TTF-1 and thyroglobulin positive
- Ki-67 usually < 5%
- p27 in most nuclei
- CD3 and CD20 in appropriate compartments of lymphoid infiltrate

DIFFERENTIAL DIAGNOSIS

Thyroid Papillary Carcinoma

- Not a diffuse process
- Complex, arborizing papillae
  - Lack of fibrovascular cores in hyperplastic papillae
- Psammoma bodies can be seen in Graves
- Has distinctive nuclear features

Chronic Lymphocytic Thyroiditis

- a.k.a. hashitoxicosis
- Hashitoxicosis exhibits follicular hyperplasia that can mimic Graves disease
- More pronounced oncocytic metaplasia
- Greater lymphocytic infiltrates and germinal centers
- Follicular atrophy and fibrosis also favor lymphocytic thyroiditis

Toxic Nodular Hyperplasia

- Must have clinical history and laboratory test results
- Grossly multinodular
- Majority of gland shows follicles with abundant colloid

Dyshormonogenetic Goiter

- Inherited disorder, affecting primarily young patients
  - Familial history usually identified
- All thyroid gland tissue is affected
- Nodules are readily identified
- Remarkably atypical nuclei in follicular epithelium limited to internodular zones
- Colloid tends to be absent or "watery"

Adenomatoid Nodules

- Multinodular goiter clinically
- Euthyroid usually
- Variably sized nodules but showing "normal" or "uninvolved" thyroid parenchyma in background or periphery
- Colloid is usually abundant and easily identified throughout
- Lacks cytologic atypia

SELECTED REFERENCES

1. Abraham P et al: Antithyroid drug regimen for treating Graves' hyperthyroidism. Cochrane Database Syst Rev. (1):CD003420, 2010
2. Brand OJ et al: Genetics of thyroid autoimmunity and the role of the TSHR. Mol Cell Endocrinol. 322(1-2):135-43, 2010
3. Davies TF et al: The genetics of the thyroid stimulating hormone receptor: history and relevance. Thyroid. 20(7):727-36, 2010
4. Lindholm J et al: Hyperthyroidism, exophthalmos, and goiter: historical notes on the orbitopathy. Thyroid. 20(3):291-300, 2010
5. Nakabayashi K et al: Recent advances in the association studies of autoimmune thyroid disease and the functional characterization of AITD-related transcription factor ZFAT. Nihon Rinsho Meneki Gakkai Kaishi. 33(2):66-72, 2010
6. Okosieme OE et al: The utility of radioiodine uptake and thyroid scintigraphy in the diagnosis and management of hyperthyroidism. Clin Endocrinol (Oxf). 72(1):122-7, 2010
7. Tomer Y: Genetic susceptibility to autoimmune thyroid disease: past, present, and future. Thyroid. 20(7):715-25, 2010
8. Hoffmann R: Thyroidectomy in Graves' disease: subtotal, near total or total? Orbit. 28(4):241-4, 2009
9. Rees Smith B et al: TSH receptor - autoantibody interactions. Horm Metab Res. 41(6):448-55, 2009
10. Khoo TK et al: Pathogenesis of Graves' ophthalmopathy: the role of autoantibodies. Thyroid. 17(10):1013-8, 2007
11. Lazarus JH et al: Significance of low thyroid-stimulating hormone in pregnancy. Curr Opin Endocrinol Diabetes Obes. 14(5):389-92, 2007
12. McLachlan SM et al: The link between Graves' disease and Hashimoto's thyroiditis: a role for regulatory T cells. Endocrinology. 148(12):5724-33, 2007
13. Rapoport B et al: The thyrotropin receptor in Graves' disease. Thyroid. 17(10):911-22, 2007
14. Smith BR et al: TSH receptor antibodies. Thyroid. 17(10):923-38, 2007
15. Das DK: Marginal vacuoles (fire-flare appearance) in fine needle aspiration smears of thyroid lesions: does it represent diffusing out of thyroid hormones at the base of follicular cells? Diagn Cytopathol. 34(4):277-83, 2006
16. Manji N et al: Influences of age, gender, smoking, and family history on autoimmune thyroid disease phenotype. J Clin Endocrinol Metab. 91(12):4873-80, 2006
17. Ban Y et al: Genetic susceptibility in thyroid autoimmunity. Pediatr Endocrinol Rev. 3(1):20-32, 2005
18. Ban Y et al: Susceptibility genes in thyroid autoimmunity. Clin Dev Immunol. 12(1):47-58, 2005
19. Lazarus JH: Thyroid disorders associated with pregnancy: etiology, diagnosis, and management. Treat Endocrinol. 4(1):31-41, 2005
20. Prummel MF et al: The environment and autoimmune thyroid diseases. Eur J Endocrinol. 150(5):605-18, 2004
21. Cooper DS: Hyperthyroidism. Lancet. 362(9382):459-68, 2003
22. Stocker DJ et al: Thyroid cancer yield in patients with Graves' disease. Minerva Endocrinol. 28(3):205-12, 2003
23. Tomer Y et al: Searching for the autoimmune thyroid disease susceptibility genes: from gene mapping to gene function. Endocr Rev. 24(5):694-717, 2003
24. Ando T et al: Intrathyroidal fetal microchimerism in Graves' disease. J Clin Endocrinol Metab. 87(7):3315-20, 2002
25. Szkudlinski MW et al: Thyroid-stimulating hormone and thyroid-stimulating hormone receptor structure-function relationships. Physiol Rev. 82(2):473-502, 2002
26. Brown TR et al: Thyroid injury, autoantigen availability, and the initiation of autoimmune thyroiditis. Autoimmunity. 27(1):1-12, 1998
27. Carnell NE et al: Thyroid nodules in Graves' disease: classification, characterization, and response to treatment. Thyroid. 8(8):647-52, 1998
28. Stanbury JB et al: Iodine-induced hyperthyroidism: occurrence and epidemiology. Thyroid. 8(1):83-100, 1998
29. Mizukami Y et al: Histologic changes in Graves' thyroid gland after 131I therapy for hyperthyroidism. Acta Pathol Jpn. 42(6):419-26, 1992
30. Winsa B et al: Stressful life events and Graves' disease. Lancet. 338(8781):1475-9, 1991
31. Brownlie BE et al: The epidemiology of thyrotoxicosis in New Zealand: incidence and geographical distribution in north Canterbury, 1983-1985. Clin Endocrinol (Oxf). 33(2):249-59, 1990
32. Margolick JB et al: Immunohistochemical analysis of intrathyroidal lymphocytes in Graves' disease: evidence of activated T cells and production of interferon-gamma. Clin Immunol Immunopathol. 47(2):208-18, 1988

GRAVES DISEASE (DIFFUSE HYPERPLASIA)

Clinical, Imaging, and Microscopic Features

*(**Left**) Clinical photograph shows Graves exophthalmus. Note the remarkable proptosis and retraction of the eyelids (lid lag). This is a very characteristic stare of patients with an infiltrative pathology of the extraocular muscles. (Courtesy K. B. Krantz, MD.) (**Right**) A graphic of the enlarged extraocular muscles juxtaposed to a computed tomography image demonstrates remarkable infiltration of the extraocular muscles ⇨ in this patient with Graves disease.*

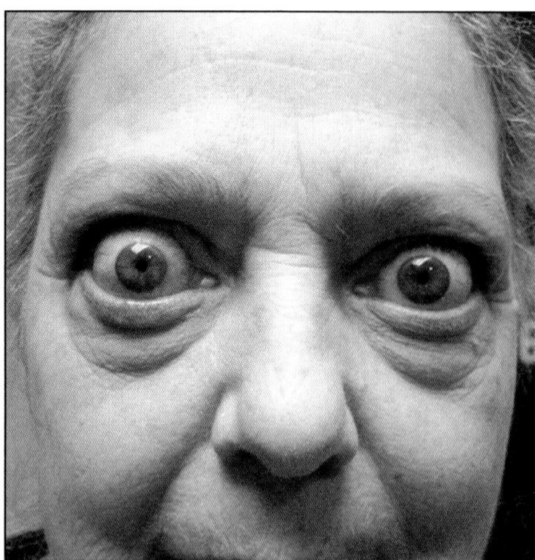

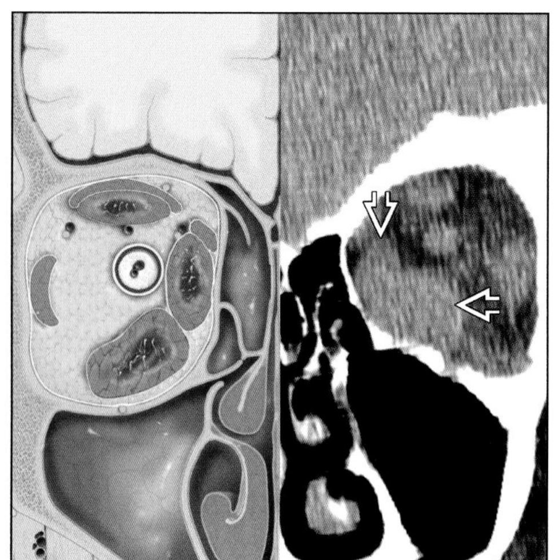

*(**Left**) Scintigraphic studies may highlight an enlarged gland. In this case, there is intense uptake in an enlarged thyroid with prominent pyramidal lobe →. It is a frequent finding in Graves disease to see the pyramidal lobe highlighted. (**Right**) Hematoxylin & eosin shows that all of the tissue in the thyroid gland is affected by the hyperplasia. The thyroid gland edge is noted at the top →. There is an accentuation of the fibrovascular septae. Very little colloid is noted.*

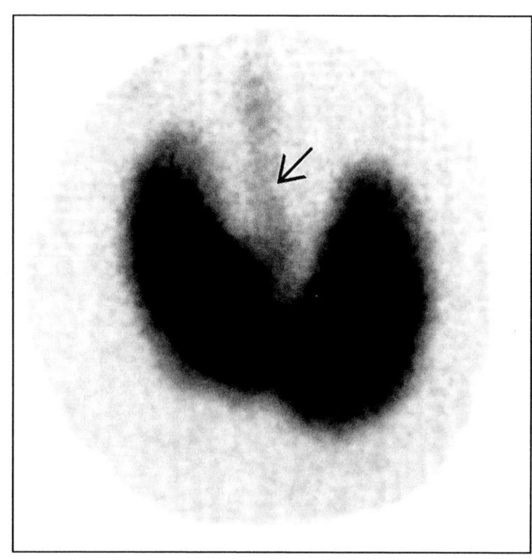

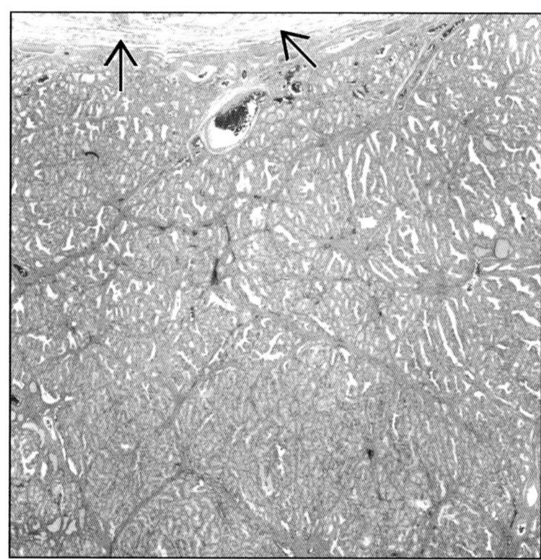

*(**Left**) Hematoxylin & eosin shows a noncomplex papillary hyperplasia into the follicle lumen. There is a lack of arborization. The fibrovascular septae separate the nodules. There is no significant colloid in this gland. (**Right**) Hematoxylin & eosin shows a number of lymphoid follicles and collections of lymphocytes in this example of diffuse hyperplasia. The low power can sometimes be confused with chronic lymphocytic thyroiditis. Germinal centers are usually absent in Graves.*

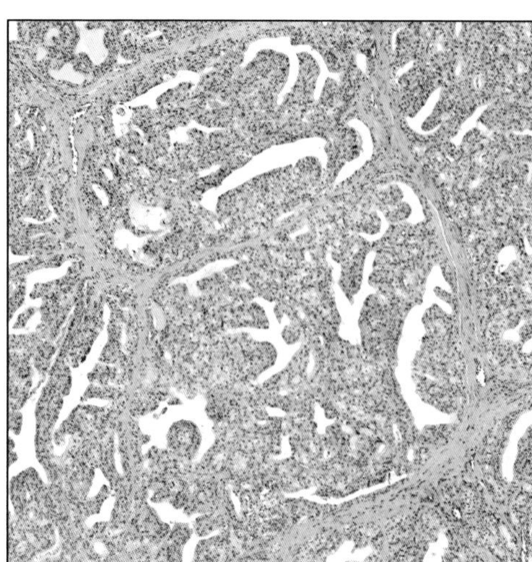

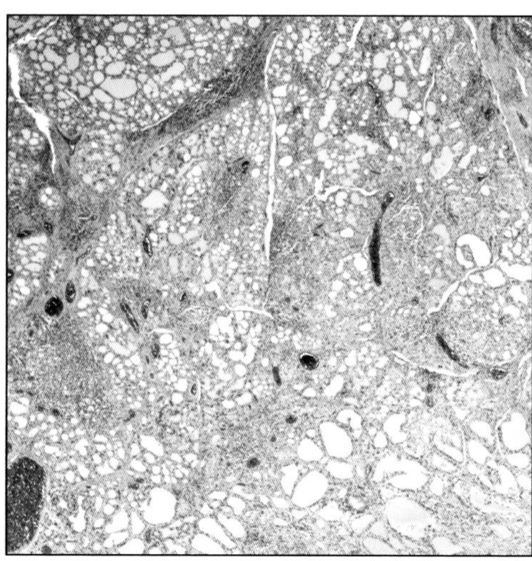

Microscopic and Cytologic Features

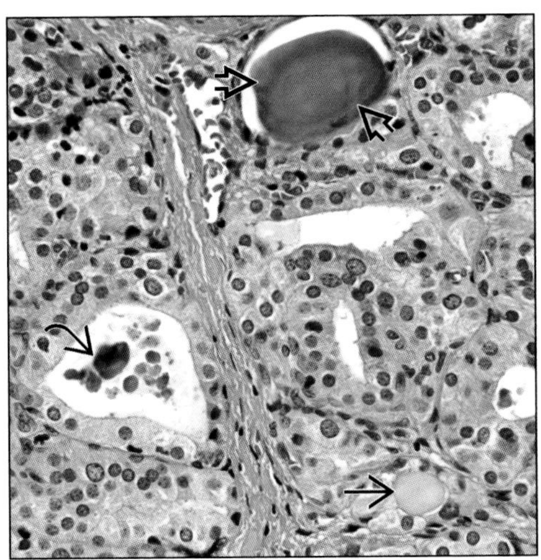
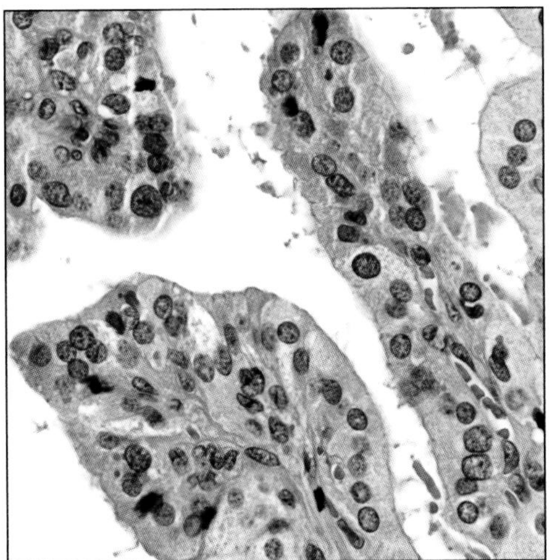

(Left) *Hematoxylin & eosin shows tall columnar cells lining the follicles. Note how thick and irregular the colloid is ⇨ in one follicle, somewhat unremarkable in another →, with isolated intraluminal calcifications in another ↷.* ***(Right)*** *Hematoxylin & eosin shows a number of simple papillae. Note the tall columnar cell containing a round, regular nucleus with coarse, heavy nuclear chromatin distribution. A delicate fibrovascular core is noted.*

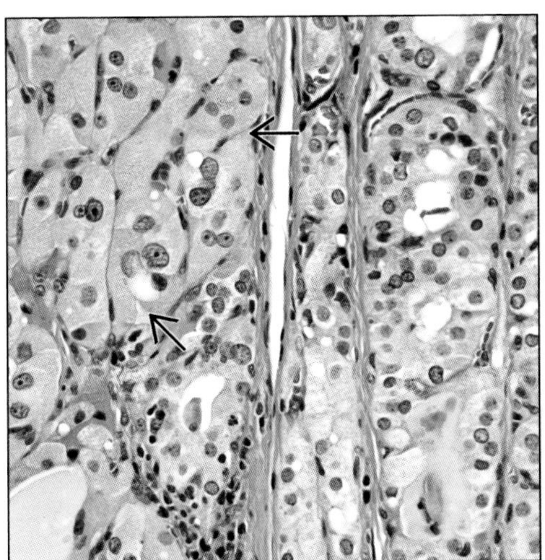
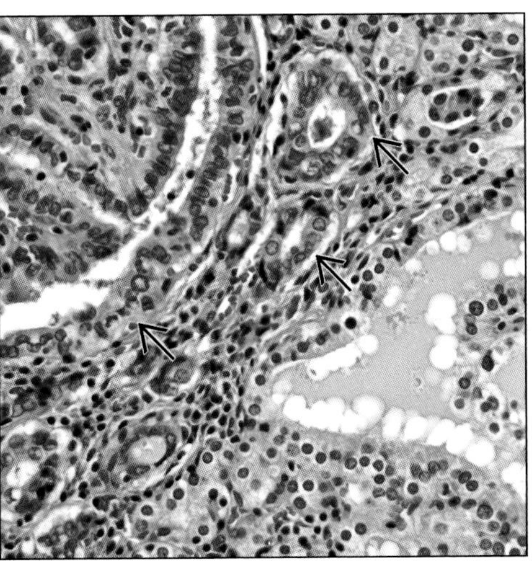

(Left) *Hematoxylin & eosin demonstrates the variability that can be seen in diffuse hyperplasia. Granular, oncocytic (Hürthle) cell changes are present → juxtaposed to the right side of the field.* ***(Right)*** *A thyroid papillary carcinoma → is present in a background of diffuse hyperplasia. There is a sharp difference between the nuclear crowding, nuclear overlapping, increased nuclear size, nuclear chromatin distribution, and optical clearing of the chromatin.*

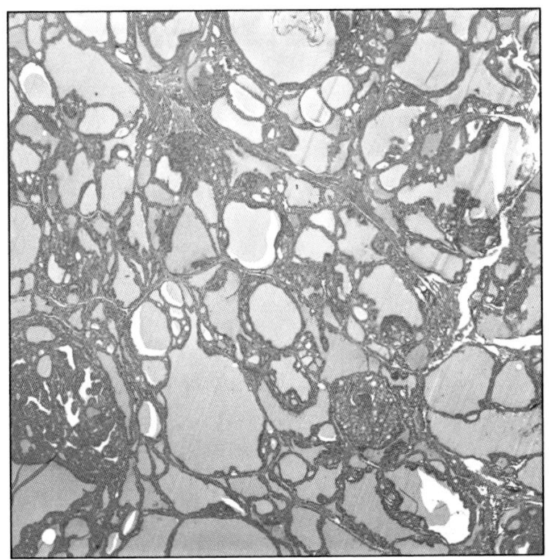
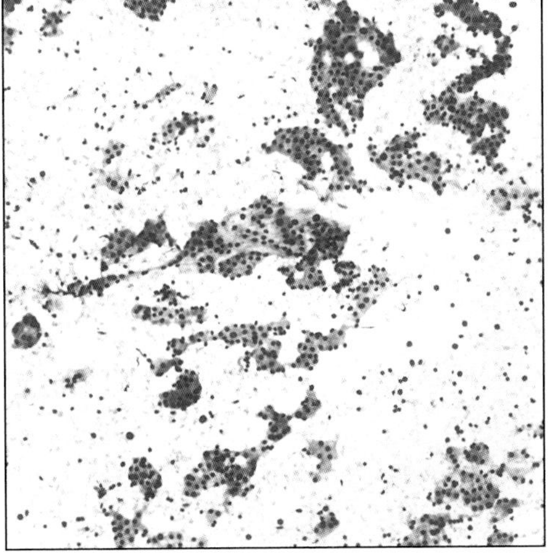

(Left) *The patient was treated medically, resulting in a remarkable increase in colloid production, although papillary projections into the lumen are still noted, just not as pronounced.* ***(Right)*** *Diff-Quik demonstrates a cellular smear. There are groups, sheets, and follicles within a background of very thin to nonexistent colloid. Note the abundant flame-type cytoplasm. Overlap with follicular tumors may be seen, requiring clinical separation.*

RIEDEL THYROIDITIS

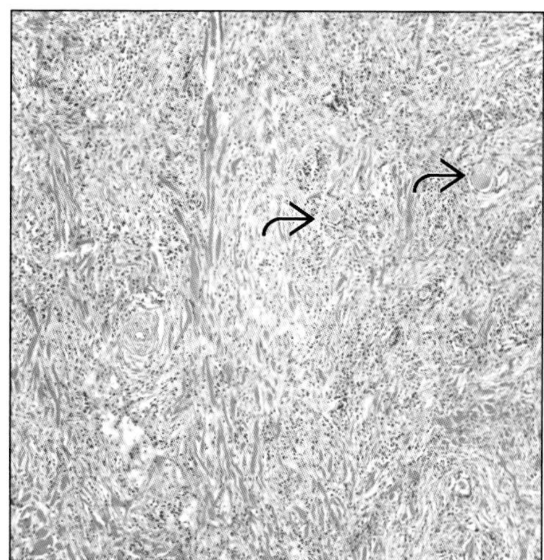

Virtually all of the thyroid tissue is replaced by dense keloid-like bands of fibrous tissue with an associated chronic inflammatory cell infiltrate. Colloid-filled follicles can be seen ⮫.

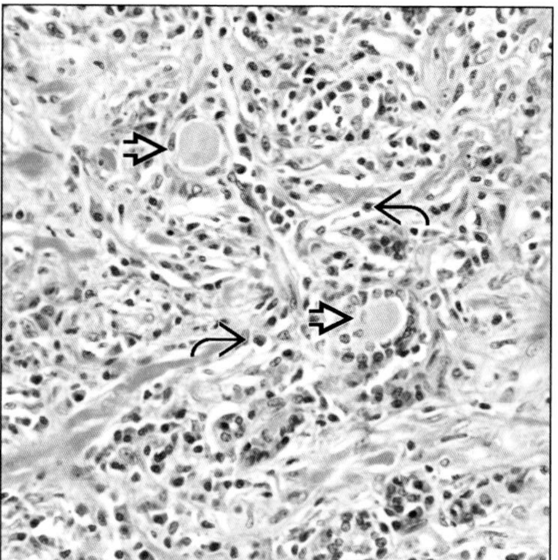

There is keloid-like fibrosis with chronic inflammation predominantly composed of plasma cells and lymphocytes, but scattered eosinophils ⮫ are present. Note colloid-filled follicles ⇨.

TERMINOLOGY

Abbreviations

- Riedel thyroiditis (RT)

Synonyms

- Invasive fibrous thyroiditis
- Ligneous thyroiditis

Definitions

- Idiopathic fibrosing process
  - Not per se an inflammatory thyroid disease (thyroiditis) of thyroid gland

ETIOLOGY/PATHOGENESIS

Autoimmune Disease

- Presence of mononuclear cells and detection of autoantibodies directed against thyroid-specific antigens favors autoimmune pathogenesis
- Association between RT and Hashimoto thyroiditis furthers supports autoimmune pathogenesis
  - RT may evolve from antecedent Graves disease
- May be associated with other autoimmune diseases including
  - Systemic lupus erythematosus, scleroderma, polyarteritis nodosa, multiple sclerosis

Systemic Fibrosing Disease/IgG4-related Systemic Disease

- RT may be part of systemic fibrosing disease (also known as inflammatory fibrosclerosis)
- Recent evidence suggests RT part of IgG4-related systemic disease spectrum
  - Characterized by IgG4(+) plasma cell infiltration and fibrosis in many organs
- Systemic disease may include
  - Retroperitoneum, mediastinum, retro-orbit, lung, sinonasal tract, parotid gland, lacrimal gland, hepatobiliary tract (sclerosing cholangitis)
  - RT may coexist with one or more of these other sites of involvement
    - Only retroperitoneal fibrosis linked to possible etiologic agent (i.e., methysergide)

CLINICAL ISSUES

Epidemiology

- Incidence
  - Uncommon disease
- Age
  - Primarily occurs in adults
- Gender
  - Female > Male

Presentation

- Painless neck mass &/or goiter
- Pressure in anterior neck often associated with dysphagia, dyspnea, stridor
- Rarely, vocal cord paralysis may occur due to recurrent laryngeal nerve involvement
- Compression and encasement of internal jugular vein and carotid artery may occur
- Thyroid is enlarged, woody or stony hard on palpation and adherent or fixed to surrounding structures in neck
  - Involvement of thyroid may be limited in extent so that 1 side is predominantly involved
  - Bilateral involvement of thyroid can also occur
- Presence of hard and fixed thyroid mass clinically simulates a neoplastic lesion (i.e., carcinoma)
  - Impression of neoplasm further suspected in cases associated with cervical lymph node involvement
- Clinically, patients present with stony hard goiter frequently associated with compressive symptoms

RIEDEL THYROIDITIS

Key Facts

Terminology
- Idiopathic fibrosing process and not per se an inflammatory (thyroiditis) thyroid disease

Etiology/Pathogenesis
- Association between RT and Hashimoto thyroiditis supports autoimmune pathogenesis
  - Presence of thyroid dysfunction, bilateral ophthalmopathy, and thyrotropin receptor stimulating autoantibodies
- RT may be part of systemic fibrosing disease (also known as inflammatory fibrosclerosis)
  - Recent evidence suggests RT part of IgG4-related systemic disease spectrum

Clinical Issues
- Painless neck mass &/or goiter
- Thyroid is enlarged, woody or stony hard on palpation and adherent or fixed to surrounding structures

Microscopic Pathology
- Destruction and replacement of thyroid parenchyma by dense collagen (keloid-like)
  - Fibrosing process is not confined to thyroid but also involves extrathyroidal connective tissues
- Vasculitis is present, primarily involving veins (phlebitis)
- Remnant of thyroid follicles may be present (but may be difficult to identify)

- Involvement of surrounding neck structures including internal jugular vein may be progressive, predisposing to cerebral venous sinus thrombosis

Laboratory Tests
- High titers of antimicrosomal and antithyroglobulin antibodies may be present
  - Reduction in levels after surgery

Treatment
- Surgical approaches
  - Wide surgical resection is indicated
    - Due to extension of fibrosis from soft tissues of neck into thyroid
    - Uninvolved thyroid need not be resected
- Drugs
  - Tamoxifen and steroid (prednisone) therapy may be effective
    - Patients who are not surgical candidates have been treated with tamoxifen and prednisone with equivocal results
  - Mycophenolate mofetil recently identified therapy for disorders associated with systemic fibrosis
    - Recent evidence suggests combined mycophenolate and prednisone may prove effective in RT
    - Improvement of compressive symptoms and decrease in mass size (small enough to allow subtotal thyroidectomy)

Prognosis
- Favorable symptomatic outcome following surgical resection

MACROSCOPIC FEATURES

General Features
- Replacement of thyroid by dense, tan-white, firm to hard tissue

MICROSCOPIC PATHOLOGY

Histologic Features
- Destruction and replacement of thyroid parenchyma by dense collagen (keloid-like bands of fibrosis)
- Fibrosing process is not confined to thyroid but also involves extrathyroidal connective tissue structures such as
  - Muscle, adipose tissue, nerves, and vascular spaces
  - Parathyroid glands can also be involved
- In addition to fibrosis, chronic inflammatory cell infiltrate is present
  - Predominantly composed of plasma cells and lymphocytes
  - Eosinophils may be present
  - Giant cells are not present
- Vasculitis is present primarily involving veins (phlebitis)
  - Characterized by adventitial inflammation that may "invade" through full thickness of vessel wall with thrombotic effect
- Remnant of thyroid follicles may be present (but may be difficult to identify)
  - Situated within dense collagen
  - Shows atrophic changes
  - Not associated with oxyphilic metaplasia (as seen in chronic lymphocytic thyroiditis) or granulomatous inflammation
- In some cases, preexisting or coexisting lesions may be present
  - e.g., adenomatoid nodule(s), follicular adenoma, follicular carcinoma, thyroid papillary carcinoma

ANCILLARY TESTS

Cytology
- Typically, aspiration generates scanty amount of cellular material ("dry tap")

Histochemistry
- Periodic acid-Schiff

- Positive staining of colloid
- May be of assistance in identification of colloid-filled follicular epithelium
- Elastic stains
  - May be helpful in identifying vasculitis

Immunohistochemistry

- Thyroglobulin and thyroid transcription factor
  - Positive in follicular epithelial cells
  - May be of assistance in identification of thyroid tissue

DIFFERENTIAL DIAGNOSIS

Hashimoto Thyroiditis, Fibrosing Variant

- Disease process confined to thyroid gland without extension of pathologic (fibroinflammatory) process outside thyroid gland
- Oxyphilic cytoplasmic change of follicular epithelial cells
- Absence of phlebitis
- Reported instances of combined RT and Hashimoto thyroiditis

Subacute Thyroiditis

- Granulomatous inflammatory condition of thyroid gland
- Clinical presentation includes
  - Neck pain localized to thyroid or radiating to jaw, ears, face, chest
  - Systemic manifestations may include malaise, fatigue, fever, chills, weight loss, anorexia, myalgia
- Laboratory findings
  - Early or hyperthyroid (thyrotoxic) phase includes
    - Elevated serum levels of T4, T3, thyroglobulin, decreased serum TSH levels
  - Later or hypothyroid phase (due to destruction of large portions of gland) includes
    - Decreased serum levels of T4, T3, thyroglobulin, increased serum TSH level
- Histologic findings change with stage of disease
  - Early phase
    - Destruction of follicular epithelial cells with extravasation and depletion of colloid
    - "Colonization" of thyroid follicles by inflammatory infiltrate (leukocytes including microabscesses, lymphocytes, histiocytes multinucleated giant cells)
  - Later phase
    - Leukocytes replaced by lymphocytes, histiocytes, giant cells, plasma cells
    - Absence of follicular epithelial cells replaced by inflammatory cells
  - Regenerative phase
    - Follicular regeneration
    - Minimal residual irregular fibrosis variably present

Anaplastic Thyroid Carcinoma, Paucicellular Variant

- Uncommon morphologic variant may resemble RT
- Clinical features those of usual anaplastic thyroid carcinoma
  - Occurrence in elderly patients, rapidly enlarging neck mass, rapidly fatal outcome
- Histologic features include
  - Acellular fibrous or infarcted tissue with central dystrophic calcification
  - Hypocellular foci comprising atypical spindle cells in at least some areas
  - Lymph-vascular invasion
  - Lymph node metastasis may be present
  - Immunoreactivity for epithelial markers (cytokeratin, epithelial membrane antigen)

SELECTED REFERENCES

1. Dahlgren M et al: Riedel's thyroiditis and multifocal fibrosclerosis are part of the IgG4-related systemic disease spectrum. Arthritis Care Res (Hoboken). 62(9):1312-8, 2010
2. Levy JM et al: Combined mycophenolate mofetil and prednisone therapy in tamoxifen- and prednisone-resistant Reidel's thyroiditis. Thyroid. 20(1):105-7, 2010
3. Lorenz K et al: Riedel's thyroiditis: impact and strategy of a challenging surgery. Langenbecks Arch Surg. 392(4):405-12, 2007
4. Kotilainen P et al: Riedel's thyroiditis in a patient with multiple sclerosis. Neuro Endocrinol Lett. 26(1):67-8, 2005
5. Harigopal M et al: Fine-needle aspiration of Riedel's disease: report of a case and review of the literature. Diagn Cytopathol. 30(3):193-7, 2004
6. Jung YJ et al: A case of Riedel's thyroiditis treated with tamoxifen: another successful outcome. Endocr Pract. 10(6):483-6, 2004
7. Moulik PK et al: Steroid responsiveness in a case of Riedel's thyroiditis and retroperitoneal fibrosis. Int J Clin Pract. 58(3):312-5, 2004
8. Papi G et al: Riedel's thyroiditis and fibrous variant of Hashimoto's thyroiditis: a clinicopathological and immunohistochemical study. J Endocrinol Invest. 26(5):444-9, 2003
9. Baloch ZW et al: Combined Riedel's Disease and Fibrosing Hashimoto's Thyroiditis: A Report of Three Cases with Two Showing Coexisting Papillary Carcinoma. Endocr Pathol. 11(2):157-163, 2000
10. Baloch ZW et al: Simultaneous involvement of thyroid by Riedel's [correction of Reidel's] disease and fibrosing Hashimoto's thyroiditis: a case report. Thyroid. 8(4):337-41, 1998
11. Vaidya B et al: Cerebral venous sinus thrombosis: a late sequel of invasive fibrous thyroiditis. Thyroid. 8(9):787-90, 1998
12. Few J et al: Riedel's thyroiditis: treatment with tamoxifen. Surgery. 120(6):993-8; discussion 998-9, 1996
13. Wan SK et al: Paucicellular variant of anaplastic thyroid carcinoma. A mimic of Reidel's thyroiditis. Am J Clin Pathol. 105(4):388-93, 1996
14. Bagnasco M et al: Fibrous invasive (Riedel's) thyroiditis with critical response to steroid treatment. J Endocrinol Invest. 18(4):305-7, 1995
15. Best TB et al: Riedel's thyroiditis associated with Hashimoto's thyroiditis, hypoparathyroidism, and retroperitoneal fibrosis. J Endocrinol Invest. 14(9):767-72, 1991

Microscopic Features and Ancillary Techniques

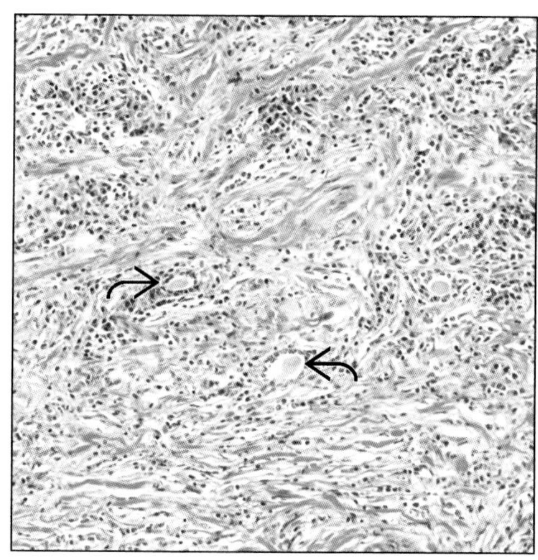

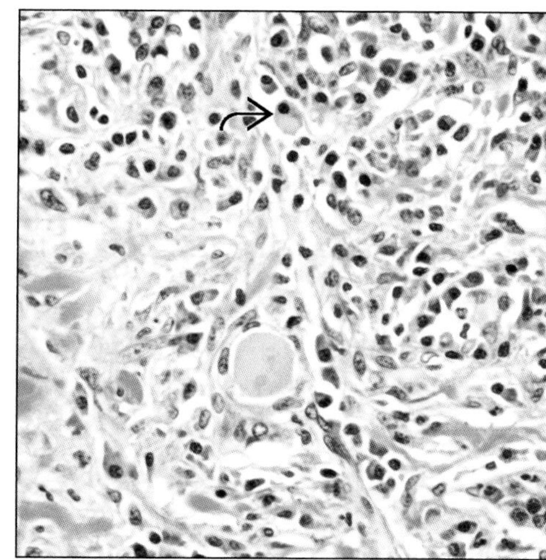

(Left) *Destruction and replacement of thyroid parenchyma by dense keloid-like bands of fibrosis with atrophic thyroid follicles are situated in the dense collagen. Follicular cells lack oncocytic metaplasia typically seen in chronic lymphocytic (Hashimoto) thyroiditis.* ***(Right)*** *Numerous plasma cells with identifiable Russell bodies are identified in RT. The plasma cells are characterized by IgG4(+) staining, which supports the idea that RT is part of IgG4-related systemic disease spectrum.*

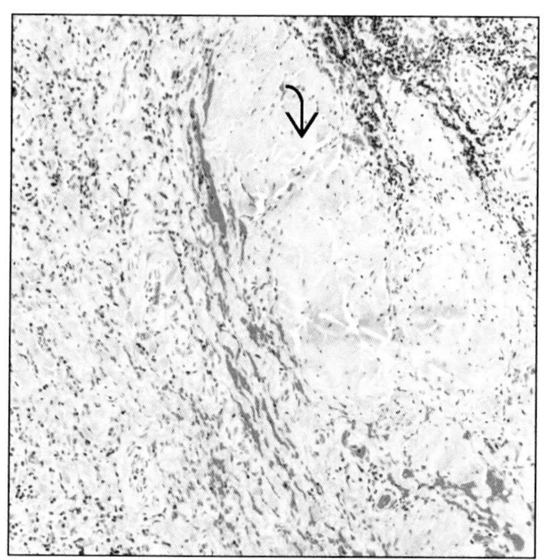

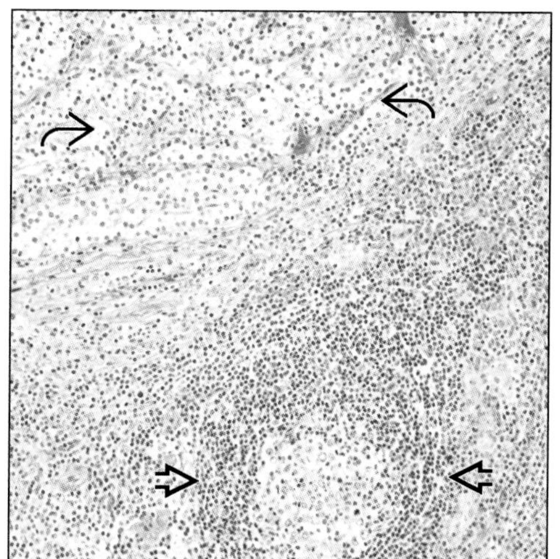

(Left) *The fibrosing process is not confined to the thyroid but may involve extrathyroidal connective tissue including skeletal muscle. Other extrathyroidal structures that may be involved include fat, nerves, and vascular spaces (not shown).* ***(Right)*** *The keloid-like fibrosing process may extend outside the thyroid gland proper to involve other structures, including the parathyroid gland. The inflammatory cell component may include lymphoid follicles with germinal centers.*

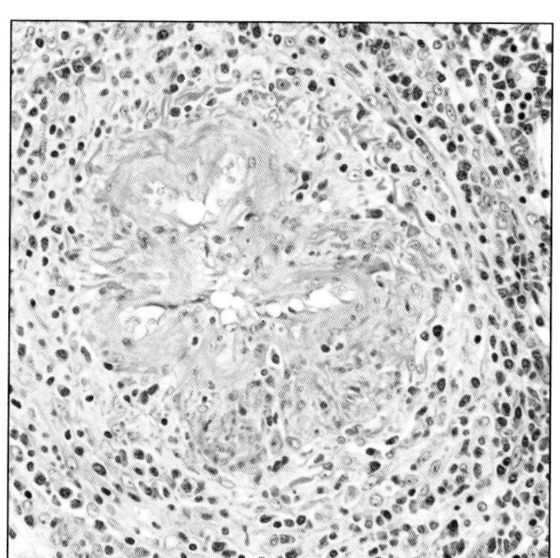

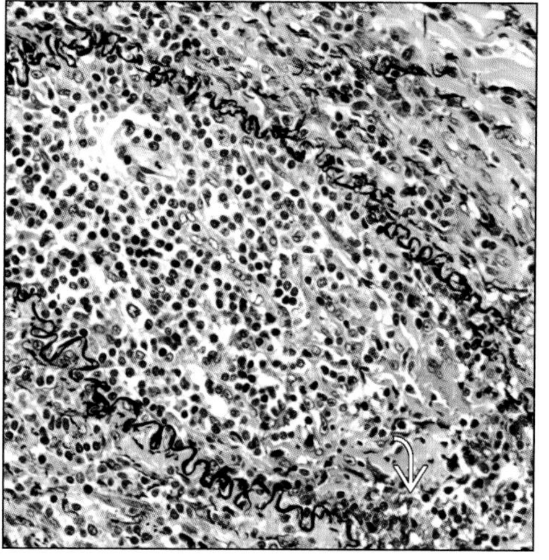

(Left) *Vasculitis (often phlebitis) is another histologic component seen in Riedel thyroiditis. The inflammatory cells composed of plasma cells and lymphocytes surround and infiltrate into endothelial-lined vascular space.* ***(Right)*** *Elastic stain shows focal disruption with discontinuation of the black-staining elastic membrane by the inflammatory cell infiltrate that is present throughout the wall as well as in the lumen (thrombus-like) of vascular spaces.*

ADENOMATOID NODULE

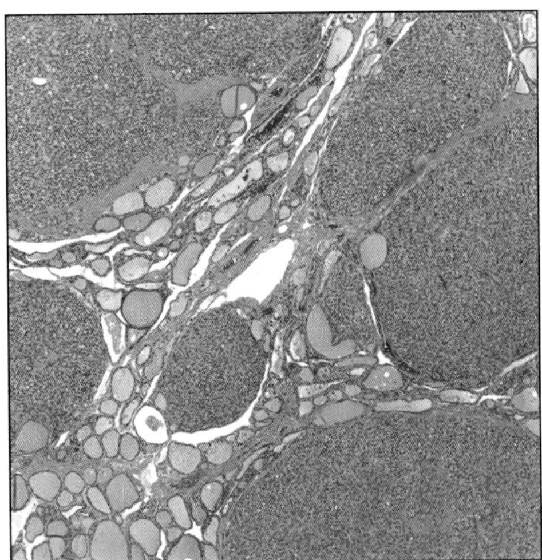

Low power shows multiple nodules separated by unremarkable thyroid parenchyma. The nodules show increased cellularity but lack a fibrous connective tissue capsule.

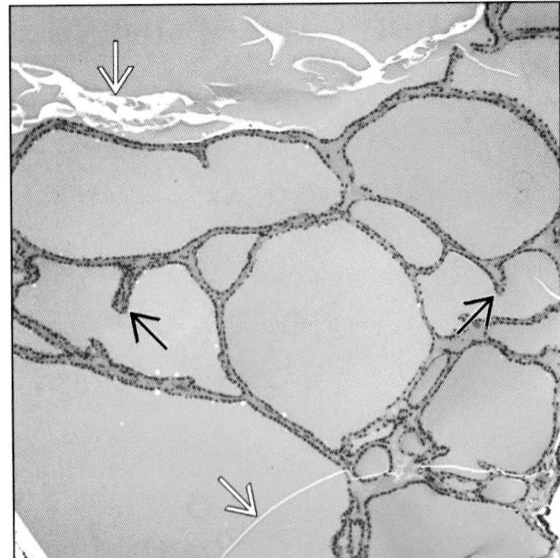

This nodule contains large follicles distended with abundant colloid. There are a number of simple papillary projections into the colloid ⇨. Note the cracking artifact in the colloid ➡.

TERMINOLOGY

Synonyms

- Multinodular goiter (MNG) (clinical term)
- Adenomatous hyperplasia
- Nontoxic nodular goiter
- Colloid goiter

Definitions

- Asymmetric, multinodular thyroid gland enlargement due to follicular epithelial hyperplasia as result of impaired thyroid hormone production &/or increased TSH secretion
  - "Goiter" is nonspecific clinical term meaning thyroid enlargement; it is not a surgical pathology diagnosis

ETIOLOGY/PATHOGENESIS

Etiology

- Multifactorial: Intrinsic thyroid follicular epithelial cell alterations with environmental and genetic factors
- Deficiency of dietary iodine
  - Amplified by tobacco use (smoking), probably thiocyanate
  - Low iodine concentration within nodules probably secondary rather than primary
  - Many facets of adenomatoid nodules are not explained by iodine deficiency
  - Many times, goiter size is inversely proportional to serum TSH
- Due to consumption of high volumes of goitrogenic foods
  - Generally raw (cooking inactivates the goitrogens)
    - **Cruciferous** vegetables (genus *Brassica*; family Brassicaceae)
- Medications, specifically those which may interfere with thyroid hormone synthesis &/or release
  - Iodine, amiodarone, lithium, thioamides (methimazole, carbimazole, propylthiouracil), thalidomide, perchlorate, rifampin, carbamazepine
- Inherited
  - Dyshormonogenetic goiter
  - Increased incidence in monozygotic compared to dizygotic twins

Pathogenesis

- Pathway of nodule production
  - Impaired thyroid hormone production: Iodine deficiency, goitrogens, medication blockage (organification of iodine is disrupted)
  - Increases secretion of TSH
    - Many paracrine and autocrine factors are also involved
  - Stimulates thyroid follicular epithelium to proliferate; remarkable functional and structural heterogeneity in thyrocytes results in profound variability
  - Results in increased thyroglobulin production
- Results in formation of adenomatoid nodule (elemental unit)
- Multiple adenomatoid nodules result in clinical goiter (aggregated units)
  - Become autonomous, TSH-independent growth

CLINICAL ISSUES

Epidemiology

- Incidence
  - Clinically detectable nodules found in < 5% of patients
    - Higher in autopsy series, especially if microscopic nodules included (up to 50%)
  - Highest incidence in areas with iodine-deficient diets; may also occur with excess iodine intake
- Age
  - Wide age range, although usually adults

ADENOMATOID NODULE

Key Facts

Terminology
- Asymmetric, multinodular thyroid gland enlargement due to follicular epithelial hyperplasia as result of impaired thyroid hormone production &/or increased TSH secretion

Clinical Issues
- Clinically detectable nodules found in < 5% of patients
- Peak: 5th to 7th decades
- Female > > > Male (5-10:1)
- Thyroid enlargement, often asymmetric and nodular
- Most patients are euthyroid
- Total thyroidectomy for symptomatic disease

Image Findings
- CT is best imaging exam for multinodular goiter
  - Ultrasound: Hypoechoic solid nodules, anechoic cysts, hyperechoic hemorrhagic regions

Microscopic Pathology
- Nodules lack a capsule, showing a pushing border that merges with surrounding follicles
- Large follicles distended with colloid, often with papillae
- Flattened, cuboidal, columnar to oncocytic cells
- Secondary and metaplastic changes are common
- FNA does not reliably separate nodules from neoplasia

Top Differential Diagnoses
- Follicular adenoma, papillary carcinoma, follicular carcinoma, dyshormonogenetic goiter

  - Peak: 5th to 7th decades
- Gender
  - Female > > > Male (5-10:1)
    - Nodules frequently detected during pregnancy

Presentation
- Thyroid enlargement, often asymmetric and nodular
- May be detected during routine physical exam
- Infrequently, stridor (tracheal compression), hoarseness (recurrent laryngeal nerve impingement), or dysphagia (interference with swallowing) may be present
- If there is mediastinal goiter, superior vena cava syndrome may be present
- Signs and symptoms usually develop gradually
  - Rapid enlargement may result from intralesional hemorrhage
- Single or dominant nodule may suggest neoplasm

Laboratory Tests
- Most patients are euthyroid
  - Few patients are hyperthyroid ("toxic nodular goiter" or Plummer disease)
- Usually normal: TSH and free T4 levels
- Low TSH level: Free T4 and free T3, if free T4 is not elevated

Treatment
- Options, risks, complications
  - Potential complications after thyroidectomy
    - Permanent hypoparathyroidism (up to 7%)
    - Transient or permanent recurrent laryngeal nerve palsy (up to 1.5%)
    - Hypothyroidism may develop, requiring lifelong replacement therapy
- Surgical approaches
  - Total thyroidectomy for symptomatic disease
  - May be used for a "dominant nodule," suspicious for neoplasm
    - Histologic examination helps to exclude unexpected malignancies (detected in up to 7-10% of cases)
- Drugs
  - TSH suppression therapy
    - Thyroxin used to suppress nodules
    - Works best for small goiters
- Radiation
  - ^{131}Iodine therapy
    - Especially in elderly patients
    - When surgery is contraindicated or in poor surgical candidates
    - Toxic nodules
    - Patients who are unwilling to have surgery
  - Reduces nodules, but changes are slow

Prognosis
- Multinodular goiters are usually treated for cosmetic or comfort reasons
  - Surgery achieves immediate and permanent cure without recurrence
- Watchful waiting if there are not changes in signs or symptoms
- No risk of malignant transformation
  - However, incidental or concurrent malignancies may be present

IMAGE FINDINGS

Radiographic Findings
- Diffusely enlarged thyroid with multiple nodules
  - Often show substernal extension (~ 1/3)
- CT is best imaging exam for multinodular goiter
  - Identifies extent and severity of airway compression
  - Presence and extent of substernal goiter

Ultrasonographic Findings
- Hypoechoic solid nodules, anechoic cysts, hyperechoic fibrotic/hemorrhagic regions
- Used to guide FNA procedure

CT Findings
- Inhomogeneous enhancement in enlarged thyroid with multiple cystic and solid masses
- Circumscribed regions of low attenuation (colloid cysts)

- High attenuation when there is hemorrhage
- Calcifications frequently noted

Nuclear Medicine

- Heterogeneous radiotracer uptake with irregular, nodular thyroid contour
- Discrete nodules may be hot (increased activity), cold (photopenic), warm, or isointense (not visualized)

MACROSCOPIC FEATURES

General Features

- Enlarged gland with multiple nodules of variable size
  - Single, dominant nodule may be seen
  - Asymmetric enlargement
  - Thyroid contour distorted
- Cut surfaces are nodular and heterogeneous
  - Gelatinous with colloid exuding from cut surface
  - Glistening and semitranslucent
  - Fleshy to beefy to firm
  - Degenerative/secondary changes
    - Hemorrhage, central scars, fibrous pseudocapsules, cystic change, calcification, and metaplastic bone formation
- Parasitic nodules attached by thin, delicate fibrous strands adjacent to "main" thyroid gland
  - Attachment may be missed intraoperatively
  - Lack lymph node architecture (subcapsular sinus, sinus histiocytosis, medullary zone)

Sections to Be Submitted

- Sample periphery of nodules for histologic sections
- Sample nodules with a different/unique appearance (to exclude malignancy)

Size

- Microscopic to enormous (> 1,000 grams; up to 35 cm)

MICROSCOPIC PATHOLOGY

Histologic Features

- Remarkable nodularity to tissue examined
  - While uncommon, compression of surrounding parenchyma may be present
- Nodules lack capsule, showing a pushing border that merges with surrounding follicles
  - "Pseudocapsule" of fibrosis lacks elastic fibers and smooth muscle-walled vessels
  - Fibrosis may be circumferential but tends to be irregular and incomplete
  - Areas of increased cellularity throughout the parenchyma
- Most nodules contain large follicles distended with colloid
  - Follicles may be small to massively distended with lakes of colloid
  - Papillary projections may be prominent
    - Papillae are simple, lacking complexity and arborization
    - Contain round, basally oriented nuclei with coarse, dense chromatin
    - Polarity of cells is maintained
  - Clusters of follicles (Sanderson polsters) may expand into colloid
- Some nodules may be dominant or cellular with increased cellularity (solid, microfollicular) and little colloid
- Lining epithelium
  - Flattened and inconspicuous epithelial cells
  - Cuboidal or columnar epithelial cells
    - Granules of hemosiderin are frequently present in cytoplasm
  - Prominent oxyphilic change
    - Oncocytic cells may have nuclear enlargement, vesicular chromatin, irregular nuclear contours, and prominent nucleoli
  - Clear cell or "signet ring" vacuoles
- Secondary changes are common
  - Hemorrhage common, with hemosiderin-laden macrophages
    - Organization shows endothelial hyperplasia (similar to intravascular papillary endothelial hyperplasia)
  - Cystic change with multiple histiocytes in background
  - Cholesterol clefts
  - Fibrosis, often in center of nodule
  - Granulation tissue reaction
  - Dystrophic calcifications
  - Fine needle aspiration site (abrupt, linear disruption) is frequently seen
- Metaplastic change can be seen
  - Osseous metaplasia, especially near dystrophic calcification
  - Cartilaginous metaplasia less common
  - Squamous metaplasia
  - Adipose metaplasia
- Chronic, acute, &/or granulomatous inflammation (due to follicle rupture) may be seen
- Concurrent, topographically distinct neoplasms may be present
  - Microscopic papillary carcinoma is most common
- Amyloid goiter is distinct entity

ANCILLARY TESTS

Cytology

- Aspirate may be scant to abundant, thin to viscous, and serosanginous to red or brown
- Usually low cellularity and abundant, thin colloid
  - Colloid yields proteinaceous film that has scratches, waves, cracks, or mosaic-like artifacts after drying
- Large, flat sheets of follicular epithelium arranged in "honeycomb pattern"
  - Monolayer sheets of evenly spaced cells
  - Microfollicular groups &/or isolated cells
  - Oncocytic cells may be present (dominant finding or isolated)
- Nuclei are small, round, with dense chromatin
  - No overlapping or crowding or contour irregularities
- Background of hemosiderin-laden macrophages or foamy histiocytes when degenerated
- Multinucleated giant cells may be seen
- Difficult to reliably predict nodules from neoplasia

- Abundant colloid favors adenomatoid nodule
- High cellularity with scant colloid favors neoplasm
- Application of molecular techniques (*BRAF* specifically) may help separate suspicious nodule from papillary carcinoma in selected FNA samples

Frozen Sections

- Seldom of value in a nodular process
  - In most cases, "deferred, follicular lesion" does not change management
  - "Follicular neoplasm" requires complete capsule evaluation for capsular or vascular invasion, a task impractical during constraints of intraoperative analysis
- If FNA was indeterminate, intraoperative assessment can be used to guide management
  - Touch preparations/smears can confirm papillary carcinoma
  - Selection of a single nodule for frozen section, only in rare instances of high clinical suspicion of malignancy

Cytogenetics

- Some susceptibility genes related to development of nodules include
  - Thyroglobulin, thyroperoxidase, sodium iodide symporter, and thyroid stimulating hormone receptor (*TSHR*)
  - Loci include *MNG1* and *TSHR* on chromosome 14q
- Occasionally, numerical &/or structural abnormalities are detected
  - Trisomy or tetrasomy 7 is most common

DIFFERENTIAL DIAGNOSIS

Follicular Adenoma

- Single nodule
- Surrounded by variably thick fibrous connective tissue capsule with smooth muscle-walled vessels
- Usually has single histologic pattern, compressing adjacent thyroid parenchyma, limited colloid
- Tends to lack degeneration and lack colloid lakes
- Both lesions may be present, but philosophically, multiple follicular nodules without invasion are within nodular hyperplasia/adenomatoid nodule category

Papillary Carcinoma

- Architecture of papillary carcinoma may overlap adenomatoid nodules
- Nuclear features of papillary are required
- In single nodule, if there are multiple topographically separate and distinct areas, especially at periphery, showing nuclear features of papillary, whole tumor should be called papillary carcinoma
- In borderline case, panel of galectin-3, CITED-1, and HBME-1 or molecular analysis (*BRAF* mutation specifically) may help with separation

Follicular Carcinoma

- Encapsulated neoplasm with variably thick capsule
- Capsular &/or vascular invasion present
- Molecular evaluation by FISH for t(2;3)(q13;p25) (fusion between *PAX8* gene on 2q13 and *PPAR*γ gene on 3p25) may be of value in some cases

Dyshormonogenetic Goiter

- Grossly similar, although colloid is usually limited to absent
- Multiple nodules histologically, but isolated pleomorphic nuclei present in internodular zones

Metastatic Carcinoma

- Parasitic adenomatoid nodules may cause confusion with metastatic papillary carcinoma
- Lymph node architecture must be identified
- Nuclear features of papillary carcinoma can usually be identified

SELECTED REFERENCES

1. Tonacchera M et al: Assessment of nodular goitre. Best Pract Res Clin Endocrinol Metab. 24(1):51-61, 2010
2. Efremidou EI et al: The efficacy and safety of total thyroidectomy in the management of benign thyroid disease: a review of 932 cases. Can J Surg. 52(1):39-44, 2009
3. Layfield LJ et al: Thyroid aspiration cytology: current status. CA Cancer J Clin. 59(2):99-110, 2009
4. Morris LF et al: Evidence-based assessment of the role of ultrasonography in the management of benign thyroid nodules. World J Surg. 32(7):1253-63, 2008
5. Baloch ZW et al: Our approach to follicular-patterned lesions of the thyroid. J Clin Pathol. 60(3):244-50, 2007
6. LiVolsi VA et al: Use and abuse of frozen section in the diagnosis of follicular thyroid lesions. Endocr Pathol. 16(4):285-93, 2005
7. Prasad ML et al: Galectin-3, fibronectin-1, CITED-1, HBME1 and cytokeratin-19 immunohistochemistry is useful for the differential diagnosis of thyroid tumors. Mod Pathol. 18(1):48-57, 2005
8. Gandolfi PP et al: The incidence of thyroid carcinoma in multinodular goiter: retrospective analysis. Acta Biomed. 75(2):114-7, 2004
9. Hegedüs L: Clinical practice. The thyroid nodule. N Engl J Med. 351(17):1764-71, 2004
10. Ko HM et al: Clinicopathologic analysis of fine needle aspiration cytology of the thyroid. A review of 1,613 cases and correlation with histopathologic diagnoses. Acta Cytol. 47(5):727-32, 2003
11. Tonacchera M et al: Gain of function TSH receptor mutations and iodine deficiency: implications in iodine prophylaxis. J Endocrinol Invest. 26(2 Suppl):2-6, 2003
12. Baloch ZW et al: Follicular-patterned lesions of the thyroid: the bane of the pathologist. Am J Clin Pathol. 117(1):143-50, 2002
13. Derwahl M et al: Nodular goiter and goiter nodules: Where iodine deficiency falls short of explaining the facts. Exp Clin Endocrinol Diabetes. 109(5):250-60, 2001
14. Salabè GB: Pathogenesis of thyroid nodules: histological classification? Biomed Pharmacother. 55(1):39-53, 2001
15. Mittendorf EA et al: Follow-up evaluation and clinical course of patients with benign nodular thyroid disease. Am Surg. 65(7):653-7; discussion 657-8, 1999
16. Oertel YC et al: Diagnosis of benign thyroid lesions: fine-needle aspiration and histopathologic correlation. Ann Diagn Pathol. 2(4):250-63, 1998

ADENOMATOID NODULE

Imaging, Gross, and Microscopic Features

(Left) Transverse grayscale US shows septations in a well-defined, cystic thyroid nodule ⇒, suggesting previous hemorrhage in a nodule in multinodular goiter (MNG). Such nodules are commonly seen in MNG. Note trachea ➡. ***(Right)*** There is a remarkably enlarged thyroid gland, showing multiple different nodules. The thyroid shows areas of calcification ➡, areas of cystic degeneration ➡, along with some areas that are more solid ➡. This is characteristic for adenomatoid nodules.

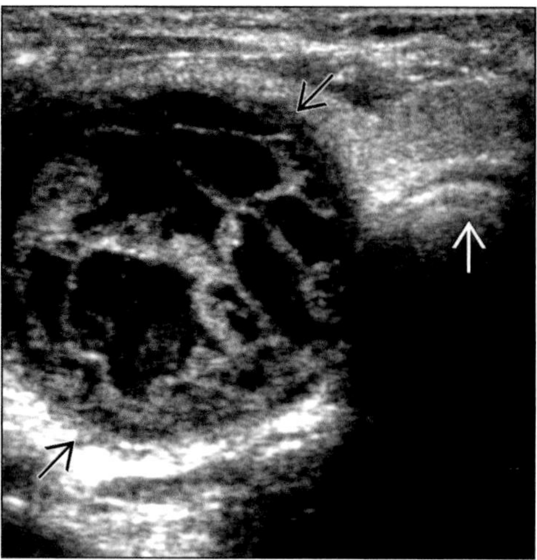

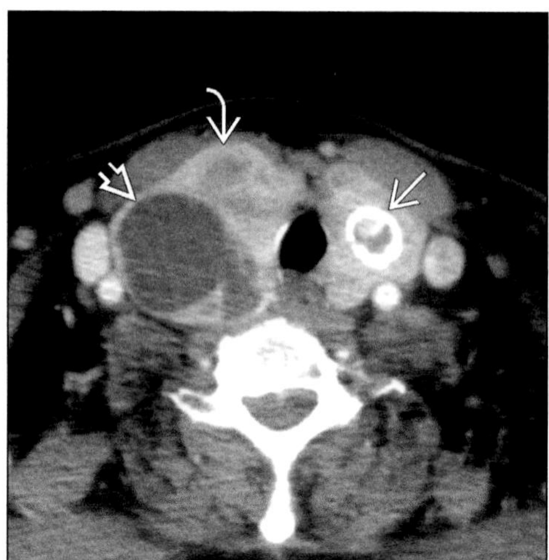

(Left) This total thyroidectomy specimen shows marked asymmetric enlargement, with multiple nodules. One nodule ➡ shows hemorrhagic degeneration in the center. The overall thyroid contour is distorted. ***(Right)*** This lobectomy specimen has been serially sectioned from top to bottom, showing a large, fleshy, and degenerated cut surface. Many times nodules will nearly completely replace the thyroid lobe.

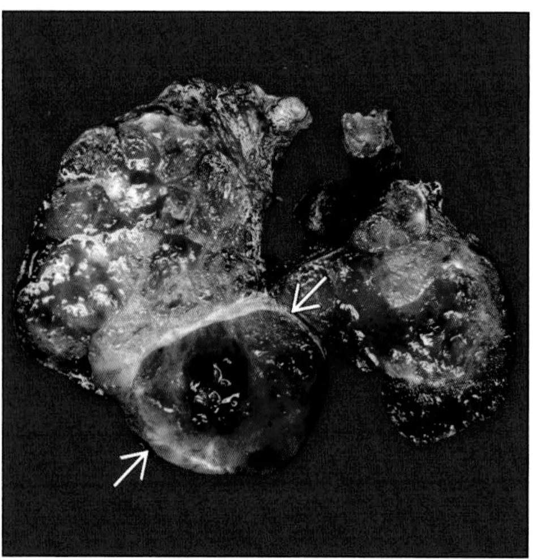

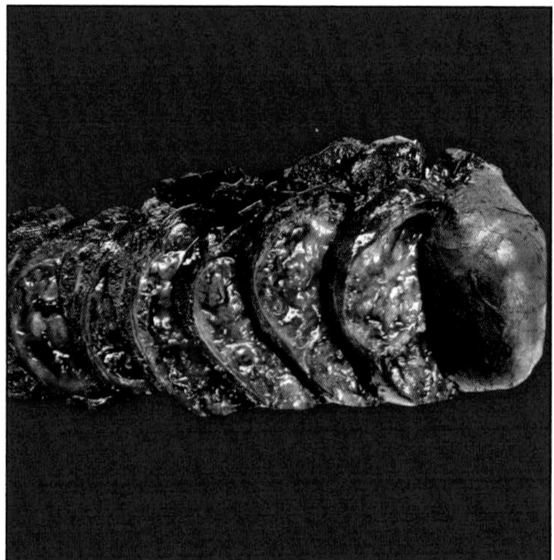

(Left) Incomplete fibrosis is noted associated with the nodules. Note the multinodular appearance, with the nodules showing variable cellularity and circumscription. Colloid is easily identified in these nodules. ***(Right)*** This nodule shows a number of papillae along with areas of granulation tissue ⇒, hemorrhage, and fatty metaplasia ➡. Nodules show variable amounts of colloid and variable cellularity.

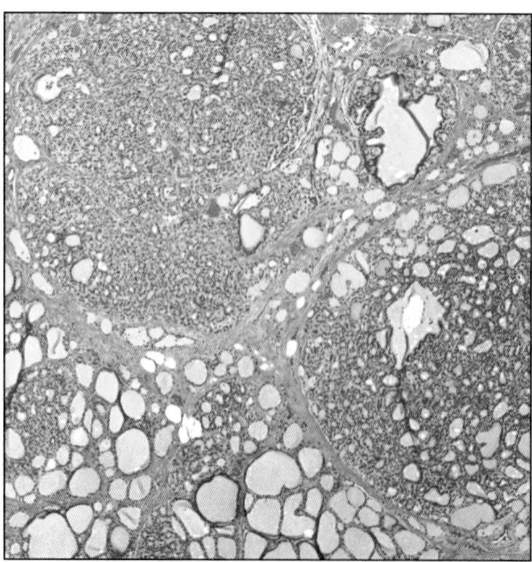

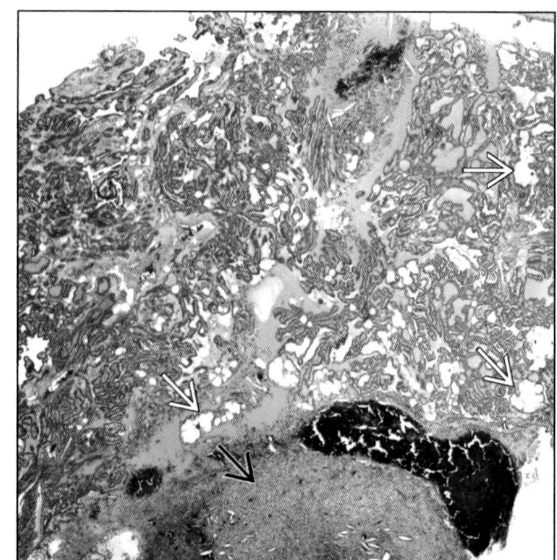

ADENOMATOID NODULE

Microscopic Features

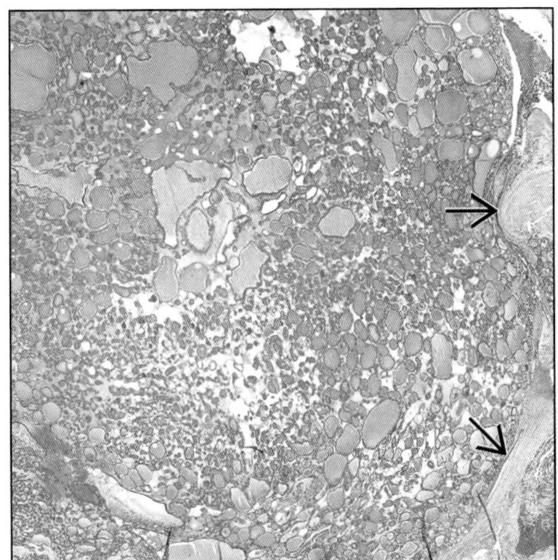

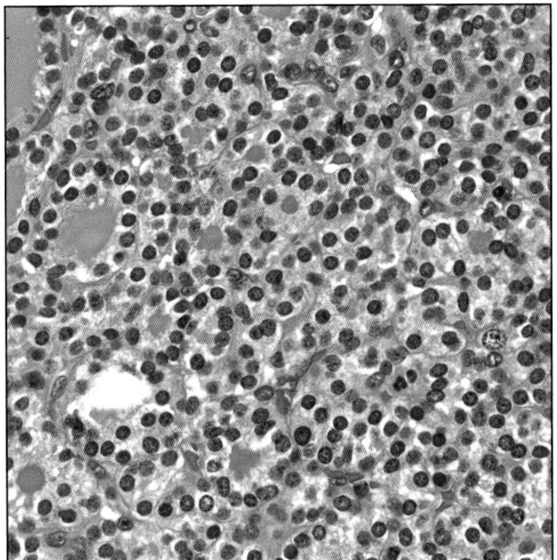

(Left) *The periphery of the nodule shows fibrous connective tissue condensation* ⇨. *The nodule shows variable cellularity, with some areas containing more colloid than others. Areas of edematous change are also present.* ***(Right)*** *Some nodules may be dominant or cellular with increased cellularity (solid, microfollicular) and little colloid, as seen in this nodule. Without examination of the periphery, this area would be indistinguishable from a follicular neoplasm.*

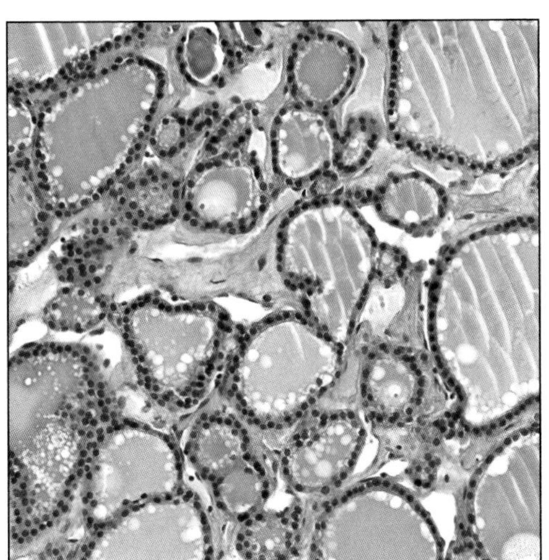

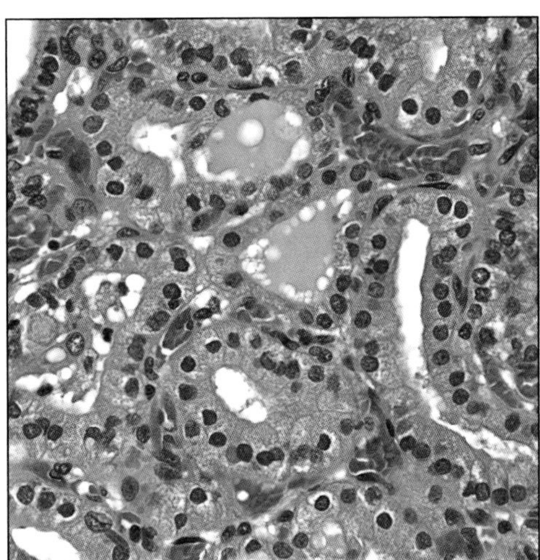

(Left) *Most nodules have abundant colloid within the expanded follicles. The follicular epithelium is low cuboidal, with dark, hyperchromatic nuclei basally polarized.* ***(Right)*** *High-power examination of nodules shows intermediate-sized cells with a low nuclear to cytoplasmic ratio and abundant cytoplasm. The cytoplasm of these cells is oncocytic or granular. The nuclei are round, regular, with dark chromatin, showing a polarized placement. Colloid is easily identified.*

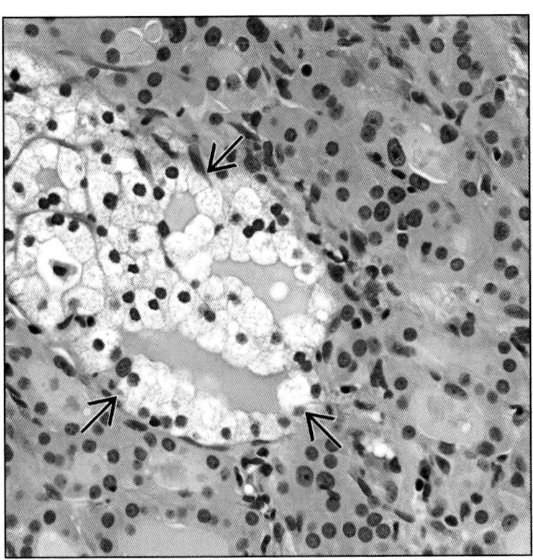

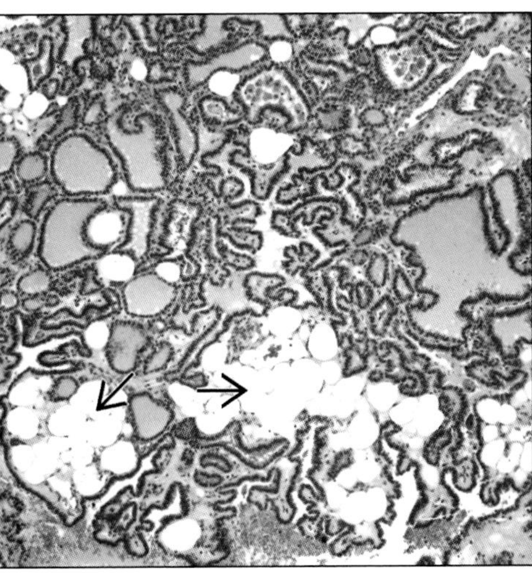

(Left) *A variety of cellular features can be seen in nodules. Here is a single focus of clear cell change* ⇨ *in a nodule that shows more of an oncocytic or oxyphilic cytoplasm in the lesional cells. Alterations like this are common.* ***(Right)*** *Colloid is easily identified in this nodule, with simple, nonarborizing papillae extending into the colloid-filled spaces. Fatty metaplasia is noted throughout this nodule* ⇨.

ADENOMATOID NODULE

Microscopic Features

(Left) Although uncommon, a signet ring-type morphology to the cytoplasm can be seen. These clear spaces would be positive with thyroglobulin, suggesting abnormal thyroglobulin production by these hyperplastic cells. Colloid is present ⇒. *(Right)* Rare, isolated cells may show nuclear pleomorphism ⇒. This isolated finding is of no clinical significance, but it is common in endocrine organ lesions. This finding is frequently present in adenomatoid nodules.

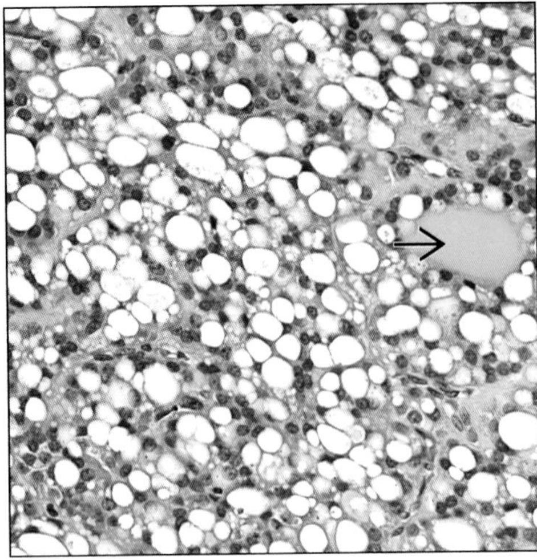

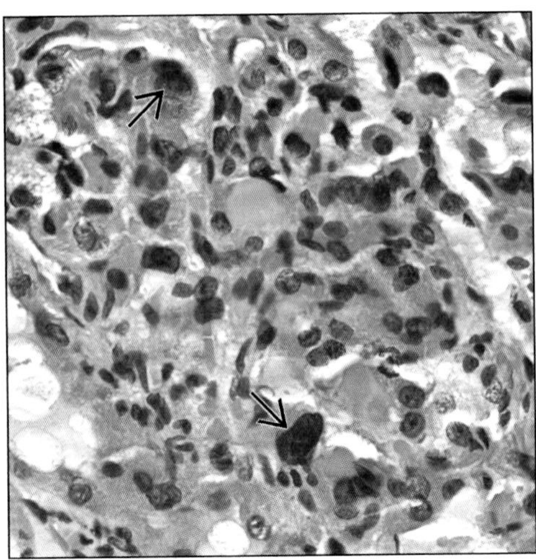

(Left) This nodule demonstrates an area of central fibrosis ⇒. Fibrosis is frequently identified in nodules as part of a degenerative or secondary change. It is often seen in the post FNA setting as well as in association with hemosiderin-laden macrophages. *(Right)* Cholesterol clefts ⇒, multinucleated giant cells ➡, and sheets of hemosiderin-laden macrophages are frequently identified degenerative changes within adenomatoid nodules.

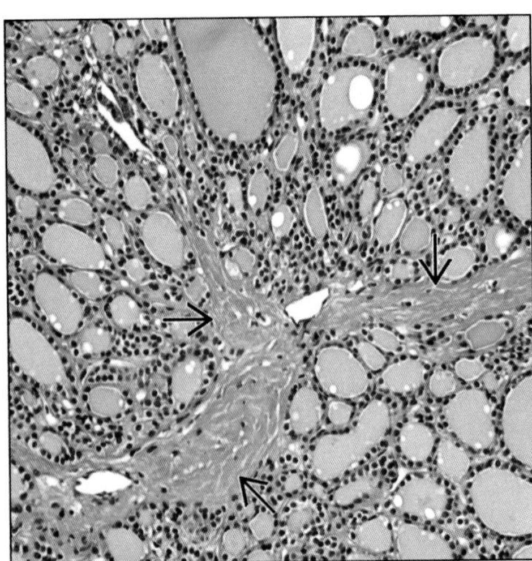

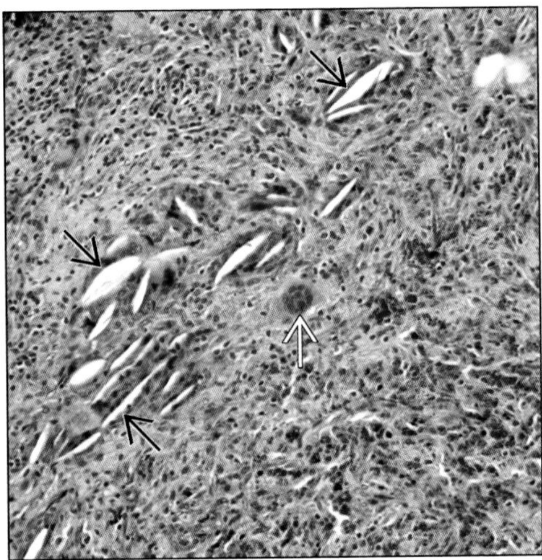

(Left) Hemosiderin-laden macrophages are present in the colloid of this nodule. Most of the follicular epithelial cells contain hemosiderin pigment within their cytoplasm, a finding frequently seen in this benign condition. This feature is vanishingly rare in neoplasms. *(Right)* Large follicles filled with colloid are shown, one of which also contains a number of macrophages/histiocytes ⇒. These cells may be identified in FNA smears, with or without hemosiderin.

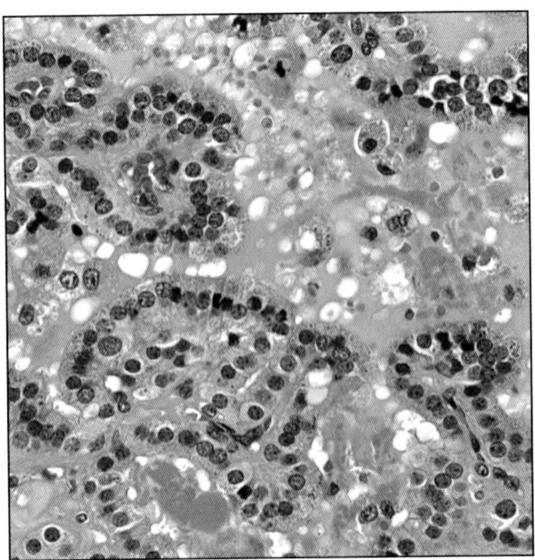

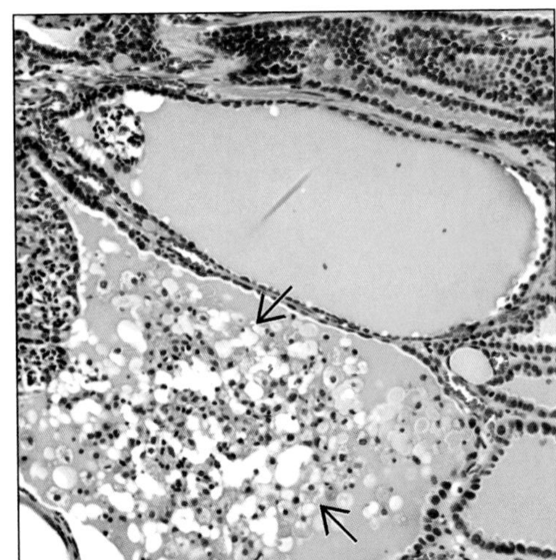

Microscopic and Cytologic Features

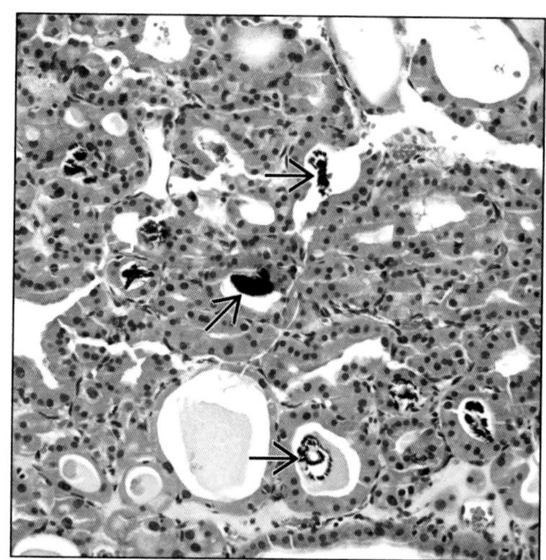

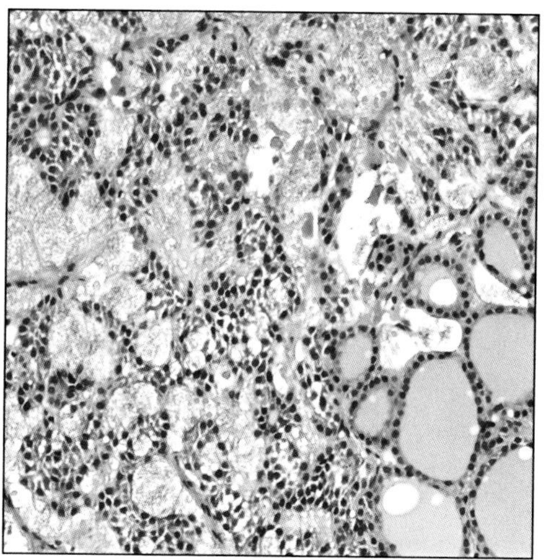

(Left) Dystrophic calcifications are often large "chunks" of calcium, but they may also be small concretions of calcium within the colloid spaces →. These mimic psammoma bodies, and are seen more frequently in oncocytic nodules than other types of nodules. **(Right)** Nodules will frequently show degenerative changes, and myxoid or edematous change is one of the most commonly seen. Here a "myxo-mucinous" change is seen within the background stroma of this nodule.

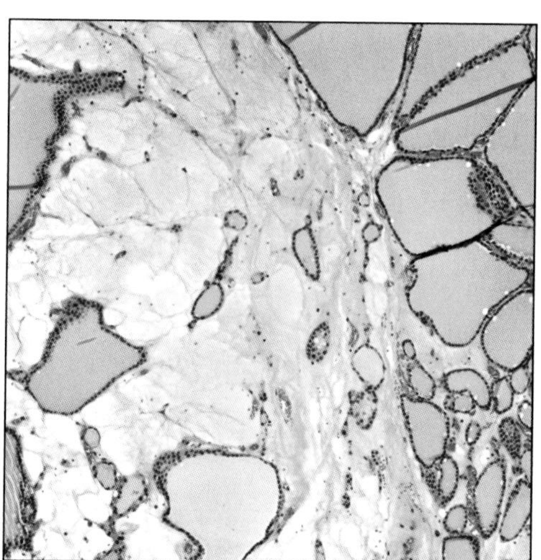

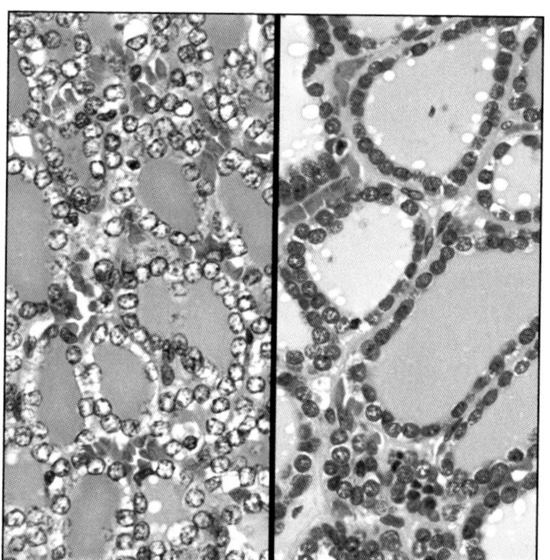

(Left) Edema or serum is present within this nodule, creating a large space. The colloid-filled follicles have a different appearance than the area of degeneration. **(Right)** Fixation artifacts are common in nodules. The left panel shows a nodule stained after drying on a heating block for 4 hours with excess water in the clearing solution. The right panel shows air drying without excess water of the exact same nodule. Processing of nodules is critical for accurate diagnosis.

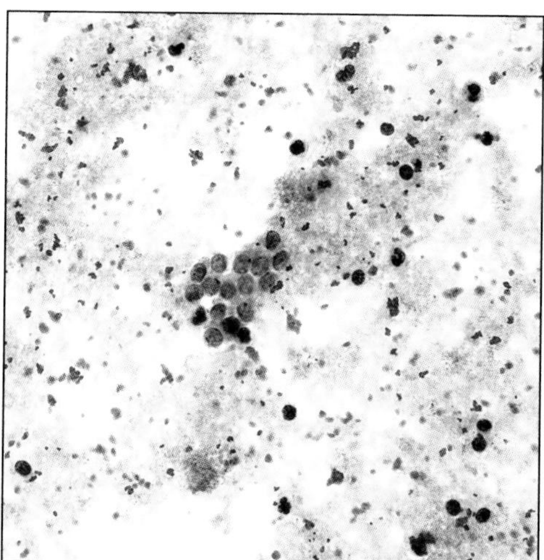

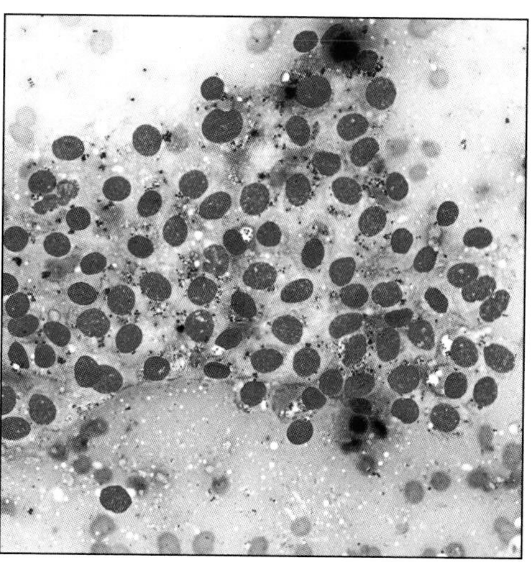

(Left) Adequacy criteria for thyroid FNA require 6-10 cells within at least 8-10 clusters per slide. Here is a single cluster of cells in a background of degenerated colloid and histiocytes. **(Right)** A large, flat sheet of follicular epithelial cells arranged in a honeycomb is quite frequently seen in adenomatoid nodules. Note the slightly "bluish" granularity of the hemosiderin pigment in the cytoplasm of these cells. This feature is more common in benign than malignant lesions.

AMYLOID GOITER

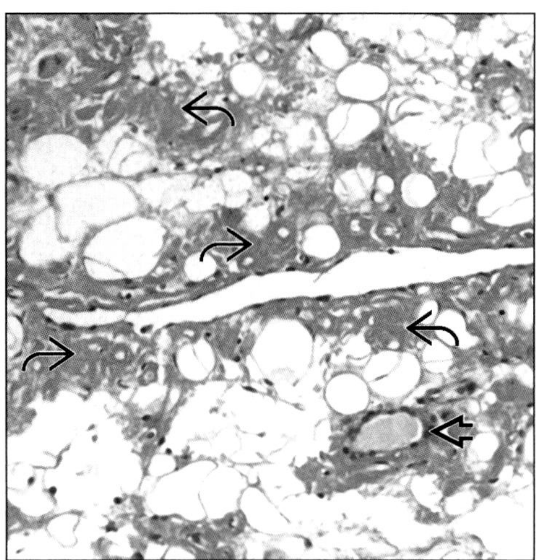

Nodular deposition of amyloid that appears eosinophilic and acellular with associated fat almost completely replaces the thyroid parenchyma, although a colloid-filled follicle is present.

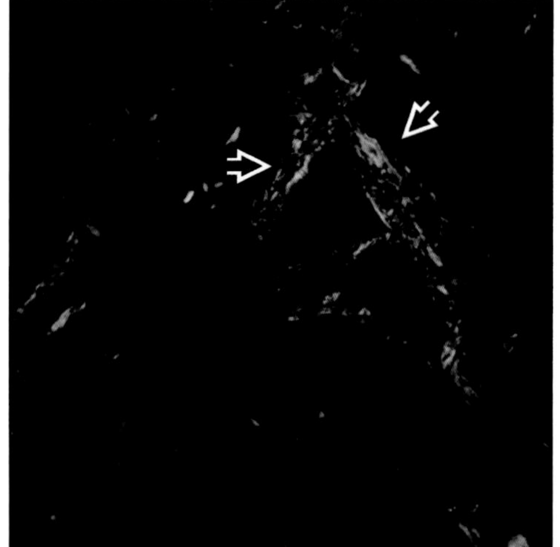

Congo red staining with polarization in amyloid goiter shows the characteristic apple-green birefringence that is associated with amyloid deposition irrespective of its site of occurrence.

TERMINOLOGY

Definitions

- Symptomatic mass or clinically detectable thyroid enlargement due to amyloid deposition
  - Amyloid deposits represent extracellular accumulation of fibrillar proteins
    - Identified in association with variety of clinical settings occurring in varied tissue sites
  - Amyloidosis may manifest in several forms including
    - Systemic amyloidosis (primary and secondary)
    - Multiple myeloma-associated amyloidosis
    - Localized or solitary amyloidosis
    - Familial amyloidosis

ETIOLOGY/PATHOGENESIS

Pathogenesis

- Classification of amyloidosis includes
  - Systemic amyloidosis (primary and secondary)
  - Multiple myeloma-associated amyloidosis
    - Chemical composition: IgG light chain (κ or λ) origin (AL)
  - Localized or solitary amyloidosis
    - Chemical composition: IgG light chain (κ or λ) origin (AL)
  - Familial Mediterranean fever
    - Chemical composition: Serum amyloid A (SAA)
  - Familial amyloidosis
    - Chemical composition: Transthyretin (TTR; prealbumin)
  - Senile amyloidosis
    - Chemical composition: Transthyretin (TTR; prealbumin)
  - Dialysis-associated amyloidosis
    - Chemical composition: B2-microglobulin (Aβ2M)
- Most common setting of amyloid in thyroid is in association with thyroid medullary carcinoma
- Amyloid deposition in thyroid can occur as part of
  - Primary amyloidosis
  - Secondary amyloidosis
- Primary amyloidosis
  - Defined as not being associated with underlying chronic disease
  - Amyloid deposition is in a variety of viscera, including heart, gastrointestinal tract, tongue
  - Chemical composition: IgG light chain (κ or λ) origin (AL)
- Secondary amyloidosis
  - Defined as being associated with underlying chronic disease
  - Amyloid deposition in kidneys, adrenal glands, liver, and spleen
  - Chemical composition: Serum amyloid A (SAA)
- More commonly seen as part of secondary systemic amyloidosis
  - In this setting, amyloid is usually found at autopsy rather than resulting in symptomatic mass
- Predisposing disorders associated with secondary systemic amyloidosis with deposition in thyroid include
  - Chronic inflammatory diseases including infections
    - Chronic osteomyelitis
    - Pulmonary tuberculosis
    - Chronic bronchitis with bronchiectasis
    - Chronic peritonitis
  - Rheumatoid arthritis
  - Familial Mediterranean fever
  - Crohn disease
  - Hodgkin disease
  - Extramedullary plasmacytoma (EMP) either as
    - Solitary plasma cell tumor (primary EMP)
    - Manifestation of multiple myeloma (secondary EMP)

AMYLOID GOITER

Key Facts

Terminology

- Symptomatic mass or clinically detectable thyroid enlargement due to amyloid deposition

Etiology/Pathogenesis

- Most common setting of amyloid in thyroid is in association with thyroid medullary carcinoma
- Amyloid deposition in thyroid can occur as part of both primary and secondary systemic amyloidosis
- More commonly seen as part of secondary systemic amyloidosis
  - In this setting, amyloid is usually found at autopsy rather than resulting in symptomatic mass

Clinical Issues

- In symptomatic amyloid goiter, clinical presentation includes
  - Nontender enlarging neck mass that may be associated with dysphagia, dyspnea, and hoarseness

Microscopic Pathology

- Diffuse amyloid deposition usually seen, but focal (nodular) deposits may occur
- Amyloid appears as extracellular eosinophilic, acellular, amorphous material
- Amyloid seen in both perifollicular and interfollicular locations compressing follicles
- Amyloid deposition seen around vascular spaces ("angiocentric")

Ancillary Tests

- Congo red, crystal violet, thioflavin-T positive
- Positive immunoreactivity with amyloid A (SAA) antibody

CLINICAL ISSUES

Epidemiology

- Incidence
  - Very rare
- Age
  - No specific age range
- Gender
  - Equal gender distribution

Site

- Anywhere in thyroid gland

Presentation

- In symptomatic amyloid goiter, clinical presentation includes
  - Nontender, rapidly enlarging neck mass
    - May be associated with dysphagia, dyspnea, and hoarseness

Laboratory Tests

- Patients are euthyroid
  - Thyroid dysfunction not generally present
- Amyloid deposition may be so extensive as to result in hypothyroidism
- May rarely be associated with hyperthyroidism
- In association with thyroid medullary carcinoma
  - Serum calcitonin levels elevated

Treatment

- Surgical approaches
  - In symptomatic patients, thyroidectomy (partial or total) is treatment of choice

Prognosis

- Prognosis in relationship to amyloid deposition in thyroid gland is excellent
  - Patient deaths may occur
    - Due to specific organ failure secondary to amyloid deposition (cardiac, renal, or hepatic failure)
- Prognosis in relationship to amyloid deposition in setting of thyroid medullary carcinoma
  - Correlates with that of medullary carcinoma

MACROSCOPIC FEATURES

General Features

- Enlarged glands with nodular to diffuse appearance
  - Weighs from 25-300 grams
- Cut surface is white to tan
  - Rubbery to firm consistency

MICROSCOPIC PATHOLOGY

Histologic Features

- Diffuse amyloid deposition usually seen, but focal (nodular) deposits may occur
- In diffuse deposition
  - Amyloid evenly distributed throughout gland
  - Replaces thyroid parenchyma
- In nodular deposition
  - Amyloid focally seen
  - Replaces gland in areas of deposition
  - Uninvolved gland appears essentially unremarkable
- Amyloid deposition
  - Amyloid appears as extracellular eosinophilic, acellular, amorphous material
  - Degree of amyloid deposition may vary from moderate to extensive
- Amyloid seen in both perifollicular and interfollicular locations compressing follicles
  - Residual follicles vary in appearance
    - From elongated with normal colloid content to slit-like atrophic follicles without colloid
  - Follicular epithelial cells generally appear as flat single cells
  - Squamous metaplasia may be seen
- Amyloid deposition seen around vascular spaces ("angiocentric")
  - Vascular-related amyloid does not result in any functional compromise of involved vascular space
  - Less often, present within walls of vascular spaces
- Additional associated findings may include
  - Chronic lymphocytic thyroiditis
  - Foreign body-type giant cell reaction

- Mature fat (focal, diffuse)
- Thyroid papillary carcinoma

ANCILLARY TESTS

Cytology

- Aspirated material contains
  - Few cells (paucicellular)
  - Small fragments of cyanophilic material (amyloid)
  - Amyloid is congophilic

Histochemistry

- Stains for amyloid
  - Congo red, crystal violet, thioflavin-T positive
    - Red appearance
    - Apple-green birefringence seen under polarized light

Immunohistochemistry

- Positive reactivity with amyloid A (SAA) antibody
- In absence of medullary carcinoma
  - Calcitonin, neuroendocrine marker reactivity not present

Electron Microscopy

- Nonbranching fibrils varying in size from 50-150 Å in diameter

DIFFERENTIAL DIAGNOSIS

Thyroid Medullary Carcinoma

- Presence of neuroendocrine neoplastic cellular proliferation
- Immunoreactivity for calcitonin, neuroendocrine markers
- Amyloid deposition limited to area(s) of neoplastic proliferation
  - Not distributed in a diffuse pattern as seen in amyloid goiter

Adenomatoid Nodules with Degenerative Changes

- Degenerative changes seen in adenomatoid nodules may include irregular fibrosis
- Fibrosis may be located
  - Within lesion (intralesional)
  - Along periphery suggesting encapsulation
  - Both intralesional and along periphery
- Amyloid may be mistaken for fibrous tissue seen in association with many thyroid diseases
- Fibrosis negative for Congo red
  - No birefringence
- Fibrosis negative for immunoreactivity associated with amyloid goiter
  - AA type

Hyalinizing Trabecular Adenoma

- Considered variant of follicular adenoma
- Characterized by presence of
  - Trabecular to organoid (paraganglioma-like) growth
  - Fibrovascular stroma
  - Extracellular hyalinization
    - May be prominent and excessive, simulating amyloid
  - Neoplastic cellular proliferation showing
    - Elongated cells with nuclei that display some morphologic similarities to papillary carcinoma
    - Orientation of nuclei perpendicular to fibrovascular stroma
    - Perinucleolar halos
    - Cytoplasmic (yellow) inclusions surrounded by clear halo
- Hyalinization negative for Congo red
  - No birefringence
- Hyalinization negative for immunoreactivity associated with amyloid goiter
  - AA type

SELECTED REFERENCES

1. Kazdaghli Lagha E et al: Amyloid goiter: First manifestation of systemic amyloidosis. Eur Ann Otorhinolaryngol Head Neck Dis. 127(3):108-10, 2010
2. Ozdemir D et al: Endocrine Involvement in Systemic Amyloidosis. Endocr Pract. Epub ahead of print, 2010
3. Villa F et al: Amyloid goiter. Int J Surg. 6 Suppl 1:S16-8, 2008
4. Himmetoglu C et al: Diffuse fatty infiltration in amyloid goiter. Pathol Int. 57(7):449-53, 2007
5. Siddiqui MA et al: Amyloid goiter as a manifestation of primary systemic amyloidosis. Thyroid. 17(1):77-80, 2007
6. Ozdemir BH et al: Diagnosing amyloid goitre with thyroid aspiration biopsy. Cytopathology. 17(5):262-6, 2006
7. Duzgün N et al: Amyloid goiter in juvenile onset rheumatoid arthritis. Scand J Rheumatol. 32(4):253-4, 2003
8. Altiparmak MR et al: Amyloid goitre in familial Mediterranean fever: report on three patients and review of the literature. Clin Rheumatol. 21(6):497-500, 2002
9. Ozdemir BH et al: Amyloid goiter in Familial Mediterranean Fever (FMF): a clinicopathologic study of 10 cases. Ren Fail. 23(5):659-67, 2001
10. Sbai A et al: Amyloid goiter as the initial manifestation of systemic amyloidosis due to familial mediterranean fever with homozygous MEFV mutation. Thyroid. 11(4):397-400, 2001
11. Bourtsos EP et al: Thyroid plasmacytoma mimicking medullary carcinoma: a potential pitfall in aspiration cytology. Diagn Cytopathol. 23(5):354-8, 2000
12. Coli A et al: Papillary carcinoma in amyloid goitre. J Exp Clin Cancer Res. 19(3):391-4, 2000
13. D'Antonio A et al: Amyloid goiter: the first evidence in secondary amyloidosis. Report of five cases and review of literature. Adv Clin Path. 4(2):99-106, 2000
14. Goldsmith JD et al: Amyloid goiter: report of two cases and review of the literature. Endocr Pract. 6(4):318-23, 2000
15. Habu S et al: A case of amyloid goiter secondary to Crohn's disease. Endocr J. 46(1):179-82, 1999
16. Sinha RN et al: Amyloid goiter due to primary systemic amyloidosis: a diagnostic challenge. Thyroid. 8(11):1051-4, 1998
17. Nijhawan VS et al: Fine needle aspiration cytology of amyloid goiter. A report of four cases. Acta Cytol. 41(3):830-4, 1997
18. Hamed G et al: Amyloid goiter. A clinicopathologic study of 14 cases and review of the literature. Am J Clin Pathol. 104(3):306-12, 1995

Microscopic Features and Ancillary Techniques

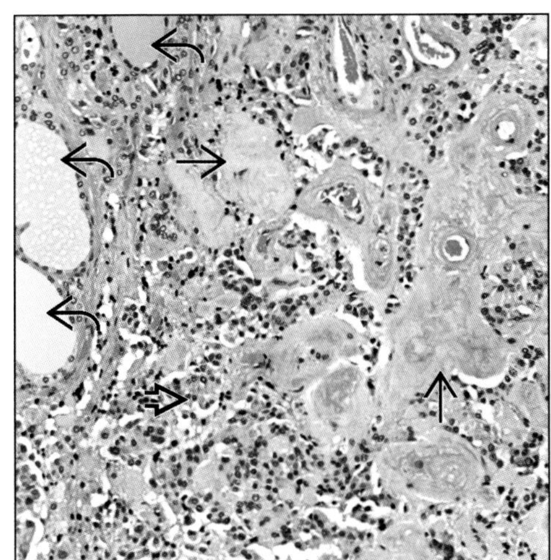

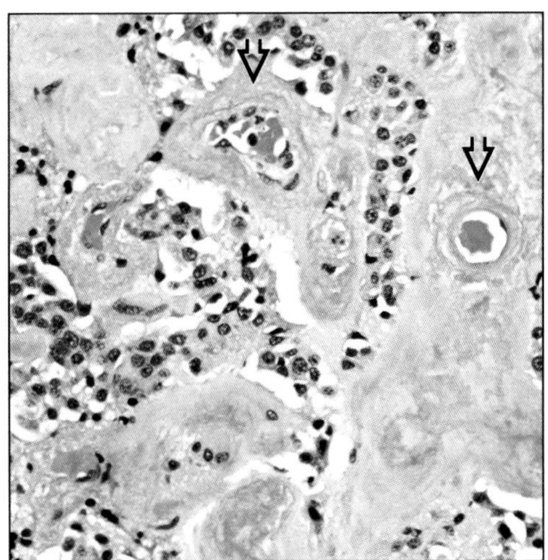

(Left) *Thyroid medullary carcinoma ⊡ with associated amyloid deposition appears as eosinophilic, acellular extracellular material ⊡. The amyloid replaces thyroid parenchyma although residual colloid-filled follicles are present ⊡.* ***(Right)*** *Amyloid deposition includes perivascular localization ⊡ intermixed with the cells of thyroid medullary carcinoma, characterized by dispersed ("salt and pepper") nuclear chromatin.*

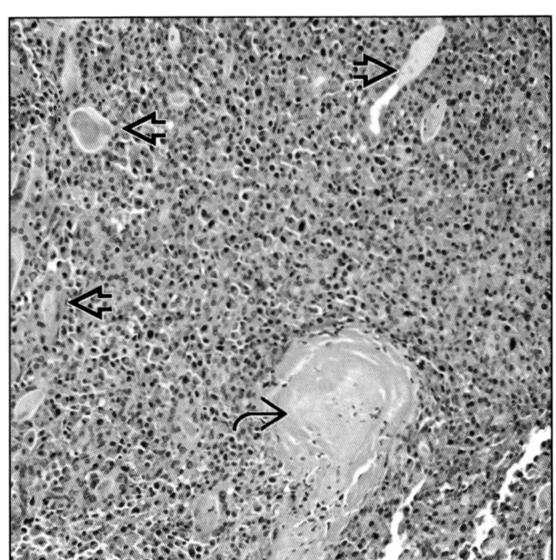

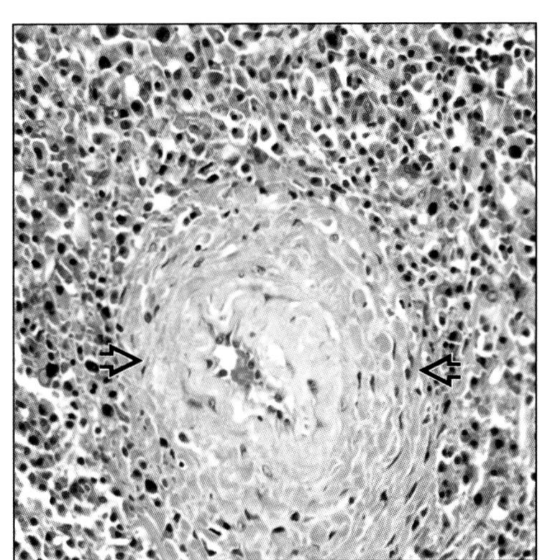

(Left) *Systemic multiple myeloma with involvement of the thyroid gland shows nodular amyloid deposition ⊡. Residual colloid-filled follicles are present ⊡, but the thyroid tissue is replaced by a hypercellular (plasma cell) infiltrate.* ***(Right)*** *The amyloid deposition occurring in association with myelomatous involvement of the thyroid gland shows perivascular localization ⊡. Congo red stain was positive and demonstrated apple-green birefringence (not shown).*

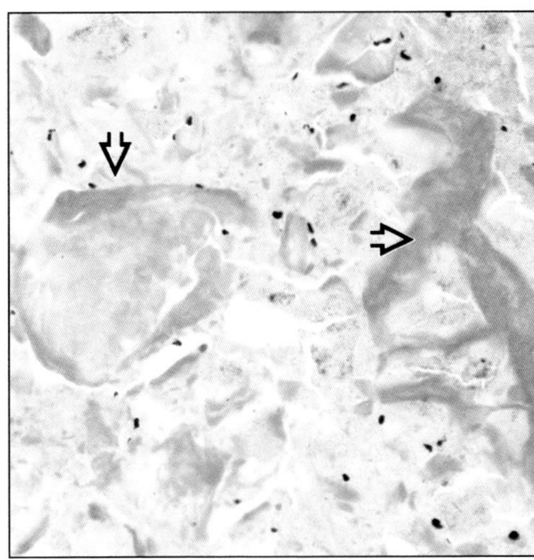

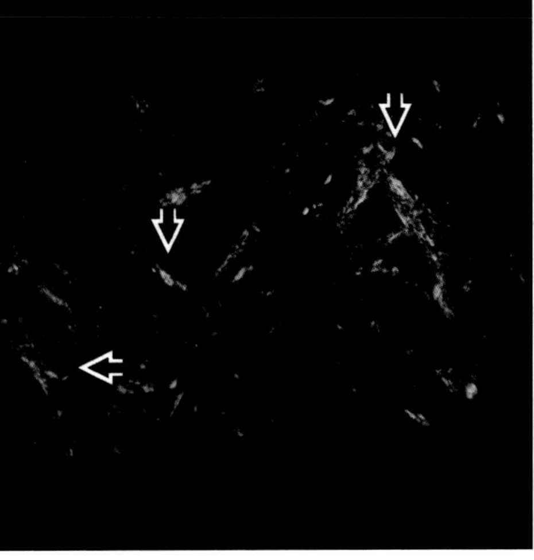

(Left) *Irrespective of the setting in which amyloid deposition occurs (e.g., primary amyloidosis, secondary amyloidosis), the staining quality of amyloid remains the same and includes Congo red positivity ⊡.* ***(Right)*** *Congo red staining with polarization shows characteristic apple-green birefringence ⊡ associated with amyloid deposition, irrespective of its site of occurrence. If needed, immunostaining for amyloid A can be used for further confirmation.*

PIGMENTS AND CRYSTALS IN THE THYROID GLAND

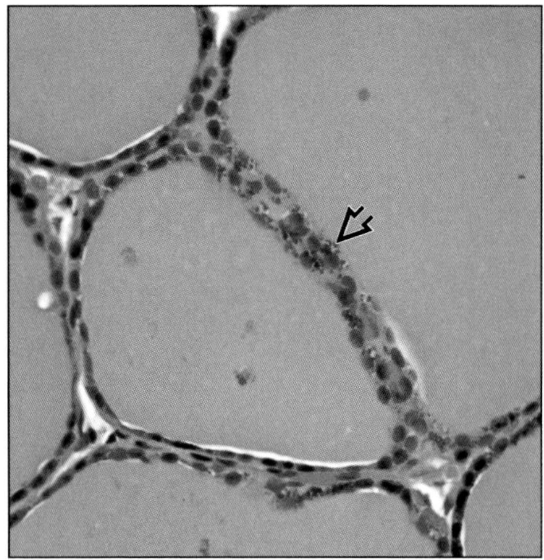

Black thyroid shows granular and black-appearing pigment in the cytoplasm of normal follicular epithelial cells ➪. The pigment can also be seen in a wide variety of pathologic thyroid lesions.

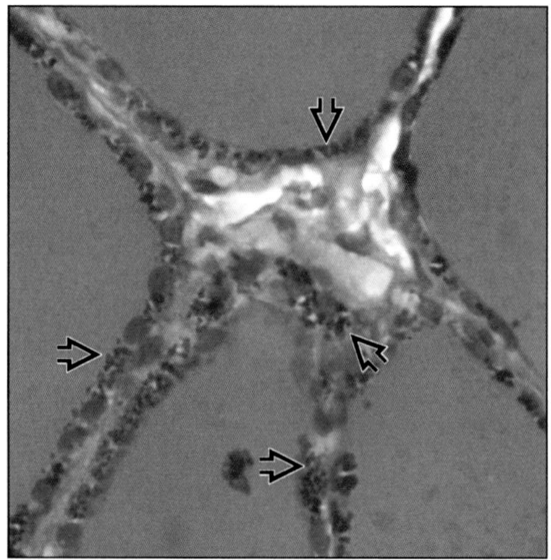

Adenomatoid nodule shows changes of black thyroid. The pigment ➪ in the thyroid epithelial cells is an incidental finding requiring clinical correlation to a history of minocycline use.

TERMINOLOGY

Synonyms

- Black thyroid
  - Specific term used to describe appearance of minocycline deposition in thyroid gland

Definitions

- Intrathyroidal deposition of endogenous or exogenous material including
  - Iron
  - Lipofuscin
  - Degradation products of minocycline
  - Crystals

ETIOLOGY/PATHOGENESIS

Environmental Exposure

- **Iron deposition**
  - Follows hemorrhage with release of iron from red blood cells
    - Resorption takes place and iron is converted to hemosiderin
    - Hemosiderin stored in cell cytoplasm of phagocytizing cells (macrophages)
  - Rarely, iron stored in thyroid as component of disorder of iron metabolism rather than secondary to hemorrhage
- **Lipofuscin**
  - Represents degenerative (aging) phenomenon
    - True nature yet to be determined
    - Contains histidine and tryptophan
- **Minocycline deposition**
  - Results from degradation products of tetracycline
  - Tetracycline derivative administered to adults for treatment of various conditions (infections, acne)
  - May cause black pigmentation and discoloration of various sites including
    - Skin
    - Thyroid gland
  - Shares histochemical, electron microscopic, and elemental analysis features with lipofuscin
  - True "makeup" not fully known; possibilities include
    - Degradation products of drug combined with lipofuscin
    - Oxidation degradation of drug itself
    - Drug interaction and alteration of tyrosine metabolism
    - Lysosomal dysfunction
- **Crystals**
  - Composed of calcium oxalate

CLINICAL ISSUES

Epidemiology

- Incidence
  - Not known
- Age
  - Typically but not exclusively in (older) adults
    - Particularly in association with iron deposition
    - Frequency of finding crystals within thyroid gland appears to increase with age
- Gender
  - Equal gender distribution

Presentation

- **Iron deposition**
  - Represents incidental finding
    - Reflects secondary phenomenon due to hemorrhage
    - Identified following traumatic (e.g., post fine needle aspiration biopsy) &/or degenerative changes
- **Lipofuscin deposition**
  - Incidental finding
- **Minocycline deposition**
  - Incidental finding

PIGMENTS AND CRYSTALS IN THE THYROID GLAND

Key Facts

Terminology
- Intrathyroidal deposition of endogenous or exogenous material
- Black thyroid
  - Specific terminology for minocycline deposition

Microscopic Pathology
- **Iron deposition**
  - Hemosiderin found in macrophages, within stromal tissues, or within follicular epithelial cells
  - Hemosiderin is readily apparent, appearing as coarse brown to yellow pigment
  - Iron stains can be used for identification and to distinguish from other pigments
- **Lipofuscin deposition**
  - Pigment seen within follicular epithelial cells
  - Intracytoplasmic accumulation of small yellow to light brown granular-appearing pigment
  - Lipid (Sudan IV), lipofuscin stains, diastase-sensitive, PAS-positive intracytoplasmic material
- **Minocycline deposition**
  - Appears within cytoplasm of follicular epithelial cells as granular and black
  - Positive staining with PAS, argentaffin stains (Fontana-Masson)
- **Crystals**
  - Intrathyroidal crystals exclusively found within colloid
  - Do not appear within cytoplasm of follicular epithelial cells or in stromal tissues

  - Not associated with glandular enlargement (hyperplasia) or functional abnormalities of gland
    - Rarely, patients may be hypothyroid but no specific link to minocycline deposition
- Crystals
  - Incidental finding
  - Increased frequency of intracolloidal crystals found in patients undergoing hemodialysis for chronic renal failure

Laboratory Tests
- Intrafollicular deposition of these pigments
  - Not associated with causing dysfunction or functional compromise of thyroid cells

Treatment
- Options, risks, complications
  - No specific treatment needed or recommended

Prognosis
- No impact on prognosis

MICROSCOPIC PATHOLOGY

Histologic Features
- **Iron deposition**
  - Hemosiderin found in macrophages, within stromal tissues, or within follicular epithelial cells
  - Hemosiderin is readily apparent, appearing as coarse brown to yellow pigment
  - If necessary, iron stains (Prussian blue, Mallory) can be used for identification and to distinguish from other pigments
- **Lipofuscin deposition**
  - Pigment seen within follicular epithelial cells
    - Intracytoplasmic accumulation of small yellow to light brown granular-appearing pigment
  - Can be an incidental finding in wide variety of thyroid pathologic conditions
    - Nonneoplastic lesions
    - Neoplastic proliferations
- **Minocycline deposition**
  - Appears within cytoplasm of follicular epithelial cells as granular and black
  - Can also be seen within follicle lumina as large black deposits admixed with colloid
  - Can be an incidental finding in wide variety of thyroid pathologic conditions
    - Nonneoplastic lesions
    - Neoplastic proliferations
  - Localization of pigment may vary including
    - In pathologic component of gland but not surrounding uninvolved thyroid
    - In nonpathologic thyroid but not in pathologic component of gland
    - In both pathologic component and surrounding uninvolved thyroid
- **Crystals**
  - Intrathyroidal crystals exclusively found within colloid
    - Do not appear within cytoplasm of follicular epithelial cells or in stromal tissues
  - Crystals readily apparent by light microscopy
    - Crystals vary in size and shape, appear in a variety of geometric shapes
    - Polarization enhances their detection
  - Finding of intracolloidal crystals is not associated with any specific diagnosis
    - May be found in virtually all thyroid abnormalities
    - Highest prevalence of crystals occurs in association with benign diseases
    - Most commonly seen in nodular goiters followed by follicular adenomas
    - May be found in association with malignant tumors (e.g., papillary carcinomas, follicular carcinomas), but prevalence is low
    - Low prevalence in association with Graves disease, lymphocytic thyroiditis, subacute thyroiditis
  - Chemical analysis shows crystals to be composed of calcium oxalate

PIGMENTS AND CRYSTALS IN THE THYROID GLAND

ANCILLARY TESTS

Cytology

- Crystals may be found by fine needle aspiration
  - Occurrence in fine needle cytology lower than that in histologic specimens

Histochemistry

- **Iron deposition**
  - Prussian blue, Mallory stains
    - Appears blue
    - Used to identify iron and distinguish it from other pigments
- **Lipofuscin deposition**
  - Lipid (Sudan IV) and lipofuscin stains
  - Diastase-sensitive, PAS-positive intracytoplasmic material
  - Iron staining is absent
- **Minocycline**
  - Positive staining with
    - Periodic acid-Schiff (PAS)
    - Lipid stains
    - Lipofuscin stains
  - Argentaffin stains (Fontana) may be positive
  - Iron staining negative

Electron Microscopy

- Lysosomes identified

DIFFERENTIAL DIAGNOSIS

Melanin

- Melanin rarely found in thyroid
- Seen in association with thyroid medullary carcinoma, melanocytic variant
  - Argentaffin(+)
  - PAS(-)
  - Neoplastic cells
    - Calcitonin(+)
    - Chromogranin(+)
    - Synaptophysin(+)
    - CD56(+)
    - Thyroid transcription factor 1 (TTF-1)(+)
    - Cytokeratins(+)
    - Thyroglobulin(-)
    - S100 protein, melanocytic markers (HMB-45, Melan-A, tyrosinase) negative
- Seen in association with metastatic malignant melanoma to thyroid
  - May be isolated metastasis or part of widespread metastatic disease
  - Argentaffin(+)
  - PAS(-)
  - Neoplastic cells immunoreactive for
    - S100 protein
    - HMB-45
    - Melan-A
    - Tyrosinase
    - Vimentin

SELECTED REFERENCES

1. Kung B et al: Malignant melanoma metastatic to the thyroid gland: a case report and review of the literature. Ear Nose Throat J. 88(1):E7, 2009
2. Singh K et al: Melanotic medullary carcinoma of thyroid--report of a rare case with brief review of literature. Diagn Pathol. 3:2, 2008
3. Oertel YC et al: Black thyroid revisited: cytologic diagnosis in fine-needle aspirates is unlikely. Diagn Cytopathol. 34(2):106-11, 2006
4. Bozbora A et al: Thyroid metastasis of malignant melanoma. Am J Clin Oncol. 28(6):642-3, 2005
5. Isotalo PA et al: Presence of birefringent crystals is useful in distinguishing thyroid from parathyroid gland tissues. Am J Surg Pathol. 26(6):813-4, 2002
6. Bell CD et al: Histologic, immunohistochemical, and ultrastructural findings in a case of minocycline-associated "black thyroid". Endocr Pathol. 12(4):443-51, 2001
7. de Lima MA et al: Cytological aspects of melanotic variant of medullary thyroid carcinoma. Diagn Cytopathol. 24(3):206-8, 2001
8. Koren R et al: Black thyroid adenoma. Clinical, histochemical, and ultrastructural features. Appl Immunohistochem Mol Morphol. 8(1):80-4, 2000
9. Hecht DA et al: Black thyroid: A collaborative series. Otolaryngol Head Neck Surg. 121(3):293-6, 1999
10. Shimizu M et al: Calcium oxalate crystals in thyroid fine needle aspiration cytology. Acta Cytol. 43(4):575-8, 1999
11. Ikeda T et al: Medullary thyroid carcinoma with a paraganglioma-like pattern and melanin production: a case report with ultrastructural and immunohistochemical studies. Arch Pathol Lab Med. 122(6):555-8, 1998
12. Katoh R et al: Birefringent (calcium oxalate) crystals in thyroid diseases. A clinicopathological study with possible implications for differential diagnosis. Am J Surg Pathol. 17(7):698-705, 1993
13. Katoh R et al: Nature and significance of calcium oxalate crystals in normal human thyroid gland. A clinicopathological and immunohistochemical study. Virchows Arch A Pathol Anat Histopathol. 422(4):301-6, 1993
14. Keyhani-Rofagha S et al: Black thyroid: a pitfall for aspiration cytology. Diagn Cytopathol. 7(6):640-3, 1991
15. Sheppard BC et al: Malignant melanoma metastatic to the thyroid as initial evidence of disseminated disease. J Surg Oncol. 43(3):196-8, 1990
16. Senba M et al: Black thyroid associated with minocycline therapy: histochemical and ultrastructural studies on the brown pigment. Isr J Med Sci. 24(1):51-3, 1988
17. Reid JD et al: Calcium oxalate crystals in the thyroid. Their identification, prevalence, origin, and possible significance. Am J Clin Pathol. 87(4):443-54, 1987
18. Alexander CB et al: Black thyroid: clinical manifestations, ultrastructural findings, and possible mechanisms. Hum Pathol. 16(1):72-8, 1985
19. Marcus JN et al: Melanin production in a medullary thyroid carcinoma. Cancer. 49(12):2518-26, 1982

Microscopic Features and Ancillary Techniques

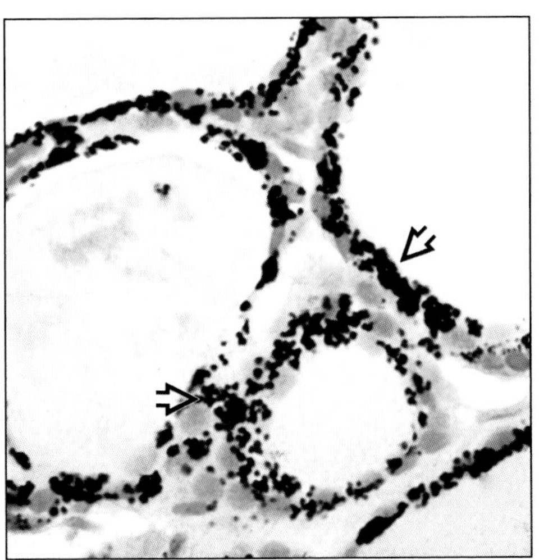

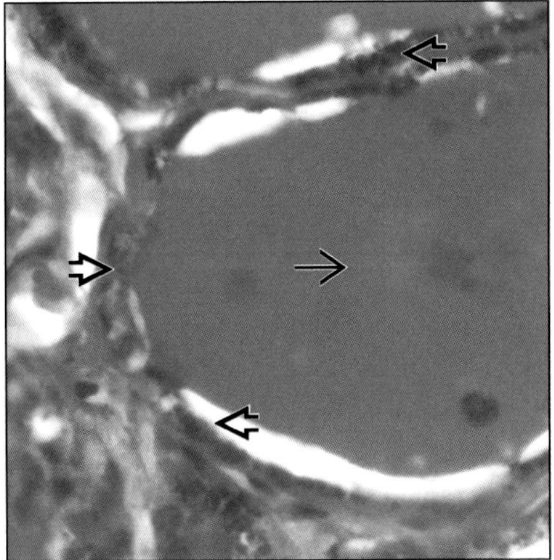

(Left) *The pigment associated with black thyroid stains with Fontana, appearing as dark black granules within the cytoplasm of follicular epithelial cells.* ***(Right)*** *The pigment associated with black thyroid stains with PAS, appearing as reddish-brown granules within the cytoplasm of follicular epithelial cells. PAS is also a good stain for colloid. Melanin may rarely be seen in the thyroid gland and will be Fontana positive but PAS negative.*

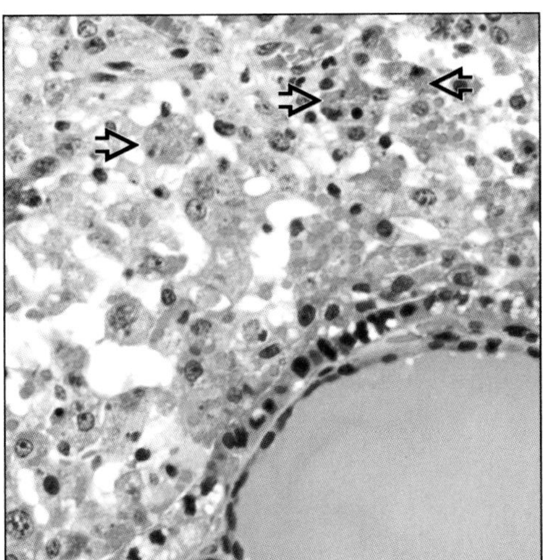

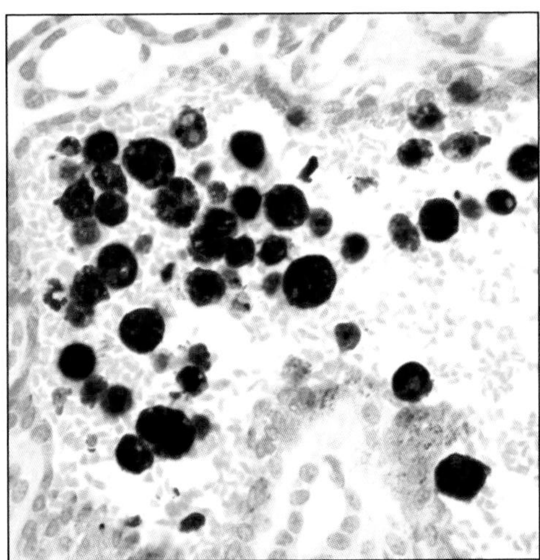

(Left) *Degenerative alterations due to trauma (e.g., post needle aspiration) or occurring spontaneously result in hemorrhage, including hemosiderin, appearing as coarse brown to yellow pigment within macrophages.* ***(Right)*** *Iron stain shows the intense blue staining of hemosiderin within the cytoplasm of macrophages found in an adenomatoid nodule that had undergone degenerative changes secondary to fine needle aspiration biopsy.*

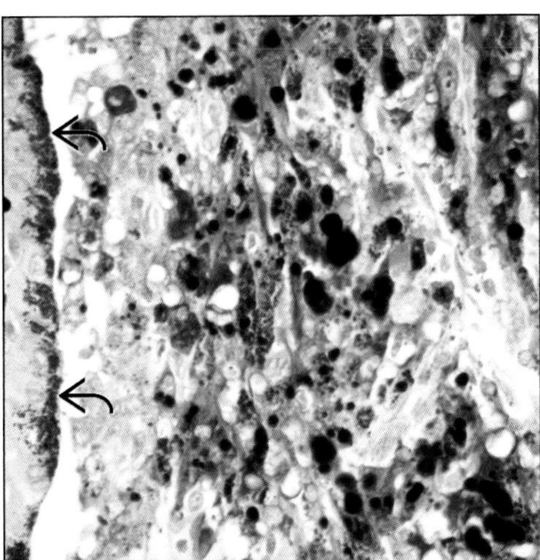

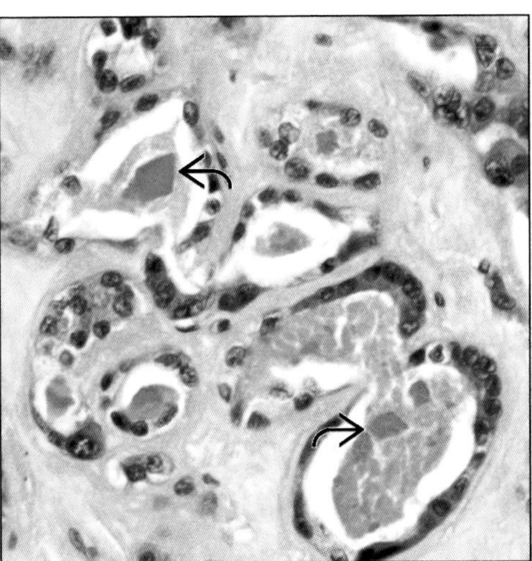

(Left) *In addition to the macrophages, iron staining shows the presence of hemosiderin within the cytoplasm of follicular epithelial cells. In spite of the intracytoplasmic pigment, there is no compromise of the functional integrity of the follicular cells.* ***(Right)*** *Intrafollicular crystals, varying in size and shape, are composed of calcium oxalate, and are exclusively found within colloid. They are most commonly found in adenomatoid nodules and follicular adenomas.*

POST FINE NEEDLE ASPIRATION CHANGES

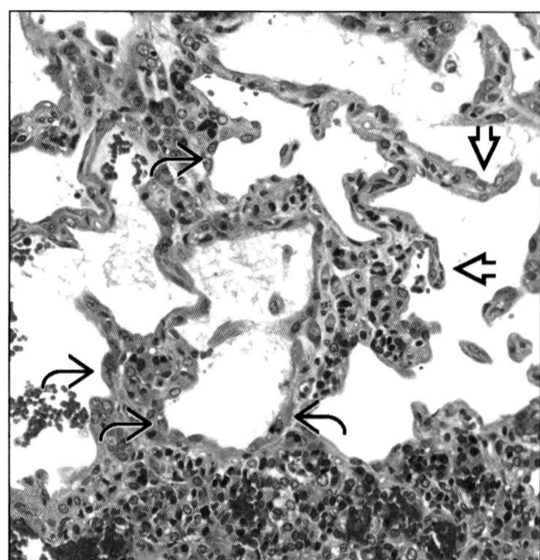

Post-aspiration alterations involve the follicular epithelial cells ⇾, including dilated and ramifying spaces, and papillations ⇨ that can be misinterpreted as a vascular neoplasm.

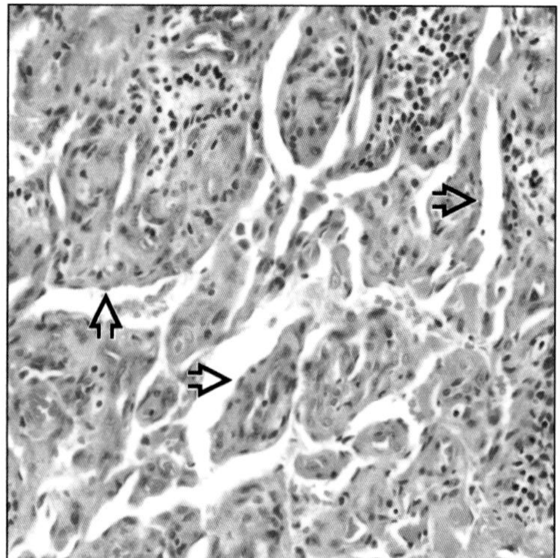

Papillary endothelial hyperplasia following FNAB shows numerous papillae projecting into the lumen composed of a layer of endothelium ⇨ surrounding a collagenized core.

TERMINOLOGY

Synonyms

- Worrisome histologic alterations following fine needle aspiration of thyroid (WHAFFT)

Definitions

- Reactive &/or degenerative morphologic alterations in thyroid lesions following fine needle aspiration biopsy

ETIOLOGY/PATHOGENESIS

Iatrogenic

- Fine needle aspiration biopsy (FNAB) has tremendous utility as 1st interventional procedure in diagnosis of thyroid masses
- Diagnostic sensitivity and specificity of FNAB for thyroid mass is high
- In most instances and with some exceptions, surgical removal is treatment for thyroid mass lesion irrespective of diagnosis by FNAB
- Post-FNAB histologic changes occur in numerous lesions including
  - Nonneoplastic lesions
    - Adenomatoid nodules
    - Hyperplastic lesions (e.g., Graves disease, others)
  - Neoplasms
    - Follicular adenoma and variants
    - Follicular carcinoma and variants
    - Papillary carcinoma and variants
    - Medullary carcinoma and variants
- Lesions/tumors with cytoplasmic oxyphilia (so-called Hürthle cells)
  - More prone than other cell types to degenerative changes following FNAB
  - Due to high content of oxygen-sensitive mitochondria, oncocytic (Hürthle cells) are more easily traumatized
    - Potentially results in infarction and additional degenerative changes

CLINICAL ISSUES

Epidemiology

- Incidence
  - Common occurrence
- Age
  - Occurs in all ages
- Gender
  - Equal gender distribution

Site

- No specific localization

Prognosis

- Dependent on nature of underlying lesion
- Histologic alterations caused by FNAB may lead to erroneous diagnosis
  - Change in interpretation from benign process to malignant one

MICROSCOPIC PATHOLOGY

Histologic Features

- FNAB may result in a number of reactive histologic changes in resected thyroid gland
- Based on type of reaction seen, post-FNAB alterations may include acute or chronic type changes
- **Acute changes**
  - Usually identified within 3 weeks following FNAB
  - Most common findings include
    - Fresh hemorrhage
    - Remote hemorrhage in form of hemosiderin-laden macrophages
    - Granulation tissue
  - Other alterations may include
    - Localized follicular destruction

POST FINE NEEDLE ASPIRATION CHANGES

Key Facts

Terminology

- Reactive &/or degenerative morphologic alterations in thyroid lesions following fine needle aspiration biopsy

Etiology/Pathogenesis

- Iatrogenically induced
  - Most often secondary to fine needle aspiration biopsy
- Lesions/tumors with cytoplasmic oxyphilia (so-called Hürthle cells) more prone to degenerative changes following FNAB

Microscopic Pathology

- **Acute changes**: Usually identified within 3 weeks following FNAB
  - Most common findings include hemorrhage, granulation tissue
- **Chronic changes**: Usually identified > 3 weeks from FNAB to surgical removal and include
  - Infarction
  - Metaplasia (squamous, oxyphilic)
  - Capsular alterations with pseudoinvasive growth
  - Vascular alterations (e.g., dilated vascular spaces with thrombosis, organization &/or papillary endothelial hyperplasia), endothelial cell atypia
- Postoperative spindle cell proliferation
  - Exuberant proliferation of spindle cells with bland cytology and numerous mitoses
  - May suggest diagnosis of anaplastic carcinoma or sarcoma

- Capsular alterations
- Reactive nuclear atypia includes enlargement with clearing of nuclear chromatin; typically occurs near needle tract
- Necrosis and mitoses

- **Chronic changes**: Usually identified > 3 weeks from FNAB to surgical removal and include
  - Fibrosis
  - Infarction
  - Metaplasia (squamous, oncocytic)
  - Capsular alterations with pseudoinvasive growth
    - May take form of needle tract with linear hemorrhagic tract
    - May suggest presence of capsular invasion
    - Key findings include absence of follicular epithelium within needle tract with associated chronic inflammatory cell infiltrate and hemorrhage (recent and remote)
  - Vascular alterations include
    - Artifactual implantation or "invasion" of tumor cells including cells floating within vascular lumens rather than adherent to vessel wall
    - Dilated vascular spaces with thrombosis, organization &/or papillary endothelial hyperplasia
    - Endothelial cell atypia
- Post-FNAB alterations of adenomatoid nodules may include
  - Cyst formation with papillary growth
  - Fibrosis and calcification
  - Cholesterol granulomas
  - Nuclear atypia
- Post-FNAB alterations of lesions with oncocytic cells (so-called Hürthle cells)
  - Oxyphilic cells occur in all settings (e.g., metaplasia, follicular adenoma, follicular carcinoma, papillary carcinoma)
    - More prone to post-FNAB degenerative changes
    - Due to oxygen-sensitive mitochondria that predominate in these cells
    - Any compromise to oxygen supply of oncocytic cells may result in degenerative changes that are not seen as readily in non-oncocytic cells
    - Changes include hemorrhage, infarction, papillary architecture
- Post-FNAB infarcted follicular adenoma
  - Infarction may be partial or complete
    - Infarction appears as coagulative necrosis with associated hemorrhage and inflammatory cell infiltrate
    - Infarction may compromise histology, making recognition of nature of lesion difficult
    - Peripheral rim of residual, viable tumor may be present, which may show marked reactive nuclear atypia
    - In infarcted foci, architectural pattern of lesion is retained despite cellular necrosis
  - With time, granulation tissue and macrophages may be present
- Postoperative spindle cell proliferation
  - Exuberant proliferation of spindle cells with bland cytology and numerous mitoses
    - May suggest diagnosis of anaplastic carcinoma, sarcoma
  - Nodular, relatively circumscribed &/or nonencapsulated
  - Often limited to central part of preexisting thyroid lesion(s)
  - Variable cellularity with mild nuclear pleomorphism, rare mitotic figures
  - Plump spindle cells with rich network of thin-walled blood vessels and chronic inflammatory cell component

ANCILLARY TESTS

Histochemistry

- Periodic acid-Schiff (PAS)
  - Stains colloid red
    - May be helpful in recognizing lesion as follicular epithelial neoplasm

POST FINE NEEDLE ASPIRATION CHANGES

Immunohistochemistry

- Thyroglobulin, TTF-1
  - Follicular epithelial cell lesion/tumor will be positive
    - In cases showing infarction, antigenicity is retained in infarcted lesional cells
- Calcitonin, neuroendocrine markers
  - C-cell derived lesions/tumor positive
  - In spite of degenerative changes, antigenicity is retained in lesional cells
- Smooth muscle actin
  - Diffusely positive in spindle cells of postoperative spindle cell proliferation
    - Suggests myofibroblastic origin

DIFFERENTIAL DIAGNOSIS

Vascular Neoplasm

- Reactive vascular alterations may suggest presence of vascular tumor
  - Post-FNAB vascular changes may include
    - Widely dilated and blood-filled spaces
    - Papillary endothelial hyperplasia
- Intrathyroidal vascular tumors may include
  - Hemangioma
  - Angiosarcoma
- Factors that may be helpful in not misdiagnosing reactive vascular alterations for a thyroid vascular neoplasm include
  - Rarity of primary vascular neoplasms occurring in thyroid gland
  - Presence of other post-FNAB reactive (nonvascular) alterations
  - Temporal sequence from FNAB to surgical removal
    - Typically relatively short interval from time of FNAB to resection
    - Knowledge that recent preoperative FNAB occurred helpful in considering changes as being reactive rather than neoplastic

Thyroid Papillary Carcinoma

- Shows constellation of nuclear alterations diagnostic for papillary carcinoma including
  - Nuclear enlargement
  - Variation in size and shape of nuclei
  - Optically clear to dispersed (very fine appearing) nuclear chromatin
  - Crowding and overlapping of nuclei
  - Nuclear grooves
  - Nuclear inclusions
- Diagnosis of papillary carcinoma predicated solely on the nuclear changes, therefore, diagnosis can be made
  - In absence of papillary architecture such as
    - Follicular variant
  - In absence of invasive growth such as
    - Capsular invasion
    - Lymph-vascular invasion

Anaplastic Carcinoma

- Densely cellular proliferation with
  - Marked nuclear pleomorphism
  - Increased mitotic activity
  - Atypical mitoses
  - Necrosis
  - Invasive growth
- Characteristic demographics and clinical history
  - Predilection for older adults
  - Clinical history of rapidly enlarging neck mass often in longstanding thyroid lesion
    - Some cases may occur in absence of longstanding thyroid lesion

Sarcoma

- Rare neoplastic type in thyroid gland that may include
  - Angiosarcoma
  - Leiomyosarcoma
  - Malignant peripheral nerve sheath tumor (malignant schwannoma)
- Sarcomas typically characterized by
  - Densely cellular proliferation with marked nuclear pleomorphism, increased mitotic activity, atypical mitoses, necrosis
- Immunohistochemical staining helpful in diagnosis including
  - Angiosarcoma
    - CD31, CD34, factor VIII-related antigen
  - Leiomyosarcoma
    - Smooth muscle actin
  - Malignant peripheral nerve sheath tumor (MPNST)
    - S100 protein variably present
    - In low-grade MPNST, S100 protein typically diffusely reactive
    - In high-grade MPNST, S100 protein typically absent to focally reactive

SELECTED REFERENCES

1. Polyzos SA et al: Histological alterations following thyroid fine needle biopsy: a systematic review. Diagn Cytopathol. 37(6):455-65, 2009
2. Baloch ZW et al: Cytologic and architectural mimics of papillary thyroid carcinoma. Diagnostic challenges in fine-needle aspiration and surgical pathology specimens. Am J Clin Pathol. 125 Suppl:S135-44, 2006
3. Pandit AA et al: Worrisome histologic alterations following fine needle aspiration of the thyroid. Acta Cytol. 45(2):173-9, 2001
4. Baloch ZW et al: Post fine-needle aspiration histologic alterations of thyroid revisited. Am J Clin Pathol. 112(3):311-6, 1999
5. Baloch ZW et al: Post-fine-needle aspiration spindle cell nodules of the thyroid (PSCNT). Am J Clin Pathol. 111(1):70-4, 1999
6. Kini SR: Post-fine-needle biopsy infarction of thyroid neoplasms: a review of 28 cases. Diagn Cytopathol. 15(3):211-20, 1996
7. Ramp U et al: Fine needle aspiration (FNA)-induced necrosis of tumours of the thyroid. Cytopathology. 6(4):248-54, 1995
8. LiVolsi VA et al: Worrisome histologic alterations following fine-needle aspiration of the thyroid (WHAFFT). Pathol Annu. 29 (Pt 2):99-120, 1994
9. Layfield LJ et al: Necrosis in thyroid nodules after fine needle aspiration biopsy. Report of two cases. Acta Cytol. 35(4):427-30, 1991

Gross and Microscopic Features

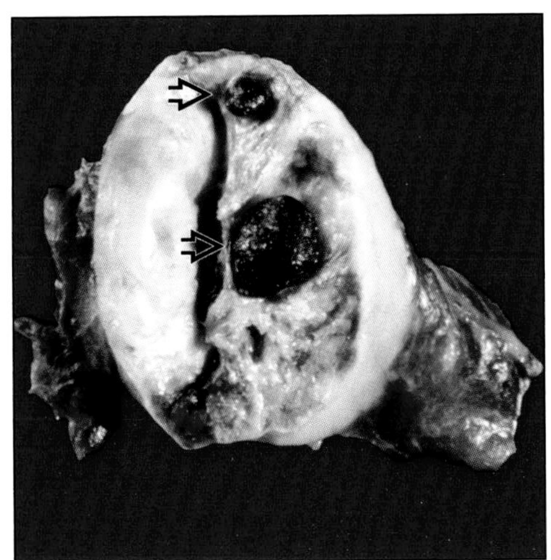

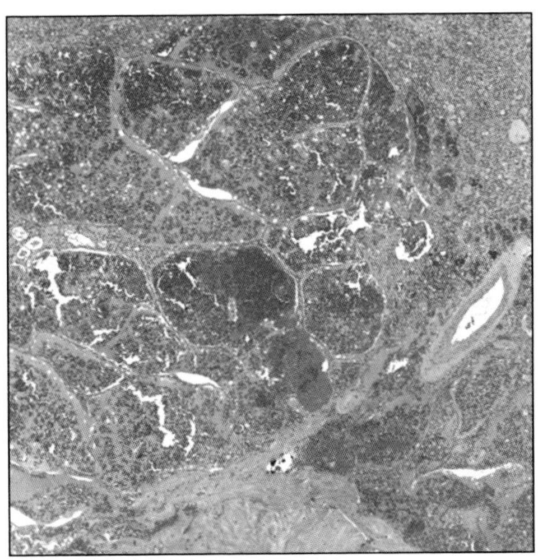

(Left) *Dominant adenomatoid nodule shows thrombi lying within cystically dilated spaces ⇨. These changes were identified in the thyroidectomy that followed a few weeks after a fine needle aspiration biopsy. The gross findings are not particularly worrisome for a vascular neoplasm.* ***(Right)*** *Post-aspiration vascular alterations include dilated and blood-filled endothelial-lined vascular spaces that suggest the possibility of a vascular neoplasm such as a hemangioma.*

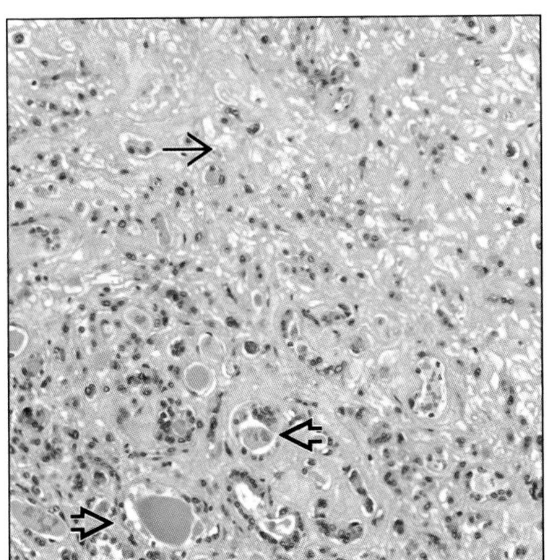

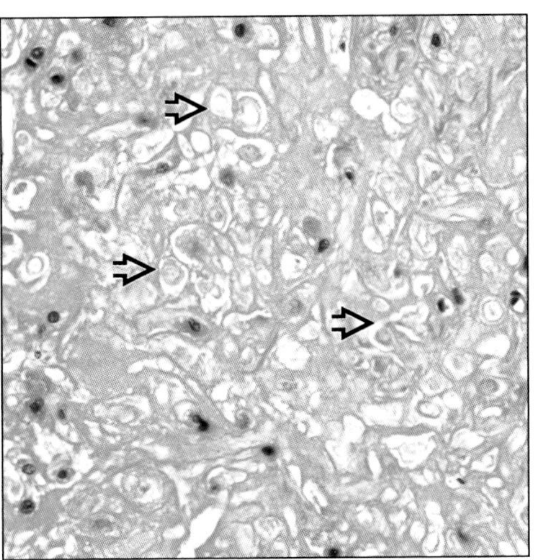

(Left) *Infarcted follicular adenoma shows residual viable colloid-filled follicles ⇨ along its peripheral aspect with the more central portion completely infarcted → with no residual viable thyroid tissue remaining.* ***(Right)*** *Infarcted follicular adenoma, oncocytic type shows loss of identifiable viable lesional cells; however, ghost outlines of the lesional cell remain ⇨. Such ghost cells retain their antigenicity and would be immunoreactive for thyroglobulin.*

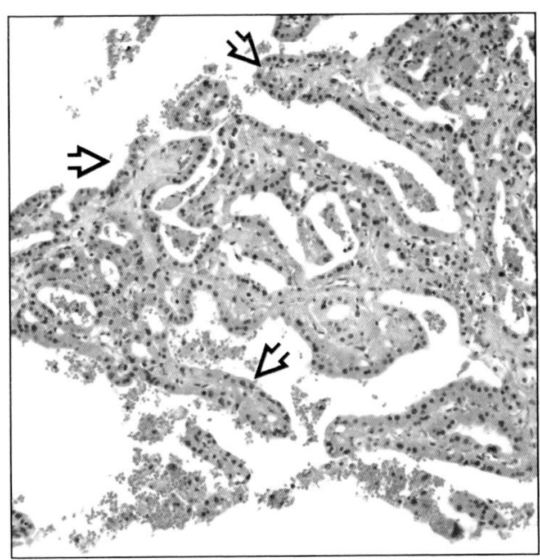

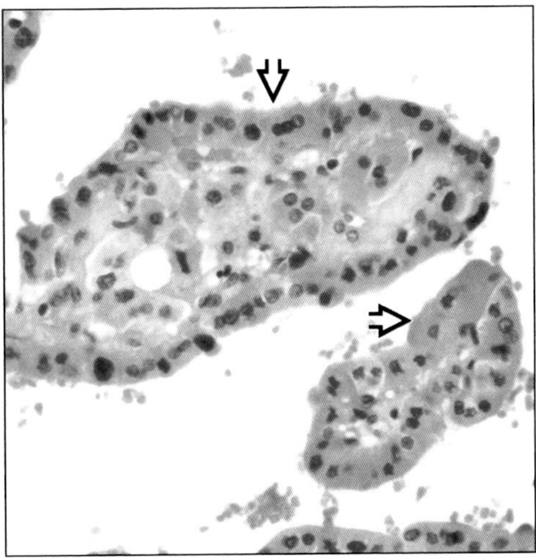

(Left) *Adenomatoid nodule with oncocytic cells shows degenerative alterations that followed a fine needle aspiration biopsy including cyst formation, hemorrhage (recent and remote), and papillary architecture ⇨.* ***(Right)*** *The papillae occurring secondary to FNAB are wider and less complex than those typically seen in papillary carcinoma and lack the diagnostic nuclear alterations of papillary carcinoma. The oncocytic cells seen ⇨ are prone to degenerative changes following FNAB.*

C-CELL HYPERPLASIA (PHYSIOLOGIC)

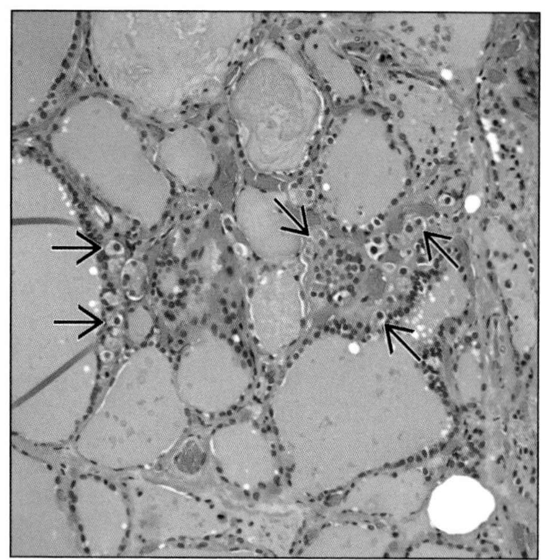

There is an increased number of C-cells ⇒ in this gland affected by adenomatoid nodules. There is no follicle destruction and no cytologic atypia. The collections are < 50 cells.

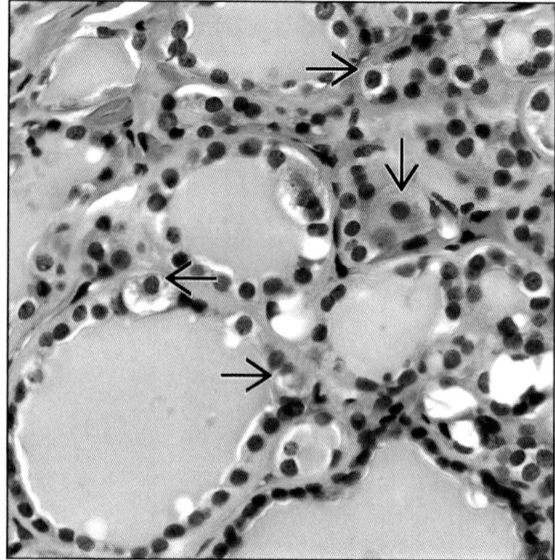

The C-cells have slightly granular, blue to cleared cytoplasm ⇒. They are usually present as single cells or in small clusters of cells in a parafollicular distribution. No cytologic atypia or destruction is present.

TERMINOLOGY

Definitions

- Benign, nonneoplastic increase in C-cells within thyroid gland parenchyma

ETIOLOGY/PATHOGENESIS

Pathogenesis

- Ultimobranchial body gives rise to C-cells
  - Identified in middle to upper thyroid lobes
    - Not identified in isthmus
  - Neuroendocrine cells with argyrophilic cytoplasmic granules
- C-cells ultimately give rise to medullary carcinoma

CLINICAL ISSUES

Epidemiology

- Incidence
  - Unknown, although common if diligently sought
- Age
  - Matches ages for underlying disease process that resulted in surgery

Site

- Most frequently concentrated in middle-upper outer zones of both thyroid lobes

Presentation

- Patients are asymptomatic

Prognosis

- No adverse outcome for this physiologic process

MACROSCOPIC FEATURES

Sections to Be Submitted

- Sections from mid-upper outer lobes maximize diagnostic opportunity

Size

- Individual cells to small clusters of cells (< 50 μm)

MICROSCOPIC PATHOLOGY

Histologic Features

- Generally easiest to find adjacent to or intermixed with solid cell nests
- Small cells in a parafollicular distribution
- Cytoplasm is clear to lightly stained
  - Cytoplasmic bluish granularity is frequently present
- Nuclei tend to be slightly larger than follicular epithelial cell nuclei
  - No nuclear atypia
- C-cell hyperplasia is separated into subtypes
  - **Physiologic or reactive**
    - Tends to be focal, with only a few cells
    - Usually, 3-5 cells in small clusters
    - 8-10 cell clusters in low power field (40x total magnification)
    - May be observed in association with other thyroid conditions or neoplasms
    - Physiologic response may be to trophic hormones, hypercalcemia, paracrine factors, or inflammation
  - **Neoplastic**
    - Nodular &/or diffuse proliferation
    - Easily identified on H&E stained sections
    - No follicle destruction
    - Not associated with amyloid or fibrosis
    - < 50 cells in an aggregate
    - Conceptually: "Medullary carcinoma in situ"
    - Seen with hereditary medullary carcinoma
    - Shows *RET* germline mutations

C-CELL HYPERPLASIA (PHYSIOLOGIC)

Key Facts

Terminology

- Benign, nonneoplastic increase in C-cells within thyroid gland parenchyma
  - Ultimobranchial body gives rise to C-cells

Microscopic Pathology

- Generally easiest to find adjacent to or intermixed with solid cell nests
- Small cells, in parafollicular distribution, with clear to lightly stained cytoplasm
- **Physiologic or reactive**
  - Tends to be focal, with only few cells
  - 8-10 cell clusters in low-power field (40x total magnification)
- **Neoplastic**
  - Nodular &/or diffuse proliferation
  - Easily identified on H&E stained sections
  - < 50 cells in an aggregate
- Calcitonin required to prove diagnosis

ANCILLARY TESTS

Immunohistochemistry

- In general, immunohistochemistry is required to highlight cells
- Cells will be positive with calcitonin
- Most cells also positive: CD56, chromogranin, &/or synaptophysin
  - Not as sensitive and specific as calcitonin

Molecular Genetics

- No *RET* mutations in physiologic C-cell hyperplasia

DIFFERENTIAL DIAGNOSIS

Microscopic Medullary Carcinoma

- Aggregates of > 50 cells
- Thyroid follicle destruction, with breaching of basement membrane
- Fibrosis &/or amyloid can be seen
- Cellular pleomorphism is more easily identified
- *RET* mutations can be detected

Palpation Thyroiditis

- Single or few follicles destroyed (follicle centric)
- Random distribution throughout gland
- Histiocytes and giant cells

Squamous Metaplasia

- Random distribution throughout gland
- Pavemented pattern
- Intercellular bridges easily identified
- No parafollicular distribution

Intraglandular Spread of Medullary Carcinoma

- Can be seen throughout gland, accentuated at periphery where vessels have their highest concentration
- Only in lymph-vascular channels
  - Not in parafollicular distribution
- Cytologic atypia seen

Microscopic Papillary Carcinoma

- Not in parafollicular distribution
- Often associated with fibrosis or stellate infiltration
- Large cells with high nuclear to cytoplasmic ratio
- Nuclear overlapping, nuclear grooves and irregularities, intranuclear cytoplasmic inclusions

SELECTED REFERENCES

1. Volante M: [Sporadic C-cell hyperplasia associated with multinodular goiter.] Pathologica. 98(2):160-3, 2006
2. Albores-Saavedra JA et al: C-cell hyperplasia and medullary thyroid microcarcinoma. Endocr Pathol. 12(4):365-77, 2001
3. Borda A et al: The C-cells: current concepts on normal histology and hyperplasia. Rom J Morphol Embryol. 45:53-61, 1999
4. Perry A et al: Physiologic versus neoplastic C-cell hyperplasia of the thyroid: separation of distinct histologic and biologic entities. Cancer. 77(4):750-6, 1996

IMAGE GALLERY

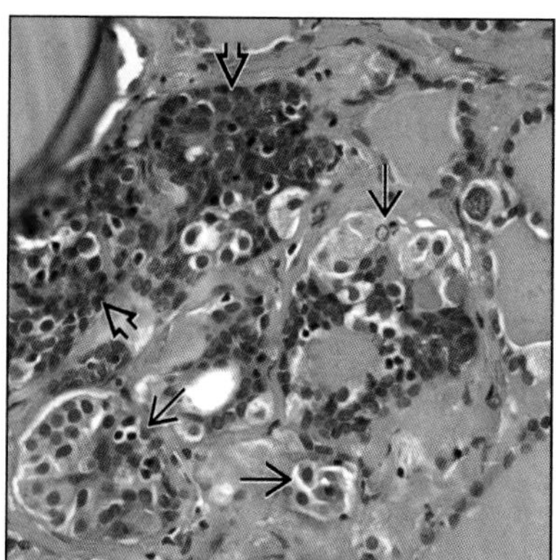

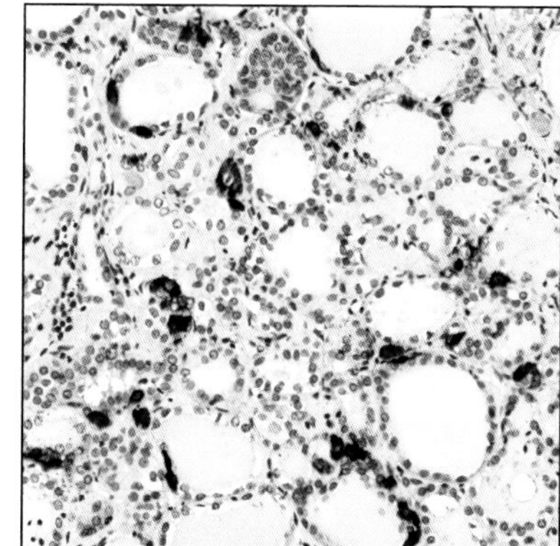

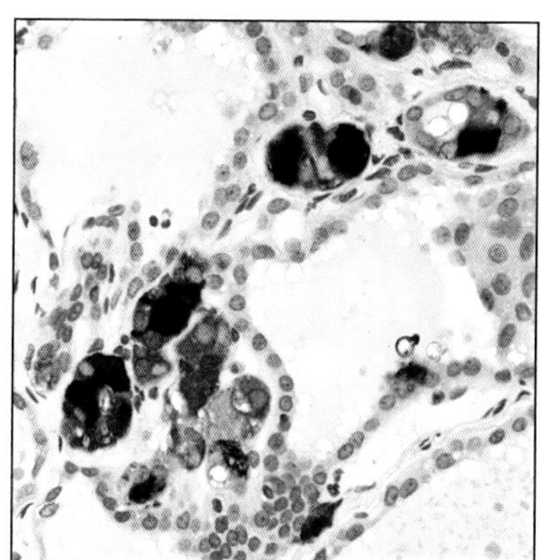

(Left) *C-cells ➔ are frequently identified in association with solid cell nests ⇒, as they are derived from these structures. While there is clustering, there is no destructive growth or amyloid.* ***(Center)*** *Calcitonin is the most reliable stain in highlighting the C-cells in physiologic C-cell hyperplasia.* ***(Right)*** *Calcitonin stain highlights the cytoplasm in a diffuse to slightly granular pattern. The follicular epithelial cells are nonreactive.*

FOLLICULAR ADENOMA

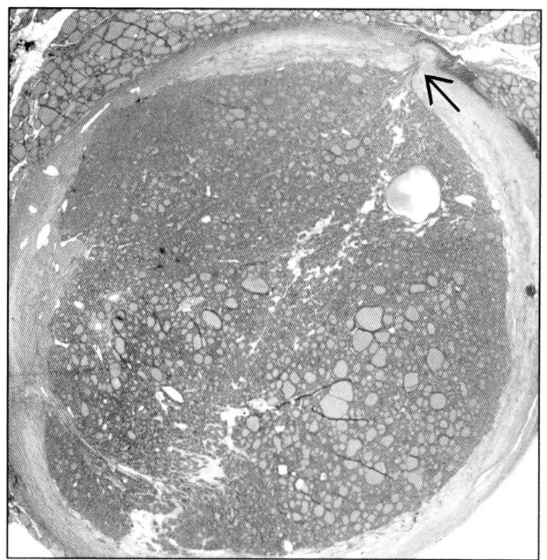

This low-power image demonstrates a follicular neoplasm surrounded by a well-formed, slightly thickened capsule. Colloid is easily identified. There is no evidence of invasion. A FNA site is present ⇒.

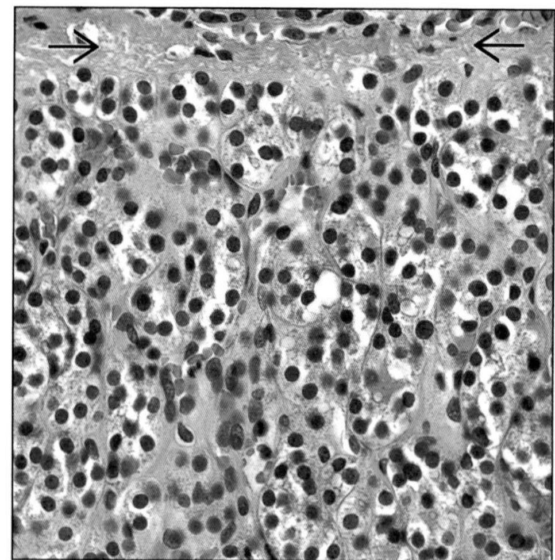

Follicles with scant colloid, surrounded by cuboidal cells with round and regular nuclei, show coarse nuclear chromatin distribution. There is ample eosinophilic cytoplasm. A capsule is noted ⇒.

TERMINOLOGY

Abbreviations

- Follicular adenoma (FA)

Definitions

- Benign, encapsulated neoplasm of thyroid follicular epithelial cells
  - Variant histologies are recognized; oncocytic type most common

ETIOLOGY/PATHOGENESIS

Environmental Exposure

- Iodine deficiency
  - Nodules are 2-3x more common in low iodine consumption areas
  - May be due to thyroid-stimulating hormone (TSH) stimulation of follicular epithelium
- Radiation (γ radiation specifically)
  - Exposure during childhood and adolescence
  - Increased risk of about 15x
  - FA develops 10-15 years after exposure

Inherited Syndrome

- Uncommon, since most adenomas are sporadic
  - Cowden disease
    - Multiple hamartoma syndrome with germline mutations of *PTEN* tumor suppressor gene, resulting in loss of *PTEN* function
    - Tumors tend to be bilateral and multiple
  - Carney complex
    - Autosomal dominant disease caused by germline mutations in the *PRKARIA* gene
    - Tumors often multiple and oncocytic

Pathogenesis

- Monoclonal proliferations, arising from a single cell

CLINICAL ISSUES

Epidemiology

- Incidence
  - Difficult to accurately determine, as cellular solitary nodules cannot be separated by noninvasive methods
  - 3-8% of adults have solitary palpable nodules
    - ~ 75% of these represent adenoma
    - Carcinoma must be excluded, which drives further evaluation
- Age
  - Broad age range
  - Most present in 5th-6th decades of life
- Gender
  - Female > > Male (4-5:1)

Site

- Any part of thyroid gland

Presentation

- Painless thyroid nodule/mass
- Identified incidentally during palpation or ultrasound of the neck for different reasons
- When large, difficulty swallowing and local compressive symptoms may be seen
- Adenomas grow slowly
- Bleeding into tumor may result in sudden pain, tenderness, and increase in size
- Mobile, discrete, smooth nodules that move with thyroid

Laboratory Tests

- Patients are usually euthyroid
- Rare adenomas are functional

Treatment

- Options, risks, complications

FOLLICULAR ADENOMA

Key Facts

Terminology
- Benign, encapsulated neoplasm of thyroid follicular epithelial cells

Clinical Issues
- 3-5% of adults
- Most present in 5th-6th decades of life
- Female > > Male (4-5:1)
- Painless thyroid nodule in euthyroid patients
- Lobectomy treatment of choice with excellent long-term prognosis

Macroscopic Features
- Solitary, well delineated from adjacent parenchyma
- Submit entire peripheral zone (parenchyma to capsule to tumor interface)

Microscopic Pathology
- Encapsulated tumor surrounded by variable thick fibrous connective tissue capsule
- Smooth muscle-walled vessels in the fibrosis help to confirm presence of capsule
- Tumor architecture and cytologic appearance distinct from surrounding parenchyma
- Cuboidal to polygonal cells, basal, round, dark nuclei

Ancillary Tests
- FNA cytology does **not** distinguish among adenomatoid nodule, follicular adenoma, or follicular carcinoma

Top Differential Diagnoses
- Follicular carcinoma, papillary carcinoma (follicular variant), medullary carcinoma

---

  - Previous radiation exposure or family history results in clinical, radiographic, and biochemical assessment
  - Fine needle aspiration is critical for initial evaluation of a thyroid nodule
  - Hypoparathyroidism and recurrent laryngeal nerve damage may result from surgery
- Surgical approaches
  - Lobectomy treatment of choice
- Drugs
  - Levothyroxine suppresses TSH, which may result in a decrease of nodule size
    - Patient should be followed at regular intervals if this method is utilized

Prognosis
- Excellent long-term prognosis
- Outcome indistinguishable among variants of adenoma
  - Specifically, oncocytic/oxyphilic variant

IMAGE FINDINGS

Radiographic Findings
- Imaging studies cannot reliably separate benign from malignant neoplasms
- Best study is ultrasound

Ultrasonographic Findings
- Identifies single or multiple nodules
  - Helps separate adenoma from adenomatoid nodules
- Solid, homogeneous mass
- Most are isoechoic
  - Can be hyperechoic or hypoechoic
- Thin, well-defined, peripheral echo-poor halo represents capsule
  - Regular margin and smooth border
- Color Doppler
  - "Spoke and wheel": Peripheral blood vessels extending toward center of lesion

MR Findings
- MR used frequently in evaluating recurrent tumors rather than primary method for thyroid nodules
- T1WI: Iso- or hypointense; decreased intensity suggests hemorrhage or degeneration
- T2WI: Typically hyperintense

CT Findings
- Findings tend to be nonspecific
  - Nodules frequently found incidentally
  - Hypodense intrathyroidal mass
  - Absence of invasion and adenopathy suggests benign diagnosis
  - Large adenomas may enhance heterogeneously due to degeneration
- Solitary, well-defined nodule compressing adjacent normal gland

Nuclear Medicine Findings
- PET: Potential pitfall when imaging, since thyroid normally takes up FDG
- Thyroid scintigraphic studies with Tc-99m pertechnetate or ^{123}I
  - Most are "cold" nodules (absent activity)
  - Rarely, hyperfunctioning adenomas will appear "hot"
    - Hot nodules are rarely malignant (< 1%)

MACROSCOPIC FEATURES

General Features
- Solitary tumor
- Well delineated from adjacent parenchyma
- Round to ovoid
- Light, whitish-gray to tan-brown tumors, depending on cellularity and histologic type
- Rubbery, fleshy, and homogeneous solid cut surface
- Secondary changes can be seen
  - Cyst formation, infarction, fibrosis, hemorrhage, and calcification

FOLLICULAR ADENOMA

Sections to Be Submitted

- Entire peripheral zone (parenchyma to capsule to tumor interface), unless nodule is large
- Sections perpendicular to capsule

Size

- Variable
  - Currently, 1-3 cm is common
    - Improved radiographic techniques and clinical surveillance help identify smaller lesions
  - Most are < 4 cm
  - Usually palpable if > 1 cm

MICROSCOPIC PATHOLOGY

Histologic Features

- Encapsulated tumor surrounded by variably thick fibrous connective tissue capsule
  - If capsule is thick, exclude carcinoma with additional sections or levels
- Smooth muscle-walled vessels in fibrosis help to confirm presence of capsule
- Reticulin and elastic fibers in fibrosis also confirm capsule
- Entrapped follicular epithelium can be seen
- Tumor architecture and cytologic appearance distinct from surrounding parenchyma
- Variable cellularity
- Variable architecture
  - Solid (embryonal), trabecular, microfollicular (fetal), normofollicular, macrofollicular, insular, and papillary patterns
  - 1 pattern typically dominates
- Colloid usually present, to a variable degree, within follicle lumen
  - May undergo calcification, resembling psammoma bodies
    - More common in oncocytic types
- Cuboidal to polygonal cells with ample cytoplasm
- Cell borders are easily identified
- Nuclei are basal (polarized), evenly spaced, round to oval, with coarse nuclear chromatin distribution
- Nucleoli tend to be small and eccentric
- Isolated "bizarre," hyperchromatic nuclei are occasionally present
- Cytoplasm ranges from cleared, eosinophilic, amphophilic, to oncocytic
  - Oncocytic type due to accumulation of abnormal mitochondria in cytoplasm
- Mitotic figures are uncommon (except in post-FNA setting)
- Delicate capillaries are present, but intratumoral fibrosis is uncommon
- Post-FNA changes (cystic degeneration, hemorrhage, hemosiderin-laden macrophages, calcifications, fibrosis) can mimic invasion

Variants

- Oncocytic (oxyphilic, Hürthle cell, Ashkenazy)
- Hyperfunctioning (toxic)
- Adenoma with papillary hyperplasia
- Adenolipoma (lipoadenoma)
- Signet ring cell-type
- Adenoma with clear cells
- Adenoma with bizarre nuclei
- Atypical follicular adenoma

ANCILLARY TESTS

Cytology

- FNA is first-line in management of solitary thyroid nodule evaluation
- FNA cytology does **not** discriminate among adenomatoid nodule, follicular adenoma, or follicular carcinoma
- Adequacy requires 5-6 follicular epithelial groups composed of at least 10 epithelial cells on smear for valid interpretation
- Usual diagnosis: "Thyroid follicular epithelial proliferation, favor neoplasm" or "follicular lesion"
- Usually cellular smears with numerous microfollicular structures
- Colloid is usually sparse
- Follicular epithelial cells are arranged in small spherical aggregates surrounding colloid droplet
- Follicular epithelial cells are round to polygonal, showing slight crowding
- Round and regular nuclei with even nuclear chromatin distribution
- Oncocytic cells have more abundant, granular cytoplasm, often associated with intranuclear cytoplasmic inclusions and nuclear irregularities

Frozen Sections

- Generally useless in accurate classification of follicular lesions
- Full capsule needs to be evaluated to exclude invasion

Histochemistry

- PAS highlights colloid

Immunohistochemistry

- Positive with keratins, TTF-1, thyroglobulin
- Oncocytic tumors must be interpreted with caution due to high background and nonspecific staining

Cytogenetics

- Numerical chromosome changes, usually gains of chromosome 7, although 12 and 5 may be gained
  - Chromosome 7 gains seen in about 15% of FA (trisomy) but in approximately 45% of oncocytic adenomas (tetrasomy)
- Translocations on 19q13 and 2p21 (approximately 10% of adenomas)

Molecular Genetics

- Activating point mutations of *RAS* genes (specifically *NRAS* and *HRAS*) are most prevalent (about 30% of cases)
- Somatic mutations in mitochondrial DNA (mtDNA) are found in oncocytic tumors
- If *PAX8/PPARγ* rearrangement is detected, submit additional sections and perform levels, as vascular or capsular invasion can usually be identified

Immunohistochemistry

Antibody	Reactivity	Staining Pattern	Comment
Thyroglobulin	Positive	Cytoplasmic	Also seen in luminal colloid; most specific marker
TTF-1	Positive	Nuclear	
pax-8	Positive	Nuclear	
CK8/18/CAM5.2	Positive	Cytoplasmic	
CK-PAN	Positive	Cytoplasmic	
CK7	Positive	Cell membrane & cytoplasm	
CK19	Positive	Cell membrane & cytoplasm	Present in about 50% of adenomas
CK-HMW-NOS	Negative		
Calcitonin	Negative		
Chromogranin-A	Negative		
CEA-M	Negative		
Galectin-3	Equivocal		About 10% of adenomas
HBME-1	Equivocal		About 10% of adenomas
MSG1	Equivocal		About 10% of adenomas

DIFFERENTIAL DIAGNOSIS

Follicular Carcinoma

- Requires identification of invasion
  - Capsular invasion
  - Vascular invasion
- Tends to have higher cellularity
- Mitotic figures are often present and increased

Papillary Carcinoma, Follicular Variant

- Capsular &/or vascular invasion can be seen
- Intratumoral fibrosis helpful
- Thick, eosinophilic colloid
  - Giant cells, crystalloids, and scalloping within colloid
- Large tumor cells with high nuclear to cytoplasmic ratio
- Loss of polarity or organization (misplaced around follicle)
- Nuclear irregularities, nuclear grooves, nuclear overlapping, intranuclear cytoplasmic inclusions, nuclear chromatin clearing
  - Sometimes identified in topographically separate foci within single tumor

Medullary Carcinoma

- Invasive growth
- Lacks colloid
- Plasmacytoid to spindled tumor cells
- Cytoplasm is slightly granular and basophilic to amphophilic
- "Salt and pepper" nuclear chromatin distribution
- Many variants may overlap with adenoma
- Calcitonin, CEA, chromogranin, synaptophysin, and TTF-1 immunoreactivity

Adenomatoid (Hyperplastic) Nodule

- Usually multiple nodules
- Lacks compression of surrounding thyroid parenchyma
- Lacks capsule, although fibrosis may mimic capsule
- Variable growth patterns within nodule
- Abundant colloid
- Degenerative changes: Cyst formation, hemosiderin-laden macrophages, blood, fibrosis, calcification, cholesterol clefts

Parathyroid Adenoma

- Cell borders tend to be more prominent
- Cytoplasm is cleared and well defined
- Nuclear chromatin is more coarse
- Chromogranin is positive, but TTF-1 and thyroglobulin are negative

SELECTED REFERENCES

1. Hunt JL: Molecular alterations in hereditary and sporadic thyroid and parathyroid diseases. Adv Anat Pathol. 16(1):23-32, 2009
2. Layfield LJ et al: Thyroid aspiration cytology: current status. CA Cancer J Clin. 59(2):99-110, 2009
3. Baloch ZW et al: Fine-needle aspiration of the thyroid: today and tomorrow. Best Pract Res Clin Endocrinol Metab. 22(6):929-39, 2008
4. Faquin WC: The thyroid gland: recurring problems in histologic and cytologic evaluation. Arch Pathol Lab Med. 132(4):622-32, 2008
5. Fischer S et al: Application of immunohistochemistry to thyroid neoplasms. Arch Pathol Lab Med. 132(3):359-72, 2008
6. Osamura RY et al: Current practices in performing frozen sections for thyroid and parathyroid pathology. Virchows Arch. 453(5):433-40, 2008
7. Serra S et al: Controversies in thyroid pathology: the diagnosis of follicular neoplasms. Endocr Pathol. 19(3):156-65, 2008
8. Yeung MJ et al: Management of the solitary thyroid nodule. Oncologist. 13(2):105-12, 2008
9. Baloch ZW et al: Our approach to follicular-patterned lesions of the thyroid. J Clin Pathol. 60(3):244-50, 2007
10. Shaha AR: TNM classification of thyroid carcinoma. World J Surg. 31(5):879-87, 2007
11. Wang TS et al: Management of follicular tumors of the thyroid. Minerva Chir. 62(5):373-82, 2007
12. Rosai J et al: Pitfalls in thyroid tumour pathology. Histopathology. 49(2):107-20, 2006

FOLLICULAR ADENOMA

Imaging, Gross, and Microscopic Features

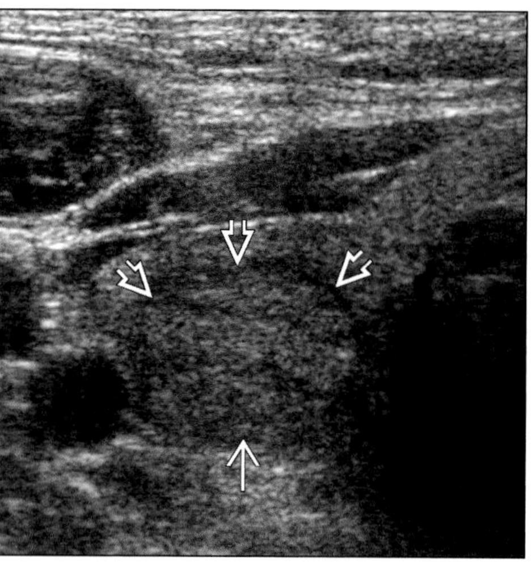

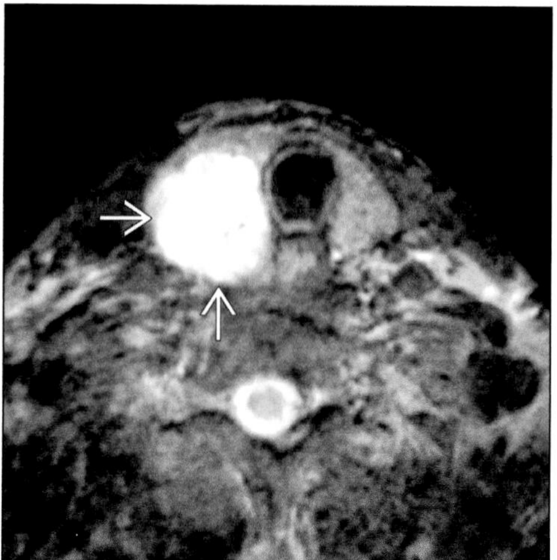

(Left) *Transverse ultrasound shows isoechoic intrathyroidal mass ➡ with echo-poor periphery ⇨. The thin, well-defined, smooth, peripheral echo-poor halo represents the capsule of this follicular adenoma.* ***(Right)*** *This T2WI MR shows a uniformly hyperintense mass within the right lobe of the thyroid ➡. The mass appears well defined and does not extend beyond the thyroid gland. There is no neck adenopathy present. While not diagnostic, the MR appearance suggests a benign diagnosis.*

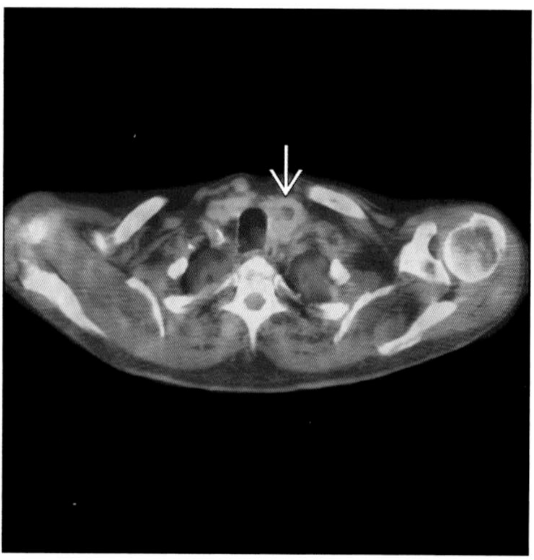

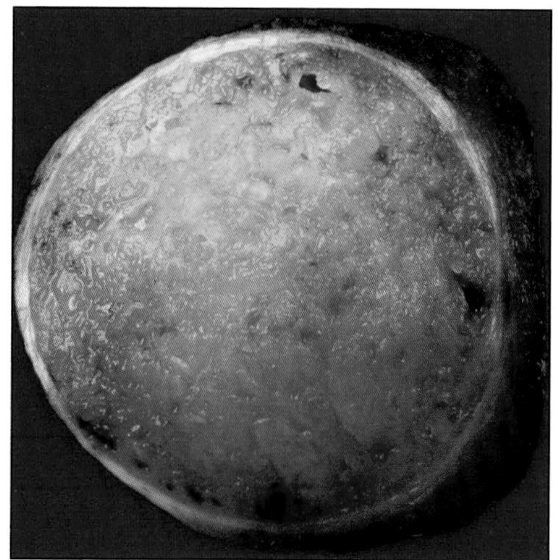

(Left) *This PET scan using FDG shows an avid thyroid nodule ➡. This finding confirms a mass but does not give a diagnosis (which proved to be adenoma in this case). PET scans frequently show thyroid uptake, but a single mass with more avid uptake requires further evaluation.* ***(Right)*** *There is a thick, well-formed fibrous connective tissue capsule separating a neoplasm from the surrounding parenchyma. There is compression of the adjacent thyroid, which is more beefy red.*

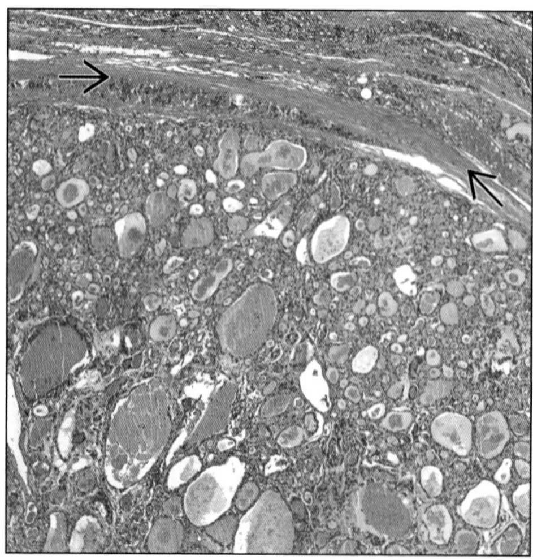

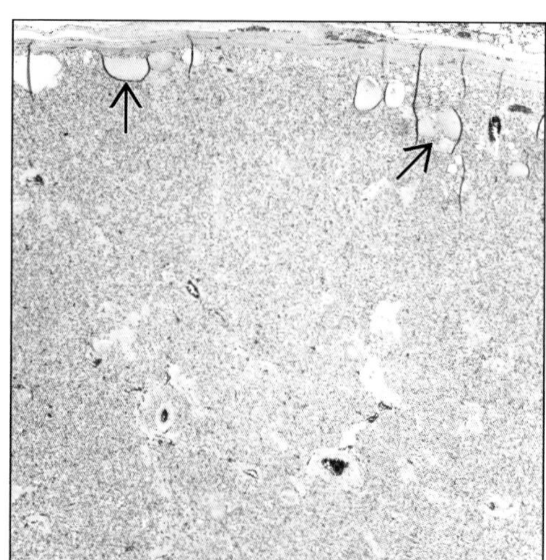

(Left) *There is a thin fibrous connective tissue capsule → surrounding a tumor whose appearance is distinct from the adjacent, compressed thyroid parenchyma. Colloid is easily identified within the follicles. This is a characteristic low-power finding of follicular adenoma.* ***(Right)*** *A thin but easily identified capsule surrounds this follicular adenoma. Colloid is present → but is not seen throughout. Adenomas can be quite cellular, as shown in this example.*

Microscopic Features

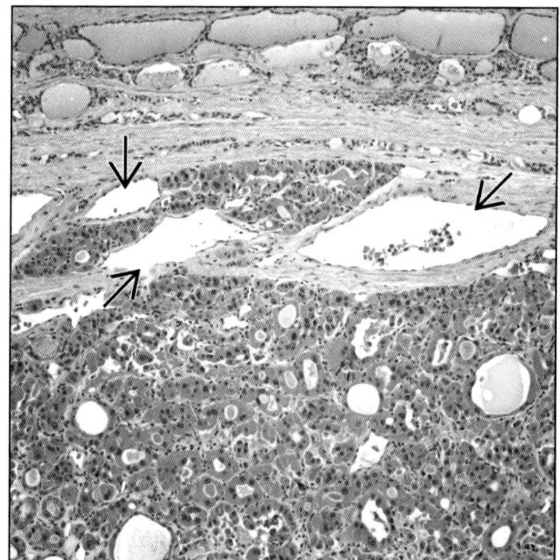

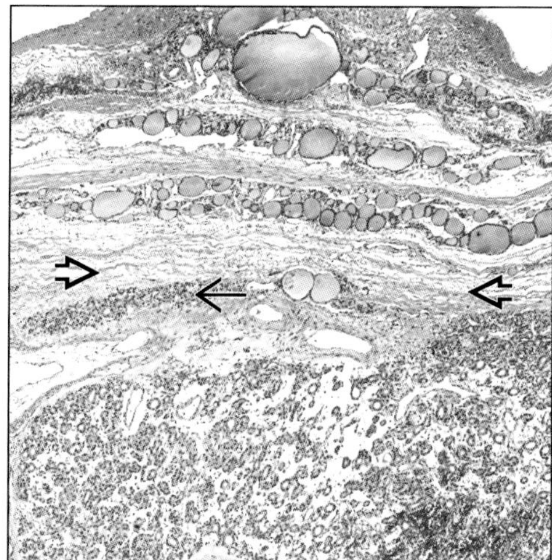

*(**Left**) The capsule is slightly irregular. Note the subcapsular vessels →, which have entrapped part of the oncocytic neoplastic cells between them. This does not represent vascular or capsular invasion. (**Right**) A thin fibrous connective tissue capsule ⇨ separates a distinct population of follicular cells from the surrounding uninvolved follicular thyroid epithelium. Entrapped follicular epithelium is identified → within secondary fibrosis at the level of the capsule.*

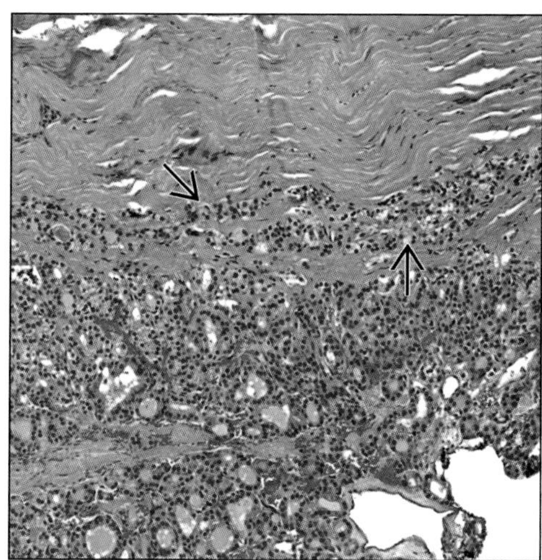

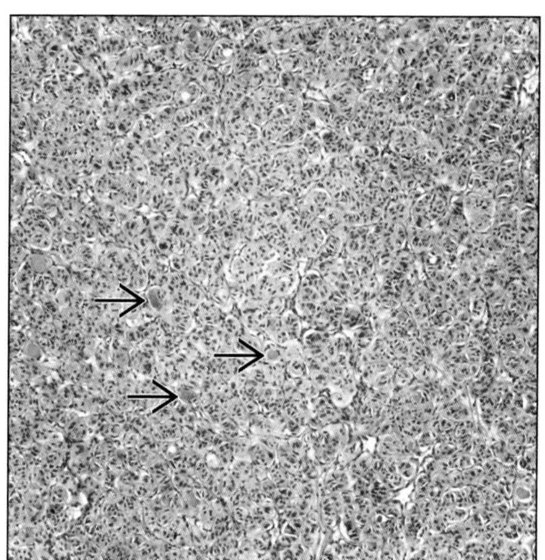

*(**Left**) Follicular neoplasms will frequently have new collagen deposition. New collagen frequently entraps the neoplastic cells →, but this does not represent invasion. The collagen often blends with the tumor cells. Careful review of these areas is required to render the correct diagnosis. (**Right**) Follicular adenomas are usually quite cellular. Colloid is easily identified →, although not abundant. The tumor has a vaguely trabecular or insular architecture.*

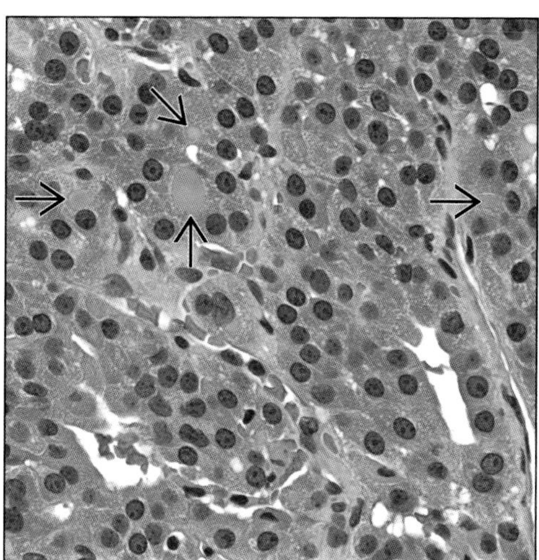

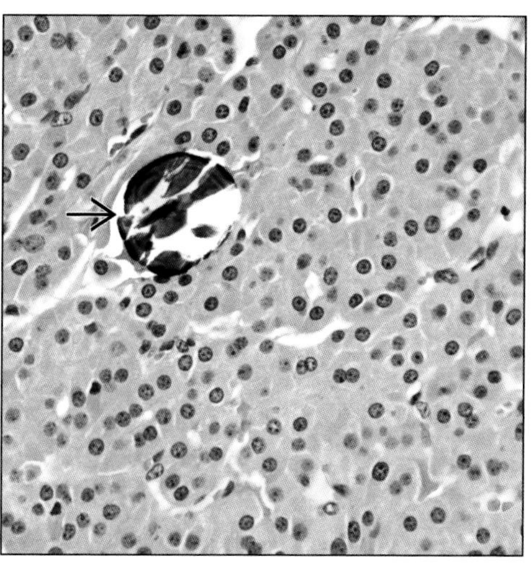

*(**Left**) Hematoxylin & eosin shows granular, opacified cytoplasm. This is on the spectrum of oxyphilia but does not change the diagnosis. Colloid is often difficult to identify →. Oncocytic tumor may require thyroglobulin to confirm the diagnosis. (**Right**) Oncocytic tumors, like this adenoma, will often have psammoma-like calcifications → within the colloid. They usually do not have laminations, although they may occasionally show laminations.*

FOLLICULAR ADENOMA

Adenoma Variants and Secondary Changes

(Left) *Sometimes adenoma will have edematous stroma, creating a pseudopapillary appearance. Note that the colloid is focally showing early calcification ➡ within the follicles.* ***(Right)*** *A variety of different patterns can be seen in follicular adenoma. This is a trabecular pattern. Note the well-formed trabeculae, separated by a delicate fibrovascular stroma. Colloid is present ➡. The nuclei are round-oval, with coarse chromatin distribution.*

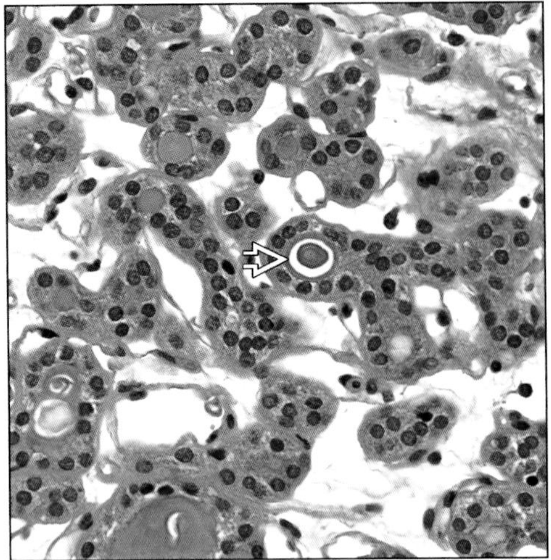

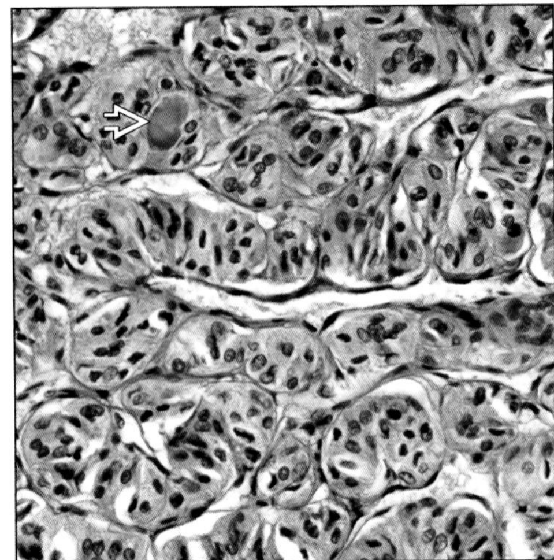

(Left) *Hematoxylin & eosin shows the signet ring morphology, a finding which can be seen in a few follicular adenomas. Thyroglobulin can be used to highlight the "signet ring" spaces.* ***(Right)*** *A slightly cleared cytoplasm can be seen in follicular adenomas, among other thyroid tumors. This tumor also has a vague paraganglioma-like growth pattern. Variant adenoma types may require ancillary techniques to confirm the diagnosis. The cells would be thyroglobulin and TTF-1 positive.*

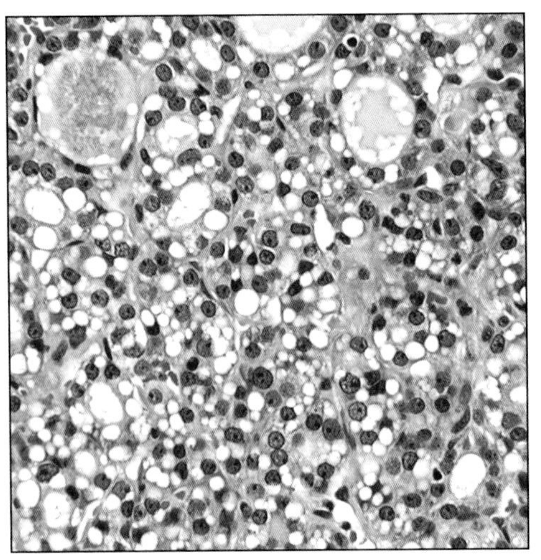

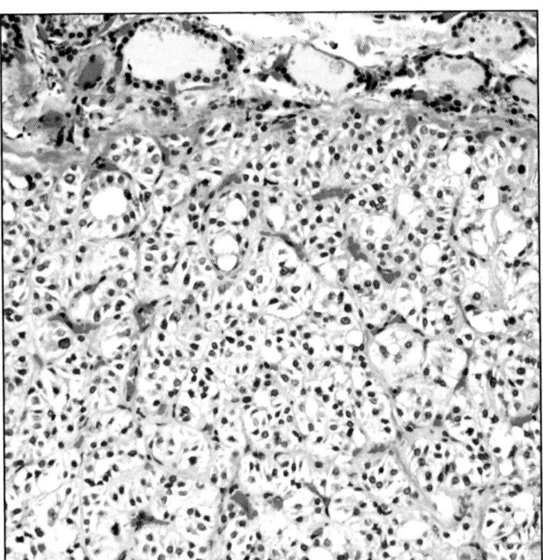

(Left) *Follicular adenomas may undergo degenerative changes, although not with the same frequency as adenomatoid nodules. There is a myxoid stroma reaction with a granulation-type tissue reaction within the tumor.* ***(Right)*** *A FNA tract can simulate invasion. However, there is an abrupt "cut" → within the capsule (caused by sharp needle point), associated with lymphocytes, extravasated erythrocytes, and reactive myxoid stroma. Tumor cells frequently "stream" through the hole.*

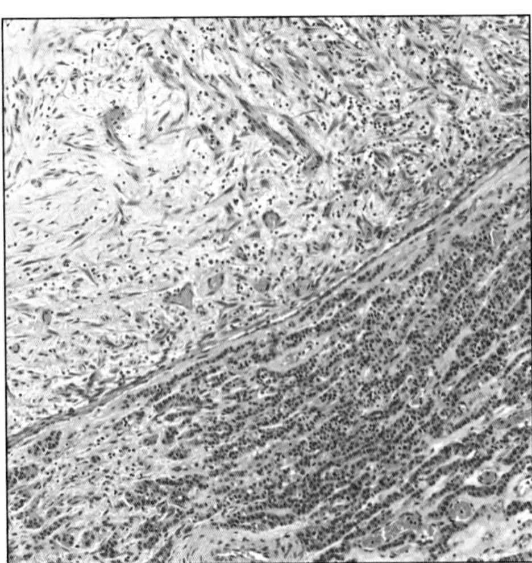

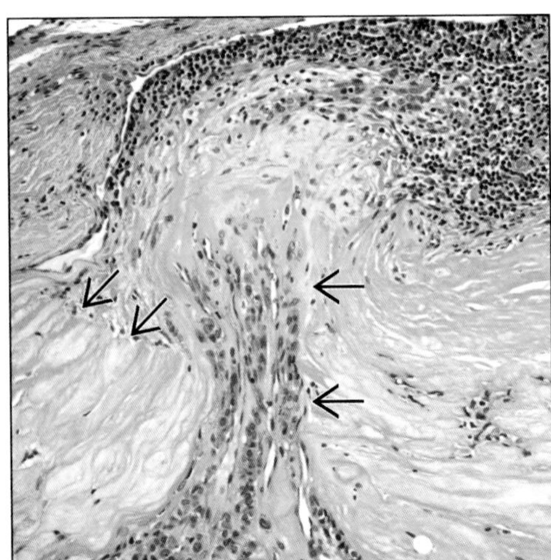

Ancillary Techniques

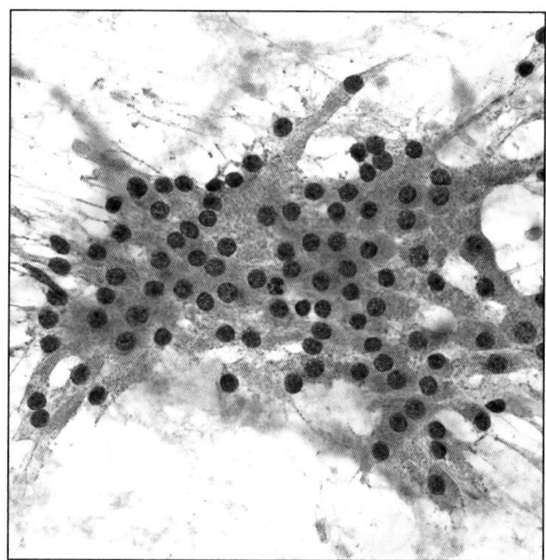

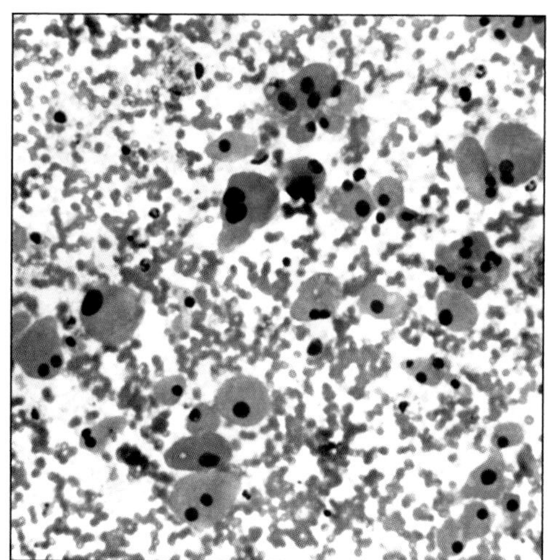

(Left) *There is a sheet of follicular epithelial cells arranged in a vague follicular appearance. The cytoplasm is abundant and granular or eosinophilic. The nuclei are round and regular with even chromatin distribution.* ***(Right)*** *Single cells or small clusters can be seen in a follicular neoplasm. There is no colloid present in the background of this image. The cells are large with abundant, granular cytoplasm. The nuclei are dark and round. These changes can be seen in an adenoma.*

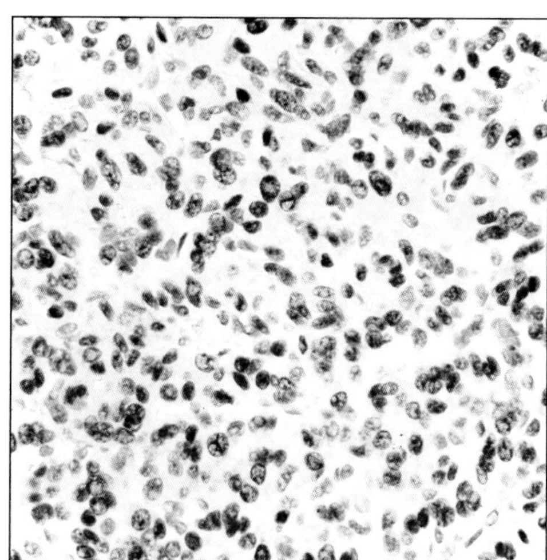

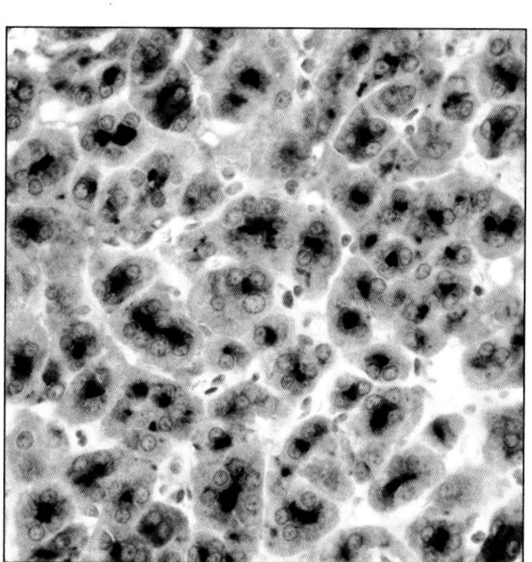

(Left) *Cellular tumors frequently show an absence of colloid. Sometimes TTF-1 can be used to highlight the nuclei of the neoplastic cells. This reaction does not separate benign from malignant lesions, although it may confirm thyroid origin.* ***(Right)*** *Oncocytic tumors especially may have very limited colloid. Thyroglobulin can be used to highlight the small globules of thyroglobulin both within the cytoplasm and within the follicular spaces.*

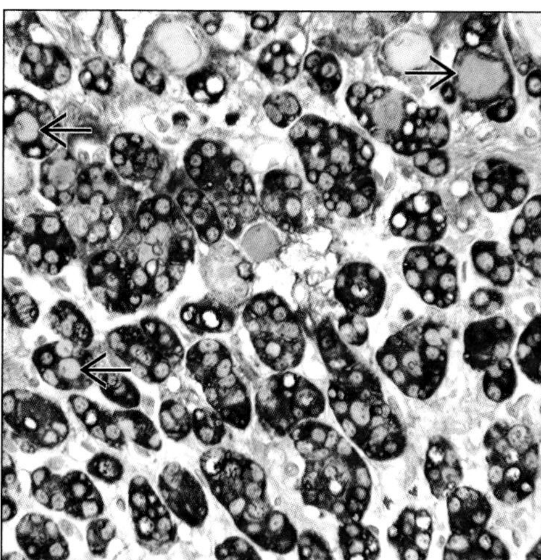

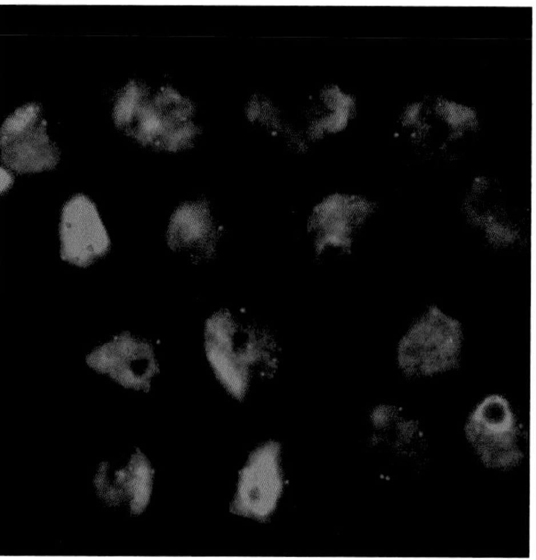

(Left) *This is an example of thyroglobulin staining in a signet ring-type of follicular adenoma. Note the strong and heavy "cytoplasmic" reaction, while the background colloid* ⇒ *stains less avidly.* ***(Right)*** *Fluorescence in situ hybridization (FISH) with a chromosome 7 centromeric probe highlights 3 copies of chromosome 7 (red dots within each nucleus). This is the most common chromosomal gain (trisomy 7) seen in adenoma.*

HYALINIZING TRABECULAR TUMOR

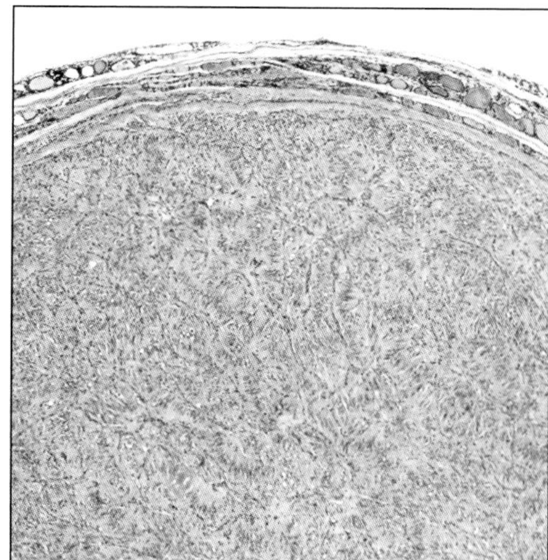

Hematoxylin & eosin shows a well-circumscribed and encapsulated neoplasm. The tumor is arranged in a trabecular architecture, with short trabeculae and "ribbons" of cells showing palisading.

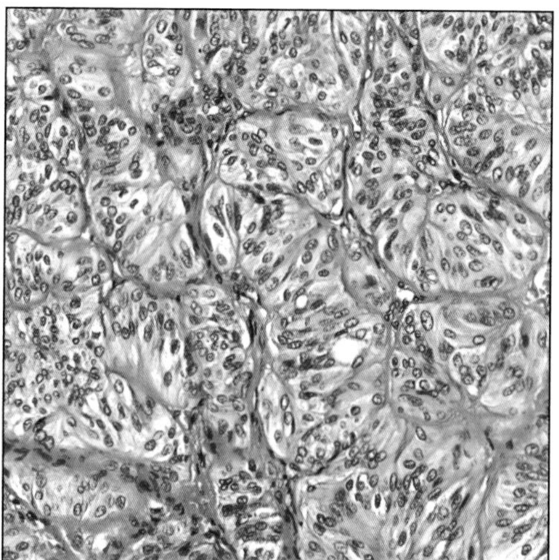

Hematoxylin & eosin shows the trabecular architecture composed by cells arranged perpendicular to the axis of the trabeculae. The cells are spindled to fusiform.

TERMINOLOGY

Synonyms

- Hyalinizing trabecular adenoma (HTA)
- Paraganglioma-like adenoma of thyroid (PLAT)

Definitions

- Rare tumor of follicular cell origin with trabecular pattern of growth and marked intratrabecular hyalinization
- Rarely, tumors show capsular or vascular invasion, develop lymph node metastases, merge with papillary carcinoma, and have *RET/PTC* rearrangements (not quantitatively analyzed), suggesting "tumor" is preferred to "adenoma"

ETIOLOGY/PATHOGENESIS

Radiation

- Several cases have occurred following radiation exposure

Related to Papillary Carcinoma

- Nuclear features suggest relationship to papillary carcinoma
- *RET/PTC* rearrangement in a number of tumors further supports this contention

CLINICAL ISSUES

Epidemiology

- Incidence
  - Very rare primary tumor type
  - < 1% of all primary thyroid gland neoplasms
- Age
  - Mean age: 50 years
  - Seldom in patients < 30 years
- Gender
  - Female > > > Male (6:1)

Site

- No specific site (i.e., **not** upper, outer lobe)

Presentation

- Usually asymptomatic and incidentally found during routine physical exam
- Palpable, solitary mass in rare cases
- May be found incidentally in multinodular glands removed for different reason
- Typically euthyroid
- Rare association with radiation

Treatment

- Surgical approaches
  - Complete, but conservative excision
    - Lobectomy is sufficient (although thyroidectomy may have been performed for different reason)

Prognosis

- Nearly all are benign with excellent long-term prognosis
- Isolated cases have developed lymph node metastases
  - Metastases develop in patients with tumors that show invasion (capsular or vascular)
  - Metastasis suggests possible relationship with papillary carcinoma
  - In review of 112 patients, only 1 developed pulmonary metastases (tumor showed invasion)

IMAGE FINDINGS

Radiographic Findings

- Ultrasonography shows solid nodule, with hypoechoic or heterogeneous echogenicity
  - High intratumoral blood flow on color Doppler
- Scintigraphy usually shows solid "cold" nodule

HYALINIZING TRABECULAR TUMOR

Key Facts

Terminology

- Rare tumor of follicular cell origin with trabecular pattern of growth and marked intratrabecular hyalinization

Clinical Issues

- Very rare primary tumor type
- Mean age: 50 years
- Female > > > Male (6:1)
- Nearly all are benign with excellent long-term prognosis after excision

Macroscopic Features

- Solitary, solid, well-circumscribed, yellow-tan tumor
- Cut surface is solid, homogeneous, lobulated
- Mean size is 2.5 cm

Microscopic Pathology

- Cellular tumors arranged in trabecular pattern
- Polygonal to fusiform cells, with oval-elongated nuclei
- Nuclei arranged perpendicular to trabeculae long axis
- Nuclear grooves, intranuclear pseudoinclusions, perinucleolar halos
- Distinctive, paranuclear, cytoplasmic yellow bodies
- Intratrabecular dense, hyalinized eosinophilic stroma
- Calcospherites may be present

Ancillary Tests

- Tumor cells show distinctive Ki-67 (MIB-1 monoclonal) **membrane** staining

Top Differential Diagnoses

- Papillary and medullary thyroid carcinomas

MACROSCOPIC FEATURES

General Features

- Solitary, solid, encapsulated or well-circumscribed tumor
- Cut surface is solid, homogeneous, delicately lobulated
- Yellow-tan or light tan with flecks and streaks
- Patulous vessels and calcifications are rare

Size

- Mean: 2.5 cm
- Range: 0.3-7 cm

MICROSCOPIC PATHOLOGY

Histologic Features

- Circumscribed with thin, irregular, and uneven fibrous connective tissue capsule
  - Vascular or capsular invasion is almost always absent
- Cellular tumors arranged in trabecular, alveolar, or insular growth
  - Straight or curvilinear bands of tumor cells 2-4 cells thick
- Scant to absent colloid
- Medium to large, polygonal to fusiform cells
- Oval to elongated nuclei arranged perpendicular to long axis of trabeculae and fibrovascular stroma
- Prominent nuclear grooves, nuclear contour irregularities, intranuclear cytoplasmic inclusions, and perinucleolar halos
- Variable cytoplasm, usually finely granular, acidophilic, amphophilic or clear
  - Tends to have homogeneous, glassy or more granular texture
- Distinctive, round, refractile, paranuclear, cytoplasmic yellow bodies/vacuoles (giant lysozymes), about 5 μm
  - Homogeneous or granular texture, occasionally surrounded by clear zone
- Tumor nests formed by intratrabecular dense, heavily hyalinized eosinophilic fibrovascular stroma
  - Hyalinization is usually more prominent at periphery of trabeculae
  - PAS-positive (diastase resistant) basement membrane material
  - May resemble amyloid but is Congo red negative
- Calcospherites (psammoma or calcific bodies) may be present
- Mitotic figures are uncommon
- Chronic lymphocytic thyroiditis may be present in surrounding thyroid parenchyma

ANCILLARY TESTS

Cytology

- Smears are frequently interpreted as papillary carcinoma or medullary carcinoma
- Cellular aspirates with bloody background
- Cohesive clusters of cells with abundant cytoplasm
- Elongated nuclei with evenly dispersed chromatin and intranuclear cytoplasmic inclusions and grooves
- Lumpy stromal deposits of basement membrane material
  - Irregularly shaped deposits between cells
  - Round, centrally located aggregates of material with radial orientation, frequently surrounding cells
- Cytoplasmic bodies (yellow bodies) are green (Papanicolaou stain) or pink (Diff-Quik stain) cytoplasmic structures
- Psammoma bodies/calcifications can be seen

Histochemistry

- PAS-positive, diastase resistant stromal matrix

Immunohistochemistry

- Positive: Thyroglobulin, TTF-1, keratin, CK7, Ki-67 (MIB-1 monoclonal) membrane staining
- Negative: Calcitonin, chromogranin, S100 protein

Flow Cytometry

- Nearly all tumors are diploid

HYALINIZING TRABECULAR TUMOR

Immunohistochemistry

Antibody	Reactivity	Staining Pattern	Comment
TTF-1	Positive	Nuclear	Nearly all tumor cells
Thyroglobulin	Positive	Cytoplasmic	Cytoplasmic and colloid-type deposition
Ki-67	Positive	Cell membrane	Strong and diffuse but only if using Dako MIB-1 antibody
CK-LMW-NOS	Positive	Cytoplasmic	Nearly all tumor cells
CK7	Positive	Cytoplasmic	Most tumor cells
Galectin-3	Positive	Cytoplasmic	About 40% of tumor cells
Laminin	Positive	Stromal matrix	Hyaline material reaction
Collagen IV	Positive	Stromal matrix	Hyaline material reaction
Calcitonin	Negative		
Chromogranin-A	Negative		
S100	Negative		

Cytogenetics

- *RET/PTC1* fusion gene by RT-PCR in few tumors
  - Performed on paraffin-embedded tumors with 35-40 cycles of amplification followed by hybridization with specific probes for qualitative result
  - Not a quantitative result: Do all cells have alteration or is a single cell's abnormality amplified?
- *RET/PTC3* fusion gene identified in rare tumors
- *BRAF, HRAS, NRAS*, and *KRAS* gene mutations absent
  - Lack of *RAS* mutations shows distinct molecular pathway for HTT

PCR

- *RET/PTC* cannot be used as diagnostic marker

Electron Microscopy

- Nests and cords of cells surrounded by basal lamina
- Polymorphic cells with short microvilli
- Nuclei have irregular contours with multiple indentations and intranuclear grooves and pseudoinclusions
- Bundles of intermediate filaments in cytoplasm
- Large, membrane-bound lysosomes, containing vacuoles, granular material, and regularly stacked membranes or "fingerprint" bodies
- Lumpy accumulation of basement membrane material

DIFFERENTIAL DIAGNOSIS

Papillary Carcinoma

- Must be excluded due to overlapping nuclear features
- Extensive intratrabecular stromal hyalinization very rare in papillary carcinoma
- Papillary and follicular pattern suggests papillary carcinoma
- Psammoma bodies (not calcified intraluminal colloid)
- Invasive growth
- Abundant nuclear grooves and pseudoinclusions
- Membranous MIB-1 antibody reactivity seen in HTT
- *BRAF* mutation confirms papillary carcinoma; *RAS* mutations excludes HTT

Follicular Adenoma/Carcinoma

- Widely invasive growth (vascular and capsular) supports follicular carcinoma
- Intertrabecular, perivascular stromal hyalinization can be seen in adenoma/carcinoma
- Perpendicular arrangement of nuclei, grooves, and pseudoinclusions more common in HTT

Medullary Thyroid Carcinoma

- Invasive tumor
- Pattern of growth can overlap
- Lack of colloid common to both
- Amyloid can mimic hyalinization but will be Congo red positive
- Strongly immunoreactive with calcitonin, chromogranin, CEA; negative for thyroglobulin

Paraganglioma

- Histology alone may not help
- Positive: Chromogranin, synaptophysin, CD56; S100 protein sustentacular reaction

SELECTED REFERENCES

1. Carney JA et al: Hyalinizing trabecular tumors of the thyroid gland are almost all benign. Am J Surg Pathol. 32(12):1877-89, 2008
2. Carney JA: Hyalinizing trabecular tumors of the thyroid gland: quadruply described but not by the discoverer. Am J Surg Pathol. 32(4):622-34, 2008
3. Nosé V et al: Hyalinizing trabecular tumor of the thyroid: an update. Endocr Pathol. 19(1):1-8, 2008
4. Casey MB et al: Hyalinizing trabecular adenoma of the thyroid gland: cytologic features in 29 cases. Am J Surg Pathol. 28(7):859-67, 2004
5. Rothenberg HJ et al: Prevalence and incidence of cytoplasmic yellow bodies in thyroid neoplasms. Arch Pathol Lab Med. 127(6):715-7, 2003
6. LiVolsi VA: Hyalinizing trabecular tumor of the thyroid: adenoma, carcinoma, or neoplasm of uncertain malignant potential? Am J Surg Pathol. 24(12):1683-4, 2000
7. Papotti M et al: RET/PTC activation in hyalinizing trabecular tumors of the thyroid. Am J Surg Pathol. 24(12):1615-21, 2000
8. Papotti M et al: Immunophenotypic heterogeneity of hyalinizing trabecular tumours of the thyroid. Histopathology. 31(6):525-33, 1997
9. Bronner MP et al: PLAT: paraganglioma-like adenomas of the thyroid. Surg Pathol. 1:383-89, 1988
10. Carney JA et al: Hyalinizing trabecular adenoma of the thyroid gland. Am J Surg Pathol. 11(8):583-91, 1987

Microscopic Features and Ancillary Techniques

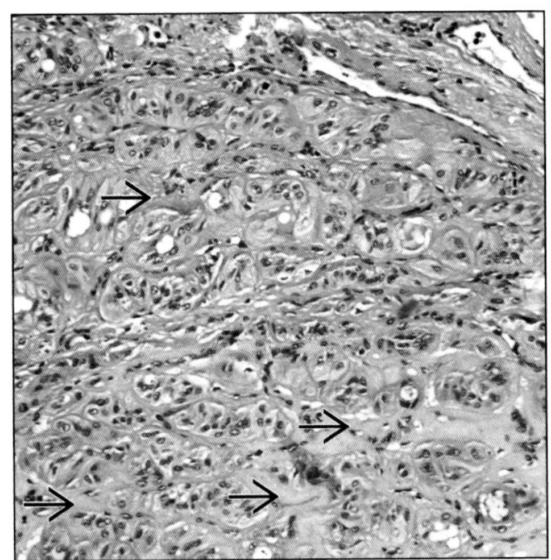

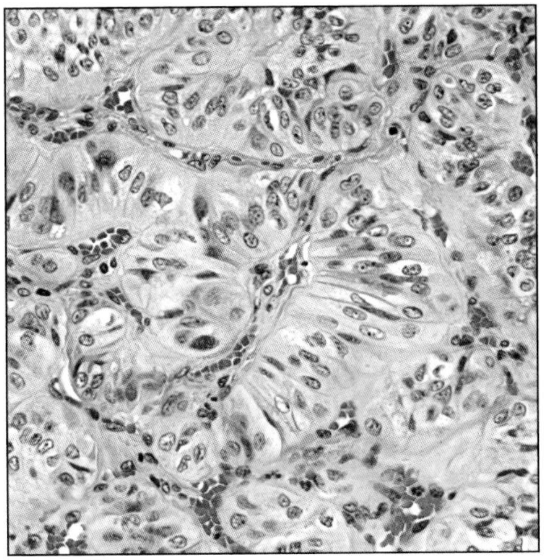

(Left) *The nested to trabecular growth pattern of the tumor is highlighted by hyalinization ➔. This hyalinization is noted within and between the trabeculae and nests. This is not intertrabecular hyalinization, which can be seen in other tumors of the thyroid gland.* ***(Right)*** *Hematoxylin & eosin high power demonstrates the spindle, fusiform cells with oval-shaped nuclei containing multiple nuclear grooves. Note the perpendicular arrangement of the nuclei to the axis of the trabeculae.*

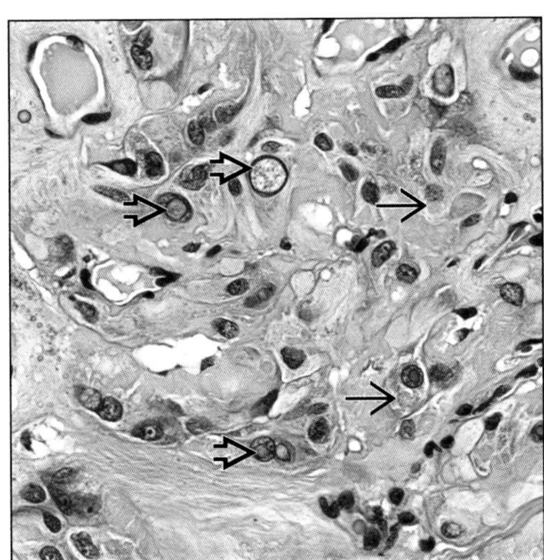

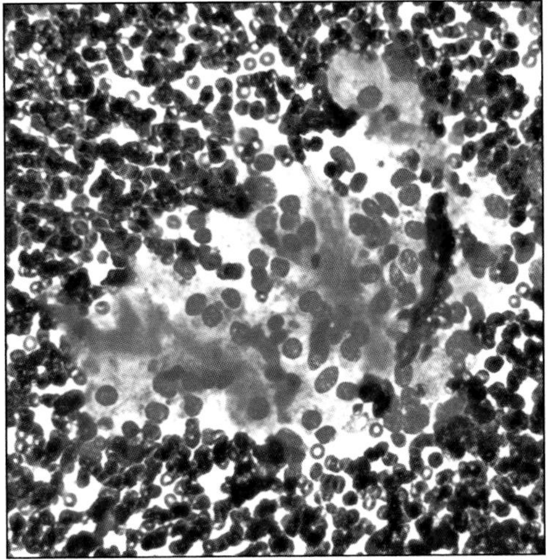

(Left) *Hematoxylin & eosin shows polygonal cells with abundant cytoplasm and frequent intranuclear pseudoinclusions ⇨ that are surrounded by a rim of nuclear membrane and stain densely eosinophilic, similar to the cytoplasm. Yellow bodies are also present ➔.* ***(Right)*** *Diff-Quik stained material shows 2 clusters of neoplastic cells immediately associated with aggregates of dense pink hyaline material. This material is the "hyalinization" characteristic for the name of the tumor.*

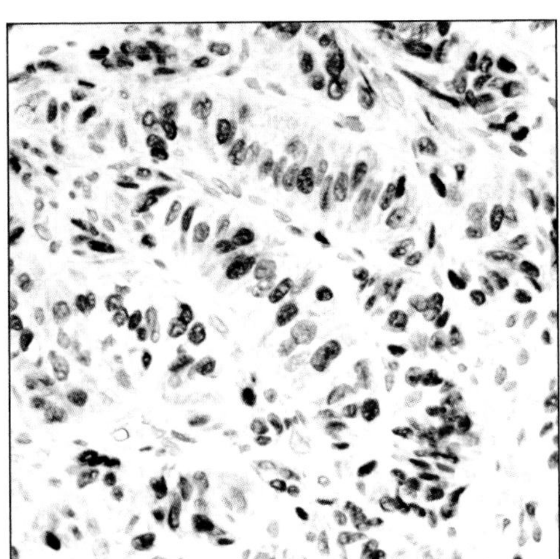

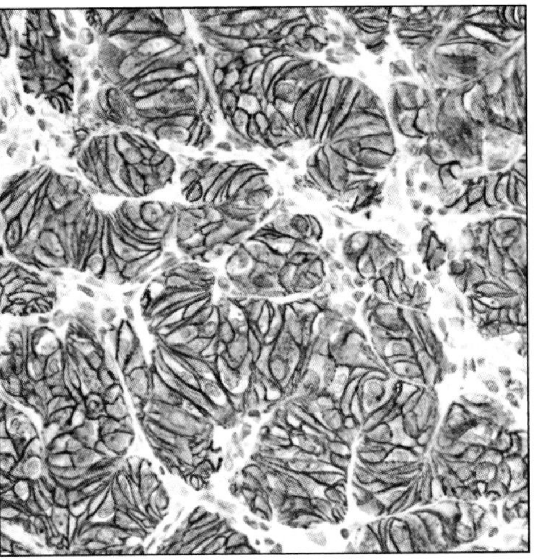

(Left) *TTF-1 highlights the nuclei of nearly all of the neoplastic cells. This stain highlights the elongated nature of the nuclei. The staining is usually strong and diffuse, without suffering from background artifacts.* ***(Right)*** *Ki-67 yields a very strong and characteristic membrane and peripheral cytoplasmic reactivity. The membranous staining is only identified with the Dako MIB-1 antibody (epitope retrieval independent) and not with other manufacturers.*

THYROID TERATOMA

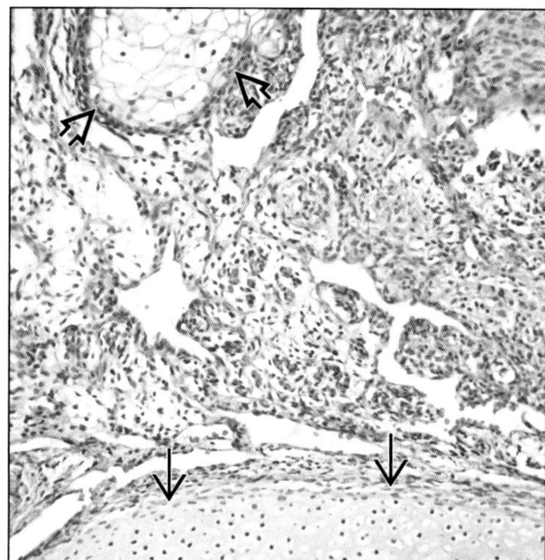

Mature elements comprise this teratoma. There is mature cartilage ⇒, with soft tissues separating squamous epithelium ⇨ in this example of a benign, mature teratoma.

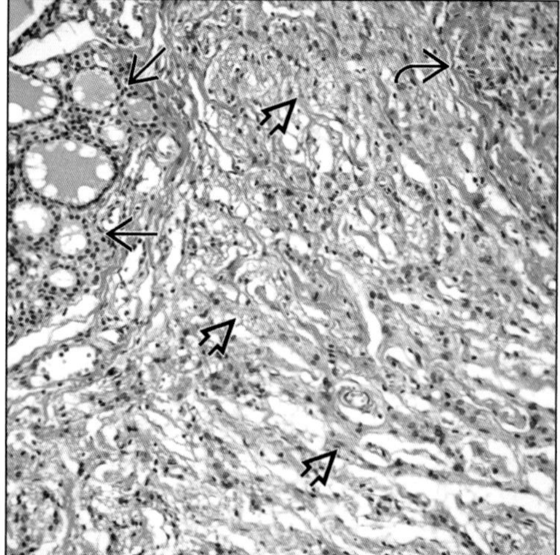

By definition, thyroid gland tissue must be present to qualify the tumor as a thyroid teratoma. The thyroid tissue ⇒ is immediately adjacent to mature glial tissue ⇨ juxtaposed to skeletal muscle ↪.

TERMINOLOGY

Synonyms

- Only **teratoma** has trilineage differentiation
- Other terms incorrectly used include
  - Choristoma
  - Hamartoma
  - Epignathus
  - Heterotopia
  - Dermoid

Definitions

- Tumor of germ cell derivation composed of mature or immature tissues derived from all 3 germ cell layers
  - Ectoderm, endoderm, and mesoderm
- Defined as **thyroid** teratomas if
  - Tumor occupies portion of thyroid gland
  - Direct continuity or close anatomic relationship between tumor and thyroid gland
  - Cervical teratoma is accompanied by complete absence of thyroid gland
    - Either total replacement of gland by tumor or thyroid anlage that failed to develop into mature thyroid gland

ETIOLOGY/PATHOGENESIS

Embryonic Developmental Abnormality

- Believed to arise from misplaced embryonic germ cells (rests) in thyroid gland that continue to develop in new location

CLINICAL ISSUES

Epidemiology

- Incidence
  - Rare
    - < 0.1% of all primary thyroid gland neoplasms
- Age
  - Broad age range: Newborn to 85 years
    - Average: < 10 years
  - Bimodal age distribution
    - Neonates and infants: > 90% are benign teratomas
    - Children and adults: ~ 50% are malignant teratomas
- Gender
  - Equal gender distribution

Site

- Anterior neck, including thyroid gland
  - Separation is difficult, especially in large neonatal tumors

Presentation

- All patients present with neck mass
  - Tumors can reach significant size
- Frequently experience
  - Dyspnea
  - Difficulty breathing
  - Stridor
- Other congenital anomalies may be present in neonatal patients

Natural History

- Neonatal cases, if untreated, will result in patient death due to airway compromise &/or mass effect
  - Irrespective of histologic grade

Treatment

- Options, risks, complications
  - Outcome depends on patient's age, tumor size at presentation, and presence and proportion of immaturity
  - Surgery must be instituted immediately in neonatal cases to avoid morbidity or mortality
- Surgical approaches
  - Surgical excision for benign or immature teratomas is treatment of choice

THYROID TERATOMA

Key Facts

Terminology
- Tumor of germ cell derivation composed of mature or immature tissues derived from all 3 germ cell layers: Ectoderm, endoderm, and mesoderm

Clinical Issues
- Bimodal age distribution
  - Neonates and infants: Nearly all are benign or immature teratomas (grade 0, 1, or 2)
  - Children and adults: Preponderance of malignant teratomas (grade 3)
- All patients present with neck mass
- Outcome depends on patient's age, tumor size, and presence and proportion of immaturity
- Surgery must be instituted immediately in neonatal cases to avoid morbidity or mortality

Macroscopic Features
- Tumor surface is smooth to bosselated or lobulated
- Firm to soft and multilocular-cystic
- Gray-tan or yellow-white to translucent cut surface

Microscopic Pathology
- Tissues from all 3 primordial layers
- By definition, thyroid parenchyma must be present
- Wide array of tissue types and growth patterns
- Variety of different epithelia, neural tissue (most common), and mesenchymal elements
- Maturation and relative proportions of immature neuroectodermal tissue determines grade
  - Completely mature (grade 0)
  - Predominantly mature (grade 1 or 2)
  - Exclusively immature (grade 3 or malignant)

  - If mass is detected in utero, consider delivering fetus by ex utero intrapartum treatment (EXIT) procedure
    - Fetus is partially delivered by cesarean section while placenta and umbilical cord remain intact
    - Uteroplacental gas exchange maintained
    - Fetus remains hemodynamically stable while airway is established
    - Avoids "crash" attempt at achieving airway at birth
- Drugs
  - Chemotherapy may be used for malignant teratoma, although often palliative
- Radiation
  - Only used for malignant teratoma, but considered palliative in most cases

Prognosis
- Age at presentation and tumor histology are strongly correlated
  - Neonates and infants: Nearly all are benign or immature teratomas (grade 0, 1, or 2)
  - Children and adults: Preponderance of malignant teratomas (grade 3)
- No patients with grade 0, 1, or 2 tumor (benign mature or benign immature) die **from** disease, although some die **with** disease
  - Death is generally direct result of significant morbidity secondary to tracheal compression or lack of development of vital structures in neck during fetal growth
  - Surgery for neonatal thyroid teratomas must be instituted immediately to avoid preoperative morbidity (mass effect) and mortality
- Malignant teratomas exhibit clinically aggressive behavior
  - May invade by direct extension into esophagus, trachea, salivary glands, &/or soft tissues of neck
  - Recurrence and dissemination (usually in lungs) occur in about 1/3 of patients
  - Many of these cases are fatal

IMAGE FINDINGS

Radiographic Findings
- Ultrasonographic images (in utero, at time of birth, or later) provide best information and are easiest to obtain
  - Most common finding is multicystic mass of thyroid gland
- Computed tomography shows inhomogeneous mass arising in thyroid gland
  - Upper airway compression can be seen no matter what the histologic findings
- Scintigraphic studies (if performed) show cold nodule or diffuse "decreased" iodine uptake

MACROSCOPIC FEATURES

General Features
- Tumor surface is smooth to bosselated or lobulated
- Tumor periphery is well circumscribed to widely infiltrative into surrounding thyroid parenchyma
- Consistency varies from firm to soft and cystic
- Multiloculated cystic spaces
  - Spaces are filled with white-tan creamy material, mucoid glairy material, or dark brown hemorrhagic fluid admixed with necrotic debris
  - Tissue resembling brain is seen, often associated with black pigmentation (retinal anlage)
  - Gritty bone or cartilage is frequently noted
- Gray-tan or yellow-white to translucent cut surface

Sections to Be Submitted
- Periphery to document thyroid gland involvement

Size
- Mean: 6-7 cm
- Range: Up to 14 cm
- Larger tumors are associated with compression symptoms (stridor, hoarseness, difficulty breathing)

THYROID TERATOMA

Histologic Grading of Thyroid Teratomas

Histologic Feature	Histologic Category and Grade
Mature elements only	Benign, mature = grade 0
≤ 1 low-power field (4x objective and 10x ocular) of immature elements	Benign, immature = grade 1
> 1 but ≤ 4 low-power fields of immature foci	Benign, immature = grade 2
> 4 low-power fields of immature elements, along with mitoses and cellular atypia	Malignant = grade 3

Based on proposed system: Thompson LD et al: Primary thyroid teratomas: a clinicopathologic study of 30 cases. Cancer. 88(5):1149-58, 2000.

MICROSCOPIC PATHOLOGY

Histologic Features

- Tissues from all 3 primordial layers
  - Ectoderm, mesoderm, and endoderm
- By definition, thyroid parenchyma should be identified
  - May be scarce or absent in malignant teratomas
- Wide array of tissue types and growth patterns
  - Inter-relationship and percentage of each element used to classify tumors into 1 of 3 types: Mature, immature, or malignant
- Small cystic spaces to solid nests
- Variety of different epithelia
  - Squamous epithelium (simple and stratified)
    - Pilosebaceous and other adnexal structures are seen
  - Pseudostratified ciliated columnar epithelium (respiratory)
  - Cuboidal glandular epithelium (with and without goblet cells)
  - Transitional epithelium
  - True organ differentiation (pancreas, liver, or lung) can be found
- Neural tissue (ectodermal derivation) is most common element
  - Mature glial tissue, choroid plexus, pigmented retinal anlage
  - Immature neuroblastomal elements
    - Immature tissues resemble embryonic tissue
    - Primitive neuroepithelial small to medium-sized cells with high nuclear to cytoplasmic ratio
    - Arranged in sheets or rosette-like structures (Homer Wright or Flexner-Wintersteiner types)
    - Nuclear chromatin is hyperchromatic
    - Mitoses are common
- Mesenchymal tissues intermixed with other components
  - Cartilage, bone, striated skeletal muscle, smooth muscle, adipose tissue, and loose myxoid to fibrous embryonic mesenchymal connective tissue
- Maturation and relative proportions of the immature neuroectodermal tissue determines grade

ANCILLARY TESTS

Cytology

- Smears are cellular, but frequently misinterpreted as "missed" or "contamination"

Immunohistochemistry

- Not used for mature or benign teratomas
- Immature components highlighted with markers specific to tissue source
  - Glial components: S100 protein, glial fibrillary acidic protein (GFAP), neuron-specific enolase (NSE), neural filament protein
  - Skeletal muscle: Desmin, MYOD1, myogenin, myoglobulin

DIFFERENTIAL DIAGNOSIS

Dermoid

- Histology limited to only skin elements

Lymphangioma

- Lateral rather than midline
- Cystically dilated vessels filled with fluid, lymphocytes, with smooth muscle walls

Small Blue Round Cell Tumor

- Only for malignant teratoma
  - Ewing sarcoma, rhabdomyosarcoma, small-cell carcinoma, lymphoma, melanoma
  - Age and histology frequently make separation
  - Immunohistochemistry useful in some cases

SELECTED REFERENCES

1. Riedlinger WF et al: Primary thyroid teratomas in children: a report of 11 cases with a proposal of criteria for their diagnosis. Am J Surg Pathol. 29(5):700-6, 2005
2. Tsang RW et al: Malignant teratoma of the thyroid: aggressive chemoradiation therapy is required after surgery. Thyroid. 13(4):401-4, 2003
3. Thompson LD et al: Primary thyroid teratomas: a clinicopathologic study of 30 cases. Cancer. 88(5):1149-58, 2000
4. Arezzo A et al: Immature malignant teratoma of the thyroid gland. J Exp Clin Cancer Res. 17(1):109-12, 1998
5. Azizkhan RG et al: Diagnosis, management, and outcome of cervicofacial teratomas in neonates: a Childrens Cancer Group study. J Pediatr Surg. 30(2):312-6, 1995
6. Zerella JT et al: Obstruction of the neonatal airway from teratomas. Surg Gynecol Obstet. 170(2):126-31, 1990
7. Buckley NJ et al: Malignant teratoma in the thyroid gland of an adult: a case report and a review of the literature. Surgery. 100(5):932-7, 1986
8. Wolvos TA et al: An unusual thyroid tumor: a comparison to a literature review of thyroid teratomas. Surgery. 97(5):613-7, 1985
9. Fisher JE et al: Teratoma of thyroid gland in infancy: review of the literature and two case reports. J Surg Oncol. 21(2):135-40, 1982

Clinical, Gross, and Microscopic Features

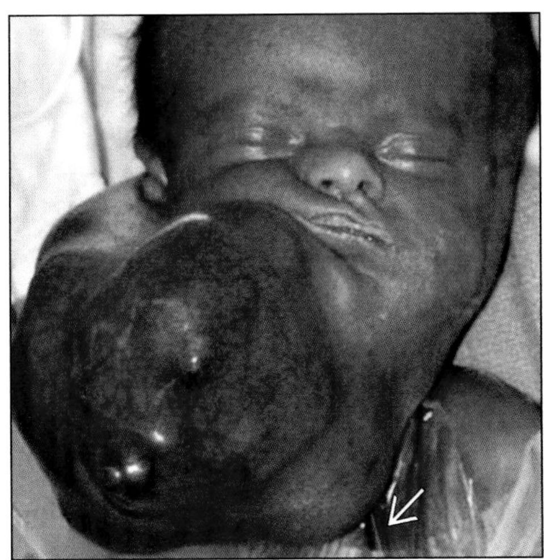

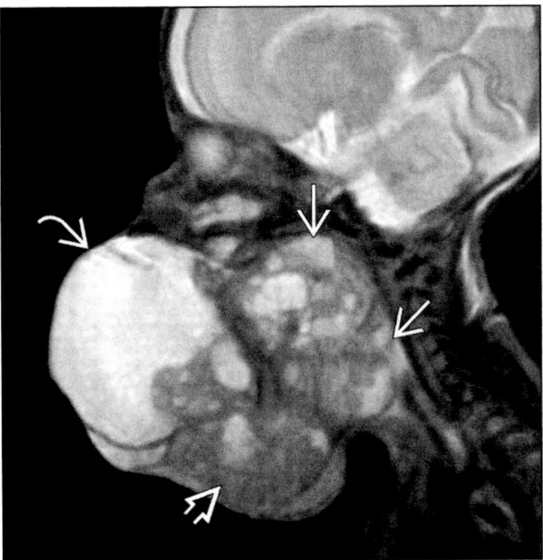

*(**Left**) Clinical photograph shows a neonate who had an anterior neck mass detected by in utero ultrasound. The airway was compromised, and a tracheostomy ➡ was placed using the EXIT procedure. (**Right**) Sagittal T2-weighted MR shows posterior extension of the mass ➡ into the airway. The mass contains both high signal cystic areas ↪ and low signal soft tissue components ⇨ typical of a teratoma. The diagnosis was an immature teratoma.*

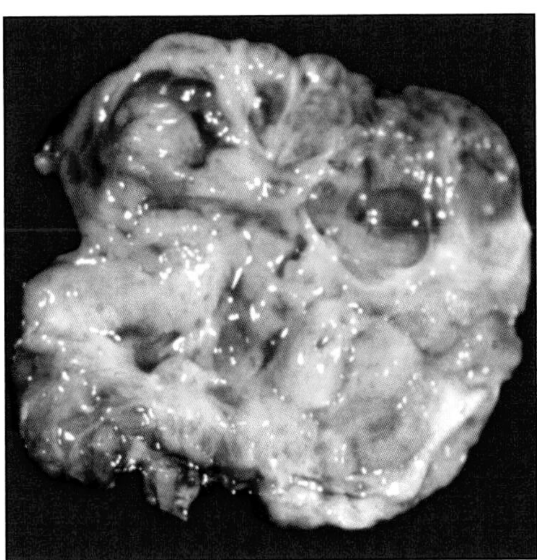

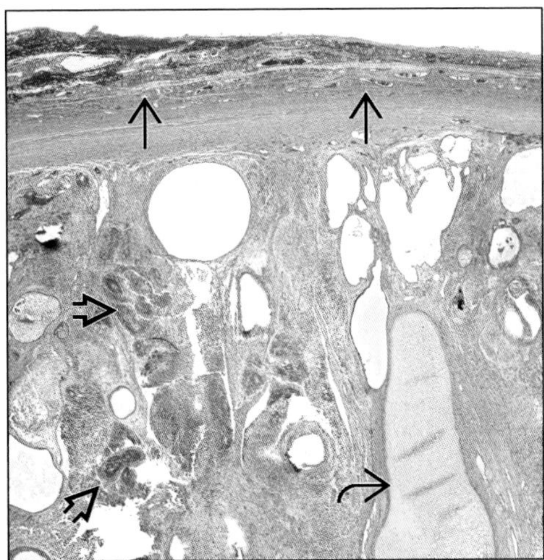

*(**Left**) Gross image shows a typical example of a thyroid teratoma. The mass was approximately the same size as the fetal head from which it was removed. Note the complex cystic and solid components typical of a teratoma. (**Right**) Thyroid gland parenchyma at the periphery → is separated from the teratoma by a fibrous capsule. There is mature cartilage ↪, immature glial tissue ⇨, and a number of cystic spaces lined by various epithelia. This is a benign, immature teratoma.*

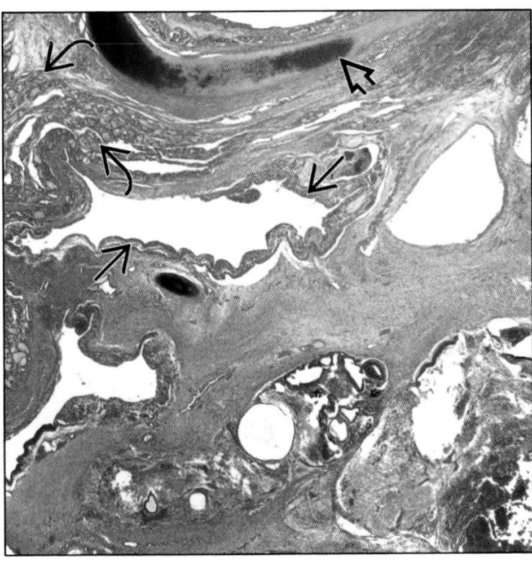

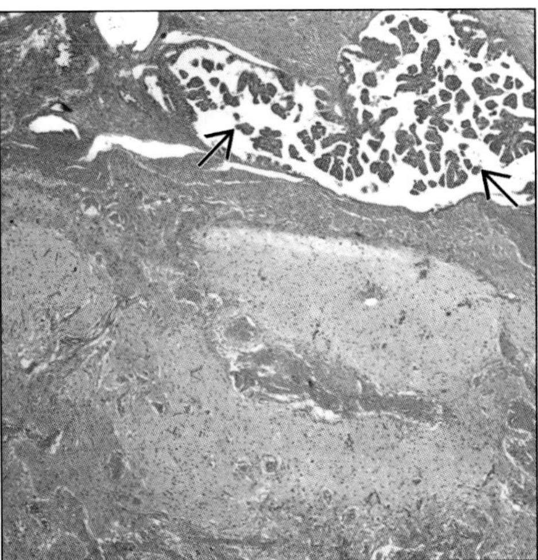

*(**Left**) There is a vague organoid appearance to this teratoma, showing a trachea ⇨ and primitive esophagus → adjacent to cystic epithelial structures, with glandular elements. Thyroid follicles ↪ are entrapped within the tumor. (**Right**) It is not uncommon for mature, benign teratoma to have mature glial tissue immediately adjacent to the choroid plexus → as shown in this teratoma. The presence of neural tissue helps to separate teratomas into various grades.*

THYROID TERATOMA

Microscopic Features

*(**Left**) This area of mature benign teratoma shows a fetal trachea. Note the cartilage, minor mucoserous glands, and respiratory type epithelium lining the lumen of the primitive structure. Thyroid follicles are noted adjacent to the cartilage. (**Right**) Pigmented retinal anlage is noted within more primitive or immature neuroblastomal tissue. The neural tissue shows a pseudorosette appearance. Note the glandular epithelium immediately adjacent to the neural tissue (immature, benign).*

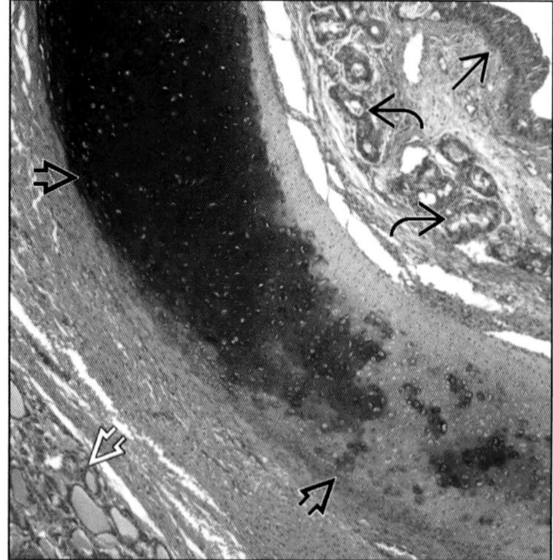

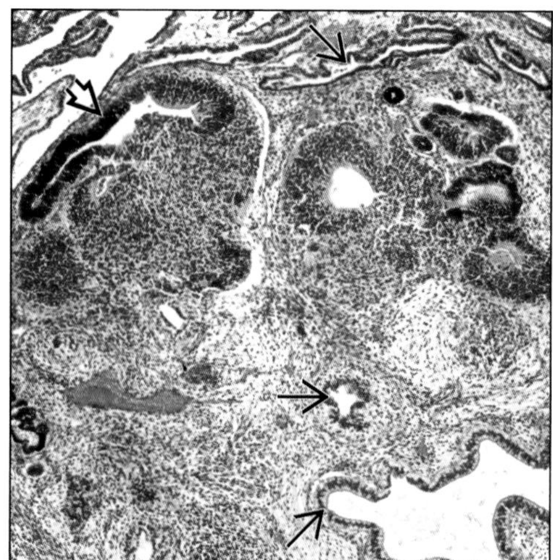

*(**Left**) Mature elements from the primordial layers are present, including cartilage, pigmented retinal anlage, respiratory epithelium, and mucinous epithelium separated by mature glial tissue. (**Right**) Fat and immature stromal elements separate the squamous epithelium from 2 large cysts lined by cuboidal epithelium and filled with debris. This type of haphazard distribution is diagnostic of a teratoma.*

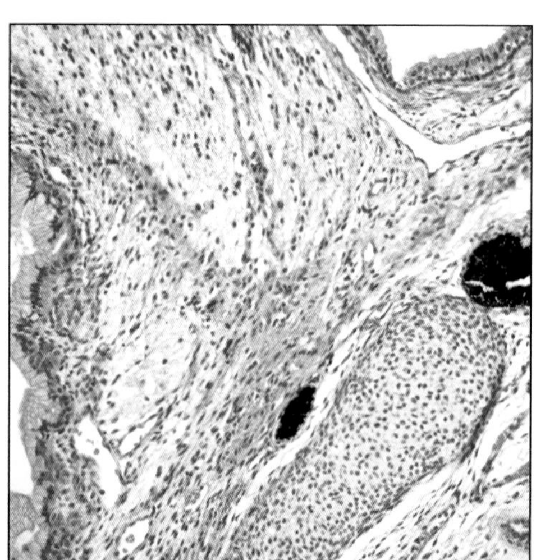

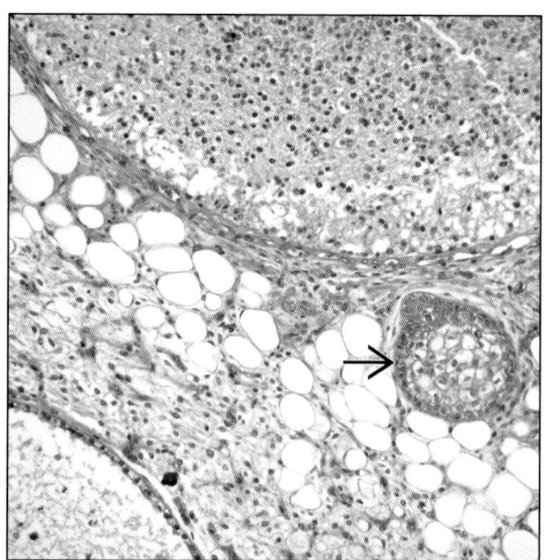

*(**Left**) Each of the 2 elements in this image are benign, mature, and "normal," although not in this arrangement: Glial tissue is noted surrounding and separating bundles of skeletal muscle. (**Right**) Primitive, immature neuroblastoma tissue fills this field, with a vague Homer Wright-type rosette created with the neural-fibrillar matrix material in the center. If this finding is dominant, the tumor is either immature or malignant, depending on the number of foci.*

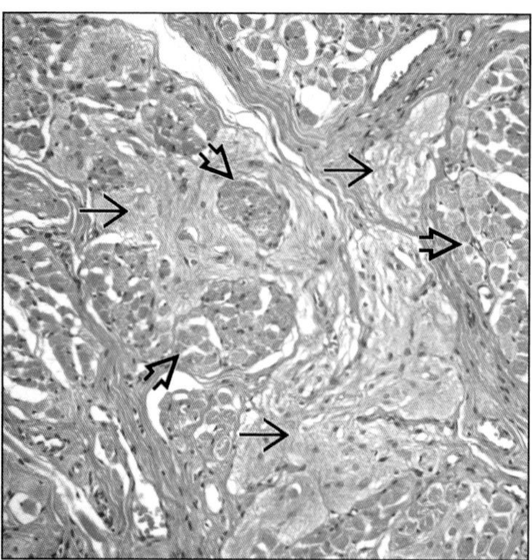

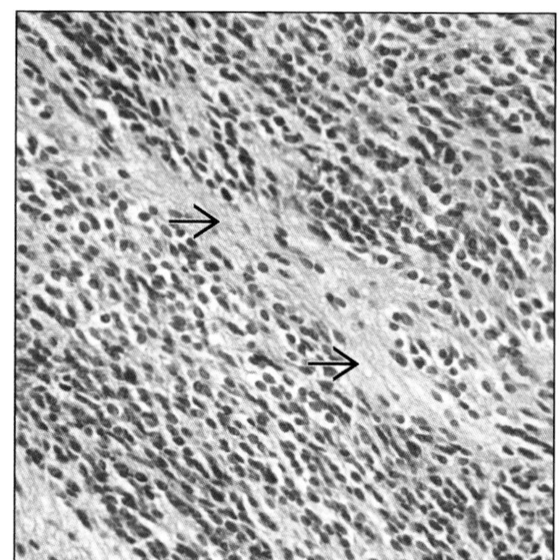

Microscopic and Immunohistochemical Features

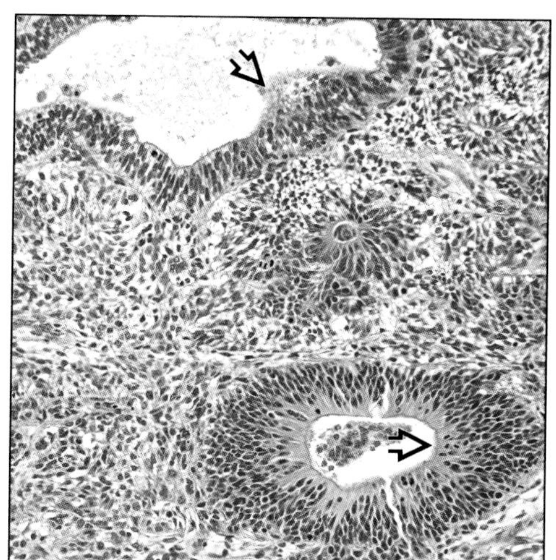

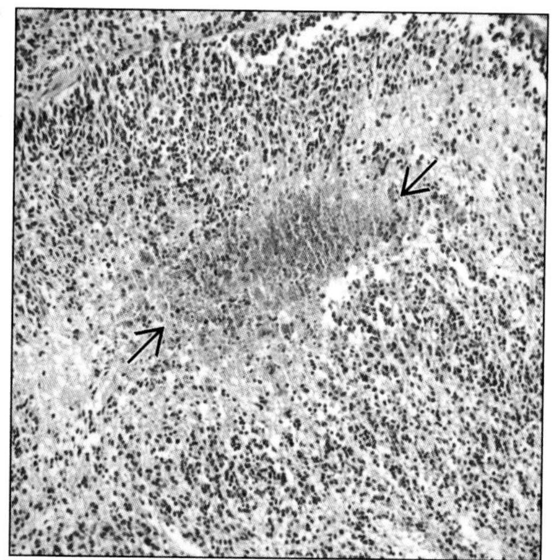

(Left) *Rosettes are usually identified within the immature neural elements. In this case, there are very characteristic Flexner-Wintersteiner rosettes ⇨, showing a well-formed gland-like lumen. Note the immature neural tissue in the rest of the field.* ***(Right)*** *The immature blastoma is surrounding an area of tumor necrosis →, a feature diagnostic for a malignant (grade 3) teratoma. Necrosis and increased mitoses are frequent in malignant teratoma.*

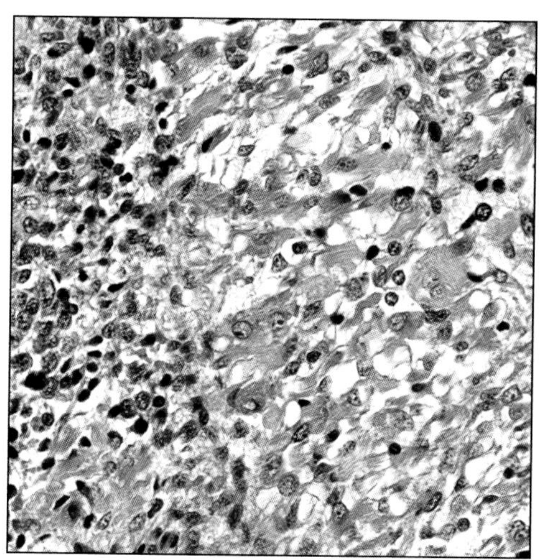

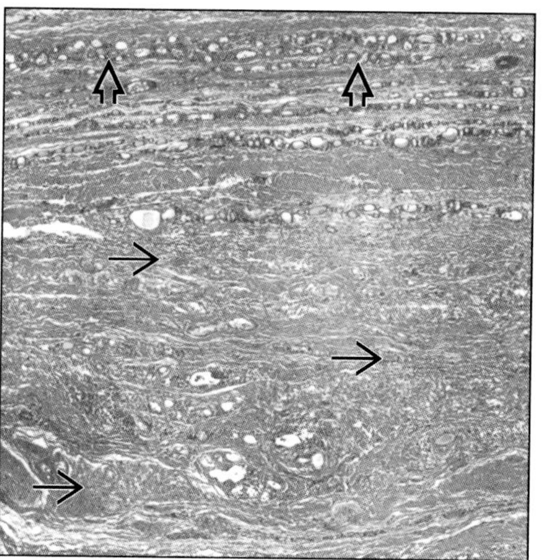

(Left) *This immature region of a malignant teratoma shows features of rhabdoid differentiation, with "strap-cell" configuration. These types of cells would be immunoreactive with myogenin or MYOD1.* ***(Right)*** *Mature glial elements → can sometimes be difficult to identify, as seen in this image. Note the areas of thyroid follicular epithelium ⇨. Immunohistochemistry can be very helpful in highlighting the various elements in the tumor.*

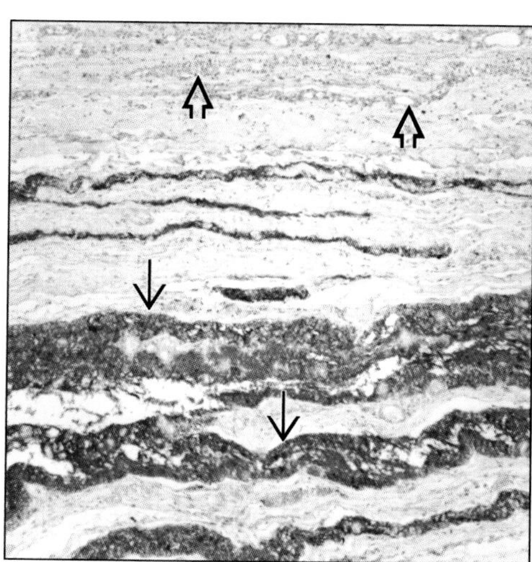

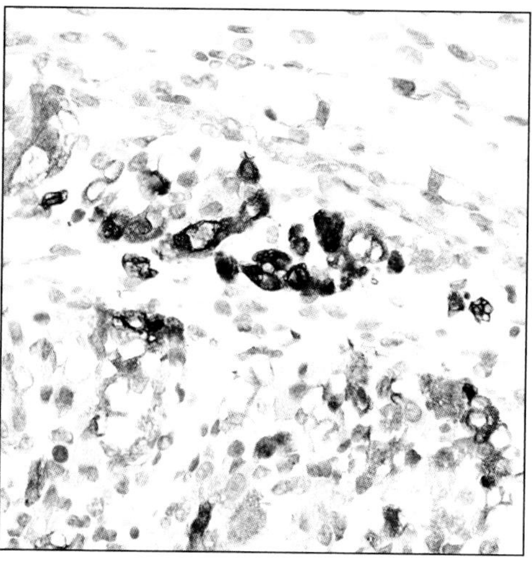

(Left) *This image shows how S100 protein highlights the mature glial elements →. These same areas would also be immunoreactive with GFAP. Note the areas of thyroid follicular epithelium ⇨, which lack S100 protein staining.* ***(Right)*** *When immature areas are evaluated, it may be necessary to confirm the nature of the cells with immunohistochemistry, as shown by the myoglobin immunoreactivity in this case. Keratin, myogenin, and CD99 among others can be useful.*

ECTOPIC HAMARTOMATOUS THYMOMA

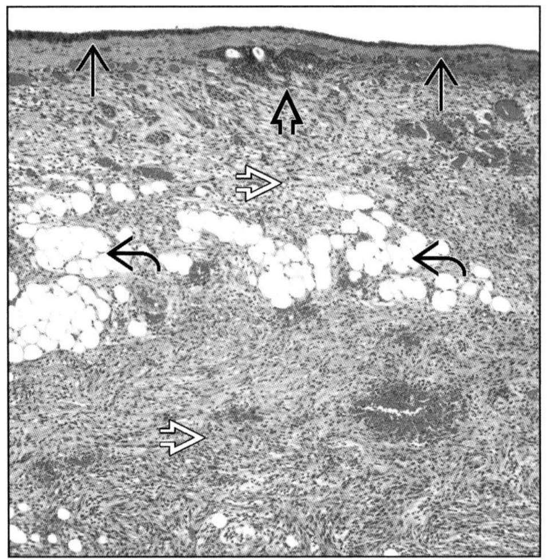

Cervical soft tissue cystic lesion is lined by epithelial cells ➙ with subjacent solid nests of squamous cells ➯ and associated spindle cells ➡, and mature adipose tissue ↗.

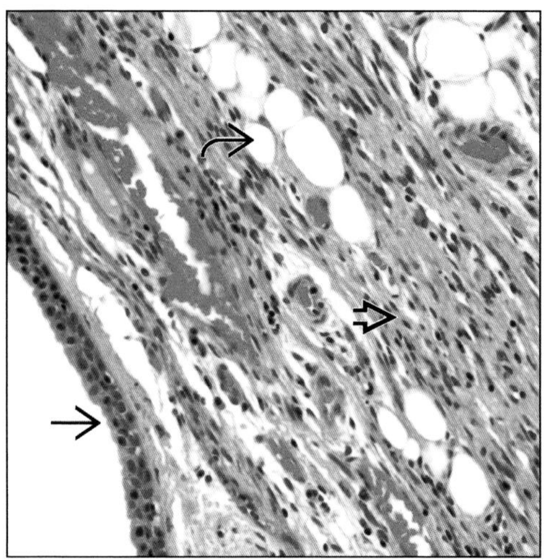

The cystic epithelial lining includes cuboidal cells ➙ with intimate admixture of slender spindle-shaped cells ➯ as well as mature adipose tissue ↗ in the cyst wall.

TERMINOLOGY

Definitions

- Benign tumor in cervical neck soft tissues exhibiting differentiation toward thymic tissue

ETIOLOGY/PATHOGENESIS

Developmental Anomaly

- Thought to arise from misplaced branchial pouch derivatives
  - Myoepithelial branchial anlage differentiation suggested but not supported
  - No compelling evidence for thymic differentiation

CLINICAL ISSUES

Epidemiology

- Incidence
  - Rare tumor
- Age
  - Range from 3rd to 8th decades (mean age: 47 years; median age: 40 years)
- Gender
  - Male > > > > > Female (approximately 20:1)

Site

- Principally involve lower neck region, usually in close proximity to sternoclavicular joint
  - May lie in proximity to thyroid gland

Presentation

- Slow growing subfascial swelling in suprasternal or supraclavicular region

Treatment

- Options, risks, complications
  - Complete surgical resection is treatment of choice

Prognosis

- Indolent behavior
- Tumors may locally recur but do not metastasize or cause tumor-related death
- Rarely, adenocarcinoma may arise in ectopic hamartomatous thymoma

MACROSCOPIC FEATURES

General Features

- Solitary, lobular or multilobular mass

Size

- Range from 2-19 cm in greatest dimension

MICROSCOPIC PATHOLOGY

Histologic Features

- Typically well marginated or circumscribed
- Composed of 3 cell types
  - Epithelial cells
    - Squamous (nonkeratinizing), cuboidal and glandular elements
    - Epithelial islands composed of solid nests, trabeculae and cysts
    - Epithelial-lined cysts may be found focally, measuring up to 2 cm in greatest dimension
  - Mature adipose tissue
  - Spindle cells
    - Plump spindled cells, delicate spindled cells with fascicular to storiform growth
- Mixed lymphocytic cell infiltrate may be identified
- Low mitotic rate
- Areas of skin adnexal differentiation reported (including sebaceous, eccrine and apocrine elements)

ECTOPIC HAMARTOMATOUS THYMOMA

Key Facts

Terminology
- Benign tumor in cervical neck soft tissues exhibiting differentiation toward thymic tissue

Clinical Issues
- Male > > > > > Female (approximately 20:1)
- Principally involve lower neck region, usually in close proximity to sternoclavicular joint
  - May lie in proximity to thyroid gland

Microscopic Pathology
- Comprised of 3 cell types
  - Epithelial cells
  - Mature adipose tissue
  - Plump to delicate spindled cells with fascicular to storiform growth

Ancillary Tests
- Epithelial and spindle cells
  - Cytokeratin, muscle specific actin positive

ANCILLARY TESTS

Immunohistochemistry
- Epithelial cells
  - Cytokeratin, muscle specific actin positive
  - Desmin, S100 protein negative
- Spindle cells
  - Cytokeratin positive (strong and diffuse), muscle specific actin, androgen receptor (nuclear) positive
    - Postulated as possible reason explaining occurrence primarily in adult men
  - Desmin, S100 protein negative

DIFFERENTIAL DIAGNOSIS

Ectopic Cervical Thymoma
- Benign tumor that can be locally invasive and exceptionally metastasize
- Histologically identical to mediastinal thymomas
  - Residual ectopic thymus not uncommonly identified in periphery of tumor

SETTLE
- Highly cellular tumors comprised of compact bundles of long spindle epithelial cells merging with tubulopapillary structures &/or mucinous glands

CASTLE
- Malignant neoplasm histologically similar to thymic carcinoma (lymphoepithelioma or squamous cell)

Synovial Sarcoma
- Limited (not diffuse and strong) cytokeratin reactivity
- Immunoreactivity for TLE1, Bcl-2, CD99, FLI-1, others

Malignant Peripheral Nerve Sheath Tumor
- S100 protein positive (limited in higher grade tumors)
- Absence of cytokeratin reactivity

SELECTED REFERENCES

1. Weinreb I et al: Ectopic hamartomatous thymoma: a case demonstrating skin adnexal differentiation with positivity for epithelial membrane antigen, androgen receptors, and BRST-2 by immunohistochemistry. Hum Pathol. 38(7):1092-5, 2007
2. Fetsch JF et al: Ectopic hamartomatous thymoma: a clinicopathologic and immunohistochemical analysis of 21 cases with data supporting reclassification as a branchial anlage mixed tumor. Am J Surg Pathol. 28(10):1360-70, 2004
3. Michal M et al: Carcinoma arising in ectopic hamartomatous thymoma. An ultrastructural study. Pathol Res Pract. 192(6):610-8; discussion 619-21, 1996
4. Chan JK et al: Tumors of the neck showing thymic or related branchial pouch differentiation: a unifying concept. Hum Pathol. 22(4):349-67, 1991
5. Fetsch JF et al: Ectopic hamartomatous thymoma: clinicopathologic, immunohistochemical, and histogenetic considerations in four new cases. Hum Pathol. 21(6):662-8, 1990
6. Rosai J et al: Ectopic hamartomatous thymoma. A distinctive benign lesion of lower neck. Am J Surg Pathol. 8(7):501-13, 1984

IMAGE GALLERY

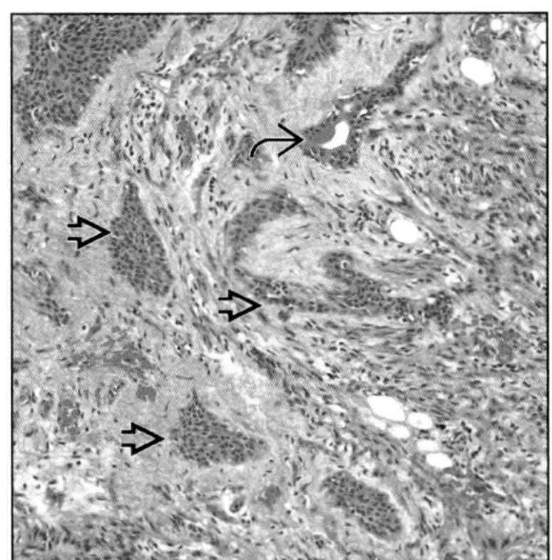

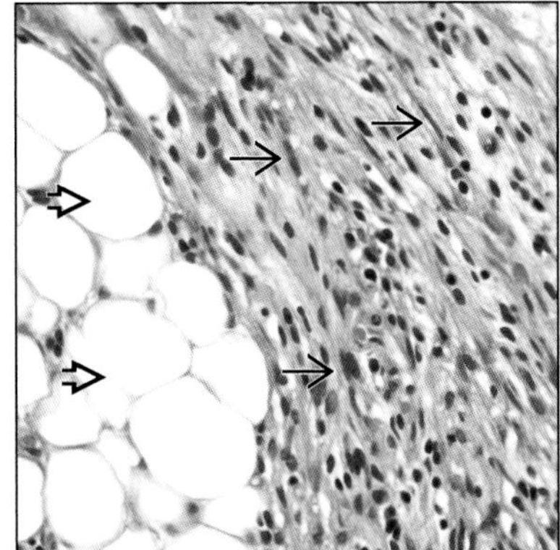

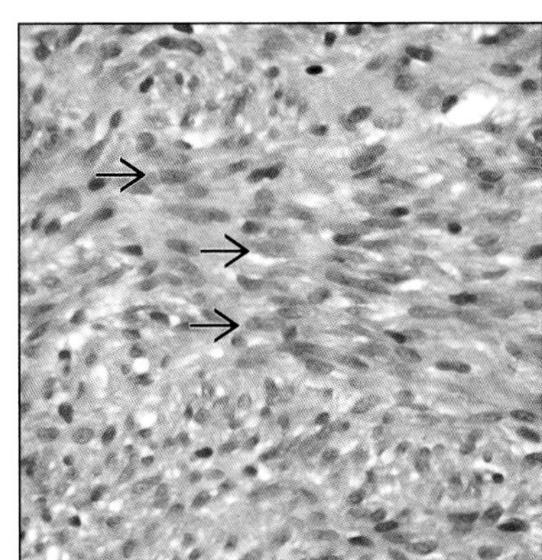

(Left) *The epithelial component also includes nests and cords of nonkeratinizing squamous epithelium ⇨ focally with cystic change ↗.* ***(Center)*** *H&E shows mature adipose tissue ⇨ intimately admixed with slender-appearing spindle cells → lacking significant pleomorphism or increase in mitotic activity. Mature lymphocytes are mixed with the spindle cells.* ***(Right)*** *Plump-appearing spindle cells → show fascicular growth and lack pleomorphism or increase in mitotic activity.*

SOLITARY FIBROUS TUMOR

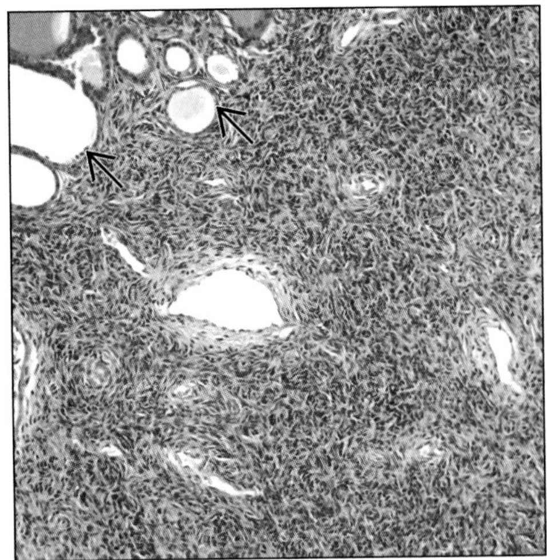

An infiltrative pattern can be seen, with trapping of thyroid follicles ⇒ as shown in this case of SFT. Note the cellular mesenchymal proliferation associated with patulous, open vessels.

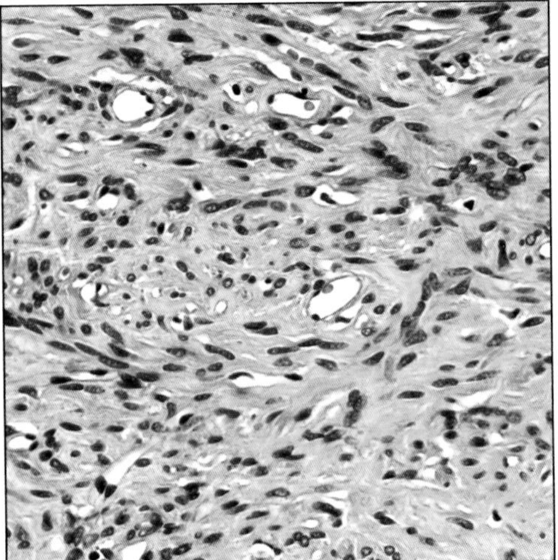

There are bland, monotonous, spindle-shaped cells without any specific growth pattern, although there is a vague fascicular appearance in this case. The cells have a syncytial appearance.

TERMINOLOGY

Abbreviations

- Solitary fibrous tumor (SFT)

Definitions

- Mesenchymal tumor composed of collagen-producing spindle cells arranged in characteristic vascular pattern
  - Identical to pleural tumors of similar nature
  - In a morphologic spectrum of solitary fibrous tumor → hemangiopericytoma

ETIOLOGY/PATHOGENESIS

Pathogenesis

- Primitive mesenchymal cell capable of myofibroblastic &/or fibroblastic differentiation

CLINICAL ISSUES

Epidemiology

- Incidence
  - Exceedingly rare thyroid neoplasm
- Age
  - Middle-aged patients; mean: 48 years
- Gender
  - Female > Male

Presentation

- Asymptomatic enlarging neck mass
- Hoarseness may be present
- Tends to be very slowly growing; present for years

Treatment

- Surgical approaches
  - Lobectomy is sufficient therapy

Prognosis

- Excellent long-term prognosis for these benign tumors
- Recurrence and metastasis are not reported
- Increased cellularity, high mitotic index, pleomorphism, necrosis, &/or invasive growth with perineural or vascular invasion suggests malignant transformation

MACROSCOPIC FEATURES

General Features

- Well circumscribed and frequently encapsulated
- Firm, solid, white-gray-tan cut appearance
- Cystic change is occasionally observed
- Necrosis and calcification is absent

Size

- Usually large; mean: ~ 4.5 cm

MICROSCOPIC PATHOLOGY

Histologic Features

- Arise within thyroid gland proper or involve immediately adjacent soft tissues
- Develops along morphologic spectrum from benign to malignant
  - Also seen along spectrum of solitary fibrous tumor to hemangiopericytoma
- Well-defined border or capsule
- Infiltrative pattern can be seen, with trapping of thyroid follicles
- Variegated, cellular, mesenchymal proliferation
- Hypocellular areas alternate with hypercellular areas
- Bland, monotonous, spindle-shaped cells without any specific growth pattern
  - Storiform, fascicular, or herringbone patterns can be seen
  - Cells are spindled with elongated, slender nuclei surrounded by scant cytoplasm
  - Cells give syncytial appearance
  - Nuclear chromatin is delicate, fine to vesicular

SOLITARY FIBROUS TUMOR

Key Facts

Terminology
- Mesenchymal tumor composed of collagen-producing spindle cells arranged in characteristic vascular pattern
- In morphologic spectrum of solitary fibrous tumor → hemangiopericytoma

Clinical Issues
- Female > Male
- Asymptomatic enlarging neck mass
- Excellent long-term prognosis

Macroscopic Features
- Well circumscribed and frequently encapsulated
- Firm, solid, white-gray-tan cut appearance
- Usually large; mean: ~ 4.5 cm

Microscopic Pathology
- Infiltrative pattern, trapping thyroid follicles
- Variegated, cellular, mesenchymal proliferation
- Hypocellular areas alternate with hypercellular areas
- Patternless proliferation of bland, monotonous, spindle-shaped cells
  - Spindled with elongated, slender nuclei surrounded by scant cytoplasm
- Cells separated by bundles of keloid-like collagen
- Delicate, open vascular spaces

Ancillary Tests
- Immunoreactive: Vimentin, CD34, CD99, Bcl-2

Top Differential Diagnoses
- Schwannoma, leiomyoma, spindle cell follicular adenoma, hyalinizing trabecular adenoma

- Cells separated by bundles of keloid-like collagen
- Background has delicate, open to patulous vascular spaces
  - Vessels are not dominant
  - Some vessels may have thick walls
- Cysts are uncommon
- Myxoid change can be seen
- Extravasated erythrocytes, inflammatory cells, and mast cells are common
- Mitoses are rare
- Necrosis is absent
- Lipomatous variant (adipocytic variant) has been reported

ANCILLARY TESTS

Cytology
- Smears tend to be paucicellular
- Dyscohesive, slender, spindle-shaped cell population
- Interspersed by fragments of collagenized stroma

Immunohistochemistry
- Immunoreactive: Vimentin, CD34, CD99, Bcl-2
  - S100 protein may highlight fat cells
  - Focal actin reactivity reported
- Negative: TTF-1, thyroglobulin, FVIIIRAg, calcitonin, HMB-45, EMA, ALK1, desmin, CD117, and keratins

DIFFERENTIAL DIAGNOSIS

Peripheral Nerve Sheath Tumors
- Antoni A and B areas, wavy nuclei, tapered cells, perivascular hyalinization
- Strong S100 protein reaction; may also have CD34 immunoreactivity

Smooth Muscle Tumors
- Short to sweeping fascicular arrangement
- Oval nuclei with blunt ends
- Tends to lack collagen deposition
- Actin immunoreactivity, but negative with CD34, Bcl-2, and CD99

Spindle Cell Follicular Adenoma
- Lacks collagen deposition, while still showing colloid production
- Immunoreactive with keratin, TTF-1, and thyroglobulin

Hyalinizing Trabecular Adenoma
- Hyalinization is intra- and intercellular
- Trabecular arrangement of follicular epithelial cells
  - Perpendicular nuclei, inclusions, and yellow bodies
- Immunoreactive with TTF-1, keratin, thyroglobulin, and Ki-67 (membranous)

Post Fine Needle Aspiration
- Localized phenomenon adjacent to nodule with hemosiderin, extravasated erythrocytes, reactive vascular pattern

Medullary Carcinoma
- Tumor cells can be spindled, but they are immunoreactive with calcitonin, CEA, chromogranin, TTF-1, and keratin

SELECTED REFERENCES

1. Farrag TY et al: Solitary fibrous tumor of the thyroid gland. Laryngoscope. 119(12):2306-8, 2009
2. Papi G et al: Solitary fibrous tumor of the thyroid gland. Thyroid. 17(2):119-26, 2007
3. Tanahashi J et al: Solitary fibrous tumor of the thyroid gland: report of two cases and review of the literature. Pathol Int. 56(8):471-7, 2006
4. Bohórquez CL et al: Solitary fibrous tumor of the thyroid with capsular invasion. Pathol Res Pract. 199(10):687-90, 2003
5. Rodriguez I et al: Solitary fibrous tumor of the thyroid gland: report of seven cases. Am J Surg Pathol. 25(11):1424-8, 2001
6. Cameselle-Teijeiro J et al: Solitary fibrous tumor of the thyroid. Am J Clin Pathol. 101(4):535-8, 1994

SOLITARY FIBROUS TUMOR

Microscopic Features

(Left) Although tumors can show well-demarcated and encapsulated lesions, an infiltrative pattern can be seen, as noted in this case with permeation between the thyroid follicles. (Right) The thyroid follicles ➞ are uninvolved. The spindled cells are arranged in a nonspecific, syncytial architecture, with a background of delicate, open to patulous vascular spaces ➪.

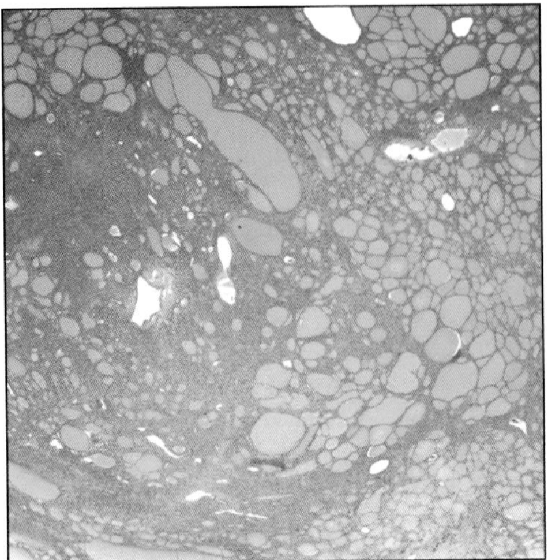

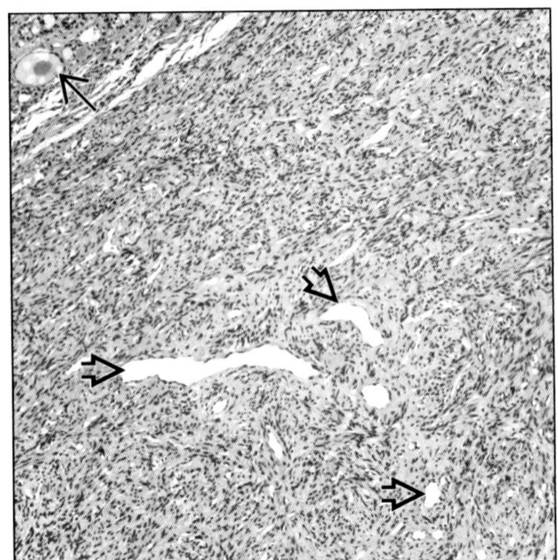

(Left) The neoplastic cells are spindled with elongated, slender nuclei surrounded by scant cytoplasm. There is a syncytial appearance to the proliferation. There is collagen deposition ➞ along with some inflammatory cells. (Right) The elongated and spindled cells are arranged in a fascicular appearance. The slender nuclei contain delicate, fine to vesicular nuclear chromatin. Extravasated erythrocytes are noted throughout. The thyroid follicle ➞ is uninvolved.

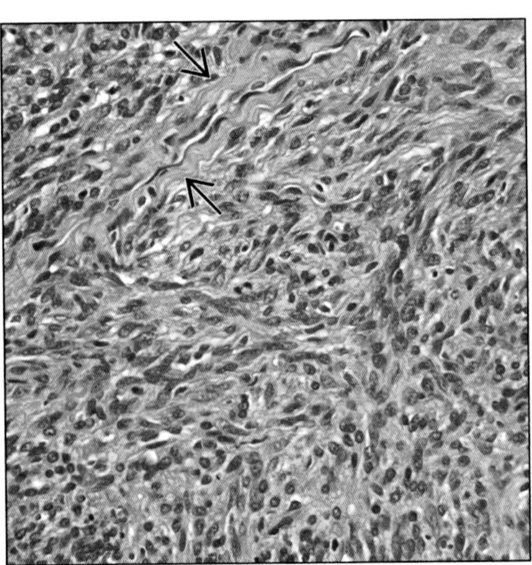

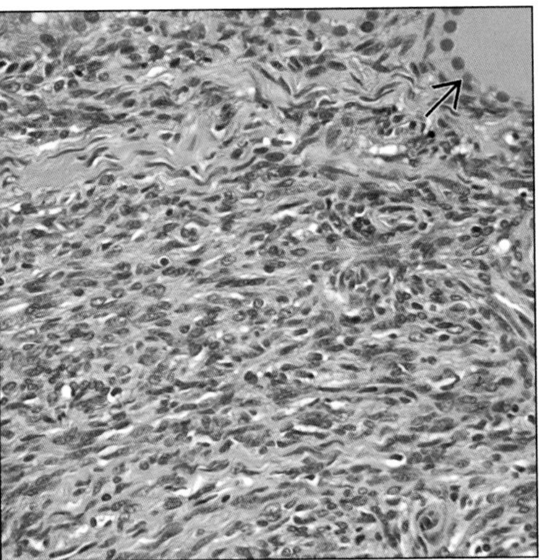

(Left) This tumor is arranged in a storiform pattern. It is hypercellular with slit-like vessels, which are quite difficult to identify ➪. The neoplastic cells are spindled and monotonous. (Right) There is a haphazard and storiform appearance to this tumor. Note the suggestion of nuclear palisading ➞ in this tumor that has a syncytial arrangement of cells. There is collagen deposition, although it is not prominent.

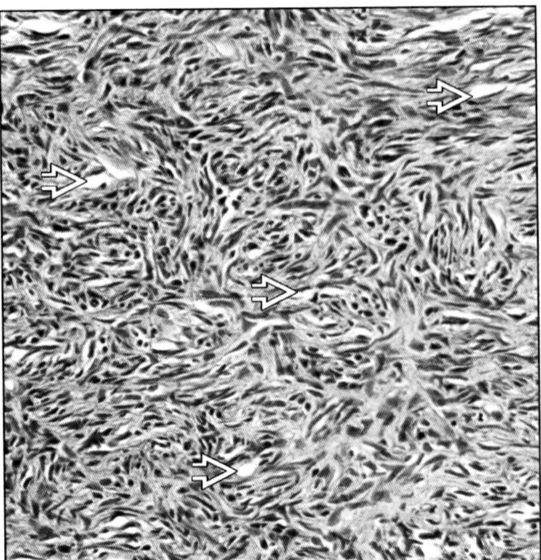

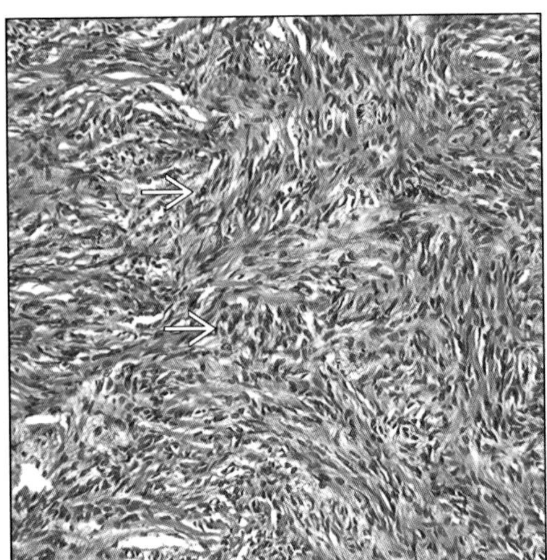

Microscopic and Immunohistochemical Features

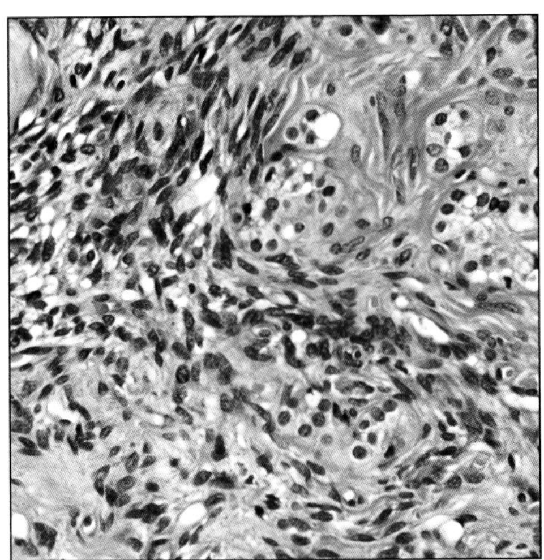

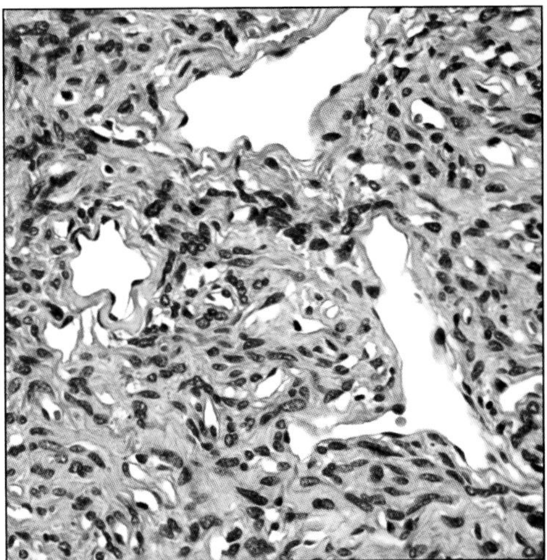

(Left) *The spindled neoplastic cells are separated by bundles of keloid-like collagen in this case. Note the areas of clear cell change. This is not a lipomatous variant.* ***(Right)*** *The vascular pattern can sometimes be more prominent, suggesting the relationship to hemangiopericytoma. The cells are noted surrounding these vessels. Mitoses are usually inconspicuous.*

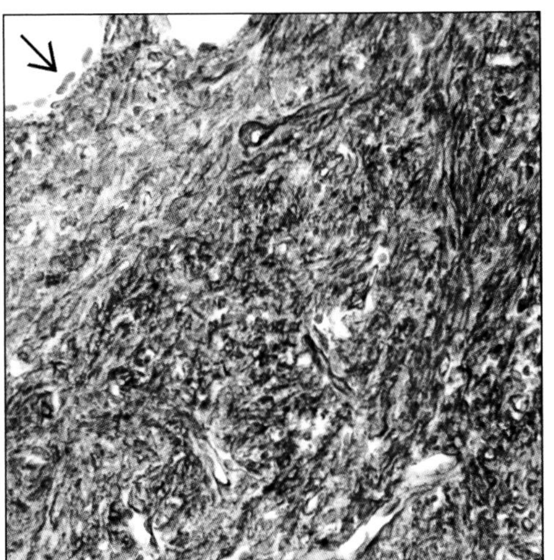

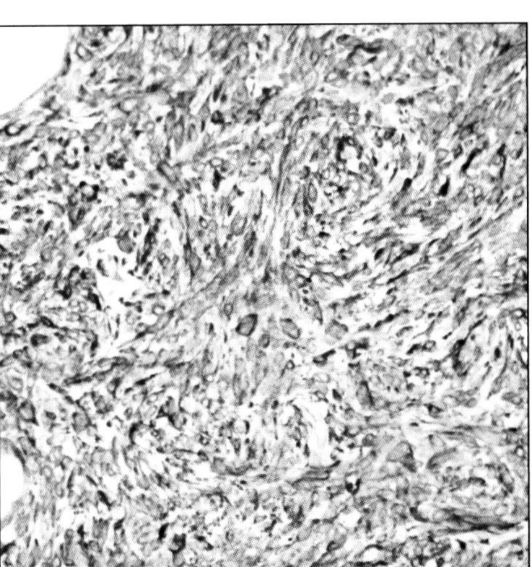

(Left) *While usually not required for the diagnosis, there is usually strong and diffuse immunoreactivity with vimentin, CD34, and Bcl-2. The CD34 is one of the most commonly immunoreactive. Note the follicle is negative* ➔. ***(Right)*** *In this case, there is strong and diffuse Bcl-2 immunoreactivity, quite similar to the previous slide with CD34. Many times these 2 stains will help to confirm the diagnosis.*

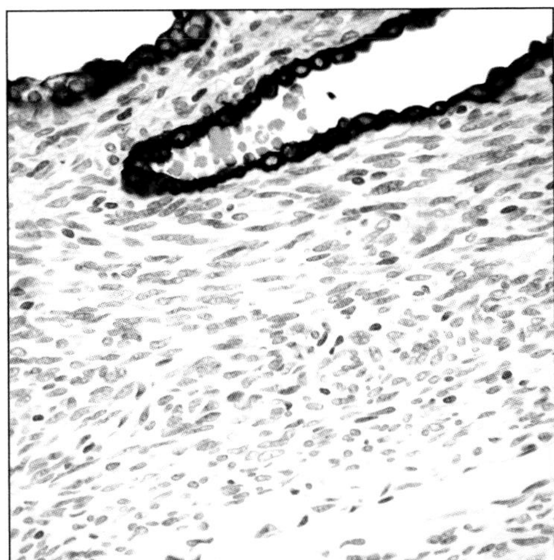

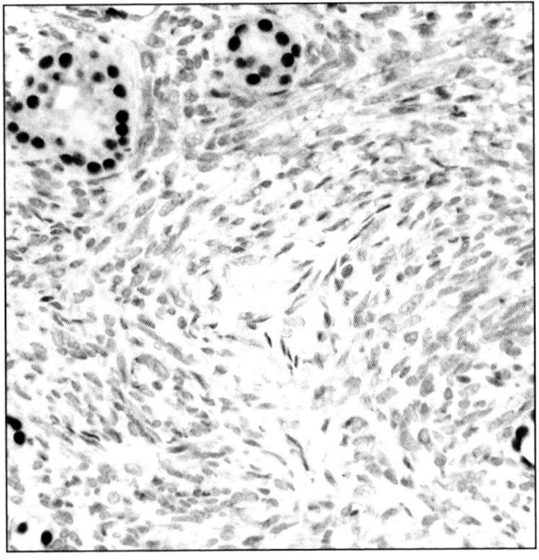

(Left) *If there is a question about the diagnosis, and the possibility of an undifferentiated or other spindled cell tumor is considered, then a negative thyroglobulin can help to support the interpretation of a mesenchymal lesion.* ***(Right)*** *The entrapped thyroid follicles show strong and diffuse nuclear immunoreactivity with TTF-1, highlighting the thyroid epithelium within the background of spindled cell population. This can be used to separate spindle cell follicular adenoma from SFT.*

PARAGANGLIOMA

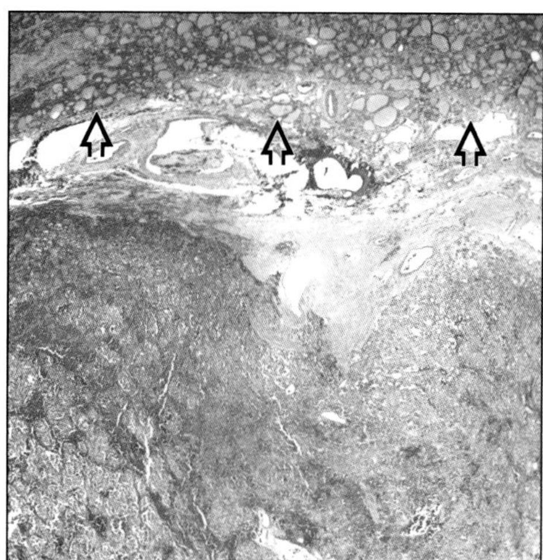

There is a well-developed capsule surrounding this paraganglioma in the thyroid gland. Note the uninvolved thyroid parenchyma ⇨. The tumor is quite vascular with extravasated erythrocytes.

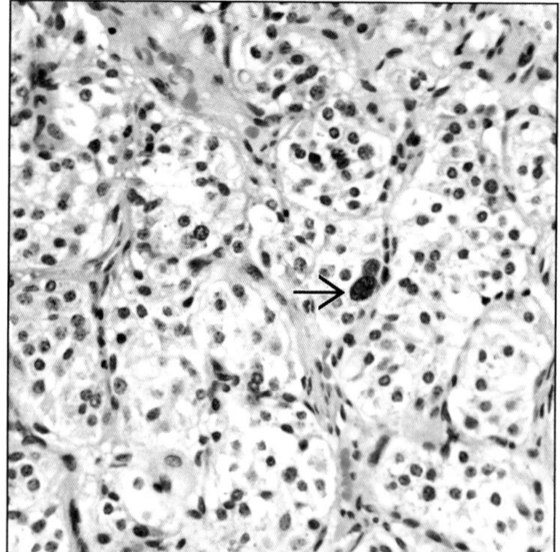

The characteristic zellballen arrangement is highlighted by delicate fibrovascular septations. The chief cells have lightly basophilic cytoplasm surrounding small nuclei. Nuclear pleomorphism is isolated →.

TERMINOLOGY

Definitions

- Thyroid gland primary paragangliomas are intrathyroidal neuroendocrine tumors of paraganglionic origin

ETIOLOGY/PATHOGENESIS

Inherited

- While familial tumors are possible, thyroid primaries appear to be sporadic

Pathogenesis

- Probably arise from inferior laryngeal paraganglia (neural crest)

CLINICAL ISSUES

Epidemiology

- Incidence
  - Exceedingly rare
- Age
  - Although wide age range, most are in 5th decade
- Gender
  - Female > > > > > Male

Presentation

- Asymptomatic neck mass
- If multifocal tumors are found, syndrome/familial association must be considered

Laboratory Tests

- Laboratory analysis to exclude MEN may be considered

Treatment

- Options, risks, complications
  - Rule out multifocal disease
- Surgical approaches
  - Surgical excision is treatment of choice

Prognosis

- Nearly all thyroid gland paragangliomas are benign
- Long-term clinical follow-up recommended, especially in multifocal disease

IMAGE FINDINGS

Radiographic Findings

- Octreotide, Sestamibi, or ^{131}I metaiodobenzylguanidine (MIBG) scintigraphy may show tumor
  - Can be used to exclude multicentric or metastatic disease

MACROSCOPIC FEATURES

General Features

- Circumscribed, gray-brown

Size

- Mean: 3 cm

MICROSCOPIC PATHOLOGY

Histologic Features

- Well-circumscribed, encapsulated intrathyroidal mass
  - Rare extrathyroidal extension reported
- Highly vascular, with rich vascular plexus
  - Fibrovascular septa are delicate and discontinuous
- Tumor cells arranged in alveolar, lobular, sheet, or zellballen pattern
- Paraganglia chief cells are polygonal with abundant, granular, amphophilic cytoplasm
- Nuclei are usually round to oval, with coarse nuclear chromatin
  - Isolated pleomorphic nuclei

PARAGANGLIOMA

Key Facts

Clinical Issues

- Thyroid gland paragangliomas are benign
- Female > > > > > Male

Microscopic Pathology

- Tumor cells arranged in zellballen pattern
- Fibrovascular septa are delicate and discontinuous
- Chief cells are polygonal with abundant, granular, amphophilic cytoplasm
- Nuclei are usually round to oval, with coarse nuclear chromatin

Ancillary Tests

- Chief cells positive: Synaptophysin, chromogranin
- Sustentacular cells positive: S100 protein

Top Differential Diagnoses

- Hyalinizing trabecular tumor, medullary thyroid carcinoma, metastatic neuroendocrine tumor

- Sustentacular supporting cells only seen with immunohistochemistry
- Necrosis and mitotic figures absent

ANCILLARY TESTS

Immunohistochemistry

- Chief cells have variety of positive reactions: Synaptophysin, chromogranin, NSE, tyrosine hydroxylase, CD56
- Sustentacular cells positive with S100 protein and glial fibrillary acidic protein
- Negative: Cytokeratins, EMA, thyroglobulin, TTF-1, calcitonin, serotonin, vimentin

Cytogenetics

- Germline mutations in several genes encoding various subunits of succinate-ubiquinone oxidoreductase gene (SDH)

Electron Microscopy

- Dense core neurosecretory granules in chief cell cytoplasm

DIFFERENTIAL DIAGNOSIS

Hyalinizing Trabecular Tumor

- Previously called "paraganglioma-like tumor"
- Well-developed intratumoral fibrosis and trabecular architecture
- Perinucleolar halos (vacuoles), intranuclear cytoplasmic inclusions, and yellow bodies
- Positive: TTF-1, thyroglobulin, MIB-1 (membranous staining)

Medullary Thyroid Carcinoma

- Invasive with fibrosis and amyloid production
- Immunoreactive with cytokeratin, calcitonin, CEA

Metastatic Neuroendocrine Tumor

- Multifocal tumor with more cytologic atypia (carcinoid, small cell carcinoma, Merkel)
- Spindled tumor cells with "salt and pepper" nuclear chromatin
- Keratin, TTF-1, and possibly CK20 immunoreactive

SELECTED REFERENCES

1. Ferri E et al: Primary paraganglioma of thyroid gland: a clinicopathologic and immunohistochemical study with review of the literature. Acta Otorhinolaryngol Ital. 29(2):97-102, 2009
2. Corrado S et al: Primary paraganglioma of the thyroid gland. J Endocrinol Invest. 27(8):788-92, 2004
3. Baloch ZW et al: Neuroendocrine tumors of the thyroid gland. Am J Clin Pathol. 115 Suppl:S56-67, 2001
4. Cayot F et al: [Multiple paragangliomas of the neck localized in the thyroid region. Papillary thyroid cancer associated with parathyroid adenoma.] Sem Hop. 58(35):2004-7, 1982
5. Buss DH et al: Paraganglioma of the thyroid gland. Am J Surg Pathol. 4(6):589-93, 1980

IMAGE GALLERY

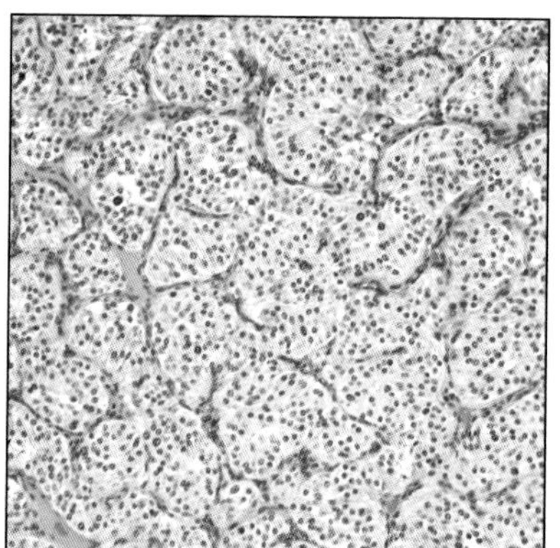

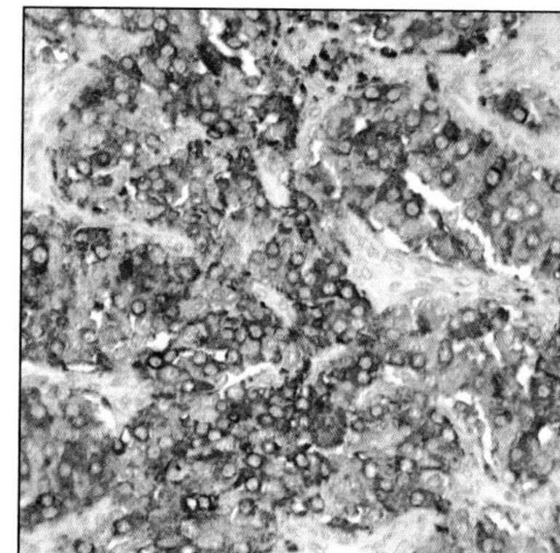

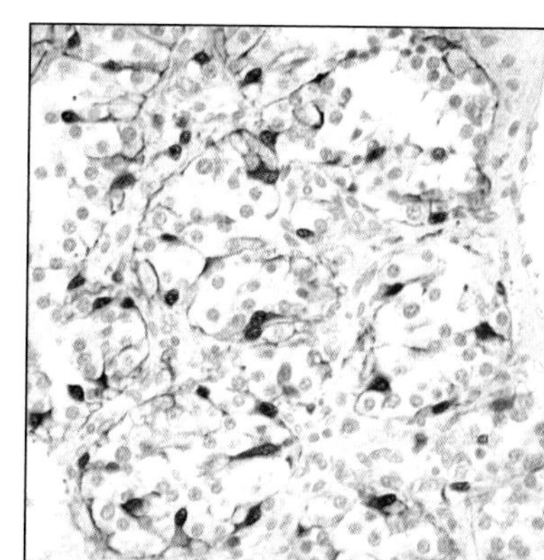

(Left) *The tumors are often quite cellular. There is a nested to zellballen architecture in this tumor. The neoplastic cells are of intermediate size with small, hyperchromatic nuclei.* ***(Center)*** *The paraganglia cells are highlighted by a variety of neuroendocrine markers. In this case, chromogranin was strongly and diffusely immunoreactive in a granular distribution.* ***(Right)*** *S100 protein highlights the sustentacular supporting cells, with a positive nuclear and cytoplasmic reaction.*

LEIOMYOMA

Key Facts

Terminology

- Benign primary thyroid neoplasm composed of cells with distinct smooth muscle differentiation histologically

Etiology/Pathogenesis

- May develop from smooth muscle-walled vessels at thyroid gland periphery

Clinical Issues

- Exceedingly rare (< 0.02% of all thyroid gland tumors)
- Younger patients with equal gender distribution
- Thyroid mass, usually slowly developing over years
- Lobectomy or thyroidectomy is curative
- Excellent prognosis without any reported cases of death from disease

Image Findings

- Thyroid scans with radioactive isotopes demonstrate a cold nodule
- Inhomogeneous low-density mass in thyroid gland

Macroscopic Features

- Well circumscribed, with smooth outer tumor surface
- Mean: 2 cm

Microscopic Pathology

- Encapsulated, with smooth, noninvasive periphery
- Arranged in bundles or fascicles of smooth muscle fibers that intersect in an orderly fashion
- Cells are spindled and blunt-ended or cigar-shaped
- Centrally placed nuclei are slightly hyperchromatic
- Perinuclear cytoplasmic vacuoles are sometimes prominent
- No pleomorphism, necrosis, or increased mitotic figures

Ancillary Tests

- Neoplastic cells positive: Vimentin, SMA, MSA, desmin

Top Differential Diagnoses

- Peripheral nerve sheath tumor, follicular spindle cell adenoma

__(Left)__ The thyroid gland parenchyma ➔ is separated from the neoplasm by a thin but well-formed fibrous connective tissue capsule. The spindled cell tumor shows short, interlacing fascicles. __(Right)__ On high power, there are interlacing bundles or fascicles of smooth muscle fibers that intersect in an orderly fashion. The spindled cells have blunt, centrally placed, hyperchromatic nuclei. Small vacuoles are noted in the cytoplasm of a few cells. There are no mitotic figures.

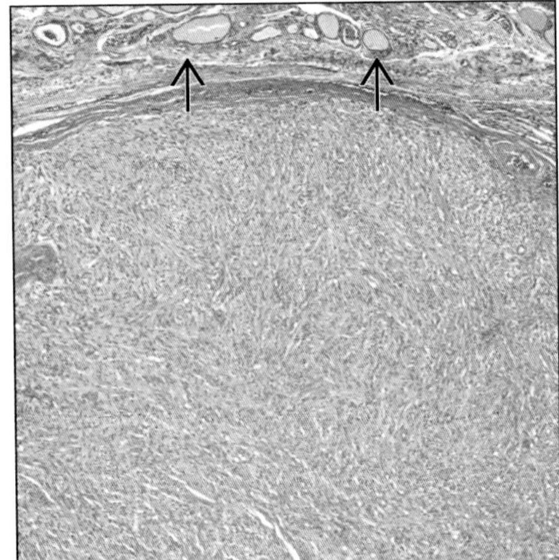

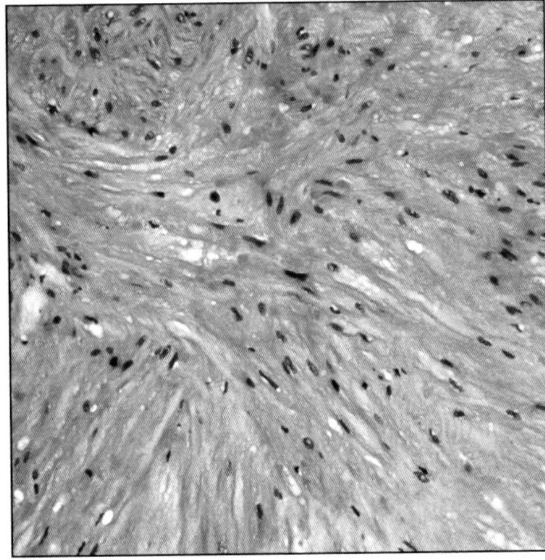

__(Left)__ The neoplastic cells of leiomyoma are strongly and diffusely immunoreactive with a variety of muscle markers, in this case a smooth muscle actin. __(Right)__ Desmin highlights the cytoplasm of these smooth muscle cells in a leiomyoma. Note the lack of cytologic atypia. Myogenin, MYOD1, and myoglobulin are generally negative in benign tumors, as are markers of thyroid derivation (TTF-1, thyroglobulin, keratin).

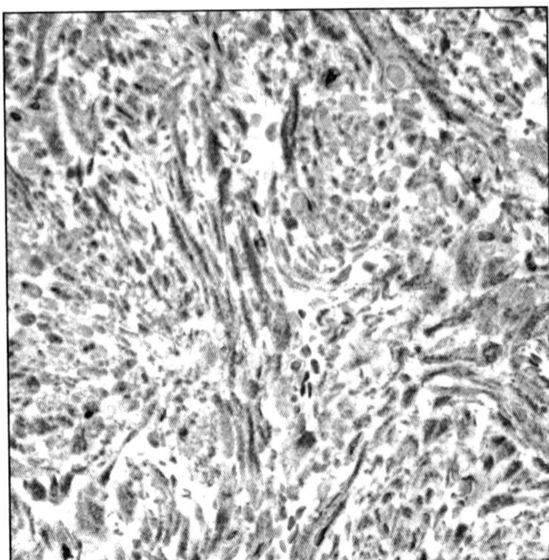

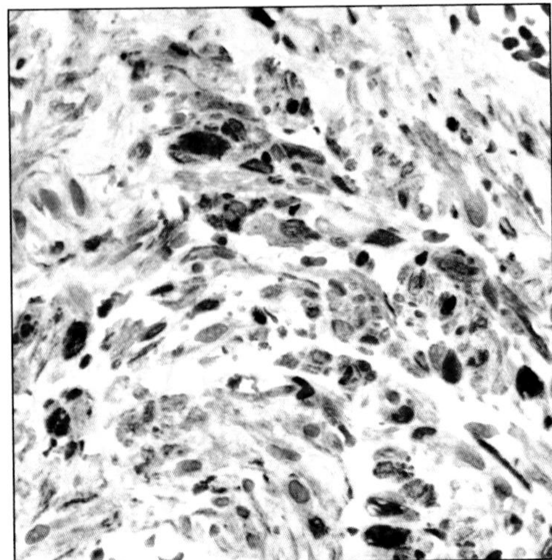

SCHWANNOMA

Key Facts

Terminology
- Benign neoplasm composed of cells with evidence of distinct peripheral nerve sheath differentiation histologically
- PNSTs include schwannoma and neurofibroma

Etiology/Pathogenesis
- May arise from sympathetic and parasympathetic or possibly sensory nerves

Clinical Issues
- Very rare (< 0.02% of all thyroid gland tumors)
- All ages affected, with equal gender distribution
- May arise from medium to large nerves at thyroid gland periphery
- Present with thyroid gland mass
- Surgical excision is curative
- Excellent long-term clinical prognosis

Image Findings
- CT images show inhomogeneous, low-density mass, identical to soft tissue

Macroscopic Features
- Smooth surface, well circumscribed or encapsulated
- Tan to white and glistening with "neural" appearance

Microscopic Pathology
- Densely packed spindle-cell areas (Antoni A)
- Loosely arranged hypocellular degenerated myxoid areas (Antoni B)
- Slender spindle cells arranged in interlacing fascicles
  - Fibrillar cytoplasmic extensions
  - Palisading of nuclei (Verocay bodies)
  - Nuclei are wavy and spindled, lacking atypia
- Small to medium-sized blood vessels may have hyalinized walls

Ancillary Tests
- Positive: S100 protein (diffuse and strong), vimentin
- Negative: TTF-1, calcitonin, actin, desmin

Top Differential Diagnoses
- Leiomyoma and soft tissue primaries

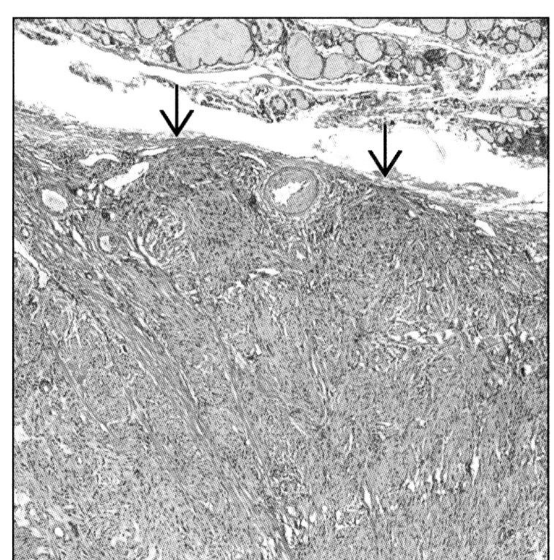

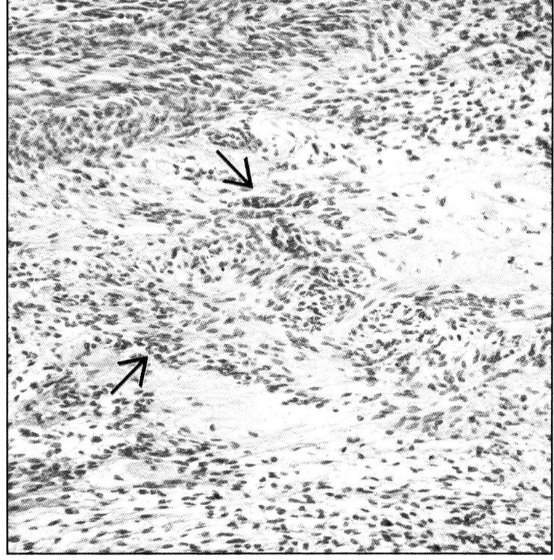

(Left) *H&E shows a very well-demarcated neoplasm* → *adjacent to the uninvolved thyroid gland parenchyma. There is an interlacing fascicular arrangement to this neoplasm at low power, showing some areas of fibrosis.* ***(Right)*** *H&E shows an alternating cellular and hypocellular area to this tumor, in which there is a palisading of the nuclei* →*, a feature seen in schwannoma. The neural matrix material is easily identified. There is no cytologic atypia.*

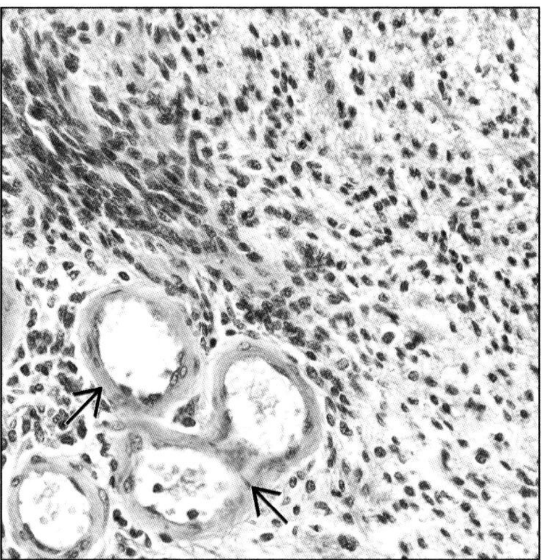

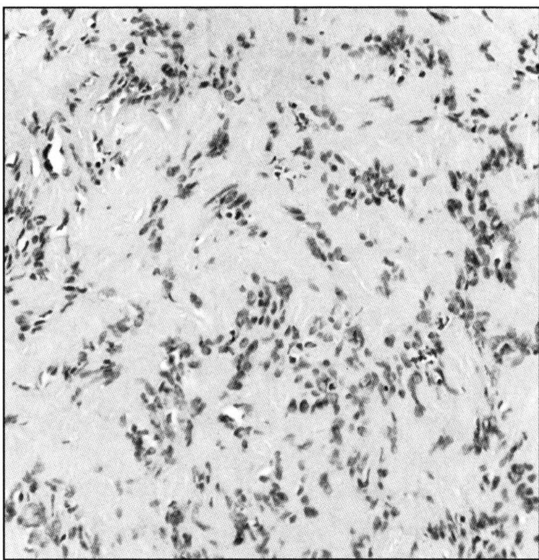

(Left) *There is a palisade of spindled to wavy nuclei in this area. Note the vessels show prominent hyalinization* →*, a feature that is quite commonly identified in schwannoma. The neural matrix is easily identified in the background of this tumor.* ***(Right)*** *The nuclei show a remarkable aggregation or palisade in this schwannoma. The neural matrix material is quite hyalinized in this example of a peripheral nerve sheath tumor. Pleomorphism, necrosis, and mitoses are absent.*

LANGERHANS CELL HISTIOCYTOSIS

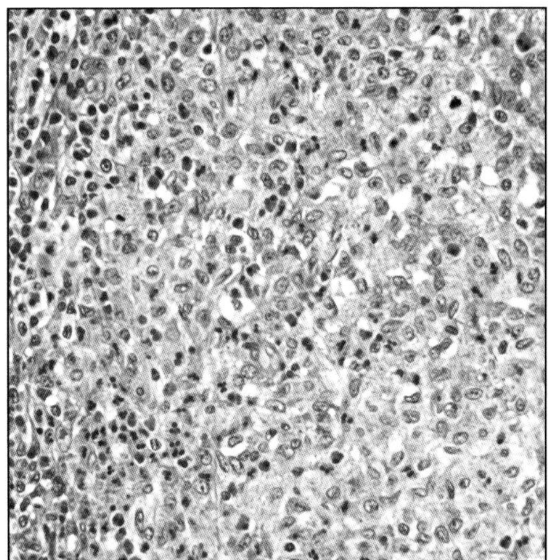

There is a sheet-like collection of enlarged cells with delicate cytoplasm surrounding vesicular nuclei. The nuclei are notched or grooved, giving a coffee bean shape. Many eosinophils are noted.

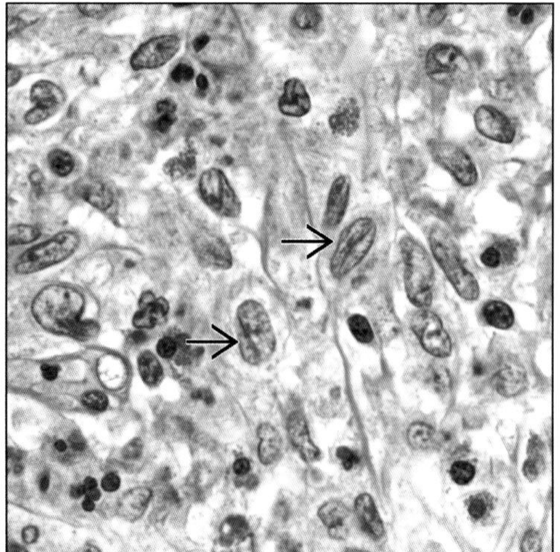

The polyhedral to spindled cells have delicate, foamy cytoplasm surrounding nuclei that are indented or folded, with longitudinal grooves ⇒. Eosinophils are noted.

TERMINOLOGY

Abbreviations

- Langerhans cell histiocytosis (LCH)

Definitions

- Increased number of Langerhans cells: Unique histiocyte containing Birbeck granules
- 3 distinct but interrelated clinical syndromes share identical histologic features
  - **Eosinophilic granuloma**: Predominantly osseous or pulmonary isolated disease
  - **Hand-Schüller-Christian**: Multiple organ systems affected, including skull base
  - **Letterer-Siwe**: Most severe form, typically involving abdominal viscera

ETIOLOGY/PATHOGENESIS

Etiology

- Although unknown, possible causes include neoplastic process, viral agent, or abnormal proliferative process

Pathogenesis

- Clonal disorder of Langerhans cells, believed to be modified histiocyte derived from dendritic system

CLINICAL ISSUES

Epidemiology

- Incidence
  - Isolated disease is exceptionally rare
    - May be more frequent as part of systemic disease
- Age
  - Wide range: Birth to old age
    - Isolated thyroid involvement more likely in older patients
    - Systemic disease more likely at young age (< 20 years)
- Gender
  - Equal gender distribution

Site

- May be focal or diffuse thyroid involvement

Presentation

- Important to identify isolated thyroid disease vs. part of more widespread disease
- Usually present with unilateral thyroid gland nodule
- Uncommonly, present with sore throat, upper respiratory tract infection, skin rash, pulmonary distress, gastrointestinal symptoms, lymph node enlargement
  - Usually in patients with systemic involvement
    - Bone, skin, liver, lymph nodes, lungs, central nervous system, spleen, gastrointestinal tract
- Duration of symptoms varies based on disease
  - Days: Systemic disease
  - Years: Isolated disease

Treatment

- Options, risks, complications
  - Treatment differs for isolated/localized vs. systemic disease
  - Must exclude systemic disease
- Surgical approaches
  - Surgery is sufficient for localized thyroid disease
- Drugs
  - Combination chemotherapy for systemic disease

Prognosis

- Closely related to extent of disease
  - Localized: Excellent
  - Systemic disease: Aggressive, with poor prognosis
- When thyroid is primary presentation, subsequent systemic disease is rare

LANGERHANS CELL HISTIOCYTOSIS

Key Facts

Terminology

- Increased number of Langerhans cells: Unique histiocyte containing Birbeck granules
  - **Eosinophilic granuloma**: Predominantly osseous or pulmonary isolated disease
  - **Hand-Schüller-Christian**: Multiple organ systems affected, including skull base
  - **Letterer-Siwe**: Most severe form, typically involving abdominal viscera

Clinical Issues

- Isolated thyroid involvement more likely in older patients
- Important to identify isolated thyroid disease vs. part of more widespread disease
- Prognosis closely related to extent of disease
  - Localized: Excellent; systemic: Aggressive, with poor prognosis

Microscopic Pathology

- Subcapsular and septal location more common
- Infiltrate frequently effaces thyroid architecture
- Collections of enlarged cells with delicate, pale or eosinophilic cytoplasm surrounding vesicular nuclei
- Nuclei have indented, notched, lobulated, folded, grooved, or coffee bean shape
- Increased number of eosinophils

Ancillary Tests

- Practical panel: S100 protein, CD1a, Langerin, CD68
- Invaginations of cell membranes (Birbeck granules)
  - Pentilaminar, with cross striations and vesicular expansions by electron microscopy

IMAGE FINDINGS

Radiographic Findings

- Nonspecific
- Scintigraphic studies show cold nodule
- Ultrasonography demonstrates mixed-density mass lesion

MACROSCOPIC FEATURES

General Features

- Nodule, usually indistinguishable from other thyroid nodules

Size

- Range: 0.2-8 cm

MICROSCOPIC PATHOLOGY

Histologic Features

- Focal or diffuse thyroid gland involvement
  - May extend beyond thyroid capsule, resulting in adherence to surrounding soft tissue or skeletal muscle
- Subcapsular and septal location more common
- Infiltrate pushes or destroys thyroid parenchyma, frequently effacing thyroid follicular architecture
- Collections of enlarged cells with delicate, pale or eosinophilic cytoplasm surrounding vesicular nuclei
- Nuclei have indented, notched, lobulated, folded, grooved, or coffee bean shape
- Cytoplasm is often finely vacuolated, with phagocytized cellular debris
- Increased number of eosinophils
  - Concentrated in collections around areas of necrosis
- Lymphocytic thyroiditis commonly present
- Adenomatoid nodules and thyroid papillary carcinoma may concurrently be present

ANCILLARY TESTS

Cytology

- Scant colloid in smears with high cellularity
- Isolated, discrete, atypical, large mononucleated cells
  - May be loosely aggregated
- Contorted nuclei with longitudinal nuclear folds/ grooves
- Abundant, foamy granular cytoplasm
- Background of eosinophils, lymphocytes, and multinucleated and foamy histiocytes
- Mitotic figures are common

Immunohistochemistry

- Langerhans cells have wide immunohistochemistry panel
  - Macrophage antigens give a concentration in perinuclear and Golgi regions
  - Negative: Cytokeratin, thyroglobulin, TTF-1
- Practical panel: S100 protein, CD1a, Langerin (CD207), CD68 sufficient for a diagnosis of LCH

Electron Microscopy

- Folded, convoluted, and lobulated nuclei
- Cytoplasmic filopodial extensions and invaginations
- Invaginations of cell membranes called Birbeck granules or Langerhans granules
  - Granules are disc-shaped, but on cross section they are rod-shaped
  - Pentilaminar, with cross striations and vesicular expansions
    - Tennis racquet appearance
  - Langerin (CD207) is protein that makes up Birbeck granules

DIFFERENTIAL DIAGNOSIS

Rosai-Dorfman Disease

- Massive lymphadenopathy with sinus histiocytosis has characteristic emperipolesis (phagocytized nuclear debris in cytoplasm of histiocyte)

LANGERHANS CELL HISTIOCYTOSIS

Immunohistochemistry

Antibody	Reactivity	Staining Pattern	Comment
S100	Positive	Nuclear & cytoplasmic	All tumor cells are positive
CD1a	Positive	Cytoplasmic	Almost all lesional cells
CD207	Positive	Cytoplasmic	Langerin gives a dot-like paranuclear positivity
CD68	Positive	Cytoplasmic	Almost all lesional cells
Lysozyme	Positive	Cytoplasmic	Most lesional cells
Fascin	Positive	Cytoplasmic	Variably positive, depending on maturation
CD15	Positive	Dot positivity	Highlights Golgi or perinuclear zone
CD30	Positive	Dot positivity	Ki-1 highlights Golgi or perinuclear zone
PLAP	Positive	Cytoplasmic	Many lesional cells reactive
PNA	Positive	Cytoplasmic	Peanut agglutinin in most lesional cells
CD2	Positive	Cytoplasmic	
CD3	Positive	Cytoplasmic	
CD4	Positive	Cytoplasmic	
CD11c	Positive	Cytoplasmic	
α-1-antichymotrypsin	Positive	Cytoplasmic	
CK-PAN	Negative		
TTF-1	Negative		
Thyroglobulin	Negative		

- Also S100 protein immunoreactivity
- Not identified in thyroid gland but in perithyroidal lymph nodes

Chronic Lymphocytic Thyroiditis

- When thyroiditis is extensive or heavy, histiocytes and eosinophils of LCH may be overlooked

Thyroid Papillary Carcinoma

- Cohesive clusters of epithelial cells with nuclear enlargement, nuclear chromatin clearing, nuclear grooves, and intranuclear cytoplasmic inclusions
- Eosinophils and histiocytes are absent

Undifferentiated Carcinoma

- Significant pleomorphism, extensive necrosis
- Lacks inflammatory infiltrate
- Different immunohistochemistry profile from LCH

DIAGNOSTIC CHECKLIST

Clinically Relevant Pathologic Features

- Recognition of disease should prompt exclusion of systemic disease

SELECTED REFERENCES

1. Jamaati HR et al: Langerhans cell histiocytosis of the lung and thyroid, co-existing with papillary thyroid cancer. Endocr Pathol. 20(2):133-6, 2009
2. Wohlschlaeger J et al: Immunocytochemical investigation of Langerin (CD207) is a valuable adjunct in the cytological diagnosis of Langerhans cell histiocytosis of the thyroid. Pathol Res Pract. 205(6):433-6, 2009
3. Burnett A et al: Thyroid involvement with Langerhans cell histiocytosis in a 3-year-old male. Pediatr Blood Cancer. 50(3):726-7, 2008
4. Lollar K et al: Langerhans cell histiocytosis of the thyroid gland. Am J Otolaryngol. 29(3):201-4, 2008
5. Ramadas PT et al: Fine needle aspiration cytology of Langerhans cell thyroid histiocytosis and its draining lymph nodes. Acta Cytol. 52(3):396-8, 2008
6. Giovanella L et al: Imaging in endocrinology: Langherans cell histiocytosis of the thyroid gland detected by 18FDG-PET/CT. J Clin Endocrinol Metab. 92(8):2866-7, 2007
7. Yağci B et al: Thyroid involvement in Langerhans cell histiocytosis: a report of two cases and review of the literature. Eur J Pediatr. 166(9):901-4, 2007
8. Elliott DD et al: Langerhans cell histiocytosis presenting as a thyroid gland mass. Ann Diagn Pathol. 9(5):267-74, 2005
9. Foulet-Rogé A et al: Incidental langerhans cell histiocytosis of thyroid: case report and review of the literature. Endocr Pathol. 13(3):227-33, 2002
10. Behrens RJ et al: Langerhans cell histiocytosis of the thyroid: a report of two cases and review of the literature. Thyroid. 11(7):697-705, 2001
11. Saiz E et al: Isolated Langerhans cell histiocytosis of the thyroid: a report of two cases with nuclear imaging-pathologic correlation. Ann Diagn Pathol. 4(1):23-8, 2000
12. Thompson LD et al: Langerhans cell histiocytosis of the thyroid: a series of seven cases and a review of the literature. Mod Pathol. 9(2):145-9, 1996
13. Thompson LD: Langerhans cell histiocytosis isolated to the thyroid gland. Eur Arch Otorhinolaryngol. 253(1-2):62-5, 1996
14. Tsang WY et al: Incidental Langerhans' cell histiocytosis of the thyroid. Histopathology. 24(4):397-9, 1994
15. Coode PE et al: Histiocytosis X of the thyroid masquerading as thyroid carcinoma. Hum Pathol. 19(2):239-41, 1988
16. Lahey ME et al: Involvement of the thyroid in histiocytosis X. Am J Pediatr Hematol Oncol. 8(3):257-9, 1986
17. Sinisi AA et al: Thyroid localization in adult histiocytosis X. J Endocrinol Invest. 9(5):417-20, 1986
18. Teja K et al: Involvement of the thyroid gland in histiocytosis X. Hum Pathol. 12(12):1137-9, 1981

Microscopic Features and Ancillary Techniques

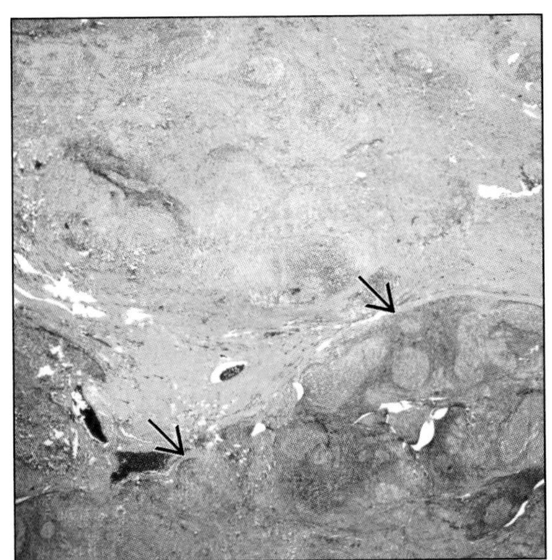

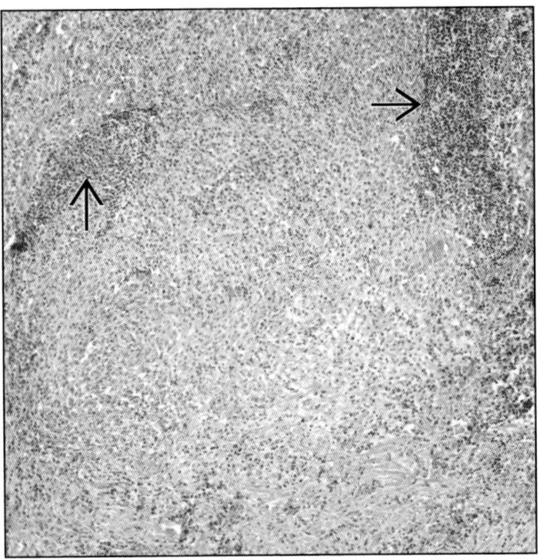

(Left) *A single focus of LCH is associated with lymphocytic thyroiditis* ⇒*. The infiltrate has effaced the thyroid follicular architecture. There is associated fibrosis in this case.* ***(Right)*** *There is a collection of "histiocytes," focally associated with lymphocytic thyroiditis* ⇒*. There is a "lightness" to the focus, as the cytoplasm is foamy. Eosinophils can be seen.*

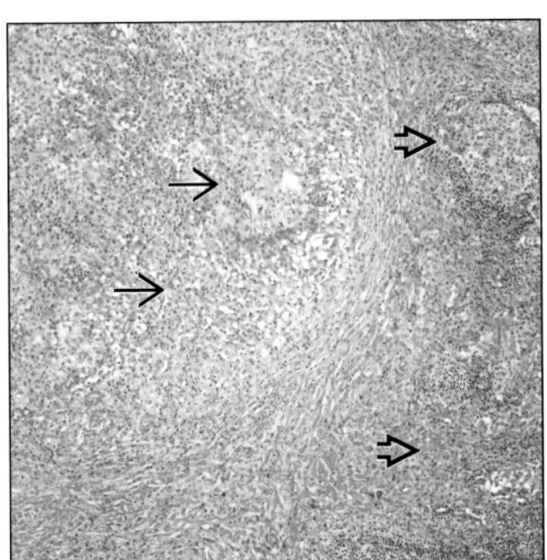

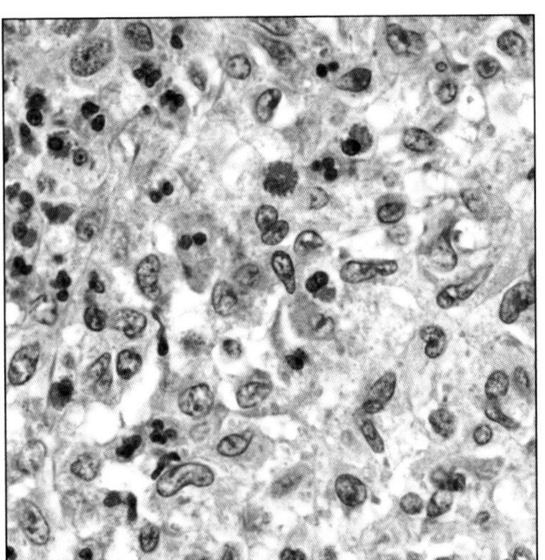

(Left) *This focus of LCH is associated with an abscess formation, in which eosinophils form the abscess* ⇒*. The thyroid parenchyma is destroyed. There is chronic lymphocytic thyroiditis at the periphery* ⇨*.* ***(Right)*** *The large cells have nuclei that give the impression of a "footprint." The nucleus is indented, notched, lobulated, folded, or grooved, yielding a coffee bean shape. Note the increased number of eosinophils in the background.*

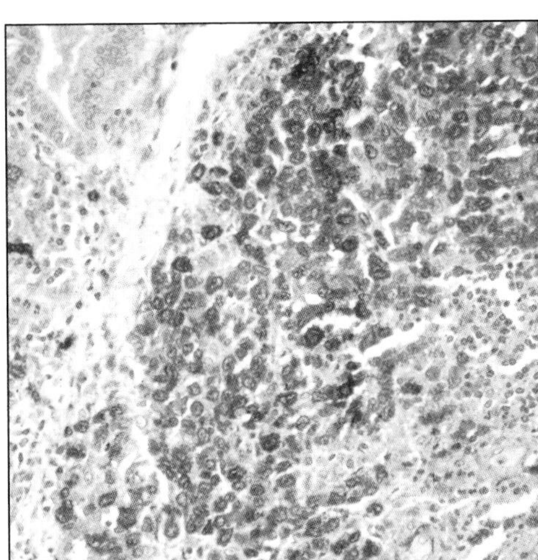

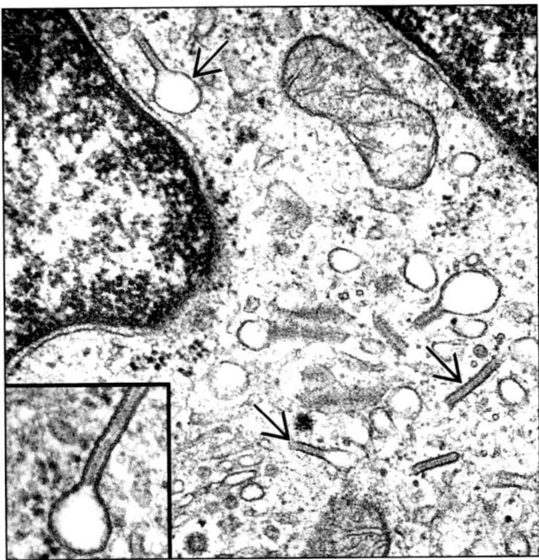

(Left) *Strong and diffuse nuclear & cytoplasmic S100 protein reactivity is noted in this collection of LCH. CD1a and CD68 would also give similar results, although only in the cytoplasm.* ***(Right)*** *The nucleus is folded and convoluted. Cell membrane invaginations result in disc-shaped granules that are rod-shaped* ⇒ *on cross section. These Birbeck or Langerhans granules are pentilaminar, with cross striations and vesicular expansions yielding a tennis racquet appearance (inset). (Courtesy S. Bhuta, MD.)*

FOLLICULAR CELL-DERIVED LESIONS IN ECTOPIC LOCATIONS (STRUMA OVARII)

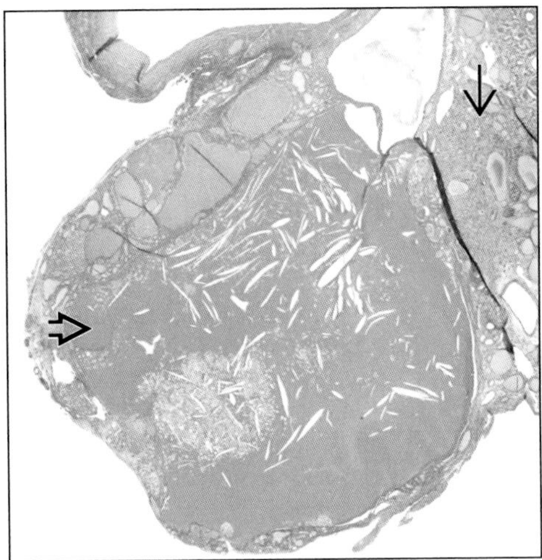

Cystic and solid ovarian lesion shows prominent thyroid tissue including normal thyroid parenchyma ⇒ and changes of adenomatoid nodule ⇒ with associated degenerative changes.

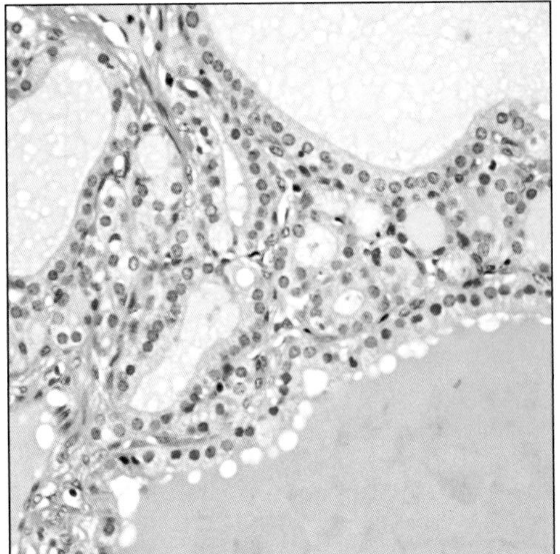

The thyroid tissue shows colloid-filled follicles composed of follicular epithelial cells with basally oriented, uniform-appearing round nuclei with coarse nuclear chromatin.

TERMINOLOGY

Definitions

- **Ovarian thyroid tissue**
  - Presence of thyroid parenchyma in setting of ovarian teratoma
  - Thyroid tissue represents only minor component of ovarian teratoma
- **Struma ovarii**
  - Ovarian teratomas in which thyroid tissue is predominant (at least 50%) or sole tissue component
- **Strumal carcinoid**
  - Ovarian tumor includes presence of thyroid tissue admixed with carcinoid tumor
    - In this setting, other teratomatous elements usually absent

ETIOLOGY/PATHOGENESIS

Idiopathic

- No known associated causes or risk factors

CLINICAL ISSUES

Epidemiology

- Incidence
  - 5-15% of mature ovarian teratomas contain thyroid tissue
    - Identification may be function of adequate sampling
- Age
  - **Struma ovarii**
    - May occur over wide range, including 2nd-9th decades of life
    - Occurs mainly over 40 years of age
  - **Strumal carcinoid**
    - Majority are postmenopausal
    - Occur over wide age range, from 3rd-8th decades of life
- Gender
  - Exclusively in women

Site

- Exclusively limited to ovary
  - Bilaterality may occur in up to 5% of cases

Presentation

- **Struma ovarii**
  - Presentation is similar to ovarian teratoma
    - Enlarging abdominal mass
    - Incidental finding on routine gynecologic (or urologic) evaluation
  - Other (uncommon) clinical presentations may include
    - Symptoms related to function of thyroid component (hyperthyroidism) occur in < 10%
    - Ascites that, in presence of ovarian mass, may be suspicious for ovarian carcinoma
    - Ascites and hydrothorax ("pseudo-Meig syndrome") may occur
- **Strumal carcinoid**
  - Presentation similar to ovarian teratoma
    - Abdominal mass
    - Acute abdominal pain
    - Incidental finding on routine gynecologic (or urologic) evaluation
    - Rarely, may initially be detected as ovarian mass complicating pregnancy
  - Other uncommon presentations may include
    - Constipation (peptide YY found in association with constipation)
    - Pain on defecation
    - Virilization, hirsutism
    - Symptoms related to hyperthyroidism rarely occur
  - Carcinoid syndrome
    - Occurs in 25-33% of cases

FOLLICULAR CELL-DERIVED LESIONS IN ECTOPIC LOCATIONS (STRUMA OVARII)

Key Facts

Terminology
- **Struma ovarii**
  - Ovarian teratomas in which thyroid tissue is predominant (at least 50%) or sole tissue component
- **Strumal carcinoid**
  - Ovarian tumor includes presence of thyroid tissue admixed with carcinoid tumor

Clinical Issues
- 5-15% of mature ovarian teratomas contain thyroid tissue
- Presentation is similar to ovarian teratoma
- Enlarging abdominal mass
- **Struma ovarii**
  - Surgical removal is curative
  - Prognosis associated with malignant thyroid tumors in struma ovarii considered good, with overall survival rates of 89% at 10 years and 84% at 25 years
- **Strumal carcinoid**
  - Prognosis considered excellent following surgical removal, even in presence of metastatic tumor

Microscopic Pathology
- **Struma ovarii**
  - Normal-appearing thyroid follicular tissue (most common finding)
  - Rarely, thyroid neoplasms arise in struma ovarii
  - Thyroid papillary carcinoma most common
- **Strumal carcinoid**
  - Characterized by presence of normal thyroid tissue admixed with carcinoid tumor

    - May include facial flushing, diarrhea, bronchospasm, hypertension
    - Rare occurrence of carcinoid heart disease reported; may include edema

Laboratory Tests
- **Struma ovarii**
  - Functional abnormalities may occur including
    - Hyperthyroidism (rarely struma ovarii may coexist with Graves disease)
    - Increased serum thyroglobulin may be present in metastatic thyroid carcinoma arising in struma ovarii
    - Increased serum CA 125 levels in "pseudo-Meig syndrome" (ascites and hydrothorax)

Treatment
- Options, risks, complications
  - **Struma ovarii**
  - Surgical excision is treatment of choice
    - Unilateral salpingo-oophorectomy or total abdominal hysterectomy and salpingo-oophorectomy (uni- or bilateral)
  - In presence of normally situated (cervical) thyroid gland without abnormalities, surgical intervention not indicated
  - Surgical excision is treatment for malignant struma ovarii
    - Unilateral salpingo-oophorectomy or total abdominal hysterectomy and salpingo-oophorectomy (uni- or bilateral)
  - Treatment for metastatic thyroid (papillary) carcinoma in struma ovarii may include
    - Surgical removal ± supplemental radioactive iodine therapy
    - Use of radioactive iodine therapy would necessitate ablation of cervical thyroid gland
  - **Strumal carcinoid**
    - Unilateral salpingo-oophorectomy in younger aged patients
    - Bilateral oophorectomy and hysterectomy in older aged patients

Prognosis
- **Struma ovarii**
  - Surgical removal is curative
- Prognosis associated with malignant thyroid tumors in struma ovarii considered good with overall survival rates of
  - 89% at 10 years
  - 84% at 25 years
  - Although unusual, fatalities secondary to widespread metastatic disease have occurred
- Metastatic disease from papillary carcinoma may occur
  - To contralateral ovary, peritoneum, regional lymph nodes, liver, and brain
- Benign stromatosis: Term used for presence of benign thyroid follicular epithelium within peritoneum
  - These foci should be considered to represent metastatic thyroid carcinoma
- Rare instances of non-Hodgkin malignant lymphomas reported in struma ovarii
- Pathologic factors predictive of poorer prognosis include
  - Large size (≥ 10 cm)
  - Strumal component > 80%
  - Extensive papillary carcinoma, especially with solid areas
  - Necrosis, ≥ 5 mitoses per 10 high-power fields
- **Strumal carcinoid**
  - Prognosis considered excellent following surgical removal, even in presence of metastatic tumor
    - Both strumal and carcinoid components capable of giving rise to metastases

IMAGE FINDINGS

MR Findings
- Presence of multilocular cystic mass with variable signal intensity within loculi
- Loculi or small cysts within septations may show
  - Low signal intensity on T1-weighted images
  - Very low signal intensity on T2-weighted images
- Gd-DTPA-enhanced T1-weighted images may show

FOLLICULAR CELL-DERIVED LESIONS IN ECTOPIC LOCATIONS (STRUMA OVARII)

- Presence of thick septations
- Locally thickened wall with marked enhancement (corresponding microscopically to thyroid tissue)

MACROSCOPIC FEATURES

General Features

- **Struma ovarii**
  - Often resembles nodular goiter appearing as multiple glistening brown nodules

MICROSCOPIC PATHOLOGY

Histologic Features

- **Struma ovarii**
  - Normal-appearing thyroid follicular tissue (most common finding)
  - Multinodular goiter with colloid-filled, variably sized follicles lined by flattened follicular epithelial cells
  - Secondary degenerative changes (e.g., fibrosis, cyst formation, hemorrhage) may be present
  - Changes of lymphocytic thyroiditis may be present
  - Other less common findings
    - Papillary hyperplasia of follicular epithelium, clear cells, signet ring cells
  - **Proliferative struma ovarii**
    - Refers to discrete mass composed of densely cellular thyroid follicles (without evidence of malignancy)
- Rarely, thyroid neoplasms arise in setting of struma ovarii
  - Thyroid papillary carcinoma (conventional or follicular variant) most common
    - Diagnosis based on cytomorphologic (i.e., nuclear) features
    - Invasive growth (vascular or stromal) not required for diagnosis of papillary carcinoma
  - Follicular carcinoma
    - Diagnosis based on presence of capsular or vascular invasion
- **Strumal carcinoid**
  - Characterized by presence of normal thyroid tissue admixed with carcinoid tumor
  - Diagnosis made as long as both components are present, not on whether one or other predominates
  - Carcinoid component shows
    - Trabecular, organoid, solid growth
    - Cells with small round to oval nuclei, dispersed ("salt and pepper") nuclear chromatin
    - Rarely, stromal amyloid deposition present
    - Rarely, carcinoid component may be mucinous type (mucus-secreting cells)
    - Birefringent calcium oxalate monohydrate crystals may be identified in colloid material

ANCILLARY TESTS

Immunohistochemistry

- **Struma ovarii**
  - Thyroglobulin reactivity positive
  - Thyroid transcription factor 1 (TTF-1)
    - Expressed in follicular epithelial cells, as well as in respiratory epithelium
  - Calcitonin, chromogranin, synaptophysin, CD56 negative
- **Strumal carcinoid**
  - Chromogranin, synaptophysin, CD56, NSE, serotonin positive
  - Calcitonin only rarely found
  - Thyroglobulin, TTF-1 negative in carcinoid component
    - Reactive in noncarcinoid component
  - Neurohormonal peptides can be present
    - Pancreatic polypeptide, vasoactive intestinal polypeptide, insulin, glucagon, substance-P, somatostatin

Molecular Genetics

- *BRAF* mutation positive (K601E)
  - Present in papillary carcinoma arising in struma ovarii

DIFFERENTIAL DIAGNOSIS

Metastatic Thyroid Carcinoma to Ovary

- Extraordinarily rare occurrence
- In presence of malignant thyroid neoplasms in struma ovarii
  - Detailed evaluation of thyroid gland proper indicated

Metastatic Carcinoid to Ovary

- Common feature from gastrointestinal carcinoids (appendix, small intestine)
- Clues in support of metastasis to ovary include bilaterality, multinodularity, presence of peritoneal metastases

SELECTED REFERENCES

1. Jiang W et al: Struma ovarii associated with pseudo-Meigs' syndrome and elevated serum CA 125: a case report and review of the literature. J Ovarian Res. 3:18, 2010
2. Shaco-Levy R et al: Natural history of biologically malignant struma ovarii: analysis of 27 cases with extraovarian spread. Int J Gynecol Pathol. 29(3):212-27, 2010
3. Wolff EF et al: Expression of benign and malignant thyroid tissue in ovarian teratomas and the importance of multimodal management as illustrated by a BRAF-positive follicular variant of papillary thyroid cancer. Thyroid. 20(9):981-7, 2010
4. Robboy SJ et al: Malignant struma ovarii: an analysis of 88 cases, including 27 with extraovarian spread. Int J Gynecol Pathol. 28(5):405-22, 2009
5. Yoo SC et al: Clinical characteristics of struma ovarii. J Gynecol Oncol. 19(2):135-8, 2008
6. Hamazaki S et al: Expression of thyroid transcription factor-1 in strumal carcinoid and struma ovarii: an immunohistochemical study. Pathol Int. 52(7):458-62, 2002

Microscopic Features and Ancillary Techniques

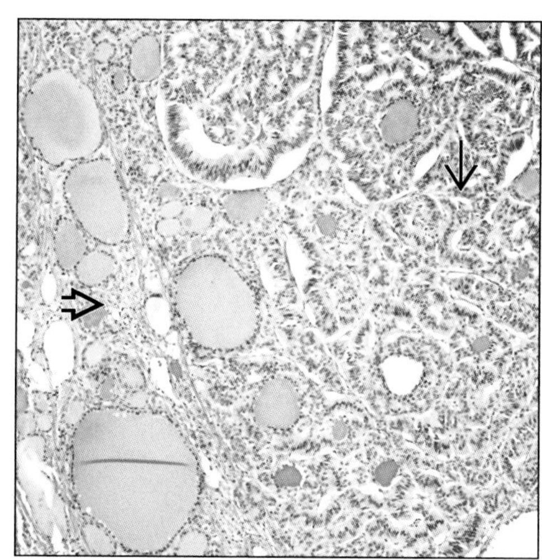

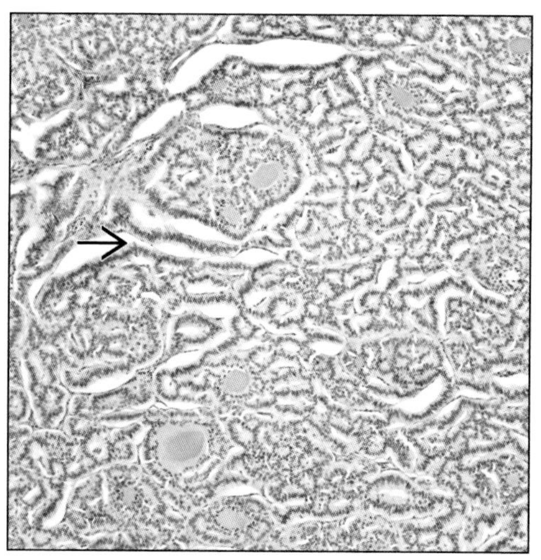

(Left) *Strumal carcinoid shows an admixture of normal thyroid tissue ⇨ and carcinoid →, the latter characterized by trabecular and organoid growth.* ***(Right)*** *Strumal carcinoid shows a portion of lesion that is entirely comprised of carcinoid tumor characterized by a cellular proliferation with complex growth, including trabecular pattern →. The diagnosis is based on finding both components, irrespective of the amount of each component in any given neoplasm.*

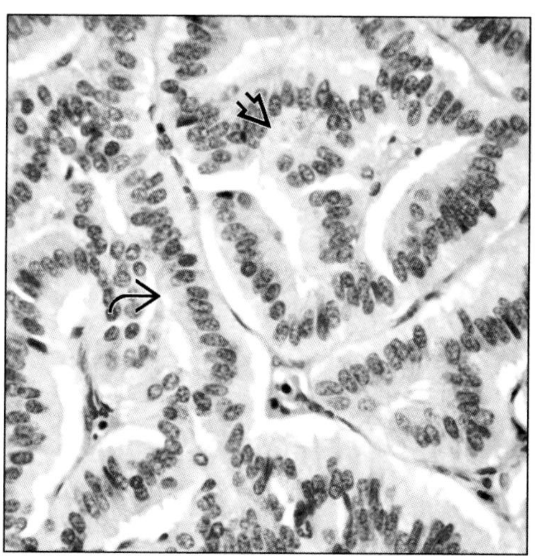

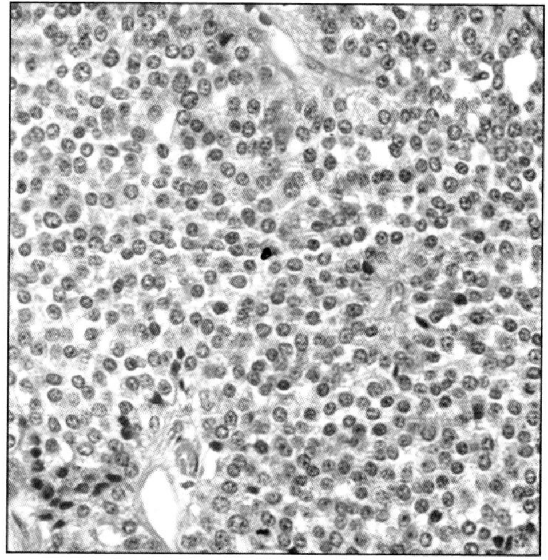

(Left) *Carcinoid shows trabecular ↗ and organoid ⇨ growth with nests separated by fibrovascular cores composed of relatively uniform-appearing cells with dispersed ("salt and pepper") nuclear chromatin characteristic of neuroendocrine lesions.* ***(Right)*** *Carcinoid shows solid growth comprised of uniform cells with dispersed ("salt and pepper") nuclear chromatin. Immunohistochemical staining to confirm the neuroendocrine differentiation is needed.*

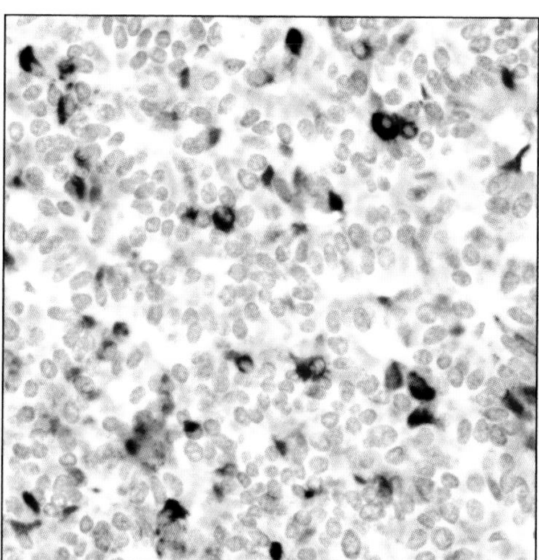

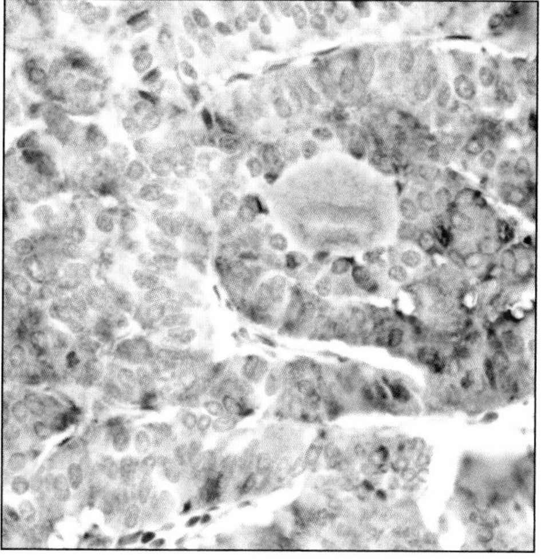

(Left) *Strumal carcinoid shows chromogranin immunoreactivity.* ***(Right)*** *Synaptophysin immunoreactivity is present. CD56 and calcitonin may be positive (not shown), but typically there is an absence of immunostaining for thyroglobulin and thyroid transcription factor 1 (TTF-1). In contrast, the thyroid tissue in strumal carcinoid will be immunoreactive for thyroglobulin and TTF-1 but negative for neuroendocrine markers.*

PAPILLARY CARCINOMA

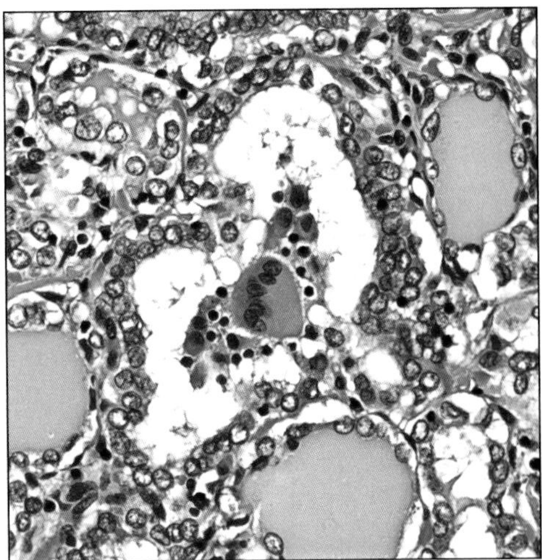

Classic cytomorphonuclear features are seen: Enlarged cells, high N:C ratio, irregular placement around follicles, nuclear grooves, nuclear contour irregularities, optical clearing, giant cells within colloid.

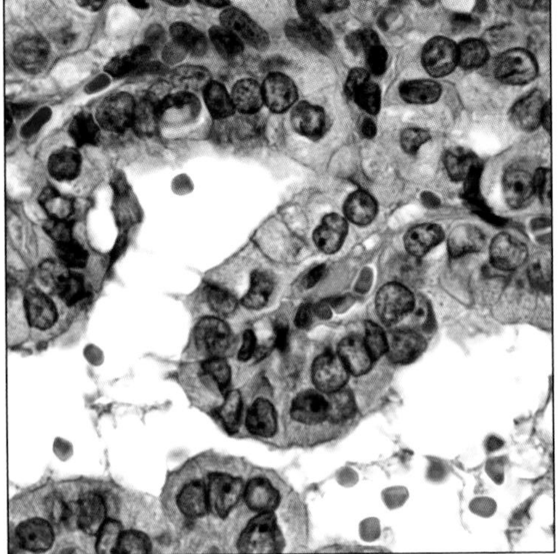

This papillary structure is lined by irregular cells, showing demilune nuclei, nuclear grooves, and delicate, even nuclear chromatin distribution. Nucleoli are noted. There is irregular placement of the nuclei.

TERMINOLOGY

Abbreviations

- Thyroid papillary carcinoma (TPC)
- Papillary thyroid carcinoma (PTC)
- Follicular variant, thyroid papillary carcinoma (FV-TPC)

Definitions

- Malignant epithelial tumor showing evidence of follicular cell differentiation and characterized by distinctive nuclear features

ETIOLOGY/PATHOGENESIS

Environmental Exposure

- Ionizing radiation exposure
  - Especially well-established relationship if exposure is in childhood
  - Especially in "solid" variant of TPC
- Iodine-rich diet
  - Higher incidence of tumor in regions with high dietary iodine intake (Iceland, Japan)

Preexisting Benign Thyroid Disease

- Nodules associated with 6x increased risk
- Solitary nodule associated with 28x increased risk

Hereditary

- 5-10x increased risk in 1st-degree relatives of patients with papillary carcinoma
- Approximately 5% of papillary carcinomas are familial
  - Familial adenomatous polyposis (FAP): *APC* gene germline mutations
  - Carney complex

Pathogenesis

- Monoclonal origin, with multifocal disease frequent

CLINICAL ISSUES

Epidemiology

- Incidence
  - Accounts for vast majority (85%) of all malignant thyroid neoplasms
  - 7.9/100,000 population
- Age
  - Usually young to middle-aged adults
    - 20-40 years for women
    - 40-60 years for men
  - Most common pediatric thyroid malignancy, although still uncommon
- Gender
  - Female > > Male (4:1)
- Ethnicity
  - Whites > blacks

Presentation

- Solitary, painless thyroid mass
- Cervical lymphadenopathy (metastatic disease) may be present (about 30%)
- Dysphagia, stridor, cough: More often in patients with large tumors (compression symptoms)
- "Incidental" tumors found during work-up for unrelated issues

Laboratory Tests

- Usually euthyroid
- Rare cases of hyper- or hypofunctional status
- Serum thyroglobulin can be used to monitor disease status (if elevated)

Natural History

- 20% prevalence of TPC at autopsy suggests indolent, nonaggressive tumors

Treatment

- Options, risks, complications

PAPILLARY CARCINOMA

Key Facts

Clinical Issues

- Accounts for vast majority (85%) of all malignant thyroid neoplasms
- Female > > Male (4:1)
- Surgery is treatment of choice
- > 98% 20-year survival
- Age (< 45 years), size, and gender (female) are most important prognostic factors

Macroscopic Features

- Discrete, ill-defined mass with irregular or infiltrative border
- Gritty, dystrophic calcification is common

Microscopic Pathology

- Multiple different patterns in same tumor
  - Papillary, solid, trabecular, micro- or macrofollicular
- Complex, arborizing, delicate, narrow papillae
- Intratumor, sclerotic eosinophilic fibrosis
- Psammoma bodies
- Nuclear enlargement, overlapping and crowding with high nuclear to cytoplasmic ratio
- Nuclear chromatin clearing, contour irregularities, nuclear grooves, intranuclear cytoplasmic inclusions
- Important variants: Follicular, macrofollicular, oncocytic, and microscopic

Ancillary Tests

- Panel: HBME-1, galectin-3, CITED-1 is more sensitive and specific for TPC
- *BRAF* gene mutations are the most common genetic alterations in TPC

  - Recurrent laryngeal nerve damage and hypoparathyroidism are known complications
- Surgical approaches
  - Surgery is treatment of choice, although extent of surgery (lobectomy, subtotal or total thyroidectomy) remains controversial
  - Lymph node sampling generally only advocated if clinical or radiographic enlargement
- Radiation
  - Radioablative iodine therapy is incorporated after total thyroidectomy
    - Tumor needs to show uptake of radiolabel to be therapeutically sensitive

Prognosis

- Excellent long-term clinical outcome
  - > 98% 20-year survival
  - < 0.2% mortality
- Spreads preferentially by lymphatic channels
  - Intraglandular spread or metastases to regional lymph nodes
- Age (< 45 years), size, and gender (female) are most important prognostic factors
  - Extrathyroidal extension and metastasis are significant for patients > 45 years
- *RET/PTC3*-positive papillary carcinomas (typically solid variant) tend to have slightly worse prognosis

IMAGE FINDINGS

Radiographic Findings

- MR scans are valuable in highlighting enlarged, cystic lymph nodes, help in identifying substernal lesions, and may define extrathyroidal extension
- MR scan shows increased signal intensity on T1-weighted images and may reveal punctate calcifications
- Radioisotope scans typically reveal "cold" nodule but are no longer used

Ultrasonographic Findings

- Valuable guide for fine needle aspiration (FNA)
- Defines size and shows if lesion is solid or cystic
- Hypoechoic or isoechoic solid nodule with ill-defined margins
- Cystic change can be seen
- Punctate microcalcifications (psammoma bodies) are frequent in papillary carcinoma
- High central blood flow within a nodule on color Doppler is common in papillary carcinoma

MACROSCOPIC FEATURES

General Features

- Discrete, ill-defined but circumscribed mass with irregular or infiltrative border
- Gritty, dystrophic calcification is common
- Extension beyond thyroid gland capsule or into adjacent thyroid parenchyma can be seen
- Cystic change is common
- Multifocality can be identified
- Cut surface is tan-brown, gray-white
- Papillary structures give a shaggy texture
- Irregular areas of fibrosis are seen and must be sampled
- Lymph nodes may contain cysts filled with hemorrhagic, brownish fluid

Sections to Be Submitted

- Must be from "tumor-to-capsule-to-parenchyma" interface
- Generally, 1 section per cm of tumor size
  - However, center of tumor is not as important as periphery

Size

- Wide range, from microscopic to 20 cm
- Mean: 1-3 cm

PAPILLARY CARCINOMA

MICROSCOPIC PATHOLOGY

Histologic Features

- Diagnostic features include growth pattern, nuclear features, psammoma bodies, and tumor fibrosis, **but** only nuclear features required for diagnosis!
  - No single feature is diagnostic
- Typically shows infiltrative growth with irregular, invasive border
- Multinodular and multifocal tumors are common
- Architectural features
  - Multiple different patterns in same tumor
  - Variable growth patterns: Papillary, solid, trabecular, micro- or macrofollicular, cystic
  - Elongated &/or twisted follicles
  - Complex, arborizing, ramifying, branching, delicate, narrow papillae
    - Finger-like projections composed of delicate fibrovascular cores covered by epithelial cells
    - Single layer of epithelial cells with nonpolar, haphazard (up and down) position of nucleus within cell
    - May have loose myxoid, edematous or hyalinized stroma
    - Lymphoid cells can be seen within papillae
- Intratumor, acellular, sclerotic, dense eosinophilic fibrosis
  - Generally found in 50-90% of all cases
  - Sometimes associated with irregular stellate fibrosis extending beyond tumor
  - Helpful at time of gross examination to determine areas to sample
  - Fibrosis is present in FV-PTC
- Mummification (peripheral cell death) very characteristic but infrequently seen
- "Bright," hypereosinophilic, intense colloid (distinct from surrounding thyroid parenchyma)
- Psammoma bodies
  - Present in up to 50% of cases
  - Generally round/spherical shape
  - Represent apoptotic cells that form nidus for concentric lamellation/layers of calcium
    - "Tombstone" of previously viable tumor cell
  - Located in association with tumor cells, in tumor stroma, or in lymphatic channel
  - Often identified within lymph-vascular channels, diagnostic of intraglandular spread
  - Inspissated and calcified colloid in lumen is different
- Crystals can be seen in colloid
- Squamous metaplasia (about 20% of cases), cyst formation, and degeneration are present, along with infarction
- Giant cells in colloid
- Chronic lymphocytic thyroiditis can be seen

Cytologic Features

- Large tumor cell size in comparison to surrounding tissue with high nuclear to cytoplasmic ratio
- Nuclear enlargement: 2-3x larger than nonneoplastic epithelium
- Nuclear overlapping and crowding: Haphazard arrangement, nuclei lack polarity, crowd out each another to give "herd," "lake," or "egg-basket" appearance
  - Cellular overlapping and multilayering is not a fixation or section thickness issue
- Chromatin clearing: Cleared chromatin with aggregation along nuclear membrane yielding accentuated nuclear membranes
  - Empty, pale, clear, ground-glass, or "Orphan Annie eye" nuclei
  - Tissue fixation is required, since clearing is not seen in frozen sections or FNA smears
    - Formalin fixation gives this clearing, but alcohol fixatives (SafeFix, HistoChoice) do not
    - May be related to heat: Sections placed on heating block before staining show this change to greater degree
- Irregularity of nuclear contours: Oval, elongated nucleus with asymmetric, angulated, crescent-moon, convoluted, and triangular shapes, and highly irregular, jagged, "rat-bites" into nuclear membrane
  - Do not assess in tissue previously frozen
- Nuclear grooves: Discrete, longitudinal folds through long axis of nucleus
  - Linear and regular ("coffee bean")
  - Curved and irregular ("popcorn")
- Nuclear pseudoinclusion: Invaginations of nuclear membrane pulling cytoplasm into nucleus
  - Rounded area within nucleus containing cytoplasmic material, sharply demarcated by thick nuclear membrane
  - Least frequently seen of nuclear features, but fixation artifacts may give this appearance in "all" cells, which should be discounted
  - Fixation "vacuoles" have empty, structureless appearance without rim of nuclear membrane
  - Nucleolus within "vacuole" shows it is not true pseudoinclusion
- High nuclear to cytoplasmic ratio
- Nucleoli: If present, seem to touch nuclear membrane rather than being centrally located
- Cytoplasmic appearance is not helpful, except for "oncocytic" and "clear" variants

Lymphatic/Vascular Invasion

- Present in many cases, lymphatics preferentially

Margins

- Must assess to exclude "extrathyroidal" extension

Lymph Nodes

- Frequently show metastatic disease
- Psammoma bodies represent metastasis
- "Benign inclusions" do not exist and should be considered metastatic carcinoma (lateral to sternocleidomastoid muscle)

Variants

- **Size variant (microscopic)**
  - a.k.a. microscopic, incidental, occult, or microcarcinoma

- By definition, any TPC or variant can be ≤ 1 cm in size
- Proclivity for subcapsular region
- Frequently sclerotic with radiating "scar-like" infiltrating edge
- Must be separated from intraglandular spread (intravascular; lacks capsule; has stellate, infiltrative growth)
- No additional therapy is necessary for tumors of this size (significant controversy exists)

- **Follicular variant**
  - Usually encapsulated
  - Exclusively composed of small, tight follicles
  - Scant, hypereosinophilic colloid
  - Papillae are absent or vanishingly rare
  - Nuclei are large with pale to powdery to cleared nuclear chromatin, nuclear grooves, and inclusions
  - Internal tumor sclerosis or fibrosis is very helpful
- **Macrofollicular variant**
  - Most difficult to recognize
  - Architectural resemblance to adenomatoid or hyperplastic nodules
  - Predominantly large/macrofollicles with subtle increased cellularity, often accentuated at periphery
  - Colloid is often scalloped or vacuolated (like Graves)
  - Nuclei are flattened and hyperchromatic with isolated classic nuclei
  - Abortive, "rigid" or straight papillary structures extend into center of colloid-filled follicle
- **Oncocytic variant**
  - Macroscopically deep "mahogany" brown, frequently cystic
  - > 70% of tumor should have complex, arborizing papillary structures
  - Enlarged cells with abundant oncocytic (oxyphilic, Askanazy, Hürthle) cytoplasm
    - Cytoplasm is compact and "glassy" (increased mitochondria)
  - Enlarged nuclei tend to be apically oriented
  - Nuclei are slightly more hyperchromatic
  - Numerous intranuclear cytoplasmic inclusions
  - Positive with CK19
  - Oncocytic cells can be seen in tall cell variant
- **Clear cell variant**
  - Very uncommon variant
  - Cells with clear cytoplasm
  - Mixture of oncocytic and clear cells may be seen
  - Must be distinguished from metastatic renal cell carcinoma or medullary carcinoma
- **Diffuse sclerosing variant** (DSV)
  - Young patients (mean: 18 years)
  - Diffuse involvement of one or both lobes with nearly 100% of patients demonstrating cervical lymph node metastasis at time of presentation
  - Firm gland with white streaks and gritty cut consistency
  - Exaggerated papillary carcinoma
    - Extensive fibrosis, innumerable psammoma bodies, extensive intravascular and extrathyroidal extension, florid squamous metaplasia, dense lymphocytic thyroiditis
  - Total thyroidectomy, lymph node dissection, and radioablative therapy gives excellent long-term prognosis
- **Columnar variant**
  - Prominent papillary growth with markedly elongated, parallel follicles ("railroad tracks")
  - Scant colloid
  - Tall cells with syncytial arrangement
  - Prominent nuclear stratification of elongated nuclei with coarse and heavy chromatin deposition (distinctive)
  - Subnuclear or supranuclear vacuolization of cytoplasm
  - Squamous metaplasia in form of "morules" is common ("endometrioid pattern")
  - Mitotic figures may be present, along with necrosis
- **Tall cell variant**
  - Tend to be older patients, more men, larger tumors (> 5 cm), with extrathyroidal extension and increased incidence of metastases
  - > 70% of tumor area must be tall cell
    - Tall cell: At least 3x as high as it is wide (plane of section must be taken into consideration)
  - Papillary structures and elongated parallel follicles with scant/absent colloid
  - Many intranuclear cytoplasmic inclusions and nuclear grooves
  - Intercellular borders are sharply demarcated
  - Nuclei are centrally located
- **Insular-solid variant**
  - Solid or insular pattern
    - Oval nests or islands with scant colloid
  - Cells with high nuclear to cytoplasmic ratio
  - Nuclear features of papillary carcinoma
- **Cribriform-morula variant**
  - Seen in patients with familial adenomatous polyposis (FAP)
    - Diagnosis should prompt colonic exam and possibly genetic testing for germline *APC* mutation
  - Multiple well-demarcated or encapsulated tumor nodules
  - Mixed patterns of growth: Cribriform, trabecular, solid, papillary, and follicular
  - Whorls or morules composed of spindle cells without keratinization
  - Classic nuclear features of TPC are rare
- **Warthin-like variant**
  - Papillary carcinoma with lymphoid stroma

ANCILLARY TESTS

Cytology

- Fine needle aspiration (FNA) is initial test of choice for thyroid nodule, with excellent sensitivity, specificity, and positive predictive value
- 25-gauge needle without suction yields excellent material uncontaminated by blood
- Adequacy: At least 6 groups of follicular cells with > 10 follicular cells per group
- Benign, indeterminate/suspicious, or malignant categories

PAPILLARY CARCINOMA

- Cellular smears with monolayered sheets (syncytium)
- 3-dimensional clusters of enlarged cells
- Nuclei are enlarged, overlap, and have irregular borders
- Powdery/dusty, delicate nuclear chromatin on alcohol-fixed preparations
- Nuclear folds or grooves and intranuclear cytoplasmic inclusions are also common
- Colloid is thickened ("chewing gum" or ropey)
- Rarely psammoma bodies will be seen

Frozen Sections

- With preoperative FNA results, use of frozen section has decreased dramatically
- Only perform frozen section if FNA was "suspicious" for papillary carcinoma
- Diagnostic confirmation is possible, but FV-TPC is still difficult

Immunohistochemistry

- Seldom of value
  - May help define thyroid origin
  - May help define malignancy (in a few cases)
- Strongly and diffusely immunoreactive with keratin, CK7, thyroglobulin, TTF-1, CK19, HBME-1, galectin-3, CITED-1
- Panel approach: HBME-1, galectin-3, CITED-1 may be more sensitive and specific for TPC

Cytogenetics

- Most commonly involve loss of chromosome 22 or Y (males) and gain of chromosome 7
- Inversion inv(10)(q11.2;q21), which leads to *RET/PTC1* rearrangement
- Translocations or inversions involving 10q11.2 (*RET* gene region), correspond to less frequent types of *RET/PTC* rearrangements
- Comparative genomic hybridization (CGH) detects losses at 22q and 9q (particularly 9q21.3-32), and gains are at 17q, 1q, and 9q33-qter

Molecular Genetics

- Dependent on technique, immunohistochemistry, in situ hybridization, whether in adults or children, radiation history, and histologic variant
- Mitogen-activated protein kinase (*MAPK*) pathway regulates cell growth, differentiation, and survival
  - Activation of this pathway by either point mutation in *BRAF* and *RAS* genes or chromosomal rearrangement involving the *RET* and *NTRK1* genes
  - Each specific mutation/rearrangement has unique effect due to distinct phenotypical and biological properties
- Mutation/rearrangements of the *BRAF* gene is most common genetic alteration in papillary carcinoma
  - T to A transversion at nucleotide 1799, which results in valine-to-glutamate substitution at residue 600 (V600E)
  - Mutations lead to constitutive activation of *BRAF* kinase, resulting in continuous stimulation of MEK, ERK, and subsequent downstream effectors of MAPK pathway
- *RET/PTC1* or *RET/PTC3* is detected in up to 80% of tumors
- *RAS* mutations are seen in up to 15% of tumors
  - Found almost exclusively in FV-TPC, in tumors that are encapsulated, and tumors with a low rate of lymph node metastases
  - Mutations are located at several specific sites (codons 12, 13, and 61) of *NRAS*, *HRAS*, and *KRAS* genes
  - Mutations stabilize protein in its active, guanosine triphosphate (GTP)-bound conformation
    - Results in chronic stimulation of several signaling pathways, most importantly the *MAPK* and *PI3K/AKT* pathways

Electron Microscopy

- Epithelial cuboidal, columnar, or polygonal cells with desmosomes and tight junctions
- Numerous microvilli and single cilia at apical pole
- Nuclear membrane showing numerous folds and indentations resulting in nuclear lobes connected by only thin channels of nuclear substance

DIFFERENTIAL DIAGNOSIS

Adenomatoid Nodules

- Multiple nodules in general, lacking a capsule
- Papillae are short, simple, nonbranching, and often "thick"
- Nuclei are round, regular, basally located, and hyperchromatic
- Intracytoplasmic hemosiderin pigment is lacking in papillary carcinoma
- Qualitative and quantitative lack of nuclear features of papillary carcinoma
- Alcohol fixatives will often cause nuclear enlargement and "optical clearing"

Diffuse Hyperplasia

- Whole gland affected (even if unevenly)
- Papillary structures are short, simple, nonbranching, and lined by single, polarized cell layer
- No nuclear features of papillary carcinoma (basal, round, hyperchromatic nuclei)

Follicular Carcinoma

- Oncocytic cytoplasm may induce nuclear enlargement
- Follicular architecture should predominate (i.e., no papillary structures)
- No nuclear features of papillary carcinoma

Medullary Carcinoma

- Follicular pattern, invasive growth, and lack of colloid
- Intranuclear cytoplasmic inclusions can be seen
- Calcitonin, chromogranin, and CEA should help

DIAGNOSTIC CHECKLIST

Pathologic Interpretation Pearls

- Papillary carcinoma is almost always there; keep looking

PAPILLARY CARCINOMA

Immunohistochemistry

Antibody	Reactivity	Staining Pattern	Comment
Galectin-3	Positive	Nuclear & cytoplasmic	Nearly all classic papillary carcinomas; important to have nuclear and cytoplasmic reactivity; not unique to TPC
HBME-1	Positive	Cell membrane & cytoplasm	Accentuated on apical surface; also stains colloid; more specific than galectin-3
MSG1	Positive	Nuclear & cytoplasmic	Equivalent to CITED-1; should be used as part of a panel: Galectin-3, HBME-1 & CITED-1
TTF-1	Positive	Nuclear	All nuclei usually strong and diffusely positive
Thyroglobulin	Positive	Cytoplasmic	Accentuated at luminal surface and also in colloid; diffusion artifact a problem
CK19	Positive	Cell membrane & cytoplasm	Low specificity for TPC
pax-8	Positive	Nuclear	While strong reaction, background follicular cells are also positive
CK7	Positive	Cytoplasmic	Nearly all cells
CK8/18/CAM5.2	Positive	Cytoplasmic	Nearly all cells
CK-PAN	Positive	Cytoplasmic	Nearly all cells
ret	Positive		Very poor correlation with *RET/PTC* rearrangements
S100-A4	Positive	Cytoplasmic	Very limited utility
Calcitonin	Negative		
CK20	Negative		

- Default diagnosis is papillary carcinoma; prove it is not

STAGING

AJCC

- T1: ≤ 2 cm, confined to thyroid
- T2: > 2 cm but ≤ 4 cm, confined to thyroid
- T3: > 4 cm, limited to thyroid or tumor showing limited extrathyroidal extension
- T4: Extending beyond thyroid gland into adjacent subcutaneous soft tissues, larynx, trachea, esophagus, recurrent laryngeal nerve, prevertebral fascia, encases carotid artery or mediastinal vessels
  - All anaplastics are by definition T4 tumors
- N1: Regional lymph nodes
- < 45 years
  - Stage I: Any T, any N, M0
  - Stage II: Any T, any N, M1
- ≥ 45 years
  - Stage I: T1, N0, M0
  - Stage II: T2, N0, M0
  - Stage III: T1-T3, N0-N1a, M0
  - Stage IV: Divided into A, B, and C, with metastases to distant sites staged as IVC

SELECTED REFERENCES

1. Chisholm EJ et al: Systematic review and meta-analysis of the adverse effects of thyroidectomy combined with central neck dissection as compared with thyroidectomy alone. Laryngoscope. 119(6):1135-9, 2009
2. Donnellan KA et al: Papillary thyroid carcinoma and familial adenomatous polyposis of the colon. Am J Otolaryngol. 30(1):58-60, 2009
3. Grodski S et al: An update on papillary microcarcinoma. Curr Opin Oncol. 21(1):1-4, 2009
4. Rosenbaum MA et al: Contemporary management of papillary carcinoma of the thyroid gland. Expert Rev Anticancer Ther. 9(3):317-29, 2009
5. Taccaliti A et al: Genetic mutations in thyroid carcinoma. Minerva Endocrinol. 34(1):11-28, 2009
6. Baloch ZW et al: Fine-needle aspiration of the thyroid: today and tomorrow. Best Pract Res Clin Endocrinol Metab. 22(6):929-39, 2008
7. Francis Z et al: Serum thyroglobulin determination in thyroid cancer patients. Best Pract Res Clin Endocrinol Metab. 22(6):1039-46, 2008
8. Nikiforova MN et al: Molecular genetics of thyroid cancer: implications for diagnosis, treatment and prognosis. Expert Rev Mol Diagn. 8(1):83-95, 2008
9. Osamura RY et al: Current practices in performing frozen sections for thyroid and parathyroid pathology. Virchows Arch. 453(5):433-40, 2008
10. Lang BH et al: Staging systems for papillary thyroid carcinoma: a review and comparison. Ann Surg. 245(3):366-78, 2007
11. Lee JH et al: Clinicopathologic significance of BRAF V600E mutation in papillary carcinomas of the thyroid: a meta-analysis. Cancer. 110(1):38-46, 2007
12. Al-Brahim N et al: Papillary thyroid carcinoma: an overview. Arch Pathol Lab Med. 130(7):1057-62, 2006
13. Albores-Saavedra J et al: The many faces and mimics of papillary thyroid carcinoma. Endocr Pathol. 17(1):1-18, 2006
14. Baloch ZW et al: Cytologic and architectural mimics of papillary thyroid carcinoma. Diagnostic challenges in fine-needle aspiration and surgical pathology specimens. Am J Clin Pathol. 125 Suppl:S135-44, 2006
15. Baloch ZW et al: Microcarcinoma of the thyroid. Adv Anat Pathol. 13(2):69-75, 2006
16. Baloch ZW et al: Pathologic diagnosis of papillary thyroid carcinoma: today and tomorrow. Expert Rev Mol Diagn. 5(4):573-84, 2005
17. Jun P et al: The sonographic features of papillary thyroid carcinomas: pictorial essay. Ultrasound Q. 21(1):39-45, 2005
18. Rosai J: Immunohistochemical markers of thyroid tumors: significance and diagnostic applications. Tumori. 89(5):517-9, 2003

PAPILLARY CARCINOMA

Imaging and Gross Features

(Left) Radiologic images show both a "cold" ➡ and a "hot" ➡ nodule in the thyroid gland. While this relates to hypo- and hyperfunctional state (respectively), it does not distinguish between benign and malignant lesions. *(Right)* MRI shows a < 0.5 cm hyperintense papillary carcinoma ➡. Much larger and more easily identified are the characteristic hyperintense metastases to the deep cervical lymph nodes ➡. This type of size disparity between the primary and metastases is common.

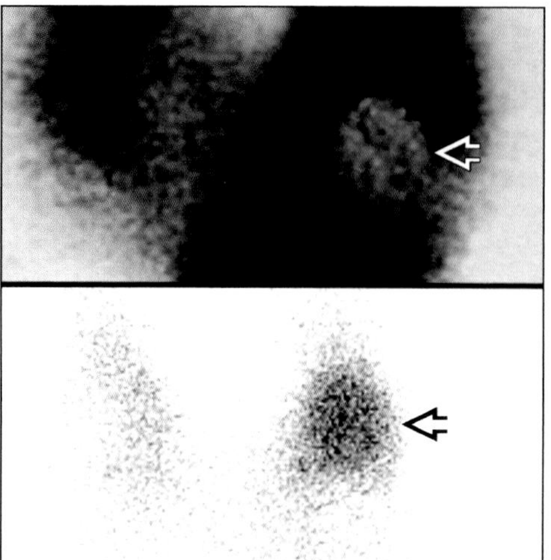

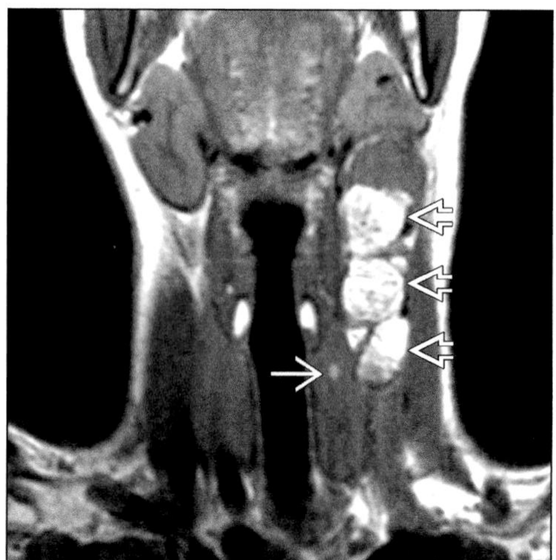

(Left) Transverse grayscale ultrasound shows a partially haloed ➡, solid, hypoechoic thyroid nodule. The halo represents the capsule. There are numerous punctate calcifications ➡, which represent psammoma bodies. The carotid artery ➡ and internal jugular vein ➡ are immediately adjacent. *(Right)* Corresponding power Doppler ultrasound shows profuse, chaotic intratumoral vascularity. This feature is more frequently seen in neoplasms than in adenomatoid nodules.

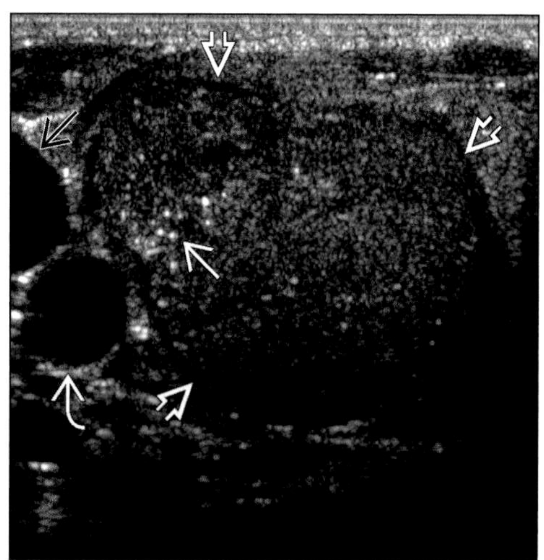

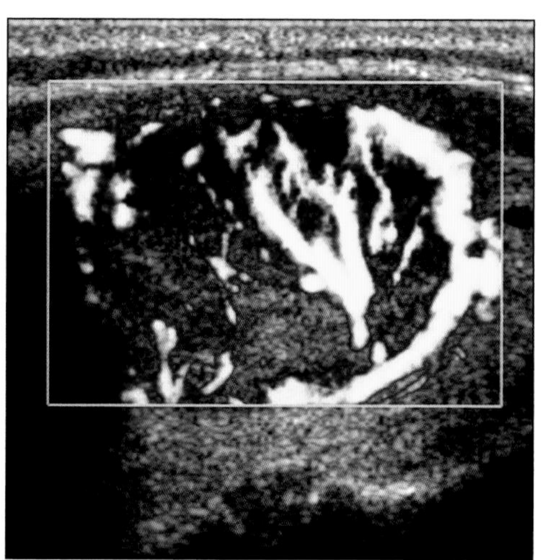

(Left) Fused PET/CT (bottom) show asymmetrical focus of FDG activity within the left lobe of the thyroid ➡ corresponding to a defined thyroid nodule ➡ in the CT (upper). *(Right)* There is a well-formed capsule ➡ surrounding the tumor, lacking areas of infiltration. However, the tumor shows numerous papillary projections, giving a pebbled appearance macroscopically. Papillary structures are frequently identified macroscopically in papillary carcinoma.

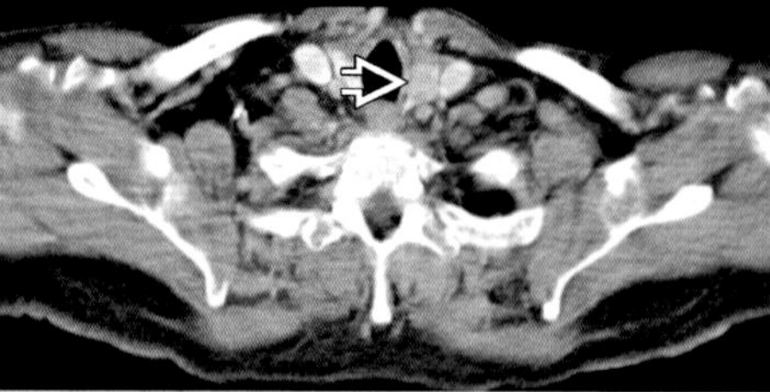

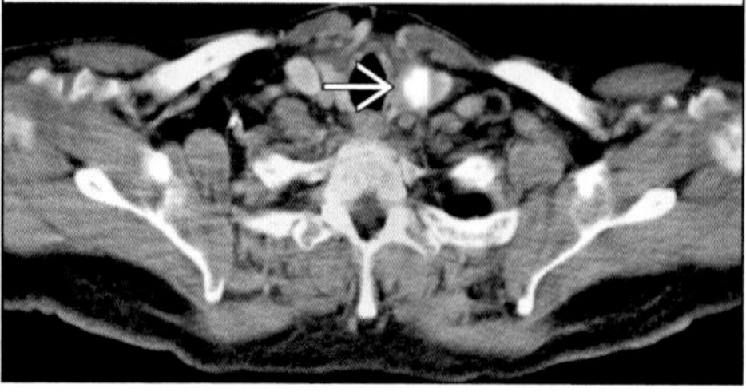

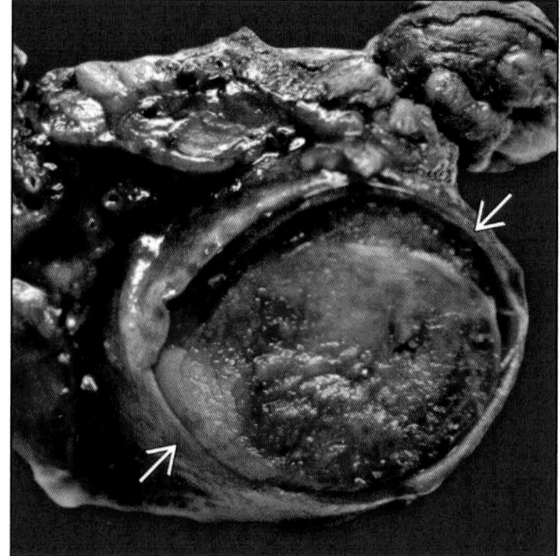

Gross and Characteristic Microscopic Features

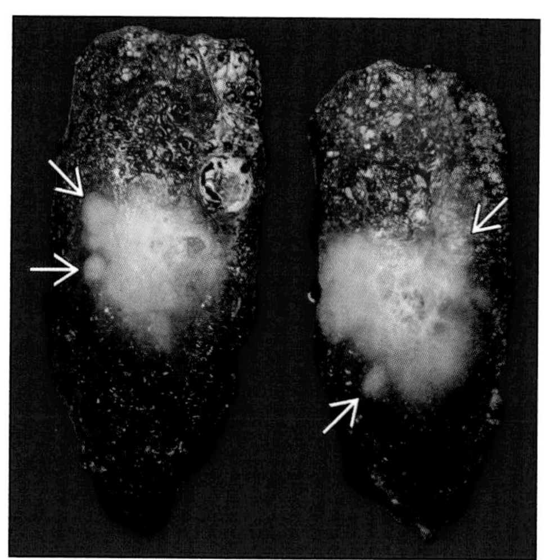

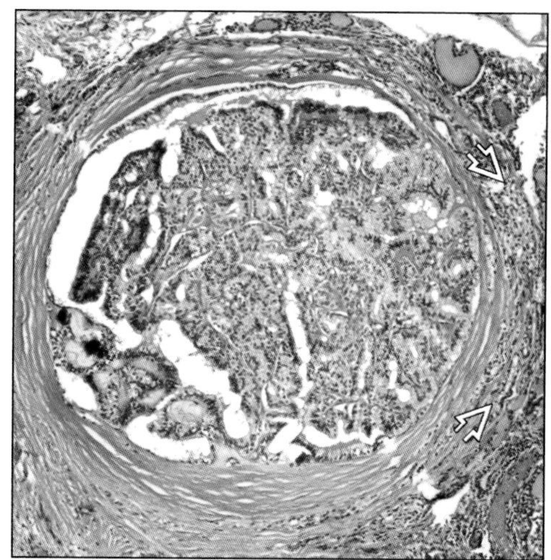

(Left) *Gross photograph shows the characteristic irregular, sclerotic, light tan appearance of a papillary carcinoma. Note small areas of invasion ➡. The thyroid parenchyma is distinctly different from the tumor.* ***(Right)*** *This tumor is surrounded by a well-formed fibrous connective capsule in which there are 2 areas of capsular invasion ➡. Invasion qualifies the tumor as a carcinoma, which can then be further classified into a specific type.*

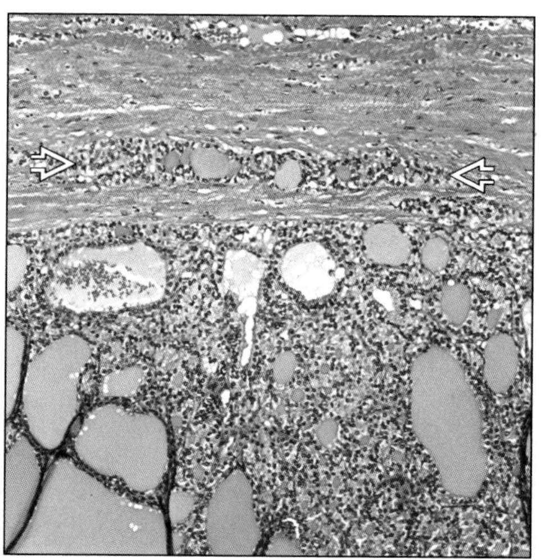

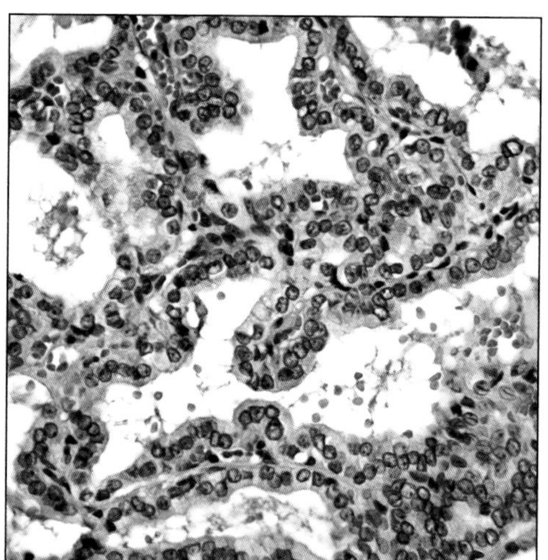

(Left) *An area of vascular invasion ➡ is easily identified within the capsule of this tumor. Capsular and vascular invasion are frequently present, but "encapsulated" tumors may lack these features, while still representing papillary carcinoma.* ***(Right)*** *There is an arborizing pattern of complex, irregular, ramifying, and overlapping papillae. The cells are enlarged and show non-polar, haphazard nuclear position within the cell. Note the lack of colloid.*

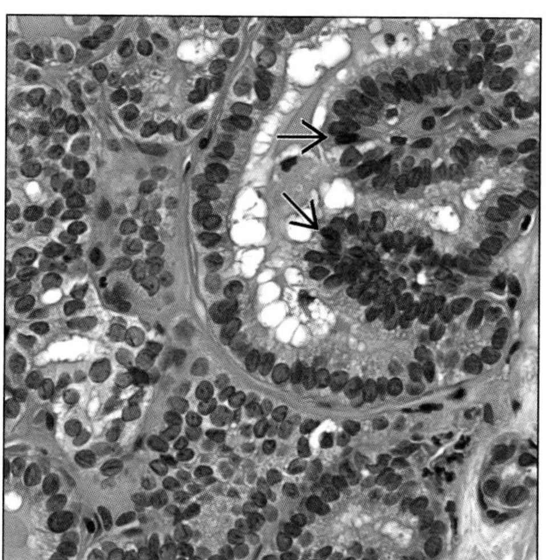

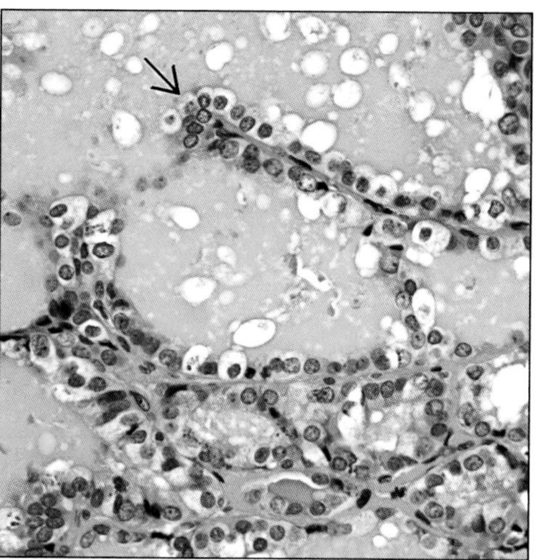

(Left) *The nuclei are frequently overlapped and jumbled or disorganized ➡. This tumor shows areas of overlapping in a lesion that is cut at 4 microns. There is colloid scalloping.* ***(Right)*** *Delicate, elongated papillae are frequently present ➡. These papillae may extend into a colloid-filled space for quite some distance (up to several hundred microns). This type of "rigid" papillary projection is more frequent in papillary carcinoma than in adenomatoid nodule.*

PAPILLARY CARCINOMA

Characteristic Microscopic Features

(Left) Intratumor, acellular, sclerotic, dense eosinophilic fibrosis is quite characteristic of papillary carcinoma, seen in up to 90% of cases. There may be irregular, stellate fibrosis extending beyond the tumor in microscopic foci. Sclerotic areas should be sampled at gross exam. ***(Right)*** *Peripheral mummification of the neoplastic cells ⇒ is a feature found at the tumor to capsule junction. This finding of cell death is not "unique" to TPC, but it is infrequently seen in other lesions.*

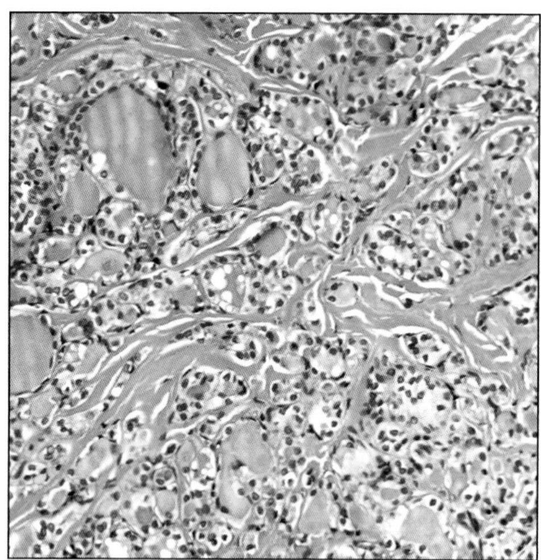

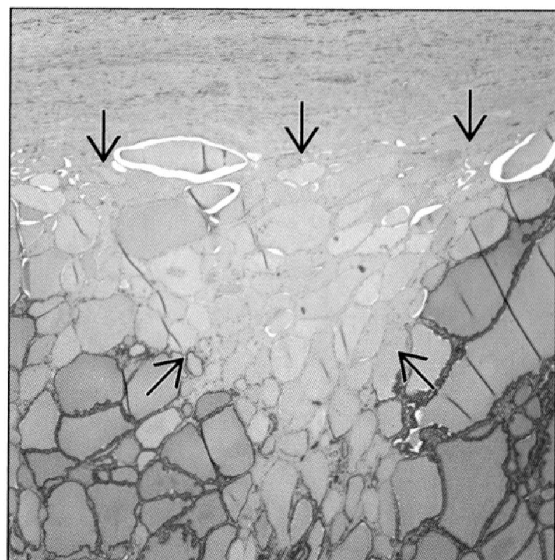

(Left) This papillary carcinoma highlights the "bright," hypereosinophilic, intense colloid within the tumor nests, which is distinct from the adjacent thyroid parenchyma ⇒. This was a focus of invasion, lacking a fibrous capsule. ***(Right)*** *Psammoma bodies can be numerous, identified within the tumor, within lymph-vascular spaces, and in lymph nodes. They are a "tombstone" of previously viable tumor cells. The inset shows a round, concentric lamellation of calcium.*

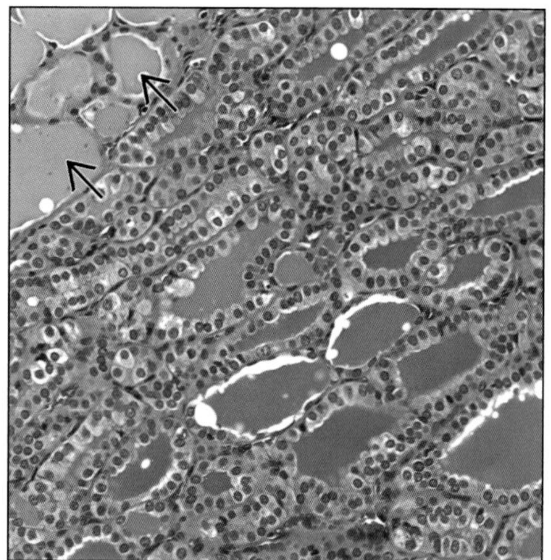

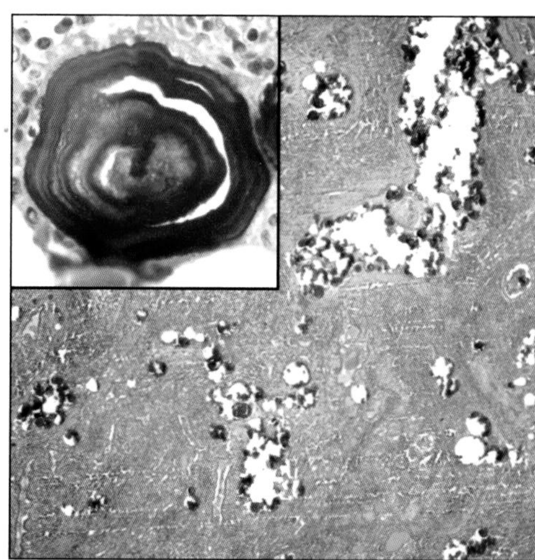

(Left) Squamous metaplasia ⇒ is seen in about 20% of cases. It may line a cystic cavity (as in this case) or be part of the tumor itself. Squamous metaplasia may be seen in adjacent lymphocytic thyroiditis. ***(Right)*** *It is not uncommon to have giant cells ⇒ in the follicle or colloid space. They are histiocytes rather than neoplastic giant cells. Although not specific, they can help in diagnostically challenging cases.*

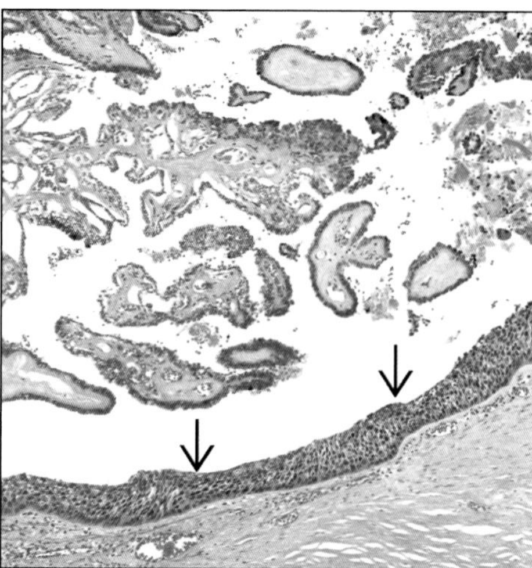

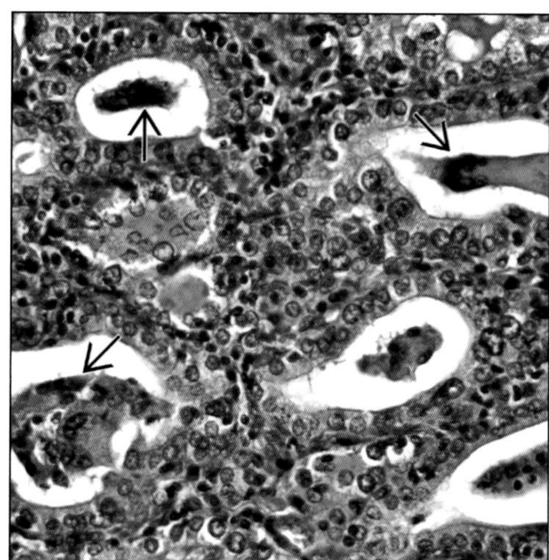

Distinctive Features of Papillary Carcinoma

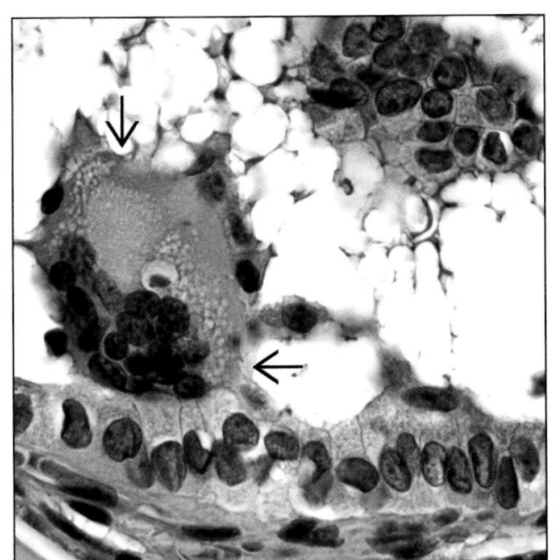

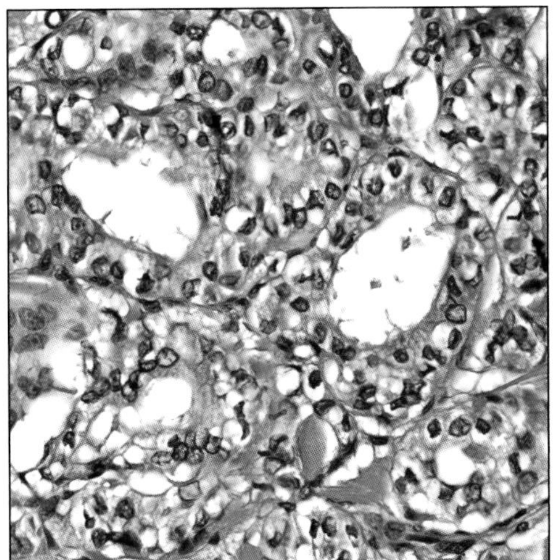

(Left) *The tumor cells are large in comparison to surrounding tissue, with a high nuclear to cytoplasmic ratio. The nuclear enlargement is about 2-3x larger than nonneoplastic epithelium. A giant cell* ⇒ *shows different nuclear features from the tumor nuclei.* ***(Right)*** *There is nuclear overlapping and crowding, with a lack of nuclear polarity. There are many contour irregularities, creating asymmetric, angulated, crescent-moon, convoluted, and triangular shapes.*

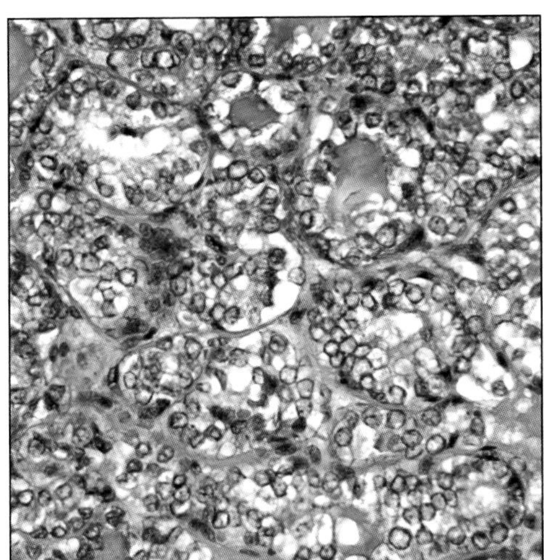

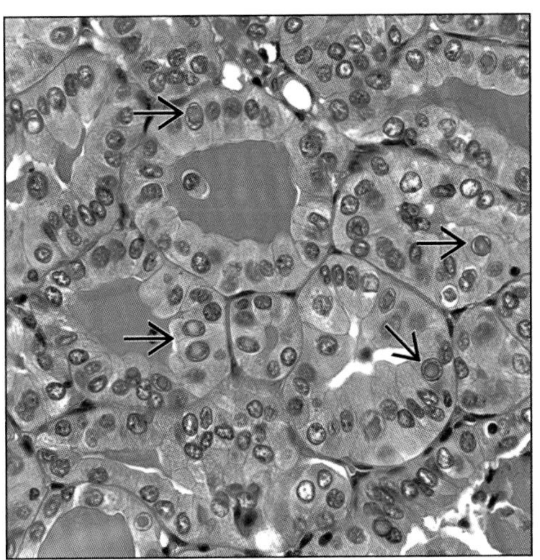

(Left) *Nuclear chromatin clearing with accumulation along the nuclear membrane yields accentuated nuclear membranes. The nuclear chromatin is empty, pale, clear, ground-glass, or "Orphan Annie eye." Note the crowding.* ***(Right)*** *Intranuclear pseudoinclusions are invaginations of the nuclear membrane pulling cytoplasm into the nucleus* ⇒*. They are sharply demarcated with a nuclear membrane, containing material with the same quality as the surrounding cytoplasm.*

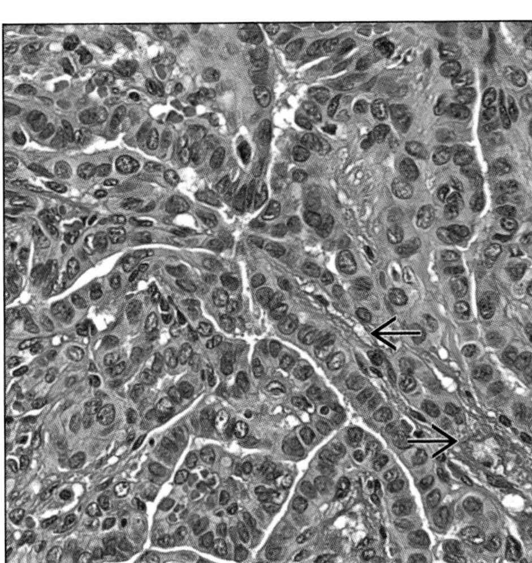

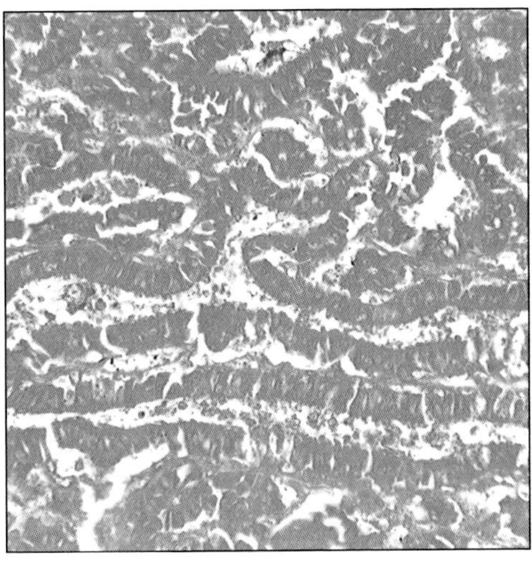

(Left) *The neoplastic cells have a high nuclear to cytoplasmic ratio, showing oval, elongated nuclei with grooves extending along the length of the nucleus. This creates a linear and regular "coffee bean" appearance. Note the loose myxoid stroma* ⇒*.* ***(Right)*** *Infarction results in the ghost outlines of the papillary projections. While this is most characteristic of a thyroid papillary carcinoma, viable tumor cells should be identified somewhere to confirm the diagnosis.*

PAPILLARY CARCINOMA

Papillary Carcinoma Variants

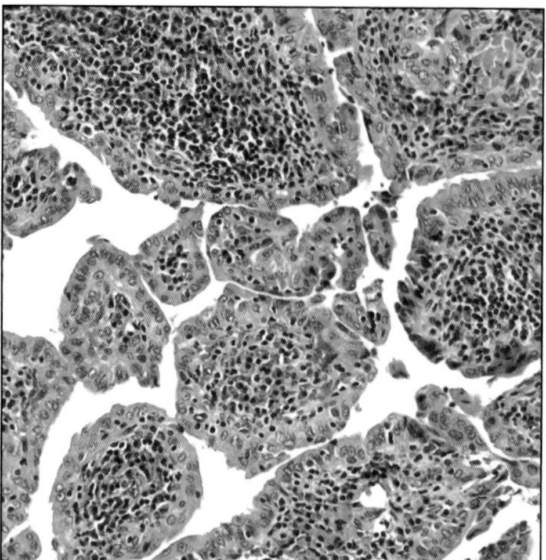

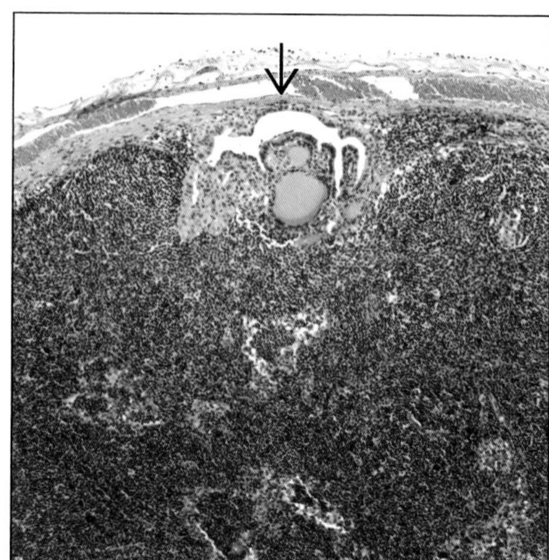

(Left) *Warthin-like variant: The papillae are expanded and filled with numerous lymphocytes and plasma cells. Lymphoid cells can be seen within the papillae of any papillary carcinoma but are accentuated in this variant.* ***(Right)*** *Metastatic disease is frequently identified. There is a collection of follicular cells within a subcapsular space* ⇒*. Psammoma bodies may be the only finding in some cases. "Benign inclusions" do not exist in cervical lymph nodes of level II-IV.*

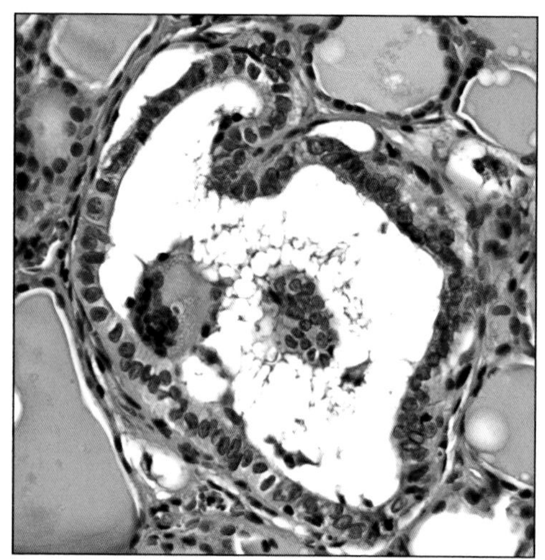

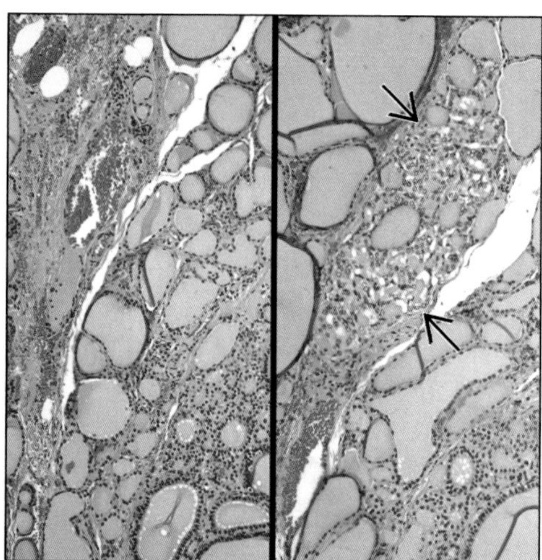

(Left) *Size variant (microscopic) papillary carcinoma range from 1 follicle up to 1 cm. Here is a single follicle papillary carcinoma, showing all of the architectural and cytomorphonuclear features of papillary carcinoma.* ***(Right)*** *This tumor was not identified on the original slide (left), but in a deeper level obtained for a different reason, a single focus of microscopic papillary carcinoma is revealed* ⇒*.*

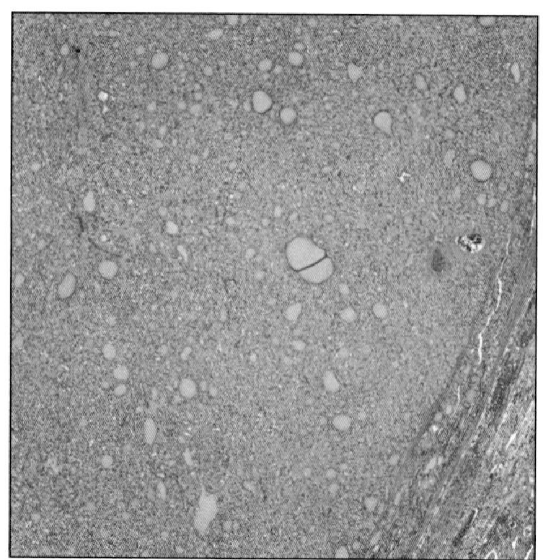

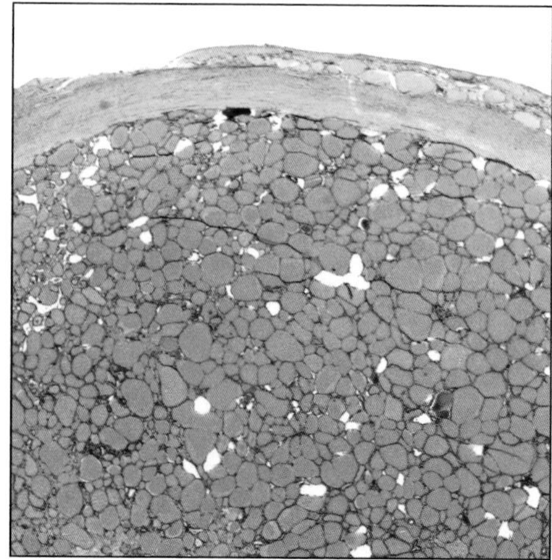

(Left) *Follicular variant: A thin capsule surrounds a tumor composed of fairly uniformly sized follicles without any papillae noted.* ***(Right)*** *Follicular variant: There is a very well-formed capsule. Nearly all of the follicles are identical, showing brightly, hypereosinophilic colloid. Papillae are absent. Internal tumor sclerosis or fibrosis is very helpful in diagnosing this variant.*

Papillary Carcinoma Variants

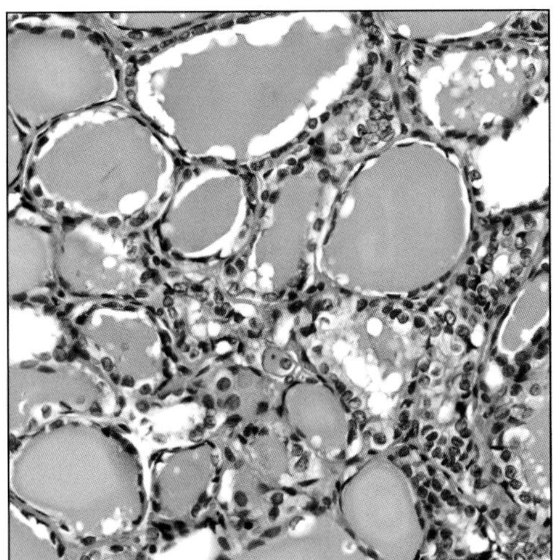

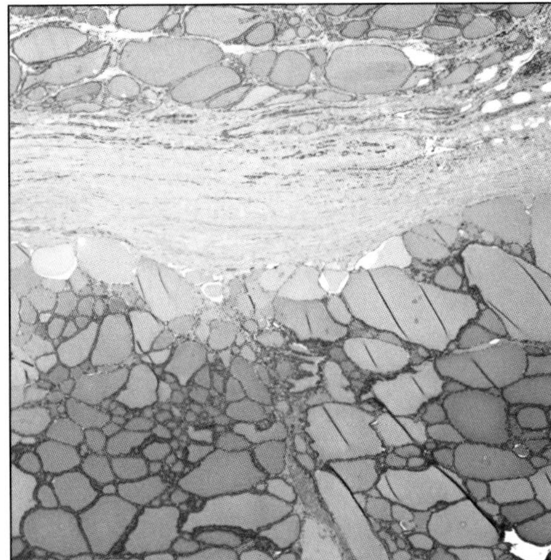

(Left) *Follicular variant: The nuclei lining the follicles show the characteristic features of papillary carcinoma. Many times, high-power examination of many fields is required to confirm this variant.* ***(Right)*** *Macrofollicular variant: There is a well-formed fibrous connective tissue capsule. The architecture mimics an adenomatoid nodule. There are macrofollicles on low power. High-power examination is required to confirm the diagnosis in this type of case.*

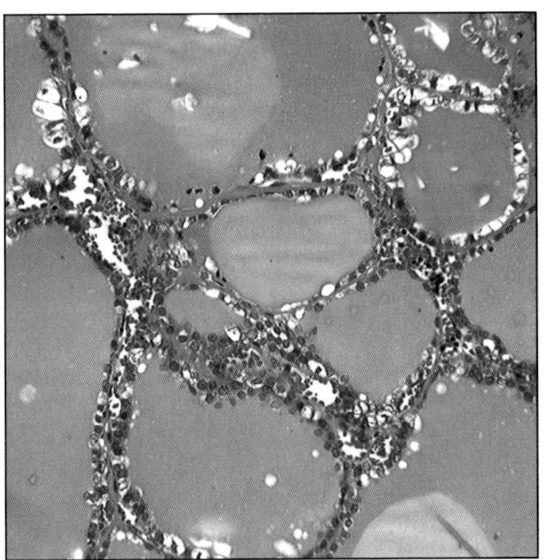

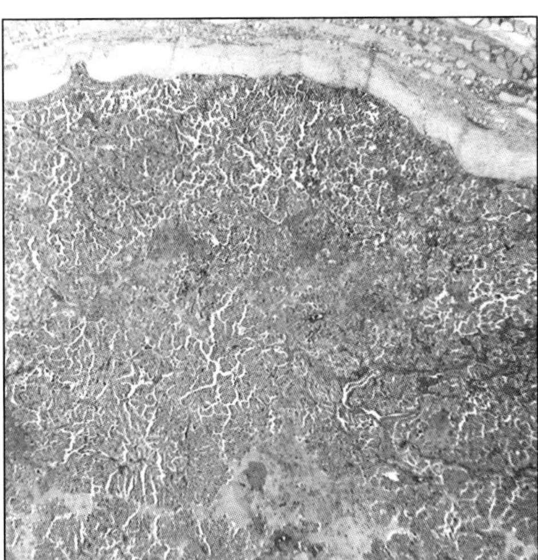

(Left) *Macrofollicular variant: The macrofollicles are lined by large cells. Frequently, scalloping or cytoplasmic clearing highlights the atypical neoplastic cells. The nuclei are flattened and hyperchromatic with only isolated classic nuclei.* ***(Right)*** *Oncocytic variant: By low-power examination, at least 70% of the tumor must show a complex, arborizing papillary architecture. Hemorrhage and degeneration are prominent. The cells have abundant oncocytic cytoplasm.*

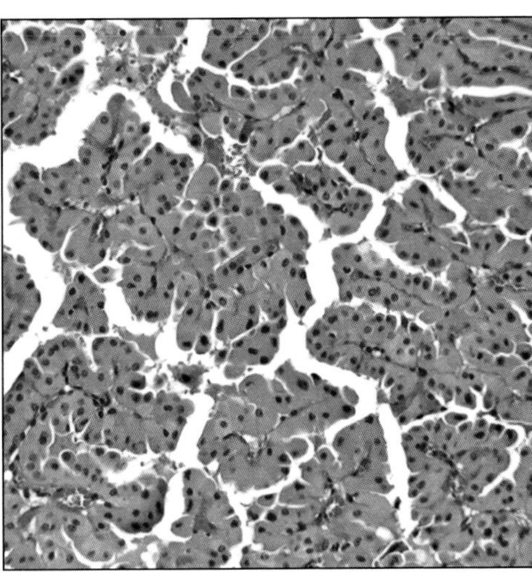

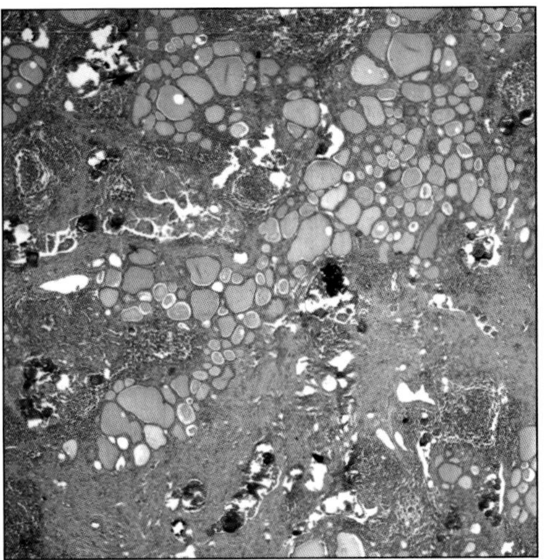

(Left) *Oncocytic variant: The cells are enlarged with abundant oncocytic (oxyphilic, Hürthle) cytoplasm. The enlarged nuclei tend to be apically oriented, appearing slightly more hyperchromatic than in conventional TPC.* ***(Right)*** *DSV: Diffuse involvement of the thyroid gland by papillary carcinoma is seen with innumerable psammoma bodies, fibrosis, chronic lymphocytic thyroiditis, and extensive lymph-vascular invasion. DSV is papillary carcinoma, raised to the 3rd power.*

Papillary Carcinoma Variants

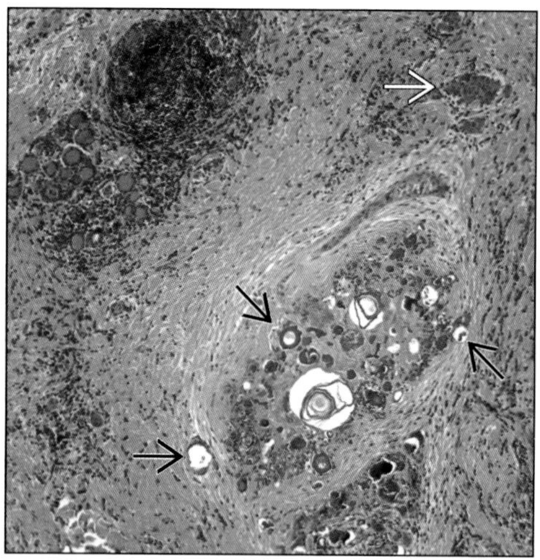

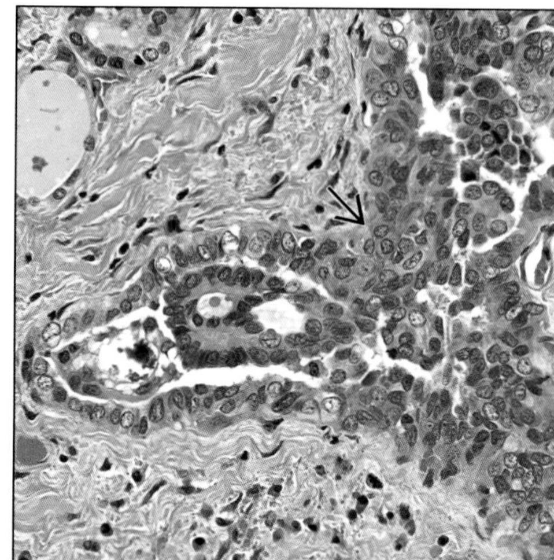

(Left) *Diffuse sclerosing variant: There is chronic lymphocytic thyroiditis associated with heavy fibrosis. Numerous psammoma bodies* ⇨ *and areas of squamous metaplasia* ➡ *comprise this variant.* ***(Right)*** *Diffuse sclerosing variant: Papillary carcinoma within a lymph-vascular space, along with areas of squamous metaplasia* ⇨*, demonstrates background fibrosis. Usually the whole lobe is affected by the neoplastic process.*

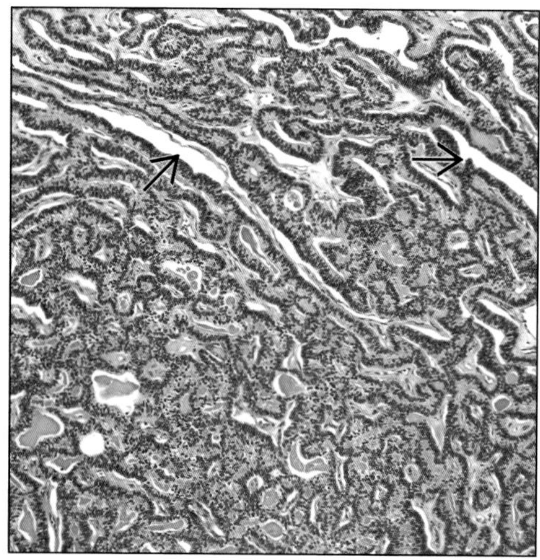

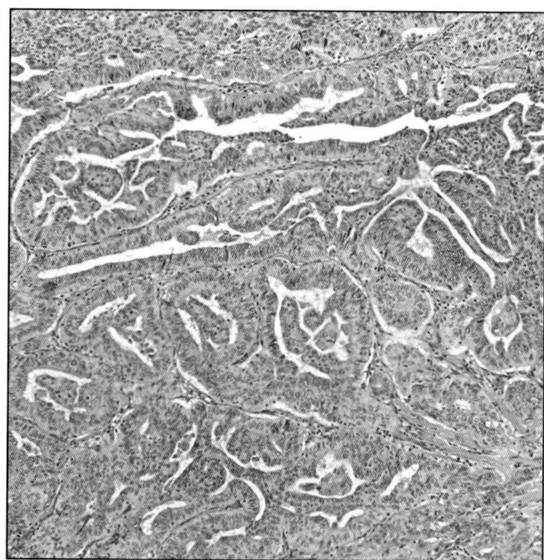

(Left) *Columnar variant: The prominent papillary growth shows markedly elongated, parallel follicles ("railroad tracks")* ⇨*. There is scant colloid. There is "hyperchromasia" created by the prominent nuclear stratification of elongated nuclei with coarse chromatin.* ***(Right)*** *Columnar variant: There is prominent papillary growth with markedly elongated, parallel follicles. The cells show stratification of the nuclei, creating a look similar to respiratory-type epithelium.*

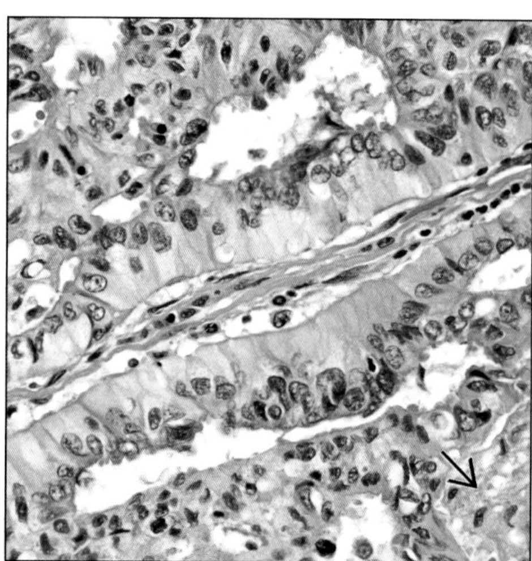

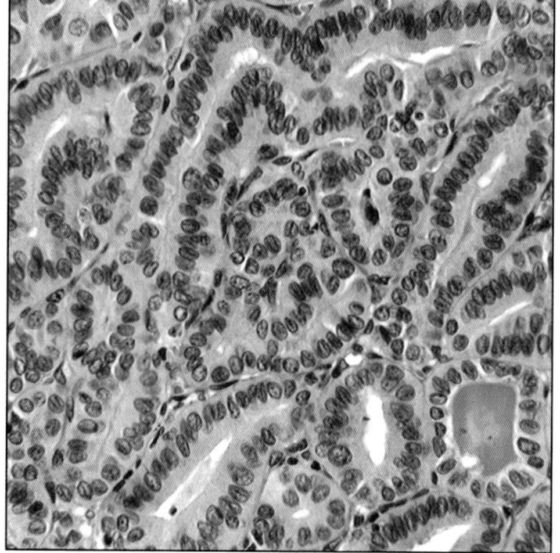

(Left) *Columnar variant: There are tall cells with a syncytial arrangement, showing subnuclear or supranuclear vacuolization of the cytoplasm. An area of necrosis is noted* ⇨*.* ***(Right)*** *Tall cell variant: The cells are tall, measuring at least 3x as high as they are wide (taking plane of section into consideration). Colloid is scant. The intercellular borders are sharply demarcated with centrally located nuclei. Intranuclear cytoplasmic inclusions and nuclear grooves are common.*

Papillary Carcinoma Variants and Ancillary Features

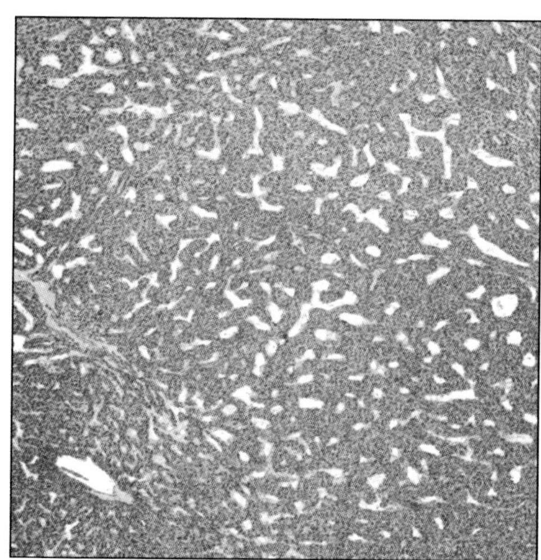

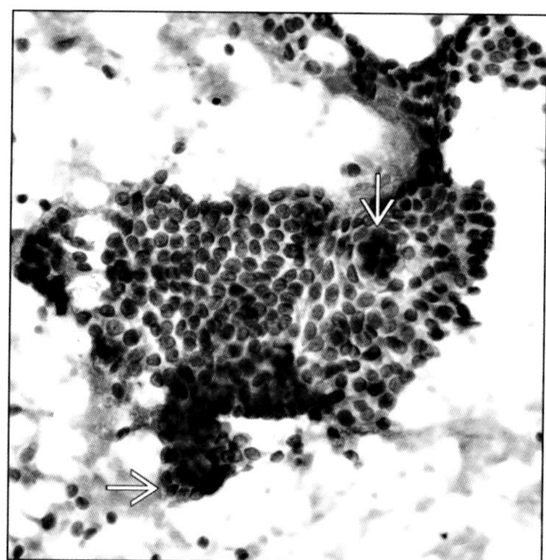

(Left) *Insular-solid variant: A variety of different patterns can be seen in papillary carcinoma. Here an insular-trabecular pattern predominates, showing scant colloid. The nuclear features are those of papillary carcinoma.* ***(Right)*** *A cellular smear with monolayered sheets (syncytium) focally shows 3-dimensional clusters of enlarged cells ➡. The nuclei are enlarged with overlapping and irregular borders.*

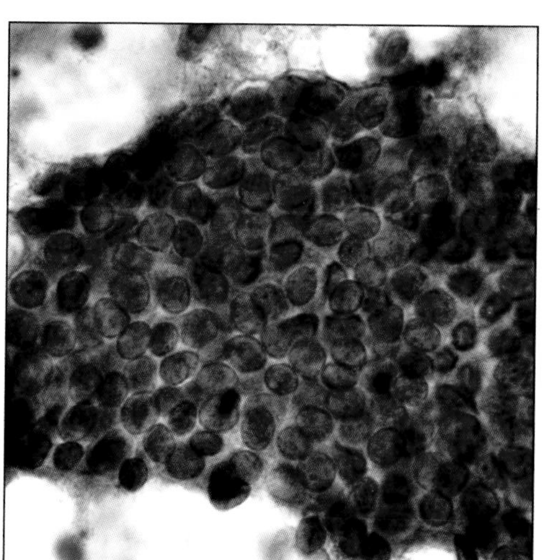

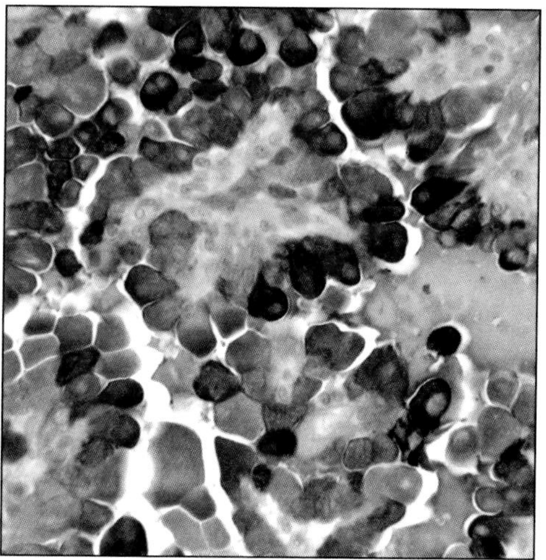

(Left) *This fine needle aspirate shows a monolayered sheet with nuclei that are greatly enlarged, overlap, and have irregular borders. There is powdery/ dusty, delicate nuclear chromatin, with some nuclear grooves.* ***(Right)*** *Immunohistochemistry is not usually required for the diagnosis, and when used, should probably incorporate several studies (panel) to confirm the diagnosis. CK19 is frequently positive in oncocytic thyroid papillary carcinoma.*

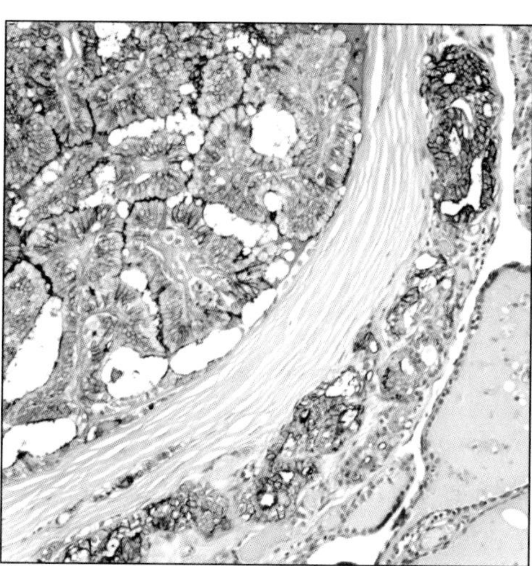

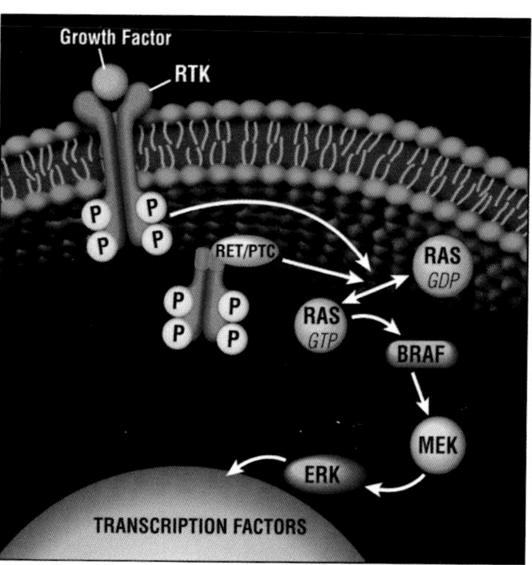

(Left) *The neoplastic tumor cells are strongly immunoreactive with HBME-1. However, an IHC panel of positive reactions for HBME-1, galectin-3, and CITED-1 may be more sensitive and specific for TPC than HBME-1 alone.* ***(Right)*** *A graphic shows the mitogen-activated protein kinase (MAPK) pathway. Activation of this pathway (point mutation in BRAF and RAS genes or rearrangement involving the RET and NTRK1 genes) is seen in papillary carcinoma.*

FOLLICULAR CARCINOMA

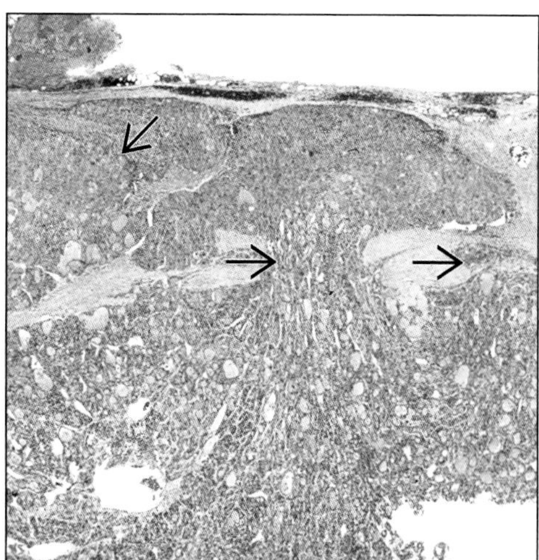

This widely invasive follicular carcinoma shows numerous areas of capsular invasion ➔, creating a mushroom-type pattern.

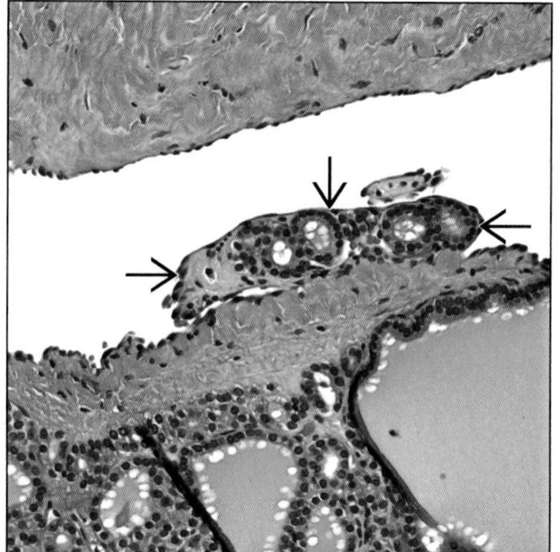

The tumor is attached to the vessel wall, associated with a delicate, discontinuous endothelial lining ➔. The tumor cells are identical to the lesional cells, helping to confirm the presence of true vascular invasion.

TERMINOLOGY

Abbreviations

- Follicular carcinoma (FC)

Synonyms

- Follicular adenocarcinoma
- Oncocytic carcinoma
- Hürthle cell carcinoma (discouraged)

Definitions

- Malignant thyroid epithelial neoplasm with follicular cell differentiation and lacking nuclear features of papillary carcinoma
  - Oncocytic (Hürthle cell) follicular carcinoma is most common variant

ETIOLOGY/PATHOGENESIS

Developmental Anomaly

- Familial syndromes: Up to 4% of FC in USA
  - Cowden disease
    - Autosomal dominant disorder caused by germline mutations in *PTEN* gene located on chromosome 10q22-23
    - Thyroid disease seen in about 2/3 of patients, with up to 20% developing FC
  - Werner syndrome
    - Autosomal recessive disease caused by germline mutations in *WRN* gene on chromosome 8p11-12
    - Thyroid disease seen in about 3%, usually FC; identified younger than nonaffected patients
  - Carney complex
    - Autosomal dominant disorder caused by germline mutations in *PRKARIA*

Environmental Exposure

- Iodine deficiency
  - Low dietary iodine intake associated with up to 3x increased risk (compared to areas with sufficient iodine consumption)
    - Low iodine associated with increased TSH stimulation, yielding goiter, promoting follicular carcinogenesis
- Radiation exposure
  - Ionizing radiation exposure results in 5.2x relative risk for developing FC (50% less than papillary carcinoma)
  - Radiation exposure history reported in ~ 4% of FC patients

Preexisting Thyroid Disease

- Identified in up to 15% of patients
- Adenoma
  - Follicular adenoma may be direct precursor lesion (progression to carcinoma)
    - Both harbor *RAS*, *PTEN*, and *PIK3CA* mutations, but carcinoma has higher frequency of mutations
  - Identical histologically except for invasion
  - Carcinomas are seldom small (< 1 cm)
  - Mean age for FC is about 8-10 years older than adenoma
- Adenomatoid nodules
  - Goiter is associated with increasing rate of cell proliferation due to prolonged TSH stimulation, which enhances chance for mutations in dividing cells
    - Increased occurrence of FC in dyshormonogenetic goiter patients (inherited defect with highly elevated TSH levels)
  - Chronic TSH stimulation needs additional mutagen (radiation or chemicals) to initiate carcinogenesis

Pathogenesis

- Cell of origin is follicular epithelial cell

FOLLICULAR CARCINOMA

Key Facts

Clinical Issues

- Accounts for ~ 10% of primary thyroid malignancies (0.8/100,000 persons per year)
- 5th and 6th decades; oncocytic: 1 decade older
- Female > Male (2-2.5:1)
- Asymptomatic, solitary, painless, slowly enlarging, palpable thyroid mass
- Surgery (lobectomy or thyroidectomy) with radioablative iodine
- 20-year survival: ~ 97% minimally invasive; 50% widely invasive
- Adverse prognostic factors
  - Age > 45 years, extrathyroidal extension, > 4 cm, presence of distant metastases

Macroscopic Features

- Thicker and more irregular capsule than adenoma
- **Parenchyma-capsule-tumor** zone should be submitted

Microscopic Pathology

- **Either** capsular or vascular invasion is sufficient for diagnosis
- Invasion of vessels within or beyond capsule, showing direct extension, attachment to wall, &/or tumor lined by endothelium
- Microfollicles, solid, cystic, trabecular, insular
- Nuclei are small, round, and regular with smooth contours
- **Variants**: Widely invasive, oncocytic, clear cell

Ancillary Tests

- **Positive**: Thyroglobulin, TTF-1, CK7
- *PPARγ* and *RAS* gene rearrangements in 50% of FC

CLINICAL ISSUES

Epidemiology

- Incidence
  - Annual incidence ~ 0.8 per 100,000 persons per year
  - ~ 10% of primary thyroid malignancies
  - 2nd most common malignancy
    - Trend is downward, as recognition of **follicular variant of papillary carcinoma** has improved
  - Increased in iodine-deficient areas
    - Dietary iodine supplementation associated with decrease in relative frequency of FC
- Age
  - Peak: 5th and 6th decades
  - Oncocytic type: Develops about 1 decade later
  - Rare in children
- Gender
  - Female > Male (2-2.5:1)
  - Oncocytic type: Female > Male (~ 1.7:1)

Site

- Any lobe, and in ectopic locations
  - Thyroglossal duct and struma ovarii
- Multifocality is uncommon

Presentation

- Usually present with an asymptomatic, solitary, painless, slowly enlarging, palpable thyroid mass
- Tend to be larger than papillary carcinomas
- Nodule usually moves with swallowing
- Lymph node and distant metastasis is uncommon
  - Ipsilateral lymphadenopathy in < 5%
    - Slightly higher in oncocytic variant (lymphatic vs. hematogenous spread)
  - Distant metastases in up to 20% of patients
    - Lungs and bone (bone pain or pathologic fracture)
- Hoarseness, dysphagia, dyspnea and stridor are rare
- Radiation exposure uncommon

Laboratory Tests

- Thyroid function tests are almost always normal

Treatment

- Options, risks, complications
  - Complications
    - Recurrent laryngeal nerve damage in up to 3%
    - Hypoparathyroidism in up to 3%
    - Hypothyroidism without replacement therapy
- Surgical approaches
  - Surgery (lobectomy vs. thyroidectomy) is treatment of choice
    - Thyroidectomy advocated only to allow subsequent radioiodine therapy and serum thyroglobulin monitoring
- Radiation
  - Radioablative iodine therapy
    - Cannot be effectively performed **without** total thyroidectomy
    - Up to 30% of tumors fail to take up ^{131}I, therefore ineffective
    - 25% failure for conventional follicular carcinomas and up to 75% failure for oncocytic carcinoma
  - External beam radiation reserved for incompletely excised tumors

Prognosis

- Excellent long-term prognosis
  - Minimally invasive: ~ 97% 20-year survival
  - Widely invasive: ~ 50% 20-year survival
- Oncocytic type has same overall outcome as conventional FC
  - Stage for stage outcome is similar
  - May be slightly higher incidence of extrathyroidal invasion and local recurrence
  - Associated with increased **lymph node** metastases
- Total thyroidectomy and lobectomy yield **identical** patient outcome
- Adverse prognostic factors
  - Age > 45 years
  - Extrathyroidal extension
  - Tumor size > 4 cm
  - Presence of distant metastases
- If metastatic, lung and bones are most common
  - Lymph nodes: Oncocytic type (10% of cases)

FOLLICULAR CARCINOMA

- *RAS* mutations correlated with tumor dedifferentiation, distant metastases, shorter survival
- Indeterminate (atypical) cases have benign outcome

IMAGE FINDINGS

Radiographic Findings

- Imaging cannot reliably distinguish between benign and malignant thyroid lesions
- MR is preferred over CT: Iodinated contrast to be avoided as it delays ^{131}I therapy
- Nuclear scintigraphy
  - Usually "cold" on scintigraphic scan
  - May be used to detect recurrence/metastasis post thyroidectomy
  - FC tend to concentrate ^{131}I less than adjacent normal thyroid parenchyma

Ultrasonographic Findings

- Used to follow nodules serially over time and for FNA guidance
- Ultrasound usually shows a solid, hypoechoic mass with peripheral nonechogenic halo (capsule)
- Irregular and poorly defined margins and turbulent intratumor blood flow suggest carcinoma

MACROSCOPIC FEATURES

General Features

- Encapsulated round to ovoid, solitary, solid tumors
- Thicker and more irregular capsule than adenoma
- Cross section has bulging, fleshy surface
- Widely invasive FC may show capsular and vascular invasion (including vena cava)
  - Sometimes encapsulation is difficult to document
- Hemorrhage, necrosis, and infarction are uncommon
- Gray-white to brown-tan or mahogany-brown (oncocytic carcinoma)

Sections to Be Submitted

- Serial sections of nodule at 2-3 mm intervals
- Unless large, entire **parenchyma-capsule-tumor** zone should be submitted
  - Minimum of 10 blocks (2-3 sections per block) from capsule-tumor interface

Size

- Most are 2-4 cm
  - Oncocytic tumors may be larger

MICROSCOPIC PATHOLOGY

Histologic Features

- Majority are conventional type (~ 20% are variants)
- Lack nuclear features of papillary carcinoma
- Tumor surrounded by capsule
  - Deposition of parallel layers of collagen fibers surrounding tumor and containing smooth muscle-walled vessels
    - Reticulin fibers within connective tissue
  - Thick and well formed (0.1-0.4 cm thick)
  - Should completely encapsulate lesion
  - Thin, irregular, attenuated, uneven and poorly formed (< 0.1 cm thick)
- **Either** capsular or vascular invasion is sufficient for diagnosis
- **Invasion** must be present
  - **Capsular invasion**
    - Penetration of > 1/2 thickness of capsule (partial thickness)
    - Beyond contour of tumor nodule
    - Unassociated with site of previous FNA
    - Direct contact of tumor cells with thyroid parenchyma is rare since new collagen is deposited around advancing edge
    - Deeper sections may show tumor connection of "satellite" nodule adjacent to parenchyma
    - Tangential sectioning frequently limits interpretation
    - **Fine needle aspiration artifact**: Abrupt capsular loss, linear architecture, reactive endothelial proliferation, hemosiderin, erythrocytes
  - **Vascular invasion**
    - Vessels are within or beyond capsule
    - **Not** within tumor
    - Direct tumor extension into a vessel
    - Tumor cells must be identical to those within main tumor
    - Lined by endothelial cells
    - Tumor thrombus **attached** to vascular spaces
    - **Not** entrapped cells with retraction artifacts
    - **Not** free-floating, nonviable cells in serum
    - Not a result of surgical or sectioning manipulation
    - Be aware of "penetrating" vessels: Tangentially sectioned vessels
- Exact number of vessels involved or areas of capsular invasion not defined
- Arranged in well-formed follicles (microfollicular), solid, cystic, trabecular and insular patterns
  - 1 pattern usually predominates
  - Macrofollicular patterns are uncommon
- Tumors are cellular, but colloid is usually easily identified
  - Oncocytic tumors may show more limited colloid
- Tumor cells are slightly larger than adjacent parenchyma, cuboidal, and regular
  - Focal tumor cell spindling can be seen
  - Cytoplasm is ample, lightly eosinophilic to amphophilic
- Nuclei are small to medium, usually round and regular with smooth contours
  - Nuclear chromatin is coarse and heavy
  - Nucleoli are small
  - Isolated nuclear pleomorphism can be seen but does not alter diagnosis
- Mitotic figures may be seen
- Degeneration and necrosis are uncommon
  - May be present in post-FNA tumors
- Direct soft tissue and tracheal extension is rare
- Intrathyroidal spread is not seen

Margins

- Surgical margins should be reported

- Extension beyond the thyroid gland "capsule" is associated with more biologically aggressive behavior

Variants

- **Widely invasive**
  - Extensive capsular invasion ("mushroom" invasion)
    - Capsule may be lost or hard to identify
  - Direct extension into adjacent thyroid parenchyma or perithyroidal soft tissue
  - Extensive vascular invasion: Large vessels and perithyroidal vessels
  - Uncommon, as result of improved physician and patient awareness, superior radiographic techniques, and advances in surgical management
- **Oncocytic variant**
  - a.k.a. Hürthle cell, Ashkenazy cell, oxyphilic cell: Due to increased accumulation of abnormal mitochondria
    - These terms are discouraged
    - Ashkenazy described cells first in 1898
    - Hürthle described C-cells in dogs!
  - Tumors tend to be larger than conventional FC
  - Macroscopically, mahogany brown appearance is distinctive
  - Invasive criteria identical to conventional FC
  - > 75% of tumor composed of oncocytic cells
    - Large, polygonal cells with well-defined cell borders
    - Abundant, fine to slightly coarse, granular, deeply eosinophilic cytoplasm
    - Opacified or smooth cytoplasm
    - Nuclei: Round and regular with coarse chromatin
    - Pleomorphism is increased in this variant
    - Frequently associated with prominent, brightly eosinophilic, centrally placed nucleoli
  - Cytoplasm is fragile, with tendency to undergo infarction, usually post FNA
    - Hemorrhage, degeneration and eventual fibrosis may result
  - Solid and trabecular patterns show scant/absent colloid
    - TTF-1 or thyroglobulin useful in these cases
  - Colloid tends to be basophilic and undergo calcification (mimic of psammoma bodies)
- **Clear cell variant**
  - Predominantly (> 75%) composed of clear cells
  - Cytoplasm is watery clear or has fine, pale eosinophilic granularity
  - Quality of cytoplasm due to accumulation of glycogen, lipid, thyroglobulin, other vesicles, or distended mitochondria
    - May be seen in oncocytic tumors especially
  - Should be separated from metastatic renal cell carcinoma and clear cell medullary carcinoma (by immunohistochemistry)
- **Signet ring variant**
  - Cells with large intracytoplasmic vacuoles that displace and compress nucleus to side
    - Material is immunoreactive for thyroglobulin and positive with PAS w/diastase
  - Invasion must be identified

ANCILLARY TESTS

Cytology

- Separation of adenoma/nodule from carcinoma cannot be reliably or predictably performed by FNA
  - Sensitivity: 78%
  - Specificity: 98%
  - Positive predictive value: 99%
- Hypercellular aspirates
- Dispersed microfollicles
  - Groups of follicular cells with 6-12 nuclei forming ring-like structure
  - Spherical, 3-dimensional aggregates
  - Enlarged cuboidal cells with uniform, round, smooth nuclei with coarse nuclear chromatin
  - Cytoplasmic borders are frequently indistinct
  - Nuclear size and shape variability
- Scant colloid
- **Oncocytic variant**: Scant colloid; dyscohesive cells; large round to oval cells; low nuclear to cytoplasmic ratio; abundant granular cytoplasm; eccentric round nuclei; bi- or multinucleation may be seen; nucleoli usually prominent; no lymphoplasmacytic infiltrate

Frozen Sections

- Nearly completely useless unless you "happen" upon the area of invasion
- If FNA has been performed, decline frozen
- If frozen is demanded, 2-3 sections of capsule sampled, before "**defer to permanent**" is used

Histochemistry

- PAS highlights colloid

Immunohistochemistry

- **Positive**: Thyroglobulin, TTF-1, CK7
  - **Panel** positive with galectin-3, HBME-1, CITED-1; may be helpful to confirm "malignancy"
  - Caution: Oncocytic tumors show nonspecific staining and high endogenous biotin activity
- **Negative**: Chromogranin, calcitonin, synaptophysin, CD56, CEA-M
- CD34, CD31, FVIII-RAg can accentuate vessels (very limited value)

Flow Cytometry

- Aneuploidy in 50-60% of FC

Cytogenetics

- High rate of loss of heterozygosity (LOH) is characteristic of FC
  - Known tumor suppressor genes: *VHL* on 3p25-26, *TP53* on 17p13, *PTEN* on 10q23

Molecular Genetics

- Rearrangements of peroxisome proliferator-activated receptor gamma (*PPARγ*) gene found in up to 50% of FC
  - t(2;3)(q13;p25) leads to fusion between *PAX8* gene on 2q13 and *PPARγ* gene on 3p25
  - FISH used for detection
  - Patients tend to be younger; tumors are smaller; solid growth pattern
  - Almost never show concurrent *RAS* mutations

FOLLICULAR CARCINOMA

Somatic Mutations in Thyroid Follicular Carcinoma

Mutation Type	Follicular Carcinoma	Oncocytic-type Follicular Carcinoma
RAS point mutations	40-50%	10-15%
*PAX8/PPAR*γ rearrangement	30-40%	0-5%
PTEN point mutations, small deletions	5-10%	NR
PI3CA point mutations	5-10%	NR

NR = not yet reported.

- *RAS* abnormal in up to 50% of FC (not carcinoma specific)
  - Activating mutations in codon 61 of *N-* and *H-RAS* genes are most common
- *GRIM-19* gene mutations recently identified in oncocytic tumors

Electron Microscopy

- Follicular cells with preserved polarity; cells resting on continuous basal lamina; microvilli on apical surface; nuclei with finely dispersed chromatin, well-developed granular endoplasmic reticulum
- Oncocytic cells filled with abnormal mitochondria showing variability in size and pleomorphism, showing disappearance of cristae

DIFFERENTIAL DIAGNOSIS

Follicular Adenoma

- Encapsulated, single tumor without invasion
- Histological features identical to carcinoma
- Periphery must be adequately sampled

Adenomatoid Nodules

- Usually multiple lesions
- Usually less cellular with more colloid than neoplasms
- Tend to have irregular fibrosis rather than a capsule
- Lack muscle-walled vessels in fibrous connective tissue
- Tangential sectioning, irregular contours, fine needle aspiration, and frozen section artifacts hamper interpretation

Papillary Carcinoma

- Specifically, FV-PTC
- Characteristic nuclear features of papillary carcinoma
  - Nuclear chromatin clearing, contour irregularities, nuclear grooves, nuclear overlapping, intratumoral fibrosis, psammoma bodies

Medullary Carcinoma

- Cellular tumors, lacking colloid
- Amyloid is often present
- Background of C-cell hyperplasia in inherited tumors
- Nesting or insular architecture
- Oval to spindled cells
- Round, eccentric nuclei with finely stippled chromatin
- Positive with chromogranin, synaptophysin, calcitonin, CEA-m, CD56

Clear Cell Tumors

- Parathyroid tumors
  - Adenoma or carcinoma show parathyroid hormone (PTH) and chromogranin reactivity
- Metastatic renal cell carcinoma
  - Immunohistochemical studies can help
  - Do not over interpret entrapped thyroid follicular cells as tumor cells positive with TTF-1 or thyroglobulin

Poorly Differentiated Carcinoma

- Solid, trabecular, and insular growth patterns require separation from poorly differentiated carcinomas
- Increased mitotic figures and necrosis with relative lack of colloid production

SELECTED REFERENCES

1. Baloch ZW et al: Fine-needle aspiration of the thyroid: today and tomorrow. Best Pract Res Clin Endocrinol Metab. 22(6):929-39, 2008
2. Nikiforov YE: Thyroid carcinoma: molecular pathways and therapeutic targets. Mod Pathol. 21 Suppl 2:S37-43, 2008
3. Baloch ZW et al: Our approach to follicular-patterned lesions of the thyroid. J Clin Pathol. 60(3):244-50, 2007
4. LiVolsi VA et al: Use and abuse of frozen section in the diagnosis of follicular thyroid lesions. Endocr Pathol. 16(4):285-93, 2005
5. Asa SL: My approach to oncocytic tumours of the thyroid. J Clin Pathol. 57(3):225-32, 2004
6. LiVolsi VA et al: Follicular neoplasms of the thyroid: view, biases, and experiences. Adv Anat Pathol. 11(6):279-87, 2004
7. Ko HM et al: Clinicopathologic analysis of fine needle aspiration cytology of the thyroid. A review of 1,613 cases and correlation with histopathologic diagnoses. Acta Cytol. 47(5):727-32, 2003
8. Rosai J: Immunohistochemical markers of thyroid tumors: significance and diagnostic applications. Tumori. 89(5):517-9, 2003
9. Thompson LD et al: A clinicopathologic study of minimally invasive follicular carcinoma of the thyroid gland with a review of the English literature. Cancer. 91(3):505-24, 2001
10. Oertel YC et al: Thyroid cytology and histology. Baillieres Best Pract Res Clin Endocrinol Metab. 14(4):541-57, 2000
11. Mazzaferri EL: An overview of the management of papillary and follicular thyroid carcinoma. Thyroid. 9(5):421-7, 1999
12. Oertel YC et al: Diagnosis of malignant epithelial thyroid lesions: fine needle aspiration and histopathologic correlation. Ann Diagn Pathol. 2(6):377-400, 1998
13. Schlumberger MJ: Papillary and follicular thyroid carcinoma. N Engl J Med. 338(5):297-306, 1998
14. Wartofsky L et al: The use of radioactive iodine in patients with papillary and follicular thyroid cancer. J Clin Endocrinol Metab. 83(12):4195-203, 1998

Imaging, Gross, and Microscopic Features

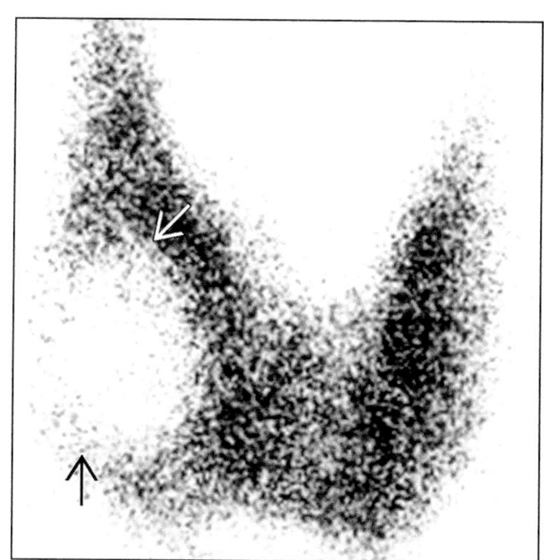

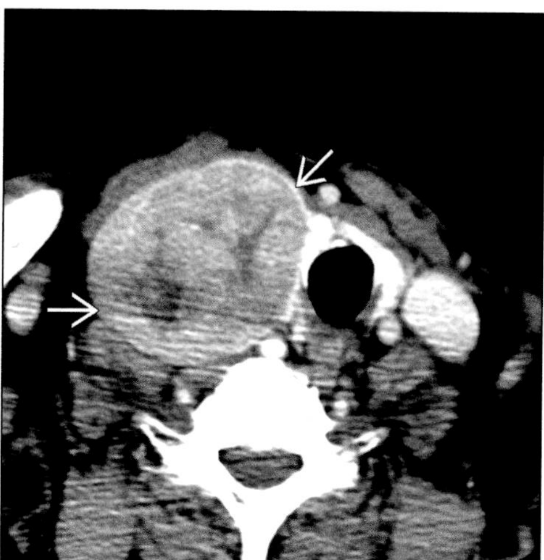

(Left) *Anterior planar ^{123}I nuclear medicine scan shows a cold nodule in the right thyroid lobe* ⇨ ➡. *A cold nodule has approximately 20% chance of being malignant. This was a case from a follicular carcinoma.* ***(Right)*** *The CT image shows a large, solid, well-circumscribed thyroid neoplasm* ➡, *lacking capsular invasion. This is a common but nonspecific finding in radiographic imaging of thyroid lesions, which may be seen with benign or malignant lesions.*

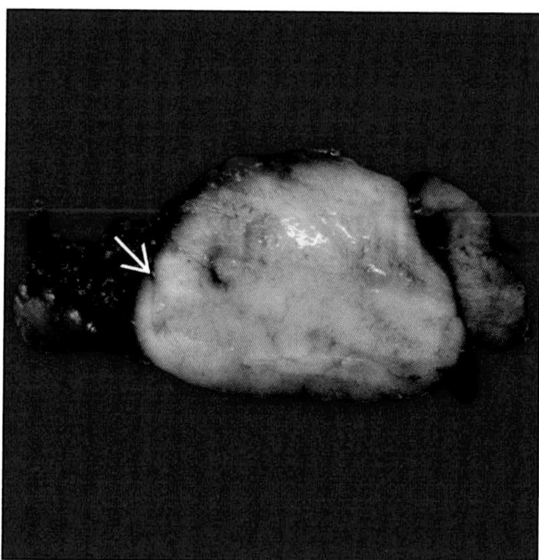

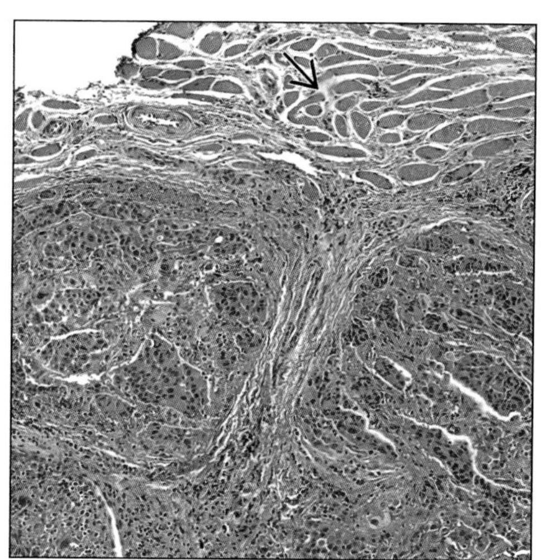

(Left) *There is a solid tumor in the thyroid gland. The cut surface appears quite light in comparison to the surrounding parenchyma. An area of extension is suggested* ➡, *although not diagnostic of capsular invasion.* ***(Right)*** *Thyroid carcinomas may demonstrate extension beyond the thyroid gland parenchyma into the adjacent soft tissue. Here, the tumor is identified blending with the skeletal muscle* ⇨. *Normal isthmus may also be blended with skeletal muscle.*

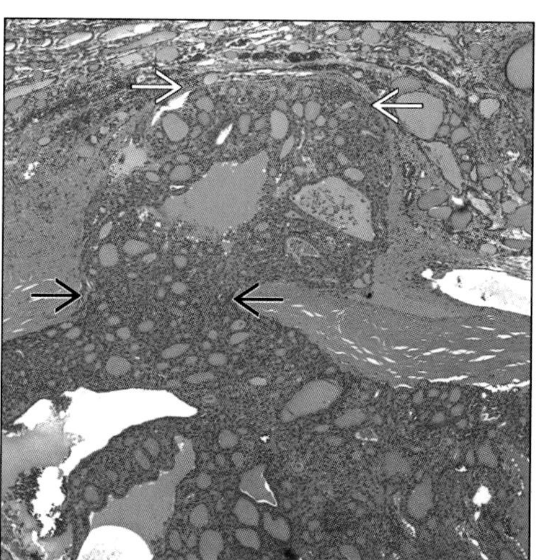

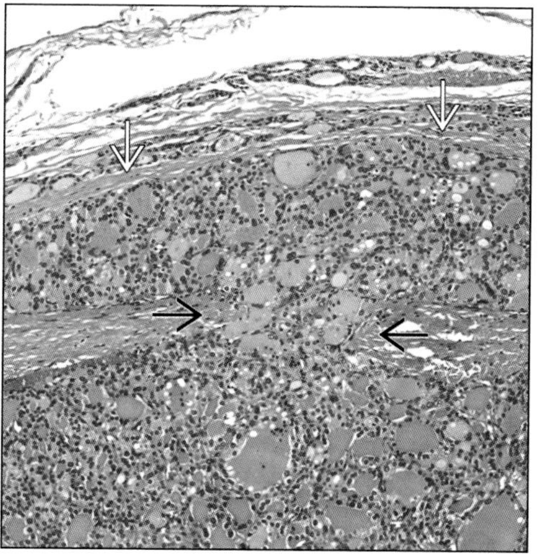

(Left) *Full penetration of the capsule is diagnostic of follicular carcinoma* ⇨. *However, sometimes the invasion is not as well developed as seen here. Note the new collagen deposition at the leading edge of the tumor nodule* ➡. ***(Right)*** *The tumor capsule is breached* ⇨ *by the neoplastic cells, which have formed a "mushroom" as it expands into the surrounding parenchyma. Note new collagen deposition* ➡ *at the leading edge of the tumor projection.*

FOLLICULAR CARCINOMA

Capsular Invasion

*(**Left**) There is a large tumor projection ⇒ beyond the tumor contour and capsule. This would categorize this tumor as a widely invasive lesion. The tumor is an oncocytic variant. (**Right**) There is a large mushroom-like projection through the tumor capsule ⇒. This is characteristic for a follicular carcinoma, and would qualify this tumor for placement in the widely invasive category. The tumor is arranged in a follicular architecture.*

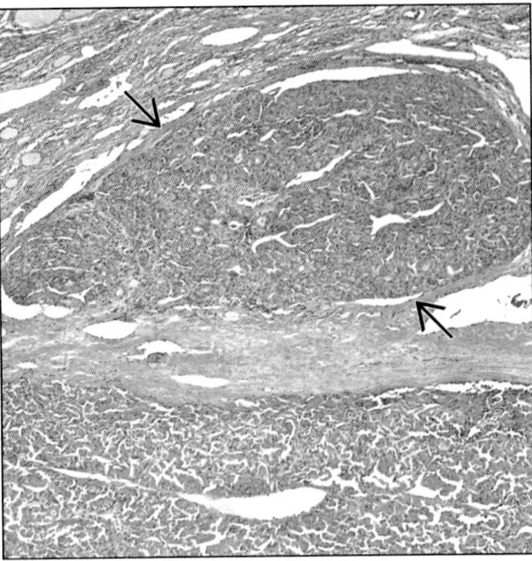

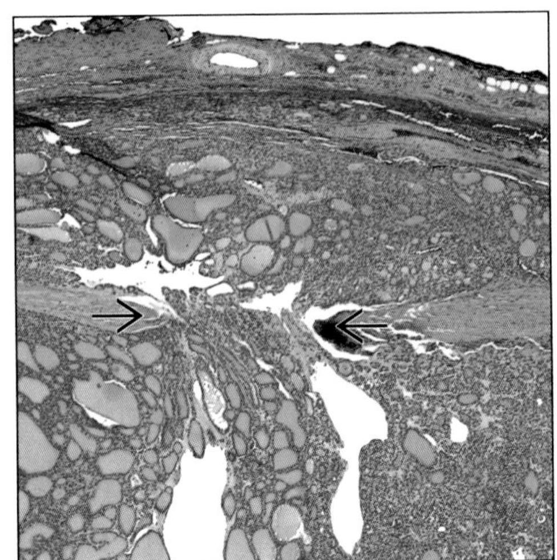

*(**Left**) In some tumors, the capsular penetration may "push" the capsule up to the point where the tumor projects well beyond the contour of the tumor ⇒. It is important to initially review the overall capsule at low power to get a sense of the tumor shape and periphery. (**Right**) H&E shows capsular extension of > 50% penetration ⇒ of the fibrous connective tissue capsule ➡ by the tumor cells. There are no features to suggest this was a site of previous FNA.*

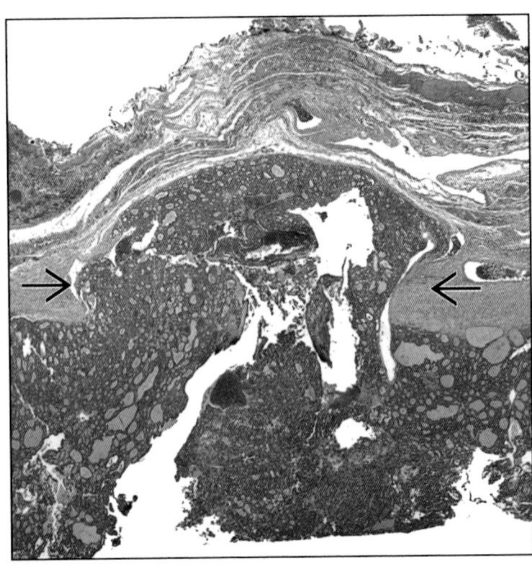

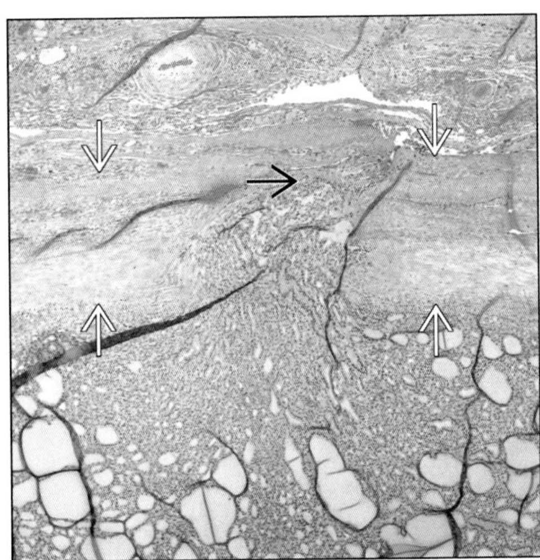

*(**Left**) This focus ⇒ is insufficient to qualify as true capsule invasion, although the capsule is partially penetrated by the neoplastic cells. In cases like this, additional levels or sections are suggested to exclude invasion. (**Right**) This was the only focus of capsular permeation ⇒ in a thoroughly sampled tumor. The capsule is very thick ➡ and the tumor is cellular. However, this area does not quite reach the threshold for capsular invasion.*

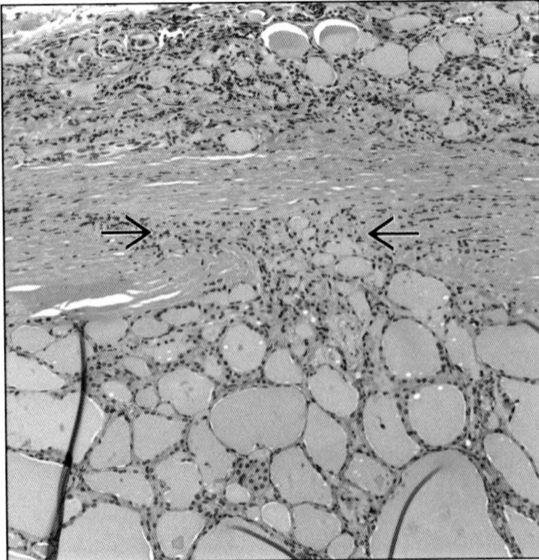

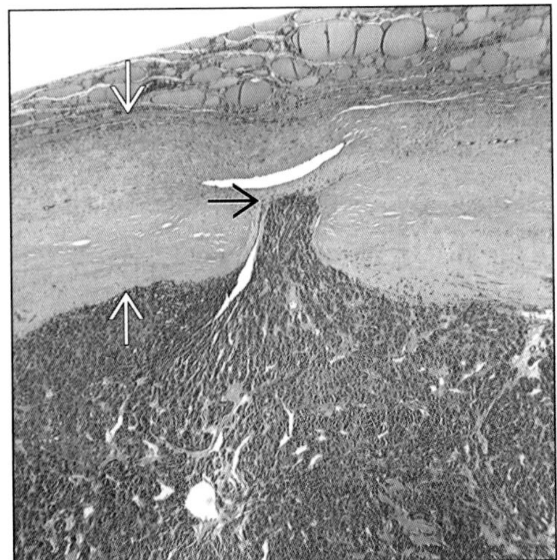

Vascular Invasion

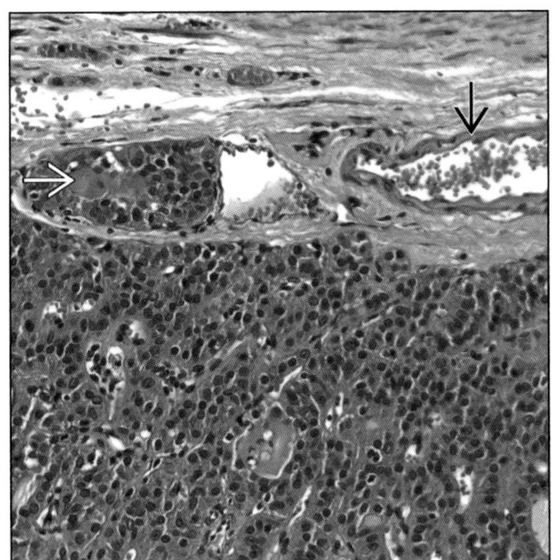

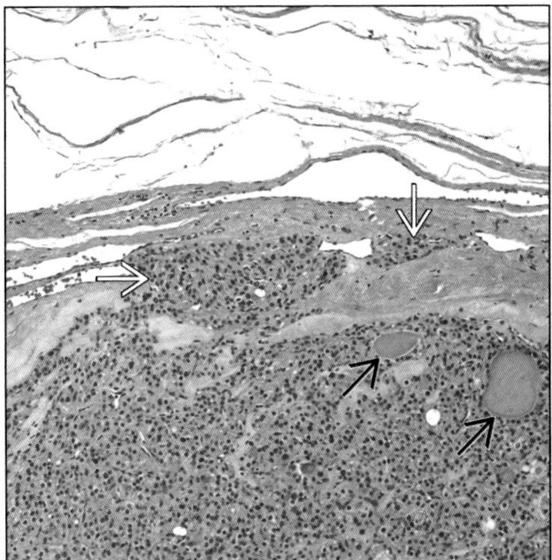

*(**Left**) The vessel is filled with tumor, including an area of colloid production ➡. The wall of the vessel is more easily identified in the continuation of the vessel in the adjacent field ⇨. (**Right**) The neoplastic cells of this follicular carcinoma are identical within the vessel ➡ as they are in the main mass. The tumor fills and expands the vessel. A delicate endothelial lining is noted. Colloid is produced ⇨ within the tumor.*

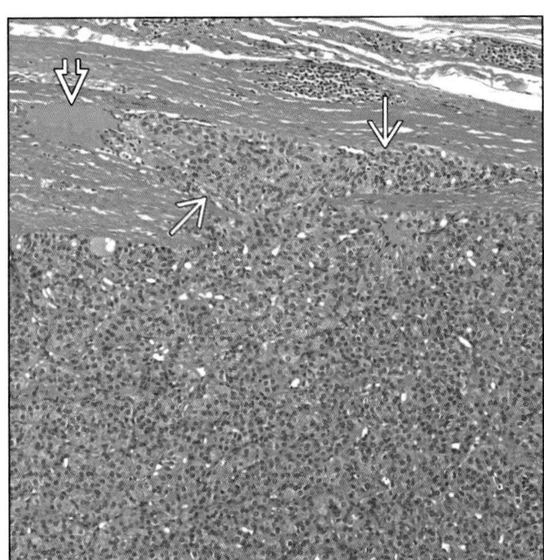

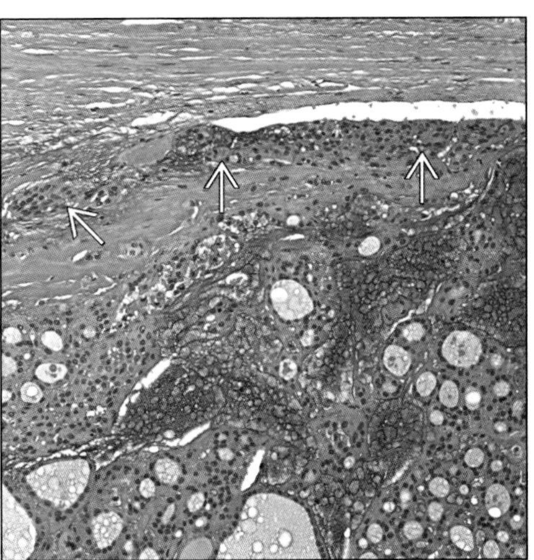

*(**Left**) The neoplastic cells have infiltrated the tumor capsule and filled into a vascular space ➡. There is a small amount of serum at one edge of the vessel ➡, helping to confirm the location of the tumor thrombus. (**Right**) Neoplastic cells line a vascular space ➡ within the tumor capsule. This is an oncocytic follicular carcinoma, associated with a mucinous material. Mucinous material is nonspecific, as it can be seen in a wide variety of thyroid lesions.*

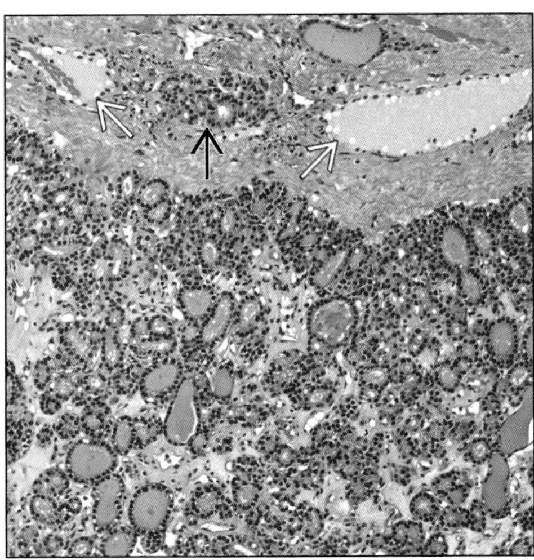

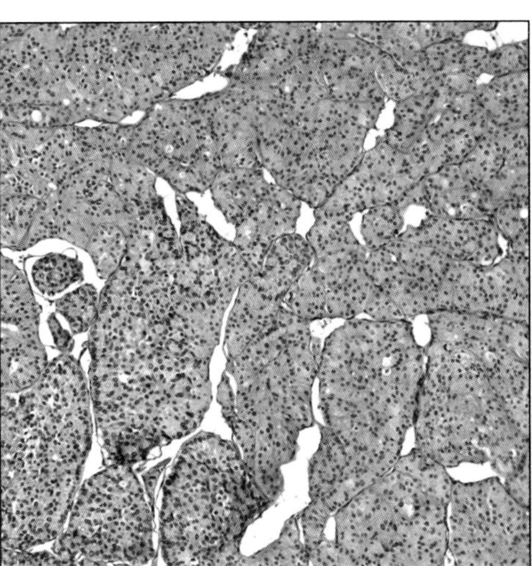

*(**Left**) This is an example of entrapment of follicular cells ⇨ between two vessels ➡. This is not invasion. There were no additional findings in this tumor, which would be diagnosed as a follicular adenoma. Entrapment is a potential pitfall in follicular tumors. (**Right**) A trabecular or insular pattern can be seen in follicular tumors. Invasion would need to be shown to diagnose carcinoma, since a trabecular or insular pattern can be seen in many different follicular lesions.*

FOLLICULAR CARCINOMA

Microscopic Features

(Left) *Tumor necrosis is present* ⇨ *in this follicular carcinoma, although it is an uncommon finding. Note the prominent nucleoli in nearly every tumor cell. Colloid is not identified in this field.* ***(Right)*** *Oncocytic (oxyphilic, Hürthle) cells are large, polygonal cells with abundant, granular, brightly eosinophilic, opacified cytoplasm. The nuclear chromatin is clear to vesicular, with prominent, brightly eosinophilic, round to irregular nucleoli seen in the center.*

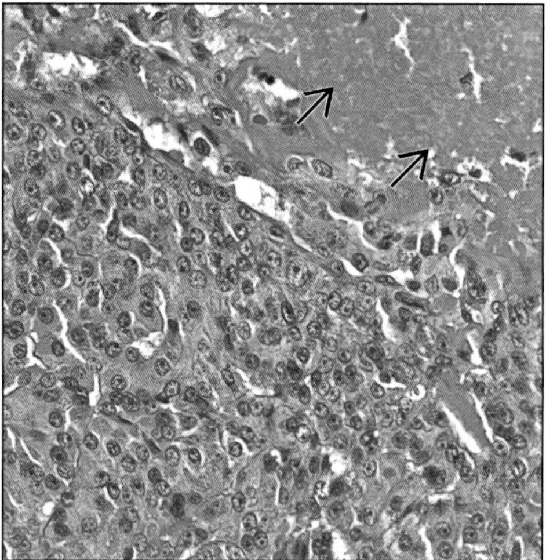

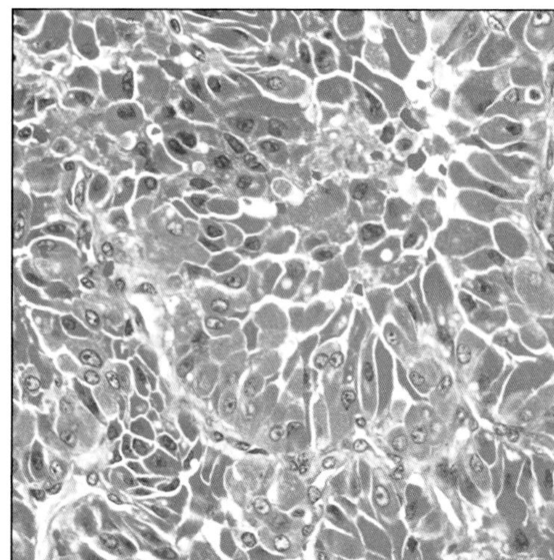

(Left) *The nuclei of follicular carcinoma are often irregular in size and shape, but the nuclear chromatin is coarse and heavy. Colloid is present throughout the tumor.* ***(Right)*** *A variety of patterns of growth can be seen in follicular carcinoma. In examples like this one, an organoid pattern can mimic a medullary carcinoma. When colloid is absent, thyroglobulin is useful in confirming the nature of the process.*

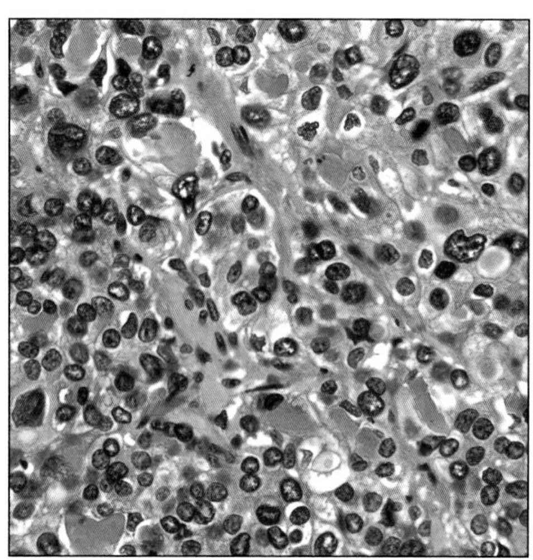

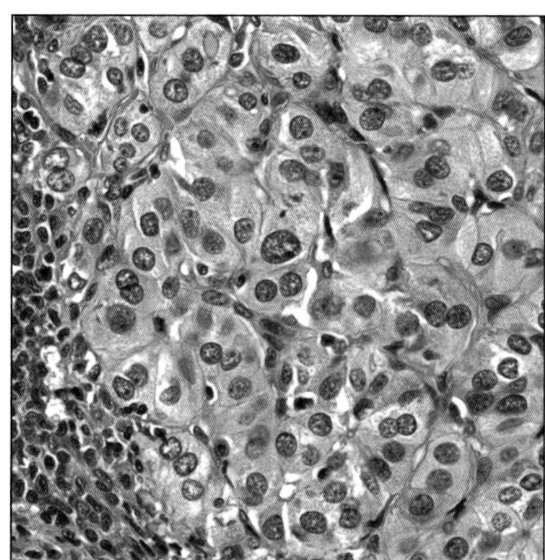

(Left) *The neoplastic cells of follicular carcinoma are frequently monotonous, with a relatively low nuclear to cytoplasmic ratio. A mitotic figure is seen* ➡*. There is abundant cytoplasm, which is often associated with intranuclear cytoplasmic inclusions* ⇨*.* ***(Right)*** *Clear cell change is frequently seen in oncocytic lesions, but can be found on its own (signet ring variant). These inclusions are usually strongly and diffusely immunoreactive with thyroglobulin.*

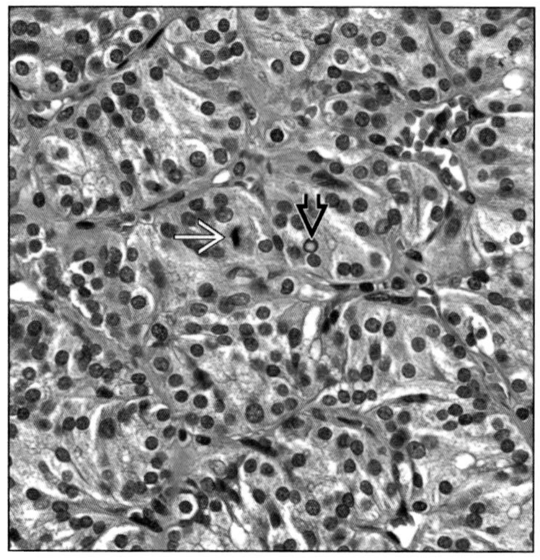

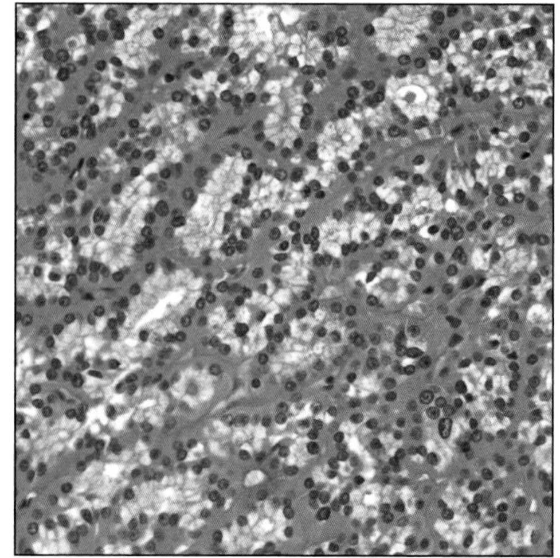

Microscopic Features and Ancillary Techniques

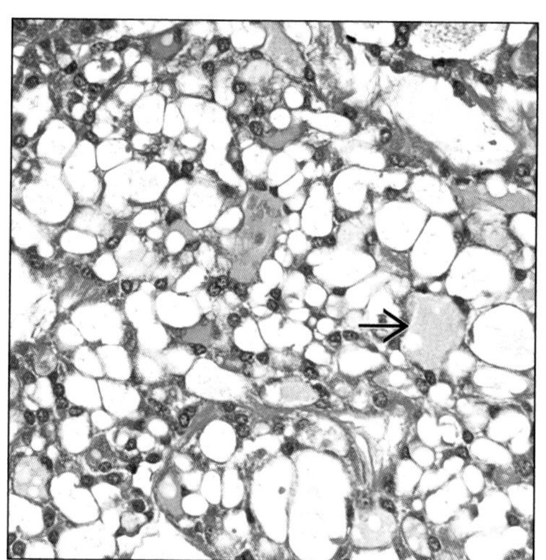

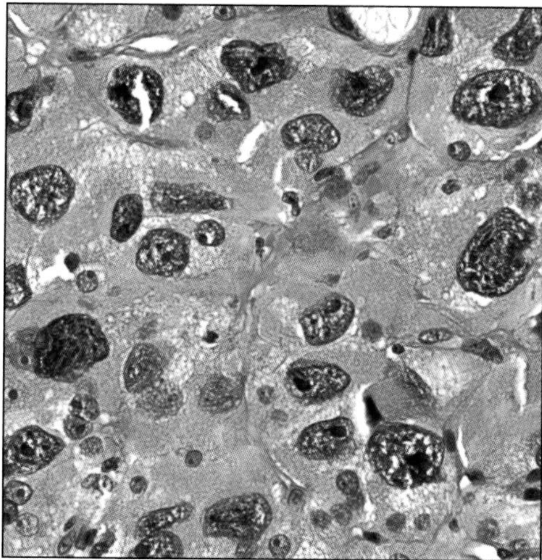

(Left) *Clear cell change creates a sieve-like appearance and focal areas of signet ring formation. There is focal colloid ➔, helping to confirm a follicular derivation to this carcinoma. This tumor showed thyroglobulin immunoreactivity.* ***(Right)*** *Isolated foci of remarkable pleomorphism can be seen within a follicular carcinoma. However, pleomorphism alone in endocrine organ tumors does not equate to malignancy.*

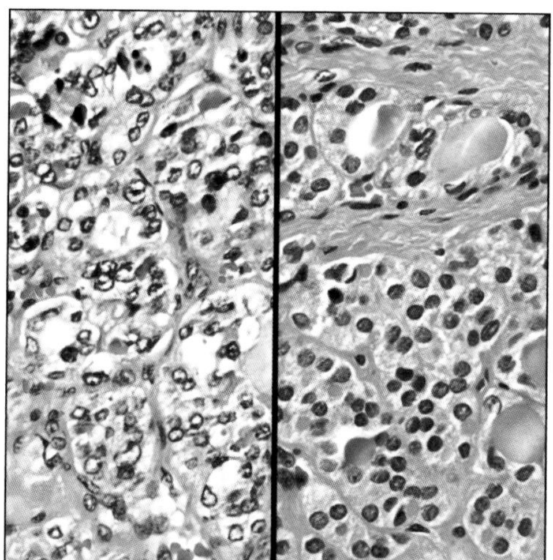

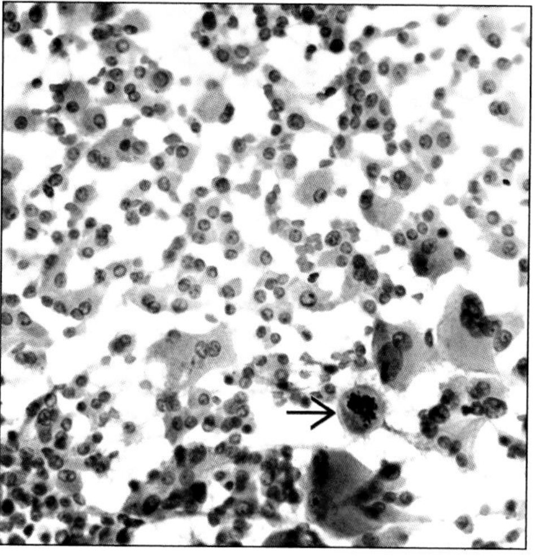

(Left) *Processing artifacts can frequently cause interpretation problems. Left: Processed on a heating plate for 2 hours without clearing the water first. Right: Re-processed without heating plate and no excess water.* ***(Right)*** *While cytology smears are unreliable in separating benign from malignant, this tumor shows increased cellularity, cytoplasmic oxyphilia, and focal cellular pleomorphism. An atypical mitotic figure ➔ suggests a tumor rather than an adenomatoid nodule.*

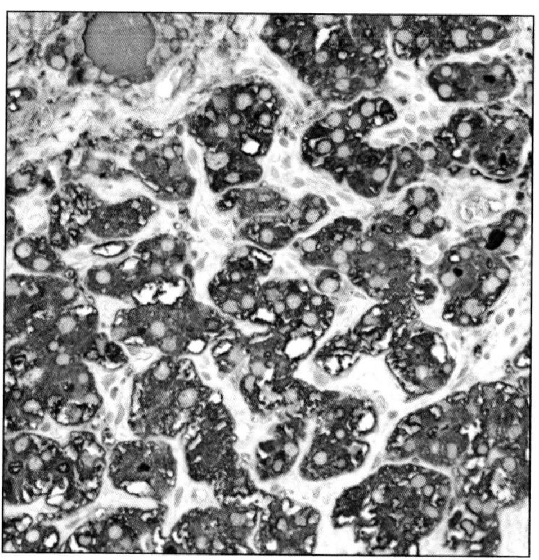

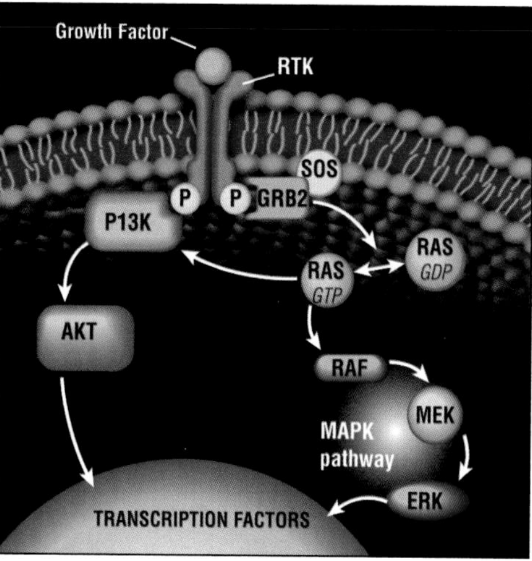

(Left) *In most FCs, immunohistochemistry is not required. Sometimes, thyroglobulin may confirm follicular cell origin.* ***(Right)*** *RAS functions as a molecular switch propagating signals from receptor tyrosine kinases. With activation, RAS shifts from an inactive, GDP-bound to active, GTP-bound form, and phosphorylates downstream cytoplasmic targets. Point mutations stabilize the protein in its active form, leading to constitutive stimulation of the MAPK and PI3K/AKT pathways.*

POORLY DIFFERENTIATED THYROID CARCINOMA

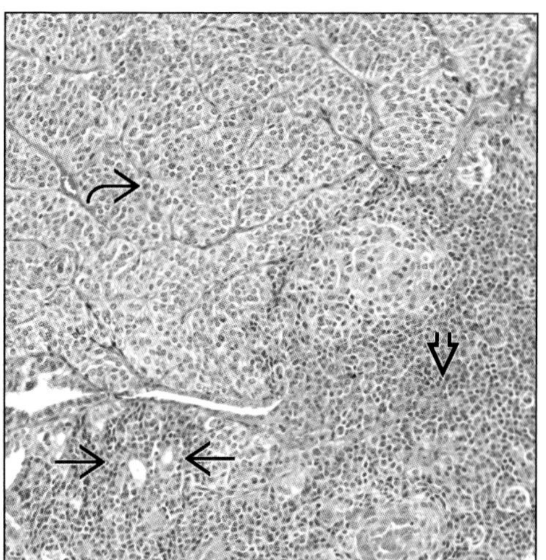

Poorly differentiated thyroid carcinoma is characterized by insular ➩ and diffuse (sheet-like) ⇨ growth patterns. Follicular growth is identified ➔, although the follicles lack colloid.

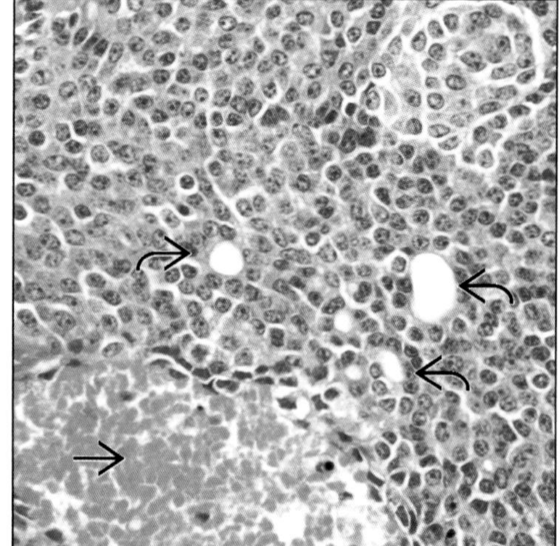

Solid growth composed of monotonous population of cells is seen with round vesicular nuclei, microfollicles ➩ without identifiable colloid, and a confluent focus of necrosis ➔.

TERMINOLOGY

Abbreviations

- Poorly differentiated thyroid carcinoma (PDTC)

Synonyms

- Insular carcinoma
- Primordial cell carcinoma
- Wuchernde struma

Definitions

- Malignant epithelial thyroid neoplasm showing histologic and biologic features intermediate between differentiated thyroid carcinomas and undifferentiated (anaplastic) carcinoma
  - Diagnosis of PDTC predicated on
    - Mitotic index
    - Presence of necrosis
  - Growth pattern alone (e.g., insular, solid, trabecular, others) not a defining criteria for classifying thyroid tumor as poorly differentiated
    - Benign tumors and differentiated thyroid carcinomas may show insular, solid, and trabecular growth; generally lack increased mitotic activity and necrosis

ETIOLOGY/PATHOGENESIS

Idiopathic

- Usually arise de novo
- May be associated with transformation from differentiated thyroid carcinomas (i.e., papillary or follicular carcinoma)

CLINICAL ISSUES

Epidemiology

- Incidence
  - Uncommon in United States
  - Represents approximately 4-7% of clinically evident thyroid carcinomas in Italy
- Age
  - Most common in 6th decade of life and later
- Gender
  - Female > Male

Site

- Anywhere in thyroid gland without specific localization

Presentation

- Thyroid mass of varying duration
  - Rapidly growing (neck) mass
  - Increasing growth in longstanding thyroid lesion
- At presentation, often locally advanced disease with extrathyroidal extension

Treatment

- Options, risks, complications
  - Treatment of choice includes
    - Total thyroidectomy, postoperative radioactive iodine, and supplemental thyroxine
  - PDTC considered advanced thyroid cancer
    - Typically resistant to conventional therapies
    - Does not respond to radioiodine
- Targeted therapy
  - Epigenetic drugs (deacetylase inhibitors and demethylating agents)
    - Target chromatin in rapidly dividing tumor cells and potentially restore normal cell functions
  - Deacetylases inhibitors modulate both epigenetic and multiple nonepigenetic mechanisms
    - Represent promising class of anticancer drugs effective against advanced thyroid cancer
  - Since multiple pathways need to be inhibited to substantially affect thyroid cancer growth
    - Likely significant increase in response rate will require combination drug therapies

POORLY DIFFERENTIATED THYROID CARCINOMA

Key Facts

Etiology/Pathogenesis

- Malignant epithelial thyroid neoplasm showing histologic and biologic features intermediate between differentiated thyroid carcinomas and undifferentiated (anaplastic) thyroid carcinoma
- Usually arise de novo but may transform from differentiated thyroid carcinomas (i.e., papillary or follicular carcinoma)

Clinical Issues

- At presentation, often locally advanced disease with extrathyroidal extension
- PDTC considered advanced thyroid cancer; typically resistant to conventional therapies and does not respond to radioiodine
- Death from disease is common but does not follow rapid demise as in undifferentiated (anaplastic) ca
  - 5-year survival rates: Approximately 50%

Microscopic Pathology

- Dominant growth patterns include insular, trabecular, solid
- Monotonous population of small cells with round hyperchromatic to vesicular nuclei, indistinct to small nucleoli, and indistinct cytoplasm
- Increased mitotic activity
- Necrosis commonly seen

Ancillary Tests

- Thyroglobulin, TTF-1, cytokeratins positive
  - Paranuclear dot-like thyroglobulin staining pattern may be present
- Calcitonin, neuroendocrine markers (chromogranin, synaptophysin, CD56) typically negative

---

  - Combination of either 2 epigenetic drugs or nonepigenetic chemotherapeutic and epigenetic drug
    - Used in attempt to increase response rates
  - Tyrosine-kinase inhibitor and inhibitors of proangiogenic factors
    - Have also shown promising results in treatment of advanced thyroid cancers

Prognosis

- Death from disease is common, but disease course does not follow rapid demise seen in association with undifferentiated (anaplastic) carcinoma
  - Death occurs after several years
    - 5-year survival rates approximately 50%
    - Few patients survive for > 5 years
    - Metastases to regional lymph nodes, lung, and bones are common
- Outcome influenced by variety of parameters including
  - Encapsulated poorly differentiated carcinomas have significantly improved overall survival compared to unencapsulated/infiltrative tumors
  - Extent of capsular invasion correlates with decreased progression-free survival
  - Tumors measuring > 4 cm have decreased progression-free survival
  - Age > 45 years associated with worse prognosis
  - Presence of extrathyroidal extension into perithyroidal soft tissues (e.g., trachea, others) correlates with decreased overall survival
  - Presence of metastatic disease to
    - Cervical lymph nodes
    - Presence of distant metastasis
  - PDTC with increased mitotic activity (≥ 5 mitoses/10 high-power fields) and necrosis found to be more aggressive than PDTC diagnosed purely on basis of growth characteristics (i.e., solid/trabecular/insular patterns)
    - Growth pattern &/or cell type have no bearing on prognosis
  - Additional adverse prognostic factors reported include
    - DNA aneuploidy and high S-phase factor significantly correlated
    - Absence of high-dose radioactive iodine (RAI) therapy
    - Advanced clinical stage
  - Expression of insulin-like growth factor II mRNA-binding protein 3 (IMP3) appears to be adverse prognostic factor

MACROSCOPIC FEATURES

General Features

- Solid and firm tumors often with associated necrosis
- Usually overtly infiltrative but may be encapsulated

Size

- Most measure > 5 cm in diameter

MICROSCOPIC PATHOLOGY

Histologic Features

- Dominant growth patterns include insular, trabecular, solid
  - Insular growth characterized by well-defined cell nests surrounded by thin fibrovascular septa
    - Nests are predominantly solid growth ± microfollicles
  - Trabecular growth characterized by cells arranged in cords or ribbons
  - Solid growth characterized by sheets of neoplastic cells
- Follicles ± colloid may be identified
  - Colloid may appear drop-like
- Monotonous population of small cells with round hyperchromatic to vesicular nuclei, indistinct to small nucleoli, and indistinct cytoplasm
- Oncocytic cytoplasmic cells may predominate (oncocytic variant)
- Increased mitotic activity identified

- Usually ≥ 3 mitoses per 10 high-power fields
- Atypical mitoses can be seen
- Necrosis commonly identified
  - May be focal or appear as confluent foci
  - May be prominent, creating peritheliomatous appearance
- Invasive growth common, including
  - Intrathyroidal invasion
  - Extrathyroidal extension
  - Angioinvasion
- Preference for diagnosing PDTC predicated on recognition of high-grade features only, including
  - Mitotic index and necrosis irrespective of growth pattern
- **Turin proposal** for diagnosis of PDTC includes
  - Presence of solid/trabecular/insular pattern of growth
  - Absence of conventional nuclear features of papillary carcinoma
  - Presence of at least one of the following features
    - Convoluted nuclei
    - Mitotic activity ≥ 3/10 high-power fields
    - Tumor necrosis
- Turin proposal might be less easily applicable for American and Japanese cases, possibly due to heterogeneous architectural and cytological features
- Minor component of differentiated thyroid carcinoma (follicular or papillary carcinoma) may be identified
- Transitional areas with undifferentiated (anaplastic) carcinoma may be present
  - In such cases, behavior may follow that of anaplastic (undifferentiated) carcinoma

ANCILLARY TESTS

Cytology

- High cellularity
- Large sheets of tumor cells showing microfollicular pattern or smaller sheets with insular, solid, or trabecular patterns
- Cellular aspirates composed of dyscohesive, small, monotonous, round to oval cells with
  - High nuclear to cytoplasmic ratio, severe crowding, nuclear hyperchromasia, coarsely or finely granular chromatin, small nucleoli, poorly outlined cytoplasm
  - Very scanty colloid
  - Plasmacytoid cells with eccentric hyperchromatic nuclei, smooth nuclear contours, small to inconspicuous nucleoli, and finely granular, ill-defined cytoplasm may be identified
  - Necrosis and mitotic figures may or may not be identified

Histochemistry

- Periodic acid-Schiff
  - May be useful in identification of colloid
  - Colloid appears red
    - Colloid may appear drop-like and be easily overlooked
    - PAS stain (&/or thyroglobulin) helpful in identification of colloid

Immunohistochemistry

- Thyroglobulin positive
  - Variable (cytoplasmic) staining
    - Positive foci adjacent to negative foci
  - May show paranuclear dot-like staining pattern
- Thyroid transcription factor 1 (TTF-1) positive
  - Diffuse and strong (nuclear) staining
- Cytokeratins (AE1/AE3, CAM5.2, others) positive
- Insulin-like growth factor II mRNA-binding protein 3 (IMP3) positive (cytoplasmic)
- Calcitonin negative
- Neuroendocrine markers (chromogranin, synaptophysin, CD56) typically negative
- Bcl-2 positive in > 80% of cases
- Ki-67 (MIB-1) shows high proliferative index

Molecular Genetics

- *TP53* and β-*catenin* mutations
  - Found with increasing incidence in poorly differentiated and undifferentiated (anaplastic) carcinomas but not in well-differentiated tumors
  - May serve as direct molecular trigger of tumor dedifferentiation
  - Found in up to 30% of PDTC
- *RAS* mutations found
  - Predominantly N-RAS
- *IMP3* expression
- *BRAF* mutations not detected
  - Supports assumption that pure insular and insular-like PDTCs more closely related to follicular carcinoma than thyroid papillary carcinoma
- No genetic mutations or chromosomal abnormalities unique for PDTC and not present in well-differentiated or undifferentiated (anaplastic) carcinomas

DIFFERENTIAL DIAGNOSIS

Thyroid Undifferentiated (Anaplastic) Carcinoma

- Clinical presentation: Rapidly enlarging neck or thyroid mass occurring over short periods of time (weeks to months)
- Growth patterns include solid, fascicular, and storiform
- Most common cell types include
  - Spindle (sarcomatoid), squamous, giant cell
  - Other less common types/variants include
    - Lymphoepithelioma-like
    - Small cell type
    - Rhabdoid cell type
    - Paucicellular
    - Angiomatoid
- Irrespective of cell type, neoplastic cellular infiltrate is poorly differentiated without evidence of colloid formation
  - Immunohistochemistry
    - Cytokeratin reactivity most useful marker with reactivity identified in majority of cases
    - Thyroglobulin and TTF-1 reactivity extremely variable, usually absent, generally not helpful in diagnosis

- Calcitonin, chromogranin, synaptophysin negative
- Vimentin reactivity usually present in all cellular components

- Extremely high mortality rates irrespective of therapy
  - Death often occurs within short periods of time (6 months)
  - 5-year survival rate < 14%
  - Median survival rates: 2.5-6 months

Papillary Carcinoma, Solid Variant

- Shows constellation of nuclear alterations diagnostic for thyroid papillary carcinoma including
  - Enlargement, variation in size and shape, clear to dispersed chromatin, crowding/overlapping, grooves and inclusions
- Diffuse thyroglobulin reactivity

Thyroid Medullary Carcinoma

- Growth patterns may include insular, trabecular, solid
- May have increased mitotic activity and necrosis
- Shows characteristic nuclear chromatin (stippled or "salt and pepper")
- Immunoreactive for calcitonin, neuroendocrine markers (chromogranin, synaptophysin, others), TTF-1, cytokeratins
- Thyroglobulin negative

SELECTED REFERENCES

1. Asioli S et al: Poorly differentiated carcinoma of the thyroid: validation of the Turin proposal and analysis of IMP3 expression. Mod Pathol. 23(9):1269-78, 2010
2. Catalano MG et al: Emerging molecular therapies of advanced thyroid cancer. Mol Aspects Med. 31(2):215-26, 2010
3. Fat I et al: An Insular Variant of Poorly Differentiated Thyroid Carcinoma. Endocr Pract. Epub ahead of print, 2010
4. Rivera M et al: Encapsulated thyroid tumors of follicular cell origin with high grade features (high mitotic rate/ tumor necrosis): a clinicopathologic and molecular study. Hum Pathol. 41(2):172-80, 2010
5. Volante M et al: Poorly differentiated thyroid carcinoma: 5 years after the 2004 WHO classification of endocrine tumours. Endocr Pathol. 21(1):1-6, 2010
6. Bongiovanni M et al: Poorly differentiated thyroid carcinoma: a cytologic-histologic review. Adv Anat Pathol. 16(5):283-9, 2009
7. Pacini F et al: Targeted therapy in radioiodine refractory thyroid cancer. Q J Nucl Med Mol Imaging. 53(5):520-5, 2009
8. Pita JM et al: Gene expression profiling associated with the progression to poorly differentiated thyroid carcinomas. Br J Cancer. 101(10):1782-91, 2009
9. Pinto AE et al: Aneuploidy and high S-phase as biomarkers of poor clinical outcome in poorly differentiated and anaplastic thyroid carcinoma. Oncol Rep. 20(4):913-9, 2008
10. Volante M et al: Poorly differentiated thyroid carcinoma: diagnostic features and controversial issues. Endocr Pathol. 19(3):150-5, 2008
11. Jung TS et al: Clinical features and prognostic factors for survival in patients with poorly differentiated thyroid carcinoma and comparison to the patients with the aggressive variants of papillary thyroid carcinoma. Endocr J. 54(2):265-74, 2007
12. Lin JD et al: Clinical characteristics of poorly differentiated thyroid carcinomas compared with those of classical papillary thyroid carcinomas. Clin Endocrinol (Oxf). 66(2):224-8, 2007
13. Sanders EM Jr et al: An evidence-based review of poorly differentiated thyroid cancer. World J Surg. 31(5):934-45, 2007
14. Volante M et al: Poorly differentiated thyroid carcinoma: the Turin proposal for the use of uniform diagnostic criteria and an algorithmic diagnostic approach. Am J Surg Pathol. 31(8):1256-64, 2007
15. Hiltzik D et al: Poorly differentiated thyroid carcinomas defined on the basis of mitosis and necrosis: a clinicopathologic study of 58 patients. Cancer. 106(6):1286-95, 2006
16. Nikiforov YE: Genetic alterations involved in the transition from well-differentiated to poorly differentiated and anaplastic thyroid carcinomas. Endocr Pathol. 15(4):319-27, 2004
17. Sakamoto A: Definition of poorly differentiated carcinoma of the thyroid: the Japanese experience. Endocr Pathol. 15(4):307-11, 2004
18. Soares P et al: BRAF mutations typical of papillary thyroid carcinoma are more frequently detected in undifferentiated than in insular and insular-like poorly differentiated carcinomas. Virchows Arch. 444(6):572-6, 2004
19. Volante M et al: Poorly differentiated carcinomas of the thyroid with trabecular, insular, and solid patterns: a clinicopathologic study of 183 patients. Cancer. 100(5):950-7, 2004
20. Volante M et al: Prognostic factors of clinical interest in poorly differentiated carcinomas of the thyroid. Endocr Pathol. 15(4):313-7, 2004
21. Sobrinho-Simões M et al: Poorly differentiated carcinomas of the thyroid gland: a review of the clinicopathologic features of a series of 28 cases of a heterogeneous, clinically aggressive group of thyroid tumors. Int J Surg Pathol. 10(2):123-31, 2002
22. Nishida T et al: Clinicopathological significance of poorly differentiated thyroid carcinoma. Am J Surg Pathol. 23(2):205-11, 1999
23. Pilotti S et al: Insular carcinoma: a distinct de novo entity among follicular carcinomas of the thyroid gland. Am J Surg Pathol. 21(12):1466-73, 1997
24. Ashfaq R et al: Papillary and follicular thyroid carcinomas with an insular component. Cancer. 73(2):416-23, 1994
25. Papotti M et al: Poorly differentiated thyroid carcinomas with primordial cell component. A group of aggressive lesions sharing insular, trabecular, and solid patterns. Am J Surg Pathol. 17(3):291-301, 1993
26. Zakowski MF et al: Cytologic features of poorly differentiated "insular" carcinoma of the thyroid. A case report. Acta Cytol. 36(4):523-6, 1992
27. Flynn SD et al: Poorly differentiated ("insular") carcinoma of the thyroid gland: an aggressive subset of differentiated thyroid neoplasms. Surgery. 104(6):963-70, 1988
28. Carcangiu ML et al: Poorly differentiated ("insular") thyroid carcinoma. A reinterpretation of Langhans' "wuchernde Struma". Am J Surg Pathol. 8(9):655-68, 1984

POORLY DIFFERENTIATED THYROID CARCINOMA

Microscopic Features and Ancillary Techniques

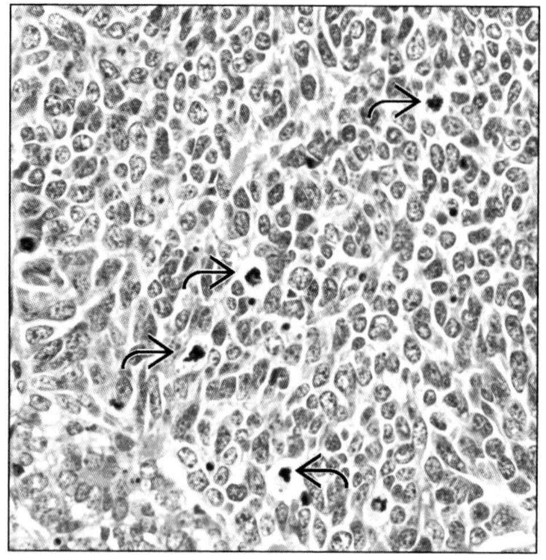

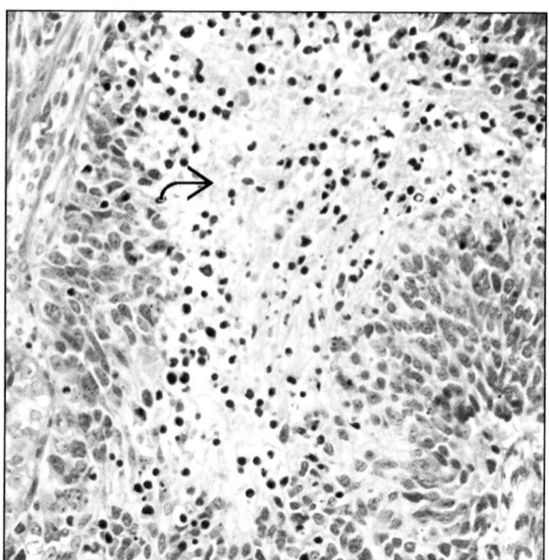

(Left) *Poorly differentiated thyroid carcinoma is characterized by diffuse (sheet-like) growth, moderate nuclear pleomorphism, and marked increase in mitotic activity ⮫.* ***(Right)*** *Confluent focus of necrosis is identified ⮫. The diagnosis of PDTC can be made in a thyroid neoplasm with increased mitotic activity and foci of necrosis irrespective of the growth patterns (e.g., insular, others). Insular growth can be seen in both benign thyroid tumors and differentiated thyroid carcinomas.*

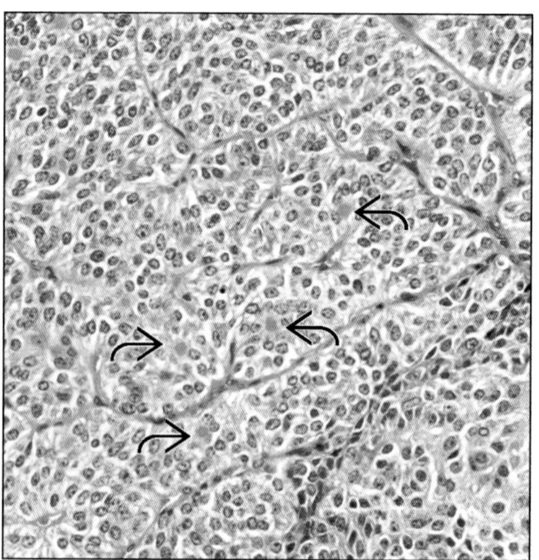

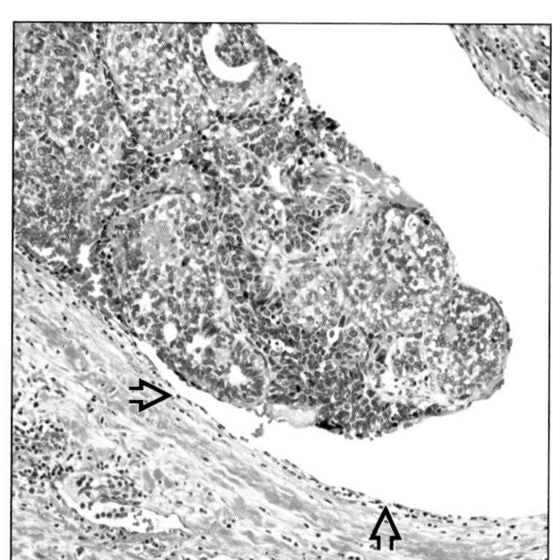

(Left) *Insular growth composed of tumor nests is separated by fibrovascular stroma. The neoplastic cells are rather monotonous appearing with scattered microfollicles containing identifiable drop-like colloid ⮫.* ***(Right)*** *Invasive growth is often present, including lymph-vascular invasion characterized by tumor colonization of endothelial-lined ⇨ vascular spaces. In addition, there often is intrathyroidal invasion; extrathyroidal invasion may be present as well (not shown).*

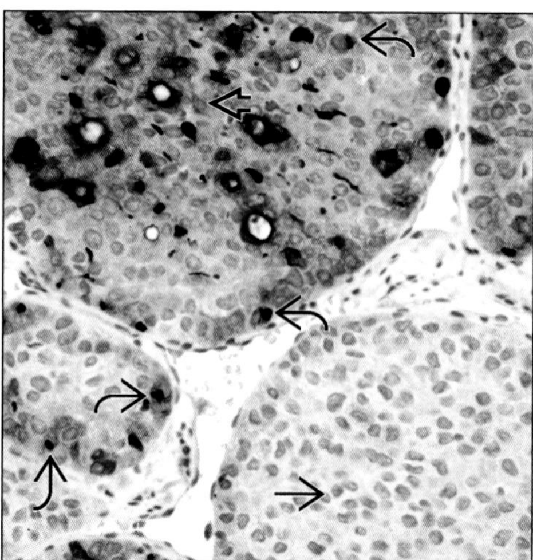

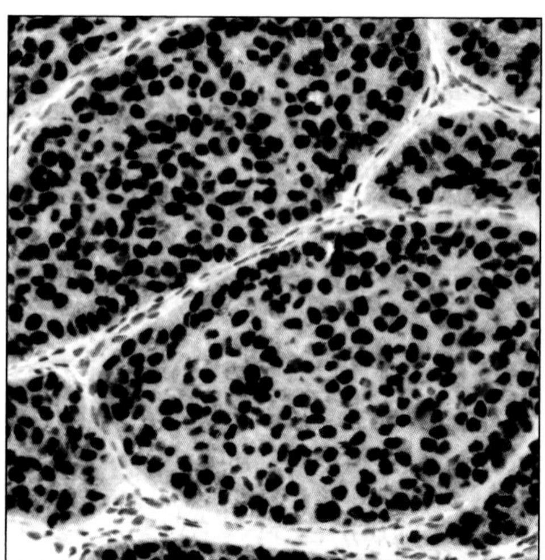

(Left) *Variable thyroglobulin immunoreactivity is present, including tumor nests with thyroglobulin staining ⇨ adjacent to tumor nests without thyroglobulin reactivity →. Dot-like paranuclear thyroglobulin staining is present ⮫, a feature seen in PDTC.* ***(Right)*** *Diffuse TTF-1 (nuclear) immunoreactivity is present. In contrast, undifferentiated (anaplastic) thyroid carcinoma typically does not express immunoreactivity for thyroglobulin and TTF-1.*

Differential Diagnosis

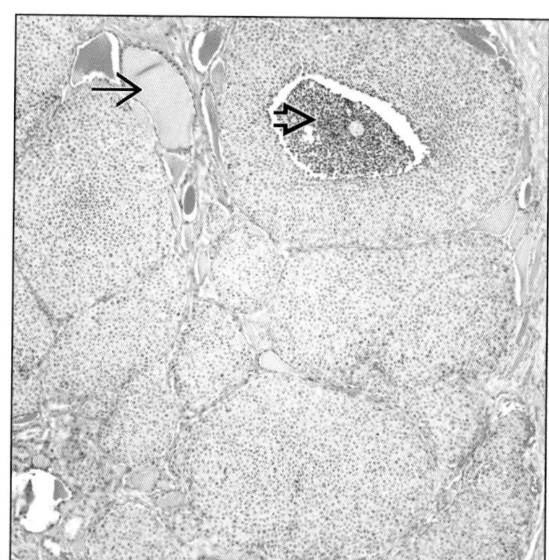

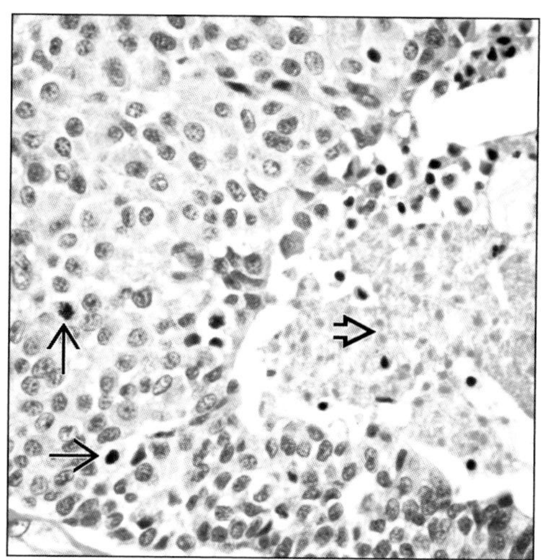

(Left) *In addition to undifferentiated (anaplastic) thyroid carcinoma, the differential diagnosis for PDTC may include thyroid medullary carcinoma, which shows cell nests and foci of necrosis* ➲*. Intervening nonneoplastic colloid-filled follicles are present* ➔*.* ***(Right)*** *Rather monotonous-appearing cell population is seen with dispersed nuclear chromatin, absence of colloid, increased mitotic activity* ➔ *and necrosis* ➲*. Differentiation requires immunohistochemical staining.*

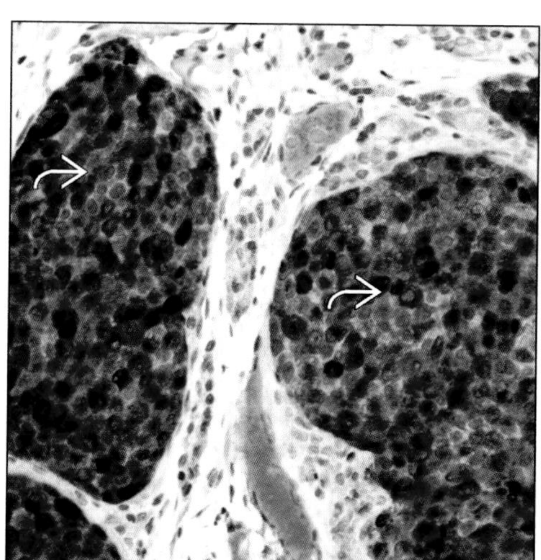

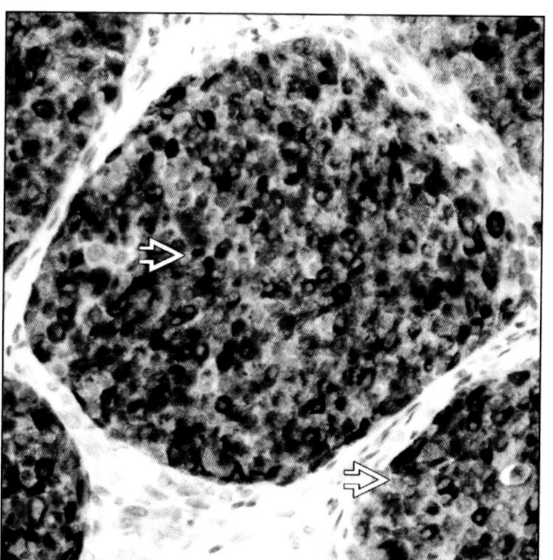

(Left) *The neoplastic cells of thyroid medullary carcinoma are calcitonin positive* ➦*.* ***(Right)*** *The neoplastic cells of thyroid medullary carcinoma are reactive for neuroendocrine markers, including chromogranin* ➲*, as well as synaptophysin (not shown). Like PDTC, thyroid medullary carcinoma will be immunoreactive for cytokeratins (not shown). The presence of calcitonin (and absence of thyroglobulin) is diagnostic for thyroid medullary carcinoma and differentiates it from PDTC.*

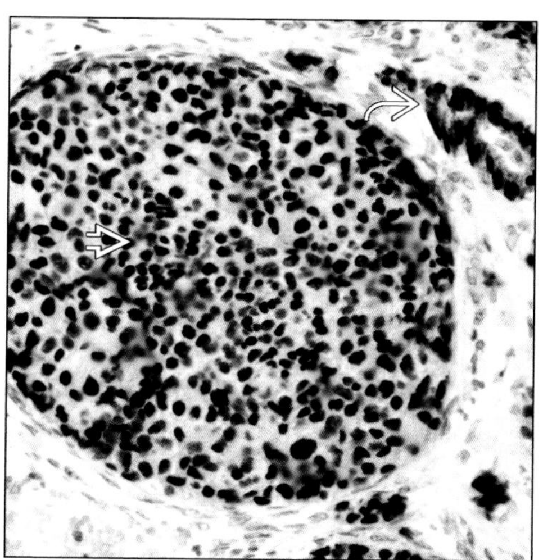

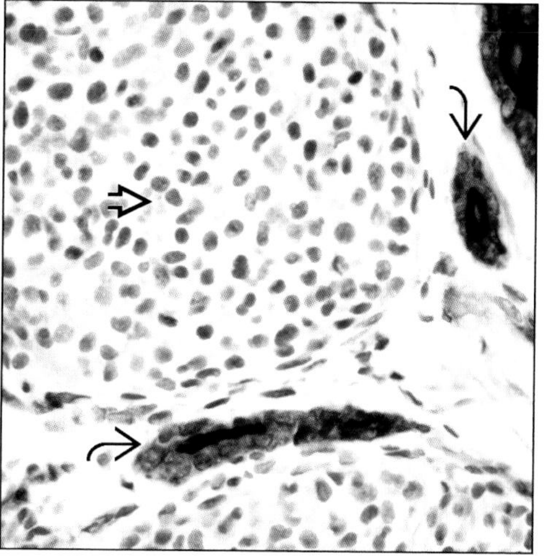

(Left) *Thyroid medullary carcinomas are (diffusely) immunoreactive for TTF-1 (nuclear)* ➲*. Similar to cytokeratin reactivity, TTF-1 immunoreactivity is present in both thyroid medullary carcinomas and PDTC and, as such, does not assist in differentiating thyroid medullary carcinoma from PDTC. Note TTF-1 reactivity in benign thyroid follicles* ➦*.* ***(Right)*** *Thyroid medullary carcinomas lack thyroglobulin immunoreactivity* ➲*, but it is present in benign thyroid follicles* ➦*.*

UNDIFFERENTIATED (ANAPLASTIC) CARCINOMA

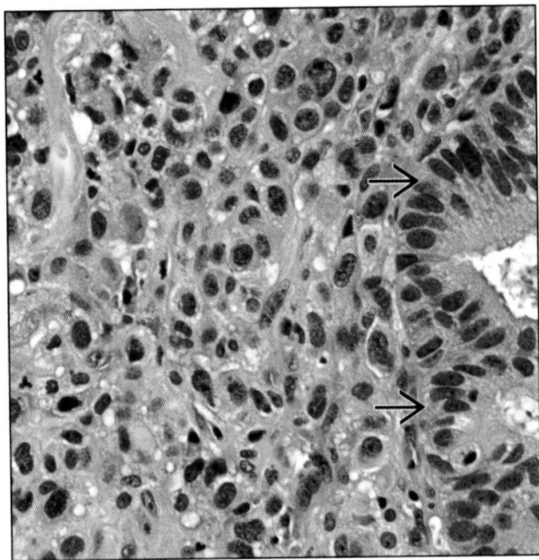

There is a pleomorphic epithelial proliferation immediately adjacent to a papillary carcinoma →. This is a typical appearance for an undifferentiated carcinoma of the thyroid.

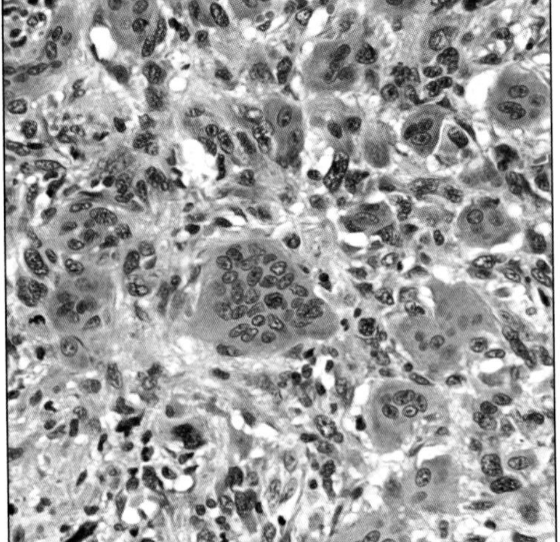

Osteoclastic-type giant cells are seen. The nuclei are relatively bland, aggregated within the cell. These cells are CD68-positive histiocytes. The malignant part is between these cells.

TERMINOLOGY

Synonyms

- Anaplastic carcinoma
- Spindle and giant cell carcinoma
- Sarcomatoid carcinoma
- Pleomorphic carcinoma
- Dedifferentiated carcinoma
- Metaplastic carcinoma
- Carcinosarcoma

Definitions

- Highly aggressive malignant thyroid neoplasm composed of undifferentiated cells that exhibit immunohistochemical or ultrastructural epithelial differentiation

ETIOLOGY/PATHOGENESIS

Environmental Exposure

- Radiation
  - ~ 10% of patients report radiation exposure
- Iodine deficiency (for at least 20 years)

Thyroid Disease

- Preexisting benign or malignant thyroid disease in nearly all cases
  - Longstanding goiter (nodules)
    - Often decades
    - Constant stimulation improves odds of transformation
- Transformation (dedifferentiation) of preexisting differentiated carcinoma
  - Papillary, follicular, or poorly differentiated carcinoma
    - Identified in up to 80% of undifferentiated carcinoma (UC)
    - Papillary carcinoma is most common (80%)

Pathogenesis

- Thyroid follicular epithelial cell origin
  - Difficult to show origin in many cases

CLINICAL ISSUES

Epidemiology

- Incidence
  - Represents ~ 2% of all thyroid gland malignancies
  - Approximately 1-2/1,000,000 population annually
  - Higher in endemic goiter regions (iodine deficiency), Europe, and low socioeconomic status
- Age
  - Elderly
  - Vast majority are > 65 years at diagnosis
- Gender
  - Female > Male (1.5:1)

Site

- Most are single (60%) lobe tumors
- Multifocal (40%) or bilateral (25%)

Presentation

- Rapidly expanding neck mass
  - Exceedingly fast tumor doubling: 1-2 weeks
  - Fixed and hard mass
- Usually long history of thyroid disease
- Hoarseness, dysphagia, vocal cord paralysis, cervical pain, and dyspnea are common
  - Invades into soft tissues (muscle, fat and nerves), esophagus, trachea
- Lymphadenopathy common
- Hyperthyroidism is uncommon; results from rapid destruction of follicles with hormone release

Laboratory Tests

- Leukocytosis can be seen (secretion of macrophage colony-stimulating factor)

UNDIFFERENTIATED (ANAPLASTIC) CARCINOMA

Key Facts

Terminology
- Highly aggressive malignancy of undifferentiated cells

Etiology/Pathogenesis
- Preexisting benign or malignant thyroid disease in nearly all cases, with transformation of preexisting carcinoma

Clinical Issues
- Majority > 65 years, present with rapidly enlarging neck mass
- Grave overall prognosis: > 95% die from disease even with multimodality therapy

Macroscopic Features
- Fleshy to firm mass, typically completely replacing thyroid parenchyma, ~ 6 cm

Microscopic Pathology
- Extrathyroidal extension, lymph-vascular invasion
- Significant necrosis and hemorrhage
- Variety of patterns: Sheet-like, storiform, fascicular, angiomatoid, meningothelial
- Poorly differentiated cells, polygonal, pleomorphic, spindle, giant, epithelioid, squamoid
- Profound pleomorphism, increased mitotic activity

Ancillary Tests
- Positive: Cytokeratin, p63, vimentin, EMA
- Negative: Thyroglobulin, TTF-1

Top Differential Diagnoses
- Metastases, primary sarcoma, melanoma, lymphoma, primary carcinoma, Riedel thyroiditis

Treatment
- Options, risks, complications
  - Multimodality therapy required
  - Targeted therapy (such as gelfitinib, an EGFR inhibitor and bevacizumab, an antibody against VEGF-R) shows promise
- Surgical approaches
  - Value of surgery is yielding diagnostic material and palliation
    - Debulking, as resectability is unlikely
  - May be valuable in limited disease cases
- Adjuvant therapy
  - Combination chemotherapy (doxorubicin, cisplatin)
  - Response is poor at best
- Radiation
  - Radiation (external beam, 3 dimensional conformal therapy, intensity modulated radiotherapy)
    - Hyperfractionation or accelerated dosing regimens improves efficacy
    - Rapid doubling rate requires accelerated dosing
    - Chemosensitization (doxorubicin) may help
    - Careful monitoring to minimize toxicity

Prognosis
- Rapidly progressive local disease
- Many patients have lymph node disease at presentation
  - Up to 50% cervical adenopathy
- Metastases to distant sites common
  - Up to 50% at presentation
    - Lungs (50%), bones (15%), brain (10%)
- Grave overall prognosis
  - > 95% die from disease
  - Median survival: 3 months
  - Accounts for > 50% of all thyroid cancer deaths
- Better prognosis in cases where anaplastic carcinoma is confined to encapsulated tumor or minor component of another tumor
- Worse prognosis if patients > 60 years, male, have tumors > 5 cm, or have extensive local disease

IMAGE FINDINGS

General Features
- Computed tomography shows extent of disease
- Infiltrative (carotid and internal jugular), heterogeneous mass with irregular borders, and necrosis
- Calcifications may be seen

MACROSCOPIC FEATURES

General Features
- Fleshy to firm mass, typically completely replacing thyroid parenchyma
- Infiltrative with irregular borders
  - Extrathyroidal extension: Soft tissue, larynx, trachea, esophagus, lymph nodes
- Pale, white-tan, brown
- Commonly variegated, with areas of necrosis and hemorrhage

Sections to Be Submitted
- Adequate sampling required to find preexisting or coexisting carcinoma

Size
- Range: 1-20 cm
- Mean: 6 cm

MICROSCOPIC PATHOLOGY

Histologic Features
- Up to 50% of tumors show extrathyroidal extension
  - Local extension into soft tissues or other organs
  - Effacement of thyroid parenchyma
- Extensive lymph-vascular invasion
  - Vessel walls invaded or colonized and destroyed
- Significant coagulative-type necrosis, hemorrhage, and degeneration
- Colloid is absent, but "entrapment" of follicles can be seen at periphery

UNDIFFERENTIATED (ANAPLASTIC) CARCINOMA

- Desmoplastic stroma may be present
- Variety of patterns: Sheet-like, storiform, fascicular, angiomatoid, meningothelial
- Poorly differentiated cells
  - Polygonal, pleomorphic, spindle, giant, epithelioid, squamoid
  - Noticeable variation within tumors and between cases
- Profound pleomorphism
- Tumor giant cells and osteoclast-like giant cells are common
- Increased mitotic figures, including atypical forms, and pyknotic cells
- Prominent acute inflammatory infiltrate may be present

Variants

- **Spindle cell variant**
  - Most common variant, with high-grade sarcoma pattern (fascicles, storiform)
- **Pleomorphic giant cell variant**
  - 2nd most common, comprised of sheets of profoundly pleomorphic/bizarre cells, often multinucleated, with intracytoplasmic hyaline globules
- **Squamoid variant**
  - Tumor shows nests and sheets of squamoid cells associated with desmoplastic stroma
  - Cytoplasm is dense, opacified, and eosinophilic, occasionally show intercellular bridges and dyskeratosis
- **Osteoclastic variant**
  - Large numbers of multinucleated, nonneoplastic, osteoclast-like giant cells (CD68-positive histiocytes)
- **Angiomatoid variant**
  - Anastomosing vascular spaces, branching "staghorn" or hemangiopericytoma-like pattern, including erythrocyte extravasation
- **Carcinosarcoma variant**
  - Carcinoma and sarcoma combined (osteosarcoma or chondrosarcoma most common)
- **Paucicellular variant**
  - Decreased cellularity with increased fibrosis and inflammation (mimic of Riedel thyroiditis)
  - Highly atypical single spindled cells
- **Rhabdoid variant**
  - Cells with dense hyaline-type cytoplasm causing eccentric nucleus placement

ANCILLARY TESTS

Cytology

- Highly cellular
- Single cells, clusters, or sheets
- Marked nuclear pleomorphism: Including squamoid, giant cell, spindle cell
  - Abundant cytoplasm
- Bizarre, single or multiple nuclei
  - Prominent nucleoli
- Mitotic figures easily identified
- Background of necrotic debris and neutrophils
  - Colloid is usually absent

- Sometimes a differentiated component may be present (dual cell pattern)

Immunohistochemistry

- Keratin in up to 80% of cases
  - Limited to focal areas of weak reactivity
  - AE1/AE3 or CAM5.2 give best results (cocktails)
- EMA in 30-50% of cases
  - Limited to focal areas of weak reactivity
- p63 positive in most cases (70%)
- Vimentin strongly and diffusely positive in nearly all cases
- CEA (~ 10% of cases), especially in squamoid areas
- Thyroglobulin and TTF-1 are rarely positive
- p53 strongly and diffusely immunoreactive
- Negative: Desmin, myogenin, MYOD1, smooth muscle actin, FVIIIRAg, CD31, CD34; S100 protein, HMB-45, Melan-A, CD45RB, ALK
- Ki-67 (MIB-1) usually high (~ 50%)

Flow Cytometry

- Nearly 100% of tumors are aneuploid
- Not technically "monoclonal," as there are many subclones that expand

Cytogenetics

- Complex and progressive accumulation of chromosomal alterations (numerical and structural aberrations)
  - Most common gains &/or losses: 1p, 3p, 5q, 8, and 5p
  - Reinforces multi-step dedifferentiation process
- Most frequent regions of LOH are 1q, 9p, 17p, 16p, 17q, and 18q
- Mutations can be seen in differentiated and dedifferentiated tumors (*BRAF*, *RAS*)
  - Early events in thyroid tumorigenesis, predisposing to additional events leading to undifferentiated transformation
  - *RAS* seen in up to 60% of tumors
    - Present in differentiated and undifferentiated portions
  - *BRAF* seen in about 25% of tumors
    - Papillary carcinoma usually found
    - Present in differentiated and undifferentiated portions
- Most common in undifferentiated tumors: *TP53* and *β-catenin*
  - *TP53* (up to 80% of tumors) but only in undifferentiated part
    - Accumulates in nucleus, showing increased immunohistochemical staining
  - *β-catenin* (up to 65% of tumors)
    - Accumulates in nucleus due to altered degradation

Electron Microscopy

- Rare tight junctions and desmosomes, complex cytoplasmic interdigitations along with tonofilaments
- Apical microvilli rare or absent
- Basal lamina is often incomplete

DIFFERENTIAL DIAGNOSIS

Metastases

- Biopsy of undifferentiated tumor, clinical history, and radiographic information helps make separation
- Metastatic tumors to thyroid gland
  - Poorly differentiated carcinoma from distant site (lung, colon, breast, gastrointestinal system)
  - Melanoma and sarcoma are considerations
- Pertinent immunohistochemical panel often helps

Primary Sarcoma

- Primary thyroid sarcomas: Leiomyosarcoma, angiosarcoma, malignant peripheral nerve sheath tumor, synovial sarcoma
  - Patterns of growth, cytologic appearance, immunohistochemistry, and molecular studies valuable

Melanoma

- Pigmentation helps, along with positive immunohistochemistry for S100 protein, HMB-45, Melan-A, tyrosinase
- Metastatic melanoma frequently positive for *BRAF* and *NRAS* mutations

Lymphoma

- Diffuse large B-cell lymphoma most common
- Lacks anaplastic appearance; is positive with CD45RB and CD20, among other hematopoietic markers

Thyroid Carcinomas

- In a tumor showing differentiated and undifferentiated foci, use undifferentiated diagnosis
- May show areas of transition from one to the other
- **Poorly differentiated carcinoma**
  - Solid, trabecular, or insular growth of monotonous, nonpleomorphic cells, showing increased mitotic figures and necrosis with relative absence of colloid
  - Keratin and TTF-1 usually maintained
- **Medullary thyroid carcinoma**
  - Young patients, often with bilateral tumors
  - May lose calcitonin and CEA reactivity but shows *RAS* mutations
- **Spindle epithelial tumor with thymus-like differentiation (SETTLE)**
  - Spindled pattern, but usually younger patients, lacks significant pleomorphism, increased mitotic figures, and necrosis
- **Carcinoma with thymus-like elements (CASTLE)**
  - Typically shows squamoid appearance within lobular or nested growth separated by fibrous stroma, lacking significant atypia; CD5(+)

Riedel Thyroiditis

- Heavy fibrosis, inflammation, and vasculitis without cellular atypia
  - p53 may be useful in highlighting scattered highly atypical cells

STAGING

Definition

- All are T4 tumors by definition
  - T4a: Intrathyroidal tumor
  - T4b: Gross extrathyroid extension
- Separated into IVA, IVB, and IVC (latter with distant metastases)

SELECTED REFERENCES

1. Smallridge RC et al: Anaplastic thyroid cancer: molecular pathogenesis and emerging therapies. Endocr Relat Cancer. 16(1):17-44, 2009
2. Chiacchio S et al: Anaplastic thyroid cancer: prevalence, diagnosis and treatment. Minerva Endocrinol. 33(4):341-57, 2008
3. Neff RL et al: Anaplastic thyroid cancer. Endocrinol Metab Clin North Am. 37(2):525-38, xi, 2008
4. Albores-Saavedra J et al: Changing patterns in the incidence and survival of thyroid cancer with follicular phenotype--papillary, follicular, and anaplastic: a morphological and epidemiological study. Endocr Pathol. 18(1):1-7, 2007
5. Cornett WR et al: Anaplastic thyroid carcinoma: an overview. Curr Oncol Rep. 9(2):152-8, 2007
6. Lang BH et al: Surgical options in undifferentiated thyroid carcinoma. World J Surg. 31(5):969-77, 2007
7. Pudney D et al: Clinical experience of the multimodality management of anaplastic thyroid cancer and literature review. Thyroid. 17(12):1243-50, 2007
8. Are C et al: Anaplastic thyroid carcinoma: biology, pathogenesis, prognostic factors, and treatment approaches. Ann Surg Oncol. 13(4):453-64, 2006
9. Jiang JY et al: Prognostic factors of anaplastic thyroid carcinoma. J Endocrinol Invest. 29(1):11-7, 2006
10. Papi G et al: Primary spindle cell lesions of the thyroid gland; an overview. Am J Clin Pathol. 125 Suppl:S95-123, 2006
11. Wang Y et al: Clinical outcome of anaplastic thyroid carcinoma treated with radiotherapy of once- and twice-daily fractionation regimens. Cancer. 107(8):1786-92, 2006
12. Goutsouliak V et al: Anaplastic thyroid cancer in British Columbia 1985-1999: a population-based study. Clin Oncol (R Coll Radiol). 17(2):75-8, 2005
13. Quiros RM et al: Evidence that one subset of anaplastic thyroid carcinomas are derived from papillary carcinomas due to BRAF and p53 mutations. Cancer. 103(11):2261-8, 2005
14. Nikiforov YE: Genetic alterations involved in the transition from well-differentiated to poorly differentiated and anaplastic thyroid carcinomas. Endocr Pathol. 15(4):319-27, 2004
15. Veness MJ et al: Anaplastic thyroid carcinoma: dismal outcome despite current treatment approach. ANZ J Surg. 74(7):559-62, 2004
16. Heron DE et al: Anaplastic thyroid carcinoma: comparison of conventional radiotherapy and hyperfractionation chemoradiotherapy in two groups. Am J Clin Oncol. 25(5):442-6, 2002
17. Fadda G et al: Histology and fine-needle aspiration cytology of malignant thyroid neoplasms. Rays. 25(2):139-50, 2000
18. al-Sobhi SS et al: Management of thyroid carcinosarcoma. Surgery. 122(3):548-52, 1997

UNDIFFERENTIATED (ANAPLASTIC) CARCINOMA

Radiographic, Gross, and Microscopic Features

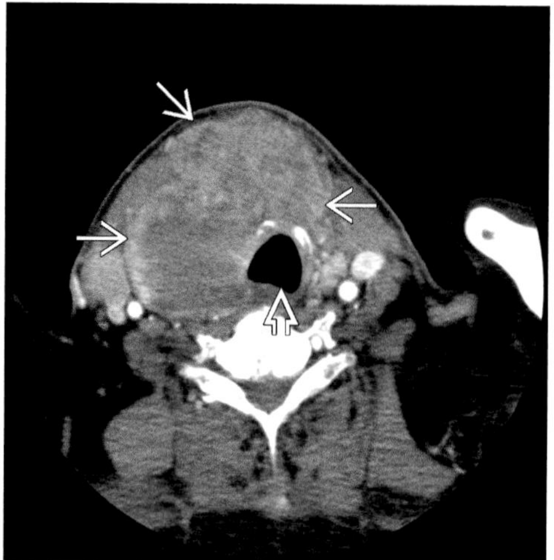

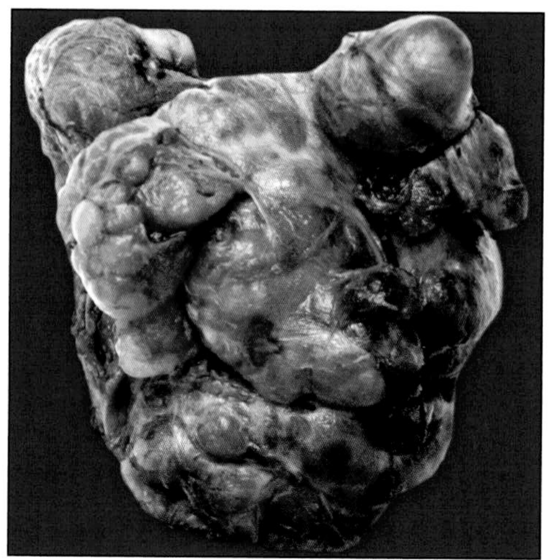

*(**Left**) There is a large mass almost entirely replacing the right thyroid lobe, expanding out into the adjacent soft tissue ➡. Note the tracheal deviation ⇨, although the lumen is free of tumor. Lymph node metastases are present. (**Right**) This lobe of the thyroid gland is greatly expanded by a multinodular and bosselated neoplasm. The tumor measures approximately 9 cm in greatest dimension.*

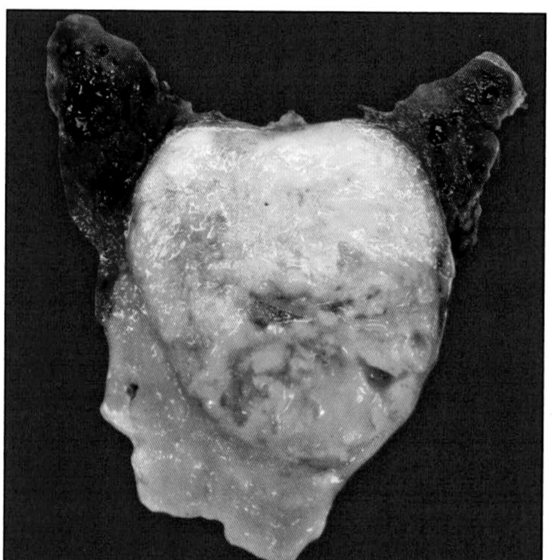

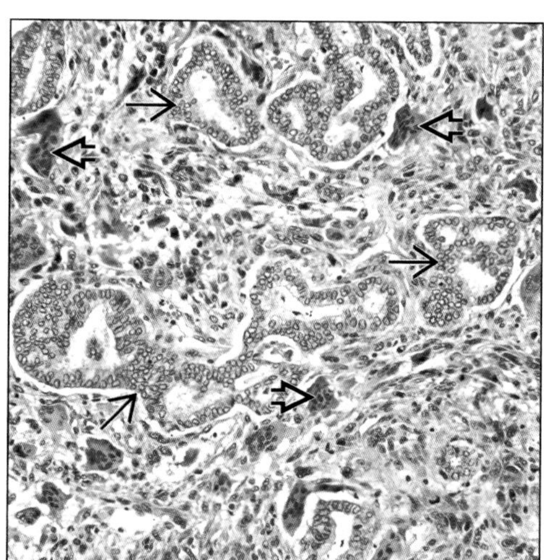

*(**Left**) The cut surface shows the thyroid parenchyma invaded by a neoplastic proliferation. The tumor is fleshy, with a yellow-tan appearance. Areas of degeneration and hemorrhage are noted. The tumor expands into the parenchyma and extends into the surrounding soft tissues. (**Right**) There are isolated areas of papillary carcinoma → juxtaposed to the pleomorphic proliferation. A number of osteoclastic-type giant cells are also present ⇨. The tumor is spindled to epithelioid.*

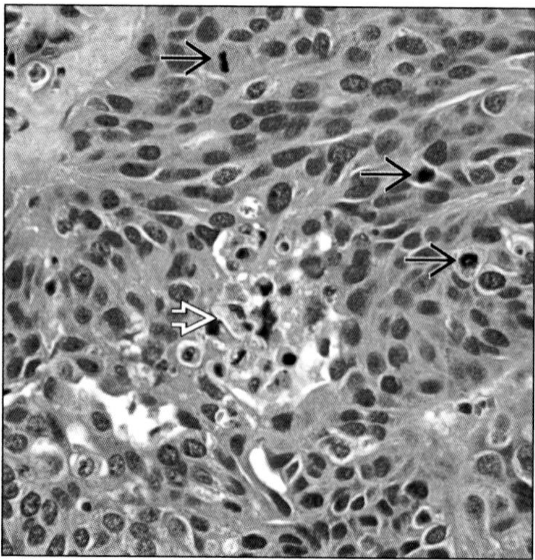

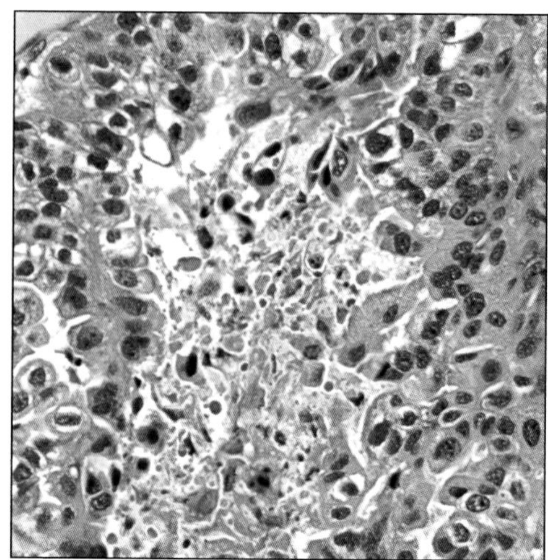

*(**Left**) An epidermoid proliferation occupies this portion of an undifferentiated carcinoma. A central area of necrosis is noted ⇨. Mitotic figures are easily identified →. (**Right**) The areas of necrosis frequently contain cells with ghost images. In this case, areas suggestive of squamous differentiation are noted. The epithelial cells in the adjacent area show moderate pleomorphism and a syncytial architecture.*

Microscopic Features and Ancillary Techniques

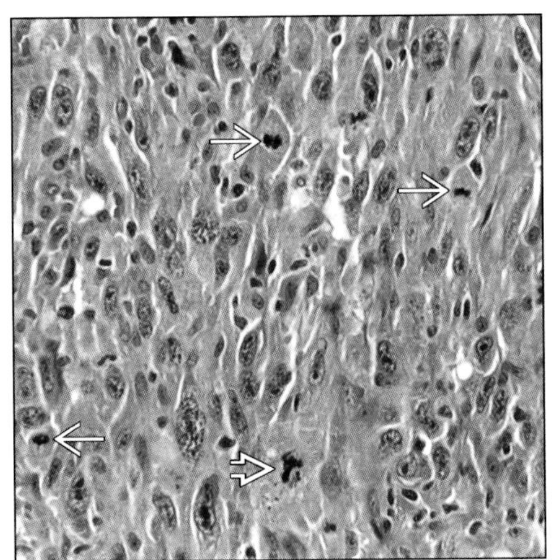

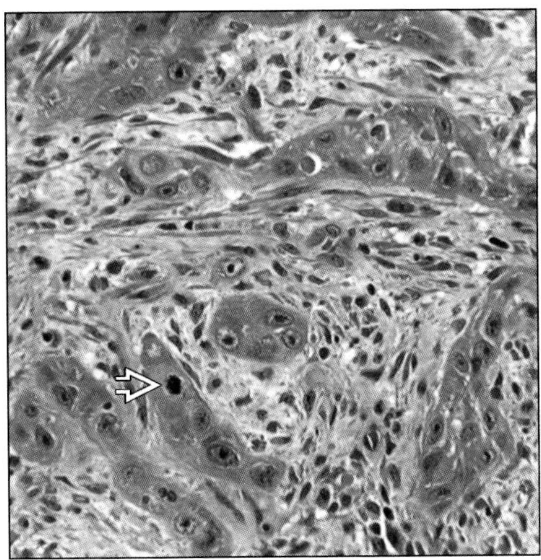

(Left) *A fascicle comprised of spindled cells is noted in this undifferentiated carcinoma. There is significant pleomorphism as well as numerous mitotic figures ➡, including atypical forms ➡.* ***(Right)*** *This epidermoid proliferation is intimately associated with a desmoplastic stroma. This is quite characteristic for this variant of undifferentiated carcinoma. Note the mitosis ➡. The cells are pleomorphic with prominent nucleoli.*

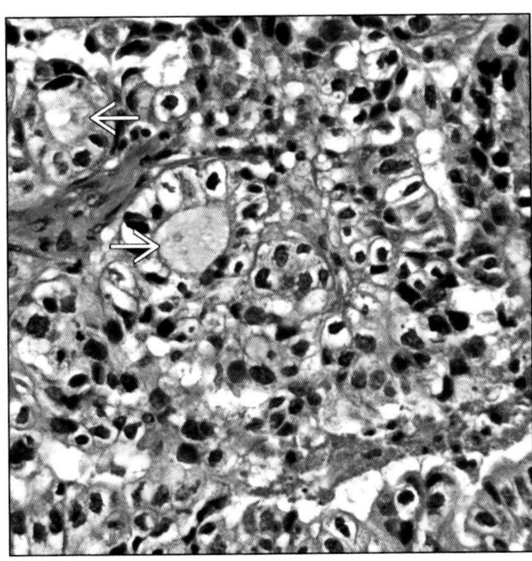

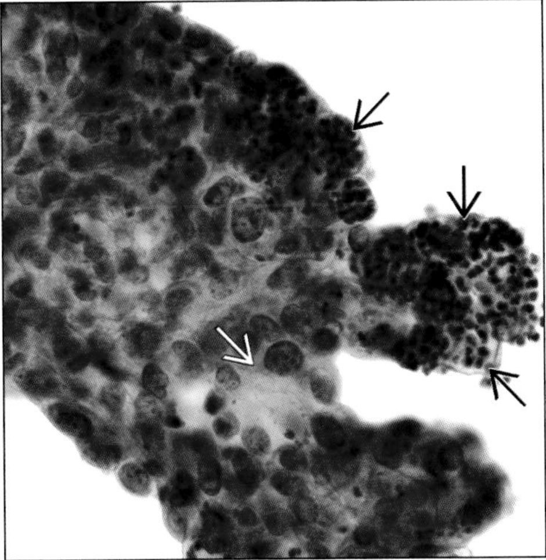

(Left) *The cells are arranged in a sheet-like distribution, with areas suggestive of mucinous production ➡. The cells are pleomorphic with an increased nuclear to cytoplasmic ratio. The nuclei are hyperchromatic and irregular.* ***(Right)*** *A fine needle aspiration demonstrates a sheet of epithelioid cells, focally suggesting a "follicle" ➡. There are numerous acute inflammatory cells (neutrophils ➡), a finding quite frequently seen in undifferentiated carcinoma.*

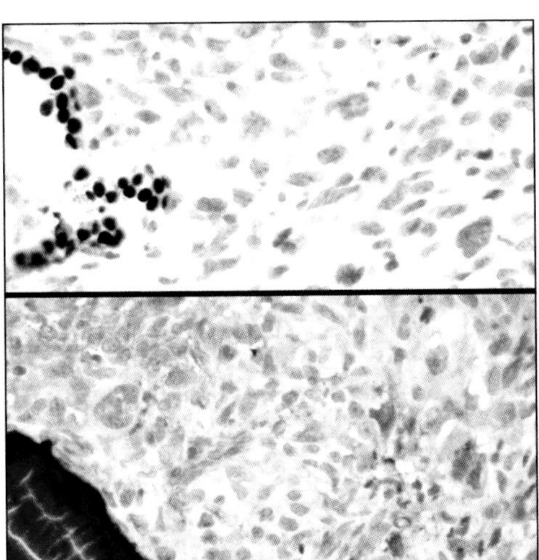

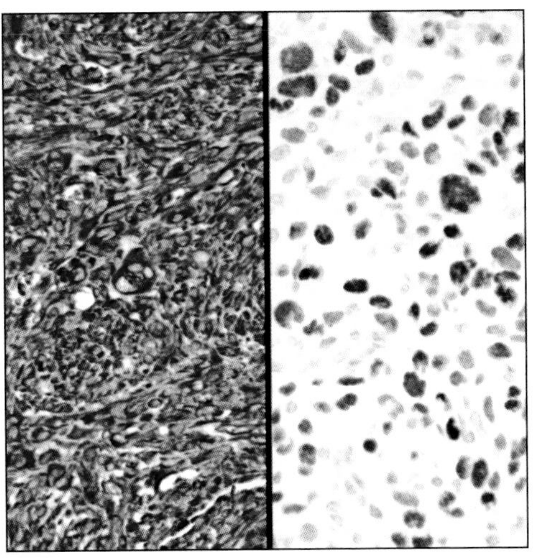

(Left) *This split-field photomicrograph includes TTF-1 (upper) and thyroglobulin (lower) in the residual thyroid follicular epithelium. A background "blush" is present with thyroglobulin. However, the pleomorphic and bizarre cells are not highlighted with either marker.* ***(Right)*** *A split field shows very strong, heavy and intense vimentin (left) immunoreactivity. Likewise, p63 highlights nearly all of the tumor cell nuclei in a very strong fashion (right).*

MEDULLARY CARCINOMA

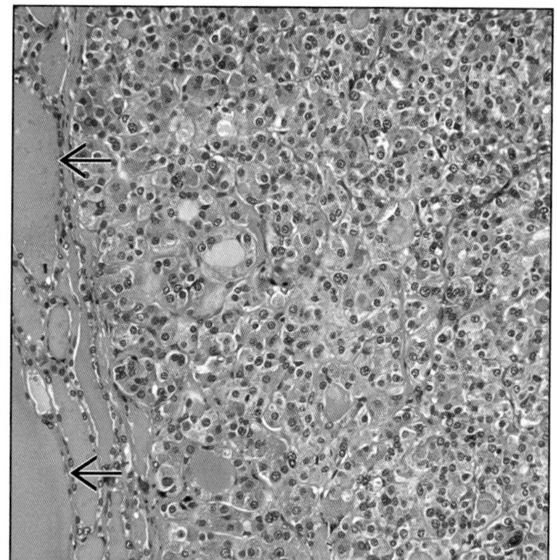

There is a proliferation of epithelial cells arranged in sheets and nests. Note the intimate association with the thyroid follicles ⇒.

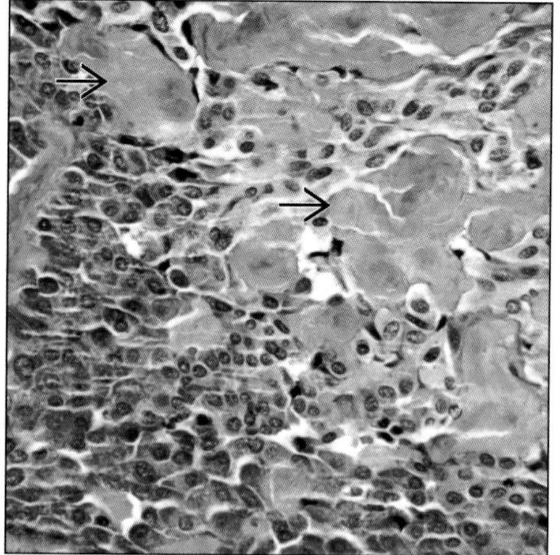

The cells of this medullary carcinoma are very plasmacytoid in appearance. The nuclei show delicate, "salt and pepper" nuclear chromatin distribution. Amyloid is quite prominent in this case ⇒.

TERMINOLOGY

Abbreviations

- Medullary thyroid carcinoma (MTC)

Synonyms

- Solid carcinoma
- Solid carcinoma with amyloid stroma
- Solid amyloidotic carcinoma
- C-cell carcinoma
- Compact cell carcinoma
- Neuroendocrine carcinoma of thyroid

Definitions

- Malignant epithelial tumor of thyroid gland exhibiting C-cell differentiation

ETIOLOGY/PATHOGENESIS

Inherited

- Strong inherited association with multiple endocrine neoplasia (MEN) syndromes
  - MEN2A (Sipple): Parathyroid hyperplasia (hyperparathyroidism), thyroid medullary carcinoma, adrenal pheochromocytoma, pancreatic endocrine tumors
  - MEN2B (Wagenmann-Froboese syndrome): As above, with soft tissue tumors present (usually mucosal)
  - Autosomal dominant inheritance, high penetrance, and variable expressivity
  - Gain of function (activating) germline mutation of *RET* gene (usually point mutation) involving 10q11.2
    - Fusion gene with portion of a gene coding for a tyrosine kinase domain, called *RET* (**RE**arranged during **T**ransfection contraction)
    - *RET* receptor activates signaling pathways responsible for cell proliferation, survival, differentiation, motility, and chemotaxis
    - *RET* has 21 exons and approximately 55,000 base pairs, coding for RET protein, member of receptor tyrosine kinase superfamily
    - Mutations of extracellular 5 cysteine codons (exon 10: 609, 611, 618, 620; exon 11: 634) collectively account for about 95% of MEN2A and 85% of FMTC kindred
    - Specifically, codon 634 is involved in 80-90% of MEN2A cases (arginine for cysteine substitution most commonly)
    - ~ 95% of MEN2B associated with point mutation in codon 918 of exon 16 (Met918Thr substitution)
    - *RET* also involved in thyroid papillary carcinoma (chromosomal rearrangement known as *RET/PTC*)
- Familial medullary thyroid carcinoma (FMTC) can be seen **without** extrathyroid associations but still with germline mutation in *RET* proto-oncogene

Sporadic

- Up to 2/3 of sporadic medullary carcinomas have somatic *RET* mutations
- Other genetic &/or epigenetic alterations are involved

Pathogenesis

- Ultimobranchial body gives rise to C-cells, which are the source of tumor development
  - C-cells (parafollicular cells) arise embryologically from 4th branchial/pharyngeal pouch
  - Found in upper and middle regions of thyroid gland lobes
    - Medullary carcinoma does not arise from isthmus
  - Calcitonin, a hormone involved in calcium homeostasis, is peptide secreted by C-cells
    - Calcitonin gene-related peptide (CGRP) tends to be seen in extrathyroidal sites
- C-cell hyperplasia is precursor of medullary carcinoma in heritable cases

MEDULLARY CARCINOMA

Key Facts

Terminology
- Malignant C-cell-derived tumor with gain of function (activating) germline mutations of *RET* gene

Etiology/Pathogenesis
- Strong inherited association with MEN2A and 2B
- C-cell hyperplasia is precursor of medullary carcinoma

Clinical Issues
- Sporadic: 5th to 6th decades; familial: 3rd decade
- Cervical lymph node metastases: ~ 50%
- Serum calcitonin and CEA levels elevated
- Total thyroidectomy (prophylactic for *RET* mutations), with neck dissection
- Overall 70-80% 10-year survival

Microscopic Pathology
- Familial tumors are multifocal and bilateral
- Many patterns: Organoid, insular, solid
- Amyloid stromal accumulation
- Round, oval, spindled to plasmacytoid cells
- Stippled, fine, uniform nuclear chromatin
- Significant lymph-vascular invasion

Ancillary Tests
- Positive: Calcitonin, chromogranin, synaptophysin, CEA-P, keratin, TTF-1

Top Differential Diagnoses
- Follicular carcinoma, papillary carcinoma, parathyroid adenoma, paraganglioma, undifferentiated carcinoma, metastatic carcinoma, hyalinizing trabecular adenoma

CLINICAL ISSUES

Epidemiology
- Incidence
  - Approximately 5-8% of all thyroid malignancies in USA
  - Majority are sporadic (80%), with remaining (20%) inherited (familial)
- Age
  - Sporadic: 5th-6th decades
  - Familial: 3rd decade
    - MEN2A: Late adolescence or early adulthood
    - MEN2B: Infant to early childhood
- Gender
  - Female > Male (1.1:1) for sporadic cases

Site
- Middle to upper part of thyroid lobes
  - Usual location for C-cells &/or ultimobranchial body
- Isthmus **not** affected

Presentation
- Sporadic
  - Painless, unilateral, solitary thyroid mass
  - Cervical lymph node enlargement in about 50%
  - Hoarseness, stridor, upper airway obstruction, or dysphagia in about 10-15%
- Inherited/familial
  - Similar thyroid/neck findings, although usually at younger age
    - Diarrhea and flushing (up to 30% of patients) related to high plasma calcitonin levels
  - Multicentric and bilateral thyroid involvement
  - Nonthyroid symptoms related to other organ disorders may dominate clinical presentation
    - Hyperparathyroidism with calcium homeostasis derangements
    - Sweating, headache, paroxysmal hypertension, palpitations, syncope, and dizziness related to pheochromocytoma
    - Cushing syndrome due to tumor ACTH production or part of pituitary adenoma peptide production
    - Gastrointestinal symptoms related to pancreatic endocrine tumor peptide secretion
    - Mucosal neuromas (oral cavity, lips, tongue, and gastrointestinal tract)
  - If part of kindred, early detection before clinical symptoms present
    - Parathyroid, adrenal, pituitary, pancreas, and gastrointestinal tract findings
    - Thyroid disease discovered incidentally during evaluation of MEN syndrome

Laboratory Tests
- Serum calcitonin levels are almost invariably increased
- CEA level elevated
- Calcium imbalances (due to calcitonin &/or parathyroid hormone abnormalities)

Treatment
- Options, risks, complications
  - Prophylactic thyroidectomy for patients with germline *RET* mutations (*RET* genotype specific)
    - Specific *RET* codon mutation will dictate recommended age at thyroidectomy
    - Codon 883, 918, & 922 mutations: Thyroidectomy before 12 months of age
    - Codon 611, 618, 620, & 634 mutations: Thyroidectomy before 5 years of age
    - Other codons: Thyroidectomy, usually after pentagastrin-stimulated calcitonin response becomes abnormal
  - Serum calcitonin and CEA levels before surgery to establish baseline for subsequent monitoring
  - Serum calcium and urinary metanephrine and catecholamines to exclude MEN-associated diseases
- Surgical approaches
  - Total thyroidectomy
  - Neck dissection
    - Central compartment (level VI)

MEDULLARY CARCINOMA

    - If central lymph nodes positive or tumor > 1 cm, ipsilateral neck dissection
    - If bilateral tumors, bilateral radical neck dissections are recommended
  - Parathyroidectomy if part of heritable disease
- Adjuvant therapy
  - Chemotherapy, somatostatin analogs, anti-CEA radioimmunotherapy is employed in some
- Radiation
  - External beam radiation for gross residual disease or palliation of distant metastases
- Additional therapies
  - Radiofrequency ablation
  - Targeted molecular therapy (tyrosine kinase inhibitors targeting *RET* kinase)

Prognosis

- Clinical stage and inherited-type dependent
  - Overall about 70-80% 10-year survival
  - Excellent prognosis for small tumors confined to thyroid, incidentally discovered and without lymph node metastases (100%)
  - Survival outcomes: Familial non-MEN > sporadic > MEN2A > MEN2B
  - Prophylactic thyroidectomy patients have best prognosis (naturally) and least likely to have lymph node metastases
- Tumor stage is most important prognostic factor (extrathyroidal extension; metastasis)
  - Stage I: 100% 10-year survival
  - Stage III: 65-85% 10-year survival
  - Stage IV: 20-50% 10-year survival
- Young patients (< 45 years) have better prognosis than older patients
- Males may have slightly worse outcome (controversial)
- Lymph node metastases common (50% at presentation)
- Distant metastases uncommon (15% at presentation)
  - Liver, lungs, bone
- Better prognosis for tumors with abundant amyloid and > 75% calcitonin-positive cells
- If somatic *RET* mutation is present, those with codon 918 mutation appear to be more aggressive
- If preoperative serum calcitonin &/or CEA levels were elevated, they can be followed to monitor disease status
- Genetic screening (biochemical or molecular) recommended for relatives of proband (found in 10-15% of cases)

IMAGE FINDINGS

General Features

- ^{131}I-meta-iodobenzylguanidine (MIBG) positive mass
  - Radiopharmaceutical and guanethidine analog confirms neuroendocrine nature of tumor
- "Cold" mass on scintigraphic scan
- Computed tomography (CT) shows extent of disease and lymph node status
- Positron emission tomography (PET) can be used to identify distant metastases
- Ultrasound shows mass lesion

MACROSCOPIC FEATURES

General Features

- Sporadic tumors are unilateral and solitary
- Familial tumors are multifocal and bilateral
- Usually well-defined, but poorly formed capsule, with infiltration
- Involve middle to upper, lateral portion of lobe(s)
- Tan-yellow, white to light gray
- Firm, rubbery cut surface; rarely soft consistency
- Gritty due to finely granular calcifications
- Hemorrhage or necrosis usually absent

Sections to Be Submitted

- If prophylactic thyroidectomy, lobes should be serially sectioned transversely and sections submitted sequentially from superior to inferior
  - Calcitonin may be necessary to highlight areas of C-cell hyperplasia or microcarcinoma

Size

- Microscopic up to 10 cm
- Large tumors may completely replace lobe

MICROSCOPIC PATHOLOGY

Histologic Features

- Broad range of histologic features
- Multitude of growth patterns
  - Solid sheets and nests, separated by heavily hyalinized fibrovascular stroma
  - Lobular, organoid, nested, insular, and trabecular tend to be more defined by stroma
    - Curvilinear anastomosing cells separated by delicate and thin to more thick and hyalinized stroma of tumor
- Amyloid stromal accumulation (70-80% of cases)
  - Homogeneous, acellular, eosinophilic, extracellular matrix material
    - Appears to be calcitonin-derived
  - May be associated with calcification
    - Calcifications may resemble psammoma bodies but without concentric laminations
  - Tumors lacking amyloid tend to have worse prognosis
- Entrapment of benign follicular epithelial cells is common
  - Can extend quite deeply into main tumor mass
- Cells are round to oval, spindled to plasmacytoid or polyhedral cells
  - Mixtures of these cell types are common
- Nuclei are round to oval nuclei with stippled, fine, uniform "salt and pepper" nuclear chromatin
  - Nucleoli are only prominent in oncocytic variant
- Intranuclear cytoplasmic inclusions common
- Cells have mild to moderate pleomorphism, although isolated bizarre nuclei are common
  - Bi- and multinucleated cells can be seen
- Cytoplasm is opaque, finely granular, and ranges from eosinophilic to clear, amphophilic, oncocytic, and pigmented

- Intracytoplasmic mucinous vacuoles with extracellular mucin accumulation can be seen
- Mitotic figures are infrequent
- Necrosis is uncommon, possibly seen in large tumors
- Significant lymph-vascular invasion
- Extensive invasion of tumor capsule, with expansion into thyroid parenchyma and extrathyroidal soft tissues
- Metastatic deposits in lymph nodes
  - Particularly central paratracheal or superior mediastinum

Precursor

- Solid cell nests are thought to be remnants of ultimobranchial body
  - Nests of pavemented cells without intercellular bridges
  - Usually seen in and around areas of C-cell proliferation
- C-cell hyperplasia: Reactive or neoplastic
- **Reactive (secondary; physiologic)**
  - Reactive increase seen in thyroids removed for other disorders (nodules, lymphocytic thyroiditis, papillary and follicular carcinoma)
  - **No** aggregates of > 50 cells; **no** destructive growth; **no** amyloid deposition; **no** fibrosis; **no** cellular pleomorphism
  - Frequently seen adjacent to solid cell nests (ultimobranchial body remnant)
  - Usually requires calcitonin &/or chromogranin to highlight
- **Neoplastic**
  - Also called C-cell carcinoma in situ or medullary carcinoma in situ
  - Seen adjacent to medullary carcinoma and in asymptomatic carriers of *RET* germline mutations
  - May be focal, diffuse, or nodular
  - Groups of C-cells surrounding or partially destroying follicles
  - Aggregates of > 50 cells
  - May be associated with amyloid deposition and fibrosis
  - Separation from "microcarcinoma" or intraglandular spread from medullary carcinoma may be challenging

Variants

- Oncocytic cell, papillary/pseudopapillary, glandular or follicular, giant cell, small cell, paraganglioma-like, spindle cell, clear cell, squamous cell, melanin-producing, angiosarcoma-like, amphicrine
  - Each of these patterns mimics other primary or secondary tumors
  - Immunohistochemical confirmation usually required

ANCILLARY TESTS

Cytology

- Frequently challenging due to wide cytologic variability
- Cellular aspirates with single cells and small, loosely cohesive clusters
- Extracellular, homogeneous, amorphous eosinophilic clumps or spheres of amyloid (up to 70% of aspirates)
  - Dark blue-purple on air-dried slides and opaque, deep green on Papanicolaou-stained slides
- Colloid absent
- Round to oval, spindle, bipolar to polygonal cells
- Rare cells with moderate pleomorphism
- Scattered bi- and multinucleated cells
- Plasmacytoid appearance with eccentric nucleus placement (plasmacytoid)
- Hyperchromatic nuclei with stippled to coarse nuclear chromatin ("salt and pepper")
- Intranuclear cytoplasmic inclusions frequent
- Abundant, eosinophilic cytoplasm
- Metachromatic red cytoplasmic granules on air-dried preparations
- Calcitonin immunostain may be helpful

Histochemistry

- Grimelius stain highlights argyrophilic granules
  - Negative with Fontana-Masson stain
- Intra- &/or extracellular mucin
  - Highlighted with mucicarmine, Alcian blue, &/or PAS
- Congo red positive in amyloid
  - Light green birefringence with polarization
- Crystal violet positive in amyloid
  - Purple metachromatic staining

Immunohistochemistry

- Positive: Calcitonin, chromogranin, synaptophysin, CEA-P, keratin, TTF-1
- Negative: Thyroglobulin

Flow Cytometry

- ~ 30% are aneuploid (possibly associated with worse prognosis)

Cytogenetics

- Germline or somatic *RET* mutations
- Can be performed on peripheral blood
  - Exons 10, 11, 13, 14, 15, and 16 of *RET* are typically analyzed
    - Restriction-fragment–length polymorphism assays, single-strand conformation polymorphism, heteroduplex techniques, or DNA sequencing

Electron Microscopy

- Neurosecretory electron dense membrane bound granules (type I and II) help to confirm neuroendocrine nature of medullary carcinoma
- Extracellular spaces contain finely fibrillar amyloid material

DIFFERENTIAL DIAGNOSIS

Follicular Carcinoma

- Trabecular and oncocytic patterns cause most quandary
- Colloid is usually difficult to detect, but nuclei tend to be more hyperchromatic

MEDULLARY CARCINOMA

- Thyroglobulin is positive
  - Calcitonin negative (sensitive and specific)

Papillary Carcinoma

- Nuclear features of papillary carcinoma are usually not seen in medullary carcinoma
- Intranuclear inclusions seen in both tumors
- Immunohistochemistry profile is different

Parathyroid Tissue

- Parathyroid tissue (normal glands or neoplasms) usually shows cleared cytoplasm, well-defined cell borders
- Parathyroid hormone positive, lacking calcitonin and thyroglobulin

Paraganglioma

- Well-defined tumor, lacking invasion
- Zellballen architecture with S100 protein(+) sustentacular cells
- Negative for calcitonin and thyroglobulin

Undifferentiated (Anaplastic) Carcinoma

- Usually older age, rapid onset of tumor
- Spindle cell pattern with pleomorphism can be difficult
- Increased mitotic figures, necrosis, hemorrhage, and association with existing thyroid lesion
- Calcitonin should help

Metastatic Carcinoma

- **Renal cell carcinoma**
  - Solitary mass but often with lymph-vascular invasion
  - Tumor cells are clear with pseudoglandular erythrocyte collections
  - Thyroglobulin, calcitonin, CD10 may help with separation, as only the latter is positive
- **Metastatic melanoma**
  - If melanin pigment is present, differential is raised
  - Melan-A, HMB-45, and tyrosinase can help (not S100 protein)
- **Metastatic neuroendocrine tumors**
  - Quite uncommon
  - Includes carcinoid, atypical carcinoid, and neuroendocrine carcinomas
  - All are typically negative for calcitonin and CEA, but require clinical-radiologic-laboratory integration
  - Direct extension from larynx must be excluded, as calcitonin can be positive

C-cell Hyperplasia vs. Intraglandular Spread

- Multifocal; aggregates of cells, often adjacent to ultimobranchial body
- Usually lacking destructive growth
- Not within lymph-vascular spaces
- Associated with possible fibrosis
- Tends to show increased calcitonin intensity over medullary carcinoma

Hyalinizing Trabecular Tumor

- Encapsulated tumor without invasion
- Trabecular growth pattern
- Intralesional hyalinization without amyloid
- Cells are spindled, arranged perpendicular to stroma
- Yellow intracytoplasmic bodies
- Thyroglobulin(+), calcitonin(-)

Amyloid Goiter

- Unencapsulated, affecting whole gland
- Fatty infiltration with squamous metaplasia and amyloid deposition (Congo red positive)

Lymphoma

- Diffuse, unencapsulated lesion
- Background of chronic lymphocytic thyroiditis (rare in medullary carcinoma)
- Spectrum of lymphoid elements (plasmacytoid cells with Dutcher bodies; immunoblasts, centrocytes, monocytoid B-cells)
- Hematologic immunohistochemistry (CD20, CD19, CD79a, CD138, κ, λ)

DIAGNOSTIC CHECKLIST

Pathologic Interpretation Pearls

- Must consider medullary in any tumor that is slightly "atypical"
- Oncocytic tumors without colloid production, must have PAS or thyroglobulin performed to confirm cell type

STAGING

Distribution

- Stage I: 20%
- Stage II: 33%
- Stage III: 32%
- Stage IV: 15%

SELECTED REFERENCES

1. Harvey A et al: Sporadic medullary thyroid cancer. Cancer Treat Res. 153:57-74, 2010
2. Milan SA et al: Current management of medullary thyroid cancer. Minerva Chir. 65(1):27-37, 2010
3. Pacini F et al: Medullary thyroid carcinoma. Clin Oncol (R Coll Radiol). 22(6):475-85, 2010
4. Sadow PM et al: Mixed Medullary-follicular-derived carcinomas of the thyroid gland. Adv Anat Pathol. 17(4):282-5, 2010
5. Tran T et al: Familial thyroid neoplasia: impact of technological advances on detection and monitoring. Curr Opin Endocrinol Diabetes Obes. 17(5):425-31, 2010
6. Ye L et al: The evolving field of tyrosine kinase inhibitors in the treatment of endocrine tumors. Endocr Rev. 31(4):578-99, 2010
7. American Thyroid Association Guidelines Task Force et al: Medullary thyroid cancer: management guidelines of the American Thyroid Association. Thyroid. 19(6):565-612, 2009
8. Moo-Young TA et al: Sporadic and familial medullary thyroid carcinoma: state of the art. Surg Clin North Am. 89(5):1193-204, 2009
9. Morrison PJ et al: Genetic aspects of familial thyroid cancer. Oncologist. 14(6):571-7, 2009

Immunohistochemistry

Antibody	Reactivity	Staining Pattern	Comment
Calcitonin	Positive	Cytoplasmic	Strong, diffuse, and most specific marker, present in ~ 95% of cases
CGRP	Positive	Cytoplasmic	May be limited to small foci within tumor
CEA-P	Positive	Cytoplasmic	Usually immunoreactive in most tumor cells, even more commonly than calcitonin
TTF-1	Positive	Nuclear	Variable intensity, slightly less than follicular tumors
Chromogranin-A	Positive	Cytoplasmic	Granular reactivity
Chromogranin-B	Positive	Cytoplasmic	Granular reactivity
Synaptophysin	Positive	Cytoplasmic	Granular to dot-like
NSE	Positive	Cytoplasmic	Most tumor cells positive but usually not helpful in diagnosis
Serotonin	Positive	Cytoplasmic	Frequently positive
Somatostatin	Positive	Cytoplasmic	Occasionally reactive
AE1/AE3	Positive	Cytoplasmic	Strong and diffusely positive
CK7	Positive	Cytoplasmic	Strong and diffuse, slightly more membrane than pan-keratin
Vimentin	Positive	Cytoplasmic	Variably positive in tumor cells
S100	Positive	Nuclear & cytoplasmic	Often in sustentacular distribution around nests
Calretinin	Positive	Nuclear & cytoplasmic	Only in about 25% of tumor cells
Galectin-3	Positive	Cytoplasmic	Variably present (45-80%) but weak and focal to strong
Thyroglobulin	Negative		
CK20	Negative		

10. Schlumberger MJ et al: Phase II study of safety and efficacy of motesanib in patients with progressive or symptomatic, advanced or metastatic medullary thyroid cancer. J Clin Oncol. 27(23):3794-801, 2009
11. Castellani MR et al: MIBG for diagnosis and therapy of medullary thyroid carcinoma: is there still a role? Q J Nucl Med Mol Imaging. 52(4):430-40, 2008
12. Dotto J et al: Familial thyroid carcinoma: a diagnostic algorithm. Adv Anat Pathol. 15(6):332-49, 2008
13. Etit D et al: Histopathologic and clinical features of medullary microcarcinoma and C-cell hyperplasia in prophylactic thyroidectomies for medullary carcinoma: a study of 42 cases. Arch Pathol Lab Med. 132(11):1767-73, 2008
14. Lodish MB et al: RET oncogene in MEN2, MEN2B, MTC and other forms of thyroid cancer. Expert Rev Anticancer Ther. 8(4):625-32, 2008
15. Nikiforova MN et al: Molecular genetics of thyroid cancer: implications for diagnosis, treatment and prognosis. Expert Rev Mol Diagn. 8(1):83-95, 2008
16. Rufini V et al: Role of PET in medullary thyroid carcinoma. Minerva Endocrinol. 33(2):67-73, 2008
17. Ball DW: Medullary thyroid cancer: monitoring and therapy. Endocrinol Metab Clin North Am. 36(3):823-37, viii, 2007
18. Bhanot P et al: Role of FNA cytology and immunochemistry in the diagnosis and management of medullary thyroid carcinoma: report of six cases and review of the literature. Diagn Cytopathol. 35(5):285-92, 2007
19. Lewiński A et al: Genetic background of carcinogenesis in the thyroid gland. Neuro Endocrinol Lett. 28(2):77-105, 2007
20. Machens A et al: Genotype-phenotype based surgical concept of hereditary medullary thyroid carcinoma. World J Surg. 31(5):957-68, 2007
21. Baloch ZW et al: Microcarcinoma of the thyroid. Adv Anat Pathol. 13(2):69-75, 2006
22. Guyétant S et al: C-cell hyperplasia. Ann Endocrinol (Paris). 67(3):190-7, 2006
23. Izikson L et al: The flushing patient: differential diagnosis, workup, and treatment. J Am Acad Dermatol. 55(2):193-208, 2006
24. Papi G et al: Primary spindle cell lesions of the thyroid gland; an overview. Am J Clin Pathol. 125 Suppl:S95-123, 2006
25. Clark JR et al: Prognostic variables and calcitonin in medullary thyroid cancer. Laryngoscope. 115(8):1445-50, 2005
26. Hunt JL: Unusual thyroid tumors: a review of pathologic and molecular diagnosis. Expert Rev Mol Diagn. 5(5):725-34, 2005
27. Ashworth M: The pathology of preclinical medullary thyroid carcinoma. Endocr Pathol. 15(3):227-31, 2004
28. Cohen EG et al: Medullary thyroid carcinoma. Acta Otolaryngol. 124(5):544-57, 2004
29. Takami H: Medullary thyroid carcinoma and multiple endocrine neoplasia type 2. Endocr Pathol. 14(2):123-31, 2003
30. Albores-Saavedra JA et al: C-cell hyperplasia and medullary thyroid microcarcinoma. Endocr Pathol. 12(4):365-77, 2001
31. Baloch ZW et al: Neuroendocrine tumors of the thyroid gland. Am J Clin Pathol. 115 Suppl:S56-67, 2001
32. Giammanco M: Medullary thyroid carcinoma. Natural history and surgical treatment. Minerva Endocrinol. 25(3-4):75-9, 2000
33. Weber AL et al: The thyroid and parathyroid glands. CT and MR imaging and correlation with pathology and clinical findings. Radiol Clin North Am. 38(5):1105-29, 2000
34. Green I et al: A spectrum of cytomorphologic variations in medullary thyroid carcinoma. Fine-needle aspiration findings in 19 cases. Cancer. 81(1):40-4, 1997
35. Komminoth P: Multiple endocrine neoplasia type 1 and 2: from morphology to molecular pathology 1997. Verh Dtsch Ges Pathol. 81:125-38, 1997

MEDULLARY CARCINOMA

Imaging and Gross Features

(Left) *It is important to realize that medullary carcinoma ➡ frequently has associated metastatic disease to the cervical and mediastinal lymph nodes ➡. Excluding parathyroid disease is important.* ***(Right)*** *Axial post-contrast CT through the neck shows marked irregularity of the thyroid gland with multiple focal areas of decreased intensity ➡. The borders of the gland are ill defined. There is an adjacent, abnormally enlarged left lymph node indicating metastatic disease ➡.*

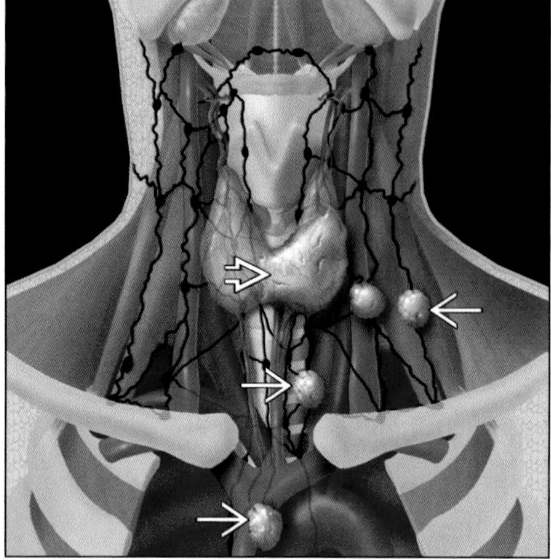

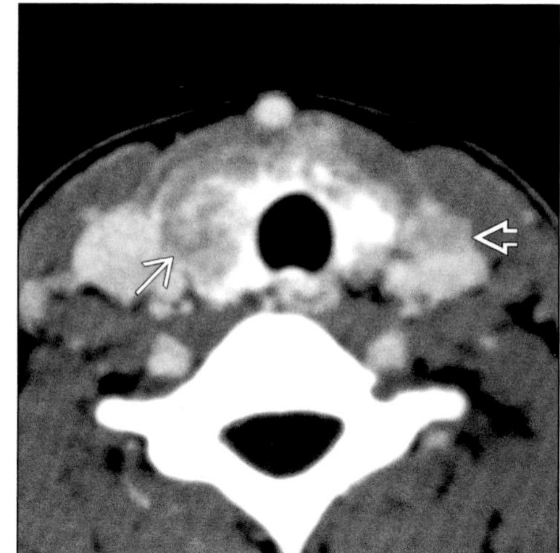

(Left) *Transverse ultrasound with power Doppler shows chaotic intralesional flow ➡ as compared to normal thyroid gland ➡. Note the internal carotid artery ➡ as a point of comparison. (Courtesy A. Ahuja, MD.)* ***(Right)*** *Serial sections of both lobes of the thyroid gland show tumors. This is an example of familial medullary carcinoma, showing bilateral and multifocal tumors. Note the areas of cystic change in the upper series.*

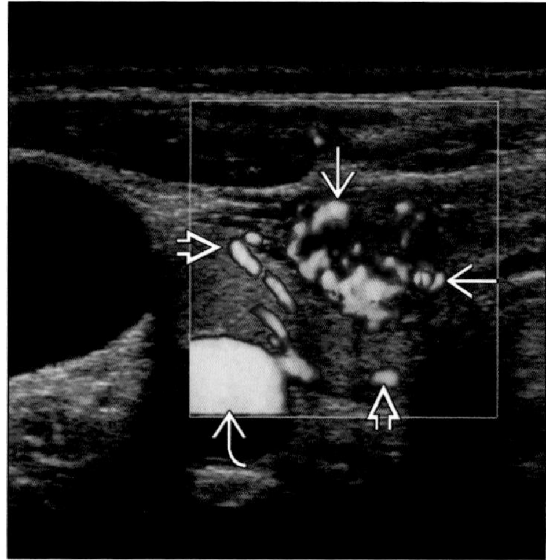

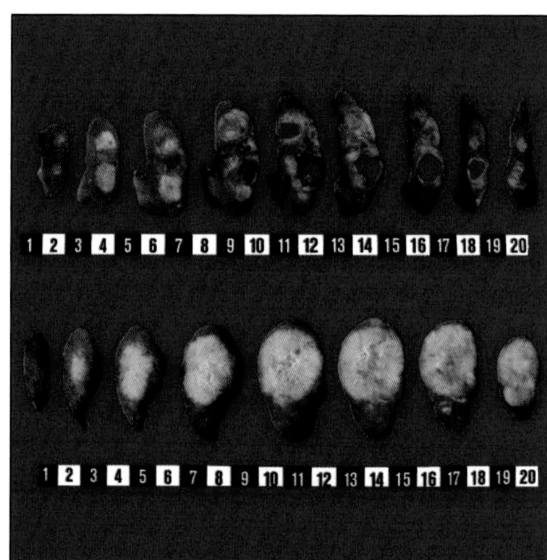

(Left) *There is a large tumor, measuring approximately 3.8 cm. The edge is infiltrative ➡, although a well-formed capsule is not present. Smaller tumor nodules are noted adjacent to the main mass ➡.* ***(Right)*** *This lobe demonstrates multifocal disease within a single lobe. The tumors are topographically separate and show different cut appearances. Multifocal disease is characteristic for inherited/familial tumors. One tumor shows an area of cystic change ➡.*

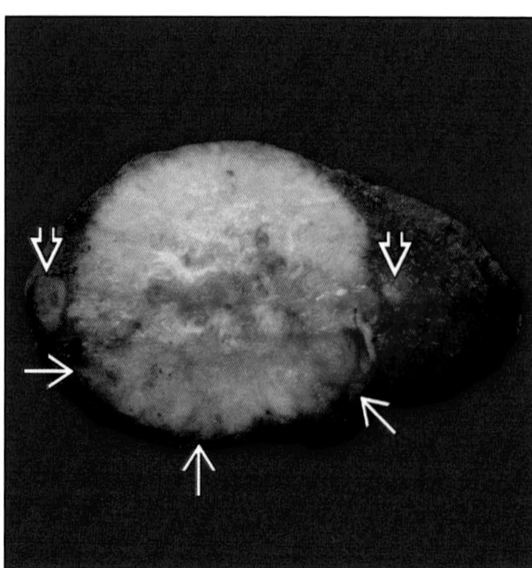

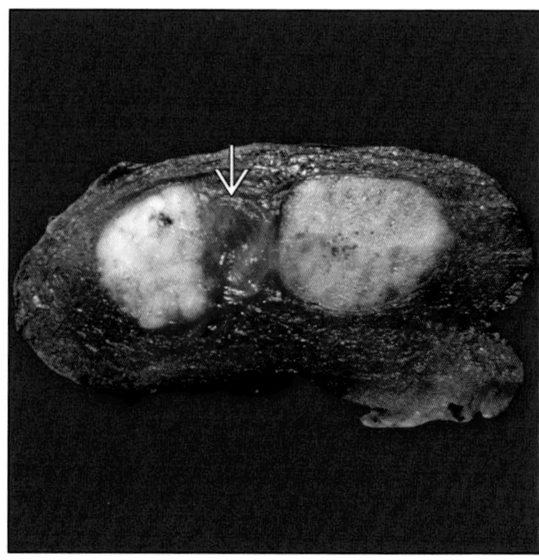

Microscopic Features

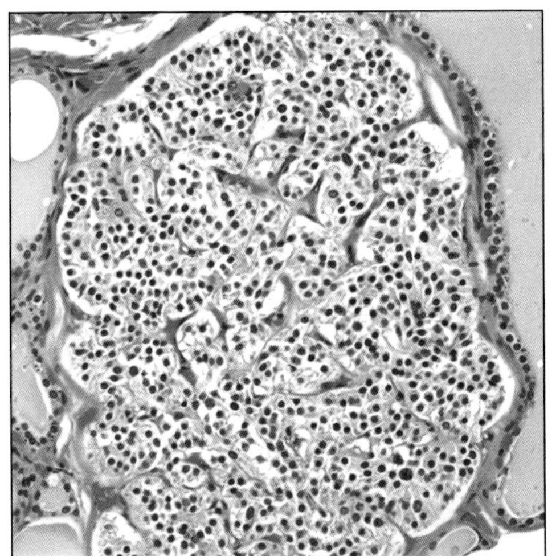

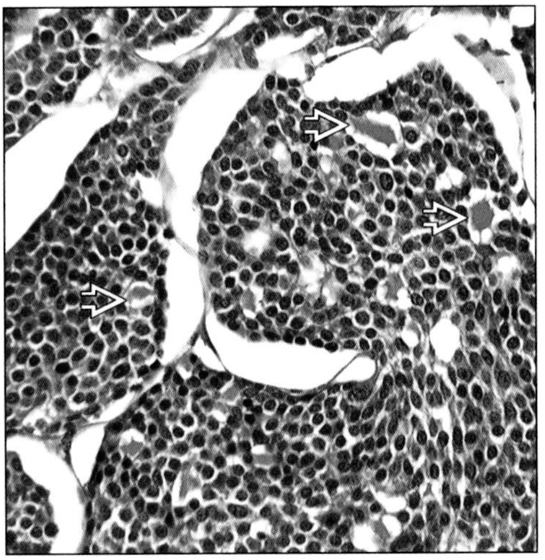

(Left) *An aggregate of C-cells forms a small nodule composed of > 50 cells. The surrounding thyroid follicles are not destroyed. There is no true fibrosis, no amyloid, and no cytologic atypia in this example of neoplastic C-cell hyperplasia.* ***(Right)*** *This tumor is arranged in a sheet-like and glandular architecture. The cells are syncytial, with a high nuclear to cytoplasmic ratio. "Glandular" lumen with secretions are noted ⮚, a pattern seen in many medullary carcinomas.*

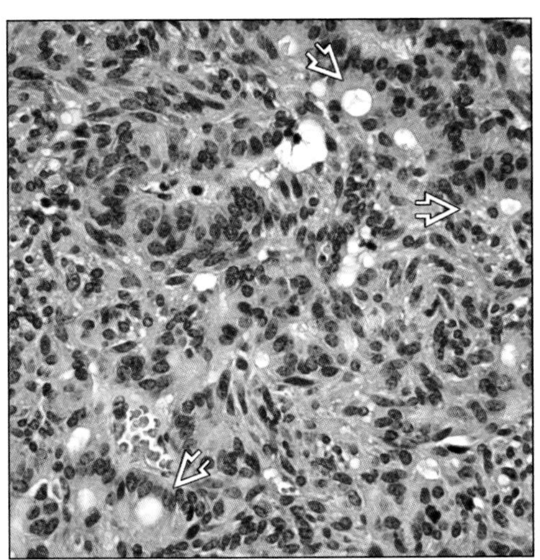

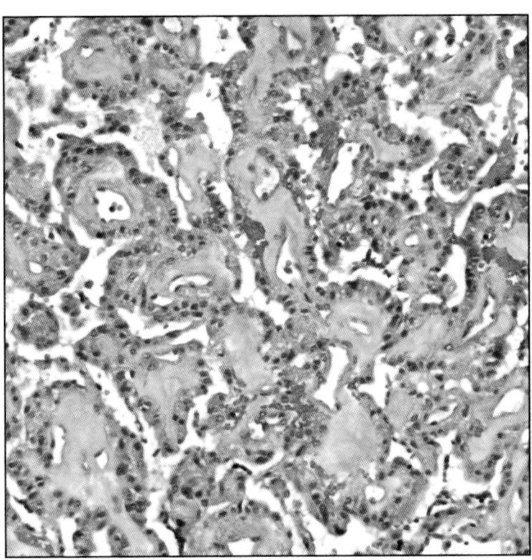

(Left) *There is a mixed glandular, insular, and spindled cell appearance to this medullary carcinoma. There is a rosette-type ⮚ pattern, lacking secretions.* ***(Right)*** *An angiomatoid or vascular pattern, mimicking what can be seen in an angiosarcoma, is present in this medullary carcinoma. Usually, a variant histology is the dominant finding, but occasionally it may be only a small fraction of the overall tumor volume. Special studies usually help to confirm the diagnosis.*

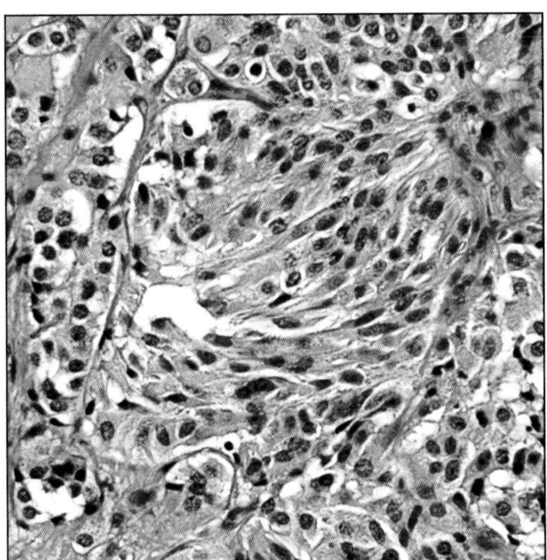

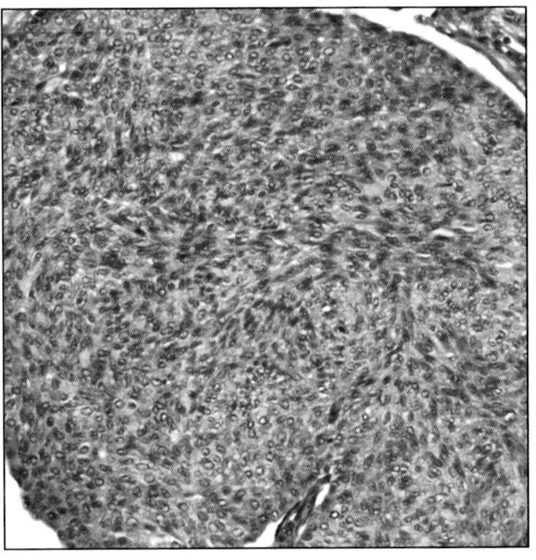

(Left) *A spindled cell appearance is frequently seen in medullary carcinoma, although it is uncommon as a dominant pattern. There is a syncytial appearance. The nuclei are spindled to oval with delicate nuclear chromatin distribution.* ***(Right)*** *A solid pattern is shown, composed of cells that have a spindled appearance. The nuclei seem to have an optical clearing. This was not the dominant finding in this medullary carcinoma but was a focal pattern, seen in < 20% of the tumor.*

MEDULLARY CARCINOMA

Microscopic Features

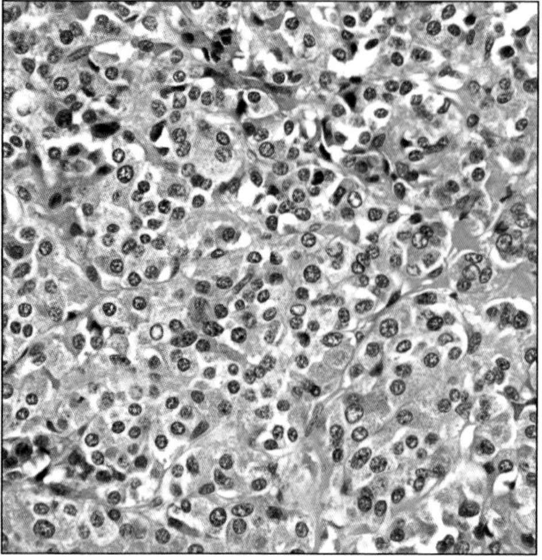
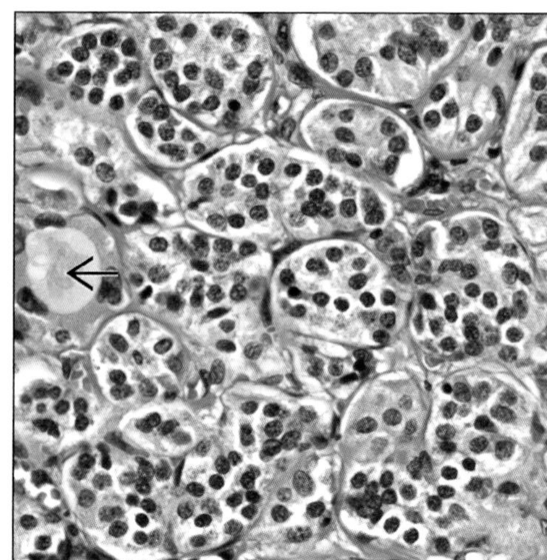

***(Left)** There is a vague nesting to this sheet of neoplastic cells. Note the granular, slightly basophilic cytoplasm surrounding nuclei that have delicate chromatin distribution. **(Right)** A characteristic nested pattern with cells that have small round nuclei and granular cytoplasm is seen in this MTC. Note the entrapped "colloid" → at the periphery. This should not be misinterpreted as follicular differentiation.*

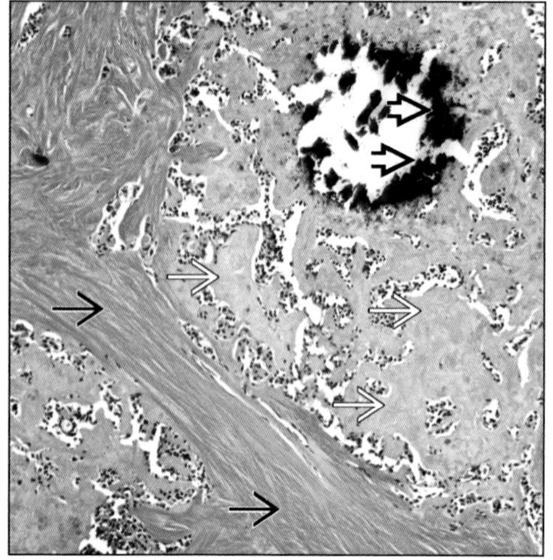
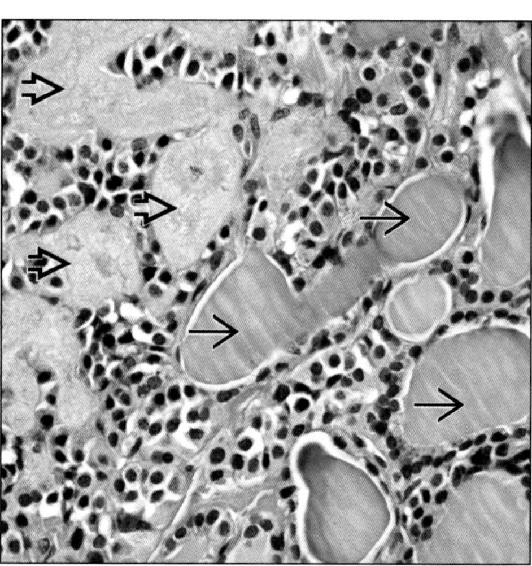

***(Left)** There are heavy bands of fibrosis (brightly eosinophilic) → separating the tumor into nodules. There is abundant amyloid: Acellular, opaque, eosinophilic, extracellular matrix material ➔. Calcification is also present within the amyloid ⇨. **(Right)** The distinction between entrapped follicular epithelium with colloid → and amyloid ⇨ can sometimes be a challenge. The tinctorial quality differences, along with the "chatter" artifacts in the colloid help.*

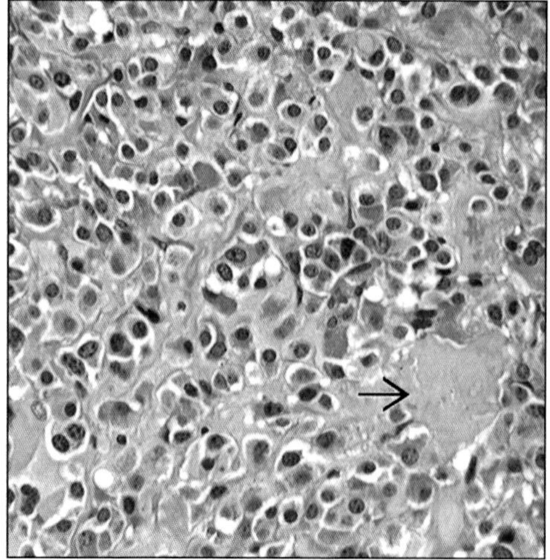
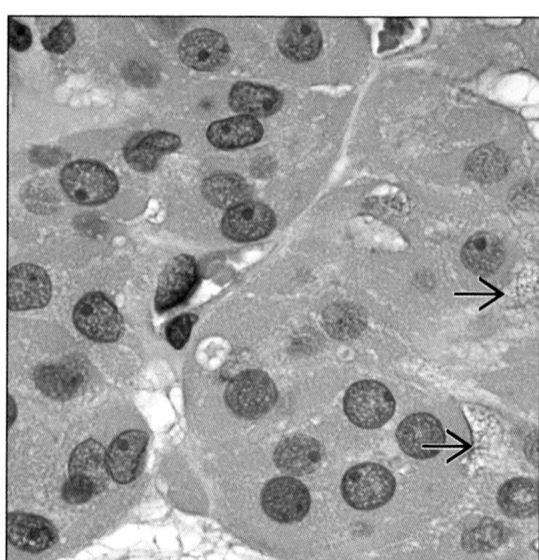

***(Left)** There is a sheet-like to organoid architecture to this medullary carcinoma.The cells have slightly bluish-granular cytoplasm. There is a plasmacytoid appearance to the cells. Amyloid is noted →. **(Right)** Oncocytic variant is quite difficult to diagnose. There are small but prominent nucleoli. Note the "mucinous" material → within the cytoplasm or between a few of the cells. Immunohistochemistry is useful in these cases to help confirm the C-cell derivation.*

Ancillary Techniques

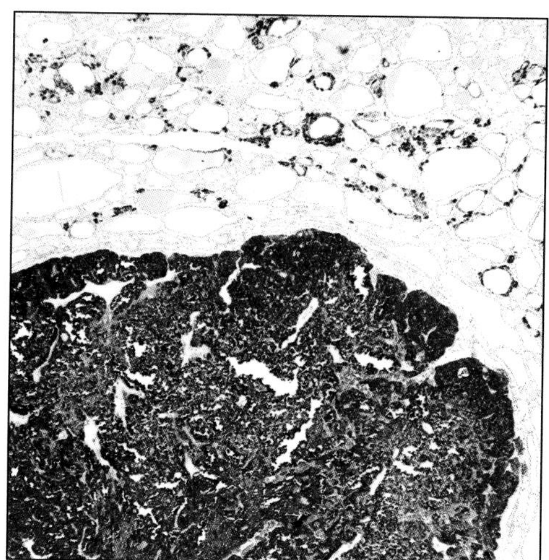

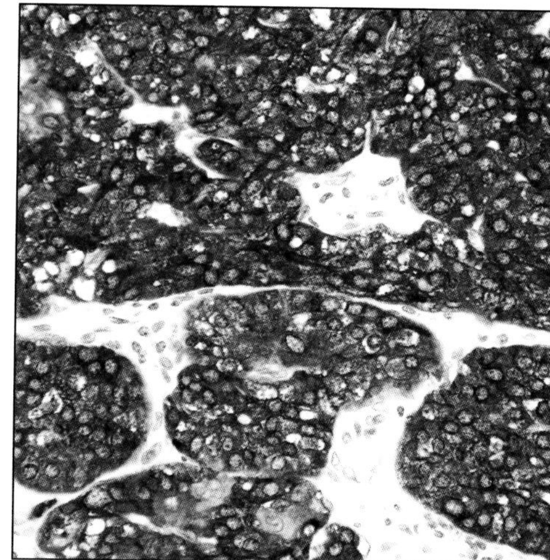

(Left) *Calcitonin is one of the most specific stains for medullary carcinoma. Note the strong and heavy deposition of chromogen within the tumor, but there is also a background of C-cell hyperplasia in the surrounding parenchyma, highlighted by the calcitonin immunohistochemistry.* ***(Right)*** *CEA usually gives a strong, heavy, cytoplasmic granular reactivity in medullary carcinoma. Polyclonal CEA is preferred to monoclonal, as there is a greater degree of sensitivity.*

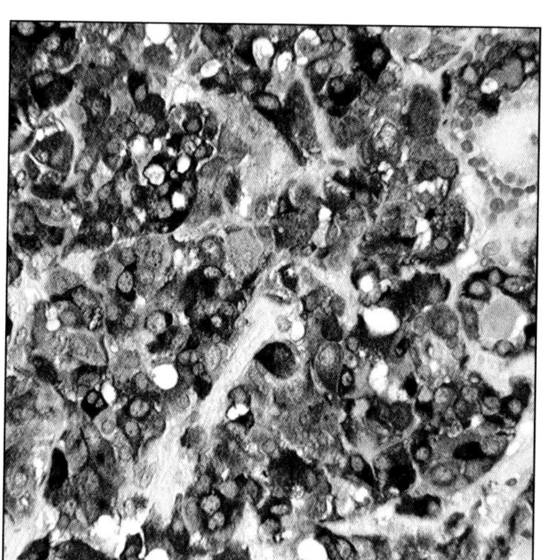

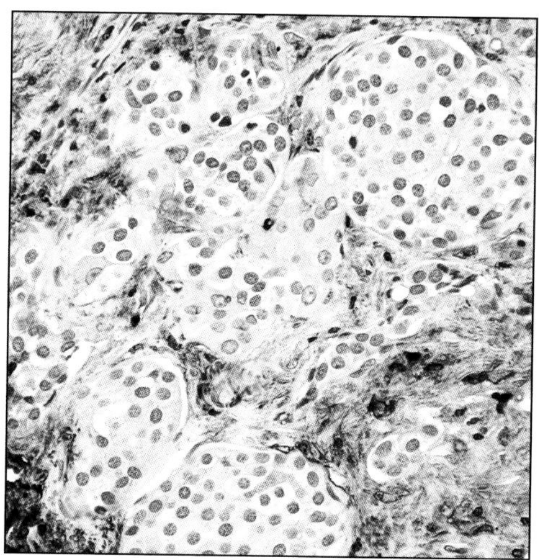

(Left) *There is a variable granular positive reaction with chromogranin. Note how some of the cells are strongly and diffusely immunoreactive, while other cells show less staining, with a weaker reaction.* ***(Right)*** *Thyroglobulin can be difficult to interpret, as there are diffusion artifacts and background reactivity from the plasma/serum. The neoplastic cells are negative in this medullary carcinoma.*

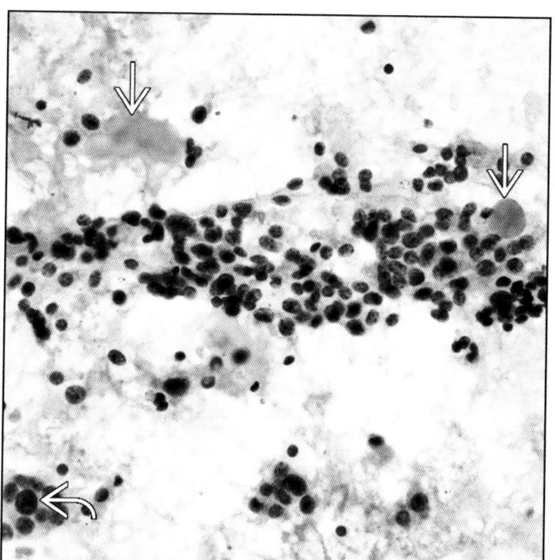

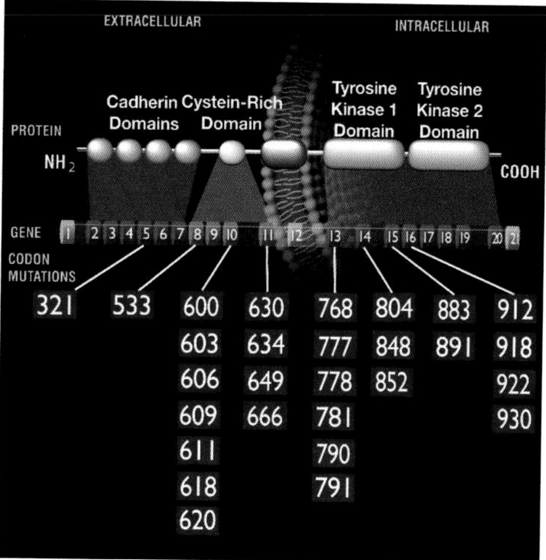

(Left) *This FNA shows dyscohesive cells with delicate nuclear chromatin distribution. Amyloid has a light green opaque appearance on PAP →. Cellular pleomorphism can be noted in isolated cells or groups →. Note the absence of colloid, although there is a vague follicular pattern.* ***(Right)*** *The RET gene is known to be associated with medullary carcinoma development. Specific codons are known to be sites of mutations resulting in hereditary medullary thyroid carcinoma, as illustrated.*

SPINDLE CELL TUMOR WITH THYMUS-LIKE DIFFERENTIATION

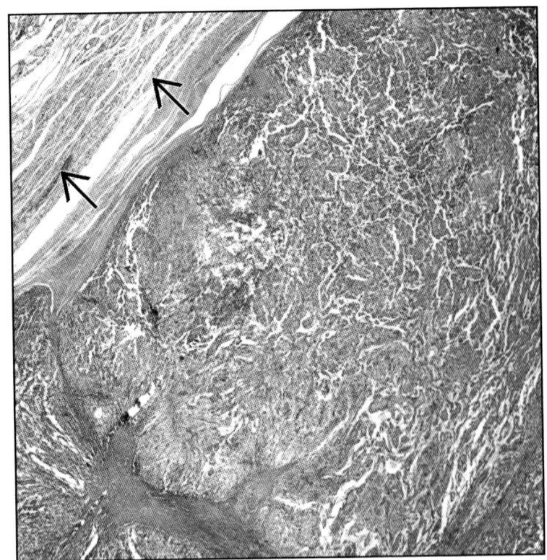

There is a very cellular tumor with lobules of tumor separated from the thyroid follicular epithelial cells ⇒ by a well-developed capsule. In this tumor there are short, intersecting and streaming bundles of tumor cells.

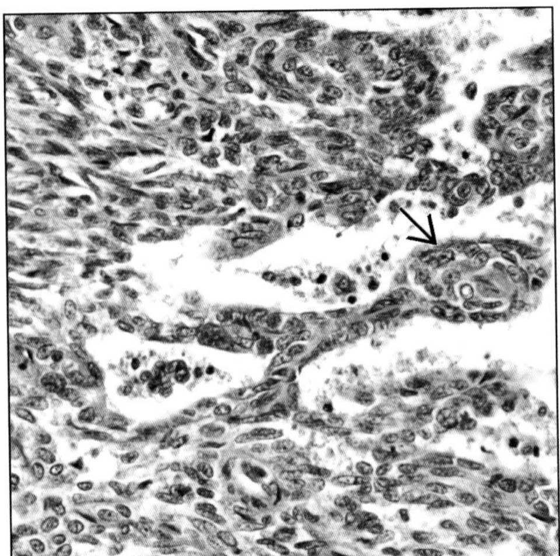

The biphasic appearance shows short, tight bundles of bland spindle cells blending with glandular and tubulopapillary structures ⇒. There is a high nuclear to cytoplasmic ratio with a syncytial appearance.

TERMINOLOGY

Abbreviations

- Spindle cell tumor with thymus-like differentiation (SETTLE)

Definitions

- Biphasic tumor showing spindle-shaped epithelial cells that blend with glandular structures, showing primitive thymic differentiation

ETIOLOGY/PATHOGENESIS

Pathogenesis

- Intrathyroidal ectopic thymic tissue
- Remnants of branchial pouches that retained ability to differentiate into thymic-type tumor

CLINICAL ISSUES

Epidemiology

- Incidence
  - Very rare
- Age
  - Most common in young patients (< 20 years)
- Gender
  - Male > Female (2:1)

Site

- Largely unilateral

Presentation

- Commonly present with painless mass
- Less frequently, patients present with
  - Rapidly enlarging neck mass
  - Localized tenderness mimicking thyroiditis
  - Tracheal compression
- Symptoms present for weeks to years

Treatment

- Options, risks, complications
  - Late metastases obligates long-term follow-up
- Surgical approaches
  - Thyroidectomy is treatment of choice
  - Resection of metastases achieves longer survival
- Drugs
  - Chemotherapy employed for metastatic disease
- Radiation
  - Used for metastatic disease

Prognosis

- Tumor has prolonged, indolent course
- ~ 90% 5-year survival
- Regional lymph node metastases can be seen at presentation
- Significant metastatic disease: 70% of cases
  - Delayed blood-borne metastases late in disease course (as many as 22 years later)
  - Frequency: Lung, lymph nodes, kidney, soft tissues
  - All metastases should be removed, since clinical course is prolonged

MACROSCOPIC FEATURES

General Features

- Variable appearance from encapsulated to partially circumscribed to infiltrative
- Vaguely lobular
- May show soft tissue adhesion (fat or skeletal muscle)
- Firm to hard, mainly solid
  - Small cysts can be seen
- Cut surface is gray-white to tan
  - Yellow areas suggest necrosis
- Gritty texture may be present

Size

- Range: 1-12 cm; mean: 3.6 cm

SPINDLE CELL TUMOR WITH THYMUS-LIKE DIFFERENTIATION

Key Facts

Terminology
- Biphasic tumor showing spindle-shaped epithelial cells that blend with glandular structures, showing primitive thymic differentiation

Clinical Issues
- Most common in young patients (< 20 years)
- Largely unilateral
- Tumor has prolonged, indolent course
- Late metastases obligates long-term follow-up
- Delayed blood-borne metastases late in disease course

Microscopic Pathology
- Very cellular tumor with primitive thymus histology
- Lobules of tumor separated by acellular, sclerotic fibrous septa
- Most tumors are biphasic
  - Short, reticulated, intersecting and streaming, tight to loose fascicles or bundles
  - Blend with glandular and tubulopapillary structures
- Long, spindled cells with scant cytoplasm
- Pale-staining cuboidal to columnar cells lining cysts

Ancillary Tests
- Spindle and glandular cells positive with
  - AE1/AE3, CAM5.2, EMA, CK7, vimentin, INI1, CD117
- Negative: Thyroglobulin, TTF-1, calcitonin, CEA, CD5, S100 protein, synaptophysin, chromogranin, CK20

Top Differential Diagnoses
- Undifferentiated carcinoma, synovial sarcoma
- Medullary carcinoma, spindled variant

MICROSCOPIC PATHOLOGY

Histologic Features
- Very cellular tumor with primitive thymus histology
- Lobules of tumor separated by acellular, sclerotic fibrous septa
- Vascular invasion may be present
- Most tumors are biphasic
  - Short, reticulated, intersecting and streaming, tight to loose fascicles or bundles
  - Blend with glandular and tubulopapillary structures
- Long, spindled cells with scant cytoplasm
  - Syncytial pattern without distinct cell borders
  - Whorling to storiform patterns
- Elongated nuclei with fine, delicate nuclear chromatin
- Nuclear pleomorphism is focal
- Glandular structures
  - Large cystic spaces lined with respiratory epithelium
  - Mucinous glands, cords, nests, Sertoli-like tubules, glomeruloid structures
  - Pale-staining cuboidal to columnar cells lining cysts
  - Cells may be goblet-like or ciliated
  - Nuclei tend to be more round than spindle cells
- Mitotic figures are scant
  - Rarely necrosis and mitoses are seen
- Intercellular fluid and mucin may be seen
- Squamous metaplasia or keratin pearls are exceptional
- Lymphocytes, often at periphery
- Calcifications are uncommon
- Rare cases are monophasic (spindle or glandular cells)

ANCILLARY TESTS

Cytology
- Smears are cellular, with cohesive clusters and single dissociated, bland spindle cells
  - Spindle cells have scant fibrillar cytoplasm and bland uniform nuclei
- Background: Red metachromatic extracellular, homogeneous material (MGG)
  - Fine, dust-like granules or irregular clumps

Immunohistochemistry
- Spindle and glandular cells: AE1/AE3, CAM5.2, EMA, CK7, vimentin, INI1, CD117
  - Some cells: SMA, MSA, CD99
- Negative: Thyroglobulin, TTF-1, calcitonin, CEA, CD5, S100 protein, synaptophysin, chromogranin, CK20

DIFFERENTIAL DIAGNOSIS

Undifferentiated Carcinoma
- Tumor of old patients with rapidly enlarged mass
- Infiltrative, marked pleomorphism, extensive necrosis
- Limited to absent keratin immunoreactivity

Synovial Sarcoma
- Also seen in young patients
- Often biphasic tumor with spindle cell population
- t(X;18) *SYT-SSX* gene fusion confirms diagnosis

Medullary Carcinoma
- Frequently contains stromal amyloid
- Nuclear chromatin is more coarse
- Positive: Calcitonin, CEA, chromogranin

Ectopic Thymoma
- Jigsaw-puzzle–like lobulation
- Rich, immature TdT-positive T-cell population

SELECTED REFERENCES

1. Folpe AL et al: Spindle epithelial tumor with thymus-like differentiation: a morphologic, immunohistochemical, and molecular genetic study of 11 cases. Am J Surg Pathol. 33(8):1179-86, 2009
2. Grushka JR et al: Spindle epithelial tumor with thymus-like elements of the thyroid: a multi-institutional case series and review of the literature. J Pediatr Surg. 44(5):944-8, 2009
3. Chan JK et al: Tumors of the neck showing thymic or related branchial pouch differentiation: a unifying concept. Hum Pathol. 22(4):349-67, 1991

SPINDLE CELL TUMOR WITH THYMUS-LIKE DIFFERENTIATION

Gross and Microscopic Features

*(**Left**) The cut surface shows a fleshy tumor with invasion of the entire thyroid gland. There are cystic spaces, with a shiny surface. (Courtesy X. Matias-Guiu, MD.) (**Right**) Sclerotic septa are noted to intersect between the lobules of tumor. A fibrous connective tissue capsule separates the tumor from the surrounding thyroid parenchyma ⇒. The spindled pattern of growth is easily identified, even at this magnification.*

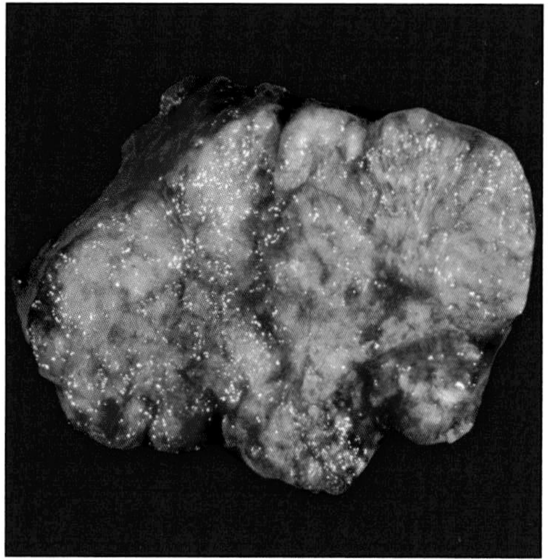

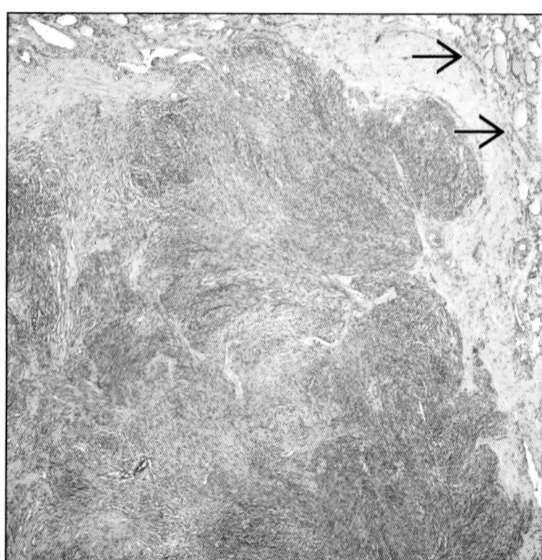

*(**Left**) Lobules of tumor are separated by acellular, sclerotic fibrous septa. In this field, there are short fascicles, juxtaposed to the thyroid gland parenchyma ⇒. (**Right**) The acellular fibrous septa separate the spindled cells into streaming tight fascicles. The cells are monotonous and bland. There is a syncytial pattern without distinct cell borders. The stroma is slightly mucinous ⇒ in this lesion.*

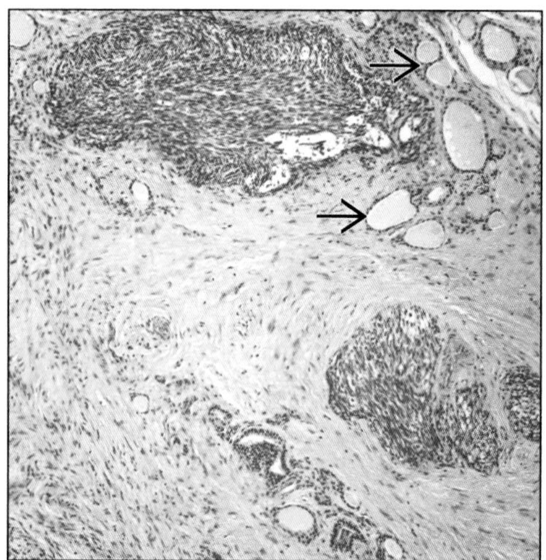

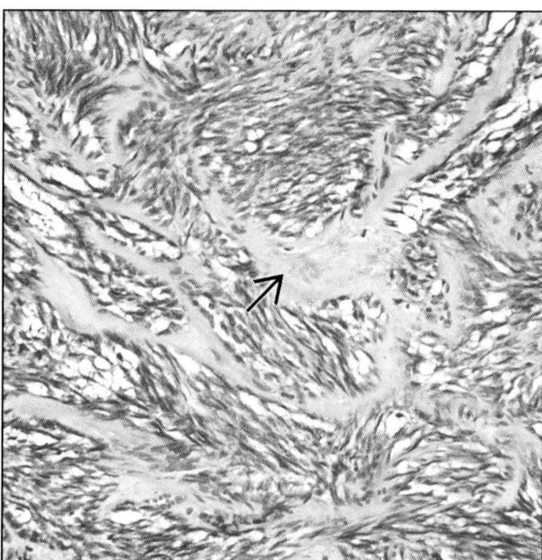

*(**Left**) In this tumor there is a more prominent epithelioid appearance to the spindled population. The syncytium shows areas of primitive glandular differentiation ⇒. The cells have a high nuclear to cytoplasmic ratio. (**Right**) This field shows short, reticulated, intersecting and streaming, tight fascicles or bundles of bland, elongated spindled cells with scant cytoplasm. There are indistinct cell borders.*

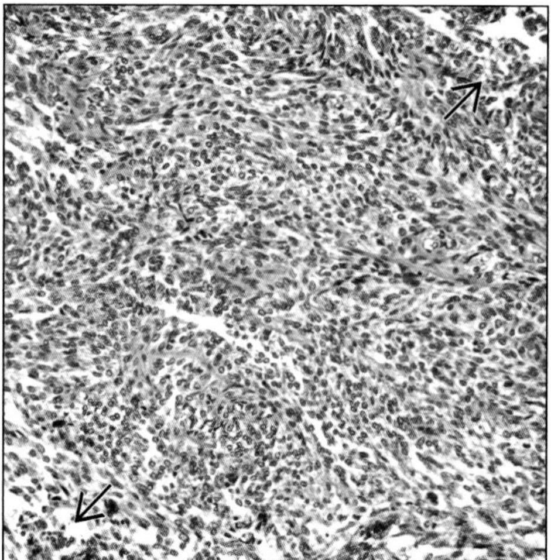

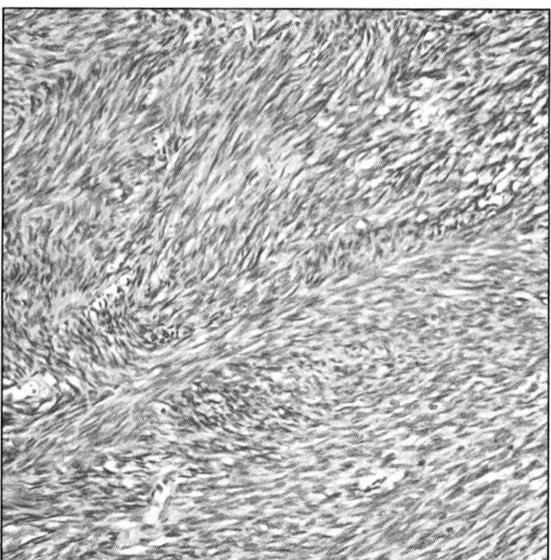

Microscopic and Immunohistochemical Features

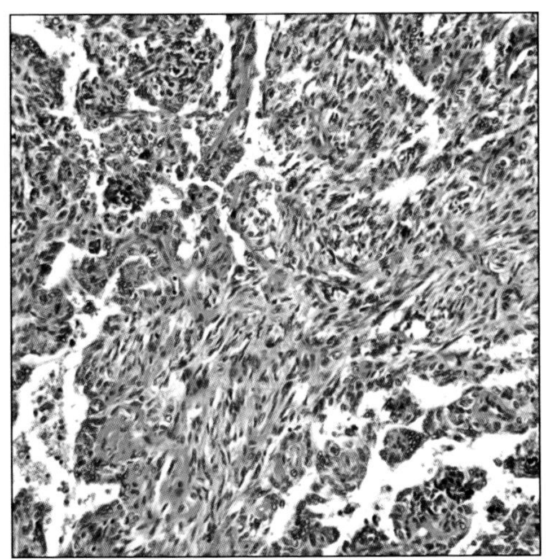

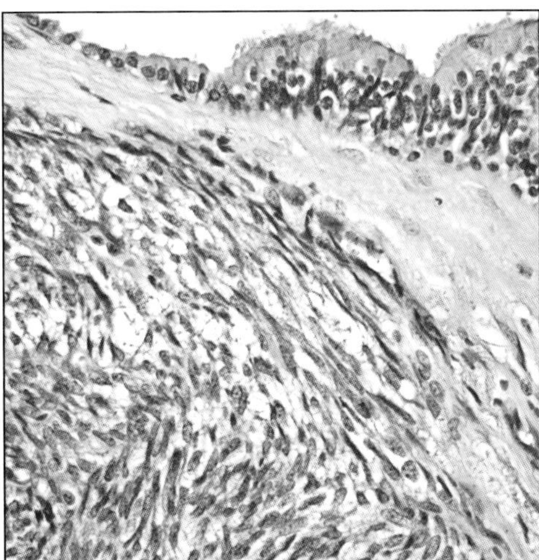

(Left) *The characteristic biphasic appearance is well developed with short fascicles blending into areas of papillary to glandular profiles. The cuboidal to columnar cells line the cystic spaces.* ***(Right)*** *Short bundles of spindled cells are separated by a mucinous material. The cystic space is lined by respiratory epithelium, showing pseudostratified columnar cells. The nuclei are rounder than the spindled population.*

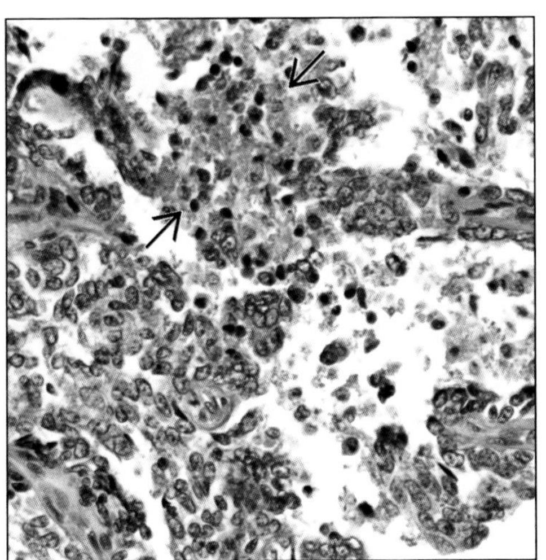

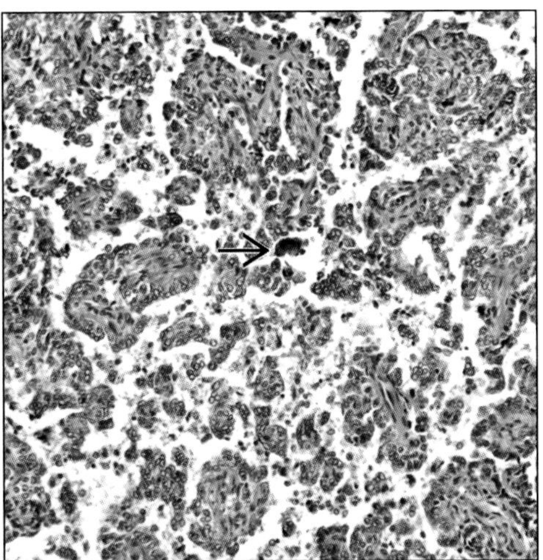

(Left) *These glandular and tubulopapillary structures show an area of necrosis* ⇒ *associated with slightly greater pleomorphism. The nuclei are still vesicular with delicate nuclear chromatin distribution.* ***(Right)*** *This area demonstrates the cystic spaces comprised of numerous tubulopapillary structures. The cells have pale-staining cuboidal to columnar cells lining the cysts. This field highlights an isolated calcification* ⇒.

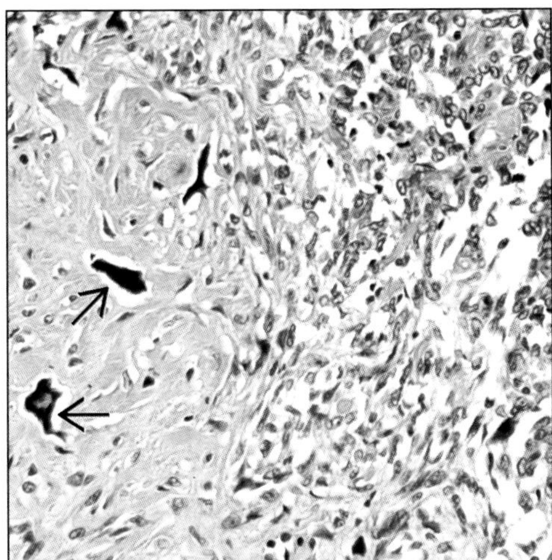

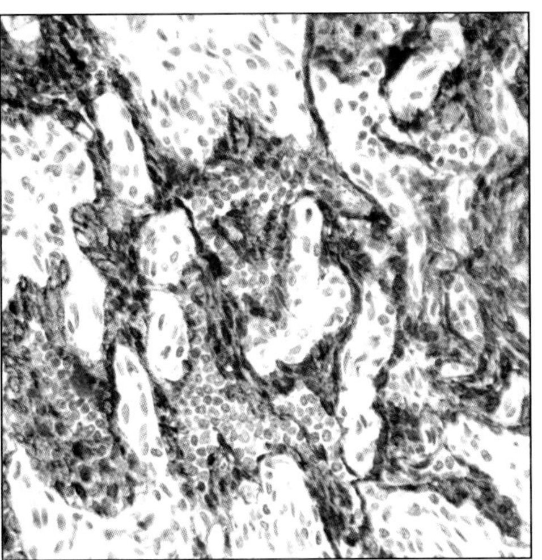

(Left) *The fibrous septa contain highly pleomorphic tumor cells* ⇒. *The remainder of the tumor shows the blending of spindled and tubulopapillary structures, showing long, spindled cells with scant cytoplasm and limited pleomorphism.* ***(Right)*** *Many different epithelial markers are positive, but keratin highlights the spindled and glandular cells. Some cells will also show reactions with actins. There is usually absent thyroglobulin, TTF-1, calcitonin, synaptophysin, and CD5.*

CARCINOMA SHOWING THYMUS-LIKE DIFFERENTIATION

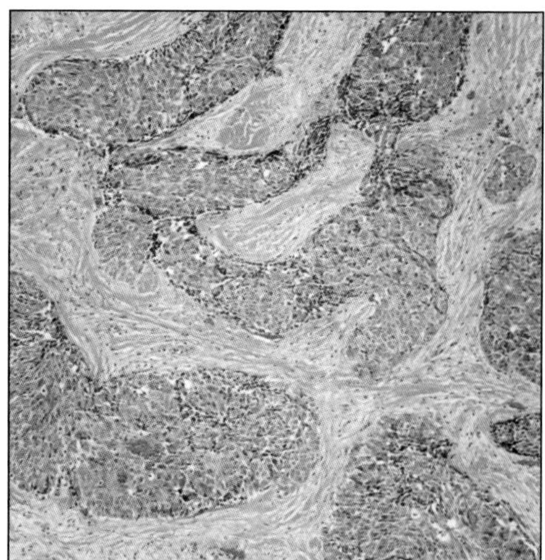

The low-power appearance of CASTLE is identical to thymic carcinoma, in which there is a distinctly lobular architecture and very heavy, dense, keloid-like collagenized fibrous bands.

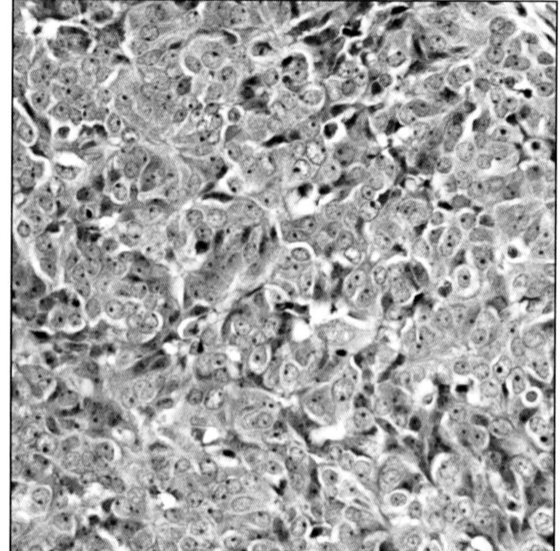

This field shows a lymphoepithelial quality that can be seen in CASTLE. The tumor is nonkeratinizing, with an undifferentiated appearance. Note the vesicular nuclear chromatin with small nucleoli.

TERMINOLOGY

Abbreviations

- Carcinoma showing thymus-like differentiation (CASTLE)

Synonyms

- Lymphoepithelioma-like carcinoma of thyroid gland
- Intrathyroid epithelial thymoma
- Primary thyroid thymoma

Definitions

- Primary thyroid gland malignancy that is architecturally and cytologically similar to thymic epithelial tumors

ETIOLOGY/PATHOGENESIS

Pathogenesis

- Arises from thymic rests adjacent to or within thyroid gland
  - Persistence of cervical thymic tissue from embryologic development
  - Branchial pouch remnants (including solid cell nests) that can differentiate along thymic lines

CLINICAL ISSUES

Epidemiology

- Incidence
  - Very rare (< 1% of all thyroid gland malignancies)
- Age
  - Most common in 5th decade
- Gender
  - Female > Male (1.3:1)

Site

- Vast majority in lower poles of thyroid gland
  - Rare cases may arise in perithyroid soft tissues

Presentation

- Commonly present with painless thyroid mass
- Less frequently, patients present with
  - Tracheal compression
  - Hoarseness
- Enlarged neck lymph nodes are seen in up to 30%
- Clinical associations with thymoma are not yet documented in CASTLE
  - These include: Myasthenia gravis, hypogammaglobulinemia, red-cell aplasia/hypoplasia, dermatomyositis

Laboratory Tests

- Thyroid function tests are normal

Treatment

- Options, risks, complications
  - Long-term clinical follow-up due to protracted clinical course
- Surgical approaches
  - Thyroidectomy is treatment of choice
  - Lymph node dissection in clinically positive neck
- Adjuvant therapy
  - Neoadjuvant chemotherapy may decrease tumor size, permitting definitive surgery
    - Etoposide and carboplatin have decreased tumor size
- Drugs
  - Chemotherapy may achieve rapid relief of symptoms, helping to decrease tumor size
- Radiation
  - Usually employed postoperatively
    - Patients receiving radiation tend not to develop locoregional recurrence

Prognosis

- Local recurrences seen in up to 30% of patients
- Cervical lymph node metastases in up to 30% of patients
  - Associated with worse prognosis

CARCINOMA SHOWING THYMUS-LIKE DIFFERENTIATION

Key Facts

Terminology
- Primary thyroid gland malignancy that is architecturally and cytologically similar to thymic epithelial tumors

Etiology/Pathogenesis
- Persistence of cervical thymic tissue from embryologic development

Clinical Issues
- Vast majority in lower poles of thyroid gland
- Commonly present with painless thyroid mass
- Protracted course requires long-term follow-up
- 10-year cause-specific survival: 82%

Microscopic Pathology
- Well circumscribed, slightly lobulated, and easily demarcated
  - Extrathyroidal extension is common
- Broad, pushing, smooth-bordered islands
- Desmoplastic cellular stroma
- Tumor cells are squamoid and syncytial to spindled
- Well-defined cell borders, intercellular bridges, and frank keratinization are uncommon
- Nuclei are oval, with vesicular chromatin
- Lymphocytes and plasma cells present
- Neoplastic cells positive: Pancytokeratin (especially HMWK), CD5, p63

Top Differential Diagnoses
- Undifferentiated carcinoma, squamous cell carcinoma, medullary carcinoma, direct extension from thymic primary

- Generally, good long-term prognosis
  - 10-year cause-specific survival: 82%
  - A few patients may experience rapidly fatal course

IMAGE FINDINGS

Radiographic Findings
- Scintigraphy shows cold nodule
- Computed tomography usually shows solid, noncalcified soft tissue density, perhaps with invasion
  - Slight enhancement with contrast material
- Appears as iso- or hypointense mass on T1-weighted magnetic resonance and hyperintense on T2-weighted imaging
- Ultrasound shows hypoechoic and heterogeneous mass

MACROSCOPIC FEATURES

General Features
- Well circumscribed, slightly lobulated, and easily demarcated
- Cut surfaces are firm to fleshy
- Mixture of yellow, gray, and tan

MICROSCOPIC PATHOLOGY

Histologic Features
- Similar to thymic carcinoma
- Extrathyroidal extension is common, including larynx and trachea
- Broad, pushing, smooth-bordered islands
  - Tumor cells are squamoid and syncytial to spindled
  - Pale to eosinophilic cytoplasm
  - Well-defined cell borders, intercellular bridges, and frank keratinization are uncommon
  - Nuclei are oval, show limited pleomorphism, and have fine pale to vesicular chromatin
  - Nucleoli are small, but easily identified
- Desmoplastic cellular stroma
- Tumor lobules associated with delicate vessels
- Lymphocytes and plasma cells present within tumor nests
- Mitotic figures are present but not increased (< 3/10 HPF)
- Hassall corpuscles may be seen (at tumor periphery)
- Granulomas are usually not identified

ANCILLARY TESTS

Cytology
- Cellular smears with atypical epithelial cells arranged in sheets and single cells
- Nuclei have vesicular chromatin and prominent nucleoli
- Lymphoid elements present in background

Immunohistochemistry
- Neoplastic cells positive: Pancytokeratin (especially HMWK), CD5, p63
- Negative: TTF-1, thyroglobulin, calcitonin, Epstein-Barr virus-encoded RNA (EBER)

Electron Microscopy
- Elongated epithelial cells with prominent desmosomes, bundles of cytoplasmic tonofilaments, lacking secretory granules and amyloid fibers

DIFFERENTIAL DIAGNOSIS

Undifferentiated (Anaplastic) Carcinoma
- Significant invasion, remarkable pleomorphism, atypical mitotic figures, tumor necrosis
- Usually shows only limited immunoreactivity, with vimentin only in many cases

Squamous Cell Carcinoma
- Significant keratinization, pearl formation, and intercellular bridges
- Invasive tumor
- Positive with S100-A9, but negative with CD5

CARCINOMA SHOWING THYMUS-LIKE DIFFERENTIATION

Immunohistochemistry

Antibody	Reactivity	Staining Pattern	Comment
CK-HMW-NOS	Positive	Cytoplasmic	All tumor cells, strong and diffuse
CK-PAN	Positive	Cytoplasmic	Nearly all tumor cells, strong and diffuse
CD5	Positive	Cytoplasmic	Nearly all tumor cells
p63	Positive	Nuclear	Most neoplastic cells
CEA-M	Positive	Cytoplasmic	Most tumor cells show reactivity
Bcl-1	Positive	Nuclear	This antiapoptosis proto-oncogene is usually positive
Mcl-1	Positive	Nuclear	Usually positive in most tumor cells
S100-A9	Positive	Nuclear & cytoplasmic	Isolated tumor cells will be positive
CD70	Positive	Cytoplasmic	Strong and diffuse positive
p53	Positive	Nuclear	Tends to be increased
TdT	Negative		In lymphoid cell compartment
CD1a	Negative		In lymphoid cell compartment
TTF-1	Negative		
Thyroglobulin	Negative		
Calcitonin	Negative		
EBER	Negative		
Chromogranin-A	Negative		

Medullary Carcinoma

- Variable morphology, including plasmacytoid and spindled cells
- Amyloid and background C-cell hyperplasia
- Positive: Calcitonin, chromogranin, CEA-M, CD56

Follicular Dendritic Cell Sarcoma

- Has lobular pattern, although infiltrating into thyroid tissue
- Extensive vascular space invasion
- Syncytial arrangement of spindled to epithelioid cells
- Nuclear chromatin is vesicular with small, well-defined nucleoli
- Positive: CD21, CD23, CD35
- Negative: Keratin, CD5

Thymic Primary

- Direct invasion into thyroid from thymic primary
- Radiographs and intraoperative findings should exclude continuity from thymic tumor

Metastatic Lymphoepithelial Carcinoma

- Primary site is most frequently nasopharynx but could be any location
- Lacks squamous differentiation, shows prominent nucleoli
- Strongly reactive with Epstein-Barr virus-encoded RNA (EBER)

Ectopic Thymoma

- Thymoma can be found in ectopic location
- Noninvasive, well circumscribed, and encapsulated
- Negative with Bcl-2 and Mcl-1, but positive with CD5 and keratin

Ectopic Hamartomatous Thymoma

- Arises in low, anterior neck, but may "appear" thyroidal
- Unique pattern with adipose tissue and haphazard distribution of thymic tissues

SELECTED REFERENCES

1. Chan LP et al: Carcinoma showing thymus-like differentiation (CASTLE) of thyroid: a case report and literature review. Kaohsiung J Med Sci. 24(11):591-7, 2008
2. Chow SM et al: Carcinoma showing thymus-like element (CASTLE) of thyroid: combined modality treatment in 3 patients with locally advanced disease. Eur J Surg Oncol. 33(1):83-5, 2007
3. Ito Y et al: Clinicopathologic significance of intrathyroidal epithelial thymoma/carcinoma showing thymus-like differentiation: a collaborative study with Member Institutes of The Japanese Society of Thyroid Surgery. Am J Clin Pathol. 127(2):230-6, 2007
4. Ito Y et al: Usefulness of S100A9 for diagnosis of intrathyroid epithelial thymoma (ITET)/carcinoma showing thymus-like differentiation (CASTLE). Pathology. 38(6):541-4, 2006
5. Papi G et al: Primary spindle cell lesions of the thyroid gland; an overview. Am J Clin Pathol. 125 Suppl:S95-123, 2006
6. Reimann JD et al: Carcinoma showing thymus-like differentiation of the thyroid (CASTLE): a comparative study: evidence of thymic differentiation and solid cell nest origin. Am J Surg Pathol. 30(8):994-1001, 2006
7. Yoneda K et al: CT and MRI findings of carcinoma showing thymus-like differentiation. Radiat Med. 23(6):451-5, 2005
8. Ahuja AT et al: Carcinoma showing thymiclike differentiation (CASTLE tumor). AJNR Am J Neuroradiol. 19(7):1225-8, 1998
9. Berezowski K et al: CD5 immunoreactivity of epithelial cells in thymic carcinoma and CASTLE using paraffin-embedded tissue. Am J Clin Pathol. 106(4):483-6, 1996
10. Chan JK et al: Tumors of the neck showing thymic or related branchial pouch differentiation: a unifying concept. Hum Pathol. 22(4):349-67, 1991

Microscopic and Immunohistochemical Features

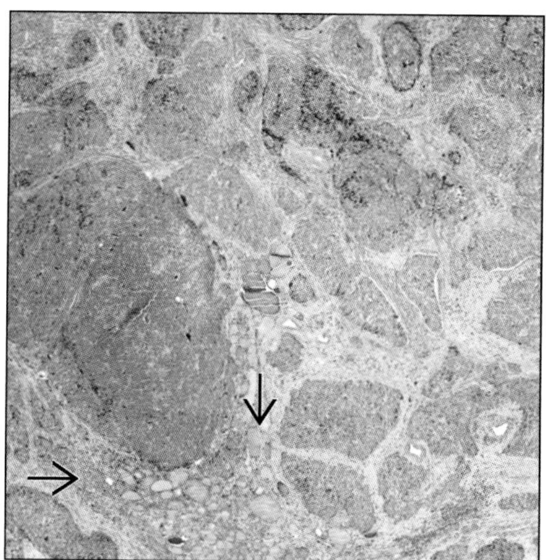

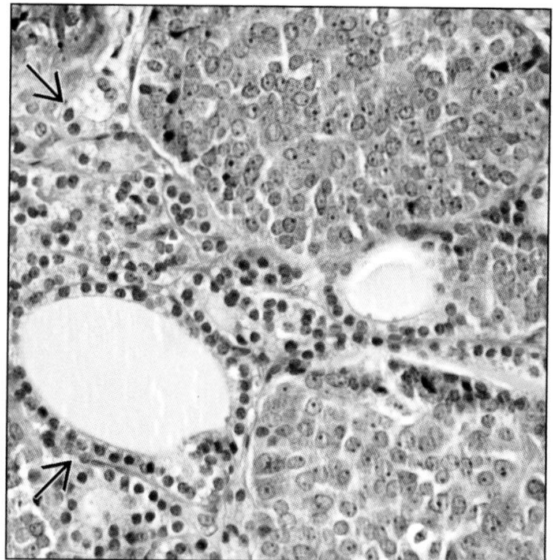

*(**Left**) The thyroid parenchyma ⇒ is infiltrated by the lobules of neoplastic epithelium. The tumor cells show well-demarcated islands separated by dense, hyalinized fibrous bands. This is a typical pattern for CASTLE. (**Right**) The lobules of neoplastic cells show a syncytial appearance. The cells have a very high nuclear to cytoplasmic ratio, vesicular nuclear chromatin, and delicate nucleoli. The thyroid follicles are surrounded by the neoplastic proliferation ⇒.*

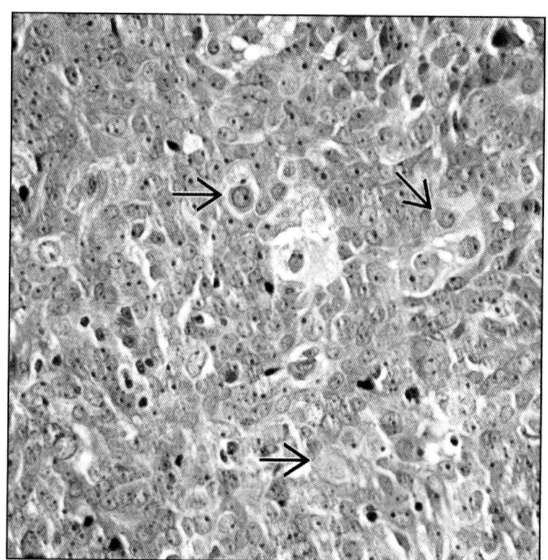

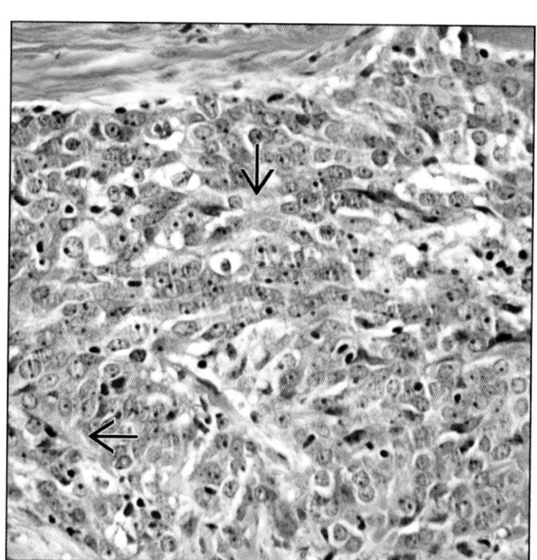

*(**Left**) There is a vague squamoid appearance to a number of the cells ⇒, which are otherwise arranged in a syncytial appearance. Intercellular borders are not prominent in this field. A few inflammatory cells are noted. (**Right**) Note the bands of fibrosis at the periphery of the tumor island. A spindled morphology is present in this area. Intercellular bridges can be appreciated ⇒, a finding that helps with the diagnosis.*

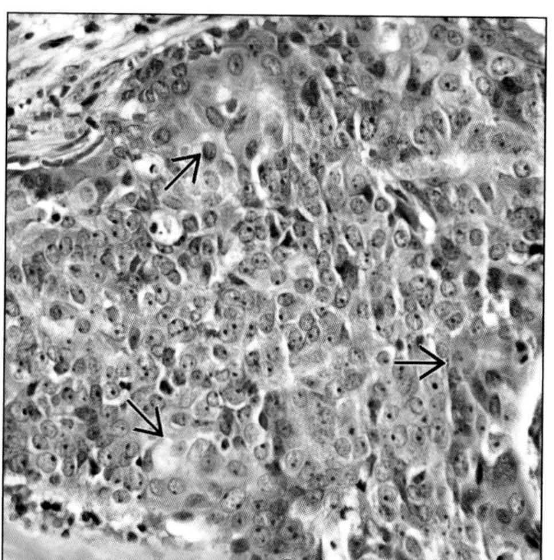

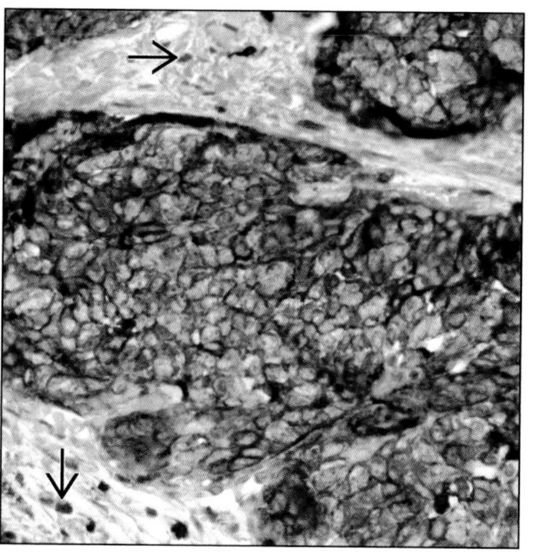

*(**Left**) Areas of squamous differentiation are sometimes quite subtle, as shown in this case. There is blending of the squamous areas ⇒ with the rest of the tumor, highlighting how difficult it can be to see these areas. (**Right**) CD5 shows a very strong and diffuse immunoreactivity in the neoplastic cells of CASTLE, a distinctive finding in the thyroid. T-cells in the fibrosis ⇒ serve as a positive internal control. CD5 is a receptor molecule that signals cell growth for T-cells.*

MUCOEPIDERMOID CARCINOMA

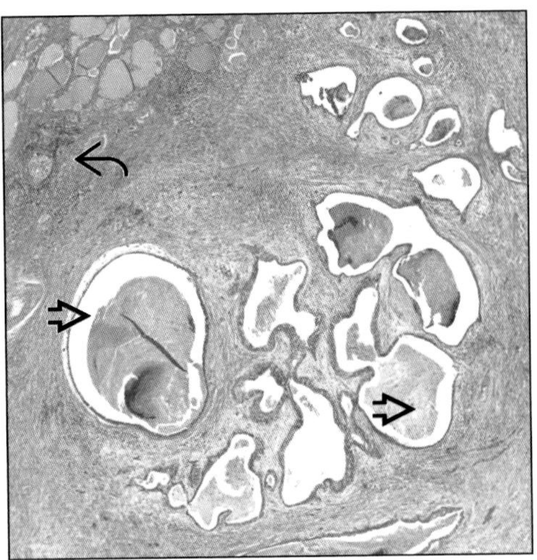

Infiltrative neoplastic proliferation shows predominantly cystic ➩ growth with associated fibrosis. Focal lymphocytic thyroiditis is present ➩ in the adjacent thyroid parenchyma.

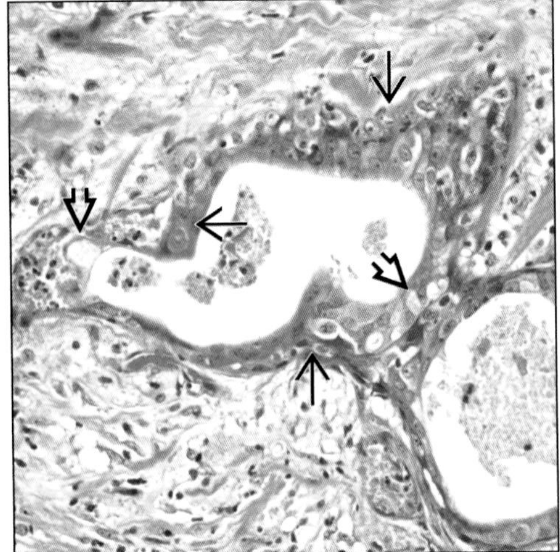

The neoplastic proliferation includes an admixture of epidermoid/squamous cells → with keratinization and mucocytes ➩ with clear appearing cytoplasm and peripherally located nucleus.

TERMINOLOGY

Abbreviations

- Mucoepidermoid carcinoma of thyroid gland (MECT)

Definitions

- Low-grade malignant thyroid tumor with histologic appearance similar to low-grade salivary gland counterpart
  - 2 histologic variants
    - Mucoepidermoid carcinoma
    - Sclerosing mucoepidermoid carcinoma with eosinophilia
  - Subclassification into 2 distinct entities appears justified based on apparent differences in light microscopic and immunohistochemical findings
  - Separation may be academic, since both tumor types share similar indolent biologic course

ETIOLOGY/PATHOGENESIS

Idiopathic

- No known etiologic factors

Histogenesis

- Cell of origin for MECT subject of debate
- Follicular epithelial cell origin favored on basis of
  - Presence of thyroglobulin, TTF-1 reactivity
  - Presence of thyroid-specific mRNAs (RT-PCR of TTF-1, TTF-2, pax-8, Na-I symporter, and thyroid peroxidase mRNA)
  - Absence of calcitonin and chromogranin
  - Association with thyroid papillary carcinoma (TPC)
    - Some authorities believe MECT represents variant of papillary carcinoma
  - Presence of keratinization, intercellular bridges
  - Presence of psammoma bodies
  - Occurrence in background of lymphocytic thyroiditis (LT), a common setting to find squamous metaplasia
    - Possible origin from squamous metaplasia
  - Indolent biology
  - Tendency to metastasize to regional lymph nodes
- Solid cell nests (SCN) of ultimobranchial origin (give rise to C-cells) considered progenitor based on some histologic, histochemical, and immunohistochemical (e.g., p63) features
  - SCN origin not favored based on
    - SCN lacking intercellular bridges
    - Absence of calcitonin, chromogranin immunoreactivity in MECT
    - Occurrence of MECT in isthmus and pyramidal lobes locations where SCNs not found

CLINICAL ISSUES

Epidemiology

- Incidence
  - Uncommon
    - Accounts for < 0.5% of all thyroid gland malignancies
- Age
  - Occurs over wide age range (2nd-8th decades)
    - Most patients in 5th-7th decades of life
- Gender
  - Female > Male

Site

- Any portion of thyroid gland including isthmus

Presentation

- Painless neck mass most common presenting complaint
- Less commonly, pain, hoarseness, vocal cord paralysis may occur

MUCOEPIDERMOID CARCINOMA

Key Facts

Terminology

- Low-grade malignant thyroid tumor with histologic appearance similar to low-grade salivary gland counterpart

Etiology/Pathogenesis

- Follicular epithelial cell origin favored

Clinical Issues

- Painless neck mass most common presenting complaint
- Surgery is treatment of choice
  - Conservative therapy (lobectomy or subtotal thyroidectomy) can be performed
- Indolent tumor with excellent prognosis

Microscopic Pathology

- Circumscribed but unencapsulated predominantly solid mass
- **Squamous or epidermoid cells**
  - Round to oval cells with round nuclei, prominent centrally located nucleoli, and eosinophilic cytoplasm
  - Horny pearl formation, individual cell keratinization, and intercellular bridges
- **Mucous cells**
  - Cells with abundant clear to foamy-appearing cytoplasm and peripherally located hyperchromatic nuclei

Laboratory Tests

- Patients are euthyroid

Treatment

- Surgical approaches
  - Surgery is treatment of choice
    - Conservative therapy (lobectomy or subtotal thyroidectomy) can be performed
    - In presence of extrathyroidal extension, total thyroidectomy advocated

Prognosis

- Indolent tumor with excellent prognosis
- Metastatic tumor to cervical lymph nodes may be seen
  - In up to 40% of patients
- Distant metastasis is uncommon but may occur (e.g., lung, bone, pleura)
- Death from tumor may occur in older patients
  - Usually limited to cases with anaplastic (undifferentiated) component

IMAGE FINDINGS

Radiographic Findings

- Hypoactive ("cold") nodule on thyroid imaging

MACROSCOPIC FEATURES

General Features

- Solitary demarcated but unencapsulated mass
  - May be infiltrative
  - Extrathyroidal extension may be identifiable
- Cut section shows
  - Solid, nodular appearance
  - Tan-brown to yellow-orange in color, rubbery to firm consistency
  - Cystic change sometimes with myxoid-mucoid appearance can be seen

Size

- May measure up to 3.5 cm in greatest dimension

MICROSCOPIC PATHOLOGY

Histologic Features

- Circumscribed but unencapsulated predominantly solid mass
  - Prominent cystic foci may be present
- Infiltrative with intertwined cords and nests of neoplastic cells in fibrous stroma
- Neoplastic proliferation includes squamous/epidermoid cells admixed with mucocytes
- **Squamous or epidermoid cells**
  - Round to oval cells with round nuclei, prominent centrally located nucleoli and eosinophilic cytoplasm
  - Horny pearl formation, individual cell keratinization and intercellular bridges
  - Mild nuclear pleomorphism, slight increase in nuclear to cytoplasmic ratio, scattered mitotic figures
- **Mucous cells**
  - Cells with abundant clear to foamy appearing cytoplasm and peripherally located hyperchromatic nuclei
  - Intimately admixed with squamous/epidermoid cells
  - Ciliated cells may be seen
  - Hyaline bodies resembling colloid may be seen in cytoplasm of mucocytes
- Mixed inflammatory cell infiltrate including mature lymphocytes and plasma cells seen within neoplastic proliferation
  - Eosinophils may predominate in any given tumor
- Intratumoral sclerosis composed of thick, acellular hyalinized bands of tissue can be seen
- Psammoma bodies occasionally present
- Nuclear grooves and intranuclear cytoplasmic inclusions can be seen
- Chronic lymphocytic thyroiditis commonly but not invariably present in surrounding nonneoplastic thyroid gland
  - May include foci of squamous metaplasia

MUCOEPIDERMOID CARCINOMA

- Foci of papillary carcinoma (separate or admixed) may be seen
  - Concurrent papillary carcinoma identified in up to 50% of cases
  - Areas of transition between MECT and papillary thyroid carcinoma can be seen
  - May rarely include tall cell features
- Generally confined to thyroid gland but extrathyroidal extension may occur
- Rarely, MEC associated with
  - Anaplastic areas
    - Transition between 2 histological patterns
  - High-grade cellular features

ANCILLARY TESTS

Cytology

- Smears are cellular with cohesive monolayered and syncytial sheets of cells
  - Background of amorphous debris and necrotic and mucinous material may be present
- Cellular sheets with microcystic-like pattern containing hyaline bodies may be identified
- Dual-cell population of
  - Mucocytes: Vacuolated to foamy cytoplasm compressing nucleus
  - Epidermoid cells: Polygonal cells with distinct cell borders, round nuclei, vesicular chromatin, prominent nucleoli, eosinophilic cytoplasm

Histochemistry

- Mucicarmine & periodic acid-Schiff (PAS) with diastase
  - Intracytoplasmic and intraluminal mucin positive material can be seen
  - Cystic spaces also show mucicarminophilic material
- Hyaline bodies PAS positive

Immunohistochemistry

- Cytokeratin (high and low molecular weight) positive
- Thyroglobulin, TTF-1 may be focally positive but often negative
- Epidermoid cells
  - p63, CK5/6 positive
- Mucocytes
  - Carcinoembryonic antigen (CEA) positive
- Calcitonin, neuroendocrine markers negative

Molecular Genetics

- Expression by RT-PCR of TTF-1, TTF-2, Pax-8, Na-I symporter and thyroid peroxidase mRNA
  - Presence of these thyroid-specific mRNAs indicative of origin from thyroid follicular epithelium
  - *BRAF* (V600E) mutation not detected
- *MECT1/TORC1/CRTC1-MAML2* fusion transcript may be identified by RT-PCR
  - Corresponds to detectable translocation t(11;19)
  - Commonly present in salivary gland MEC
- Marked abnormalities of cadherin/catenin complex
  - Consistent neoexpression of P-cadherin
  - Major alterations in expression of E-cadherin

DIFFERENTIAL DIAGNOSIS

Squamous Metaplasia in Lymphocytic Thyroiditis

- Does not produce mass
- Absence of mucocytes

Epithelial Cysts in Lymphocytic Thyroiditis

- Predominantly lined by squamous epithelium
- Columnar (respiratory-type) epithelium can be seen, which may contain mucocytes that stain for mucin
- Almost invariably described in association with chronic lymphocytic thyroiditis
- Unifocal or multifocal without infiltrative growth or associated desmoplasia

TPC with Squamous Metaplasia

- Characteristic nuclear features diagnostic for papillary carcinoma
- Absence of mucocytes

Medullary Carcinoma with Squamous Differentiation

- Presence of calcitonin, neuroendocrine markers

Primary Thyroid Squamous Cell Carcinoma

- Characterized by marked cytologic atypia
- Absence of mucocytes

SELECTED REFERENCES

1. Tirado Y et al: CRTC1/MAML2 fusion transcript in high grade mucoepidermoid carcinomas of salivary and thyroid glands and Warthin's tumors: implications for histogenesis and biologic behavior. Genes Chromosomes Cancer. 46(7):708-15, 2007
2. Hunt JL et al: p63 expression in sclerosing mucoepidermoid carcinomas with eosinophilia arising in the thyroid. Mod Pathol. 17(5):526-9, 2004
3. Minagawa A et al: A case of primary mucoepidermoid carcinoma of the thyroid: molecular evidence of its origin. Clin Endocrinol (Oxf). 2002 Oct;57(4):551-6. Erratum in: Clin Endocrinol (Oxf). 58(1):114, 2003
4. Rocha AS et al: Mucoepidermoid carcinoma of the thyroid: a tumour histotype characterised by P-cadherin neoexpression and marked abnormalities of E-cadherin/catenins complex. Virchows Arch. 440(5):498-504, 2002
5. Baloch ZW et al: Primary mucoepidermoid carcinoma and sclerosing mucoepidermoid carcinoma with eosinophilia of the thyroid gland: a report of nine cases. Mod Pathol. 13(7):802-7, 2000
6. Cameselle-Teijeiro J et al: Papillary and mucoepidermoid carcinoma of the thyroid with anaplastic transformation: a case report with histologic and immunohistochemical findings that support a provocative histogenetic hypothesis. Pathol Res Pract. 191(12):1214-21, 1995
7. Wenig BM et al: Primary mucoepidermoid carcinoma of the thyroid gland: a report of six cases and a review of the literature of a follicular epithelial-derived tumor. Hum Pathol. 26(10):1099-108, 1995
8. Larson RS et al: Primary mucoepidermoid carcinoma of the thyroid: diagnosis by fine-needle aspiration biopsy. Diagn Cytopathol. 9(4):438-43, 1993

Microscopic Features and Ancillary Techniques

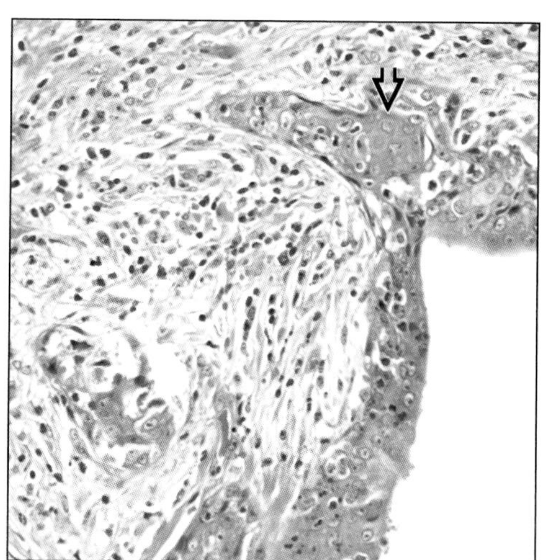

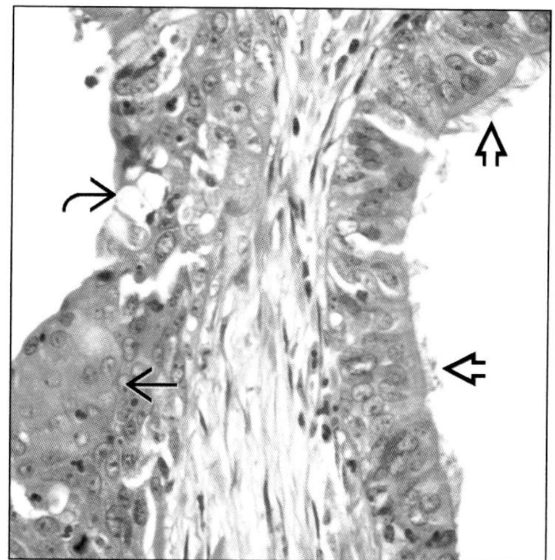

(Left) *Cystic and solid area of neoplasm exclusively comprised of the squamous or epidermoid cell component shows individual cell keratinization ⇨. Scattered mucocytes were present in other areas of the neoplasm (not shown).* ***(Right)*** *Cystic foci show squamous/epidermoid cells → and admixed mucocytes ↷. The presence of ciliated cells ⇨ has raised a possible (although unproven) branchial cleft derivation for MECT given histologic similarities to branchial cleft cysts.*

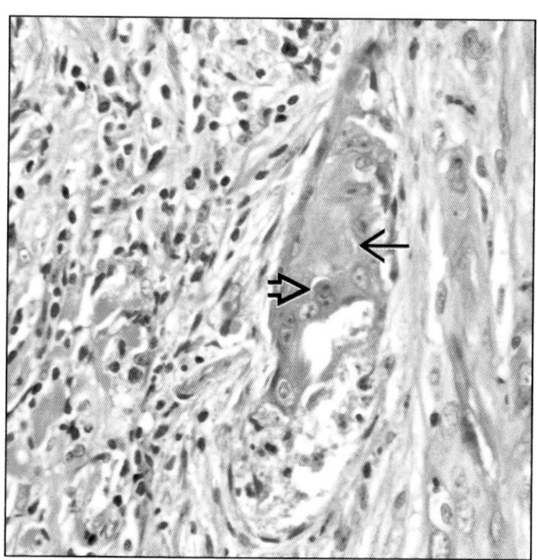

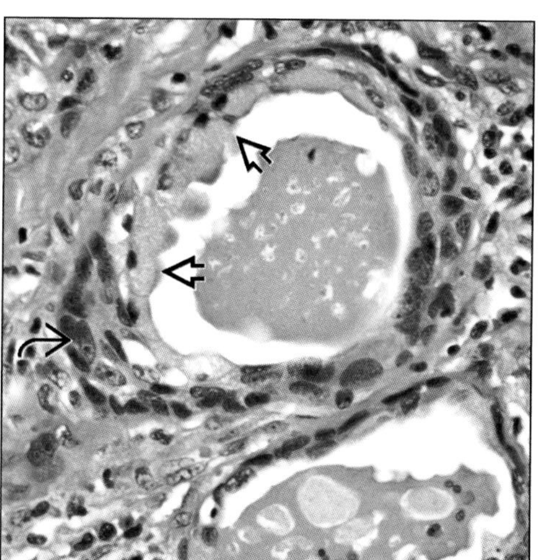

(Left) *H&E shows infiltrative solid focus of tumor composed of squamous/epidermoid cells with keratinization, dyskeratotic cell ⇨, and intercellular bridges → with surrounding inflammatory cells. Scattered mucocytes were present in other areas of the neoplasm (not shown).* ***(Right)*** *Tumor nest comprised of a greater number of mucocytes ⇨ is characterized by abundant basophilic-appearing cytoplasm and peripherally placed nuclei. Squamous/epidermoid cells are seen along the periphery ↷.*

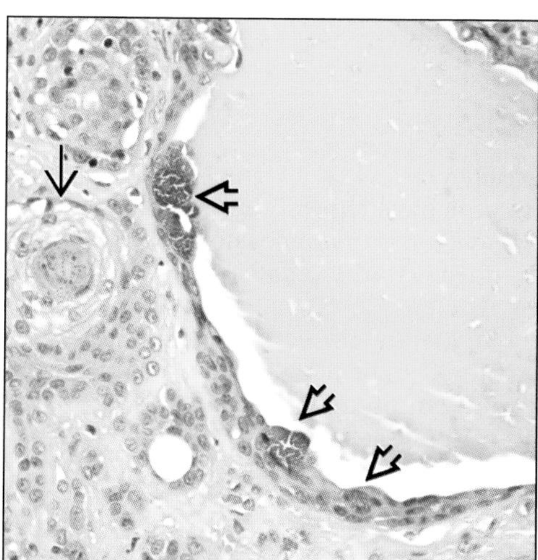

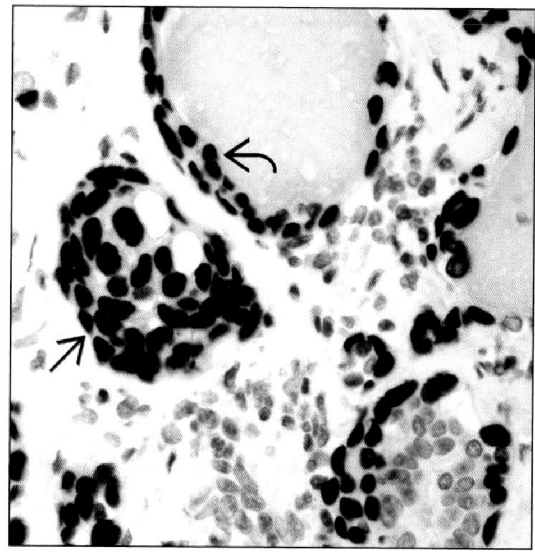

(Left) *Intracytoplasmic mucin positive material ⇨ can be utilized in the identification &/or confirmation of mucocytes; adjacent solid tumor nests of squamous/epidermoid cells are mucicarmine negative →.* ***(Right)*** *The cyst lining cells ↷ and cells of the solid tumor nests → show TTF-1 (nuclear) immunoreactivity. This finding along with thyroglobulin staining (not shown) support a follicular epithelial cell origin for MECT.*

SCLEROSING MUCOEPIDERMOID CARCINOMA WITH EOSINOPHILIA

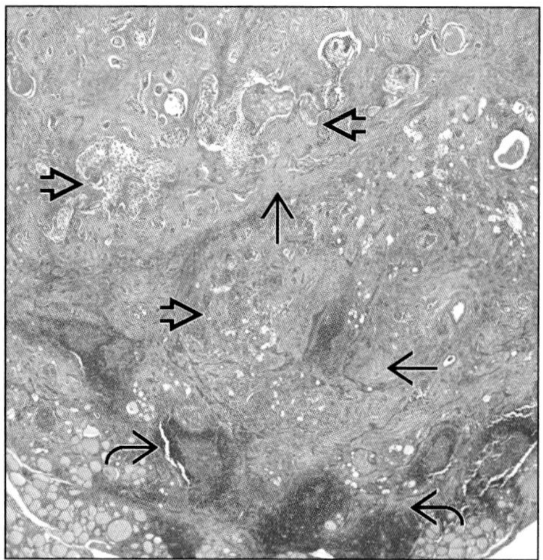

The tumor is unencapsulated and infiltrative, composed of tumor nests ➪ with an associated sclerotic stroma →, and occurs in the background of chronic lymphocytic thyroiditis ↪.

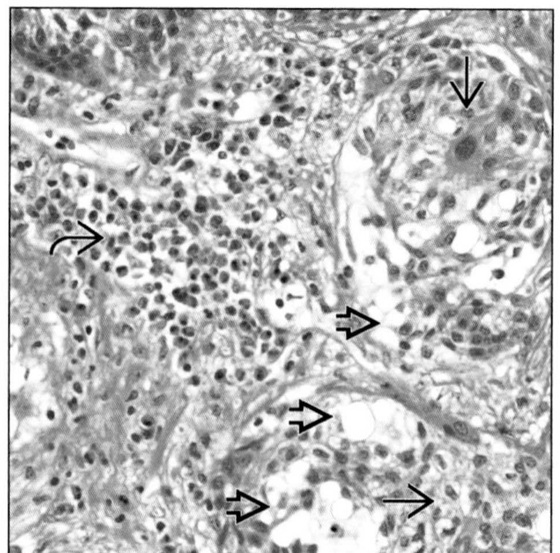

The neoplastic foci include an admixture of squamous/epidermoid cells → and mucocytes ➪ with an associated inflammatory cell infiltrate dominated by eosinophils ↪.

TERMINOLOGY

Abbreviations

- Sclerosing mucoepidermoid carcinoma with eosinophilia of thyroid gland (SMECET)

Definitions

- Low-grade malignant thyroid tumor with histologic appearance similar to low-grade salivary gland counterpart including
  - Squamous/epidermoid cells and mucous cell differentiation
  - Plus presence of prominent sclerotic stroma with eosinophil-rich inflammatory cell component

ETIOLOGY/PATHOGENESIS

Idiopathic

- No known etiologic agent

Histogenesis

- Presumed to arise from squamous metaplasia of thyroid follicular epithelium
  - Usually occurs in setting of chronic lymphocytic (Hashimoto) thyroiditis
- Origin from ultimobranchial body (solid cell nests) suggested as possible origin for SMECET
  - Some histologic, histochemical, and immunohistochemical features suggest possible origin from SCN
  - However, origin from follicular epithelial cell origin supported by
    - Presence of keratinization, intercellular bridges, and thyroglobulin reactivity
    - Absence of calcitonin and chromogranin reactivity
  - Presence of thyroid specific mRNAs by RT-PCR in thyroid mucoepidermoid carcinoma including
    - TTF-1, TTF-2, pax-8, Na-I symporter, and thyroid peroxidase mRNA supports origin from thyroid follicular epithelium

CLINICAL ISSUES

Epidemiology

- Incidence
  - Rare
    - Fewer than 50 cases reported
- Age
  - Occurs over wide age range (2nd-8th decades)
    - Most patients in 5th-7th decades of life
- Gender
  - Female > Male

Presentation

- Slowly growing, painless neck mass
- Rarely presents with rapid enlargement, hoarseness, or vocal fold paralysis

Laboratory Tests

- Euthyroid

Treatment

- Surgical approaches
  - Surgery is treatment of choice
    - Total thyroidectomy treatment of choice, especially since extrathyroidal extension is common
    - Conservative therapy (lobectomy or subtotal thyroidectomy) can be performed
  - Selected cervical lymph node sampling recommended in presence of clinically enlarged nodes

Prognosis

- Excellent prognosis
  - Generally follows indolent course

SCLEROSING MUCOEPIDERMOID CARCINOMA WITH EOSINOPHILIA

Key Facts

Terminology
- Low-grade malignant thyroid tumor with histologic appearance similar to low-grade salivary gland counterpart including
  - Squamous/epidermoid cells and mucous cell differentiation
  - Plus presence of prominent sclerotic stroma with eosinophil-rich inflammatory cell component

Etiology/Pathogenesis
- Presumed to arise from squamous metaplasia of thyroid follicular epithelium
  - Usually occurs in setting of chronic lymphocytic (Hashimoto) thyroiditis

Clinical Issues
- Slowly growing, painless neck mass
- Rarely presents with rapid enlargement, hoarseness, or vocal fold paralysis
- Surgery is treatment of choice
  - Total thyroidectomy treatment of choice, especially since extrathyroidal extension common
- Excellent prognosis
  - Generally follows indolent course

Microscopic Pathology
- Circumscribed but unencapsulated to infiltrative
- **Squamous or epidermoid cells**
  - Keratinization (keratin pearls, keratin debris) and intercellular bridges present
- **Mucous cells**
  - Occasional mucocytes &/or mucin pools
- Associated mixed inflammatory cell infiltrate that includes prominent eosinophilic cell component

---

- Metastatic tumor to cervical lymph nodes may be present
  - Occurs in up to 30% of cases at presentation
- Distant metastasis is uncommon
  - May occur (e.g., lung, liver, and bone)
- Extrathyroidal extension may occur
- Specific prognostic factors are unknown

IMAGE FINDINGS

Radiographic Findings
- Hypoactive ("cold") nodule on thyroid imaging

MACROSCOPIC FEATURES

General Features
- Tumors usually appear as ill-defined, white to yellow, firm, solid masses
- Cystic change may occur, but this is uncommon

Size
- Range: 1-13 cm

MICROSCOPIC PATHOLOGY

Histologic Features
- Circumscribed but unencapsulated to infiltrative
- Anastomosing cords and narrow strands of tumor cells infiltrating sclerotic stroma
- Neoplastic cells include
  - **Squamous or epidermoid cells**
    - Keratinization (keratin pearls, keratin debris) and intercellular bridges present
  - **Mucous cells**
    - Occasional mucocytes &/or mucin pools
- Clear cells may be seen
  - Represent minor component (10-30%)
  - Appear to be glycogen-rich squamous cells
- Associated mixed inflammatory cell infiltrate that includes prominent eosinophilic cell component
- Chronic lymphocytic thyroiditis commonly present in surrounding nonneoplastic thyroid gland
  - Arises in thyroid glands affected by Hashimoto thyroiditis, particularly fibrous variant
  - May include foci of squamous metaplasia
- Papillary carcinoma may be identified
  - Transition between SMECET and papillary carcinoma less common than in mucoepidermoid carcinoma of thyroid gland (MECT)
- Perineural and vascular invasion may be present
- Neoplastic infiltrate generally confined to thyroid gland
  - Extrathyroidal extension may occur

ANCILLARY TESTS

Cytology
- Definitive diagnosis by fine needle aspiration cytology is difficult due to nonspecific nature of findings
- Findings include combination of malignant epithelial cells set in mucinous stroma with eosinophils
- Cohesive clusters of cells with
  - Either epidermoid or glandular differentiation
- Findings suggest malignancy but may also raise possibility of metastatic tumor or Hashimoto thyroiditis

Histochemistry
- Mucin stains (mucicarmine and periodic acid-Schiff with diastase)
  - Intracytoplasmic and intraluminal mucin positive material
  - Cystic spaces show mucicarminophilic material

Immunohistochemistry
- Cytokeratins, TTF-1 positive
- Thyroglobulin negative
- Carcinoembryonic antigen
  - Sometimes expressed in mucocytes
  - Negative in squamous/epidermoid cells
- Calcitonin, chromogranin negative
- p63 strongly stains squamous/epidermoid cells

SCLEROSING MUCOEPIDERMOID CARCINOMA WITH EOSINOPHILIA

- p53 staining occasionally seen in squamous/ epidermoid cells

Molecular Genetics

- *BRAF* mutations not identified

DIFFERENTIAL DIAGNOSIS

Chronic Lymphocytic Thyroiditis with Squamous Metaplasia

- Tends not to form mass
- Lacks mucocytes, mucin pools, significant eosinophil cell component

Direct Extension of Carcinoma from Adjacent Organ

- Primary squamous cell carcinomas of larynx and esophagus can invade thyroid gland
- In general, clinical &/or radiographic evidence confirms presence of extrathyroidal cancer invading thyroid gland
- Absence of mucocytes &/or glandular differentiation

Undifferentiated (Anaplastic) Thyroid Carcinoma

- Characteristic demographics and clinical presentation
  - Most often occurs in older adults
  - Typically occurs as rapidly enlarging neck mass in presence of longstanding history of thyroid lesion
    - May occur as rapidly enlarging neck mass without history of longstanding history of thyroid lesion
- Histology characterized by presence of
  - Sheet-like growth
  - Marked pleomorphism
  - Increased mitotic activity, atypical mitoses
  - Necrosis
  - Lymph-vascular invasion
  - Extensively infiltrative including
    - Intrathyroidal &/or extrathyroidal
- Lacks mucocytes, mucin pools, significant eosinophil component

Squamous Cell Carcinoma

- Rare type of primary thyroid carcinoma
- Lacks mucocytes, mucin pools, significant eosinophil cell component

Carcinoma Showing Thymus-like Differentiation (CASTLE)

- Architecture shows some resemblance to lobulated appearance seen in thymic tumors (thymoma or thymic carcinoma) including
  - Solid nests or lobules with expansile or infiltrative growth into thyroid tissue in broad fronts
  - Dense fibrous bands creating lobulated or septated appearance
- Cellular composition similar to nasopharyngeal carcinoma, nonkeratinizing undifferentiated type including
  - Epithelioid cells with large, pleomorphic nuclei with vesicular chromatin, small distinct nucleoli, abundant eosinophilic cytoplasm with indistinct cell borders
- Mitotic activity seen on order of 1-2 mitoses per 10 high-power fields
- Squamous differentiation may be present including
  - Keratinization, intercellular bridges, foci of abrupt keratinization (resembling Hassall corpuscle)
- May have mucinous material
- Lacks mucocytes, mucin pools, and significant eosinophilic component
- Unique immunohistochemical profile including
  - Cytokeratin positive
  - Thyroglobulin, TTF-1, calcitonin negative
  - Immunoreactivity for markers associated with thymic carcinoma including
    - CD5, Bcl-2, Mcl-1 may be present
  - CD117 (CKIT) reactivity also present
  - EBV negative

Hodgkin Lymphoma

- Rarely, primary Hodgkin disease of thyroid may occur
  - Hodgkin disease involving thyroid usually occurs secondary to cervical or mediastinal nodal disease
- Nodular sclerosing most common histologic type

SELECTED REFERENCES

1. Das S et al: Sclerosing mucoepidermoid carcinoma with eosinophilia of the thyroid. Indian J Pathol Microbiol. 51(1):34-6, 2008
2. Musso-Lassalle S et al: A diagnostic pitfall: nodular tumor-like squamous metaplasia with Hashimoto's thyroiditis mimicking a sclerosing mucoepidermoid carcinoma with eosinophilia. Pathol Res Pract. 202(5):379-83, 2006
3. Hunt JL et al: p63 expression in sclerosing mucoepidermoid carcinomas with eosinophilia arising in the thyroid. Mod Pathol. 17(5):526-9, 2004
4. Shehadeh NJ et al: Sclerosing mucoepidermoid carcinoma with eosinophilia of the thyroid: a case report and review of the literature. Am J Otolaryngol. 25(1):48-53, 2004
5. Albores-Saavedra J et al: Clear cells and thyroid transcription factor I reactivity in sclerosing mucoepidermoid carcinoma of the thyroid gland. Ann Diagn Pathol. 7(6):348-53, 2003
6. Baloch ZW et al: Primary mucoepidermoid carcinoma and sclerosing mucoepidermoid carcinoma with eosinophilia of the thyroid gland: a report of nine cases. Mod Pathol. 13(7):802-7, 2000
7. Solomon AC et al: Thyroid sclerosing mucoepidermoid carcinoma with eosinophilia: mimic of Hodgkin disease in nodal metastases. Arch Pathol Lab Med. 124(3):446-9, 2000
8. Geisinger KR et al: The cytomorphologic features of sclerosing mucoepidermoid carcinoma of the thyroid gland with eosinophilia. Am J Clin Pathol. 109(3):294-301, 1998
9. Sim SJ et al: Sclerosing mucoepidermoid carcinoma with eosinophilia of the thyroid: report of two patients, one with distant metastasis, and review of the literature. Hum Pathol. 28(9):1091-6, 1997
10. Bondeson L et al: Cytologic features in fine-needle aspirates from a sclerosing mucoepidermoid thyroid carcinoma with eosinophilia. Diagn Cytopathol. 15(4):301-5, 1996
11. Chan JK et al: Sclerosing mucoepidermoid thyroid carcinoma with eosinophilia. A distinctive low-grade malignancy arising from the metaplastic follicles of Hashimoto's thyroiditis. Am J Surg Pathol. 15(5):438-48, 1991

Microscopic Features and Ancillary Techniques

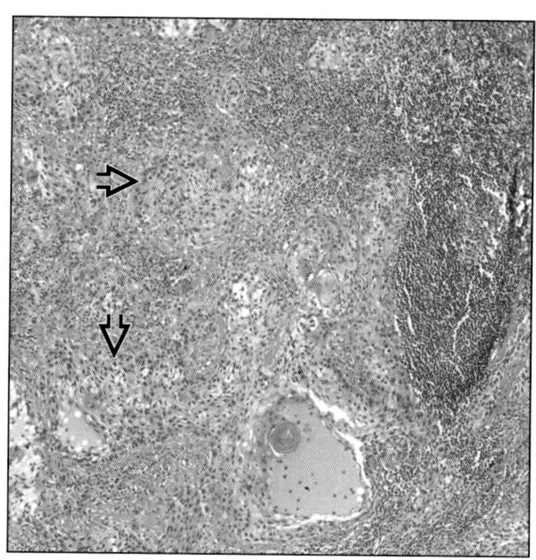

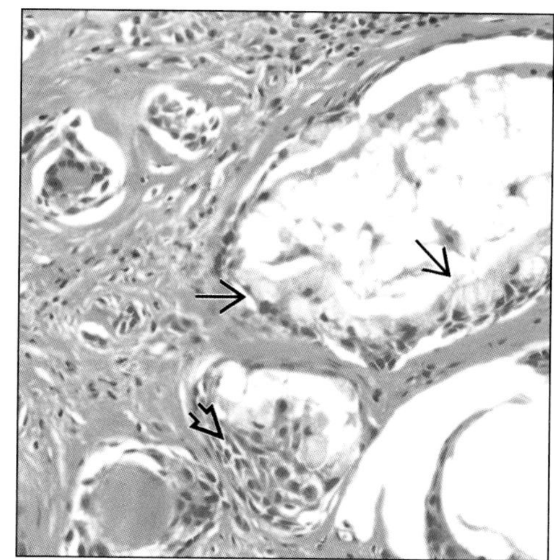

(Left) *Infiltrative tumor is predominantly composed of solid tumor nests of squamous/epidermoid cells ➲ with sclerotic stroma, associated chronic inflammation, and background of chronic lymphocytic thyroiditis.* ***(Right)*** *The neoplastic cellular infiltrate shows solid and cystic growth composed of an admixture of squamous/epidermoid cells ➲ and mucocytes → with associated sclerosis and chronic inflammatory cells, including eosinophils.*

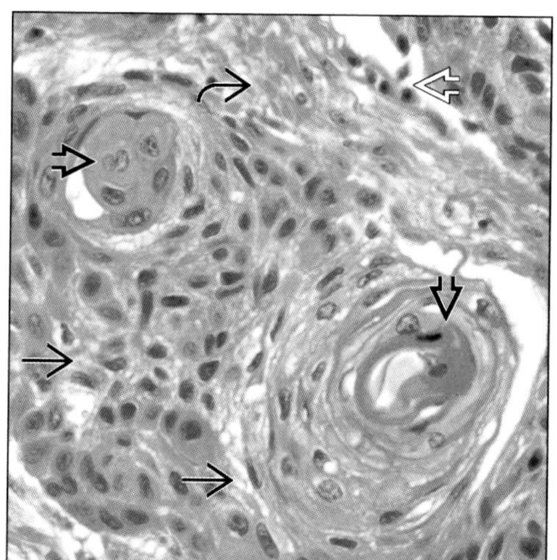

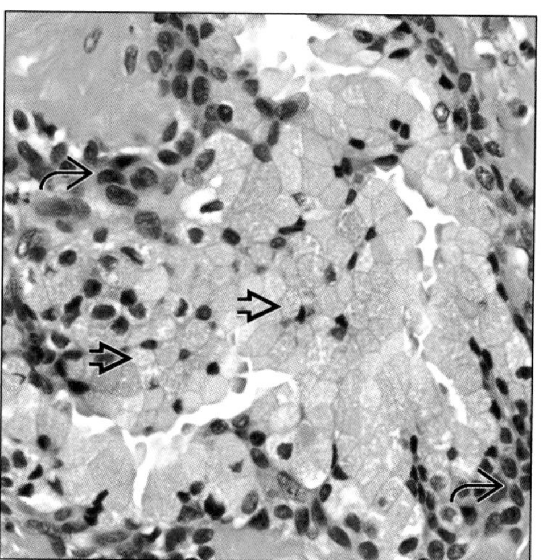

(Left) *Solid tumor nest is entirely composed of squamous/epidermoid cells characterized by keratinization ➲ and intercellular bridges →; associated sclerosis ↷ and eosinophils ➲ are present.* ***(Right)*** *Area of tumor is almost entirely composed of mucocytes characterized by cells with abundant basophilic-appearing cytoplasm ➲ that displaces the nucleus to the peripheral aspect of the cell. Along the outer aspect of the cell nest are squamous/ epidermoid cells ↷.*

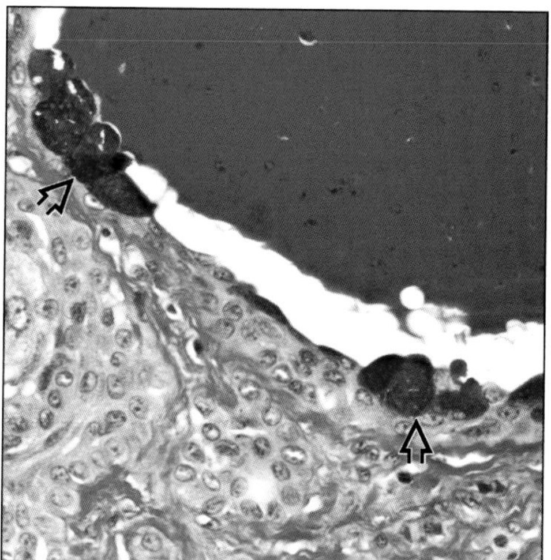

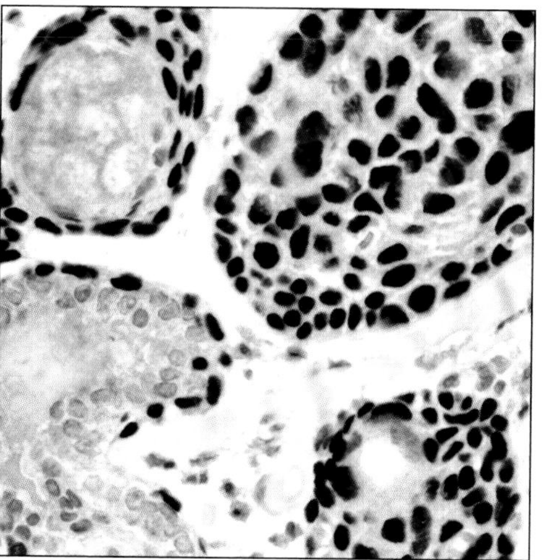

(Left) *Periodic acid-Schiff with diastase staining assists in identifying and confirming the presence of mucocytes as evidenced by the presence of intracytoplasmic diastase-resistant, PAS-positive material ➲.* ***(Right)*** *Tumor nests of squamous/ epidermoid cells are p63 (nuclear) immunoreactive. The tumor cells were also variably immunoreactive for thyroglobulin and TTF-1 (not shown), supporting the theory that SMECET originates from follicular epithelial cells.*

SQUAMOUS CELL CARCINOMA

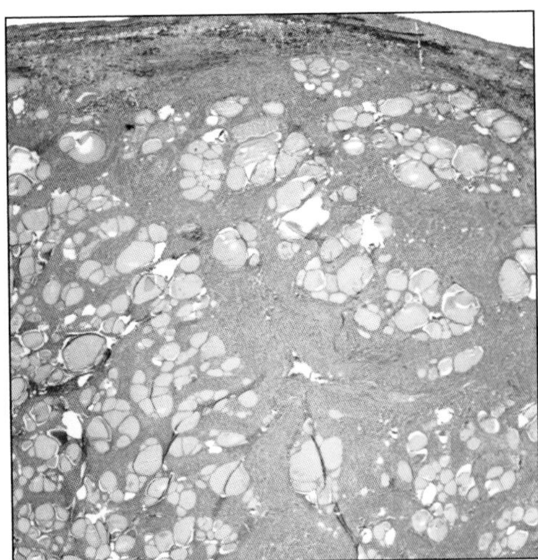

The thyroid gland is nearly completely replaced by a widely infiltrating tumor. The tumor type is not identifiable at this magnification, but effacement of the thyroid gland is obvious.

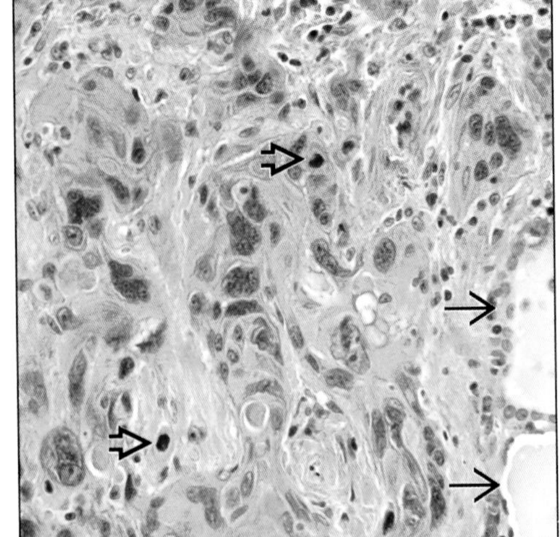

The squamous epithelium shows profound nuclear pleomorphism. There is dyskeratosis and keratinization. Thyroid follicles are noted at the periphery ⇒. Mitotic figures are present ⇨.

TERMINOLOGY

Abbreviations

- Squamous cell carcinoma (SCC)

Definitions

- Thyroid primary squamous cell carcinoma is composed entirely of squamous cells without mucocytes and without direct invasion from adjacent organs (larynx, esophagus)

ETIOLOGY/PATHOGENESIS

Environmental Exposure

- Radiation history is occasionally present

Pathogenesis

- Derived from thyroid follicular epithelium
  - Directly or via squamous metaplasia, then additional alterations to reach malignant tumor
- Persistence of thyroglossal duct or branchial pouch embryonic remnants

CLINICAL ISSUES

Epidemiology

- Incidence
  - Rare: < 1% of malignant thyroid tumors
- Age
  - Mean: 6th and 7th decades
- Gender
  - Female > Male (3:1)

Site

- Affects one or both lobes of thyroid gland

Presentation

- Patients present with rapidly enlarging neck mass
  - Many have preexisting thyroid disease
- Frequent recurrent laryngeal nerve compression and pressure symptoms
  - Airway obstruction, dyspnea, dysphagia
  - Direct involvement of nerves, vessels, and soft tissues
- Cervical lymph node enlargement is common
- Hashimoto thyroiditis is concurrently identified in a few patients
- Paraneoplastic syndrome is rare
  - Hypercalcemia, fever, and leukocytosis
  - Probably develops as result of tumor-derived humoral mediators

Endoscopic Findings

- Endoscopic evaluation (laryngoscopy, esophagoscopy, bronchoscopy) to exclude direct extension

Treatment

- Options, risks, complications
  - Airway collapse and esophagotracheal fistula may complicate course
- Surgical approaches
  - Early radical resection yields best prognosis
    - Debulking if clear margins cannot be achieved
- Drugs
  - Thyroid hormone suppression may help
    - Thyroid-stimulating hormone may be a growth factor
  - Chemotherapy does **not** alter disease course
- Radiation
  - Radical-dose radiotherapy is part of initial treatment
  - Radiation alone for unresectable tumors &/or poor surgical candidates
  - Radioiodine therapy does **not** work

Prognosis

- Nearly all patients present with advanced disease
- Tumors follow rapidly fulminant course
  - Prognosis is poor; mean survival: < 1 year; 5-year survival: < 10%

SQUAMOUS CELL CARCINOMA

Key Facts

Terminology

- Thyroid primary squamous cell carcinoma is composed entirely of squamous cells without mucocytes and without direct invasion from adjacent organs (larynx, esophagus)

Clinical Issues

- Mean: 6th and 7th decades
- Female > Male (3:1)
- Patients present with rapidly enlarging neck mass
- Early radical resection yields best prognosis
- Radical-dose radiotherapy is part of initial treatment
- Prognosis is poor; mean survival: < 1 year; 5-year survival: < 10%

Microscopic Pathology

- Must 1st exclude direct extension: Larynx, esophagus
- Widely invasive tumor, destroying thyroid parenchyma
- Cohesive cells arranged in sheets, ribbons, nests
  - Polygonal, polyhedral, and spindle tumor cells
- Keratinization and keratin pearl formation
- High mitotic index, including atypical forms
- Classified as keratinizing or nonkeratinizing

Ancillary Tests

- Positive: Keratin, CK5/6, CK19, p63
- Negative: Thyroglobulin, CEA, calcitonin, CD5

Top Differential Diagnoses

- Direct extension from adjacent organs
- Metastatic squamous cell carcinoma
- Extensive squamous metaplasia
- CASTLE

  - Localized disease only; managed aggressively, patients may survive longer
  - Airway compromise results in death
- Local invasion and lymph node metastases is common
- Distant metastasis (lung) is less common (~ 30%)

IMAGE FINDINGS

Radiographic Findings

- Large mass, often showing necrosis
- Radiographic studies exclude direct invasion from contiguous organs

MACROSCOPIC FEATURES

General Features

- Involves one or both lobes
  - Multiple nodules of tumor can be seen
- Extrathyroidal extension is frequent
- Necrosis is common
- Firm, tan-white mass

Size

- Large: Up to 12 cm

MICROSCOPIC PATHOLOGY

Histologic Features

- Must 1st exclude direct extension (larynx, esophagus)
- Widely invasive tumor, destroying thyroid parenchyma
- Vascular and perineural invasion is common
- Cohesive cells arranged in sheets, ribbons, nests
- There is variable pleomorphism
- Polygonal, polyhedral, and spindle tumor cells
- Keratinization and keratin pearl formation
- High mitotic index, including atypical forms
- Classified as keratinizing or nonkeratinizing
- Inflammatory infiltrate and stromal fibroplasia often present
  - Association with Hashimoto thyroiditis is known
- Other tumors may be present: Papillary carcinoma, follicular carcinoma, follicular adenoma
  - By convention, if another tumor is present, it is diagnosed with "squamous differentiation" incorporated into diagnosis

ANCILLARY TESTS

Cytology

- Confirm site of FNA (thyroid, larynx, lymph node, esophagus, metastasis) before diagnosis
- Background filled with necrotic and granular, eosinophilic keratin debris
- Cellular smears contain cohesive clusters and isolated cells
- Irregular shapes (tadpole cells), nuclear hyperchromasia, and cytoplasmic orangeophilia and dyskeratosis

Immunohistochemistry

- Positive: Keratin, CK5/6, CK19, p63
- Negative: Thyroglobulin, CEA, calcitonin, CD5

Molecular Genetics

- Abnormal p53 expression and loss of p21 expression
  - p53 expression is greater in tumors with less squamous differentiation

DIFFERENTIAL DIAGNOSIS

Direct Extension from Adjacent Organs

- Much more frequent than primary thyroid SCC
- Tumor or bulk of tumor is centered in larynx, esophagus, or trachea
  - Up to 25% of radical laryngectomies show direct thyroid invasion, especially if true vocal cord fixation
  - Also show cricothyroid membrane, anterior commissure, laryngeal ventricle, and thyroid cartilage invasion

SQUAMOUS CELL CARCINOMA

Immunohistochemistry

Antibody	Reactivity	Staining Pattern	Comment
CK-PAN	Positive	Cytoplasmic	All tumor cells
CK5/6	Positive	Cytoplasmic	Nearly all tumor cells
CK19	Positive	Cytoplasmic	Nearly all tumor cells
p63	Positive	Nuclear	Most tumor cells
CK7	Positive	Cytoplasmic	Weak and focal or patchy reactivity
CK18	Positive	Cytoplasmic	Weak and focal or patchy reactivity
EMA	Positive	Cytoplasmic	Weak and focal or patchy reactivity
TTF-1	Positive	Nuclear	Strong, but only focal tumor nuclei reactivity
S100-A9	Positive	Cytoplasmic	Diffuse, laminated positive in most tumor cells
Ki-67	Positive	Nuclear	High index (usually > 50%)
p53	Positive	Nuclear	Increased reactivity as tumor becomes less differentiated
Thyroglobulin	Negative		
Calcitonin	Negative		
CEA-M	Negative		
CK1	Negative		
CK4	Negative		
CK10/13	Negative		
CK20	Negative		
CD5	Negative		
Galectin-3	Negative		
p21	Negative		

- Confirmed endoscopically, radiographically, or during surgery
- Primary thyroid SCC have much worse prognosis than tumors with direct extension
- Primary malignancy detected before thyroid involvement

Metastatic Squamous Cell Carcinoma

- Different primary site known clinically
  - Usually develops within 3 years of primary site documentation
- Tend to be multifocal, with high lymph-vascular invasion

Extensive Squamous Metaplasia

- Squamous differentiation can be seen in lymphocytic thyroiditis, adenomatoid nodules, papillary carcinoma (diffuse sclerosing variant), undifferentiated carcinoma
- Tends to be focal, does not form mass clinically; lacks "infiltration," cytologic atypia, and necrosis
- Squamous metaplasia does not predispose to developing SCC

CASTLE

- a.k.a. carcinoma showing thymus-like differentiation
- Greater degree of tumor spindling, has more keloid-like collagen deposition, and inflammatory cells
- Positive with CD5, S100-A9

GRADING

3 Grades

- Well, moderately, poorly differentiated
  - Most thyroid tumors are poorly differentiated

STAGING

Same as Undifferentiated Carcinoma

- By convention, SCC is staging as if it were undifferentiated carcinoma

SELECTED REFERENCES

1. Fassan M et al: Primary squamous cell carcinoma of the thyroid: immunohistochemical profile and literature review. Tumori. 93(5):518-21, 2007
2. Ryska A et al: Massive squamous metaplasia of the thyroid gland-- report of three cases. Pathol Res Pract. 202(2):99-106, 2006
3. Sparano A et al: Predictors of thyroid gland invasion in glottic squamous cell carcinoma. Laryngoscope. 115(7):1247-50, 2005
4. Sahoo M et al: Primary squamous-cell carcinoma of the thyroid gland: new evidence in support of follicular epithelial cell origin. Diagn Cytopathol. 27(4):227-31, 2002
5. Lam KY et al: Primary squamous cell carcinoma of the thyroid gland: an entity with aggressive clinical behaviour and distinctive cytokeratin expression profiles. Histopathology. 39(3):279-86, 2001
6. Nakhjavani M et al: Direct extension of malignant lesions to the thyroid gland from adjacent organs: report of 17 cases. Endocr Pract. 5(2):69-71, 1999
7. Burman KD et al: Unusual types of thyroid neoplasms. Endocrinol Metab Clin North Am. 25(1):49-68, 1996
8. Tsuchiya A et al: Squamous cell carcinoma of the thyroid--a report of three cases. Jpn J Surg. 20(3):341-5, 1990
9. Simpson WJ et al: Squamous cell carcinoma of the thyroid gland. Am J Surg. 156(1):44-6, 1988
10. Lee JR et al: Squamous cell carcinoma of the thyroid gland. J Med Assoc Ga. 69(9):755-8, 1980

Microscopic Features and Ancillary Techniques

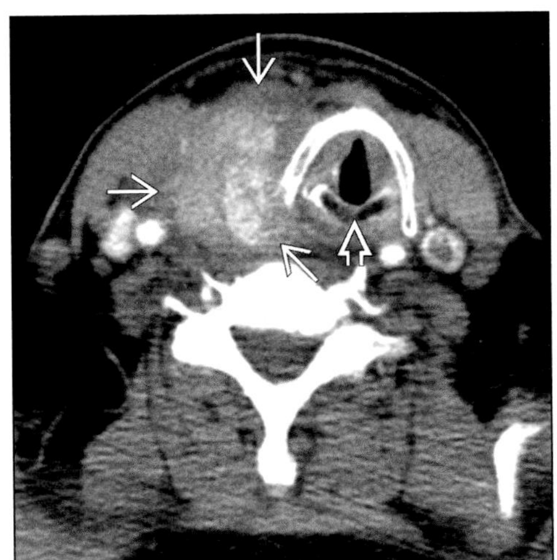

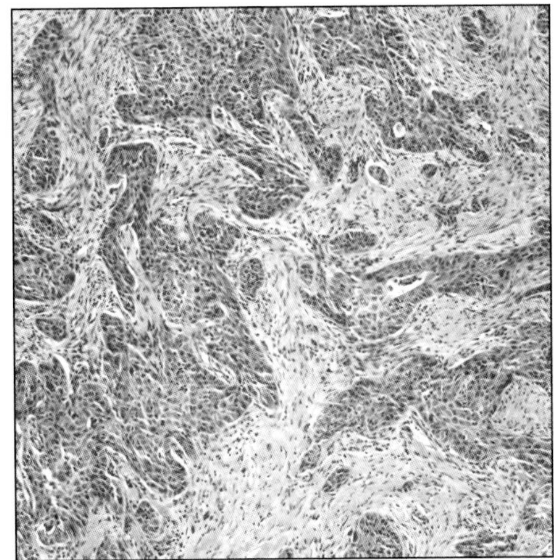

(Left) *Radiographic images are used to highlight the extent of tumor and specifically to exclude invasion from the adjacent larynx ➡ or esophagus. In this case, there is a large mass ➡ replacing the right thyroid lobe.* ***(Right)*** *There is a desmoplastic stroma separating the neoplastic islands of this SCC of the thyroid. There is a nested, sheet-like, and individual cell infiltration by the neoplastic cells.*

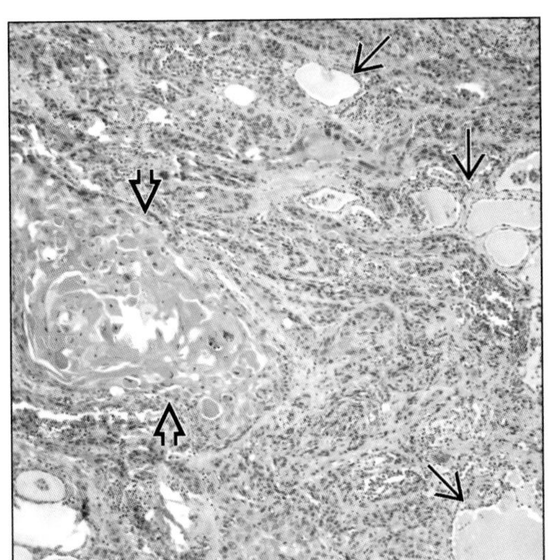

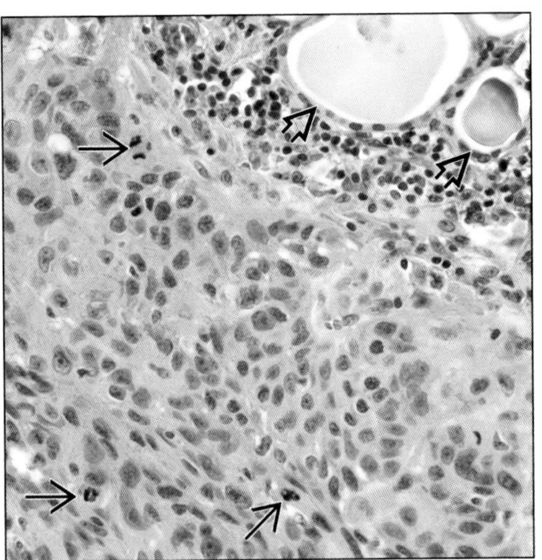

(Left) *Keratin pearl formation with keratinaceous debris ➡ is noted within this squamous cell carcinoma. There is extensive infiltration and destruction of the follicular epithelium ➡.* ***(Right)*** *There is a pavemented appearance to the squamous epithelium in this SCC. There are a number of mitotic figures ➡ within the sheet of neoplastic cells. The thyroid follicles are uninvolved ➡.*

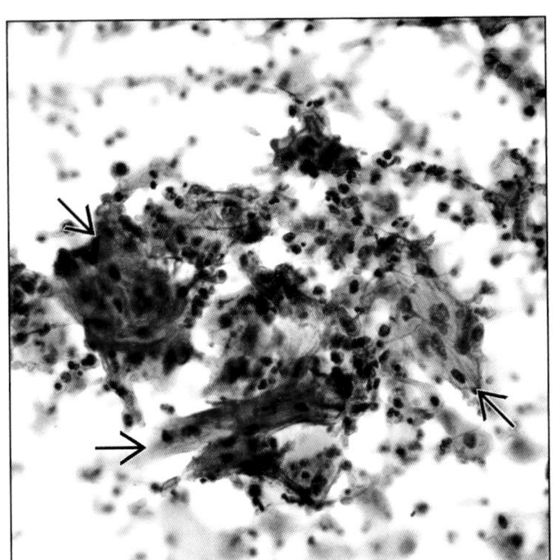

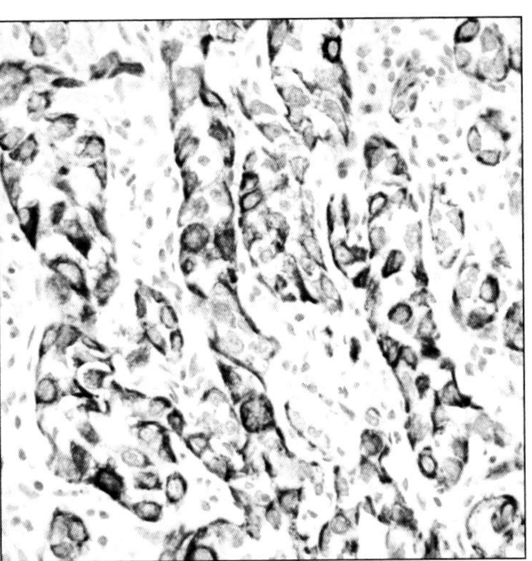

(Left) *Smears show marked variation in cellular size and shape with spindled and tadpole cells showing dense orangeophilic cytoplasm ➡, characteristic of squamous differentiation. The cells contain nuclei with dense chromatin. There is a background of inflammatory elements. Confirmation of the site of the sample is required.* ***(Right)*** *The neoplastic cells are strongly and diffusely highlighted with CK5/6, although in general immunohistochemistry is not required for the diagnosis.*

LYMPHOMA

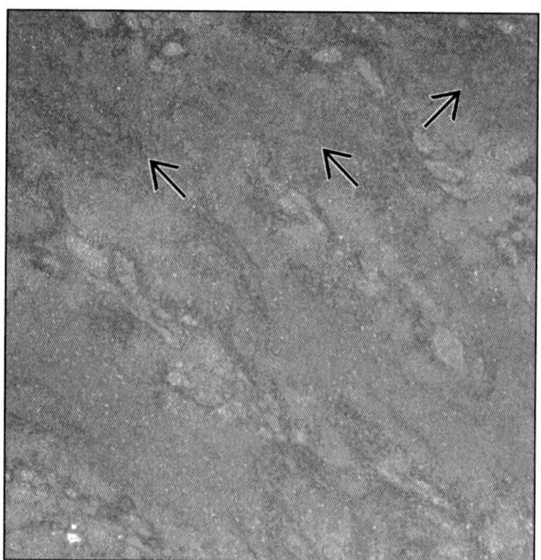

This EMZBCL shows a vague nodularity or "follicular" effacement of the thyroid parenchyma. The multifocal zones begin to show aggregation. There is a background of chronic lymphocytic thyroiditis ⇒.

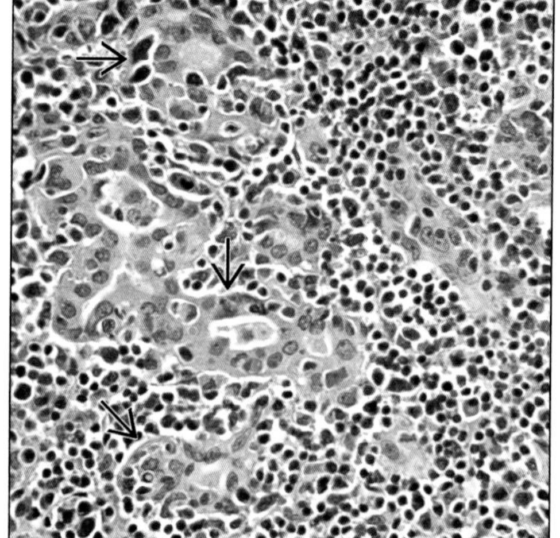

Lymphoepithelial lesions (LELs) are one of the best diagnostic features of thyroid lymphomas. They are comprised of atypical lymphoid cells infiltrating and destroying the thyroid follicular epithelium ⇒.

TERMINOLOGY

Abbreviations

- Diffuse large B-cell lymphoma (DLBCL)
- Extranodal marginal zone B-cell lymphoma (EMZBCL)

Synonyms

- WHO terminology is used
  - Past lymphoma classifications systems are not to be used

Definitions

- Primary lymphoma arising within thyroid gland, usually associated with lymphocytic thyroiditis, comprising a heterogeneous group of tumors
  - Mucosa-associated lymphoid tissue (MALT) is setting for development of extranodal marginal zone B-cell lymphoma, which may transform into diffuse large B-cell lymphoma
  - Lack systemic involvement
    - Regional lymph nodes may occasionally be affected
  - Rare: Follicular lymphoma (FL), extraosseous (extramedullary) plasmacytoma, Hodgkin lymphoma

ETIOLOGY/PATHOGENESIS

Pathogenesis

- Carcinogenesis is multistep, multifactorial process with progressive accumulation of genetic changes
- Nearly all lymphomas arise in setting of chronic lymphocytic thyroiditis (Hashimoto disease)
- Acquired MALT from autoimmune, immune deficiency or inflammatory process
  - Nodular or diffuse infiltrate of lymphoid cells, frequently with follicles and germinal centers, and oncocytic metaplasia of thyroid epithelium
  - Fibrosis and epithelial atrophy supports chronicity
- MALT lymphoma shows increased ratio of CD8(+) cells (suppressor/cytotoxic cell) to CD4(+) cells (helper/inducer cell) as compared to lymphocytic thyroiditis
- MALT lymphoma cell of origin is from post germinal center, marginal zone B-cells

CLINICAL ISSUES

Epidemiology

- Incidence
  - Uncommon
    - ~ 2-5% of all thyroid gland neoplasms
    - ~ 5% of all extranodal lymphomas
    - EMZBCL: < 2% of all extranodal lymphomas; DLBCL: ~ 15%
  - Relative risk of developing a lymphoma is **80x** greater in patients with chronic lymphocytic thyroiditis (compared to age- and sex-matched controls)
- Age
  - Mean: 65 years
    - Wide age range (14-90 years)
- Gender
  - Female > > Male (3-7:1)

Site

- Must exclude secondary involvement of thyroid gland
  - Neck or mediastinal lymph nodes affected by lymphoma directly extending into thyroid gland
  - Relates to different staging and management

Presentation

- Mass or goiter, often with recent rapid enlargement
  - Causes obstructive symptoms related to compression
- Pain
- Dysphagia, dyspnea, and hoarseness
  - ~ 30% of patients
- Hypothyroidism (associated with Hashimoto thyroiditis)
  - Rarely, hyperthyroidism due to follicle destruction

LYMPHOMA

Key Facts

Terminology

- Primary thyroid lymphoma comprising heterogeneous group of tumors
  - Nearly all arise within chronic lymphocytic thyroiditis (80x increased risk)

Clinical Issues

- ~ 2-5% of all thyroid gland neoplasms
- Mean age: 65 years
- Female > > Male (3-7:1)
- Patients usually present with stage IE or IIE
- Adjuvant chemotherapy and radiation
- Mortality is grade and stage dependent (overall, 60% 5-year survival)

Microscopic Pathology

- Soft to firm, lobular, bulging cut surface, "fish flesh"
- Thyroid gland effaced by atypical lymphoid cells
- Lymphoepithelial lesions (LELs) are diagnostic
- **EMZBCL**: Vague nodularity to diffuse effacement
  - Colonization or follicle lysis by neoplastic B-cells
  - Atypical small lymphocytes, marginal zone cells, monocytoid B-cells, immunoblasts and centroblast-like cells, plasma cells
- **DLBCL**: Diffuse, large, atypical cells with increased mitotic figures

Ancillary Tests

- Usually B-cell immunophenotype (CD20, CD79a)
- Keratin highlights lymphoepithelial lesions

Top Differential Diagnoses

- Chronic lymphocytic thyroiditis, undifferentiated carcinoma

---

- Associated cervical adenopathy in some cases
- Choking, coughing, and hemoptysis are uncommon
- Symptoms are usually present for short duration
  - EMZBCL: Mean: 6-12 months
  - DLBCL: Mean: 4 months
- Patients usually present with stage IE or IIE
- Patients usually lack B symptoms
  - Fever, profound night sweats, weight loss, anorexia

Laboratory Tests

- Antithyroid serum antibodies usually present
- Most patients are euthyroid

Treatment

- Options, risks, complications
  - Surgery for debulking and tissue diagnosis
  - Radiation may result in mucositis, hypothyroidism, and radiation pneumonitis
- Surgical approaches
  - Obtain tissue for diagnosis: Core needle or partial lobectomy
  - Previously, surgery included lobectomy or thyroidectomy with lymph node dissection
  - Surgery is used to debulk or decompress
- Adjuvant therapy
  - Adjuvant chemotherapy and radiation after appropriate classification through needle biopsy
  - DLBCL: Combined modality therapy
- Drugs
  - Chemotherapy regimens based on histologic type, grade, and stage
    - EMZBCL: Oral chlorambucil or intravenous chemotherapy
    - DLBCL: Cyclophosphamide, doxorubicin, vincristine, and prednisone (CHOP) chemotherapy
- Radiation
  - Based on histologic type, grade, and stage
    - EMZBCL: Single modality radiation therapy (usually up to 40 Gy)
    - "Involved field only" or "extended field radiotherapy"; latter associated with lower rates of local recurrence or relapse
    - DLBCL: Hyperfractionated radiation
- New modalities
  - Anti-CD20 therapy and new forms of immunotherapy are experimental but hold promise

Prognosis

- Mortality is grade and stage dependent
- Overall, approximately 60% 5-year disease-specific survival (DSS), although grade and stage dependent
  - Stage IE or IIE, low-grade histology: > 95% 5-year DSS
  - Stage IE or IIE, DLBCL: 50-70% 5-yr DSS
  - Stage IVE: ~ 30% 5-yr DSS
- Poor prognostic features include
  - Age > 65 years
  - Male
  - High stage (IIIE, IVE)
  - Dysphagia (vocal cord paralysis)
  - Extrathyroidal extension
  - Tumor histology (DLBCL > FL > EMZBCL)
  - Diffuse architecture
  - Vascular invasion
  - High mitotic rate
- Combined conservative treatment: Lower relapse rate, reduced distant recurrence, least side effects
- Most patients present at stage IE or IIE (extranodal)
  - DLBCL: More likely to have stage IIIE or IVE
- If disseminated, most frequently involved sites are
  - Regional (cervical), mediastinal, and abdominal lymph nodes
  - Less common: Bone marrow, gastrointestinal tract, lung, bladder, and liver

IMAGE FINDINGS

Radiographic Findings

- Ultrasound
  - Marked hypoechoic, asymmetrical pseudocystic mass compared with residual thyroid tissue

LYMPHOMA

- Computed tomography
  - Heterogeneous mass, sometimes with cystic change
- Radioisotopic scan
  - ^{131}I scan: Lymphoma usually "cold"
  - Tc-99m pertechnetate scintigraphy: Possible "warm" nodule

MACROSCOPIC FEATURES

General Features

- May affect one or both lobes
- Soft to firm, lobular and multinodular appearance
- Effacement of normal thyroid
- Solid and cystic areas
- Cut surface: Bulging, smooth, pale-tan, "fish flesh"
- Usually homogeneous or mottled
- Extension into perithyroidal soft tissues

Size

- Wide variation
- Range up to 20 cm

MICROSCOPIC PATHOLOGY

Histologic Features

- Nearly constant background of chronic lymphocytic thyroiditis
- Effacement of normal thyroid gland parenchyma
  - Ranges from vague nodularity to diffuse effacement
- Extension beyond thyroid gland into fat and skeletal muscle in about 50% of cases
- Lymphoepithelial lesions (LELs) are diagnostic
  - Atypical lymphoid cells infiltrating **and** destroying thyroid follicular epithelium
  - 2 types
    - **MALT balls**: Rounded balls or masses, filling and distending lumen of thyroid follicles
    - **Lymphoepithelial lesion**: Single or aggregated lymphocytes within or between follicular epithelial cells
- Lymph-vascular invasion common in high-grade tumors
- Atrophy of residual thyroid parenchyma and fibrosis
- Uninvolved thyroid parenchyma: May have adenomatoid nodules, adenomas, or foci of carcinoma (papillary > > > follicular > medullary)
- Vast majority are B-cell lymphomas: EMZBCL and DLBCL with transitions between the two
  - Single or multifocal areas of large cell transformation adjacent to low-grade component

Extranodal Marginal Zone B-cell Lymphoma

- Extranodal marginal zone B-cell lymphoma (EMZBCL) of mucosa-associated lymphoid tissue (MALT) ± large cell component
  - Low-grade tumor by definition
  - Composed of heterogeneous population of B-cells
  - Vague nodularity to diffuse effacement
    - Single or multifocal zones of large cell transformation
    - Transition from low- to high-grade morphology is easy to identify in most cases
- 20-30% of all thyroid gland lymphomas
- Background of chronic lymphocytic thyroiditis in almost all cases
- Reactive germinal centers, ± follicle colonization, are invariably present
  - Colonization or follicle lysis by neoplastic B-cells
  - These cells yield darker zone within follicles on low power
  - Follicular architecture may mimic follicle center cell lymphoma
- Heterogeneous B-cells include
  - Atypical small lymphocytes, marginal zone (centrocyte-like) small cleaved cells, monocytoid B-cells, scattered large immunoblasts and centroblast-like cells, and plasma cells
    - Monocytoid B-cells are monotonous population of atypical lymphoid cells with abundant, pale cytoplasm with lobulated or kidney-shaped nuclei
    - Small collections of monocytoid cells can be seen
- Dutcher bodies and Russell bodies easily identified
  - Cytoplasmic immunoglobulin ("Mott cells") and striking plasmacytoid differentiation may simulate plasmacytoma
  - Crystal-storing histiocytes may be seen
- LELs easily identified
  - Keratin(s) highlights LELs
- Increased proliferation index usually within germinal center regions
- Infrequently, concurrent disease of gastrointestinal tract, salivary gland, orbit, lung, skin, or breast

Diffuse Large B-cell Lymphoma

- Diffuse, large, atypical cells with increased mitotic figures suggests transformation into diffuse large B-cell lymphoma
- 60-70% of all thyroid gland lymphomas
- Perithyroidal extension into fat or skeletal muscle
- Vascular invasion is often seen
- Sheets of large, atypical lymphoid cells destroying the thyroid parenchyma
  - Transitions between EMZBCL and DLBCL are common
  - However, may occur in absence of low-grade areas
- Large cells have spectrum of cytologic features
  - Centroblasts, immunoblasts, monocytoid B-cells, and plasmacytoid cells
  - Focal Reed-Sternberg-like cells can be seen
  - Burkitt-like growth with brisk mitotic activity, apoptosis, "starry sky" pattern
- Atrophy of residual thyroid parenchyma and fibrosis are often noted

Extramedullary Plasmacytoma

- Solitary extramedullary plasmacytoma (EMP)
  - No evidence of bone marrow involvement (excludes multiple myeloma)
- EMP very rare in thyroid
  - Most cases are probably EMZBCL with extensive plasma cell differentiation
- Sheets of plasma cells that may form nodules
  - Germinal center colonization or diffuse sheets of plasma cells around follicles
- Light chain restriction demonstrates monoclonality

Hodgkin Lymphoma
- Classical Hodgkin lymphoma, nodular sclerosis subtype is only one identified in thyroid gland
- Exceedingly rare
- Classic Hodgkin-Reed-Sternberg (HRS) cells identified in variably cellular background diathesis of plasma cells, eosinophils, and neutrophils
  - Lacunar and mummified variant HRS cells
- Birefringent collagen banding (stromal fibrosis), nodular pattern, and epithelioid histiocytes
- HRS cells: CD45RB negative, CD30 and CD15 positive
  - May coexpress B-cell markers (CD20), follicle center cell markers (CD10, Bcl-x, Bcl-2), and fascin, CD138, Bcl-6 and EMA
- HRS-like cells can be seen in DLBCL (but lack specific immunohistochemistry profile)

Follicular Lymphoma (FL)
- Considered primarily nodal-based lymphoma
- Exceedingly rare
  - Follicular pattern in EMZBCL: Current classification probably excludes FL
- Thyroid effacement by back to back neoplastic germinal centers with attenuated/absent mantle zones
- Monotonous population of centrocytes &/or centroblasts without tingible body macrophages
- CD10 and Bcl-6 highlight neoplastic germinal centers and possible diffuse component

Primary Peripheral T-cell Lymphoma
- Exceedingly rare
- Monoclonal gene rearrangements for T-cell receptor β- and γ-specific primers can be seen in chronic lymphocytic thyroiditis
  - Reactive phenomenon, especially when patients are HTLV-1 serologically negative
- Histologic, immunophenotypic, and molecular support required for diagnosis

ANCILLARY TESTS

Cytology
- Fine needle aspiration (FNA) may not work as well for diffuse thyroid enlargement
- Cellular aspirates, which may resemble chronic lymphocytic thyroiditis
  - Thyroid follicular epithelium is usually absent
- Dispersed, noncohesive admixture of lymphocytes, centrocytes, monocytoid B-cells, immunoblasts, plasma cells, and histiocytes
  - Cytologic atypia may be present but tends to be "limited" in EMZBCL
  - No tingible body macrophages
- Monotonously atypical population of large cells with vesicular nuclear chromatin and prominent nucleoli and background lymphoglandular bodies suggests DLBCL
  - Cells are 2-3x size of mature lymphocytes
  - Necrosis is infrequently present
- Immunohistochemistry, flow cytometry, &/or Ig heavy chain gene rearrangements can be performed on aspiration material

Immunohistochemistry
- Usually B-cell immunophenotype (CD20, CD79a)
  - κ or λ light chain restriction
- Keratin highlights lymphoepithelial lesions
- Germinal center follicular dendritic cells are disrupted or abortive

Flow Cytometry
- May be used to separate specific lymphoid populations

Cytogenetics
- Constitutive activation of nuclear factor (NF-κB) oncogenic pathway
- t(1;14)(p22;q32), t(14;18)(q32;q21), and t(3;14)(p14.1;q32) are detected in a few cases, mutually exclusive
- Immunoglobulin heavy chain locus (IgH) is rearranged on chromosome 14, with partner gene on another chromosome
- Aberrant p15, p16, and p73 promoter methylation is quite common
- *TP53* mutation followed by complete inactivation by loss of 2nd allele may be associated with high-grade transformation
- CD40 signaling in combination with Th2 cytokines are necessary for development and progression of low-grade MALT-type B-cell lymphoma
  - T-cells, which activate B-cells in a CD40-dependent fashion, may contribute to lymphoma pathogenesis and may be identified in lymphocytic thyroiditis

Molecular Genetics
- Different B-cell clones dominating at different times, suggesting oligoclonal B-cell proliferation
  - Immunoglobulin heavy and light chain variable genes (*VH* and *VL*) expressed by MALT lymphomas show numerous point mutations in both *VH* and *VL* genes that are different relative to germline genes
  - Intraclonal sequence heterogeneity, indicating ongoing somatic hypermutation
  - *Ig* gene hypermutation occurs at post germinal center stage of B-cell development
- Gene rearrangements for *Ig VH* and *VL*, and for T-cell receptor β-chain genes are detected in lymphocytic thyroiditis
  - Different families of *VH* genes are detected in different lymphoma types
    - DLBCL shows *VH3*
    - EMZBCL shows *VH4* and *VH3*

DIFFERENTIAL DIAGNOSIS

Chronic Lymphocytic Thyroiditis
- No lymphoepithelial lesions (MALT balls)
- Not a diffuse process, although usually multifocal
- No germinal center colonization or destruction
  - Perifollicular Bcl-2 reaction
- Oncocytic change in thyroid follicular epithelium
- No cytologic atypia
- Lack of Dutcher bodies
- In rare cases, IHC, flow cytometric, or molecular genetic analyses may be required

LYMPHOMA

Immunohistochemistry

Antibody	Reactivity	Staining Pattern	Comment
CD20	Positive	Cytoplasmic	Dominant reaction in atypical lymphocytes
CD79-α	Positive	Cytoplasmic	Especially in plasmacytoid cells
CD138	Positive	Cytoplasmic	May highlight plasmacytoid cells
κ light chain	Positive	Cytoplasmic	Restriction of either κ **or** λ in EMZBCL
λ light chain	Positive	Cytoplasmic	Restriction of either κ **or** λ in EMZBCL
Bcl-2	Positive	Cytoplasmic	In neoplastic, colonizing cells (negative image of normal germinal centers)
Bcl-10	Positive	Nuclear & cytoplasmic	May be present in neoplastic lymphocytes
CD43	Positive	Cytoplasmic	Coexpressed with CD20 in selected cases
CD45RA	Positive	Cytoplasmic	Coexpressed with CD20 in selected cases
Bcl-6	Positive	Nuclear	Identified more often in DLBCL
Ki-67	Positive	Nuclear	Variable, although highest in DLBCL
CK-PAN	Positive	Cytoplasmic	Highlights destroyed thyroid follicular epithelium, especially "lymphoepithelial lesions"
CD3	Negative		

  - No light chain restriction
  - Lacks CD10 and Bcl-6

Undifferentiated (Anaplastic) Carcinoma
- Cohesive to dyscohesive highly atypical infiltrate
- Epithelioid appearance
- May have concurrent epithelial tumor present (papillary or follicular carcinoma)
- Distinction from DLBCL may require immunohistochemistry
  - Cytokeratin, TTF-1, thyroglobulin, CD45RB, CD20

Ectopic Thymoma
- Combination of epithelial and lymphoid elements
  - Not lymphoepithelial lesion
  - Nondestructive pattern
- Neoplastic cells with epithelial and T-cell antigens (CD5)

Melanoma
- Rare to have melanoma metastasize to thyroid
- Pigment, if present, is helpful
  - Melanin: Also in pigmented medullary carcinoma
- Dyscohesive cells, spindled morphology, intranuclear cytoplasmic inclusions
- Positive: S100 protein, HMB-45, Melan-A, tyrosinase

Sclerosing Mucoepidermoid Carcinoma with Eosinophilia
- Epithelial islands with heavy fibrosis
- Mucin production can be seen
- Eosinophils are prominent
- May mimic Hodgkin lymphoma
  - Immunohistochemistry (CD15, CD30, EBER) helps with separation

STAGING

Lymphoma in General
- "E" is added because they are extranodal
  - Perithyroidal lymph nodes may be involved
  - Other lymph nodes (mediastinal, abdominal) &/or bone marrow may then be affected
  - Gastrointestinal tract, lung, bladder, and liver
- Most are IE or IIE disease at presentation
- DLBCL tend to be higher stage (IIIE or IVE)

SELECTED REFERENCES

1. Graff-Baker A et al: Primary thyroid lymphoma: a review of recent developments in diagnosis and histology-driven treatment. Curr Opin Oncol. 22(1):17-22, 2010
2. Koida S et al: Primary T-cell lymphoma of the thyroid gland with chemokine receptors of Th1 phenotype complicating autoimmune thyroiditis. Haematologica. 92(3):e37-40, 2007
3. Mack LA et al: An evidence-based approach to the treatment of thyroid lymphoma. World J Surg. 31(5):978-86, 2007
4. Green LD et al: Anaplastic thyroid cancer and primary thyroid lymphoma: a review of these rare thyroid malignancies. J Surg Oncol. 94(8):725-36, 2006
5. Wang SA et al: Hodgkin's lymphoma of the thyroid: a clinicopathologic study of five cases and review of the literature. Mod Pathol. 18(12):1577-84, 2005
6. Derringer GA et al: Malignant lymphoma of the thyroid gland: a clinicopathologic study of 108 cases. Am J Surg Pathol. 24(5):623-39, 2000
7. Ansell SM et al: Primary thyroid lymphoma. Semin Oncol. 26(3):316-23, 1999
8. Fonseca E et al: Primary lymphomas of the thyroid gland: a review with emphasis on diagnostic features. Arch Anat Cytol Pathol. 46(1-2):94-9, 1998
9. Stone CW et al: Thyroid lymphoma with gastrointestinal involvement: report of three cases. Am J Hematol. 21(4):357-65, 1986
10. Anscombe AM et al: Primary malignant lymphoma of the thyroid--a tumour of mucosa-associated lymphoid tissue: review of seventy-six cases. Histopathology. 9(1):81-97, 1985
11. Devine RM et al: Primary lymphoma of the thyroid: A review of the Mayo Clinic experience through 1978. World J Surg. 5(1):33-8, 1981
12. Woolner LB et al: Primary malignant lymphoma of the thyroid. Review of forty-six cases. Am J Surg. 111(4):502-23, 1966

Radiographic, Gross, and Microscopic Features

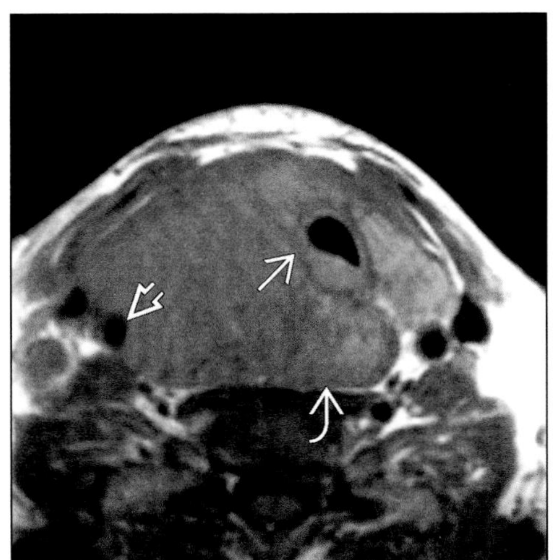

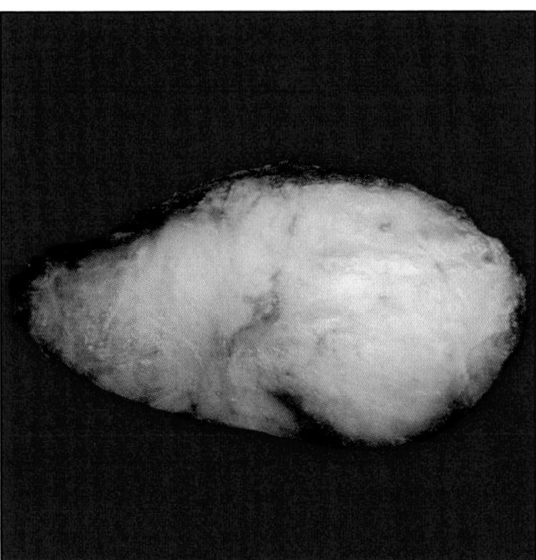

(Left) *Axial T1WI MR shows thyroid lymphoma as a homogeneous, circumscribed, solid thyroid mass. There is tracheal and carotid space displacement with concurrent invasion of the esophagus.* ***(Right)*** *This lobe of the thyroid gland shows a firm, slightly lobular mass, with effacement of the normal thyroid gland. The cut surface is bulging, smooth, pale-tan, and "fish flesh" with a homogeneous appearance. Extrathyroidal extension is frequently present.*

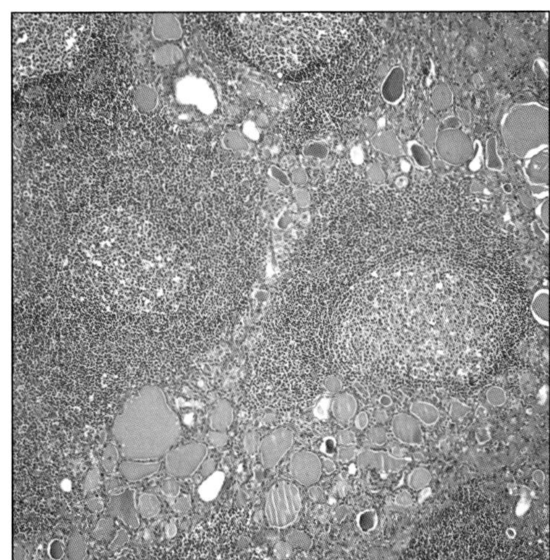

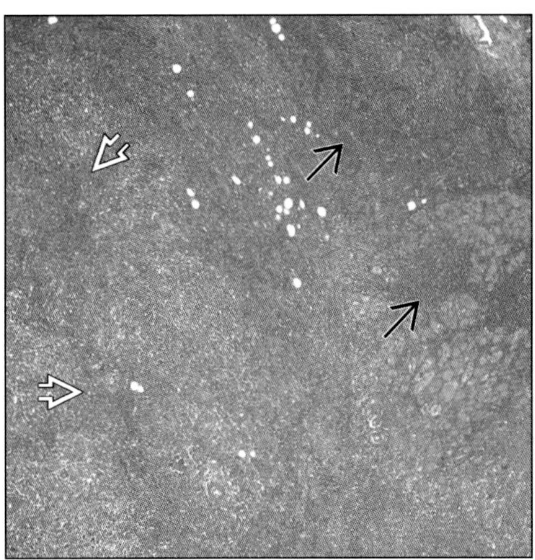

(Left) *Although it may not always be identified, chronic lymphocytic thyroiditis is nearly always present in the background of all patients with primary thyroid lymphoma. In cases where it is absent, it is presumed to be overtaken by the lymphoma.* ***(Right)*** *A multinodular or "follicular" pattern is seen in this EMZBCL. Chronic lymphocytic thyroiditis is noted in the background. Follicle colonization can be seen in lymphoma, yielding a darker zone within the follicles on low power.*

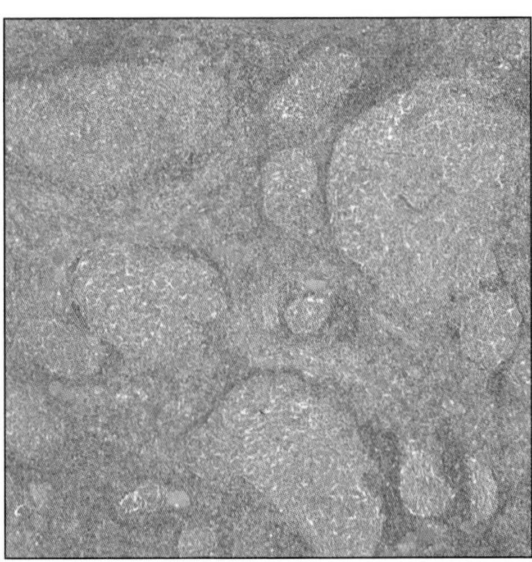

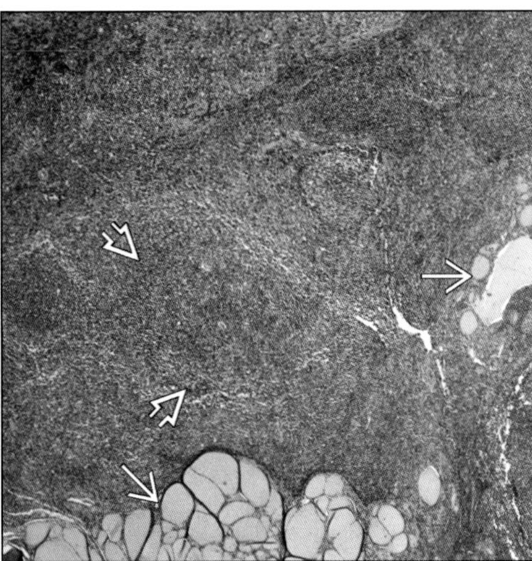

(Left) *Greatly enlarged germinal centers create a nodular or follicular pattern to this EMZBCL, with effacement of the thyroid parenchyma. It is easy to see how this pattern mimics a follicle center cell lymphoma.* ***(Right)*** *There is a vague nodularity to this lymphoma, which has effaced the thyroid parenchyma. Follicle lysis and involution with colonization by the neoplastic cells is present, creating a darker zone within the follicles.*

LYMPHOMA

Common Microscopic Features

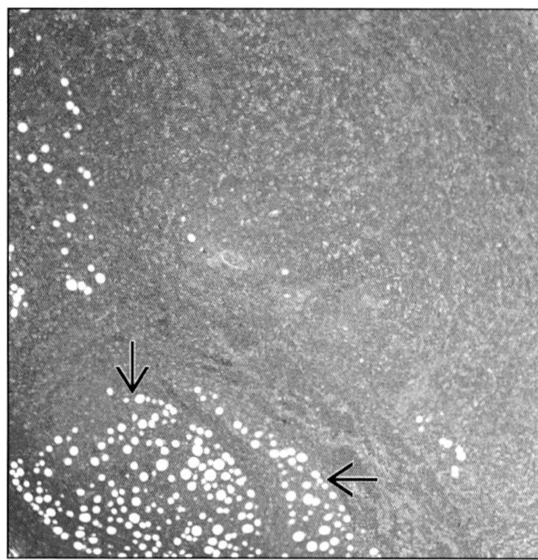

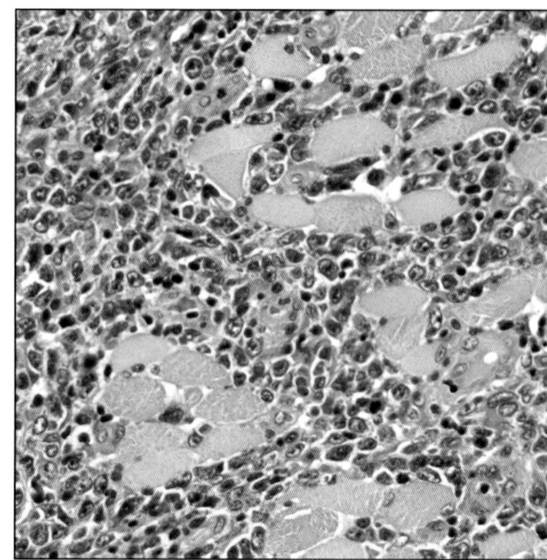

(Left) *There is complete effacement of normal thyroid gland parenchyma, showing vague nodularity and diffuse patterns. There is extension of the process into the adjacent adipose tissue ➔.* ***(Right)*** *The cells of a DLBCL have expanded into the perithyroidal skeletal muscle. This is a frequent finding in high-grade lymphomas. Note the plasmacytoid appearance of many of the neoplastic cells.*

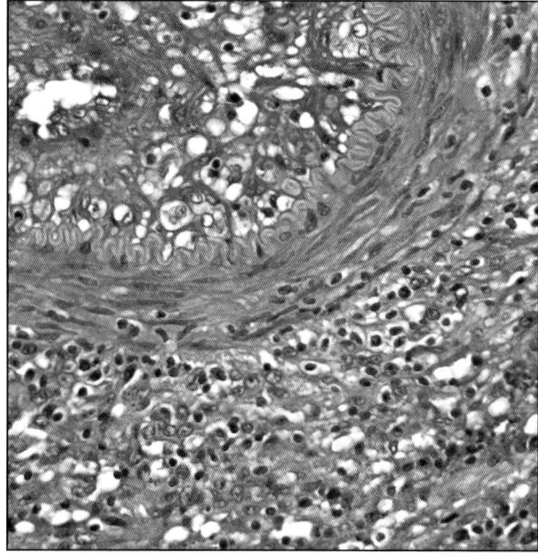

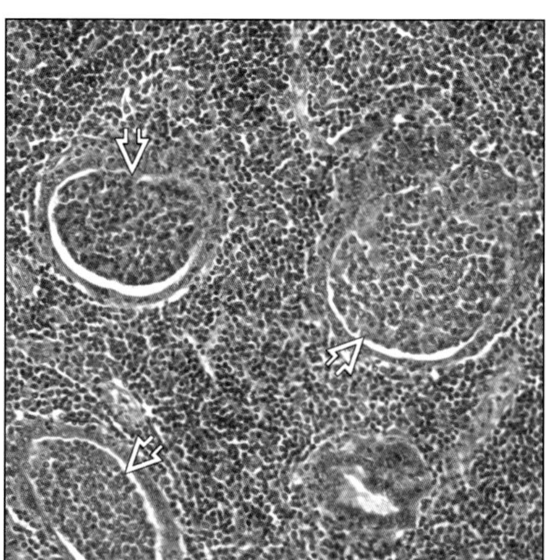

(Left) *Atypical lymphoid cells are noted in the wall of the vessel and continuing into the sub-intimal space. Vascular invasion is most common in high-grade tumors.* ***(Right)*** *Lymphoepithelial lesions (LELs) are one of the best features to confirm a lymphoma. Atypical lymphoid cells infiltrate into and destroy the thyroid follicular epithelium. Of the 2 types, "MALT balls" are unique ➔: Rounded balls or masses, filling and distending the lumen of the thyroid follicles.*

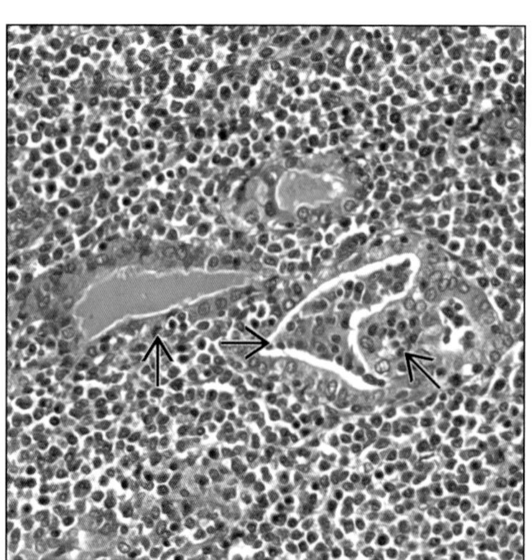

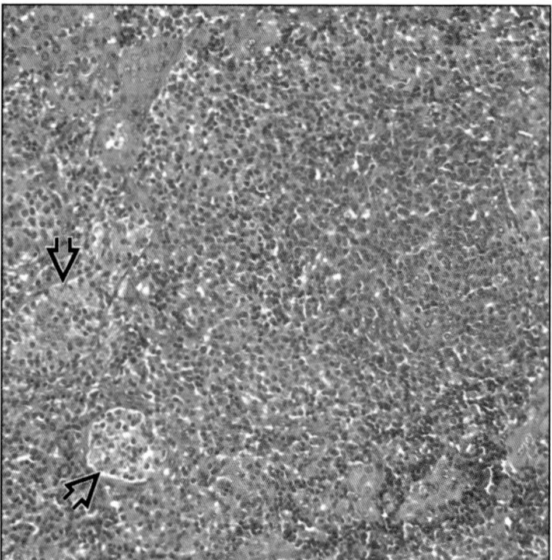

(Left) *LELs are atypical lymphoid cells that infiltrate into and destroy the thyroid follicular epithelium. Here, there are single and aggregated lymphocytes within ➔ or between the follicular epithelial cells.* ***(Right)*** *EMZBCL have a heterogeneous population of B-cells, including marginal zone cells, monocytoid B-cells, and plasma cells. The monocytoid B-cells ➔ are a monotonous population of atypical lymphoid cells with abundant, pale cytoplasm and lobulated or kidney-shaped nuclei.*

EMZBCL Microscopic Features; Uncommon Lymphomas

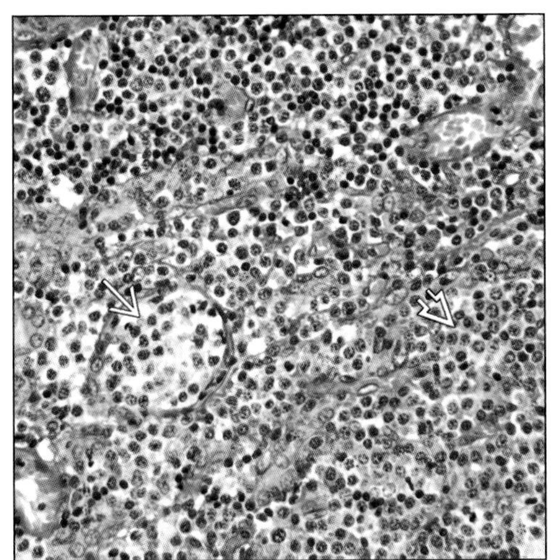

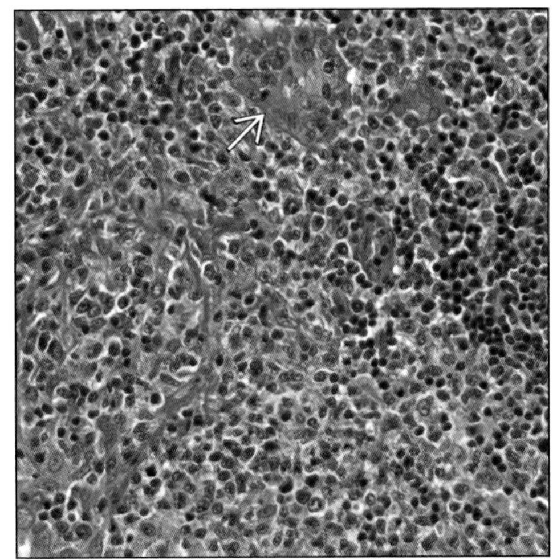

(Left) *There are atypical small lymphocytes, marginal zone (centrocyte-like) small cleaved cells, monocytoid B-cells ➡, and plasma cells ➡. They are frequently blended with one another as in this example.* ***(Right)*** *It is important to remember that EMZBCL are heterogeneous, in this field showing eosinophils, mature lymphocytes, plasma cells, and monocytoid B-cells. A partially destroyed thyroid epithelial follicle is present ➡.*

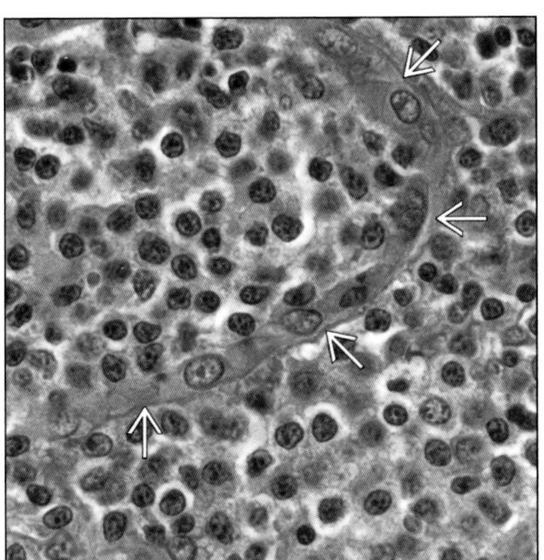

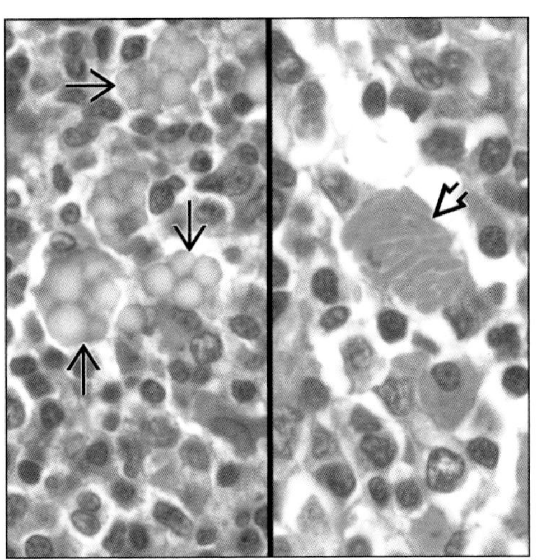

(Left) *The monocytoid B-cells are a monotonous population of atypical lymphoid cells with abundant, pale cytoplasm with lobulated or kidney-shaped nuclei. They frequently show grooves or cleaves. They frequently aggregate, as they are within this thyroid follicle ➡.* ***(Right)*** *Cytoplasmic immunoglobulin ("Mott cells" ➡) accentuates the plasmacytoid differentiation. Uncommonly, crystal-storing histiocytes ➡ may be seen. Dutcher and Russell bodies are usually easy to find.*

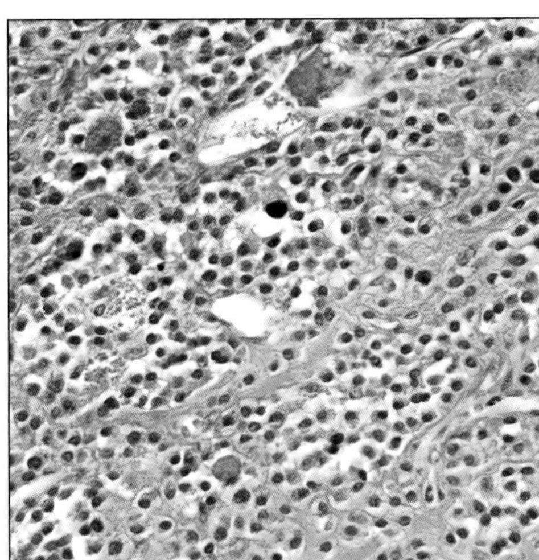

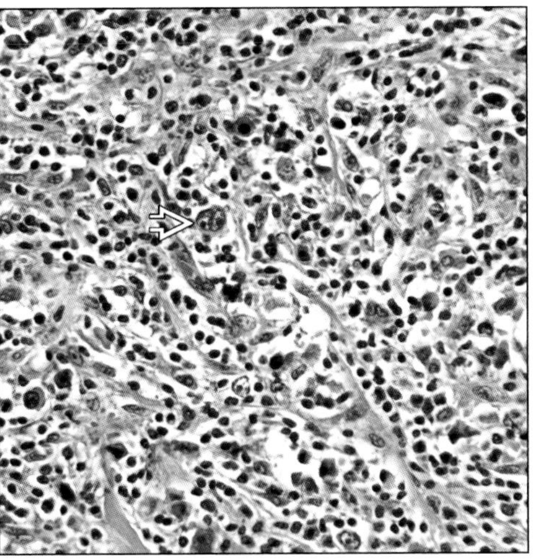

(Left) *Sometimes, EMZBCL can show such extensive plasma cell differentiation (sheets of plasma cells) that it simulates a plasmacytoma. Light chain restriction demonstrates monoclonality.* ***(Right)*** *Classical Hodgkin lymphoma, nodular sclerosis subtype is the only one identified in thyroid. Classic Hodgkin-Reed-Sternberg (HRS) cells ➡ are noted in a variably cellular background diathesis of plasma cells, eosinophils, and neutrophils. Appropriate immunohistochemistries are necessary for the diagnosis.*

Diffuse Large B-cell Lymphoma Features

*(**Left**) There is a zone of transition from EMZBCL ➯ to DLBCL ➔. It is not uncommon to see areas of transition between these 2 tumor types. Pattern of growth, atypia, and increased mitoses can help with this separation. (**Right**) In this field, there is a plasmacytoid appearance to the lymphoid population. However, it is a diffuse, sheet-like growth. There is a vaguely plasmacytoid appearance to the cells.*

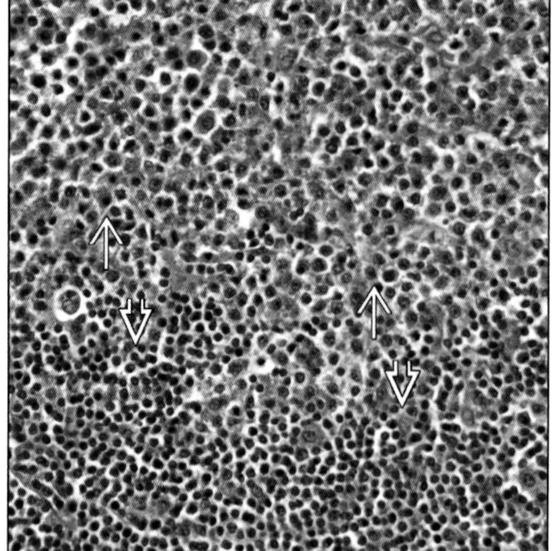

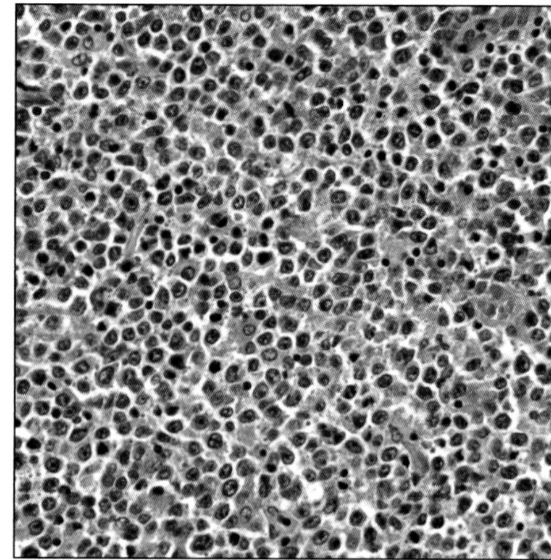

*(**Left**) This high-power view shows large cells that demonstrate a spectrum of features, with centroblasts, immunoblasts, monocytoid B-cells, and plasmacytoid cells. Focal necrosis ➯ is easily identified. (**Right**) Sheets of a single type of large cell can be seen in DLBCL. While uncommon, these cells have a monocytoid B-cell appearance. Mitotic figures are noted, and cytologic pleomorphism is moderate.*

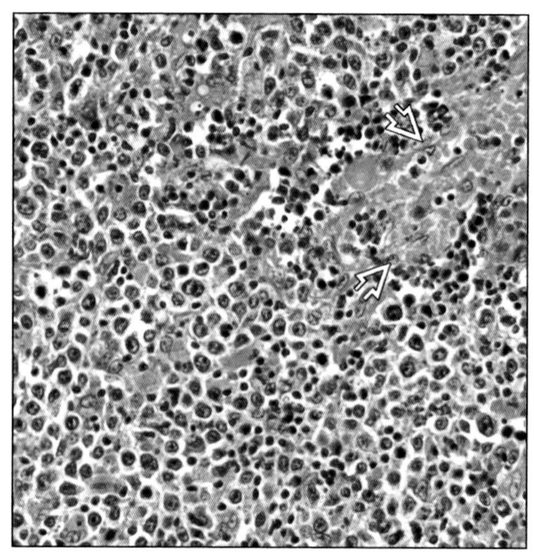

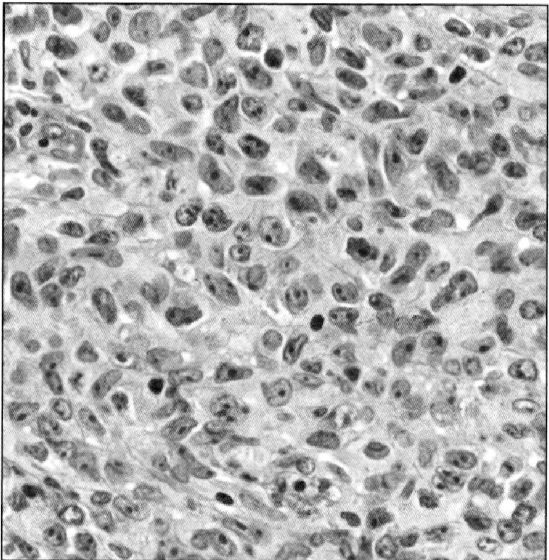

*(**Left**) Occasionally the tumor is arranged in a Burkitt-like pattern, with brisk mitotic activity, apoptosis, and a "starry sky" pattern. A residual thyroid follicle is present ➔. (**Right**) The tumor shows a sheet-like appearance of large centroblast-like cells in association with a large, multinucleated, Reed-Sternberg-like cell ➔. These features are quite frequently present in a DLBCL.*

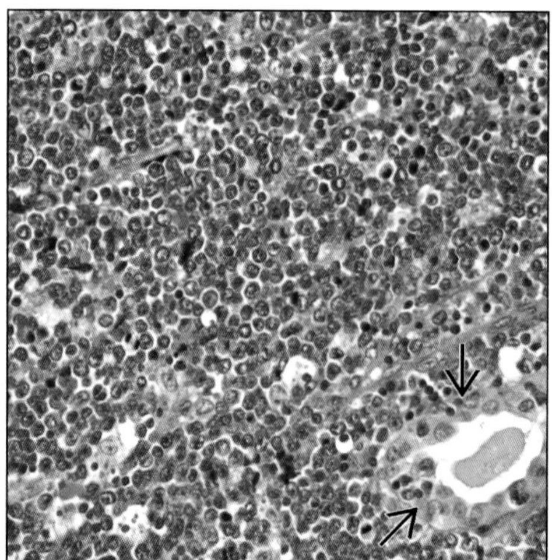

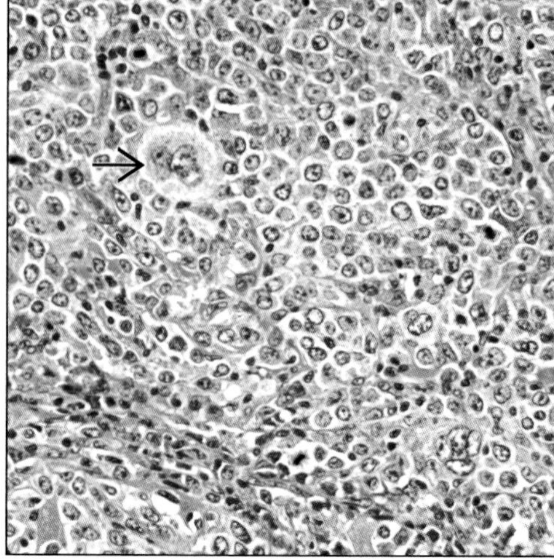

Ancillary Techniques

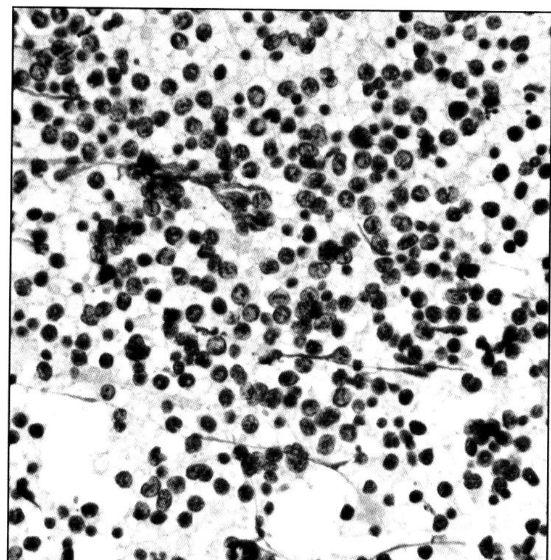

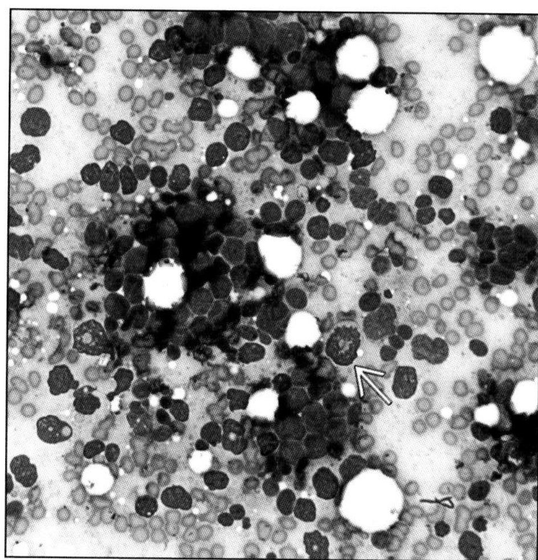

(Left) *There is a cellular aspirate without thyroid follicular epithelium. The cells are monotonous, slightly enlarged, and show a background of lymphoglandular bodies. The chromatin is slightly vesicular. This pattern can mimic a chronic lymphocytic thyroiditis.* ***(Right)*** *Smears show a noncohesive admixture of atypical, large (3x erythrocyte size) cells, with lymphoglandular bodies and mitotic figures ➡. Thyroid epithelium and tingible body macrophages are absent.*

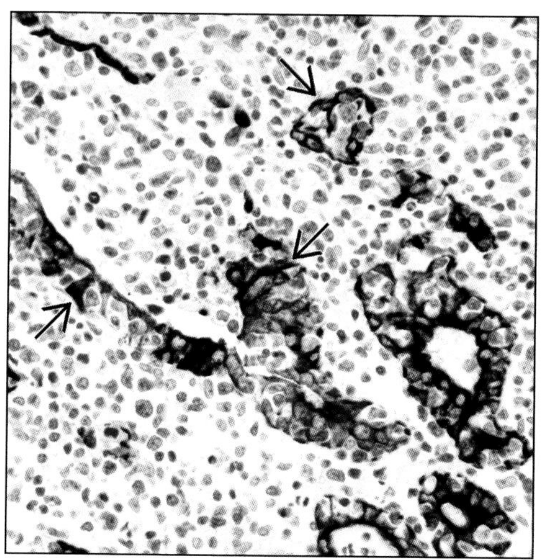

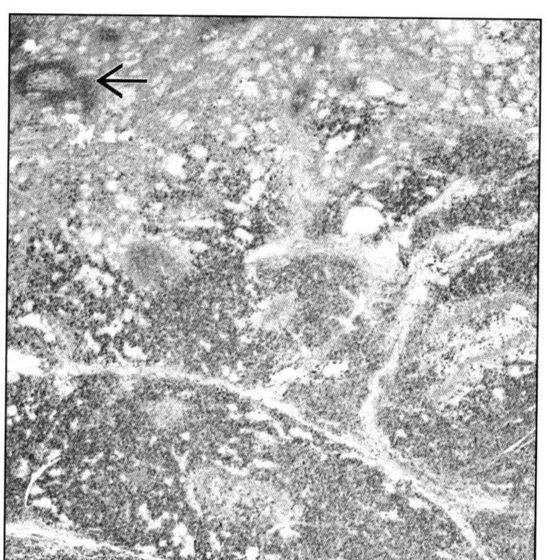

(Left) *Keratin can be used to highlight ➡ the residual thyroid follicular epithelium, especially in lymphoepithelial lesions, where atypical lymphocytes invade and destroy the follicles.* ***(Right)*** *Either CD79-α or CD138 can be used to highlight the plasmacytoid cells within an EMZBCL. In this case, plasmacytoid cells are also highlighted in the background germinal centers ➡. Location is important in lymphoma immunohistochemistry interpretation.*

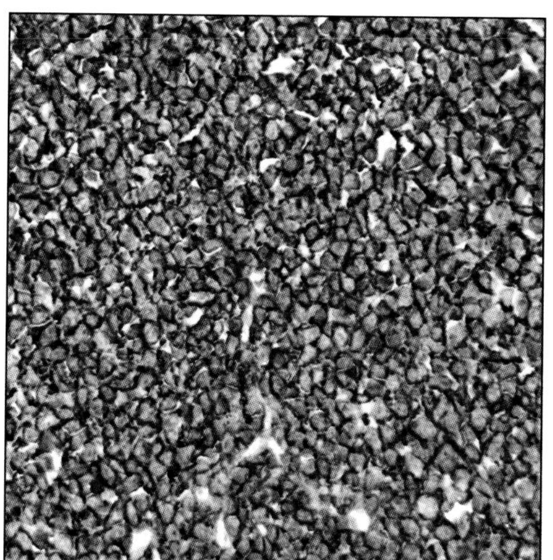

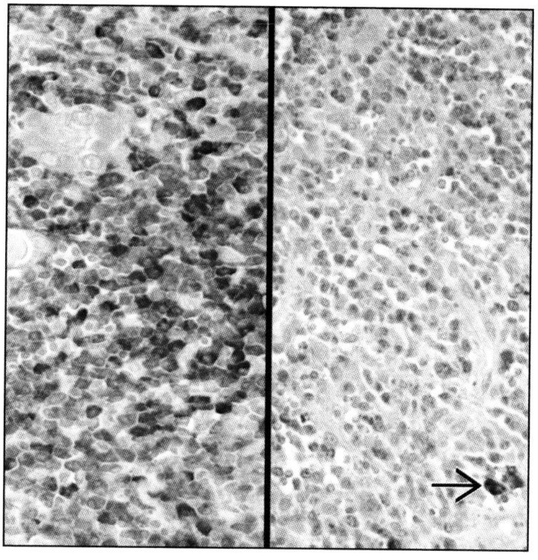

(Left) *Nearly all primary thyroid gland lymphomas are immunoreactive with CD20, giving a strong and diffuse cytoplasmic reaction in the atypical lymphocytes. By contrast, CD3 will be positive in chronic lymphocytic thyroiditis or only in isolated cells in the tumor.* ***(Right)*** *This EMZBCL demonstrates a remarkable restriction with κ light chain (left), while only isolated nonneoplastic cells are positive with λ light chain ➡ (right).*

ANGIOSARCOMA

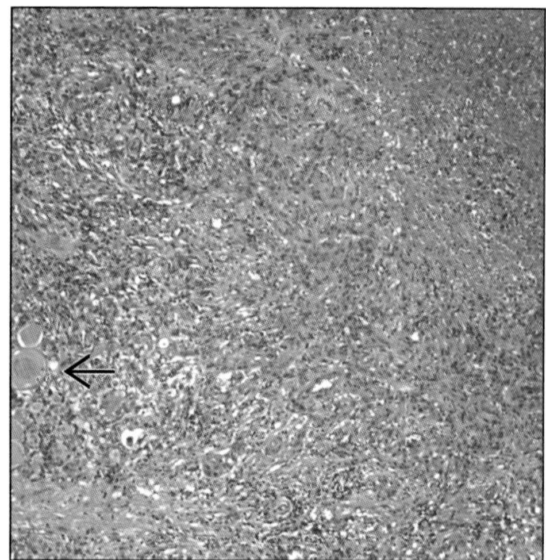

There are isolated thyroid gland follicles ⇒ surrounded by a vascular proliferation. There is extensive necrosis associated with the proliferation. This is a common finding for angiosarcoma.

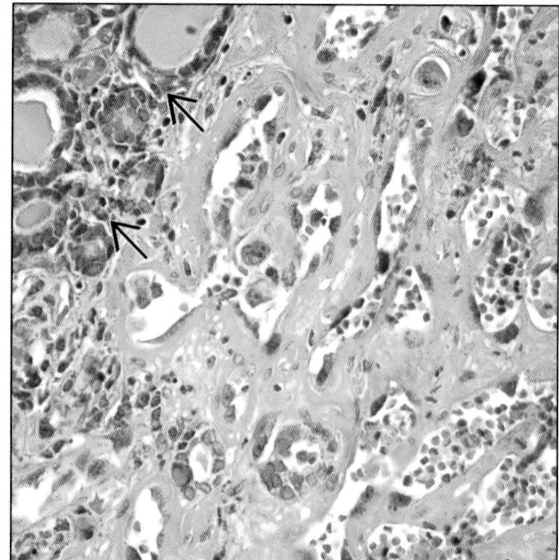

A freely anastomosing vascular proliferation is separated by a desmoplastic stroma adjacent to thyroid follicles ⇒. Erythrocytes are noted within the channels lined by atypical endothelial cells.

TERMINOLOGY

Definitions

- Primary thyroid gland angiosarcoma is a malignant tumor of endothelial cell differentiation

ETIOLOGY/PATHOGENESIS

Environmental Exposure

- Dietary iodine deficiency, especially in alpine areas of central Europe
  - Prevalence reduced with iodized salt prophylaxis
- Significant occupational exposure to industrial vinyl chloride and other polymeric materials

Multifactorial

- Other factors considered etiologic

Pathogenesis

- Endothelial origin seems supported
  - No thyroglobulin mRNA expression (tested by radioactive in situ hybridization)

CLINICAL ISSUES

Epidemiology

- Incidence
  - Uncommon
  - < 2% of all thyroid gland malignancies
- Age
  - Usually in 7th decade of life
- Gender
  - Female > > Male (4:1)
- Ethnicity
  - Increased in inhabitants of central Europe (alpine areas)

Presentation

- Painless mass
  - Often seen in setting of longstanding goiter
- May have dyspnea, asthenia, weight loss
- Rarely: Rapidly growing mass with pressure symptoms
- Hyperthyroidism is rare
  - Angiosarcoma may have trophic effect on follicular epithelium

Treatment

- Options, risks, complications
  - Severe bleeding at primary or metastatic sites may complicate surgery
- Surgical approaches
  - Radical surgery (total thyroidectomy)
- Drugs
  - Chemotherapy can be used but may be palliative
- Radiation
  - Adjuvant radiotherapy, frequently administered as brachytherapy
    - Razoxane may benefit patients as a radiation sensitizer

Prognosis

- Overall poor prognosis
- Majority of patients die from disease (< 6 months)
- Rarely, patients may survive > 5 years
- Distant metastases may cause fatal bleeding
  - Most common sites: Lung, gastrointestinal tract, bone

MACROSCOPIC FEATURES

General Features

- Macroscopically they appear circumscribed, but microscopically they are invasive
- Cut surface is variegated with extensive hemorrhage and necrosis

Size

- Tend to be large; range up to 10-12 cm

ANGIOSARCOMA

Key Facts

Terminology
- Primary thyroid gland angiosarcoma is a malignant tumor of endothelial cell differentiation

Clinical Issues
- Increased in inhabitants of Europe (alpine areas)
- Female > > Male (4:1)
- Severe bleeding at primary or metastatic sites may complicate surgery
- Overall poor prognosis

Macroscopic Features
- Variegated with extensive hemorrhage and necrosis
- Tend to be large (up to 12 cm)

Microscopic Pathology
- Irregular periphery, invading thyroid parenchyma
- Tumor necrosis and hemorrhage throughout
- Freely anastomosing vascular channels
- Irregular, cleft-like to patulous vascular channels
- Large, epithelioid polygonal cells lining vessels
- Neolumen formation with erythrocytes

Ancillary Tests
- Positive: Vascular endothelial markers (CD31, FVIIIRAg, CD34), vimentin, and keratin
- EM: Membrane-bound, rod-shaped cytoplasmic Weibel-Palade bodies

Top Differential Diagnoses
- Undifferentiated carcinoma
- Degenerative adenomatoid nodules
- Post fine needle aspiration changes
- Metastatic angiosarcoma

MICROSCOPIC PATHOLOGY

Histologic Features
- Irregular periphery, with blending and invasion of thyroid parenchyma
- Freely anastomosing vascular channels
  - Many patterns: Solid, spindled, papillary, pseudoglandular
- Tumor necrosis and hemorrhage throughout
- Increased mitotic figures, including atypical forms
- Irregular, cleft-like to patulous vascular channels
- Hemosiderin-laden macrophages common
- Large, epithelioid polygonal cells lining vascular channels
  - Abundant eosinophilic to vacuolated cytoplasm surrounding round nuclei with vesicular chromatin
  - Prominent macronucleoli
  - Neolumen formation with erythrocytes
  - Multinucleated tumor giant cells are rare

ANCILLARY TESTS

Cytology
- Diagnostic cytology material is difficult to interpret
- Background of necrotic material and blood

Immunohistochemistry
- Positive with vascular endothelial markers: CD31, FVIIIRAg, CD34, ULEX-1
  - Avoid overinterpretation of diffusion artifacts
- Positive: Vimentin, occasionally keratin
- Negative: TTF-1, thyroglobulin, calcitonin

DIFFERENTIAL DIAGNOSIS

Undifferentiated (Anaplastic) Carcinoma
- Pseudoangiomatous pattern can be seen in undifferentiated carcinoma
- Usually greater degree of pleomorphism, tumor giant cells, and solid pattern
- Undifferentiated (anaplastic) carcinoma frequently has concurrent thyroid gland disease (nodules, tumor)
- Immunohistochemistry may help, but results must be interpreted with caution

Degenerative Adenomatoid Nodules
- Nodules frequently undergo degenerative/retrogressive changes, with hemorrhage followed by organization
  - Granulation-type tissue, blood, hemosiderin-laden macrophages, cyst formation and calcification
- No cytologic atypia, freely anastomosing vessels, atypical mitoses, necrosis

Post Fine Needle Aspiration
- Common to have a "Masson papillary endothelial hyperplasia" type reaction
- Single area of involvement, with breached capsule, hemosiderin-laden macrophages, extravasated erythrocytes
- No cytologic atypia, no freely anastomosing vessels

Metastatic Angiosarcoma
- Highly vascular; metastases to thyroid may be seen
- Must use past history, clinical exam, radiology
- Direct invasion (soft tissue or skin) into thyroid

SELECTED REFERENCES

1. Papotti M et al: Diagnostic controversies in vascular proliferations of the thyroid gland. Endocr Pathol. 19(3):175-83, 2008
2. Ryska A et al: Epithelioid haemangiosarcoma of the thyroid gland. Report of six cases from a non-Alpine region. Histopathology. 44(1):40-6, 2004
3. Cutlan RT et al: Immunohistochemical characterization of thyroid gland angiomatoid tumors. Exp Mol Pathol. 69(2):159-64, 2000
4. Maiorana A et al: Epithelioid angiosarcoma of the thyroid. Clinicopathological analysis of seven cases from non-Alpine areas. Virchows Arch. 429(2-3):131-7, 1996
5. Eusebi V et al: Keratin-positive epithelioid angiosarcoma of thyroid. A report of four cases. Am J Surg Pathol. 14(8):737-47, 1990

ANGIOSARCOMA

Gross and Microscopic Features

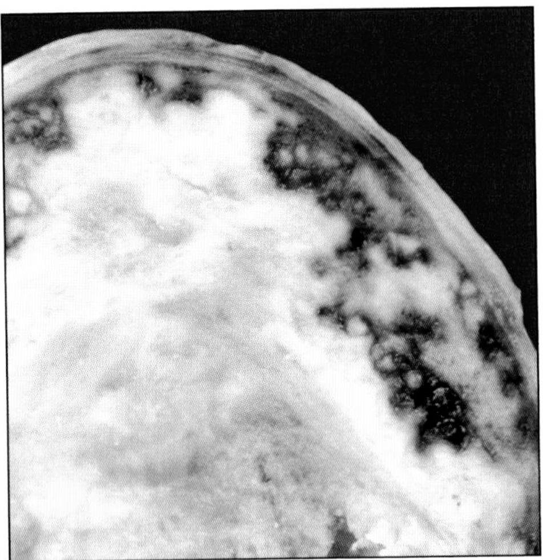

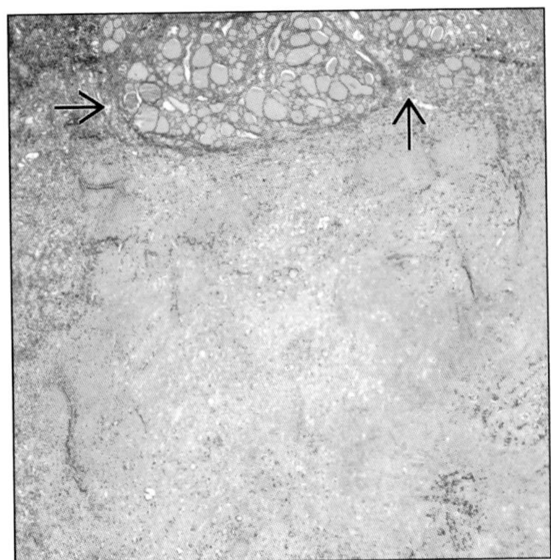

(Left) *The cut section of the thyroid shows areas of hemorrhage and necrosis within an encapsulated mass. (Courtesy A. Ryška, MD.)* ***(Right)*** *A low-power magnification shows a degenerative neoplastic proliferation immediately adjacent to and involving the thyroid gland parenchyma ⇒. Areas of necrosis are present. At this power, a vascular neoplasm may not be considered; however, extensive necrosis is present.*

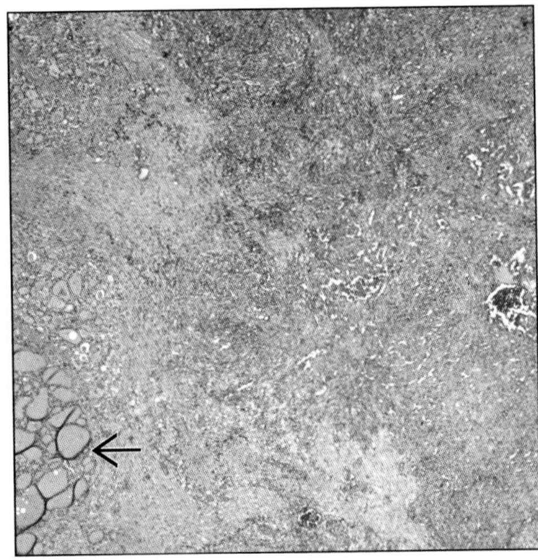

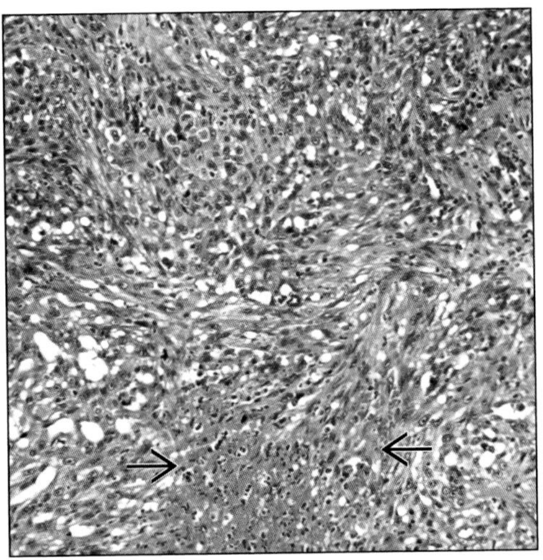

(Left) *Open, freely anastomosing vascular channels can be detected in this angiosarcoma. The tumor is cellular, showing an infiltrative growth into the adjacent thyroid gland parenchyma ⇒. Extravasated erythrocytes are plentiful.* ***(Right)*** *Interlacing fascicles of spindled tumor cells are noted in this angiosarcoma. There is still a vascular quality with open vascular spaces and lumen formations. There is also tumor necrosis ⇒, a frequent finding in angiosarcoma.*

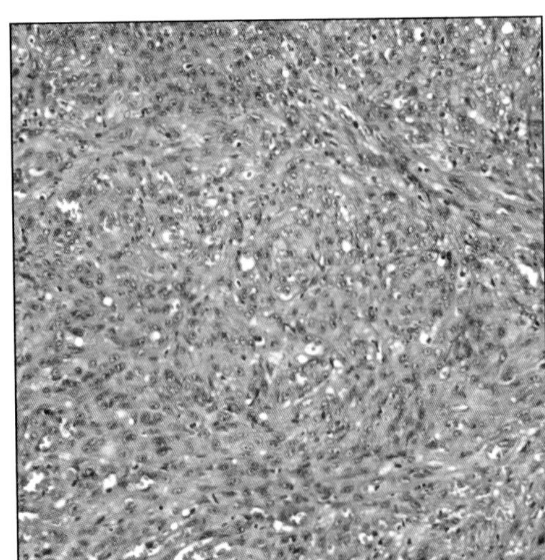

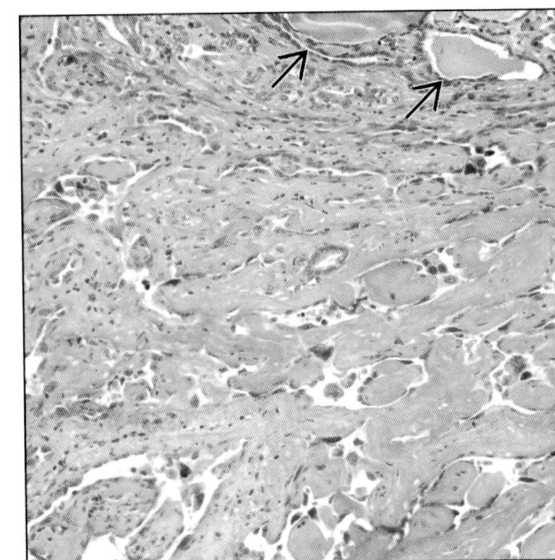

(Left) *This tumor shows the characteristic epithelioid to spindled appearance of many primary thyroid angiosarcomas. The nuclei are vesicular and open. Thyroid parenchyma is not identified in this field. Vessels are slit-like spaces.* ***(Right)*** *Heavy, collagenized stroma can be seen separating the tumor vessels. In this case, there are open vascular channels lined by remarkably atypical epithelioid endothelial cells. A few thyroid follicles are noted ⇒.*

Microscopic Features and Ancillary Techniques

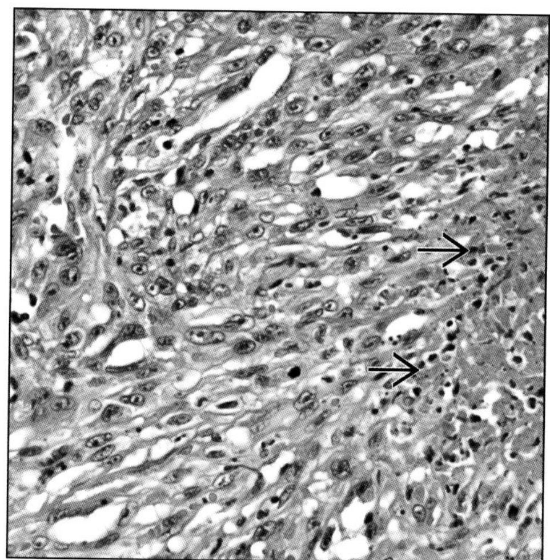

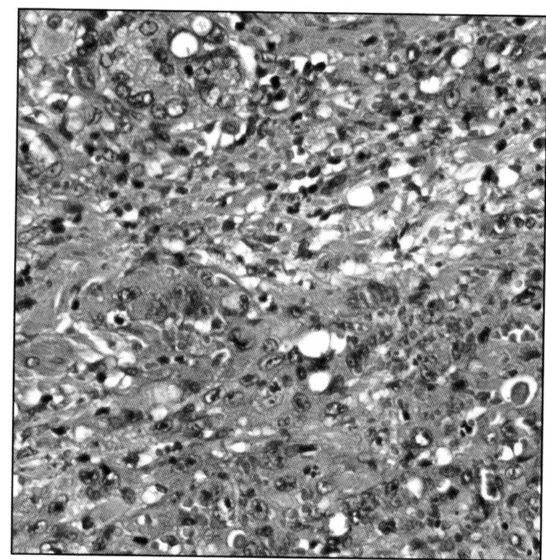

(Left) *Necrosis → blends into the neoplastic proliferation of irregular, cleft-like vascular channels. The cells are large and epithelioid, with prominent nucleoli easily identified. Extravasated erythrocytes are easily identified throughout the lesion.* ***(Right)*** *Abundant extravasated erythrocytes are present throughout this tumor. Note the vacuolization of the cytoplasm. Nucleoli are easily identified even at this intermediate magnification. The cells have a syncytial quality.*

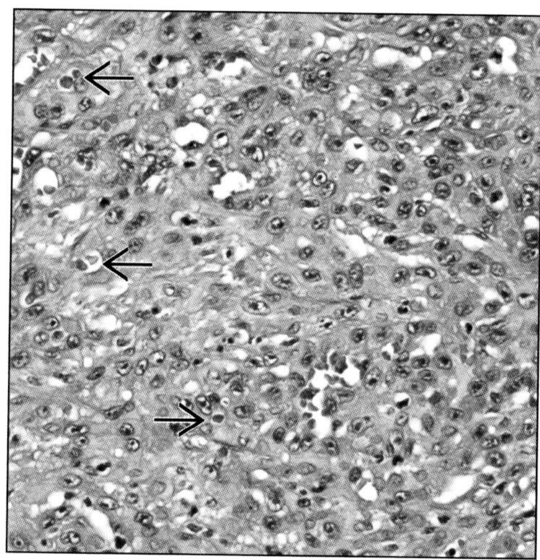

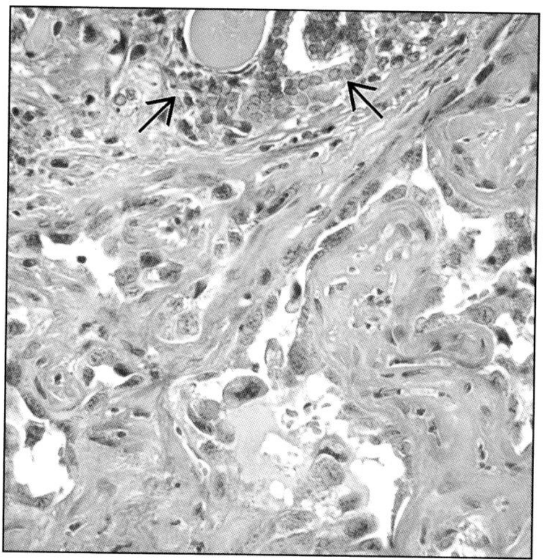

(Left) *Prominent macronucleoli are present within a number of epithelioid to polygonal neoplastic cells. Areas of neolumen formation → can help to confirm the true nature of the neoplasm as an angiosarcoma. Erythrocytes are noted within the lumen.* ***(Right)*** *The epithelioid neoplastic cells are large and polygonal and line the patulous vascular spaces. The nuclei are vesicular. Thyroid follicular epithelium can be seen as a point of comparison →.*

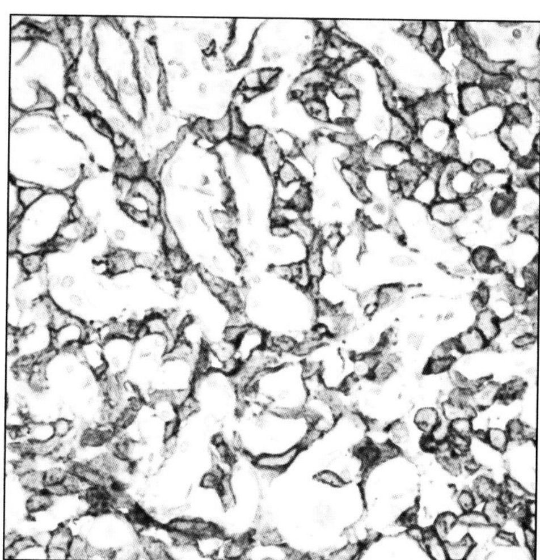

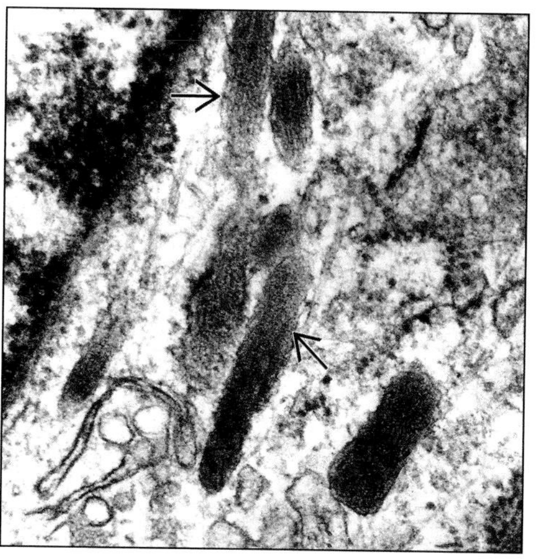

(Left) *The neoplastic endothelial cells are immunoreactive with a variety of vascular markers (CD31, CD34, FVIIIRAg), but are also keratin immunoreactive, as seen in this thyroid angiosarcoma.* ***(Right)*** *Weibel-Palade bodies contain fine tubules → and are the intracytoplasmic storage granules of endothelial cells. The structures contain von Willebrand factor and P-selectin, molecules involved in homeostasis. (Courtesy S. Bhuta, MD.)*

LEIOMYOSARCOMA

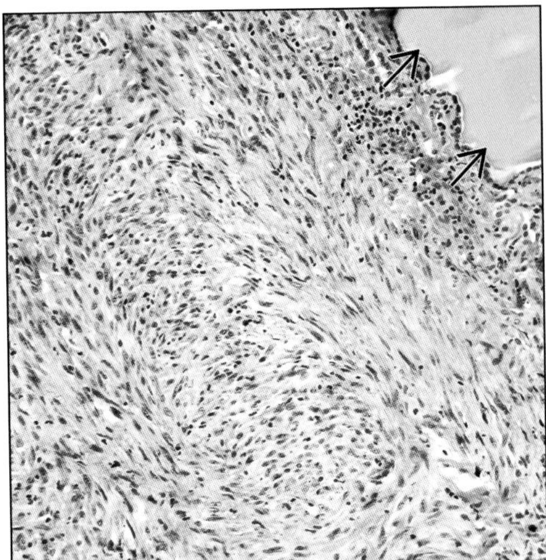

A highly cellular neoplasm is seen, arranged in short, interlacing disordered fascicles. The tumor cells are spindled with spindled, hyperchromatic nuclei. The thyroid follicle is entrapped at the edge ➔.

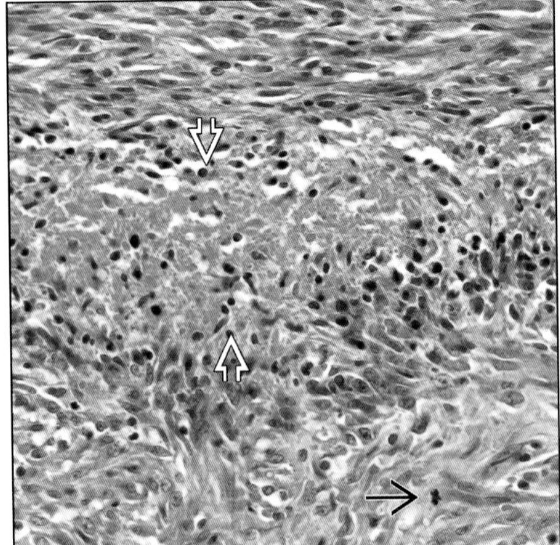

There is a haphazard distribution of neoplastic spindled cells. The tumor cells are associated with an area of tumor necrosis ➔. Mitotic figures are easily identified ➔.

TERMINOLOGY

Abbreviations

- Leiomyosarcoma (LMS)

Definitions

- Malignant primary thyroid neoplasm composed of cells with distinct smooth muscle differentiation histologically

ETIOLOGY/PATHOGENESIS

Histogenesis

- Postulated to arise from smooth muscle-walled vessels at thyroid gland periphery

CLINICAL ISSUES

Epidemiology

- Incidence
  - Exceedingly rare; < 0.02% of all thyroid gland tumors
- Age
  - Older age patients
- Gender
  - Equal gender distribution

Site

- Often thyroid gland periphery

Presentation

- Nonspecific signs and symptoms
- Thyroid mass, usually increasing in size
- May be associated with dyspnea, difficulty breathing, &/or stridor

Treatment

- Surgical approaches
  - Complete, radical surgical removal
- Drugs
  - Chemotherapy may be of value
- Radiation
  - Does not show significant benefit

Prognosis

- Poor, with all reported patients dying from disease

IMAGE FINDINGS

Radiographic Findings

- Inhomogeneous low-density mass in thyroid gland by CT evaluation
  - Signal intensity similar to surrounding soft tissue
  - May have calcifications
- Features suggestive of malignancy but not diagnostic of tumor type
  - Compression of upper airway, infiltration into soft tissues or thyroid cartilage, thyroid destruction, and necrosis

MACROSCOPIC FEATURES

General Features

- Nodular to bosselated outer surface
- Periphery tends to show widely invasive appearance into surrounding soft tissue

Size

- Range: Up to 12 cm
- Mean: 6 cm

MICROSCOPIC PATHOLOGY

Histologic Features

- Irregular, invasive periphery
  - Encapsulation may be seen, although invasion is common
- Entrapment and destruction of thyroid follicles

LEIOMYOSARCOMA

Key Facts

Terminology
- Malignant primary thyroid neoplasm composed of cells with distinct smooth muscle differentiation histologically

Etiology/Pathogenesis
- Postulated to arise from smooth muscle-walled vessels

Clinical Issues
- Typically affects older age patients
- Poor prognosis, with all patients dying from disease

Microscopic Pathology
- Nodular to bosselated outer surface
- Irregular, invasive periphery
- Entrapment and destruction of thyroid follicles
- Origin from smooth-muscle-walled vessels
- Tumor necrosis usually present
- Highly cellular tumors, arranged in bundles or disordered fascicles
- Spindled tumor cells
- Centrally placed, hyperchromatic, blunt-ended, cigar-shaped nuclei
- Perinuclear cytoplasmic vacuoles quite characteristic
- Nuclear pleomorphism is pronounced
- Increased mitoses (> 5/10 HPF), including atypical

Ancillary Tests
- Positive: Vimentin, SMA, MSA, desmin

Top Differential Diagnoses
- Medullary carcinoma, undifferentiated carcinoma, metastatic leiomyosarcoma

---

- Origin from smooth muscle-walled vessels may be seen
- Vascular and perineural invasion frequently present
- Tumor necrosis usually present
- Highly cellular tumors, arranged in bundles or disordered fascicles
- Spindled tumor cells
  - Centrally placed, hyperchromatic, blunt-ended, cigar-shaped nuclei
  - Perinuclear cytoplasmic vacuoles quite characteristic
  - Nuclear pleomorphism is easily identified
- Increased mitoses (> 5/10 HPF), including atypical

ANCILLARY TESTS

Immunohistochemistry
- Neoplastic cells positive: Vimentin, SMA, MSA, desmin
  - Focal immunoreactivity: MYOD1, myogenin, CD117
- Increased to high Ki-67 labeling index
- Neoplastic cells negative: Thyroglobulin, cytokeratin, S100 protein, chromogranin, and calcitonin

Electron Microscopy
- Cytoplasmic thin myofilaments with dense bodies and discontinuous basal lamina

DIFFERENTIAL DIAGNOSIS

Medullary Carcinoma
- Spindled cell morphology can be seen
- Plasmacytoid growth, "salt and pepper" nuclear chromatin distribution, amyloid, and background of C-cell hyperplasia
- Immunoreactive: TTF-1, calcitonin, chromogranin, CD56, CEA-M

Undifferentiated Carcinoma
- Significant overlap clinically, radiographically, and histologically between LMS and UC
- Usually have longstanding history of preexisting thyroid lesion that has rapidly enlarged
- Presence of residual well-differentiated thyroid carcinoma favors undifferentiated carcinoma
- May show epithelial differentiation (histologic, immunophenotypic, ultrastructural), but lacks myoid markers (desmin, actins)

Metastatic Leiomyosarcoma
- Direct extension and metastatic leiomyosarcoma to thyroid gland must be excluded
- Clinical and radiographic correlation required
- Most common primary sites: Uterus, gastrointestinal tract, soft tissue
- Metastatic disease tends to be multifocal in thyroid
  - Rarely isolated to thyroid gland only

GRADING

Not Performed
- Not used, but nuclear anaplasia, increased mitotic figures, and tumor necrosis would be included

SELECTED REFERENCES

1. Just PA et al: An unusual clinical presentation of a rare tumor of the thyroid gland: report on one case of leiomyosarcoma and review of literature. Ann Diagn Pathol. 12(1):50-6, 2008
2. Wang TS et al: Primary leiomyosarcoma of the thyroid gland. Thyroid. 18(4):425-8, 2008
3. Eloy JA et al: Metastasis of uterine leiomyosarcoma to the thyroid gland: case report and review of the literature. Thyroid. 17(12):1295-7, 2007
4. Tulbah A et al: Epstein-Barr virus-associated leiomyosarcoma of the thyroid in a child with congenital immunodeficiency: a case report. Am J Surg Pathol. 23(4):473-6, 1999
5. Thompson LD et al: Primary smooth muscle tumors of the thyroid gland. Cancer. 79(3):579-87, 1997
6. Chetty R et al: Leiomyosarcoma of the thyroid: immunohistochemical and ultrastructural study. Pathology. 25(2):203-5, 1993
7. Kawahara E et al: Leiomyosarcoma of the thyroid gland. A case report with a comparative study of five cases of anaplastic carcinoma. Cancer. 62(12):2558-63, 1988

LEIOMYOSARCOMA

Imaging and Microscopic Features

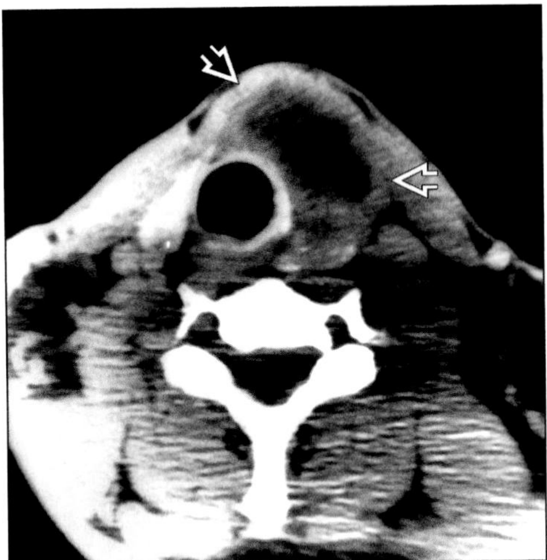

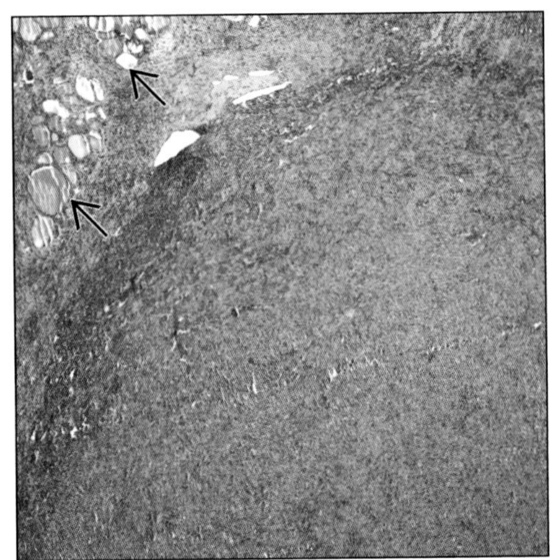

(Left) *A computed tomography scan demonstrates a large tumor replacing the left lobe of the thyroid gland ➲. There is central necrosis. Lymphadenopathy is absent.* ***(Right)*** *There are a number of thyroid follicles entrapped and destroyed ➙ at the periphery of the irregular, invasive neoplasm. There is no encapsulation identified. While it is a spindled cell tumor, the specific type cannot be determined from this magnification.*

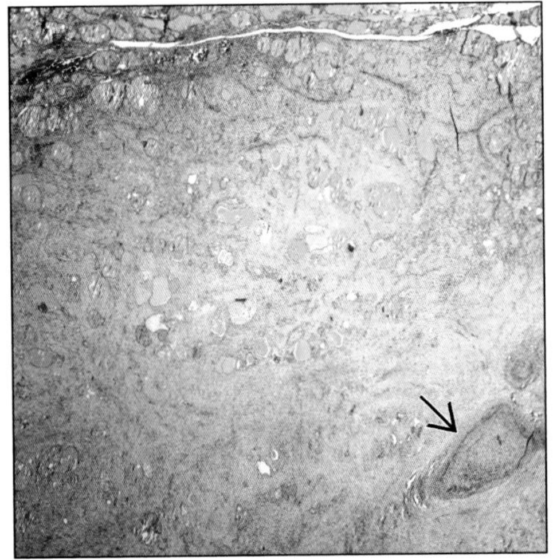

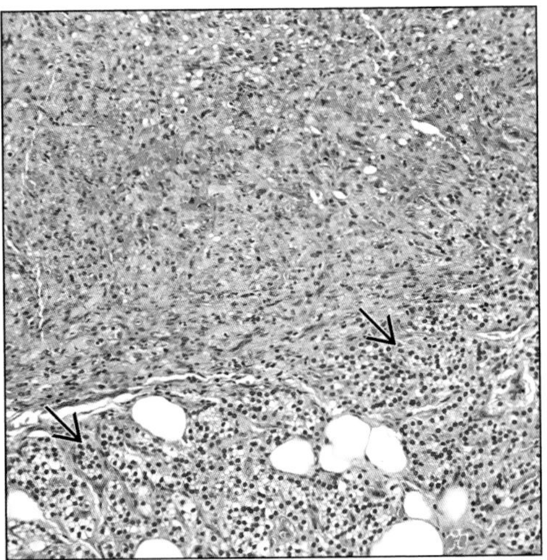

(Left) *There is no encapsulation of this tumor; rather, it is an irregular invasive neoplasm. Entrapment and destruction of thyroid follicles is noted as the tumor invades. Note the large vessel ➙ giving rise to the tumor.* ***(Right)*** *The spindled cell neoplastic population is noted invading into and destroying the parathyroid tissue ➙ identified adjacent to the thyroid. Extravasated erythrocytes are noted within the tumor.*

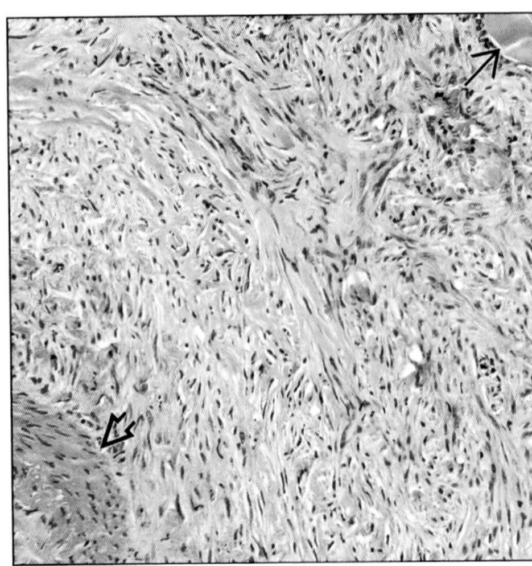

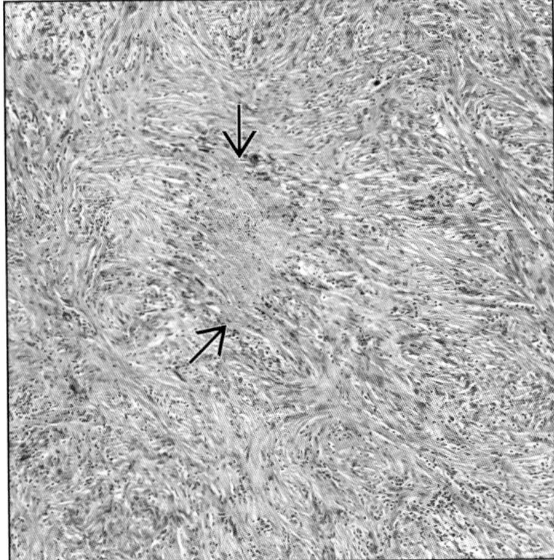

(Left) *Origin from a smooth-muscle-walled vessel ➲ is noted in this leiomyosarcoma. The tumor cells scroll off the wall of the vessel and blend into the surrounding thyroid parenchyma ➙.* ***(Right)*** *Tumor necrosis is usually present ➙ in a leiomyosarcoma. There is a disordered arrangement to the spindle cells, which show irregular short bundles that intersect at acute angles. This is a characteristic pattern for leiomyosarcoma of the thyroid gland.*

Microscopic and Immunohistochemical Features

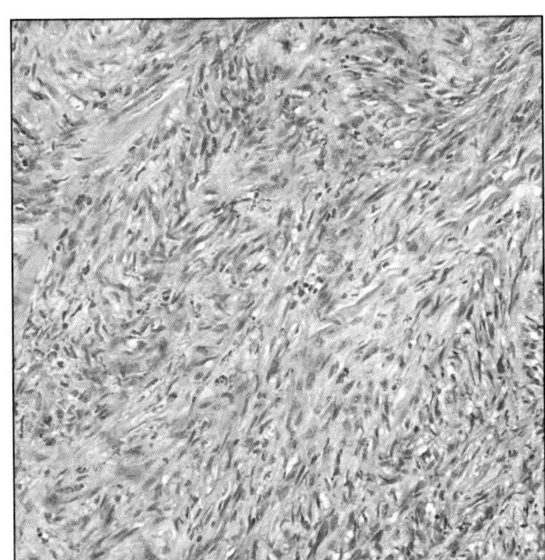

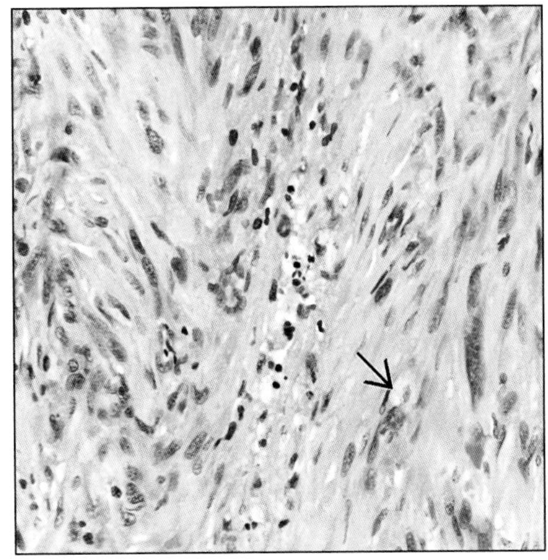

(Left) *There is a cellular spindled cell neoplastic proliferation arranged in interlacing bundles. The spindled cells show only limited pleomorphism in this intermediate-power field.* ***(Right)*** *The interlocking bundles show neoplastic spindle cells with moderate pleomorphism. The nuclei are centrally placed, hyperchromatic, and blunt-ended. A suggestion of a perinuclear cytoplasmic vacuole is seen* ⇒.

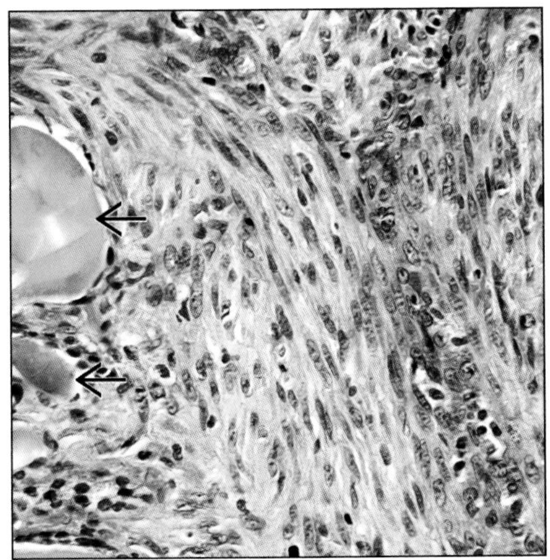

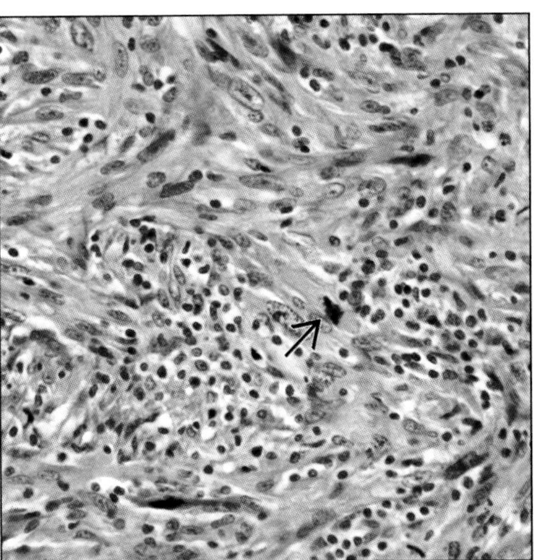

(Left) *The neoplastic spindle cell tumor shows blunt, cigar-shaped nuclei within the spindled cells. Entrapment of the thyroid follicular epithelium* ⇒ *is noted. The nuclear pleomorphism is mild to moderate in this field.* ***(Right)*** *This tumor demonstrates the interlacing fascicular architecture of spindled cells with moderate pleomorphism. Note the mitotic figure* ⇒*, along with areas of numerous inflammatory cells.*

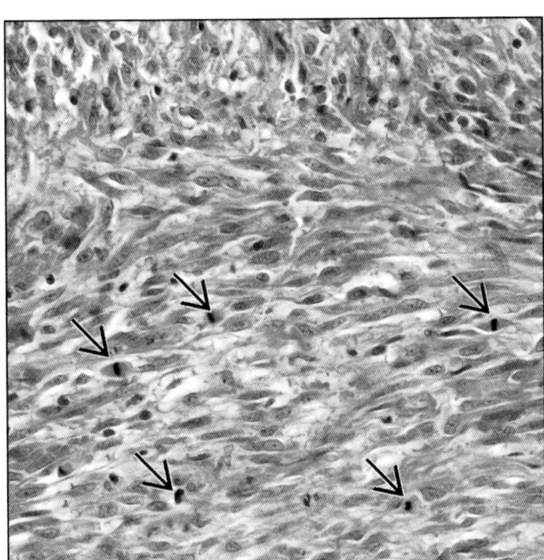

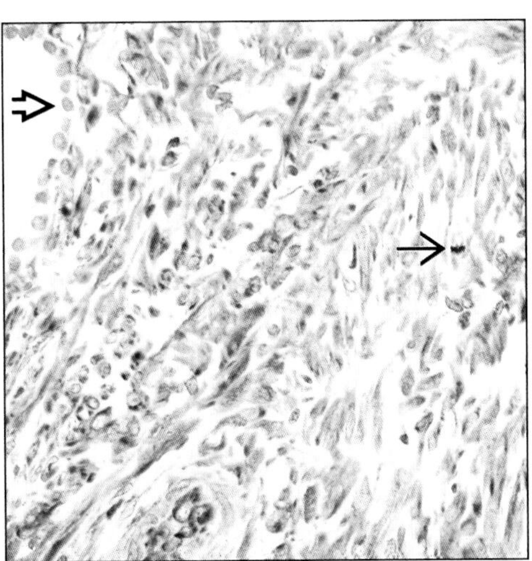

(Left) *The bundles of neoplastic cells clearly demonstrate a large number of mitotic figures* ⇒*, a feature that would not be seen in a benign neoplasm. Cytoplasmic perinuclear clearing is also present.* ***(Right)*** *The neoplastic cells are strongly and diffusely immunoreactive with desmin. The thyroid follicle is negative* ⇨*. Note the mitotic figure* ⇒*. Neoplastic cells are positive with a variety of markers, including vimentin, SMA, MSA, and CD117.*

MALIGNANT PERIPHERAL NERVE SHEATH TUMOR

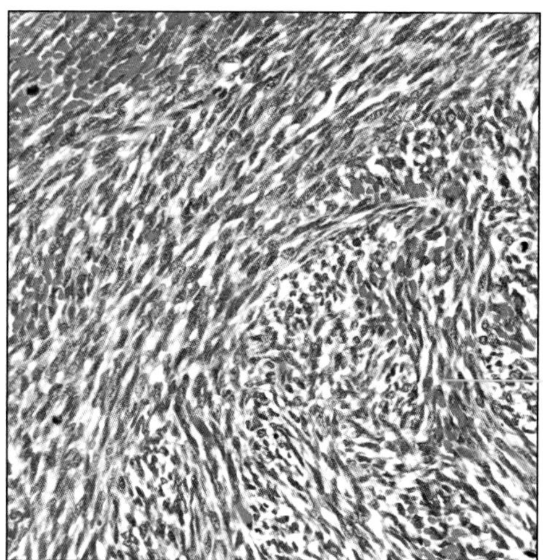

This is a highly cellular tumor, showing compact spindled cells arranged in interlacing fascicles. There is mild pleomorphism. There is no cytoplasmic vacuolization.

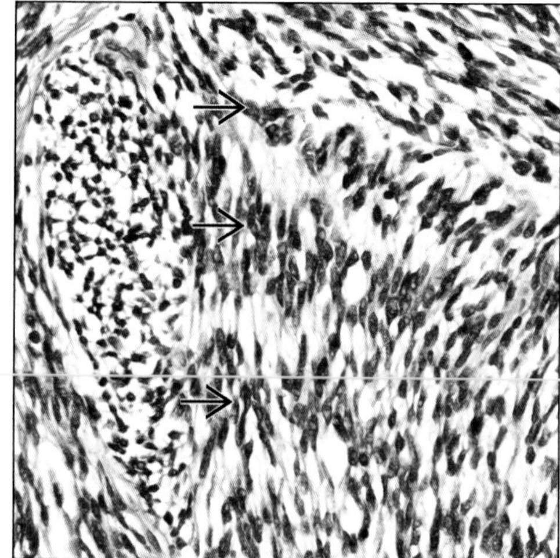

There is well-developed palisading ⇨ in this malignant peripheral nerve sheath tumor. The spindled cells show a Verocay body-type formation. There is limited pleomorphism in this field.

TERMINOLOGY

Abbreviations

- Malignant peripheral nerve sheath tumors (MPNST)
- Peripheral nerve sheath tumor (PNST)

Definitions

- Malignant neoplasm composed of cells with evidence of distinct peripheral nerve sheath differentiation histologically
  - Must arise within thyroid parenchyma or be contained within capsule of thyroid gland

ETIOLOGY/PATHOGENESIS

Histogenesis

- May arise from sympathetic and parasympathetic or possibly sensory nerves

CLINICAL ISSUES

Epidemiology

- Incidence
  - Very rare, representing < 0.02% of all thyroid gland tumors
  - Prevalence of PNSTs is higher among kindred with von Recklinghausen disease and neurofibromatosis, although not detected in thyroid gland disease
- Age
  - All ages affected, although usually older at initial presentation
    - Syndrome-associated tumors tend to develop in patients of younger age
- Gender
  - Equal gender distribution

Site

- Although not specific site, development from medium to large nerves at periphery of gland is common

Presentation

- Signs and symptoms are nonspecific
- Thyroid gland mass, usually increasing in size
- May have associated dyspnea, difficulty breathing, and weight loss

Treatment

- Surgical approaches
  - Excision
    - Usually lobectomy or thyroidectomy
- Radiation
  - Radiotherapy of limited palliative value

Prognosis

- Poor clinical outcome irrespective of clinical features, size, grade, or stage of tumor
- Staging is not applied, but local effects are more prognostically significant than other features
- All patients reported die from disease

IMAGE FINDINGS

Radiographic Findings

- CT images show inhomogeneous, low-density mass
  - Signal density is similar to that of surrounding soft tissue
  - May show
    - Compression of upper airway
    - Infiltration into soft tissues
    - Destruction of thyroid gland
    - Necrosis
- Scintigraphic scans demonstrate a cold nodule
- In general, lymphadenopathy is absent

MACROSCOPIC FEATURES

General Features

- Tumors are tan to white and glistening with "neural" appearance

MALIGNANT PERIPHERAL NERVE SHEATH TUMOR

Key Facts

Terminology
- Malignant neoplasm composed of cells with evidence of distinct peripheral nerve sheath differentiation histologically

Clinical Issues
- May develop from medium to large nerves at periphery of gland
- Poor clinical outcome irrespective of clinical features, size, grade, or stage of tumor

Macroscopic Features
- Tumors are tan to white and glistening with "neural" appearance
- Range: Up to 7 cm

Microscopic Pathology
- Arranged in tightly packed fascicles
- Woven into vague herringbone pattern
- High cellularity with fusiform to spindled cells
- Fibrillar cytoplasmic extensions
- Cellular pleomorphism and necrosis
- Increased mitotic figures, including atypical forms

Ancillary Tests
- Positive: S100 protein (may be focal), vimentin, p53
- Negative: Thyroglobulin, TTF-1, calcitonin, actin, desmin

Top Differential Diagnoses
- Undifferentiated carcinoma, medullary thyroid carcinoma, Reidel thyroiditis
- Primary or metastatic fibrosarcoma, leiomyosarcoma, rhabdomyosarcoma, malignant fibrous histiocytoma, angiosarcoma, melanoma

- Cut surface may focally appear cystic with yellow fluid
- Effacement of thyroid parenchyma and invasion beyond tumor capsule is common
- Tend to arise from medium to large nerves at thyroid gland periphery

Size
- Range: Up to 7 cm

MICROSCOPIC PATHOLOGY

Histologic Features
- Absence of direct extension from perithyroidal neoplasm
- Thyroid gland infiltration
  - Invasion
  - Entrapment
  - Destruction
- Origin from large nerves identified at thyroid gland periphery
- Vascular invasion can be seen
- Arranged in tightly packed fascicles that are woven into vague herringbone pattern
- High cellularity with fusiform cells
- Antoni B hypocellular areas can be seen
- Neoplastic cells are spindled
- Fibrillar cytoplasmic extensions arranged in loose background
- Cellular pleomorphism
- Increased mitotic figures
- Atypical mitoses
- Necrosis
- Hemorrhage

ANCILLARY TESTS

Cytology
- Soft tissue neck tumors may present as thyroid primary: Know anatomic site
- Cellular, highly atypical spindled to epithelioid tumor cells
- Elongated, slender, and wavy nuclei
- Fibrillary metachromatic stroma (on air-dried Romanowsky-stained slides) may be present
- Necrosis and mitoses may be seen
- No colloid or thyroid follicular epithelial cells
- S100 protein may confirm neural differentiation

Immunohistochemistry
- **Positive**
  - S100 protein (may be focal)
  - Vimentin
  - p53
- **Negative**
  - Thyroglobulin
  - TTF-1
  - Calcitonin
  - Actin
  - Desmin

Flow Cytometry
- Triploidy or tetraploidy associated with high-grade tumors

Cytogenetics
- Chromosome loss of 22q
- Monosomy 17
- Trisomy 7

Electron Microscopy
- Narrow to broad, entangled cell processes
- Processes covered by discrete basement membrane substance
- Fibrous long-spacing collagen, with its distinct periodicity
- Cytoplasmic intermediate filaments
- Primitive cellular junctions
- Collagen fibers are banded together and inserted into basal lamina

MALIGNANT PERIPHERAL NERVE SHEATH TUMOR

Immunohistochemistry

Antibody	Reactivity	Staining Pattern	Comment
S100	Positive	Nuclear & cytoplasmic	Tends to be focal and only a limited number of cells, although strong and diffuse reactions can be seen
Vimentin	Positive	Cytoplasmic	Nearly all tumor cells (but nonspecific reaction)
p53	Positive	Nuclear	Can be high
CK-PAN	Positive	Cytoplasmic	Only in rare and isolated tumor cells, in a limited number of cases
Thyroglobulin	Negative		
TTF-1	Negative		
Chromogranin-A	Negative		
Calcitonin	Negative		
Actin-sm	Negative		
Desmin	Negative		

DIFFERENTIAL DIAGNOSIS

Undifferentiated (Anaplastic) Carcinoma

- Spindle cell type specifically
- Based purely on treatment and prognosis considerations, separation from primary MPNST is not clinically significant
- Often associated with preexisting thyroid disease
- Often lacks all thyroid and epithelial markers but also lacks neural markers
  - MPNST must have definite evidence of specific Schwann cell derivation histologically, immunophenotypically, &/or ultrastructurally

Other Sarcomas

- Both primary and metastatic sarcomas must be excluded
- Malignant triton tumor (malignant schwannoma with rhabdomyoblastic differentiation) is vanishingly rare
- Fibrosarcoma, leiomyosarcoma, rhabdomyosarcoma, malignant fibrous histiocytoma, or angiosarcoma
  - Direct extension from soft tissue primary
  - Metastatic disease from distant primary
  - Primary thyroid gland tumor
- Each tumor usually has specific growth pattern and distinctive immunohistochemical features
- Metastatic spindle cell melanoma is also S100 protein positive
  - HMB-45, Melan-A, and tyrosinase reactions would help to separate from MPNST

Medullary Thyroid Carcinoma

- Spindle cell variant specifically
- Usually has plasmacytoid cells, spindled cells, "salt and pepper" nuclear chromatin pattern, and amyloid
- Positive: Calcitonin, chromogranin, CEA, TTF-1

Riedel Thyroiditis

- Spindled population is associated with inflammatory cells
- Associated with vasculitis and long-term clinical thyroid disorder
- Histologically, not associated with a "mass" per se
- Lacks neural markers

GRADING

Not Used

- While not used, features include
  - Nuclear anaplasia
  - Increased mitotic figures
  - Tumor necrosis
  - Vascular invasion

STAGING

Not Used

- Although not approved, staging as undifferentiated carcinoma may be meaningful in management

SELECTED REFERENCES

1. Kandil E et al: Primary peripheral nerve sheath tumors of the thyroid gland. Thyroid. 20(6):583-6, 2010
2. Yildirim G et al: Concurrent epithelioid malignant peripheral nerve sheath tumor and papillary thyroid carcinoma in the treated field of Hodgkin's disease. Head Neck. 30(5):675-9, 2008
3. Lucioni M et al: Paediatric laryngeal malignant nerve sheath tumour. Int J Pediatr Otorhinolaryngol. 71(12):1917-20, 2007
4. Papi G et al: Primary spindle cell lesions of the thyroid gland; an overview. Am J Clin Pathol. 125 Suppl:S95-123, 2006
5. Aron M et al: Neural tumours of the neck presenting as thyroid nodules: a report of three cases. Cytopathology. 16(4):206-9, 2005
6. Pallares J et al: Malignant peripheral nerve sheath tumor of the thyroid: a clinicopathological and ultrastructural study of one case. Endocr Pathol. 15(2):167-74, 2004
7. Thompson LD et al: Peripheral Nerve Sheath Tumors of the Thyroid Gland: A Series of Four Cases and a Review of the Literature. Endocr Pathol. 7(4):309-318, 1996

Microscopic and Immunohistochemical Features

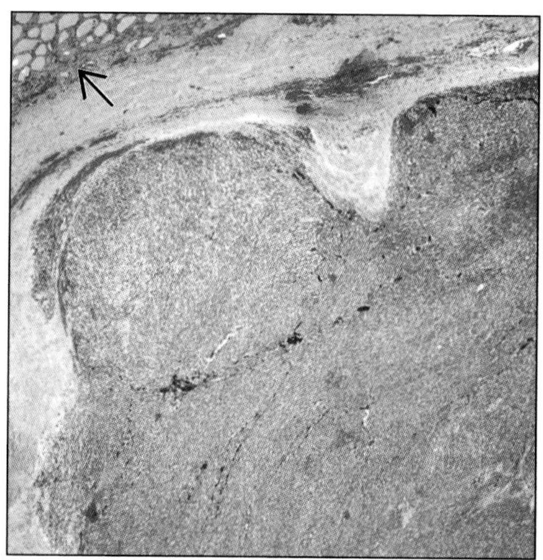

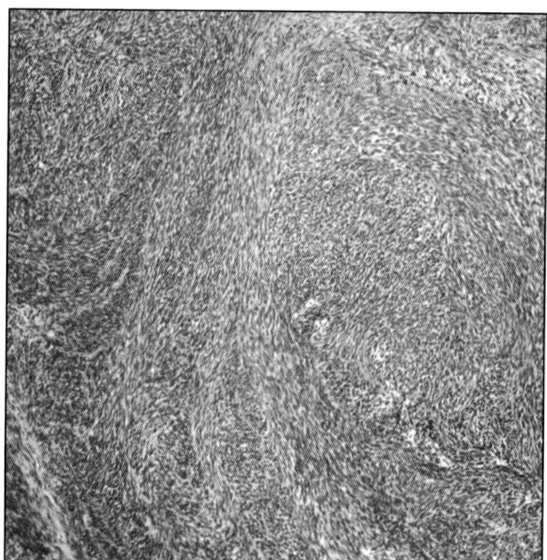

(Left) *The thyroid gland parenchyma ⇒ is separated from the tumor by a very thick and well-developed fibrous connective tissue capsule. The tumor is highly cellular, showing a pushing border. A vague fascicular arrangement is noted.* ***(Right)*** *This tumor is arranged in tightly packed fascicles that are woven into a vague herringbone pattern. There is high cellularity comprised of fusiform cells. A slightly more hypocellular area is noted.*

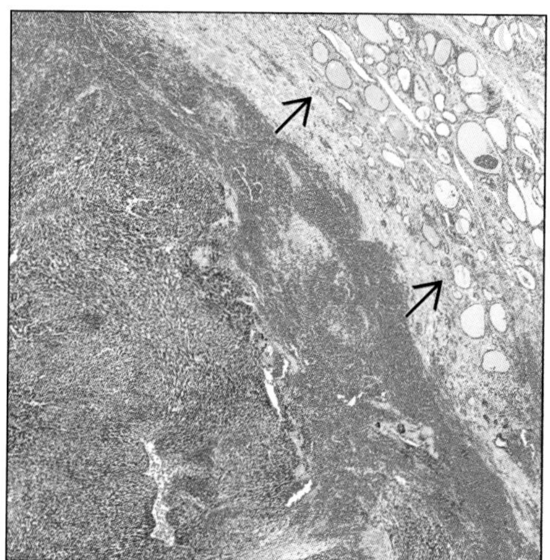

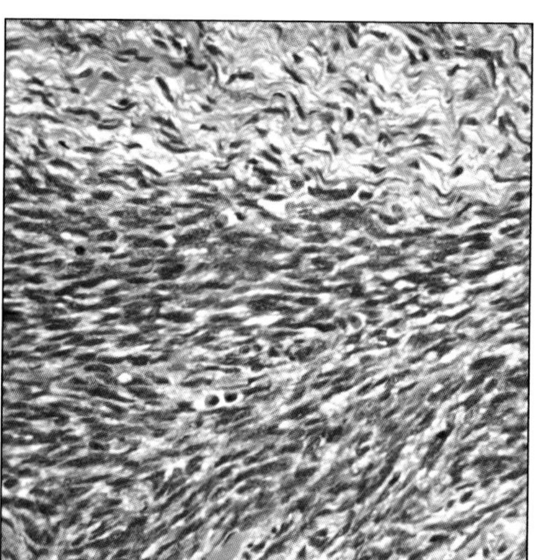

(Left) *The tumor abuts the thyroid gland parenchyma ⇒. Hemorrhage is noted at the leading edge of this tumor. The neoplasm is quite cellular, although a specific histology cannot be determined from this low power.* ***(Right)*** *The tumor cells are arranged in a tightly packed fascicle, composed of fusiform to spindled cells. At the periphery, the fibrillar cytoplasmic extensions arranged in a loose background are more easily identified. There is cytologic atypia, although it is not well developed.*

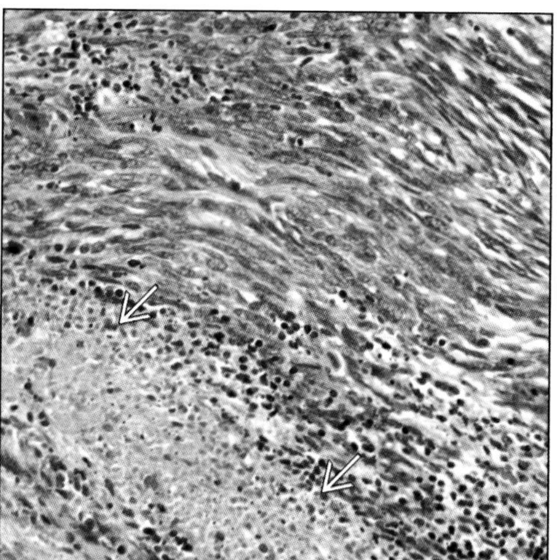

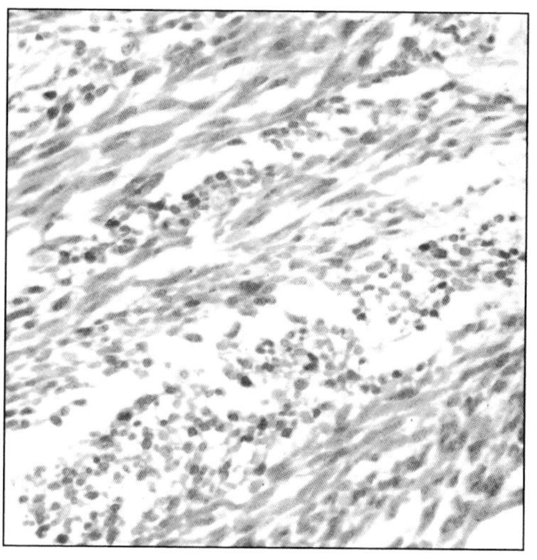

(Left) *This highly cellular tumor is arranged in tightly packed fascicles composed of spindled tumor cells. There is an almost syncytial quality to this tumor. Note the remarkable necrosis ➡ in this tumor. Mitotic figures are increased.* ***(Right)*** *It is unusual to have a malignant peripheral nerve sheath tumor show such strong and diffuse nuclear and cytoplasmic reactivity with S100 protein. However, this particular area was identified in a tumor that otherwise showed only focal immunoreactivity.*

FOLLICULAR DENDRITIC CELL TUMOR

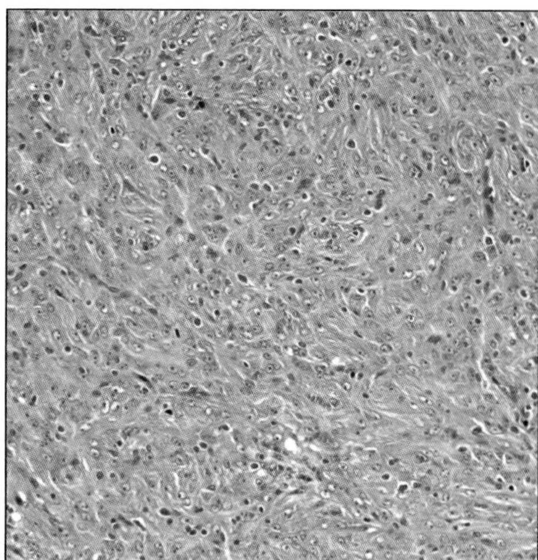

The tumor has a sheet-like pattern of growth, giving a diffuse appearance. The neoplastic cells are slightly spindled, with a vaguely syncytial architecture.

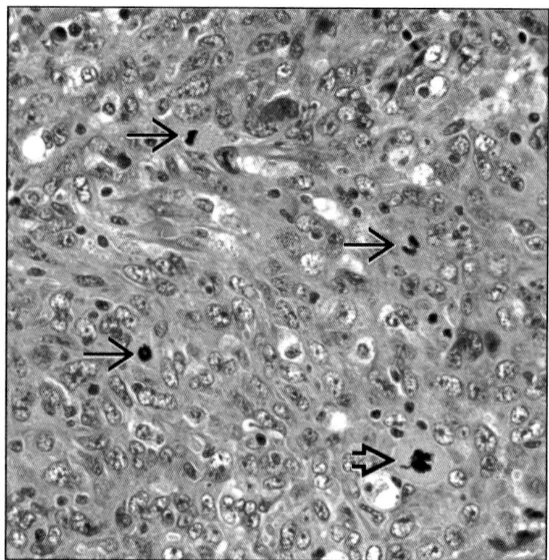

The syncytial arrangement of spindled to epithelioid cells shows ample eosinophilic cytoplasm surrounding vesicular nuclei. Note the numerous mitotic figures ⇒, including atypical forms ⇒.

TERMINOLOGY

Abbreviations

- Follicular dendritic cell (FDC) tumor

Synonyms

- Follicular dendritic cell sarcoma (FDCS)
- Reticulum cell sarcoma

Definitions

- Primary thyroid gland neoplasm composed of follicular dendritic cells

ETIOLOGY/PATHOGENESIS

Etiology

- Possible association with hyaline vascular-type Castleman disease

Histogenesis

- Follicular dendritic cells are antigen-presenting cells, identified in primary and secondary germinal centers
- Putative cell of origin for follicular dendritic cell tumor

CLINICAL ISSUES

Epidemiology

- Incidence
  - Very rare
- Age
  - Develops in older patients
- Gender
  - Equal gender distribution

Presentation

- Present with slowly growing painless mass
- Cervical lymph nodes may show alterations of hyaline vascular-type Castleman disease
  - Up to 20% of cases

Treatment

- Surgical approaches
  - Complete surgical excision
- Drugs
  - Chemotherapy has been employed
- Radiation
  - Provides some improved outcome

Prognosis

- Rarity makes predictions about prognosis difficult
- Recurrence and metastases frequent
- Cervical lymph node metastases may develop
- Secondary thyroid involvement may also be seen

MACROSCOPIC FEATURES

General Features

- Well circumscribed, solid, tan-gray
- In larger tumors, necrosis and hemorrhage may be seen

MICROSCOPIC PATHOLOGY

Histologic Features

- Tumors are unencapsulated
- Invades into and blends with thyroid gland parenchyma
- Lymphatic and blood vessel invasion is common
- Tumors are cellular
- Arranged in diffuse, fascicular, and whorled patterns
- Syncytial arrangement of spindled to epithelioid cells
  - Ample eosinophilic cytoplasm surrounds round to spindled nuclei
  - Nuclear chromatin is open (vesicular)
  - Small, well-defined nucleoli
- Mitoses are usually easily identified, sometimes increased

FOLLICULAR DENDRITIC CELL TUMOR

Key Facts

Terminology

- Primary thyroid gland neoplasm composed of follicular dendritic cells
- Follicular dendritic cells are antigen-presenting cells, identified in primary and secondary germinal centers

Clinical Issues

- Cervical lymph nodes may show alterations of hyaline vascular-type Castleman disease
- Rarity makes predictions about prognosis difficult

Microscopic Pathology

- Well circumscribed, solid, tan-gray
- Invades into and blends with thyroid gland parenchyma
- Lymphatic and blood vessel invasion is common
- Arranged in diffuse, fascicular, and whorled patterns
- Syncytial arrangement of spindled to epithelioid cells
- Ample eosinophilic cytoplasm surrounds round to spindled nuclei
- Nuclear chromatin is open (vesicular)
- Mitoses are usually easily identified, sometimes increased

Ancillary Tests

- Lesional cells strongly positive with
  - CD21, CD35, CD23, fascin, clusterin, and vimentin

Top Differential Diagnoses

- Undifferentiated (anaplastic) carcinoma, medullary carcinoma, SETTLE, CASTLE
- Leiomyosarcoma, malignant peripheral nerve sheath tumor

Immunohistochemistry

Antibody	Reactivity	Staining Pattern	Comment
CD21	Positive	Cytoplasmic	Nearly all tumor cells; weak-patchy staining of thyroid follicular epithelium may be seen as background staining
CD23	Positive	Cytoplasmic	Nearly all tumor cells; lymphoid germinal centers will be highlighted as internal control
CD35	Positive	Cytoplasmic	Most tumor cells
Fascin	Positive	Cytoplasmic	Most tumor cells
Clusterin	Positive	Cytoplasmic	Most tumor cells
Vimentin	Positive	Cytoplasmic	Nearly all tumor cells
CD68	Positive	Cytoplasmic	Variably present
EMA	Positive	Cytoplasmic	Variably present
S100	Positive	Nuclear & cytoplasmic	Variably present, but usually limited
CD45RB	Positive	Cytoplasmic	Only isolated cells
CD20	Positive	Cytoplasmic	Only isolated cells
EBV-LMP	Negative		
CK-PAN	Negative		
CK8/18/CAM5.2	Negative		

- Uncommonly, grape-like clusters of nuclei create giant cells, resembling Warthin-Finkeldey cells
- Lymphocytes are seen within tumor
  - Perivascular lymphoid cuffing may be seen
- Chronic lymphocytic thyroiditis often present

ANCILLARY TESTS

Immunohistochemistry

- Lesional cells strongly positive with CD21, CD35, CD23, fascin, clusterin, and vimentin

DIFFERENTIAL DIAGNOSIS

Spindled Tumors

- Generally, unique histologic and immunohistochemical profile allows for separation
- Requires high index of suspicion
- Undifferentiated carcinoma, medullary carcinoma, SETTLE, CASTLE, leiomyosarcoma, malignant peripheral nerve sheath tumors

SELECTED REFERENCES

1. Yu L et al: Primary Follicular Dendritic Cell Sarcoma of the Thyroid Gland Coexisting With Hashimoto's Thyroiditis. Int J Surg Pathol. Epub ahead of print, 2009
2. Papi G et al: Primary spindle cell lesions of the thyroid gland; an overview. Am J Clin Pathol. 125 Suppl:S95-123, 2006
3. Moz U et al: Follicular dendritic cell tumour of the cervical lymph node: case report and brief review of literature. Acta Otorhinolaryngol Ital. 24(4):223-5, 2004
4. Biddle DA et al: Extranodal follicular dendritic cell sarcoma of the head and neck region: three new cases, with a review of the literature. Mod Pathol. 15(1):50-8, 2002
5. Vargas H et al: Follicular dendritic cell tumor: an aggressive head and neck tumor. Am J Otolaryngol. 23(2):93-8, 2002
6. Galati LT et al: Dendritic cell sarcoma of the thyroid. Head Neck. 21(3):273-5, 1999

FOLLICULAR DENDRITIC CELL TUMOR

Microscopic Features

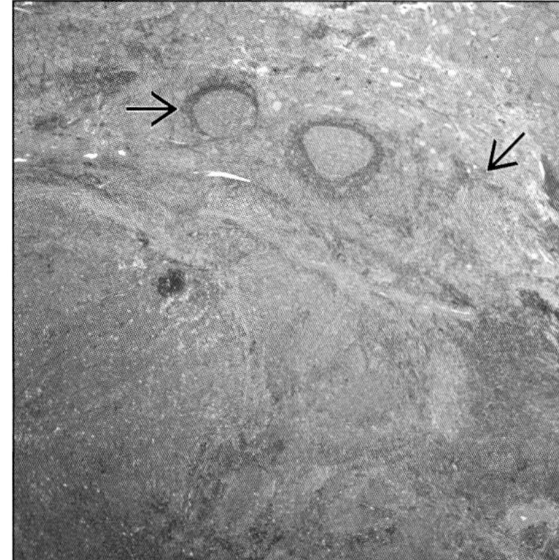

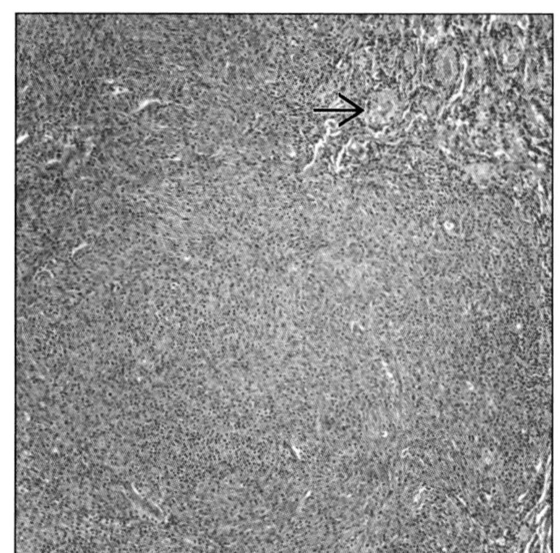

(Left) *In this focus, the chronic lymphocytic thyroiditis is quite prominent at the leading edge of the tumor ⇒. The neoplasm is unencapsulated, arranged in a lobular to sheet-like distribution.* **(Right)** *Thyroid follicles ⇒ are entrapped by the neoplastic proliferation. The tumor is arranged in a diffuse sheet, lacking any specific architecture.*

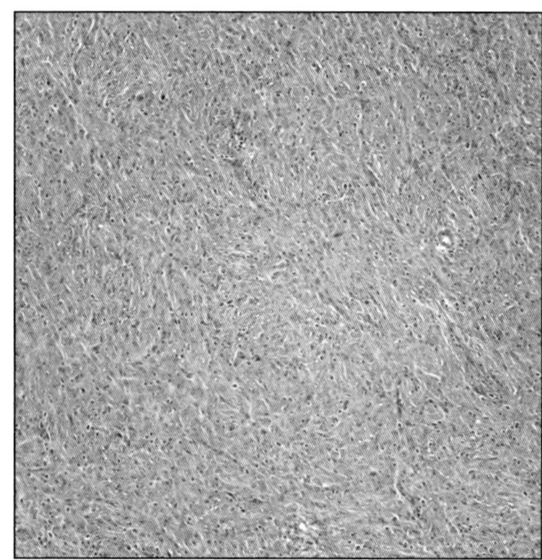

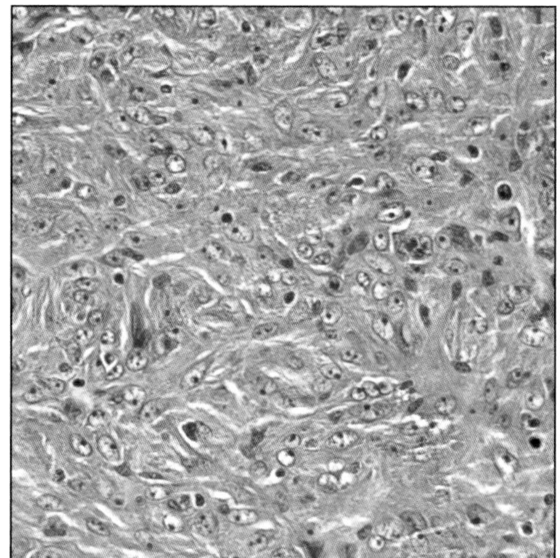

(Left) *The tumors are cellular, showing a whorled pattern. The tumor cells are spindled to epithelioid. There is some connective tissue, but it is not well developed.* **(Right)** *The tumor cells form short fascicles to whorls. This syncytium shows abundant eosinophilic cytoplasm surrounding oval nuclei. The nuclear chromatin is vesicular and open, with small but well-defined nucleoli.*

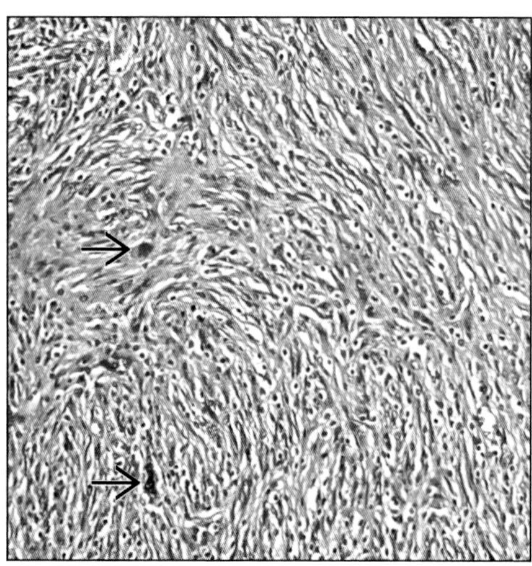

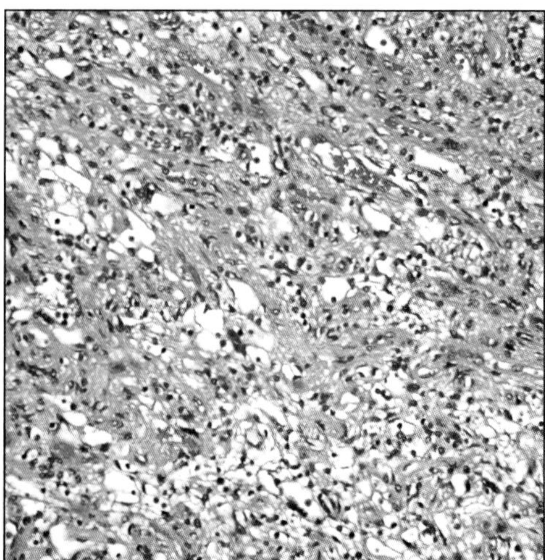

(Left) *A storiform-type architecture can sometimes be seen, with the neoplastic cells separated by delicate collagen. There are numerous lymphocytes sprinkled throughout the tumor. There are isolated "tumor giant cells" ⇒ in this lesion.* **(Right)** *At the edge of some tumors, areas of degeneration are noted, creating clear cytoplasm. Inflammatory cells are noted throughout. This high-power field shows prominent vascularity.*

Microscopic and Immunohistochemical Features

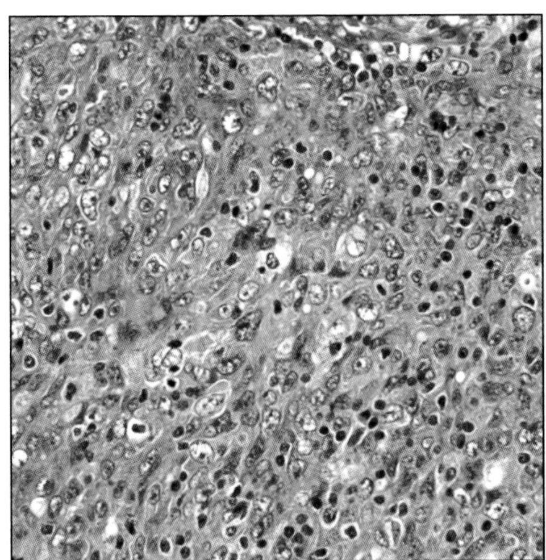

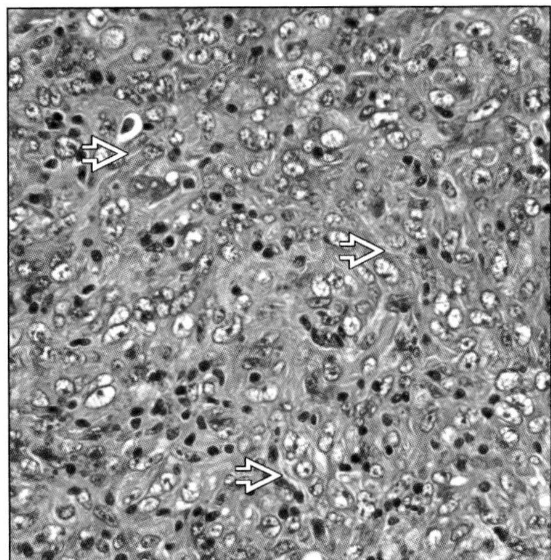

(Left) *The sheet-like growth of epithelioid cells intimately associated with lymphocytes gives an appearance similar to metastatic lymphoepithelial carcinoma. Note the prominent nucleoli within vesicular nuclei.* ***(Right)*** *There is a suggestion of epithelioid growth in this tumor. Note the "cell borders" ➡ that hint at squamoid differentiation. The nuclei, however, are vesicular with prominent nucleoli. There are inflammatory elements throughout.*

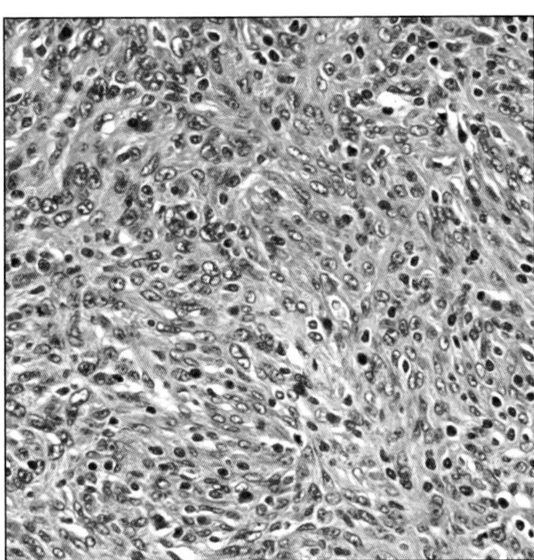

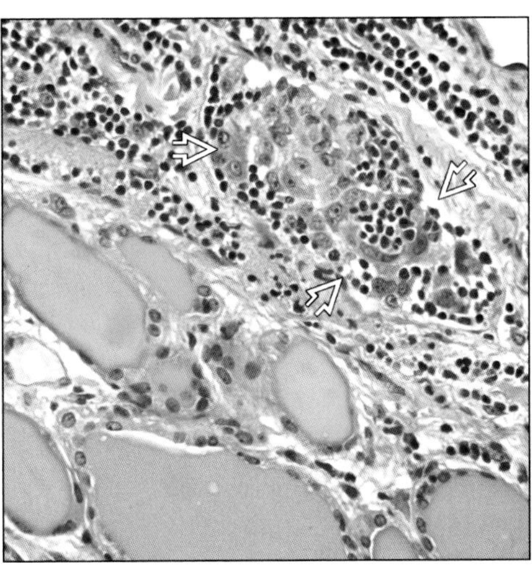

(Left) *The high cellularity, with poorly differentiated tumor cells and inflammatory elements, may mimic undifferentiated carcinoma. It is in cases like this that immunohistochemistry becomes useful.* ***(Right)*** *The thyroid gland follicles are unremarkable, although associated with a chronic inflammatory infiltrate. Note the tumor thrombus filling a vascular space ➡. It is very common to see lymphatic or vascular space invasion in FDC tumors.*

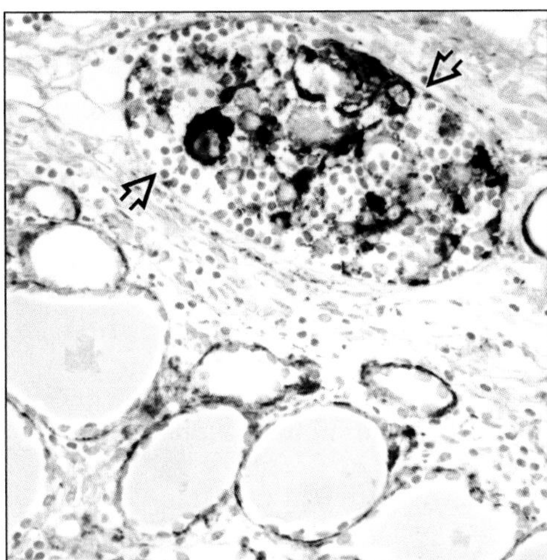

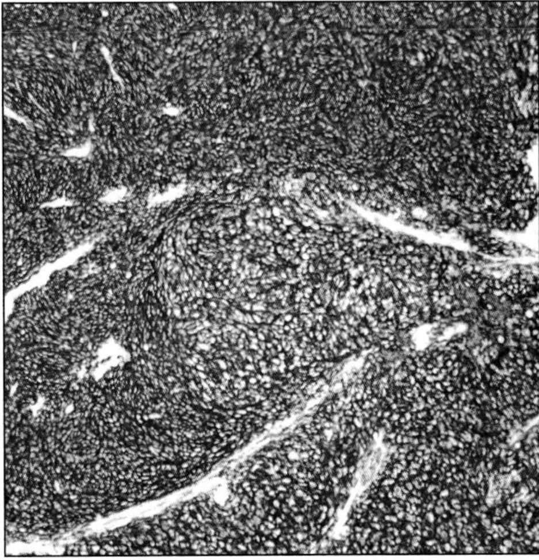

(Left) *The neoplastic cells within the vascular space are strongly and diffusely highlighted with CD21 ➡. Note the background staining of the thyroid follicles.* ***(Right)*** *There is a diffuse, sheet-like, strong membrane immunoreactivity with CD23. A similar reactivity can be seen with CD35 in FDC tumors. Similar reactivity can be found in the germinal centers of lymphocytic thyroiditis, although highlighting only the follicular dendritic cells.*

METASTATIC/SECONDARY TUMORS

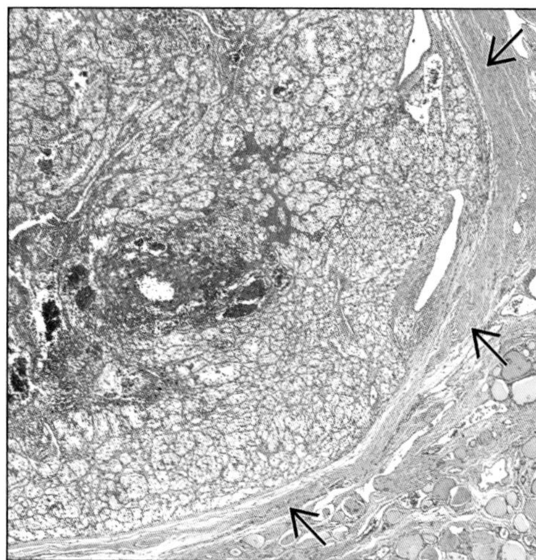

Metastatic renal cell carcinoma frequently presents as a solitary nodule or mass. There is a well-defined capsule ➔. The tumor is composed of clear cells with extravasated erythrocytes.

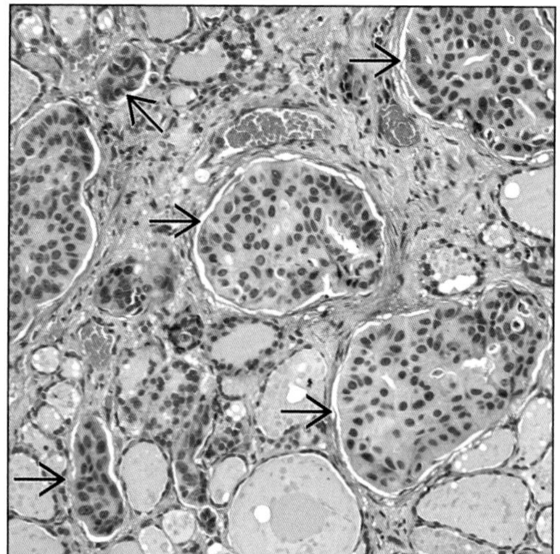

Metastatic breast carcinoma is most frequently identified within lymphatics ➔. The cells can be quite variable, showing glandular profiles. H&E alone may not allow separation from other adenocarcinomas.

TERMINOLOGY

Definitions

- Tumors secondarily involving the thyroid gland as a result of hematogenous/lymphatic spread from primary malignancies of distant sites
  - Direct extension from contiguous structures (larynx, trachea, pharynx, esophagus, lymph nodes, neck soft tissues, mediastinum) is excluded
- Lymphomas and leukemias are excluded

ETIOLOGY/PATHOGENESIS

Pathogenesis

- Thyroid gland is richly vascularized, predisposing to relatively high frequency of metastases
- Abnormal thyroid tissue (adenomatoid nodules, thyroiditis, neoplasms) contains metastases more frequently than normal tissue
  - Alterations in vascularity or blood flow may contribute to development of metastatic disease

CLINICAL ISSUES

Epidemiology

- Incidence
  - Depends on underlying frequency of primary tumor
  - Seen in up to 7.5% of surgically removed thyroid glands
  - Potential increased incidence related to
    - Advances in radiographic techniques
    - Improved treatments, resulting in prolonged survival
    - Increased frequency of fine needle aspiration (FNA) for thyroid gland nodules
  - Up to 25% in autopsied patients with disseminated malignancies
- Age
  - All ages affected
  - Mean: 62 years
- Gender
  - Female > Male (1.2:1)
    - Increased metastases of breast and gynecologic primaries compared to prostate primaries

Site

- Any region of thyroid can be affected
- Majority present with unilateral involvement (80%)
- Predilection for larger vessels at thyroid periphery
- Posterior region (if direct extension is considered)

Presentation

- Underlying thyroid disease results in clinical presentation in most patients
- Patients present with thyroid gland mass
  - Occasionally, rapidly enlarging thyroid mass
- Hoarseness, dysphagia, dysphonia, neck pain, hemoptysis uncommonly identified
- Hyperthyroidism due to thyroid parenchymal destruction and hormone release
- Thyroid gland metastases are initial manifestation of occult primary in up to 40% of patients
  - Most frequently noted in kidney primaries
- Development of metastasis to thyroid has taken up to 22 years
  - Approximately 80% of metastases develop within 3 years of primary tumor resection (majority in < 9 months)
  - Renal cell carcinoma tends to have long latency period
- Primary site depends on age and gender
  - Carcinomas are most common: Kidney and lung most common
  - All anatomic sites are potential candidates

Treatment

- Options, risks, complications
  - Postoperative hypothyroidism, recurrent laryngeal nerve damage, hypoparathyroidism

METASTATIC/SECONDARY TUMORS

Key Facts

Terminology
- Tumors secondarily involving the thyroid gland as a result of hematogenous/lymphatic spread from primary malignancies of distant sites

Clinical Issues
- Thyroid is richly vascularized, predisposing to relatively high frequency of metastases
- Thyroid metastases are initial manifestation of occult primary in up to 40%
- Underlying thyroid disease results in clinical presentation in most patients
- Usually multifocal and bilateral
  - Surgical series, unilateral solitary mass

Microscopic Pathology
- Usually resemble primary tumor although dedifferentiation can occur
- Presents as small deposits within lymph-vascular spaces or as solitary mass
- Interlobar fibrous septations widened, with tumor filling lymphatic channels
  - Predilection for larger vessels at thyroid periphery
- Carcinomas are most common (approximately 80%)
- Distinctly different architecture and histology from primary thyroid neoplasms

Ancillary Tests
- Smears are cellular, with 2 distinct populations
- Metastases have unique immunohistochemical profiles (thyroglobulin negative)

- Surgical approaches
  - Specific procedure dictated by primary thyroid disease (in most cases)
  - Surgery advocated if tumor is slow growing or it is an isolated metastasis

Prognosis
- Usually poor clinically outcome, determined by primary type, although exceptions occur
- Prognosis is determined by underlying primary
  - Metastasis to thyroid gland correlates with poor prognosis
  - If metastatic disease is limited to thyroid, surgery can result in prolonged survival
    - Specifically for renal cell carcinoma

IMAGE FINDINGS

Radiographic Findings
- Ultrasound shows unilateral or bilateral, multiple, ill-defined, infiltrating, hypoechoic nodules with heterogeneous texture
  - Bilateral, multiple nodules without microcalcifications suggest metastatic disease, especially in patients with known primary tumor
- May be useful in directing biopsy or FNA

MACROSCOPIC FEATURES

General Features
- Usually multifocal and bilateral
  - However, in surgical series, unilateral solitary mass is more likely
  - Renal cell carcinoma is most common tumor to present with unilateral, solitary mass
- Can metastasize to preexisting thyroid lesions

Size
- Wide range, from microscopic up to 15 cm
  - Up to 50% are macroscopic lesions

MICROSCOPIC PATHOLOGY

Histologic Features
- Usually resemble primary tumor although dedifferentiation can occur
- Fibrous septations within gland are frequently widened, with tumor filling lymphatic channels
- Carcinomas are most common (approximately 80%)
  - Leiomyosarcoma and skin melanoma are most common noncarcinomas
- Separated into 2 forms
  - Small deposits within lymph-vascular spaces
    - Peripheral lymph-vascular channels show tumor most frequently
  - Solitary mass
- Distinctly different architecture and histology from primary thyroid neoplasms
  - Primary lung adenocarcinomas
    - Glands, large cells, high N:C ratio, coarse chromatin, prominent nucleoli
  - Metastatic clear cell renal cell carcinoma
    - Polygonal cells with clear cytoplasm, distinct cell membranes, small nuclei
    - Rich vascular network, pseudoalveolar pattern, extravasated erythrocytes filling spaces
  - Metastatic neuroendocrine carcinomas mainly in fibrous septa
- Sarcomas can be primary or metastatic
  - Leiomyosarcoma, angiosarcoma, malignant peripheral nerve sheath tumors
  - Clinical, radiographic, histologic, and immunohistochemical features used in aggregate
- Metastases to thyroid primary tumors are uncommon

ANCILLARY TESTS

Cytology
- FNA or core needle biopsy is initial study of choice
  - FNA confirms malignancy but is frequently misinterpreted as to type

METASTATIC/SECONDARY TUMORS

Primary Sites Metastatic to Thyroid Gland

Primary Site	Approximate Frequency
Kidney (renal cell carcinoma)	25%
Lung (squamous cell, adenocarcinoma, neuroendocrine)	25%
Breast	12%
Esophagus (squamous cell, adenocarcinoma)	4%
Stomach	4%
Skin (melanoma usually)	4%
Uterus (leiomyosarcoma, cervix squamous cell carcinoma)	3%
Colon	3%
Miscellaneous	20%

Based on review of approximately 314 cases reported in the medical literature.

- Smears are cellular, often showing 2 distinct cell populations
  - One is uninvolved thyroid gland parenchyma
  - Other is metastatic neoplastic population
- Renal cell carcinoma has a bloody background, lacks colloid, and shows stripped nuclei or rare cells with clear cytoplasm
- Adenocarcinoma: Gland formation, well-developed cell borders, and coarse, heavy nuclear chromatin with prominent nucleoli
  - Necrosis and mitotic figures are frequently noted
- Metastatic poorly differentiated carcinoma can mimic primary undifferentiated thyroid carcinoma
- Clinical and radiographic findings, cytology, and immunohistochemistry combined to yield diagnosis

Immunohistochemistry

- Metastatic tumors have unique immunohistochemical profiles, distinctly different from thyroid primaries
- Exceptions include
  - Lung adenocarcinoma: TTF-1, CEA-M, CK7 positive; thyroglobulin negative
  - Small cell carcinoma: Chromogranin, synaptophysin, TTF-1 positive; calcitonin and CEA-M negative
- Thyroglobulin may diffuse into adjacent tissue or be "entrapped" within metastatic deposits

Cytogenetics

- Can be helpful (*RET/PTC*, *PAX8/PPARγ*), although there are overlapping results with other mutations
- *BRAF*
  - Identified in papillary thyroid carcinoma, melanoma, colorectal carcinoma, ovarian carcinoma, and even lung adenocarcinomas
- *KRAS*
  - Codon 12/13 mutations much more likely in lung, colon, and other sites than thyroid primaries

DIFFERENTIAL DIAGNOSIS

Follicular Adenoma/Carcinoma

- Specifically, clear cell adenoma and carcinoma
- Single, unilateral mass with well-defined capsule
- Colloid usually identified
- Lacks prominent vascularity and extravasated erythrocytes
- Positive with TTF-1, thyroglobulin, and pax-8

Metastatic Tumors to Primary Neoplasms

- Both tumors are concurrently present
- Usually interspersed, although occasionally as single tumor deposits

Direct Extension

- Direct extension from adjacent organs usually radiographically and clinically distinctive
- Squamous cell carcinoma is rare as primary thyroid gland tumor, so direct extension must be excluded

Medullary Carcinoma

- Solitary, solid mass, often with background of C-cell hyperplasia
- Lacks prominent interstitial disease
- Strongly positive with calcitonin, CEA-M, chromogranin, synaptophysin, and TTF-1

SELECTED REFERENCES

1. Nabili V et al: Collision tumor of thyroid: metastatic lung adenocarcinoma plus papillary thyroid carcinoma. Am J Otolaryngol. 28(3):218-20, 2007
2. Papi G et al: Metastases to the thyroid gland: prevalence, clinicopathological aspects and prognosis: a 10-year experience. Clin Endocrinol (Oxf). 66(4):565-71, 2007
3. Kim TY et al: Metastasis to the thyroid diagnosed by fine-needle aspiration biopsy. Clin Endocrinol (Oxf). 62(2):236-41, 2005
4. Wood K et al: Metastases to the thyroid gland: the Royal Marsden experience. Eur J Surg Oncol. 30(6):583-8, 2004
5. Heffess CS et al: Metastatic renal cell carcinoma to the thyroid gland: a clinicopathologic study of 36 cases. Cancer. 95(9):1869-78, 2002
6. Chen H et al: Clinically significant, isolated metastatic disease to the thyroid gland. World J Surg. 23(2):177-80; discussion 181, 1999
7. Nakhjavani M et al: Direct extension of malignant lesions to the thyroid gland from adjacent organs: report of 17 cases. Endocr Pract. 5(2):69-71, 1999
8. Lam KY et al: Metastatic tumors of the thyroid gland: a study of 79 cases in Chinese patients. Arch Pathol Lab Med. 122(1):37-41, 1998
9. Nakhjavani MK et al: Metastasis to the thyroid gland. A report of 43 cases. Cancer. 79(3):574-8, 1997

Radiographic, Gross, and Microscopic Features

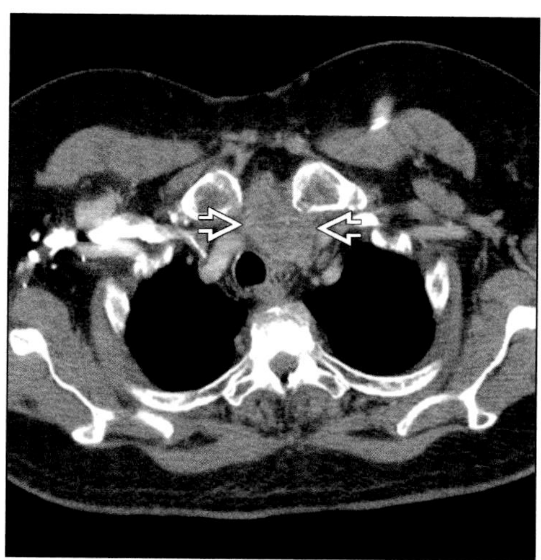

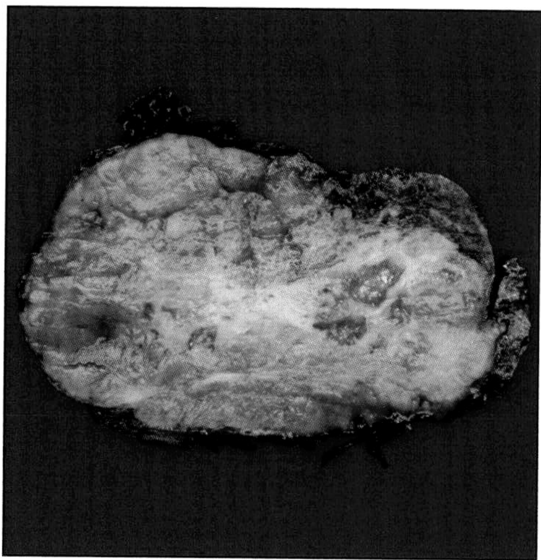

(Left) *The radiographic findings are often difficult to interpret. In this case, there is enlargement of the thyroid gland, with a mass identified within a mediastinal extension of the enlarged gland ⇨. This was an example of metastatic urothelial carcinoma to thyroid.* ***(Right)*** *The thyroid lobe has a fleshy appearance, with multiple nodules and areas of degeneration. No well-defined masses are identified. The histology showed a metastatic lung adenocarcinoma.*

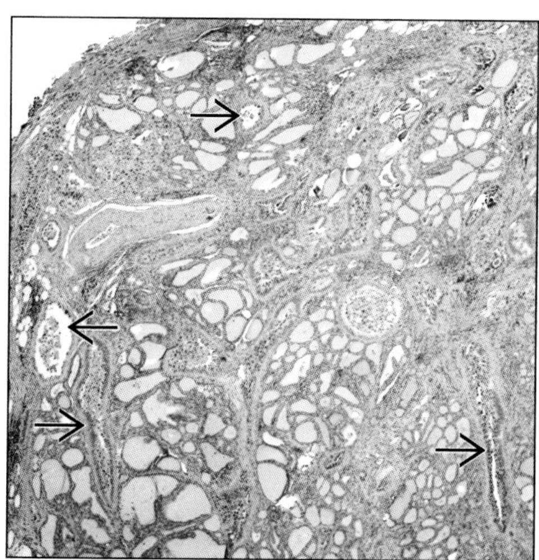

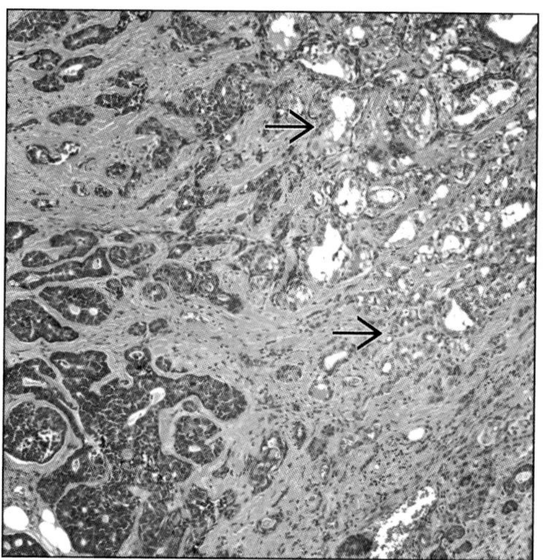

(Left) *The thyroid shows a background of adenomatoid nodules and focal chronic lymphocytic thyroiditis. There are numerous lymphatics filled with tumor emboli → from a lung adenocarcinoma.* ***(Right)*** *Tumor-to-tumor metastases are not uncommon. This is an example of a metastatic adenoid cystic carcinoma (parotid gland) to a thyroid papillary carcinoma →. Papillary carcinoma is the most common primary thyroid tumor type affected by metastases. Note the blending.*

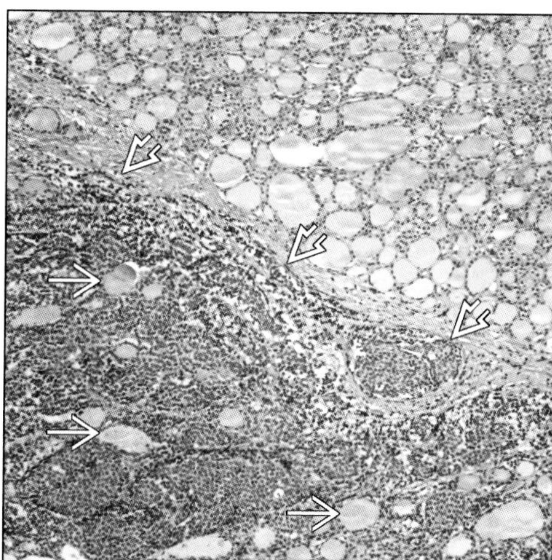

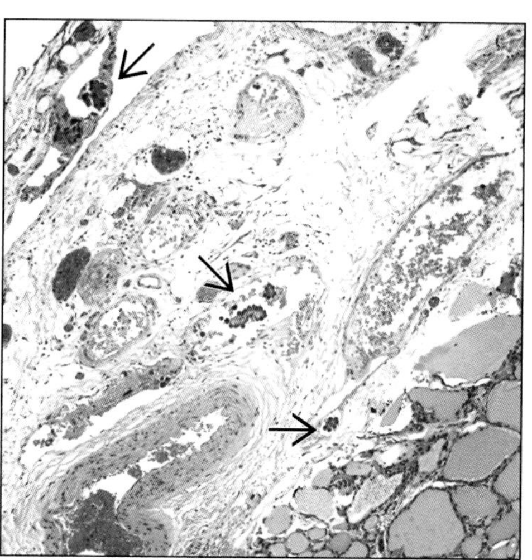

(Left) *There is a mass ⇨ appearance to this metastatic breast ductal carcinoma. Note the entrapped thyroid epithelium ⇨, an important consideration when interpreting follow-up immunohistochemistry.* ***(Right)*** *Multiple small lymphatic channels at the thyroid gland periphery contain small foci of metastatic lung adenocarcinoma →. These foci have a "papillary" configuration, but this is an artifact of their intravascular location.*

METASTATIC/SECONDARY TUMORS

Microscopic Features

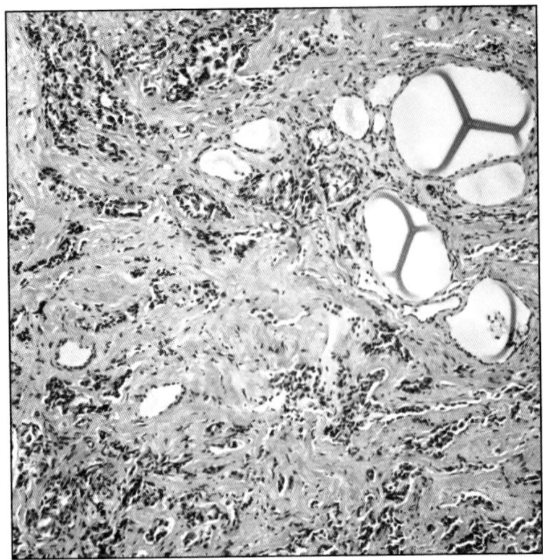

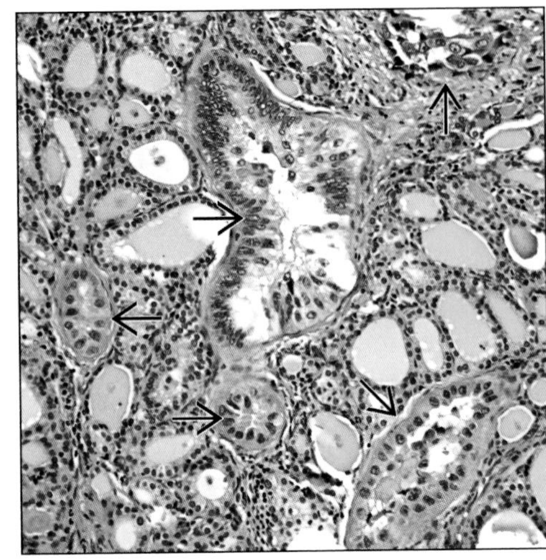

(Left) *The fibrous septa of the thyroid gland are widened, with the tumor cells filling the lymphatic spaces. This creates a sclerotic appearance to this metastatic lung adenocarcinoma. This may mimic a primary papillary carcinoma.* ***(Right)*** *Metastatic adenocarcinoma is confined to the lymphatic spaces ➔, but the widened lymphatic spaces separate between the residual thyroid follicles. At low power, this often creates a "cellular" appearance to the thyroid gland.*

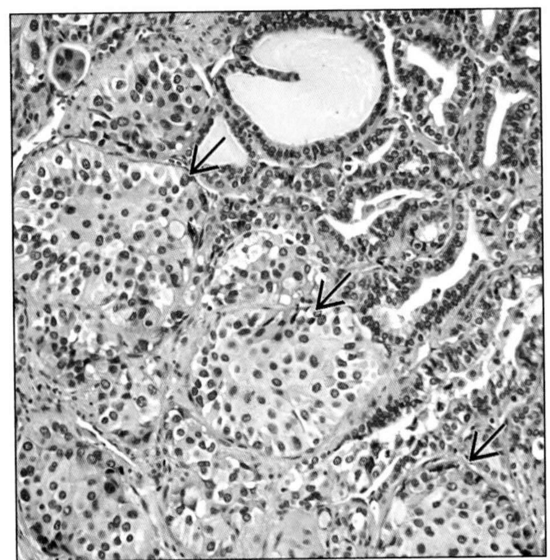

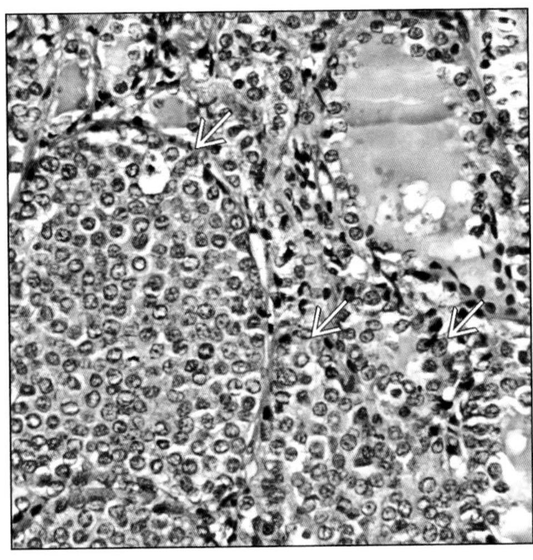

(Left) *This metastatic urothelial carcinoma has an opacified cytoplasm, with a well-developed pavemented appearance ➔. This tumor has metastasized to a thyroid papillary carcinoma. There is intimate blending between the tumors.* ***(Right)*** *There is blending between the metastatic breast carcinoma cells ➔ and the background thyroid gland parenchyma. In cases like this, the separation between a primary vs. metastatic tumor can be quite challenging, though frequently made easier by immunohistochemistry.*

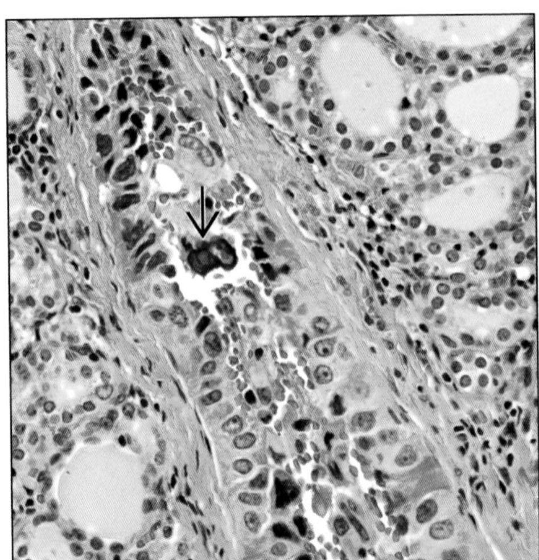

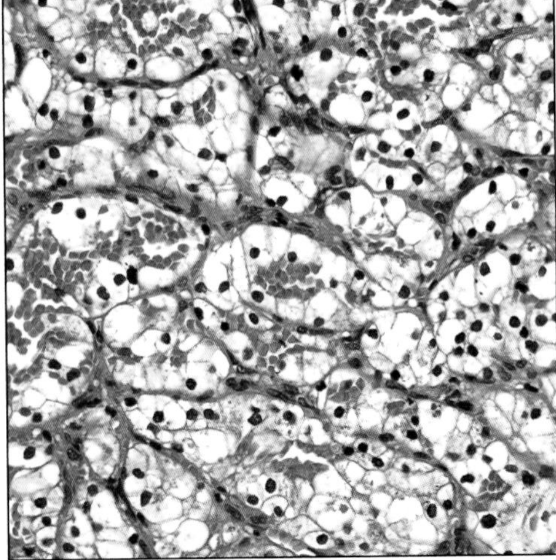

(Left) *The interlobar septum is widened, with metastatic lung adenocarcinoma filling the lymphatic channel. Note the calcification ➔ as well as tall cell appearance of these neoplastic cells, a mimic of thyroid papillary carcinoma.* ***(Right)*** *A rich vascular network divides this metastatic clear cell renal cell carcinoma into a pseudoalveolar pattern with extravasated erythrocytes filling the spaces. There are very distinct cell membranes and small nuclei.*

Ancillary Techniques

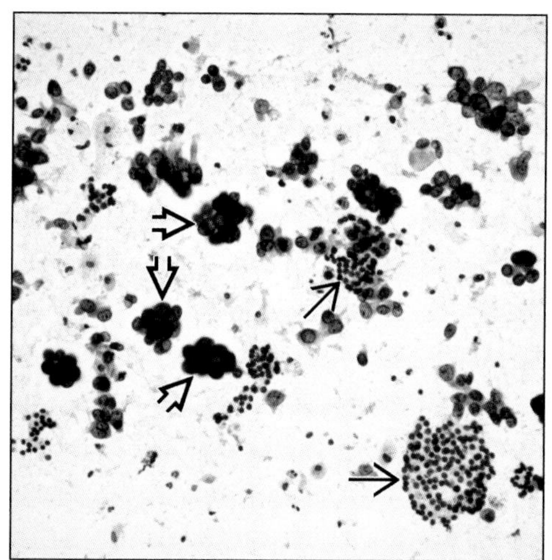

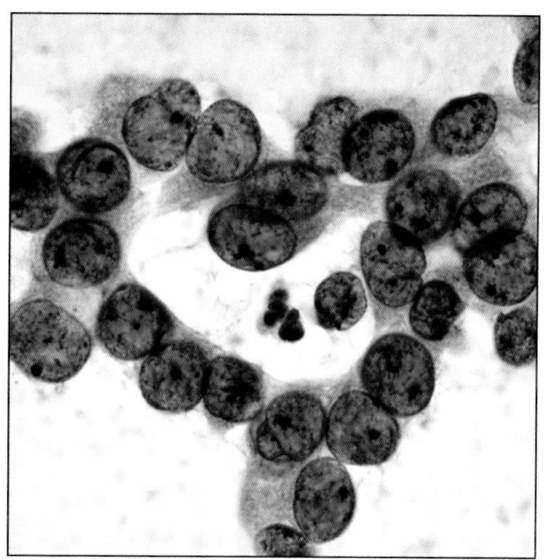

(Left) *A cellular smear shows 2 distinct cell populations. The uninvolved thyroid epithelium ⇨ is interspersed between metastatic adenocarcinoma ⇨ from the lung. While there is a papillary appearance, there are also glands and coarse nuclear chromatin.* ***(Right)*** *A high power shows "gland" formation. The chromatin is quite delicate with small nucleoli. It is easy to see how this could be a mimic of thyroid papillary carcinoma.*

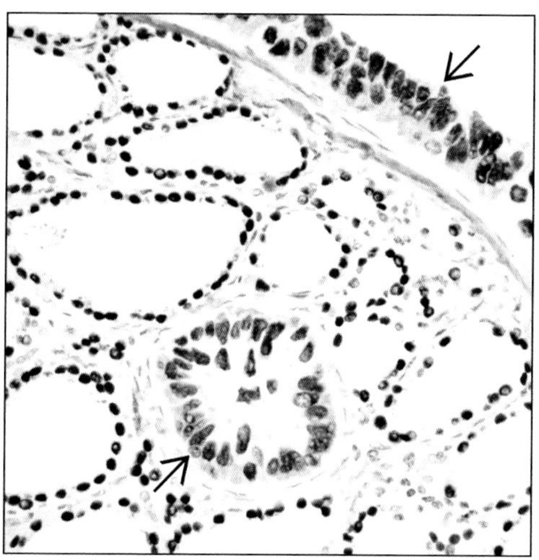

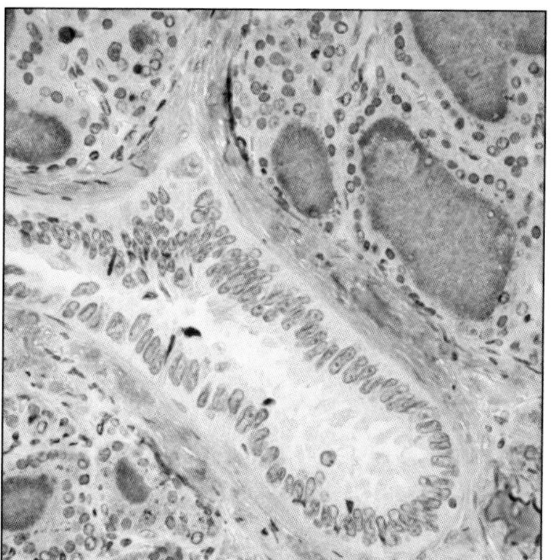

(Left) *An example of the different staining appearance with TTF-1 highlights the metastatic lung adenocarcinoma ⇨ with a different intensity than the uninvolved thyroid parenchyma. However, this marker must be interpreted with caution.* ***(Right)*** *Thyroglobulin highlights the native thyroid follicles but does not stain the metastatic lung adenocarcinoma within the lymphatic channel. Negative staining for thyroglobulin can be quite helpful in separating primary from metastatic tumors.*

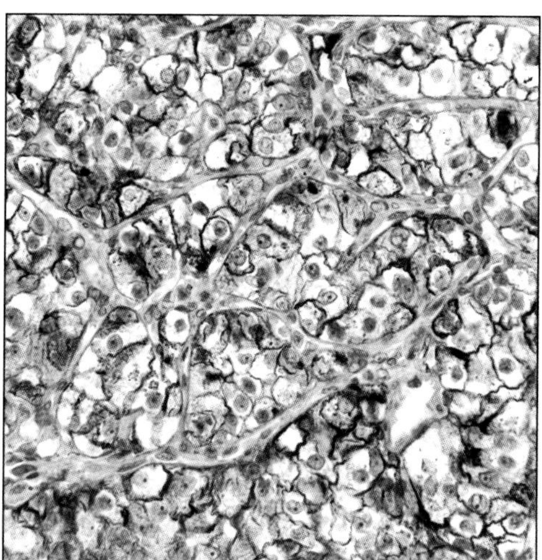

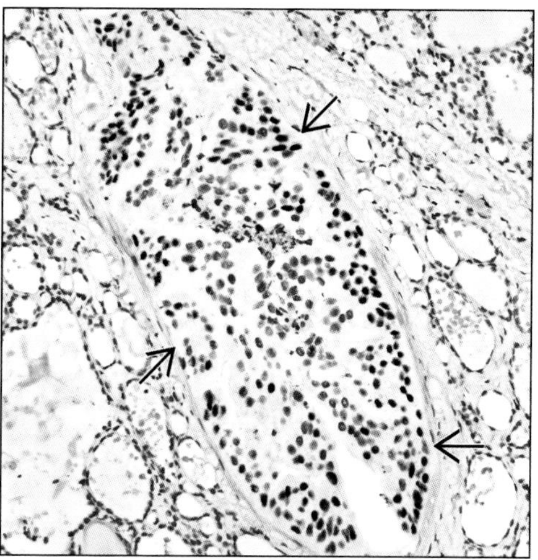

(Left) *Metastatic renal cell carcinoma is strongly and diffusely immunoreactive with RCC, highlighting the membranous reactivity. This stain is not unique to renal cell carcinoma but is usually nonreactive in primary thyroid gland lesions.* ***(Right)*** *Estrogen receptor highlights a tumor embolism within a lymphatic space ⇨. Note the negative thyroid parenchyma surrounding the lymphatic space. Differential immunoreactivity for selected antibodies is very useful in this setting.*

PROTOCOL FOR THE EXAMINATION OF THYROID GLAND SPECIMENS

Examination of Thyroid Gland Carcinoma Specimens

Resection

Procedure

___ Thyroid lobectomy
 ___ Right
 ___ Left
___ Partial thyroidectomy (anything less than a lobectomy)
 ___ Right
 ___ Left
___ Total thyroidectomy
___ Total thyroidectomy with central compartment dissection
___ Total thyroidectomy with right neck dissection
___ Total thyroidectomy with left neck dissection
___ Total thyroidectomy with bilateral neck dissection
___ Other (specify): ______________________
___ Not specified

*Received

*___ Fresh
*___ In formalin
*___ Other

Specimen Integrity

___ Intact
___ Fragmented

Specimen Size

Right lobe: ________ x ________ x ________ cm
Left lobe: ________ x ________ x ________ cm
Isthmus ± pyramidal lobe: ________ x ________ x ________ cm
Central compartment: ________ x ________ x ________ cm
Right neck dissection: ________ x ________ x ________ cm
Left neck dissection: ________ x ________ x ________ cm
*Additional dimensions (specify): ________ x ________ x ________ cm

*Specimen Weight

*Specify: ________ g

Tumor Focality (select all that apply)

___ Unifocal
___ Multifocal (specify)
 ___ Ipsilateral
 ___ Bilateral
 ___ Midline (isthmus)

Dominant Tumor

Tumor laterality
 ___ Right lobe
 ___ Left lobe
 ___ Isthmus
 ___ Not specified

Tumor size
 Greatest dimension: ________ cm
 *Additional dimensions: ________ x ________ cm
 ___ Cannot be determined

Histologic type (select all that apply)
 ___ Papillary carcinoma

Variant, specify
- ____ Classical (usual)
- ____ Clear cell variant
- ____ Columnar cell variant
- ____ Cribriform-morular variant
- ____ Diffuse sclerosing variant
- ____ Follicular variant
- ____ Macrofollicular variant
- ____ Microcarcinoma (occult, latent, small, papillary microtumor)
- ____ Oncocytic or oxyphilic variant
- ____ Solid variant
- ____ Tall cell variant
- ____ Warthin-like variant
- ____ Other (specify): ____________________________

Architecture
- ____ Classical (papillary)
- ____ Cribriform-morular
- ____ Diffuse sclerosing
- ____ Follicular
- ____ Macrofollicular
- ____ Solid
- ____ Other (specify): ____________________________

Cytomorphology
- ____ Classical
- ____ Clear cell
- ____ Columnar cell
- ____ Oncocytic or oxyphilic
- ____ Tall cell

____ Follicular carcinoma

Variant, specify
- ____ Clear cell
- ____ Oncocytic (Hürthle cell)
- ____ Other (specify): ____________________________

____ Poorly differentiated thyroid carcinomas, including insular carcinoma

____ Medullary carcinoma

____ Undifferentiated (anaplastic) carcinoma

____ Other (specify): ____________________________

____ Carcinoma, type cannot be determined

*Histologic grade
- *____ Not applicable
- *____ GX: Cannot be assessed
- *____ G1: Well differentiated
- *____ G2: Moderately differentiated
- *____ G3: Poorly differentiated
- *____ G4: Undifferentiated
- *____ Other (specify): ____________________________

Margins
- ____ Cannot be assessed
- ____ Margins uninvolved by carcinoma
  - *Distance of invasive carcinoma to closest margin: _________ mm
- ____ Margin(s) involved by carcinoma
  - *Site(s) of involvement: ____________________________

Tumor capsule
- ____ Cannot be assessed

PROTOCOL FOR THE EXAMINATION OF THYROID GLAND SPECIMENS

____ Totally encapsulated
____ Partially encapsulated
____ None

Tumor capsular invasion
____ Cannot be assessed
____ Not identified
____ Present
Extent
____ Minimal
____ Widely invasive
____ Indeterminate

Lymph-vascular invasion
____ Cannot be assessed
____ Not identified
____ Present
Extent
____ Focal (< 4 vessels)
____ Extensive (≥ 4 vessels)
____ Indeterminate

*Perineural invasion
*____ Not identified
*____ Present
*____ Indeterminate

Extrathyroidal extension
____ Cannot be assessed
____ Not identified
____ Present
Extent
____ Minimal
____ Extensive

Second Tumor (for multifocal tumors only)

Tumor laterality (select all that apply)
____ Right lobe
____ Left lobe
____ Isthmus
____ Not specified

Tumor size
Greatest dimension: __________ cm
*Additional dimensions: __________ x __________ cm
____ Cannot be determined

Histologic type (select all that apply)
____ Papillary carcinoma
Variant, specify
____ Classical (usual)
____ Clear cell variant
____ Cribriform-morular variant
____ Diffuse sclerosing variant
____ Follicular variant
____ Macrofollicular variant
____ Microcarcinoma (occult, latent, small, papillary microtumor)
____ Oncocytic or oxyphilic variant
____ Solid variant
____ Tall cell variant
____ Warthin-like variant

____Other (specify): ____________________

Architecture

____ Classical (papillary)

____ Cribriform-morular

____ Diffuse sclerosing

____ Follicular

____ Macrofollicular

____ Solid

____ Other (specify): ____________________

Cytomorphology

____ Classical

____ Clear cell

____ Columnar cell

____ Oncocytic or oxyphilic

____Tall cell

____ Follicular carcinoma

Variant, specify

____ Clear cell

____ Oncocytic (Hürthle cell)

____ Other (specify): ____________________

____ Poorly differentiated thyroid carcinomas, including insular carcinoma

____ Medullary carcinoma

____ Undifferentiated (anaplastic) carcinoma

____ Other (specify): ____________________

____ Carcinoma, type cannot be determined

*Histologic grade

*____ Not applicable

*____ GX: Cannot be assessed

*____ G1: Well differentiated

*____ G2: Moderately differentiated

*____ G3: Poorly differentiated

*____ G4: Undifferentiated

*____ Other (specify): ____________________

Margins

____ Cannot be assessed

____ Totally encapsulated

____ Partially encapsulated

____ None

Tumor capsular invasion

____ Cannot be assessed

____ Not identified

____ Present

Extent

____ Minimally

____ Widely invasive

____ Indeterminate

Lymph-vascular invasion

____ Cannot be assessed

____ Not identified

____ Present

Extent

____ Focal (< 4 vessels)

____ Extensive (≥ 4 vessels)

____ Indeterminate

PROTOCOL FOR THE EXAMINATION OF THYROID GLAND SPECIMENS

*Perineural invasion

*____ Not identified

*____ Present

*____ Indeterminate

Extrathyroidal extension

____ Cannot be assessed

____ Not identified

____ Present

Extent

____ Minimal

____ Extensive

Pathologic Staging (pTNM)

TNM descriptors (required only if applicable) (select all that apply)

____ m (multiple primary tumors)

____ r (recurrent)

____ y (post-treatment)

Primary tumor (pT)†

____ pTX: Cannot be assessed

____ pT0: No evidence of primary tumor

____ pT1: Tumor size ≤ 2 cm, limited to thyroid

____ pT1a: Tumor ≤ 1 cm in greatest dimension, limited to thyroid

____pT1b: Tumor > 1 cm but ≤ 2 cm in greatest dimension, limited to thyroid

____ pT2: Tumor > 2 cm, but ≤ 4 cm, limited to thyroid

____ pT3: Tumor > 4 cm limited to thyroid, or any tumor with minimal extrathyroid extension (e.g., extension to sternothyroid muscle or perithyroid soft tissues)

____ pT4a: Moderately advanced disease.

Tumor of any size extending beyond thyroid capsule to invade subcutaneous soft tissues, larynx, trachea, esophagus, or recurrent laryngeal nerve

____ pT4b: Very advanced disease. Tumor invades prevertebral fascia or encases carotid artery or mediastinal vessels

Undifferentiated (anaplastic) carcinoma

____ pT4a: Intrathyroidal undifferentiated carcinoma, surgically resectable

____ pT4b: Extrathyroidal undifferentiated carcinoma, surgically unresectable

Regional lymph nodes (pN)††

____ pNX: Cannot be assessed

____ pN0: No regional lymph node metastasis

____ pN1a: Nodal metastases to level VI (pretracheal, paratracheal, and prelaryngeal/Delphian) lymph nodes

____ pN1b: Metastases to unilateral, bilateral, or contralateral cervical (levels I, II, III, IV, V) or retropharyngeal or superior mediastinal lymph nodes (level VII)

Specify: Number examined: ________

Number involved: ________

*Lymph node, extranodal extension

*____ Not identified

*____ Present

*____ Indeterminate

Distant metastasis (pM)

____ Not applicable

____ pM1: Distant metastasis

*Specify site(s), if known: ______________________

*Source of pathologic metastatic specimen (specify): ______________________

**Additional Pathologic Findings (select all that apply)*

*____Adenoma

*____Adenomatoid nodule(s) or nodular follicular disease (e.g., nodular hyperplasia, goitrous thyroid)

*____Diffuse hyperplasia (Graves disease)

*____Thyroiditis

*____ Advanced
*____ Focal (nonspecific)
*____ Palpation
*____ Other (specify): ____________________
*____ Parathyroid gland(s)
*____ Within normal limits
*____ Hypercellular
*____ Other (specify): ____________________
*____ C-cell hyperplasia
*____ Other (specify): ____________________
*____ None identified

*Ancillary Studies

*Specify type (e.g., histochemistry, immunohistochemistry, DNA analysis): ____________________

*Specify results: ____________________

*Clinical History (select all that apply)

*____ Radiation exposure
*____ Yes (specify type): ____________________
*____ No
*____ Indeterminate
*____ Family history
*____ Other (specify): ____________________

**Data elements with asterisks are not required. However, these elements may be clinically important but are not yet validated or regularly used in patient management. †Note: There is no category of carcinoma in situ (pTis) relative to carcinomas of thyroid gland. ††Superior mediastinal lymph nodes are considered regional lymph nodes (level VII). Midline nodes are considered ipsilateral nodes. Adapted with permission from College of American Pathologists, "Protocol for the Examination of Specimens from Patients with Carcinoma of the Thyroid Gland." Web posting date October 2009, www.cap.org.*

Stage Groupings: Papillary or Follicular Carcinoma

Stage	T	N	M
Under 45 Years of Age			
Stage I	Any T	Any N	M0
Stage II	Any T	Any N	M1
45 Years or Older			
Stage I	T1	N0	M0
Stage II	T2	N0	M0
Stage III	T1, T2	N1a	M0
	T3	N0, N1a	M0
Stage IVA	T1, T2, T3	N1b	M0
	T4a	N0, N1a, N1b	M0
Stage IVB	T4b	Any N	M0
Stage IVC	Any T	Any N	M1

Adapted from 7th edition AJCC Staging Forms.

Stage Groupings: Medullary Carcinoma (All Age Groups)

Stage	T	N	M
Stage I	T1	N0	M0
Stage II	T2, T3	N0	M0
Stage III	T1	N1a	M0
	T2, T3	N1a	M0
Stage IVA	T1, T2, T3	N1b	M0
	T4a	N0, N1a, N1b	M0
Stage IVB	T4b	Any N	M0
Stage IVC	Any T	Any N	M1

Adapted from 7th edition AJCC Staging Forms.

Stage Groupings: Undifferentiated (Anaplastic) Carcinoma

Stage	T	N	M
Stage IVA	T4a	Any N	M0
Stage IVB	T4b	Any N	M0
Stage IVC	Any T	Any N	M1

Note: All anaplastic carcinomas are considered Stage IV. Adapted from 7th edition AJCC Staging Forms.

Anatomic and Tumor Staging Graphics

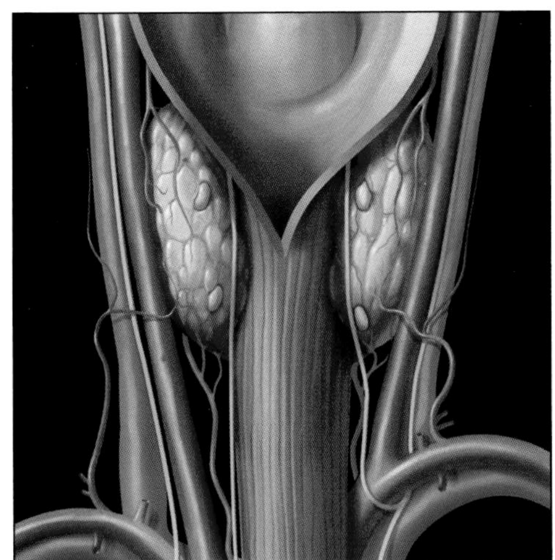

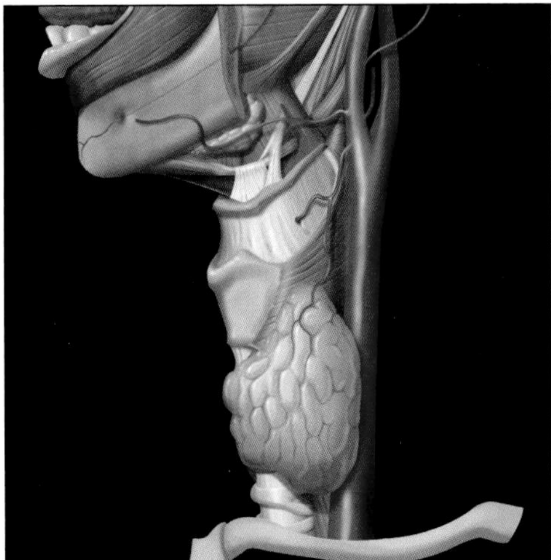

(Left) *A coronal posterior graphic demonstrates the thyroid gland lobes along with the embedded parathyroid glands. The relationship to the larynx and vessels, along with the nerves is illustrated.* ***(Right)*** *This sagittal view highlights the left lobe of the thyroid gland, and its relationship to the laryngeal cartilages, membranes, and vessels of the neck. These anatomic landmarks are helpful in the staging of tumors.*

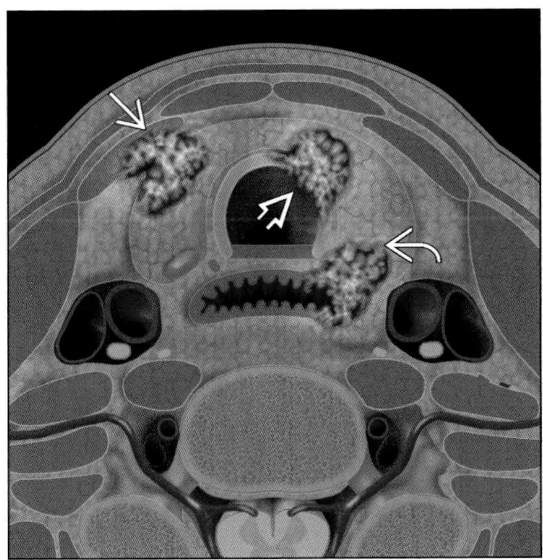

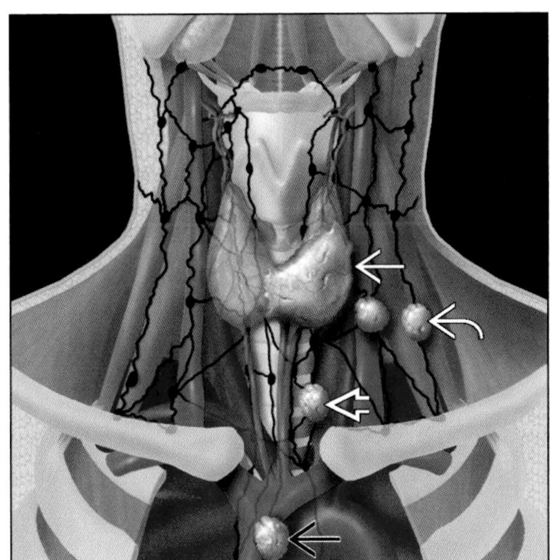

(Left) *An axial graphic shows 3 separate tumors within the thyroid gland. The right lobe tumor ➡ shows extrathyroidal soft tissue invasion; the anterior left lobe tumor ➡ shows larynx invasion, while the posterior left lobe tumor ➡ shows esophagus involvement.* ***(Right)*** *A coronal graphic shows a left lobe thyroid carcinoma ➡, with multiple paratracheal ➡, low jugular/spinal accessory ➡ and superior mediastinal ➡ lymph node metastases.*

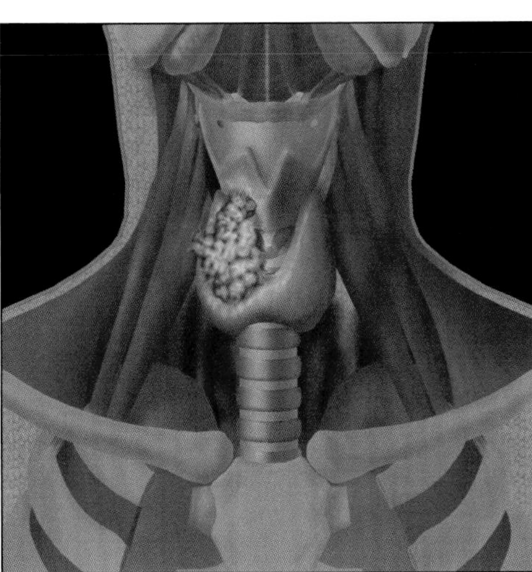

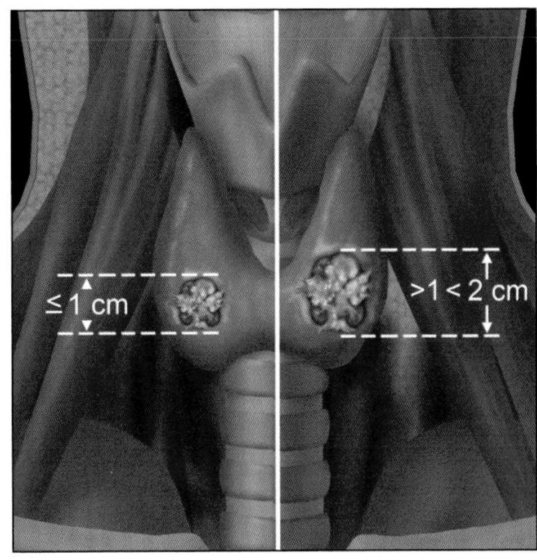

(Left) *The right lobe of the thyroid gland shows a neoplastic proliferation that extends beyond the thyroid gland macroscopically into the adjacent skeletal muscle. This would be a pT3 tumor for a differentiated carcinoma.* ***(Right)*** *There is a neoplasm in both lobes of the thyroid gland. 1 tumor is called "microscopic" since it is < 1 cm (right). The presence of bilateral disease is given an (m) designation in the staging system to represent bilateral tumors.*

Parathyroid Glands

Nonneoplastic

Benign Neoplasm

Malignant Neoplasm

PARATHYROID HYPERPLASIA

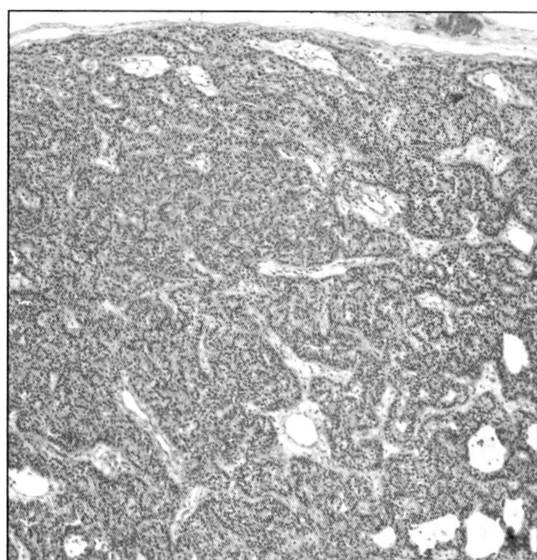

Diffuse proliferation without stromal fat and absent rim of normal gland is shown. These findings could also be those of an adenoma, requiring biopsy of another gland to determine if more than 1 gland is involved.

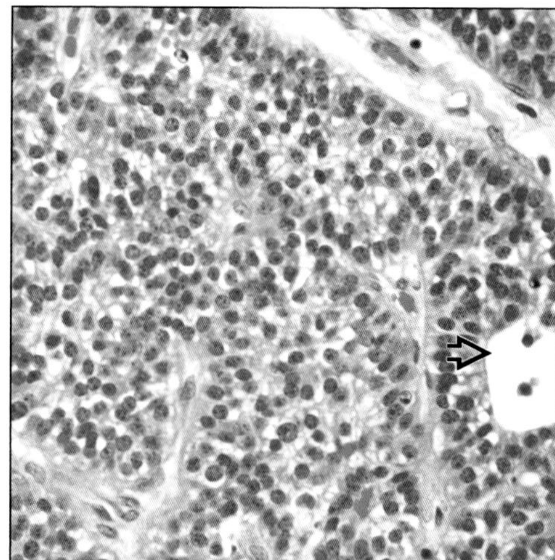

The cellular proliferation shows a predominance of chief cells arranged in solid sheets and cords focally with a follicular-appearing structure ⇨. There is an absence of stromal fat.

TERMINOLOGY

Synonyms

- Wasserhelle cell hyperplasia (for water-clear cell hyperplasia)

Definitions

- Nonneoplastic increase in parenchymal cell mass
  - Involves multiple parathyroid glands
  - Occurs in absence of known clinical stimulus for increased secretion of parathyroid hormone (PTH)
- Includes
  - Primary chief cell hyperplasia
  - Water-clear cell hyperplasia

ETIOLOGY/PATHOGENESIS

Idiopathic

- Sporadic cases represent 80% of patients with primary chief cell hyperplasia

Familial

- 20% have familial disease
  - Usually associated with one of the multiple endocrine neoplasia (MEN) syndromes
  - May occur in familial parathyroid hyperplasia without other endocrine abnormalities
- Approximately 20% of patients with primary chief cell hyperplasia have MEN
  - Association most frequent in MEN type 1 (Wermer syndrome)
    - Autosomal dominant transmission with variable penetrance
    - 90% have parathyroid hyperplasia
    - Less often associated with parathyroid neoplasms (adenoma and carcinoma)
    - Pancreatic or duodenal endocrine tumors (gastrinoma, insulinoma, glucagonoma)
    - Gastrointestinal endocrine cell hyperplasia or neoplasia (functioning and nonfunctioning)
    - Anterior pituitary adenoma (functioning and nonfunctioning)
    - Some patients also develop pulmonary and thymic neuroendocrine neoplasms, adrenal cortical neoplasms, and thyroid follicular neoplasms
    - *MEN1* gene localized on chromosome 11q13
  - Parathyroid proliferative disease seen in 30-40% of patients with MEN 2A (Sipple syndrome) but rare in MEN 2B

Hyperparathyroidism (HPT)

- Represents state of elevated serum PTH as a result of excessive secretion
- HPT divided into primary, secondary, and tertiary
- **Primary hyperparathyroidism**
  - Inappropriately increased PTH secretion due to intrinsic abnormality of parathyroid gland(s)
    - Occurs in absence of known stimulus for PTH secretion
    - Causes elevation of serum calcium (hypercalcemia) with decreased serum phosphate (hypophosphatemia)
- **Secondary hyperparathyroidism**: Increase in parathyroid parenchymal cell mass of multiple glands in response to known clinical stimulus for increased secretion of PTH
  - Usually characterized by hypocalcemia and hyperphosphatemia
  - Causes include
    - Chronic renal failure (most common)
    - Dietary vitamin D deficiency or abnormalities of vitamin D metabolism
    - Malabsorption
    - Pseudohypoparathyroidism
  - Symptoms primarily related to PTH-mediated bone resorption, which results in
    - Osteomalacia and osteitis fibrosa cystica

PARATHYROID HYPERPLASIA

Key Facts

Terminology

- Nonneoplastic increase in parenchymal cell mass
  - Involves multiple parathyroid glands
  - Occurs in absence of known clinical stimulus for increased secretion of parathyroid hormone
- Includes
  - Primary chief cell hyperplasia
  - Water-clear cell hyperplasia

Etiology/Pathogenesis

- Sporadic cases represent 80% of patients with primary chief cell hyperplasia
- 20% have familial disease
  - Usually associated with one of the multiple endocrine neoplasia (MEN) syndromes

Microscopic Pathology

- **Primary chief cell hyperplasia**
  - Increase in parenchymal cell mass
  - Predominantly composed of chief cells
  - Oncocytic cells may be present
  - May be diffuse or nodular
  - Stromal fat cells absent or markedly decreased in most areas
- **Water-clear cell hyperplasia**
  - Composed of cells with clear cytoplasm
- **Parathyromatosis**
  - Nests of hyperplastic parathyroid tissue in soft tissue of neck or mediastinum in primary chief cell hyperplasia

- **Tertiary hyperparathyroidism**: Absolute increase in parathyroid parenchymal cell mass associated with autonomous hyperfunction
  - Results in hypercalcemia in patients with known secondary HPT following implementation of dialysis or renal transplantation
    - Hypercalcemia usually develops several years after diagnosis of renal disease
    - Hypercalcemia due to tertiary HPT represents serious threat to renal grafts and requires prompt surgical therapy
  - Laboratory findings similar to those of primary HPT
    - Usually characterized by hypocalcemia and hyperphosphatemia
  - Causes of autonomous hyperfunction of parathyroids in patients with treated renal failure are unknown
    - Elevation of "set point" for serum calcium postulated
    - Would result in stimulation of parathyroid tissue in spite of normal serum calcium levels
  - Evidence that sheer mass of parathyroid tissue in patients with tertiary HPT may cause autonomous function
  - Removal of bulk of hyperplastic tissue results in readily suppressible remnant
- **Parathyroid proliferative disease (PPD)**
  - Parathyroid gland histopathologic lesions causing HPT collectively referred to as PPD
  - PPD classification includes the following
  - Parathyroid adenoma
    - Causes ~ 85% of HPT cases
  - Parathyroid hyperplasia
    - Causes ~ 13-15% of HPT cases
  - Parathyroid carcinoma
    - Causes ~ 1-2% of HPT cases

CLINICAL ISSUES

Epidemiology

- Incidence
  - Current reported annual incidence of HPT 0.04 per 1,000 persons
- Age
  - May occur over wide age range from 2nd to 9th decades
    - Mean: 6th decade
    - Incidence increases with age
    - Primarily occurs in middle and older ages
- Gender
  - Female > Male (3:1)

Site

- No specific localization

Presentation

- HPT secondary to parathyroid hyperplasia may be caused by
  - Chief cell hyperplasia
  - Water-clear cell hyperplasia
- **Chief cell hyperplasia**
  - Most common type of hyperplasia causing HPT
  - Symptoms related to level and duration of serum calcium elevation
  - Patients commonly asymptomatic or present with vague complaints
    - e.g., lethargy, weakness, polyuria, polydipsia, arthralgia, constipation, depression
  - Nonspecific presentation encountered more often in past 2 decades due to
    - Routine biochemical testing resulting overall in increased prevalence in clinically silent cases
  - Signs and symptoms of severe classical primary hyperparathyroidism are uncommon compared to incidence 2-3 decades ago
    - Severe bone disease, once common complication, now rare
  - Bone manifestations more commonly seen may include
    - Diffuse osteopenia ± compression fractures
    - Articular chondrocalcinosis and other joint disorders (e.g., pseudogout, true gout)
  - Renal manifestations also uncommon, may include

PARATHYROID HYPERPLASIA

- Nephrolithiasis: Recurrent and severe; stones composed of calcium phosphate
- Nephrocalcinosis: Presence of bilateral, extensive mineralization in renal pyramids and medullary regions

- **Water-clear cell hyperplasia**
  - Rare cause of HPT
    - Water-clear cell hyperplasia may represent advanced form of chief cell hyperplasia
  - Nephrolithiasis occurs in 90% of patients (vs. 53% in chief cell hyperplasia patients)
  - Overall incidence of bone disease similar to that of chief cell hyperplasia
    - Occasional presentation with osteitis fibrosa generalisata
  - No documented association with multiple endocrine neoplasia or other familial syndromes

Laboratory Tests

- Elevated serum calcium
  - Most accurately reflected by serum ionized calcium value
  - Regulated fraction of calcium not bound to plasma proteins
- Elevated serum PTH levels
  - Normal serum intact PTH levels 210-310 pg/mL
  - Elevations vary depending on type of assay
- Decrease in serum inorganic phosphorus
  - Results from increased urinary loss of phosphates induced by action of PTH at renal tubular level
  - Reflected by decreased tubular reabsorption of phosphate or by increased renal phosphate clearance
  - Corresponding increase in urinary cyclic AMP usually accompanies PTH-induced alterations in urinary phosphate metabolism

Treatment

- Surgical approaches
  - **Primary hyperparathyroidism**
    - Most widely accepted therapy: Subtotal parathyroidectomy with complete removal of 3 glands, leaving remnant of 4th
    - Total parathyroidectomy with autotransplantation of remnants of parathyroid tissue in forearm also common surgical therapy
  - **Secondary hyperparathyroidism**
  - Subtotal parathyroidectomy is treatment of choice
    - Remnant of parathyroid gland may be left in situ or transplanted to soft tissue of forearm
  - Autotransplantation of parathyroid tissue into forearm musculature following total parathyroidectomy may be associated with
    - Graft failure and hypoparathyroidism
    - Recurrent HPT due to hyperplasia of transplanted remnant of parathyroid
  - Recurrence of HPT common problem in patients with chronic renal failure
    - Stimulus for hypersecretion of parathyroid hormone frequently not correctable
  - Recurrent hyperplasia may be associated with
    - Multifocal proliferation of islands of parathyroid tissue in adipose tissue and skeletal muscle
    - Parathyroid proliferation may be widely separated from original site of transplantation
    - Hyperplastic cells may be more pleomorphic than original parathyroid proliferation
    - Hyperplastic cells may be mitotically active
    - Should not be interpreted as evidence of malignancy
  - **Tertiary hyperparathyroidism**
    - Subtotal parathyroidectomy is preferred therapy
    - Recurrent HPT in approximately 8% of patients after surgery

Prognosis

- Recurrence rate of HPT following subtotal parathyroidectomy: Approximately 16%
- Recurrences may not be evident for several years
- Recurrences may be due to inadequate neck exploration
  - May result from diagnosis of "adenoma" in cases of asymmetrical hyperplasia
- Less frequent causes of recurrence include
  - Failure to recognize supernumerary or ectopic glands
  - Parathyromatosis
  - Surgical implantation of hyperplastic tissue in soft tissue of neck

IMAGE FINDINGS

Radiographic Findings

- Imaging procedures less effective in localizing glands in hyperplasia as compared to adenomas or carcinomas
- Tc-99m sestamibi effective in localizing up to 60% of hyperplastic glands
  - Widely utilized in recurrent hyperparathyroidism after parathyroid resection

MACROSCOPIC FEATURES

General Features

- Distinction between hyperplastic and adenomatous glands generally not made by gross exam
  - Glands with minimal enlargement may be indistinguishable from normal glands
- All 4 glands may be enlarged but
  - Not uncommon for hyperplasia to be asymmetrical with enlargement of only 1, 2, or 3 glands
  - 1 gland may be enlarged, suggesting adenoma
  - Emphasizes need to biopsy grossly "normal" glands to facilitate discrimination between hyperplasia and adenoma
- Diffuse or nodular enlargement
- Soft, tan-brown
- Cystic change may be present but is not common

Size

- Total gland weight in primary chief cell hyperplasia variable
  - < 1 g in approximately 50%
  - 1-5 g in approximately 30%
  - 5-10 g in approximately 20%

MICROSCOPIC PATHOLOGY

Primary Chief Cell Hyperplasia

- Increase in parenchymal cell mass
  - Predominantly composed of chief cells
  - Oncocytic cells may be present
- May be diffuse or nodular
  - Arranged in solid sheets, cords, acinar-like or follicular structures, or commonly mixed patterns identified
  - Variable nodularity; nodules may be small (micronodular), solitary or multiple
  - Chief cells
    - Polyhedral cells
    - Round, centrally located nuclei with coarse chromatin and well-defined nuclear membrane
    - Cytoplasm is eosinophilic to amphophilic to clear and vacuolated
  - Oncocytic cells
    - Characterized by striking eosinophilic granular cytoplasm
    - Nuclei larger than those in chief cells
- Stromal fat cells absent or markedly decreased in most areas
  - Areas with residual fat may simulate appearance of "normal" gland
    - When identified adjacent to large nodules devoid of fat, may suggest diagnosis of adenoma
  - Lipohyperplasia: Term used in cases of hyperplastic glands with abundant fat
    - Presence of fat in this setting makes diagnosis of hyperplasia challenging
    - Biopsies may contain only fat or predominantly fat with limited parenchymal cells
    - Clinical setting and enlargement of multiple glands is of importance in diagnosis of lipohyperplasia
- Mitotic figures may be seen
  - Usually number < 1 per 10 high-power fields (HPF)
  - May be increased mitotic rates of 1-5 per HPF
  - Atypical mitoses not present

Water-Clear Cell Hyperplasia

- Very rare cause of HPT
- Composed of cells with clear cytoplasm
- May contain multiple cytoplasmic vacuoles

Parathyromatosis

- Nests of hyperplastic parathyroid tissue in soft tissue of neck or mediastinum in primary chief cell hyperplasia
- Probably results from stimulation of embryonic rests of parathyroid cells in primary HPT
- Should not be mistaken for "invasion"
  - Lack of fibroblastic reaction or infiltrative contour
  - Absence of intravascular location
  - Lack of histologic features of carcinoma
- May be cause of recurrent HPT after apparently complete resection of grossly evident hyperplastic glands

Secondary Hyperparathyroidism

- Proliferation includes chief cells, oxyphilic cells, and transitional cells
- Increased parenchymal cell mass varies depending on duration of disease
  - Parenchymal cells may grow in sheets, cords, or acinar structures
  - Nodular aggregates of chief cells or oxyphilic cells common in very enlarged glands
  - Oncocytic cells more common component than in primary chief cell hyperplasia
- Presence of residual stromal fat cells varies depending on duration of disease
  - In advanced disease, fat cells are absent
- Areas of fibrosis, cystic change, and calcification may be present

Tertiary Hyperparathyroidism

- 95% of patients have hyperplasia
  - Chief cells predominate in hyperplasia
  - Oncocytic cells may be seen in either diffuse or nodular hyperplasia
  - Rarely, areas with water-clear cells may be present
  - Areas of hemorrhage, fibrosis, and calcification common
  - Mitotic figures, nuclear pleomorphism uncommon
  - Stromal fat cells are sparse but more often present in areas between nodules
  - Distribution may suggest diagnosis of "adenoma"; however, multinodularity more consistent with hyperplasia
- Only 5% found to have adenomas

ANCILLARY TESTS

Cytology

- Smears indistinguishable from adenoma

Histochemistry

- Periodic acid-Schiff
  - Small follicular structures may contain PAS-positive material
    - Resembles colloid
    - Thyroglobulin negative
- Fat stains (oil red O, Sudan black)
  - Hyperplastic cells
    - Usually contain less intracytoplasmic fat than normal or atrophic parathyroid tissue
    - May contain abundant intracytoplasmic fat
    - Intracytoplasmic fat may be more abundant in chief cells between hyperplastic nodules while usually absent in cells within nodules

Immunohistochemistry

- Chief cells
  - Cytokeratins, neuroendocrine markers (chromogranin, synaptophysin)
    - Positive (cytoplasmic)
    - Stain less intensely than normal gland
    - Chief cells stain more intensely than oncocytic cells
  - Parathyroid hormone

PARATHYROID HYPERPLASIA

    - Positive (cytoplasmic)
  - CD4
    - Positive (cell surface staining)
    - Restricted to chief cells
    - Oncocytic cells nonreactive
  - Renal cell carcinoma antigen may be positive
  - CD10 negative
  - Negative for thyroglobulin, TTF-1
- Clear cells
  - Cytokeratin, chromogranin positive
  - Calcitonin, calcitonin gene-related peptide (CGRP) positivity may be present
- Ki-67 (MIB-1) proliferative index is low

Electron Microscopy

- Chief cells
  - Characteristic secretory granules
  - Abundant mitochondria, endoplasmic reticulum, large Golgi areas
- Clear cells
  - Contain numerous membrane-bound vacuoles, many appear "empty"
  - Some contain intracytoplasmic electron-dense material similar to typical secretory granules seen in chief cells

DIFFERENTIAL DIAGNOSIS

Parathyroid Adenoma

- Almost always solitary
- Encapsulated to circumscribed
- Absence of stromal fat
- Remnant of normal or atrophic gland may be identified
  - Includes stromal fat

Parathyroid Carcinoma

- Associated with higher levels of serum calcium and parathyroid hormone
- Single enlarged gland
  - Often adherent to surrounding anatomic structures
- Invasion present in approximately 2/3 of cases, may include
  - Angioinvasion
  - Neurotropism
  - Invasion into adjacent tissues (e.g., thyroid)
- May metastasize

Thyroid Follicular Neoplasm

- Thyroglobulin positive
- Parathyroid hormone immunostaining negative

Metastatic Renal Cell Carcinoma

- May metastasize to cervical lymph nodes
- May share features with water-clear cell hyperplasia
- Immunoreactive for CD10, renal cell carcinoma antigen
- Negative immunostaining for parathyroid hormone

Lithium Therapy

- Associated with form of HPT similar to primary HPT
  - Hypercalcemia, elevated serum parathormone levels
- Both chief cell hyperplasia and "adenomas" described in these patients
- HPT resolves after discontinuing lithium therapy
- Patients requiring lithium may be treated successfully with subtotal parathyroidectomy

Humoral Hypercalcemia of Malignancy

- Important clinical differential diagnostic consideration in patients suspected of primary HPT
- Independent of extent of metastatic disease involving bone
- Characterized by hypercalcemia, hypophosphatemia, elevated urinary cyclic AMP levels
- Unlike HPT
  - Serum parathormone and 1,25-dihydroxyvitamin D suppressed
- Mechanism for hypercalcemia appears to be increased bone resorption
  - Due to humoral factor known as parathyroid hormone-related protein
- This form of hypercalcemia most frequent in patients with squamous cell carcinoma
  - Lung, upper aerodigestive tract, female genital tract
  - Renal cell carcinoma
  - Urothelial (transitional) cell carcinoma
- 2nd mechanism of hypercalcemia associated with malignancy related directly to osteolytic effect of bone metastases
  - This form of hypercalcemia more common in patients with breast carcinoma and hematologic malignancies
  - Patients have suppressed levels of parathormone but
    - Urinary cyclic AMP not elevated
    - Parathyroid hormone-related protein not implicated

SELECTED REFERENCES

1. Alabdulkarim Y et al: Sestamibi (99mTc) scan as a single localization modality in primary hyperparathyroidism and factors impacting its accuracy. Indian J Nucl Med. 25(1):6-9, 2010
2. Melck AL et al: Recurrent hyperparathyroidism and forearm parathyromatosis after total parathyroidectomy. Surgery. 148(4):867-73; discussion 873-5, 2010
3. Santarpia L et al: Hypercalcemia in cancer patients: pathobiology and management. Horm Metab Res. 42(3):153-64, 2010
4. Lew JI et al: Surgical management of primary hyperparathyroidism: state of the art. Surg Clin North Am. 89(5):1205-25, 2009
5. Szalat A et al: Lithium-associated hyperparathyroidism: report of four cases and review of the literature. Eur J Endocrinol. 160(2):317-23, 2009
6. DeLellis RA et al: Primary hyperparathyroidism: a current perspective. Arch Pathol Lab Med. 132(8):1251-62, 2008
7. Seethala RR et al: Parathyroid lipoadenomas and lipohyperplasias: clinicopathologic correlations. Am J Surg Pathol. 32(12):1854-67, 2008
8. Falchetti A, Marini F, Brandi ML. Multiple Endocrine Neoplasia Type 1. 1993-, 2005
9. Castleman B et al: Parathyroid hyperplasia in primary hyperparathyroidism: a review of 85 cases. Cancer. 38(4):1668-75, 1976

Diagrammatic and Microscopic Features

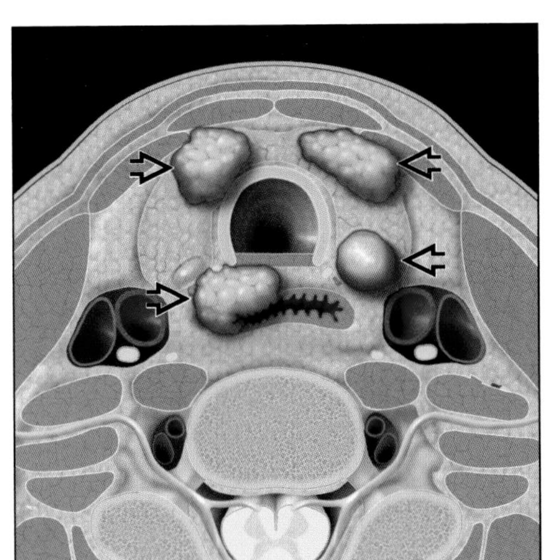

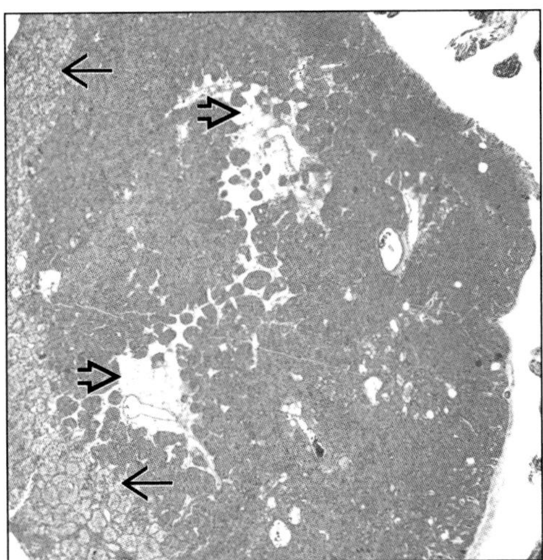

(Left) *Graphic depicts enlargement of all 4 parathyroid glands* ➩*. More commonly, glandular enlargement is limited to 2 or possibly 3 glands but may only involve 1 gland, making distinction from an adenoma problematic.* ***(Right)*** *Hyperplastic gland shows nodular appearance with limited but identifiable stromal fat* ➩ *predominantly composed of oxyphilic cells, although chief cells are present* →*. There is an absence of a rim of normal parathyroid tissue.*

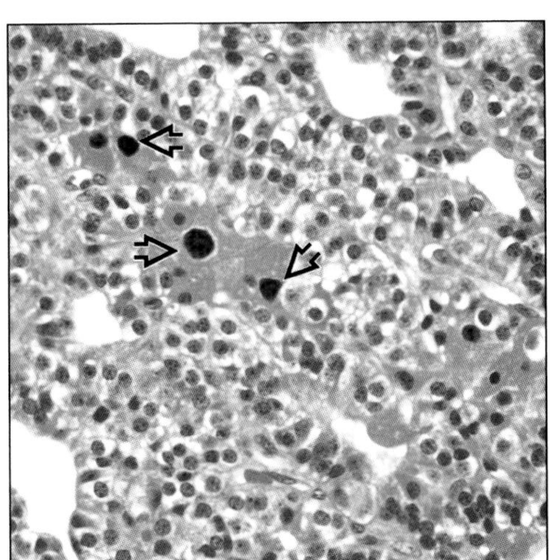

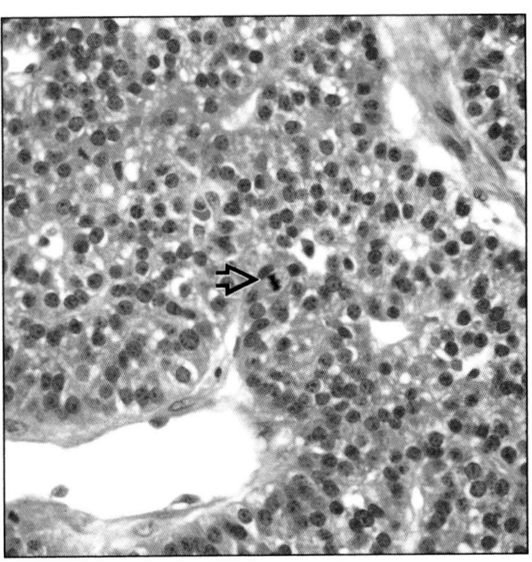

(Left) *Diffuse cellular proliferation shows an admixture of chief cells and oxyphilic cells; the oxyphilic cells have enlarged pleomorphic and hyperchromatic nuclei* ➩*. The presence of nuclear atypia is not a diagnostic feature for parathyroid carcinoma.* ***(Right)*** *Parathyroid hyperplasia shows a mitotic figure* ➩*. Increased mitotic figures are not, in and of themselves, diagnostic for parathyroid carcinoma and can be identified in parathyroid hyperplasia and adenoma.*

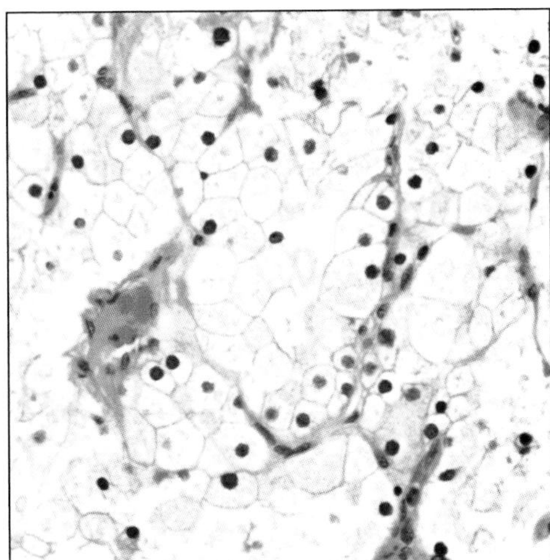

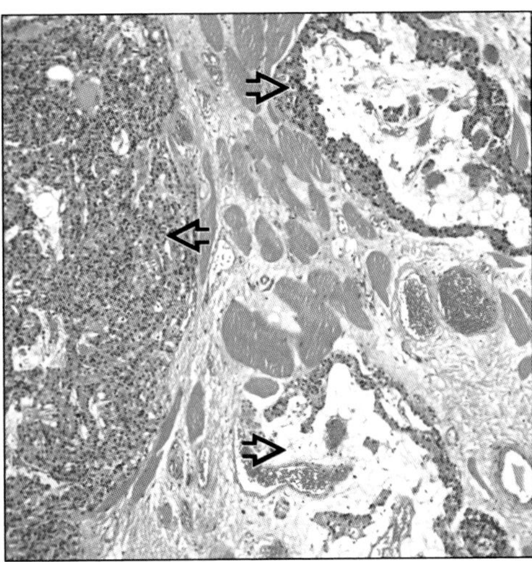

(Left) *Water-clear cell hyperplasia shows cells with clear cytoplasm and represents a rare cause of HPT.* ***(Right)*** *Parathyromatosis shows nests of hyperplastic parathyroid tissue* ➩ *in soft tissue of neck that should not be mistaken for "invasion" lacking fibroblastic reaction, infiltrative contour, and histologic features of carcinoma. It probably results from stimulation of embryonic rests and may be the cause of recurrent HPT after resection of grossly evident hyperplastic glands.*

CHRONIC PARATHYROIDITIS

Key Facts

Terminology
- Inflammatory infiltrate within parathyroid parenchyma, possibly related to autoimmunity

Etiology/Pathogenesis
- Poorly understood condition, although thought to be autoimmune
- Lymphocytic infiltration is ongoing destructive process

Clinical Issues
- Extremely rare
- Older aged patients
- Female > Male
- > 1 parathyroid gland may be involved
  - Multifocal disease seen in Sjögren disease (or other autoimmune disorders)
- Most patients are asymptomatic
- Slightly enlarged gland (not usually clinically detected)
- May occur in patients with
  - Hypoparathyroidism
  - Hyperparathyroidism
- Antibodies to parathyroid tissue are seen in only a few cases
- Management is supportive, if clinically necessary
- Significance is unknown

Macroscopic Features
- Slightly enlarged gland
- Appearance is not specific

Microscopic Pathology
- Aggregates of mature lymphocytes within parathyroid parenchyma
- Parenchyma may be normal or show hyperplasia
- Lymphoid follicle formation may be seen, with germinal centers
- Plasma cells predominate
- Fibrosis separates gland into lobules
- Atrophy may be seen
- Destruction of parenchyma has been reported

Top Differential Diagnoses
- **Parathyroid infection**
  - Predominantly mature lymphocytes may be seen in viral process
  - Sparse infiltrate with perivascular distribution
- **Parathyroid carcinoma**
  - Significant acellular, eosinophilic fibrosis
  - Invasion of the following
  - Parenchyma
  - Adipose tissue outside the gland
  - Perineural invasion
  - Vascular invasion
  - Presence of necrosis
  - Profound pleomorphism
  - Increased mitoses
- **Lymphoma**
  - May involve parathyroid glands as part of systemic disease
  - Histologic features include the following: Cellular monotony, mitoses, tingible body macrophages, immunohistochemical clonality

*(**Left**) A low-power micrograph shows sheets ⇒ of inflammatory cells within the cellular parathyroid gland parenchyma. While there is no well-developed germinal center formation in this case, it is frequently seen in this entity. (**Right**) There are sheets of lymphoid cells and plasma cells identified immediately adjacent to and intimately involved with the parathyroid parenchyma cells. Note the isolated stromal adipocytes ⇒.*

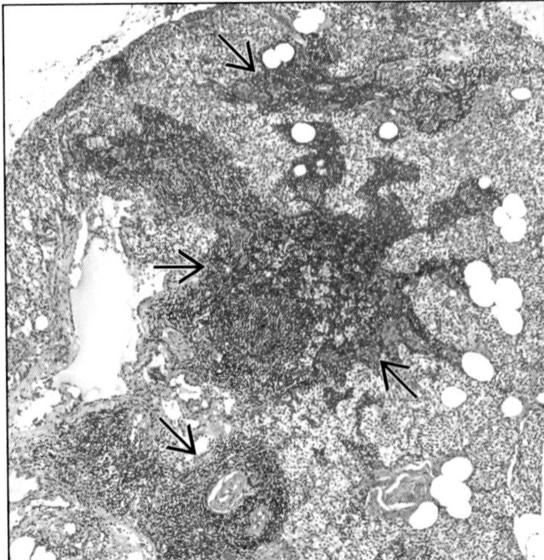

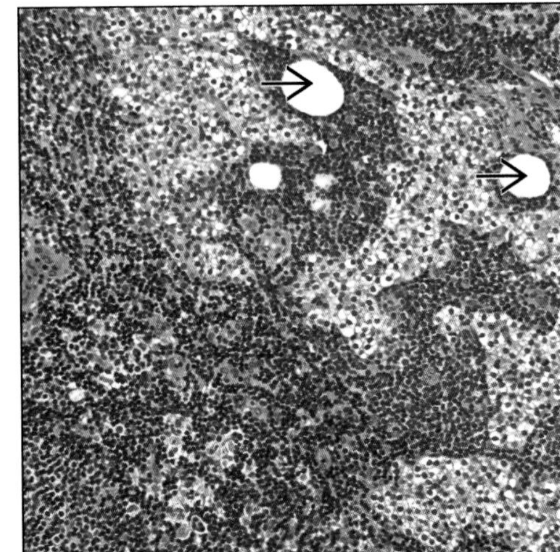

TERTIARY HYPERPARATHYROIDISM

Key Facts

Terminology

- Absolute increase in parathyroid parenchymal mass associated with autonomous hyperfunction
- Hypercalcemia in patient with known secondary hyperparathyroidism following dialysis or renal transplantation

Etiology/Pathogenesis

- Exact cause of autonomous parathyroid gland hyperfunction is unknown
  - Increase in "set point" of calcium is proposed
  - Parathyroid glands are stimulated in spite of normal serum calcium levels
  - Greatly increased parathyroid parenchymal mass might cause autonomous function
  - If bulk of hyperplastic tissue is removed, remnant seems to be suppressible

Clinical Issues

- Uncommon
- Wide age range, based on incidence of chronic renal failure
- Equal gender distribution
- Parathyroid gland enlargement
- Hypercalcemia usually develops years after diagnosis of renal disease
  - Hypercalcemia is usually a significant threat to renal grafts, requiring prompt surgical therapy
- Laboratory values
  - Elevated ionized calcium
  - Elevated intact parathyroid hormone level
  - May have hypophosphatemia
- Treatment
  - Renal graft may fail if therapy is delayed
  - Subtotal parathyroidectomy is required
- Recurrent hyperparathyroidism can be seen
  - Recurrence of hypercalcemia may be seen in up to 10% of patients

Macroscopic Features

- Diffuse or nodular enlarged glands
  - May be asymmetric enlargement
- Diffuse hyperplasia: 10-20x normal size
- Nodular hyperplasia: 20-40x normal size

Microscopic Pathology

- Hyperplastic glands is most common presentation (95%)
  - Adenoma accounts for < 5% of tertiary hyperparathyroidism
- Chief cell hyperplasia accounts for majority of parenchyma
  - May have isolated oxyphilic, transitional, or clear cells
- Hemorrhage and fibrosis, ± calcifications, is common
- Nearly absent mitoses and pleomorphism
- Stromal fat is greatly decreased
  - When present, distributed between nodules

Top Differential Diagnoses

- **Parathyroid adenoma**
  - Single gland enlargement
  - Atrophic or compressed rim of normal parenchyma at periphery
  - Capsule separating fatless tumor from adjacent parenchyma
  - Usually a single tumor cell type, glandular architecture

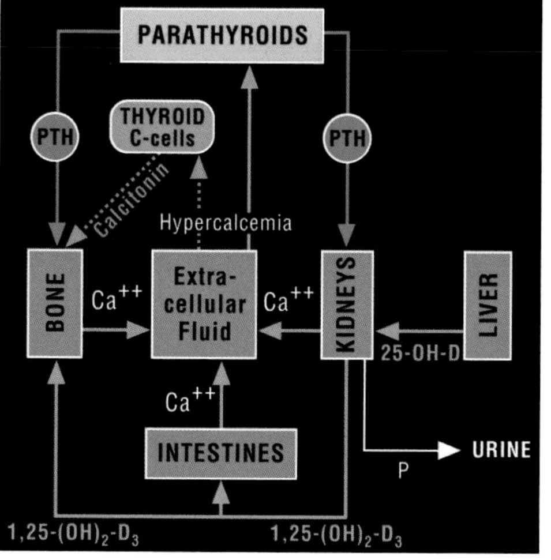

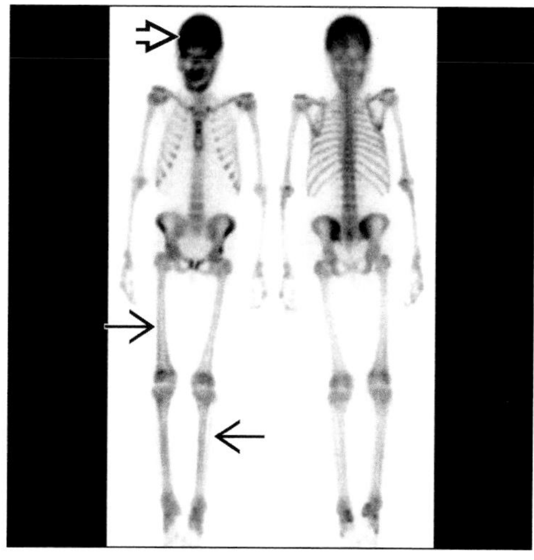

*(**Left**) Calcium metabolism is controlled by a complex biofeedback mechanism which involves several organs. PTH affects kidney and bone to control serum calcium levels. Vitamin D (1,25-(OH)2-D3) is also involved in calcium metabolism and includes various conversions in the liver, skin, and intestines. (**Right**) Anterior and posterior bone scans show diffusely increased uptake in calvarium ⇨, axial and appendicular skeleton → with absent soft tissue and renal activity, typical of secondary or tertiary hyperparathyroidism.*

PARATHYROID ADENOMA

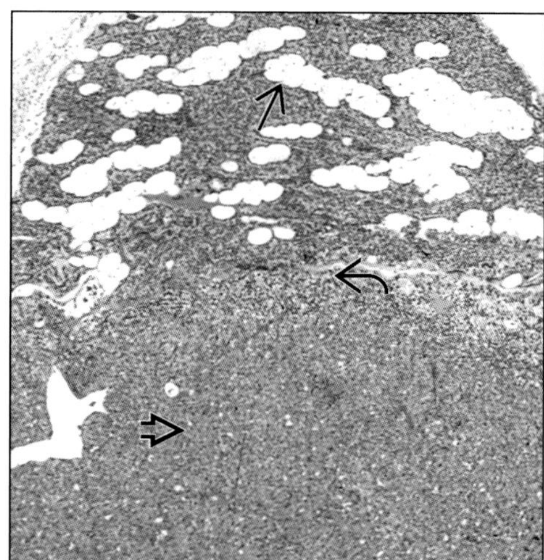

Parathyroid adenoma is characterized by increased cells and absent intraparenchymal fat ⊳. Here, it is demarcated ↶ from the normal parathyroid gland, which shows the presence of stromal fat →.

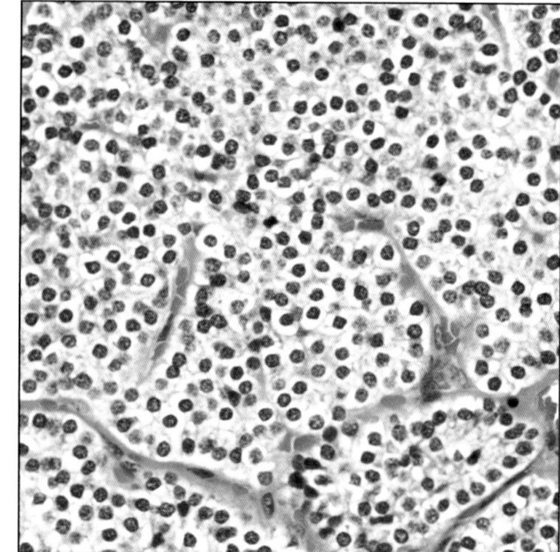

This image shows adenoma exclusively composed of chief cells that resemble those of the normal gland but typically have larger nuclei than normal chief cells. Stromal fat is absent.

TERMINOLOGY

Definitions

- Benign neoplasm of parathyroid parenchymal cells

ETIOLOGY/PATHOGENESIS

Idiopathic

- No specific link to any cause
- Some evidence supports role of ionizing radiation in development of adenoma

Genetic

- May be associated with hyperparathyroidism-jaw tumor syndrome (HPT-JT)
  - Autosomal dominant disorder
  - Characterized by parathyroid adenoma or carcinoma
  - Fibroosseous lesions of jaw (e.g., ossifying fibroma of mandible or maxilla)
  - Renal cysts or tumors
    - Approximately 80% of patients develop HPT
    - Renal lesions may include renal cysts, polycystic renal disease, renal hamartoma
    - Papillary renal cell carcinoma, renal cortical adenomas, Wilms tumor
    - *HRPT2* gene mapped to 1q25-q31

CLINICAL ISSUES

Epidemiology

- Incidence
  - Considerable variation in incidence
    - Due to lack of uniformity of diagnostic criteria
  - Single most common cause of hyperparathyroidism (HPT)
- Age
  - Occurs over broad range
    - Most frequently discovered in 4th-5th decades
- Gender
  - Female > Male (3-4:1)

Site

- 90% of cases affect glands in their usual anatomic location
  - Lower glands are more commonly involved
- Less commonly occur in any location where parathyroid tissue may be found
  - Includes ectopic sites such as mediastinum, retroesophageal soft tissue, within thyroid gland, in thymic tissue
- Reports of occurrence in supernumerary glands arising in vagus nerve, pericardium, or other soft tissue sites in neck

Presentation

- Clinical findings are essentially similar to those of primary HPT due to hyperplasia
- Symptomatology changing as result of routine biochemical screening and early detection
  - Hypercalcemia may be incidentally discovered in asymptomatic patients
  - Many patients complain only of fatigue, weakness, or depression
- Nephrolithiasis documented in 69% of men and 36% of women, but incidence decreasing in recent years to 5-20%
- Severe bone disease, once common complication, now rare
  - Osteopenia (with or without compression fractures) often present
  - Articular chondrocalcinosis and other joint disorders (e.g., pseudogout, true gout)
- Rarely presents as palpable mass

Laboratory Tests

- Serum calcium levels generally higher than in patients with primary chief cell hyperplasia
- Elevated serum parathyroid hormone (PTH) levels
  - Normal serum intact PTH levels 210-310 pg/mL

PARATHYROID ADENOMA

Key Facts

Terminology
- Benign neoplasm of parathyroid parenchymal cells
- No specific link to any cause
- May be associated with hyperparathyroidism-jaw tumor syndrome (HPT-JT)

Clinical Issues
- Single most common cause of hyperparathyroidism
- Clinical findings are essentially similar to those of primary HPT due to hyperplasia
  - Serum calcium levels generally higher than in patients with primary chief cell hyperplasia

Microscopic Pathology
- Most are predominantly composed of chief cells
- Oncocytic cells may be present in variable numbers
- Rim of nonneoplastic parathyroid tissue found in association with only about 50% of cases
- Oxyphilic adenoma composed of large cells with abundant eosinophilic granular cytoplasm and hyperchromatic nuclei
- Lipoadenoma: Rare benign neoplasm characterized by proliferation of parenchymal and stromal fat cells
- Atypical adenoma: Tumor that shares some features of parathyroid carcinoma but lacks definitive evidence of invasive growth

Ancillary Tests
- Parafibromin
  - Positive (nuclear staining)
  - Diminished to absent staining in parathyroid carcinoma

  - Elevations vary depending on type of assay
- Hypophosphatemia, hyperphosphaturia

Treatment
- Surgical approaches
  - Most widely accepted therapy includes
    - Excision of adenomatous gland
    - Biopsy of at least 1 additional gland "normal" in size

Prognosis
- Recurrent HPT following surgery may result from
  - Incomplete excision
  - Rupture of tumor capsule with spillage into operative field
  - Hyperfunction of autografted parathyroid tissue following subtotal parathyroidectomy
- Recurrence rates vary significantly and may reflect problems in classification
  - Particularly in cases of hyperplasia with nodules, which may erroneously be diagnosed as adenoma
- Most atypical adenomas prove to be benign tumors in long-term follow-up
  - Treatment similar to typical parathyroid adenoma
  - Patients should be followed for potential
    - Recurrent hyperparathyroidism
    - Local recurrence of tumor
    - Evidence of aggressive behavior (e.g., metastasis)
- Osteitis fibrosa cystica
  - Also known as "brown tumors"
  - May occur in patients with HPT of any etiology
    - Related to degree and duration of serum calcium elevation
  - Lesions characterized by resorption of bone with replacement by fibrous tissue
  - Histology includes
    - Proliferation of multinucleated giant cells and osteoclasts with hemorrhage and hemosiderin deposition
    - Over time degenerative changes occur including cyst formation
    - Cannot be distinguished histologically from giant cell (reparative) granuloma
  - Clinical information is essential in diagnosis

IMAGE FINDINGS

Radiographic Findings
- Several imaging methods used for localization of hyperfunctioning parathyroid tissue, including
  - Retrograde phlebotomy for determination of serum parathormone levels
  - CT scanning, ultrasonography, MRI, thallium subtraction scanning, and ^{99}mTc sestamibi imaging
- Tc-99m sestamibi imaging appears to be most useful
  - Localization of > 90% of adenomas

MACROSCOPIC FEATURES

General Features
- Almost always solitary
- Most "multiple adenomas" probably represent cases of asymmetrical or nodular hyperplasia
- Rounded borders, firm, brown to tan, contained within delicate capsule
  - May be ovoid or lobulated
- Remnant of uninvolved parathyroid tissue at periphery of tumor may be visible
- Cystic change may be present
  - When prominent, may mask neoplastic nature of proliferation
  - Marked cystic degeneration frequently associated with scarring and calcification

Size
- Significant variation in weight with most 0.3-1.0 g

MICROSCOPIC PATHOLOGY

Histologic Features
- Most are predominantly composed of chief cells

PARATHYROID ADENOMA

- Cells tend to be larger than nonneoplastic chief cells in uninvolved rim of parathyroid tissue (if present)
- Nuclei usually slightly larger than those of normal chief cells
- Nuclei typically round, central to slightly basal location within cell, inconspicuous nucleoli
- Cytoplasm is typically slightly eosinophilic but may be clear
- Cells with hyperchromatic enlarged nuclei; multinucleated cells commonly found scattered or clustered in small foci
  - Not an indicator of malignancy in absence of other evidence
- Usually have less intracellular fat than do cells in uninvolved (or suppressed) parathyroid tissue
- Oncocytic cells may be present in variable numbers
  - Either focally admixed with chief cells or as nodular aggregates
  - Some adenomas composed entirely of oncocytic cells
    - Referred to as "oxyphilic" or "oncocytic" adenomas
- Cells arranged in sheets, cords, nests, or glandular structures
  - Glandular formations may contain eosinophilic "colloid-like" material
  - Distinct trabecular pattern uncommon
- Mitotic figures can be found in adenomas
  - Usually number fewer than 1 per 10 high-power fields (HPF)
  - Mitotic rates as high as 4 mitoses per 10 HPF reported
  - Atypical mitoses not present
- Rim of nonneoplastic parathyroid tissue found in association with only about 50% of cases
  - If present, this finding is very helpful in making distinction between adenoma and hyperplasia
  - Generally contains abundant stromal fat cells
  - Parenchymal cells smaller than neoplastic cells
  - Generally separated from neoplasm by connective tissue capsule
    - Capsule may be indistinct or absent
- Histologic variants include
  - Oxyphilic adenoma
  - Lipoadenoma
  - Atypical adenoma

Variants

- Oxyphilic adenoma
  - Composed of large cells with abundant eosinophilic granular cytoplasm and hyperchromatic nuclei
  - Scattered large atypical nuclei or multinucleated cells may be seen
- Lipoadenoma
  - Referred to as parathyroid hamartoma
  - Rare benign neoplasm characterized by proliferation of parenchymal and stromal fat cells
  - Encapsulated
  - May be associated with compressed rim of "normal" gland
  - May be difficult to recognize as "abnormal" parathyroid tissue in small biopsy specimens
    - Easily mistaken for normal parathyroid tissue due to abundance of stromal fat
    - Stromal fat often contains areas of fibrosis or myxoid alteration
    - Most associated with HPT
- Atypical adenoma
  - Shares some features of parathyroid carcinoma but lack definitive evidence of invasive growth
  - Atypical histologic features may include
    - Capsular irregularities without infiltration of adjacent soft tissues
    - Growth characteristics worrisome for but not diagnostic of invasion (angioinvasion, soft tissue invasion)
    - Increased mitotic activity but < 5 per 10 HPF, absence of atypical mitoses
    - Trabecular growth, intralesional fibrotic bands, spindle-shaped nuclei
- Double (multiple) adenomas
  - Controversial issue whether > 1 adenoma occurs
    - Some data to support such an occurrence
    - Probably represents asymmetric hyperplasia

ANCILLARY TESTS

Cytology

- Occasionally enlarged parathyroid glands have been subjected to fine needle aspiration as clinically suspected "solitary thyroid nodule"
- Aspirates of parathyroid tissue typically contain
  - Numerous naked nuclei, as well as as small sheets of cells, sometimes forming acinar or follicular structures
  - Small aggregates of dense colloid-like material may be seen but are not numerous
  - Cells generally small with predominantly round nuclei
    - Nuclei generally hyperchromatic with coarse chromatin typical of neuroendocrine cells
    - Anisonucleosis in scattered cells and occasional large atypical naked nuclei common
  - May-Grünwald-Giemsa or Romanowsky stain
    - Cytoplasm is granular and may exhibit scattered large metachromatic granules
  - Papanicolaou stain
    - Cells have clear to finely granular cytoplasm
  - Distinction from follicular epithelium of thyroid may be difficult
    - Cells are usually smaller than those of thyroid origin
    - Immunohistochemistry helpful in differential diagnosis

Histochemistry

- Fat stains (oil red O, Sudan black)
  - Considerable variation in literature regarding utility of fat stains in diagnosis
  - Generally hyperfunctioning cells have significantly decreased amount of intracellular fat compared to normal or suppressed parenchymal cells

Immunohistochemistry

- Cytokeratin, neuroendocrine markers (chromogranin, synaptophysin)

- Positive (cytoplasmic staining)
- Parathyroid hormone
  - Positive (cytoplasmic staining)
- Parafibromin
  - Represents protein product of *HRPT2* gene responsible for hyperparathyroidism-jaw tumor (HPT-JT) syndrome
  - Positive (nuclear staining)
  - Uniformly expressed in adenoma
  - Diminished to absent staining in
    - Parathyroid carcinoma (but may be present)
    - HPT-JT-associated adenomas (but may be present)
- CD4 positive
  - Cell surface staining
  - Restricted to chief cells
  - Oncocytic cells nonreactive
- Negative for thyroglobulin, TTF-1
- Ki-67 (MIB-1) proliferative index is low
  - Index > 5% raises suspicion for carcinoma, but diagnosis of carcinoma requires confirmatory findings
  - Proliferative indices in differentiating adenoma from carcinoma of limited utility

Molecular Genetics

- Alterations in cyclin-D1
- Loss of heterozygosity of chromosome 11q
- Adenomatous polyposis coli (APC) expression
  - Reduced expression or loss of tumor suppressor protein APC associated with parathyroid malignancy
    - Adenomas express APC
    - Loss of APC frequent molecular event in carcinomas but not adenomas
    - Loss of APC expression in atypical adenoma may be indicative of carcinoma

Electron Microscopy

- May have large number of microvilli
  - Thought to reflect higher level of endocrine activity
- More abundant rough endoplasmic reticulum and Golgi apparatus than nonneoplastic cells
- Annulate lamellae may be seen

DIFFERENTIAL DIAGNOSIS

Parathyroid Hyperplasia

- Multiple glands enlarged
- Histomorphologic changes of PPD in multiple glands
- Absent rim of normal &/or atrophic parathyroid

Parathyroid Carcinoma

- Typically associated with higher levels of serum calcium and PTH (than adenoma and hyperplasia)
- Clinically may be adherent to surrounding tissues
  - Per surgeon, difficulties in resection due to adhesions
  - Adenomas (and hyperplasias) not adherent to surrounding tissues
    - Exceptions occur in presence of prior trauma (e.g., prior surgery, post FNA)
    - Prior procedures may produce fibrosis resulting in adherence to surrounding structures
    - Histologic evidence may include hemosiderin deposition, cholesterol granulomas, foreign body giant cell reaction
- Diagnostic histologic features, including
  - Angioinvasion, invasion of adjacent structures (e.g., thyroid, others), neurotropism, metastasis
- Reduced expression or loss of tumor suppressor proteins parafibromin and APC
  - Diminished to absent parafibromin (nuclear) staining
    - Some carcinomas may be positive
  - Loss of APC expression frequent molecular event in carcinomas

SELECTED REFERENCES

1. Juhlin CC et al: Parafibromin and APC as screening markers for malignant potential in atypical parathyroid adenomas. Endocr Pathol. 21(3):166-77, 2010
2. Lieu D: Cytopathologist-performed ultrasound-guided fine-needle aspiration of parathyroid lesions. Diagn Cytopathol. 38(5):327-32, 2010
3. Iacobone M et al: Hyperparathyroidism-jaw tumor syndrome: a report of three large kindred. Langenbecks Arch Surg. 394(5):817-25, 2009
4. Mihai R et al: Surgical strategy for sporadic primary hyperparathyroidism an evidence-based approach to surgical strategy, patient selection, surgical access, and reoperations. Langenbecks Arch Surg. 394(5):785-98, 2009
5. DeLellis RA et al: Primary hyperparathyroidism: a current perspective. Arch Pathol Lab Med. 132(8):1251-62, 2008
6. Delellis RA: Challenging lesions in the differential diagnosis of endocrine tumors: parathyroid carcinoma. Endocr Pathol. 19(4):221-5, 2008
7. Gill AJ et al: Loss of nuclear expression of parafibromin distinguishes parathyroid carcinomas and hyperparathyroidism-jaw tumor (HPT-JT) syndrome-related adenomas from sporadic parathyroid adenomas and hyperplasias. Am J Surg Pathol. 30(9):1140-9, 2006
8. Simonds WF et al: Familial isolated hyperparathyroidism is rarely caused by germline mutation in HRPT2, the gene for the hyperparathyroidism-jaw tumor syndrome. J Clin Endocrinol Metab. 89(1):96-102, 2004
9. Tan MH et al: Loss of parafibromin immunoreactivity is a distinguishing feature of parathyroid carcinoma. Clin Cancer Res. 10(19):6629-37, 2004
10. Shattuck TM et al: Somatic and germ-line mutations of the HRPT2 gene in sporadic parathyroid carcinoma. N Engl J Med. 349(18):1722-9, 2003
11. Carpten JD et al: HRPT2, encoding parafibromin, is mutated in hyperparathyroidism-jaw tumor syndrome. Nat Genet. 32(4):676-80, 2002
12. Snover DC et al: Mitotic activity in benign parathyroid disease. Am J Clin Pathol. 75(3):345-7, 1981
13. Weiland LH et al: Lipoadenoma of the parathyroid gland. Am J Surg Pathol. 2(1):3-7, 1978

PARATHYROID ADENOMA

Imaging and Microscopic Features

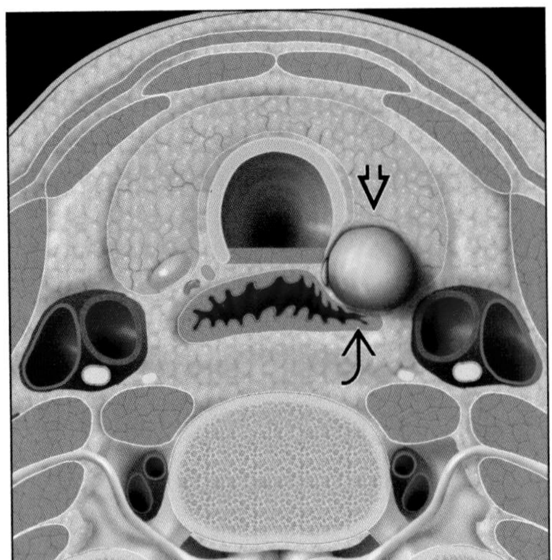

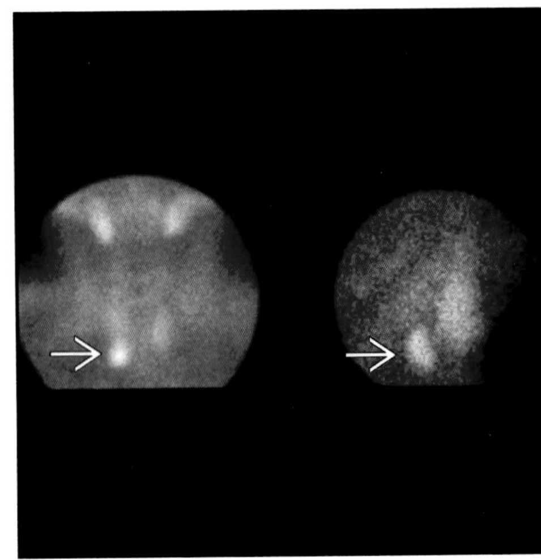

(Left) *Graphic depicts a solitary enlarged parathyroid gland ⇨ characterized by rounded borders. There is compression of the esophagus ➙ but absence of infiltrative growth, which might be of concern for a parathyroid carcinoma. Typically, adenomas are easily excised.* ***(Right)*** *Anterior (left) and right lateral (right) Tc-99m MIBI scan of the neck at 90 minutes post injection shows parathyroid adenoma ➡ posterior to the inferior aspect of the right thyroid lobe.*

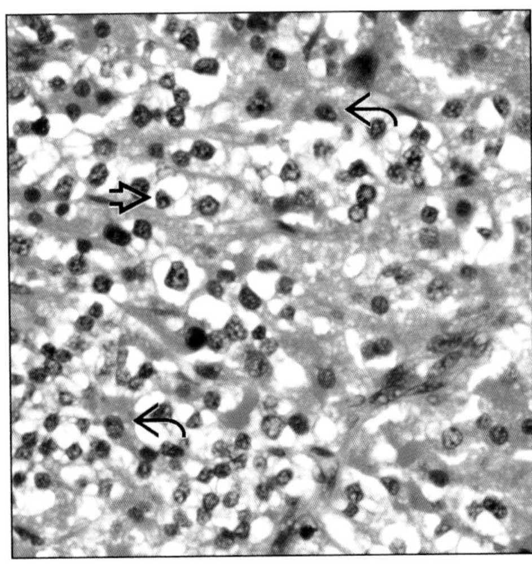

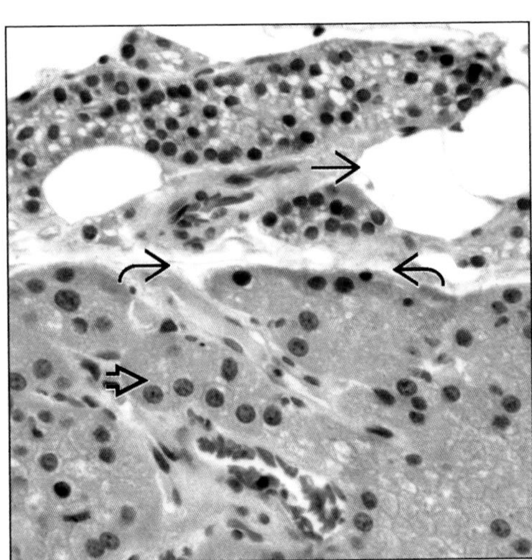

(Left) *Admixture of cell types includes chief cells with amphophilic to clear cytoplasm ⇨ and intermixed cells with oncocytic cytoplasmic changes ➙.* ***(Right)*** *Parathyroid oncocytic adenoma is entirely composed of oncocytic cells ⇨ with absent stromal fat. The adenoma is demarcated ➙ from a rim of normal parathyroid gland with stromal fat ➡. The nuclei of the adenoma are larger than the nuclei of the nonneoplastic parathyroid cells.*

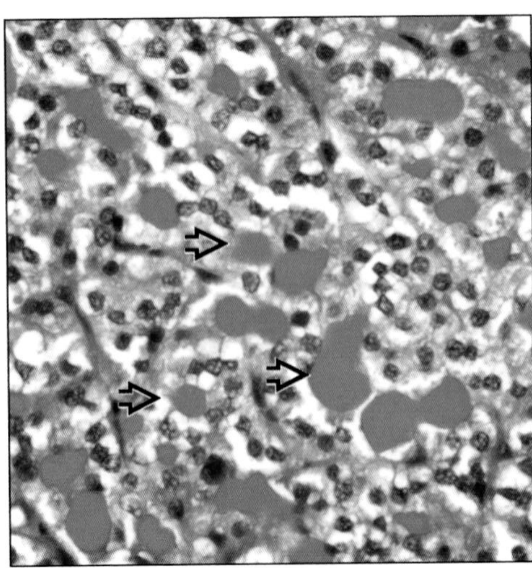

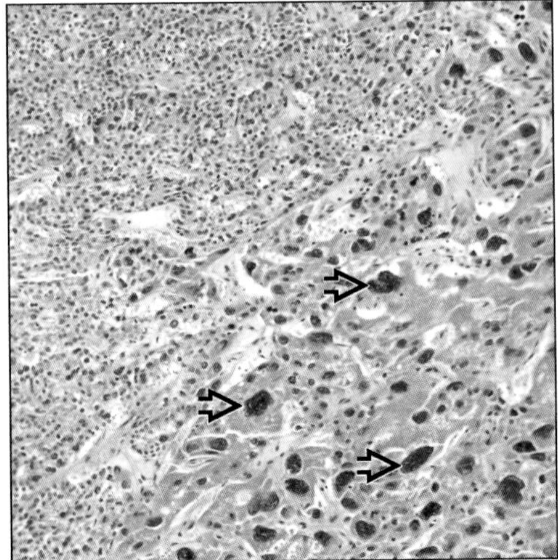

(Left) *Parathyroid adenoma (PA) shows a follicular growth pattern that may be confused with thyroid follicular neoplasms. Eosinophilic material in follicles resembles colloid ⇨ and is PAS(+) like colloid but, unlike colloid, is negative for thyroglobulin immunostaining (not shown).* ***(Right)*** *PA shows marked nuclear atypia with markedly enlarged, pleomorphic, and hyperchromatic nuclei ⇨. Nuclear pleomorphism raises concern for a diagnosis of carcinoma but is not a diagnostic feature of parathyroid carcinoma.*

Microscopic Features and Ancillary Techniques

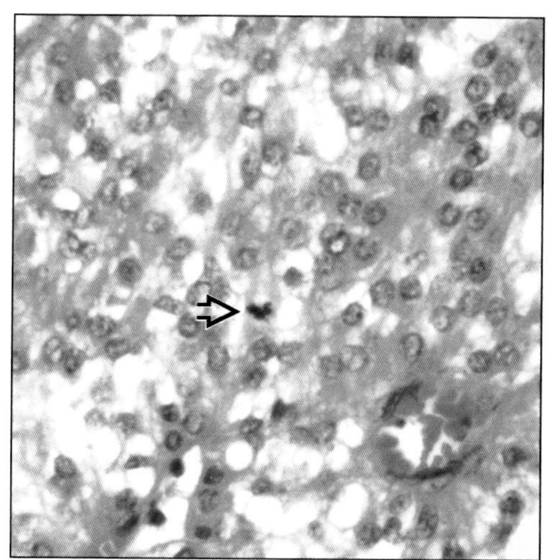

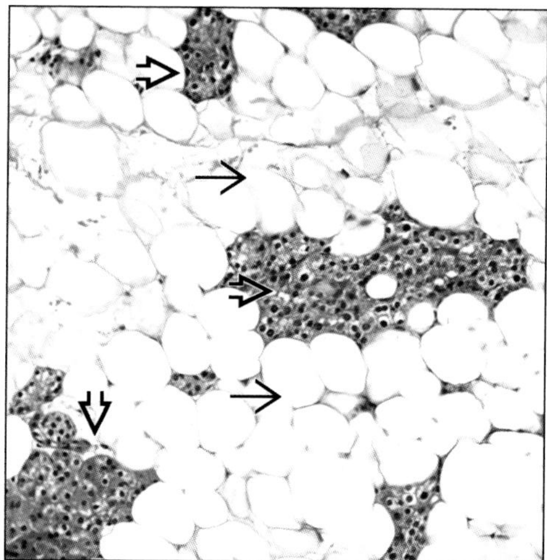

(Left) *Parathyroid adenoma shows a mitotic figure ➩. Mitoses can be identified in benign parathyroid proliferations (i.e., hyperplasia, adenoma) and are not, in and of themselves, diagnostic of a parathyroid carcinoma.* ***(Right)*** *Lipoadenomas are distinct parathyroid tumors associated with hyperparathyroidism and composed of a proliferation of parenchymal chief cells ➩ and abundant stromal fat cells ➔.*

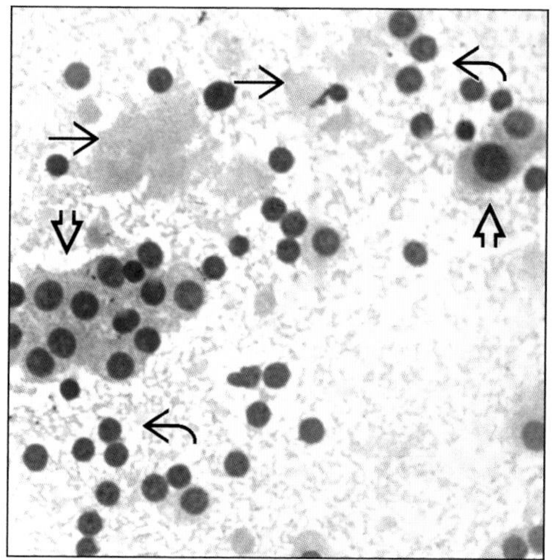

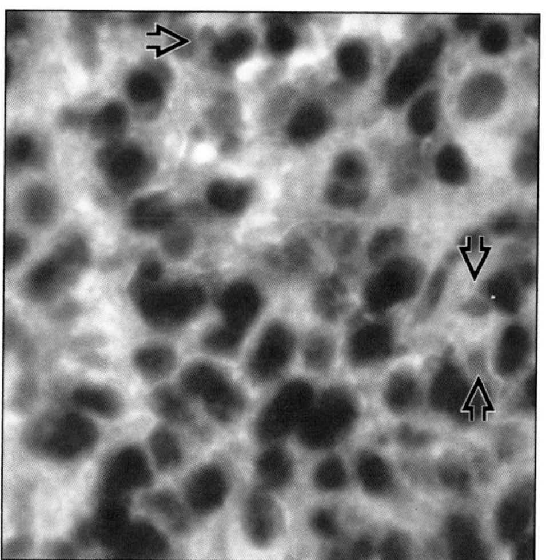

(Left) *Smear of a neck mass shows cohesive groups of small epithelial cells ➩ as well as fragments of pink colloid-like material ➔ suggesting a thyroid follicular lesion. The colloid-like material is sparse and the cells are fragile, yielding smears with numerous naked nuclei ↶, findings in support of a parathyroid lesion.* ***(Right)*** *Frozen section shows a small amount of fat within adenoma cells ➩. Decreased lipid is indicative of a hyperfunctioning lesion, as normal cells contain abundant lipid.*

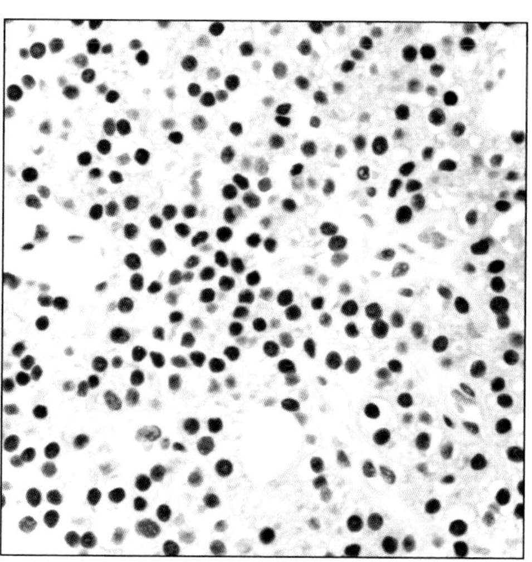

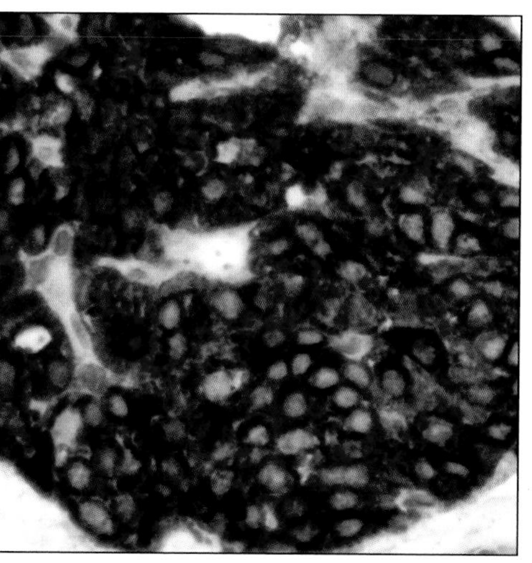

(Left) *Parathyroid adenoma shows diffuse parafibromin (nuclear) staining. The expression of parafibromin is believed to assist in differentiating adenoma from carcinoma. Parathyroid carcinomas show reduced to absent expression of parafibromin.* ***(Right)*** *Parathyroid adenoma shows cytoplasmic reactivity for parathyroid hormone (PTH). If there is uncertainty whether a lesion is of parathyroid origin, the expression of PTH is confirmatory of a parathyroid proliferation.*

PARATHYROID CARCINOMA

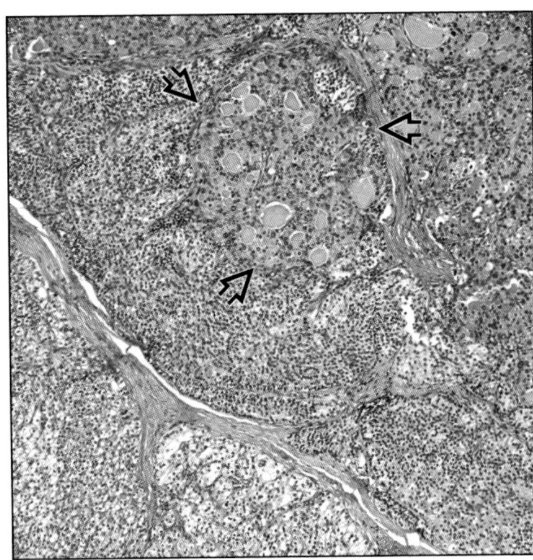

Hematoxylin & eosin shows an invasive parathyroid carcinoma nearly completely surrounding thyroid gland tissue ⊳. Adherence to the thyroid gland is one of the histologic features of malignancy.

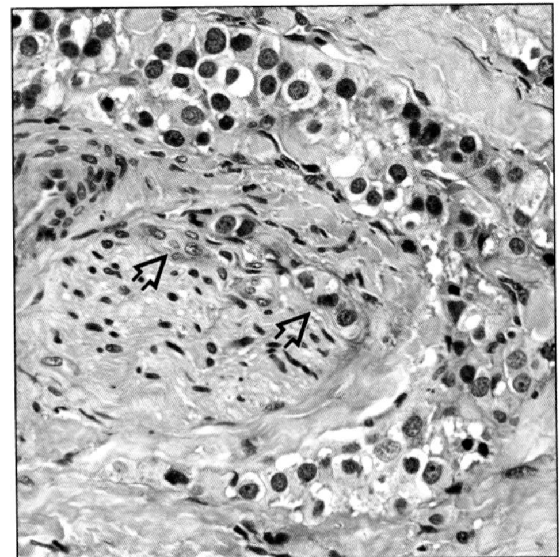

No one histologic feature is diagnostic for parathyroid carcinoma; intraneural ⊳ or perineural invasion is a feature only seen in carcinoma, although only present in about 5% of tumors.

TERMINOLOGY

Abbreviations

- Parathyroid hormone (PTH)
- Hereditary hyperparathyroidism-jaw tumor syndrome (HPT-JT)

Definitions

- Malignant neoplasm of parathyroid parenchymal cells
  - No malignant adipose tumors are recognized in parathyroid

ETIOLOGY/PATHOGENESIS

Irradiation

- Neck irradiation has been suggested as etiologic factor

Inherited

- Hyperparathyroidism-jaw tumor syndrome (*HRPT2* locus on chromosome 1)

Hyperplasia

- Secondary parathyroid hyperplasia is possible risk factor

CLINICAL ISSUES

Epidemiology

- Incidence
  - Accounts for < 2% of primary hyperparathyroidism in Western countries
- Age
  - Develops in wide age range, but predominantly in older adults
- Gender
  - Equal gender distribution
    - Distinctly different from marked female predominance among patients with parathyroid adenomas
    - Further support for de novo development of carcinoma instead of from adenoma
- Ethnicity
  - Japanese patients tend to have higher incidence of carcinoma (~ 5% of primary hyperparathyroidism)

Site

- Arises in any site in which parathyroid tissue may be found
  - Slightly more common in lower parathyroid glands

Presentation

- Effects of excessive parathyroid hormone secretion (PTH) and hypercalcemia dictate signs and symptoms
- Nonspecific symptoms include weakness, fatigue, anorexia, weight loss, nausea, vomiting, polyuria, polydipsia
- Nephrolithiasis, nephrocalcinosis, renal insufficiency and bone "brown tumors" generally develop in patients with high serum calcium levels; feature more common in carcinoma
  - Concomitant bone and stone disease is more frequent in parathyroid carcinoma than parathyroid adenoma
- Palpable neck mass, often difficult to excise
  - Due to adherence to soft tissues, nerves (recurrent laryngeal nerve) &/or thyroid gland
  - Identified in up to 75% of patients with carcinoma
- Hoarseness is common with recurrent laryngeal nerve involvement
  - Recurrent laryngeal nerve palsy in patient with primary hyperparathyroidism should suggest possibility of parathyroid carcinoma

Laboratory Tests

- Excessively high serum calcium levels (> 16 mg/dL) are more common in carcinoma
- Extremely high PTH levels (> 1,000 ng/L)
- Frankly elevated serum alkaline phosphatase activity (> 200 IU/L)

PARATHYROID CARCINOMA

Key Facts

Terminology
- Malignant neoplasm of parathyroid parenchymal cells

Clinical Issues
- Accounts for < 2% of primary hyperparathyroidism
- Effects of excessive PTH secretion and hypercalcemia create signs and symptoms
- Simultaneous bone and kidney stone disease more frequent in carcinoma
- Palpable neck mass, often difficult to excise
- Serum calcium > 16 mg/dL, PTH levels > 1,000 ng/L suggests carcinoma
- Recurrences develop in up to 60% of patients
- Disruption of capsule during surgery can result in parathyromatosis

Microscopic Pathology
- Large tumors with capsular and vascular invasion
- Perineural invasion is nearly pathognomonic
- Prominent, eosinophilic, irregular macronucleoli
- Tumor cell necrosis (comedonecrosis)
- Trabecular growth separated by thick, acellular, band-forming fibrosis

Ancillary Tests
- Mutations of *HRPT2* is associated with carcinoma development

Top Differential Diagnoses
- Parathyroid adenoma
- Medullary thyroid carcinoma
- Thyroid follicular neoplasms
- Metastatic renal cell carcinoma

Treatment
- Options, risks, complications
  - Must manage metabolic effects of PTH and hypercalcemia
    - Calcium metabolism adversely affects cardiovascular system
  - Recurrent laryngeal nerve damage/involvement can render hoarseness
- Surgical approaches
  - Best outcome when there is complete radical resection at first surgery

Prognosis
- Overall, indolent tumor with 5-year survival up to 85%
  - 10-year survival of approximately 50%
- Recurrences develop in up to 60% of patients
  - Documented by localization studies in patient with recurrent hypercalcemia
  - Once recurrence is present, cure is unlikely, although palliative surgery gives prolonged survival
  - Average time between surgery and first recurrence is usually < 3 years
- Disruption of capsule during surgery may cause seeding of parathyroid tissue (parathyromatosis)
  - Incisional biopsy is discouraged to prevent tumor cell seeding
- When metastatic disease develops, lung, bone, cervical and mediastinal lymph nodes, and liver are most frequently affected
  - If metastases are found, these patients eventually die from disease
  - Benign "brown tumors" (caused by profound hyperparathyroidism) can mimic bone metastases
  - Ossifying fibromas, component of HPT-JT syndrome, may also mimic bone metastases

IMAGE FINDINGS

General Features
- Tc-99m sestamibi scintigraphy is positive, documenting location, but does not separate adenoma from carcinoma
- Mass is frequently noted, but CT and MR do not have specific features

MACROSCOPIC FEATURES

General Features
- Large tumors
- Adherent to soft tissues, thyroid gland and nerves
- Firm, gray-white cut surface
- Central necrosis may be present
- Must use caution if there has been previous surgery, as scarring and hemorrhage may simulate "invasion"

Size
- Range: 1.5-6.0 cm
- Mean: 3 cm

MICROSCOPIC PATHOLOGY

Histologic Features
- No one histologic feature, other than metastatic disease, is considered diagnostic for parathyroid carcinoma
- Constellation of features can usually support diagnosis
- Perineural invasion is nearly pathognomonic
  - Present in only about 5% of cases
- Tumor cell necrosis (comedonecrosis)
- Chief cell neoplasms are more common than oncocytic neoplasms
- Adherence to thyroid gland
- Soft tissue extension
- Capsular invasion
  - Entrapped epithelium in degenerative fibrosis can mimic invasion

PARATHYROID CARCINOMA

- Autotransplanted hyperplastic parathyroid tissue may give seemingly invasive growth pattern
- Vascular invasion
  - Endothelial-lined space invasion or tumor thrombus in vessel
  - Identified in tumor capsule or in surrounding soft tissue rather than within tumor
- Thick, acellular, band-forming fibrosis between tumor cells
  - Proclivity for perivascular distribution or origin
  - Can be mixed with hemosiderin and hemorrhage
- Trabecular growth is most suggestive of malignancy
  - Solid, diffuse or organoid is suggestive, but not diagnostic
- Perivascular reserve-palisading of tumor cells
- Tumor cell monotony, although profound pleomorphism can be seen
- High nuclear to cytoplasmic ratio
- Spindling of tumor cells
- Prominent, eosinophilic, irregular macronucleoli
- Increased mitotic figures, including atypical forms
  - > 5/50 HPF is worrisome for carcinoma
- Tumor cell spindling, "watermelon seeds," and pyknosis suggest malignancy

Atypical Adenoma

- Intermediate category between adenoma and carcinoma
- Use for parathyroid neoplasm lacking unequivocal evidence of invasiveness, but showing some other feature(s) suspicious for malignancy
- Uncertain malignant potential, requiring close clinical follow-up
  - Long-term follow-up usually shows benign course

ANCILLARY TESTS

Cytology

- Separation of thyroid from parathyroid may be difficult
- Does not separate benign from malignant primary tumors
- Positive immunoreactions with chromogranin, parathyroid hormone, and keratins

Frozen Sections

- Of no value in separating benign from malignant disease

Flow Cytometry

- Unhelpful: Adenomas can be aneuploid and carcinomas are often diploid

Cytogenetics

- Significantly, many genomic alterations in parathyroid adenomas, including 11q (location of *MEN1* gene), are rarely identified in carcinomas
  - Supports de novo development of parathyroid carcinoma (not from adenoma)
  - Parathyroid carcinoma is not proven neoplasm of *MEN1*
- Mutations of *HRPT2* (inactivating germline mutations of this tumor suppressor gene), located on1q25, cause HPT-JT and some sporadic parathyroid carcinomas
  - Gene encodes parafibromin, which is lost in carcinoma (lack of nuclear staining)
- Cyclin-D1 appears to be overexpressed in carcinoma
- Recurrent losses of chromosome 13q in parathyroid carcinomas (CGH and molecular allelotyping)
  - 13q is region known to contain retinoblastoma (*RB1*) and *BRCA2* tumor suppressor genes
- LOH in 1p32.3-36.2
- Decreased *Rb* protein expression

DIFFERENTIAL DIAGNOSIS

Parathyroid Adenoma

- Setting of previous surgery or neck manipulation makes separation difficult
- Adenomas are usually smaller, but when adenomas are larger, they tend to have fibrosis, hemosiderin deposits, and cystic degeneration
- Rim of uninvolved/normal parathyroid parenchyma is rarely seen in parathyroid carcinoma
- Cells of adenoma are greatly enlarged and lack conspicuous nucleoli
- Mitotic activity is usually low (> 5% Ki-67 labeling index is worrisome for carcinoma)
- Adenomas **positive** with
  - p27
  - Bcl-2
  - MDM2
  - Parafibromin

Medullary Thyroid Carcinoma

- Direct extension or metastasis
- Chromogranin positive, but also calcitonin and CEA-m positive

Thyroid Follicular Neoplasms

- "**Follicular**" pattern can be seen in both tumor types
- Thyroid tumors have eosinophilic cytoplasm
  - Parathyroid tumors tend to have clear(er) cytoplasm and prominent cell borders
- TTF-1 and thyroglobulin will be positive

Metastatic Renal Cell Carcinoma

- May present as clear cell neoplasm in parathyroid gland
- Vascular pattern and sinusoidal growth
- Extravasated erythrocytes may help
- Immunoreactivity with vimentin, RCC, CD10, and EMA does not help
  - Positive in renal and parathyroid tumors

GRADING

System

- No grading used

PARATHYROID CARCINOMA

Immunohistochemistry

Antibody	Reactivity	Staining Pattern	Comment
Chromogranin-A	Positive	Cytoplasmic	Nearly all tumor cells
PTH	Positive	Cytoplasmic	Nearly all tumor cells
CK-PAN	Positive	Cytoplasmic	
CK7	Positive	Cytoplasmic	
CK18	Positive	Cytoplasmic	
RCC	Positive	Cell membrane & cytoplasm	Delicate staining, usually only focal
CD10	Positive	Cell membrane & cytoplasm	Positive in most tumors
EMA	Positive	Cytoplasmic	Reactive in most tumor cells
p16	Positive	Nuclear	
Cyclin-D1	Positive	Nuclear	Overexpressed in most carcinomas
Ki-67	Positive	Nuclear	> 5% may help separate between benign and malignant
S100	Positive		Highlights nerves (not tumor cells) which allow for the detection of perineural invasion
Parafibromin	Negative	Nuclear	Usually positive in adenoma but negative in carcinoma
TTF-1	Negative		
Thyroglobulin	Negative		

STAGING

System

- No AJCC staging criteria

SELECTED REFERENCES

1. Owen RP et al: Parathyroid carcinoma: A review. Head Neck. Epub ahead of print, 2010
2. Thompson LD: Parathyroid carcinoma. Ear Nose Throat J. 88(1):722-4, 2009
3. Delellis RA: Challenging lesions in the differential diagnosis of endocrine tumors: parathyroid carcinoma. Endocr Pathol. 19(4):221-5, 2008
4. Fakhran S et al: Parathyroid imaging. Neuroimaging Clin N Am. 18(3):537-49, ix, 2008
5. Marcocci C et al: Parathyroid carcinoma. J Bone Miner Res. 23(12):1869-80, 2008
6. DeLellis RA: Parathyroid carcinoma: an overview. Adv Anat Pathol. 12(2):53-61, 2005
7. Woodard GE et al: Parafibromin, product of the hyperparathyroidism-jaw tumor syndrome gene HRPT2, regulates cyclin D1/PRAD1 expression. Oncogene. 24(7):1272-6, 2005
8. Erickson LA et al: Oxyphil parathyroid carcinomas: a clinicopathologic and immunohistochemical study of 10 cases. Am J Surg Pathol. 26(3):344-9, 2002
9. Isotalo PA et al: Presence of birefringent crystals is useful in distinguishing thyroid from parathyroid gland tissues. Am J Surg Pathol. 26(6):813-4, 2002
10. Kameyama K et al: Parathyroid carcinomas: can clinical outcomes for parathyroid carcinomas be determined by histologic evaluation alone? Endocr Pathol. 13(2):135-9, 2002
11. Gupta A et al: Disseminated brown tumors from hyperparathyroidism masquerading as metastatic cancer: a complication of parathyroid carcinoma. Am Surg. 67(10):951-5, 2001
12. Shane E: Clinical review 122: Parathyroid carcinoma. J Clin Endocrinol Metab. 86(2):485-93, 2001
13. Kytölä S et al: Patterns of chromosomal imbalances in parathyroid carcinomas. Am J Pathol. 157(2):579-86, 2000
14. Farnebo F et al: Evaluation of retinoblastoma and Ki-67 immunostaining as diagnostic markers of benign and malignant parathyroid disease. World J Surg. 23(1):68-74, 1999
15. Vasef MA et al: Expression of cyclin D1 in parathyroid carcinomas, adenomas, and hyperplasias: a paraffin immunohistochemical study. Mod Pathol. 12(4):412-6, 1999
16. Agarwal SK et al: Comparative genomic hybridization analysis of human parathyroid tumors. Cancer Genet Cytogenet. 106(1):30-6, 1998
17. Carling T et al: Parathyroid MEN1 gene mutations in relation to clinical characteristics of nonfamilial primary hyperparathyroidism. J Clin Endocrinol Metab. 83(8):2960-3, 1998
18. Bondeson L et al: Cytopathological variables in parathyroid lesions: a study based on 1,600 cases of hyperparathyroidism. Diagn Cytopathol. 16(6):476-82, 1997
19. Vargas MP et al: The role of prognostic markers (MiB-1, RB, and bcl-2) in the diagnosis of parathyroid tumors. Mod Pathol. 10(1):12-7, 1997
20. Cinti S et al: Ultrastructure of human parathyroid cells in health and disease. Microsc Res Tech. 32(2):164-79, 1995
21. Lloyd RV et al: Immunohistochemical Analysis of the Cell Cycle-Associated Antigens Ki-67 and Retinoblastoma Protein in Parathyroid Carcinomas and Adenomas. Endocr Pathol. 6(4):279-287, 1995
22. Hakaim AG et al: Parathyroid carcinoma: 50-year experience at The Cleveland Clinic Foundation. Cleve Clin J Med. 60(4):331-5, 1993
23. Smith JF: The pathological diagnosis of carcinoma of the parathyroid. Clin Endocrinol (Oxf). 38(6):662, 1993
24. Mallette LE: DNA quantitation in the study of parathyroid lesions. A review. Am J Clin Pathol. 98(3):305-11, 1992
25. Sandelin K et al: Prognostic factors in parathyroid cancer: a review of 95 cases. World J Surg. 16(4):724-31, 1992
26. Wynne AG et al: Parathyroid carcinoma: clinical and pathologic features in 43 patients. Medicine (Baltimore). 71(4):197-205, 1992
27. Bondeson AG et al: Fat staining in parathyroid disease--diagnostic value and impact on surgical strategy: clinicopathologic analysis of 191 cases. Hum Pathol. 16(12):1255-63, 1985

PARATHYROID CARCINOMA

Radiographic and Microscopic Features

*(**Left**) A radionucleotide scan (Sestamibi) at 4-hour delay shows a single mass in the neck. This test does not separate between benign and malignant parathyroid tumors but does suggest a neoplasm vs. hyperplasia as the potential cause of hyperparathyroidism. (**Right**) Islands of tumor have invaded beyond the capsule of the neoplasm. This is a finding most suggestive of parathyroid carcinoma.*

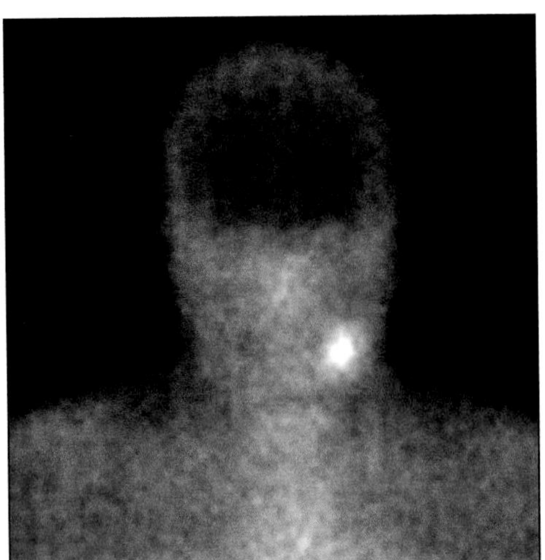

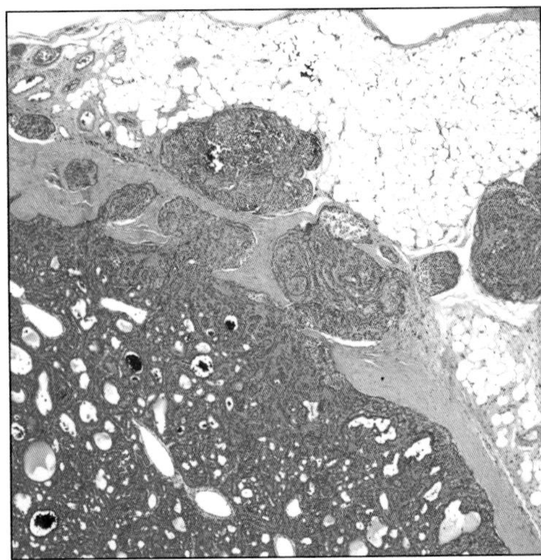

*(**Left**) Hematoxylin & eosin demonstrates a vessel with the lumen filled with tumor cells. Thrombus of tumor, like this, is not a feature seen in benign lesions. (**Right**) The neoplastic cells are arranged in a trabecular architecture, separated by delicate fibrous connective tissue bands. Trabeculae are usually 8-10 cells wide. This is usually not a feature seen in adenoma, although focal trabeculae can be seen.*

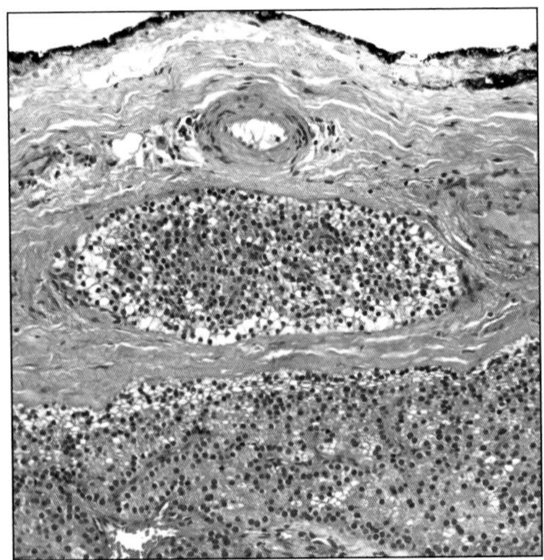

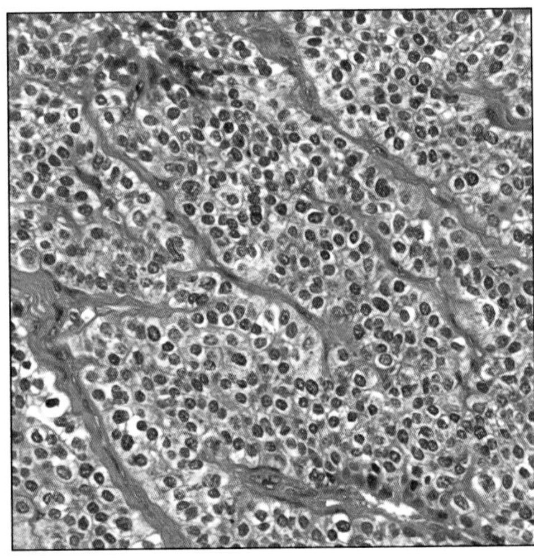

*(**Left**) Heavy, dense, acellular eosinophilic fibrosis is frequently seen in carcinoma. The fibrosis often begins around vessels ⇨. There is no associated hemosiderin or degeneration. (**Right**) This tumor shows an abrupt transition from one pattern to another, showing completely different histologic appearance. The lower portion of the field → shows a neoplastic population that has a significantly higher nuclear to cytoplasmic ratio and a more glandular architecture than the top.*

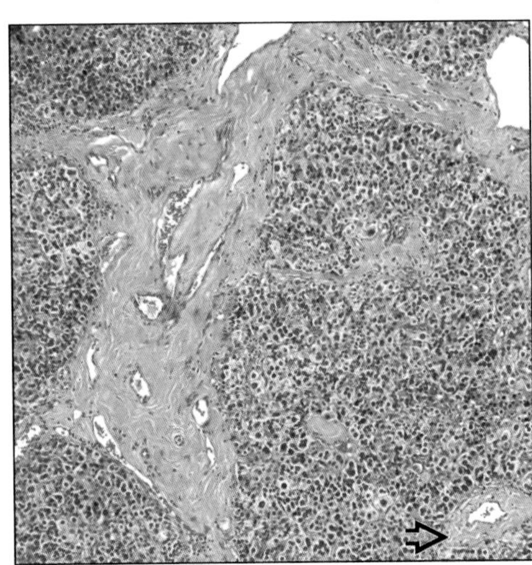

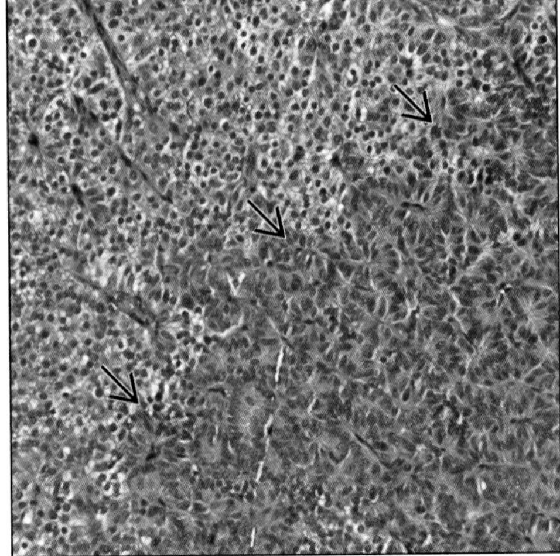

Microscopic and Immunohistochemical Features

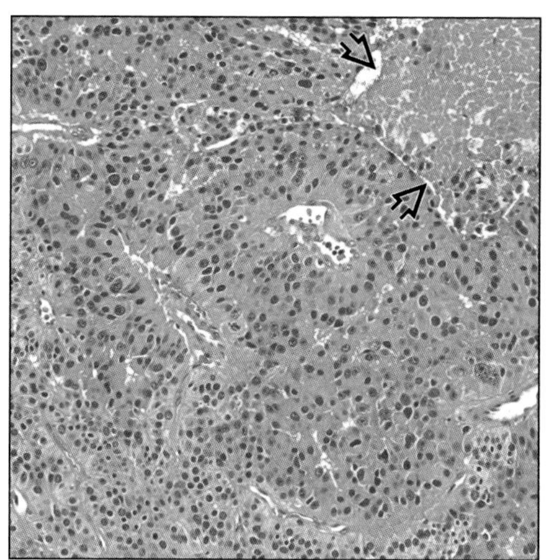

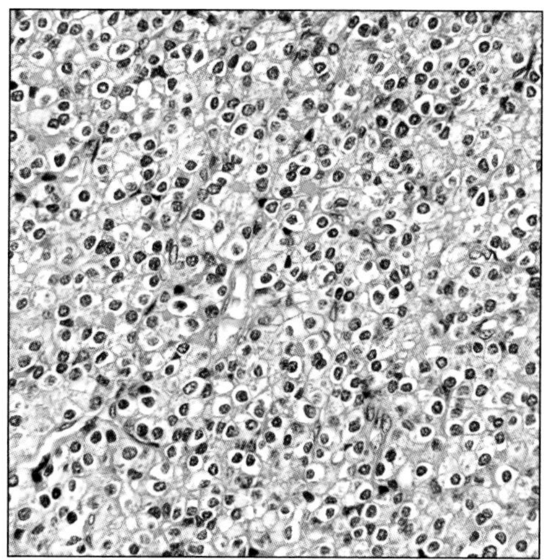

(Left) *Hematoxylin & eosin demonstrates an oncocytic or oxyphilic neoplastic population. The cells are greatly enlarged. Tumor cell necrosis ➪ is identified. Genuine tumor cell necrosis is not present in benign lesions.* ***(Right)*** *There is a sheet-like distribution of these neoplastic cells. They possess a high nuclear to cytoplasmic ratio, hyperchromatic nuclei, and a perinuclear halo, highlighting the cellular borders.*

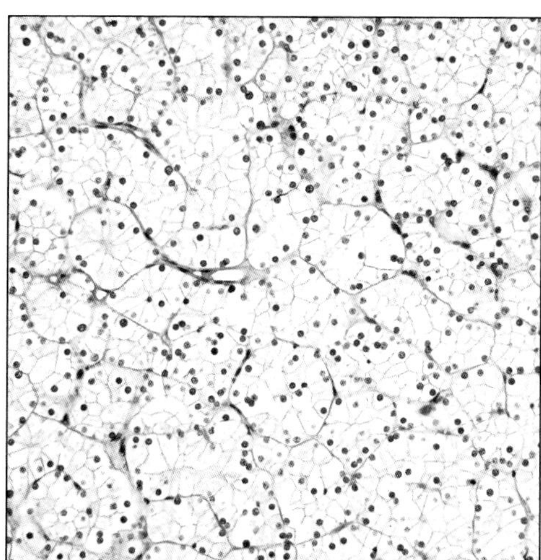

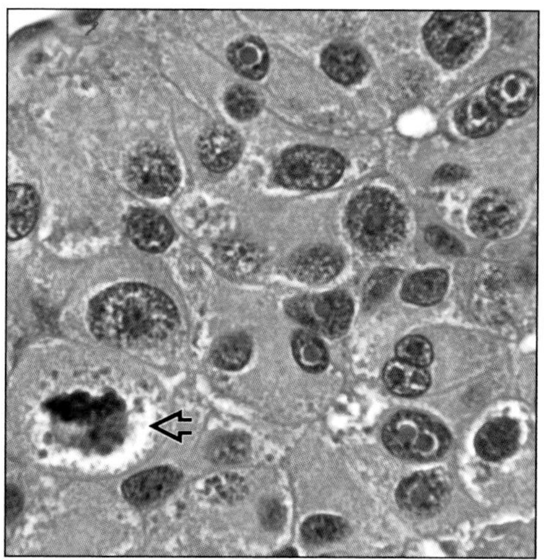

(Left) *Clear cell change is not a common finding in parathyroid carcinoma. This tumor, if viewed on high power only, does not show the characteristics of parathyroid carcinoma, even though the tumor had necrosis and perineural invasion elsewhere.* ***(Right)*** *Very large neoplastic cells with prominent, brightly eosinophilic, and irregular nucleoli are shown. There is a perinucleolar halo, a finding seen in carcinoma. Note the atypical mitotic figure ➪.*

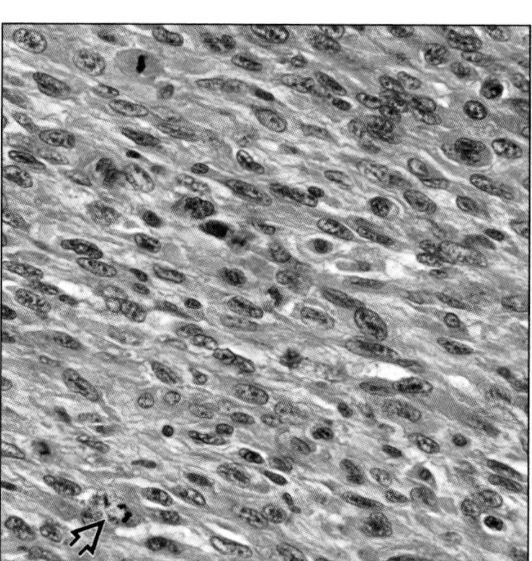

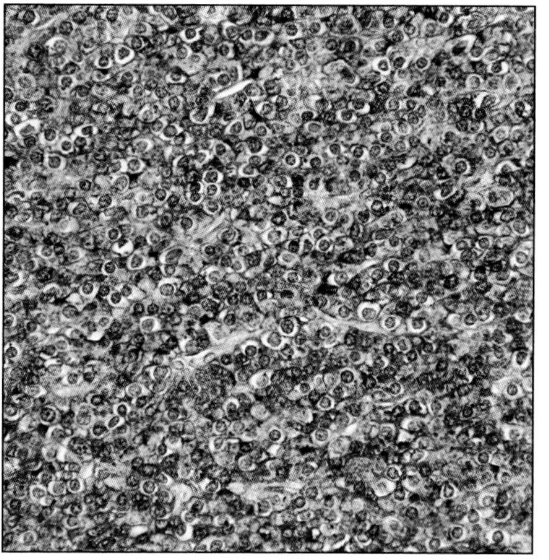

(Left) *Although uncommon, a predominantly or focally spindle cell pattern can be seen in carcinoma. There are mitotic figures, including an atypical form ➪. Typical glandular features of parathyroid tissue are usually identified somewhere within the tumor.* ***(Right)*** *Chromogranin is generally positive in parathyroid tissue. In this case, there is a membrane reactivity, although often a granular cytoplasmic reaction is present. Immunohistochemistry alone does not confirm carcinoma.*

METASTATIC/SECONDARY TUMORS

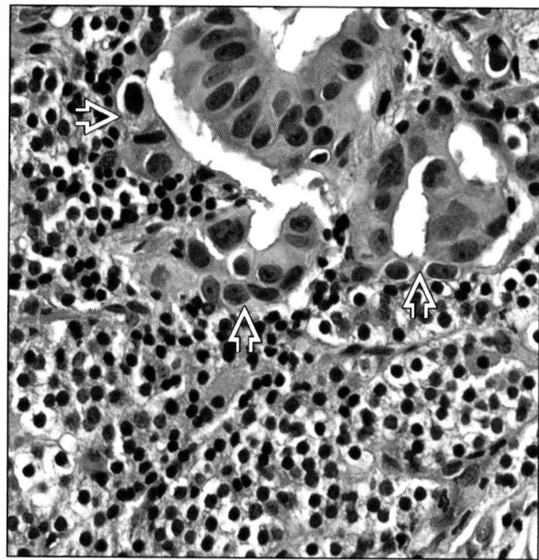

A metastatic breast adenocarcinoma ➡ is identified within the parenchyma of a parathyroid adenoma. Metastases are identified in abnormal parathyroid tissue more often than normal tissue.

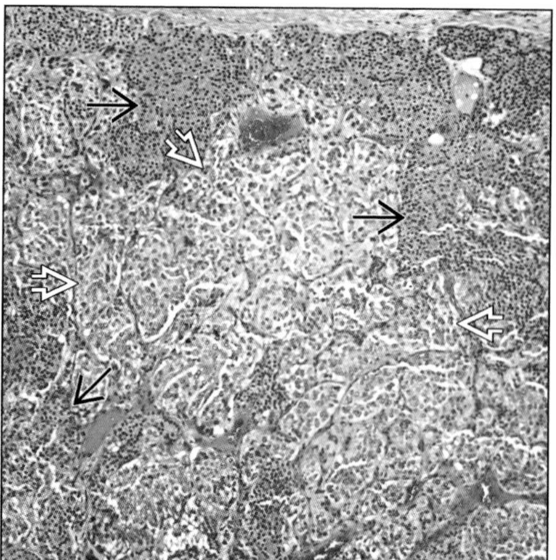

There is an intimate relationship between the parathyroid parenchyma ➡ and the paraganglioma ➡. Separation of these 2 elements would require immunohistochemical evaluation.

TERMINOLOGY

Definitions

- Tumors secondarily involving parathyroid gland as result of hematogenous/lymphatic spread from primary malignancies of distant sites
  - Direct extension from contiguous structures (larynx, trachea, pharynx, thyroid, esophagus, lymph nodes, neck soft tissues, mediastinum) is excluded
- Lymphomas and leukemias are excluded

ETIOLOGY/PATHOGENESIS

Pathogenesis

- Parathyroid gland is richly vascularized, but tends not to have high frequency of metastases
- Abnormal parathyroid tissue (hyperplasia, adenoma, carcinoma) seem to contain metastases more frequently than normal tissue
  - Alterations in vascularity or blood flow may contribute to metastatic disease development

CLINICAL ISSUES

Epidemiology

- Incidence
  - Depends on underlying frequency of primary tumor
  - < 0.1% of parathyroid glands removed surgically
  - ~ 1% in autopsied patients with disseminated malignancies
- Age
  - All ages affected
  - Tend to be older (mean: 7th decade)
- Gender
  - Female > Male (1.2:1)
    - Increased metastases of breast and gynecologic primaries compared to prostate primaries

Site

- Unknown due to asymptomatic presentation
- Involves multiple glands (if removed)

Presentation

- Vast majority of patients are asymptomatic
- Occasionally mass in neck
- Hyper- or hypoparathyroidism are exceptionally rare
- Primary site depends on age and gender
  - Carcinomas are most common
    - Breast (lobular > ductal), lung, kidney
    - Melanoma, soft tissue sarcomas
    - All anatomic sites are potential candidates
- Direct extension from laryngeal or esophageal squamous cell carcinoma may be identified
- Paraganglioma or soft tissue tumors rarely affect parathyroid tissue

Laboratory Tests

- Generally, no parathyroid hormone or calcium abnormalities
- Primary hyperparathyroidism may be present

Treatment

- Surgical approaches
  - Parathyroidectomy, especially if slow-growing tumor or isolated metastasis

Prognosis

- Usually poor outcome, determined by primary type
- Metastases to parathyroid gland correlate with poor prognosis
  - Seldom isolated parathyroid metastases; usually extensive multiorgan metastases
- Management is usually symptomatic or palliative

MACROSCOPIC FEATURES

General Features

- Gland may be slightly enlarged

METASTATIC/SECONDARY TUMORS

Key Facts

Terminology
- Tumors secondarily involving parathyroid gland as result of hematogenous/lymphatic spread from primary malignancies of distant sites

Clinical Issues
- < 0.1% of parathyroid glands removed surgically
- Carcinomas are most common
  - Breast (lobular > ductal), lung, kidney
- Metastases to parathyroid gland correlate with poor prognosis

Microscopic Pathology
- Features of primary tumor are usually maintained
- Lymphatic or vascular location of tumor emboli

Ancillary Tests
- Metastatic tumors have unique immunohistochemical profiles, distinct from parathyroid primaries, except renal cell carcinoma

  - Metastases not usually identified grossly
- Direct extension may result in "attachment" to thyroid, larynx, or esophagus
- Metastases may be multifocal

Size
- Wide range, but vast majority are "microscopic"

MICROSCOPIC PATHOLOGY

Histologic Features
- Features of primary tumor are usually maintained
- Lymphatic or vascular location of tumor emboli
- If direct extension, tumor is usually large, incidentally encompassing parathyroid
- Lymphomas and squamous cell carcinomas are easy to distinguish from primary lesions
- Secondary tumors have unique morphology (lymphoma, paraganglioma)

ANCILLARY TESTS

Immunohistochemistry
- Metastatic tumors have unique immunohistochemical profiles, distinct from parathyroid primaries
  - Exceptions are known
  - Renal cell carcinoma and primary parathyroid lesions are EMA, RCC, CD10 immunoreactive

DIFFERENTIAL DIAGNOSIS

Clear Cell Adenoma
- Distinct population of cells that compress surrounding parathyroid parenchyma
- Lacks lymph-vascular invasion
- Lacks vascular pattern, extravasated erythrocytes

Medullary Carcinoma
- May directly invade into parathyroid tissue
- Positive with calcitonin, CEA-M, TTF-1, along with chromogranin, synaptophysin, and CD56

SELECTED REFERENCES

1. Levy MT et al: Primary paraganglioma of the parathyroid: a case report and clinicopathologic review. Head Neck Pathol. 4(1):37-43, 2010
2. Boggess MA et al: Renal clear cell carcinoma appearing as a left neck mass. Ear Nose Throat J. 75(9):620-22, 1996
3. Bumpers HL et al: Endocrine organ metastases in subjects with lobular carcinoma of the breast. Arch Surg. 128(12):1344-7, 1993
4. Benisovich VI et al: A case of adenocarcinoma of the lung associated with a neck mass and hypercalcemia. Cancer. 68(5):1106-8, 1991
5. Goddard CJ et al: Symptomatic hypocalcaemia associated with metastatic invasion of the parathyroid glands. Br J Hosp Med. 43(1):72, 1990
6. Horwitz CA et al: Secondary malignant tumors of the parathyroid glands. Report of two cases with associated hypoparathyroidism. Am J Med. 52(6):797-808, 1972

IMAGE GALLERY

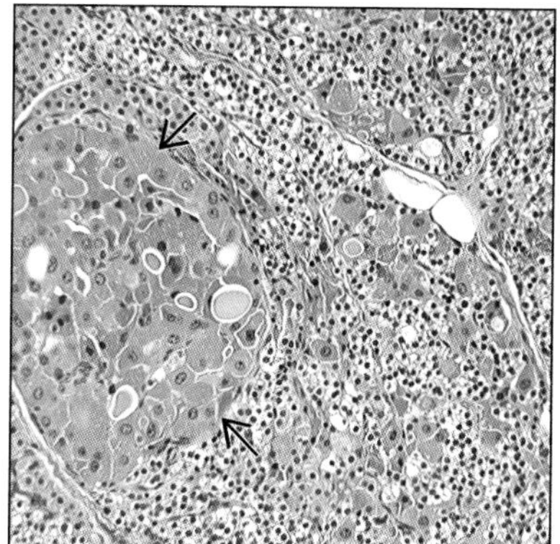

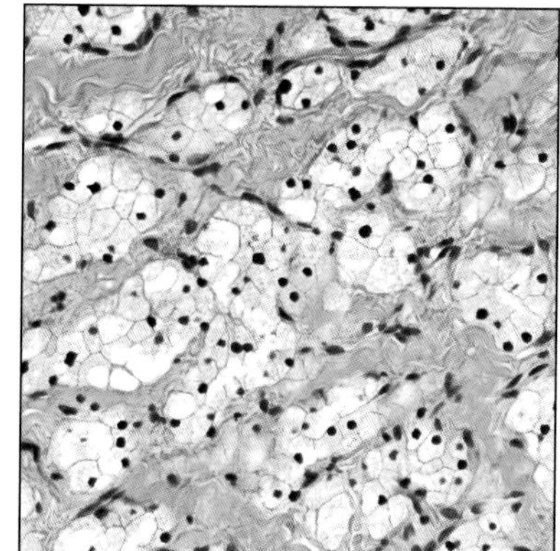

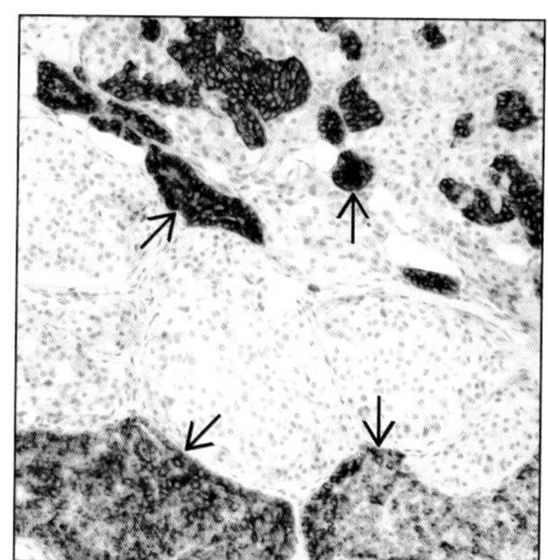

(Left) *This is an example of metastatic thyroid follicular carcinoma (oncocytic type) ⇒ to the parathyroid gland. There is a distinct "nodule" of tumor that is morphologically malignant, distinct from the surrounding parathyroid tissue.* ***(Center)*** *A clear cell parathyroid adenoma can morphologically mimic a metastatic clear cell renal cell carcinoma. However, the cytoplasm is slightly oxyphilia, and there are no pseudoalveolar erythrocyte collections.* ***(Right)*** *Parathyroid hormone ⇒ can help to separate parathyroid tissue from metastatic tumor.*

Antibody Index

ANTIBODY INDEX

Antibodies Discussed

Antibody Name/Symbol	Antibody Description	Clones/Alternative Names
α-1-antichromotrypsin	alpha 1 antichromotrypsin	A1ACT
α-1-antitrypsin	alpha 1 antitrypsin	A1AT
α-amylase	alpha amylase	A-amylase
α-fetoprotein	alpha 1 fetoprotein	AFP, Z5A06, Clone C3
β-catenin	beta catenin; involved in regulation of cell adhesion and in signal transduction through Wnt pathway	B-catenin, CLONE 14, E-5, RB-9035Po, 17C2, 5H10
β-catenin cytoplasm		B-caten-cyt
β-tubulin	beta tubulin	B-tubulin, TUJ1
κ light chain	kappa light chain	KAPPA
λ light chain	lambda light chain	LAMBDA
12C3	early malignant change in ovary, non-commercial	
34βE12	cytokeratin -high molecular weight (34bE12- CK 1, 5, 10, 14)	MA-903, CK903
ACTH	adrenocorticotropic hormone	
Actin-HHF-35	actin, muscle (HHF35)	MSA, HHF-35
Actin-SM	actin, smooth muscle	SMA, ASM-1, CGA7, 1A4, HUC1-1
AE1/AE3	AE1/AE3; mixture of 2 anticytokeratin clones that detect a variety of both high-and low- molecular weight cytokeratins	
AFP	Alpha 1 fetoprotein	α-fetoprotein, Z5A06, Clone C3
ALK	anaplastic lymphoma kinase 1	ALK1, 5A4, ALKC
Amylase		
Androgen receptor	Dihydrotestosterone receptor; nuclear receptor subfamily 3, group C, member 4	AR441, F39.4.1, AR-N20, AR27
APC	adenomatous polyposis coliprotein	
B72.3	tumor-associated glycoprotein 72	TAG72, CC49, TAG-72, BRST-3
BCL-2	B-cell lymphoma 2; suppresses apoptosis in a variety of cell systems	ONCL2, BCL2/100/D5, 124, 124.3
BCL-6	B-cell CLL /lymphoma 6	LN22, GI191E/A8, N-3, PG-B6P, P1F6, 3FR-1
BCL-10	B-cell CLL/lymphoma 10	151, 331.3
BER-EP4	epithelial cell adhesion molecule	AUA1, VU-1D9, EPCAM, C10, HEA125
Brachyury	crucial regulator of notochordal development and biomarker for chordomas	
BRST-2	gross cystic fluid protein 15	GCDFP-15, 23A3, D6, AB-1, SABP, GPIP4, Gp17
CA125	Mucin 16	OV185:1, OC125, MUC16
Calcitonin	polypeptide hormone produced by parafollicular cells (C cells) of the thyroid	CALBINDIN28
Calponin	thin filament-associated protein that is implicated in regulation and modulation of smooth muscle contraction	N3, 26A11, CALP, CNN1, SMCC, Sm Calp
Calretinin	29 kDa calcium binding protein that is expressed in central and peripheral nervous system and in many normal and pathological tissues	DAK-CALRET, 5A5, CAL 3F5, DC8, AB149
CAM5.2	cytokeratin 8/18 (CAM5.2)	5D3, Zym5.2, 5D3, CAM 5.2, KER 10.11, NCL-5D3
CD1a	T-cell surface glycoprotein	JPM30, CD1A, O10, NA1/34
CD2	T-cell surface antigen, LFA2	271, MT910, AB75, LFA-2
CD3	T-cell receptor	F7238, A0452, CD3-P, CD3-M, SP7, PS1
CD4	T-cell surface glycoprotein L3T4	IF6, 1290, 4B12, CD4
CD5	T-cell surface glycoprotein Leu1, T1	NCL-CD5 4C7 54/B4 54/F6
CD8	T-cell coreceptor antigen, Leu2, T-cytotoxic cells	M7103, C8/144, C8/144B
CD10	neutral endopeptidase	CALLA, neprilysin, neutral endopeptidase, NEP
CD11c	integrin alpha X chain protein	LEU-M5
CD15	reacts with Reed-Sternberg cells of Hodgkin disease and with granulocytes	VIM-2,3C4, LEU-M1, TU9, VIM-D5, MY1, CBD1, MMA, 3CD1, C3D1, Lewis x, SSEA-1

ANTIBODY INDEX

CD20	membrane spanning 4 domains of B-lymphocytes	FB1, B1, L26, MS4A1
CD21	CR2, complement component receptor 2, Epstein-Barr virus receptor	IF8
CD23	Fc ϵ RII, low-affinity IgE receptor, IGEBF	1B12, MHM6BU38
CD24	sialic acid epitope of B lymphocytes	BA-1
CD30	tumor necrosis factor receptor SF8	BER-H2, KI-1, TNFRSF8
CD31	PECAM-1, platelet endothelial cell adhesion molecule	JC/70, JC/70A, PECAM-1
CD34	hematopoietic progenitor cell antigen	MY10, IOM34, QBEND10, 8G12, 1309, HPCA-1, HPCA, NU-4A1, TUK4, clone 581, BI-3c5
CD35	erythrocyte complement receptor 1, CR1, immune adherence receptor, C3b/C4b receptor	CR1, BER-MAC-DRC, TO5, CD35, E11
CD38	acute lymphoblastic leukemia cell antigen, T 10	SPC32, VS38, T10
CD43	Major sialoglycoprotein on surface of human T-lymphocytes, monocytes, granulocytes, and some B-lymphocytes	LEU-22, DF-T1, L60, MT1, sialophorin, leukosialin, SPN
CD45	leukocyte common antigen	LCA, PD7/26, 1.22/4.14, T29/33, RP2/18, PD7, 2D1, 2B11+PD7/26
CD45RA	isoform of CD45 expressed by naive T cells	4KB5, MT2, CD45RA, MB1
CD45RB	isoform of CD45 expressed by naive and memory T cells	
CD56	NCAM (neutral cellular adhesion molecule)	MAB 735, ERIC-1, 25-KD11, 123C3, 24-MB2, BC56C04, 1B6, 14-MAB735, NCC-LU-243, MOC-1, NCAM
CD57	β-1,3-glucuronyltransferase 1 (glucuronosyltransferase P)	LEU-7, NK1, HNK-1, TB01, B3GAT1
CD68	cytoplasmic granule protein of monocytes, macrophages	PG-M1, KP-1, LN5
CD70	cellular ligand of TNF receptor family member CD27 that is expressed transiently on activated T and B cells	
CD79-α	immunoglobulin-associated alpha, MB1	MB-1, 11D10, 11E3, CD79A, HM47/A9, HM57, JCB117
CD99	cell surface glycoprotein for migration, T cell adhesion, MIC2	CD99-MEMB, MIC2, 12E7, HBA71, O13, P30/32MIC2, M3601
CD117	C-kit; tyrosine-protein kinase activity	C-19 (C-KIT), 104D2, 2E4, C-KIT, A4502, H300, CMA-767
CD138	syndecan; a useful marker for plasma cells	B-B4, AM411-10M, MI15
CD163	Macrophage hemoglobin scavenging system	10D6
CD207	type II transmembrane cell surface receptor produced by Langerhans cells	langerin
CDK4	Cyclin dependent kinase 4	DCS-31
CDX-2	caudal-type homeobox transcription factor 2	AMT28, 7C7/D4, CDX-2-88
CEA-M	carcinoembryonic antigen, monoclonal	mCEA, CEA-B18, CEA-D14, CEA-GOLD 1, T84.6, CEA-GOLD 2, CEA 11, CEA-GOLD 3, CEA 27, CEA-GOLD 4, CEA 41, CEA-GOLD 5, T84.1, CEA-M, A5B7, CEJ065, IL-7, T84.66, TF3H8-1, 0062, D14, alpha-7, PARLAM 1, ZC23, CEM010, A115, COL-1, AF4, 12.140.10, 11-7, M773, CEA-M431_31, CEJO65
CEA-P	carcinoembryonic antigen, polyclonal	
CGRP	calcitonin gene related peptide	
Chromogranin-A	pituitary secretory protein 1	PHE-5, PHE5, E001, DAK-A3
Chromogranin-B	Secretogranin 1	PE-11, SECRETONEUR
CITED-1	melanocyte specific gene 1 antibody, CBP/P300-interacting transactivator 1	J72220K, MSG1
CK1	cytokeratin 1	CK 01, 34BB4
CK4	cytokeratin 4	215B8, 6B10
CK5/6	cytokeratin 5/6, high molecular weight cytokeratins	D5/16 B4
CK7	cytokeratin 7, low molecular weight cytokeratin	K72.7, KS7.18, OVTL 12/30, LDS-68, CK 07
CK8	cytokeratin 8	K8.8, 4.1.18, TS1, C-51, M20
CK10	cytokeratin 10	LHP1, DE-K10, RKSE60
CK10/13	cytokeratin 10/13	DE-K13, A3.3
CK13	cytokeratin 13	KS13.1, KS-1A3, AE8, 2D7

ANTIBODY INDEX

CK14	cytokeratin 14, high molecular weight cytokeratin	LL002
CK17	cytokeratin 17	E3
CK18	cytokeratin 18	M9, DC-10, CY-90, KS18.04
CK19	cytokeratin 19, low molecular weight cytokeratin	BA17, RCK108, LP2K, B170, A53-BA2, KS19.1, 170.2.14
CK20	cytokeratin 20, low molecular weight cytokeratin	KS20.8
CK8/18/CAM5.2	cytokeratin 8/18; simple epithelial-type cytokeratins	5D3, Zym5.2, CAM 5.2, KER 10.11, NCL-5D3, cytokeratin LMW
CK-HMW-NOS	high molecular weight cytokeratin, not otherwise specified	
C-KIT	C-kit; tyrosine-protein kinase activity	CD117, C-19 (C-KIT), 104D2, 2E4, C-KIT, A4502, H300, CMA-767
CK-LMW-NOS	low molecular weight cytokeratin, not otherwise specified	
CK-PAN	cytokeratin-pan (AE1/AE3/LP34); cocktail of high and low molecular weight cytokeratins	keratin pan, MAK-6, K576, LU-5, KL-1, KC-8, MNF 116, pankeratin, pancytokeratin
Claudin-1	senescence-associated epithelial membrane protein	JAD.8
Clusterin	clusterin, alpha chain specific	41D, E5
CMV	cytomegalovirus	
Collagen IV	major constituent of the basement membranes along with laminins, proteoglycans, and enactins	CIV22, COL4A [1-5], collagen α-1(IV) chain
Cyclin-D1	protein with important cell cycle regulatory functions	bcl-1 (cyclin D1) A-12, PRAD1, AM29, DCS-6, SP4, 5D4, D1GM, P2D11F11, CCND1Cyl-1
Desmin	class III intermediate filaments found in muscle cells	M760, DE-R-11, D33, DE5, DE-U-10, ZC18
EBER	Epstein-Barr virus encoded RNA	
EBV-LMP	Epstein-Barr virus latent membrane protein	LMP1, CS 1-4
E-cadherin	epithelial calcium dependent adhesion molecule	36B5, ECH-6, ECCD-2, CDH1, 5H9, NCH 38, CLONE 36, 4A2 C7, E9, 67A4, HECD-1, SC-8426
EGFR	v-erb-b1 erythroblastic leukemia viral gene,epidermal growth factor receptor	2-18C9, EGFR1, EGFR PHRMDX, NCL-R1, H11, C-ERBB-1, E30, EGFR, EGFR.113, 31G7, 3C6
EMA	epithelial membrane antigen	GP1.4, 214D4, MC5, E29
EpCam/BER-EP4/CD326	epithelial cell adhesion molecule	AUA1, VU-1D9, EPCAM, C10, HEA125, BER-EP4
ER	estrogen receptor protein	1D5, 6F11, SP1, 15D, H222, TE111, ERP, ER1D5, NCLER611, NCL-ER-LH2, PGP-1A6
ERP-β	estrogen receptor protein beta	ER-BETA, 14C8, 57/3, PPG5/10
Fascin	marker for Reed-Sternberg cells of Hodgkin disease	55K2
FLI-1	Friend leukemia virus integration 1	GI146-222, SC356
FVIIIRAg	factor VIII-related antigen	F8/86, von Willebrand factor
FXIIIA	factor-XIIIA (fibrin stabilizing factor)	
Galectin-3		NCL-GAL3, B2C10, 9C4
GCDFP-15	gross cystic fluid protein 15	23A3, BRST-2, D6, SABP, GPIP4, Gp17
GFAP	glial fibrillary acidic protein	6F2, M761, GA-51, GFAP, GFP-8A
GH	growth hormone	HGH, hGH
GLUT1-cytoplasm	glucose transporter 1-cytoplasmic	GLUT1-CYT
HAM56	Fc receptor for IgG antibodies, high affinity	CD64
HBME-1	mesothelioma antibody	
HER2	v-erb-b2 erythroblastic leukemia viral gene protein, human epidermal growth factor receptor 2	Her2/neu, NEU, Her2, NCL-CBE1, 10A7, 9G6.10, SP3, 4B5, P185, 9G6.20, A0485, C-ERBB-2, CB11, ERBB-2, 3B5, TAB250, HERCEPTEST, E2-4001, HER-2_NEU
HHV8	human herpes virus 8	13B10, LNA-1
HMB-45	monoclonal antibody that reacts against an antigen present in melanocytic tumors	
HMFG	human milk fat globule 1	HMFG-2
HMGA2	high mobility group chromatin protein A2	HMGI-C

ANTIBODY INDEX

HPP	human pancreatic peptide	
HPV	human papilloma virus	
HPV 16	human papilloma virus 16	
IgA	immunoglobin A	
IGF-2	insulin growth factor-like 2	W2-H1
IgG	immunoglobulin G	IGG
IgM	immunoglobin M	
IL-15	interleukin 15	
IMP3	insulin-like growth factor II MRNA-binding protein 3	L523S
Inhibin-α	produced by ovarian granulosa cells; inhibits production or secretion of pituitary gonadotropins, a sensitive marker for majority of sex cord-stromal tumors	
Keratin-Pan	cytokeratin-pan (AE1/AE3/LP34); cocktail of high and low molecular weight cytokeratins	keratin pan, MAK-6, K576, LU-5, KL-1, KC-8, MNF 116, pankeratin, pancytokeratin
KI-67	marker of cell proliferation	MMI, KI88, IVAK-2, MIB1
Laminin	major protein in basal lamina	LAMININ-4C7, 4C12.8, LAM-89
Langerin	CD207 molecule	CD207
LCA	leukocyte common antigen	PD7/26, 1.22/4.14, T29/33, CD45RB, RP2/18, CD45, PD7, 2D1, 2B11+PD7/26
LF	lactoferrin	
LH	Luteinizing hormone	beta-LH
LMP1	Epstein-Barr virus latent membrane protein	EBV-LMP, CS 1-4
Lysozyme	1,4-beta N-acetylmuramidase C	Lyz, Lzm, Ec3.2.1.17
MAC387	macrophage antibody	
MBP	major basic protein	
mCEA	carcinoembryonic antigen, monoclonal	CEA-M, CEA-B18, CEA-D14, CEA-GOLD 1, T84.6, CEA-GOLD 2, CEA 11, CEA-GOLD 3, CEA 27, CEA-GOLD 4, CEA 41, CEA-GOLD 5, T84.1, CEA-M, A5B7, CEJ065, IL-7, T84.66, TF3H8-1, 0062, D14, alpha-7, PARLAM 1, ZC23, CEM010, A115, COL-1, AF4, 12.140.10, 11-7, M773, CEA-M431_31, CEJO65
Mcl-1	myeloid cell leukemia	38G3, MCL-1, S-19
MCM2	Microsome maintenance protein 2	
MDM2	murine double minute oncogene (mdm2)	HDM2, IF2, 2A10, 1B10, SMP14, MDM-2
Melan-A	melanoma antigen recognized by T cells 1 (MART-1); protein found on melanocytes; melanocyte differentiation antigen	M2-7C10, CK-MM
Melan-A103	clone of Melan-A	A103
MIB1	KI-67 (MIB1); marker of cell proliferation	MMI, KI88, IVAK-2, MIB1
MIC2	cell surface glycoprotein for migration, T cell adhesion, MIC2	CD99, CD99-MEMB, MIC2, 12E7, HBA71, O13, P30/32MIC2, M3601
MITF	Microphthalmia-associated transcription factor	34CA5, D5, C5+D5
MK	neurite growth promoting factor 2	MIDKINE, MK1
MSA	muscle-specific actin	ACTIN-SM, ASM-1, CGA7, 1A4, HUC1-1
MSG1	melanocyte specific gene 1 antibody	CITED-1, J72220K
MSH2	mutS homolog 2	FE11
MT	metallothionein	CLONE E9
MUC1	epithelial membrane antigen	LICR-LON-M8, BC3, DF3, VU3D1, MUSEII, RD-1, MA695, MA552, PS2P446, 115D8
MUC2	mucin 1, intestinal	CCP58, MUC2-P, M53, MRP, LUM2-3, LDQ10
MYOD1	myogenic differentiation 1	5.8A, 5.2F
Myogenin	myogenic factor 4; class C basic helix-loop-helix protein 3	F5D, MYF3, MYF4, LO26, BHLHc3, cb553, MYF4, MYOG

ANTIBODY INDEX

Myoglobin	Iron and oxygen-binding protein found in muscle tissue	MG-1
Myosin	Motor proteins responsible for actin-based motility in striated and smooth muscle cels	
N3	calponin	26A11, CALP
NFP	neurofilament H/M phosphorylated protein	TPNFP-1A3, SMI31, SMI33, NFP, SMI32, TA-51, 2F11
NGFR	nerve growth factor receptor	
NSE	neuron specific enolase	BSS/H14
p14	cyclin dependent kinase 4 inhibitor A	P14_ARF
p16	cyclin dependent kinase 4 inhibitor 2A	P16_INK4A, E6H4, sc1661, JC8, ZJ11, P16, G175-405, F-12, DCS-50, 6H12, 16P07, 16P04
p21	Cyclin Dependent Kinase Inhibitor 1A	WAF1, DCS-60.2, EA10, 6B6, 4D10, SX118, P21, P21_WAF1, WAFT
p27	Cyclin Dependent Kinase Inhibitor 1B	P27_KIP1, 57, 1B4, DCS-72.F6, SX53G8, P27, K25020, DCS72, KIP-1
p53	p53 tumor suppressor gene protein	DO7, 21N, BP53-12-1, AB6, CM1, PAB1801, DO1, BP53-11, PAB240, RSP53, MU195, P53
p63	tumor protein p63	H-137, 7JUL
p73	tumor protein p73	AB7824
p80	anaplastic lymphoma kinase-1	KU
Parafibromin	tumor suppressor that is associated with hyperparathyroidism-jaw tumor syndrome	2H1
pax-2	paired box gene 2	Z-RX2, PAX-2
pax-8	paired box gene 8	PAX-8
P-cadherin	placental dependent adhesion protein	56, clone 56
PCNA	proliferating cell nuclear antigen	19 A2, PC10
PDGF-B	platelet derived growth factor B	
PGP9.5	protein gene product 9.5	13C4
PLAP	placental alkaline phosphatase	228M, 8A9, 88B
PNA	peanut agglutinin	
Podoplanin	marker for reactive follicular dendritic cells and follicular dendritic cell sarcomas	D2-40, M2A
PR	progesterone receptor protein	10A9, PGR-1A6, KD68, PGR-ICA, PRP-P, PRP, PRI, 1A6, 1AR, HPRA3, PGR-636, 636, PR88, NCL-PGR
PRL	prolactin	
PSA	prostate specific antigen	PSA-M, PSA, ER-PR8, PSA-P, F5
PTEN	phosphatase and tensin homolog	PN37
PTH	parathyroid hormone	
Rb	retinoblastoma associated protein	3C8, 3H9, PRB1, G3-245, RB1, RB-WL 1, RB-1, 1F8, RB
RCC	renal cell carcinoma	66.4C2, PN-15, RCC, RCC MA
ret	Multiple endocrine neoplasia and medullary thyroid carcinoma 1	3F8
S100	Low molecular weight protein normally present in cells derived from neural crest (Schwann cells, melanocytes, and glial cells), chondrocytes, adipocytes, myoepithelial cells, macrophages, Langerhans cells, dendritic cells, and keratinocytes	S-100, A6, 15E2E2, Z311, 4C4.9
S100-A4	S100 calcium binding protein A4	
S100-A9	S100 calcium binding protein A9	MRP14
SCC	squamous cell carcinoma-related antigen	F2H7C
Serotonin	5-hydroxytryptamine (5-HT), a monoamine neurotransmitter	5-HT, 5HT-H209
SMHC	myosin heavy chain smooth muscle	ID8, SM_MYOSIN_H, HSM-V, SMMS-1
SNF5	member of SWI/SNF chromatin remodeling complex	BAF47/SNF5, INI1
Somatostatin	somatotropin release-inhibiting factor	
Synaptophysin	major synaptic vesicle protein p38 antibody	SVP38, SY38, SNP-88, SYP, SYPH, Sypl, Syn p38
SYT	SYT homolog 1	

ANTIBODY INDEX

Tag72	tumor-associated glycoprotein-72	CC49, B72.3, BRST-3
TCR	T-cell antigen receptor	T_CELL_AG_R, BETA-F1, 8A3, BF1
TdT	terminal deoxynucleotidyl transferase	SEN 28
Tenascin	Extracellular matrix glycoprotein	DB7, TN2
TF	Thomsen-Friedrenreich blood group antigen	HB-T1, TF ANTIGEN
Thyroglobulin	dimetric protein specific to thyroid gland	DAK-TG6
TIA	T-cell intracellular antigen 1	NS/1-AG4, 2G9, TIA-1
TLE1	transducer-like enhancer 1	
TNF-α	gamma catenin	G-catenin, TNF alpha, alpha alpha
TPO	thyroid peroxidase	THYROPEROX
TSH	thyroid stimulating hormone	beta-TSH
TTF-1	transcription termination factor	8G7G3/1, SPT-24, SC-13040
Tyrosinase	Catalyzes production of melanin	NCL-TYROS, T311
ULEX-1	Ulex europaeus agglutinin-1	ULEX, UEA1
VCA	Epstein Barr virus- viral capsid antigen	EBV-VCA
Villin	protein binding the actin filaments of microvillar cores	1D2C3
Vimentin	major subunit protein of intermediate filaments of mesenchymal cells	43BE8, 3B4, V10, V9, VIM-B34, VIM
Von Willebrand factor	factor VIII-related antigen	FVIIIRAg, F*/86
WT1	Wilms tumor gene-1	6F-H2, C-19

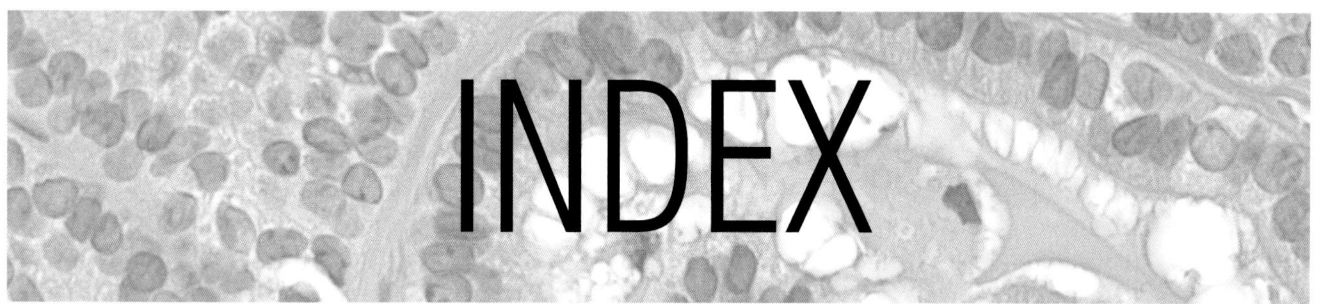

A

INDEX

INDEX

INDEX

B

INDEX

INDEX

INDEX

INDEX

INDEX

D

E

INDEX

INDEX

F

INDEX

INDEX

H

INDEX

INDEX

I

J

INDEX

K

L

INDEX

INDEX

INDEX

M

INDEX

INDEX

INDEX

N

Index

INDEX

INDEX

INDEX

O

INDEX

INDEX

P

INDEX

R

INDEX

S

Index

INDEX

INDEX

INDEX

INDEX

INDEX

INDEX

T

INDEX

INDEX

INDEX

INDEX

INDEX

U

V

INDEX

W

X